Essentials of Surgery

SCIENTIFIC PRINCIPLES
AND PRACTICE

D1495427

Essentials of Surgery

SCIENTIFIC PRINCIPLES AND PRACTICE

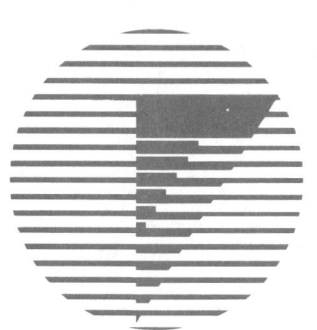

EDITOR-IN-CHIEF

Lazar J. Greenfield, MD
Frederick A. Coller Professor of Surgery
Chairman, Department of Surgery
University of Michigan Medical School
Surgeon-in-Chief
University of Michigan Hospitals
Ann Arbor, Michigan

ASSOCIATE EDITORS

Michael W. Mulholland, MD, PhD
Professor and Associate Chairman
Department of Surgery
University of Michigan Medical School
University of Michigan Hospitals
Ann Arbor, Michigan

Keith T. Oldham, MD
Professor of Surgery and Pediatrics
Duke University School of Medicine
Chief, Division of Pediatric Surgery
Duke University Medical Center
Durham, North Carolina

Gerald B. Zelenock, MD
Professor of Surgery
Section of Vascular Surgery
University of Michigan Medical School
University of Michigan Hospitals
Ann Arbor, Michigan

Keith D. Lillemoe, MD
Associate Professor of Surgery
Johns Hopkins University School of Medicine
Johns Hopkins Hospital
Baltimore, Maryland

With 183 contributors

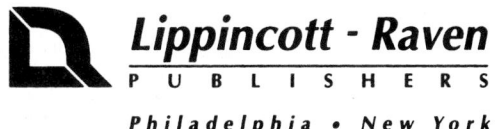

Lippincott - Raven
PUBLISHERS

Philadelphia • New York

Acquisitions Editor: Lisa McAllister
Developmental Editor: Anne Sydor
Manufacturing Manager: Dennis Teston
Production Manager: Maxine Langweil
Production Editor: Jonathan Geffner
Cover Designer: Patty Gast
Indexer: Elizabeth Babcock-Atkinson
Compositor: Tapsco, Inc.
Printer: Courier-Kendallville

Printed in the United States of American

Library of Congress Cataloging-in-Publication Data

Essentials of Surgery—scientific principles and practice/editor-in-chief, Lazar J.
  Greenfield; associate editors, Michael W. Mulholland . . . [et al.]; with 183
  contributors.
        p.   cm.
      Condensed version of: Surgery—scientific principles and practice. 2nd ed. ©1997.
      Includes bibliographical references and index.
      ISBN 0-397-51532-4
      1. Surgery—Handbooks, manuals, etc.   2. Medicine—Handbooks, manuals, etc.
I. Greenfield, Lazar J., 1934–   . II. Mulholland, Michael W.   III. Surgery—scientific
principles and practice, second edition.
      [DNLM: 1.   Surgery—handbooks.   2.   Surgery, Operative—handbooks.   WO 39 E78
1997]
  RD37.E88   1997
  617—dc21
  DNLM/DLC
  for Library of Congress   97-2444
                                                                                CIP

Care has been taken to confirm the accuracy of the information presented and to describe
generally accepted practices. However, the authors, editors, and publisher are not responsible for errors or omissions or for any consequences from application of the information in
this book and make no warranty, express or implied, with respect to the contents of the
publication.
      The authors, editors, and publisher have exerted every effort to ensure that drug selec-
tion and dosage set forth in this text are in accordance with current recommendations
and practice at the time of publication. However, in view of ongoing research, changes in
government regulations, and the constant flow of information relating to drug therapy and
drug reactions, the reader is urged to check the package insert for each drug for any change
in indications and dosage and for added warnings and precautions. This is particularly
important when the recommended agent is a new or infrequently employed drug.
      Some drugs and medical devices presented in this publication have Food and Drug
Administration (FDA) clearance for limited use in restricted research settings. It is the
responsibility of the health care provider to ascertain the FDA status of each drug or device
planned for use in their clinical practice.

9   8   7   6   5   4   3   2   1

Contents

SECTION I   HERNIA, MESENTERY, AND RETROPERITONEUM

SECTION J   SURGICAL ENDOCRINOLOGY

SECTION K   THORAX

Occlusive Disease Involving Specific Vascular Territories

Aneurysmal Disease

SECTION N   VENOUS AND LYMPHATIC SYSTEMS

Contributors

Dana K. Andersen, MD
Professor and Vice Chairman
Department of Surgery
Yale University School of Medicine
Chief, General Surgery Service
Yale–New Haven Hospital
New Haven, Connecticut

W. Scott Arnold, MD
Chief Resident in Surgery
University of Virginia Health Sciences Center
Charlottesville, Virginia

David A. August, MD
Associate Professor of Surgery
Cancer Institute of New Jersey
University of Medicine and Dentistry of New Jersey
Robert Wood Johnson Medical School
New Brunswick, New Jersey

William G. Austen, Jr., AB, MD
Research Fellow in Surgery
Department of Surgery
Brigham and Women's Hospital
Boston, Massachusetts

Dennis F. Bandyk, MD, FACS
Professor of Surgery
Director, Vascular Surgery Division
University of South Florida College of Medicine
Tampa, Florida

Robert H. Bartlett, MD
Professor of Surgery
University of Michigan Medical School
University of Michigan Medical Center
Ann Arbor, Michigan

James M. Becker, MD
James Utley Professor and Chairman of Surgery
Boston University School of Medicine
Boston City Hospital
Surgeon-in-Chief
Boston University Medical Center Hospital
Boston, Massachusetts

Richard H. Bell, Jr., MD
Professor and Vice Chairman
Department of Surgery
University of Washington School of Medicine
Chief, Surgical Service
VA Puget Sound Health Care System
Seattle, Washington

William D. Belville, MD
Associate Professor of Surgery
Section of Urology
University of Michigan Medical Center
Ann Arbor, Michigan

David A. Bloom, MD
Professor, Department of Surgery
University of Michigan Medical School
Chief, Pediatric Urology
C.S. Mott Children's Hospital
Ann Arbor, Michigan

C. Richard Boland, MD
Professor of Medicine
Chief, Division of Gastroenterology
University of California, San Diego, School of Medicine
UCSD Hospitals
Veterans Affairs Medical Center
La Jolla, California

Michael F. Boland, MD
Neurosurgeon
Neurosurgical Associates, Incorporated
St Louis, Missouri

Steven F. Bolling, MD
Associate Professor of Surgery
University of Michigan Medical School
Section of Thoracic Surgery
University of Michigan Hospitals
Ann Arbor, Michigan

R. Morton Bolman III, MD
Professor and Chief
Department of Surgery
Division of Cardiovascular and Thoracic Surgery
Fairview–University Hospital
Minneapolis, Minnesota

Edward L. Bove, MD
Professor of Surgery
University of Michigan Medical School
Chief, Pediatric Cardiac Surgery
C.S. Mott Children's Hospital
Ann Arbor, Michigan

Robert S. Bresalier, MD
Associate Professor of Medicine
University of Michigan Medical School
Ann Arbor, Michigan
Director, Gastrointestinal Oncology
Henry Ford Health Sciences Center
Detroit, Michigan

David C. Brewster, MD
Clinical Professor of Surgery
Harvard Medical School
Massachusetts General Hospital
Boston, Massachusetts

Jonathan S. Bromberg, MD, PhD
Associate Professor of Surgery and Microbiology
    and Immunology
Transplant Surgeon
University of Michigan Medical Center
Ann Arbor, Michigan

F. Charles Brunicardi, MD
George Jordan Professor
Department of Surgery
Chief, Section of General Surgery
Baylor University College of Medicine
Houston, Texas

David R. Byrd, MD
Assistant Professor of Surgery
Chief, Surgical Oncology
Department of General Surgery
University of Washington School of Medicine
Seattle, Washington

Darrell A. Campbell, Jr., MD
Professor of Surgery
Head, Section of General Surgery
Associate Chairman for Hospital Affairs
University of Michigan Medical Center
Ann Arbor, Michigan

Howard R. Champion, FRCS (Edin), FACS
Professor of Surgery
Chief, Division of Surgery for Trauma
Department of Surgery
Uniformed Services University of the Health Sciences
Bethesda, Maryland
Research Professor of Surgery
National Study Center for Trauma and EMS
University of Maryland at Baltimore
Baltimore, Maryland

William F. Chandler, MD
Professor of Surgery
Section of Neurosurgery
University of Michigan Medical School
Ann Arbor, Michigan

Alfred E. Chang, MD
Professor of Surgery
University of Michigan Medical School
Chief, Division of Surgical Oncology
University of Michigan Medical Center
Ann Arbor, Michigan

Randall M. Chesnut, MD
Associate Professor of Neurosurgery
Department of Surgery
Division of Neurosurgery
Oregon Health Sciences University
Portland, Oregon

Paul J. Chiao, PhD
Assistant Professor of Surgical Oncology and Tumor
    Biology
University of Texas M.D. Anderson Cancer Center
Houston, Texas

Kyung J. Cho, MD
Professor of Radiology
University of Michigan Medical School
University of Michigan Hospital
Ann Arbor, Michigan

G. Patrick Clagett, Jr., MD
Professor and Chairman
Department of Surgery
Division of Vascular Surgery
University of Texas Southwestern Medical Center
Dallas, Texas

Alexander W. Clowes, MD
Professor of Surgery
University of Washington School of Medicine
Chief, Division of Vascular Surgery
University of Washington Medical Center
Seattle, Washington

Lisa M. Colletti, MD
Associate Professor of Surgery
University of Michigan Medical School
University of Michigan Hospitals
Ann Arbor, Michigan

Robert L. Conter, MD
Associate Professor of Surgery
Department of Surgery
Pennsylvania State University
Hershey, Pennsylvania

Arnold G. Coran, MD
Professor of Surgery
Head, Section of Pediatric Surgery
University of Michigan Medical School
Surgeon-in-Chief
C.S. Mott Children's Hospital
University of Michigan Medical Center
Ann Arbor, Michigan

Jack L. Cronenwett, MD
Associate Professor of Surgery
Dartmouth Medical School
Chief, Section of Vascular Surgery
Dartmouth-Hitchcock Medical Center
Lebanon, New Hampshire

Peter F. Crookes, MD
Assistant Professor of Surgery
University of Southern California School of Medicine
Attending Physician
Los Angeles County–University of Southern California
    Medical Center
University of Southern California University Hospital
Los Angeles, California

H. Gill Cryer, MD
Associate Professor of Surgery
University of California, Los Angeles, UCLA School
    of Medicine
Chief, Trauma and Emergency Surgery Service
UCLA Medical Center
Los Angeles, California

Louis G. D'Alecy, DMD, PhD
Professor of Physiology
Departments of Physiology and Surgery
Section of Vascular Surgery
University of Michigan Medical School
Ann Arbor, Michigan

James W. Davis, MD, FACS
Associate Professor of Surgery
Department of Surgery
Division of Trauma
University of South Florida
Tampa General Hospital
Tampa, Florida

Lillian G. Dawes, MD
Associate Professor of Surgery
Northwestern University/VA Lakeside
Chicago, Illinois

David C. Dawson, PhD
Professor and Associate Chair
Department of Physiology
University of Michigan Medical School
Ann Arbor, Michigan

Tom R. DeMeester, MD
Professor and Chairman
Department of Surgery
University of Southern California School of Medicine
Chief of Surgery
University of Southern California Hospital
Los Angeles, California

Verdi J. DiSesa, MD
Professor of Medicine and Cardiothoracic Surgery
Allegheny University of the Health Sciences
Allegheny University Hospitals, MCP Division
Hahnemann University Hospital
Philadelphia, Pennsylvania

Gerard M. Doherty, MD
Assistant Professor of Surgery
Washington University School of Medicine
St Louis, Missouri

Lisa S. Dresner, MD
Assistant Professor of Surgery
State University of New York Health Science Center
    at Brooklyn
Brooklyn, New York

David L. Dunn, MD, PhD
Jay Phillips Professor and Head
Department of Surgery
University of Minnesota Medical School—Minneapolis
Minneapolis, Minnesota

Frederic E. Eckhauser, MD
Professor of Surgery
University of Michigan Medical School
Chief, Division of Gastrointestinal Surgery
University of Michigan Medical Center
Ann Arbor, Michigan

Lee M. Ellis, MD
Assistant Professor of Surgery and Cell Biology
University of Texas M.D. Anderson Cancer Center
Houston, Texas

Calvin B. Ernst, MD
Clinical Professor of Surgery
University of Michigan Medical School
Ann Arbor, Michigan
Head, Division of Vascular Surgery
Henry Ford Hospital
Detroit, Michigan

Steve Eubanks, MD
Assistant Professor of Surgery
Director, Surgical Endoscopy
Duke University Medical Center
Durham, North Carolina

Gary J. Faerber, MD
Assistant Professor of Surgery
Section of Urology
University of Michigan Medical Center
Ann Arbor, Michigan

F. Robert Fekety, MD
Professor Emeritus of Internal Medicine
Division of Infectious Diseases
University of Michigan Medical School
University of Michigan Hospitals
Ann Arbor, Michigan

Ronald M. Ferguson, MD, PhD
Professor and Chairman
Department of Surgery
Ohio State University College of Medicine
Chief, Division of Transplantation
Ohio State University Hospital
Columbus, Ohio

Mark F. Fillinger, MD
Assistant Professor of Surgery
Dartmouth Medical School
Dartmouth-Hitchcock Medical Center
Lebanon, New Hampshire

Neil A. Fine, MD
Assistant Professor of Surgery
Division of Plastic and Reconstructive Surgery
Northwestern University Medical School
Northwestern University Memorial Hospital
Chicago, Illinois

Heidi L. Frankel, MD
Assistant Professor of Surgery
Hospital of the University of Pennsylvania
Division of Traumatology, Surgical Critical Care
Philadelphia, Pennsylvania

Larry M. Gentilello, MD
Associate Professor of Surgery
University of Washington School of Medicine
Associate Director, Trauma Intensive Care Unit
Harborview Medical Center
Seattle, Washington

Dan I.N. Giurgiu, MD
Research Fellow in Surgery
Medical College of Pennsylvania and Hahnemann
    University School of Medicine
Philadelphia, Pennsylvania

Steven A. Goldstein, MD
Professor of Surgery
Section of Orthopaedic Surgery
University of Michigan
Ann Arbor, Michigan

Jerry Goldstone, MD
Professor of Surgery
University of California, San Francisco, School
    of Medicine
UCSF Medical Center
San Francisco, California

Linda M. Graham, MD
Professor of Surgery
University of Michigan Medical Center
Ann Arbor, Michigan

Lazar J. Greenfield, MD
Frederick A. Coller Professor of Surgery
Chairman, Department of Surgery
University of Michigan Medical School
Surgeon-in-Chief
University of Michigan Hospitals
Ann Arbor, Michigan

Anita K. Gregory, MD
Chief Resident in General Surgery
St Luke's–Roosevelt Hospital Center
Columbia University College of Physicians and Surgeons
New York, New York

H. Barton Grossman, MD
Professor of Urology and Cell Biology
W.A. "Tex" and Deborah Moncrief, Jr., Chair in Urology
University of Texas M.D. Anderson Cancer Center
Houston, Texas

Karen S. Guice, MD
Professor of Surgery
Duke University Medical Center
Durham, North Carolina

John M. Ham, MD
Assistant Professor of Surgery
Medical College of Virginia
Virginia Commonwealth University
Richmond, Virginia

John B. Hanks, MD
C. Bruce Morton Professor of Surgery
Chief, Division of General Surgery
University of Virginia Health Sciences Center
Charlottesville, Virginia

E. John Harris, Jr., MD
Assistant Professor of Surgery
Division of Vascular Surgery
Stanford University School of Medicine
Stanford, California

Mark A. Healey, BSc, MD, FRCSC
Assistant Professor
Department of Surgery
University of Saskatchewan
Royal University Hospital
Saskatoon, Canada

Mitchell L. Henry, MD
Associate Professor of Surgery
Ohio State University College of Medicine
Director, Clinical Transplantation
Ohio State University Medical Center
Columbus, Ohio

Anil P. Hingorani, MD
Resident
Columbia University College of Physicians and Surgeons
St Luke's–Roosevelt Hospital Center
New York, New York

Daniel B. Hinshaw, MD
Associate Professor of Surgery
University of Michigan Medical School
Chief of Staff
Ann Arbor Veterans Affairs Medical Center
Ann Arbor, Michigan

Julian T. Hoff, MD
Professor of Surgery
University of Michigan Medical School
Head, Section of Neurosurgery
University of Michigan Medical Hospitals
Ann Arbor, Michigan

David B. Hoyt, MD, FACS
Professor of Surgery
University of California, San Diego, School of Medicine
Chief, Division of Trauma
Director, Surgical Intensive Care Unit
UCSD Medical Center
San Diego, California

Thomas S. Huber, MD, PhD
Assistant Professor of Surgery
University of Florida College of Medicine
Shands Teaching Hospital
Veterans Affairs Medical Center
Gainesville, Florida

W. Glenn Hurt, MD
Professor of Obstetrics and Gynecology
Virginia Commonwealth University
Medical College of Virginia
Richmond, Virginia

Mark D. Iannettoni, MD
Assistant Professor of Surgery
University of Michigan Medical School
University of Michigan Medical Center
Ann Arbor, Michigan

O. Wayne Isom, MD
Professor of Cardiothoracic Surgery
Cornell University Medical Center
Cardiothoracic Surgeon-in-Chief
New York Hospital
New York, New York

Lloyd A. Jacobs, MD
Associate Professor of Surgery
University of Michigan Medical School
University of Michigan Hospitals
Ann Arbor, Michigan

Timothy M. Johnson, MD
Assistant Professor
University of Michigan Health System
Ann Arbor, Michigan

Dennie V. Jones, Jr., MD
Assistant Professor of Medicine
University of Texas M.D. Anderson Cancer Center
Houston, Texas

Gregory J. Jurkovich, MD
Professor of Surgery
University of Washington School of Medicine
Chief of Trauma
Director, Emergency Surgical Services
Harborview Medical Center
Seattle, Washington

Kim U. Kahng, MD
Associate Professor of Surgery
Vice Chairman, Administrative Affairs
Medical College of Pennsylvania and Hahnemann
   University School of Medicine
Philadelphia, Pennsylvania

Larry R. Kaiser, MD
Professor of Surgery
Hospital of the University of Pennsylvania
Philadelphia, Pennsylvania

Gordon L. Kauffman, Jr., MD
Professor of Surgery and Cellular and Molecular
   Physiology
Departments of Surgery and Cellular and Molecular
   Physiology
Milton S. Hershey Medical Center of the Pennsylvania
   State University
Hershey, Pennsylvania

James A. Knol, MD
Associate Professor of Surgery
University of Michigan Medical School
University of Michigan Hospitals
Ann Arbor, Michigan

M. Margaret Knudson, MD
Associate Professor of Surgery
Department of Surgery
University of California, San Francisco
San Francisco, California

Walter A. Koltun, MD
Assistant Professor of Surgery
Pennsylvania State University College of Medicine
Milton S. Hershey Medical Center of the Pennsylvania
   State University
Hershey, Pennsylvania

John W. Konnak, BS, MD
Professor of Surgery and Urology
University of Michigan Medical School
University of Michigan Hospitals
Ann Arbor, Michigan

William C. Krupski, MD
Professor of Surgery
Chief, Vascular Surgery Section
University of Colorado Health Sciences Center
Denver, Colorado

Steven L. Kunkel, MS, PhD
Professor of Pathology
University of Michigan Medical School
Ann Arbor, Michigan

Michael P. LaQuaglia, BS, MD
Associate Professor of Surgery
Cornell University Medical College
Chief, Pediatric Surgery
Memorial Sloan-Kettering Cancer Center
New York, New York

Baxter Larmon, PhD, MICP
Associate Professor of Medicine
Emergency Medicine Center
University of California, Los Angeles, UCLA School
   of Medicine
Los Angeles, California

Raymond W. Lee, MD
Fellow in Vascular Surgery
Division of Vascular Surgery
Oregon Health Sciences University
Portland, Oregon

L. Scott Levin, MD
Associate Professor of Plastic and Reconstructive Surgery
   and Orthopaedic Surgery
Duke University Medical Center
Durham, North Carolina

Keith D. Lillemoe, MD
Professor of Surgery
The Johns Hopkins Hospital Medical Institutions
Baltimore, Maryland

S. Martin Lindenauer, MD
Professor of Surgery
Department of Surgery
University of Michigan Medical Center
Ann Arbor, Michigan

Carson D. Liu, MD
Clinical Instructor of General Surgery
UCLA Medical Center
Los Angeles, California

Ricardo V. Lloyd, MD, PhD
Professor of Pathology
Mayo Clinic
Rochester, Minnesota

Michael R. Lucey, MD, FRCPI
Associate Professor of Medicine
University of Pennsylvania School of Medicine
Associate Chief, Division of Gastroenterology
Director, Division of Hepatology
Medical Director, Liver Transplant Program
Hospital of the University of Pennsylvania
Philadelphia, Pennsylvania

Flavian M. Lupinetti, MD
Associate Professor of Surgery
University of Washington School of Medicine
Seattle, Washington

Robert C. Mackersie, MD, FACS
Associate Professor of Surgery
University of California, San Francisco, School
    of Medicine
Director, Trauma and Surgical Critical Care
San Francisco General Hospital
San Francisco, California

Samuel M. Mahaffey, MD
Assistant Professor
Division of Pediatric Surgery
Department of Surgery
Duke University Medical Center
Durham, North Carolina

Ronald V. Maier, BS, MD
Professor and Vice Chair
Department of Surgery
University of Washington School of Medicine
Surgeon-in-Chief
Harborview Medical Center
Seattle, Washington

Philippe A. Masser, MD
Staff Surgeon
Salem Memorial Hospital
Salem, Oregon

Larry S. Matthews, MD
Professor and Program Director
Department of Surgery
Section of Orthopaedic Surgery
University of Michigan Medical Center
Ann Arbor, Michigan

David W. McFadden, MD
Associate Professor and Chief
Division of General Surgery
University of California, Los Angeles, UCLA School
    of Medicine
Los Angeles, California

David S. Medich, MD
Director, Division of Colon and Rectal Surgery
Allegheny General Hospital
Pittsburgh, Pennsylvania

Robert M. Merion, MD
Associate Professor of Surgery
Department of General Surgery–Transplant
University of Michigan Medical Center
Ann Arbor, Michigan

Charles L. Mesh, MD
Teaching Staff
Jewish Hospital of Cincinnati
Cincinnati, Ohio

Louis M. Messina, MD
Professor of Surgery
Chief, Division of Vascular Surgery
University of California, San Francisco, School
    of Medicine
San Francisco, California

Anthony A. Meyer, MD, PhD
Professor of Surgery
Chief, Division of General Surgery
University of North Carolina at Chapel Hill School
    of Medicine
Medical Director, Critical Care Services
Assistant Director, North Carolina Jaycee Burn Center
University of North Carolina Hospitals and Clinics
Chapel Hill, North Carolina

Thomas A. Miller, MD, FACS
C. Rollins Hanlon Professor and Chairman
Department of Surgery
St Louis University Medical School
Chief of Surgery
St Louis University Hospital
St Louis, Missouri

R. Scott Mitchell, MD
Associate Professor of Cardiovascular and Thoracic
    Surgery
Stanford University Medical Center
Stanford, California

Ralph S. Mosca, MD
Assistant Professor of Surgery
C.S. Mott Children's Hospital
University of Michigan Medical Center
Ann Arbor, Michigan

Michael W. Mulholland, MD, PhD
Professor and Associate Chairman
Department of Surgery
University of Michigan Medical School
University of Michigan Hospitals
Ann Arbor, Michigan

Michel M. Murr, MD
Research Fellow in Gastrointestinal Surgery
Mayo Clinic and Foundation
Rochester, Minnesota

Thomas A. Mustoe, MD
Professor of Surgery
Chief, Division of Plastic Surgery
Northwestern University Medical School
Northwestern University Hospital
Chicago, Illinois

David L. Nahrwold, AB, MD
Loyal and Edith Davis Professor and Chairman
Department of Surgery
Northwestern University Medical School
Surgeon-in-Chief
Northwestern Memorial Hospital
Chicago, Illinois

James P. Neifeld, MD
Professor of Surgery
Division of Surgical Oncology
Virginia Commonwealth University
Medical College of Virginia
Richmond, Virginia

H.H. Newsome, Jr., MD
Professor of Surgery
Virginia Commonwealth University
Medical College of Virginia
Medical College of Virginia Hospitals
Richmond, Virginia

Santhat Nivatvongs, MD
Professor of Surgery
Mayo Medical School
Consultant, Colon and Rectal Surgery
Mayo Clinic
Rochester, Minnesota

Patrick J. O'Hara, MD
Associate Professor of Surgery
Ohio State University College of Medicine
Department of Vascular Surgery
Cleveland Clinic Foundation
Cleveland, Ohio

Dana A. Ohl, MD
Associate Professor of Surgery
Section of Urology
University of Michigan Medical School
Ann Arbor, Michigan

Keith T. Oldham, MD
Professor of Surgery and Pediatrics
Duke University School of Medicine
Chief, Division of Pediatric Surgery
Duke University Medical Center
Durham, North Carolina

Geneva M. Omann, PhD
Associate Professor of Surgery and Biological Chemistry
Departments of Surgery and Biological Chemistry
University of Michigan Medical School
Research Chemist
Veterans Affairs Medical Center
Ann Arbor, Michigan

Lisa A. Orloff, MD
Assistant Professor of Surgery
Department of Surgery
Division of Otolaryngology
University of California, San Diego, School of Medicine
UCSD Medical Center
San Diego, California

Mark B. Orringer, MD
Professor of Surgery
Head, Section of Thoracic Surgery
University of Michigan Medical Center
Ann Arbor, Michigan

Mary F. Otterson, MD, MS, FACS
Associate Professor of Surgery
Medical College of Wisconsin
Milwaukee, Wisconsin

Theodore N. Pappas, MD
Professor of Surgery
Chief, Gastrointestinal Surgery
Duke University Medical Center
Durham, North Carolina

Neal R. Pellis, PhD
Associate Professor of Surgery and Immunology
University of Texas Graduate School of Biomedical
    Sciences
Adjunct Associate Professor of Immunology and Surgical
    Oncology
University of Texas M.D. Anderson Cancer Center
Program Manager, Biotechnology Program
NASA-Johnson Space Center
Houston, Texas

William S. Pierce, MD
Professor of Surgery
Director of Surgical Research
Pennsylvania State University College of Medicine
Milton S. Hershey Medical Center
Hershey, Pennsylvania

John M. Porter, MD
Professor of Surgery
Head, Division of Vascular Surgery
Oregon Health Sciences University
Portland, Oregon

Bruce M. Potenza, MD, MPH
Instructor in Surgery
University of Massachusetts Medical Center
Worcester, Massachusetts

Jeffrey D. Punch, MD
Associate Professor of Surgery
University of Michigan Medical School
University of Michigan Hospitals
Ann Arbor, Michigan

Steven E. Raper, MD
Associate Professor of Surgery
Institute for Human Gene Therapy
University of Pennsylvania School of Medicine
Philadelphia, Pennsylvania

Joseph H. Rapp, MD
Professor in Residence of Surgery
University of California, San Francisco, School
  of Medicine
Chief, Vascular Surgery Service
San Francisco Veterans Affairs Medical Center
San Francisco, California

Daniel J. Reddy, MD
Clinical Associate Professor of Surgery
Division of Vascular Surgery
University of Michigan Medical School
Henry Ford Hospital
Detroit, Michigan

Riley S. Rees, MD
Professor of Surgery and Plastic and Reconstructive
  Surgery
University of Michigan Medical School
Ann Arbor, Michigan

Linda M. Reilly, MD
Associate Professor of Surgery
University of California, San Francisco, School
  of Medicine
San Francisco Veteran's Affairs Medical Center
San Francisco, California

Michael L. Ritchey, MD, FAAP, FACS
Associate Professor
University of Texas Health Science Center
Chief, Pediatric Urology
Departments of Surgery and Pediatrics
Hermann Children's Hospital
Houston, Texas

Lawrence Rosenberg, MD, PhD
Professor of Surgery
McGill University Faculty of Medicine
Associate Surgeon
Montreal General Hospital
Montreal, Quebec, Canada

Todd K. Rosengart, MD
Associate Professor of Cardiothoracic Surgery
Cornell University Medical College
New York Hospital
New York, New York

Joel J. Roslyn, MD
Professor and Chairman
Alma Dea Morani Department of Surgery
Allegheny University of the Health Sciences
Medical College of Pennsylvania and Hahnemann
  University School of Medicine
Philadelphia, Pennsylvania

Grace S. Rozycki, MD
Associate Professor of Surgery
Emory University School of Medicine
Atlanta, Georgia

Valerie W. Rusch, MD
Professor of Surgery
Cornell University Medical College
Member and Attending Surgeon, Thoracic Service
Memorial Sloan-Kettering Cancer Center
New York, New York

Timothy W. Rutter, BSc Hon, MB, BS, LRCP, MRCS,
FRCA
Associate Professor of Anesthesiology
University of Michigan Medical School
Clinical Director and Associate Chair, Department
  of Anesthesiology
University of Michigan Hospitals
Ann Arbor, Michigan

John S. Sapirstein, MD
General Surgery Resident
Department of Surgery
University of Chicago Hospitals
Chicago, Illinois

Michael G. Sarr, MD
Professor of Surgery
Mayo Medical School
Chairman, Division of General and Gastroenterologic
  Surgery
Mayo Clinic and Mayo Foundation
Rochester, Minnesota

Felix H. Savoie III, MD
Co-Director of Upper Extremity Service
Mississippi Sports Medicine and Orthopaedic Center
Jackson, Mississippi

Wolfgang H. Schraut, MD, PhD, FACS
Professor of Surgery
University of Pittsburgh School of Medicine
Chief, Gastrointestinal Surgery
Presbyterian University Hospital
Pittsburgh, Pennsylvania

Arnold W. Scott, MD
Chief Resident
Department of Surgery
University of Virginia Health Sciences Center
Charlottesville, Virginia

Brian J. Sennett, MD
Clinical Instructor of Orthopaedic Surgery
Medical College of Pennsylvania and Hahnemann
    University School of Medicine
Associate Director, Joe Torg Center for Sports Medicine
Philadelphia, Pennsylvania

Steven R. Shackford, MD, FACS
Professor and Chairman
Department of Surgery
University of Vermont
Fletcher Allen Health Care
Burlington, Vermont

Alexander D. Shepard, MD
Clinical Associate Professor of Surgery
University of Michigan Medical School
Ann Arbor, Michigan
Senior Staff Surgeon
Medical Director, Vascular Laboratory
Henry Ford Hospital
Detroit, Michigan

Robert L. Sheridan, MD
Assistant Professor of Surgery: Trauma and Burns
Harvard Medical School/Massachusetts General Hospital
Assistant Chief of Staff
Shriners Burns Institute
Boston, Massachusetts

Sara J. Shumway, MD
Professor of Surgery
University of Minnesota Medical School—Minneapolis
Surgical Director, Heart Transplantation
University of Minnesota Hospital and Clinics
Minneapolis, Minnesota

Richard Keith Simons, MB, BChir, FRCS, FRCS(C)
Associate Professor of Surgery
University of British Columbia
Vancouver, British Columbia
Canada

Michael J. Sise, MD
Associate Clinical Professor of Surgery
University of California, San Diego, School of Medicine
Chief, Division of Trauma
Mercy Hospital and Medical Center
San Diego, California

Vernon K. Sondak, MD
Associate Professor of Surgery
University of Michigan Medical School
Director, Sarcoma Program
University of Michigan Comprehensive Cancer Center
Ann Arbor, Michigan

David E. Soper, MD
Professor of Obstetrics and Gynecology
Director, Division of Benign Gynecology
Medical University of South Carolina College
    of Medicine
Charleston, South Carolina

Nathaniel J. Soper, MD
Professor of Surgery
Washington University School of Medicine
Barnes Hospital
St Louis, Missouri

Wiley W. Souba, MD, ScD
Professor of Surgery
Harvard Medical School
Professor of Nutrition
Harvard School of Public Health
Chief, Division of Surgical Oncology
Massachusetts General Hospital
Boston, Massachusetts

David I. Soybel, MD
Associate Professor of Surgery
Department of General Surgery
West Roxbury Veterans Administration Medical Center
West Roxbury, Massachusetts

James C. Stanley, MD
Professor of Surgery
Section of Vascular Surgery
University Hospital
Ann Arbor, Michigan

Thomas Ray Stevenson, MD
Professor of Surgery
Chief, Division of Plastic and Reconstructive Surgery
University of California, Davis, School of Medicine
Sacramento, California

James R. Stewart, MD
Associate Professor of Surgery
Department of Cardiac and Thoracic Surgery
Vanderbilt University School of Medicine
Vanderbilt University Medical Center
Veterans Affairs Medical Center
Nashville, Tennessee

Robert M. Strieter, MD
Professor of Internal Medicine
Department of Internal Medicine
Division of Pulmonary and Critical Care Medicine
University of Michigan Medical School
Ann Arbor, Michigan

Harvey J. Sugerman, MD
David M. Hume Professor of Surgery
Vice-Chairman, Department of Surgery
Virginia Commonwealth University
Medical College of Virginia
Richmond, Virginia

David S. Sumner, MD
Distinguished Professor of Surgery
Chief, Section of Peripheral Vascular Surgery
Southern Illinois University School of Medicine
Springfield, Illinois

Lloyd M. Taylor, Jr., MD
Professor of Surgery
Department of Vascular Surgery
Oregon Health Sciences University
Portland, Oregon

Gordon L. Telford, MD
Professor of Surgery
Medical College of Wisconsin
Froedtert Memorial Lutheran Hospital
Milwaukee, Wisconsin

Norman W. Thompson, MD, PhD
Henry King Ransom Professor of Surgery
University of Michigan Medical School
Chief, Division of Endocrine Surgery
University of Michigan Hospitals
Ann Arbor, Michigan

M. David Tilson, MD
Alisa Mellon Bruce Professor of Surgery
Columbia University College of Physicians and Surgeons
Professor of Surgery
St Luke's–Roosevelt Hospital Center
New York, New York

Ronald G. Tompkins, MD, ScD
John Francis Burke Professor of Surgery
Department of Surgery
Massachusetts General Hospital
Boston, Massachusetts

Kevin K. Tremper, PhD, MD
Professor and Chair
Department of Anesthesiology
University of Michigan Medical School
University of Michigan Medical Center
Ann Arbor, Michigan

Jeremiah G. Turcotte, MD
Professor of Surgery
University of Michigan Medical School
Director, Organ Transplantation Center
University of Michigan Hospitals
Ann Arbor, Michigan

Richard H. Turnage, MD
Assistant Professor of Surgery
University of Texas Southwestern Medical School
Dallas, Texas

Richard B. Wait, MD, PhD
Professor and Chairman
Department of Surgery
State University of New York Health Sciences Center
   at Brooklyn
Brooklyn, New York

Thomas W. Wakefield, MD
Associate Professor of Surgery
University of Michigan Medical School
University of Michigan Medical Center
Veterans Affairs Medical Center
Ann Arbor, Michigan

Samuel A. Wells, Jr., MD
Bixby Professor of Surgery
Chairman, Department of Surgery
Washington University School of Medicine
St Louis, Missouri

John R. Wesley, MD
Clinical Professor of Surgery
University of California, Davis, School of Medicine
Chief, Pediatric Surgery
UCD Medical Center
Sacramento, California

Rodney A. White, MD
Professor of Surgery
University of California, Los Angeles, UCLA School
   of Medicine
Chief, Vascular Surgery
Associate Chairman, Department of Surgery
Harbor-UCLA Medical Center
Torrance, California

Glenn J.R. Whitman, MD
Professor of Surgery
Department of Cardiothoracic Surgery
Allegheny University of the Health Sciences
Philadelphia, Pennsylvania

David M. Williams, MD
Associate Professor of Radiology
University of Michigan Medical Center
Ann Arbor, Michigan

John A. Williams, MD, PhD
Professor of Physiology and Internal Medicine
Chair, Department of Physiology
University of Michigan Medical School
Ann Arbor, Michigan

Robert J. Winchell, MD
Assistant Professor of Surgery
Division of Trauma
University of California, San Diego, Medical Center
San Diego, California

David H. Wisner, MD
Professor of Surgery
University of California, Davis, School of Medicine
Department of Surgery
University of California, Davis, Medical Center
Sacramento, California

James S.T. Yao, MD, PhD
Magerstadt Professor of Surgery
Northwestern University Medical School
Chief, Division of Vascular Surgery
Vice Chair, Department of Surgery
Northwestern Memorial Hospital
Chicago, Illinois

Charles J. Yeo, MD
Associate Professor of Surgery and Oncology
Johns Hopkins University School of Medicine
Johns Hopkins Hospital
Baltmore, Maryland

Gerald B. Zelenock
Professor of Surgery
Section of Vascular Surgery
University of Michigan Medical School
University of Michigan Hospitals
Ann Arbor, Michigan

Preface

Along with the practice of medicine, medical education is changing to a greater emphasis on ambulatory care. With fewer patients in hospitals, shorter stays, and more limited time for contact with surgical problems, students need a portable source of information to understand the rationale for the diagnostic and therapeutic efforts they observe. To fill this need, we accepted the responsibility of defining the "essentials" of each of the topics detailed in the second edition of our textbook *Surgery: Scientific Principles and Practice*. It is our hope and expectation that the readers of this Essentials book will seek the more complete review of the topic to be found in the textbook. Although intended for students, this book should also be of value to the house officer or medical practitioner seeking a quick, practical, and reliable overview of a common surgical problem for rounds, conferences, and consultations.

The editors wish to acknowledge the outstanding work of Catherine Judge Allen who drafted the initial condensation of the chapters. We are also grateful to Anne Sydor who served as Developmental Editor, to Paula Callaghan for her efforts as Associated Medical Editor, and to our Editor, Lisa McAllister, whose vision of this project has been invaluable. Above all, we are grateful to the authors whose original contribution to the second edition of *Surgery: Scientific Principles and Practice* made it possible for us to distill this work.

LAZAR J. GREENFIELD, MD
Editor-in-Chief

Essentials
of Surgery

SCIENTIFIC PRINCIPLES
AND PRACTICE

ONE

SCIENTIFIC PRINCIPLES

ESSENTIALS OF SURGERY: SCIENTIFIC PRINCIPLES AND PRACTICE,
edited by Lazar J. Greenfield, Michael W. Mulholland, Keith T. Oldham, Gerald B. Zelenock,
and Keith D. Lillemoe. Lippincott–Raven Publishers, Philadelphia, © 1997.

CHAPTER 1

CELL STRUCTURE AND FUNCTION

JOHN A. WILLIAMS AND DAVID C. DAWSON

CELL STRUCTURE

Membranes and Organelles

Plasma Membrane

The plasma membrane defines the boundary of the cell and contains and concentrates enzymes and other macromolecules (Fig. 1-1). The membrane is composed of phospholipids and proteins that contain regions that are insoluble (hydrophobic) or soluble in water (hydrophilic). By orienting themselves so that their hydrophobic portions contact each other, phospholipids form lipid bilayers, within which proteins and hydrophobic components such as cholesterol are embedded (Fig. 1-2). The plasma membrane forms a continuous barrier between the extracellular and intracellular fluids. Besides restraining macromolecules within a cell, the hydrophobic core of the lipid bilayer presents a barrier to small, charged molecules, such as ions and adenosine triphosphate (ATP).

Nucleus

The largest of the cellular organelles is the *nucleus,* which is defined by inner and outer nuclear membranes. The outer membrane is continuous with the rough endoplasmic reticulum (ER) and is studded with ribosomes. All chromosomal DNA is contained within the nucleus in association with acidic proteins called *histones.* Histones and DNA exist together as *chromatin fibers.* The contents of the nucleus communicate with the cytoplasm through *nuclear pores,* which are composed of proteins that function as channels to regulate the movement of material between nucleus and cytoplasm. The nucleus also contains the *nucleolus,* where ribosomes are assembled.

The *cytoplasm* is the portion of the cell outside the nucleus but within the plasma membrane. Cytoplasm is composed of cytosol, a number of membranous organelles, and the cytoskeleton.

Mitochondria

Mitochondria are oblong organelles defined by a smooth outer membrane and an inner membrane with infoldings, or cristae, that protrude into the central matrix. Mitochondria are the most important source of energy production. Enzymes involved with electron transport and oxidative phosphorylation exist in an array of small, stalked particles that protrude inward from the inner membrane. Enzymes involved in oxidation of sugars and lipids are present in the matrix space, which contains granules of mitochondrial DNA and a few ribosomes. Oxidative phosphorylation at the inner mitochondrial membrane generates an electrochemical proton gradient, and the downhill movement of H^+ through adenosine triphosphatase (ATPase) molecules provides energy to synthesize ATP.

Endoplasmic Reticulum

The ER is a network of interconnected membranes that form closed vesicles, tubules, and saccules. The ER is involved in the synthesis of protein and lipids. It is divided into rough ER, which is studded with ribosomes and involved in the synthesis of exportable proteins, and smooth ER, which lacks ribosomes and is involved in the synthesis of fatty acids and lipids.

Golgi Complex

Adjacent to the rough ER and involved in the sorting and packaging of secreted protein is the Golgi complex. Each complex consists of a series of flattened membrane sacs, or cisternae, surrounded by a number of vesicles. These vesicles shuttle secretory proteins from the rough ER to the Golgi bodies. The Golgi complex directs secretory proteins to either lysosomes or secretory granules.

Cytoskeleton

The cytoskeleton is a collection of filamentous proteins that allow cells to assume and maintain a variety of shapes, to move organelles within the cell, and to move the entire cell relative to other cells.

CELL-CELL INTERACTION

The cells in a tissue contact the extracellular matrix. In connective tissue, the matrix surrounds the cells. In other tissues, epithelial cells are directly attached to each other, and the extracellular matrix is a thin layer under the cellular sheet. Some cells, such as neurons and endocrine cells, influence others by means of specialized secretions.

Cell Junctions

Cell junctions can be classified as follows:
Occluding junctions connect cells in epithelium and allow the epithelium to serve as a selective permeability barrier
Anchoring junctions connect the cytoskeleton to the extracellular matrix or neighboring cells
Communicating junctions, or gap junctions, mediate electrical and chemical coupling

Cell-Matrix Adhesion

The extracellular matrix is a meshwork of negatively charged polysaccharide glycosaminoglycan chains and protein fibers. The protein fibers are structural or adhesive. The principle protein molecules in the plasma membrane, the *integrins,* integrate the extracellular matrix with the cytoskeleton.

MEMBRANE TRANSPORT

The cell and its environment are not in equilibrium. For example, the concentration of Ca^{2+} in the extracellular fluid is about 10^{-3} M (1 mmol) but in the cytosol it is about 10^{-7} M (10^{-4} mmol), a 10,000-fold gradient. The ability of a cell to maintain its composition in the absence of equilibrium is the result of two properties of the plasma membrane—selectivity and energy conversion.

Selectivity and Its Modulation

The plasma membrane is leaky to a variety of substances, but it selects one substance over another. For example, the plasma membrane of many cells is 10 to 100 times more leaky to K^+ than to Na^+. Membrane-spanning proteins exhibit an enzyme-like specificity for particular molecules and can catalyze their selective transport across the plasma membrane. In nerve and muscle cells, for example, the selectivity of the resting membrane for K over Na can be completely reversed so that the membrane becomes 100-fold selective for Na over K.

3

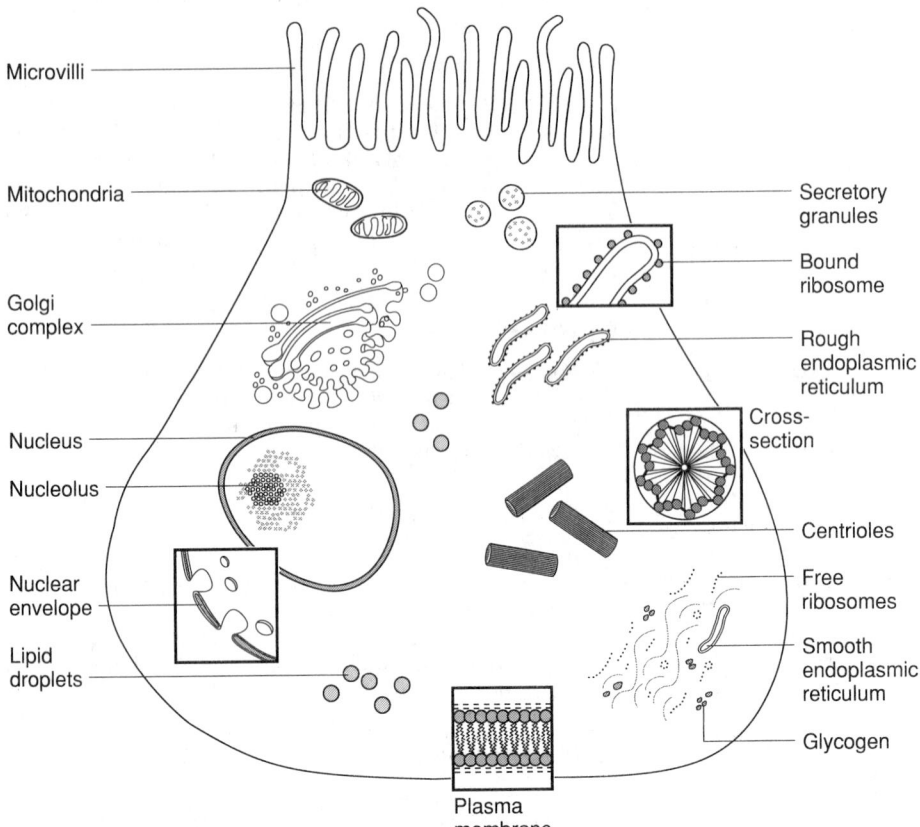

Microvilli

Mitochondria

Golgi complex

Nucleus

Nucleolus

Nuclear envelope

Lipid droplets

Secretory granules

Bound ribosome

Rough endoplasmic reticulum

Cross-section

Centrioles

Free ribosomes

Smooth endoplasmic reticulum

Glycogen

Plasma membrane

Figure 1-1. Schematic diagram of a typical epithelial cell, showing the common internal organelles.

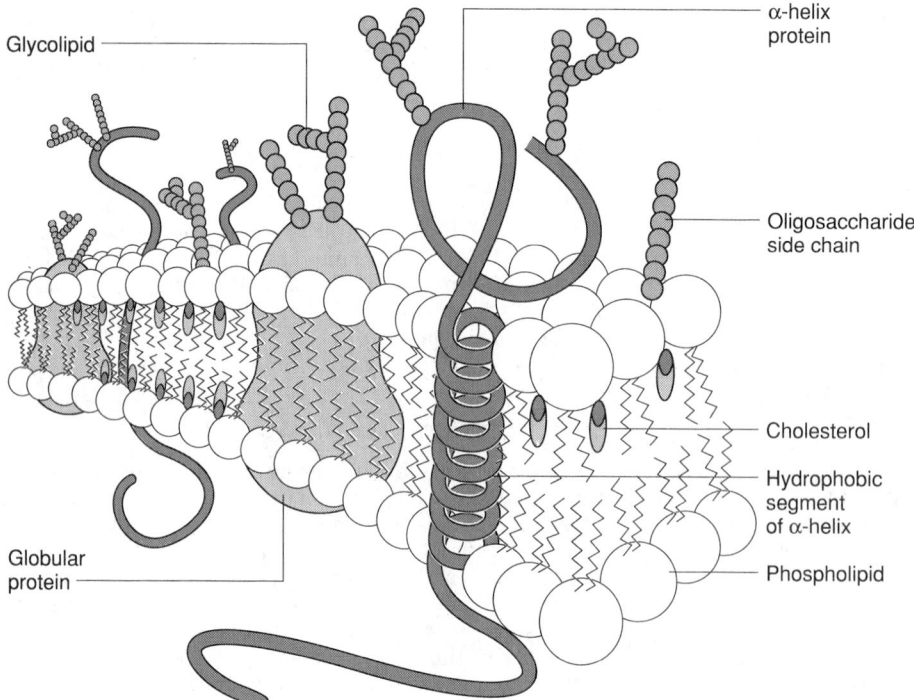

Glycolipid

α-helix protein

Oligosaccharide side chain

Cholesterol

Hydrophobic segment of α-helix

Phospholipid

Globular protein

Figure 1-2. Structure of the cell membrane as a fluid mosaic consisting of a phospholipid bilayer that contains cholesterol and embedded proteins.

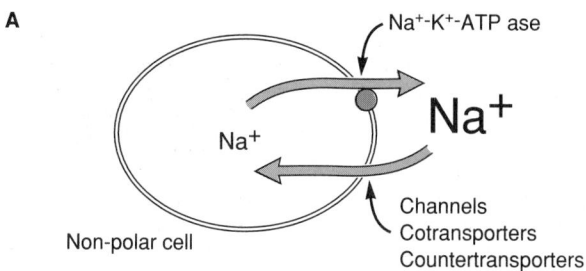

A

Non-polar cell

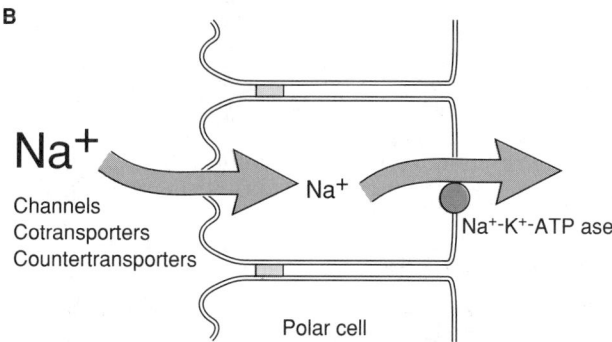

B

Polar cell

Figure 1-3. Cytosolic composition is maintained in a steady state by balancing pumps and leaks. Shown here are mechanisms that maintain low intracellular Na^+ concentration in two cells, one a symmetric cell (*A*) and the other a polar, epithelial cell (*B*). In the symmetric cell, Na^+ efflux by the pump is balanced by the sum of all the Na^+ leaks into the cell. In the polar cell, Na^+ influx at the apical (lumen-facing) side is balanced by active Na^+ efflux at the basolateral (blood-facing) side. The rates of Na^+ transport are typically much greater for the polar cell, which is designed to effect the net transcellular movement of Na^+ that is important for the function of the kidney and gastrointestinal tract.

Membrane Proteins: Specific Transport Pathways

The movement of substances like glucose and ions across the plasma membrane requires permeation pathways formed by membrane-spanning proteins. These transport proteins are divided into two broad categories: ion channels and carriers. In ion channels, the protein forms a pore that can open and close to provide a mechanism for passive flow of ions across membranes. In carriers, the protein forms a pore-like structure, but translocation occurs by means of conformational changes in the protein. To perform transport, membrane-spanning proteins interact with the hydrocarbon of the bilayer and with the transported substrate. Such proteins have a hydrophobic portion that allows the protein to pass through the lipid layer and hydrophilic portions that are stable in the cytoplasm and the extracellular fluid.

Transport: Energetics and Mechanism

All transport mechanisms consist of the following three steps: 1. Entry of the substance into the membrane on one side, 2. Translocation that conveys the substance to the other side, and 3. Exit of the substance from the membrane into the aqueous compartment. If the distribution of any substance is not at equilibrium, flow of that substance is expected to be in a direction that restores equilibrium. If the distribution is maintained away from equilibrium, a process that involves energy conversion is moving the substance against a gradient (Fig. 1-4). Ion flow through a channel can be driven by an ion concentration gradient or by an electrical potential difference (Fig. 1-5).

Energy-Converting Transport

A cell can be maintained in a lack of equilibrium only with the continuous expenditure of energy. The plasma membrane is the site of energy converters, membrane proteins that function as biologic transporters using energy from metabolism. *Na^+-K^+-ATPase* is a membrane protein that hydrolyzes cytosolic ATP and couples the resulting free energy to the transport of Na^+ and K^+. The energy conversion that occurs in Na^+-K^+-ATPase is an example of primary active transport, in which energy is derived directly from ATP hydrolysis. Secondary active transport allows energy that has been invested in the transmembrane Na gradient by Na^+-K^+-ATPase to be used to perform various kinds of transport (Fig. 1-3).

Membrane Composition: Implications for Selectivity and Energy Conversion

Plasma membranes consist of a matrix of lipids in which are embedded the membrane proteins responsible for the transport properties of the cell interface. Lipid is an important component of the plasma membrane. Membrane phospholipids exhibit a strong tendency to organize into a stable, bimolecular layer. The hydrocarbon layer formed by the fatty acid tails of phospholipids has the transport properties of a layer of oil. Substances can penetrate this layer by means of solubility-diffusion. That is, they dissolve into the hydrocarbon and diffuse across the membrane.

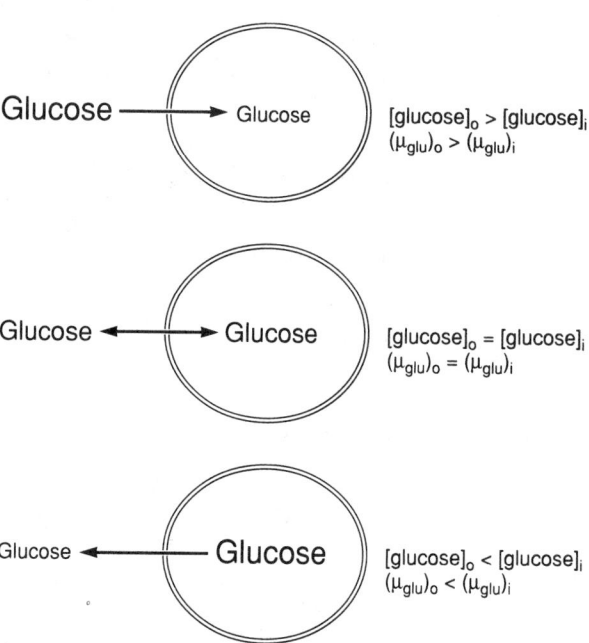

Figure 1-4. For a substance that moves by a non–energy-dependent transport mechanism, the direction of the net flow is determined by the passive driving force. In this example, the movement of glucose is determined by the orientation of the concentration gradient (the chemical potential gradient).

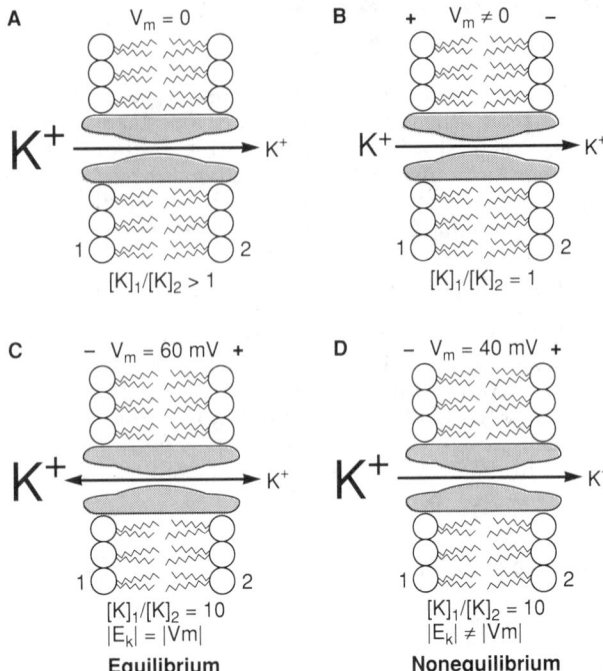

Figure 1-5. The direction of passive ion flow is determined by the *electrochemical potential gradient*. The total driving force is the sum of that due to the K concentration gradient (*A*) and that due to the electrical potential difference (*B*). If the driving force due to the concentration gradient is equal in magnitude and opposite in direction to the electrical potential (*C*), the total passive force is zero (ie, the ion is distributed at equilibrium). (*D*) A net driving force exists because there is an imbalance between E_k and V_m.

Driving Force for Water Flow

Water moves across cell membranes only passively because of gradients of hydrostatic pressure or water concentration. Hydrostatic pressure is an important driving force only for specialized cells—the capillary endothelium and the glomeruli of the kidney. For most cells in the body, the transmembrane hydrostatic pressure is zero, because of membrane elasticity, and water moves only in response to water concentration gradients. Because the concentration of water is determined by the amount of dissolved solute, the difference in water concentration is expressed as a function of the difference in solute concentration, or osmotic pressure difference (Fig. 1-6). Because there are no specialized, energy-converting transport mechanisms for water, water is distributed at equilibrium. If a cell gains solute, it swells by gaining water. If a cell loses solute, it shrinks because of efflux of water.

Transport Mechanisms

Transport is classified in terms of equality between work available and work done. For most cells, water movement across the plasma membrane is by solubility–diffusion across the lipid bilayer. To penetrate the lipid bilayer, a substance must dissolve into it. Movement across the bilayer occurs by diffusion. Some cells may also have transport proteins that function as water channels.

Ion Channels

Ion channels are transmembrane proteins that form pores that conduct ions across the plasma membrane. The lipid portion of the plasma membrane is virtually imper-

meable to small ions such as Na^+, K^+, Cl^-, and Ca^{2+}. The ions cannot cross a hydrophobic layer because of the enormous amount of energy required to move an ion from a highly polar aqueous environment into the relatively nonpolar region formed by the hydrocarbon tails of the phospholipids. These polar groups take the place of the water of hydration, which stabilizes an ion in an aqueous solution. The polar groups produce a water-like environment into which the ion can partition and move in the presence of an appropriate driving force. The channel protein undergoes conformational changes, called *gating*, between conducting (open) states and nonconducting (closed) states. Gating of ion channels is crucial to the survival of cells and organisms. Two of the most important mechanisms that regulate ion channels are *voltage gating* (Fig. 1-7) and *ligand gating* (Fig. 1-8). Conduction can be blocked by ions or organic compounds that enter the channel, bind there, and occlude the pore. Channel blockade is a reversible binding reaction, so the efficacy of the blocker is determined by the affinity of the blocker for the binding site.

Water Channels

The plasma membrane of most cells is highly permeable to water. A few cells, however, such as epithelial cells in the distal renal tubule, exhibit a highly regulated water permeability. In such cells, water permeability is regulated by antidiuretic hormone (ADH). Regulated water permeability requires that two conditions be met: (1) there must be a regulatable pathway for water transport (ie, water

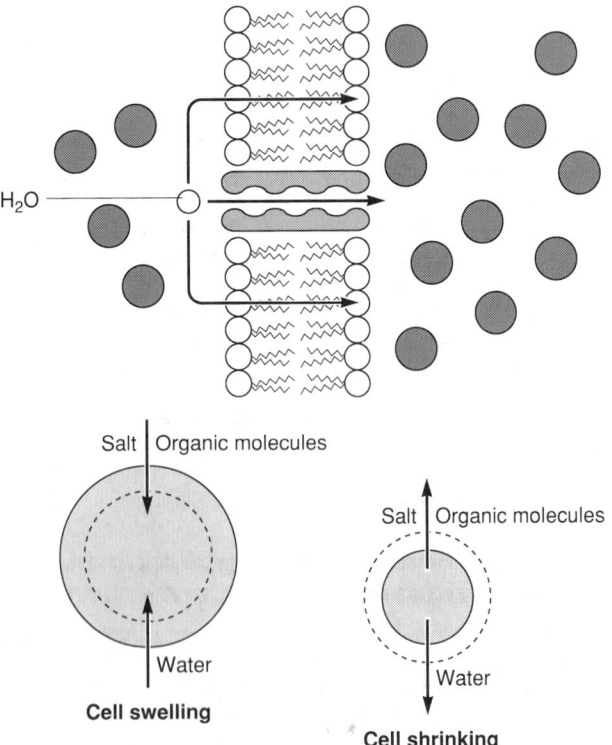

Figure 1-6. Water permeates the plasma membrane by means of *solubility–diffusion* through the lipid bilayer and, in some cells, through specialized water channels. Cell volume is normally determined by *solute* distribution because plasma membrane water permeability is high and cells tend to approach osmotic equilibrium.

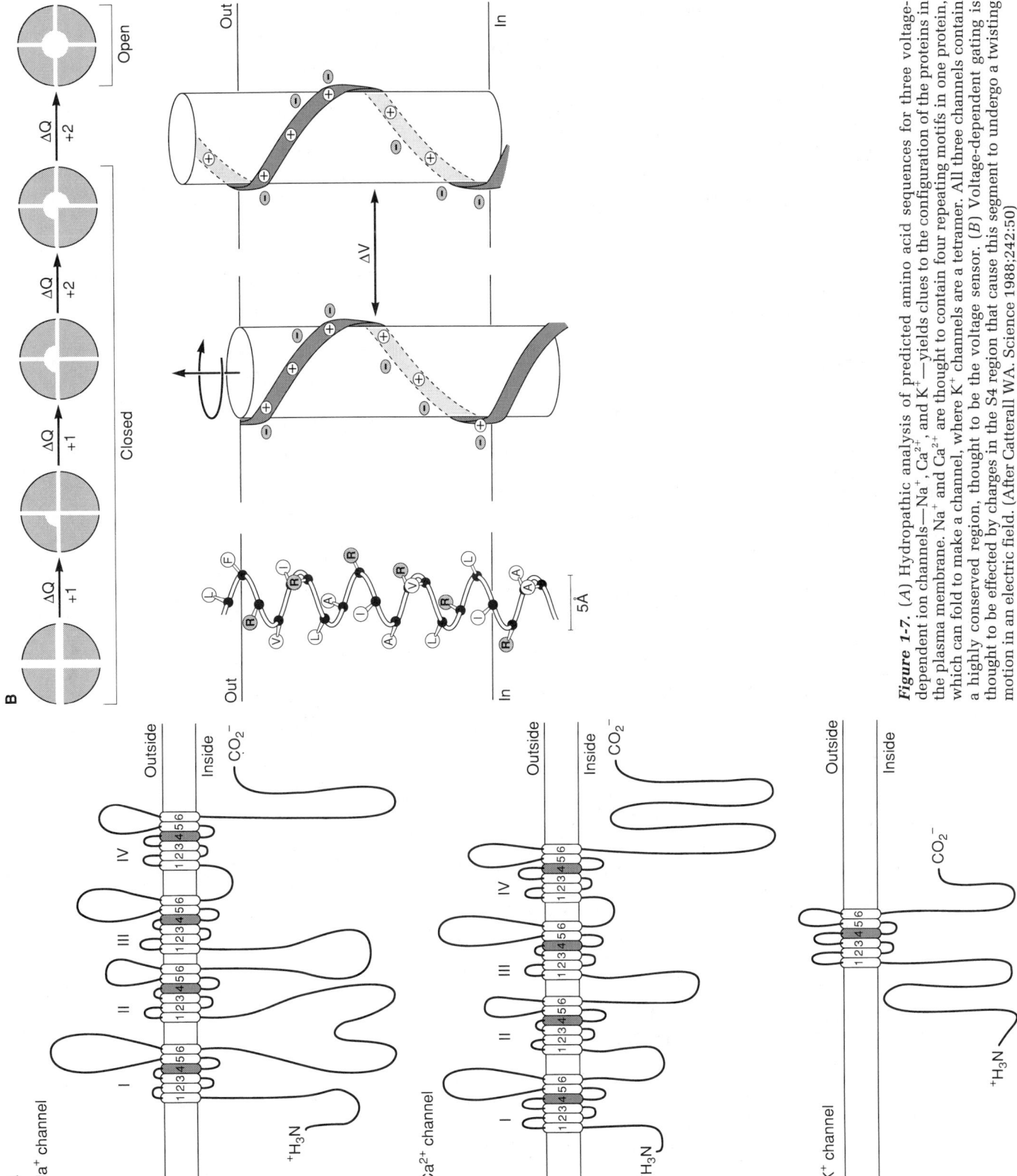

Figure 1-7. (*A*) Hydropathic analysis of predicted amino acid sequences for three voltage-dependent ion channels—Na^+, Ca^{2+}, and K^+—yields clues to the configuration of the proteins in the plasma membrane. Na^+ and Ca^{2+} are thought to contain four repeating motifs in one protein, which can fold to make a channel, where K^+ channels are a tetramer. All three channels contain a highly conserved region, thought to be the voltage sensor. (*B*) Voltage-dependent gating is thought to be effected by charges in the S4 region that cause this segment to undergo a twisting motion in an electric field. (After Catterall WA. Science 1988;242:50)

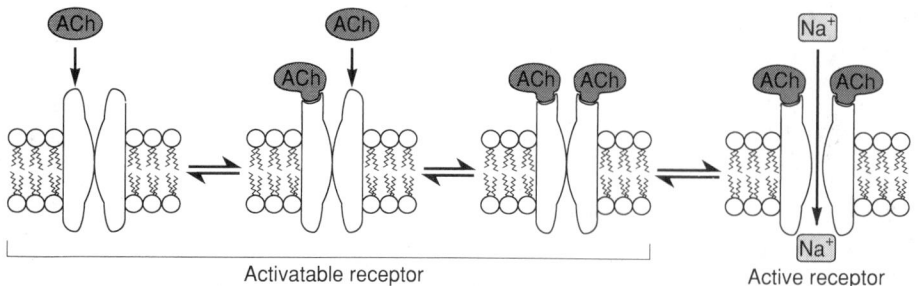

Figure 1-8. The acetylcholine receptor is an example of a ligand-gated channel. Two molecules of acetylcholine must bind before the channel can reach the open (conducting) conformation.

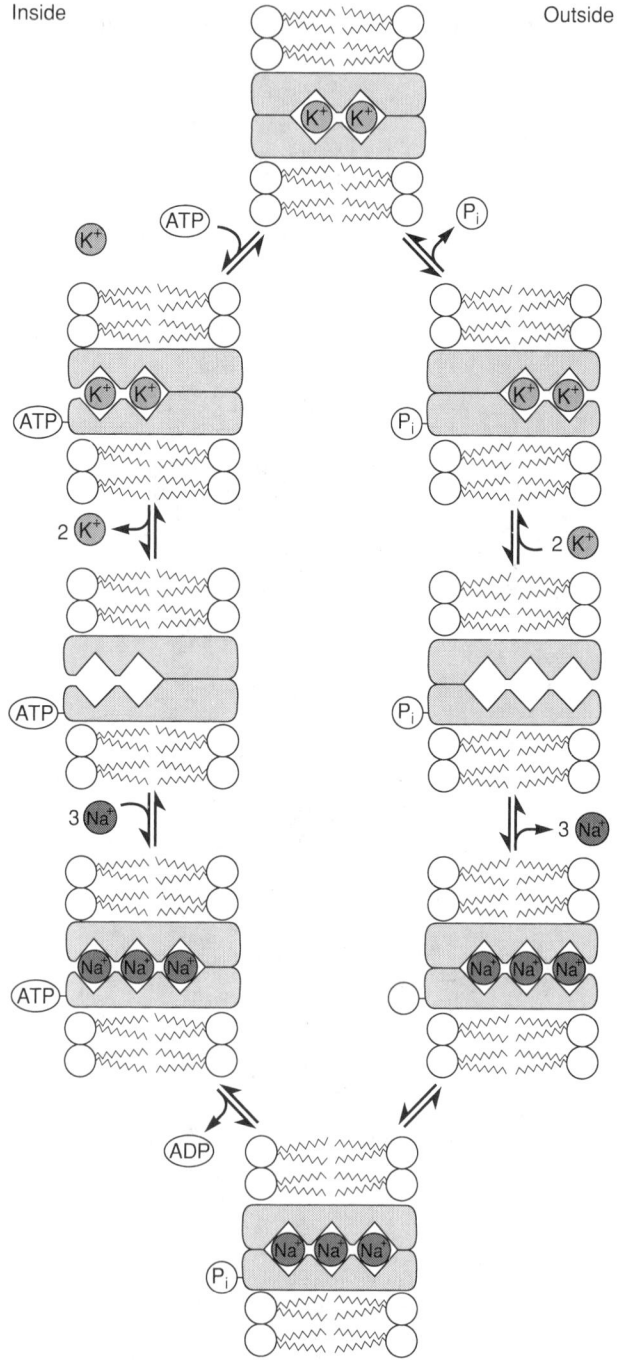

Figure 1-9. The Na^+-K^+-ATPase has a complicated catalytic cycle that involves not only the binding and unbinding of Na^+ and K^+ but also the binding of ATP, phosphorylation of the protein, and subsequent dephosphorylation, so that one ATP is hydrolyzed per transport cycle.

channels), and (2) the non–ADH-dependent water permeability of the membrane must be low.

Carrier Proteins

Membrane carriers are a broad class of transmembrane proteins that include simple leaks as well as energy-converting mechanisms such as ATPase, countertransporters, and cotransporters. The most important difference between a channel mechanism and a carrier mechanism is that in a channel, gating involves a conformational change between open and closed states. Conduction is associated with an open channel, and gating is not coupled to translocation. In a carrier mechanism, translocation is directly linked to a conformational change in the membrane protein. One consequence of the cyclic nature of carrier transport is that it is slower than channel transport. Another is that the conformation of the carrier can be influenced by the transmembrane distribution of the transported substrate. This produces a mechanism for coupling of the flows of two substrates. The archetype for biologic pumps is Na^+-K^+-ATPase (Fig. 1-9).

Volume Regulation

The functions of the solute transport mechanisms in the plasma membrane are maintenance and regulation of cell volume. Water distribution in most cells is determined entirely by solute distribution. The volume of a cell is determined by the same mechanisms that maintain the steady-state solute composition of the cell. Many if not all cells are capable of volume regulation. Volume regulatory responses are based on membrane transporters that enable the cell to undergo a net loss or a net gain of solute and hence loss or gain of water (Fig. 1-10).

INTRACELLULAR SYNTHESIS, TRANSPORT, AND ORGANIZATION OF MACROMOLECULES

DNA, RNA, and Protein Synthesis

The genetic code of an organism is contained in the nucleus of every cell. A sequence of four bases—adenine (A), guanine (G), cytosine (C), and thymine (T)—makes up two long chains bound by hydrogen bonds to form a DNA double helix. A is paired with T by two hydrogen bonds, and C is paired with G by three hydrogen bonds. This base-pair configuration is the basis of DNA replication, RNA transcription, and protein synthesis.

A gene is a segment of DNA that is transcribed into an RNA molecule, which either codes for a protein or forms a structural RNA molecule (Fig. 1-11). Genes are 10,000 to 100,000 base pairs long and include, in addition to the coding sequence, flanking regions and intervening se-

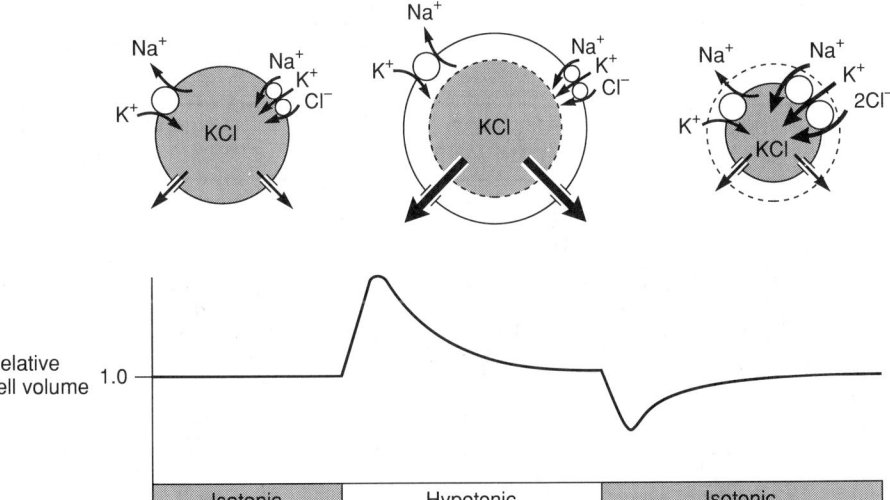

Figure 1-10. Many cells actively regulate their volume by turning on and off specific transport pathways. A hypotonic solution is shown here as causing cell swelling and activating channels for K^+ and Cl^+ so that salt leaves the cell, promoting shrinkage. A return to isotonic conditions leads to water efflux and cell shrinkage, which activates a coupled, Na^+-K^+-$2Cl^-$ entry process that results in a gain of salt and water and a return to normal volume.

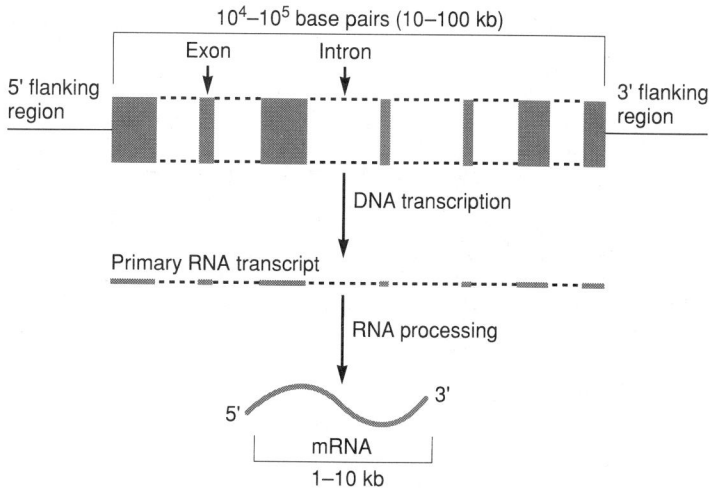

Figure 1-11. Structure of a typical gene, its primary RNA transcript, and the resulting mature mRNA. The entire coding region of the gene is initially transcribed, and the regions coded for introns are then spliced out during processing. The mature mRNA is then an RNA copy of the exon regions of the gene.

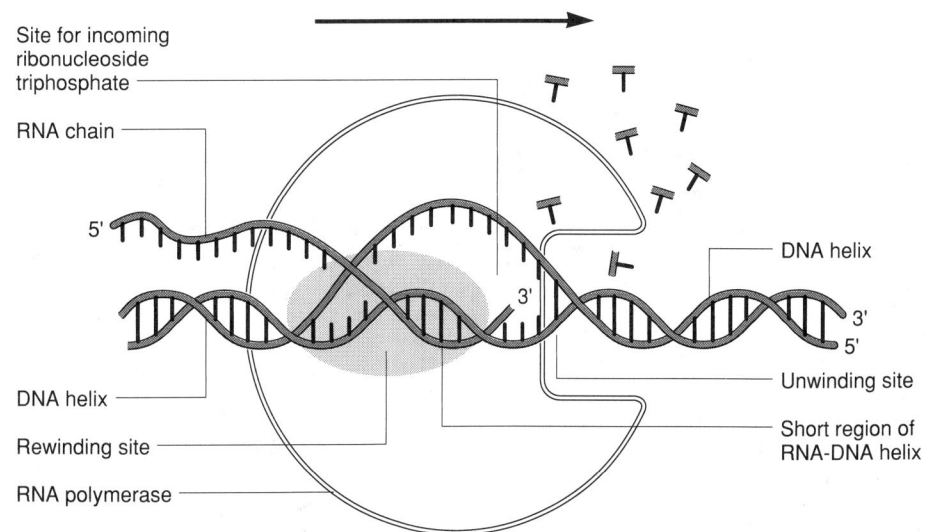

Figure 1-12. Transcription of DNA. RNA polymerase acts to unwind the DNA helix, catalyzes the formation of a transient RNA–DNA helix, and then releases the RNA as a single-strand copy while the DNA rewinds. In the process, the polymerase moves along the DNA from a start sequence to a stop sequence.

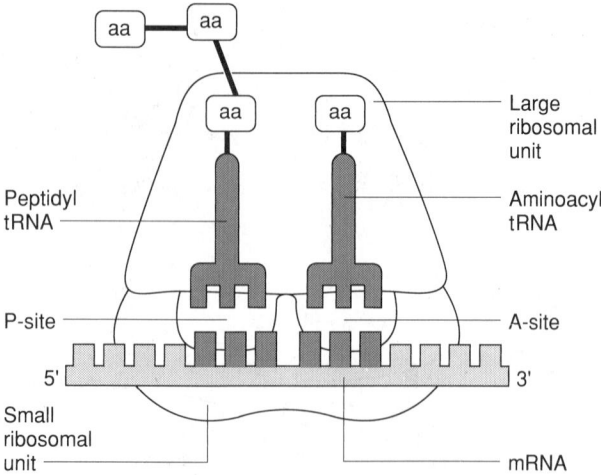

Figure 1-13. Schematic view of the elongation phase of protein synthesis on a ribosome. As the ribosome moves along the mRNA, incoming aminoacyl–tRNA complexes bind to the A-site on the ribosome, after which a new peptide bond is formed with the nascent polypeptide chain previously attached to the peptide tRNA. The ribosome then moves, ejecting the now-empty tRNA and opening the A-site for the next aminoacyl–tRNA complex.

quences, called *introns.* Introns are removed from the primary RNA transcript by *splicing.*

When cells divide, the two DNA chains of the double helix separate, and each serves as a template for synthesis of a complementary strand directed by the enzyme DNA polymerase. One of the new double helices goes to each daughter cell. The amount and sequence of DNA in each new cell is the same as that of the parent cell. To direct the synthesis of protein, the DNA sequence has to be tran-

scribed into three types of RNA—messenger RNA (mRNA), transfer RNA (tRNA), and ribosomal RNA (rRNA). RNA synthesis is directed by an RNA polymerase enzyme that makes an RNA copy of DNA.

Transcription of a gene begins at an initiation site associated with a specific DNA sequence, a *promotor region.* Recognition of this region by the polymerase is aided by proteins, *transcription factors,* which bind to DNA, and by *initiation factors,* which bind to the polymerase. After binding to DNA, RNA polymerase opens a short region of the double helix to expose the nucleotides. Once the two strands of DNA are separated, the strand containing the promoter becomes a template to which ribonucleoside triphosphates form base pairs by means of hydrogen bonds. Nucleotides are then joined together as the RNA polymerase moves stepwise along the DNA (Fig. 1-12). Behind the polymerase, the DNA double helix re-forms, displacing the RNA polymer. When a termination signal is reached, the polymerase releases both the template and the newly made RNA strand and is free to rebind to another promoter region.

The synthesis of protein involves translation from a four-letter nucleotide language to one of 20 chemically distinct amino acids. There is no mechanism for direct chemical recognition between specific nucleic acid bases and specific amino acids. Instead, an adapter molecule, tRNA, is used. Covalent attachment to tRNA allows amino acids to be added to a growing protein in the sequence specified by the nucleic acid code. Protein synthesis occurs by formation of a peptide bond between the carboxyl terminal of the growing polypeptide chain and the free amino group of the activated amino acid tRNA. This process occurs within ribosomes (Fig. 1-13).

Targeting of Newly Synthesized Protein

After synthesis, a new protein molecule must be targeted to its location in the cell. During targeting, all except cytosolic proteins must be inserted into or cross a membrane.

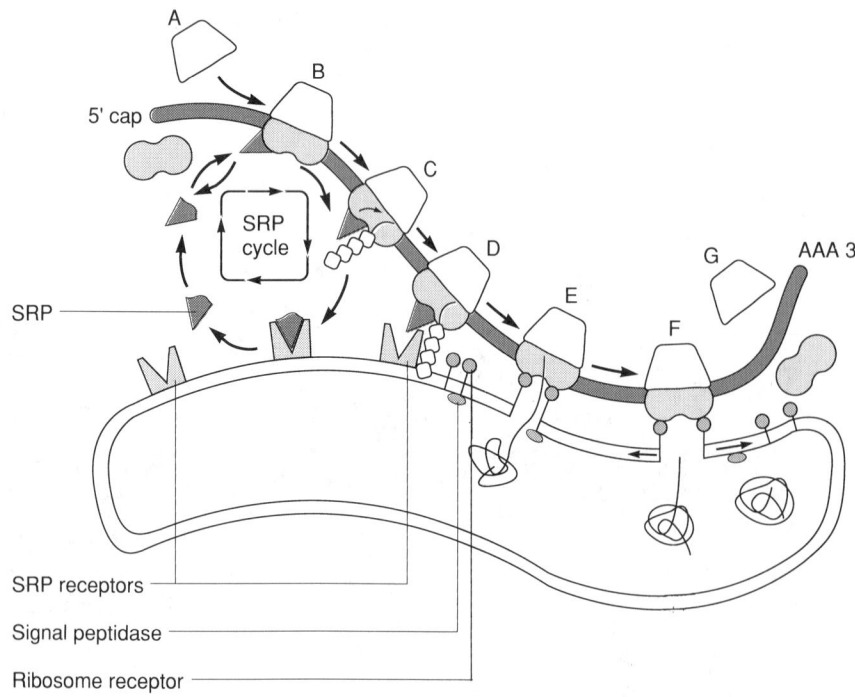

Figure 1-14. Synthesis and sequestration of secretory protein. Synthesis begins on the left as ribosomal subunits aggregate (*A*) and begin to translate mRNA (*B*). The signal-recognition particle (SRP) binds to the complex (*C*) and arrests peptide-chain elongation until SRP binds to a receptor in the endoplasmic reticulum membrane (*D*). The nascent polypeptide is then extruded into the lumen (*E* and *F*) with the aid of ribosome receptors, and SRP is released to recycle. The amino-terminal sequence may be cleaved by a signal peptidase. On chain termination, the ribosome dissociates (*G*), and its subunits can recycle.

After protein synthesis, a newly synthesized protein either enters the secretory pathway or remains in the cytoplasm or other organelles.

All protein synthesis originates on ribosomes in the cytosol, but proteins that take the secretory pathway rapidly bind to the ER (Fig. 1-14). Nuclear proteins such as histones, DNA and RNA polymerases, and gene regulatory proteins are synthesized on cytoplasmic-free ribosomes and enter the nucleus through the nuclear pores. Mitochondria contain DNA and synthesize some proteins, but most mitochondrial proteins are imported from the cytoplasm.

Secretory Pathway

Once they have been translocated across a lipid bilayer into the lumen of the ER, secretory proteins pass through a number of compartments, including the Golgi bodies, where they are processed and end up in a secretory vesicle or lysosome (Fig. 1-15). This process involves vesicular transport, in which the proteins do not cross membranes but are transferred between lumens of compartments. A small vesicle buds from one compartment, such as ER, and fuses with another, such as a Golgi body. The biosynthesis of lysosomes involves production of lysosomal enzymes and lysosomal membrane proteins that separate from other secretory proteins in the trans-Golgi network.

Transport to the Cell Surface: Exocytosis

Transport vesicles that bud off from the trans-Golgi network carry both material to be secreted from the cell and proteins that become components of the plasma membrane. This process, *exocytosis*, results in the re-

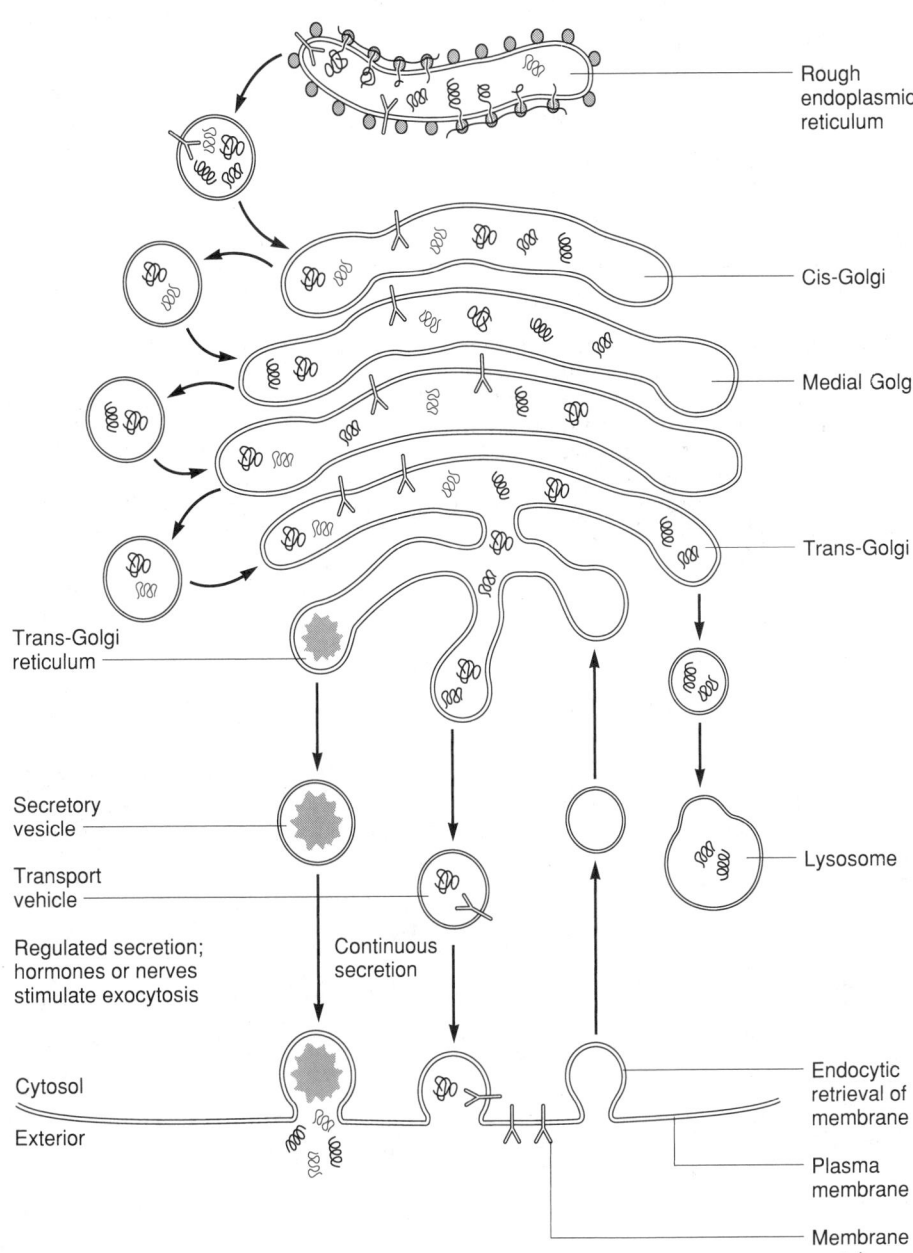

Figure 1-15. Intracellular transport and sorting of proteins destined for secretion, insertion into the plasma membrane, or targeting to the lysosome. After insertion into the endoplasmic reticulum lumen, movement from one compartment to another is by vesicular transport, which buds off one compartment and fuses with the next. Sorting signals intrinsic to the newly synthesized proteins specify the pathway to be taken.

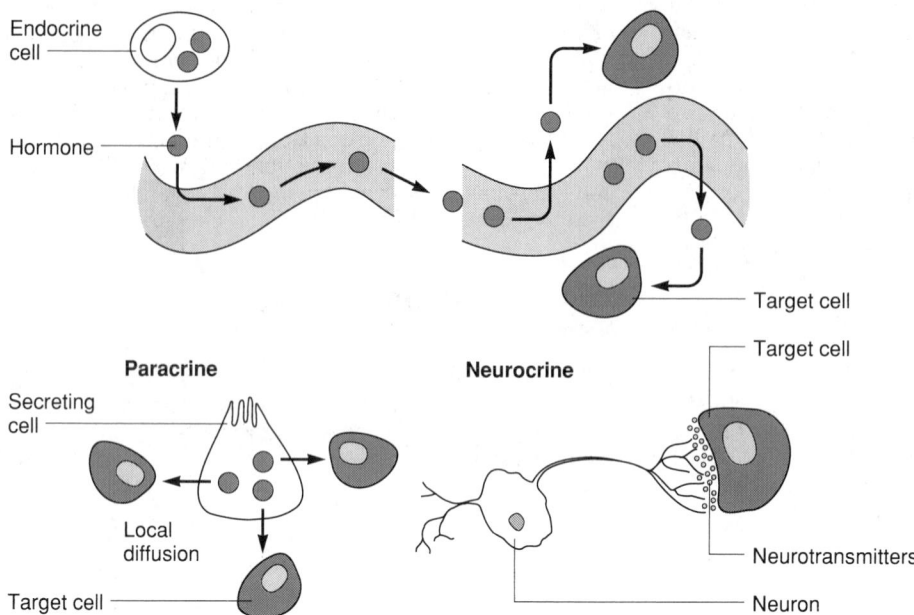

Figure 1-16. Endocrine, paracrine, and neurocrine modes of cell-to-cell communication.

lease of the content of the vesicle and the incorporation of the vesicle membrane into the plasma membrane. The former internal surface of the vesicle now faces the outside of the cell.

Vesicular transport to the cell surface can be divided into two components. *Constitutive secretion* involves small, coated vesicles that move rapidly to the plasma membrane and fuse. Secretory and plasma membrane proteins take this route. This pathway transports basement membrane components secreted by all cells and delivers membrane proteins such as Na^+-K^+-ATPase to the plasma membrane. *Regulated secretion* occurs in

cells that secrete digestive enzymes, hormones, and other regulatory molecules and neurotransmitters. The material to be secreted is sorted into a storage vesicle or granule. Fusion with the plasma membrane and exocytosis then take place in response to external stimulation.

Digestive enzymes and protein and polypeptide hormones have a signal sequence on the molecules that directs the molecules into the regulated pathway. The production of secretory granules involves budding of clathrin-coated vesicles from the trans-Golgi network. These vesicles fuse to form a large vesicle of dilute

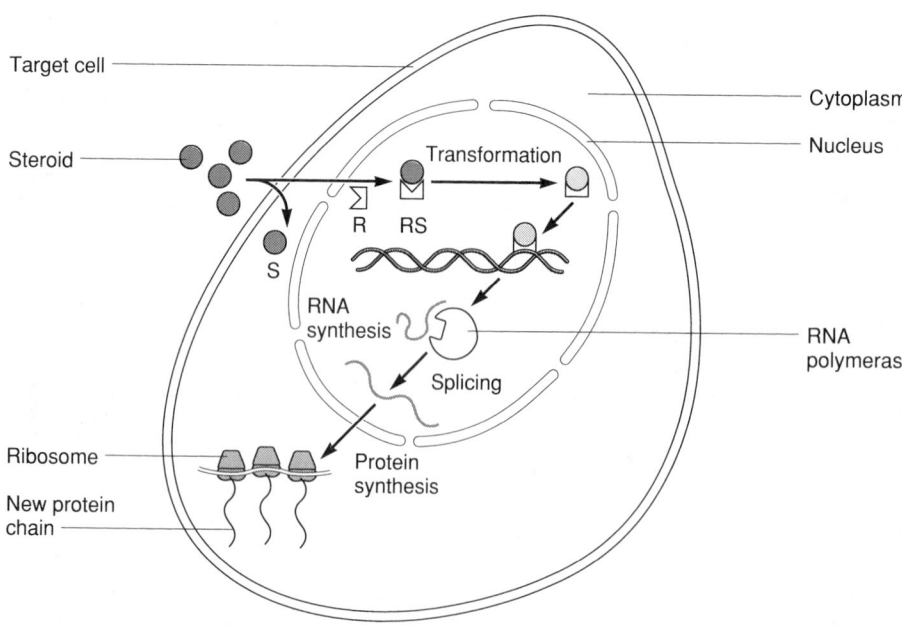

Figure 1-17. Schematic diagram of steroid hormone action. Steroids (S) enter the target cell and bind to a receptor (R), which is then transformed and binds to DNA in the nucleus, where it acts as a transcription factor to regulate the binding of RNA polymerase and the synthesis of new mRNA.

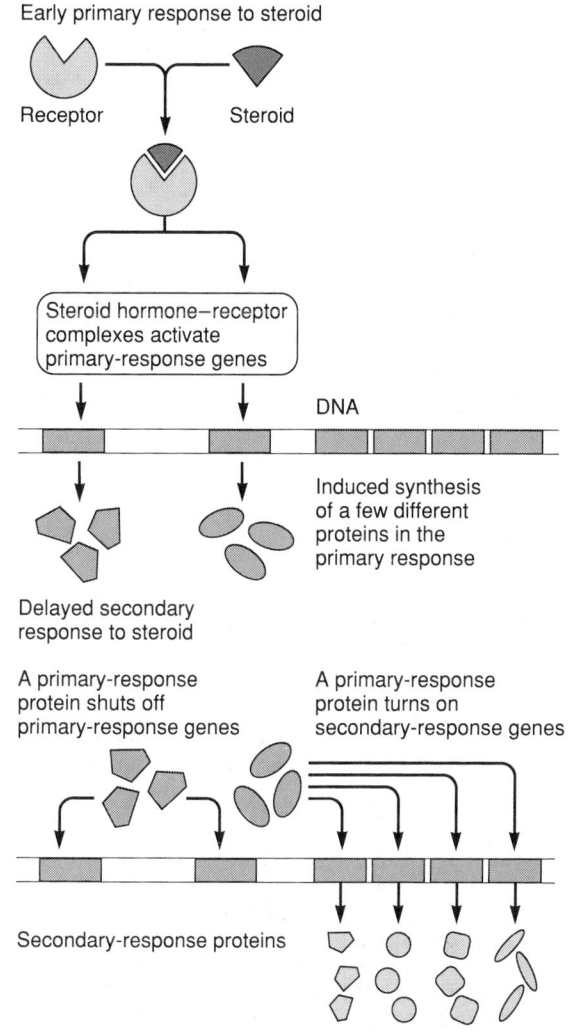

Figure 1-18. Pattern of gene expression in response to steroid hormone, whereby a few different primary-response genes are activated, and their products then regulate the expression of secondary-response genes.

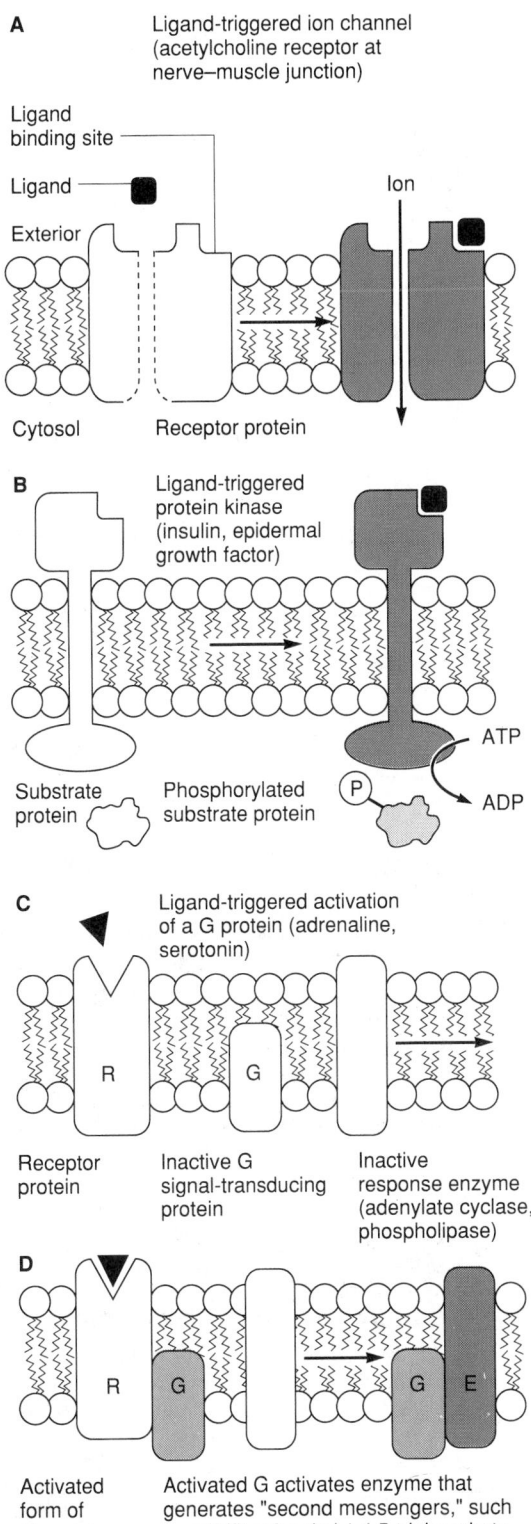

Figure 1-19. Types of cell-surface receptors. (*A*) Ligand-activated ion channel; binding results in a conformational change, opening or activating the channel. (*B*) Ligand-activated protein kinase; binding activates the kinase domain, which phosphorylates substrate proteins. (*C* and *D*) Ligand activation of a G protein, which then activates an enzyme that generates second, or intracellular, messengers.

content. This vesicle concentrates secretory proteins and, in some cells, completes processing of the secretory protein.

In some neurons and mast cells, newly formed secretory granules do not contain secretory material, but do contain transporters and enzymes necessary for the uptake or synthesis of small molecules such as histamine and norepinephrine. These molecules are condensed with counterions and proteins and are stored until regulated secretion is triggered. Regulated secretion is usually triggered by a hormone or neurotransmitter.

Endocytosis and Phagocytosis

Opposite in direction to secretion of macromolecules but occurring by similar mechanisms is *endocytosis.* The membrane invaginates and pinches off to form an intracellular vesicle that contains both membrane proteins and ingested material. The ingested macromolecules do not mix with the cytoplasm and are transferred within the cell by budding and fusion of vesicles. Endocytosis is distinct from *phagocytosis,* by which specialized cells take up

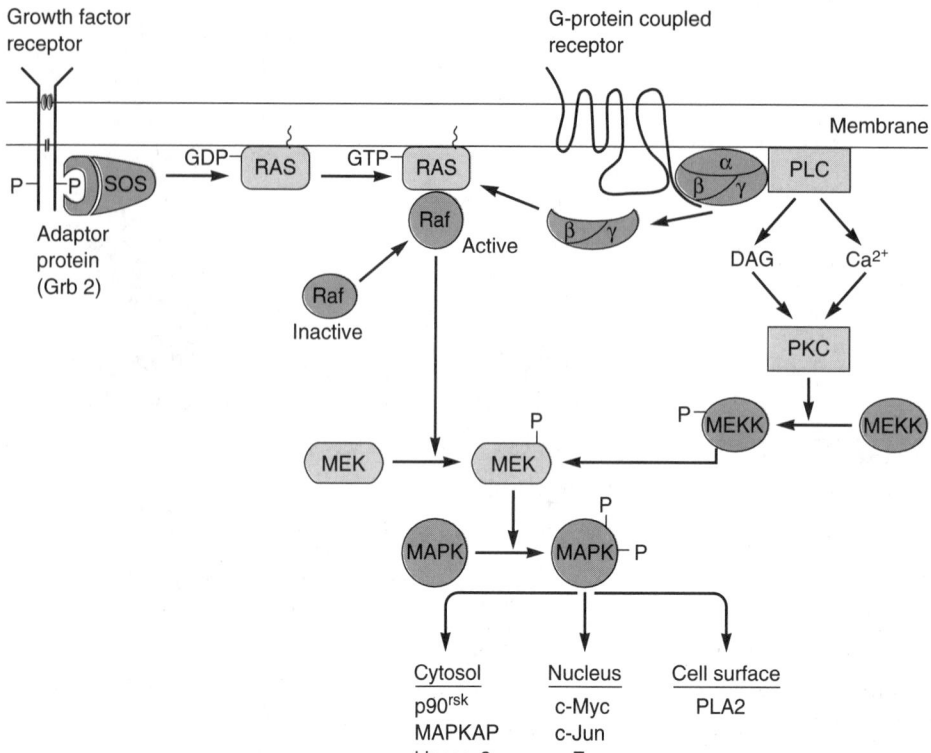

Figure 1-20. Schematic diagram for activation of the MAP kinase cascade.

larger particles, such as bacteria or erythrocytes. *Pinocytosis* is the capture of fluid.

REGULATION OF CELL FUNCTION

The growth, differentiation, and function of all cells are highly regulated. Most regulation occurs by means of extracellular chemical messengers. Depending on how the extracellular messenger arrives, cell regulation can be classified as follows (Fig. 1-16): *Paracrine regulation*—a chemical messenger or mediator is produced and acts locally; *Endocrine regulation*—extracellular messengers (hormones) are released into the blood and act on target cells that possess appropriate receptors; *Neurocrine regulation*—neurons secrete transmitters into the synaptic cleft to produce a connection between the neuron and the target cell.

Intracellular Receptors and the Control of Gene Expression

Receptors for steroid hormones, thyroid hormones, vitamin D, and retinoic acid form a superfamily of receptors that bind DNA and also bind a particular ligand (hormone). Most cells contain about 10,000 receptors for one or more steroid hormones or other similar receptors. Once a ligand binds, a receptor undergoes activation, which allows cytoplasmic receptors to move into the nucleus and bind to DNA. Receptors already in the nucleus increase their affinity for DNA. Activated steroid and thyroid receptors bind to specific regions of DNA and influence the synthesis of mRNA, regulating the production of proteins that mediate the cellular response to the hormone (Figs. 1-17, 1-18).

Transduction by Cell Surface Receptors

All water-soluble regulatory molecules, including peptide and protein hormones and smaller neurotransmitters, bind to cell surface receptor proteins. Binding of the ligand

evokes an intracellular signal, which regulates enzyme activity, membrane transport, or gene expression. Most cell surface receptors belong to one of the following classes (Fig. 1-19): *Ion channel receptors*—multisubunit assemblies in which each subunit has multiple membrane-spanning segments. These subunits form an ion-selective pore that can be gated by a change in the transmembrane electrical potential or by binding of a ligand to one of the subunits; *Catalytic receptors*—membrane proteins with enzymatic activity; *G-protein–linked receptors*—structures that interact with proteins that activate production of the intracellular message and influence the affinity of the receptor (Fig. 1-20).

Intracellular Messengers

The prototypic intracellular messenger is cAMP. Most, if not all, actions of cAMP are mediated by activation of cAMP-dependent protein kinase A. cAMP binds to the regulatory subunit, causing it to release the active catalytic subunit. The active kinase then catalyzes the phosphorylation from ATP of residues of target proteins.

Intracellular calcium ions function as second messengers. The intracellular concentration of Ca^{2+} increases as a result of the enzymatic hydrolysis of phosphatidyl inositol bisphosphate (PIP_2). Both Ca^{2+} and diacylglycerol exert many of their effects by altering protein phosphorylation.

SUGGESTED READING

Aberts B, Bray D, Lewis J, Raff M, Roberts K, Watson JD. Molecular biology of the cell, ed 3. New York, Garland, 1994.

Berridge MJ. Inositol trisphosphate and calcium signalling. Nature 1993;361:315.

Blenis J. Signal transduction via the MAP kinases: proceed at your own RSK. Proc Natl Acad Sci USA 1993;90:5889.

Bourne HR, Saunders DA, McCormick F. The GTPase superfamily:

conserved structure and molecular mechanism. Nature 1991;349:117.

Fantl WJ, Johnson DE, Williams LT. Signaling by receptor tyrosine kinases. Annu Rev Biochem 1993;62:453.

Nishizuka Y. Intracellular signaling by hydrolysis of phospholipids and activation of protein kinase C. Science 1992;258:607.

Rothman JE. Mechanisms of intracellular protein transport. Nature 1994;372:55.

ESSENTIALS OF SURGERY: SCIENTIFIC PRINCIPLES AND PRACTICE, edited by Lazar J. Greenfield, Michael W. Mulholland, Keith T. Oldham, Gerald B. Zelenock, and Keith D. Lillemoe. Lippincott–Raven Publishers, Philadelphia, © 1997.

CHAPTER 2

NUTRITION AND METABOLISM

WILEY W. SOUBA AND WILLIAM G. AUSTEN, JR.

Many patients lose weight during hospitalization. Patients can tolerate limited weight loss because short-term caloric shortfall does not prolong illness, nor does it complicate convalescence after an operation or other therapy. Other patients, such as those with severe injuries or life-threatening complications such as sepsis, need vigorous nutritional care.

BASIC NUTRITIONAL BIOCHEMISTRY

Body Composition

Total body mass has an aqueous component and a nonaqueous component. The nonaqueous portion is bone, tendon, mineral mass, and adipose tissue. The aqueous component is fluid in circulating blood cells and the cells that compose skeletal muscle, abdominal and thoracic organs, and skin; interstitial fluid; and intravascular volume. Total body water in a 70-kg man is 55% to 60% (almost 40 L) of total body mass. About 22 L is intracellular fluid, 14 L interstitial fluid, and 3-3.5 L plasma volume.

Body composition varies with age and sex and in response to injury or an operation. These changes are characterized by a loss of lean body mass, a loss of body fat, expansion of the extracellular fluid compartment, and a decrease in the metabolically active body mass.

The body contains fuel reserves that are used during starvation and stress. The greatest energy component is fat, which provides about 9 kilocalories per gram. Body protein is the next largest mass of usable energy, but amino acids yield only about 4 kilocalories per gram. Body protein is not a storage form of energy but is a structural and functional component. A chronic catabolic state can lead to erosion of body protein stores that makes one susceptible to infection and impaired wound healing.

Energy Metabolism

The body burns fuel to generate energy, which is used to perform work. The body performs mechanical work (locomotion, breathing), transport work (carrier-mediated uptake of nutrients into cells), and synthetic work (biosynthesis of proteins and other complex molecules). The energy to perform work comes from the chemical bonds of nutrients. The body converts this energy into internal work (eg, enzymatic catalysis) and external work (eg, muscular contraction for locomotion).

Sources of Energy

Amino acids, glucose, and fatty acids are the energy sources the body uses to perform work. *Amino acids* are derived from endogenous or dietary protein or are provided for IV administration as crystalline L-amino acids. *Glucose* is produced when carbohydrates are broken down in the intestinal lumen or is generated in the liver from other sugars. *Fatty acids* are derived from the hydrolysis of triglycerides.

Caloric Requirements

A *calorie* is the amount of heat required to raise the temperature of 1 g of water from 14.5°C to 15.5°C at a pressure of 1 standard atmosphere. A kilocalorie (1000 calories) is the unit of energy used in the United States. Basal energy requirements are measured with the person at rest (ie, no external work is being done).

Caloric requirements (metabolic rate) are related to oxygen consumption with the following formula:

$$\text{Metabolic rate} = 4.83 \times O_2 \text{ consumption}$$

where metabolic rate is expressed in kilocalories per unit time and O_2 consumption is expressed in liters of oxygen consumed per unit time. For example, a resting 70-kg man consumes about 200 mL of oxygen per minute, or 288 L a day. This is ≈1450 kcal/day.

For most adult surgical patients, energy requirements are estimated. Basal metabolic rate (BMR) is estimated from body weight (Table 2-1). Energy needs increase as the severity of illness increases (Table 2-2). After an elective operation, the expenditure of kilocalories increases only minimally. The largest increase occurs after severe multiple trauma or thermal injury.

Glucose in TPN solutions is in the form of dextrose, which provides 3.4 kcal/g. One liter of D_5W contains 50 g of dextrose, or 170 kcal. The usual surgical patient given IV glucose solution at 125 mL/h receives approximately 500 kcal/day, far less than the number of kilocalories needed to meet energy requirements. It is, however, enough to stimulate release of insulin, which stimulates amino-acid uptake and protein synthesis.

When high carbohydrate loads are given, respiratory quotient may increase in such a way that some infused glucose is converted to fat, producing large amounts of CO_2. Under normal circumstances, extra CO_2 is removed from the body during breathing. Patients with pulmonary insufficiency, however, may experience CO_2 retention during high-glucose feedings, necessitating a decrease in glucose calories to prevent acid–base abnormalities.

Table 2-1. **APPROXIMATE BASAL METABOLIC RATES IN ADULTS**

Weight (kg)	Basal Metabolic Rate (kcal/d)
50	1300
60	1450
70	1600
80	1750
90	1900
100	2050

Table 2-2. CALORIC REQUIREMENTS FOR AN AVERAGE (70-KG) ADULT MAN

Disease Process	kcal/d
Basal	1450
Postoperative (uncomplicated)	1500–1700
Sepsis	2000–2400
Multiple trauma (ventilator)	2200–2600
Major burn	2500–3000

Protein and Amino Acid Metabolism

About 15% of total body weight is protein, half of which is intracellular and half extracellular. Extracellular proteins are those that circulate in the bloodstream (eg, albumin, transferrin, hemoglobin) and those that compose the intracellular matrix (eg, collagen and other fibrous proteins).

Dietary protein is the source of most amino acids. Digestion of protein provides free amino acids that are absorbed by the small intestine and delivered to the body, where they are incorporated into new proteins or other biosynthetic products. Excess amino acids are degraded, and their carbon skeleton is oxidized to produce energy, or it is incorporated into glycogen or free fatty acids. While dietary amino acids are being metabolized, proteins that exist in the cell are being recycled. Total body protein turnover is about 300 g/d.

Urinary nitrogen losses decrease in patients fed a protein-free diet but never become zero. In stressed patients, this ability to adapt to starvation is compromised in such a way that proteolysis of body proteins continues at a high rate. Net proteolysis occurs in skeletal muscle and organs such as the intestine and liver. Compromise of the ability to synthesize protein, as in malnutrition or disease, results in a reduction in function, such as impaired wound healing, decreased immunocompetence, or breakdown of the GI mucosal barrier.

Nitrogen (N) balance is calculated from the difference between the amount of nitrogen taken in and the amount of nitrogen lost in the urine, stool, skin, wounds, and fistula drainage

$$N_{balance} = N_{intake} - N_{output}$$

Positive nitrogen balance means intake is greater than output, as in postoperative anabolism and a child's growth. *Negative nitrogen balance* means intake is less than output, as in starvation, injury, and severe infection. Over long periods, healthy adults stay in nitrogen equilibrium (zero nitrogen balance). Surgical patients are prone to negative nitrogen balance because of their underlying disease. This is most often manifested as wasting of skeletal muscle.

Metabolism of amino acids generates ammonia, a toxic physiologic compound. In healthy people, ammonia levels in the blood are kept at nontoxic concentrations, primarily by the liver, which converts ammonia to urea. Urea is a highly soluble, nontoxic molecule with a high nitrogen content. Healthy people excrete about 30 g of urea daily. This may increase to >60 g per day in catabolic surgical patients. Urea accounts for 85% of total urinary nitrogen; the other 15% is ammonia and creatinine.

Because nitrogen losses are accentuated in catabolic disease, surgical patients have increased energy and nitrogen needs. The recommended daily allowance for protein is 0.8 g/kg per day. This requirement may triple in critically ill patients. One gram of nitrogen is equivalent to 6.25 g of protein.

After an overnight fast, the intestinal lumen is empty of ingested protein. Therefore, the rate of absorption of luminal amino acids is low. Circulating amino acid levels are maintained by the release of preformed amino acid pools and the breakdown of cellular proteins. In catabolic surgical patients, protein synthesis in skeletal muscle increases but so does breakdown, and to a greater extent than synthesis. This is manifested as loss of lean body mass and negative nitrogen balance.

Thermoregulation

Alterations in the central thermostat in the hypothalamus almost always occur in patients with systemic infections. Core temperature reflects the balance between heat production and heat loss, both of which may be altered in surgical patients. Most of the heat produced in the postabsorptive basal state occurs in the brain and the abdominal organs. Increases in heat production occur after an infectious challenge and are caused by re-setting of the hypothalamic setpoint, which is mediated by cytokines such as interleukin-1. Metabolic rate increases about 10% for each degree (C) increase in temperature. Heat loss is regulated by perspiration and adjustments in skin blood flow.

HOMEOSTATIC RESPONSES AND ADJUSTMENTS TO STRESS

The body's defense mechanisms are initiated within moments of injury. These mechanisms are essential for survival—they are designed to maintain body homeostasis at a time when key physiologic processes are threatened. The

Table 2-3. DIFFERENCES IN BODILY RESPONSES TO ELECTIVE SURGERY AND TO ACCIDENTAL INJURY

Insult	Elective Operation	Accidental Injury (Trauma)
Tissue damage	Minimal; tissues are dissected with care and reapproximated	Can be substantial; tissues usually torn or ripped; débridement often necessary
Hypotension	Uncommon; preoperative hydration is employed and fluid status is carefully monitored intraoperatively	Fluid resuscitation often not immediate; blood loss can be substantial, leading to shock
Pain, fear, anxiety	Generally can be alleviated with preoperative medication	Generally present
Infectious complications	Uncommon; prophylactic antibiotics often administered	More common as the result of contamination, hypotension, and tissue devitalization
Overall stress response	Controlled and of lesser magnitude; starvation better tolerated	Uncontrolled; proportional to the magnitude of the injury; malnutrition poorly tolerated

mechanisms involve responses to stimuli such as volume loss, tissue damage, fear, or pain. The greater the insult, the more pronounced the response. Invasive infection and starvation perpetuate the responses. Whether the injury is accidental or surgical, the responses to trauma are similar. The differences that do exist are shown in Table 2-3.

Components of the Stress Response

Volume Loss and Tissue Underperfusion

When circulating blood volume decreases, the body begins to compensate to maintain organ perfusion. Pressure receptors in the aortic arch and carotid artery and volume receptors in the wall of the left atrium detect the decrease in blood volume and immediately respond by signaling the brain. Heart rate and stroke volume increase. Afferent nerve signals are initiated that stimulate the release of both antidiuretic hormone (ADH) and aldosterone.

ADH increases water reabsorption in the kidney. Aldosterone increases renal sodium reabsorption, conserving intravascular water. These mechanisms are only partially effective, and severe hemorrhage, without adequate resuscitation, often leads to a prolonged low-flow state. Under these circumstances, oxygen delivery is inadequate to meet tissue demands, and the cell switches to anaerobic metabolism, which leads to lactic acidosis.

Tissue Damage

Injury to body tissues appears to be the most important factor that sets the stress response in motion. Afferent neural pathways from the wound signal the hypothalamus that injury has occurred, and tissue destruction is sensed as pain. Efferent pathways from the brain are immediately triggered to stimulate the responses designed to maintain homeostasis.

Pain and Fear

Pain and fear lead to excessive production of catecholamines, which prepares the body for the fight-or-flight response.

Lack of Nutrient Intake

The metabolic response to injury or an operation causes an increase in energy expenditure. In many surgical patients, nutrient intake is inadequate for 1 to 5 days after the operation. If energy intake is less than expenditure, body fat stores are oxidized and lean body mass is eroded; the patient loses weight. Body glycogen stores are depleted within 24 to 36 hours. Then glucose, which is required by the central nervous system and white blood cells, must be synthesized de novo. Amino acids, which are released principally by skeletal muscle, are the precursors of gluconeogenesis.

Most injured patients tolerate a loss of 15% of normal weight without a marked increase in surgical risk. When weight loss exceeds 15% of body weight, the complications of undernutrition interact with stress and may impair the ability of the body to respond to injury and complications such as infection.

Invasive Infection

A serious complication for surgical patients is infection. The normal barrier defense mechanisms are disrupted by indwelling catheters, nasotracheal and nasogastric tubes, and breakdown of skin and mucous membranes. Infection alone initiates catabolic responses such as fever, hyperventilation, tachycardia, accelerated gluconeogenesis, increased proteolysis, and lipolysis. Inflammatory cells release a variety of soluble mediators

that aid host resistance and wound repair. Undernutrition may compromise the host defense mechanisms and increase the likelihood of invasive sepsis, multiple-system organ failure, and death.

Determinants of the Host Response to Surgical Stress

The body must be capable of transmitting and integrating injury signals, both neural and humoral, and mounting an appropriate response, which requires the interaction of a number of organ systems. The nature, intensity, and duration of the stress determine the host mediators activated and the physiologic changes that occur. Responses to a minor elective operation are similar to those during a comparable, brief period of fasting and bed rest. There are profound metabolic differences, however, between the response to simple starvation and the response to injury (Table 2-4).

Body Composition

Posttraumatic nitrogen excretion is directly related to body protein mass. The net loss of nitrogen from the body indicates the net breakdown of the corresponding amount of protein.

Nutritional Status

Patients in a state of nutritional depletion who undergo elective operations experience decreased nitrogen losses. Protein-depleted patients have lower preoperative respiratory muscle strength and vital capacity, an increased incidence of postoperative pneumonia, and longer postoperative hospital stays.

Age

Many of the changes in the metabolic responses to surgical illness that occur with aging can be attributed to alterations in body composition and to long-standing patterns of physical activity. Although weight is stable, fat mass increases with age, and muscle mass decreases. The loss of strength that accompanies immobility, starvation, and acute surgical illness may have marked functional consequences.

Sex

Differences between the metabolic responses of men and those of women reflect differences in body composition. Lean body mass is lower in women than in men. This may

Table 2-4. METABOLIC DIFFERENCES IN BODILY RESPONSES TO SIMPLE STARVATION AND TO INJURY

Parameter	Simple Starvation	Severe Injury
Basal metabolic rate	−	++
Presence of mediators	−	+++
Major fuel oxidized	Fat	Mixed
Ketone body production	+++	±
Hepatic ureagenesis	+	+++
Negative nitrogen balance	+	+++
Gluconeogenesis	+	+++
Muscle proteolysis	+	+++
Hepatic protein synthesis	+	+++

be why the net loss of nitrogen after elective abdominal operations is lower in women than in men.

MEDIATORS OF THE STRESS RESPONSE

The response to surgical stress or accidental injury has two components—neurohormonal and inflammatory. The principal *hormones* are catecholamines, corticosteroids, and glucagon. The *inflammatory* component involves the local elaboration of cytokines and the systemic activation of humoral cascades involving complement, eicosanoids, and platelet-activating factor. These mediators promote wound healing by stimulating angiogenesis, white cell migration, and ingrowth of fibroblasts.

During elective operations, the inflammatory response is confined to the wound, and large amounts of mediators do not gain access to the systemic circulation. After accidental injury in which there is massive tissue destruction or prolonged hypotension that leads to cell injury, these mediators may be produced in the wound in excessive amounts. The excess spills over into the systemic circulation, and cells in other tissues may become activated to produce the mediators. A systemic response may follow in which the mediators cause detrimental effects, such as hypotension and organ dysfunction.

THE GASTROINTESTINAL MUCOSAL BARRIER AND THE STRESS RESPONSE

Under some circumstances the intestine may become a source of sepsis. Maintenance of an intact brush border and intercellular tight junctions prevents the movement of toxic substances into the intestinal lymphatic vessels and the circulation. These functions may become altered in critically ill patients. Maintenance of a GI mucosal barrier that excludes luminal bacteria and toxins requires an intact epithelium and normal mucosal immune mechanisms.

Microbial translocation is the process by which microorganisms cross the mucosal barrier and invade the host. Translocation is promoted in three ways:

1. Altered permeability of the intestinal mucosa (as in hemorrhagic shock or sepsis or administration of cell toxins)
2. Decreased host defense (due to glucocorticoid administration, immunosuppression, or protein depletion)
3. An increased number of bacteria within the intestine (as in bacterial overgrowth or intestinal stasis)

Infection is associated with bacterial invasion from the intestine. Because many of the factors that facilitate bacterial translocation occur simultaneously in surgical patients and the effects may be additive or cumulative, patients in an ICU may be extremely vulnerable to the invasion of enteric bacteria or to the absorption of their toxins. Such patients usually do not receive enteral feedings, and parenteral therapy leads to intestinal atrophy.

NUTRITION AND METABOLISM AFTER ELECTIVE OPERATIONS

Physiologic Response to Surgical Stress

The physiologic responses to surgical stress are summarized in Figure 2-1. The period of catabolism initiated by an operation, a combination of inadequate nutrition and alteration of the hormonal environment, lasts 1 to 3 days. The withdrawal phase, which lasts another 1 to 3 days, is followed by the onset of anabolism, which often begins with the start of oral feeding. A prolonged period of early anabolism is characterized by positive nitrogen balance and weight gain. Protein synthesis increases as a result of sustained enteral feedings, and this change is related to the return of lean body mass and muscular strength.

Nutritional Support

Most patients who undergo elective operations are adequately nourished. Unless the patient has suffered marked preoperative malnutrition or a severe intraoperative or postoperative complication, solutions that contain 5% dextrose may be administered for 5 to 7 days before enteral nutrition is begun.

Nutritional Assessment

The objectives of nutritional assessment are:

1. Determine the patient's nutritional status
2. Determine energy, protein, and other nutrient requirements

The medical history and physical examination emphasize associated diseases and weight loss. They are used to establish the diagnosis of cachexia, protein-energy malnutrition, or specific nutrient deficiencies. Measurements of skinfold thickness are helpful to determine fat mass, and a 24-hour urine collection with measurement of creatine allows determination of the creatine-height index, which is proportional to muscle mass.

Immunologic status is used to evaluate nutritional status. Total peripheral lymphocyte count, delayed hypersensitivity with a skin-test response to common antigens, and lymphocyte transformation are used as indicators of immunocompetence. Depressed immune function often returns to normal with nutritional repletion.

Determination of Nutritional Requirements

Total energy requirements are based on:

1. BMR
2. The degree of stress imposed by the disease
3. The amount of energy expended with activity

Nomograms relate normal metabolic requirements to a person's age, sex, height, and weight. The principal determinants of nitrogen requirements in surgical patients are total energy intake, nitrogen intake, and the metabolic state of the patient. Malnourished patients with intact protein-conserving mechanisms can achieve nitrogen equilibrium when 7% to 8% of the total caloric needs are provided as protein. This translates into a calorie-to-nitrogen ratio of 350:1. A hypermetabolic, catabolic state necessitates provision of more protein.

Route of Feeding

For patients who can eat and who have a functional GI tract, adequate nutrition is provided with a regular hospital diet. Patients with a functional intestinal tract who cannot eat receive nasogastric or nasojejunal feedings. Patients with a diseased or nonfunctional GI tract may need parenteral nutrition. Peripheral venous feedings provide dilute nutrients in a large fluid volume and rely on fat emulsions as a principal calorie source. Central venous feedings consist of hypertonic glucose and amino acid solutions infused through a catheter in the superior vena cava.

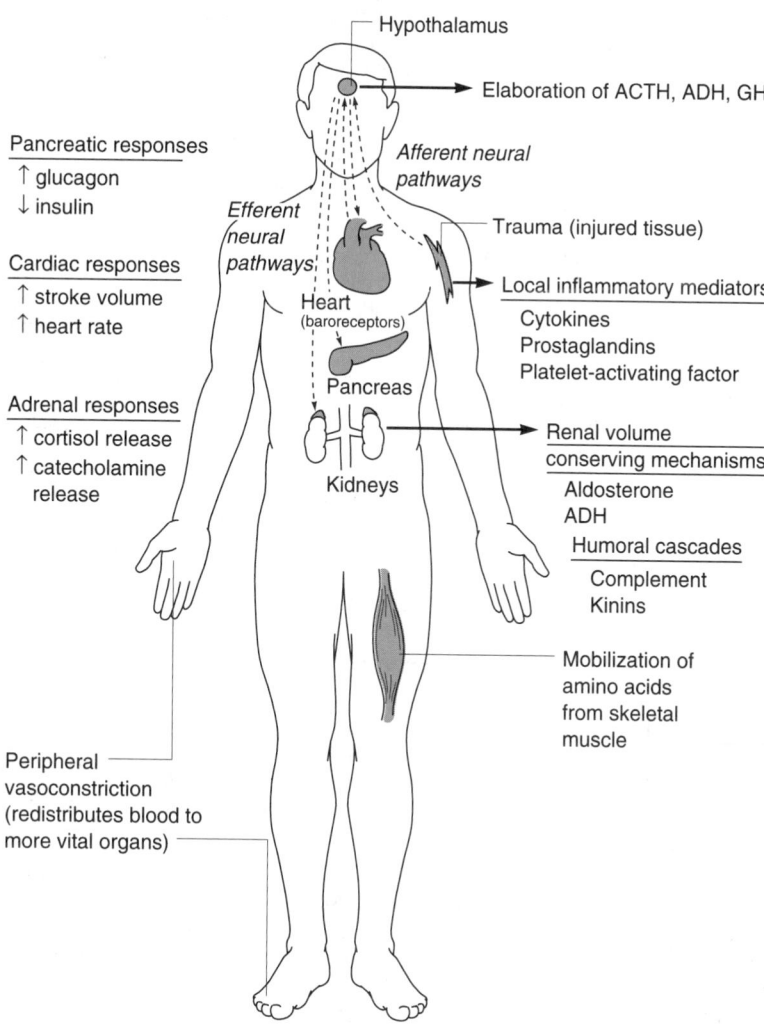

Figure 2-1. Homeostatic adjustments initiated after injury.

NUTRITION AND METABOLISM IN TRAUMA

Consequences of Malnutrition

Goals of Nutritional Support

Increased metabolic demands after injury quickly lead to malnutrition if the patient does not receive nutritional support. As soon as the patient's condition is stabilized, nutritional support is gradually initiated. The goal of nutritional support is maintenance of body cell mass and limitation of weight loss to less than 10% of preinjury weight. The nutritional requirements of trauma patients are determined as follows:

1. Determine BMR for age, sex, and body surface area (result is kcal/day)
2. Determine percentage increase in metabolic rate from the injury
3. Add 25% × BMR for hospital activity (walking, physical therapy, sitting, treatment)
4. Add the values obtained in steps 1, 2, and 3 to find estimated daily caloric requirement for maintenance of body weight
5. Divide the value obtained in step 4 by 150 to determine nitrogen requirements (protein = 6.25 × nitrogen).

6. Give approximately 70% of caloric requirement as glucose. Give the other 30% as fat. Reassess energy and nitrogen needs at least twice a week
7. If nutritional support seems inadequate because of progressive weight loss, consider direct measurement of oxygen consumption or measurement of nitrogen balance

NUTRITION AND METABOLISM IN SEPSIS

The response patterns to infection are less predictable than those after elective operations and trauma. Invasion of the body by microorganisms initiates many host responses, such as mobilization of phagocytes, inflammation at the site, fever, and tachycardia. Systemic events during the hyperdynamic phase of sepsis are related to host immunologic defenses and to metabolic and circulatory adjustments to infection. Changes in metabolism relate to alterations in glucose, nitrogen, and fat metabolism and redistribution of trace metals.

Nutritional Requirements

The objectives of nutritional assessment are to evaluate the patient's present nutritional status and to determine energy, protein, and macro- and micronutrient require-

Table 2-5. INDICATIONS FOR AND CONTRAINDICATIONS TO USE OF TPN BY PATIENTS WITH CANCER

Length of Hospital Stay	Contraindications	Indications
7–14 d	Good nutrition or mild malnutrition	Severe malnutrition
	Rapidly progressive malignant disease that does not respond to antitumor treatment	GI or other toxicity that precludes enteral intake for ≥7 d (TPN is administered before or in conjunction with antitumor therapy)
> wk 2 or home TPN	Rapidly progressive malignant disease that does not respond to antitumor treatment	Treatment-associated toxicity that precludes enteral nutrition
		Malnutrition in patients with disease that allows normal or near-normal performance status

ments. Total energy requirements are calculated with the stress equation (metabolic rate = $4.83 \times O_2$ consumption). Mild-to-moderate infections increase energy requirements 20% to 30%, and severe infection increases caloric needs 50% above basal levels.

Special Feeding Problems in Sepsis

Respiratory Insufficiency

A common problem associated with systemic infection is oxygenation and elimination of CO_2. Patients often require intubation and vigorous ventilatory support. Most of the enteral and parenteral formulas used to provide nutritional support for critically ill patients contain large amounts of carbohydrate, which generate large quantities of CO_2 after oxidation. The large CO_2 load may worsen pulmonary function or delay weaning from the ventilator. If this factor becomes a problem, the carbohydrate load is reduced to 50% of metabolic requirement, and fat emulsion is administered to provide additional calories.

Renal Failure

Hemodialysis minimizes the effects of uremia superimposed on the metabolism of sepsis. Proteins of high biologic value, in much smaller quantities than usually given, are administered along with adequate calories, usually in the form of glucose. When enteral feeding is not feasible, a central venous infusion of essential amino acid solution and hypertonic dextrose provides calories and a small quantity of nitrogen.

Gastrointestinal Dysfunction

The most common GI abnormality in sepsis is ileus, which results from intra-abdominal disease or the effects of bacteria elsewhere in the body. Breakdown of the GI mucosal barrier with translocation of luminal bacteria and their toxins initiates a prolonged hypermetabolic state. Treatment involves provision of appropriate nutrition and maintenance of mucosal structure and function with enteral feeding, intestine-specific nutrients such as glutamine and short-chain fatty acids, and growth factors.

Hepatic Failure

Hepatic dysfunction is a common manifestation of septicemia. The dysfunction may appear early as a slight elevation of liver enzymes, or it may cause severe jaundice and hyperbilirubinemia. Hepatic dysfunction resolves when the sepsis resolves, but if the inflammation persists, the feeding formulation must be adjusted. The carbohydrate load is usually reduced to no more than 50% of metabolic requirements, and the additional calories are provided as fat emulsion. If encephalopathy occurs, the protein load is reduced.

Cardiac Dysfunction

The myocardial dysfunction that occurs in sepsis may be due to the elaboration of cytokines or to heart failure due to pulmonary insufficiency. Malnourished patients with sepsis may be sensitive to volume overload. Use of a concentrated solution of hypertonic dextrose mixed with amino acids may be indicated to maximize calories and minimize volume. Twenty percent fat emulsion provides additional energy.

NUTRITION AND METABOLISM IN PATIENTS WITH CANCER

Malnutrition in patients with cancer is associated with an increase in the rate of postoperative complications, including sepsis, ileus, and wound dehiscence. It has adverse effects on immune function and tolerance of treatment. The rationale for providing nutritional support is to prevent or reverse host tissue wasting, broaden the spectrum of therapeutic options, improve clinical course, and prolong patient survival. If a patient has a functional GI tract and can consume adequate calories by mouth, a regular hospital diet is provided, and no specialized nutritional support is necessary.

Table 2-6. COMPOSITION OF A STANDARD CENTRAL VENOUS SOLUTION

VOLUME

10% amino acid solution	500 mL
50% dextrose solution	500 mL
Fat emulsion	—
Electrolytes + vitamins + minerals	~50 mL
Total volume	~1050 mL

COMPOSITION

Amino acids	50 g
Dextrose	250 g
Total potassium	50/6.25 = 8 g
Dextrose kcal	250 g × 3.4 kcal/g = 840 kcal
mOsm/L	~2000

Electrolytes Added to TPN Solutions	Usual Concentration (mEq/L)	Range of Concentrations (mEq/L)
Sodium	60	0–150
Potassium	40	0–80
Acetate	50	50–150
Chloride	50	0–150
Phosphate	15	0–30
Calcium*	4.5	0–20
Magnesium	5	5–15

* Generally added as calcium gluconate or calcium chloride. One ampule of calcium gluconate = 1 g of calcium = 4.5 mEq.

Enteral Nutrition

For patients with cancer who need nutritional support, enteral nutrition is always preferred if the GI tract is functional. Nutrition is provided with between-meal supplements, a soft nasogastric feeding tube, or a gastrostomy or jejunostomy feeding catheter. Infusion into the GI tract allows processing and absorption of nutrients in a normal physiologic manner. Enteral feeding maintains the integrity of the mucosal lining, providing a barrier to intraluminal enteric organisms that might translocate into the systemic circulation.

Total Parenteral Nutrition

The most important factor to consider about the use of TPN in patients with cancer is how the tumor will respond to antineoplastic therapy. Table 2-5 presents the indications for and contraindications to the use of TPN by patients with cancer.

ENTERAL VS TOTAL PARENTERAL NUTRITION

Enteral nutrition is provided to malnourished patients if feasible. The patient should have a functional GI tract and must be able to receive adequate amounts of calories and nitrogen.

TPN is used as primary therapy for the following conditions:

- Enterocutaneous fistula
- Short-bowel syndrome
- Hepatic failure
- Thermal injury
- Acute renal failure

TPN is used as secondary therapy for the following conditions:

- Prolonged ileus
- Acute enteritis after radiation therapy or chemotherapy
- Preoperative nutrition

Because of the risk of infectious complications, such as pneumonia, abscess, and line sepsis, preoperative TPN should be provided only to severely malnourished patients who cannot be nourished via the enteral route.

TPN Formulations

TPN solutions are administered through a central venous catheter inserted into the subclavian vein. The composition of a standard TPN solution is shown in Table 2-6. Blood sugar and serum electrolyte levels are monitored, and liver function tests are performed regularly. Elevations in serum glucose are common in surgical patients who receive TPN, especially if the patient is under stress and has glucose intolerance. Hyperglycemia is controlled with the addition of insulin to the TPN formulation or with a reduction in the amount of glucose in the solution.

Table 2-7. COMPLICATIONS ASSOCIATED WITH THE USE OF TOTAL PARENTERAL NUTRITION (TPN)

Complication	Cause	Treatment
MECHANICAL		
Pneumothorax	Puncture or laceration of lung pleura	Serial chest radiographs; chest tube if indicated
Subclavian artery injury	Penetration of subclavian artery during needlestick	Chest radiograph; serial monitoring of vital signs
Air embolism	Aspiration of air into the subclavian vein and right side of heart	Place patient in Trendelenberg and left lateral decubitus positions; aspirate air
Catheter embolization	Shearing off the tip when withdrawing catheter	Retrieve catheter transvenously under fluoroscopic guidance
Venous thrombosis	Clot formation in great vein secondary to catheter	Heparinization if clinically significant
Catheter malposition	Tip of catheter directed outside of superior vena cava or right atrium	Reposition under fluoroscopy
METABOLIC		
Hyperglycemia	Excessive glucose calories or glucose intolerance	Decrease glucose calories; administer insulin
Hypoglycemia	Sudden cessation of TPN	Bolus 50% glucose solution; monitor blood glucose
Carbon dioxide retention	Infusion of glucose calories in excess of energy needs	Decrease glucose calories and replace with fat
Hyperglycemic, hyperosmolar, nonketotic coma	Dehydration from excessive diuresis	Discontinue TPN immediately; give insulin; monitor glucose and electrolytes
Hyperchloremic metabolic acidosis	Excessive chloride administration	Give sodium and potassium as acetate salts
Azotemia	Excessive amino acid administration with inadequate calories	Decrease amino acids; increase glucose calories
Essential fatty acid deficiency	Inadequate essential fatty acid administration	Administer fat solution
Hypertriglyceridemia	Rapid fat infusion of decreased fat clearance	Slow rate of fat infusion
Hypophosphatemia, hypocalcemia, hypomagnesemia, hypokalemia	Inadequate administration of electrolyte in question	Increase administration
Bleeding	Vitamin K deficiency	Administer vitamin K
SEPTIC		
Line sepsis	Catheter tip infected	Remove catheter; antibiotics
Infection at skin site	Bacteria at site of catheter entry into skin	Remove catheter; local wound care

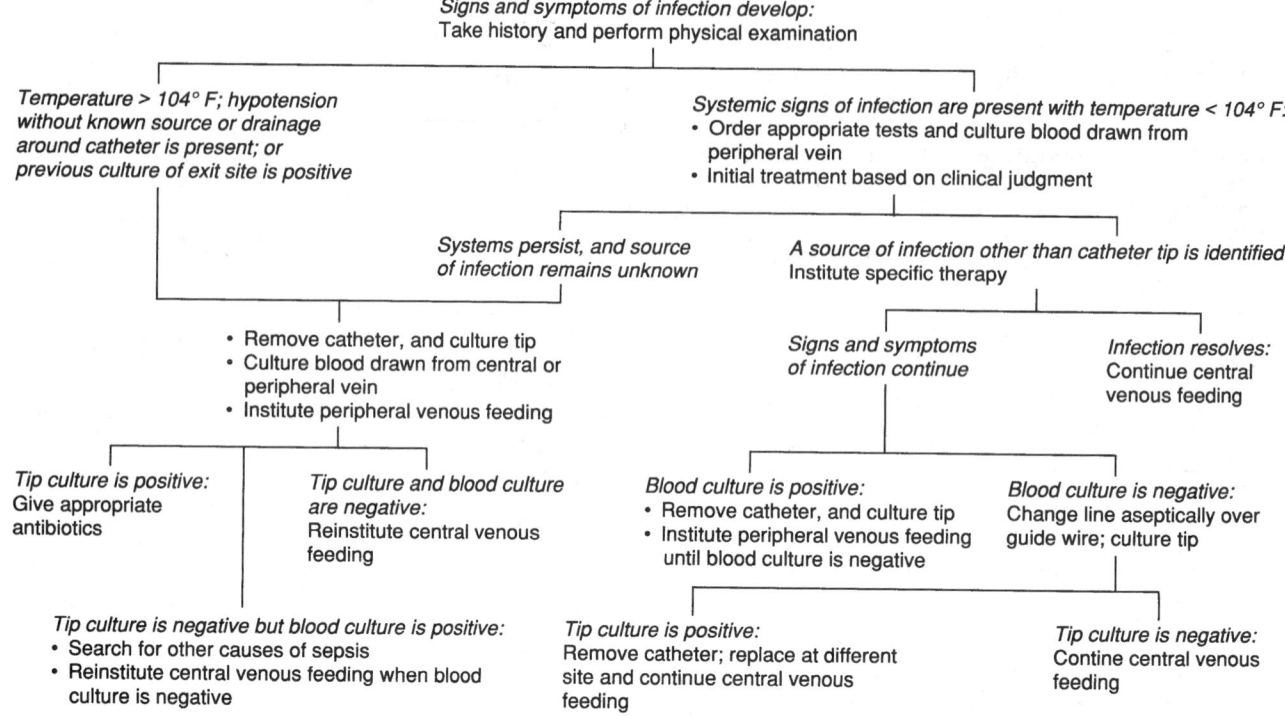

Figure 2-2. Treatment of a patient receiving total parenteral nutrition who becomes septic.

The amounts of electrolytes provided vary with factors such as previous nutritional and hydration status. Monitoring is critical because as new cell mass accrues, intracellular accumulation of potassium and phosphate ions may lead to severe hypokalemia or hypophosphatemia. These electrolyte disturbances develop rapidly and are life-threatening. Vitamin and trace mineral requirements also are taken into consideration.

Because of the complications associated with infusion of large amounts of dextrose, lipids are used in TPN solutions to meet linoleic acid requirements and full caloric needs in hypermetabolic patients. IV fat emulsions are composed of soy or safflower oil.

Complications of TPN

Complications of TPN are of three types: mechanical, metabolic, and infectious (Table 2-7). The main disadvantage of TPN is related to intestinal disuse, which may predispose a patient to infectious complications. Figure 2-2 is an algorithm for the management of sepsis during TPN.

SUGGESTED READING

Brennan MF, Pisters PWT, Posner M, et al. A prospective randomized trial of total parenteral nutrition after major pancreatic resection for malignancy. Ann Surg 1994;220:436.

Buzby GP and The Veterans Affairs Total Parenteral Nutrition Cooperative Study Group. Perioperative total parenteral nutrition in surgical patients. N Engl J Med 1991;325:525.

Fan ST, Lo CM, Lai ECS, et al. Perioperative nutritional support in patients undergoing hepatectomy for hepatocellular carcinoma. N Engl J Med 1994;331:1547.

Fong Y, Marano MA, Barber A, et al. Total parenteral nutrition and bowel rest modify the metabolic response to endotoxin in humans. Ann Surg 1989;210:449.

Jiang ZM, He GZ, Zhang SY, et al. Low-dose growth hormone and hypocaloric nutrition attenuates the protein-catabolic response after major operation. Ann Surg 1989;210:514.

Scheltinga MR, Young LS, Benfell K, et al. Glutamine-enriched intravenous feedings attenuate extracellular fluid expansion after standard stress. Ann Surg 1991;214:385.

Shils M, Young V (eds). Modern nutrition in health and disease. 8th ed. Philadelphia, Lea & Febiger, 1994.

Souba W. Cytokines: Key regulators of the nutritional/metabolic response to critical illness. Curr Probl Surg 1994;31:577.

van der Hulst RRWJ, van Kreel BK, von Meyenfeldt MF, et al. Glutamine and the preservation of gut integrity. Lancet 1993;341:1363.

ESSENTIALS OF SURGERY: SCIENTIFIC PRINCIPLES AND PRACTICE, edited by Lazar J. Greenfield, Michael W. Mulholland, Keith T. Oldham, Gerald B. Zelenock, and Keith D. Lillemoe. Lippincott–Raven Publishers, Philadelphia, © 1997.

CHAPTER 3

WOUND HEALING

NEIL A. FINE AND THOMAS A. MUSTOE

PRINCIPLES OF WOUND HEALING

A full-thickness injury to the skin sets in motion the following sequence of wound repair (Fig. 3-1).

Inflammation

The inflammatory phase begins immediately after wounding. The initial response is bleeding. The homeostatic response that stops the bleeding is clot formation,

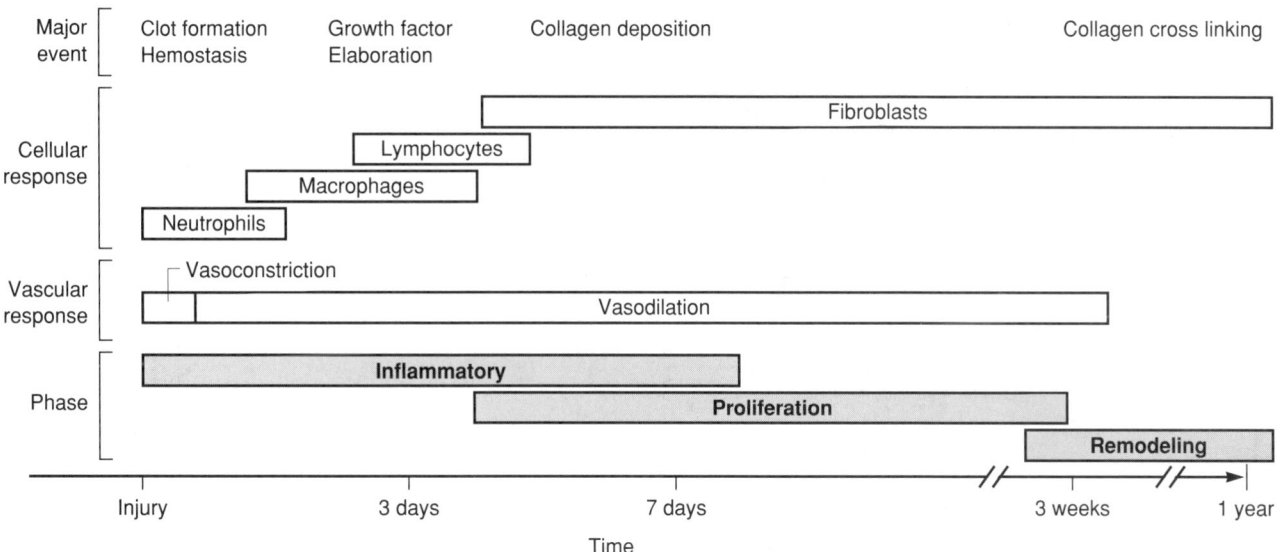

Figure 3-1. Time line of phases of wound healing with dominant cell types and major physiologic events.

in which a platelet plug held together by fibrin provides a framework for the cellular response that follows.

After wounding, transient *vasoconstriction* is mediated by catecholamines, thromboxane, and prostaglandin $F_{2\alpha}$. Platelets degranulate, releasing the contents of their α and dense granules, most notably platelet-derived growth factor and transforming growth factor-β (Table 3-1). These substances initiate chemotaxis and proliferation of inflammatory cells. Transient vasoconstriction decreases blood loss at the time of wounding, allowing the clot to form. This period of vasoconstriction lasts for 5 to 10 minutes.

After a clot forms and bleeding stops, *vasodilatation* occurs in and around the wound, increasing blood flow to the area to supply cells and substrate necessary for repair. Vascular endothelial cells deform, increasing in permeability. These responses are mediated by histamine, prostaglandin E_2, prostacyclin, and vascular endothelial cell growth factor (Fig. 3-2).

Table 3-1. **PLATELET GRANULES AND MEDIATORS OF PLATELET AGGREGATION**

PLATELET GRANULES

α **Granules: Contain Platelet-Specific Proteins**

Platelet factor 4
β-Thromboglobulin
Platelet-derived growth factor
Transforming growth factor β

Dense Granules

Adenosine diphosphate
Serotonin
Calcium

MEDIATORS OF PLATELET AGGREGATION

Thromboxane A_2
Thrombin
Platelet factor 4

In the inflammatory phase, the wound is full of debris from the initial injury: a mixture of injured, devitalized tissue (fat, muscle, epithelium), clot (platelets, red blood cells [RBCs], fibrinogen), bacteria (from the skin surface and external environment), extravasated serum proteins (glycoproteins and mucopolysaccharides), and foreign material (suture, dirt). Over the next several days, the wound is cleared of bacteria, devitalized tissue, and foreign material by an influx of phagocytic cells:

1. *Polymorphonuclear leukocytes* (PMNs) begin to arrive immediately, reaching large numbers within 24 hours.
2. The PMNs are soon followed by *macrophages,* which are present in large numbers within 2 to 3 days. Macrophages complete the process of removing all material not necessary for wound healing. Macrophages also release more than 30 growth factors and cytokines. These growth factors induce fibroblast proliferation, endothelial cell proliferation (angiogenesis), matrix production, and recruitment and activation of more macrophages.
3. *Lymphocytes* appear during the inflammatory phase but in small numbers. They seem to be more important in chronic inflammation than in the initial stages of wound healing.

Proliferation (Matrix Deposition and Scar Formation)

The proliferative phase of wound healing begins with a *provisional matrix* of fibrin and fibronectin derived from serum as part of the initial clot formation. At first, the provisional matrix is populated by macrophages. About 3 days after injury, *fibroblasts* begin to migrate along the fibronectin–fibrin framework to initiate collagen synthesis. Fibroblasts proliferate in response to growth factors to become the dominant cell type. At the same time, growth factors produced by macrophages induce the growth and proliferation of *endothelial cells,* which form new *capillaries* in the wounded area (angiogenesis). This vascularity is visible through the epithelium and gives the wound a

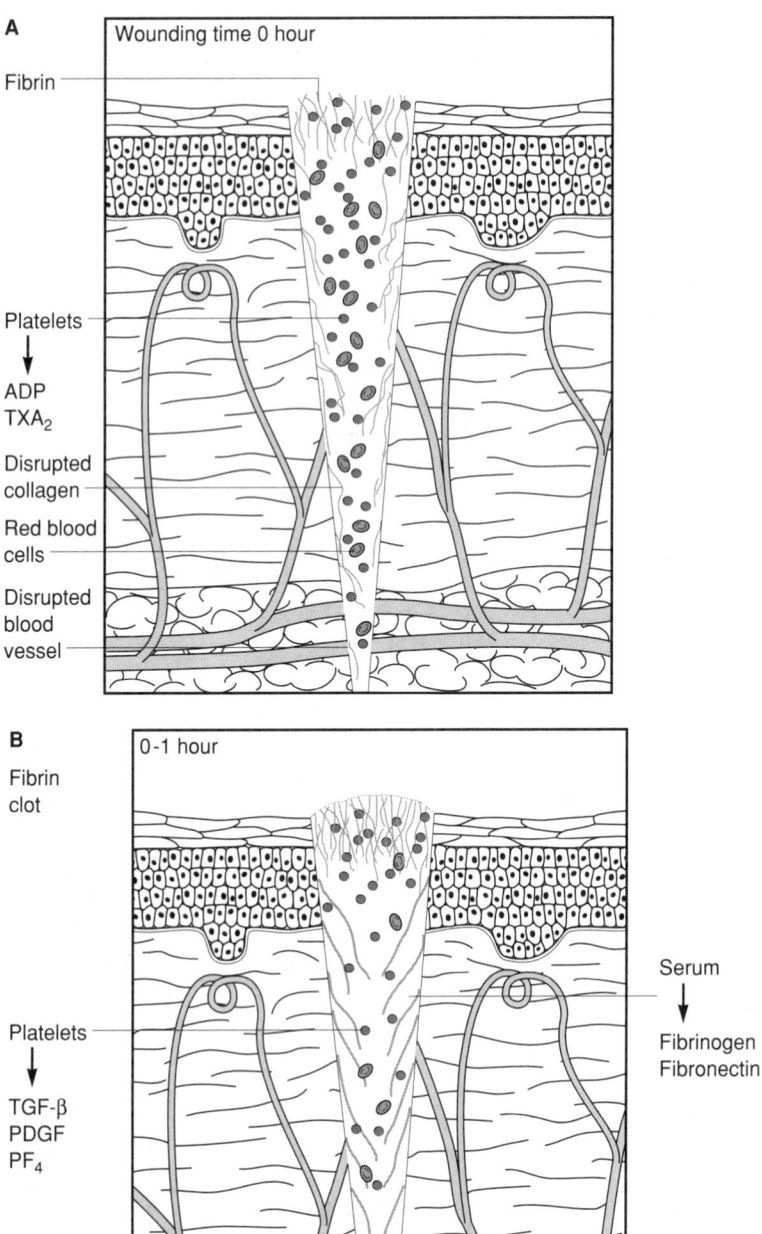

A

Wounding time 0 hour

Fibrin

Platelets
↓
ADP
TXA$_2$

Disrupted
collagen

Red blood
cells

Disrupted
blood
vessel

B

0-1 hour

Fibrin
clot

Platelets
↓
TGF-β
PDGF
PF$_4$

Serum
↓
Fibrinogen
Fibronectin

Figure 3-2. Schematic representation of wound healing processes. ADP, adenosine diphosphate; TXA$_2$, thromboxane A$_2$; TGF, transforming growth factor; PDGF, platelet-derived growth factor; PF$_4$, platelet factor 4; TNF-α, tumor necrosis factor α; FGF, fibroblast growth factor; PAF, platelet-activating factor; KGF, keratinocyte growth factor. *(continues)*

pink or purple appearance. This capillary ingrowth provides the fibroblasts with oxygen and nutrients for proliferation and production of a *permanent matrix* of collagen and proteoglycans.

Collagen is the dominant molecule in the wound matrix and in the final scar. It is synthesized into an organized cable-like network in a process that ends with formation of stable, cross-linked collagen fibrils (Fig. 3-3). These intra- and intermolecular bonds provide strength and stability to the wound. As the wound matures, fibrils cross link to form large cables of collagen that increase tensile strength. The wound is now a scar.

Proteoglycans, also called *ground substance*, are composed of a protein backbone and long carbohydrate side chains. The hydrophilic nature of these molecules is responsible for much of the water content of scar tissue. Immature wounds contain a disproportionately large amount of proteoglycans, particularly hyaluronic acid.

Remodeling

The transition from the proliferative phase to the remodeling phase is defined by collagen equilibrium, which occurs 2 to 3 weeks after wounding. Production of new colla-

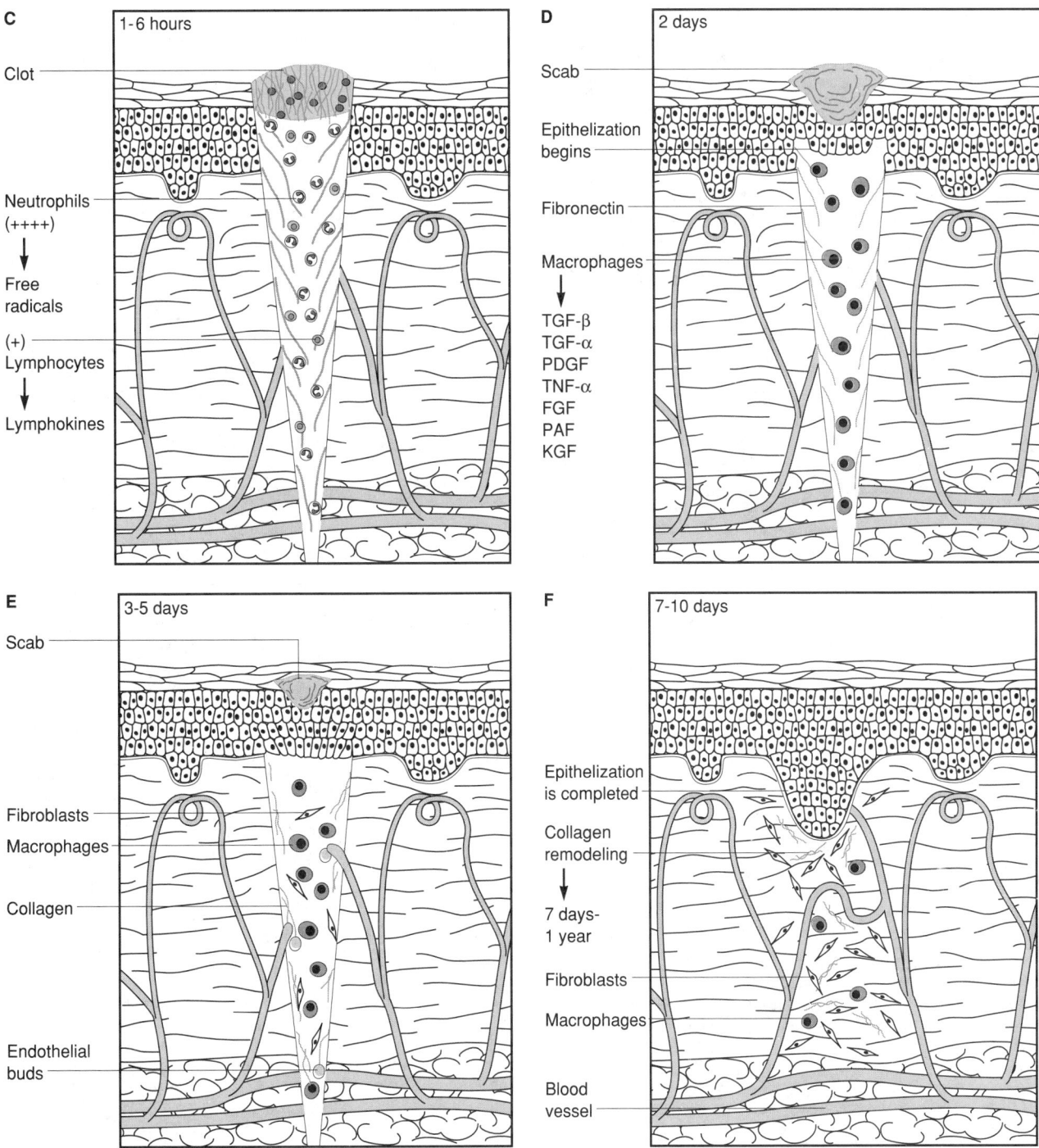

C | 1-6 hours

Clot

Neutrophils
(++++)

↓

Free
radicals

(+)
Lymphocytes

↓

Lymphokines

D | 2 days

Scab

Epithelization
begins

Fibronectin

Macrophages

↓

TGF-β
TGF-α
PDGF
TNF-α
FGF
PAF
KGF

E | 3-5 days

Scab

Fibroblasts

Macrophages

Collagen

Endothelial
buds

F | 7-10 days

Epithelization
is completed

Collagen
remodeling

↓

7 days-
1 year

Fibroblasts

Macrophages

Blood
vessel

Figure 3-2. (Continued)

gen and degradation of collagen by collagenases reach a steady state. During achievement of this equilibrium, collagen fibrils become aligned longitudinally in a configuration dictated by the stresses on the wound. Capillary density and the number of fibroblasts decrease, and the wound loses its pink or purple color. Tensile strength gradually increases as haphazard collagen fibrils are replaced by orderly collagen fibrils with strong intermolecular bonds. Strengthening continues for at least 6 months, and the scar eventually reaches 70% of the strength of unwounded skin.

Epithelialization

Reconstitution of the epithelial barrier begins within hours of injury. Epithelial cells from the basal layer at the wound edge flatten and migrate across the wound. The cells along the margin divide to reform the multilayered mature epithelium. Epithelial cells continue to migrate across a bed until a single continuous layer is formed. In migration, the epithelial cells send out pseudopods that allow the cells to attach to the extracellular matrix by means of integrin receptors. Bacteria, large amounts of pro-

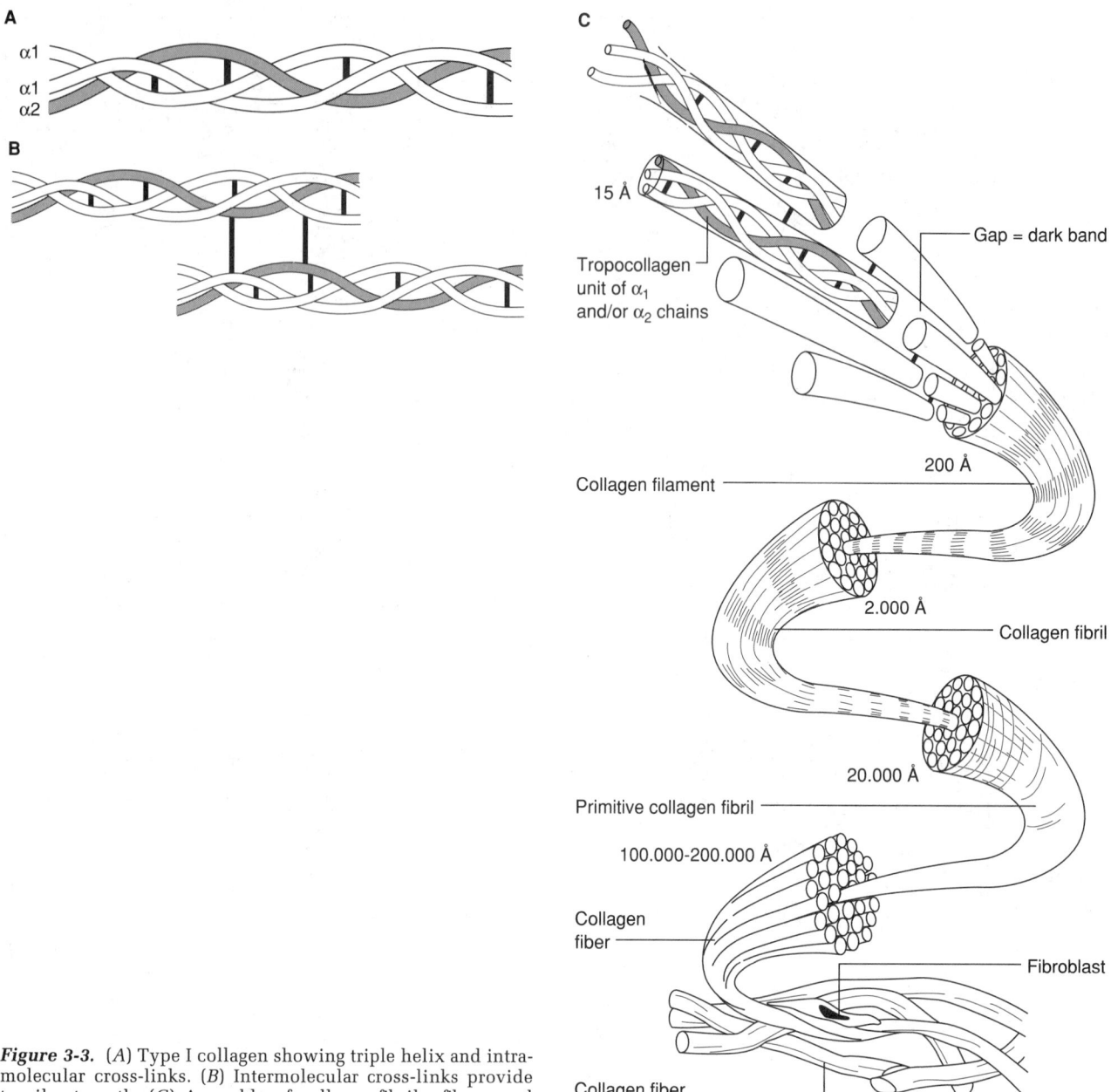

A

α1
α1
α2

B

C

15 Å

Tropocollagen
unit of α₁
and/or α₂ chains

Gap = dark band

Collagen filament

200 Å

2.000 Å

Collagen fibril

20.000 Å

Primitive collagen fibril

100.000-200.000 Å

Collagen
fiber

Fibroblast

Collagen fiber
bundle

Figure 3-3. (*A*) Type I collagen showing triple helix and intra-molecular cross-links. (*B*) Intermolecular cross-links provide tensile strength. (*C*) Assembly of collagen fibrils, fibers, and fiber bundles.

tein exudate from leaky capillaries, and necrotic tissue all compromise this process, delaying epithelialization. A delay in epithelialization leads to increased and prolonged inflammation, which can lead to unsatisfactory scar formation.

In *full-thickness wounds,* the dermis is destroyed or removed. Epithelialization occurs from the edge of the wound at the rate of 1 to 2 mm/day at the most. In an open wound, the rate of epithelialization depends on the vascularity and health of the granulation tissue (neodermis) across which it migrates. Epithelial cells provide little strength when not anchored to dermis and are prone to injury. The basal layer is attached to the dermis by *hemidesmosomes,* which are attached to *keratin filaments,* the underlying structural elements of epithelial cells. The hemidesmosomes connect by means of a series of interme-

diate proteins to anchoring filaments, long proteins that intertwine with the collagen network of the dermis. The epithelium resists sheer forces because of these strong dermal attachments. Without an adequate dermal base, epidermis provides unstable wound coverage and is subject to chronic breakdown.

In *partial-thickness wounds* the dermis is not destroyed. Epithelialization is the result of migration of epithelial cells from remaining dermal appendages (sweat glands and hair follicles) (Fig. 3-4). After the first layer of cells has completed restoration of the epithelial barrier, additional layers are added, restoring basilar to apical order. As the cells mature, they resume keratin formation. This regenerates the stratum corneum layer of the epidermis and completes epithelialization. The process usually takes 7 to 10 days.

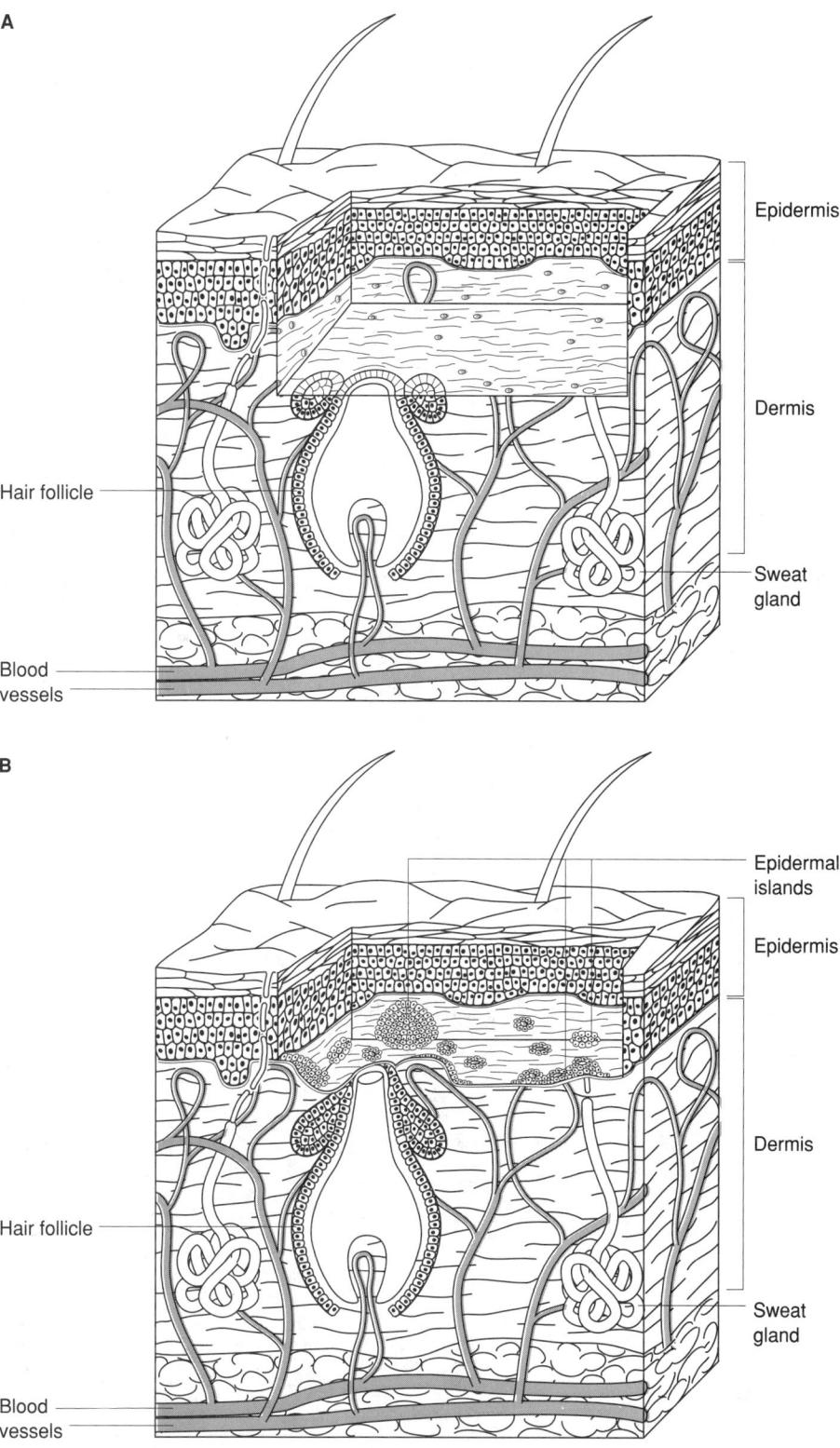

A

B

Epidermis

Dermis

Hair follicle

Sweat gland

Blood vessels

Epidermal islands

Epidermis

Hair follicle

Dermis

Sweat gland

Blood vessels

Figure 3-4. Reepithilialization of a partial-thickness wound. *(continues)*

INCISIONS

The most important factor in the healing of incisions is the gain in tensile strength of the wound. The rate of collagen synthesis determines the initial strength. Ultimate strength is determined by the degree of collagen organization and cross linking.

Intraoperative Considerations

Meticulous hemostasis prevents hematoma formation. When a hematoma forms, toxic metabolites of hemoglobin are released, and inflammation and phagocytosis increase to clear the wound of blood, impairing wound healing.

Rough handling of tissue must be avoided to decrease

C

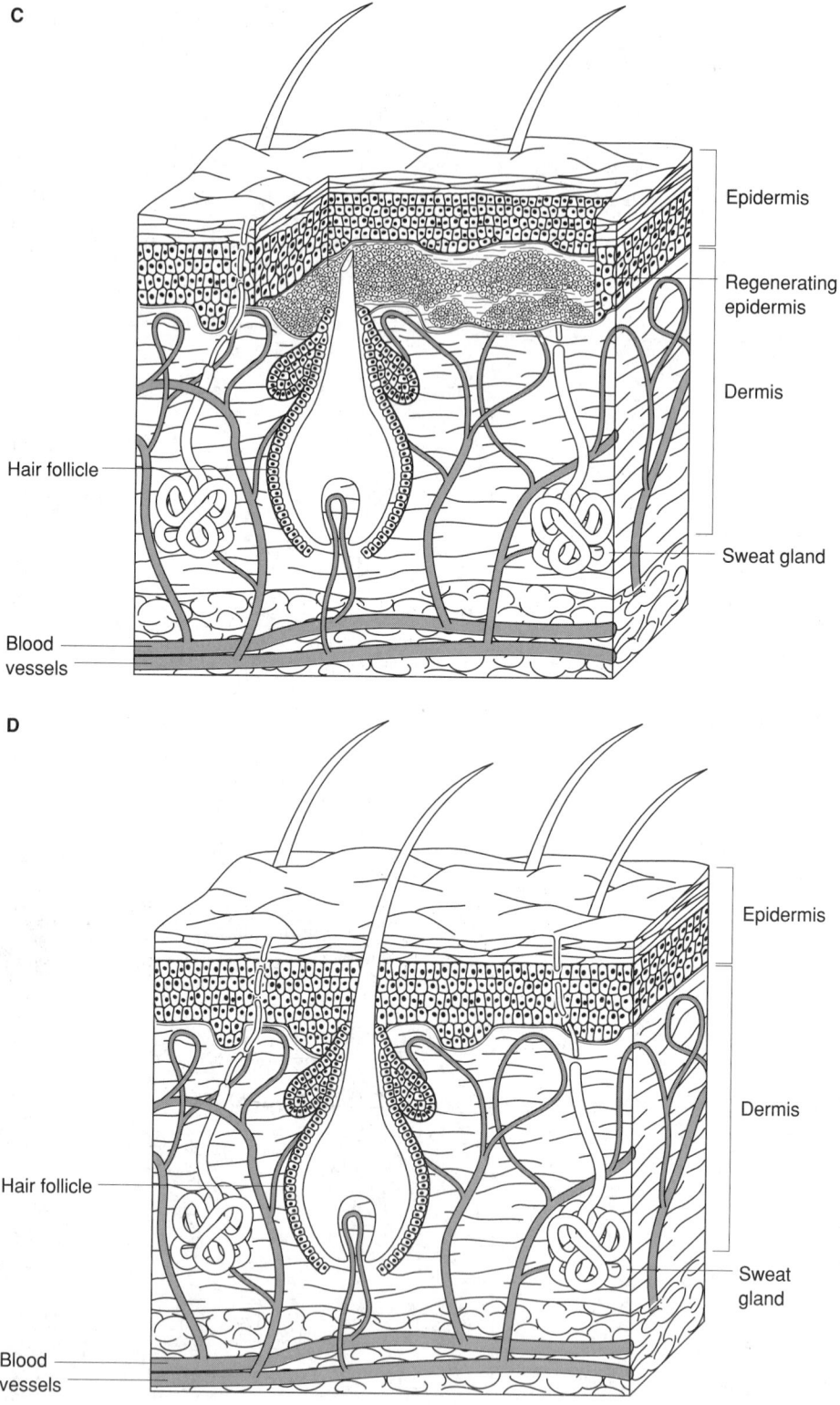

D

Figure 3-4. (Continued)

the volume of necrotic or nonviable cells at the wound margin. Tissue is best handled with fine forceps or skin hooks for retraction and coaptation of the dermis. Crush injury to the epidermis with forceps must be avoided.

Deep sutures are placed only into structures that hold tension, such as dermis, intestinal submucosa, muscular fascia, tendon, ligament, Scarpa fascia, and blood vessel wall. These tissues contain organized collagen and have the tensile strength to hold sutures under tension. The sutures used are usually of absorbable material, such as polyglycolic acid (Dexon) or polyglactin (Vicryl), and retain their tensile strength for about 3 weeks. Sutures used in tendon and abdominal fascia usually are permanent; if absorbable, they ideally retain their tensile strength for close to 6 weeks.

Fat does not contain collagen and does not hold tension, so fatty tissue is sutured as a separate layer. Closure of a laparotomy incision is limited to the abdominal fascia, the skin, and sometimes Scarpa fascia. Additional sutures pull through fat, increasing tissue damage and serving as a nidus for infection.

Obliteration of dead space and fluid evacuation are best achieved with suction drainage rather than suturing, which introduces a foreign body (the suture material) into the wound.

Wound Care

Because epithelialization usually is complete in 24 to 48 hours, an incision does not have to be protected from water longer than that. A shower 1 to 2 days after an operation gently debrides the incision and keeps it clean by rinsing away surface bacteria and debris. This cleaning reduces the risk for bacterial accumulation in surface crust along the incision and on sutures. Reducing bacterial contamination decreases inflammation and prevents breakdown of the fragile epithelial layer over the incision, allowing good scar formation.

One to two weeks after an operation, the time when most sutures are removed, the wound has a small fraction of its eventual strength and can tear or spread with even modest stress. It takes at least 3 weeks for collagen to undergo sufficient remodeling and cross linking to attain moderate strength. After 6 weeks, the wounded tissue has gained approximately 50% of its eventual strength. To prevent hernia formation or tendon disruption, the patient is instructed to avoid heavy lifting for 6 weeks after a major abdominal operation. Tendon repairs are splinted to avoid full tension for a similar period of time.

OPEN WOUNDS

In an open wound, such as an ulcer or an incision left to heal by secondary intention, the events in healing (inflammation, matrix deposition, epithelialization, and scar maturation) lead to formation of granulation tissue—the pebbly pink surface of healthy new tissue.

The Healing Process

Granulation

In the center of a healing wound, a bed of granulation tissue forms over the exposed subcutaneous tissue. The granulation tissue is made up of new capillaries, proliferating fibroblasts, and an immature matrix of collagen, proteoglycans, substrate adhesion molecules (fibronectin, laminin, and tenascin), and acute and chronic inflammatory cells. Variable amounts of bacteria and protein exudate are present, depending on care of the wound.

At the advancing edge of epithelium, acute inflammation is present. Behind the advancing edge is a proliferative area. Behind the area of proliferation, the scar is maturing and remodeling. The ability of an open wound to form granulation tissue is governed by the blood supply to the tissue (for oxygen and nutrient delivery) and the relative absence of devitalized tissue and bacteria.

Epithelialization

Successful healing of an open wound relies more on maintaining epithelial integrity than on maintaining the tensile strength of a scar. At the edge of a healing wound, the basal epithelial cells flatten out, lose their hemidesmosome attachments, and migrate over the wound base. The speed of epithelialization is limited by the rate of migration of the proliferating epithelial edge. Rapid epithelialization depends on an optimal matrix manufactured by the underlying granulation tissue and on delivery of an adequate blood supply, which provides nutrients and oxygen to the healing tissue.

Wound Contraction

When an open wound contracts, the surrounding skin is pulled over the wound, reducing its size. Contraction occurs much faster than epithelialization. At the cellular level, the force that generates wound contraction comes from fibroblasts, which like muscle cells contain actin microfilaments. Contraction accelerates wound closure and resurfaces an open wound with normal sensate skin from around the wound. The skin becomes tightly adherent and inelastic. In areas with a large amount of skin, such as the perineum, contraction may account for 90% of the reduction in wound size. On the lower leg, however, contraction accounts for only 30% to 40% of the healing of an ulcer (one reason why leg ulcers are so slow to heal).

Bacterial Colonization

All open wounds, unless produced and dressed under sterile conditions, are contaminated by bacteria from the surrounding skin and the environment. Bacterial *colonization* of a wound is normal and is not deleterious to healing. Bacterial *infection* is deleterious and can delay or prevent healing. If the bacteria count is too high in wound granulation tissue, excessive proteases and endotoxins delay epithelialization. Capillary leakage occurs when vascular endothelial cells deform, increasing in permeability. The increased permeability is mediated by histamine, kinins (arachidonic acid derivatives), complement, prostaglandin E_2, and prostacyclin. This exudate of serum proteins and inflammatory cells serves as a rich culture medium for bacteria.

Role of Moisture

Epithelialization is faster under moist conditions than dry conditions (Fig. 3-5).

Role of Oxygen

PMNs need PO_2 levels of 25 mmHg to produce superoxide radicals and effectively kill bacteria. Collagen synthesis is oxygen dependent. A fresh wound is initially avascular and is always hypoxic relative to the surrounding tissues; in the center of a new wound, PO_2 can drop to near zero.

Role of Edema

In normal tissue, each cell is only a few cell diameters away from the nearest capillary and receives nutrients and oxygen by diffusion. In the presence of inflammation, venous insufficiency, or extremity dependency, the amount of extracellular and extravascular fluid increases, increasing the diffusion distance for oxygen and lowering tissue PO_2.

Role of Tissue Necrosis and Exudate

The presence of a large amount or even a small amount of necrotic tissue or fibrinous exudate impairs or delays healing. The exudate of serum protein and dead inflammatory cells produced by an open wound increases in the presence of devitalized tissue.

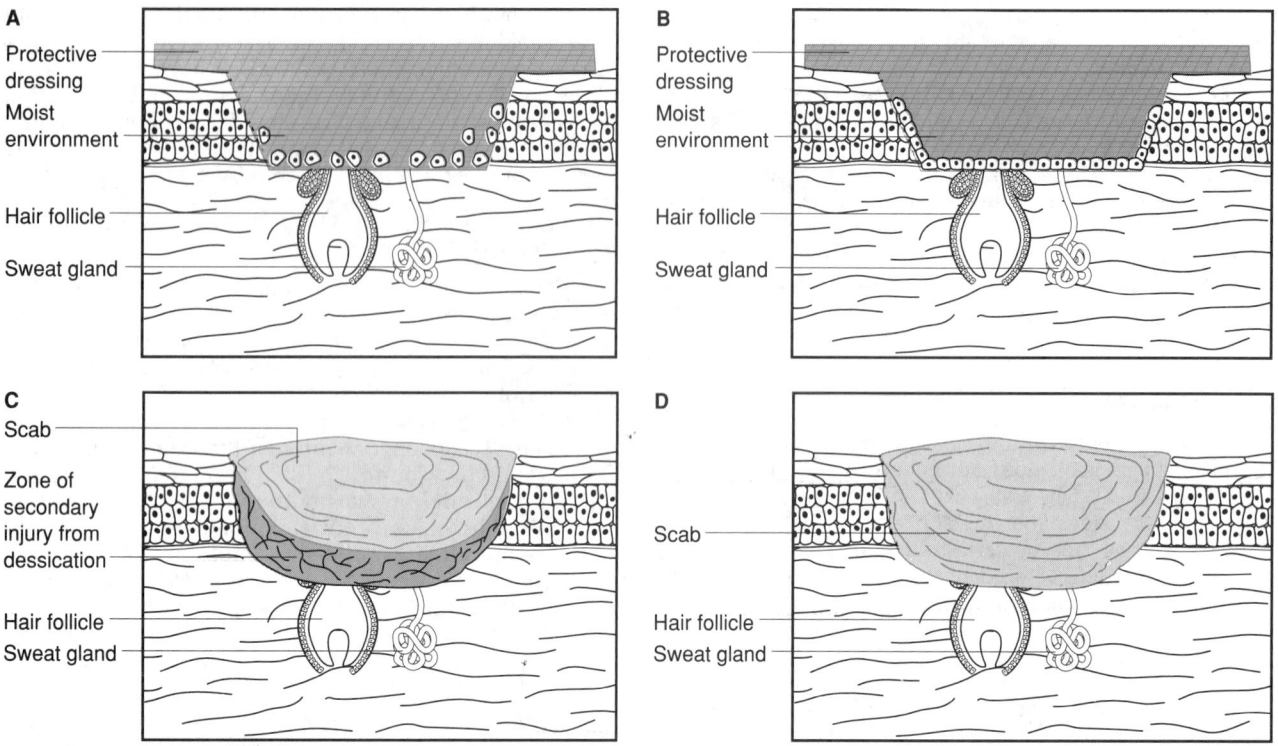

Figure 3-5. Rapid epithilialization occurs in a moist environment. Desiccation delays healing by causing tissue necrosis in the exposed wound. The scab ultimately forms a moisture barrier, and epithilialization occurs from the wound edge and any remaining dermal appendages (see Fig. 3-4).

Wound Care

Care of an open wound involves:

1. Cleaning
2. Débridement
3. Edema control
4. Avoidance and treatment of ischemia
5. Achievement of a moist wound healing environment

Unless large amounts of necrotic tissue are present, surgical débridement is not necessary. Simple application of moist dressings, however, may not be adequate to remove proteinaceous exudate. Irrigation either in a whirlpool or with water from a handheld shower spray or dental water-cleaning device can be gentle, yet generate enough power for effective débridement. Frequent changes of moist dressings serve the same purpose. In some wounds, occlusive absorptive dressings can generate enough tissue proteases to effectively degrade proteins, which the absorptive dressings remove.

The detrimental effect of edema on healing is often underestimated. Patient education about the importance of avoiding leg swelling is critical. Many patients have habits that are difficult to break, such as sitting with legs dependent most of the day, and need to be taught ways to modify their behavior. Many patients also object to wearing compression stockings, the most effective method for limiting edema. Patients must modify their behavior to treat this problem.

Supplemental O_2, optimal fluid administration, pain control, and revascularization, if necessary, all enhance tissue blood flow.

Large amounts of devitalized tissue, especially dermis, are removed by means of surgical excision, although enzymatic débridement with collagenases may be acceptable. If the necrotic dermis is left in place, the underlying subcutaneous tissue (fat), which is less vascular, becomes infected, forming an abscess or even producing systemic sepsis.

CHRONIC WOUNDS

A chronic wound is one that has not healed in 3 months. Almost all chronic wounds are leg ulcers, pressure sores, or diabetic foot ulcers. The lack of healing is usually due to inadequate attention to the principles of wound care. However, the wound environment of many chronic wounds does appear to be different from that of wounds that heal normally. Chronic wounds appear to have a large amount of proteases and collagenases that degrade matrix proteins (ie, collagen) and growth factors, inhibiting proliferation and chemotaxis.

Wound Care

Chronic wounds are débrided, and topical and systemic antibiotics are administered for bacterial infection or overpopulation. Arterial revascularization increases oxygenation in the wound, and elevation and compression dressings decrease edema. If the factors that caused the wound and allow it to persist are identified and treated, many chronic wounds can be closed, and they remain closed after treatment.

Often the underlying cause of a chronic wound cannot be corrected, such as diabetes with neuropathy or venous insufficiency with secondary venous hypertension. Patient education to avoid leg edema with compression garments, or orthotic shoes and avoidance of prolonged pressure are necessary before treatments, such as skin grafts which do not address the underlying condition, are performed.

SYSTEMIC FACTORS THAT AFFECT WOUND HEALING

Nutrition

Wound healing requires energy. Patients who are severely malnourished or whose condition is catabolic have delayed or impaired healing. Serum albumin level is the most useful measurement of nutritional status. A serum albumin >3.5 g/dL suggests adequate protein stores and nitrogen balance. An albumin level <3.0 g/dL indicates potential wound healing problems and an increased risk for postsurgical breakdown. Most surgeons avoid trying to close chronic wounds surgically until nutritional levels are considered acceptable.

Vitamins and minerals are necessary for wound healing. Deficiencies are rare, however, unless parenteral nutrition or other extreme dietary restrictions are being used. High-dose supplementation, especially with fat-soluble vitamins, has no known benefit and may have serious complications.

Aging

Elderly people heal more slowly and with less scarring than younger people because the inflammatory response decreases with age. This decrease in inflammation and proliferation results in finer scars. Sutures are left in place longer in elderly patients, though, to allow for a slow gain in tensile strength.

Chemotherapy and Steroid Use

Any chemotherapeutic agent that suppresses the bone marrow impairs wound healing. A decrease in lymphocytes and monocytes impairs cellular proliferation in the inflammatory phase of wound healing. The impairment resolves when the chemotherapy is discontinued. Adrenocortical steroids inhibit wound healing because of their anti-inflammatory and immunosuppressive effects. These drugs reduce the synthesis of procollagen by fibroblasts, delaying wound contraction. Even after wounds heal, tensile strength is weaker than in patients not taking steroids. In patients who take systemic steroids over long periods, the dermis thins and becomes highly susceptible to injury.

Ischemia

Adequate oxygenation is critical to wound healing. Oxygen is needed for aerobic metabolism and for neutrophil function, especially in bacterial killing. Oxygen also is needed for the hydroxylation of proline and lysine to form stable collagen fibrils. The following factors contribute to wound ischemia:

- Smoking and use of nicotine patches
- Radiation
- Edema
- Diabetes
- Atherosclerosis
- Vasculitis
- Prolonged pressure
- Venous insufficiency
- Tissue fibrosis in chronically scarred wounds

EXCESSIVE SCARRING: HYPERTROPHIC SCARS AND KELOIDS

The most important factors in the formation of an ideal scar are:

1. Accurate alignment of sharply incised tissue parallel to the natural lines of resting skin tension
2. Closure of the wound without tension on the epidermis and without underlying dead space
3. Primary healing without complications such as infection or dehiscence
4. The person's genetic composition
5. The location of the scar on the body

Keloids and hypertrophic scars are histologically similar. They both contain an overabundance of dermal collagen. The difference is that keloids extend beyond the boundary of the original wound and hypertrophic scars do not. Keloids develop several months after the injury and, rarely, if ever, subside. Hypertrophic scars often occur on the upper torso and across flexor surfaces. They usually develop within 1 month of wounding and gradually subside.

The treatment of keloids is difficult. Excision followed by intralesional steroid injection may be helpful. For severe keloids, excision may be followed by a short course of radiation therapy. However, the scar is sometimes unchanged or even made worse. Hypertrophic scars may be improved with pressure garments, topical silicone sheeting, or re-excision and closure.

SUGGESTED READING

Ahn ST, Monafo WW, Mustoe TA. Topical silicone gel: A new treatment for hypertrophic scars. Surgery 1989;106:781.

Brown GL, et al. Enhancement of wound healing by topical treatment with epidermal growth factor. N Engl J Med 1989; 321:76.

Carver N, Leigh IM. Synthetic dressings. Int J Dermatol 1992; 31:10.

Jonsson K, et al. Tissue oxygenation, anemia, and perfusion in relation to wound healing in surgical patients. Ann Surg 1991;214:605.

LaVan FB, Hunt TK. Oxygen and wound healing. Clin Plast Surg 1990;17:463.

Lawrence WT. In search of the optimal treatment of keloids: Report of a series and a review of the literature. Ann Plast Surg 1991;27:164.

Rockwell WB, Cohen IK, Ehrlich HP. Keloids and hypertrophic scars: A comprehensive review. Plast Reconstr Surg 1989; 84:827.

Siebert JW, et al. Fetal wound healing: A biochemical study of scarless healing. Plast Reconstr Surg 1990;85:503.

ESSENTIALS OF SURGERY: SCIENTIFIC PRINCIPLES AND PRACTICE,
edited by Lazar J. Greenfield, Michael W. Mulholland, Keith T. Oldham, Gerald B. Zelenock,
and Keith D. Lillemoe. Lippincott–Raven Publishers, Philadelphia, © 1997.

CHAPTER 4

HEMOSTASIS

THOMAS W. WAKEFIELD

BASIC CONSIDERATIONS

Coagulation-related systems include ongoing thrombus formation, inhibition of thrombus formation, and thrombus dissolution. Abnormalities in coagulation occur when one of the processes overcomes the others.

Extrinsic Pathway

Interaction between platelets and coagulation complexes leads to clot formation. Tissue factor released from injured cells activates the extrinsic pathway of coagulation. Disruption of the endothelium of blood vessels exposes the underlying collagen to platelets, activating them. In blood, tissue factor forms a complex with activated factor VII, activating factors IX and X to factors IXa and Xa. At the same time, activated platelets spread in shape and their procoagulant phospholipid (platelet factor 3) is externalized. This allows proteins to assemble on the surface of platelets, accelerating coagulation.

Platelet membranes contribute critical surfaces for assembly of the coagulation complex. Activated, but not resting, platelets express binding sites for coagulation factors. Once the platelet plug has formed, coagulation protein assembly begins. Factors Xa and Va, ionized calcium, and factor II (prothrombin) form on the platelet phospholipid surface to initiate the prothrombinase complex. When the amount of tissue factor is limited, activation of factor IX allows tissue factor activation in the presence of low tissue factor concentration.

Thrombin is central to all coagulation. It cleaves fibrinopeptide A (FPA) from the α chain of fibrinogen and fibrinopeptide B (FPB) from the β chain. This leads to release of fibrinopeptides and formation of new fibrin monomers, which cross-link, resulting in fibrin polymerization. Thrombin activates factor XIII, which catalyzes the cross-linking of fibrin to make the clot firm, and activates platelets and factors V and VIII. Only activated factors V and VIII (Va, VIIIa) are involved in coagulation. Factor XIIIa also cross-links other plasma proteins, incorporating them into clot.

Intrinsic Pathway

The intrinsic pathway of coagulation requires activation of factor XI. This occurs by means of the contact activation system through factor XII, plasma prekallikrein, high-molecular-weight kininogen, and thrombin.

NATURAL ANTICOAGULANT MECHANISMS

While thrombin forms, natural anticoagulant systems oppose thrombus formation.

Antithrombin III, the most important natural anticoagulant protein, binds to thrombin, preventing removal of FPA and FPB from fibrinogen and activation of factors V and VIII, and inhibiting activation and aggregation of platelets. Antithrombin III inhibits factors IXa, Xa, and XIa.

Activated protein C inactivates factors Va and VIIIa, reducing the ability of the Xase and prothrombinase complexes to accelerate thrombin formation. Protein C is activated on endothelial cell surfaces by thrombin complexed with one of its receptors, thrombomodulin. Protein S is a cofactor for protein Ca.

Heparin cofactor II helps regulate thrombin formation in extravascular tissues. Thrombin is inactivated when it becomes incorporated into the clot itself.

FIBRINOLYSIS

During thrombus formation, a constant process of clot lysis prevents unphysiologic thrombus formation from leading to pathologic intravascular thrombosis. Plasminogen, tissue plasminogen activator (tPA), and α_2-antiplasmin (α-2-AP) become incorporated into the fibrin clot as it forms. Thrombin promotes release of tPA from endothelial cells and production of plasminogen activator inhibitor (PAI-1) from endothelial cells.

tPA converts plasminogen to plasmin, the main fibrinolytic enzyme. The natural inhibitor of excess plasmin, α-2-AP, is released by endothelial cells. In fibrinolysis, α-2-AP is bound to fibrin, and excess plasmin is inactivated. In fibrinolytic states and during treatment with fibrinolytic agents, circulating fibrinogen and clot-bound fibrin are degraded by circulating plasmin. Plasminogen activators include exogenous factors such as streptokinase, endogenous factors such as tPA and urokinase, and intrinsic factors such as factor XII, prekallikrein, and high–molecular-weight kininogen. The factors of the contact system are more important in clot lysis than in thrombus formation. The endothelial cell itself can act as a nonthrombogenic surface. It has three systems for promotion of a nonthrombotic surface: thrombin–thrombomodulin interaction, heparin–antithrombin III binding, and a membrane-bound fibrinolytic system.

THROMBOSIS AND INFLAMMATION

Thrombosis and inflammation are closely linked (Fig. 4-1). Vascular injury causes margination of circulating platelets along the vessel wall. Platelets then activate and aggregate in an interaction mediated by fibrinogen, producing a platelet plug. Blood clotting is stimulated by expression of tissue factor; the clotting complexes are propagated on the activated platelets, producing a fibrin clot. Circulating neutrophils and monocytes interact with the platelets, leading to interaction between leukocytes and platelets at the thrombus-wall interface.

In the venous circulation, thrombus formation involving platelets, neutrophils, and monocytes is initiated at venous confluences, saccules, and valve pockets. Adherent neutrophils and platelets are activated, releasing substances that activate and attract more platelets and neutrophils. Coagulation is initiated on the phospholipid surface of the platelets. New layers of neutrophils and platelets form on the surface of fibrin, activate, and begin another round of clotting. Leukocytes extravasate into the vein wall via a chemotactic gradient that develops in the wall in response to venous thrombosis.

PROCOAGULANT STATES

Procoagulant screening includes (1) coagulation tests: aPTT, platelet count, antithrombin III activity and antigen assay, protein C antigen and activity levels, protein S antigen level, mixing studies to identify a lupus anticoagulant,

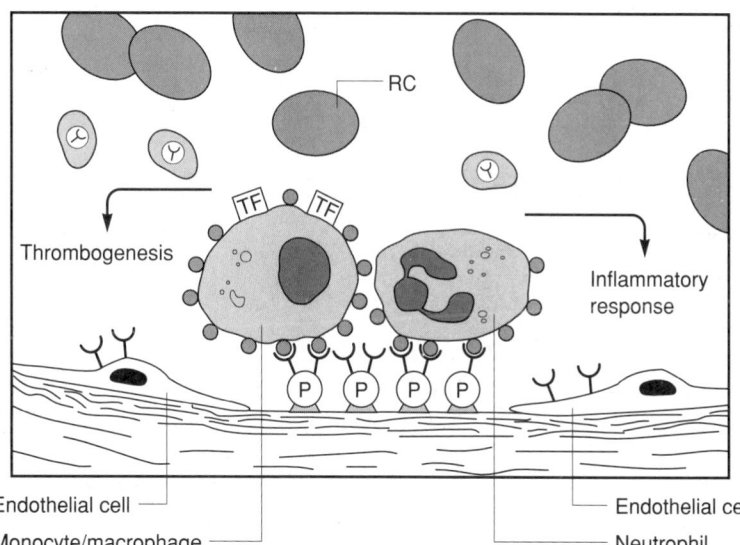

Figure 4-1. Cellular basis for blood coagulation, including platelets (P), neutrophils, monocytes, P-selectin (Y), and red blood cells (RC). (After Furie B, Furie BC. Molecular and cellular biology of blood coagulation. N Engl J Med 1992;326:803)

(2) an antiphospholipid antibody screen: anticardiolipin antibody, fibrinogen level, functional plasminogen assay, and platelet aggregation. Only patients with a family history of thrombosis, young patients with arterial and venous thrombosis without obvious cause, and patients with multiple episodes of thrombosis without underlying anatomic abnormality need screening.

Heparin-Associated Thrombocytopenia

Thrombocytopenia may be present when thrombosis occurs during heparin administration or when platelet count decreases to <100,000/mm³. The syndrome usually begins 5 to 15 days after initiation of heparin administration. Even minimal exposure, such as heparin coating on pulmonary artery catheters, may cause this syndrome. The laboratory diagnosis is suggested by demonstration of at least 20% platelet aggregation within 15 minutes or ≥6% ¹⁴C serotonin release within 45 minutes when heparin is added to donor platelets and the patient's own platelet-poor plasma. Other coagulation tests are usually normal. Treatment is cautious administration of protamine sulfate for heparin reversal if active thrombosis has occurred or discontinuation of heparin and administration of another anticoagulant after the effects of heparin have worn off.

Antithrombin III Deficiency

Antithrombin III deficiency accounts for about 2% of venous thrombotic events and a small number of cases of arterial thrombosis. Patients usually have thrombosis despite the use of heparin. The deficiency may be congenital or acquired. People with a homozygous congenital deficiency usually die in infancy. Acquired deficiencies occur with inadequate antithrombin III production due to liver disease, malignant tumors, nephrotic syndrome, disseminated intravascular coagulation (DIC), malnutrition, or increased protein catabolism. Thrombotic episodes often are related to operations, childbirth, and infections; recurrent episodes are common. The diagnosis is made with measurement of antithrombin III levels, preferably while the patient is not taking anticoagulants. Both antigen and activity levels are assessed. Treatment is with fresh

frozen plasma followed by warfarin or antithrombin III concentrates.

Protein C and S Deficiencies

Protein C and S deficiencies can be congenital or acquired. People with homozygous congenital deficiencies usually die in infancy. Acquired protein C and S deficiencies usually occur after conditions that interfere with hepatic synthesis. Antigen levels and activity of protein C can be measured, but only antigen levels of protein S can be measured. Treatment is lifelong anticoagulant therapy with warfarin. Not all patients with these deficiencies experience thrombosis. Low levels of either protein C or protein S factor by themselves in a patient without thrombosis are not an indication for anticoagulation.

Resistance to Activated Protein C

Resistance to activated protein C occurs in some patients with idiopathic venous thrombosis. It is one of the most common congenital conditions responsible for a progoagulant state. In this syndrome, aPTT is measured with the addition of activated protein C and calcium chloride to the patient's serum. The result is compared with the results of the same test without the addition of activated protein C. Genetic analysis can be used to confirm the diagnosis.

Lupus Anticoagulant–Antiphospholipid Syndrome

This entity is not an anticoagulant but is associated with the procoagulant state. The lupus anticoagulant–antiphospholipid syndrome (APS) consists of the presence of an antiphospholipid antibody or the lupus anticoagulant with recurrent thromboses, recurrent spontaneous abortions, thrombocytopenia, or livido reticularis. A prolonged aPTT not corrected with normal plasma in the presence of normal results of other coagulation tests is indicative of this problem, as is prolongation of the Russell viper venom time. One can also measure antiphospholipid and anticardiolipin antibody. Although the lupus anticoagulant exists in 5% to 40% of patients with systemic lupus erythematosus (SLE), the condition can exist in patients without SLE. Treatment of thrombosis associated with APS includes heparin followed by long-term warfarin therapy.

Defective Fibrinolytic Activity

Abnormal plasminogen activity is evident only after a thrombosis-prone event occurs. Treatment is long-term warfarin therapy. Defective fibrinolytic activity may be caused by a decreased content or release of plasminogen activators or increased activation of the inhibitor of plasminogen. Fibrinolytic activity is reduced for 7 to 10 days after an operation because of an altered relation between tPA and its inhibitor. Pneumatic compression devices probably exert part of their antithrombotic effect through prevention of fibrinolytic shutdown.

Abnormal Platelet Aggregation

Abnormal platelet aggregation has been associated with

- Advanced malignant tumors, especially of the lung and uterus
- Thrombosis at the site of carotid endarterectomy
- Arterial graft thrombosis in patients undergoing peripheral vascular reconstruction

Platelet function may depend more on external factors such as the circulating level of fibrinogen or production of thrombin, than on an intrinsic feature of the platelets themselves. Antiplatelet agents alone are unlikely to eliminate thrombogenic potential.

Disseminated Intravascular Coagulation

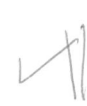

DIC is the primary form of acute thrombosis. Causes of DIC include abruptio placenta, gram-positive and gram-negative sepsis, malignant tumors, pelvic operations, some snake bites, malignant hematologic disease, and hepatic failure. Coagulation is activated by the release into the circulation of tissue factor, which activates factor VII, leading to massive thrombin production and fibrin generation. Fibrinolysis is activated, causing bleeding in the later stages of the syndrome. Laboratory values in DIC show a decline in platelet count and fibrinogen level with a concomitant elevation in split products.

BLEEDING DISORDERS

Although surgeons deal with procoagulant states more often than with bleeding disorders, it is important to recognize the following disorders when they occur:

Disorders of blood vessels

- Abnormal blood vessel growth and development
- Increase in vascular permeability and fragility
- Coagulation factor deficiency states
- Factor VIII (hemophilia A)
- Factor IX (hemophilia B)
- Von Willebrand disease
- Factor XI, V, VII, X, II deficiency
- Fibrinogen deficiency
- Platelet disorders
- Receptor defects
- Organelle zone abnormalities
- Abnormalities in fibrinolysis
- α_2-Antiplasmin deficiency
- Factor XIII deficiency
- PAI deficiency

PHARMACOLOGIC AND NONPHARMACOLOGIC INTERVENTION

Heparin

Heparin is used to manage and prevent venous thrombosis and to manage pulmonary embolism. It accelerates the reaction between thrombin and antithrombin III, accelerating inhibition of thrombin and other serine proteases by antithrombin III. It also binds and inhibits coagulation proteases. Heparin is cleared through the reticuloendothelial system and does not cross the placental barrier. A lower frequency of bleeding complications occurs with continuous infusion than with bolus injection.

In monitoring heparin effect, an aPTT 1.5 times control, a thrombin clotting time (TCT) 2 times control, or an activated clotting time (ACT) of 150–200 sec suggests adequate anticoagulation. Direct measurement of heparin levels does not always correlate with the level of anticoagulation measured with aPTT. Patients who undergo heparin therapy and are known to have taken heparin in the past should have a platelet count every other day after the fourth day of therapy. The most common complication of heparin therapy is bleeding.

Reversal of heparin anticoagulation with protamine sulfate is often associated with adverse hemodynamic and hematologic side effects. Immunologic reactions may occur in patients with previous exposure to protamine, especially those with diabetes who use NPH insulin. No other agent for heparin neutralization is approved for general use. When heparin must be neutralized, use of protamine cannot be avoided.

Warfarin

Oral anticoagulant therapy is recommended for long-term management of venous thromboembolism. Warfarin interferes with the vitamin K-dependent factors II, VII, IX, and X and proteins C and S. The complications of warfarin therapy are recurrent thrombosis, bleeding, and skin necrosis. Warfarin therapy should be continued for 4-6 mo after an initial episode of deep venous thrombosis (DVT). In recurrent DVT, however, the thrombotic risk is high, and sustained anticoagulation is appropriate.

Antiplatelet Agents

Antiplatelet agents are used to prevent cardiovascular disorders such as coronary thrombosis and neointimal hyperplasia. Platelet aggregation can be inhibited with agents that

1. Block cyclooxygenase
2. Block thromboxane synthase
3. Block the thromboxane A_2 receptor
4. Increase intraplatelet levels of cyclic AMP or cyclic GMP
5. Block GP IIb/IIIa

Fibrinolytic Agents

Fibrinolytic agents are direct or indirect activators of plasminogen. Platelets are both inhibited and stimulated by fibrinolytic agents. Although they decrease the ability of blood to clot during therapy, fibrinolytic agents may promote reocclusion soon after lysis. Indications for thrombolytic therapy are controversial. Contraindications are listed in Table 4-1.

In *DVT*, fibrinolytic agents allow complete clot lysis more frequently than heparin therapy and help preserve valve function, but at the risk of a higher degree of bleeding complications. Fibrinolytic therapy is used to manage *upper extremity venous thrombosis;* it is followed by correction of the venous compression site and oral anticoagulant therapy for 3 months. Thrombolytic therapy for *pulmonary embolism* is considered when angiographically documented lobar or greater pulmonary embolism causes acute pulmonary hypertension and shock. Lesser degrees of pulmonary embolism are treated with standard heparin anticoagulation. Any benefit of lytic therapy is expected only early in the course of events.

Thrombolytic therapy for *peripheral arterial disease* involves passing a guide wire through the thrombus and then infusing a high dose of urokinase directly into the clot. If progress is made, further fibrinolytic therapy is given for 6 to 12 h or until complete clot lysis. The incidence of bleeding complications is low. After thrombolytic therapy has been used to reopen an occluded vessel or graft, radiologic or surgical correction of the lesion responsible for the thrombosis must be performed for long-term success. Complications associated with thrombolytic therapy for arterial thrombosis include bleeding, rethrombosis, embolization treated with additional thrombolytic therapy, and sepsis due to prolonged catheter placement. The use of tPA in peripheral vascular disease has had promising results, but tPA can still induce systemic thrombolytic effects.

Intraoperative thrombolytic therapy can be used when complete clot evacuation cannot be accomplished or when the distal vasculature is occluded. One method involves infusion of urokinase and heparin distal to an occluding clamp. For patients who have multivessel occlusions or for whom any degree of systemic fibrinolysis would be a risk, a high-dose, isolated limb perfusion technique involves anticoagulation, limb exsanguination, application of a proximal tourniquet, and direct arterial infusion of urokinase with direct drainage of the venous effluent below the tourniquet.

The use of thrombolytic agents in *acute myocardial infarction* is being investigated. The clinical benefits of coronary thrombolysis are determinutesed by the rapidity of coronary artery reperfusion. Platelet-mediated thrombotic events may be responsible for the reocclusion associated with currently used agents and protocols. Adding heparin to tPA improves the efficacy of tPA during coronary thrombolysis and helps prevent reocclusion after thrombolysis.

Dextran

Dextran-40 is a volume-expanding agent. It causes hemodilution, decreases blood viscosity, decreases platelet adhesiveness, reduces factor VIII activity, and increases the lysability of clot. Dextran-40 increases the patency of femorotibial bypasses and all infrainguinal bypasses in which autologous vein is not used. Dextran-40 may be used to treat vascular trauma and in endarterectomy, arterial and venous thrombectomy, venous reconstruction, and prophylaxis of venous thrombosis.

Mechanical Measures

Mechanical measures for the prevention of DVT during surgical procedures or in patients who cannot take pharmacologic agents include early ambulation, elastic stockings, electrical calf-muscle stimulation, and external pneumatic compression with uniform-pressure or graded-pressure stockings. Intermittent pneumatic compression is as effective as low-dose heparin therapy. Besides augmenting venous return, these devices appear to stimulate local and systemic fibrinolysis, even in areas remote from the application of compression.

Vena caval interruption for venous thromboembolism is used if traditional methods of anticoagulation fail or if anticoagulant agents are contraindicated. The Greenfield vena caval filter is a cone-shaped device in which 85% of the filter can be filled with clot while blood flows around the periphery, allowing natural fibrinolysis and 95% long-term patency. Percutaneous insertion, rather than direct surgical technique, offers a number of advantages to this filter, including increased patient comfort, shorter time of insertion, and less cost.

In *catheter pulmonary embolectomy,* a cup catheter is inserted through the jugular or common femoral vein and guided by means of fluoroscopy through the right side of the heart into the pulmonary artery. The cup is juxtaposed to the embolus, syringe suction is used to aspirate the clot into the cup, and the entire catheter and clot are withdrawn.

Surgical approaches to pulmonary embolism are indicated for patients who have massive embolism with hypotension and who require massive doses of vasopressors. Open pulmonary embolectomy is reserved for patients who require manual cardiac massage for hypotension or in whom catheter pulmonary embolectomy fails.

LABORATORY MONITORING OF COAGULATION AND ANTICOAGULATION
Tests of Platelet Function

Peripheral platelet counts
Bleeding time assays
Platelet aggregation tests (not performed in most labora-

Table 4-1. CONTRAINDICATIONS TO THROMBOLYTIC THERAPY

ABSOLUTE
Active internal bleeding
Recent (<2 mo) cerebrovascular accident
Intracranial pathology

RELATIVE
Major
Recent (<10 d) major surgery, obstetric delivery, or organ biopsy
Left heart thrombus
Active peptic ulcer or gastrointestinal abnormality
Recent major trauma
Uncontrolled hypertension

Minor
Minor surgery or trauma
Recent cardiopulmonary resuscitation
Atrial fibrillation with mitral valve disease
Bacterial endocarditis
Hemostatic defects (ie, renal or liver disease)
Diabetic hemorrhagic retinopathy
Pregnancy

CONTRAINDICATIONS FOR STREPTOKINASE
Known allergy
Recent streptococcal infection
Previous therapy within 6 mo

(Data from NIH Consensus Development Conference. Thrombolytic therapy in treatment. Ann Intern Med 1980;93:141)

tories, probably because of the observer-dependent nature of the test)

Coagulation Tests

Prothrombin Time

The only abnormality that causes an isolated elevation in prothrombin time (PT) when all other tests are normal is factor VII deficiency. PT also is sensitive to small decreases in factor V. PT is the most common way to measure levels of oral anticoagulant therapy.

Activated Partial Thromboplastin Time

Conditions that cause a prolongation of aPTT include the presence of heparin, deficiencies in factors VIII, IX, and XII, and the presence of lupus-like anticoagulants. Values of aPTT have been shown to correlate with heparin dosages and serum heparin levels. Heparin levels 0.2 IU/mL or greater usually correlate with an aPTT 1.5 times control or greater.

Thrombin Clotting Time

The time it takes exogenously added thrombin to convert plasma fibrinogen into fibrin clot (TCT) is an excellent way to measure the level of heparin-induced anticoagulation. Because TCT is not specific for any disease, it may be used to differentiate factor deficiencies from the presence of heparin or lupus anticoagulant from abnormalities in fibrinogen levels.

Activated Clotting Time

Measurement of the ability of whole blood to clot (ACT) is used to monitor intraoperative heparin levels. ACT responds to increasing heparin doses in a linear manner and correlates with observed clinical anticoagulation (thrombus-free surface on cardiopulmonary bypass devices). ACT may be affected by hemodilution, cardioplegia solutions, hypothermia, platelet dysfunction, hypofibrinogenemia and other coagulopathies, medications, and excess protamine administration.

Tests of Fibrinolysis

Euglobulin lysis time is a crude but effective screening test for problems with fibrinolysis. Other tests include α_2-antiplasmin, plasminogen activator inhibitor, and D-dimer levels.

RISKS OF BLOOD TRANSFUSION

The risks of blood transfusions are as follows:

- Immediate hemolytic reactions
- Delayed hemolytic reactions
- Nonhemolytic reactions
- Allergic reactions
- Infectious disease transmission
- Massive transfusion complications

Autotransfusion devices decrease the amount of nonautologous blood transfused and the overall risk for complications. Patients may donate their own blood as often as every 4 days up to 14 days before an operation. Because directed relative donation does not enhance the safety of blood, autologous programs are of far greater clinical use.

SUGGESTED READING

Coller BS. Platelets and thrombolytic therapy. N Engl J Med 1990;322:33.

Comerota AJ, Aldridge SC. Thrombolytic therapy for acute deep vein thrombosis. Seminutes Vasc Surg 1992;5:76.

Davie EW, Fujikawa K, Kisiel W. The coagulation cascade: initiation, maintenance, and regulation. Biochemistry 1991;30:1036.

Furie B, Furie BC. Molecular and cell biology of blood coagulation. N Engl J Med 1992;326:800.

Greenfield LJ, Proctor MC, Williams DM, et al. Long-term experience with transvenous catheter pulmonary embolectomy. J Vasc Surg 1993:18:450.

Hirsh J. Heparin. N Engl J Med 1991;324:1565.

Hirsh J. Oral anticoagulant drugs. N Engl J Med 1991;324:1865.

Penner JA, Hassouna HI (eds). Coagulation disorders II. Hematol Oncol Clin North Am 1993, volume 6.

Stewart GJ. Neutrophils and deep venous thrombosis. Haemostasis 1993;23:127.

Turpie AGG. Thrombolytic agents in venous thrombosis. J Vasc Surg 1990;12:196.

ESSENTIALS OF SURGERY: SCIENTIFIC PRINCIPLES AND PRACTICE, edited by Lazar J. Greenfield, Michael W. Mulholland, Keith T. Oldham, Gerald B. Zelenock, and Keith D. Lillemoe. Lippincott–Raven Publishers, Philadelphia, © 1997.

CHAPTER 5

CYTOKINES

LISA M. COLLETTI, STEVEN L. KUNKEL, AND ROBERT M. STRIETER

Cytokines are intercellular polypeptides involved in a large number of normal and pathologic conditions. The early host response to infection, trauma, and acute surgical injury is mediated through the release of cytokines. An orchestrated cytokine cascade is essential for normal immune function.

Increased local or systemic levels of the early response cytokines—tumor necrosis factor (TNF), interleukin (IL)-1, and IL-6—trigger a cascade of additional cytokines and mediators, which perpetuate the inflammatory response (Fig. 5-1). Alterations in the vascular endothelium and leukocytes are critical to the migration of leukocytes into the area of injury. TNF, interleukins, and chemokines contribute to this process. This integrated response leads to the organized cascade of mediators and the localization of cells to an area of injury or infection. Tissue repair then restores the organism to a functional, uninjured state.

Excessive amounts of cytokines, especially the early response cytokines and those responsible for tissue repair and scarring, may perpetuate or even exacerbate the abnormality they were designed to repair, resulting in life-threatening syndromes such as multisystem organ failure (MSOF). Excessive amounts of the cytokines that orchestrate wound healing also contribute to tissue fibrosis and scarring, as in pulmonary fibrosis, liver cirrhosis, and scleroderma. Although cytokines are important in host defense and tissue repair, they must be tightly regulated to prevent the pathologic processes that occur with overexpression of the molecules.

Cytokine production at tissue sites depends, in part, on the proximity of the site to the injurious stimulus. Cytokines function in an autocrine and paracrine manner to signal the presence of local, rather than systemic, inflammation. TNF and IL-1 trigger host responses, including an increase in neutrophil margination; activation of the antimicrobial activity of monocytes, macrophages, neutrophils, and eosinophils; induction of the acute-phase response; and increased degradation of skeletal muscle to

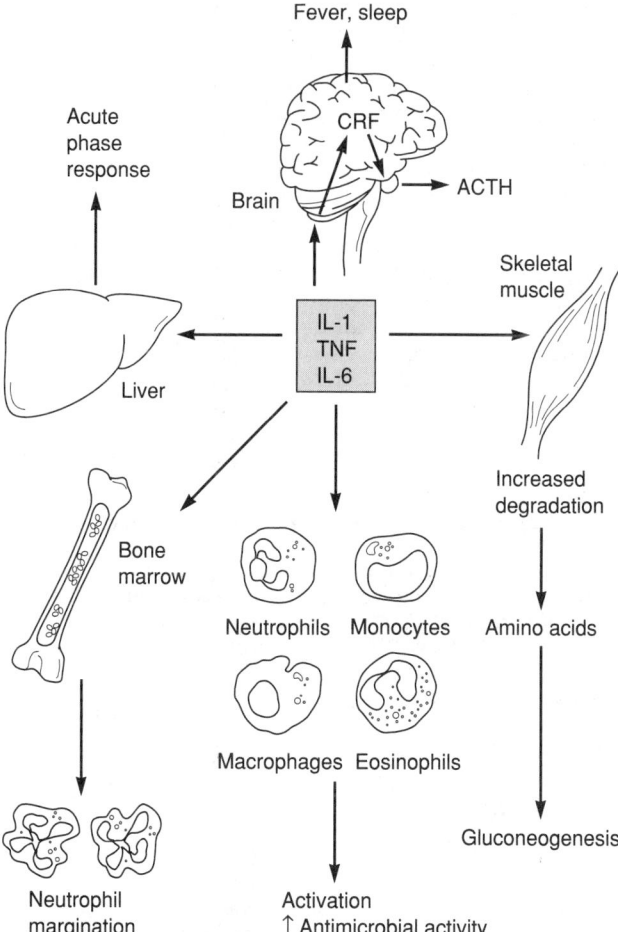

Figure 5-1. Early-response cytokines and the initiation of inflammation. TNF, IL-1, and IL-6 have a multitude of effects in the initiation of the inflammatory response, including the increased breakdown of skeletal muscle to yield amino acids for gluconeogenesis; the activation of monocytes, macrophages, neutrophils, and eosinophils, with an increase in neutrophil margination and an overall increase in leukocyte antimicrobial activity; and the induction of the acute-phase response. In the brain, these molecules cause changes that induce fever and sleep. In addition, they up-regulate corticotropin-releasing factor, which stimulates the production of ACTH.

yield amino acids for gluconeogenesis. During wound repair, these same molecules help regulate vascular proliferation, fibroblast and osteoclast activity, and collagen synthesis.

INFLAMMATION

Early Response Cytokines

In addition to being triggers for the induction of other cytokines in the inflammatory network, TNF and IL-1 appear to promote adherence of inflammatory cells to the endothelium, enhancing the movement of immunologically active cells into an area of injury or infection. The interaction between the endothelium and neutrophils is critical in initiation of the inflammatory response and is responsible for the localization of inflammatory cells to an injured area (Fig. 5-2). Three classes of adhesion molecules are important for leukocyte–endothelial interactions: (1) the immunoglobulin G (IgG) superfamily, (2) the selectins, and (3) the integrins.

Tumor Necrosis Factor

At *local* sites of inflammation, TNF mediates the normal initiation, maintenance, and repair of tissue injury. High *systemic* levels of TNF, however, can lead to MSOF and death.

TNF is involved in the pathogenesis of septic shock, which is characterized by circulatory failure and collapse. It is also associated with acute respiratory distress syndrome (ARDS) and MSOF, which if unchecked cause death. The interaction among monocytes, tissue macrophages, neutrophils, and endothelial cells appears to be important in this process. At the cellular level, septic shock is associated with hypermetabolism and an energy deficit, which leads to cellular injury and death. The cascade of events that culminates in MOSF is initiated by trauma, microorganisms, microbial byproducts, and cytokines.

Although MOSF can occur in an aseptic state, the initiating agent is not known. In the septic state, endotoxin triggers the expression of a number of cytokines, especially TNF and IL-1, which orchestrate the inflammatory response. Cells of the monocyte–macrophage lineage are the principal cellular sources of TNF.

Mechanism of TNF-Induced Injury

TNF has a *procoagulant* effect on endothelial cells; it precipitates intravascular thrombosis (Fig. 5-3). TNF causes endothelial cells to release tissue factor, platelet-

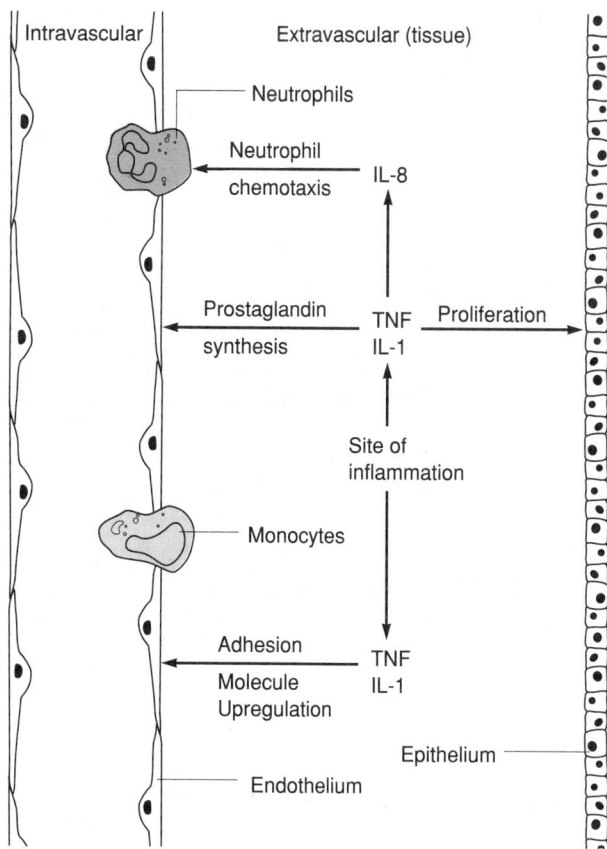

Figure 5-2. Initial interaction between leukocytes and the endothelium. TNF and IL-1 are important early mediators in the initial interaction between the endothelium and leukocytes. The early adherence of leukocytes to the endothelium is an important first step in the elicitation of leukocytes into an area of injury or inflammation, and TNF and IL-1 are critical mediators in this process, since they are capable of up-regulating endothelial and leukocyte adhesion molecules. TNF and IL-1 can also induce IL-8, a powerful neutrophil chemotactic agent.

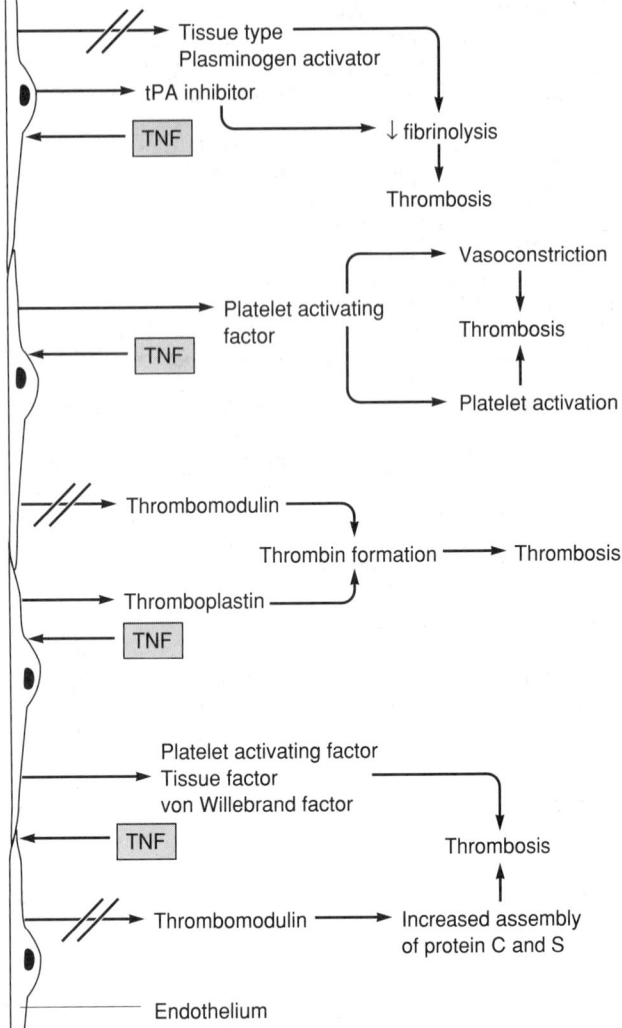

Figure 5-3. Actions of TNF favoring thrombosis. TNF has numerous procoagulant effects, favoring intravascular thrombosis. TNF causes endothelial cells to release a variety of factors with procoagulant properties including tissue factor, platelet-activating factor, von Willebrand factor, thromboplastin, and tissue-type plasminogen-activator inhibitor. It also inhibits the formation of tissue-type plasminogen activator and thrombomodulin. The inhibition of thrombomodulin increases coagulation through two mechanisms. A decrease in thrombomodulin allows both an increase in the assembly of protein C and S complexes, as well as increasing thrombin formation. In addition, both the decrease in thrombomodulin and the increase in thromboplastin further facilitate thrombin formation. Similarly, the decrease in tissue-type plasminogen activator and the increase in tissue-type plasminogen-activator inhibitor decrease overall fibrinolysis, again favoring thrombosis. The TNF-mediated increase in platelet-activating factor favors thrombosis through platelet activation and vasoconstriction.

activating factor, and von Willebrand factor, which promote thrombosis. TNF down-regulates the expression of thrombomodulin, which blocks assembly of protein C and protein S, decreasing the anticoagulant properties of the endothelial cell surfaces. TNF influences fibrinolysis by modulating tissue plasminogen activator (tPA) and tPA inhibitors.

The *antithrombotic* properties of the vascular endothelium are altered by exposure to TNF (Table 5-1). TNF enhances thrombin formation on the endothelial surface by inducing synthesis of thromboplastin and suppressing

thrombomodulin gene expression. TNF also induces synthesis of platelet-activating factor. In addition, TNF stimulates endothelial synthesis of prostacyclin and urokinase-type plasminogen activator (Fig. 5-4). The increase in prostacyclin causes vasodilation at sites of inflammation and hypotension associated with systemic cytokine release, ie, septic shock. The net effect of TNF may depend on the location and the quantity in which it is produced and the vascular bed with which it interacts.

TNF alters cell-surface molecule expression on neutrophils and endothelial cells. It does so by stimulating endothelial–neutrophil adhesion and altering chemotaxis and procoagulant and antimicrobial neutrophil activity through the up-regulation of distal inflammatory cytokines, particularly IL-8 and other chemokines. TNF activates PMNs directly and indirectly through the release of

Table 5-1. PRIMARY EFFECTS OF TNF AND IL-1 ON THE VASCULAR ENDOTHELIUM

INCREASE LEUKOCYTE ADHESION BY INCREASING THE EXPRESSION OF ENDOTHELIAL ADHESION MOLECULES; FACILITATES EXTRAVASATION OF NEUTROPHILS

ICAM-1
PECAM-1
VCAM-1
E-selectin
P-selectin

INCREASE THROMBOGENICITY

Increases tissue factor
Decreases thrombomodulin
   Blocks assembly of protein C and S complexes
Increases synthesis of thromboplastin
   Increase in thromboplastin plus a decrease in thrombomodulin
     results in an increase in thrombin formation at the endothelial
     surface
Decreases fibrinolysis
   Increases tissue-type plasminogen activator inhibitor
   Decreases tissue-type plasminogen activator
Increases platelet-activating factor
   Potent platelet and leukocyte activator
   Powerful vasoconstrictor
Increases von Willebrand factor

DECREASE THROMBOGENICITY

Increases prostacyclin synthesis
   Powerful vasodilator
   Inhibits platelet aggregation
Increases urokinase-type plasminogen activator
   Activates fibrinolysis
Increases nitric oxide synthesis
   Inhibits platelet aggregation
Causes release of many substances that increase vasodilation
   Prostaglandin E_2
   Prostacyclin
   Thromboxane A_2
   Nitric oxide

STIMULATE CYTOKINE EXPRESSION AND SECRETION THAT RESULT IN LEUKOCYTE RECRUITMENT AND ACTIVATION

IL-1
IL-6
GM-CSF
G-CSF
IL-8
MCP-1

INCREASE PDGF

CAUSE MORPHOLOGIC CHANGE

STIMULATE ANGIOGENESIS

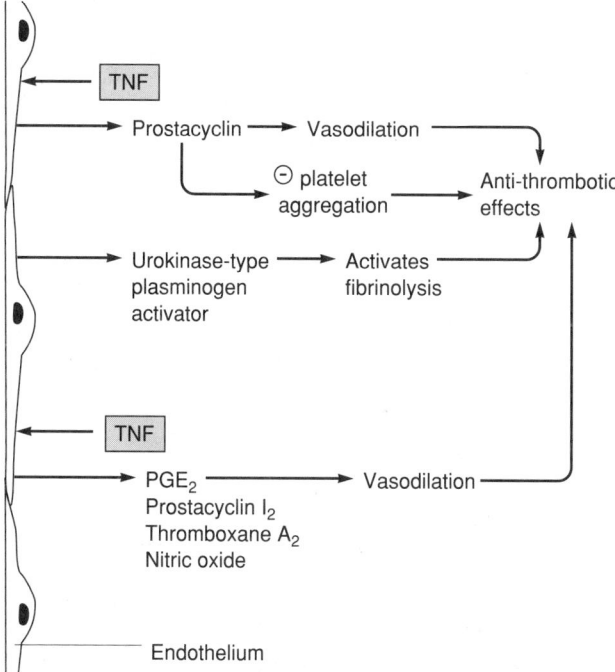

Figure 5-4. Anticoagulant effects of TNF. Although most TNF-induced effects on the endothelium favor thrombosis, this cytokine also has antithrombotic actions. These include an increase in endothelial synthesis of prostacyclin and urokinase-type plasminogen activator. Prostacyclin inhibits platelet aggregation and is a potent vasodilator. Urokinase-type plasminogen activator induces fibrinolysis. TNF also up-regulates endothelial production of PGE_2, prostacyclin I_2, thromboxane A_2, and nitric oxide, which are all powerful vasodilators.

distal inflammatory cytokines, inducing the production and release of reactive oxygen metabolites and the production of additional cytokines.

Metabolic Effects of TNF

TNF regulates cellular metabolism. Some chronic infections and malignant diseases are associated with *cachexia,* a syndrome of weight loss, wasting, anorexia, and muscle weakness that appears to be mediated by TNF.

TNF Kinetics and Tolerance

Systemic TNF levels increase within 1 hour and then return to baseline within 3 hours of endotoxin administration. Even though TNF levels peak and return to baseline within a short time, systemic levels precipitate a vigorous inflammatory cascade, which continues despite the absence of detectable TNF.

Interleukin-1

The effects of TNF and IL-1 overlap. TNF stimulates the production of IL-1, and the effects of the two cytokines together are far greater than those of either alone. IL-1 is produced in sepsis in concert with TNF. However, the mechanism of IL-1–induced shock appears to be related to the release of other small mediator molecules, such as platelet-activating factor, prostaglandins, and nitric oxide. Antigen presentation by macrophages to T cells requires participation and synthesis of macrophage-derived IL-1. In contrast to TNF, small doses of endotoxin or other cytokines have no mitigating effect on IL-1 production.

The proinflammatory effects of IL-1 include effects on

fibroblasts, synovial cells, chondrocytes, endothelial cells, hepatocytes, and osteoclasts. IL-1 stimulates arachidonic acid metabolism and secretion of inflammatory proteins, including other cytokines and proteases. IL-1 stimulates the release of pituitary stress hormones, increases the synthesis of collagenases, resulting in the destruction of cartilage, and stimulates prostaglandin production.

IL-1 also induces fever. There is no evidence that IL-1 crosses the blood-brain barrier. The pyrogenic action probably is due to interaction between IL-1 and endothelial cells of the hypothalamic-pituitary portal venous system, resulting in the generation of prostaglandin E (PGE). PGE then acts on the hypothalamus to alter the firing rates of the thermosensitive neurons, resulting in fever. Antipyretic drugs, such as aspirin, are effective because they inhibit the cyclooxygenase enzyme involved in the conversion of arachidonic acid to prostaglandin. Other cytokines also induce an elevation in body temperature.

An increase in the synthesis of hepatic acute-phase proteins (Table 5-2) accompanied by a decrease in albumin synthesis is a sign of inflammation. Whereas IL-1 appears to induce acute-phase proteins, IL-6 is responsible for direct stimulation of hepatic acute-phase proteins.

IL-1 interacts with the vascular endothelium, overlapping the action of TNF. By inducing the expression of intracellular adhesion molecule (ICAM)-1, E-selectin, and vascular cell adhesion molecule (VCAM)-1 on endothelial cells, IL-1 provides a key step in the extravasation of leukocytes to sites of local inflammation and injury. Many cells synthesize and release IL-1 in response to a variety of stimuli (Fig. 5-5). Cells considered to be involved in the immune response produce IL-1, most importantly the monocyte–macrophage cell line, including blood monocytes, alveolar and peritoneal macrophages, Kupffer cells, and synovial macrophages. Lymphocytes, including natural killer (NK) cells, B cells, and helper T cells also are sources of IL-1. The following nonimmune cells produce IL-1: astrocytes, microglia, and glioma cells; vascular smooth muscle cells and endothelial cells; neutrophils; fibroblasts; chondrocytes; epithelial cells; keratinocytes; Langerhans cells; and renal mesangial cells.

Manifestations of IL-1–endothelial cell interactions include production prostaglandin, of platelet-activating fac-

Table 5-2. ACUTE-PHASE PROTEINS REGULATED BY CYTOKINES

INDUCED BY IL-6

C-reactive protein
α_2-macroglobulin
α_1 Acid glycoprotein
Fibrinogen
α_1-Proteinase inhibitor
α_1-Antichymotrypsin
Haptoglobin
Hemopexin
Ceruloplasmin
Complement C_3
Serum amyloid P
Serum amyloid A

INDUCED BY IL-1

C-reactive protein
α_1 Acid glycoprotein
Complement C3
Serum amyloid P
Serum amyloid A
Haptoglobin
Hemopexin

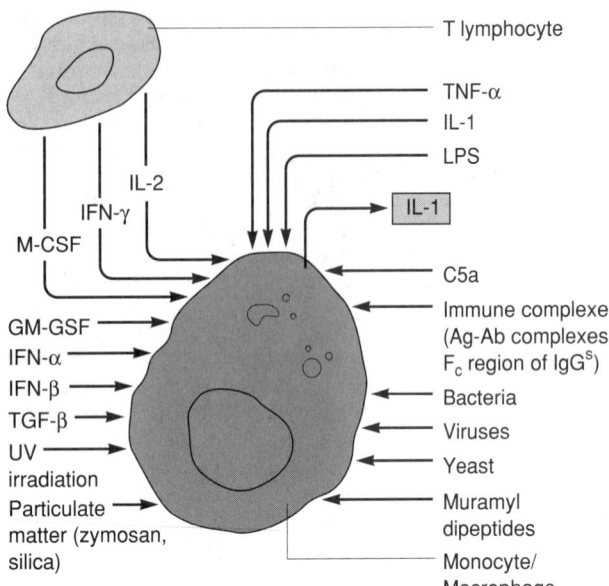

Figure 5-5. Stimuli for IL-1 production in cells of the monocyte/macrophage lineage. The macrophage is the most important cellular source of IL-1 in vivo.

tor, and of a variety of colony-stimulating factors. These responses mobilize and activate specific leukocyte populations for localized immune responses. Other effects of IL-1 on the vascular endothelium are to shift the balance toward thrombosis and a procoagulant state by down-regulating the fibrinolytic system and enhancing the activity of plasminogen activator inhibitor (PAI) and tissue-factor–like procoagulant and of thrombomodulin and the protein C system. IL-1 shifts the fibrinolytic properties of the endothelium by increasing PAI-1 production while leaving unchanged or decreasing tPA. IL-1 enhances thrombin formation on the endothelial surface by inducing synthesis of thromboplastin and suppressing thrombomodulin gene expression. IL-1 also induces synthesis of platelet-activating factor. This phospholipid is a potent platelet and leukocyte activator and a powerful vasoconstrictor.

Although most IL-1–induced changes facilitate a hypercoagulable state, like TNF, this cytokine can also stimulate endothelial synthesis of prostacyclin and urokinase-type plasminogen activator, facilitating antithrombotic tendencies.

Interleukin-6

The most important function of IL-6 appears to be regulation of the hepatic acute-phase response—a series of homeostatic responses induced by injury or infection. After an injury or infection, physiologic changes occur within several hours. These changes reflect alterations in the set point of a variety of functions, including thermoregulation, manifest by fever; nitrogen balance, manifest by a catabolic state; and circulating levels of acute-phase proteins. All these changes are designed to allow the host to recover from the injury or infection.

IL-6 expression is stimulated by a large number of cytokines and growth factors and by bacterial endotoxins. In monocytes and macrophages, lipopolysaccharide (LPS) is the most potent stimulus of IL-6 production. The most potent stimuli for fibroblast-derived IL-6 are IL-1 and TNF. Platelet-derived growth factor (PDGF) and fibro-

blast growth factor (FGF) also induce IL-6 in fibroblasts (Fig. 5-6).

Macrophage-derived IL-1 or TNF can activate fibroblasts and endothelial cells to release high levels of IL-6. This cascade results in increased plasma levels of IL-6 and stimulation of the hepatic acute-phase response.

Leukocyte–Endothelial Cell Interactions

Cytokines allow communication between leukocytes and endothelial cells in the initiation of the hemostatic, inflammatory, and immune response to injury and infection. The expression of a receptor and a counterreceptor on the surface of these cells also allows physical interaction and communication between the cells. Binding of inflammatory cells to the endothelium localizes the cells to an area of inflammation, infection, or injury.

Leukocyte–endothelial adherence must be strong enough to allow leukocytes to attach to the endothelium, but must allow the adherence to be transient and reversible. Once adherence occurs, a chemotactic signal elicits transmigration of the inflammatory cells across the basement membrane and into the interstitium.

Leukocyte and Endothelial Adhesion Molecules

The events that initiate and propagate neutrophil recruitment are shown in Figure 5-7. The initial neutrophil–endothelial cell adhesion is required for successful neutrophil extravasation at sites of inflammation. The following three families of adhesion molecules are expressed on the surface of leukocytes and endothelial cells and are important for leukocyte–endothelial interactions:

1. Immunoglobulin supergene family (ICAM-1, VCAM-1, and platelet–endothelial cell adhesion molecule [PECAM-1])
2. Selectin family—E-selectin and P-selectin, expressed on the surface of endothelial cells, are important for leukocyte adherence. L-selectin, expressed on the cell surface of all leukocytes, is important for the early adherence of polymorphonuclear leukocytes (PMNs) to the activated endothelium
3. Integrin family: b_1 (VLA antigens 1 through 6)—Primarily distributed on T lymphocytes, b_2 (CD11a, CD11b, CD11c)—Expressed on the cell surface of leukocytes, probably the most important subgroup with respect to leukocyte–endothelial interactions, b_3 (GPIIb, GPIIb/IIIa)—Expressed on platelets and endothelium.

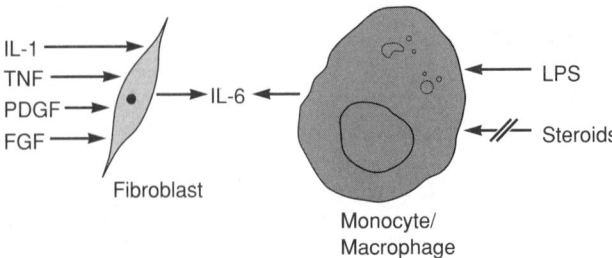

Figure 5-6. Stimuli for IL-6 production in fibroblasts and cells of the monocyte/macrophage lineage. In vivo, TNF and IL-1 are the most potent stimuli for fibroblast IL-6 production, while LPS is the most potent stimulus for monocyte/macrophage IL-6 production. Steroids inhibit monocyte/macrophage IL-6 production and release. PDGF and FGF are also capable of inducing fibroblast IL-6 production in vivo.

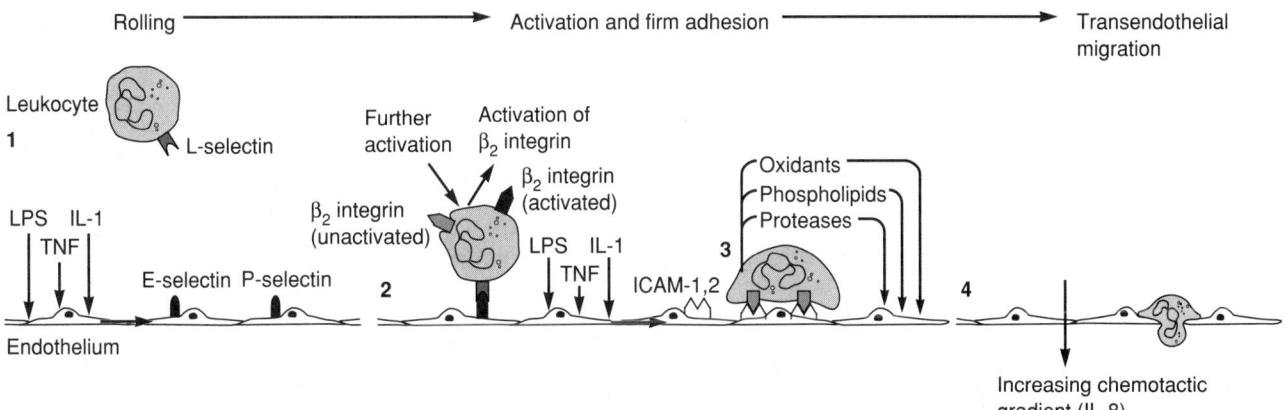

Figure 5-7. Neutrophil recruitment and activation into areas of inflammation. (1) Selectins mediate early loose adhesion or "rolling." This is a low-affinity adherence between constituitively expressed L-selectin on the neutrophil and E-selectin or P-selectin on the activated vascular endothelium. (2) This rolling slows the neutrophil enough to allow it to be activated, with expression and activation of β_2-integrins on the cell surface. Further activation of the endothelium by TNF, IL-1 or LPS leads to increased expression of ICAM-1 and ICAM-2, with subsequent firm adherence of the neutrophil to the endothelium. This is mediated through ICAM-β_2-integrin interactions. (3) The activated adherent neutrophil can then release proteases, oxidants, and phospholipids, resulting in endothelial cell injury and increased microvascular permeability. (4) Neutrophils then diapedese into the extravascular space via established chemotactic gradients. PECAM-1 may be important in transendothelial migration.

Adhesion Molecules and Wound Repair

The β_1 and β_3 integrins help generate a wound matrix after tissue injury. After the injury, platelets bind to the exposed matrix (Fig. 5-7). This requires interaction between β_1 and β_3 integrins and collagen, laminin, and fibronectin receptors. Activation of the coagulation cascade generates thrombin, which activates platelet GPIIb/IIIa, promoting further platelet aggregation. A wound matrix forms that contains platelets, fibrinogen, fibrin, and fibronectin. The activated platelets within the wound matrix elaborate TGF-β, PDGF, and thrombin.

TGF-β is strongly chemotactic for neutrophils, macrophages, and fibroblasts. As these inflammatory cells migrate

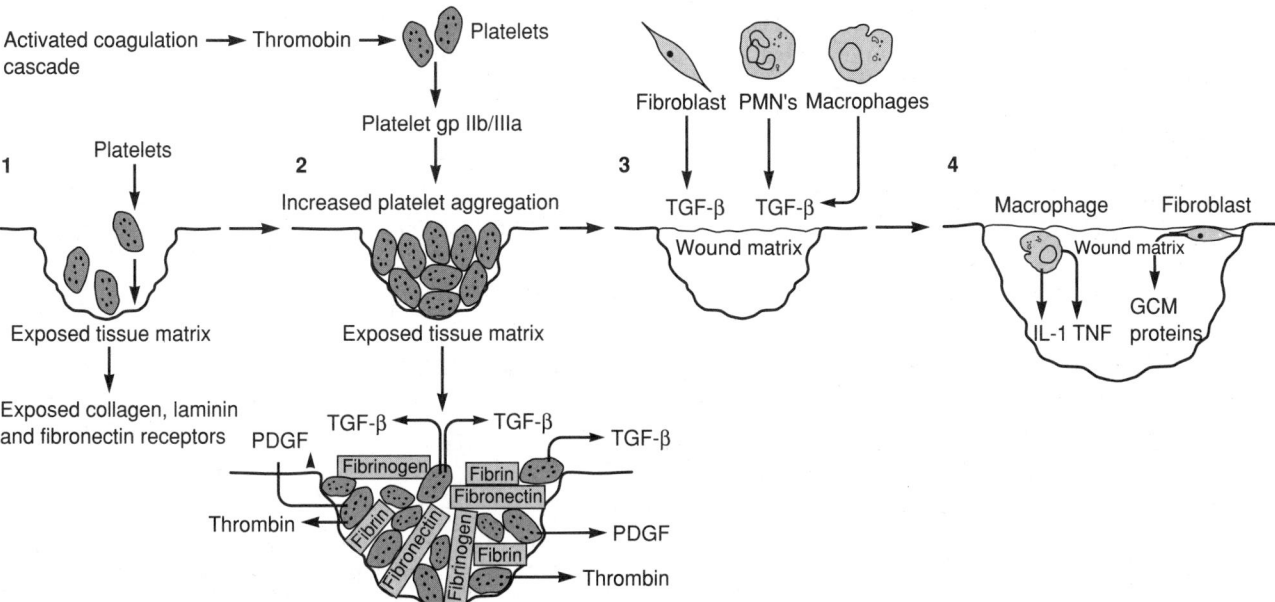

Figure 5-8. Establishment of a provisional wound matrix. (1) Platelets bind to exposed wound matrix via interaction of β_1 and β_3 integrins and collagen, laminin, and fibronectin receptors. (2) Following wounding, the coagulation cascade is activated, generating thrombin, which activates platelet gp IIb/IIIa and increases platelet aggregation. A provisional wound matrix is formed and is made up of platelets, fibrin, fibrinogen, and fibronectin. The activated platelets in the wound generate TGF-β, PDGF, and thrombin. (3) TGF-β is strongly chemotactic for neutrophils, macrophages, and fibroblasts, recruiting these cells into the provisional wound matrix, where they are also subsequently activated by TGF-β. (4) Increasing concentrations of TGF-β result in macrophage activation, producing increased amounts of TNF and IL-1. TGF-β also stimulates fibroblast production of extracellular matrix proteins. These reactions further enhance migration of macrophages and fibroblasts into the wound, facilitating tissue repair.

into the wound, they encounter increasing concentrations of TGF-β, which activates the cells. Macrophages increase their synthesis of TNF and IL-1, and fibroblasts increase their synthesis of extracellular matrix proteins. These reactions stimulate macrophage and fibroblast integrins, which promote further migration of inflammatory cells into the wound site and increase deposition of the provisional matrix.

Chemotactic Factors

TNF, IL-1, and LPS are not directly chemotactic for neutrophils. Cytokine networks may depend on the initial expression of TNF and IL-1. This initial interaction is followed by generation of distal inflammatory mediators that have a direct influence on neutrophil chemotaxis and activation.

One important group of chemotactic cytokines is called the *C-X-C chemokine family* because of its structure. These chemokines are all clustered on human chromosome 4.

WOUND HEALING

Normal wound healing rapidly restores tissue integrity and function after trauma, burns, and infection (Fig. 5-8). Healing involves a complex interaction among humoral, cellular, and extracellular matrix networks, yet it occurs in a controlled, sequential manner. It depends on the ability of cells to communicate with one another. Although cellular communication is often accomplished through direct cell-to-cell contact by means of cellular adhesion molecules, cells may also signal one another through soluble mediators, such as cytokines. Chemokines are chemotactic factors, but they also appear to have reparative capabilities. These molecules are important in angiogenesis, which is important in tissue repair and wound healing.

After injury, repair begins immediately with hemorrhage and extravasation of plasma into the wound. This activates the intrinsic and extrinsic coagulation pathways, leading to fibrin deposition and establishment of a provisional matrix. Platelet activation and degranulation also occur during coagulation, leading to the deposition of a number of cytokines into the provisional matrix (Fig. 5-9).

Neutrophils are the first leukocytes to arrive at a wound. Their primary function is phagocytosis of debris. These cells also produce a number of cytokines instrumental in orchestrating the progression of wound repair. Although neutrophils are important for initial host defense, the second wave of leukocytes consists of mononuclear phagocytes that generate a number of inflammatory mediators to help transform the provisional matrix to mature granulation tissue.

Cytokines and Angiogenesis

The ingrowth of new blood vessels is critical to the continued supply of oxygen and nutrients to regenerating tissues. An imbalance in the production of angiogenic and angiostatic factors may lead to diseases associated with an overexpression of angiogenic activity, such as rheumatoid arthritis, scleroderma, psoriasis, atherosclerosis, and idiopathic pulmonary fibrosis. Persistent neovascularization in these disorders allows continual fibroproliferation.

IL-8 is a potent neutrophil chemotaxin and activator. It is also a potent *angiogenic* factor. Another C-X-C chemokine, platelet factor (PF)-4, has angiostatic properties.

Cytokines and Fibroblasts

Because fibroblasts are present in almost all tissues, cytokine production by fibroblasts is important in most tissues. Fibroblasts are involved in many functions, including regulation of tissue repair and fibrosis, hematopoiesis, bone metabolism, inflammation, and immune response.

Tissue levels of IL-1 peak within the first day after a wound occurs, as do levels of TNF. IL-1 appears to have multiple effects on soft-tissue wound healing and to have important modulating effects on bone and cartilage. In addition to regulating fibroblast collagen synthesis, IL-1 controls some aspects of fibroblast cytokine production.

The effects of TNF on fibroblasts are difficult to separate from the influence of other cytokines, especially IL-1. TNF appears to be important in the early inflammatory response to wounding and the later tissue repair. Tissue levels of TNF peak the first day after a wound occurs. Abnormal levels of TNF or the continued presence of TNF in a wound may inhibit healing by inhibiting ingrowth of granulation tissue, retarding the accumulation of collagen hydroxyproline, and down-regulating collagen synthesis.

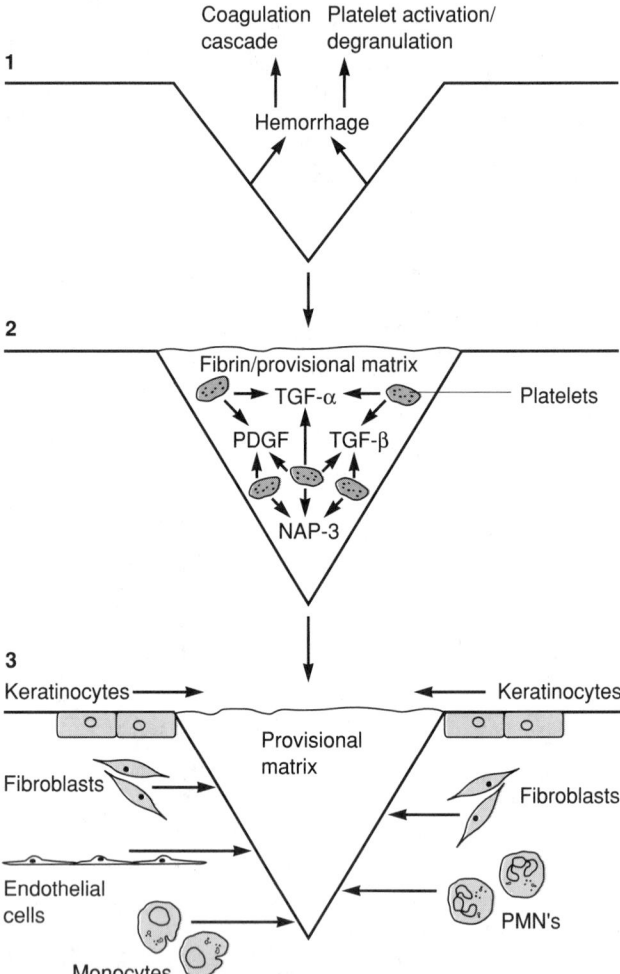

Figure 5-9. The wound matrix. (1) Following injury, hemorrhage occurs, with activation of coagulation and deposition of fibrin in the wound. (2) Concurrently, platelets are activated, resulting in degranulation, with the deposition of TGF-α, TGF-β, PDGF, and NAP-2 within the provisional wound matrix. (3) TGF-α, TGF-β, PDGF, and NAP-2 are important growth factors and chemotaxins for recruiting or activating fibroblasts, endothelial cells, monocytes, and neutrophils into the wound. Neutrophils are typically the first cells recruited into a site of injury, and produce a number of cytokines that are important for initiating wound repair. While neutrophils are important in initial host defense, the monocyte/macrophage is recruited into the wound after inflammation is established and is important in converting the provisional wound matrix into mature granulation tissue. Thus, coagulation and platelet degranulation are key processes for the subsequent cellular recruitment and activation necessary for wound healing.

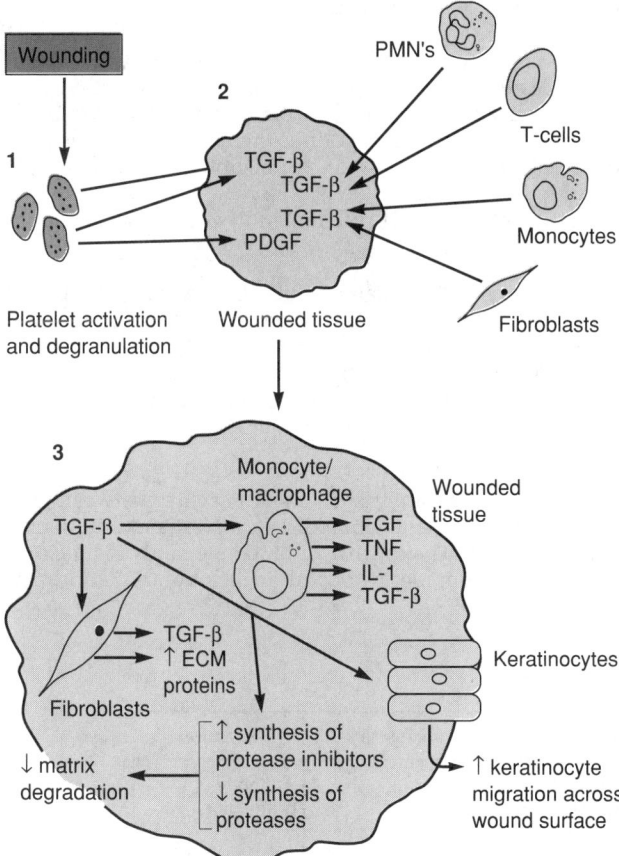

Figure 5-10. TGF-β in wound healing. TGF-β is one of the key cytokines in the orchestration of tissue repair. Immediately after wounding, platelets are activated and degranulated, releasing large amounts of TGF-β and PDGF into the wounded tissue. TGF-β is a powerful chemotactic agent for neutrophils, T-lymphocytes, monocytes, and macrophages, which are all recruited into the wound. As these cells encounter increasing concentrations of TGF-β, they become activated and release a variety of other factors that are important for perpetuating wound healing. Monocytes and macrophages release FGF, TNF, IL-1, and additional TGF-β. Fibroblasts also generate more TGF-β and increase their synthesis of extracellular matrix proteins. TGF-β inhibits matrix degradation by increasing the synthesis of extracellular matrix proteins, as well as increasing the synthesis of protease inhibitors, and decreasing protease synthesis. TGF-β also increases keratinocyte migration across the wound surface, facilitating reepithelialization.

TNF has no chemotactic effect on fibroblasts and does not alter fibroblast response to other chemoattractants. TNF does, however, stimulate the production of fibroblast PGE_2 and enhance transcription and translation of IL-6. IL-6 may facilitate metabolism of the extracellular matrix of the fibroblast. TNF acting locally may inhibit wound healing by inhibiting the expression of the gene for Type I collagen. TNF also stimulates cartilage resorption, stimulates release of proteoglycans from cartilage, and inhibits proteoglycan synthesis. These phenomena may be mediated and promoted by collagenase and PGE_2, since both are up-regulated in fibroblasts and macrophages by TNF and are involved in the degradation of collagen matrix and stimulation of the intracellular proteases responsible for tissue remodeling.

Topical epithelial growth factor (EGF) enhances soft-tissue wound healing by means of soft-tissue neovascularization. EGF accelerates epidermal regeneration in cutaneous wounds. It is also a chemoattractant for granulation-tissue fibroblasts. Cells at all stages of wound repair are responsive to EGF.

Sustained production of TGF-β has been implicated in tissue fibrosis in a variety of chronic diseases. Wound healing begins with platelet-induced hemostasis, followed by an influx of inflammatory cells and fibroblasts, deposition of extracellular matrix and neovascularization, and proliferation of the cells that reconstitute the injured tissue. TGF-β is involved in each of these events (Fig. 5-10). Topical application of TGF-β accelerates wound healing. TGF-β enhances collagen synthesis, deposition, and maturation. These actions have many clinical applications, including surgical wound healing in debilitated patients or those undergoing chemotherapy or treatment of burns or diabetic, decubitus, or varicose ulcers.

PDGF is synthesized by megakaryocytes, fibroblasts, endothelial cells, macrophages, and smooth muscle cells. The molecule is a chemotactic and activating factor for neutrophils, smooth muscle cells, and fibroblasts. It is also a fibroblast chemoattractant, the chemotactic response being inversely related to the rate of cellular proliferation. PDGF may accelerate normal wound healing by as much as 30%. The accelerated healing is associated with an enhanced influx and activation of macrophages, followed by the accumulation, activation, and proliferation of fibroblasts. Extracellular matrix deposition increases and re-epithelialization accelerates.

SUGGESTED READING

Bussolino F, Breviario F, Tetta C, Aglietta M, Mantovani A, Dejana E. Interleukin 1 stimulates platelet activating factor production in cultured human endothelial cells. J Clin Invest 1986;77:2027.

Cerami A. Inflammatory cytokines. Clin Immunol Immunopathol 1992;62:S3.

Koch AE, Polverini PJ, Kunkel SL, et al. Interleukin-8 (IL-8) as a macrophage-derived mediator of angiogenesis. Science 1992; 258:1798.

Lynch SE, Colvin RB, Antoniades NH. Growth factors in wound healing. J Clin Invest 1989;84:640.

Mustoe TA, Cutler NR, Allman RM, et al. A phase II study to evaluate recombinant platelet-derived growth factor-BB in the treatment of stage 3 and 4 pressure ulcers. Arch Surg 1994; 150:213.

Remick DJ, Kunkel RG, Larrick JW, Kunkel SL. Acute in vivo effects of human recombinant tumor necrosis factor. Lab Invest 1987;56:583.

Sehgal PB. Interleukin-6: a regulator of plasma protein gene expression in hepatic and non-hepatic tissues. Mol Biol Med 1990;7:117.

Springer TA. Adhesion receptors of the immune system. Nature 1990;346:425.

Strieter RM, Kunkel SL, Showell HJ, et al. Endothelial cell gene expression of a neutrophil chemotactic factor by TNF-alpha, LPS, and IL-1 beta. Science 1989;243:1467.

Tracey KJ, Wei H, Manogue KR, et al. Cachectin/tumor necrosis factor induces cachexia, anemia and inflammation. J Exp Med 1988;167:1211.

ESSENTIALS OF SURGERY: SCIENTIFIC PRINCIPLES AND PRACTICE,
edited by Lazar J. Greenfield, Michael W. Mulholland, Keith T. Oldham, Gerald B. Zelenock,
and Keith D. Lillemoe. Lippincott–Raven Publishers, Philadelphia, © 1997.

CHAPTER 6

INFLAMMATION

GENEVA M. OMANN AND DANIEL B. HINSHAW

Inflammation is the result of a complex series of the immune reactions. It occurs when an invading organism is present in large quantity or when tissue injury and cell death occur. The classic symptoms are swelling, redness, local heat, pain, and altered function.

Within minutes of injury, mediators are released that cause vasodilatation (resulting in redness) and increased vascular permeability, leading to accumulation of fluid (swelling) at the site of injury. Within 30 to 60 minutes, neutrophils marginate, extravasate, and accumulate at the site of injury, where they perform nonspecific phagocytosis and release oxidants and proteinases. Within 4 to 5 hours, monocytes and lymphocytes accumulate. Monocytes participate in nonspecific phagocytosis, and lymphocytes orchestrate specific, antibody-dependent cell lysis (Fig. 6-1). These processes limit the site of injury, destroy injurious agents, and remove necrotic tissue to allow healing.

The development of inflammation at a site of tissue injury involves the following:

1. Release of chemoattractants that recruit cells to the site of injury and induce the release of proteinases, toxic oxidants, and cytotoxic cationic proteins
2. Release of priming agents that enhance the ability of cells to respond to the chemoattractants
3. Release of growth factors that increase production of leukocytes

Figure 6-2 summarizes the interplay between the humoral and cellular components of inflammation in a clinical situation—exposure of blood elements to an extracorporeal membrane, as occurs in hemodialysis and car-

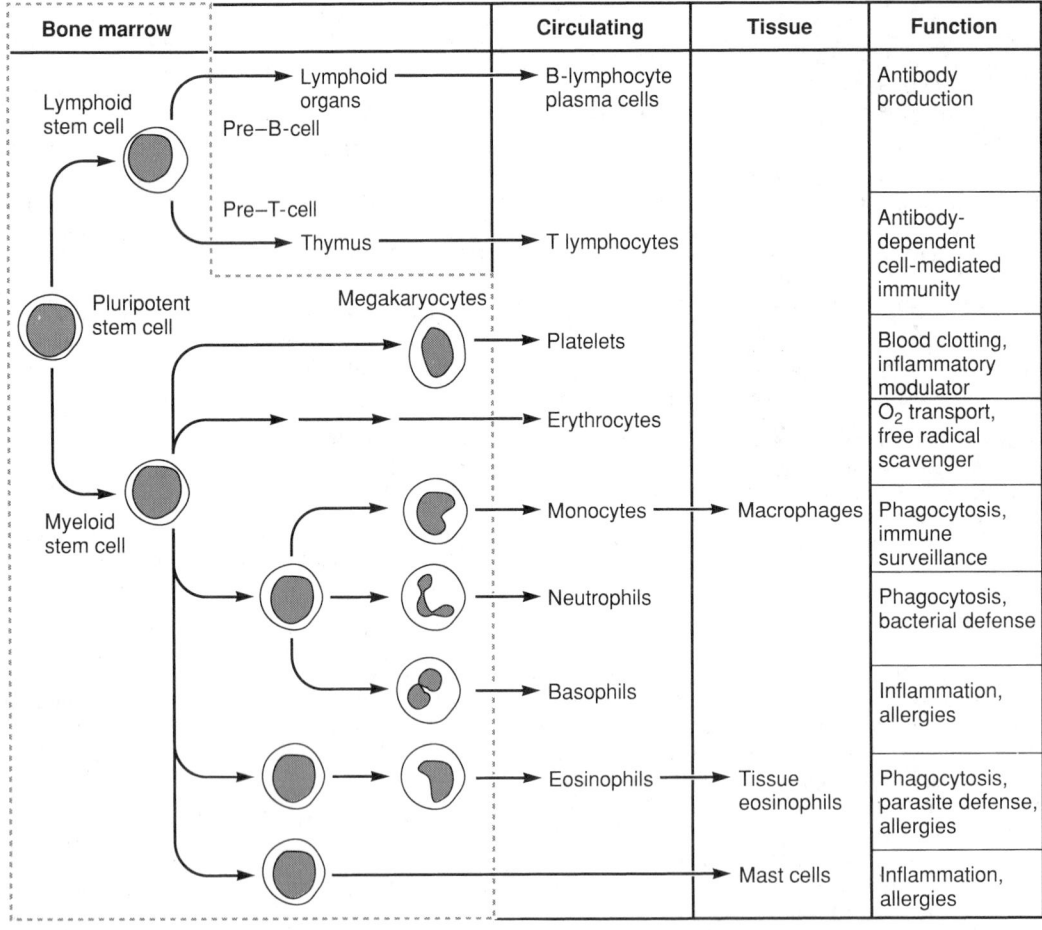

Figure 6-1. Cells of the hemopoietic cell system. Pluripotent stem cells in the bone marrow differentiate into lymphoid or myeloid stem cells. Lymphoid stem cells differentiate into pre–B cells or pre–T cells. In lymphoid organs, pre–B cells differentiate into B cells, which are released into the circulation. B cells further develop in the lymphoid organs into plasma cells, the antibody-producing cells of the immune system. Myeloid stem cells further differentiate in the bone marrow to produce mature cells. These mature cells are released into the circulation with the exception of mast cells, which are not found in the circulation. Circulating monocytes migrate into tissues, where they develop into macrophages.

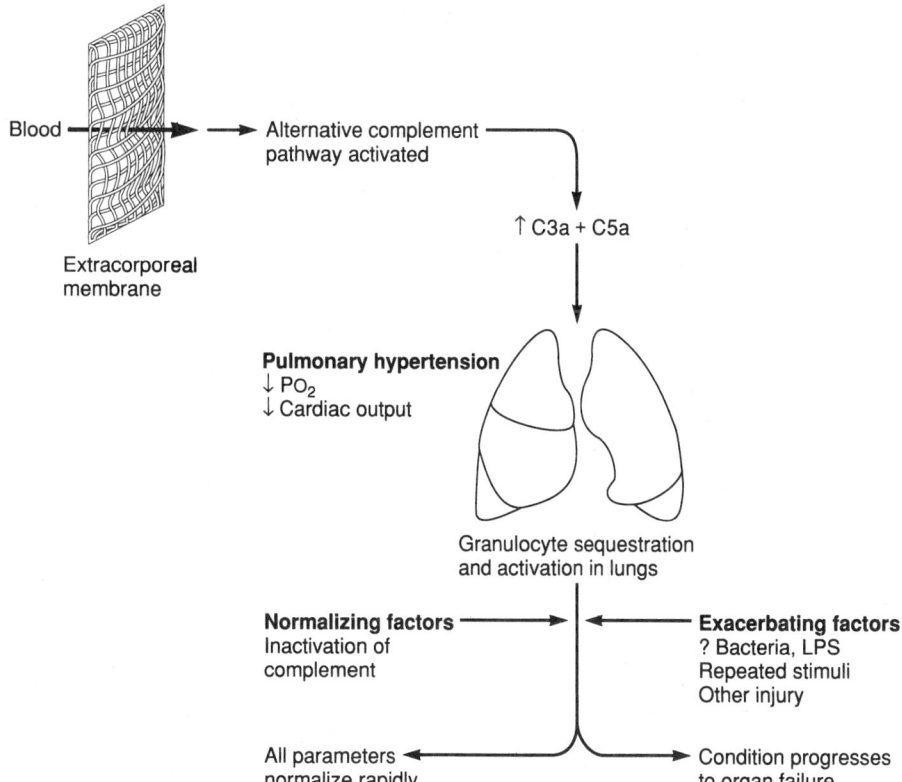

Figure 6-2. Homeostasis of inflammatory mediators. Many relatively common clinical situations, such as exposure of blood to extracorporeal membranes (eg, dialysis, cardiopulmonary bypass), lead to activation of inflammatory pathways (eg, the alternative complement pathway). Activation of these pathways results in the generation of mediators (eg, anaphylatoxins) that produce a number of physiologic and cellular effects. Under most circumstances, all affected parameters normalize rapidly, with no persistent adverse effect on the organism. The actual determinants that convert typically transient phenomena into persistent responses leading to organ dysfunction and failure are still poorly understood. LPS, lipopolysaccharide.

diopulmonary bypass. Under these circumstances, the inflammatory cascade is usually limited and does not result in progressive tissue injury.

ACUTE-PHASE RESPONSE AND INFLAMMATION

The acute-phase response (Fig. 6-3) is a series of homeostatic responses to tissue injury in infection and inflammation. After an inflammatory stimulus occurs, physiologic

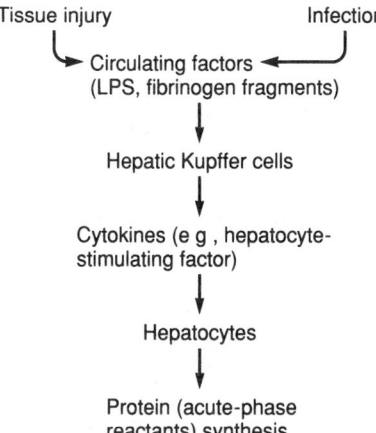

Figure 6-3. Acute-phase response. Certain soluble factors, such as the lipopolysaccharide (LPS) component of bacterial endotoxin or fibrinogen fragments, are released into the circulation after tissue injury or during infection. These factors stimulate Kupffer cells in the liver to secrete cytokines, which may in turn stimulate or inhibit the synthesis of certain proteins (acute-phase reactants) by hepatocytes.

changes take place within a few hours. These changes reflect altered setpoints for processes such as thermoregulation (fever), nitrogen balance, and modulation of plasma proteins.

HUMORAL COMPONENTS OF INFLAMMATION
Complement

The complement system comprises classic and alternative pathways (Fig. 6-4). The pathways involve serum proteins that amplify the inflammatory-immune response and mediate tissue injury. Complement activation stimulates a large number of physiologic and pathologic effects by activating leukocytes. This complement-dependent activation of leukocytes may be important in remote organ injury and dysfunction during inflammation. The adult respiratory distress syndrome (ARDS) that develops after a severe burn is an example of this phenomenon.

Kinins

Kinins modulate the inflammatory response by localizing and often amplifying the effects of inflammation. Kinins are generated at the site of inflammation by three mechanisms involving plasma proteins, tissue proteins, or cellular proteinases. Kinin formation is linked to activation of the clotting cascade. Pain and vascular congestion at the site of injury notify the organism of the location of the injury and direct blood to the area so that inflammatory cells can respond to chemoattractants in the vicinity.

Eicosanoids

The eicosanoids are prostaglandins, thromboxanes, leukotrienes, and lipoxins (Table 6-1). Eicosanoids are not stored in cells. Rather, they are rapidly synthesized in re-

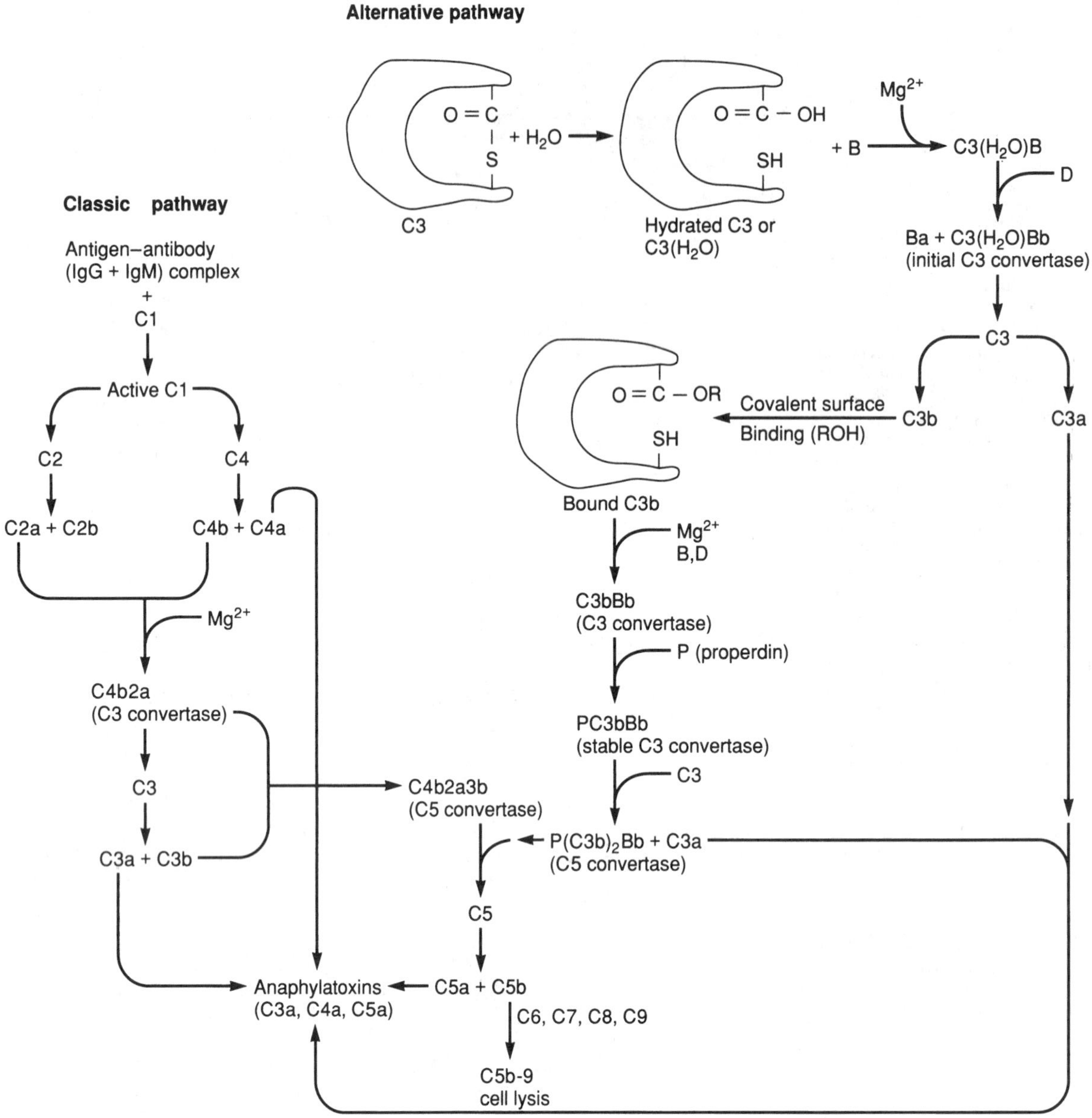

Alternative pathway

C3　+ H₂O →　Hydrated C3 or C3(H₂O)

O = C | S　　O = C — OH | SH

+ B →　C3(H₂O)B　　Mg²⁺

→ D

Ba + C3(H₂O)Bb (initial C3 convertase)

→ C3

Classic pathway

Antigen–antibody (IgG + IgM) complex
+
C1
↓
Active C1
↓　　↓
C2　　C4
↓　　↓
C2a + C2b　　C4b + C4a
↓
C4b2a (C3 convertase) — Mg²⁺
↓
C3
↓
C3a + C3b

O = C — OR | SH　Covalent surface Binding (ROH) ← C3b　　C3a

Bound C3b
↓ Mg²⁺ B,D
C3bBb (C3 convertase)
↓ P (properdin)
PC3bBb (stable C3 convertase)
↓ C3

C4b2a3b (C5 convertase)
↓
P(C3b)₂Bb + C3a (C5 convertase)
↓
C5
↓
C5a + C5b → Anaphylatoxins (C3a, C4a, C5a)
↓ C6, C7, C8, C9
C5b-9 cell lysis

Figure 6-4. The classic and alternative pathways of complement activation.

sponse to a variety of stimuli such as mechanical forces, tissue injury, and chemical mediators.

Eicosanoids are rapidly metabolized or are so chemically unstable that they exert their effects mostly near the site of synthesis. The first step in production of eicosanoids is action of phospholipase, which liberates arachidonic acid. Depending on cell type, the arachidonic acid has several fates.

A large number of antiinflammatory drugs disrupt eicosanoid synthetic pathways. Corticosteroids inhibit inflammation, at least in part, by inhibiting the release of arachidonic acid from phospholipids. Nonsteroidal antiinflammatory drugs (NSAIDs), such as aspirin, inhibit cyclooxygenase activity and block synthesis of prostaglandins and thromboxanes.

Platelet-Activating Factor

Platelet-activating factor (PAF) is not stored in cells but is produced rapidly during inflammation by activated leukocytes, mast cells, and vascular endothelium. Pathophys-

iologic effects include bronchoconstriction, hypotension, and increased vascular permeability. PAF is chemotactic for leukocytes and enhances neutrophil oxidant production in response to other stimuli. PAF is synthesized at activation by a variety of inflammatory cells including platelets, neutrophils, basophils, mast cells, mononuclear phagocytes, eosinophils, and vascular endothelium.

- PAF stimulates many of the inflammatory cells, smooth muscle cells, renal mesangial cells, epithelial cells, and vascular endothelium to release additional modulators of cellular behavior
- is chemotactic for migratory inflammatory cells and helps these cells adhere to the vascular endothelium
- induces secretion and oxidant production by cells that can perform those functions (mononuclear phagocytes, neutrophils, eosinophils)
- enhances the ability of neutrophils to respond to challenge with N-formylpeptides (bacterial peptides) and leukotriene LTB₄

Table 6-1. SOME EFFECTS OF EICOSANOIDS IN INFLAMMATION

PROSTAGLANDINS

PGE_2, PGI_2	Bronchodilation
	Vasodilation
	Potentiate effect of other mediators (eg, histamine, bradykinin, C5a) that increase vascular permeability
	Block platelet aggregation
	Stimulate bone resorption by osteoclasts
PGD_2	Bronchoconstriction
	Vasodilation
	Potentiates effect of other mediators (eg, histamine, bradykinin) that increase vascular permeability
	Stimulates random movement (chemokinesis) of neutrophils and eosinophils

LEUKOTRIENES

LTC_4, LTD_4, LTE_4	Account for the slow-reacting substance of anaphylaxis
	Bronchoconstriction (more severe in distal airways than in proximal airways)
	Increased secretion of bronchial mucus
	Vasoconstriction and increased vascular permeability
	Produce wheal and flare reaction in skin
LTB_4	Induces chemotaxis (directed movement) and chemokinesis of neutrophils, eosinophils, and monocytes
	Promotes adhesion of leukocytes especially to endothelium
	Stimulates production of $O_2^{\bullet-}$ and release of hydrolytic enzymes by neutrophils

LIPOXINS

LXA_4, LXB_4	Vasoactive
	Inhibit inflammatory response

Cytokines and Growth Factors

Cytokines induce activation of other cells (Table 6-2; see Chapter 5). On an immediate time scale, cytokines enhance activation of existing leukocytes. Over a longer time, cytokines increase differentiation and production of hemopoietic cells. Some cytokines do both.

CELLULAR COMPONENTS

Granulocytes

The three types of granulocytes (polymorphonuclear leukocytes [PMNs]) are neutrophils, basophils, and eosinophils. All these cells are migratory and contain numerous granules in the cytoplasm. The granules usually contain cytotoxic compounds and proteinases that degrade phagocytosed material; they also mediate inflammatory responses. Neutrophils are 60% of the circulating leukocyte population, basophils 0.1% to 0.5%, and eosinophils 1% to 3%.

Neutrophils

Neutrophils are a migratory, phagocytic cells that defend a host against bacteria and eliminutesate necrotic tissue. Neutrophils mature in the bone marrow and are released to the circulation as fully differentiated cells. Neutrophils are loaded with granules that contain a variety of proteinases, hydrolases, and antimicrobial agents. The neutrophils phagocytose material, and the granules fuse with the phagocytic vacuoles to degrade the foreign material. When neutrophils are challenged with a large amount of material, the granule contents may be released into the extracellular space, where damage to surrounding tissue occurs. Figure 6-5 summarizes the balance of forces that influence neutrophil behavior during inflammation.

Neutrophils circulate in the blood for 7 to 10 hours. Then they move into tissues, where they stay for 1 to 2 days before being cleared from the system. Spent granules are not replenished once the cells are in the circulation, and tissue neutrophils do not reenter the circulation. Neutrophils are poised to respond rapidly to stimuli, but they are rapidly spent in the process. Neutrophil function is replenished only by the formation of new neutrophils.

Eosinophils

Eosinophils constitute a small percentage of leukocytes in the bloodstream. They also exist in tissue; for every circulating eosinophil, there are 100 tissue eosinophils. Eosinophils exist outside the circulation for several days, and may later reenter the circulation. They exhibit phagocytic capabilities and contain granules with peroxisome-like proteins, lysophospholipase, and cytotoxic proteins, including major basic protein, eosinophil cationic protein, eosinophil-derived neurotoxin, and eosinophil peroxidase. Eosinophils are less effective as bactericidal agents than neutrophils, but may be important in defense against parasites.

Eosinophils are primary effectors in allergic reactions because they have immunoglobulin E (IgE) receptors, which do not exist on neutrophils. Eosinophils contain histaminase, and the major basic protein causes release of histamine from basophils and mast cells. Eosinophils may release prostaglandins that inhibit mast cell function by cyclic adenosine monophosphate (cAMP)-dependent pathways. Eosinophils also produce LTC4 and PAF, which increase vascular permeability.

Basophils

Basophils are fully differentiated cells released into the circulation from the bone marrow. Their granules contain histamine, proteoglycans, proteinases, acid hydrolases, eosinophil chemotactic factor, and neutrophil chemotactic factor. Basophils contain the main source of histamine in the blood. Basophils may be involved in defense against parasites. Besides the release of granule constituents, activation of basophils results in production of leukotrienes and PAF.

Mast Cells

Mast cells are formed from bone marrow precursors that differentiate and proliferate in connective tissue. Mast cells and basophils are similar, but mast cells do not enter

Table 6-2. CYTOKINES IN INFLAMMATION

Component	Sources*	Role in Inflammatory Response
Granulocyte-macrophage colony-stimulating factor	T lymphocytes, fibroblasts, endothelial cells	Increased production of granulocyte and mononuclear phagocytes; enhanced function of granulocytes and mononuclear phagocytes
Macrophage colony-stimulating factor	Lymphocytes (and others?)	Increased production of mononuclear phagocytes; enhanced function of mononuclear phagocytes
Granulocyte colony-stimulating factor	Lymphocytes?	Increased production of granulocytes; enhanced function of granulocytes
Platelet-derived growth factor	Platelets, macrophages	Leukocyte chemoattractant
Transforming growth factor β (TGF-β)	Platelets, lymphocytes, macrophages	Mononuclear phagocyte chemoattractant
Interleukin-1 (IL-1)†	Mononuclear phagocytes, fibroblasts, endothelial cells, keratinocytes, smooth muscle cells	Lymphocyte differentiation and activation; production of lymphokines; production of hepatic acute-phase proteins
IL-2	Lymphocytes	Lymphocyte differentiation; antiinflammatory effects on monocytes and macrophages; regulation of B-cell function and endothelial cell expression of adhesion molecules
IL-3	T lymphocytes	Early myeloid and lymphoid differentiation
IL-4	T lymphocytes	Lymphocyte proliferation and priming; enhanced myeloid differentaition (with other growth factors)
IL-5	Lymphocytes	B-cell activation; eosinophil differentiation
IL-6	Fibroblasts, mononuclear phagocytes, endothelial cells, T and B cells, mesangial cells, keratinocytes	Synergistic with IL-1 in lymphocyte proliferation, induction of hepatic acute-phase proteins
IL-7	Thymic stromal cells; bone marrow	Early B-cell precursor differentiation; induces lymphokine-activated killer cell activity; promotes tumor-specific, tumor-infiltrating lymphocytes
IL-8	Mononuclear phagocytes, endothelial cells, fibroblasts, epithelial cells	Neutrophil chemotactic factor
IL-9	T cells; peripheral blood mononuclear cells	Increases mast cell proliferation; increases IgE and IgG production by B cells; supports erythropoiesis
IL-10	T cells; macrophages; others	Inhibits monocyte and macrophage secretion of several interleukins; inhibits antigen-presenting capabilities of monocytes; increases IL-2 and IL-4 proliferative action on T cells
IL-11	Stromal cells	Stimulatory for lymphopoietic and myeloid and erythroid systems
IL-12	Monocytes	Growth factor for T cells and natural killer cells; promotes Th1 cell differentiation
IL-13	T cells	Antiinflammatory effects on monocytes and macrophages; regulation of B-cell function and endothelial cell expression of adhesion molecules
Tumor necrosis factor‡ (TNF)	Macrophage (TNF-α), lymphocytes (TNF-β)	Induction of hepatic acute proteins; enhances leukocyte function
Interferon-γ	T cells, macrophage?	B- and T-cell activation; enhances neutrophil and mononuclear phagocyte function

* These sources must be activated to release these compounds. Activation can result from injury, autoimmune reactions, antigen challenge, or activation by cytokines.

† IL-1 and TNF share many biologic properties, but they are coded on separate genes, and TNF does not promote cell growth.

‡ TNF has two components. TNF-β is derived from lymphocytes and is also known as *lymphocytoxin*. TNF-α is derived from macrophages. These two compounds both appear to bind to the same cell receptor and induce similar physiologic responses, although they share only a 30% sequence homology. Because TNF-α has been cloned, more work has been done with this compound.

the circulation, and basophils do not populate tissues. Mast cell granules contain histamine and proteoglycans. They are the main source of histamine in tissues except the stomach and central nervous system. Mast cells release histamine when injured. Histamine appears to activate xanthine oxidase, which increases production of toxic oxygen radicals.

Monocytes and Macrophages

The monocyte–macrophage system (mononuclear phagocytes) consists of phagocytic cells scattered throughout the body. *Monocytes* are derived from precursors that mature in the bone marrow and are released into the circulation. Monocytes migrate into tissue, where they differentiate into mature *macrophages*. Macrophages have various forms, depending on the tissue in which they differentiate: Kupffer cells in the liver, alveolar macrophages in the lung, and microglial cells in the brain.

Mononuclear phagocytes have numerous effector and modulatory roles in immunity and inflammation (Fig. 6-6). The phagocytic function of macrophages is crucial to removal of senescent cells and cell debris. The release of lysosomal enzymes and oxidants (including the free radical nitric oxide) during this process may contribute to inflammation. Mononuclear phagocytes are antigen-

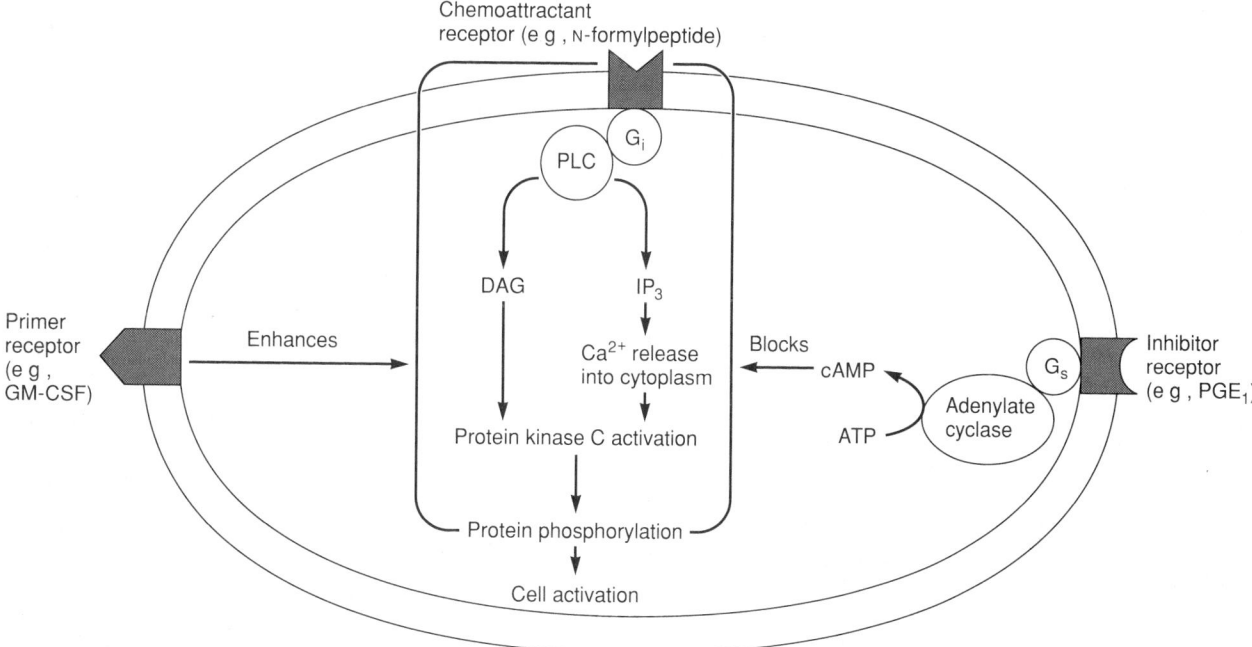

Figure 6-5. Modulation of neutrophil signal transduction pathways. The chemoattractant-mediated signal transduction pathway is enhanced by priming agents, such as granulocyte-macrophage colony-stimulating factor (GM-CSF). The mechanism is not clearly defined, but it may involve an enhanced expression of chemoattractant receptors on the cell surface. The chemoattractant-mediated signal transduction pathway is inhibited by agents such as PGE_1 and β-adrenergic agonists that cause G_s-mediated activation of adenylcyclase. This inhibition is thought to occur by way of cyclic AMP (cAMP)-mediated phosphorylation events. G_i, G protein that mediates phospholipase C (PLC) activation by chemoattractants; G_s, G protein that stimulates adenylate cyclase; DAG, diacylglycerol; IP_3, inositol 1,4,5-trisphosphate.

presenting cells (APCs) that take up and process foreign proteins, and make the processed epitopes available at the cell surface for recognition by and activation of T lymphocytes.

During acute inflammation, monocytes respond to chemoattractants released during the inflammatory response (eg, PAF, C5a) and are recruited to the site of inflammation. Mononuclear phagocytes respond to inflammatory stimuli by releasing macrophage colony-stimulating factor, GM-CSF, IL-1, and TNF (in addition to a variety of growth factors). These factors allow fibroblasts and endothelial cells to produce cytokines. The growth factors ultimately increase the production of mononuclear phagocytes. Several of these factors enhance the ability of effector cells (eg, neutrophils and mononuclear phagocytes) to respond to chemotactic stimuli released at the site of injury. Mononuclear phagocytes also produce chemoattractants, such as neutrophil-activating peptide 1, PAF, and LTB_4, which recruit more leukocytes.

Lymphocytes

The lymphocyte response in inflammation is slower than the response of other inflammatory effector cells (eg, neutrophils), which occurs within seconds of exposure to a noxious stimulus. The primary role of lymphocytes in inflammation is orchestration of chronic inflammatory processes. Presentation of processed antigen (eg, digested bacterial products), primarily by macrophages or other APCs to T lymphocytes, sets the stage for chronic inflammation. The stimulated T lymphocytes produce cytokines, which further enhance the activity of the APCs. Cytokines stimu-

late differentiation and proliferation of B lymphocytes and can make antigen-specific antibodies. Stimulated T lymphocytes injure target cells at sites of inflammation.

Platelets

Few of the factors released or the functions performed by platelets during inflammation are unique to platelets. Other inflammatory cells often have the same capabilities. Platelets have the following functions in inflammation:

- Synthesis and release of vasoactive eicosanoids
- Release of chemotactic factors
- Interaction with other inflammatory cells
- Interaction with endothelial cells
- Adherence to and coating of bacterial and tumor cells
- Increase of vascular permeability

Contact between platelets and abnormal vascular surfaces (injured or activated endothelium and exposed basement membrane) leads to platelet activation and release of factors that modulate or amplify the inflammatory event. Once platelets are activated by thrombin or an abnormal endothelial surface, they release chemotactic factors (Table 6-3) that recruit other inflammatory cells (eg, neutrophils, eosinophils, and monocytes).

Erythrocytes

At sites of acute inflammation where oxidant generation occurs in the presence of hemorrhage, the presence of erythrocytes may help attenuate the deleterious effects of the oxidants on the surrounding tissue. Another possible

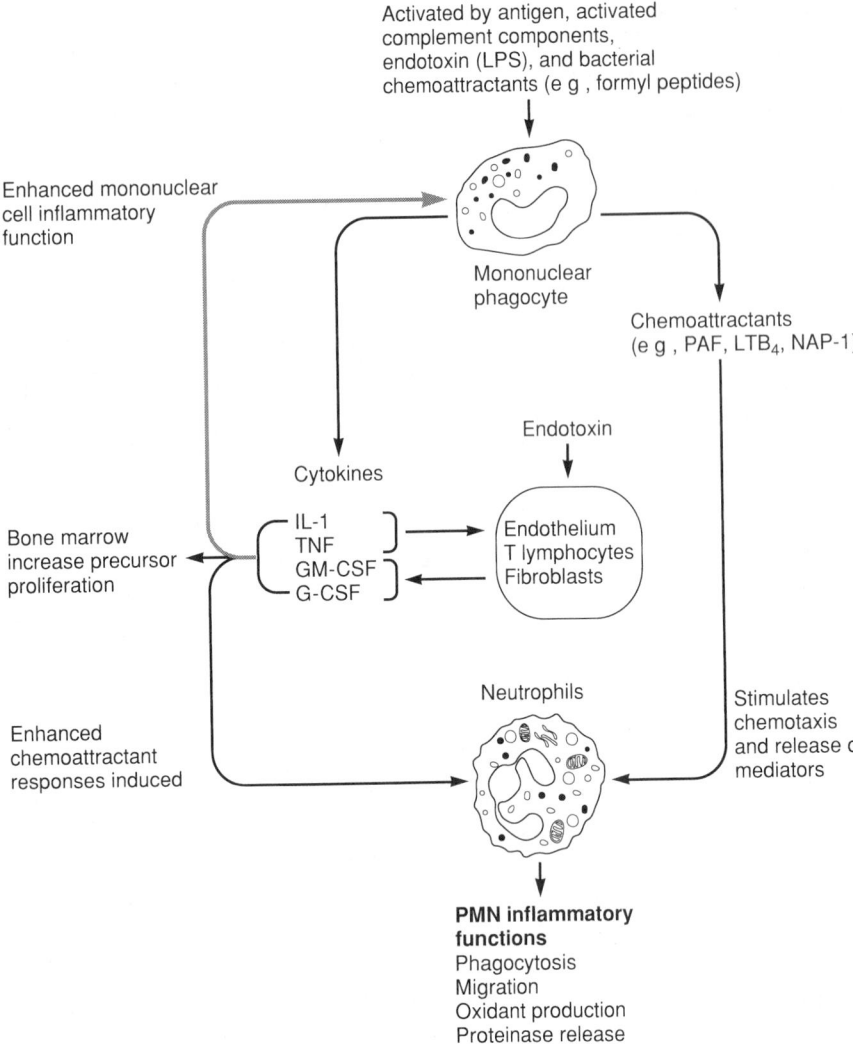

Activated by antigen, activated
complement components,
endotoxin (LPS), and bacterial
chemoattractants (e g , formyl peptides)

Enhanced mononuclear
cell inflammatory
function

Mononuclear
phagocyte

Chemoattractants
(e g , PAF, LTB$_4$, NAP-1)

Endotoxin

Cytokines

IL-1
TNF
GM-CSF
G-CSF

Bone marrow
increase precursor
proliferation

Endothelium
T lymphocytes
Fibroblasts

Neutrophils

Stimulates
chemotaxis
and release of
mediators

Enhanced
chemoattractant
responses induced

**PMN inflammatory
functions**
Phagocytosis
Migration
Oxidant production
Proteinase release

Figure 6-6. The central role of the mononuclear phagocyte in initiating and augmenting the inflammatory response. Activation of mononuclear phagocytes results in the release of neutrophil chemoattractants, growth factors, and interleukins, enhancing the ability of neutrophils to respond to the chemoattractants. In addition, these growth factors and interleukins can modulate the release of additional growth factors from the vascular endothelium, T lymphocytes, and fibroblasts. This function is also produced by endotoxin acting directly on these cells. The growth factors feed back to enhance mononuclear phagocyte function. On a longer time scale, they stimulate myeloid cell differentiation in the bone marrow. LPS, lipopolysaccharide; PAF, platelet-activating factor; NAP-1, neutrophil-activating protein 1; IL-1, interleukin-1; TNF, tumor necrosis factor; GM-CSF, granulocyte macrophage colony-stimulating factor; G-CSF, granulocyte colony-stimulating factor; PMN, polymorphonuclear leukocyte.

role for erythrocytes in the acute inflammatory response after ischemia–reperfusion injury involves adenosine deaminase, the erythrocyte enzyme.

Vascular Endothelium

Endothelial cells are not passive participants in inflammation; they direct and focus many aspects of an inflammatory event.

Leukocyte Adhesion to Endothelial Cells

PMNs adhere to endothelial cells as an early event in inflammation. Cytokines (IL-1, tumor necrosis factor [TNF], lymphotoxin) and bacterial LPS induce an activated state in endothelial cells. These agents cause endothelial cells to express an adhesion molecule (endothelial-leukocyte adhesion molecule 1 [ELAM-1]) on their surfaces, markedly enhancing PMN adhesion. Peak expression occurs about 4 h after exposure to IL-1 or the other cytokines.

High Endothelial Venules and Lymphocytes

High endothelial venules are specialized postcapillary venules that contain enlarged, cuboidal (high) endothelial cells. High endothelial venules may be central to lymphocyte homing to lymph nodes and lymphoid

tissues. Exposure of endothelial cells to cytokines enhances their adherence to lymphocytes. High endothelial venule patterns of endothelium occur in postcapillary venules near sites of chronic inflammation; they probably are the main portal of entry for lymphocytes into inflammatory lesions.

Other Endothelial Functions in Inflammation

IL-1, TNF, lymphotoxin, interferon-γ, LPS, and thrombin may induce synthesis and release of prostaglandin I$_2$ (PGI$_2$), PAF, GM-CSF, and growth factors for endothelial cells, fibroblasts, and smooth muscle cells. Endothelial cells can produce IL-1 after activation and produce and remodel their own basal laminutesa (basement membrane). At stimulation, endothelial cells release collagenases that partially digest the basal lamina and allow new vessel growth. This function may enhance egress of inflammatory cells from the circulation through the endothelium during acute inflammation.

Endothelial cells are important in regulation of vascular tone. ACE is present on the surface of endothelial cells. It converts angiotensin I to the active vasoconstrictor angiotensin II and inactivates the potent inflammogen, bradykinin.

Endothelial cells exert regulatory effects on the underlying smooth muscle by means of endothelium-derived

Table 6-3. FACTORS DERIVED FROM PLATELET ACTIVATION

CHEMOATTRACTANTS DERIVED FROM PLATELET ACTIVITY

C5a derived from complement cleavage by neutral proteinases
    released from activated platelets
Lipids
    12-Hydroxy eicosatetraenoic acid (12-HETE)
    Platelet-activating factor
α-Granule proteins
    Platelet-derived growth factor
    Platelet factor 4

GROWTH FACTORS PRODUCED BY PLATELETS

Transforming growth factors α and β
Fibroblast growth factor
Platelet-derived growth factor

ANTIMICROBIAL ACTIVITY FROM PLATELETS

Cationic bactericidal protein (β lysin)
IgE-mediated oxidant production by platelets directed at
    schistosomes

VASOACTIVE SUBSTANCES FROM PLATELETS

Vasodilators
    Prostaglandin E_2
    Prostaglandin I_2
Vasoconstrictors
    Prostaglandin $F_{2\alpha}$
    Serotonin
    Platelet-derived growth factor

AGENTS RELEASED BY PLATELETS AND THAT INCREASE VASCULAR PERMEABILITY

Serotonin
Platelet-activating factor
Prostaglandin E_2
Cationic proteins (eg, prostaglandin F_4)

relaxing factor (EDRF) and endothelin, a peptide. Both agents are important in determination of distribution of blood flow, which can affect the magnitude of a local inflammatory response.

Under unusual circumstances, endothelial cells exhibit macrophage-like properties, in that they can act as APCs and phagocytose particles. They may be a source of oxidants in inflammatory reactions after ischemic insults.

CELLULAR INJURY IN INFLAMMATION

One effect of the inflammatory cascade is cellular injury and death. This may be beneficial, as in neutrophil-mediated destruction of invading bacteria or phagocytic killing of tumor cells. The effect is harmful if the main force of the inflammatory response is directed at host tissues. Figure 6-7 shows the cycle of organ dysfunction in inflammatory tissue injury.

Necrosis and Apoptosis

Cell death usually results from one of two processes: necrosis or apoptosis. *Apoptosis* is a morphologic pattern of nuclear fragmentation and condensation associated with cell shrinkage. This leads to fragmentation of the cell into many small, membrane-enclosed fragments (apoptotic bodies) that contain portions of fragmented chromatin. The apoptotic bodies retain intact plasma membranes for some time and are phagocytized by neighboring cells. A wide variety of stimuli can induce the apoptotic process (Table 6-4).

Many pathologic agents that at low concentrations induce apoptosis in a cell, cause *necrosis* in the same cell at higher concentrations. Injury leading to necrosis is associated with cellular swelling and loss of plasma membrane

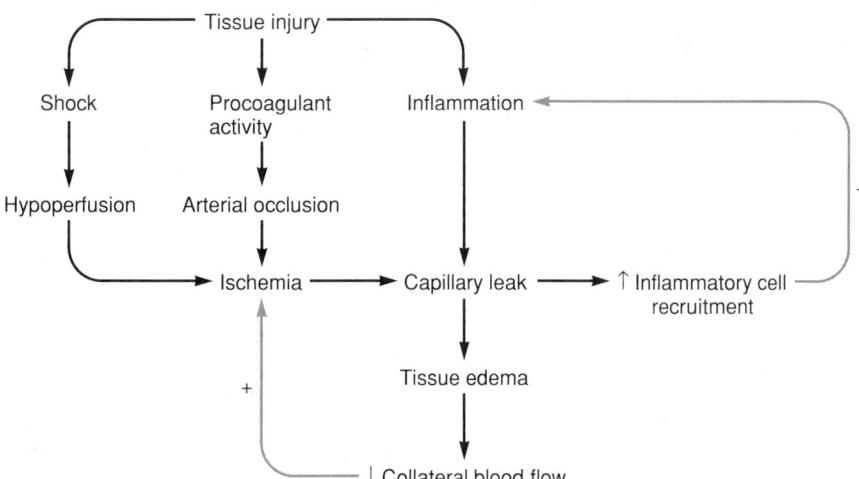

Figure 6-7. Cycle of organ dysfunction in inflammatory tissue injury. Tissue injury can lead to the expression of procoagulant (tissue factor) activity, followed by activation of the coagulation cascade and subsequent vascular occlusion. Ischemia may then develop, leading to capillary leak. Massive tissue injury with shock can produce global ischemic changes associated with hypoperfusion of multiple organs. Concomitant activation of inflammatory cascades (eg, complement activation, kinin formation, and generation and release of cytokines) can also lead to capillary leak secondary to the various mediators described in the text. The capillary leak in turn accentuates the inflammatory process by allowing greater accumulation of inflammatory cells at the site of the leak. Also, the associated tissue edema further exacerbates the hypoperfusion and ischemia by compromising collateral blood flow, establishing a vicious cycle.

Table 6-4. STIMULI OF APOPTOSIS

PHYSIOLOGIC
Normal development
Removal of trophic factors
Steroid hormones
Spontaneous (some tumors)
Cytotoxic T lymphocytes
Tumor necrosis factor

PATHOLOGIC
Ischemia, oxidant stress
Ultraviolet and x-irradiation
Thermal stress (hyperthermia and hypothermia)
Anticancer agents
Agents that disrupt the cytoskeleton
Human immunodeficiency virus infection (lymphocytes)

integrity. Failure of ATP synthesis in injured cells limits energy available for biosynthetic and repair processes and limits the function of the membrane ATPases that maintain the ion gradients. The transmembrane electrical potential collapses and membrane integrity is destroyed. The result is cell death.

Molecular lesions (eg, denatured proteins) are produced in cells as a result of thermal stress or other forms of injury (eg, oxidant stress), and the cellular response to this stress involves coordinated synthesis of proteins that helps confer protection from later stress. Although the specific proteins induced vary with the particular stress (eg, heat shock vs oxidant exposure or hypoxia), features common to the responses allow cross protection (Table 6-5). Some antioxidant proteins are induced as part of the stress response. Under ATP-depleted conditions, a stressed cell seems to perceive a decrease in the level of free, unassociated stress protein, and this leads to initiation of the stress response.

Oxidants and Cellular Injury

Humans live by oxygen-dependent cellular respiration. Yet, oxygen, the central element of aerobic life, also may provide the means of death. Several reactive species of oxygen (oxidants) are sources of tissue injury in inflammation.

Some oxidants are free radicals, which are chemical species that have an unpaired electron, usually designated $\bullet$. For example, superoxide anion, a one-electron reduction product of oxygen, is designated $O_2^{\bullet-}$. Oxidants that are free radicals may be initiators of free radical chain reactions

Table 6-5. STRESS PROTEINS AND THEIR PRIMARY INDUCERS

Stress Proteins	Inducers
Heat-shock protein (HSP) groups HSP (110, 90, 70, 65 kd) Small HSPs (20–28 kd)	Thermal stress
Glucose-regulated proteins (GRPs) GRP (78, 96 kd)	Glucose starvation
Ubiquitin (8 kd)	Degraded proteins
Metallothioneins	Heavy metals (eg, Zn^{2+}, Ca^{2+}, Hg^{2+}, cd^{2+})
Oxidant-related stress proteins Superoxide dismutase (Mn-SOD; 90 kd)	Oxidant stress (also thermal stress)
Heme oxygenase (32 kd)	

that involve unsaturated fatty acids in the lipid bilayer of cell membranes. This series of lipid oxidations can disrupt the lipid bilayer by means of cell lysis. Oxidants attack many molecular targets, including amino acids in proteins and DNA.

SUGGESTED READING

Baumann H, Gauldie J. The acute phase response. Immunol Today 1994;15:74.
Deitch EA, Mancini MC. Complement receptors in shock and transplantation. Arch Surg 1993;128:1222.
Gallin JI, Goldstein IM, Snyderman R, eds. Inflammation: basic principles and clinical correlates. New York, Raven, 1988.
Gerschenson LE, Rotello RJ. Apoptosis: a different type of cell death. FASEB J 1992;6:2450.
Hart CM, Tolson JK, Black ER. Supplemental fatty acids alter lipid peroxidation and oxidant injury in endothelial cells. Am J Physiol 1991;(Lung Cell Mol Physiol 4):L481.
Serhan CN. Lipoxin biosynthesis and its impact in inflammatory and vascular events. Biochim Biophys Acta 1994;1212:1.
Williams WJ, Beutler E, Ersley A, Lichtman MA, eds. Hematology. New York, McGraw-Hill, 1990.
Zelenock G, D'Alecy L, Fantone J III, et al, eds. Clinical ischemic syndromes: mechanisms and consequences of tissue injury. St Louis, Mosby, 1990.

ESSENTIALS OF SURGERY: SCIENTIFIC PRINCIPLES AND PRACTICE, edited by Lazar J. Greenfield, Michael W. Mulholland, Keith T. Oldham, Gerald B. Zelenock, and Keith D. Lillemoe. Lippincott–Raven Publishers, Philadelphia, © 1997.

CHAPTER 7

INFECTION
DAVID L. DUNN

HOST DEFENSES

Host defenses prevent microbes from causing infection, and they contain and eradicate infection if it occurs. Host defenses are barriers, endogenous microbial flora, cellular elements, and humoral factors, including cytokines. Although individual host defenses provide a series of barriers to infection, these components also act in synergy. Individual components of the host defense system also have deleterious potential for the host.

Barriers

Barrier defenses separate sterile body tissues from the external environment and from portions of the body (eg, oropharynx, intestine) that contain resident microbial flora. The skin, mucous membranes, and epithelial layers of some organs constitute physical barriers against microbial invasion.

Microbial Flora

Anaerobic organisms are found in greatest quantity at each end of the gastrointestinal (GI) tract, but each end contains different types of organisms (Fig. 7-1). The GI microflora contributes chemical and physical barriers at the mucous membrane level by (1) occupying potential

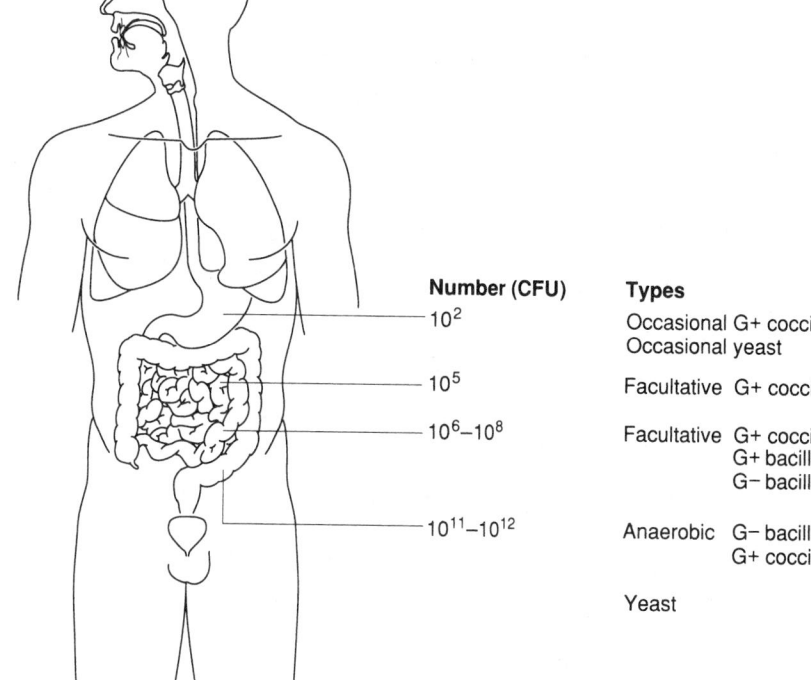

Number (CFU)	Types
10^2	Occasional G+ cocci Occasional yeast
10^5	Facultative G+ cocci
$10^6 - 10^8$	Facultative G+ cocci G+ bacilli G− bacilli
$10^{11} - 10^{12}$	Anaerobic G− bacilli G+ cocci
	Yeast

Figure 7-1. Autochthonous microflora of the gastrointestinal tract. Large numbers and different types of anaerobic bacteria are present in both the oropharynx and distal gut. The stomach is virtually sterile in normal individuals, but the number of microorganisms increases in an aboral direction. These organisms provide the initial inoculum of microorganisms when perforation of a viscus occurs. G+, grampositive; G−, gram-negative.

binding sites for pathogens, a phenomenon called *colonization resistance,* and (2) providing a physical barrier composed of mucus and bacteria.

Because of its low pH, the *stomach* keeps oropharyngeal microbes from passing into the intestine. Gastric acid kills most microbes unless they occur in very large numbers or are acid-resistant (eg, *Mycobacterium*). This function, coupled with rapid transit in the stomach and upper small intestine, probably explains why so few microbes are present in the *upper small intestine*. The *lower small intestine* contains large numbers of aerobes and anaerobes, especially in patients in whom the ileocecal valve allows backwash of cecal contents into the terminal ileum. The *colon* contains a wide diversity and large number of facultative and strict anaerobic isolates. Only a small number of aerobes (eg, *Streptococcus faecalis, Escherichia coli*) are present. Microbes constitute as much as one-third of the dry weight of feces.

Humoral Defenses

Humoral defenses include antibody (primarily immunoglobulins G, M, and A), complement (Fig. 7-2), and cytokines. The immune system is stimulated after phagocytic cells engulf, process, and present antigen to T lymphocytes of the helper lineage. These T lymphocytes stimulate B lymphocytes to produce antibody against specific antigen. Complement is a relatively primitive but effective family of proteins that opsonize foreign antigen and lyse certain cell membranes.

Cytokines

Macrophages, endothelial cells, lymphocytes, and other cells secrete a large number of cytokines. Cytokines may act on the cell itself to increase secretion of the same cytokine, or on other cells in the area to secrete other cytokines.

Examples of cytokines are interferon, tumor necrosis factor (TNF), and interleukin (IL) (Fig. 7-3). During overwhelming infection, the body's attempt to contain infection with humoral, cellular, and cytokine defenses after physical barriers are breached limits infection. In extreme cases, however, the defenses limit infection, but allow cytokines into the systemic circulation, triggering tissue injury throughout the body. This process may explain why the systemic inflammatory response syndrome occurs in patients in whom no active infection is identified.

Cellular Defenses

Macrophages present antigen to helper T cells, initiating the immune response. In the process of engulfing and processing antigen, macrophages may become activated and secrete cytokines. *Polymorphonuclear leukocytes (PMNs)* enter an area of infection after chemotactic stimuli are generated by macrophages and other cells. Bacterial breakdown products and complement activation products also are chemotactic agents. Excessive activation of the endogenous inflammatory response can injure host tissues as well as foreign pathogens in the generation of lysosomal enzymes, oxygen free radicals, nitric oxide, and cytokines by macrophages and PMNs. These substances can injure both local cells and tissues remote from the site of infection.

Interactions Among the Components of Host Defense

Invading microorganisms encounter antibody and complement, as well as PMNs and macrophages. These first-line, or resident, host defenses work together as second-line, or activation, host defenses become operative (Fig. 7-4).

(text continues on page 56)

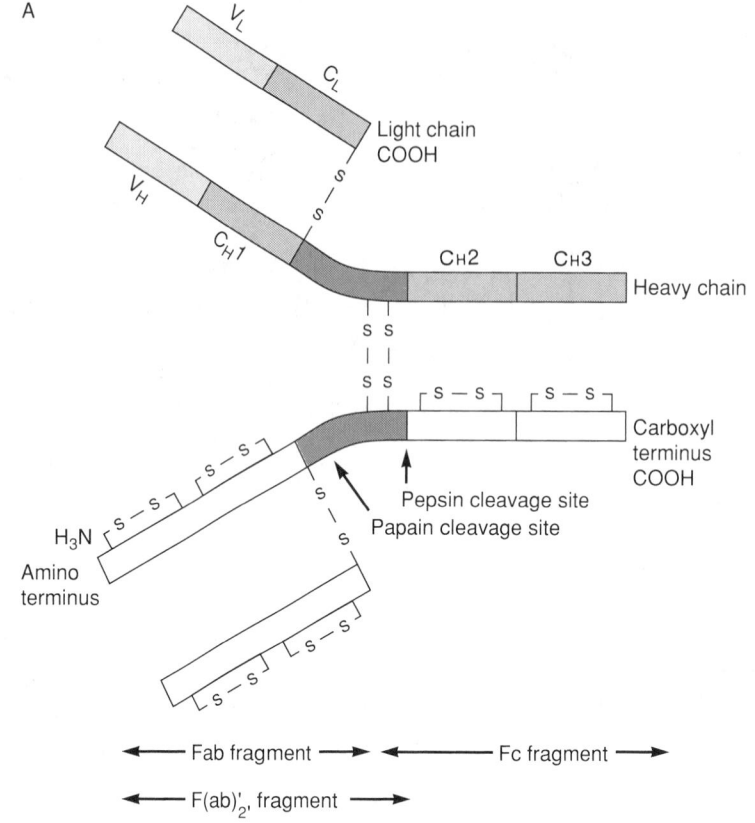

A

V_L

C_L

Light chain
COOH

V_H

C_H1

C_H2 C_H3

Heavy chain

Carboxyl
terminus
COOH

Pepsin cleavage site
Papain cleavage site

H_3N

Amino
terminus

Fab fragment — Fc fragment

$F(ab)'_2$, fragment

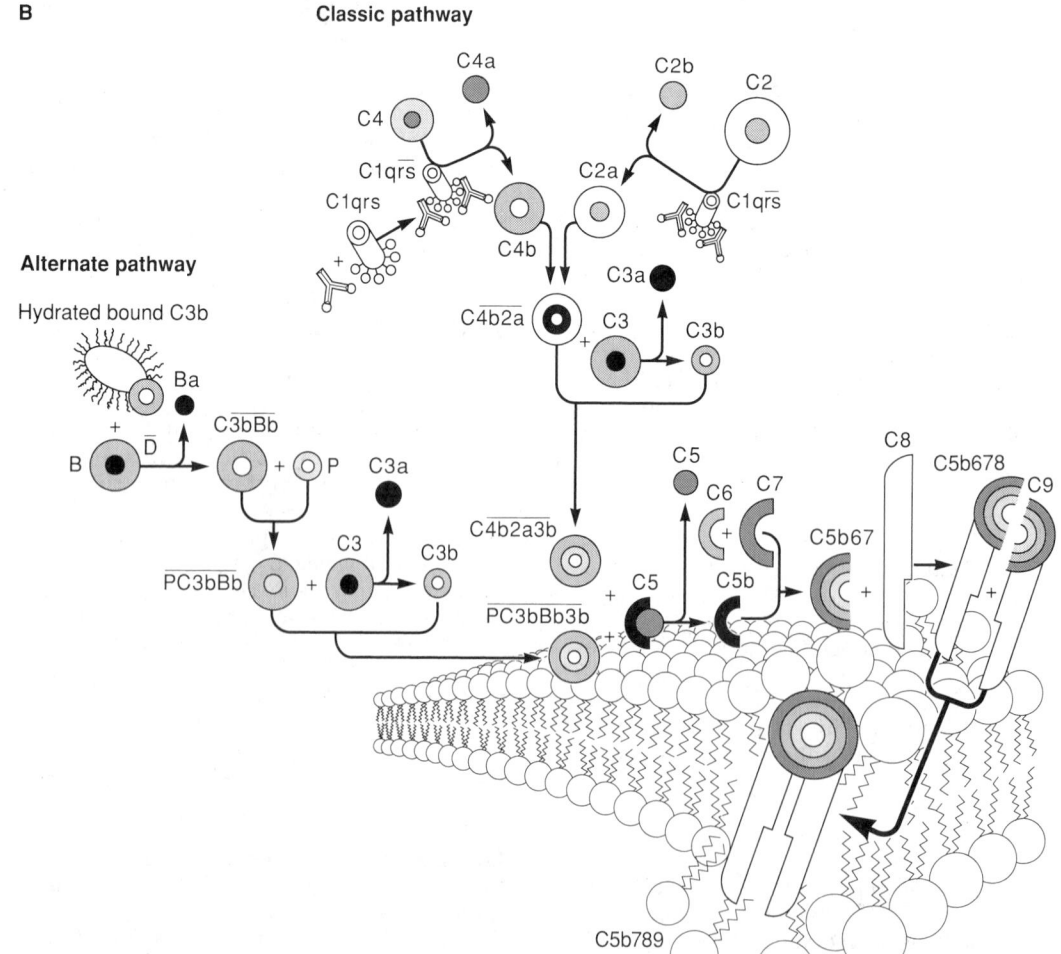

B

Classic pathway

C4a

C2b   C2

C4

C1qrs̄

C2a   C1qr̄s̄

C1qrs

+

C4b   C3a

C4̄b2̄a   C3   C3b

Alternate pathway

Hydrated bound C3b

Ba

C3b̄B̄b̄

+   P   C3a

B   +   D̄

C8   C5b678

C5   C9

C6   C7

C5b67

C4̄b2̄a3̄b̄

C3   C3b   C5   C5b

P̄C3bB̄b̄   +

P̄C3bB̄b3̄b̄   +   C5

C5b789

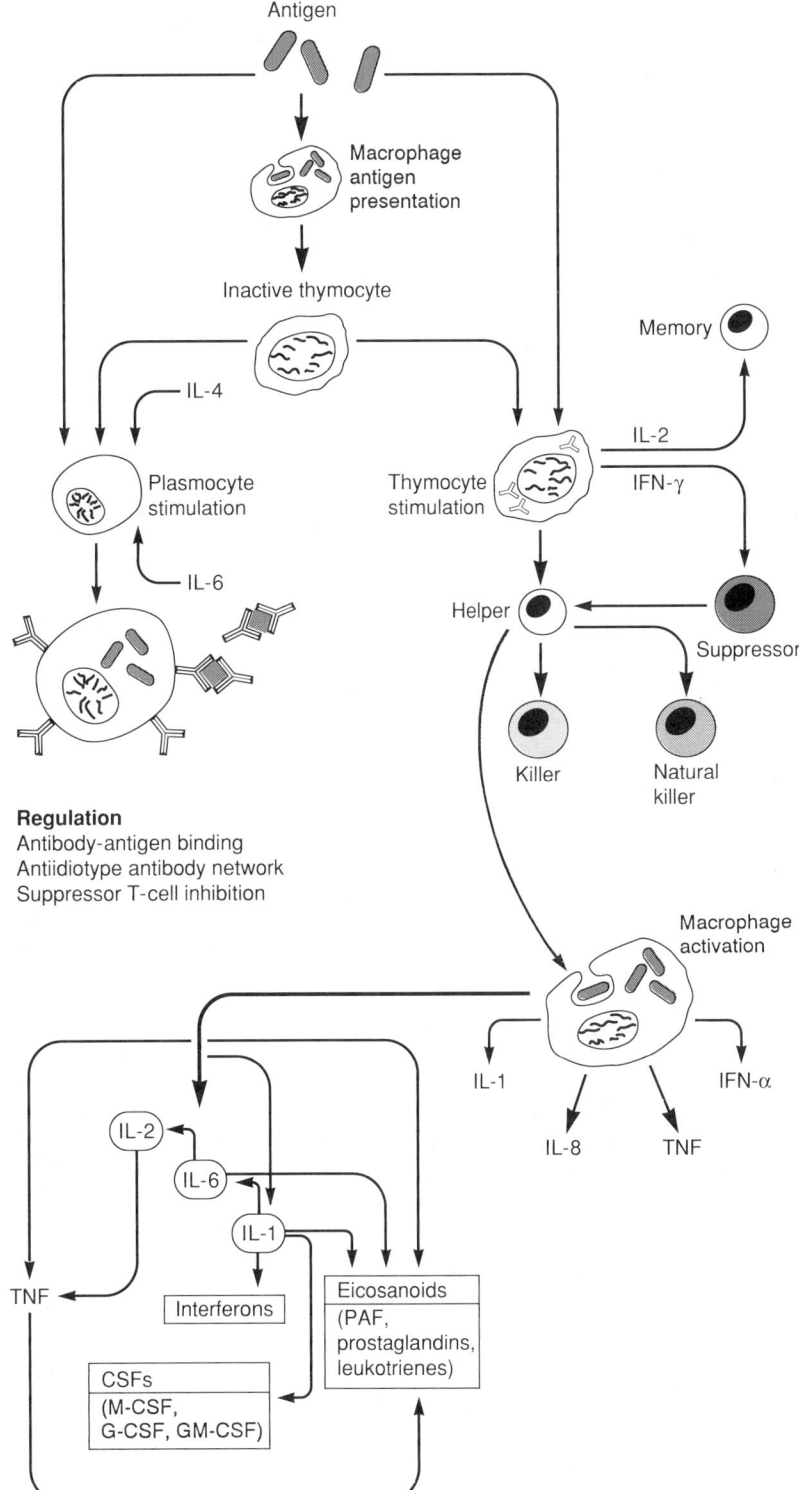

Figure 7-3. Inflammatory and immune response cytokine cascade. After initial antigen processing and presentation by macrophages and other cells, T lymphocytes act to stimulate B lymphocytes to become mature plasmacytes through secretion of cytokines such as IL-4 and IL-6, dedicated to the production of antibody directed against a specific antigen. Initial macrophage stimulation in response to bacterial products, interferon-γ (IFN-γ) release by T cells, and IL-1 release by macrophages themselves may be followed by macrophage tumor necrosis factor-α (TNF-α) production and subsequent secretion of IL-6 and other cytokines.

◀ **Figure 7-2.** Humoral defenses consist of immunoglobulin (*A*) and complement (*B*). (*A*) All Ig classes and IgG subclasses are composed of one type (M, G, A, E, D) of heavy (H) and one type (κ or γ) of light (L) protein chains. The complement system consists of a series of serum proteins that may become activated through either a classic pathway or alternate (properdin) pathways, both of which eventuate in deposition of terminal complement pathway components on the antigenic cell surface.

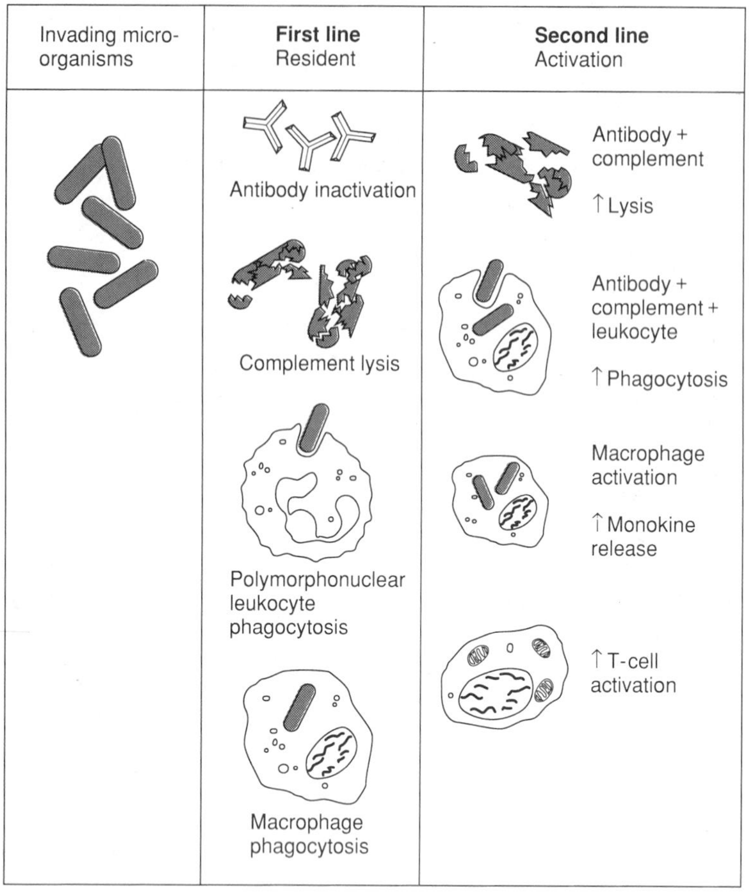

Figure 7-4. Interactions of various portions of mammalian host defenses. Antibody and complement act in concert to enhance bacteriolysis and phagocytosis, simultaneously recruiting additional humoral and cellular components to the site of infection. Macrophages act as pluripotent cells involved in first-line (resident) host defense, antigen presentation and T-cell activation, and subsequent activation and cytokine secretion.

MICROBIOLOGIC DIAGNOSTIC TECHNIQUES

Staining Techniques

Gram stain—Gram-positive organisms stain dark blue; gram-negative microorganisms stain red

High-power oil immersion light microscopy—The criteria for infection are (1) more than two bacteria per 1000X field, equivalent to 5×10^4 to 10^5 colony-forming units (cfu) per milliliter within the specimen, and (2) the presence of white blood cells (WBCs)

Potassium hydroxide stain—Allows detection of yeast or mycelia

Gomori methenamine-silver stain, Giemsa stain—Used to detect fungal hyphae or spores and protozoa within tissue

Ziehl–Neelsen stain—Used to identify acid-fast bacteria

Culture Techniques and Sensitivity Determinations

Specimens are collected for culture of aerobic and anaerobic bacteria and fungi. Isolation of single colonies on plates allows growth and identification of a specific organism. Automated detection systems are used to perform biochemical tests that allow precise identification of a specific pathogen and determination of sensitivity patterns of antimicrobial agents.

Once an microorganism is identified, a sample is inoculated on a broth containing varying amounts of an antibi-

otic. After 18–24 hours, the tube or well that exhibits no visible growth is identified, and the reciprocal of this dilution is the *minimal inhibitory concentration* (MIC). This value is compared with achievable serum levels of a particular antimicrobial agent.

Determination of the *serum bactericidal level* involves obtaining serum from a patient after administration of an antimicrobial agent. This serum is used to determine inhibitory concentrations against a specific pathogen or series of pathogens.

If an initial lack of response to therapy is coupled with evidence of microorganisms resistant to the antimicrobial agents initially chosen, the surgeon can change or add agents once the microbiologic results are available.

Newer Detection Methods

Increasing reliance is being placed on assays that do not use culture data. The antibody and cytokine host response is being studied, and extremely sensitive amplified assays that rely on antigen, antibody, or microbial DNA detection are being used in the clinical setting. Examples are enzyme-linked immunosorbent assay (ELISA), Southern immunotransblot to detect DNA, Northern immunotransblot to detect RNA, Western immunotransblot to detect protein, and polymerase chain reaction (PCR).

ANTIMICROBIAL AGENTS

Antimicrobial agents do not supplant but are adjuncts to débridement of devitalized tissue and drainage of infected material. Use of antimicrobial agents involves prophylaxis,

Table 7-1. MECHANISM OF ACTION OF ANTIMICROBIAL AGENTS

Agent	Mechanism of Action
Penicillins, cephalosporins, carbapenems, monobactams	Bind to bacterial division-plate proteins, inhibiting cell-wall peptidoglycan synthesis and inducing autolytic bacteriolysis
Tetracyclines, chloramphenicol, macrolides (eg, erythromycin)	Inhibit bacterial ribosomal activity and overall protein synthesis
Aminoglycosides	Inhibit protein synthesis and presumably act on a second target site, a supposition based on the fact that aminoglycosides are bacteriolytic and the other agents are bacteriostatic
Vancomycin	Inhibits assembly of peptidoglycan polymers
Quinolones	Bind to DNA helicase proteins and inhibit bacterial DNA synthesis
Sulfonamides	Inhibit incorporation of paraaminobenzoic acid into dihydropteroic acid, reducing folic acid and purine synthesis
Trimethoprim	Inhibits dihydrofolate reductase, an enzyme in the purine synthesis pathway, such that these two agents in combination act synergistically
Rifampin	Binds to bacterial RNA polymerase, directly inhibiting bacterial replication

empiric therapy, and directed therapy. There is frequently no need to alter antimicrobial therapy in the face of clinical improvement, despite information obtained with cultures.

Antibacterial agents are categorized according to structure, mechanism of action, and activity pattern (Table 7-1; Fig. 7-5).

Prophylaxis

The benefits of antimicrobial prophylaxis depend on the initial numbers and types of pathogens within the skin and body site, the degree of contamination during the procedure, the activity of local and systemic host defenses, and the tissue level and activity of the antimicrobial agent against specific pathogens.

Empiric Therapy

Empiric antimicrobial therapy is drug administration based on clinical course without microbiologic confirmation. The principles are (1) a search for a septic source (cultures, diagnostic imaging); (2) reevaluation of therapy

Antimicrobial agent	Gram-Positive Streptococci	Staphylococci	Enterococi	Gram-Negative Enterics	Pseudomonas	Anaerobic Cocci	Bacteroides
Penicillins							
Penicillin G	3	1	1	0	0	2	1
Ampicillin	2	1	3	1	0	1	0
Carboxypenicillins	1	1	1	3	2	1	1
Ureidopenicillins	2	2	3	3	3	1	2
Ampicillin + β-lactamase inhibitor	2	2	3	2	1	2	2
Carboxypenicillins + β-lactamase inhibitor	2	2	2	3	2	2	3
Cephalosporins							
First generation	2	3	0	1	0	2	0
Second generation*	1	2	0	2	1	1	2
Third generation*	0	0	0	3	3	1	1
Monobactams	0	0	0	3	2	0	0
Carbapenems	3	3	0	3	3	2	3
Aminoglycosides	0	1	1	3	3	0	0
Vancomycin	3	3	3	0	0	3	0
Erythromycin	2	2	2	0	0	2	0
Quinolones*	2	1	1	3	2	1	0
Tetracyclines	2	1	1	1	0	1	2
Chloramphenicol	2	2	1	1	0	2	2
Clindamycin	2	1	2	0	0	2	3
Metronidazole	0	0	0	0	0	1	3
Trimethoprim-sulfamethoxazole	2	1	0	3	2	1	0

Figure 7-5. General spectrum of activity of commonly used antimicrobial agents. Higher numbers correspond to higher sensitivity of the organism to the antibiotic. *Specific agents vary markedly with respect to spectrum of activity.

according to clinical findings; (3) drug selection based on activity patterns in the institution. Controversy in the use of empiric therapy involves the use of multiple-agent regimens in which each agent is aimed at a specific class of pathogens, as opposed to the use of broad-spectrum agents aimed at several groups of pathogens but that may not be specific for an individual pathogen.

Directed Therapy

Directed antimicrobial therapy consists of aiming specific antibacterial agents at identified pathogens once sensitivity reports are available. The agents administered exhibit activity against various components of an infection. This is achieved with extended-spectrum penicillins or second- or third-generation cephalosporins combined with other agents, or with carbapenem agents alone. Single-agent therapy is equivalent to combined therapy in the treatment of peritoneal contamination as long as the spectrum of activity includes aerobes and anaerobes. Extended-spectrum agents are not used for prophylaxis or when routine agents can be aimed at a specific pathogen.

TYPES OF INFECTIONS
Clinical Manifestations of Infection

The symptoms and signs of infection are pain, swelling, and redness at the site and fever. Absence of these signs and symptoms does not exclude infection, particularly in an immunocompromised host. Severe systemic infections may produce confusion, ileus, hypotension, and profound shock.

The patient's history, surgical reports, physical findings, and laboratory and physiologic data are studied. Blood, urine, sputum, and any obviously infected site are cultured for bacteria, fungi, and viruses. Diseases not related to infection cause fever in the immediately postoperative period (atelectasis, thrombophlebitis, pulmonary embolism, drug allergy), and these must be included in the differential diagnosis.

Wound Infection

A surgical wound encompasses both the superficial (extrafascial skin and subcutaneous tissue) and deep (body cavity) compartments. Operations are classified on the basis of the likelihood of bacterial contamination of the wound:

Clean—No viscus entered, as in herniorrhaphy

Clean-contaminated. Minimal contamination, as in elective colonic resection with adequate mechanical and antimicrobial preparation

Contaminated. Heavy contamination, as in resection of unprepared, obstructed intestine with spillage of intestinal contents, drainage of abscesses, or débridement of neglected traumatic wounds

Antimicrobial agents are administered before clean-contaminated and contaminated operations. The wounds of most patients undergoing contaminated operations are managed without initial closure. Healing occurs by delayed primary closure (5 to 7 days after the initial operation) or by secondary intention.

Intraabdominal Infection

Intraabdominal infection usually results from perforation of a hollow viscus and contamination of the peritoneal cavity (*secondary microbial peritonitis*). *Primary microbial peritonitis* occurs when no viscus is perforated, as when microorganisms are introduced during peritoneal dialysis. Persistent or *tertiary microbial peritonitis* occurs when the microbial flora in patients with secondary microbial peritonitis changes, so that ongoing infection with normally low-virulence pathogens occurs. Peritonitis often is accompanied by bacteremia and intraabdominal abscesses.

An average of four or five species of bacteria, more than half of them anaerobes, are isolated from intraabdominal infections. Both aerobes and anaerobes are found in almost all specimens. Empiric antimicrobial therapy for secondary microbial peritonitis is directed against both aerobes and anaerobes.

Evaluation of a suspected intraabdominal infection begins with a physical examination and a flat plate and upright or decubitus radiograph of the abdomen. If no visceral perforation is detected and there is no obvious need for emergency laparotomy (ie, acute abdomen), an ultrasound or computed tomographic (CT) scan of the abdomen is performed to exclude biliary tract disease or an intraabdominal abscess. intraabdominal fluid collections may be sampled with a small needle and drained with a percutaneous catheter if purulent material is aspirated or if the initial Gram stain or potassium hydroxide preparation is positive. Culture specimens are obtained at the time of percutaneous aspiration or laparotomy, and the results are used to direct therapy, perhaps through alteration in the empiric antimicrobial regimen. If the condition of a patient who undergoes percutaneous drainage of an intraabdominal abscess deteriorates, a laparotomy is performed.

Necrotizing Soft-Tissue Infections

Necrotizing soft-tissue infections involve the skeletal muscles, the deep muscular fascia, the superficial fascia, or a combination of these tissues. The form usually seen by surgeons is necrotizing fasciitis, which has a mortality as high as 40%. Three factors predispose to necrotizing infections: (1) an impaired immune system due to, for example, diabetes mellitus, malignant tumor, or alcoholism; (2) compromise of the fascial blood supply; and (3) the presence of microorganisms that proliferate in the area.

These infections are usually polymicrobial, which probably accounts for their severity. Gram-positive organisms such as staphylococci and streptococci (aerobic and anaerobic), gram-negative enteric bacteria, and gram-negative anaerobes are identified. Some microorganisms, such as *Clostridium, Pseudomonas,* and *Aeromonas* sp, are so virulent that they can cause the disease alone.

The clinical signs of necrotizing soft-tissue infections are skin discoloration or necrosis; blebs; drainage of thin, watery, grayish, foul-smelling fluid; and subcutaneous crepitus. Early recognition based on clinical signs, exploration of the local site, and CT findings; prompt débridement that removes all devitalized and infected tissue; administration of broad-spectrum antibiotics; fluid resuscitation; hemodynamic monitoring; and nutritional support afford the best chance of survival.

Gram-Negative Bacterial Sepsis, Shock, and Multiple-System Organ Failure

Gram-negative bacterial sepsis is one of the most severe infections in a surgical patient. Although many different organisms cause gram-negative sepsis, *E coli* predominates. Also common are isolates of *Klebsiella, Enterobacter,* and *Serratia* sp. The initial host septic response to gram-negative bacterial infection is fever, systemic acidosis, arterial hypoxemia, disordered substrate and oxygen usage, abnormal metabolism, hyperkalemia, hyperglycemia, decreased systemic vascular resistance, elevated cardiac output, and hypotension. This may lead to failure of organs away from the infected site and, possibly, death—apparently due to an overexuberant host inflammatory response. Gram-negative bacterial lipopolysaccharide (LPS) appears to be the portion of the gram-negative bacterial cell membrane responsible for the toxic effects of gram-negative bacterial sepsis.

The diagnosis of systemic sepsis is suspected when physiologic alterations occur after a source of infection is identified, but the diagnosis is confirmed only after blood cultures become positive for a specific microorganism. During the time it takes to establish a diagnosis, clinical deterioration may occur, and therapy must be begun before the culture results are available.

Infections of Catheters and Prosthetic Devices

Infections associated with prosthetic devices or catheters usually are caused by low-virulence gram-positive organisms. Gram-positive organisms adhere to synthetic polymers with great avidity, forming an exopolysaccharide slime layer that inhibits penetration by an antimicrobial agent. Treatment is removal of the device and administration of antimicrobial agents directed against the infecting organism.

Urinary Tract Infections

Urinary tract infections are the most common cause of gram-negative bacterial sepsis. Because many antimicrobial agents concentrate in urine, most urinary tract infections are quickly eradicated.

Nosocomial Pneumonia

Nosocomial pneumonia occurs in patients with sepsis who require prolonged endotracheal intubation and mechanical ventilation. Chest radiographs are difficult to interpret. Bronchoscopy may be needed to obtain samples for diagnosis. Stains and cultures are performed for bacteria, fungi, acid-fast bacteria, viruses, and protozoa. Gram-negative bacilli, including *Pseudomonas aeruginosa,* are commonly isolated, but gram-positive bacteria and yeast also are common.

Other Site-Specific Infections

Other surgical infections include parotitis, sinusitis, and pseudomembranous colitis (Table 7-2).

FUNGAL INFECTIONS

Fungal infections occur in patients with prolonged stays in surgical intensive care units and in immunocompromised patients. Diagnosis involves assessment of depth of infection and laboratory evaluation of sensitivity patterns. Superficial infections and infections with organisms of low virulence (*Candida* esophagitis or sepsis) are treated with systemic amphotericin B. Agents such as fluconazole may be effective. Aggressive *Candida* infections and infections with organisms with high invasive potential, such as *Cryptococcus neoformans,* necessitate a prolonged course of fluconazole and, often, use of a second agent, such as 5-fluorocytosine. Infections due to *Aspergillus* sp and *Mucor* sp necessitate prolonged treatment with amphotericin B and 5-fluorocytosine. The addition of a third agent, such as rifampin, may be beneficial. Ketoconazole, fluconazole, or itraconazole may be used in selected patients. Drug dosage is reduced in patients receiving exogenous immunosuppressive agents, and, if possible, these agents are discontinued until the infection is controlled or eradicated.

VIRAL INFECTIONS
Herpesvirus Infections
Cytomegalovirus Infection

Factors associated with *CMV infection* include antirejection therapy, advanced age, or receiving a cadaveric transplant. The infection presents as fever, leukopenia, cough, diffuse interstitial infiltrates on a chest radiograph, and hypoxia. The diagnosis is based on the symptoms and signs and is confirmed with serologic and culture evidence. CMV also can be detected with fluorescence techniques, direct nucleic acid blotting, and PCR analysis. Although CMV disease is associated with decreased patient and allograft survival, prophylactic administration of ganciclovir (GCV), acyclovir (ACV), anti-CMV immune globulin, or a combination may reduce the incidence of the disease. It may be possible to treat mild CMV disease with GCV and concurrently treat rejection.

HSV infection causes painful oropharyngeal ulcerations, but sporadic cases of disseminated disease have occurred. Although HSV alone does not seem to have an adverse effect on patient or allograft survival, combined HSV and

Table 7-2. SITE-SPECIFIC SURGICAL INFECTIONS

Infection	Predisposing Factors	Therapy
Parotitis	Advanced age Dehydration	Rehydration Enhancement of salivation Removal of obstruction of the Stensen duct Stains and cultures Antibiotics against *S aureus,*
Sinusitis	Prolonged nasal intubation	Radiographs, CT scans Aspiration and drainage to obtain material for stain and culture
Pseudomembranous colitis	*Clostridium difficile* overgrowth and toxin secretion in colon Alterations in colonic microflora during administration of antimicrobial agents or debilitating illness	Oral metronidazole or vancomycin Discontinuation of intravenous antimicrobial therapy

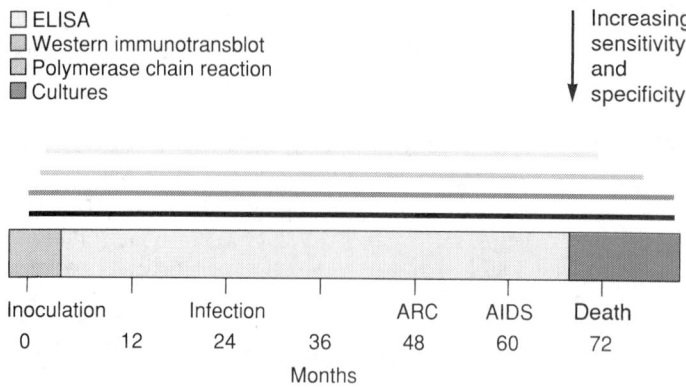

□ ELISA
▨ Western immunotransblot
□ Polymerase chain reaction
▨ Cultures

Increasing
sensitivity
and
specificity

Inoculation   Infection   ARC   AIDS   Death

0   12   24   36   48   60   72

Months

Figure 7-6. Diagnostic tests used to identify the human immunodeficiency virus (HIV) and the general time courses during infection in which they may be positive. The enzyme-linked immunosorbent assay (ELISA) has a 0.1% false-positive rate, whereas the Western immunotransblot is more sensitive and specific. The polymerase chain reaction test is also used for HIV detection and may become increasingly important in the diagnosis of HIV because many patients who are infected with HIV may not exhibit an initial antibody response, so that the infection is undetected by either ELISA or Western immunotransblot analysis.

CMV infection is worse than CMV infection alone. *EBV infection* causes a mononucleosis-type syndrome and may lead to posttransplantation lymphoma. *Varicella-zoster virus (VZV) infection* presents as disseminated and occasionally life-threatening infection in transplant patients who are not immune to the virus, or as painful herpes zoster in patients who have had chicken pox. *HV-6 infection* causes malaise, fever, and lethargy.

Primary HSV, EBV, and VZV infections are treated with ACV. Life-threatening disease or rapid disease progression mandates hospitalization, reduction in immunosuppression, and intravenous administration of ACV. VZV hyperimmune globulin may be used as prophylaxis in VZV-seronegative patients who have been exposed to VZV, or in conjunction with ACV as treatment of severe infection.

Acquired Immunodeficiency Syndrome

AIDS is caused by a retrovirus (human immunodeficiency virus [HIV]-1) that infects T lymphocytes and causes severe immunosuppression. Infection is through parenteral or sexual transmission. HIV detection consists of ELISA screening, Western immunotransblot analysis, and culture after the latent period has elapsed, when anti-HIV antibody becomes detectable. Direct Southern transblot detection and amplified PCR analysis also can be used (Fig. 7-6).

HIV infection progresses from asymptomatic infection, to AIDS-related complex (ARC), to AIDS itself. Those infected with HIV are predisposed to infections (Table 7-3) and malignant tumors.

It is not yet possible to eradicate HIV infection. Treat-

ment is aggressive antiinfective therapy once a specific infection occurs and use of zidovudine. This drug appears to prolong survival when given early in the course of disease. Identification of CD3 antigen as the target molecule for HIV on the human T cell has led to proposals for drugs that mimic this receptor and prevent binding. This approach holds much promise, but prevention of disease transmission is the most important treatment.

Because of concerns over HIV disease transmission, most institutions use universal blood and body substance precautions. A person exposed to HIV may consider use of prophylactic zidovudine or sequential serologic testing.

Hepatitis Viruses

Five hepatitis viruses have been identified—A, B, C (formerly non-A, non-B), D (δ), and E. *Hepatitis A* is usually spread through the fecal–oral route and only occasionally comes to the attention of a surgeon. *Hepatitis C* causes acute elevations in hepatic enzymes and chronic antigenemia. Transmission occurs through blood products. Identification is possible with ELISA, recombinant immunoblot assays, and PCR. *Hepatitis D* virus cannot cause disease but acts as a secondary virus to HBV. The disease caused by both together is worse than that caused by HBV alone. Little is known about *hepatitis E.*

Hepatitis B usually is transmitted through the parenteral route, although oral or sexual transmission may occur. Infection may lead to asymptomatic or symptomatic disease, depending on the extent of infection within the liver. Symptoms and signs are jaundice, lethargy, malaise, and acute hepatic transaminase elevations that persist for several weeks. During this stage, IgM antibody is directed against surface and, subsequently, core antigens, followed by the development of IgG antibody production.

Acute HBV infection usually resolves without further sequelae, but 10–15% of patients experience chronic active or chronic persistent hepatitis with evidence of chronic antigenemia. Rarely, acute hepatitis may progress to fulminant hepatic failure, coma, and death.

Patients at high risk (eg, those undergoing hemodialysis or transplantation and those with hemophilia) and health care workers (surgeons, dentists, hemodialysis unit personnel) receive three vaccinations of the recombinant DNA hepatitis B vaccine if they have had no previous exposure. Vaccination is not recommended for people with anti–hepatitis B antibody. Those not immune to HBV are given anti–hepatitis B immunoglobulin and are vaccinated if they are exposed to the virus.

Table 7-3. INFECTIONS THAT COMMONLY OCCUR IN PATIENTS WITH AIDS

Pneumocystis carinii pneumonia
CMV pneumonitis
Gastroenteritis
Hepatitis
Maningitis due to *Cryptococcus* neoformans
Pneumonia and disseminated infection due to atypical mycobacteria such as *Mycobacterium avium-intracellulare, M. kansasii,* and *M. chelonei*
Gastrointestinal infections due to *Cryptosporidium* and *Campylobacter jejuni*

PROTOZOAN PATHOGENS

Patients who receive solid-organ transplants and patients with AIDS may contract infections caused by *Pneumocystis carinii* and *Toxoplasma gondii*. *P carinii* infection causes cough, tachypnea, and mild fever. Bilateral diffuse alveolar infiltrates and signs of interstitial pneumonia are seen on chest radiographs. The diagnosis often is established with bronchoscopy, but some patients need open lung biopsy. Treatment is with parenteral trimethoprim-sulfamethoxazole, trimethoprim-dapsone, or pentamidine, even if the diagnosis is presumptive. The disease rarely occurs in patients who receive trimethoprim-sulfamethoxazole prophylaxis.

T gondii causes a mononucleosis-like syndrome. In immunosuppressed patients, necrotizing encephalitis, myocarditis, pneumonitis, and death may occur. Patients who do not carry *Toxoplasma* organisms are prone to infection if they receive organs from donors with evidence of previous *Toxoplasma* infection. Treatment is with pyrimethamine and sulfadiazine.

TREATMENT MODALITIES UNDER INVESTIGATION

Selective *intestinal decontamination* involves the oral administration of antimicrobial agents to achieve a high intraluminal level against gram-negative aerobes and yeast but leaves the host anaerobic intestinal microflora relatively undisrupted. *LPS-neutralizing agents* bind against the LPS of the outer membrane of gram-negative bacteria, reducing the mortality of sepsis due to these bacteria. *Immunostimulating agents* enhance the state of activation of host defenses.

SUGGESTED READING

Bartlett JG, Condon RE, Gorbach S, et al. Veterans Administration Cooperative Study on Bowel Preparation for Elective Colorectal Operations: impact of oral antibiotic regimen on colonic flora, wound irrigation cultures and bacteriology of septic complications. Ann Surg 1978;188:249.

Burke JF. Preventing bacterial infection by coordinating antibiotic and host activity: a time-dependent activity. South Med J 1977;1:24.

Dunn DL. Immunotherapeutic advances in the treatment of gram-negative bacterial sepsis. World J Surg 1987;11:233.

Dunn DL. The role of infection and use of antimicrobial agents during multiple system organ failure. In: Deitch EA, ed. Multiple organ failure: pathophysiology and basic concepts of therapy. New York, Thieme, 1990:150.

Dunn DL. Autochthonous microflora of the gastrointestinal tract. Perspect Colon Rectal Surg 1990;2:105.

Dunn DL, Barke RA, Knight NB, et al. The role of resident macrophages, peripheral neutrophils, and translymphatic absorption in bacterial clearance from the peritoneal cavity. Infect Immun 1985;49:257.

Dunn DL, Meakins JL. Humoral immunity to infection and the complement system. In: Howard RJ, Simmons RL, eds. Surgical infectious diseases. Norwalk, CT, Appleton & Lange, 1988:175.

Dunn DL, Najarian JS. Infectious complications in transplant surgery. In: Shires GT, Davis J, eds. Principles and management of surgical infection. Philadelphia, JB Lippincott, 1990:425.

Dunn DL, Simmons RL. The role of anaerobic bacteria in intraabdominal infections. Rev Infect Dis 1984;6:S139.

Durum SK, Oppenheim JJ. Macrophage-derived mediators: interleukin-1, tumor necrosis factor, interleukin-6, interferon, and related cytokines. In: Paul WE, ed. Fundamental immunology, ed 2. New York, Raven Press, 1989:639.

Rotstein OD, Pruett TL, Simmons RL. Microbiologic features and treatment of persistent peritonitis in patients in the intensive care unit. Can J Surg 1986;29:247.

ESSENTIALS OF SURGERY: SCIENTIFIC PRINCIPLES AND PRACTICE, edited by Lazar J. Greenfield, Michael W. Mulholland, Keith T. Oldham, Gerald B. Zelenock, and Keith D. Lillemoe. Lippincott–Raven Publishers, Philadelphia, © 1997.

CHAPTER 8

SHOCK
RONALD V. MAIER

Shock is a syndrome of inadequate tissue perfusion characterized by an imbalance between delivery of metabolic substrate and cellular metabolic needs. Progression of shock results in loss of homeostasis (decompensation) and inability to maintain mean arterial pressure, producing organ dysfunction and hypotension.

MANAGEMENT

Patients in shock who do not need emergency surgical treatment are cared for in a critical care setting. Blood pressure, pulse, and respiration are monitored. Resuscitation is assessed on the basis of urine output and mental status. Aggressive monitoring involves invasive techniques such as pulmonary artery catheterization (Tables 8-1 through 8-4) and gastric tonometry.

Hypovolemic Shock

Any process that contributes to intravascular volume depletion can cause hypovolemic shock. Such processes include hemorrhage, extravascular fluid sequestration, gastrointestinal and urinary losses, or insensible loss. The physiologic response to hypovolemic shock is to maintain central perfusion and restore effective circulating blood volume. The stages of hemorrhagic shock are based on the volume of blood lost (Table 8-5). Mild volume loss can be tolerated with relatively few external signs, especially in a supine, resting patient (Table 8-6).

Diagnosis

Hypovolemic shock is readily diagnosed when there is an obvious source of volume loss and when overt signs of hemodynamic instability and increased adrenergic output are present. The diagnosis is difficult when the source of volume loss is occult. Profuse blood loss into the chest, abdomen, retroperitoneum, pelvis, and thigh can occur with few specific findings. Plasma losses from tissue trauma or burns, free water deficit, or unreplaced insensible loss also cause hypovolemia.

Invasive monitoring with a pulmonary arterial catheter provides information about the degree of hypovolemia and

Table 8-1. NORMAL CARDIOVASCULAR PRESSURES

Pressures	Values (mm Hg)
Right atrium or central venous	0–6
Right ventricle	20–30/0–6
Pulmonary artery	20–30/6–12
Pulmonary artery mean	12–18
Pulmonary capillary wedge	6–12
Left atrium	4–12
Left ventricle	100–140/5–14
Arterial (systolic/diastolic)	100–140/60–80
Mean arterial	75–100

Table 8-2. NORMAL HEMODYNAMIC PARAMETERS

Parameter	Calculation	Normal Values
Cardiac output (CO)	$SV \times HR$	4–8 L/min
Cardiac index (CI)	CO/BSA	2.5–4 L/min/m²
Stroke volume (SV)	CO/HR × 1000	60–100 mL/beat
Systemic vascular resistance (SVR)	(MAP − RAP)/CO × 80	800–1400 dynes/s/cm⁻⁵
Systemic vascular resistance index (SVRI)	SVR × BSA	1500–2400 dynes/s/cm⁻⁵/m²
Pulmonary vascular resistance (PVR)	(PAPₘ − PCWP)/CO × 80	100–150 dynes/s/cm¹⁵
Pulmonary vascular resistance index (PVRI)	PVR × BSA	200–400 dynes/s/cm⁻⁵/m²
Left ventricular stroke work (LVSW)	SV/(MAP − PCWP) × 0.0136	60–80 g-m/beat
Left ventricular stroke work index (LVSWI)	LVSW/BSA	45–60 g-m/beat/m²
Right ventricular stroke work (RVSW)	SV (PAPₘ − PAP) × 0.0136	10–15 g-m/beat
Right ventricular stroke work index (RVSWI)	RVSW/BSA	6–10 g-m/beat/m²

cardiac dysfunction. Diminished cardiac filling pressures (CVP, PCWP) and a low cardiac output responsive to volume resuscitation occur with hypovolemia (Table 8-5).

Management

Restoration of perfusion in hypovolemic shock involves reexpansion of the circulating blood volume with intervention to control ongoing volume loss. Vigorous volume resuscitation is crucial. Even after resuscitation, diastolic compliance may be abnormal for some time and necessitate relatively high filling pressures to maintain ventricular performance. In severe, prolonged hypovolemia, ventricular contractile function may become depressed, and inotropic support may be needed to maintain ventricular performance.

Measures to increase central blood pressure by increasing resistance to flow may temporarily maintain cerebral and coronary perfusion. These temporizing measures include use of a pneumatic antishock garment (PASG), aortic cross-clamping, and infusion of α-adrenergic agents.

A result of hypoperfusion is diminished transport of oxygen to tissues and ineffective removal of toxic wastes. Resuscitation entails restitution of tissue oxygenation. Initial therapy is directed at support of respiratory and circulatory function. Immediate concerns are establishment of an airway, ventilation, and intravenous access. Supplementary oxygen is provided. If ventilatory function is in question, mechanical assistance is instituted. Endotracheal intubation is desirable if the airway is tenuous because of obtundation or injury, or if ventilation is needed for more than a short time. The presence or possibility of cervical spinal fracture or instability necessitates measures to attain airway control with as little manipulation of the neck as possible. In these circumstances, nasotracheal intubation, tracheostomy, or cricothyroidotomy may be life-saving.

Volume resuscitation is initiated through peripheral intravenous lines during the initial stages of evaluation. Rapid infusion of isotonic saline or balanced salt solution is of diagnostic value and therapeutic benefit. Infusion of 2 to 3 L of crystalloid for 10 to 30 minutes restores blood pressure in most instances. Continued hemodynamic instability implies that shock is not reversed or that there is ongoing blood or volume loss. Further volume resuscitation includes simultaneous transfusion of fully cross-matched blood or, in dire circumstances, type-specific or O-negative packed cells (O-positive blood is acceptable for patients older than 50 years of age). Measures are taken after resuscitation to avoid hypothermia and its consequences.

Hypovolemic shock poorly responsive to volume resuscitation suggests ongoing volume loss. It also raises concern that other causes of instability, such as pericardial tamponade, tension pneumothorax, or ventricular dysfunction, are present. In the first two settings, prompt treatment is essential; although invasive monitoring is indicated, it must not delay treatment.

Traumatic Shock

Tissue injury evokes a broader pathophysiologic immunoinflammatory response and potentially more devastating degree of shock than that produced by hypovolemia alone.

Initial management involves assurance of airway, breathing, and circulation. Assurance of circulation involves volume resuscitation and control of ongoing losses. Control of hemorrhage demands priority over attention to all other injuries. After resuscitation and control of volume losses, efforts to minutesimize lethal postshock sequelae, including multiple organ failure syndrome (MOFS), are undertaken. These include restoration of perfusion to isch-

Table 8-3. OXYGEN TRANSPORT CALCULATIONS

Parameters	Calculation	Normal Values
Oxygen-carrying capacity of Hgb		= 1.38 mL O₂/g Hgb
Plasma O₂ content		= PO₂ × 0.0031
Arterial O₂ content (CaO₂)	= SaO₂ (range, 0–1.00) × Hgb (g/dL) × 1.38 (mL/g)	20 vol%
Venous O₂ content (CVO₂)	= SvO₂ × Hgb × 1.38	15.5 vol%
Arteriovenous O₂ difference (AV O₂ difference)	= CaO₂ − CvO₂	3.5 vol%
	= (SaO₂ − SvO₂) × Hgb × 1.38	
Systemic oxygen delivery (DO₂)	= CaO₂ × CO (L/min) × 10 L/dL	800–1600 mL/min
	= SaO₂ × Hgb × 1.38 × CO × 10	
Systemic oxygen consumption (VO₂)	= (AV)O₂ difference × CO × 10	150–400 mL/min
	= (SaO₂ − SvO₂) × Hgb × 1.38 × CO × 10	
Oxygen consumption index (VO₂I)	= VO₂/BSA	115–165 mL/m²/min

Table 8-4. PHYSIOLOGIC CHARACTERISTICS OF THE VARIOUS FORMS OF SHOCK

Type of Shock	CVP and PCWP	Cardiac Output	Systemic Vascular Resistance	Venous O$_2$ Saturation
Hypovolemic	↓	↓	↑	↓
Cardiogenic	↑	↓	↑	↓
Septic				
Hyperdynamic	↓↑	↑	↓	↑
Hypodynamic	↓↑	↓	↑	↑↓
Traumatic	↓	↓↑	↑↓	↓
Neurogenic	↓	↓	↓	↓
Hypoadrenal	↓↑	↓	↑↓	↓

CVP, central venous pressure; PCWP, pulmonary capillary wedge pressure.

emic areas, stabilization of fractures, débridement of devitalized or contaminated tissues, and evacuation of hematomas.

Postresuscitation hypermetabolism driven by systemic inflammatory response syndrome (SIRS) exists even in the absence of bacterial contamination or infection. This common process contributes to the development of organ dysfunction and MOFS. It is not unusual for a patient to have a temperature of 38.8°C (102°F), tachycardia, and a widened pulse pressure, reflecting elevated cardiac output. Other findings include transient increases in serum lactate, oxygen consumption, and aminuteso acid clearance. Fluid sequestration and salt and water retention are common and contribute to weight gain. These effects of the local and systemic inflammatory response resolve as hemodynamic stability is maintained and repair follows. Persistence of SIRS with progression to MOFS may be related to a persistent inflammatory focus, intercurrent infection, or ongoing perfusion deficit.

Cardiogenic Shock

Intrinsic Cardiogenic Shock

Intrinsic cardiogenic shock results from failure of the heart as an effective pump.

Any history of cardiac disease is of diagnostic value. Associated physical findings include those of hemodynamic instability, peripheral vasoconstriction, and congestive fluid accumulation and findings specific to the cardiac abnormality. Tachycardia, tachypnea, hypotension, and cool, pale, mottled, or cyanotic extremities in an agitated oliguric patient are typical. With severe or progressive shock, the level of consciousness may deteriorate from agitation to obtundation. The posture of a conscious patient with congestive heart failure is typically upright; collapse occurs once the hypotension of cardiogenic shock develops. Rales and an S$_3$ gallop rhythm may be appreciated. Jugular venous distention and peripheral edema occur in right-sided or biventricular failure.

An electrocardiogram (ECG) may provide evidence of preexisting cardiac disease and any acute changes. Chest radiographs may contain signs of the specific heart disease, pulmonary vascular congestion, pulmonary edema, pleural effusions, or cardiomegaly. Surface or transesophageal echocardiograms may demonstrate structural abnormalities or the functional impairment of cardiac contractility. Cardiac enzyme determinations may provide evidence of acute myocardial injury. Arterial blood gas determinations confirm the presence of hypoxia and provide information about the adequacy of ventilation and acid–base status. Urinary indices suggest prerenal azotemia.

Sometimes it is difficult to ascertain the role of cardiac dysfunction in shock. Pulmonary edema associated with increased pulmonary capillary permeability may have noncardiac causes. Pulmonary disease and mechanical ventilation may obscure or otherwise alter the findings of cardiogenic failure. A sudden cardiac event may lead to a fall, a motor vehicle accident, or another type of trauma.

Table 8-5. CLASSIFICATION OF HEMORRHAGIC SHOCK

Class	Percentage of Blood Volume Lost	Amount of Blood Lost (mL in a 70-kg person)	Characteristics
I	10–15	500–750	Minimal change in clinical condition Little or no alteration in blood pressure and heart rate Pallor, diaphoresis, diminished capillary refill due to adrenergic discharge Decrease in prominence of subcutaneous veins because of collapse
II	20–30	1000–1500	Anxiety Mild tachycardia Normal blood pressure Prominent skin changes Oliguria due to adrenergic-mediated renal arteriolar constriction and production vasopressin and aldosterone
III	30–40	1500–2000	Postural changes in heart rate and blood pressure Extreme tachycardia, oliguria, agitation or confusion
IV	≥40	>2000	Progressive tachycardia Profound hypotension even in supine position Progress of mental status changes from restlessness and agitation to listlessness and obtundation (blood flow to the brain is insufficient to maintain function)

Table 8-6. PHYSICAL FINDINGS IN HEMORRHAGIC SHOCK*

Mild (<20% Blood Volume)	Moderate (20%–40% Blood Volume)	Severe (>40% Blood Volume)
Pallor	Pallor	Pallor
Cool extremities	Cool extremities	Cool extremities
Diminished capillary refill	Diminished capillary refill	Diminished capillary refill
Diaphoresis	Diaphoresis	Diaphoresis
Collapsed subcutaneous veins	Collapsed subcutaneous veins	Collapsed subcutaneous veins
	Tachycardia	Tachycardia
	Oliguria	Oliguria
	Postural hypotension	Hypotension
		Mental status changes

* Alcohol or drug intoxication may alter physical findings.

The shock apparent in the emergency department may be mistakenly ascribed to traumatic, rather than cardiac causes and vice versa.

Invasive hemodynamic monitoring often establishes the specific nature of shock and allows expedient treatment. Hemodynamic findings of cardiogenic shock include low cardiac output (cardiac index <2.2 L/min/m^2) and high systemic vascular resistance (SVR) despite elevated cardiac filling pressures (pulmonary capillary wedge pressure [PCWP] ≥18 mmHg). Tissues compensate for diminished oxygen delivery with an increased oxygen extraction; the mixed venous oxygen saturation is decreased and the arteriovenous oxygen difference increased. An increased plasma lactate concentration is common, indicating a shift to anaerobic metabolism in principal tissue beds.

Management of shock of cardiac origin involves the principles used in treating other forms of shock. Peripheral perfusion is restored by means of optimizing cardiovascular and respiratory dynamics. Initial measures include administration of supplemental oxygen, mechanical ventilation (as needed), and treatment of dysrhythmias. Cardiopulmonary resuscitation may be needed. When acute myocardial infarction is the cause of shock, coronary angiography and aggressive therapy with thrombolytic agents, balloon dilation, or a surgical procedure may be needed.

Any patient in shock, especially with compromised cardiac function, may need mechanical ventilation. The work of breathing can be considerable, especially for patients in a state of agitation or distress or with decreased compliance. The patient can be sedated with a secure airway, the work of breathing is undertaken by the ventilator, and gas exchange can be optimized.

Systematic manipulation of preload, afterload, and contractility with information from pulmonary artery catheterization allows optimization of cardiac dynamics. A PCWP of 15 to 20 mmHg is the initial goal and is achieved with manipulation of intravascular volume or capacitance or with increases in contractile activity. During cardiogenic shock, wedge pressure is not typically <18 mmHg. Because of inadequate homeostatic responses, filling pressures may not be optimal, and intravascular hypovolemia may exist. If it does, volume expansion is accomplished with infusion of crystalloid, colloid, or blood products. Packed cells provide volume expansion and increased oxygen-carrying capacity.

After correction of preexisting or relative hypovolemia,

the mainstay of management of cardiogenic shock is inotropic support with drugs such as dopaminen and dobutamine.

Patients with cardiogenic shock and an inadequate response to volume expansion and drug therapy can be supported for long periods with intraaortic balloon counterpulsation (IABC). This involves placement of a balloon in the descending thoracic aorta via a peripheral artery. Inflation of the balloon during diastole augments diastolic pressure and improves coronary perfusion; deflation during systole provides afterload reduction. After myocardial infarction, use of an IABC pump to manage cardiogenic shock provides hemodynamic support. Objective findings include immediate increases in cardiac index, stroke volume, and diastolic pressure–stroke work index. In 12 to 24 hours, decreases in PCWP and SVR and improved maintenance of systemic pressure occur.

Additional measures to manage refractory cardiogenic shock include placement of ventricular assist devices, urgent myocardial revascularization, correction of other anatomic cardiac defects, or urgent cardiac transplantation.

Compressive Cardiogenic Shock

Shock from cardiac compression occurs when external pressure on the heart impairs ventricular filling. The diagnosis of hypotension due to compressive cardiogenic shock is made largely on the basis of clinical findings and a chest radiograph.

Physical findings of tension pneumothorax include ipsilateral decreased breath sounds, tracheal deviation away from the affected thorax, and jugular venous distention. Radiographic findings are those of a pneumothorax with signs of increased intrathoracic volume in the affected hemithorax, including tracheal and mediastinal deviation to the contralateral side, splaying of the ipsilateral ribs, and depression of the diaphragm. Absence of those findings in the presence of pneumothorax does not exclude tension pneumothorax.

All patients need urgent chest decompression. Release of air with tube thoracotomy restores normal cardiovascular dynamics. If chest tube placement cannot be immediately accomplished, tension may be relieved by placement of a 14-gauge needle over the third rib in the midclavicular line. Establishment of an open pneumothorax by making a defect in an interspace for chest tube placement relieves the hemodynamic abnormality while materials for tube thoracostomy are gathered.

The clinical findings of pericardial tamponade are the Beck triad: hypotension, neck vein distention, and muffled heart sounds. Pulsus paradoxus also may be present. Tachycardia and peripheral vasoconstriction are always present but are nonspecific signs. Placement of a central venous pressure (CVP) catheter confirms the elevation in right-sided filling pressure. If a pulmonary artery catheter is in place, findings of tamponade are a trend toward equalization of chamber pressures as hypotension progresses. For patients at risk, echocardiography is used to demonstrate pericardial fluid and need for operation.

A diaphragmatic hernia can cause cardiac compression. Signs of a hernia are distended neck veins and decreased breath sounds on the affected side. A chest radiograph may establish the diagnosis, demonstrating abdominal viscera or a radiopaque nasogastric tube within the chest. Peritoneal lavage fluid exiting through a chest tube establishes the diagnosis, as does palpation of a defect or intrathoracic position of abdominal organs during chest tube placement.

After trauma, hypotension associated with distended neck veins or a wound close to the heart is considered to be compressive cardiogenic shock until proved otherwise. Chest tube placement (or bilateral chest tube placement) resolves potential tension pneumothorax. Pericardial tamponade must be relieved, and cardiac injuries necessitate emergency sternotomy. Traumatic diaphragmatic defects necessitate surgical repair to avoid cardiac compression and other complications.

Septic Shock

Septic shock is caused by the combination of metabolic and circulatory derangements that accompany systemic infection. Local responses include redness (rubor), warmth (calor), pain (dolor), and swelling (tumor). Generalized findings in sepsis include fever, tachypnea, tachycardia, or end-organ dysfunction. Hemodynamic instability is associated with these findings.

The hemodynamic changes in septic shock consist of two characteristic patterns/hyperdynamic and hypodynamic. *Hyperdynamic,* or warm, septic shock is marked by peripheral vasodilation, increased cardiac output, and warm extremities.

The *hypodynamic* response of cold septic shock is accompanied by inadequate cardiac output, peripheral vasoconstriction, mottling, and cool extremities. A hypodynamic response results from inadequate effective circulating blood volume and depressed cardiac function, which promotes a tissue perfusion deficit. Hypoperfusion then enhances the elaboration of additional inflammatory mediators initiated by products of infection. The inflammatory response causes further microvascular compromise, progression of shock, and secondary organ dysfunction. The targets of the pathophysiologic process are the heart, vascular endothelium, and metabolic machinery of the peripheral tissues. Progression from hyperdynamic to hypodynamic sepsis signals collapse of adaptive homeostatic mechanisms.

Management

Whether septic shock causes a hyperdynamic or a hypodynamic response, the measures to reverse shock are based on the following three principles: 1) Restoration of tissue perfusion and oxygen delivery to a level that meets metabolic demands, 2) Correction or control of the source of sepsis, and 3) Supportive care to ensure the optimal environment for maintaining functional reserves, healing, and recovery (Fig. 8-1).

In sepsis, resuscitation and restoration of nutrient flow to tissues is accomplished before a complex operation is performed for source control. This differs from management of hemorrhagic or cardiac compression shock, in which immediate intervention is accomplished with resuscitation. In septic shock, priorities are shifted toward alleviation of the perfusion deficit and restoration of oxygen transport, avoiding the dangerous combination of sepsis and microcirculatory hypoperfusion. Propagation of shock and the development of postshock organ dysfunction are caused by increased activation of inflammatory cells and elaboration of mediators in areas of hypoperfusion. Restoration of perfusion may break the cycle of shock, inflammation, and more shock. Intervention then can be undertaken to manage the sepsis in a patient whose condition is stable.

Initial therapy for septic shock includes volume resuscitation, placement of invasive monitoring lines (Swan–Ganz catheter, arterial line, and Foley catheter), administration of antibiotics, and respiratory support as indicated. Immediate laboratory studies include arterial blood gases, serum electrolytes, blood urea nitrogen (BUN), creatinine, lactate, and complete blood count with differential. Blood, sputum, urine, and other cultures are obtained. If the source of sepsis is obvious but would necessitate a complex operation for control, surgical intervention is deferred until resuscitation is complete. If the source is not obvious, additional diagnostic studies are undertaken, including lumbar puncture and computed tomography (CT). Unusual sites, such as the facial sinuses, may be the source of sepsis.

Venodilatation and vasodilatation in sepsis may limit effective venous return and ventricular end-diastolic volume even if the true circulating blood volume is not depleted. To restore effective circulating blood volume, aggressive fluid resuscitation is needed. Optimal end-diastolic volume and pressure to support a dysfunctional myocardium may necessitate an increase in circulating blood volume. Resuscitation to a PCWP of 15 mmHg is the initial goal. This may be accomplished with isotonic crystalloid, colloid, or blood products. Further intervention may be needed to achieve hemodynamic stability and flow-independent oxygen consumption. If hemoglobin level is <13 g/dL, oxygen transport may be restored with red-cell transfusion.

If septic shock is accompanied by a hypodynamic response, augmentation of cardiac output may necessitate inotropic support, use of vasodilators, or a combination of the two.

If surgical intervention is needed for control of sepsis, it is undertaken when hemodynamic status is optimal. Control of the septic focus with restoration of perfusion decreases risk for persistent hypermetabolism and MOFS.

Neurogenic Shock

Neurogenic shock results from interruption of sympathetic vasomotor input and develops after spinal cord injury, spinal anesthesia, and severe head injury. Patients usually have clear signs of neurologic injury. Hypotension and tachycardia may be present, but the extremities are warm and appear well-perfused. With high cervical lesions, bradycardia inappropriate for the degree of hypotension is present. CVP, PCWP, stroke volume, and SVR are decreased; cardiac output is decreased. Blood pressure is usually responsive to postural changes.

Restoration of effective, albeit expanded, intravascular volume may necessitate administration of extremely large volumes of resuscitation fluid to restore normal cardiac filling pressures. This restores cardiac output and reverses hypotension. Pharmacologic intervention with vasoactive agents may be necessary, and this is preferable to excessive volume resuscitation. There is marked hypotension with neurogenic shock but little, if any, hypoperfusion.

A problem in the management of neurogenic shock is unappreciated coexistent hemorrhage or ongoing volume loss. If hemodynamic instability persists after initial trauma resuscitation, the cause is probably not neurogenic, and occult blood loss or cardiogenic causes of shock are explored.

A brain injured severely enough to sustain acute loss of sympathetic tone is virtually nonsalvageable. Despite concerns about cerebral edema formation, volume administration is still the initial therapy. After the acute phase, severe head injury may exacerbate hypovolemia by means of other mechanisms. Head injury and loss of antidiuretic hormone (ADH) from the posterior pituitary gland can allow excessive urinary-free water loss. Brain injury also can initiate or contribute to generalized severe coagulopathy, leading to increased hemorrhage from multiple sites.

Hypoadrenal Shock

Shock of a dramatic nature that is poorly responsive to resuscitation may be caused by adrenal insufficiency. Adrenal insufficiency is caused by long-term therapeutic adminis-

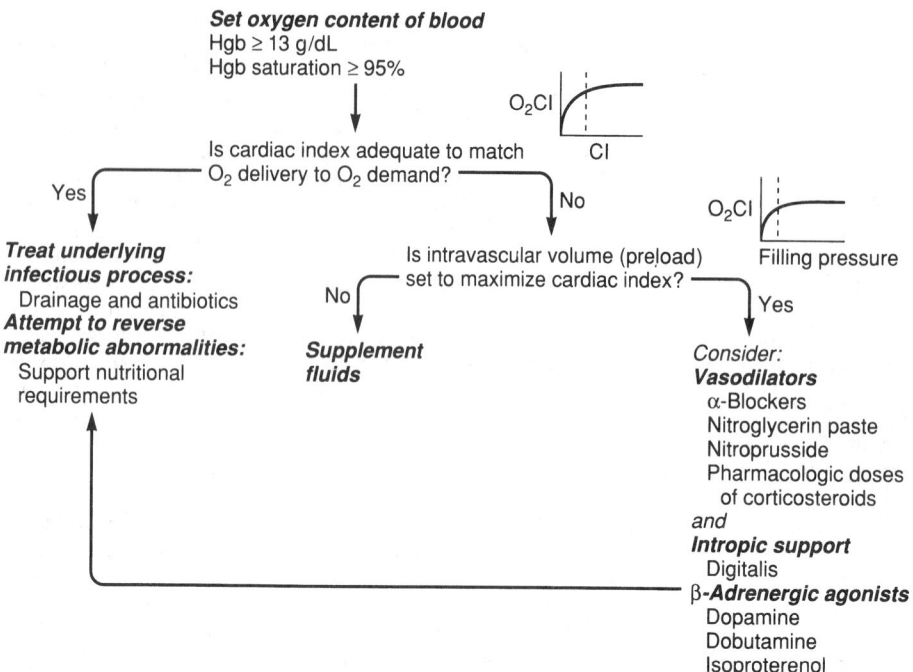

Figure 8-1. The basic algorithm for resuscitation. The goal is to match oxygen delivery with oxygen demand. The outcome variable is oxygen consumption; the managed variables are preload, afterload, and contractile function. (After Stahl TJ, Cerra FB. Hemodynamic and metabolic responses. In: Howard RJ, Simmons RL, eds. Surgical infectious diseases, ed 2. Norwalk, CT, Appleton & Lange, 1988:209)

tration of high-dose exogenous corticosteroids, idiopathic adrenal atrophy (Addison disease), tuberculosis, metastatic disease, bilateral hemorrhage, or amyloidosis. The stress of illness, operation, or trauma requires that the adrenal glands secrete cortisol in excess of that needed in the nonstressed state.

Findings associated with adrenal insufficiency include weakness, fatigue, anorexia, abdominal pain, nausea, vomiting, and weight loss. In Addison disease, there may be hyperpigmentation of the skin and mucous membranes. Hyponatremia, hypochloremia, and hyperkalemia are signs of decreased minuteseralocorticoid activity. Adrenal insufficiency may present acutely as fever, hypotension, and an acute abdomen.

Surgical patients with adrenal insufficiency may not have the typical findings. They may have refractory shock, often with hyperthermia, in the course of injury or illness. Hypotension can be dramatic despite massive volume resuscitation and pressor support. There may be no findings to suggest the diagnosis other than lack of response to therapy. Whenever shock does not respond to therapy, the diagnosis of adrenal insufficiency is considered.

The diagnosis of adrenal insufficiency may be confirmed or excluded by means of an ACTH stimulation test. A measurable cortisol response must be elicited with ACTH administration. Confirming the diagnosis does not impede therapy, and dexamethasone may be given if exogenous corticosteroids are necessary while the test is being administered.

Therapy for addisonian crisis often necessitates cardiovascular support and stress doses of corticosteroids. Hydrocortisone is given with a rapid taper to maintenance level. Volume resuscitation and pressor support may be needed for hours to days after therapy is initiated. Monitoring with a pulmonary artery catheter is maintained until the hemodynamic instability resolves. The patient is treated for the precipitating illness.

ADJUNCTIVE MEASURES IN THERAPY FOR SHOCK
Inotropic Agents

Inotropic agents are used in the management of shock when there is inadequate cardiac output despite adequate circulating blood volume. Inotropic support is indicated for persistent shock and when, despite apparent hemodynamic stability, there is evidence of a perfusion deficit. Agents used include dopamine, dobutamine, epinephrine, norepinephrine, isoproterenol, and amrinone.

Vasodilators

Vasodilators are used to augment cardiac function by means of optimization of ventricular filling pressures (preload) and SVR (afterload), both of which reduce demands on the myocardium. Vasodilators include nitroprusside, nitroglycerin, and captopril.

Pneumatic Antishock Garment

PASGs are used at a trauma scene to provide temporary support of the central hemodynamics of patients in shock. A PASG in place when a patient arrives at the hospital is deflated sequentially beginning with the abdominal compartment. Ongoing volume resuscitation may be needed. In the hospital the most appropriate use of a PASG is to tamponade bleeding and augment hemostasis. A PASG can be used if shock is *noncardiogenic* or systolic blood pressure is <80 mmHg. Use of the abdominal compartment of a PASG is contraindicated in pregnancy, esophageal variceal bleeding, diaphragmatic herniation, and evisceration.

Hypothermia and Rewarming

A risk of massive volume resuscitation is hypothermia. The use of refrigerated banked blood and room-temperature crystalloid solutions rapidly drops core temperatures if caution is not exercised to run all solutions through warming devices. Rapid rewarming decreases the requirement for blood products and improves the cardiac function of hypovolemic, hypothermic patients. Rewarming is conducted with extracorporeal counter-current warmers via femoral artery and vein cannulas.

COMPLICATIONS OF SHOCK

The complications of shock include: ischemia-reperfusion injury, abdominal compartment syndrome, immune suppression, and multiple organ failure syndrome.

SUGGESTED READING

Bickwell WH, Wall MJ, Pepe PE, et al. Immediate versus delayed fluid resuscitation for hypotensive patients with penetrating torso injuries. N Engl J Med 1994;331:1105.

Bone RC, Sibbald WJ, Sprung CL. The ACCP SCCM consensus conference on sepsis and organ failure. Chest 1992;101:1481.

Boyd O, Grounds RM, Bennett ED. A randomized clinical trial of the effect of deliberate increase of oxygen delivery on mortality in high risk surgical patients. JAMA 1993;270:2699.

Eastridge BJ, Darlington DN, Evans JA, et al. A circulating shock protein depolarizes cells in hemorrhage and sepsis. Ann Surg 1994;219:298.

Gattinoni L, Brazzi L, Pelosi P, et al. A trial of goal-oriented hemodynamic therapy in critically ill patients. N Engl J Med 1995;333:1025.

Gentilello LM, Cobean RA, Offner PJ, Soderberg RW, Jurkovich GJ. Continuous arteriovenous rewarminutesg: rapid reversal of hypothermia in critically ill patients. J Trauma 1992; 32:316.

Gubler KG, Hassantash SA, Gentilello LM, Maier RV. The impact of hypothermia on dilutional coagulopathy. J Trauma 1994;36:847.

Hayes MA, Timminutess AC, Yau EHS, Palazzo M, Hinds CJ, Watson D. Elevation of systemic oxygen delivery in the treatment of critically ill patients. N Engl J Med 1994;330:1717.

Schein M, Wittman DH, Aprahamian CC, Condon RE. The abdominutesal compartment syndrome: the physiological and clinical consequences of elevated intra-abdominutesal pressure. J Am Coll Surg 1995;180:745.

ESSENTIALS OF SURGERY: SCIENTIFIC PRINCIPLES AND PRACTICE, edited by Lazar J. Greenfield, Michael W. Mulholland, Keith T. Oldham, Gerald B. Zelenock, and Keith D. Lillemoe. Lippincott–Raven Publishers, Philadelphia, © 1997.

CHAPTER 9
CRITICAL CARE
ROBERT H. BARTLETT

MANAGEMENT OF RESPIRATORY FAILURE

Severe Respiratory Failure

An algorithm for management of severe respiratory failure is shown in Fig. 9-1. *Severe respiratory failure* means intubation, mechanical ventilation, and supplemental inspired oxygen are needed. Although patients undergoing routine ventilation can be treated without one, a pulmonary artery catheter device provides essential information. Whenever a pulmonary artery catheter is placed, a fiberoptic oximetry catheter provides continuous measurement of mixed venous saturation.

Although the cause of respiratory failure is usually in the lung interstitium and parenchyma, it is important not to overlook simple mechanical causes such as pneumothorax, hydrothorax, plugged endotracheal tubes, occluded airways, or ascites. *Bronchoscopy* is performed if there is any possibility of aspiration or if there is any evidence of mucous plugging or impaction in the airways.

Tracheostomy rather than long-term intubation is used in the treatment of patients with severe respiratory failure. Pulmonary embolism may be a cause of respiratory failure if pulmonary artery systolic pressure is >40 mmHg.

Optimization of Oxygen Delivery

Optimizing systemic oxygen delivery in relation to oxygen requirement is the primary goal of management. Oxygenation of the blood is improved by means of improving alveolar inflation, managing anemia, and/or optimizing cardiac output. Most patients in an intensive care unit (ICU) are anemic, and oxygen delivery is maintained by means of increasing cardiac output. Since patients with severe respiratory failure are at risk for death due to decreased oxygen delivery (or related multiple organ failure), transfusion should be performed. Oxygen delivery is optimized first with maintenance of a normal hematocrit.

Cardiac output is optimized to maintain delivery at four to five times consumption. It is better to *avoid situations that decrease cardiac output* rather than actively trying to increase cardiac output. This means keeping airway pressure as low as possible to maximize venous return, avoiding abdominal distention, maintaining blood volume based on pulmonary capillary wedge pressure of about 15 mmHg, and maintaining blood pressure high enough to provide coronary perfusion (mean arterial pressure >50 mmHg), but not so high as to limit left ventricular function (mean arterial pressure >90 mmHg). If all of these steps are taken, cardiac output usually autoregulates to maintain delivery at four to five times consumption.

If myocardial contractility is inadequate, *inotropic drugs* such as dopamine or dobutamine are used. These drugs, however, increase oxygen consumption in addition to increasing contractility. The titration of inotropes to achieve maximum benefit is based on mixed venous saturation measurements.

Oxygen delivery can be maintained by ensuring adequate saturation of arterial blood. This is done by supplying *supplemental oxygen* to the airway and improving inflation of collapsed or poorly ventilated alveoli. Alveolar collapse is managed by cleaning airways, avoiding 100% oxygen, removing fluid from the lung or chest, and using positive end-expiratory pressure (PEEP) to hold open alveoli opened by other measures. The optimal PEEP is that which maintains arterial oxygenation but does not decrease venous return or cardiac output. This level is best determined with monitoring of mixed venous saturation. When PEEP is varied, the patient's position on the pressure–volume curve is recorded, and volume is decreased if peak airway pressure is >40 cm H_2O.

Another step in optimizing lung function is to take advantage of the gravitational effects on pulmonary blood flow by *turning the patient prone* or to a full lateral position to direct blood flow to areas of optimal alveolar inflation. This step often opens posterior alveoli compressed by the weight of fluid in the lung.

While oxygen delivery is being optimized, *oxygen consumption is decreased* to normal or even below normal if necessary. Managing infection, providing adequate sedation, and establishing muscular paralysis decrease oxygen consumption and decrease the need for oxygen delivery. The degree of sedation or paralysis is based on mixed venous saturation. If oxygen delivery is still inadequate for metabolic needs despite these measures (venous saturation <70%), oxygen consumption can be further decreased by active cooling of the patient.

Removal of Carbon Dioxide

Optimizing CO_2 removal is usually easier than optimizing oxygen delivery. Ventilator rate and tidal volume are adjusted to achieve normal arterial P_{CO_2}. Peak airway pressure >40 cm H_2O is avoided. If P_aCO_2 is >45 mmHg, tidal volume, rate, or both are increased until P_{CO_2} is normal. CO_2 production can be minimized by means of sedation, paralysis, treat-

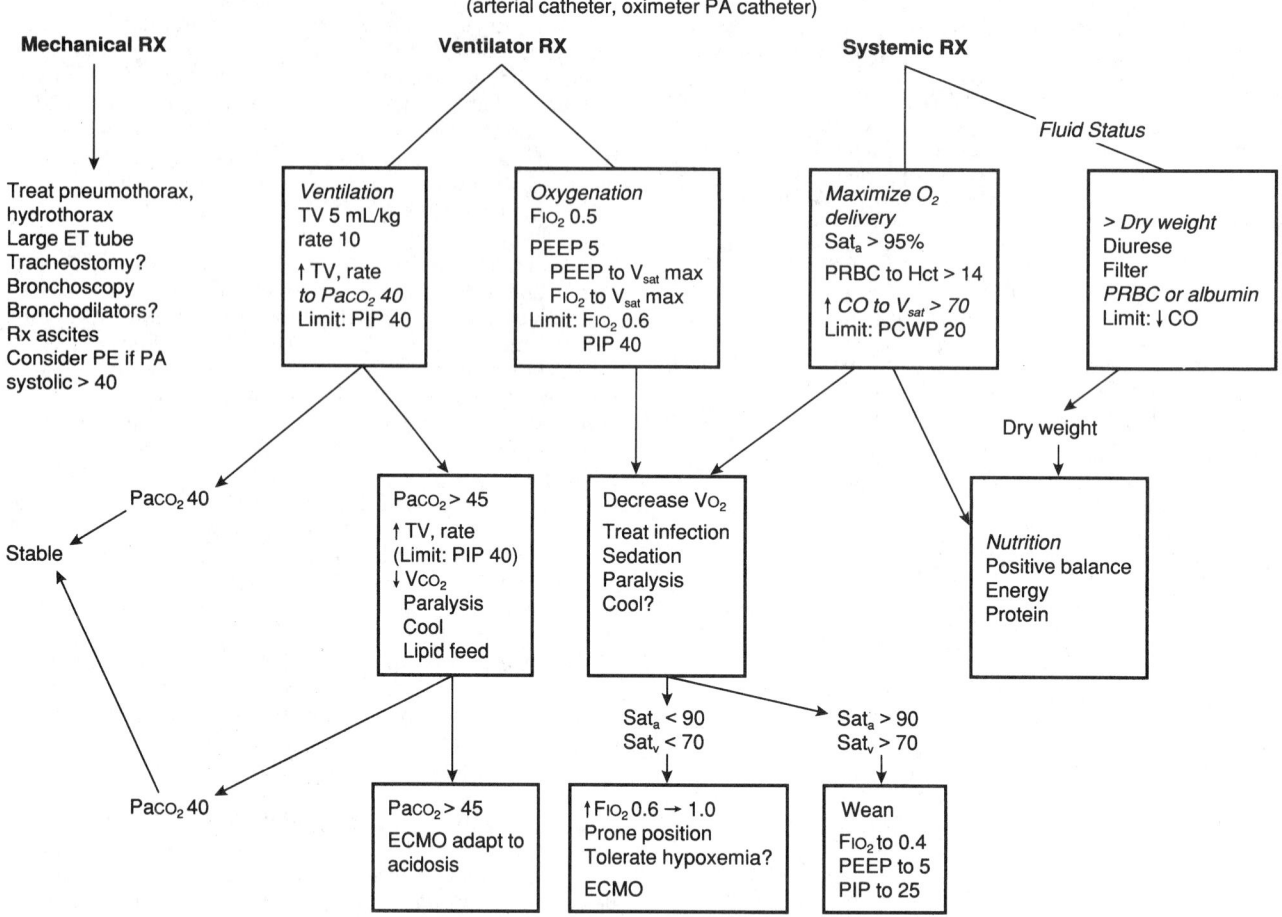

Figure 9-1. Respiratory failure algorithm. ET, endotrachial; PE, pulmonary embolism; PA, pulmonary artery; PEEP, positive end-expiratory pressure; PIP, peak inspiratory pressure; ECMO, extracorporeal membrane oxygenation; PRBC, packed red blood cells; PCWP, pulmonary capillary wedge pressure. (After Bartlett RH. University of Michigan critical care handbook. 1991)

ing infection, avoiding heavy carbohydrate loads, and cooling the patient. If P_aCO_2 is >45 mmHg despite these measures (and tube or airway occlusion is ruled out), it is permissible to tolerate hypercarbia and achieve acid–base balance with bicarbonate or Tham buffer solution.

Extracorporeal Membrane Oxygenation

If oxygen delivery or CO_2 excretion is inadequate despite all measures, the patient is not likely to live. Extracorporeal membrane (ECMO) can be used in this situation.

General Steps

Fluid overload is managed with diuresis or hemofiltration until the patient returns to dry weight. Cardiac output must be supported. The combination of diuresis and packed red blood cell (RBC) transfusion is used to maintain normal blood volume in the early stages of severe respiratory failure.

Mechanical Ventilation

Mechanical ventilation is considered when spontaneous breathing is inadequate to maintain gas exchange or when the effort required to maintain gas exchange is exhausting the patient. Tracheostomy is preferred for long-term management.

The ventilator is set on the assist–control mode at a low sensitivity. The patient breathes at a rate that regulates P_aCO_2 to normal, but each breath is mechanically assisted, providing maximal inflation. The volume of each breath is set by limiting the maximal pressure or maximal volume of each breath. Whichever method is used, peak inspiratory pressure (PIP) should not be >40 cm H_2O. If the patient is comatose or paralyzed, the assist mode cannot be used, and rate as well as volume is set (controlled mechanical ventilation or intermittent mechanical ventilation).

Adequate indices for discontinuation of ventilation are: inspiratory force >20 cm H_2O, vital capacity twice the tidal volume, adequate gas exchange on assisted ventilation at FIO_2 of 0.3 and 5 cm H_2O of PEEP, and minute ventilation <10 L/min.

Discontinuation of mechanical ventilation is accomplished by means of an immediate change from assist–control mode to spontaneous breathing with continuous gas flow. Spontaneous breathing is associated with adequate gas exchange, adequate tidal volume, respiratory rate <20 breaths/min, and pulse rate <120 beats/min. If the patient is hypermetabolic or is receiving excess carbohydrate, minute ventilation is elevated, even during assisted mechanical ventilation. The patient tires rapidly during spontaneous breaths. The primary problem must be managed before discontinuation of ventilation is attempted.

Treatment of the Interstitial Space

Therapy for interstitial edema is to maintain hydrostatic pressure as low as is compatible with adequate cardiac output and raise the oncotic pressure selectively in the vascular space. These measures, combined with fluid restriction and diuresis, decrease the amount of pulmonary edema. Regulation of hydrostatic pressure and cardiac output requires the use of a pulmonary artery catheter and frequent determination of cardiac output.

Inotropic drugs can be used to improve left ventricular contractility. Isoproterenol or dopamine is used with serial cardiac output and filling pressure measurements. A Starling curve can be constructed and the optimal combination of filling pressure and inotropic drug determined.

The first step in decreasing pulmonary edema is to decrease the pulmonary capillary hydrostatic pressure as low as is compatible with adequate cardiac output. This is done by means of diuresis and fluid restriction. Blood volume is replenished with a fluid that stays in the vascular space, such as packed RBCs. When hematocrit is normal, concentrated salt-poor albumin is used.

MANAGEMENT OF HYPOTENSION AND HYPOPERFUSION

A hemodynamics algorithm is presented in Fig. 9-2. The first sign of hemodynamic problems often is low blood pressure. If a patient with low blood pressure or tachycardia, confusion, syncope, or narrow pulse pressure appears to have inadequate systemic oxygen delivery to meet metabolic needs (shock), the first response is to assess venous pressure by means of physical examination.

If venous pressure is high, the problem is presumed to be related to the heart or mechanical obstruction to blood flow. If venous pressure is low, the problem is presumed to be hypovolemia or systemic vasodilation. If the patient does not respond promptly to initial management, central venous pressure or pulmonary artery catheter monitoring is needed. If this level of monitoring provides a diagnosis, treatment is started. If signs of inadequate blood flow persist despite treatment based on central venous pressure measurement, direct monitoring of pulmonary arterial pressure, saturation, and cardiac output is required.

With pulmonary artery catheter monitoring, one can determine whether delivery is adequate to meet metabolic needs (venous saturation >65% assuming arterial saturation is >95%). If delivery is adequate, no further treatment is needed. If delivery is not adequate, a blood volume expander is given until wedge pressure is >10 mmHg or central venous pressure is >5 mmHg. The volume expander may be blood, crystalloid, or plasma, depending on the type of fluid loss that caused hypovolemia.

If despite adequate filling pressure, cardiac output is low or venous saturation is <65%, the cause is probably cardiac dysfunction, and treatment is begun. Once mechanical factors are ruled out and contractility is shown to be the limiting factor, inotropic drugs are given (Fig. 9-3). If cardiac output is high and hypotension persists, the cause may be systemic vasodilatation (due to sepsis, paralysis, or vasodilating drugs) or metabolic (hypoglycemia, hypocalcemia, or Addison disease). If blood pressure is normal or high and cardiac output is decreased despite adequate filling pressure, the problem may be systemic hypertension or systemic hypertension combined with decreased contractility. Only then are systemic vasodilating drugs used.

METABOLISM AND NUTRITION

Every patient admitted to an ICU undergoes an evaluation of nutritional status. Patients with evidence of malnutrition begin a feeding regimen soon after admission. During critical illness, nutritional and metabolic status is assessed daily. An algorithm is shown in Fig. 9-4.

Metabolic Requirements

Energy expenditure is measured in terms of basal metabolic rate or *basal energy expenditure* (BEE). BEE is properly expressed in joules, the standard unit of energy, but is practically expressed in calories. BEE decreases with advancing age and varies with sex and body size. It is a function of cellular metabolism and body cell mass. BEE is usually estimated from a chart combining age, sex, and body size.

The metabolic rate of any given patient can be estimated by modifying the predicted basal rate according to the clinical condition. For example, metabolic rate is decreased by 10% in a starving person and increased by 10% with minimal activity. This further estimation of metabolic activity in the resting (as opposed to basal state) is *resting energy expenditure*. Trauma, stress, sepsis, and operations all increase metabolic rate. Metabolic rate is expressed in calories per day and is normalized to body surface area (m²). These units do not account for body composition. Reporting results per square meter underestimates metabolism in a fat person and overestimates it in a lean person.

Actual measurement of energy expenditure is better than estimation. The most commonly used method is *indirect calorimetry*. In this method, the amount of oxygen absorbed across the lungs into the pulmonary blood is measured over a given period of time.

Energy Sources

The main sources of energy are carbohydrate (including ketones and alcohols) and fat. Protein can be oxidized through gluconeogenesis and is often an important source of energy for critically ill patients. Nutritional therapy supplies energy from nonprotein sources, allowing the use of endogenous and exogenous protein for anabolism, rather than catabolism. Protein breakdown decreases with administration of exogenous fuel, be it glucose, fat, or xylitol (*protein-sparing effect*).

Carbohydrate is the main source of energy during normal, nonstarving existence. Carbohydrate produces 4 cal of energy per gram of substrate, 5 cal of energy per liter of oxygen consumed, and one molecule of CO_2 for each molecule of oxygen consumed. The latter ratio is the respiratory quotient (RQ), which is 1 for carbohydrate (Table 9-1).

Fat is the most efficient source of energy. Fat produces 9 cal of energy per gram of substrate metabolized, produces 4.7 cal per liter of oxygen consumed in this oxidation, and has an RQ of 0.7. Fat is stored as triglyceride. For every three molecules of fatty acid oxidized to produce energy, one molecule of glycerol is also oxidized. Endogenous fat is the main source of energy during starvation. Glycogen stores are depleted after 1 day of fasting. Protein breakdown supplies some glucose through gluconeogenesis.

Protein Metabolism

Estimating and Measuring Protein Requirements

In normal protein metabolism, continuous excretion of nitrogen (mostly as urea) is equivalent to about 50 g of protein each day, matched by protein intake of 50 g/d. The protein synthesis and breakdown rate is about 300 g/d, most endogenous amino acids being recycled into new protein.

(text continues on page 72)

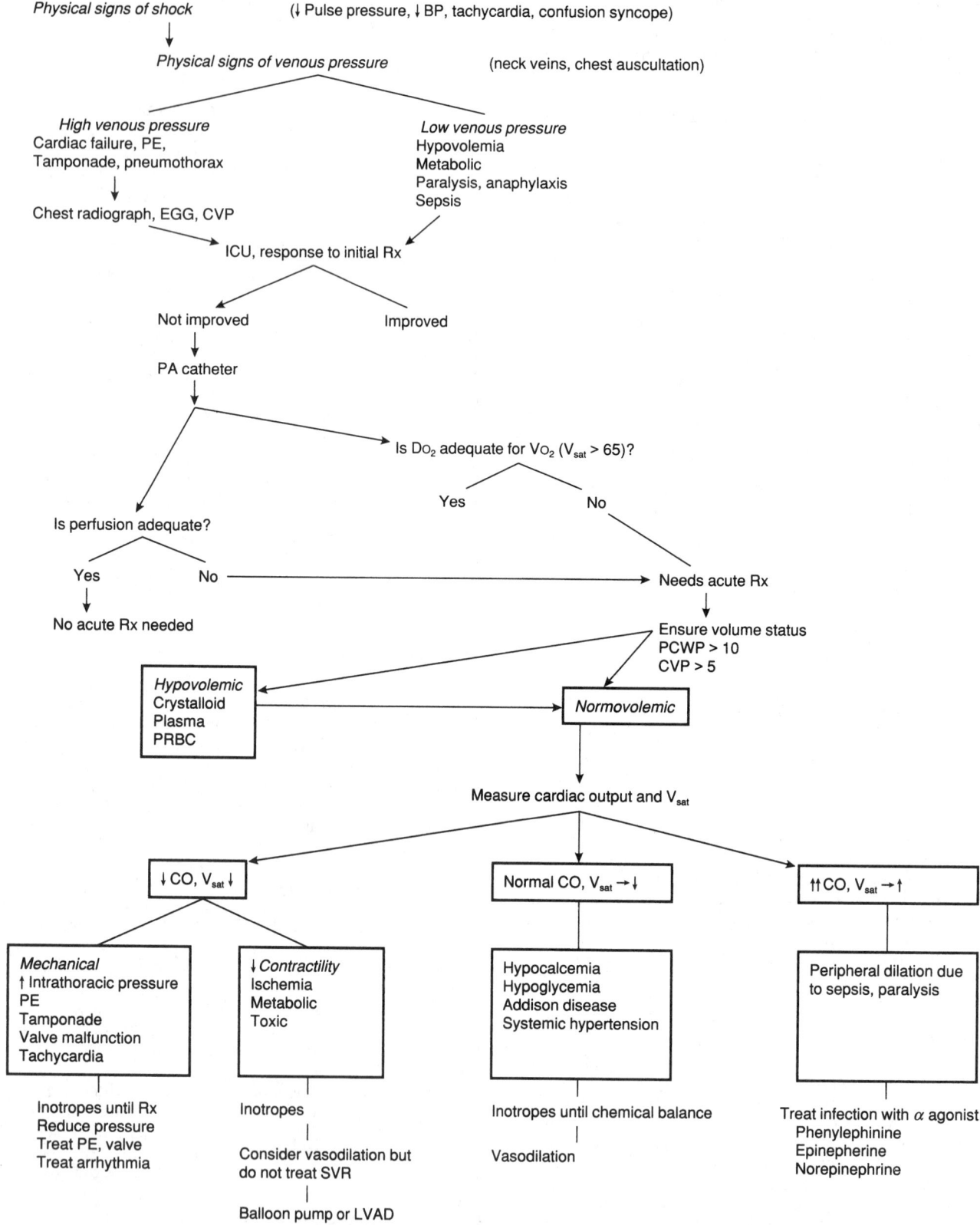

Figure 9-2. Hemodynamic algorithm. (After Bartlett RH. University of Michigan critical care handbook. 1991)

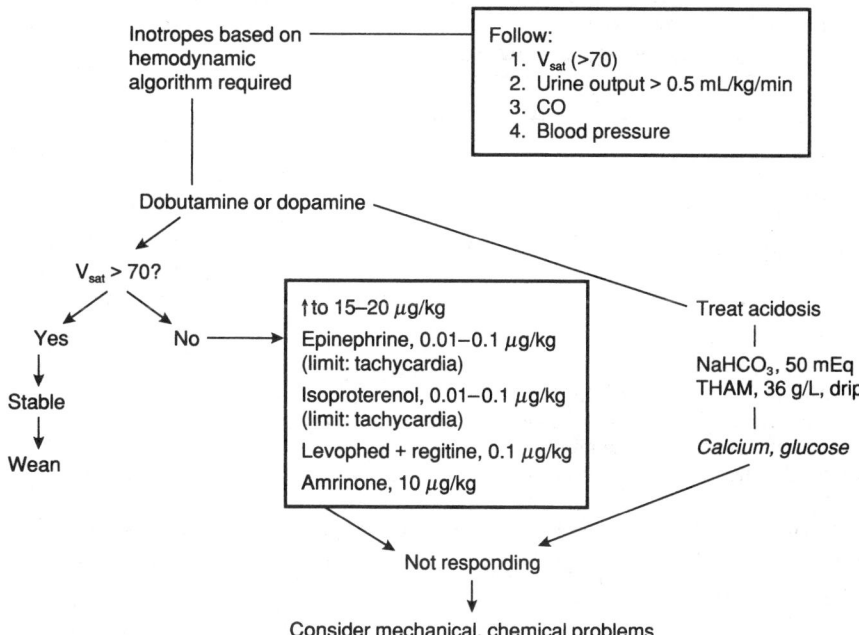

Figure 9-3. Commonly used inotropic drugs.

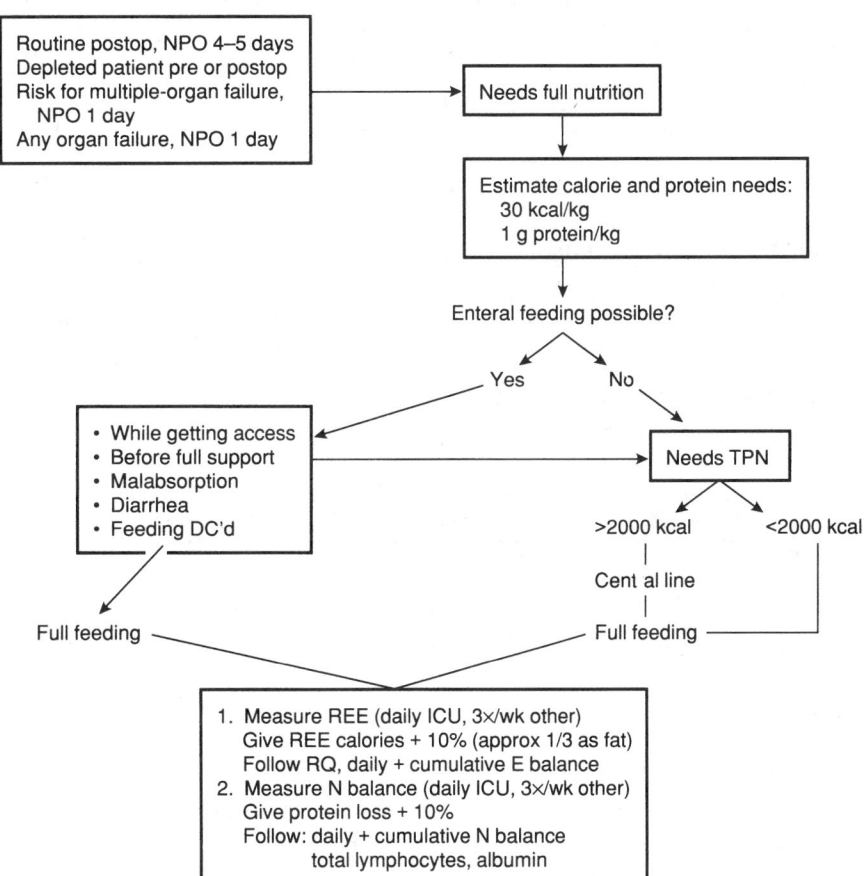

Figure 9-4. Nutritional management algorithm. TPN, total parenteral nutrition; REE, resting energy expenditure; RQ, respiratory quotient. (After Bartlett RH. University of Michigan critical care handbook. 1991)

Table 9-1. CALORIC VALUE OF METABOLIC SUBSTRATES

	kcal/g	kcal/L O$_2$	RQ
Carbohydrate	4.0	5.0	1.0
Fat	9.5	4.7	0.7
Protein	4.8	4.5	0.8
Carbohydrate → fat	—	—	8.0

RQ, respiratory quotient.

In starvation, protein catabolism continues (although at a slower rate) without corresponding protein intake, leaving the patient in a negative protein balance. This protein flux is measured as nitrogen flux (negative nitrogen balance). During critical illness, the rate of protein catabolism increases while intake stops, resulting in negative nitrogen balance. This protein breakdown is necessary to produce glucose when other carbohydrate stores are exhausted.

Protein Sources

Negative nitrogen balance does not mean protein synthesis stops or slows. Synthesis of new cells, inflammatory cells, collagen, coagulation factors, antibodies, and other proteins is accelerated during critical illness. Amino acids derived from muscle tissue or other somatic and visceral proteins become the building blocks for protein in healing tissue and host defenses.

The site of a traumatic or surgical wound or an area of acute inflammation becomes a protein parasite. This parasite may overwhelm the host. Part of nutritional management is to provide energy sources so that endogenous proteins are not needed for energy and to supply exogenous proteins so that all needs of protein synthesis can be met without breaking down endogenous sources. Basal protein requirement is 1 g/kg/d (40 g/m^2/d).

Vitamins and Minerals

Vitamin stores are plentiful, and deficiency states develop slowly, so vitamin loss is not a concern during the early days of critical illness. High doses of vitamins A and C may be beneficial to patients with injuries.

Trace metals must be managed more carefully than vitamins. Calcium, phosphorous, magnesium, and sulfur are lost continuously in urine, stool, gastric juices, and other drainage. Deficiency can develop rapidly. Enteral and parenteral feeding must include these elements. Zinc, copper, chromium, selenium, and manganese must be supplied to patients who are taking enteral or parenteral feeding for >2 weeks.

Endogenous Sources of Energy and Protein

In a healthy 80-kg man, about 1000 cal are available as glycogen and other stored carbohydrates. About 140,000 cal are stored as fat. The body contains about 6 kg of protein, which can be consumed as an energy source or maintained to do work. Nutritional assessment is the process of measuring the amount of these energy and protein reserves. Nutritional assessment is used to classify the nutritional status of patients at the time of injury, operation, or critical illness (Table 9-2).

Energy Reserves

The simplest measurement of nutritional status is body weight in relation to body height. Changes in weight not caused by fluid shifts are related to changes in body fat. Energy reserves are estimates of body fat. One way to measure energy reserve is to estimate caloric balance. Daily resting energy expenditure is estimated, and daily energy intake is estimated from the caloric value of nutrients.

A 10,000-cal deficit in a critically ill patient is a severe, acute energy deficit. The problem associated with a 10,000-cal deficit is not loss of a few pounds of fat but protein catabolism commonly associated with this amount of energy deficit. Fat reserves can be estimated with triceps skinfold measurement or change in body weight corrected for fluid balance.

Protein Reserves

The creatinine–height index is a measurement of creatinine excreted normalized for body size. Because muscle is an important source of endogenous protein, muscle wasting is characteristic of the malnourished state. This can be detected with muscle strength and endurance testing.

Actual nitrogen balance can be measured with measurement of the amount of nitrogen excreted. This is done by

Table 9-2. ASSESSMENT OF ENERGY AND PROTEIN STORES

	Excess	Normal	Depletion Mild (kcal)	Depletion Severe (kcal)
Energy reserves				
Cumulative caloric balance	+	0	−5000	−10,000
Triceps skinfold	−	Per table	−5%	−40%
Arm circumference	−	Per table	−5%	−30%
Weight change	−	Variable		−20%
Protein reserves				
Creatinine/height index		Per table	−5%	−30%
Lymphocyte count	>2000	1800/µL	1600	500
Cumulative nitrogen balance	+	0	−30 g	−300 g
Albumin	>3	3 g/dL	2.5	1.5
Total protein	>8	6 g/dL	5.5	4.0
Muscle strength				
Inspiratory force	>100	100 cm H$_2$O	50	20
Maximal volume ventilation	>120	100% Predicted	60	30
Skin test reactivity		Reactive	Anergic	

Table 9-3. COMPONENTS OF COMMONLY USED ENTERAL FEEDING FORMULAS

Name	Nonprotein Calories			Protein (g)	Osmolarity (mOsm/kg)
	Total	Fat	Carbohydrate		
Milk	565	369	196	33	277
Eggnog	881	297	584	58	480
Isocal	924	396	528	34	300
Ensure	909	333	576	37	450
Vivonex	913	9	904	21	550
Vivonex HN	845	9	844	43	810
Magnacal	1720	720	1000	70	590

measuring the amount of urea excreted in the urine, assuming urea constitutes 85% of total nitrogen excretion. When nitrogen excretion is known, the amount of protein catabolized can be estimated and compared with the amount of protein ingested.

Energy Balance

Energy expenditure is measured with respirometry and indirect calorimetry.

Nutrition Supplies

Energy and Protein

The goals of nutritional therapy in critically ill patients are to maintain a positive nitrogen balance and to avoid endogenous protein breakdown. Exogenous protein can be given through the gastrointestinal tract or parenterally. Parenteral nutrition is amino acid solutions.

In the steady state, a 70-kg adult consumes 1800 cal and 60 g of protein each day, a ratio of 30 cal/g of protein or 187 cal/g nitrogen. This is the amount of nutrients for a patient who is not nutritionally depleted and is not hypermetabolic (eg, a patient using ventilator support for Guillain–Barré syndrome).

If the patient is nutritionally depleted but not hypermetabolic (eg, a patient with esophageal cancer being prepared for an operation), the maximal amount of protein that can be introduced into the active body cell mass is given. The actual amount depends on caloric support. Such a patient receives 150 g of protein and 2500 cal daily (13 cal/g protein or 85 cal/g N).

A patient who is actively catabolizing protein because of depleted carbohydrate energy stores combined with a hypermetabolic state (eg, a patient with a severe burn) requires an energy supply to match the hypermetabolic losses (3500 cal for a burn patient who is metabolizing 3000 cal/d). An exogenous supply of energy may or may not reduce or turn off protein catabolism. Therefore, it is common practice to provide gross excesses of protein to these patients. Such a patient receives 3500 mL of a 4% protein formula; 140 g of protein with 3500 cal, or a ratio of 25 cal/g of protein (160 cal/g N).

Methods of Supplying Nutrition

Feeding by mouth is the most efficient way of providing energy and protein and is feasible for many critically ill patients.

If the patient cannot or will not take food by mouth, liquid food is administered directly into the stomach or intestine through a feeding tube. Formulas for enteral feeding are listed in Table 9-3. Feedings are given by continuous infusion into the stomach rather than large boluses.

Commercial preparations for parenteral feeding are limited to glucose (5% to 45%) and fat (10% to 20%) as energy sources and amino acid or peptide solutions (2% to 10%) as protein sources. Both parenteral and tube feedings are planned so total energy requirements can be met through fat, carbohydrate, or both. Any protein administered is available for anabolic processes.

The standard solution for total parenteral nutrition (TPN) is equal amounts of 50% glucose and 9% amino acids. This solution contains the equivalent of 1 carbohydrate calorie per milliliter at a ratio of 25 cal/g of protein. The osmolarity of this solution is 1800 mOsm/L, and it must be given into an area of rapidly flowing blood. TPN formulas are shown in Table 9-4.

MANAGEMENT OF ACUTE RENAL FAILURE

Acute renal failure (ARF) can occur alone or as a component of multiple organ failure syndrome (MOF) and often is accompanied by infection. Management involves therapy for the underlying disease. This includes surgical drainage of a septic focus, excision of necrotic tissue, early implementation of renal replacement therapy, and nutritional support. Measurements in the evaluation of renal failure are shown in Table 9-5.

Table 9-4. COMPONENTS OF COMMONLY USED PARENTERAL FEEDING FORMULAS*

	Glucose		Amino Acid (g)	mOsm	Calories: Gram of Nitrogen
	Grams	Calories			
Peripheral vein	100	400	25	880	85:1
Plus 500 mL 10% fat	100	900	25	880	222:1
Standard central	250	1000	45	1750	140:1
Concentrated cardiac	350	1400	45	2250	200:1

* Values per liter of solution.

Table 9-5. STANDARD MEASUREMENTS IN THE DIAGNOSIS OF RENAL FAILURE

Test	Prerenal	Parenchymal
Urine osmolarity (mOsm)	>500	250–350
U/P osmolality	>1.5	<1.1
U/P creatinine	>20	<10
Urine sodium	<20	>40
FE$_{Na}$	<1%	>3%

FE$_{NA}$, fraction of excreted sodium; U/P, urine-to-plasma ratio.

General Care

An algorithm for evaluation and management of renal failure is shown in Fig. 9-5. With nonoliguric ARF, treatment may differ little from that of patients with normal renal function. Oliguria and anuria pose management difficulties. In the absence of normal urine output, problems of fluid overload can lead to anasarca, pulmonary edema, and congestive heart failure. The pharmacokinetics of drugs becomes difficult to predict as a result of decreased elimination and increased volume of distribution. The volume status of patients with ARF must be carefully monitored. Fluid intake and output are tabulated, and body weight is measured daily. Pulmonary arterial catheterization may be necessary to monitor the fluid status of these patients. Management of hypervolemia is fluid restriction or fluid removal with artificial kidney techniques.

Serum electrolytes are measured daily. Hyperkalemia is the most serious abnormality. Treatment consists of additions or restrictions of i.v. solutions and use of an artificial kidney.

Platelet dysfunction and coagulopathy also are associated with ARF. Anemia also accompanies ARF in surgical patients. In addition to blood loss due to hemorrhage or operation, erythropoietin production decreases in direct proportion to decreasing renal function.

Nutrition

In *chronic* renal failure, patients are generally healthy and have energy requirements that differ little from those without chronic renal failure. Protein intake is required only for metabolic turnover and is restricted to minimize production of urea and other products of protein metabolism. The metabolic requirements of a patient with *acute* renal failure are those of a critically ill hospitalized patient.

Renal Replacement Therapy

Indications for use of renal replacement therapy include fluid overload (pulmonary edema, congestive heart failure), hyperkalemia, metabolic acidosis, uremic encepha-

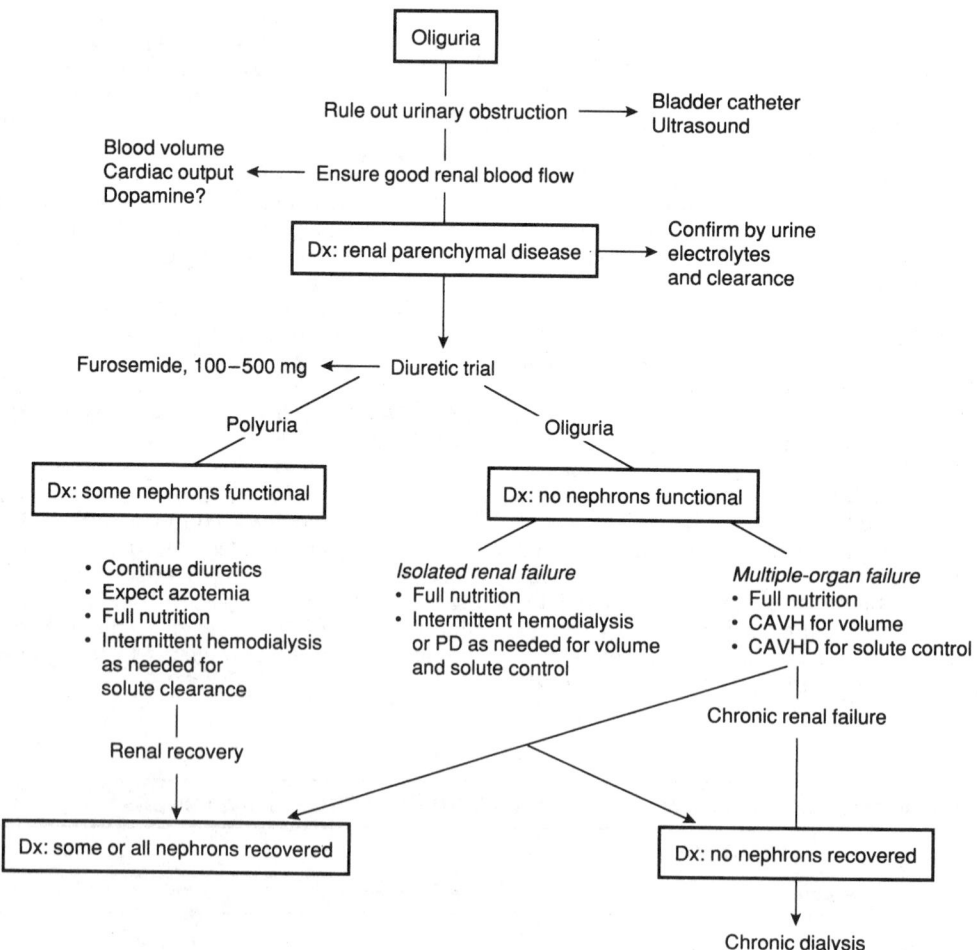

Figure 9-5. Acute renal failure management algorithm. PD, peritoneal dialysis; CAVH, continuous arteriovenous hemofiltration; CAVHD, continous arteriovenous hemodialysis. (After Mault JR, Bartlett RH. Acute renal failure. In: Greenfield LJ, ed. Complications in surgery and trauma, ed 2. Philadelphia, JB Lippincott, 1989:149)

Table 9-6. COMPARISON OF RENAL REPLACEMENT THERAPIES

	Hemodialysis	Peritoneal Dialysis	CAVH/CAVHD
Description	Rapid, intermittent	Slow, intermittent	Slow, continuous
Access	Arteriovenous or venovenous	Abdominal catheter	Arteriovenous
Anticoagulation	Required	None required	Required
Solute removal	Excellent	Excellent	Good with standard CAVH; excellent with CAVHD
Fluid removal	Good to excellent	Good	Excellent
Hemodynamic instability	Significant	None	None
Risks of procedure	Hypotension/hypoxemia, dysequilibrium syndrome	Infection or peritonitis; intraabdominal adhesions; respiratory distress	Dehydration; hemorrhage; electrolyte imbalance
Overall appraisal	Useful for urgent removal of solutes or poisons	Contraindicated with abdominal operation	Allows great flexibility with fluid and electrolyte balance
	Hemodynamic instability limits use in intensive care patients	Useful in burn patients and poor vascular access	Solute removal enhanced with CAVHD

CAVH, continuous arteriovenous hemofiltration; CAVHD, continuous arteriovenous hemodialysis.

lopathy, coagulopathy, and acute poisoning. The modalities of renal replacement therapy are hemodialysis, peritoneal dialysis, and continuous arteriovenous hemofiltration (CAVH) (Table 9-6).

The guidelines for renal replacement therapy in ARF are:

1. Volume (IV fluids, TPN) is supplemented as needed, independent of method of renal replacement.
2. Renal replacement therapy is begun early in the course of ARF, before hypervolemia, azotemia, or hyperkalemia occurs.
3. For severely ill patients with ARF, CAVH is used.
4. If solute clearance is insufficient with CAVH, therapy is converted to CAVHD or conventional hemodialysis is provided.
5. Peritoneal dialysis is used when vascular access is unavailable or when risk for hemorrhage is prohibitive.
6. Patients in hemodynamically stable condition with isolated ARF receive intermittent hemodialysis or peritoneal dialysis.

MULTIPLE ORGAN FAILURE

MOF is dysfunction of two or more of the six vital organ systems: cardiovascular, respiratory, nervous system, renal, liver, and host defenses. Failure of other organs (skin, coagulation, digestive system) may occur, but these are of secondary importance. Table 9-7 list the criteria for organ system failure.

The phases of MOF are:

Phase I—Generalized increased capillary permeability resulting in edema, weight gain, IV volume requirement, and increased protein concentration in urine and lymph. The lung is the most obvious end organ in a generalized permeability defect.

Phase II—A hypermetabolic state with increased VO_2 and a compensatory increase in oxygen delivery characterized by tachycardia and high cardiac output.

Phase III—Organ malfunction due to localized edema (particularly of the lung and heart) and cellular injury (particularly to the kidney, liver, brain, and host defense system). Hemorrhagic shock predisposes to bacterial translocation and endotoxin absorption from the intestine.

Phase IV—In the absence of systemic sepsis, organs recover to normalcy, or they are irreversibly damaged, leading to the need for chronic support (eg, of the kidney). If the organ failure phases lead to systemic infection or irreversible tissue damage in the lung or brain, death of the entire organ is likely.

Management principles are to avoid further local or systemic ischemia and keep the brain viable with drug or mechanical support of the failing organs until organ recovery occurs.

Table 9-7. CRITERIA FOR ORGAN FAILURE*

Cardiovascular	Cardiac index <2.5 L/m^2/min with left atrial pressure >10 mmHg
	Inotropic or vasopressor drugs required to maintain adequate perfusion
Respiratory	Alveoloarterial O_2 gradient >300 mmHg
Nervous	Glasgow coma score <10
Renal	Creatinine >3 mg/dL
Liver	Bilirubin >5 mg/dL
Host defenses	Positive blood culture
	Invasive tissue infection
	Anergic to common antigens

* Arbitrary definitions of the University of Michigan Surgical Intensive Care Unit.

SUGGESTED READING

Bernard GR, Artigas A, Brigham KL, et al. The American–European consensus conference on ARDS: definitions, mechanisms, relative outcomes, and clinical trial coordination. Am J Respir Crit Care Med 1994;149:818.

Fleming A, Bishop M, Shoemaker W, et al. Prospective trial of supranormal values as goals of resuscitation in severe trauma. Arch Surg 1992;127:1175.

Gattinoni L, Bombino M, Pelosi P, et al. Lung structure and function in different stages of severe adult respiratory distress syndrome. JAMA 1994;271:1772.

Hickling KG, Walsh J, Henderson S, Jackson R. Low mortality rate in ARDS using low volume, pressure-limited ventilation with permissive hypercapnia: a prospective study. Crit Care Med 1994;22:1568.

Moore FA, Moore EE, Kudsk KA, et al. Clinical benefits of an immune-enhancing diet for early postinjury enteral feeding. J Trauma 1994;37:607.

Russel JA, Phang PT. Oxygen delivery/consumption controversy:

approaches to management of critically ill. Am J Respir Crit Care Med 1994;149:533.

Shoemaker W, Appel PL, Kram HB. Hemodynamic and oxygen transport responses in survivors and nonsurvivors of high-risk surgery. Crit Care Med 1993;21:977.

ESSENTIALS OF SURGERY: SCIENTIFIC PRINCIPLES AND PRACTICE, edited by Lazar J. Greenfield, Michael W. Mulholland, Keith T. Oldham, Gerald B. Zelenock, and Keith D. Lillemoe. Lippincott–Raven Publishers, Philadelphia, © 1997.

CHAPTER 10

FLUIDS AND ELECTROLYTES AND ACID–BASE BALANCE

RICHARD B. WAIT, KIM U. KAHNG, AND LISA S. DRESNER

TOTAL BODY WATER AND THE FLUID COMPARTMENTS

The total volume of water within the body is total body water (TBW). The relation between TBW and body weight depends on the amount of fat in the body. Because fat contains little water, TBW as a percentage of body weight decreases with increasing body fat. Average TBW in men is 60% of body weight. In women, who have more adipose tissue, estimated average TBW is 50% of body weight.

The percentage of body weight accounted for by water also varies with age. Water makes up about 80% of the body weight of infants. This value decreases to about 65% by 1 year. Throughout adult life, TBW gradually decreases because the amount of fat in the body increases. Among obese people, estimates of TBW are 10% to 20% lower than the norm, and for very lean people, TBW is about 10% higher.

TBW is contained in intracellular, intravascular, and interstitial compartments (Table 10-1). These three compartments are in dynamic equilibrium. Alterations in one lead to compensatory changes in the others.

COMPOSITION OF BODY FLUIDS

Sodium and potassium are the dominant cations in the body. Sodium is mainly restricted to the extracellular fluid (ECF) and potassium to the intracellular fluid (ICF). Sodium content in the average adult is about 60 mEq/kg. About 25% of this sodium is nonexchangeable because it is confined to bone. Of the exchangeable fraction, about

Table 10-1. BODY FLUID COMPARTMENTS

Total Body Water	Body Weight (%)	Total Body Water (%)
Total	60	100
Intracellular	40	67
Extracellular	20	33
Intravascular	5	8
Interstitial	15	25

Table 10-2. ELECTROLYTE CONCENTRATIONS OF INTRACELLULAR AND EXTRACELLULAR FLUID COMPARTMENTS

	Extracellular Fluid (mEq/L)		
	Plasma	Interstitial Fluid	Intracellular Fluid
CATIONS			
Na^+	140	146	12
K^+	4	4	150
Ca^{2+}	5	3	10^{-7}
Mg^{2+}	2	1	7
ANIONS			
Cl^-	103	114	3
HCO_3^-	24	27	10
SO_4^{2-}	1	1	—
HPO_4^{3-}	2	2	116
Protein	16	5	40
Organic anions	5	5	—

85% is in the ECF. Small amounts of potassium, calcium, and magnesium constitute the rest of the cations in the ECF (Table 10-2).

Effective Circulating Volume

Effective circulating volume is the portion of extracellular volume that perfuses the organs and affects the baroreceptors. Effective circulating volume normally corresponds to intravascular volume, but in disease, the two can be substantially different. An example of this is congestive heart failure in the presence of high intravascular volume; effective circulating volume is low because of cardiac failure.

Effective circulating volume is usually in a state of equilibrium with the rest of the extracellular volume, so changes in total extracellular volume are reflected by changes in effective circulating volume.

Abnormal shifts of fluid from the intravascular space to the tissues are *third-space fluid losses*. An example of a disorder that causes third-space fluid loss is intestinal obstruction, which causes edema of the intestinal wall and transudation of fluid into the intestinal lumen. This fluid stays in the extracellular compartment, but it is poorly exchangeable while the disease persists. In this situation, total ECF remains constant or increases, and interstitial water increases at the expense of intravascular volume.

Volume Control

Changes in volume are detected by osmoreceptors, which detect changes in plasma osmolality, and baroreceptors, which are sensitive to changes in pressure. Osmoreceptors are responsible for day-to-day fine-tuning of volume. Baroreceptors contribute little to control of fluid balance under normal conditions. Large changes in circulating volume can modify osmoregulation of secretion of antidiuretic hormone (ADH).

Hormonal Mediators of Volume Control

Renin-Angiotensin System. The key to much of the volume and pressure control exerted by the kidneys is release of renin from the juxtaglomerular cells of the afferent arterioles. Renin is released in response to changes in arterial pressure, changes in sodium delivery to the macula densa of the distal convoluted tubule, increases in β-adrenergic activity, and increases in cellular cAMP, which may be stimulated by prostaglandins, histamine, glucagon, and other hormonal influences.

Renin cleaves angiotensin I from angiotensinogen and α_2-globulin. Angiotensin I is further cleaved to angiotensin II by angiotensin-converting enzyme, which is produced by vascular endothelial cells. One pass through the pulmonary microvasculature converts most angiotensin I to angiotensin II. The actions of angiotensin II are summarized in Fig. 10-1.

Aldosterone. Aldosterone is a mineralocorticoid produced in the adrenal cortex. This hormone influences sodium balance by increasing renal tubular reabsorption of sodium. Aldosterone acts directly on the distal tubular segments, predominantly on the collecting tubules. By increasing protein production in the tubular cells, aldosterone induces an influx of sodium, which causes an increase in cellular Na^+-K^+-ATPase activity. The result is an increase in sodium reabsorption and potassium excretion. Aldosterone secretion is regulated by angiotensin II, increased potassium levels, ACTH, and prostaglandins.

NORMAL WATER AND ELECTROLYTE EXCHANGE

Normal Water Exchange

Water losses are both sensible (measurable) and insensible.

Sensible Water Loss

Sensible losses occurs in urine, stool, and sweat. Table 10-3 summarizes normal daily sensible and insensible losses.

Insensible Water Loss

Insensible water loss is the evaporatory loss of water from the skin and the respiratory tract (Table 10-3). Evaporatory *skin losses* depend on body surface area, body temperature, and relative humidity of the environment. Evapo-

Table 10-3. WATER LOSSES IN A 60- TO 80-kg MAN

	Average Daily Volume (mL)	Minimal Daily Volume (mL)
Sensible losses		
Urinary	800–1500	300
Intestinal	0–250	0
Sweat	0	0
Insensible losses		
Lungs and skin	600–900	600–900

(Adapted from Shires GT, Canizaro PC. Fluid and electrolyte management of the surgical patient. In: Sabiston DC, ed. Textbook of surgery. Philadelphia, WB Saunders, 1986:77)

ration through the skin is a mechanism for heat loss and is proportional to calories expended. About 30 mL of water is lost for every 100 kcal expended. *Respiratory* exchange depends on ambient temperature, relative humidity, and rate of air exchange. At normal respiratory rates, 13 mL of water is lost for every 100 kcal expended.

Normal insensible water losses average 8 to 12 mL/kg/d. Insensible water loss increases 10% for each degree of body temperature >37.2°C (99°F). Patients with tracheostomies who breathe unhumidified air lose additional free water. Patients who use respirators, or who breathe air that is 100% humidified, have no respiratory losses and may gain free water.

Normal water consumption is about 2000 mL/d. About one third of this amount comes from water bound to food; the rest is from free water intake. Water is gained when carbohydrates and proteins, which are kept in solution by water in the cell, are metabolized. Although this gain is usually minimal, catabolic states may increase the amount of oxidative free water gain to about 500 mL/d. To maintain proper fluid volume, intake and excretion are balanced through thirst and changes in renal excretion.

Normal Salt Exchange

Salt intake averages 100 to 250 mEq/d Na^+ (6 to 15 g/d NaCl). This intake is balanced by losses through sweat, stool, and urine. Renal sodium excretion is the mechanism by which sodium balance is controlled. In hyponatremia, the kidney can conserve sodium with urinary losses <1 mEq/d. Urinary excretion can be maximized up to 5000 mEq/d if necessary to achieve sodium balance. Normal sodium requirement is 1 to 2 mEq/kg/d.

Because most potassium remains in the intracellular compartment, potassium homeostasis is maintained by a balance between intake and GI and renal losses and a balance between extracellular and intracellular potassium. In a normal diet, 40 to 120 mEq of potassium is ingested daily. Of this potassium, 10% to 15% is excreted in the feces, and the rest is excreted in the urine. Normal daily potassium requirements are 0.5 to 1 mEq/kg/d. Abnormal renal function changes this figure; potassium intake must be minimized for patients with renal failure.

FLUID AND ELECTROLYTE THERAPY

Parenteral Solutions

Selection of the electrolyte solutions is determined by maintenance fluid requirements, existing fluid deficits, and ongoing fluid losses. Table 10-4 lists electrolyte solutions. In some situations a particular solution does not

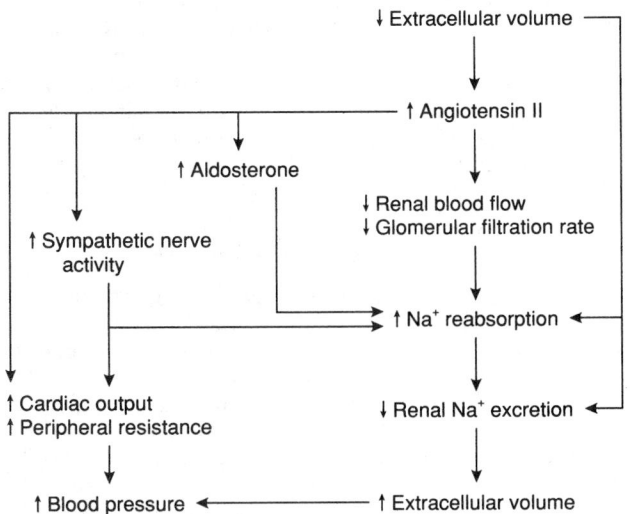

Figure 10-1. Multiple effects of increased angiotensin II release in response to the stimulus of decreased extracellular volume.

accurately replace the electrolyte components of the losses or deficits, and more than one type of solution may be used. Potassium, magnesium, and calcium can be added to parenteral solutions.

Lactated Ringer solution is used to replace losses of fluid with the ionic composition of plasma, such as edema fluid and small-intestinal losses. It is ideal for replacement of existing fluid deficits when serum electrolyte concentrations are normal.

Isotonic saline (0.9% or normal saline) contains 154 mEq of both sodium and chloride. Although this solution can be useful to patients with hyponatremia or hypochloremia, the excess of both sodium and chloride can cause electrolyte and acid–base disturbances. Infusion of large volumes of 0.9% saline can cause total body sodium overload and hyperchloremia. The added chloride load can result in hyperchloremic metabolic acidosis or aggravate preexisting acidosis. The pH of this solution and of the related solutions (0.45%, 0.33%, and 0.2% saline) is 4.0 to 5.0.

Less-concentrated saline solutions are used to replace ongoing fluid losses, such as nasogastric tube losses, and are used in maintenance fluid therapy.

Hypertonic saline solutions (3% NaCl, 5% NaCl) are not often used and reserved for unusual circumstances such as replacement of sodium in patients with symptomatic hyponatremia.

Plasma expanders are used to treat surgical patients (Table 10-5).

Goals of Fluid and Electrolyte Therapy

Correction of Existing Volume Abnormalities

Volume Deficit. Symptoms of chronic volume deficits are decreased skin turgor, weight loss, sunken eyes, hypothermia, oliguria, orthostatic hypotension, and tachycardia. Serum blood urea nitrogen (BUN) and creatinine may be elevated with a high BUN-to-creatinine ratio (>15:1). If there is no change in RBC mass, hematocrit increases 6 to 8 points for each liter deficit in intravascular volume. Urine concentration is high, and urine sodium excretion is low (<20 mEq/L Na+). Plasma sodium is not an indicator of intravascular volume; if the fluid losses are isotonic, plasma sodium concentration is normal.

Acute volume losses are manifested by changes in vital signs without concomitant tissue changes. If organ perfu-

Table 10-4. ELECTROLYTE CONTENT OF COMMONLY USED INTRAVENOUS ELECTROLYTE SOLUTIONS

Solution	Electrolyte (mEq/L)					
	Na+	K+	Ca2+	Mg2+	Cl-	HCO3-
0.9% NaCl (normal saline)	154	—	—	—	154	—
0.45% NaCl	77	—	—	—	77	—
0.33% NaCl	56	—	—	—	56	—
0.2% NaCl	34	—	—	—	34	—
Lactated Ringer solution	130	4	4	—	109	28
3.0% NaCl	513	—	—	—	513	—
5.0% NaCl	855	—	—	—	855	—

Table 10-5. PLASMA EXPANDERS

Solution	Concentration (%)
HUMAN ALBUMIN	
Albutein 5% (Alpha Therapeutic)	5
Albutein 25% (Alpha Therapeutic)	25
Albuminar-5 (Armour)	5
Albuminar-25 (Armour)	25
Buminate 5% (Hyland)	5
Buminate 25% (Hyland)	25
PLASMA PROTEIN FRACTIONS: ALBUMIN 4.4%	
Plasmanate (Cutter)	
Plasmatein (Alpha Therapeutic)	
Plasma-Plex (Armour)	
Proteinate (Hyland)	
DEXTRANS AND STARCH	
Dextran 40 (Rheomacrodex)	10
Dextran 70 (Macrodex)	6
Hetastarch (Hespan)	6

(Adapted from Carroll HJ, Oh MS. Water, electrolyte and acid–base metabolism. Philadelphia, JB Lippincott, 1989:82)

sion is compromised, urine output may be low. Oliguria and hypovolemia may be caused by intrinsic renal dysfunction. Attempts to quantify volume deficits are of little value. All deficits are addressed immediately. Volume resuscitation is continued until hemodynamic values are normal. The volume of fluid needed for resuscitation is the best estimate of the volume deficit.

Fluid resuscitation for hypovolemia is initiated with an isotonic solution such as lactated Ringer solution. Urine flow in critically ill patients is monitored with an indwelling Foley catheter. Urine output >0.5 mL/kg/h is desirable. After fluid resuscitation is initiated, history and physical examination help determine the origins of the volume deficit, and the cause is addressed. Central venous pressure may be monitored with a central venous catheter or pulmonary artery catheter.

Volume Excess. Large volumes of fluid can be sequestered in extravascular spaces (third-space losses) as a consequence of surgical intervention, trauma, and disease. With resolution of the pathologic condition and normalization of microvascular permeability, these fluid losses stop and eventually reverse. The sequestered fluid is autotransfused at variable rates. This may lead to volume overload if fluid management is not adjusted. Manifestations of volume overload are weight gain, elevated central venous pressure, pulmonary edema, peripheral edema, and an S3 gallop. Therapy for intravascular volume excess is volume restriction and use of loop diuretics if acute symptoms occur.

Maintenance Fluid Therapy

Maintenance fluid replacement is aimed at replacing fluids normally lost during the course of a day. Maintenance fluid replacement begins after reestablishment of normal hemodynamic status with resuscitation fluids.

Basal requirements for water and electrolytes are determined on the basis of sensible and insensible losses. Insensible water loss averages 8 to 12 mL/kg/d and increases 10% for every degree of body temperature >37.2°C (99°F). A 70-kg man without a fever has a daily insensible water loss of about 840 mL. Urinary and stool losses must be added to this figure. A formula for calcula-

Table 10-6. CALCULATION OF MAINTENANCE FLUID REQUIREMENTS

Body Weight	Fluid Requirement*	
For 0–10 kg	Give 100 mL/kg/d	A
For the next 10–20 kg	Give an additional 50 mL/kg/d	B
For weight > 20 kg†	Give 20 mL/kg/d	C

* Maintenance fluid requirements = sum of A + B + C.
† For elderly patients or patients with cardiac disease, this amount should be reduced to 15 mL/kg/d.

tion of maintenance water requirements is provided in Table 10-6.

Sodium requirements are variable, and excess sodium administration is usually balanced by increased urinary sodium excretion. An estimated 1 to 2 mEq/kg/d of sodium is needed for maintenance therapy. Potassium requirement is about half that of sodium (0.5 to 1 mEq/kg/d).

Replacement of calcium, phosphate, or magnesium is not necessary for patients who need short-term therapy. Critically ill patients, however, have deficits of these electrolytes, which must be replaced. For patients who need long-term fluid replacement, addition of these electrolytes and trace elements, vitamins, protein, and calories is essential. Administration of parenteral nutrition solutions is started as soon as possible for all patients not expected to resume full enteral nutrition or expected to need fluid replacement for >1 week.

Replacement of Ongoing Fluid Losses

Once volume deficits are replaced and maintenance fluids calculated and given, fluid balance is maintained by means of replacement of any fluid losses greater than maintenance. Intraoperative and postoperative losses and third-space fluid losses are estimated. Ongoing losses from nasogastric tubes, ileostomies, and fistulas can be easily measured and quantitated. The electrolyte content of these fluids can be predicted (Table 10-7) and the exact electrolyte content replaced.

Ongoing losses are documented by recording intake and output of all fluids. Patients who need an emergency operation need preoperative fluid resuscitation, unless they have uncontrolled hemorrhage, for which surgical intervention is the only means of stabilizing the volume loss.

Intraoperative Fluid Therapy

During surgical procedures, fluid losses result from blood loss, third-space sequestration due to trauma to or manipulation of tissues, and evaporative losses from the wound itself. Blood loss is quantified by direct measurement and estimation during an operation. Most patients can tolerate an unreplaced blood loss of 500 mL, but losses greater than this must be replaced during the operation.

Shifts of fluid from the intravascular space to the extravascular space (third-space volume losses) due to surgical manipulation, tissue trauma, and evaporation cannot be measured but are anticipated. Isotonic solutions, such as lactated Ringer solution, are given at 500 to 1000 mL/h during the operation. Intraoperative monitoring of blood pressure and urine output aids the surgeon and anesthesiologist in avoiding periods of hypotension due to volume depletion.

Central venous pressure is monitored for patients undergoing complex procedures. In critically ill patients or patients at high risk for cardiac or fluid balance abnormalities during an operation, cardiac output and pulmonary artery wedge pressures are used to gauge the adequacy of fluid resuscitation. Elderly patients and patients at high risk also may benefit from preoperative placement of a pulmonary artery catheter to optimize preoperative, surgical, and postoperative cardiac function and fluid resuscitation.

Postoperative Fluid Therapy and Monitoring

Postoperative fluid therapy depends on the adequacy of volume status at the end of the surgical procedure and on ongoing fluid losses. Maintenance fluid therapy is supplemented with additional fluids to replace ongoing third-space losses and losses from tubes and drains. Isotonic solutions are used for volume resuscitation during the early postoperative period. Potassium supplements are not given during this period unless they are indicated by serum electrolyte measurements.

During the postoperative period fluid status is monitored with vital signs, urinary output, and central venous pressure if necessary. Urine output is maintained at >0.5 mL/kg/h. Urine specific gravity serves as an indicator of volume status and renal ability to concentrate and dilute urine. Urine specific gravity >1.010 to 1.012 indicates that the urine is being concentrated, and a urine specific gravity <1.010 indicates that dilute urine is being produced.

Both short-term and long-term fluid management are facilitated by daily measurement of body weight and fluid intake and output. Insensible fluid losses are estimated and added to total output. Daily intake and output must be balanced with fluid management. Weight gain usually indicates increases in TBW rather than in protein or fat content.

CONCENTRATION CHANGES IN BODY FLUIDS

Hyponatremia

Most surgical patients with hyponatremia are euvolemic or hypervolemic. Patients without symptoms are treated with free water restriction. Patients with hypovolemia benefit from rehydration because their symptoms often are caused by dehydration rather than hyponatremia. Isotonic saline or lactated Ringer solution can be used to normalize volume. Because rapid normalization of volume may lead to hypernatremia, serial monitoring of serum $[Na^+]$ is per-

Table 10-7. ELECTROLYTE CONCENTRATIONS IN GASTROINTESTINAL SECRETIONS

Secretion	Electrolyte (mEq/L)					Rate (mL/d)
	Na^+	K^+	Cl^-	HCO_3^-	H^+	
Salivary	50	20	40	30	—	100–1000
Gastric						
Basal	100	10	140	—	30	1000
Stimulated	30	10	140	—	100	4200
Bile	140	5	100	60	—	500–1000
Pancreatic	140	5	75	100	—	1000
Duodenum	140	5	80	—	—	100–2000
Ileum	140	5	70	50	—	100–2000
Colon	60	70	15	30	—	—

formed during judicious volume replacement. Patients with symptomatic hyponatremia need aggressive treatment tempered by the duration of the hyponatremia. Because risk for central pontine myelinolysis is greatest among patients hyponatremic >48 h, 5% or 3% saline solution is given slowly to increase serum $[Na^+]$ at a rate not >0.5 mEq/L/h. For acute hyponatremia (<48 h), therapy is more rapid. Symptomatic acute hyponatremia may be treated with hypertonic saline to correct serum $[Na^+]$ at a rate of 1 to 2 mEq/L/h.

Hypernatremia

Once hypernatremia becomes symptomatic, it has a high morbidity and mortality. Prompt treatment is essential. Rapid correction of hypernatremia, however, is associated with high risk for cerebral edema and herniation. In chronic hypernatremia, the cells in the brain gradually adapt by increasing intracellular osmotic solute content, regaining cellular volume. These cellular changes are not readily reversed. A sudden decrease in extracellular sodium concentration and osmolality causes cell swelling. Because chronic hypernatremia is well-tolerated, there are few advantages to rapid correction of the free water deficit. Free water is administered to correct serum $[Na^+]$ at a rate not >0.7 mEq/L/h. The amount of water depends on free water deficit, insensible free water losses, and urinary free water excretion rate.

COMPOSITIONAL CHANGES
Potassium

Hyperkalemia

Therapy for hyperkalemia is dictated by serum level and ECG changes or symptoms. Severe hyperkalemia with ECG abnormalities necessitates urgent treatment. The effects of hyperkalemia on membrane potentials can be reduced by increasing calcium levels. Rapid infusion of 10% to 20% calcium gluconate may be life-saving. The effects are transient and usually last about 30 minutes. Administration of sodium bicarbonate is another temporary measure. Movement of potassium into the intracellular compartment can be achieved by giving 25 to 50 g of glucose (50 to 100 mL of 50% glucose solution) with 10 to 20 units of regular insulin.

Definitive therapy for hyperkalemia involves increasing potassium excretion. This may be accomplished with administration of K^+-Na^+ exchange resins such as sodium polystyrene sulfonate (Kayexalate). The usual oral dose is 40 g dissolved in 20 to 100 mL of sorbitol. Each gram removes about 1 mEq of potassium. Kayexalate also can be given as a retention enema in a dose of 50 to 100 g in 200 mL of water. Each gram removes about 0.5 mEq of potassium. Peritoneal dialysis or hemodialysis is indicated for severe hyperkalemia and renal failure.

Hypokalemia

Therapy for hypokalemia is potassium replacement; acid–base balance must be considered before therapy. The route and rate of potassium replacement depend on the presence and severity of symptoms. A reduction in serum potassium of 1 mEq/L represents a total body potassium deficiency of 100 to 200 mEq. Potassium is administered intravenously (IV) if the symptoms are severe, if serum concentration is <2 mEq/L, or if the patient is unable to take oral potassium. IV potassium can be administered at a rate of about 10 mEq/h, and the concentration of potassium is ≤40 mEq/L. If less fluid is desired, up to 20 mEq in 100 mL of IV solution can be given, although no more

than 40 mEq is administered per hour. Potassium is given orally if possible. Oral formulations include potassium salts such as potassium chloride, potassium phosphate, and potassium bicarbonate.

Calcium

The regulation of calcium homeostasis is depicted in Fig. 10-2.

Hypercalcemia

Elevation of total serum calcium concentrations to >14 mg/dL necessitates prompt treatment to prevent potentially lethal complications. Immediate measures are directed at maximizing renal excretion of calcium. Because these patients are often dehydrated, 0.9% or 0.45% saline solution with 20 to 30 mEq/L of potassium is administered IV. Hydration proceeds at 200 to 300 mL/h to promote diuresis. Furosemide may be given to enhance calcium excretion, but hydration is performed first.

Long-term treatment depends on the cause of the hypercalcemia. Therapy for primary hyperparathyroidism is resection of the parathyroid abnormality (adenoma or hyperplasia). Definitive treatment of secondary or tertiary hyperparathyroidism may be subtotal parathyroidectomy or total parathyroidectomy with autonomous parathyroid transplantation. Hypercalcemia due to tumor secretion of hormonal mediators may be controlled with extirpation of the tumor. In the presence of metastatic bone disease, therapy is inhibition of bone resorption with mithramycin or calcitonin.

Hypocalcemia

Asymptomatic hypocalcemia, which may be due to low protein or albumin levels with normal ionized calcium levels, need not be treated. Symptomatic hypocalcemia is treated with IV infusion of calcium gluconate or calcium chloride. Calcium is administered at a rate not exceeding 50 mg/min (2.5 mEq/min). Long-term calcium replacement is oral calcium lactate, calcium citrate, or calcium carbonate. Vitamin D_3 (calcitriol) increases intestinal absorption of calcium.

Magnesium

Hypermagnesemia

Hypermagnesemia is rare. In the presence of renal failure, withholding magnesium-containing drugs usually prevents magnesium excess. Calcium antagonizes the effects of magnesium, so infusion of 5-10 mEq of calcium by slow IV injection is used as emergency treatment.

Hypomagnesemia

Magnesium may be administered orally to manage mild cases of hypomagnesemia, but large oral doses can cause diarrhea. Correction of deficits is managed with IV administration of magnesium sulfate 50-100 mEq/d.

ACID–BASE DISTURBANCES
Metabolic Acidosis

Three mechanisms result in a decrease in extracellular bicarbonate concentration and metabolic acidosis:

1. Dilutional acidosis. Rapid infusion of an alkali-free solution results in dilution of the bicarbonate concentration.
2. Cellular retention of K^+ in exchange for Na^+ and H^+.

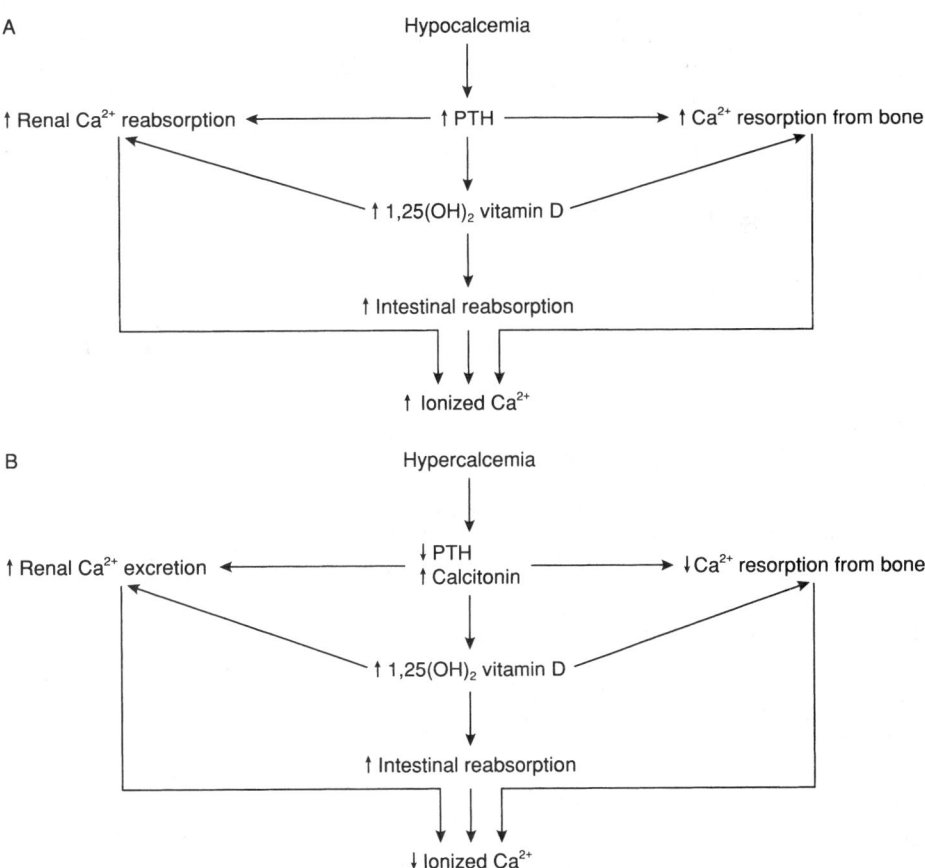

Figure 10-2. Effects of hypocalcemia (*A*) and hypercalcemia (*B*) on the mediators of calcium homeostasis. PTH, parathyroid hormone.

Buffering of the H$^+$ may result in a transient decrease in extracellular bicarbonate concentration.

3. Decreased body bicarbonate content. Net loss of bicarbonate exceeds bicarbonate generation.

The first two mechanisms are infrequent and produce only mild, self-limiting metabolic acidosis. Most clinically significant metabolic acidosis is related to net loss of bicarbonate, which occurs when loss or consumption due to titration is greater than bicarbonate generation.

Under normal circumstances, about 70 mEq of acid is generated daily. Acid gain is partially offset by GI absorption of metabolizable anions, such as citrate, which are metabolized to yield bicarbonate. The rest of the excess acid is balanced by renal excretion of acid with generation of bicarbonate. A decrease in body bicarbonate content may be the result of an increase in net acid generation (*extrarenal acidosis*) or a reduction in renal acid excretion (*renal acidosis*).

Treatment

Acute Metabolic Acidosis. Management of mild-to-moderate acute metabolic acidosis is correction of the cause. For surgical and trauma patients, metabolic acidosis is often the result of hypoxia due to inadequate tissue perfusion and lactic acidosis. Volume and blood resuscitation alone may be enough to correct acidosis.

Bicarbonate is reserved for cases of metabolic acidosis that are not easily reversed; the purpose is to prevent cardiovascular collapse. Bicarbonate is not administered until pH falls to 7.1 to 7.2. The amount of bicarbonate needed to increase serum concentration to any given level cannot be precisely calculated. The goal is to increase pH to 7.2 to 7.3 with initial administration of one or two ampules of bicarbonate (44.5 to 50 mEq/amp). The need for more bicarbonate is based on repeated arterial blood gas results. Rapid correction to achieve normal serum bicarbonate concentration may be *harmful* because organic anions are precursors of bicarbonate, and their eventual metabolism combined with administered bicarbonate may result in metabolic alkalosis.

Chronic Acidosis. Therapy for distal renal tubular acidosis (RTA) is daily doses of alkali to correct acidosis and prevent nephrocalcinosis and nephrolithiasis. Patients with distal RTA and hypokalemia need potassium supplementation. Mild cases of proximal RTA do not require specific therapy. Severe cases are managed with thiazide diuretics and a low-salt diet to achieve a modest degree of volume depletion, which reduces the requirement for bicarbonate supplementation.

Diabetic Ketoacidosis. Acidosis and hyperglycemia are corrected with administration of insulin. Metabolism of the anions of the ketoacids begins promptly and results in generation of bicarbonate. Insulin inhibits ketone formation and gluconeogenesis and stimulates peripheral use of ketones and glucose. A loading dose of 20 IU of regular insulin is administered IV followed by continuous IV infusion of 5 to 10 IU/h. Infusion of small amounts of insulin (1 to 3 IU/h) is continued until acidosis clears. Volume resuscitation is needed (4 to 5 L in the first 24 hours). Liters of normal and half-normal saline are alternated to minimize risk for cerebral edema. Potassium replacement is essential. Unrecognized hypokalemia can cause death due to diabetic ketoacidosis.

Hyperosmolar Nonketotic Acidosis. Therapy is correction of the cause of the hyperosmolar nonketotic hyperglycemia, such as gram-negative sepsis. Hyperglycemia is corrected with administration of insulin. Volume depletion can be more severe than with diabetic ketoacidosis. Potassium supplementation must be provided.

Metabolic Alkalosis

Correction of potassium depletion and volume depletion corrects metabolic alkalosis. Volume depletion is corrected with chloride-containing solutions. For patients without intravascular volume deficits, renal excretion of bicarbonate can be enhanced with administration of acetazolamide. If renal excretion of bicarbonate cannot be increased because of renal insufficiency, or if the metabolic alkalosis is severe, acid may be administered to titrate the excess extracellular bicarbonate. Partial correction of the alkalosis is the initial goal. A guide is that 2.2 mEq/kg decreases serum bicarbonate by about 5 mEq/L. Dialysis may be necessary to remove excess bicarbonate.

Respiratory Alkalosis and Acidosis

Respiratory alkalosis is an increase in extracellular pH due to a decrease in P_{CO_2}. Causes of hyperventilation and the fall in P_{CO_2} include hypoxia, reflex stimulation from decreased pulmonary compliance, drugs, or mechanical ventilation. Therapy is management of the stimulus of hyperventilation. The cause of hypoxemia is determined and corrected. In acute symptomatic respiratory alkalosis, rebreathing or breathing 5% CO_2 temporarily relieves the symptoms. If the condition is due to mechanical ventilation, adjustment of tidal volume or respiratory rate resolves the respiratory alkalosis.

Respiratory acidosis is a decrease in extracellular pH due to an increase in P_{CO_2}. The cause is inadequate ventilation. Although pulmonary disease commonly causes hypoxemia, respiratory acidosis is uncommon because diffusion of O_2 is more readily impaired than diffusion of CO_2. The causes of hypoventilation include depression of the respiratory center, impaired respiratory excursion of the thorax, airway obstruction, chronic obstructive pulmonary disease, and inappropriate ventilatory settings.

Endotracheal intubation to achieve adequate ventilation is key to management of acute respiratory acidosis. Therapy for chronic, compensated respiratory acidosis may be complicated by hypoxemia. Complete correction of the hypoxemia may further suppress respiration and worsen the respiratory acidosis. P_{CO_2} must not be normalized rapidly. Reequilibration of cerebral bicarbonate concentration lags behind systemic changes.

SUGGESTED READING

Bachman S, Mundel P. Nitric oxide and the kidney: synthesis, localization and function. Am J Kid Dis 1994:24:112.

Briggs JP, Sawaya BE, Schnerman J. Disorders of salt balance. In: Kokko JP, Tannen RL, eds. Fluid and electrolytes. Philadelphia, WB Saunders, 1990:70.

Carroll HJ, Oh MS. Water, electrolyte and acid–base metabolism. Philadelphia, JB Lippincott, 1989:206.

Foster DW, McGarry JD. The metabolic derangements and treatment of diabetic ketoacidosis. N Engl J Med 1983;309:159.

Goetz KL. Renal natriuretic peptide (urodilatin?) and atriopeptin: evolving concepts. Am J Physiol 1991;261:F921.

Reuzzi G, Benigni A. Endothelins in the control of cardiovascular and renal function. Nature 1993:342:589.

Rodeberg DA, Chaet MS, Bass RC, Arkovitz MS, Garcia VF. Nitric oxide: an overview, Am J Surg 1995:170:292.

Wait RB, Kahng KU. Renal failure complicating obstructive jaundice. Am J Surg 1989;157:256.

ESSENTIALS OF SURGERY: SCIENTIFIC PRINCIPLES AND PRACTICE, edited by Lazar J. Greenfield, Michael W. Mulholland, Keith T. Oldham, Gerald B. Zelenock, and Keith D. Lillemoe. Lippincott–Raven Publishers, Philadelphia, © 1997.

CHAPTER 11

TRAUMA

DAVID B. HOYT, BRUCE M. POTENZA, H. GILL CRYER, BAXTER LARMON, JAMES W. DAVIS, RANDALL M. CHESNUT, LISA A. ORLOFF, GREGORY J. JURKOVICH, ROBERT J. WINCHELL, DAVID H. WISNER, ROBERT C. MACKERSIE, MICHAEL J. SISE, STEVEN R. SHACKFORD, MARK A. HEALEY, M. MARGARET KNUDSON, HEIDI L. FRANKEL, GRACE S. ROZYCKI, HOWARD R. CHAMPION, RICHARD K. SIMONS, AND LARRY M. GENTILELLO

Trauma is categorized as penetrating or blunt. Blunt trauma produces injury as the tissues are compressed or deceleration occurs. Penetrating trauma produces injury by crushing and separation of tissues along the path of the penetrating object.

MECHANICS OF INJURY

Blunt Trauma

The first and second ribs, sternum, scapula, and femur are the strongest and least vulnerable bones in the body. Fractures of these bones indicate severe trauma (Table 11-1).

Motor Vehicle Collisions

The patterns in motor vehicle collisions include head-on or frontal impact, rear impact, lateral or side impact, rotational impact, and rollover. As an automobile collides with an object, passengers collide with the interior of the automobile, and the internal organs collide with the body

Table 11-1. PATTERNS OF INJURY TO THE HEAD, NECK, TRUNK, AND EXTREMITIES ASSOCIATED WITH ORTHOPEDIC INJURIES

Diagnosed Injury	Associated Injury
Fracture—temporal, parietal bone	Epidural hematoma
Maxillofacial fracture	Cervical spine fracture
Sternal fracture	Cardiac contusion
First and second rib fracture	Descending thoracic aorta, intraabdominal bleeding
Fractured scapula	Pulmonary contusion
Fractured ribs 8–12, right	Lacerated liver
Fractured ribs 8–12, left	Lacerated spleen
Fractured pelvis	Ruptured bladder, urethral transection
Fractured humerus	Radial nerve injury
Supracondylar humerus	Brachial artery injury
Distal radius fracture	Median nerve compression
Supracondylar femur fracture	Thrombosis popliteal artery
Anterior dislocation shoulder	Axillary nerve injury
Posterior dislocation of hip	Sciatic nerve injury
Posterior dislocation of knee	Popliteal artery thrombosis

wall or are sheared from anatomic attachment. Each type of collision causes a different kind of damage.

Restraint Device Injury

Kinetic energy transfer from impact is absorbed by the bony pelvis and chest when three-point passenger restraints are used. If improperly positioned, lap belts rise above the pelvis, delivering this compression force to the soft tissues of the abdomen or retroperitoneum. Injuries associated with shoulder straps include clavicle and rib fractures and carotid artery injuries.

Motorcycles

Motorcycle trauma involves four types of impact: frontal, angular, ejection, and rear end collision. Each involves different types of injury.

Pedestrians

The initial impact between an adult and a vehicle is often from the car bumper, fracturing the tibia and fibula. A second strike may fracture the femur or pelvis and cause abdominal or thoracic injury. Head injury depends on whether the head strikes the car hood or is protected by the arms. A third impact occurs as the person falls away, striking the ground. This impact often causes head injury.

The initial impact between a child and a car bumper may injure the pelvis or upper femur. The second impact is when the front of the hood strikes the thorax. The final impact occurs as the child is dragged under the vehicle.

Falls

Falls result in multiple impacts. Energy transfer is due to the velocity achieved during the fall; the height of the fall determines the magnitude of injury. The surface on which the victim lands (eg, water vs concrete) affects energy transfer and the types of shear and tensile strain.

Penetrating Injuries

Penetrating trauma involves transfer of energy to a small tissue area. The kinetic energy of a bullet disrupts and fragments cells and tissues, moving them away from the path of the bullet. The actual size of the area of missile impact is determined by three factors: profile (cross-sectional area), tumble (spin and yaw), and fragmentation.

Evaluation of entrance and exit wounds is essential to assess the number of projectiles, their course, and which organs are at risk for injury. Once a missile penetrates tissue, the energy is distributed within a closed space and, depending on the organs that receive the impact and the type of tissue traversed, certain injuries can be anticipated. For example, in the thorax, lung parenchyma has low mass and sustains less damage from penetrating injury than other thoracic tissues.

Blood vessels that are not fixed may be pushed aside without marked damage. Large fixed vessels, such as the aorta and vena cava, are susceptible to fatal injury. When bones are penetrated, fragments may become secondary missiles that can lacerate the surrounding tissues. Low-velocity bullets may not follow a straight path, but rather ricochet through a body cavity, injuring organs. Muscles may expand out of the path of a missile, but this can result in stretching and hemorrhage. Injury to adjacent blood vessels can cause intimal damage and thrombosis even if most of the vessel is intact.

Penetrating injuries are evaluated with regard to topography. For example, in penetrating wounds of the abdomen, the possibility of vascular injury, particularly to the aorta and vena cava, must be considered. Associated abdominal injuries include hepatic and splenic, diaphragmatic, pulmonary, and gastric injuries. Duodenal and pancreatic injuries are common with injuries to the liver, inferior vena cava, stomach, and colon.

SCORING SYSTEMS AND INJURY ASSESSMENT

One way to classify trauma is to classify severity of injury: (1) injuries that are rapidly fatal, (2) injuries that may be fatal, and (3) injuries that are not fatal. The first group are exsanguinating injuries, massive head injuries, transection of the cervical spinal cord, or airway disruption; the victim dies in <10 minutes. The third group, affecting 80% of trauma patients, are minor soft tissue injuries or isolated extremity fractures. The following scoring systems were developed for patients with the second type of injury:(1) Revised Trauma Score (RTS) and triage (Table 11-2; Fig. 11-1); (2) Abbreviated Injury Scale (AIS) (Table 11-3); (3) Injury Severity Score (ISS) calculated by assigning AIS values to each injury in six body areas: (a) head and neck, (b) face, (c) chest, (d) abdomen and pelvic contents, (e) extremities and pelvis, and (f) general and cutaneous; (4) TRISS combines the trauma score, or physiologic component, and the ISS, or anatomic component. It also incorporates the patients' ages.

PREHOSPITAL AND RESUSCITATION CARE

Management of immediately life-threatening injuries begins during transport and continues after arrival at the trauma center. Rapid initial evaluation is followed by a detailed secondary survey. The management priorities are to identify and treat in the following order:

1. Airway obstruction
2. Inadequate ventilation
3. Free hemorrhage (external, intrapleural, intraperitoneal)
4. Epidural or subdural hematoma
5. Contained hemorrhage (retroperitoneal, transected aorta)
6. Peripheral vascular injury
7. Nonbleeding visceral injury
8. Long bone fracture

The secondary survey is interrupted as necessary to treat life- and limb-threatening injuries as they are identified.

Prehospital Care

Assessment and Management Priorities

Airway. Loss of airway patency is the priority of the response team on arrival at the injury site. Suctioning, placement of oropharyngeal airways, and use of bag mask

Table 11-2. REVISED TRAUMA SCORE COMPONENTS

Glasgow Coma Scale	Systolic Blood Pressure (mmHg)	Respiratory Rate (breaths/min)	Coded Value
13–15	>89	10–29	4
9–12	76–89	>29	3
6–8	50–75	6–9	2
4–5	1–49	1–5	1
3	0	0	0

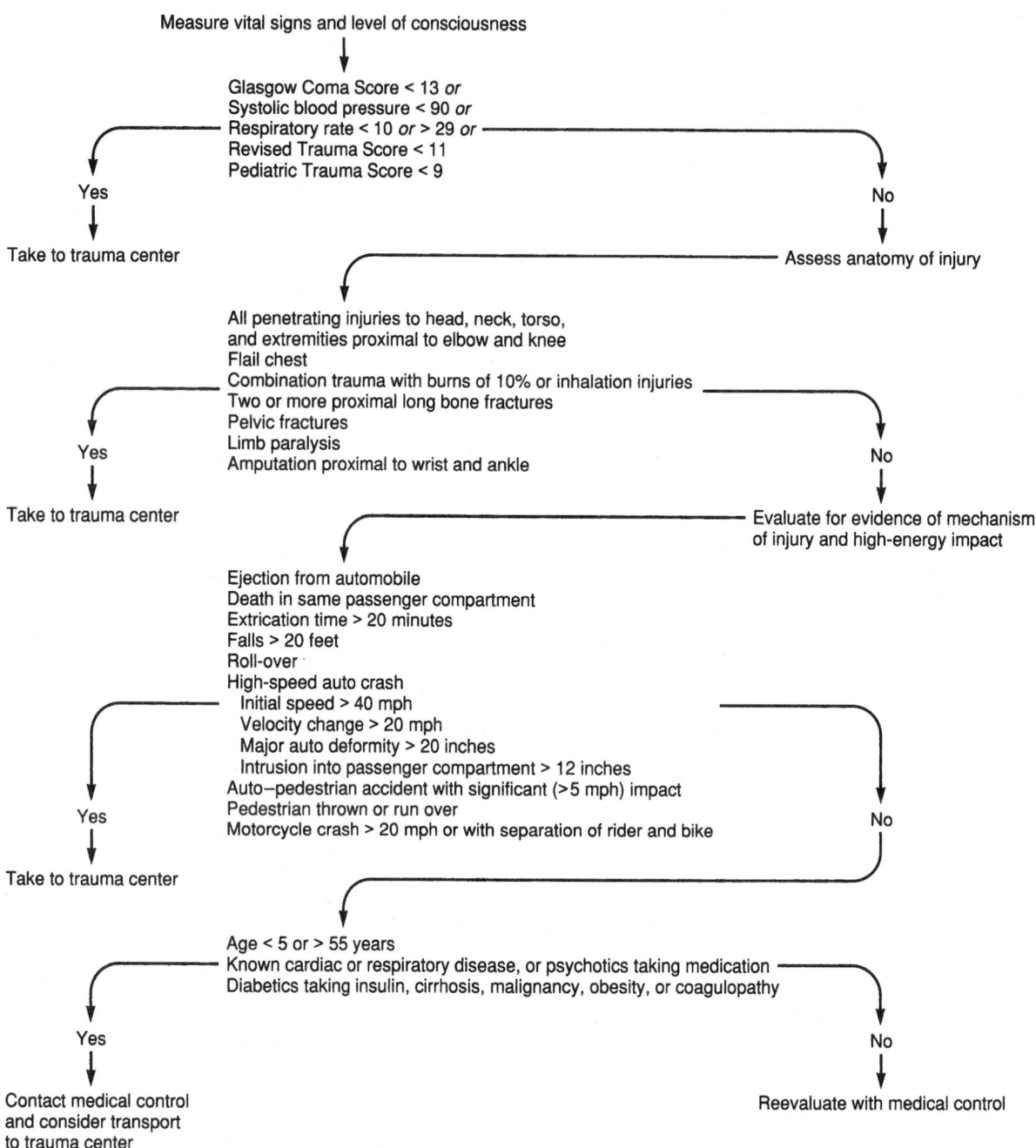

Figure 11-1. Field triage decision scheme as recommended by the American College of Surgeons.

devices temporarily restore oxygenation at the injury scene.

Indications for endotracheal intubation in the field include respiratory distress, hypovolemic shock, unconsciousness, severe head injury, and severe chest injury.

Breathing. After establishment of an airway, the next step is to ensure that air exchange is taking place. Problems with breathing are handled by means of endotracheal intubation, assisted ventilation, and rapid transport to a trauma center.

Circulation. The most common cause of death during the first hour after injury is hemorrhage. After establishment of a patent airway and adequate air exchange, the next step is support of the circulation. Direct pressure con-

trols obvious external hemorrhage. The placement of one or two large-bore IV lines in the upper extremities en route to the trauma center facilitates resuscitation. The standard of care in the prehospital setting for hypotensive patients is volume replacement and application of a pneumatic antishock garment (PASG).

Resuscitation Phase

Primary Survey

The trauma team receives the patient from the transport team in a specially equipped resuscitation room. The priority is simultaneous assessment of airway, blood pressure, and level of consciousness. This examination begins with

Table 11-3. ABBREVIATED INJURY SCALE SCORING SYSTEM FOR ABDOMINAL INJURIES

Score	Injury Examples
1	Abdominal wall abrasion
2	Liver, stomach, colon, mesentery contusion
3	Minor liver or spleen laceration
	Bowel laceration without perforation
4	Major liver or spleen laceration
	Bowel laceration with perforation
5	Major liver or spleen laceration with tissue loss
	Bowel laceration with tissue loss

observation of ability to talk and breathe and palpation of the wrist for a pulse.

Airway obstruction often responds to simple maneuvers such as suctioning, chin lift jaw thrust, and placement of an oropharyngeal airway. Protection of the cervical spine with inline immobilization is imperative during these maneuvers. Persistence of respiratory insufficiency necessitates endotracheal intubation. Unsuccessful intubation necessitates cricothyroidotomy. When cricothyroidotomy cannot be performed, tracheotomy must be. After intubation, auscultation of the chest is performed to confirm air exchange. A chest radiograph ensures proper tube position.

After establishment of an airway, *ventilatory exchange* is assessed by means of rapid auscultation of both lung fields and assessment for mechanical factors that may interfere with breathing. These include compression of the lung from hemothorax, pneumothorax, or visceral herniation; loss of chest wall stability from flail chest; lung damage from pulmonary contusion; and airway obstruction from aspiration. Cyanosis, intense respiratory effort without air movement, distended neck veins, and lack of breath sounds on chest auscultation indicate tension pneumothorax. The diagnosis is confirmed with immediate needle thoracostomy followed by chest tube thoracostomy.

Sucking chest wounds are sealed with an occlusive dressing secured on three sides to function as a flap valve. Most other problems become evident on the initial chest radiograph and are relieved by chest tube insertion, suctioning, or repositioning of the endotracheal tube.

The third step is to assess *circulatory status* by estimating blood volume and cardiac function. Blood pressure, pulse, skin perfusion and capillary refill, mental status, breath sounds, and neck vein distention are clinical indicators of hemodynamic status. The first step is to establish whether a patient is in hypovolemic shock and, if so, the magnitude of shock. Management of hypotension is volume resuscitation with crystalloid solution and packed red blood cells (RBCs).

The final step in the primary survey is a brief *neurologic evaluation* with the Glasgow Coma Scale (see Table 104-1). A patient with a GCS 8 is assumed to have a brain injury. In this situation, aggressive brain resuscitation, including hyperventilation, restoration of circulating volume, and provision of adequate oxygenation is essential.

Secondary Survey

The secondary survey is directed at identification of suspected and unsuspected injuries. It consists of observation and palpation of the entire body for evidence of injury. The priorities of the secondary survey depend on the results of the primary survey and response to initial resuscitative efforts. For example, the secondary survey for a patient in

hemorrhagic shock and unresponsive to initial resuscitative efforts during the primary survey consists only of rapid identification of the bleeding site and rapid transport to the operating room for definitive control of hemorrhage. A completely stable patient with relatively minor injuries undergoes a complete physical examination with confirmatory laboratory and radiographic tests before initiation of treatment:

Head and face
  Palpation of the skull and the head
  Testing of visual acuity, pupillary function, and ocular range of motion, fundoscopic examination
  Palpation of the facial bones
  Reassessment of the airway
Neck
  Examination for tracheal deviation, subcutaneous emphysema, hematomas, or distended jugular veins
  Palpation of posterior cervical spine to elicit tenderness or other signs of obvious fractures
  Determination and documentation of cranial nerve function
  Assessment of carotid pulses
  No probing, cannulation, or exploration past the platysma muscle. [For wounds that penetrate the platysma, surgical neck exploration or a combination of angiography, endoscopy, contrast radiography, computed tomography (CT), and observation
  CT evaluation of bone and ligament injuries]
Chest
  Chest wall inspection for instability (flail chest) and lacerations, sucking chest wounds, abrasions, and contusions
  Auscultation
  Chest radiograph
  Electrocardiogram (ECG)
  Echocardiography
  Arch aortography, spiral dynamic CT, transesophageal echocardiography
  Chest tube placement
  Bronchoscopy, esophagoscopy, aortography, and pericardial window
Abdomen
  Diagnostic peritoneal lavage (DPL)
  CT
  Serum amylase
  Ultrasound (US) examination
  Local exploration of wound
  Laparoscopy
  Exploratory laparotomy
Pelvis
  Palpation
  Inspection of the genitalia
  Bimanual pelvic examination
  Rectal examination
  Urethrography
  Radiographs of the pelvis
  Angiography
Extremities
  Examination for open wounds and open fracture
  Evaluation of pulses, auscultation for bruits, recognition of expanding hematomas
  Palpation and passive range of motion tests
  Duplex scanning or arteriography

SHOCK

Shock can result from a variety of insults, including hypovolemic, septic, cardiac, or neurologic compromise. It is defined by blood flow that is insufficient to meet the metabolic demands of organs and tissues. Shock is covered in Chapter 8.

HEAD INJURIES

Complications of closed head injuries are the single largest cause of morbidity and mortality among patients who reach the hospital alive. Most injuries are a result of blunt trauma, and motor vehicle accidents (MVAs) are the most frequent cause. Nervous system injury is covered in Chapter 104.

MAXILLOFACIAL INJURIES

The main causes of maxillofacial trauma are MVAs, direct assault, industrial and sports-related injuries, and low- and high-velocity GSWs. Airway compromise and hemorrhage are immediate concerns. Associated brain and cervical spine injuries must be recognized, and timing of treatment must be coordinated with care of torso and extremity injuries.

Early Considerations

Maxillofacial injuries usually are identified while the airway is being secured. Until proved otherwise, a patient with maxillofacial injuries is treated as if the cervical spine is unstable. Direct pressure is applied to external sites of bleeding; packing is used for nasal and pharyngeal hemorrhage.

Definitive Care

Infection Prophylaxis

Contaminated wounds are managed with prophylactic antibiotics until definitive treatment is delivered. Oral hygiene also is extremely important.

Management of Soft Tissue Injuries

Foreign bodies, gross debris, and bacterial contamination are scrubbed and rinsed from the wound. Antiseptic solutions are followed by copious irrigation with sterile saline solution. Tissues are kept moist with saline solution until they are closed.

Before wound closure, tissue is assessed for damage and loss. Small amounts of tissue that are abraded or crushed are excised. Larger areas are allowed to heal, and scar revision is performed later. Jagged wound edges are reapproximated without trimming. Avulsion wounds and defects with tissue loss are closed. Large defects are closed with flaps or grafts. Lacerations of the facial nerve are repaired at the time of soft tissue repair.

Management of Bony Injuries

Facial fractures are treated with closed or open reduction, with or without wire or rigid fixation. Nondisplaced fractures may require no treatment at all. Displaced fractures necessitate reduction and stabilization and management of injuries to the facial soft tissues and intracranial structures.

NECK INJURIES
Initial Management

After initial resuscitation, a physical examination is performed to detect associated injuries and define the extent of neck trauma. Neck wounds are *not probed* because they may dislodge a clot and reinstitute hemorrhage. The neck is palpated, and normal anatomic landmarks and areas of tenderness are recorded. Crepitus of subcutaneous emphysema indicates injury to the trachea, esophagus or lung until proved otherwise. If the patient is able to talk, the presence of hoarseness, dysphagia, or dysphonia is determined. Hemoptysis and hematemesis are signs of tracheal or esophageal injury. Table 11-4 lists the signs of injury that mandate neck exploration.

All patients with blunt or penetrating neck trauma undergo chest radiography to rule out thoracic trauma. Patients in stable condition undergo soft tissue neck radiography to rule out retropharyngeal hematoma, tracheal narrowing or deviation, retained missile fragments and pathways, and subcutaneous or retropharyngeal air. Neck CT is used in blunt trauma to evaluate the larynx. Patients with blunt neck trauma with inconsistent neurologic and CT findings undergo cerebral angiography.

Neck exploration is performed in the operating room under general endotracheal anesthesia. Extension of the neck incision into a median sternotomy allows exposure of the thoracic great vessels. The injury is followed to its depth, and each structure in or near the track is systematically examined. Surgical management depends on the extent of the injury and the structure involved carotid and vertebral arteries, trachea and larynx, pharynx and esophagus.

CHEST INJURIES

Blunt injuries to the chest are more common than penetrating injuries, except in urban areas. Most injuries to the chest can be managed without surgical intervention. Tube thoracostomy is used to manage hemothorax and pneumothorax. Thoracotomy is needed to control massive bleeding or bleeding that persists despite tube thoracostomy.

ABDOMINAL INJURIES
Hospital Resuscitation and Diagnosis

Figures 11-2 and 11-3 are diagnostic algorithms for abdominal trauma. Indications for laparotomy include signs of peritonitis, unexplained shock, evisceration, uncontrolled hemorrhage, clinical deterioration during observation, and DPL consistent with hemoperitoneum. In preparation for laparotomy, the patient must be protected from hypotension during the early stages of surgical exploration. Vascular access must be secure. Femoral venous lines or large-bore catheters placed by means of saphenous cutdown at the ankle are options for rapid infusion of large volumes of fluid. If the patient has lost large amounts of blood, central venous catheterization is performed.

Table 11-4. CLINICAL SIGNS OF SIGNIFICANT INJURY IN PENETRATING NECK TRAUMA

VASCULAR	DIGESTIVE TRACT
Shock	Hemoptysis
Active bleeding	Dysphagia or odynophagia
Large or expanding hematoma	Hematemesis
Pulse deficit	Subcutaneous emphysema

AIRWAY	NEUROLOGIC
Dyspnea	Focal or lateralized neurologic deficit
Stridor	
Hoarseness	
Dysphonia or voice change	
Subcutaneous emphysema	

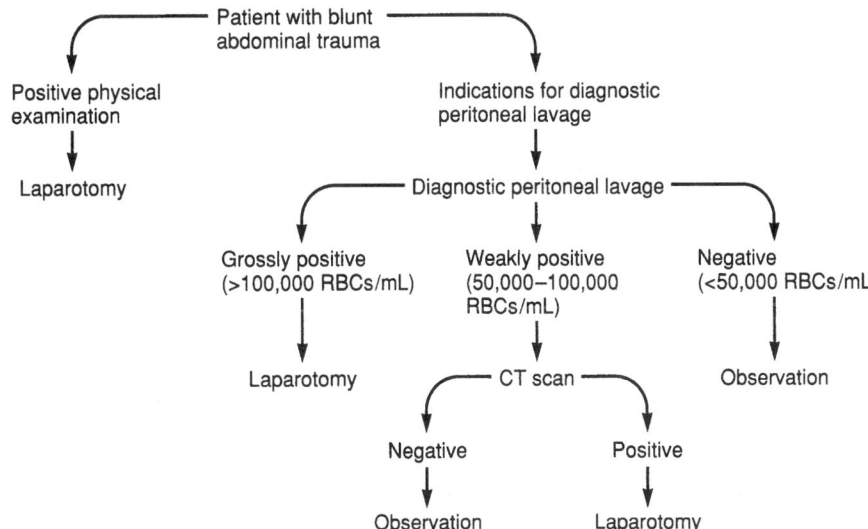

Figure 11-2. Diagnostic algorithm for blunt abdominal trauma.

Broad-spectrum antibiotics are given as soon as the decision to perform a laparotomy is made. The postoperative use of antibiotics is dictated by the surgical findings. Tetanus prophylaxis is administered.

The patient is prepared from sternal notch to midthigh to allow harvesting of saphenous vein if necessary, and a midline incision is made. Once the abdomen is opened, obvious blood and clot are removed from the lower abdomen and the upper abdomen by means of packing of all four quadrants of the abdomen. If the peritoneal cavity is full of blood, the location of clot is often a clue to the site of bleeding. Any source of hemorrhage can be repacked. Inflow occlusion can be accomplished if needed by clamping the aorta at the diaphragmatic hiatus.

Obvious hollow viscus wounds are rapidly sutured. This initial closure does not have to be definitive and is done primarily to minimize contamination during the operation.

Retroperitoneal hematomas may be the source of exsanguinating hemorrhage if rupture into the free peritoneal cavity has occurred. If not, they can be left for later examination, depending on location. Hematomas of the pelvis associated with pelvic fractures and stable hematomas in the perinephric space lateral to the midline are not disturbed. Central hematomas that may involve injury to large blood vessels, pancreas, or duodenum are explored after control of injuries in the peritoneal cavity.

Once hemorrhage is controlled with packing and ongoing contamination is stopped, time is taken to allow resuscitation of circulating blood volume. Warming may be performed at this time if massive blood loss has occurred. Once the abdominal injuries are repaired, the contents of the abdomen are explored.

RETROPERITONEAL INJURIES
Pelvic Fractures

The spectrum of pelvic fracture injuries ranges from minor isolated nondisplaced fractures of the pubic rami to severe injuries with multiple fractures that may be rapidly lethal. The proximity of adjacent organs presents high risk for genitourinary (GU) and abdominal injuries. Screening radiographs of the pelvis are obtained for all patients with severe blunt injuries or hypotension from any blunt mechanism.

Massive hemorrhage is the main cause of early death among patients with pelvic fractures. Survival depends on rapid identification and control (Fig. 11-4). Grossly positive DPL is considered an indication for exploratory laparotomy in adults.

At laparotomy, once thorough abdominal exploration is performed and injuries repaired, the size of the pelvic he-

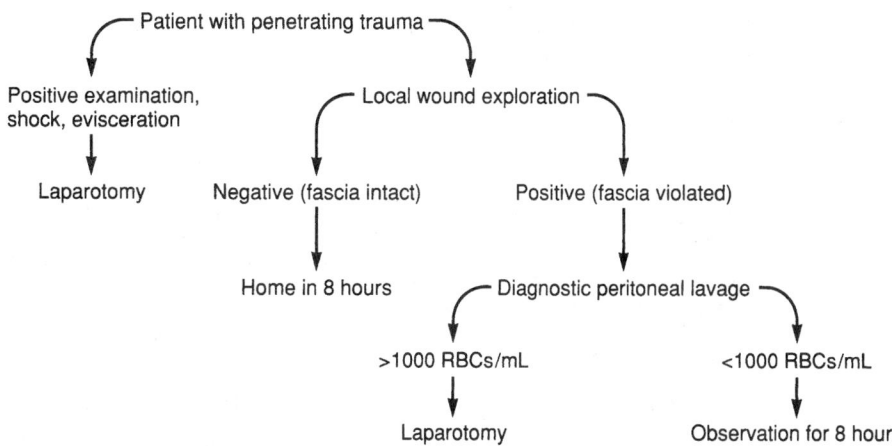

Figure 11-3. Diagnostic algorithm for low-velocity penetrating abdominal trauma.

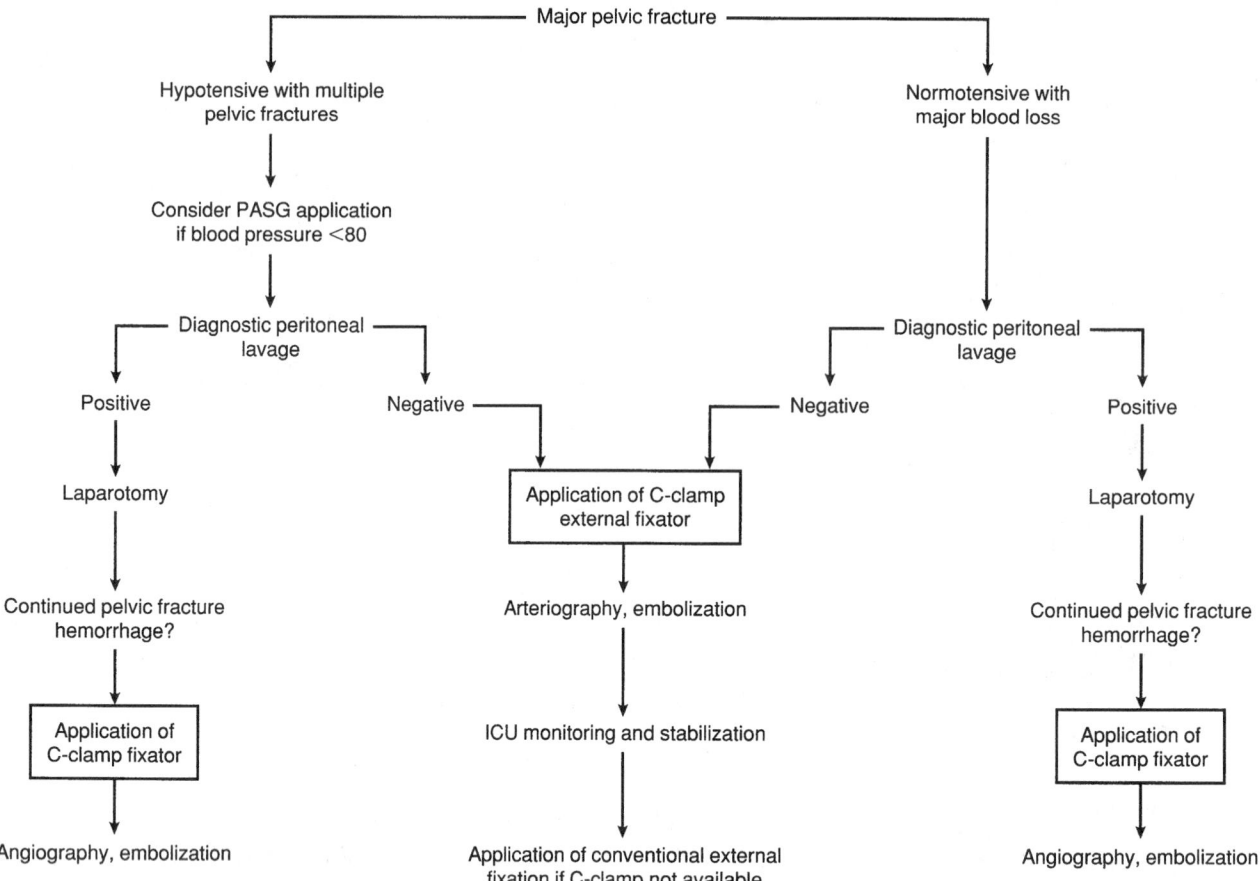

Figure 11-4. Algorithm for the initial management of abdominal and pelvic hemorrhage. External pelvic fixation should precede arteriography only if it is immediately available. PASG, pneumatic antishock garment.

matoma may be assessed. Pelvic fracture hemorrhage rarely can be controlled surgically, and decompression of the hematoma may exacerbate bleeding. For rapidly expanding pelvic hematomas, placement of laparotomy packs in the pelvis to aid in tamponade may provide effective temporary control. Rapid closure of the abdominal wound is followed immediately by pelvic angiography and embolization of active arterial bleeding.

After control of hemorrhage, management of pelvic fractures involves orthopedic stabilization of the fracture sites. An exception is open pelvic fractures with extensive soft tissue injury to the perineum or rectum. For these fractures fecal diversion is undertaken after control of hemorrhage and other life-threatening injuries and correction of hypothermia, coagulopathy, and acidosis.

Renal Injuries

Three factors suggest renal trauma shock, gross hematuria, and serious associated injuries (pelvic fracture, spinal or abdominal injuries). Intravenous pyelography (IVP) is indicated for all stab wounds or GSWs to the flank or upper abdomen if clinical status allows the time. IVP abnormalities that suggest renal injury prompt CT evaluation.

Most blunt renal injuries diagnosed with preoperative CT are contusions and minor lacerations and may be treated nonsurgically with close monitoring and follow-up CT. Patients with evidence of ongoing hemorrhage, large or expanding perinephric hematomas, collecting system disruptions, or persistent hemorrhage into the collecting system undergo early surgical treatment.

The goal of renal exploration is to control hemorrhage and salvage the kidney. GSWs necessitate exploratory laparotomy because of risk for other abdominal injuries and complex renal injury. Some stab wounds produce only minor isolated renal lacerations without hilar or collecting system involvement and minimal hematomas. Some patients can be treated nonsurgically.

The surgical approach to renal trauma includes proximal control of the renal artery and vein. Once control of the renal hilum is obtained, the kidney is explored. The surgical approach depends on the injury. The objectives are to control hemorrhage, repair injuries to the collecting system, and revascularize or remove nonperfused renal tissue. Options include simple suture repair of lacerations with or without pedicle flap coverage, partial nephrectomy with oversewing of vessels and repair of the collecting system, and total nephrectomy. Repair must be performed within 8 hours of injury if ischemic kidney parenchyma is to be salvaged. Postoperative complications of renal trauma include recurrent hemorrhage, arteriovenous fistula, and urinary extravasation with fistula or urinoma.

Bladder Injuries

Most blunt bladder injuries occur in association with pelvic fractures. The most common mechanism is laceration of the extraperitoneal bladder. Severe deceleration can burst the dome of the bladder. Penetrating injuries to the bladder usually are associated with other abdominal injuries. Cystography is performed on any patient with visible blood in the urine in association with a pelvic fracture. Small retroperitoneal perforations may be missed, so the bladder must be emptied and a postvoid radiograph obtained. All male patients are examined for scrotal or urethral hematoma, free-floating prostate, or blood at the meatus. Retrograde urethrography is performed before urinary catheters are placed.

Intraperitoneal bladder ruptures require prompt surgical repair. After bladder repair a simple urethral catheter is left in place. Most extraperitoneal bladder injuries can be managed nonsurgically by means of urethral catheter drainage. Patients with extraperitoneal bladder rupture are given antibiotics for the duration of urinary catheter placement.

Ureteral Injuries

Ureteral injuries occur less frequently than injuries to the bladder or kidney. They are most often caused by GSWs and stab wounds. A search for ureteral injury is required for any penetrating trauma.

The diagnosis of a ureteral injury after trauma usually can be made if an IVP shows a cutoff in ureteral drainage or contrast extravasation. About 15% of ureteral injuries are not evident initially on IVP, so retrograde ureterography is necessary to confirm the diagnosis.

Ureteral injuries must be excluded at operation. Exploration of the wound tract excludes or confirms ureteral injury. With massive retroperitoneal hematomas or multiple penetrating injuries, direct inspection of the entire ureter may not be feasible, so intraoperative IVP or chromopyelography is performed.

Ureteral injuries are managed at the time of initial injury. In penetrating trauma, short segments of ureter are involved, and there is little, if any, loss of length. Primary ureteroureterostomy with stenting or reimplantation of the distal ureter into the bladder can be performed. For ureteral injuries involving loss of a long segment, as with shotgun injuries, the problem is complex. Lower ureteral injuries may be repaired by means of reimplantation of the distal ureter into the bladder. Transureteroureterostomy is an option for lower and middle ureteral injuries.

Urethral Injuries

Any male patient with a pelvic fracture may have a urethral tear. These patients are examined for signs of urethral injury, including scrotal or perineal hematomas, blood at the urethral meatus, or anterior displacement of the prostate during rectal examination. Any of these findings is a *contraindication* to immediate placement of a urethral catheter. A retrograde urethrogram is obtained.

Initial management of urethral tears consists of suprapubic cystostomy for urinary drainage. Because of risk for impotence and urinary stricture, immediate repair or reconstruction of the urethra is not attempted. Formal reconstruction of urethral tears is performed several months after the injury.

VASCULAR INJURIES
Diagnosis

Vascular trauma frequently is occult. The history is noteworthy if the presence of arterial bleeding (pulsatile, oxygenated blood) or severe venous bleeding (dark blood flowing from the wound) can be obtained. The presence of hypotension also is an important observation.

Abdominal or thoracic vascular injury is likely when penetrating torso trauma is associated with hypovolemic shock. Blunt injury to the great vessels is likely whenever there is external evidence of thoracic trauma, such as a steering wheel imprint on the anterior chest. Other signs of thoracic vascular trauma are a widened mediastinum, thoracic outlet hematoma, upper extremity hypotension, and diminished lower-extremity pulse. A history of altered mental status or intermittent paralysis suggests aortic or arch vessel disruption.

The course of a penetrating injury is estimated visually and with plain radiographs with radiopaque markers of entrance and exit sites. Patients with blunt injuries need a complete examination with emphasis on examination of the pulses. Once fluid resuscitation is complete, peripheral pulses should be palpable. Doppler US and duplex scanning can be used to evaluate extremity vascular trauma. Complete proximal occlusion or arterial disruption results in distal ischemia (Table 11-5).

Arteriography is used to rule out the presence of occult vascular injury in patients with a suggestive history or physical examination and to establish the anatomy and location of an injury. In the absence of signs of vascular injury, patients with penetrating wounds close to large vessels may undergo observation without arteriography. If the patient's condition is unstable, there are other injuries, and occult extremity arterial trauma is suspected, arteriography may be performed in the emergency department or on the operating table.

Surgical Management

The goal of surgical management of vascular injuries is rapid control of hemorrhage and restoration of perfusion with salvage of the extremity or organ in jeopardy. IV broad-spectrum antibiotics are administered. For injury to an isolated extremity with arterial occlusion, systemic heparin is administered. *In the presence of multiple injuries, especially if there is CNS trauma, heparin is inappropriate.* Tetanus prophylaxis is administered.

A wide sterile surgical field is prepared to allow exposure of vessels with proximal and distal control. A lower extremity always is prepared as a site for saphenous vein harvest. In patients with lower-extremity injury, the contralateral limb is prepared for vein harvest. For patients with possible neck or abdominal sites of vascular trauma, the chest is prepared to allow access to the aorta and its branches.

If there are skeletal injuries, vascular repair is performed first, followed by stabilization of the skeletal injuries. Proximal and distal control of the injured vessel is accomplished through uninjured areas adjacent to the injury.

Table 11-5. PHYSICAL FINDINGS ASSOCIATED WITH EXTREMITY VASCULAR INJURY

Classic Signs	Signs of Occult Injury
Pulsatile bleeding	History of significant hemorrhage
Thrill or bruit	Proximity wounds
Pain	Peripheral nerve deficit
Pulselessness	Diminished pulse
Pallor	Fracture dislocation (knee, elbow)
Paresthesias	Unexplained shock
Paralysis	
Poikilothermia	

Balloon-tipped catheters can be inserted through the site of injury and inflated if necessary.

Once control is established, thrombectomy of the proximal and distal arteries is performed until there is no evidence of thrombus. Heparinized saline solution is flushed proximally and distally into the lumen of the artery. The artery is repaired, usually by means of end-to-end anastomosis.

In the repair of extensive arterial injuries, reversed saphenous vein from an uninjured lower extremity is the first choice for interposition graft. Intraoperative completion angiography is mandatory to determine the adequacy of repair, confirm patency, and visualize distal arterial runoff.

Proximal extremity veins and the great veins are repaired whenever feasible to avoid the sequelae of venous occlusion. Techniques of repair vary from simple suture closure to saphenous vein patch or graft interposition. Venous repair is not attempted if the patient's condition is hemodynamically unstable.

Wound management is essential to limb salvage after vascular trauma to the extremities. Débridement and pulse irrigation with copious amounts of antibiotic solution are performed. Coverage of the vascular repair with viable muscle or fascia and subcutaneous tissue is essential to prevent desiccation and infection. Monitoring for compartment syndrome is essential if ischemia has been prolonged. Primary skin closure is delayed except for injuries that involve minimal trauma or surgical dissection.

ORTHOPAEDIC AND SPINAL INJURIES

Orthopedic Injuries in the Primary Survey

Injuries to the axial spine and pelvis and multiple long-bone fractures can affect hemodynamic stability and ability to assess other injuries. It is important to assess bleeding due to orthopedic injuries. For example, a closed femoral fracture, simple or complex, causes 1 to 2 units of blood loss. Multiple fractures can produce shock.

Pain from multiple orthopedic injuries can complicate assessment of injuries at other locations. Physical examination of the chest, abdomen, and cervical spine often re-

lies on the patient's ability to react to pain during palpation, and pelvic or rib fractures may produce such pain during abdominal palpation. Radiographs, DPL, CT, or US are objective screening tools for abdominal injuries. The following are true orthopedic emergencies and necessitate immediate intervention: pelvic fracture, spinal injury with neurologic compromise, open fractures, dislocations with potential for neurovascular compromise.

Compartment Syndrome

When bleeding or edema occurs inside a closed fascial compartment, the pressures within that compartment may become high enough to impair blood flow and lower oxygen tension, resulting in impaired cellular metabolism, and cell death. This syndrome occurs commonly after crush injury to an extremity with or without fractures, and also after a period of ischemia followed by reperfusion. Compartment syndrome may be present during the initial assessment, or it may not appear until the postoperative or postresuscitative period. If there has been prolonged elevation of the limb on a fracture table or prolonged use of a PASG, this complication can occur on the uninjured side. It must be diagnosed and managed early to avoid loss of a functional limb. For patients with multiple injuries, this involves measurement of compartment pressures and early surgical release if needed.

PEDIATRIC TRAUMA
Anatomic and Physiologic Considerations in Children

The small size of pediatric patients increases the likelihood of multiple system trauma because the force of impact is dissipated over a small area. The higher frequency of head injuries among children than adults is partially explained by the greater head-to-body ratio, thin skull, and weaker supporting cervical musculature. In infants with unfused cranial sutures and open fontanels, intracranial hemorrhage can be profuse and cause shock. The mediastinum is mobile in childhood, and intrapleural pressure increases due to hemothorax or pneumothorax cause mediastinal shift and obstruction of venous return more readily

Table 11-6. TRAUMA SCORING SYSTEMS

Revised Trauma Score*			
Glasgow Coma Scale Score	Systolic Blood Pressure (mmHg)	Respiratory Rate	Coded Value
13–15	>89	10–29	4
9–12	76–89	>29	3
6–8	50–75	6–9	2
4–5	1–49	1–5	1
3	0	0	0

Pediatric Trauma Score†						
Size (kg)	Airway	Blood Pressure (mmHg)	CNS	Open Wound	Skeletal Wound	Score
>20	Normal	>90	Awake	None	None	+2
10–20	Maintained	50–90	Obtunded	Minor	Closed	+1
<10	Required	<50	Coma	Major	Multiple	−1

* An RTS of 11 or less predicts increased mortality and can be used as a triage index. (Boyd CR, Tolson MA, Cope WS. Evaluating trauma care: the TRISS method. J Trauma 1987;27:370).
† A PTS of 8 or less is associated with increased mortality.
(Tepas JJ, Ramenofsky ML, Mollit DL, Gaus BM, DiScala C. The Pediatric Trauma Score as a predictor of injury severity. J Pediatr Surg 1987;22:14)

than in adults. The protuberant abdomen of a child is not protected by the thoracic cage or pelvis, making abdominal injuries more likely. The bones of young children are not completely calcified, and bending can occur without fracture (buckle fractures), or only one cortex may be involved (greenstick fractures). Fractures through immature epiphyses can present long-term growth problems.

The physiologic response to hypovolemia after pediatric trauma is immediate constriction of small and medium-sized arteries, in order to maintain normal blood pressure. Tachycardia, tachypnea, diminished peripheral perfusion, and change in level of consciousness are better indicators of early shock than blood pressure. The thin skin, lack of subcutaneous fat, and large surface area to body weight ratio contribute to the propensity of young children for hypothermia. Hypothermia can induce pulmonary hypertension, increase hypoxia, and exacerbate metabolic acidosis, rendering the child unresponsive to resuscitation.

Triage and Prehospital Care

The prehospital care of an injured child is limited to assessing and securing the airway and stabilization of the spine and obvious fractures. During short transport times, IV access is not necessary. For longer transport times (>20 min), intraosseous infusion is begun, especially for children in shock. Children with minor injuries are cared for in the emergency department of the local hospital, close to family and pediatrician. Children with life-threatening injuries go to a trauma center. The trauma scores used for children are shown in Table 11-6.

Initial Evaluation and Resuscitation

Figure 11-5 shows the pediatric resuscitation algorithm.

Child Abuse

The physical signs of child abuse include periorbital injuries; retinal hemorrhage; multiple subdural hematomas without a fresh skull fracture; genital or perianal injuries; burns in unusual areas; and radiographic evidence of multiple old or healed fractures. When abuse is suspected, hospital admission is mandatory. All who care for injured children have the ethical and legal responsibility to report the possibility of child abuse.

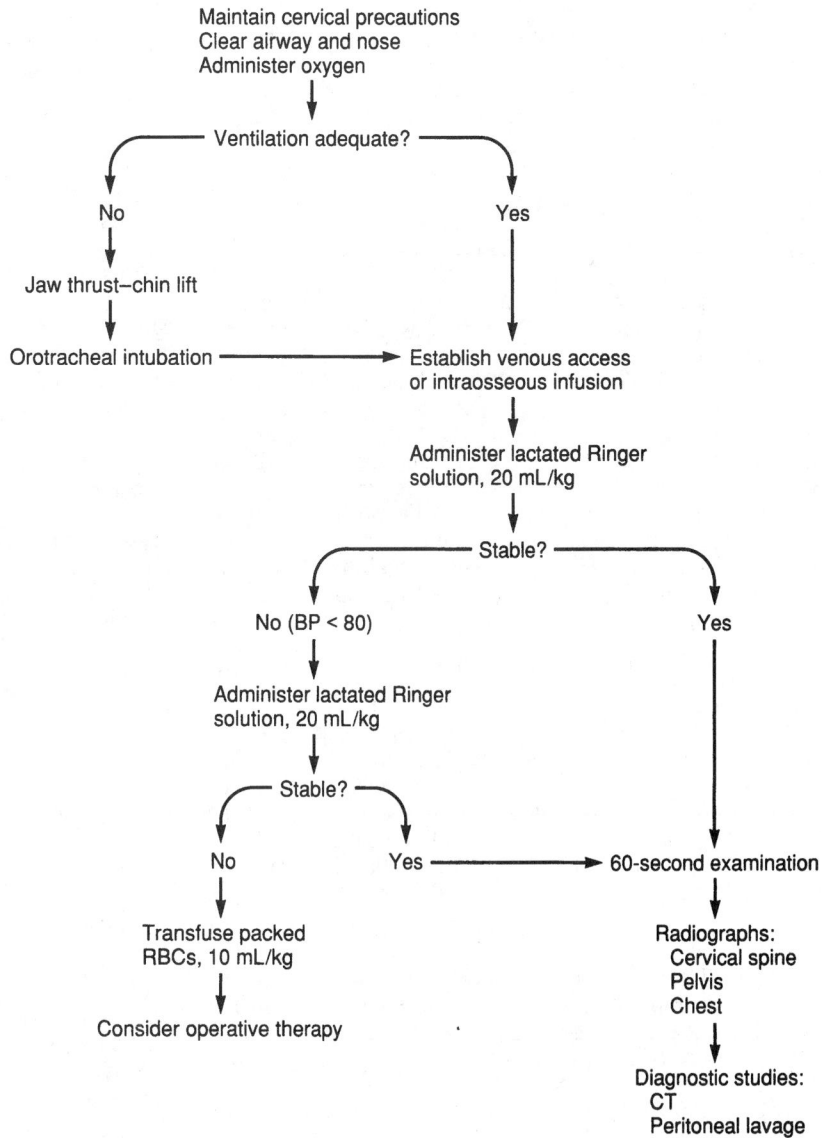

Figure 11-5. Pediatric resuscitation algorithm.

GERIATRIC TRAUMA

Initial Evaluation and Resuscitation

The initial resuscitation of the elderly injured patient follows the basic principles of trauma care with special considerations based on physiologic alterations. Elderly people are likely to be accustomed to higher than normal blood pressures. Fluid resuscitation therapy must be precise. Geriatric trauma patients with an ISS >9, evidence of shock or hypoperfusion, or a history of intercurrent disease may undergo monitoring with pulmonary artery and intraarterial catheters during the initial resuscitation.

After the initial resuscitation efforts and the primary survey, it is important to obtain a detailed account of the events surrounding the trauma. A heart attack or stroke may have preceded a fall or MVA. The history includes questions about medications used. For example, long-term diuretic therapy can lead to intravascular volume and electrolyte deficiencies, contributing to development of shock after trauma.

Radiographs of the chest, spine, and pelvis are obtained in the trauma resuscitation room. Degenerative changes in the cervical spine increase the likelihood of spinal cord injury after trauma. The sclerotic changes and the osteophytes present on the bones of elderly patients make plain radiographs difficult to interpret. CT may be needed to delineate spinal fractures.

Cerebral atrophy accompanies aging. The cerebral vasculature is fragile, particularly the veins. The combination of these factors makes elderly people prone to subdural hematoma. CT of the head is used liberally in the treatment of elderly patients.

TRAUMA IN PREGNANCY

Initial Assessment and Management

The best treatment of the unborn child is expedient resuscitation of the mother. An airway with supplemental oxygenation is essential to prevent fetal hypoxemia. Maternal hemorrhagic shock, with its resultant catecholamine release, causes uterine artery vasoconstriction, reducing uterine perfusion and compromising fetal viability. Vigorous crystalloid resuscitation is provided, even for patients who appear normotensive. An NG tube is inserted because of pregnant patients' propensity toward vomiting and aspiration. Urinary volume per hour is monitored to evaluate perfusion status. If a PASG is used to stabilize fractures or control hemorrhage; the abdominal component is *not* inflated.

History and Physical Examination

The secondary survey consists of a history (including obstetric history), physical examination, and fetal monitoring. Gestational age (fetal maturity) is estimated with measurements of fundal height at palpation. Pelvic and rectal examinations are performed, with special attention to vaginal discharge (amniotic fluid or blood), effacement, dilatation, and fetal station. The Kliehaure–Betke (KB) test detects fetal cells in the maternal circulation.

Fetal Assessment and Monitoring

Fetal evaluation consists of uterine assessment, fundal height measurement, and recording of heart tones, heart rate (100 beats/min or less is considered bradycardia), and movement. Uterine tenderness and contraction may be related to abruptio placentae, which may occur in the absence of vaginal bleeding. Auscultation for 1 minute determines regularity (acceleration–deceleration). Continuous fetal monitoring is used to evaluate fetal response (healthy vs distressed). A guideline for fetal monitoring of patients with severe injuries, including shock, is to provide continuous fetal monitoring for 48 hours after stabilization.

Fetal heart rate and uterine activity may be monitored with external (indirect) or internal (direct) methods. Normal fetal heart rate is 120 to 160 beats/min. Abnormalities in variability may signal hypoxia or dysrhythmia in the fetus. US is used to determine fetal viability.

Management

Blunt Trauma

Pelvic fractures, usually incurred in MVAs, in a pregnant patient cause extensive retroperitoneal hemorrhage because the pelvic veins are engorged. These fractures often cause direct fetal injury, usually skull fracture or intracerebral hemorrhage. Uterine rupture due to blunt trauma occurs most often at the site of prior cesarean section or at the posterior fundus. It can present with massive hemorrhage or with minimal vaginal bleeding if rupture occurs at the fundus. Repair can be primary in two layers or with a prosthetic patch.

Placental abruption occurs within 48 h after trauma. Separation >50% invariably results in fetal death. Placental abruption may occur in the absence of obvious abdominal injury. Maternal shock is a far greater stimulus for abruption than mechanical forces. Pregnant patients who are at risk are monitored accordingly.

Surgical Care

General anesthesia is used for pregnant patients with multisystem injury. Intraoperative fetal monitoring is imperative. A vertical midline incision is used. The pregnant uterus does not affect the need for exploration or repair of an injury. Indications for cesarean section are: maternal shock, pregnancy near term; threat to life from exsanguination (injury or DIC); mechanical limitation for maternal repair; risk for fetal distress exceeding risk for prematurity; unstable thoracolumbar spinal injury.

SUGGESTED READING

Dennis JW, Menawat S, Von Thron J, et al. Efficacy of deep venous thrombosis prophylaxis in trauma patients and identification of high-risk groups. J Trauma 1993;35:132.

Eichelberger MR, ed. Pediatric trauma: prevention, acute care, rehabilitation. Chicago, Mosby Year Book, 1993.

Fabian TC, Croce MA, Stewart RM, et al. A prospective analysis of diagnostic laparoscopy in trauma. Ann Surg 1993;217:557.

Gentilello L, Moujaes S. Treatment of hypothermia in trauma victims: thermodynamic considerations. J Intensive Care Med 1995;10:5.

Mattox KL, ed. Complications of trauma. New York, Churchill Livingstone, 1994.

Mattox KL, Moore EE, Feliciano DV, eds. Trauma, ed 2. Norwalk, CT, Appleton & Lange, 1991.

Mendez C, Gubler KD, Maier RV. Diagnostic accuracy of peritoneal lavage in patients with pelvic fractures. Arch Surg 1994;129:477.

Sampalis JS, Lavoie A, Williams JI. Impact of on-site care, prehospital time, and level of in-hospital care on survival in severely injured patients. J Trauma 1993;34:252.

Santora TA, Schinco MA, Trooskin SZ. Management of trauma in elderly patients. Surg Clin North Am 1994;74:163.

Shackford SR, Mackersie RC, Hollingsworth-Fridlund P, Hollbrook TL, Wolf PL, Hoyt DB. The epidemiology and pathology of traumatic death: a population-based analysis. Arch Surg 1993;128:571.

ESSENTIALS OF SURGERY: SCIENTIFIC PRINCIPLES AND PRACTICE,
edited by Lazar J. Greenfield, Michael W. Mulholland, Keith T. Oldham, Gerald B. Zelenock,
and Keith D. Lillemoe. Lippincott–Raven Publishers, Philadelphia, © 1997.

CHAPTER 12

BURNS

ROBERT L. SHERIDAN AND RONALD G. TOMPKINS

EPIDEMIOLOGY

Each year, approximately 2 million people in the United States require medical attention for burn injuries. Children 6 months to 2 years of age and the elderly are at high risk for sustaining burns in cooking and bathing accidents. Young adults are injured in the workplace. Structural fires spare no age group. As in motor-vehicle trauma, alcohol use frequently contributes to these injuries. Although the life-threatening nature of large injuries usually draws the most attention, poorly managed small burns have a potentially devastating impact.

A great deal of effort has been exerted to diminish the incidence of pediatric burn injury through public education. For example, legislation mandating lower temperatures for hot-water heaters has decreased the incidence of hot-water injuries to children. However, inconsistent application of laws remains a problem.

A systematic approach to burn care includes the following:

- With rare exception, resuscitation of all patients regardless of severity of injury
- Early excision and biologic closure of deep wounds
- Continuous rehabilitation
- Judicious use of broad-spectrum antibiotics with early detection and specific treatment of septic foci
- Intensive patient and family psychosocial support
- Long-term follow-up with ongoing rehabilitation and reconstruction

NATURAL HISTORY

The epidermis provides vapor and bacterial barriers, and the dermis provides flexibility and strength to the skin. Dermal appendages prevent desiccation of the skin by producing oils. The dermal microvasculature provides heat dissipation and conservation (Fig. 12-1). These functions are compromised or lost when the skin is burned.

Local Response to Burn Injury

The local response to thermal injury involves destruction and thrombosis of vessels in the dermis. Progressive vasoconstriction and thrombosis in the surrounding dermis vary according to the severity of the initial injury.

Systemic Response to Burn Injury

Loss of the barrier function of the skin results in:

- Accelerated fluid loss and decreased host resistance to infection
- Release of mediators from the injured tissue with microvascular and end-organ dysfunction
- Bacterial overgrowth within the eschar, which leads to systemic infection

The physiologic challenge of a burn of >20% of the total body surface area (TBSA) frequently causes an initial decrease in cardiac output and metabolic rate. A hypermetabolic response follows in which cardiac output and resting energy expenditure nearly double over the next 24 to 48 hours in patients who are successfully resuscitated. The magnitude of this response peaks in injuries of ≥60% TBSA, in which the metabolic rate more than doubles resting levels.

Treatment of patients with large burns is to support the hypermetabolic response with provision of adequate quantity and quality of substrate. Although limited modification of the hypermetabolic response by means of administration of antipyretic agents is widely used, elimination of this response is of unknown value and may be harmful.

The cause of the hypermetabolic response is not understood, but it is assumed to involve the following:

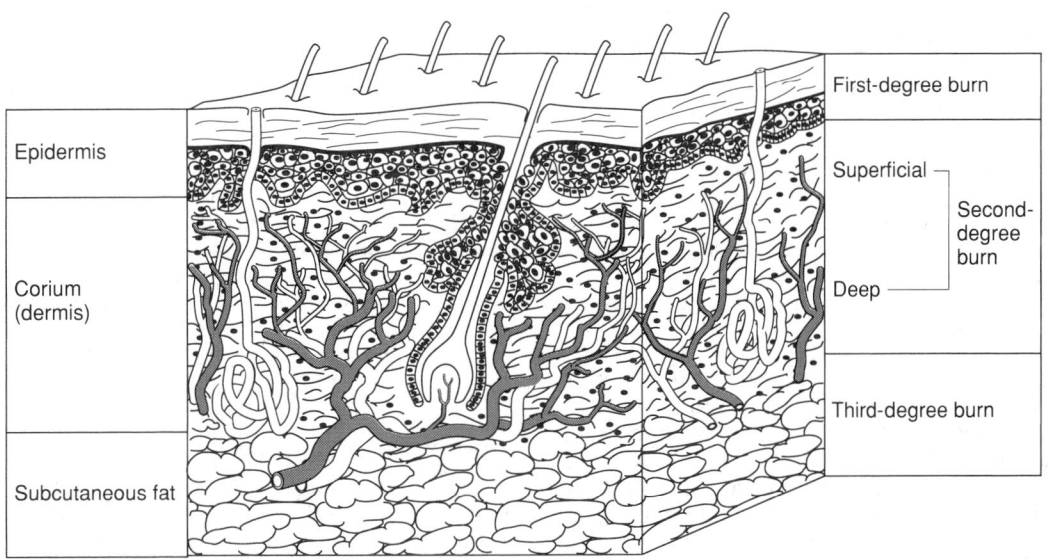

Figure 12-1. Schematic depiction of skin.

- A change in hypothalamic function with increases in glucagon, cortisol, and catecholamine secretion
- Deficient gastrointestinal barrier function with translocation of bacteria and their byproducts
- Bacterial contamination of the burn wound with systemic release of bacterial products
- Enhanced heat loss through transeschar evaporation of fluid

EVALUATION

Primary Survey

Many burn patients sustain other injuries. The initial evaluation is as for any patient with multiple trauma. One must:

1. Maintain control of the cervical spine while evaluating and securing the airway
2. Assess breathing mechanics
3. Estimate circulating blood volume
4. Document level of consciousness
5. Remove the patient's clothes in a warm environment to avoid hypothermia

A secure airway and vascular access are crucial and are achieved early in the evaluation. A badly burned face makes tape ineffective in securing the endotracheal tube, so an umbilical-tie harness is used. Secure venous access is achieved with a central line, although two peripheral intravenous lines are a reasonable option. In a child with hypovolemia, intraosseous resuscitation can be life-saving; however, the intraosseous catheter is replaced with a venous cannula as soon as is practical.

All patients should have a nasogastric tube placed, particularly if transported by air, because gas filling the stomach may cause emesis and aspiration. A bladder catheter facilitates fluid resuscitation. Continuous temperature monitoring with rectal or esophageal probes and arterial access is helpful. If ventilation is restricted by overlying circumferential eschar, torso escharotomies are made with electrocautery to minimize blood loss (Fig. 12-2)..

Secondary Survey

The burn-specific secondary survey (Table 12-1) includes a complete history, vital signs, a detailed physical examination, and laboratory and radiographic studies appropriate for the mechanism of injury. Resuscitation status is evaluated according to age-specific norms (Table 12-2).

The history, particularly details regarding the mechanism of injury, is obtained from witnesses, rescue personnel, and family members. The mechanism of injury often determines the need for special studies, such as computed tomography (CT) of the head and abdomen or radiographs of the cervical spine.

A complete physical examination proceeds in an organized manner. The presence of the burn should not distract the examiner from a complete assessment. Evaluation of the wound is deferred until higher-priority evaluations are complete.

An accurate determination of *burn depth is not necessary* to proceed with initial wound management or fluid resuscitation. In contrast, an accurate assessment of *burn size is important* because resuscitative fluid administration is determined on the basis of overall burn size. Burn size in children is best estimated with an age-specific chart (Fig. 12-3), because body proportions change with growth. It is helpful to check one's estimate of TBSA burned by also calculating the areas not burned. The sum of both areas never exceeds 100%.

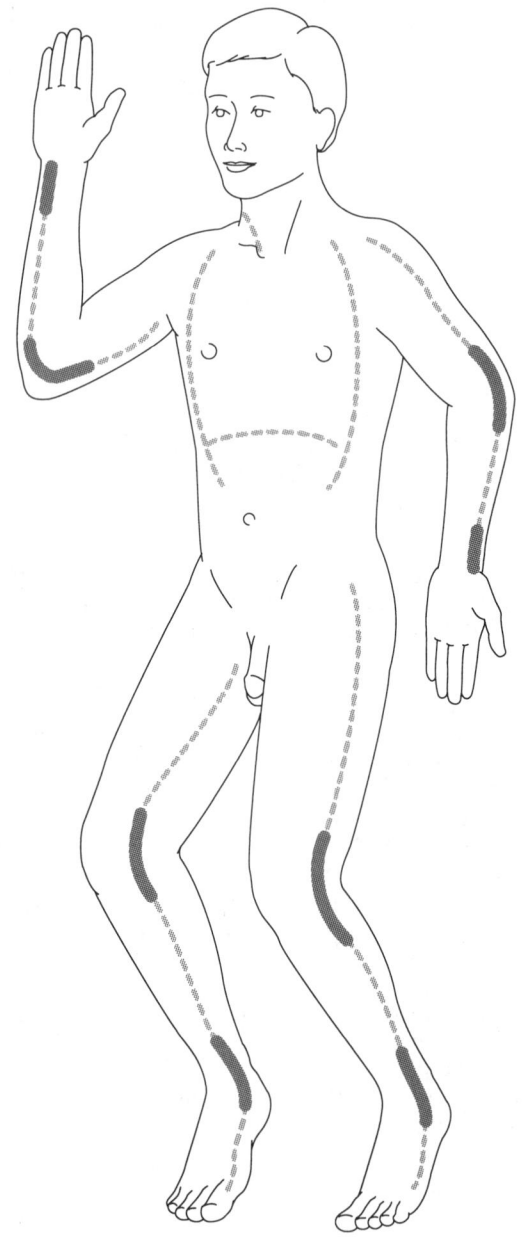

Figure 12-2. Preferred sites of escharotomy. Connecting lateral axial incisions across the midline facilitates ventilation with low inflating pressures. Extremity escharotomies are performed using medial and lateral axial incisions.

Relatively few laboratory studies are essential during the initial evaluation (see Table 12-1). Patients with electrical or very deep thermal injuries often require blood products during the initial resuscitation. For such patients, collection of a blood-bank specimen is routine. Routine hematology and chemistry profiles are of limited usefulness at first, but they do establish a baseline.

Electrical Injuries

Low-voltage contact may cause locally destructive injuries without systemic sequelae. High-voltage (> 1000 volts) contact causes a combination of deep-tissue injury due to the passage of current, locally destructive entrance and exit wounds, deep wounds where current arches

Table 12-1. IMPORTANT ASPECTS OF THE BURN-SPECIFIC SECONDARY SURVEY

HISTORY

Closed-space exposure
Extrication time
Delay in seeking attention
Fluid given during transport
Previous illnesses and injuries

HEAD, EYES, EARS, NOSE, AND THROAT

The globes should be examined and corneal epithelium stained with fluorescein before adnexal swelling makes examination difficult. Adnexal swelling provides excellent coverage and protection during the first days after injury. Tarsorrhaphy is virtually never indicated acutely.

Corneal epithelial loss can be overt, giving a clouded appearance to the cornea, but it is more often subtle, requiring fluorescein staining for documentation. Topical ophthalmic antibiotics constitute optimal initial treatment.

Signs of airway involvement include perioral and intraoral burns or carbonaceous material and progressive hoarseness.

Hot liquid can be aspirated with a facial scald injury and result in acute airway compromise requiring urgent intubation.

Endotracheal tube security is crucial and is best maintained with an umbilical tape harness, rather than adhesive tape, on the burned face.

NECK

The radiographic evaluation is driven by the mechanism of injury.

Neck escharotomies are rarely needed to facilitate venous drainage of the head.

CARDIAC

Cardiac rhythm should be monitored for 24 to 72 hours in electrical injury.

Elderly patients may experience transient atrial fibrillation if modestly overresuscitated.

Significant arrhythmias are unusual if intravascular volume and oxygenation are adequately supported.

History of myocardial infarction increases the risk of new infarct with the stress of burn injury, and appropriate monitoring is necessary.

PULMONARY

Inflating pressures should be kept below 40 cm H_2O by the performance of chest escharotomies when needed.

Severe inhalation injury may lead to slough of endobronchial mucosa and thick endobronchial secretions. Sudden endotracheal tube occlusions may occur.

VASCULAR

Burned extremities should be vigilantly monitored by serial examinations. Indications for escharotomy include decreasing temperature, increasing consistency, slowed capillary refill and diminished Doppler flow in the digital vessels. One should not wait until flow in named vessels is compromised to decompress the extremity.

Fasciotomy is indicated after electrical or deep thermal injury when distal flow is compromised. Compartment pressure measurement can be helpful, but clinical examination is an indication for decompression regardless of compartment pressure readings.

ABDOMEN

Nasogastric tubes should be placed and their function verified, particularly before air transport in unpressurized helicopters.

An inappropriate resuscitative volume requirement may be a sign of an occult intraabdominal injury.

Torso escharotomies may be required to facilitate ventilation of deep circumferential abdominal wall burns.

Immediate stress ulcer prophylaxis with histamine-receptor blockers and antacids is indicated with serious burns.

GENITOURINARY

Bladder catheterization is appropriate in all who require fluid resuscitation and urine output monitoring.

The foreskin should be reduced over the bladder catheter after insertion, since progressive swelling may otherwise result in paraphimosis.

NEUROLOGIC

Early neurologic evaluation is important, since the sensorium is altered by medication or hemodynamic instability during the hours after injury. CT scanning is appropriate if possible for head trauma.

Patients who require neuromuscular blockade for transport should also receive adequate sedation and analgesia.

EXTREMITIES

Extremities with circumferential thermal burns or electrical injury should be promptly decompressed by escharotomy or fasciotomy when clinical examination reveals diminished distal perfusion. Limbs at risk should be dressed so they can be frequently examined.

The need for escharotomy usually becomes evident during the early resuscitation. Most escharotomies can be delayed until transport has been effected if this is less than 6 hours.

Burned extremities should be elevated and splinted in a position of function.

WOUNDS

Wounds are often underestimated in depth and overestimated in size on initial examination.

Size, depth, and the presence of circumferential components are important issues.

LABORATORY TESTS

Arterial blood gas analysis is important when airway compromise or inhalation injury is present.

Normal carboxyhemoglobin concentration on admission does not eliminate the possibility of a significant exposure as the half-life of carboxyhemoglobin is 30 to 40 minutes in those effectively ventilated with 100% oxygen.

Baseline hemoglobin and electrolytes can be helpful later during resuscitation.

Urinalysis for occult blood should be performed with deep thermal or electrical injuries.

RADIOGRAPHIC EVALUATIONS

Radiographic evaluation is driven by the mechanism of injury and the need to document placement of supportive cannulae.

(continued)

Table 12-1. IMPORTANT ASPECTS OF THE BURN-SPECIFIC SECONDARY SURVEY (Continued)

ELECTRICAL BURNS

Cardiac rhythm should be monitored in high (greater than 1000 volts) or intermediate (greater that 220 volts) voltage exposures for 24 to 72 hours.

Low and intermediate voltage exposures can cause locally destructive injuries but uncommonly result in systemic sequelae.

After high-voltage exposures, delayed neurologic and ocular sequelae can occur, so a carefully documented admission examination is important.

Injured extremities should be serially evaluated for intracompartmental edema and promptly decompressed when necessary.

Bladder catheters are required for high-voltage exposure to assess the possibility of pigmenturia. This is treated adequately with volume loading in most patients.

CHEMICAL BURNS

Wounds should be irrigated with tapwater for at least 30 minutes. The globe is irrigated with isotonic crystalloid solution. Blepharospasm may require ocular anesthetic administration.

Exposure to hydrofluoric acid may be complicated by life-threatening hypocalcemia, particularly exposures to concentrated or anhydrous solutions. Close monitoring and supplementation of serum calcium is necessary. Subeschar injection of 10% calcium gluconate solution is appropriate after exposure to highly concentrated or anhydrous solutions.

TAR BURNS

Tar should be initially cooled with tapwater irrigation, then removed with a lipophyllic solvent.

---

across flexed joints, flame burns due to clothing ignition, flash burns, fractures of the spine due to tetanic contraction of paravertebral muscles, and other injuries related to the fall or blast that commonly accompanies high-voltage injury.

Chemical and Tar Injuries

After initial irrigation, chemical and tar burns are managed surgically as indicated by depth, which is frequently underestimated at initial examination. Chemical burns are first managed with at least 30 min of copious tap-water irrigation. Ocular injuries are irrigated with saline solution. Tar is often heated to >300°F, and contact commonly causes a deep burn.

Injuries of Abuse

All burned children should be examined for abuse or neglect (Table 12-3). It is an ethical and legal mandate that reports of suspicious injuries be filed with the appropriate local agency.

FLUID RESUSCITATION

Formulas for estimating fluid resuscitation requirements are helpful (Table 12-4). However, no formula can replace a physician at the bedside repeatedly evaluating the pa-

Table 12-2. Age-Specific Resuscitation Endpoints

Evaluation	Target
Sensorium	Comfortable, arousable
Urine output	
Infants	1–2 mL/kg/h
Children	0.5–1 mL/kg/h
All others	0.5 mL/kg/h
Base deficit	<2 mEq/dL
Systolic blood pressure	
Infants	60–70 mmHg
Children	70–90 + (twice age in years) mmHg
Adolescents and adults	90–120 mmHg

tient's physiologic needs throughout the resuscitative period.

INITIAL WOUND EXCISION AND BIOLOGIC CLOSURE

Early removal of extensive areas of devitalized tissue with immediate biologic closure of the wounds is the surgical objective during the first postburn week. The entire wound is excised coincident with fluid resuscitation, or, more commonly, staged excision of all deep partial and full-thickness components of the wound is performed. Wounds of the face, palms, soles, and genitals usually are not excised.

The advantages of early excision include an improved survival rate among patients with injuries involving >30% to 40% TBSA, truncated hospital stays, fewer painful dressing changes, and lower cost. Although not proved, it appears that a decrease in the duration and intensity of the hypermetabolic response, improved immunologic function, and less hypertrophic scarring may result from early excision.

Estimation of Burn Depth

Only deep partial or full-thickness burns are treated with early excision. It is difficult to determine burn depth at initial examination. No technical aid equals in accuracy or practicality the eye of an experienced examiner. Differentiation between superficial burns that heal within 3 weeks with topical antimicrobial treatment and deep injuries that require excision can be made at clinical examinations during the first days after injury. In general, if overall wound size is <15% TBSA, the wound can be treated with topical antimicrobial agents until the portion that requires grafting becomes evident.

Topical Antimicrobial Agents

Topical antimicrobial agents that delay wound colonization and infection are used until excision and grafting.

Techniques of Excision

Tissue viability is assessed on the basis of color and texture rather than the presence of diffuse bleeding. The principle is to excise nonviable tissue and conserve viable

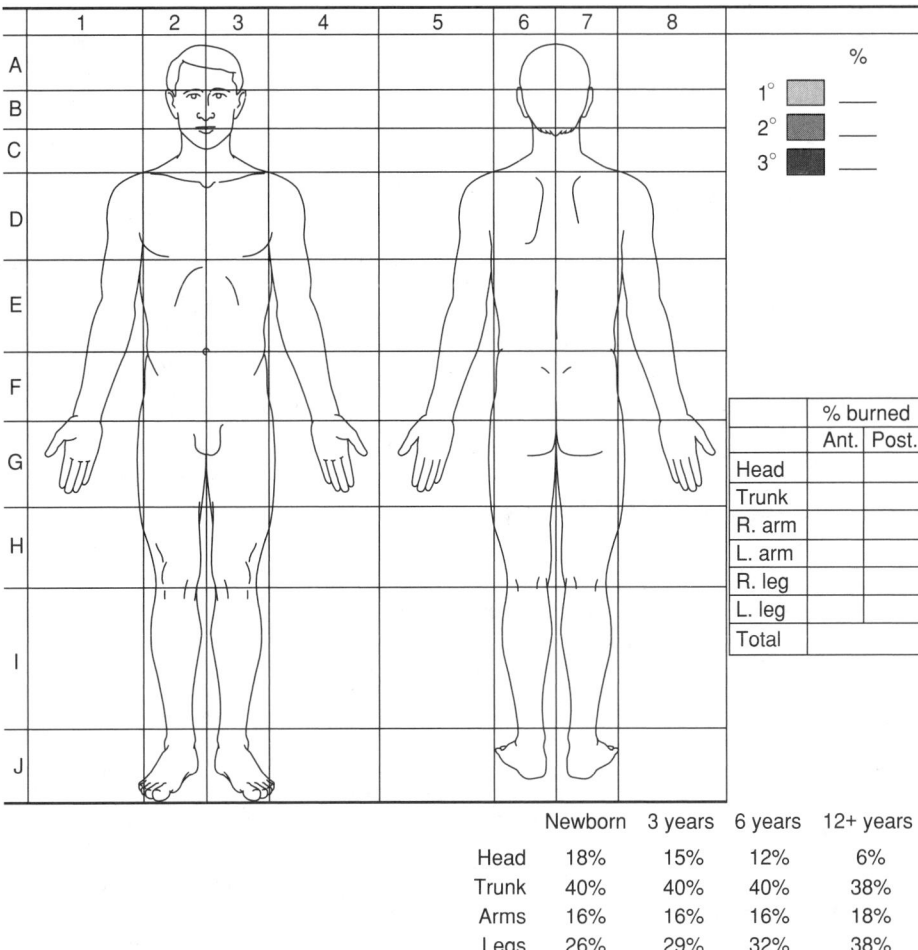

	% burned	
	Ant.	Post.
Head		
Trunk		
R. arm		
L. arm		
R. leg		
L. leg		
Total		

	Newborn	3 years	6 years	12+ years
Head	18%	15%	12%	6%
Trunk	40%	40%	40%	38%
Arms	16%	16%	16%	18%
Legs	26%	29%	32%	38%

Figure 12-3. An age-specific chart facilitates accurate estimation of burn size over a broad range of ages.

tissue. Tangential excisions of the torso, neck, and head are performed after subeschar injection of dilute epinephrine solutions. Tangential excisions of the extremities are performed after exsanguination and inflation of a pneumatic tourniquet.

Instruments used for tangential excision of burned tissue include hand, compressed-gas, and electric dermatomes. When required, excisions to the underlying fascia are performed with a coagulating electrocautery. Although such

Table 12-3. IMPORTANT POINTS OF HISTORY AND PHYSICAL EXAMINATION THAT SUGGEST ABUSE OR NEGLECT

HISTORY

Delayed presentation for medical care
Conflicting histories
Previous injuries

SUSPICIOUS BURN PATTERNS

Sharply demarcated margins
Uniform depth
Absence of splash marks
Stocking or glove patterns
Flexor sparing
Porcelain contact sparing
Dorsal location of contact injury of the hands
Very deep localized contact injury

procedures have traditionally been limited to 2 hours of operating time or 20% TBSA, far larger procedures can be performed safely if blood-conserving practices are followed rigorously and patients are kept warm with operating-room temperatures higher than 90°F.

Temporary Alternatives to Wound Closure

Once necrotic eschar is excised to a bed of viable tissue, immediate biologic closure is mandatory. Immediate autografting is ideal. When donor sites are insufficient for this purpose, a temporary biologic cover must be chosen while donor sites heal. Such covers prevent desiccation and provide a vapor and bacterial barrier over the excised wound. Fresh or cryopreserved human allograft is most appropriate for this purpose. It is placed meshed but unexpanded, exactly as one would place autograft. When placed on a viable wound bed, the graft vascularizes and provides physiologic wound closure until rejected 2 to 4 weeks later, when it is replaced with autograft.

DEFINITIVE WOUND CLOSURE

During definitive wound closure, allograft is replaced with autograft, and burns of specialized areas are addressed (Table 12-5). This phase usually begins one week after injury and lasts for several weeks thereafter, depending on the extent of burn and the availability of suitable donor sites.

CRITICAL CARE

Inhalation Injury and Respiratory Failure

Points in the patient's history that suggest inhalation injury are entrapment within a closed space or a prolonged extrication time. Physical signs are singed nasal vibrissae and facial hair, burns of the central face, intraoral burns, carbonaceous debris in the oropharynx, and diffuse wheezing. Management is aggressive pulmonary toilet by means of frequent chest physiotherapy and bronchoscopic suctioning and lavage. Positive pressure ventilation facilitates the care of patients with large shunts or compliance poor enough to result in an excessive work of breathing.

Carbon Monoxide and Cyanide Exposure

Both carbon monoxide and cyanide are commonly inhaled by people caught in closed-space fires. Patients who are well-ventilated with high concentrations of oxygen from the time of extrication, commonly have normal carboxyhemoglobin values at initial evaluation despite exposure to carbon monoxide at the time of injury. *Hyperbaric oxygen is not used* unless the patient can be placed in the chamber before the carboxyhemoglobin level has normalized. With proper ventilation and fluid resuscitation, cyanide-induced acidosis corrects rapidly in most patients, and specific treatment is not usually required.

Vascular Access Techniques

Peripheral vascular access is often impractical in burn patients and is associated with unacceptable rates of suppurative thrombophlebitis. For this reason, central access is routine, except in patients with small injuries who require venous access for only a few days. Arterial access can be safely maintained if the radial or femoral artery is

Table 12-4. MODIFIED BROOKE FORMULA

FIRST 24 HOURS
Adults and Children >10 kg
Lactated Ringer solution: 2–4 mL/kg/% burn/24 h
(first half in first 8 h)
Colloid: none

Children <10 kg
Lactated Ringer Solution: 2–3 mL/kg/% burn/24 h
(first half in first 8 h)
Lactated Ringer solution with 5% dextrose: 4 mL/kg/h
Colloid: none

SECOND 24 HOURS
All Patients
Crystalloid: to maintain urine output. If silver nitrate is used, sodium leeching will mandate continued isotonic crystalloid. If topical is used, free water requirement is significant. Serum sodium should be monitored closely. Nutritional support should begin, ideally by the enteral route.
Colloid (5% albumin in lactated Ringer solution)
0%–30% burn: none
30%–50% burn: 0.3 mL/kg/% burn/24 h
50%–70% burn: 0.4 mL/kg/% burn/24 h
>70% burn: 0.5 mL/kg/% burn/24 h

Table 12-5. WOUND MANAGEMENT ACCORDING TO AREA BURNED

FACE
Administer topical antimicrobial agents for 2 wk
Excise and close with thick-sheet autograft areas that remain unhealed
Place autografts on full-thickness facial wounds in cosmetic units

OCULAR ADNEXAE
Provide ocular lubrication when wound contracture occurs
Perform surgical release of the lid if necessary

EXTERNAL EAR
Clean wound and apply mafenide acetate twice a day
Avoid pressure on burned auricle (eg, from pillows)
Perform immediate débridement of infected cartilage if acute suppurative chondritis occurs

HANDS
Examine hands for perfusion
Perform prompt escharotomy if perfusion is poor
Perform urgent fasciotomy in high-voltage electrical injury or deep thermal burns if there is progressive firmness of the compartments of the hand and forearm, progressive neurologic impairment, or pain. In equivocal cases, perform prompt decompression.

Superficial Burns
Elevate hand
Administer topical antimicrobial agents
Move each joint through full passive range of motion twice a day
Split hand in functional position if there is marked edema

Deep Partial and Full-Thickness Burns
Excise wound and provide sheet graft as soon as practical
Immobilize hand in functional position for 7 days after operation
Administer physical therapy

Fourth-Degree Hand Burns
(Burns that involve the underlying extensor mechanism, joint capsules, or bone)
Perform staged sheet autografting
Provide temporay axial Kirschner-wire fixation of open and unstable interphalangeal or metacarpophalangeal joints
Perform débridement and provide groin or abdominal flap coverage if burn covers small area
Administer physical therapy

Burns of Palm
Preserve specialized attachment of the palmar skin to the underlying fascia
Graft full-thickness injuries with full-thickness or thick split-thickness sheet grafts and splint hand in extension

FEET
Dorsum: Perform prompt excision and grafting of deep dermal and full-thickness injuries
Plantar surface: Provide full- or thick split-thickness sheet grafts if wound does not heal within 3 weeks

GENITAL AREA
Reduce burned foreskin into a normal position
Place bladder catheter only to facilitate resuscitation; remove catheter when genital edema resolves and close monitoring of urine output is no longer required
Do not perform diversion of the intestinal tract
When débriding the deeply burned foreskin, preserve any viable remnant for reconstruction
Deep burns: Provide topical therapy for 2–3 wk unless the wounds are extremely deep
Unhealed injuries: Debride wound and provide sheet autograft

Table 12-6. COMMON COMPLICATIONS AFTER BURN INJURY

NEUROLOGIC

Transient delirium occurs in up to 30% of patients and generally resolves with supportive therapy. Evaluation is for anoxia, metabolic disturbance and structural lesions.

Seizures most commonly result from hyponatremia or abrupt benzodiazepine withdrawal.

Peripheral nerve injuries occur from direct thermal injury, compression from compartment syndrome or overlying nonelastic eschar, major metabolic disturbances, or improper splinting techniques.

Delayed peripheral nerve and spinal cord deficits develop weeks or months after high-voltage injury secondary to small vessel injury and demyelinization.

RENAL

Early acute renal failure follows inadequate perfusion during resuscitation or myoglobinuria.

Late renal failure complicates sepsis and multiple organ failure or the use of nephrotoxic agents.

ADRENAL

Acute adrenal insufficiency secondary to adrenal hemorrhage presents with hypotension, fever, hyponatremia, and hyperkalemia.

CARDIOVASCULAR

Endocarditis and suppurative thrombophlebitis typically present with fever and bacteremia without signs of local infection.

Hypertension occurs in up to 20% of children and is best managed with β-adrenergic blockers.

Venous thromboembolic complications are so infrequent in patients with large burns that prophylaxis is not currently routine.

Iatrogenic catheter insertion complications are minimized by meticulous technique.

PULMONARY

Carbon monoxide intoxication is best managed acutely with ventilation with pure oxygen. It can be associated with delayed neurologic sequelae.

Pneumonia may occur with or without inhalation injury and is treated with pulmonary toilet and antibiotics.

Early respiratory failure may occur secondary to inhalation of noxious chemicals. Later respiratory failure may occur secondary to sepsis or pneumonia.

HEMATOLOGIC

Neutropenia and thrombocytopenia, as well as disseminated intravascular coagulation, are common indicators of impending sepsis.

Systemic immunologic deficits contribute to a high rate of infectious complications.

OTOLOGIC

Auricular chondritis secondary to bacterial infection results in rapid loss of viable cartilage. It is preventable by the routine use of topical mafenide acetate on all burned ears.

Sinusitis and otitis media can be caused by transnasal instrumentation and are treated by relocation of tubes, antibiotics, and judicious surgical drainage.

Complications of endotracheal intubation include nasal alar and septal necrosis, vocal cord erosions and ulcerations, tracheal stenosis and tracheoesophageal and trachoinnominate artery fistulae. Complications are minimized by compulsive attention to tube position, avoidance of oversized tubes, and attention to cuff pressures.

ENTERIC

Hepatic dysfunction, secondary to transient hepatic blood flow deficits and manifested as hepatocellular enzyme (AST, ALT) elevations, is extremely common. Late hepatic failure begins with elevations of cholestatic enzymes and may progress through coagulopathy and hepatic failure. It is associated with sepsis and multiple organ failure.

Pancreatitis is generally coincident with splanchnic flow deficits early and sepsis induced organ failures later.

Acalculous cholecystitis can present as sepsis without localized symptoms or signs. Radiographic evaluation can be followed by bedside percutaneous cholecystostomy in unstable patients.

Gastroduodenal ulceration, secondary to splanchnic flow deficits that degrade mucosal defenses, is common and potentially life threatening if routine histamine-receptor blockers and antacids are not administered.

Intestinal ischemia is possible if it is secondary to inadequate resuscitation and splanchnic flow deficits.

OPHTHALMIC

Ectopia, from progressive contraction of burned ocular adnexae, results in exposure of the globe. This requires acute eyelid release. Tarsorrhaphy is rarely helpful, more often resulting in injury to the tarsal plate as contraction forces pull out tarsorrhaphy sutures.

Corneal ulceration can progress to full-thickness corneal destruction if secondary infection occurs. This is prevented by careful globe lubrication with topical antibiotics and possibly acute lid release for ectropion.

Symblepharon, or scarring of the lid to the denuded conjunctiva, occurs following chemical burns or corneal epithelial defects complicating toxic epidermal necrolysis. It is prevented by daily examination and adhesion disruption with a fine glass rod.

GENITOURINARY

Urinary tract infections are minimized by maintaining bladder catheters only when required. Neither bladder catheterization nor colonic diversion is required for management of perineal and genital burns.

Candidal cystitis occurs with bladder catheters and broad-spectrum antibiotics. Catheter change and Amphotericin B irrigation for 5 days is generally therapeutic. If infections are recurrent, the upper tracts should be screened ultrasonographically.

(continued)

Table 12-6. COMMON COMPLICATIONS AFTER BURN INJURY (Continued)

MUSCULOSKELETAL

Burned exposed bone is generally débrided with a drill until viable cortical bone is reached. This is allowed to granulate and is autografted. Patients whose overall condition and wounds are appropriate are treated with local or distant flaps.

Fractured and burned extremities are best immobilized with external fixators while overlying burns are grafted. Burn patients with coincident fractures in unburned extremities benefit from prompt internal fixation.

Heterotopic ossification develops weeks after injury and is seen most commonly around deeply burned major joints such as the triceps tendon. It presents with pain and decreased range of motion. Most patients respond to physical therapy, but some require excision of heterotopic bone to achieve full function.

SOFT TISSUE

Hypertrophic scar formation is a major cause of long-term functional and cosmetic deformities. It heralded by a secondary increase in neovascularity 9 to 13 weeks after epithelialization. Management options include grafting of deep dermal and full-thickness wounds, compression garments, judicious steroid injections, topical silicone products, and scar release and resurfacing procedures.

used. The femoral artery is usually best in children. A transmission oximetry probe and central venous line are used for blood gases in patients intubated for airway protection only and who have no substantial intrapulmonary shunt or dead space.

Line care includes inserting the catheter through unburned tissue, insertion-site cleaning every 4 hours, and changing catheters at least once a week.

Nutritional Support

Accurate nutritional support is essential because overfeeding is associated with hepatic steatosis, hepatic dysfunction, and increased CO_2 production, which exacerbates respiratory insufficiency. Underfeeding leads to inanition and poor wound healing. Standard formulas are poorly predictive of actual energy requirements in patients. Therefore, indirect calorimetry is commonly used to guide nutritional support. Total energy expenditure can be roughly estimated with expired-gas indirect calorimetry to determine resting energy expenditure (REE) and then multiplying REE by a factor of 1.3-1.7. Protein loads of 2.5-3.0 g/kg per day are recommended to support the requirements of the seriously burned. Recombinant human growth hormone can be used, but prompt donor-site healing and positive nitrogen balance usually can be achieved without this therapy.

Multiple Organ Failure and Other Complications of Thermal Injury

Care of patients with large burns necessitates identification and management of a series of complications while the wound is progressively closed (Table 12-6).

A burn patient whose condition is deteriorating commonly displays early evidence of multiple organ dysfunction in a predictable sequence—increasing obtundation followed by progressive intrapulmonary shunting with hypoxia, ileus, nonoliguric renal failure, cholestasis, and thrombocytopenia. The most common initiating event is one of the many infections to which burn patients are prone. When an underlying infectious focus can be identified and addressed, organ function improves. If not, the organ failures progress to death.

REHABILITATION

Early therapy may be limited to antideformity positioning and splinting of the hands and extremities with twice-daily range of motion exercises of all joints. In patients whose condition is stable, and in those with large injuries nearing wound closure, therapy sessions involve strengthening, ambulation, active and passive range of motion, development of adaptive skills with modified utensils, activities of daily living and, in older adolescents and adults, development of work-related skills. These activities are continued after discharge from the hospital.

The coordinated involvement of psychiatric, psychologic, and social work staff facilitates psychologic recovery and social reintegration. These staff members are actively involved with the patient, family, and local outpatient support services throughout the hospitalization. Planning for discharge and arrangements and funding for outpatient services begins at the time of admission. The expectation for every burn patient is a return to family and community life.

RECONSTRUCTION

Any wound is subject to hypertrophy. However, those most likely to undergo hypertrophy are deep dermal burns that heal in ≥ 3 weeks, full-thickness wounds that heal by contraction and epithelial spread from wound edges, and wounds on which there is much tension, as across flexor surfaces. Surgeons have limited ability to influence the development of hypertrophic scars. Tools include compression garments, topical silicone sheets, steroid injections, and release or excision and autografting. Recalcitrant areas of hypertrophic scarring often are best treated with release or excision. Resultant wounds are covered with sheet autograft or flaps. Tissue expanders can be helpful, particularly for closure of defects of the hair-bearing scalp.

When function is not limited, it is ideal to wait 2 years for full scar maturation before reconstruction is undertaken. However, when function is threatened, prompt surgical intervention is indicated. Patients who survive large injuries commonly require a series of reconstructive procedures over the first few postinjury years to attain optimal cosmetic and functional results.

ADJUNCTIVE THERAPY

Adjunctive measures are as follows:

1. Support, rather than modification, of the hypermetabolic response. The adverse aspects of the hypermetabolic response are best obviated by minimizing release of inflammatory mediators from the wound by prompt excision and biologic closure. Support of gastrointestinal barrier function is ensured by establishment of splanchnic blood flow by means of normalization of hemodynamics and providing enteral nutritional support as soon as possible after injury. Early detection and elimination of infectious foci are

fundamental. Research with blocking antibodies and recombinant mediators related to TNFα, IL-1, IL-2, IL-6 and others promises to enhance understanding of the hypermetabolic response to injury.

2. Growth factors. Topical epidermal growth factor and systemic human growth hormone have been associated with shortened donor-site healing times in burn patients. However, any potential benefit should be weighed against the financial and, as yet, undefined long-term physiologic costs of these therapies. Other growth factors are being studied to enhance understanding of wound healing.

3. Wound management. The ability to determine the depth of wounds at initial presentation may shorten hospital stays by eliminating the period of wound observation that is commonly used to facilitate accurate predictions of wound healing in patients with small burns of indeterminate depth. Although several such technical adjuncts, such as laser Doppler flow meters, high-resolution ultrasound, and low-power laser fluorescence are promising, none is of clinical utility. Wound débridement with a scanning CO_2 laser or débriding enzymes may facilitate both wound-depth evaluation and blood-conserving removal of eschar.

4. Critical care technologies. New modes of ventilation emphasize avoidance of high inflating pressures and techniques of extracorporeal support. Nitric oxide, delivered by aerosol into the ventilator circuit, has been shown to decrease intrapulmonary shunting by increasing pulmonary blood flow to well-ventilated lung segments and to decrease pulmonary vascular resistance in patients with respiratory failure.

5. Permanent skin substitutes. Substitutes under development include epidermal analogs, dermal analogs, and composite substitutes. Experience with these substitutes is limited and their general use cannot be recommended.

SUGGESTED READING

Aggarwal SJ, Diller KR, Blake GK, Baxter CR. Burn-induced alterations in vasoactive function of the peripheral cutaneous microcirculation. J Burn Care Rehabil 1994;15:1.

Carlson DE, Cioffi WG Jr, Mason AD Jr, McManus WF, Pruitt BA Jr. Resting energy expenditure in patients with thermal injuries. Surg Gynecol Obstet 1992;174:270.

Heimbach D, Engrav L, Grube B, Marvin J. Burn depth: A review. World J Surg 1992;16:10.

Heimbach D, Luterman A, Burke J, et al. Artificial dermis for major burns: A multi-center randomized clinical trial. Ann Surg 1988;208:313.

Rue LW III, Cioffi WG, Mason AD, McManus WF, Pruitt BA Jr. Improved survival of burned patients with inhalation injury. Arch Surg 1993;128:772.

Sheridan RL, Tompkins RG, Burke JF. Management of burn wounds with prompt excision and immediate closure. J Intensive Care Med 1994;9:6.

Sheridan RL, Tompkins RG, McManus WF, Pruitt BA Jr. Intracompartmental sepsis in burn patients. J Trauma 1994;36:301.

Zapol WM, Falke KJ, Hurford WE, Roberts JD Jr. Inhaling nitric oxide: A selective pulmonary vasodilator and bronchodilator. Chest 1994;105:87S.

ESSENTIALS OF SURGERY: SCIENTIFIC PRINCIPLES AND PRACTICE,
edited by Lazar J. Greenfield, Michael W. Mulholland, Keith T. Oldham, Gerald B. Zelenock, and Keith D. Lillemoe. Lippincott–Raven Publishers, Philadelphia, © 1997.

CHAPTER 13

ANESTHESIOLOGY AND PAIN MANAGEMENT

TIMOTHY W. RUTTER AND KEVIN K. TREMPER

Anesthesia is a combination of amnesia, analgesia and muscle relaxation. The goals of anesthesia are (1) to achieve this state quickly and safely by choosing the appropriate techniques and agents considering the patient's medical condition; (2) to maintain this state throughout the surgical procedure while compensating the effects of painful stimuli and blood and fluid loss; and (3) to reverse muscle relaxation and amnesia, bringing the patient back to physiologic control while maintaining sufficient analgesia to minimize postoperative pain.

ANESTHETIC AGENTS AND THEIR EFFECTS

Inhalation Agents

Inhalation agents (halothane, enflurane, isoflurane) produce their anesthetic effects in a dose-dependent manner with approximately 1% inhaled concentration. The measurement used to compare potency of inhalation agents is the minimum alveolar concentration (MAC, expressed as a percentage) that prevents movement on painful stimulation (incision) in 50% of patients. Table 13-1 lists the commonly used inhalation agents.

All inhalation agents depress blood pressure by means of myocardial depression and vasodilation. There is a generalized depression of cerebral function and cerebral metabolic rate of oxygen consumption, although cerebral blood flow may increase because of vascular dilatation and a loss of autoregulation. Renal blood flow and glomerular filtration rate decrease 20% to 50%. Blood flow to the skin increases, which impairs the ability to conserve heat. The combination of these effects, the cold environment of the operating room, and open body cavities make patients extremely vulnerable to hypothermia.

Muscle Relaxants

Neuromuscular blocking agents (Tables 13-2 and 13-3) are used to prevent movement and to facilitate surgical exposure. These drugs are competitive or noncompetitive inhibitors of the neurotransmitter acetylcholine at the neuromuscular junction.

The only *noncompetitive inhibitor* in clinical use is *succinylcholine*. This drug rapidly binds to the neuromuscular junction and produces depolarization, clinically apparent as fine-muscle fasciculations that occur approximately 60 seconds after injection. The effects of succinylcholine cannot be reversed, but they are short-acting. Because of its rapid onset, succinylcholine is frequently used to facilitate endotracheal intubation when it must be accomplished quickly.

All muscle relaxants besides succinylcholine are *competitive inhibitors* and do cause depolarization when they attach at the neuromuscular junction. Because these agents compete with acetylcholine, the block produced is propor-

Table 13-1. COMMON INHALATION AGENTS: MINIMUM ALVEOLAR CONCENTRATIONS AND EFFECTS

Agent	Minimum Alveolar Concentration (%)	Strengths	Weaknesses
Nitrous oxide	105	Analgesia Rapid uptake and elimination Little cardiac or respiratory depression	Sympathetic stimulation Expansion of closed air spaces Interference with vitamin B_{12} metabolism Limitation of Fio_2
Halothane	0.75	Low cost Effectiveness in low concentrations Little airway irritability Uterine relaxation	Less chemical stability Slow uptake and elimination Biodegradablility Hepatic necrosis Cardiac depression and arrhythmias
Enflurane	1.68	Good muscle relaxation Stable cardiac rate and rhythm	Pungent odor Seizure activity on electroencephalography
Isoflurane	1.15	Good muscle relaxation Stable cardiac rate and rhythm Usability in neurosurgery	Pungent odor High cost

(Adapted from Miller FL, Marshall BE. The inhaled anesthetics. In: Longnecker DE, Murphy FL, eds. Introduction to anesthesia, ed 8. Philadelphia, WB Saunders, 1992:77)

tional to the concentration of the agent relative to the concentration of acetylcholine. If the ratio is low, competitive relaxants can be reversed if the concentration of acetylcholine is elevated with an anticholinesterase, such as neostigmine. There is a ceiling to which an anticholinesterase can elevate acetylcholine; high levels of nondepolarizing relaxants cannot be reversed.

There are undesirable systemic consequences of increasing the plasma concentration of acetylcholine. Acetylcholine is the predominant neurotransmitter in the preganglionic sympathetic and parasympathetic nervous systems and in the postganglionic parasympathetic nervous sys-

tem. For this reason, an anticholinergic drug (atropine or glycopyrrolate) must be given with the anticholinesterase.

Neuromuscular blocking agents have no analgesic or amnesic properties and only prevent motion of voluntary muscles. *These drugs must be given in conjunction with analgesic and amnesic agents.* When prolonged muscle relaxation is required, it is best to administer the relaxant in continuous infusion and to monitor effect with a nerve stimulator.

All muscles in the body do not have equal sensitivity to muscle relaxants. The diaphragm is most resistant to neuromuscular blockade, whereas the neck and pharyn-

Table 13-2. COMMON NEUROMUSCULAR BLOCKING DRUGS AND REVERSAL AGENTS

Muscle Relaxant	Intubating Dose (mg/kg)	Infusion Dose (μg/kg/min)	Strengths	Weaknesses
DEPOLARIZING				
Succinylcholine	1.0	100*	Fastest onset (30 to 60 s) Short duration† (5 min)	Associated with malignant hyperthermia, dysrhythmias, bradycardia, and hyperkalemia, especially in patients with burns or neurologic injury
NONDEPOLARIZING				
Long Acting (>1 h)				
Pancuronium	0.1	0.3	No histamine release	Tachycardia Slow onset Long duration
Pipecuronium	0.08	—	Similar to pancuronium, no cardiovascular effects	—
Doxacurium	0.07	—	Similar to pancuronium, minimal cardiovascular effects	—
Intermediate Acting ($\approx$1 h)				
Atracurium	0.5	10	Spontaneous breakdown in plasma	Histamine release
Vecuronium	0.1	1	No cardiovascular effects	—
Rocuronium	0.8	10	Fast onset, no cardiovascular effects	—
Short Acting (10 min)				
Mivacurium	0.2	10	Fast onset, short duration	Histamine release

* This should not be used for longer than 1 hour.
† Duration is dramatically increased in patients with abnormal plasma pseudocholinesterase.

Table 13-3. DRUGS FOR ANTAGONIZING NONDEPOLARIZING NEUROMUSCULAR BLOCKADE*

Dose	Time to Peak Effect (min)	Dose	Use With
ANTICHOLINESTERASES			
Edrophonium	1–2	0.5–1.0 mg/kg	—
Neostigmine	3–5	0.04–0.07 mg/kg	—
Pyridostigmine	10–12	0.2–0.3 mg/kg	—
ANTICHOLINERGICS			
Glycopyrrolate	—	0.008 mg/kg (0.5–0.6 mg/70 kg)	Neostigmine Pyridostigmine
Atropine	—	0.007–0.02 mg/kg (0.05–1.5 mg/70 kg)	Edrophonium Neostigmine

* For reliable results in reversing the effects of nondepolarizing muscle relaxants, administration of anticholinesterases is delayed until spontaneous recovery permits three of four responses to a train-of-four stimulus. For patients with more profound blockade, larger amounts of anticholinesterases may be required, but doses of neostigmine higher than 0.14 mg/kg are unlikely to produce additional improvement.
(Adapted from Watling SM, Dasta JF. Prolonged paralysis in intensive care unit patients after the use of neuromuscular blocking agents: a review of the literature. Crit Care Med 1994;22:884)

geal muscles that support the airway are most sensitive. The clinical test for complete reversal of neuromuscular blockade is the ability of the patient to sustain a head lift from the bed for 5 seconds.

Narcotics

Narcotics and synthetic analogs belong to the class of drugs called *opioids* (Table 13-4). The most commonly used narcotics are morphine, meperidine, codeine, and fentanyl. Narcotics produce profound analgesia and respiratory depression. They have no amnesic properties, no direct myocardial depressive effect, and no muscle-relaxant properties. Patients may be totally aware and have substantial recall of conversations although they appear completely anesthetized.

Narcotics may produce hemodynamic effects indirectly through the release of histamine and blunting of the patient's sympathetic vascular tone. Because patients with acute injuries can experience dramatic drops in systemic blood pressure with minimal doses of opioids, it is important to titrate narcotics in small, incremental doses. Because of the lack of direct myocardial depression and the absence of histamine release with the synthetic opioids, these drugs are frequently used as the primary anesthetic in combination with an amnesic agent and a muscle relaxant in patients with myocardial dysfunction.

When opioids are titrated intravenously, patients become apneic because of respiratory depression but still breathe on command. As the dose increases, patients become unresponsive. An unusual side-effect of high-dose IV opioids is rigidity of the chest-wall muscles, which may make it extremely difficult to ventilate a patient without the aid of a muscle relaxant.

All opioids are reversed with naloxone. The duration of action of naloxone may be shorter than that of the narcotic, and patients must be observed carefully after they have been treated with naloxone. Naloxone reversal of opioids can be dangerous because the agent reverses not only the analgesic effects of the opioid, but also the analgesic effects of native endorphins. Naloxone is not used electively to reverse a narcotic. It is used in emergencies when the airway is not controlled and the patient is not ventilating because of a narcotic overdose.

Propofol

Propofol (Table 13-4) produces rapid induction of anesthesia. IV administration of propofol produces total anesthesia, that is, amnesia, analgesia, and some muscle relaxation. This agent is rapidly cleared through hepatic metabolism, so the patient becomes alert very soon after cessation of infusion. Propofol causes less nausea and vomiting than opioids or inhalation anesthetics. It is useful in intensive care units as a continuous-infusion sedative. Propofol may produce marked hypotension when IV induction doses are administered. It also produces pain on injection. The pain can be diminished or eliminated by means of pretreatment with IV lidocaine.

Table 13-4. ANALGESICS

	Potency	Sedation Dose	Duration	Infusion Dose
OPIOIDS				
Morphine	1	0.02–0.1 mg/kg IV	2–7 h	—
Meperidine	0.1	0.2–1 mg/kg IV	2–4 h	—
Fentanyl	100	0.5–1 μg/kg IV	30–60 min	—
Sufentanil	1000	Not recommended		
Alfentanil	25	10–20 μg/kg IV	10–15 min	—
OTHER ANALGESICS AND ANESTHETICS				
Propofol		0.5–1 mg/kg IV		25–50 μg/kg/min
Ketamine		0.5–1 mg/kg IV		15–80 μg/kg/min

Table 13-5. **ANXIOLYTICS AND AMNESICS (BENZODIAZEPINES)**

Name	Dose	Duration (h)	Strengths	Weaknesses
Midazolam (Versed)	0.05 (infusion dose 0.25 μg/kg/min)	0.5	Water soluble Short duration Good for sedation for short procedures	Acute respiratory depression
Diazepam (Valium)	0.1	1	Intermediate duration	Irritation on IV injection Phlebitis Acute respiratory depression after IV overdose
Lorazepam (Ativan)	0.02–0.08	6–8	Long duration	—
BENZODIAZEPINE REVERSAL				
Flumazenil (Romazicon)	4–20 μg/kg (0.2 mg repeated every 2 to 10 min until reversal is achieved) Maximum dose 1 mg	45 to 90 min	—	May produce seizures, panic, arrhythmias

Ketamine

Ketamine (Table 13-4) produces anesthesia characterized by dissociation between the thalamus and limbic systems. Patients appear to be in a cataleptic state in which their eyes remain open with a slow nystagmic gaze. The drug produces amnesia and analgesia but has been associated with unpleasant visual and auditory hallucinations. The incidence of these problems is reduced if benzodiazepines are administered with the ketamine.

Amnesics and Anxiolytics

Benzodiazepines (Table 13-5) are the primary class of agents used as amnesics and anxiolytics. The prototype, diazepam, is being replaced by its water-soluble analog, midazolam, which is of shorter duration. Benzodiazepines produce anxiolysis and some degree of amnesia but have no analgesic properties. Intraoperatively, midazolam is always used in conjunction with an opioid or inhalation agent. Midazolam is used with fentanyl to produce conscious sedation for minor procedures.

Benzodiazepines can produce apnea and have synergistic effects with narcotics. Small doses of midazolam and fentanyl quickly produce unconsciousness and apnea. For IV sedation, benzodiazepines are given in small, incremental doses. Flumazenil is the reversal agent for benzodiazepines.

Local Anesthetics

Local anesthetics (Table 13-6) produce temporary blockade of nerve conduction. As the concentration of the local anesthetic increases around a nerve, autonomic transmission is blocked first, then sensory transmission, then motor nerve transmission. These drugs can be injected into tissue to produce a field block, around peripheral nerves to produce a dermatome block, or into the spinal or epidural space to produce a conduction block.

Adverse consequences of the use of local anesthetics are:

- Acute central nervous system toxicity due to excessive plasma concentration
- Hemodynamic and respiratory problems due to excessive conduction block of the sympathetic or motor nerves
- Allergic reactions

Whenever a local anesthetic is injected, there is a risk for unintentional injection into a blood vessel or an overdose of the drug due to rapid uptake from the tissues. Both may produce seizures. One may minimize these complications by withdrawing the needle before injecting the agent if the needle is in a blood vessel and by limiting doses to the safe range.

When local anesthetics are administered for a spinal or epidural block, *total sympathectomy*—profound systemic vasodilatation and bradycardia—may occur. The hypotension that ensues is usually below the minimal cerebral perfusion pressure required to maintain consciousness. This disastrous situation is remedied if treated quickly with a vasopressor (phenylephrine or ephedrine) and atropine. If not treated promptly, the situation proceeds to cardiac arrest.

PREOPERATIVE EVALUATION

The anesthesiologist must do the following before the patient enters the operating room:

1. Take a history and perform a physical examination
2. Review the results of laboratory studies and conduct medical consultations

Table 13-6. **LOCAL ANESTHETICS**

	Maximum Single Dose (mg)	Duration (h)	Comments
AMIDES			
Lidocaine	500	1*	Fast onset Exaggerated cardiotoxicity with IV injection
Bupivacaine	200	4–12*	Slow onset Long duration
ESTERS†			
2-Chloroprocaine	1000	0.5–1*	Fast onset Lowest toxicity
Tetracaine	80	0.5–1	Slow onset

* Addition of 100 μg of epinephrine (0.1 mL of 1:1000) lowers the toxicity and increases the duration of the local anesthetic.
† Metabolism to para-aminobenzoic acid may cause allergic reactions.

3. Evaluate the patient's condition and assign an American Society of Anesthesiologists (ASA) physical status (Table 13-7)
4. Discuss options and risks with the patient
5. Develop an anesthetic plan

The history and physical examination are the most valuable parts of the preoperative assessment. The surgeon's history-taking includes questions about current medical conditions, current medication, previous operations, and experiences with anesthesia. Questions the anesthesiologist asks involve previous problems with anesthesia, anesthesia problems in blood relatives, and exercise tolerance. ASA physical status (Table 13-7) is a measure of the state of well-being of the patient. It takes into account all problems the patient brings to the operating room, including systemic disturbances caused by the surgical illness. Laboratory tests are ordered only if indicated by the history and physical findings.

The following examination enables one to determine if intubation may be difficult. Intubation should proceed smoothly if:

1. The patient has a normal mouth opening
2. The patient has normal neck flexion and extension
3. The examiner can fit three fingerwidths under the patient's chin between the thyroid cartilage and the mentum

Table 13-7. PHYSICAL STATUS CLASSIFICATION OF THE AMERICAN SOCIETY OF ANESTHESIOLOGISTS

Physical Status Classification	Description
PS-1	A normal healthy patient
PS-2	A patient with mild systemic disease that results in no functional limitation *Examples:* Hypertension, diabetes mellitus, chronic bronchitis, morbid obesity, extremes of age
PS-3	A patient with severe systemic disease that results in functional limitation *Examples:* Poorly controlled hypertension, diabetes mellitus with vascular complications, angina pectoris, prior myocardial infarction, pulmonary disease that limits activity
PS-4	A patient with severe systemic disease that is a constant threat to life *Examples:* Congestive heart failure, unstable angina pectoris, advanced pulmonary, renal, or hepatic dysfunction
PS-5	A moribund patient who is not expected to survive without the operation *Examples:* Ruptured abdominal aneurysm, pulmonary embolus, head injury with increased intracranial pressure
PS-6	A declared brain-dead patient whose organs are being removed for donor purposes
Emergency operation (E)	Any patient in whom an emergency operation is required *Example:* An otherwise healthy 30-year-old woman who requires dilation and curettage for moderate but persistent vaginal bleeding (PS-1E)

4. When the patient opens his or her mouth and sticks out the tongue, the uvula can be completely seen (class 1). If only part of the uvula can be seen (class 2) or if the uvula cannot be seen and only the hard and soft palate is visible (class 3), intubation may be difficult.

MONITORING SURGICAL PATIENTS

Monitors of Oxygenation

Pulse oximetry is used to measure arterial hemoglobin saturation (S_aO_2) and peripheral pulse by measuring light absorption. The oximeter uses two wavelengths of light, one red and one infrared, that shine through a tissue bed, usually a finger. The oximeter measures the ratio of the pulsatile component of red light absorbed to the pulsatile component of infrared light absorbed. This ratio changes with S_aO_2.

Pulse oximetry does not measures arterial oxygen tension (P_aO_2), although it can be estimated. As S_aO_2 drops below 90%, P_aO_2 can be estimated by subtracting 30 points from S_aO_2. For example, an S_aO_2 of 85% corresponds to a P_aO_2 of 55 mmHg. Pulse oximetry also can be used to estimate arterial oxygen content (C_aO_2), which is directly proportional to S_aO_2 and hemoglobin concentration (Hgb). Because Hgb is about one-third of hematocrit (Hct), the following equation can be used to estimate C_aO_2:

$$C_aO_2 = 0.45 \text{ Hct} \times S_aO_2$$

or if

$$S_aO_2 = 100\%$$

$$C_aO_2 \approx 1/2 \text{ Hct}$$

One can quickly assess the O_2-carrying capacity of blood by spinning an Hct and measuring S_aO_2 with a pulse oximeter.

Ventilation Monitors

Capnography, or end tidal CO_2 monitoring, is the visual display of carbon dioxide concentration at the airway. A patient is appropriately ventilated when arterial carbon dioxide tension (P_aCO_2) is 40 mmHg. The presence of a capnogram implies there is metabolism (production of CO_2), circulation (blood flow to the lungs), and ventilation (respiratory rate and an intact ventilator circuit). On a breath-to-breath basis, a continuous capnogram is useful as a surveillance monitor of both the respiratory circuit and the cardiovascular system. Any acute decrease in cardiac output causes an acute drop in end tidal CO_2. This principle allows detection of pulmonary emboli or acute drops in cardiac output.

The only acute catastrophic cardiopulmonary problem not detected with capnography is arterial desaturation. Therefore, the combination of capnography and pulse oximetry allows beat-to-beat and breath-to-breath surveillance of metabolism, circulation, ventilation, and oxygenation.

Circulation Monitors

The most basic way to monitor hemodynamic stability is to measure systemic arterial blood pressure with an oscillometric blood pressure cuff. When tighter control is required in patients with hypertension or serious heart disease or when an operation may cause acute blood loss, invasive arterial monitoring is performed. A continuous invasive arterial tracing can be used to assess the adequacy of fluid resuscitation.

Central venous pressure monitoring is frequently used in patients without left ventricular dysfunction who are undergoing extended surgical procedures with substantial fluid shifts and possible blood loss. Pulmonary arterial catheter monitoring is reserved for critically ill patients and for those with marked left ventricular dysfunction. Adequacy of circulation can be documented with thermo-dilution cardiac output measurements and mixed venous oxygen saturation monitoring.

Transesophageal echocardiography is used to assess cardiac function. This technique is easily used in anesthe-

tized, intubated patients and can be used for quick assessment of systolic and diastolic function and valvular dysfunction.

COMMON PROBLEMS IN THE POSTOPERATIVE PERIOD

Table 13-8 lists standards for postanesthesia care. The postanesthesia recovery score is used to evaluate postanesthesia status (Table 13-9). Figure 13-1 is an algorithm for the treatment of postoperative *nausea and vomiting. Hypothermia* alters drug metabolism and delays recovery. It also causes shivering, which increases the metabolic demand for oxygen.

Table 13-8. STANDARDS FOR POSTANESTHESIA CARE*

	Standards	Criteria to Be Fulfilled
Standard I†	All patients who have received general, regional, or monitored anesthesia care shall receive appropriate postanesthesia management.	1. A PACU or an area that provides equivalent postanesthesia care shall be available to receive patients after anesthesia care. All patients who receive anesthesia care shall be admitted to the PACU or its equivalent *except* by specific order of the anesthesiologist responsible for the patient's care. 2. The medical aspects of care in the PACU shall be governed by policies and procedures that have been reviewed and approved by the department of anesthesiology. 3. The design, equipment, and staffing of the PACU shall meet requirements of the facility's accrediting and licensing bodies.
Standard II	A patient transported to the PACU shall be accompanied by a member of the anesthesia care team who is knowledgeable about the patient's condition. The patient shall be continually evaluated and treated during transport with monitoring and support appropriate to the patient's condition.	
Standard III	On arrival in the PACU, the patient shall be reevaluated and a verbal report provided to the responsible PACU nurse by the member of the anesthesia care team who accompanies the patient.	1. The patient's status on arrival in the PACU shall be documented. 2. Information concerning the preoperative condition and the surgical/anesthetic course shall be transmitted to the PACU nurse. 3. The member of the anesthesia care team shall remain in the PACU until the PACU nurse accepts responsibility for the nursing care of the patient.
Standard IV	The patient's condition shall be evaluated continually in the PCAU.	1. The patient shall be observed and monitored by the methods appropriate to the patient's medical condition. Particular attention shall be given to monitoring oxygenation, ventilation, circulation, and temperature. During recovery from all anesthetics, a quantitative method of assessing oxygenation such as pulse oximetry shall be employed in the initial phase of recovery. This is not intended for application during the recovery of the obstetric patient in whom regional anesthesia was used for labor and vaginal delivery. 2. An accurate written report of the PACU period shall be maintained. Use of an appropriate PACU scoring system is encouraged for each patient on admission, at appropriate intervals prior to discharge, and at the time of discharge. 3. General medical supervision and coordination of patient care in the PACU should be the responsibility of an anesthesiologist. 4. There shall be a policy to ensure the availability in the facility of a physician capable of managing complications and providing cardiopulmonary resuscitation for patients in the PACU.
Standard V	A physician is responsible for discharging the patient from the PACU.	1. When discharge criteria are used, they must be approved by the department of anesthesiology and the medical staff. They may vary depending on whether the patient is discharged to a hospital room, to the ICU, to a short stay unit, or home. 2. In the absence of the physician responsible for the discharge, the PACU nurse shall determine that the patient meets the discharge criteria. The name of the physician accepting responsibility for discharge shall be noted on the record.

* Based on ASA's Standards for Postanesthesia Care. A copy of the full text can be obtained from ASA, 520 N. Northwest Highway, Park Ridge, IL 60068-2573.
† For nursing care issues, refer to Standards of Postanesthesia Nursing Practice, published by the American Society of Postanesthesia Nurses.

Table 13-9. POSTANESTHESIA RECOVERY SCORE*

Parameter	Score
ACTIVITY	
Voluntary movement of all limbs to command	2
Voluntary movement of 2 extremities to command	1
Unable to move	0
RESPIRATION	
Breathes deeply and coughs	2
Dyspnea, hypoventilation	1
Apneic	0
CIRCULATION	
Blood pressure equals 80% of preanesthetic level	2
Blood pressure equals 50%–80% of preanesthetic level	1
Blood pressure equals <50% of preanesthetic level	0
CONSCIOUSNESS	
Fully awake	2
Arousable	1
Unresponsive	0
COLOR	
Pink	2
Pale, blotchy	1
Cyanotic	0

* Patients should score at least 7 before discharge from the postanesthesia care unit.

Table 13-10. DIFFERENTIAL DIAGNOSIS OF DELAYED EMERGENCE

NEUROLOGIC INJURY
Ischemia
Mass lesions
Seizure disorders

METABOLIC ABNORMALITIES
Hypoglycemia
Diabetic ketoacidosis
Nonketotic hyperosmolar hyperglycemic coma
Hepatic dysfunction
Electrolyte disturbances
Renal dysfunction
Thyroid dysfunction
Adrenocortical dysfunction
Cardiorespiratory failure
Hypothermia
Malignant hyperthermia

DRUG EFFECTS
Inhalational anesthetics
Opioids
Barbiturates
Benzodiazepines
Ketamine
Antichlorinergics
Muscle relaxants

The most serious cardiovascular complication is *myocardial ischemia.* Only 10% to 30% of patients with documented myocardial infarction have pain, and postoperative ECG T-wave changes are often nonspecific. One must identify secondary signs of ongoing ischemia, such as hypotension, arrhythmias, elevated filling pressures, or postoperative oliguria.

The most common cause of *delayed emergence* is the residual effects of anesthesia. A differential diagnosis of delayed emergence is presented in Table 13-10.

MANAGEMENT OF ACUTE POSTOPERATIVE PAIN

Postoperative pain is inevitable. Its severity depends on the site of the operation (Table 13-11). Superficial somatic pain is well-localized and serves a protective function. It is readily treated with common analgesic techniques. Deep somatic pain may not be well-localized, may have some protective function, and is fairly responsive to a variety of

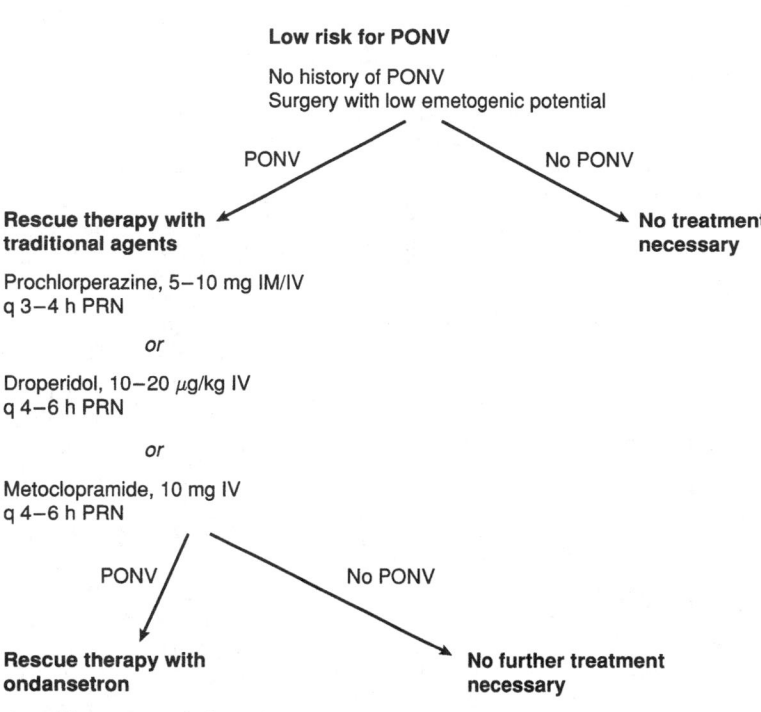

Figure 13-1. Algorithm for preventing and treating postoperative nausea and vomiting (PONV) in adults.

Table 13-11. PERCENTAGE OF PATIENTS WHO REQUIRE ANALGESIC INJECTIONS

Operation	No Analgesic Needed (%)	Three or More Analgesic Injections (%)
Minor chest wall	82	0
Inguinal hernia	52	0
Appendicectomy	25	10
Lower abdominal surgery	18	40
Upper abdominal surgery	10	45–65

analgesic agents. Visceral pain is poorly localized, often referred, and difficult to treat.

The use of nonsteroidal anti-inflammatory drugs (*NSAIDs*) with or without injection of local anesthetics into the wound is effective treatment of postoperative pain. *Opioids* are used to treat deep pain, both somatic and visceral. However, the responses to standard regimens are unreliable.

Patient-controlled analgesia (PCA) provides prompt and painless analgesia that matches the patient's need over time. PCA is as safe as conventional IM medication. Morphine and meperidine are the drugs in common use.

Transdermal narcotic delivery maintains continuous delivery and constant blood levels. Fentanyl is the drug most frequently used. The method appears to be safe, but considerable time elapses between application and attainment of therapeutic blood levels.

In *epidural opiate analgesia* (EOA), opioids are applied directly to pain receptors on the spinal cord. Morphine and fentanyl, sometimes combined with a dilute local anesthetic, are most often prescribed.

RISKS ASSOCIATED WITH ANESTHESIA

Patients with pre-existing medical conditions are at greater risk than other patients when they undergo a surgical procedure.

Hypertension

Hypertension is treated with medication before an elective operation. The medication is continued throughout the perioperative period. Patients with untreated hypertension are at risk for intraoperative hypotension and myocardial ischemia. Patients with inadequately treated hypertension who undergo carotid endarterectomy are at high risk for neurologic deficit, and those with a history of myocardial infarction are at risk for reinfarction. Patients with hypertension may have exaggerated responses to painful stimuli and are more likely than other patients to have perioperative ischemia.

Congestive Heart Failure

All elective operations should be deferred until CHF is treated. If the operation cannot be deferred, the goal of perioperative management is to optimize cardiac output.

Coronary Artery Disease

Patients at high risk (men >40 years, women >50 years) undergo a preoperative ECG exercise tolerance test. In patients without pulmonary disease, the ability to climb two flights of stairs without stopping or experiencing angina or shortness of breath is considered good cardiac reserve. Unfortunately, many patients with ischemic heart disease have pulmonary disease or other problems that limit their activity. A resting 12-lead ECG is an alternative for these patients.

A history of *myocardial infarction* is important. Mortality due to reinfarction among patients undergoing noncardiac operations is 20% to 50%. Most reinfarction occurs within 3 months of an operation. Hemodynamic monitoring with a pulmonary artery catheter and aggressive pharmacologic intervention reduce the risk for reinfarction. Prophylactic therapy with beta-blockers, calcium channel agents, and nitrates has not proved beneficial. However, withdrawal of these agents is associated with perioperative ischemia, myocardial infarction, and death.

Pulmonary Disease

Pulmonary disease is restrictive or obstructive. *Restrictive diseases,* such as ARDS, chest-wall defects, or obesity, reduce lung volume. These diseases produce pulmonary dysfunction, but they do not necessitate complicated anesthetic preparation. *Obstructive disease* is characterized by reduced flow rates on pulmonary function tests. It is either chronic (COPD) or acute (asthma). Any reversible component is reversed before an elective operation. Patients are given bronchodilator medication; those with chronic secretions are hydrated and receive therapy to mobilize secretions.

In patients with reactive airway disease, the endotracheal tube may induce severe bronchospasm. Even in patients who receive adequate preoperative therapy, reactive bronchospasm may complicate anesthetic induction and emergence from anesthesia. Bronchospasm is prevented or diminished with intubation at a deep level of anesthesia when reflexes are blunted.

For elective operations, patients should not be wheezing, and patients with chronic disease should not have any signs of bacterial infection, such as purulent sputum.

Obesity

The primary concern of an anesthesiologist caring for an obese patient is gaining adequate control of the airway. For this reason, one may consider nasal or oral awake intubation. All patients should receive prophylactic administration of H_2 receptor antagonists and metoclopramide to decrease the volume of gastric content. To prevent aspiration at emergence, obese patients are extubated when fully awake, preferably in the sitting position.

Obese patients may experience pulmonary failure just by lying flat, making it difficult to use epidural or spinal anesthesia for abdominal procedures. Epidural analgesics for postoperative pain management allow early extubation and ambulation.

Multiple Chronic Diseases

Overall hospital mortality increases when a patients has more than one chronic diseases. Renal failure and CHF are associated with the highest hospital mortality, especially among elderly patients who undergo emergency operations.

SUGGESTED READING

Blitt CD, Hines RL. Monitoring in Anesthesia and Critical Care Medicine (3d ed). New York: Churchill Livingston, 1994.

Breslow MJ, et al. Changes in T-wave morphology following anesthesia and surgery: A common recovery-room phenomenon. Anesth 1986;64:398.

Coriat P, Vrillon M, Perel A, et al. A comparison of systolic pressure variations and echo cardiographic estimates of end diastolic left ventricular size in patients after aortic surgery. Anesth Analg 1994;78:46.

Mallampati SR, Gatt SP, Guigino LD, et al. A clinical sign to predict difficult trachael intubation: A prospective study. Can Anesth Soc J 1985;32:429.

Mangao DT, et al. Association of perioperative myocardial ischemia with cardiac morbidity and mortality in men undergoing noncardiac surgery. N Engl J Med 1990;323:1781.

Marks RM, Sacher EJ. Undertreatment of medical inpatients with narcotic analgesics. Ann Intern Med 1973;78:173.

Stoelting RK, Dierdorf SF. Anesthesia and Co-Existing Disease (3rd ed). New York: Churchill Livingstone, 1993.

Tverskoy M, et al. Post-operative pain after inguinal herniorthaphy with different types of anesthesia. Anesth Analg 1990;70:29.

Yaeger M, Glass D, Neff R, Brink-Johnsed T. Epidural anesthesia and analgesia in high risk surgical patients. Anesthesiology 1987;66:729.

ESSENTIALS OF SURGERY: SCIENTIFIC PRINCIPLES AND PRACTICE, edited by Lazar J. Greenfield, Michael W. Mulholland, Keith T. Oldham, Gerald B. Zelenock, and Keith D. Lillemoe. Lippincott–Raven Publishers, Philadelphia, © 1997.

CHAPTER 14

TUMOR BIOLOGY

NEAL R. PELLIS, DENNIE V. JONES, JR., PAUL J. CHIAO, LEE M. ELLIS, AND CHARLES M. BALCH

DEFINITIONS

Neoplasia means "new growth." Neoplastic cells proliferate more rapidly than normal cells and do not respond to cessation of a growth stimulus or endogenous inhibitors of proliferation. Neoplastic growth frequently results in an abnormal swelling or tumor. Neoplasm and tumor are interchangeable.

Benign or malignant indicates the clinical behavior of a neoplasm, not merely the presence of abnormal growth. Malignancy is uncontrollable growth or dissemination.

Cancer is malignant neoplasia with a tendency toward local recurrence and dissemination.

Hyperplasia is an increase in cell number in both normal and neoplastic tissues. High basal growth rates are normal for some tissues.

Metaplasia is reversible transformation of one mature cell type to another. Metaplasia occurs when the replacing mature cell type is present in tissue where it is not normally present.

Dysplasia is alteration in cell size, shape, and organization, usually of epithelial tissues. Carcinoma in situ is the most disordered form of dysplasia. Although dysplasia may be associated with invasive carcinoma, not all dysplastic tissue progresses to carcinoma.

ETIOLOGY

The causes of neoplastic disease include familial and ethnic influences, as in familial breast cancer and hereditary nonpolyposis colorectal cancer (HNPCC)

- Carcinogenesis
- Viruses
- Immunodeficiency

Carcinogenesis can be physical or chemical. Tumor induction by physical agents occurs by one of two mechanisms: (1) The presence of a foreign body, such as asbestos,

induces cell proliferation over an extended period, increasing the opportunity for transformation. (2) An agent such as ionizing radiation or ultraviolet light damages or changes DNA replication.

Carcinogenesis may occur as a result of external contact with or ingestion or inhalation of a chemical. Chemical carcinogens can be organic, such as polycyclic hydrocarbons and nitrosamines, or inorganic, such as heavy-metal compounds that result from fossil fuel combustion or industrial processes such as smelting.

BIOLOGY OF ONCOGENESIS

Characteristics of the Transformed Cell

Most hematopoietic and solid tumors originate from a single transformed cell (Fig. 14-1). Not all cells exposed to a causative agent undergo transformation, and most transforming events are lethal. From the small surviving population of transformed cells, some cells progress to terminal differentiation or are recognized as altered-self and are eliminated by the host (Fig. 14-2).

The characteristics of neoplastic tissue are (1) heritable alterations in the genome and (2) loss of regulation of growth. Malignant or neoplastic transformation requires demonstration of tumorigenicity when transformed cells are inoculated into a living host.

Cellular transformation has many phenotypic, biochemical, and immunologic characteristics (Fig. 14-3). Transformed cells may exhibit changes in cellular morphology, such as cellular and nuclear pleomorphism, disordered arrangement of microfilament formation, and a variety of changes in cell surface characteristics. Karyotypic changes often evident in transformed cells are an increase in aneuploid populations, monosomy, trisomy, and other chromosomal aberrations. Cells transformed by chemicals or ultraviolet irradiation exhibit more antigenicity than spontaneously transformed cells.

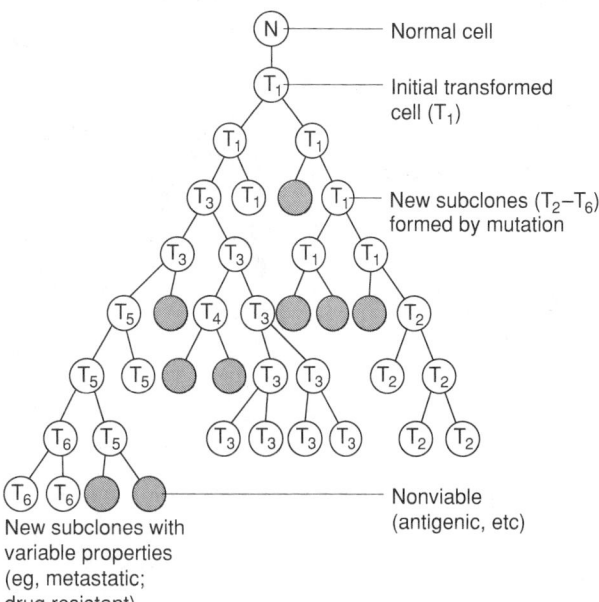

N — Normal cell

T₁ — Initial transformed cell (T₁)

New subclones (T₂–T₆) formed by mutation

Nonviable (antigenic, etc)

New subclones with variable properties (eg, metastatic; drug resistant)

Figure 14-1. Clonal evolution of tumors. New subclones can emerge by mutation. Many mutations are fatal, and the subclones become extinct (*colored areas*); others provide growth advantages, and the subclones become dominant. (After Nowell PC. The clonal evolution of tumor cell populations. Science 1976;194:23)

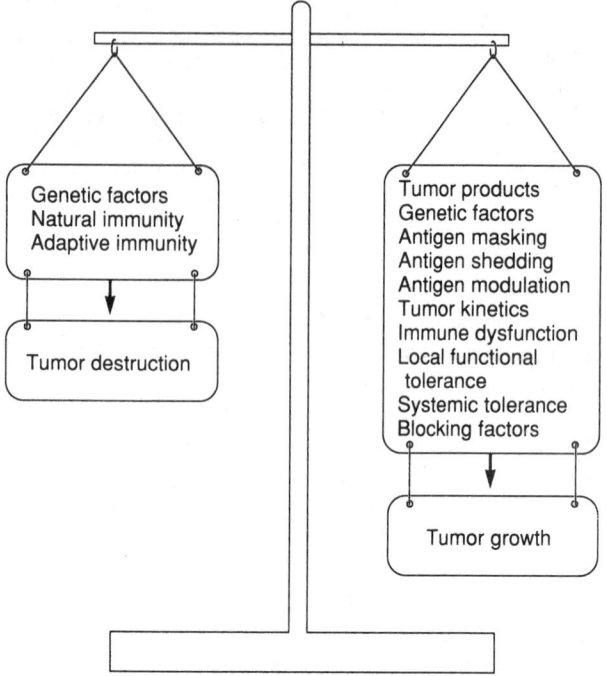

Figure 14-2. Tumor growth or destruction depends on a balance of factors within the host. (After Roitt IM, Brostoff J, Male DK. Immunology. St Louis, CV Mosby, 1985)

Growth and Proliferation of Neoplastic Cells

Measurement of tumor growth involves calculation of the time required to increase the volume of the tumor cell mass twofold (volume doubling time [T_D]). Methods to obtain this value are

1. Serial caliper measurement of skin, subcutaneous, breast, and other body surface tumors
2. Serial chest radiography or computed tomography (CT) of primary or metastatic pulmonary nodules, intraabdominal lesions, or lesions of other internal structures
3. Comparison of the product of the maximal perpendicular tumor diameters
4. Computerized measurement of tumor volume with CT and magnetic resonance imaging (MRI)

Tumor Volume Doubling Time

A solid tumor that originates from a single cell has undergone about 30 volume doublings to reach 1 cm³ (1 g), the smallest clinically detectable size. Most tumors become lethal at a mass of about 1 kg, which requires only ten additional doublings of cell mass (Fig. 14-4). The length of time a tumor is clinically apparent is only a fraction of the natural history. Most solid tumors do not exhibit exponential growth; growth slows in later stages. Tumor volume doubling time provides only a gross, and often late, estimate of tumor cell kinetics.

Flow Cytometry

Flow cytometry (FCM) allows analysis and sorting of individual cells. It is used for rapid measurement of DNA content and estimation of the proliferative rate of normal cells and populations of cells that compose solid or hematopoietic malignant tumors. FCM allows quantification and graphic display of the DNA content of a tumor.

Factors That Affect Tissue Growth

Tumor Growth Fraction

The growth fraction is the proportion of the total cell mass undergoing replication at one point in time. Primary tumors often consist of many cell types in addition to tu-

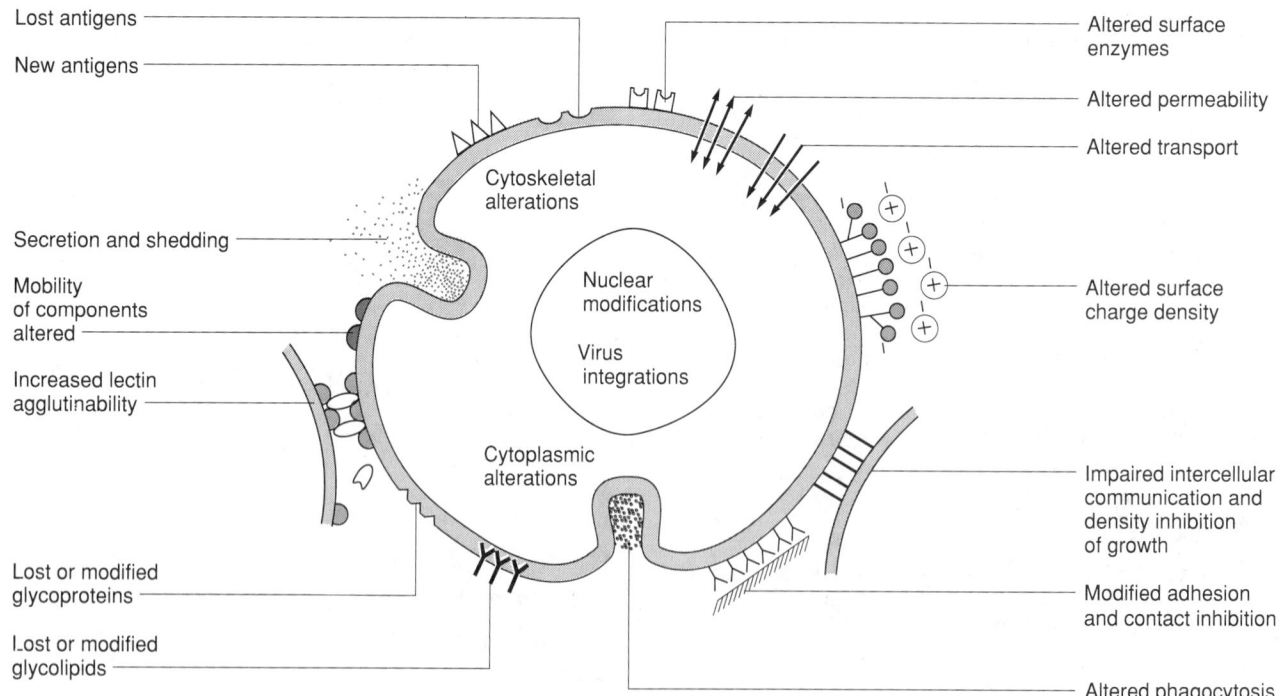

Figure 14-3. Alterations of cell structure and function that have been noted with neoplastic transformation. (After Nicolson GL. Trans-membrane control of the receptors on normal and tumor cells. II. Surface changes associated with transformation and malignancy. Biochim Biophys Acta 1976;458:1)

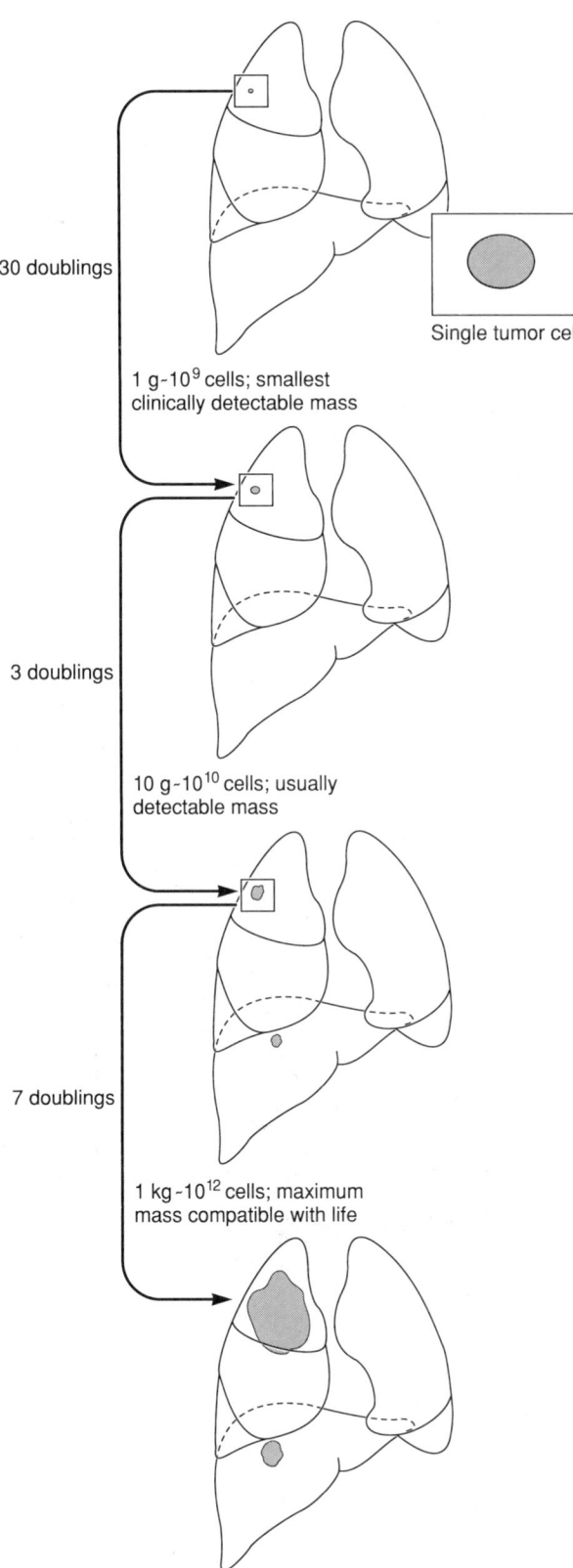

30 doublings

Single tumor cell

1 g-10^9 cells; smallest
clinically detectable mass

3 doublings

10 g-10^{10} cells; usually
detectable mass

7 doublings

1 kg-10^{12} cells; maximum
mass compatible with life

Figure 14-4. Growth of a solid tumor from a single transformed cell into a lethal tumor mass. (After Tannock IF. Biology of tumor growth. Hosp Pract 1983;18:81)

mor cells, and most cells that compose neoplasms do not undergo cell division. The growth fraction may be measured with FCM. Even in clinically aggressive solid tumors, a growth fraction of only 10% is not uncommon. The growth fraction does not fluctuate over the natural history of most solid tumors.

Tumor Cell Cycle

The cell cycle is the sequence of events involved in the growth and division of one cell into two daughter cells with identical chromosomal number and composition. The fate of these daughter cells may take three directions: (1) reentry into a new cell cycle resulting in two new identical progeny; (2) early cell death; or (3) entry into a permanent or reversible quiescent phase with no increase in cell number. Cells participating in the cell cycle are proliferating.

The cell cycle is defined by time intervals involved in DNA synthesis (S phase), mitosis (M phase), and the gaps of time between these events (G_1 before DNA synthesis; G_2 between DNA synthesis and mitosis; G_0, for cells not actively proliferating but capable of cellular division at the appropriate signal). The duration of the cell cycle is 2 to 4.5 days for most tumors.

Tumor Cell Death or Cell Loss

The primary determinant of neoplastic tissue growth and progression is a discordance between the growth fraction and the cell-loss fraction. In tumors, a slight increase in growth fraction is not compensated by a proportional increase in cell death or cell loss. The loss of growth regulation is linked to abnormalities in growth factor expression and alterations in specific cellular growth-regulatory genes (protooncogenes).

ONCOGENES

Oncogenes and tumor-suppressor genes are important in the pathogenesis of neoplastic cells and in the development, differentiation, and growth of normal cells. Oncogenesis occurs in three steps initiation, promotion, and progression. Each stage is the result of a series of changes in the molecular mechanisms that govern cellular differentiation and growth.

Retroviruses

Many advances in molecular oncology stem from the discovery of tumor viruses and retroviral oncogenes (Fig. 14-5). Viral gene expression results in neoplastic transformation of cells in vitro and tumor induction in vivo. All transforming retroviruses contain at least one gene that is not involved in viral replication but participates in transformation.

Retroviral oncogenes are designated by three-letter names that represent the tumors induced or the cell line from which the oncogene was isolated. For example, Rous sarcoma virus contains the src gene, which encodes a membrane-associated enzyme responsible for phosphorylation of cellular proteins. Oncogenes isolated from viruses have the prefix v (v-erb) and oncogenes isolated from host cellular DNA the prefix c (c-myc).

The products of oncogenes differ in cellular location, function, and mechanism of transformation. In some systems, the genes are expressed as a distinct translational product with transforming potential or as fusion of a viral replicative sequence and a transforming sequence. In all retroviruses, oncogenes are a part of the viral genome not involved in replication but essential for the malignant potential of the virus.

Retroviral oncogenes originate from normal cellular

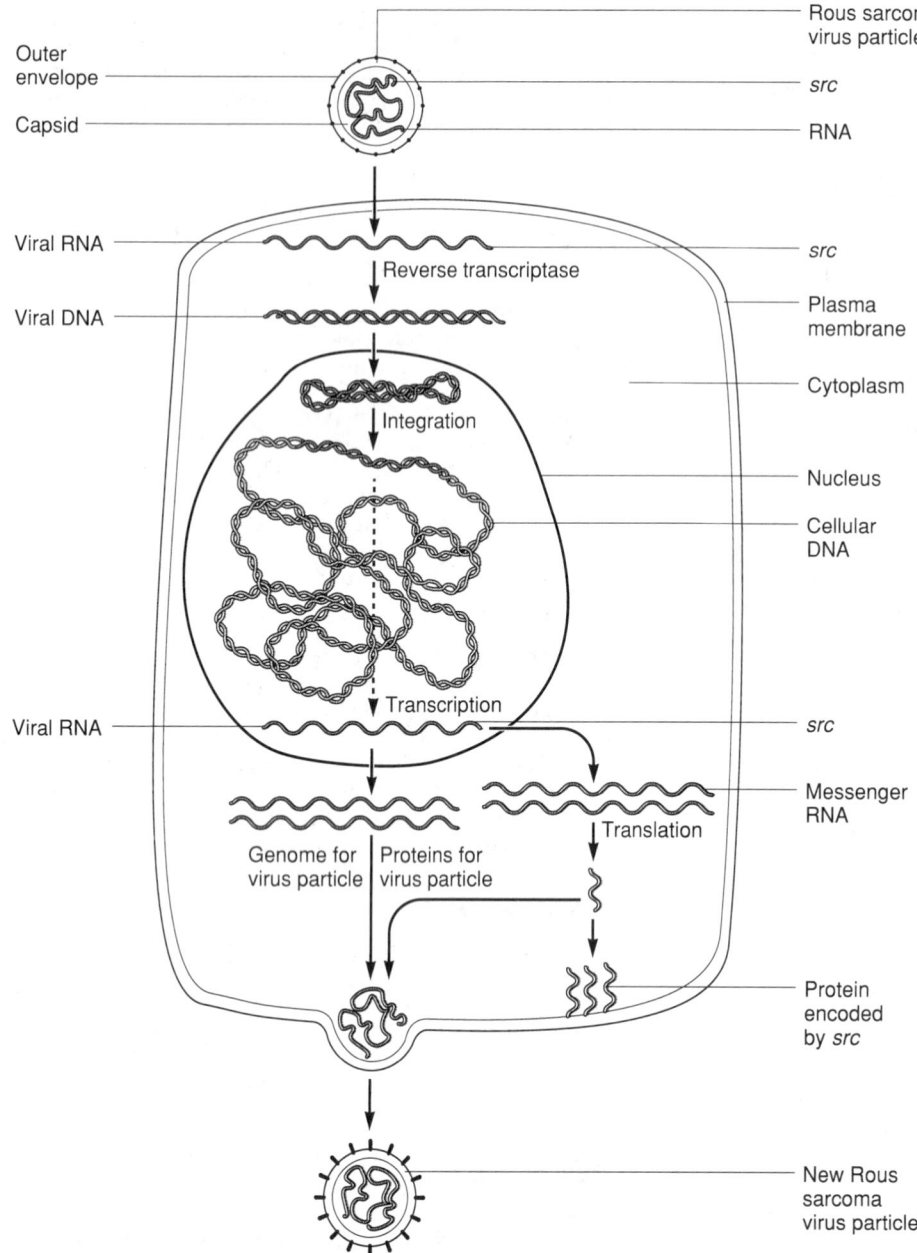

Figure 14-5. Neoplastic transformation by Rous sarcoma virus. When the Rous sarcoma retrovirus infects a cell, viral RNA is copied into double-stranded DNA by viral reverse transcriptase. After forming a circle, the viral DNA becomes integrated into the host cell DNA. Transcription of host DNA also results in transcription of viral DNA. Some viral RNA copies are included in new viral particles. Translation of viral RNA provides several proteins for inclusion into virus particles. Translation of viral RNA also produces the V-*src* gene product, which is not a component of the virus particle. The *src* gene product is a protein kinase, localized to the inner surface of the plasma cell membrane, which phosphorylates intracellular proteins. Protein phosphorylation results in cellular proliferation. (After Bishop JM. Oncogenes. Sci Am 1982;246:80)

genes called protooncogenes. Protooncogenes are incorporated into the viral genome during recombination events between the virus and host DNA. During transduction, normal genes may be rearranged or mutated. The altered forms of the protooncogenes may differ in regulatory or protein-coding sequences. These alterations produce the transforming potential of retroviruses.

Activation

The following mechanisms can change a normal gene to an oncogene:

- Point mutation (single nucleotide changes in DNA)
- Translocation, the shifting of a segment of one chromosome to another chromosome
- Amplification, the presence of an oncogene in a large number of gene copies per cell (Fig. 14-6)

Table 14-1 lists oncogenes and their mechanisms of activation.

Tumor-Suppressor Genes

Tumor-suppressor genes function as governors of growth and proliferative signals and suppress malignant transformation (Fig. 14-7). A loss of these genes appears to have a role in the development of neoplasia. The lost genes are presumed to encode growth-inhibitory signals. A mutation in the normal allele causes transformation to the cancerous phenotype. Oncogenes are classified according to the actions of their encoded proteins. The loss of tumor-suppressor genes is a recessive change in that the loss of function leads to the loss of normal growth-inhibitory signals (Table 14-2).

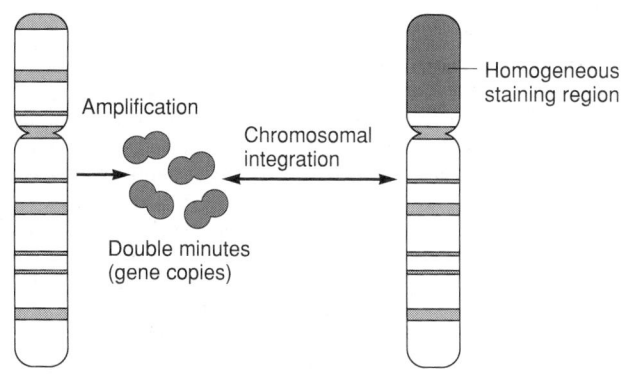

Figure 14-6. Oncogene activation through amplification. A gene locus can be amplified by repeated DNA replication. Recombination yields tandem arrays of amplified DNA, which form double minutes when excised from the chromosome. Integration of the double minutes into another chromosome forms a homogeneous staining region. (After Cooper GM. Oncogenes. Boston, Jones & Bartlett, 1990)

Table 14-1. ONCOGENE ACTIVATION ASSOCIATED WITH HUMAN NEOPLASMS

Neoplasm	Oncogene	Activation Mechanism
Burkitt lymphoma	c-myc	Translocation
Breast and lung carcinoma	c-myc	Amplification
Neuroblastoma, lung carcinoma	N-myc	Amplification
Lung carcinoma	L-myc	Amplification
Chronic myelogenous and acute lymphocytic leukemia	abl	Translocation
Follicular B-cell lymphoma	bcl-2	Translocation
Breast and ovarian carcinoma	erb B-2	Amplification
Colon and pancreatic carcinoma	K-ras	Point mutation
Acute myeloid and lymphoid leukemia	N-ras	Point mutation

(Adapted from Cooper GM. Oncogenes. Boston, Jones & Bartlett, 1990)

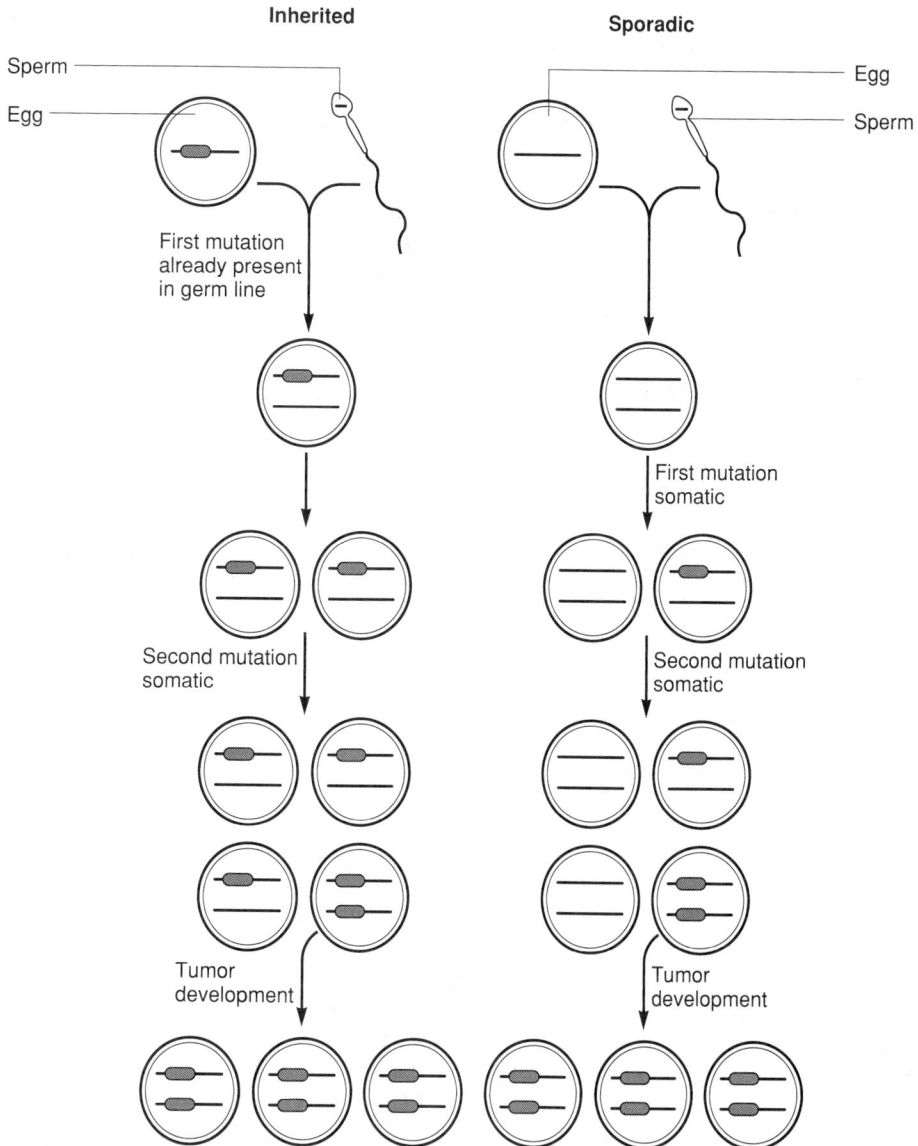

Figure 14-7. The model for development of retinoblastoma has served as a model for tumor-suppressor gene function. In inherited retinoblastoma, a mutation is transmitted through the gene line of the affected parent. The second mutation occurs somatically in a retinal cell. The second mutation leads to the development of a tumor. In sporadic retinoblastoma, two somatic mutations precede tumor development. (After Cooper GM. Oncogenes. Boston, Jones & Bartlett, 1990)

Table 14-2. TUMOR-SUPPRESSOR GENE LOSS REPORTED IN HUMAN NEOPLASMS

Tumor-Suppressor Gene or Chromosome	Neoplasm
Rb (Chromosome 13)	Retinoblastoma; osteosarcoma; breast, bladder, and small cell lung carcinoma
p53 (Chromosome 17)	Lung and colon carcinoma
Chromsome 1	Neuroblastoma
Chromosome 3	Lung and renal cell carcinoma
Chromosome 5	Colon carcinoma
Chromosome 11	Wilms tumor, hepatoblastoma, adrenal carcinoma, rhabdomyosarcoma, bladder and breast carcinoma
Chromosome 18	Colon carcinoma
Chromosome 22	Acoustic neuroma, meningioma

(Adapted from Cooper GM. Oncogenes. Boston, Jones & Bartlett, 1990)

Growth Factors

Growth factors are small peptides that bind to cellular receptors to produce intracellular responses that lead to proliferation or differentiation. Several growth factors function as transforming agents (Table 14-3). Growth factors and oncogenes interact on several levels. Oncogenes may (1) encode proteins that function in an autocrine manner to stimulate cell proliferation or (2) cause expression of altered growth factor receptors with abnormal signal transduction activity. Growth factors may act through activation of protooncogenes.

Signal Transduction

The generation of intracellular signals in response to extracellular factors at the cell surface is called signal transduction. The src and ras families of oncogenes are membrane-associated proteins involved in signal transduction.

In a normal cell, phosphorylation of an enzyme is a transient, regulatory event. In an oncoprotein, the enzyme may be activated, producing unregulated transfer of phosphate to tyrosine residues on targeted proteins. These targets, or effector proteins, may be responsible for sending abnormal or uncontrolled mitogenic signals to the cell nucleus.

Proteins known to bind guanosine triphosphate (GTP) are G proteins. Binding of GTP results in elevated enzyme activity. Enzyme activity is regulated by the length of time GTP remains bound before it is degraded to guanosine diphosphate (GDP). The principal G proteins belong to the ras family of protooncogenes. These genes encode related proteins localized to the inner surface of the cell membrane. Abnormal expression or activation of cell-surface receptors or any of the molecules in the signal system may be responsible for transformation of the cell.

Many protooncogenes function normally as integrated members of precise signal transduction pathways. Malignant transformation must involve abnormal mitogenic signals transmitted to the cell nucleus and loss of normal gene expression.

Transcription of Target Genes

In a regulated cell, binding of extracellular ligands by specific cell membrane receptors is transmitted as a mitogenic signal to the cell nucleus (Table 14-4). The final response involves increased transcription of target genes, DNA synthesis, and cell proliferation. Many protooncogenes act in a cooperative way that involves signal transduction. For example, binding of platelet-derived growth factor (PDGF) at its receptor on fibroblasts results in increased transcription of the c-myc gene.

Table 14-3. ONCOGENES AND ASSOCIATED NEOPLASMS

Category	Oncogene	Homologous Cellular Gene	Associated Neoplasm
Growth factors	*sis*	PDGF	
	int-2	FGF	Breast carcinoma
Transmembrane growth factor receptors	*erbB*	EGF receptor	
	neu		Breast carcinoma
	fms	M-CSF receptor	
	ros, kit		
Membrane-associated tyrosine kinases	*abl*		Chronic myelogenous leukemia, acute lymphocytic leukemia, acute myelogenous leukemia
	src		
	fes, fps		
Cytoplasmic serine and threonine kinases	*raf/mil, mos*		
Cytoplasmic hormone receptors	*erb A*	Thyroid hormone receptor	
Nuclear factors	*c-myc*		Burkitt lymphoma
	N-myc		Neuroblastoma
	L-myc		Small cell lung carcinoma
	fos		Osteosarcoma
	jun		
	myb, ets, ski		
Antioncogenes	*Rb, p53, p21, pcc, mcc*		Retinoblastoma
Others	*bcl-2*		Non-Hodgkin lymphomas
	bcl-1, int-1		Breast carcinoma

PDGF, platelet-derived growth factor; FGF, fibroblast growth factor; EGF, epidermal growth factor; M-CSF, mononuclear colony-stimulating factor.
(Adapted from Ducker BJ, Mamon HV, Roberts U. Oncogenes, growth factors and signal transduction. N Engl J Med 1989;321:1383)

Table 14-4. NUCLEAR ONCOGENE PRODUCTS

Protooncogene	Protein Molecular Weight
Thyroid hormone receptor (erb)	52,000
myc Family	
c-myc	64,000
L-myc	66,000
N-myc	64,000
Transcription factor AP-1 components	
c-jun	47,000
jun-B	40,000
jun-D	40,000
c-fos	62,000
fra-1	38,000
fos-B	45,000
Other nuclear oncogenes	
myb	75,000
ets-1	51,000
ets-2	56,000
ski	60,000
rel	68,000

(Adapted from Cooper GM. Oncogenes. Boston, Jones & Bartlett, 1990)

Tumorigenesis

Genetic events that lead to activation of oncogenes increase gene expression or increase activity of the oncoprotein. These genes appear to act in a dominant, positive regulatory manner. In other words, introduction of the altered genes into cells causes malignant transformation. A genetic model for colorectal tumorigenesis is shown in Figure 14-8. Mutations in at least four genes are required for full malignant transformation. The total accumulation of changes rather than the sequence of accumulation is important.

BIOLOGY OF METASTASIS

Metastasis is the active or passive dissemination of neoplastic disease from the site of origin to a distant site or organ in the host. The primary site undergoes changes that enable tumor cells to enter the microcirculation (intravasation) and increase the possibility for seeding distal sites. Seeding follows, and seeding is followed by adherence of tumor cells to endothelial walls, extravasation, and invasion of the stroma (Fig. 14-9).

Invasion

The ability of a tumor to dissociate cells that initiate neoplastic outgrowth is a direct measure of malignant potential. Distribution of tumor cells from the primary site may occur by direct spread or seeding. The routes of dissemination are determined by the histologic characteristics and the location of the primary tumor.

Dissemination frequently occurs as hematogenous or lymphatic metastasis. Invasion and infiltration into host tissues around the primary tumor eventually penetrate blood vessels, lymph vessels, or both, and provide access for widespread dispersion. Mechanical pressure produced by the rapid proliferation of neoplasms may force fingerlike projections of tumor cells along lines of least resistance.

Many highly invasive tumors grow slowly. Intrinsic cell motility may have a role in tumor cell invasion. Tumor cells possess the organelles necessary for active locomotion and can form cellular cytoplasmic processes, indicative of motility, during invasion.

Invasion of normal tissues, intercellular matrices, and vascular basement membranes by metastatic cells requires hydrolytic enzymes. Connective tissue proteins are classified into four groups: collagen, elastin, glycoproteins, and proteoglycans. The distribution of each protein varies among different tissues. The constituents of the extracellular matrix are stabilized and organized by interactions among the tissue proteins. The stability is easily disordered by degradative enzymes released from tumor cells. Table 14-5 lists factors involved in metastasis formation.

Lymphatic and Hematogenous Spread

Clinical observations give the erroneous impression that carcinomas spread by the lymphatic route and mesenchymal tumors spread via the bloodstream. Lymphatic and vascular systems have numerous connections, and disseminating tumor cells may pass from one system to another.

Lymphatic Dissemination

Infiltration and expansion into host tissues results in penetration of small lymphatic vessels by tumor cells. Tumor cell emboli in the vessels are responsible for initiation of lymphatic metastases. Tumor emboli may be trapped in the first lymph node encountered, or metastatic emboli may traverse lymph nodes or even bypass them to form distant nodal metastases (skip metastasis).

Lymph nodes are immunologically responsive in patients with neoplasms. Lymph nodes in the area of a primary neoplasm are often enlarged and palpable, indicating hyperplasia of lymph node follicles accompanied by proliferation of reticulum cells and sinus endothelium or growth of tumor cells. The presence of a tumor stimulates the activation, proliferation, and release of immunocompetent cells in the lymphoreticular system. The reaction begins in the regional lymph nodes and proceeds to distant nodes and the spleen. Proliferative changes in the regional

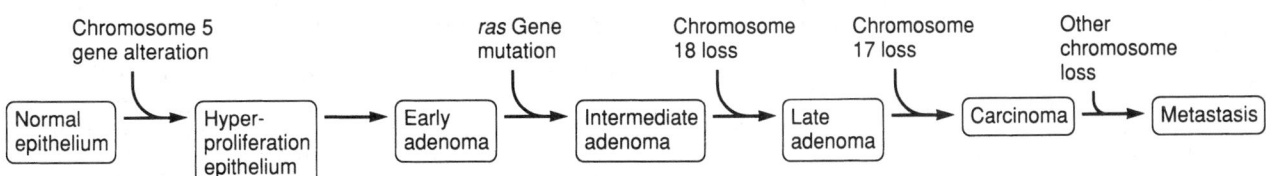

Figure 14-8. Model of colorectal tumorigenesis proposed by Vogelstein. Oncogenesis is postulated to be a multistep process involving a series of genetic alterations. The cumulative effects of oncogene activation and tumor-suppressor gene loss, but not the order of the alteration, are proposed to be crucial for neoplastic transformation. (After Fearen ER, Vogelstein B. A genetic marker for colorectal tumorigenesis. Cell 1990;61:759)

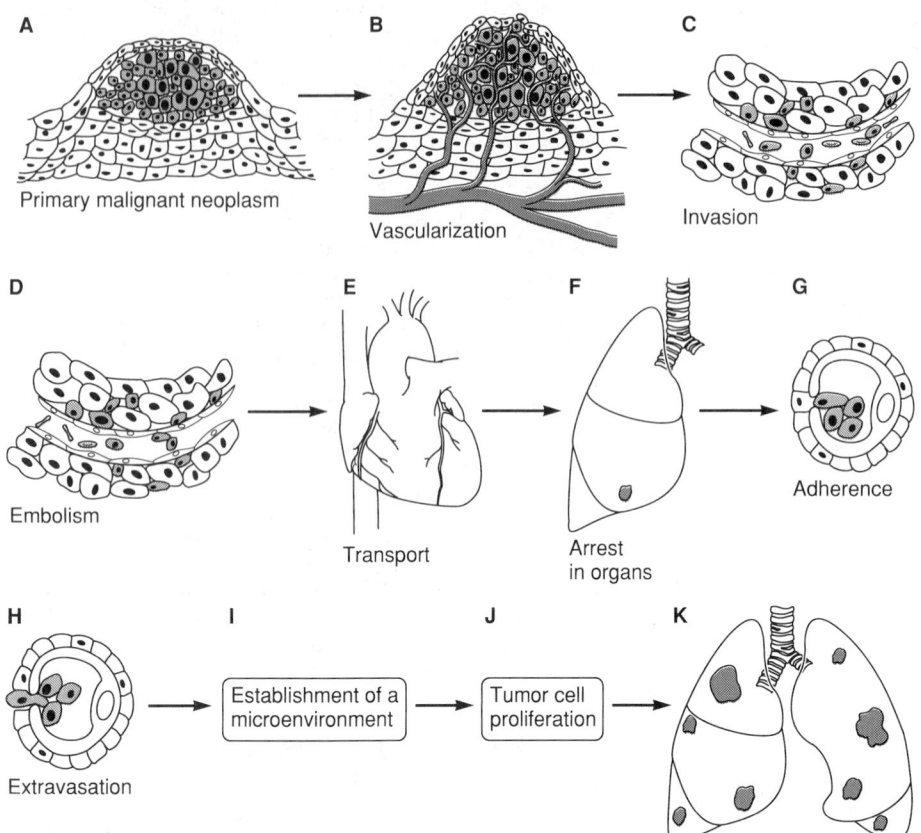

A Primary malignant neoplasm
B Vascularization
C Invasion
D Embolism
E Transport
F Arrest in organs
G Adherence
H Extravasation
I Establishment of a microenvironment
J Tumor cell proliferation
K Metastases

Figure 14-9. Steps in the formation of metastatic cancer. (After Fidler IJ, Balch CM. The biology of cancer metastasis and implications for therapy. Curr Probl Surg 1987;24:136)

lymph nodes often precede the spread and growth of tumor emboli within them.

Lymph nodes may serve as a temporary filter for metastatic tumor cells. Although lymph nodes are an effective, but temporary, barrier to tumor spread, they may be a repository for immunoselected, resistant tumor cells. The filtration capacity of lymph nodes is reduced by tumor growth, acute or chronic inflammatory reactions, and fibrosis due to local irradiation.

Hematogenous Metastasis

The Metastatic Cascade. Metastasis is a series of linked, sequential steps that favor survival of a subpopulation of metastatic cells in the primary tumor mass. Failure to complete one or more steps of the process eliminates the cells. The mere presence of tumor cells in the circulation does not mean metastasis will occur; most tumor cells that enter the blood stream are rapidly destroyed. Continued metastatic growth requires acquisition of a blood supply. To produce clinically relevant metastases, a successful metastatic cell must exhibit a complex phenotype regulated by transient or permanent changes in different genes at the DNA or mRNA level.

The Role of Angiogenesis in Metastasis. Tumor angiogenesis (vessel counts or density) is essential for both primary and metastatic growth. The greater the vascularization of a tumor, the greater is the likelihood of distant metastases.

Tumor angiogenesis is not passive. Specific factors must be expressed, and the appropriate receptors must be present on the target endothelium to initiate basement membrane degradation, endothelial cell proliferation and mi-

gration, and capillary tubule formation. Although tumor cells are constantly shed from a primary tumor and enter the circulation, only a small percentage actually form a metastasis. The greater the number of cells released into the circulation, the greater is the likelihood a cell may possess the phenotype necessary to form a metastasis. As tumors grow, they shed more cells into the circulation.

Host Factors and Metastasis

Two arguments are used to explain organ-specific metastasis:

1. The growth of metastases is influenced by the interaction of particular tumor cells (seed) with unique organ environments (soil). Metastases occur only when seed and soil are compatible.
2. Metastatic dissemination occurs by means of mechanical factors determined by the anatomic structure of the vascular system.

Heterogeneity of Metastasis

At diagnosis, many neoplasms are composed of subpopulations of cells with different biologic properties. Cells isolated from individual neoplasms differ in morphology, karyotype, growth rate, antigenicity-immunogenicity, cell surface receptors for lectins, hormone receptors, response to therapy, and potential for invasion and metastasis.

To produce a clinically apparent metastasis, malignant tumor cells must pass through a sequence of potentially lethal interactions with host homeostatic mechanisms, not the least of which is avoidance of recognition and destruction by host

Table 14-5. FACTORS INVOLVED IN METASTASIS FORMATION

DEGRADATIVE ENZYMES
Metalloproteinases
    Collagenases
    Transin and stromelysin
Tissue inhibitors of metalloproteinases (TIMP) I, II, III
Serine proteases
    Plasminogen activators
        Urokinase
        Tissue plasminogen activator
Cysteine Proteases
    Cathepsins

MOTILITY FACTORS
Autocrine motility factor
Hepatocyte growth factor and scatter factor

ANGIOGENIC FACTORS
Acidic fibroblast growth factor
Angiogenin
Basic fibroblast growth factor
Hepatocyte growth factor
Interleukin-8
Placenta growth factor
Platelet-derived endothelial cell growth factor
Pleotropin
Prostaglandin E_1 and E_2
Transforming growth factor α
Transforming growth factor β
Tumor necrosis factor α
Vascular endothelial growth factor and vascular permeability factor

ENDOGENOUS INHIBITORS OF ANGIOGENESIS
Angiostatin
Cartilage-derived inhibitor
Heparinase
Interferon
Platelet factor 4
Prolactin fragment
Protamine
Thrombospondin
Tissue inhibitor of metalloproteinase

ADHESION MOLECULES
Carcinoembryonic antigen
Proteoglycans
Intercellular adhesion molecule 1
Selectins
CD43
CD44
E-cadherin
P-cadherin
Selectins
Integrins

defenses. Failure to complete any step in the metastatic process results in elimination of the errant tumor cell.

There are three important principles for metastatic development:

1. The process of metastasis is not random
2. Neoplasms are not uniform entities but rather contain cells exhibiting heterogeneous metastatic capabilities
3. The outcome of metastasis depends on the properties of both tumor cells and host factors; the balance of the contributions varies among tumors that originate in different tissues and even among tumors of similar histologic origin in different patients

Origin of Cellular Diversity

Tumors undergo a series of changes as part of the natural history of the disease. For example, tumors initially diagnosed as benign may, over a period of many months or even years, assume a malignant phenotype. Acquired genetic variability in developing clones of tumors coupled with host selection pressures results in new clonal sublines of increased growth autonomy or malignancy.

The hypothesis of cellular diversity poses that progression toward malignancy is accompanied by increased genetic instability of malignant cells. The rapid generation of diversity is presumed to be the product of increased genetic instability. Highly metastatic clones exhibit a higher rate of spontaneous mutation than cells from poorly metastatic lines. The more metastatic a tumor cell population, the greater is the likelihood that the constituent cells will undergo spontaneous mutations that cause rapid phenotypic diversification and increased opportunities for escape from therapy. Diversification may be exaggerated by the mutagenic action of many of the cytotoxic antineoplastic drugs used in therapy.

The hypothesis of cellular diversity applies to tumors of multicellular origin. Tumors of unicellular origin, however, may exhibit metastatic heterogeneity early in development.

Origin of Heterogeneity in Metastases

Certain tumors metastasize to specific sites. For example, renal cell carcinoma tends to metastasize to the lung, colon cancer to the liver, and breast and prostate cancer to bone. Although the site of metastasis may seem to be determined by venous drainage patterns, environment is important in the metastatic process. The environment in the organ of metastasis must express growth factors that are ligands for specific growth factor receptors on the membrane of tumor cells.

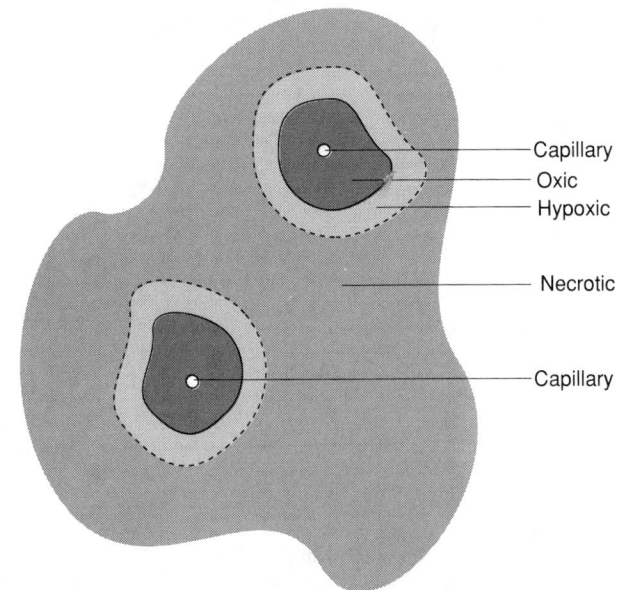

Figure 14-10. Tumors contain regions that are anoxic, hypoxic, and well-oxygenated and that vary with the distance from capillaries. The response to ionizing radiation varies with the degree of tissue oxygenation. (After Hellman S. Principles of radiation therapy. In: DeVita VT, Hellman S, Rosenberg SA, eds. Cancer: principles and practice of oncology, ed 3. Philadelphia, JB Lippincott, 1989:247)

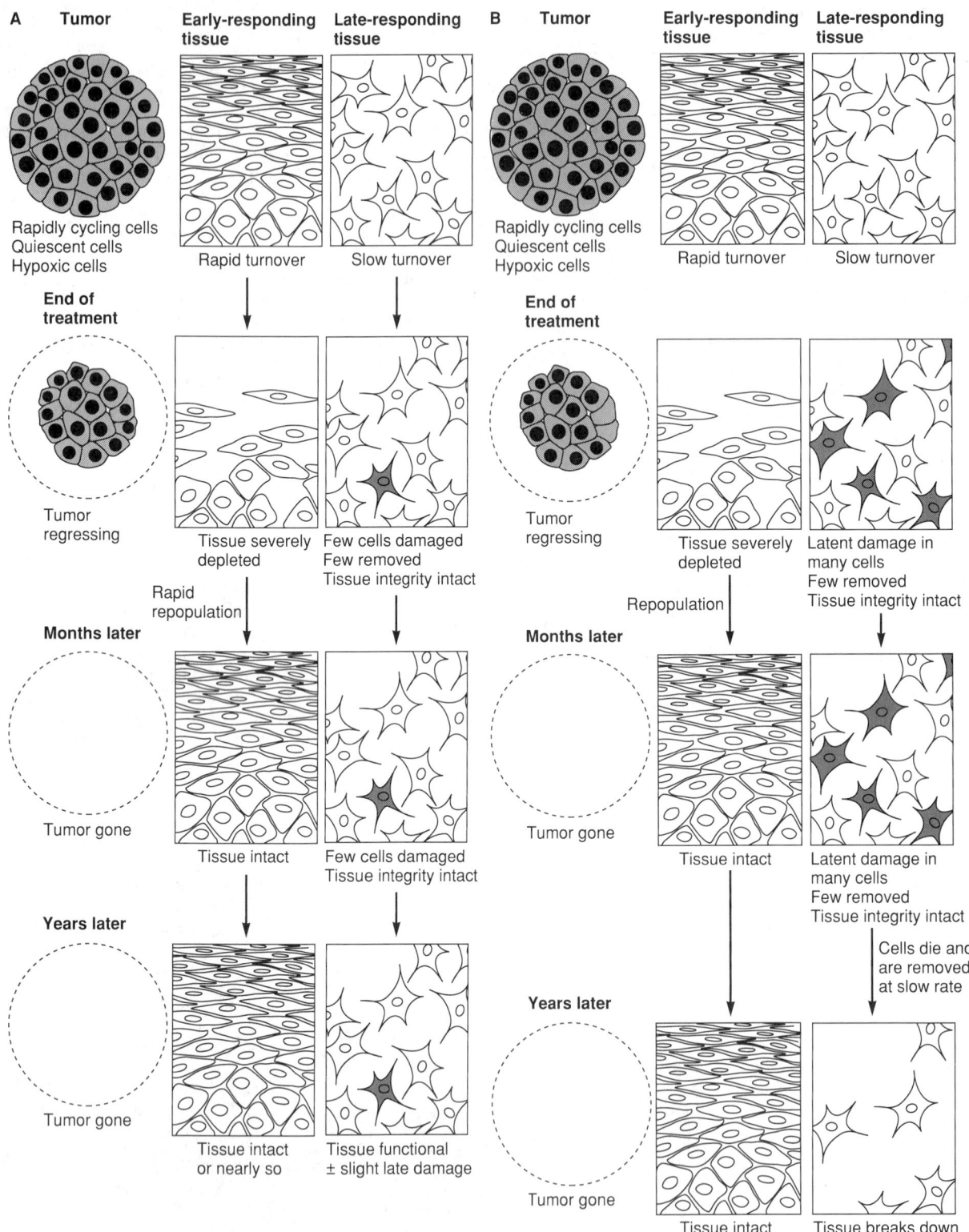

Figure 14-11. Patterns observed after delivery of radiation dose in many small fractions (*A*) and a few large fractions (*B*). Smaller dose fractions produce less damage to late-responding tissues than to early-responding tissues; larger fractions produce relatively more damage to late-responding tissues than to early-responding tissues. With smaller fractions, early-responding tissues can repair and repopulate by cell division. With larger-dose fractions, early-responding tissues repair and repopulate as with smaller fractions. However, late-responding tissues are damaged to a greater extent and exhibit this damage after a latent period when cells in these tissues begin to turn over. (After Hall EJ. Radiation biology. CA 1985;55:2051)

RADIATION BIOLOGY AND RADIATION THERAPY

The goal of radiation therapy is to control the tumor while minimizing the adverse effects on normal tissue.

Ionizing Radiation

Ionizing radiation is energy absorbed by tissue. Absorption of the energy causes excitation and ejection of an orbital electron, producing ionized atoms and molecules. Particulate radiation consists of subatomic particles such as electrons, protons, and neutrons. Electromagnetic radiation is derived from electrical machines and linear accelerators (x rays) or from the decay of radioisotopes (γ rays). The energy released by electromagnetic radiation has the characteristics of a wave or a packet of energy, the photon.

The intensity of radiation can be quantified to provide information about tissue absorption and penetration. As the energy of radiation increases, the depth of penetration through tissue increases. The absorption mechanisms differ at varying intensities. At supervoltage or megavoltage, the full energy of the radiation is not transferred to the tissue until some distance is reached. Therefore, high-energy radiation penetrates skin and other superficial structures and reaches its full ionizing potential when it reaches the deeper target tissues (skin-sparing effect).

The clinical description of absorbed energy is based on the amount of energy absorbed per unit mass. Dosages are measured in grays (1 Gy = 1 joule/kg).

Radiation Techniques

Brachytherapy

The source of radiation is adjacent to or within the targeted tissue. Isotopes such as ^{198}Au and ^{125}I are placed in special catheters, the positioning of which is based on precise geometric considerations. The placement of the radiation source is critical because a high dose of energy is aimed directly at the target, and the dose decreases rapidly with distance. The advantage of this technique is the ability to deliver high, concentrated doses to the target while limiting damage to nearby normal tissue.

Teletherapy

Orthovoltage or supervoltage machines, such as cobalt machines, electrical machines, and linear accelerators are used to deliver high-energy electromagnetic beams. The source of the radiation is not in direct contact with the target. The absorbed dose is determined by the geometric and tissue characteristics of the target and the energy of the radiation. The radiation beam can be modified to deliver a maximum dose to targeted tissues while minimizing the effects on normal tissue.

Radiation Biology

Radiation therapy renders malignant cells incapable of further proliferation. This is accomplished by causing irreparable damage to key biologic molecules in the cell. High-energy radiation can cause direct breaks in chromosomal DNA, rendering it incapable of replication. Most of the biologic effects, however, are due to an indirect action mediated by free radicals generated by the interaction between ionizing radiation and water. The free radicals have an extremely short half-life but while present can damage DNA and other key intracellular molecules.

Adverse Effects and Biology of Normal Tissue

The radiosensitivity of cells depends on their position in the cell cycle. Cells in the M phase (mitotic phase) are most sensitive. During irradiation, only a fraction of cells are in a vulnerable position in the cell cycle. The sensitivity of the tumor in contrast to normal tissue depends on the ability of cells to redistribute and repopulate in the radiated volume. In tumors that are particularly radiosensitive, this balance between cell killing and repopulation favors normal tissue over the tumor. The ability to recruit cells from adjacent undamaged areas also favors normal tissue.

The presence or absence of molecular oxygen greatly influences the proportion of cells killed by a given dose of radiation. It is the most important biologic response modifier for enhancing formation of and prolonging the survival of free radicals. Therefore, radiosensitivity of cells in a tumor varies according to location relative to oxygen-carrying capillaries (Fig. 14-10). Cells in hypoxic regions of a tumor may escape the effects of radiation. As conditions change with progressive cell killing, fewer cells exist in hypoxic regions, and oxygen may become more evenly distributed in the tumor volume.

Pharmacologic Modification

The response of cells and tissues is altered by chemical agents. Some agents substitute for molecular oxygen and serve as hypoxic cell sensitizers. Others are incorporated

Table 14-6. MECHANISMS OF DRUG RESISTANCE

Mechanism	Agent
Multidrug resistance	Vinca sp alkaloids
	Antitumor antibiotics
	Etoposide
Transport defect	Methotrexate
	Melphalan
	Nitrogen mustard
	Cytosine arabinoside
Poor activation	Cytosine arabinoside
	5-Azacitidine
	5-Fluorouracil
	6-Thioguanine
	6-Mercaptopurine
	Methotrexate
	Doxorubicin
Drug inactivation	Cytosine arabinoside
	Alkylating agents
	6-Thioguanine
	6-Mercaptopurine
Improved DNA repair	Alkylating agents
	Antitumor antibiotics
	Cisplatin
Gene amplification	Methotrexate
	2-Deoxycoformycin
	5-Fluorouracil
Alternate pathways	Methotrexate
	5-Fluorouracil
Altered pools of competing substrate	Cytosine arabinoside
	5-Fluorouracil
Target alterations	Vincristine
	Methotrexate
	5-Fluorouracil
	Hydroxyurea
	Steroids

(Adapted from DeVita VT. Principles of chemotherapy. In: DeVita VT, Hellman S, Rosenberg SA, eds. Cancer: principles and practice of oncology, ed 3. Philadelphia, JB Lippincott, 1989:279)

into DNA and increase sensitivity to the ionizing effects of radiation.

Tumor Biology

The risk for serious complications is related to total radiation dose. There is a range in which tumor control improves with increasing total dose and the probability of serious complications is low. At progressively higher doses, little is gained in tumor control, and the risk for serious complications is high. The adverse effects on organ function of normal tissue depend on the reproductive requirements of the irradiated cells. The following techniques are used to improve therapeutic gain while minimizing complications.

Fractionation

The total dose of radiation is given in a series of small fractions rather than a single large dose. Normal tissues are spared because time is allowed for repopulation. The effect on the tumor is greater than if the same amount of radiation were delivered in a single exposure because reoxygenation occurs between dose fractions (Fig. 14-11).

High Linear Energy Transfer Radiation

High LET radiation is produced with large atomic particles, such as neutrons, which are densely ionizing. (Conventional radiation uses photons and electrons, which are sparsely ionizing.) The biologic effectiveness of LET radiation is higher than that of conventional radiation at any given dose.

Radiation Therapy Combined With Surgical Therapy

Surgical excision removes the principal tumor mass but is limited in the extent of peripheral margins obtainable. Radiation therapy rarely fails at the periphery of tumors. Its use is limited in the management of large tumors because of the large number of cells in various stages of the cell cycle and because the environment is relatively hypoxic. Macroscopic tumor control often requires high doses

---

Table 14-7. CHEMOTHERAPEUTIC AGENTS AND THEIR COMMON ABBREVIATIONS

ALKYLATING AGENTS

Nitrogen mustards
  Mechlorethamine
  Cyclophosphamide
  Ifosfamide
  Phenylalanine mustard
  Chlorambucil
Ethylenimine derivatives
  Triethylenethiophosphoramide
Alkyl sulfonates
  Busulfan
Nitrosoureas
  Cyclohexyl-chloroethyl nitrosourea
  1,3-Bis-[2-chloroethyl]-1-nitrosourea
  Streptozotocin
Triazenes
  Dimethyl triazenoimidazole carboxamide

ANTIMETABOLITES

Folic acid analogues
  Methotrexate
Pyrimidine analogues
  5-Fluorouracil
  Cytosine arabinoside
Purine Analogues
  6-Mercaptopurine
  6-Thioguanine
  Deoxycoformycin

NATURAL OR SEMISYNTHETIC PRODUCTS

Vinca alkaloid
  Vinblastine
  Vincristine
Antibiotics
  Doxorubicin
  Mitoxantrone
  Daunorubicin
  Bleomycin
  Dactinomycin
  Mithramycin
  Mitomycin C
Enzymes
  L-Asparaginace
Epipodophyllotoxins
  Etoposide
  Teniposide

MISCELLANEOUS

Platinum coordination complexes
  Cis-Diamminedichloroplatinum II
  Cisplatin (Platinol)
  Carboplatin
Substituted urea
  Hydroxyurea
Methylhydrazine derivative
  Procarbazine
Estramustine phosphate
Acridine derivative
  Amsacrine

HORMONES AND HORMONE INHIBITORS

Estrogens
  Diethylstilbestrol
  Conjugated estrogens
  Ethinyl estradiol
Androgens
  Testosterone propionate
  Fluoxymesterone
Progestins
  17-Hydroxyprogesterone caproate
  Medroxyprogesterone acetate
  Magestrol acetate
Leuprolide
  Goserelin acetate
Adrenocorticosteroids
Antiestrogens
  Tamoxifen
Hormone Synthesis Inhibitors
  Aminoglutethimide
Antiandrogens
  Flutamide

Table 14-8. COMMON CHEMOTHERAPEUTIC AGENTS

Drug	Indication	Toxicities
ALKYLATING AGENTS: transfer alkyl groups to nucleic acids and other biologically important molecules		
Busulfan	Chronic myelogenous leukemia, myeloproliferative disorders	Myelosuppression, pulmonary fibrosis, gonadal dysfunction, marrow failure
Chlorambucil	Chronic lymphocytic leukemia, Waldenström macroglobulinemia	Myelosuppression, gonadal dysfunction, secondary leukemia
Cyclophosphamide	Hematologic malignancies, Hodgkin's disease, non-Hodgkin's lymphomas, carcinomas of the breast and ovary, sarcomas, small cell lung cancer, pediatric malignancies	Leukopenia, cystitis, nausea and vomiting, alopecia, cardiac necrosis, gonadal dysfunction, SIADH
Ifosfamide	Carcinomas of the breast, ovaries, lung, testicles; lymphomas; sarcomas	Myelosuppression, cystitis, nephrotoxicity, hepatoxicity, lethargy and confusion
Dacarbazine	Hodgkin's disease, non-Hodgkin's lymphomas, melanoma, sarcomas	Nausea and vomiting, flu-like syndrome, myelosuppression, hepatotoxicity
Cisplatin	Carcinomas of the ovary, testis, cervix, head and neck, bladder, lung (small and non–small cell), esophagus; lymphomas	Nausea and vomiting, nephrotoxicity, neurotoxicity, hearing loss, electrolyte imbalance
Carboplatin	Carcinoma of the ovary, bone marrow transplantation	Myelosuppression, nausea and vomiting
Melphalan	Multiple myeloma, ovarian cancer	Myelosuppression, anorexia, nausea and vomiting
Mechlorethamine	Lymphomas, Hodgkin's disease	Myelosuppression, secondary leukemia, severe vesicant, nausea and vomiting, alopecia, rash, gonadal dysfunction, neurotoxicity
Nitrosoureas (Carmustine, BCNU; lomustine, CCNU)	Lymphomas, Hodgkin's disease, brain cancer, bone marrow transplantation	Myelosuppression, secondary leukemia, hepatotoxicity, pulmonary fibrosis, nausea and vomiting, nephrotoxicity, confusion
Streptozocin	Neuroendocrine tumors	Nephrotoxicity, nausea and vomiting, myelosuppression, hepatotoxicity, hypoglycemia
Procarbazine	Hodgkin's disease, lymphomas, brain cancer	Myelosuppression, monoamine oxidase inhibition, nausea and vomiting, lethargy, myalgias, arthralgias, neurotoxicity, dermatitis
Mitomycin C	Carcinomas of the breast, lung, gastrointestinal tract, cervix, bladder	Myelosuppression, severe vesicant, weakness, anorexia, hemolytic anemia, renal insufficiency, nausea and vomiting
ANTIMETABOLITES: interfere with nucleic acid synthesis and are cell cycle specific		
Cytosine arabionoside	Acute myelogenous leukemia, leptomeningeal carcinomatosis, lymphomas	Myelosuppression, ischemic bowel, stomatitis, nausea and vomiting, hepatotoxicity, cerebellar toxicity
5-Fluorouracil	Carcinomas of the breast, cervix, head and neck, gastrointestinal tract; nonmelanoma skin cancer	Mucositis, diarrhea, myelosuppression, dermatitis, hepatotoxicity (intraarterial therapy), nausea and vomiting
Floxuridine	Hepatic arterial therapy	Mucositis, biliary sclerosis, nausea and vomiting, abdominal pain
6-Mercaptopurine	Acute lymphoblastic leukemia	Myelosuppression, cholestasis, rash, anorexia, nausea and vomiting
Methotrexate	Carcinomas of the breast, head and neck, esophagus; choriocarcinoma; leptomeningeal carcinomatosis; osteogenic sarcoma	Myelosuppression, stomatitis, diarrhea, intestinal bleeding and perforation, arachnoiditis, hepatic dysfunction, cirrhosis, radiation recall, pneumonitis, renal dysfunction
Gemcitabine (Difluorodeoxycytidine)	Experimental	Myelosuppression, weakness
Pentostatin	Hairy cell leukemia, T-cell lymphomas	Nephrotoxicity, risk of severe infections without neutropenia, lethargy, hepatotoxicity, mild myelosuppression
Fludarabine	B-cell chronic lymphocytic leukemia	Myelosuppression, tumor lysis syndrome, weakness, neurotoxicity, edema, pneumonitis, nausea and vomiting, anorexia, gastrointestinal bleeding, stomatitis, diarrhea
PLANT ALKALOIDS		
Epipodophylotoxins: topoisomerase II inhibition		
Etoposide (VP-16)	Acute myelogenous leukemia, testicular cancer, small cell lung cancer	Myelosuppression, nausea and vomiting, alopecia, ileus, hypotension
Teniposide (VM-26)	Pediatric leukemia	Same as etoposide
Taxanes: excessive microtubule polymerization		
Paclitaxel (Taxol)	Carcinomas of the breast, ovary, head and neck, esophagus; lymphomas	Myelosuppression, alopecia, cardiac arrhythmias, neurotoxicity, abdominal pain, muscular cramps and myalgias
Docetaxel (Taxotere)	Experimental	Same as paclitaxel, fluid third spacing (vascular leak syndrome)

(continued)

Table 14-8. **COMMON CHEMOTHERAPEUTIC AGENTS** (Continued)

Drug	Indication	Toxicities
Vinca Alkaloids: microtubule disruption		
Vincristine	Acute lymphocytic leukemia; Hodgkin disease; lymphomas; sarcomas; carcinomas of the breast, bladder, lung; Wilms tumor	Mild myelosuppression, neuropathy, ileus, SIADH
Vinblastine	Carcinomas of the breast and testis, Hodgkin's disease, lymphomas, neuroblastoma, choriocarcinoma	Myelosuppression, mild neuropathy, ileus, abdominal pain, nausea and vomiting
Camptothecins: topoisomerase I inhibition		
Topotecan Irnotecan (CPT-11) 9-Aminocamptothecin	Experimental	Myelosuppression, diarrhea (CPT-11), nausea and vomiting, pulmonary toxicity, weakness
ANTIBIOTICS		
Anthracyclines: Topoisomerase II inhibition		
Doxorubicin Daunorubicin Idarubicin	Acute leukemias (daunorubicin, idarubicin); multiple myeloma; lymphomas; Hodgkin's disease; carcinomas of the breast, liver, stomach, bladder, lung (small cell); sarcomas; neuroblastoma; Wilms tumor	Myelosuppression, cardiomyopathy, alopecia, nausea and vomiting, mucositis, radiation recall, severe vesicant
Bleomycin: DNA strand scission	Lymphomas; Hodgkin's disease; carcinomas of the head and neck, testis	Pneumonitis, pulmonary fibrosis, fever and chills, anaphylaxis, dermatitis, mild myelosuppression
Actinomycin D: RNA synthesis inhibition	Choriocarcinoma, sarcomas, neuroblastoma, Wilms tumor	Myelosuppression, nausea and vomiting, mucositis, dermatitis, alopecia, diarrhea, severe vesicant, radiation recall
MISCELLANEOUS AGENTS		
Mitoxantrone—*topoisomerase II inhibitor*	Acute leukemias, lymphomas	Myelosuppression, nausea and vomiting (mild), minimal cardiotoxicity, alopecia (mild), blue sclera and nails
Mitotane—*blocks adrenocorticoid synthesis*	Adrenal carcinoma	Nausea and vomiting, depression, dermatitis, lethargy
Hydroxyurea—*blocks nucleotide reductase, inhibits DNA synthesis*	Chronic myelogenous leukemia	Myelosuppression, nausea and vomiting, increased blood urea nitrogen, headaches, dermatitis
Amsacrine—*Topoisomerase II inhibition*	Acute myelogenous leukemia	Myelosuppression, vesicant, phlebitis, alopecia, stomatitis, hepatotoxicity, neurotoxicity
L-Asparaginase—*depletes extracellular asparagine stores*	Acute lymphoblastic leukemia	Allergic reactions, nausea and vomiting, anorexia, hepatitis, pancreatitis, coagulopathy (usually subclinical), lethargy, depression, glucose intolerance
Tamoxifen—*estrogen receptor antagonist*	Breast carcinoma	Thrombophlebitis, vaginal bleeding, endometrial carcinoma, tumor flare, nausea, hot flashes
Estrogens—*androgen antagonists*	Prostate carcinoma, breast carcinoma	Thromboembolic events, gynecomastia, fluid retention, vaginal bleeding, increased cardiovascular deaths, hypercalcemic flare
Aminoglutethimide—*aromatase inhibitor*	Breast carcinoma	Dermatitis, somnolence, ataxia, nystagmus

SIADH, syndrome of inappropriate antidiuretic hormone secretion.

of radiation applied in a wide area. This results in a high rate of complications. The rationale for combination therapy is that lower doses of radiation can be used to eradicate microscopic tumor extensions while surgical excision is performed to remove the principal mass.

ANTINEOPLASTIC CHEMOTHERAPY

For a chemotherapeutic regimen to work perfectly,

1. All tumor cells are progressing through the cell cycle
2. All tumor cells are equally sensitive to the regimen
3. The patient finds the regimen tolerable enough to undergo six cycles of therapy

Such a situation is unrealistic. Not all cells in tumors are continuously cycling, and not all cells are equally sen-

sitive to therapy. Malignant cells are often inherently resistant to chemotherapeutic agents. This resistance usually causes the treatment regimen to fail (Table 14-6).

Because cells resistant to an agent are likely to be present in a malignant neoplasm at diagnosis, combination chemotherapy is used to provide antineoplastic therapy that encompasses all potential tumor clones while minimizing toxic adverse effects.

Dose Intensity

It important to deliver adequate drug doses with each treatment cycle and to deliver them in a timely manner. The interval between treatment cycles is determined by the toxic effects experienced by normal tissues and the amount of time required for resolution of the effects. The

Table 14-9. GENE DELIVERY SYSTEMS

Method	Ex Vivo	In Vivo	Expression
Direct injection of DNA	+	++	Transient
Electroporation	++	—	Stable after selection
Calcium phosphate precipitation	+	—	Stable after selection
Liposomes	+	++	Transient
Ligand DNA conjugates	—	++	Transient
Complex ligand DNA conjugates	—	++	Transient
Viral delivery			
Retrovirus	++	++/?	Stable
Adenovirus	+	++	Transient
Adeno-associated virus	++	?	Stable
Vaccinia virus	+	++	Transient
Herpesvirus	+	++	?

(After Lyerly HK, Dimaio MJ. Gene delivery systems in surgery. Arch Surg 1993;128:1197)

scheduling of treatment courses is crucial. If a course follows too closely on the preceding one, additive toxicities occur, and often the ability to deliver further therapy is at least temporarily compromised. For most agents, the dose-limiting toxicity is myelosuppression, usually leukopenia or thrombocytopenia.

Administration of Chemotherapy

Table 14-7 lists the common chemotherapeutic agents. Most chemotherapy is administered IV, though some drugs, such as tamoxifen and hydroxyurea, are absorbed well enough to be administered orally. Systemic administration of chemotherapy addresses metastatic disease throughout the body, though cytotoxic concentrations may not be achieved in all areas.

Malignant disease often is limited to one organ or site. Techniques can be used to deliver therapy solely or predominately to the affected area. Examples are intra-arterial chemotherapy for neoplasms limited to the liver; chemotherapy administered into the abdominal cavity to manage peritoneal disease; and intrathecal therapy to manage leptomeningeal carcinomatosis.

Adjuvant Chemotherapy

Administered after surgical resection or irradiation of gross disease. The goal is not palliation of symptoms or reduction of a mass but prolongation of survival and reduction of the likelihood of relapse.

Neoadjuvant or Primary Chemotherapy

Administered before definitive local therapy. May reduce the primary lesion and allow less extensive resection. Also may eliminate micrometastatic disease before it is clinically apparent.

Induction or First-Line Chemotherapy

Administered as the only treatment for advanced disease (metastases in multiple sites that cannot be resected for cure or safely encompassed in a radiation therapy port).

Salvage Regimens

Administered if disease progresses after induction chemotherapy. Less active than first-line regimens, and responses have a shorter duration.

Therapeutic Responses and Toxicity

A partial response is regarded as 50% to 99% reduction in all bidimensionally measurable disease that lasts at least 4 weeks or one treatment cycle. A complete response is disappearance of all signs and symptoms associated with all malignant lesions and complete resolution of all abnormal laboratory values that lasts at least 4 weeks or one treatment cycle. A minor response is a reduction of <50% of all bidimensionally measurable disease or a reduction of ≥50% that does not last at least 4 weeks or a treatment cycle. A minor response is not considered statistically significant, though it may indicate potential biologic activity. Table 14-8 provides indications for and toxicities of chemotherapeutic agents.

IMMUNOTHERAPY

Biologic Therapy

The premises of biologic therapy are:

1. Cancer progression occurs because host immune defenses do not recognize and reject the tumor
2. Biologic agents may augment the immune response

Table 14-10. CHARACTERISTICS OF VIRAL VECTORS FOR GENE THERAPY

Virus	Advantages	Disadvantages
Retrovirus	Extensive experience using this virus is available; efficient; integrates genome	Need for active cell replication; potential risk of insertional mutagenesis; potential for development of replication-competent (helper) virus (depending on the construct)
Adenovirus	Able to concentrate to high titers; can infect nonreplicating cells; no packaging cell lines	Presence of many adenoviral genes in vectors can stimulate immunity, affecting ability to give repeated doses
Adeno-associated virus	Less risk of insertional mutagenesis; nonpathogenic (ubiquitous in humans); can infect nonreplicating cells	Lack of information on long-term consequences of integration and gene expression from the adeno-associated virus provirus; requires coinfection with helper adenovirus or herpesvirus for replication
Herpesvirus	Can infect nonreplicating cells; large genome (150 kb), can potentially transfer large, intact genes	Little information on long-term fate or stability of gene expression; could potentially become latent in neural cells
Hepatitis B virus (hepadnavirus)	Hepatotropic; tendency to integrate *in vivo*	Little information or experience with its usage

(After Chang AGY, Wu GY. Gene therapy: applications to the treatment of gastrointestinal and liver diseases. Gastroenterology 1994;106:1076)

and elicit a rejection response that reverses the imbalance in tumor–host relations and blunts tumor progression

A variety of biologic therapy agents are being used in clinical trials. The objective of the trials is to stimulate function of effector cells, including T lymphocytes, NK cells and cytotoxic macrophages, and B lymphocytes. Techniques include

- Tumor-cell vaccination
- Administration of recombinant cytokines (interleukins and interferons)
- Adoptive cellular therapy, in which lymphokine-activated killer (LAK) cells are administered with high doses of interleukin-2
- Multiagent biologic therapy

Considerable toxicity is associated with IV administration of cytokines to patients with cancer. Cytokines must be administered frequently because of their short half-life in blood. Cytokines are not always distributed to all areas of the body and often do not traverse the blood–brain barrier. One method of delivery is incorporation of interferon and adjuvants into liposomes, directing the cytokine to a specific host cell population.

Gene Therapy

Multiple genetic aberrations are necessary for a cell to become malignant. Correction of any one of these aberrations may return the cell to the normal state. Methods to correct genetic aberrations in tumor cells involve delivery of normal genes to the cells. In vitro gene therapy involves the removal of cells from the patient (Table 14-9). In vivo gene therapy involves the use of viral vectors (Table 14-10). The viral vectors used are not considered dangerous outside the host.

SUGGESTED READING

Cantley LC, Auger KR, Carpenter C, et al. Oncogenes and signal transduction. Cell 1991;64:281.

Cross M, Dexter TM. Growth factors in development, transformation, and tumorigenesis. Cell 1991;64:271.

Fearon ER, Vogelstein B. A genetic model for colorectal tumorigenesis. Cell 1990;61:759.

Graham CH, Rivers J, Kerbel RS, Stankiewicz KS, White WL. Extent of vascularization as a prognostic indicator in thin (<0.76) malignant melanomas. Am J Pathol 1994;145:510.

Kerbel RS. Growth dominance of the metastatic cancer cell: Cellular and molecular aspects. Adv Cancer Res 1990;55:87.

Liotta LA, Steeg PS, Stetler-Stevenson WG. Cancer metastasis and angiogenesis: An imbalance of positive and negative regulation. Cell 1991;64:327-336.

Marshall CJ. Tumor suppressor genes. Cell 1991;64:313-326.

Takahashi Y, Kitadai Y, Bucana C, Cleary KR, Ellis LM. Expression of vascular endothelial growth factor and its receptor (KDR) correlates with vascularity, metastasis and proliferation of human colon cancer. Cancer Res 1995; 55:3964.

Weidner N, Carroll PR, Flax J. Tumor angiogenesis correlates with metastasis in invasive prostate carcinoma. Am J Pathol 1993;143:401.

ESSENTIALS OF SURGERY: SCIENTIFIC PRINCIPLES AND PRACTICE, edited by Lazar J. Greenfield, Michael W. Mulholland, Keith T. Oldham, Gerald B. Zelenock, and Keith D. Lillemoe. Lippincott–Raven Publishers, Philadelphia, © 1997.

CHAPTER 15
HUMAN GENE THERAPY

STEVEN E. RAPER

The new disciplines of molecular medicine and gene therapy are now clinical realities that will revolutionize the practice of medicine. Only a fraction of the human genome (genetic material) has been cloned, sequenced, and mapped to individual chromosomes. As genes become known, their role in the pathogenesis of disease can be studied, and preventive, diagnostic, and therapeutic strategies can be developed. The first gene therapy protocols are being directed at the hematopoietic system, the liver, and the respiratory tract. Other organs and organ systems are probably amenable to such treatments, including heart, skeletal muscle, skin, kidney, and pancreas.

The identification of enzymes that precisely cut DNA molecules at defined locations made it possible to recombine DNA fragments. In addition, the ability of tumor viruses to transform cells to a malignant phenotype was found to be the result of stable, heritable integration of viral genes into the host cell genome.

The first gene-marking study, to evaluate the presence of tumor-infiltrating lymphocytes transduced with a retrovirus containing a neomycin resistance gene (neo[r]), was begun in 1989. The first therapeutic protocol, treatment of children with severe combined immunodeficiency by transducing autologous lymphocytes with a retrovirus containing the gene adenosine deaminase (ADA), was begun in 1990. Before they begin, all gene therapy protocols are reviewed for safety (Fig. 15-1).

The US Human Genome Project is part of an international effort to identify all human genes. One question is how many genes the genome contains. If a gene is defined as a distinct transcriptional unit that may be translated into one or a set of proteins, the number is 60,000-70,000. Other important aspects of the US Human Genome Project include development of computer technology to help store the massive amounts of data generated; analysis of the ethical, social, and legal implications of the genetic data base; and education of new investigators. Genes associated with hypertension, diabetes, Alzheimer disease, and cancers of the colon and breast, have been identified.

GENERAL APPROACHES TO GENE THERAPY

Ex vivo gene therapy involves harvesting autologous cells, modifying the cells ex vivo, and transplanting genetically modified autologous cells back into the patient from whom they are derived. Somatic cells studied for ex vivo somatic gene transfer include hematopoietic stem cells, lymphocytes, hepatocytes, endothelial cells, and fibroblasts. Two advantages to this approach are that gene transfer can be accomplished in vitro and the genetically modified cells can be characterized before transplantation. Ex vivo gene therapy requires two invasive procedures: target cell harvest and reinfusion of the genetically altered cells. Efficacy depends on the number of cells harvested and the titer and efficiency of infection of the target cells by the

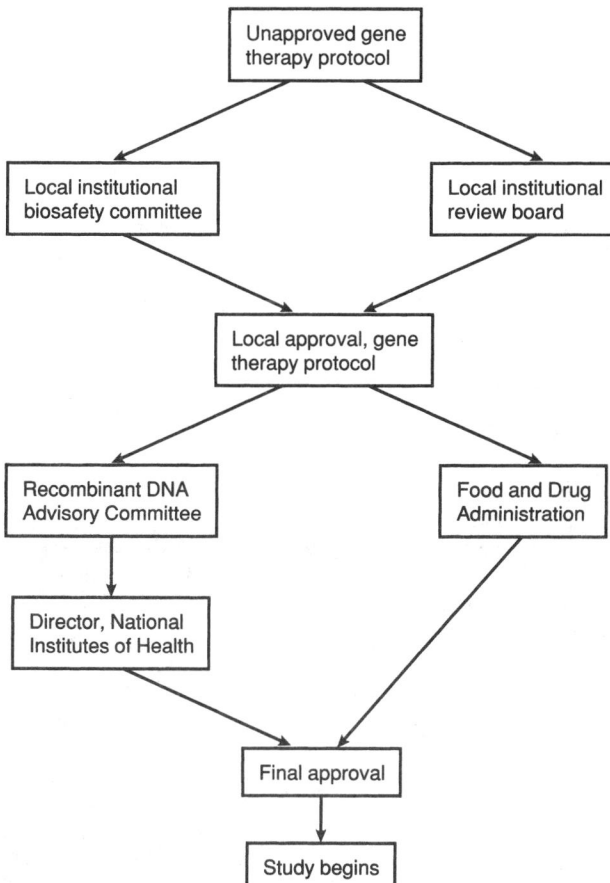

Figure 15-1. Pathway taken for approval of gene therapy protocols. On May 9, 1996, the RAC was dissolved. Gene therapy protocols no longer require sign-off by the Director of NIH. These responsibilities were assumed by the FDA.

chosen vector. Recombinant retroviruses are the vectors in most ex vivo gene therapy trials.

In vivo gene therapy involves direct delivery of therapeutic genes to cells. This approach requires gene transfer vectors that target the correct cell type and transport the gene to the nucleus, where it is expressed. Gene transfer substrates include respiratory epithelial cells, myocytes, synovium, and brain. Vectors include adenoviruses, adeno-associated viruses, herpes simplex virus, hybrid viruses, and nonviral substrates, such as liposomes and DNA-protein complexes (Table 15-1).

THE HEMATOPOIETIC SYSTEM
Recombinant Retroviruses

Recombinant retroviruses are used for almost all trials of hematopoietic gene transfer, both to mark cells and to treat diseases. Retroviruses are important in gene therapy trials for two reasons—the genome is relatively easy to manipulate, and the virally encoded genes integrate into host chromosomes. Retrovirus particles are composed of an RNA genome encapsulated into a particle that contains viral and cellular components (Fig. 15-2).

The virus enters cells during interactions between viral coat proteins and complementary proteins on the host cell membrane. Once internalized, the viral RNA is converted to a double-stranded DNA sequence, the provirus. The proviral DNA is integrated into the host chromosome by an integrase protein. An important point is that host–cell replication is required for successful proviral DNA integration.

Retroviruses used in gene therapy protocols must be replication-defective, that is, they should be able to infect host cells and produce the protein of interest, but not produce more retroviruses. These replication-defective retroviruses are produced by a packaging cell line (Fig. 15-2D) engineered to produce proteins necessary to assemble retroviral particles.

The following limitations of recombinant retroviruses make them unsuitable for some gene transfer protocols:

1. Retrovirus entry requires that target cells contain the appropriate viral receptor. In many cases, these receptors are not known.
2. Retroviral gene integration requires cell proliferation. The dependence of integration on mitosis is thought to be due to the need for nuclear membrane breakdown to enable the viral integration complex to enter the nucleus.
3. Production is a problem because retrovirus particles are labile. Retroviruses usually cannot be purified without loss of infectivity.

Gene Transfer Strategies in the Hematopoietic System

The first approved gene transfer protocol involved a marker study of tumor infiltrating lymphocytes (TILs) and their trafficking patterns in vivo. TILs are lymphocytes in tumors that are believed to facilitate immune-mediated tumor destruction. In the trial, TILs from five patients with advanced melanoma were transduced in vitro with an antibiotic resistance gene and reinfused back into patients. Some cells isolated from subsequent tumor biopsies of these patients were TILs that had antibiotic resistance. Transduced cells were demonstrated in the tumor for up to 64 days and in the peripheral circulation for up to 189 days. Similar marker studies have been performed in patients with lymphoma who underwent intensive chemotherapy and autologous bone marrow transplantation. Marker studies have been used for studies of relapse of a variety of lymphoid tumors (Fig. 15-3).

GENE THERAPY FOR CANCER

Given the diversity of proposed targets for cancer therapy, opportunities for cancer gene therapy trials abound (Table 15-2).

(text continues on page 128)

Table 15-1. VECTORS IN GENE THERAPY

Vector	Application to Gene Therapy		
	Ex Vivo	In Situ	Expression
Retrovirus	Yes	No	Stable
Adenovirus	No	Yes	Transient
Adeno-associated virus	Yes	Yes	Stable
Herpes simplex virus	No	Yes	Latent
Vaccinia virus	No	Yes	Transient
Liposomes	Yes	Yes	Transient
DNA–protein complexes	No	Yes	Transient
DNA injection	No	Yes	Transient
CaPO$_4$ precipitation	Yes	No	Transient
DEAE dextran	Yes	No	Stable

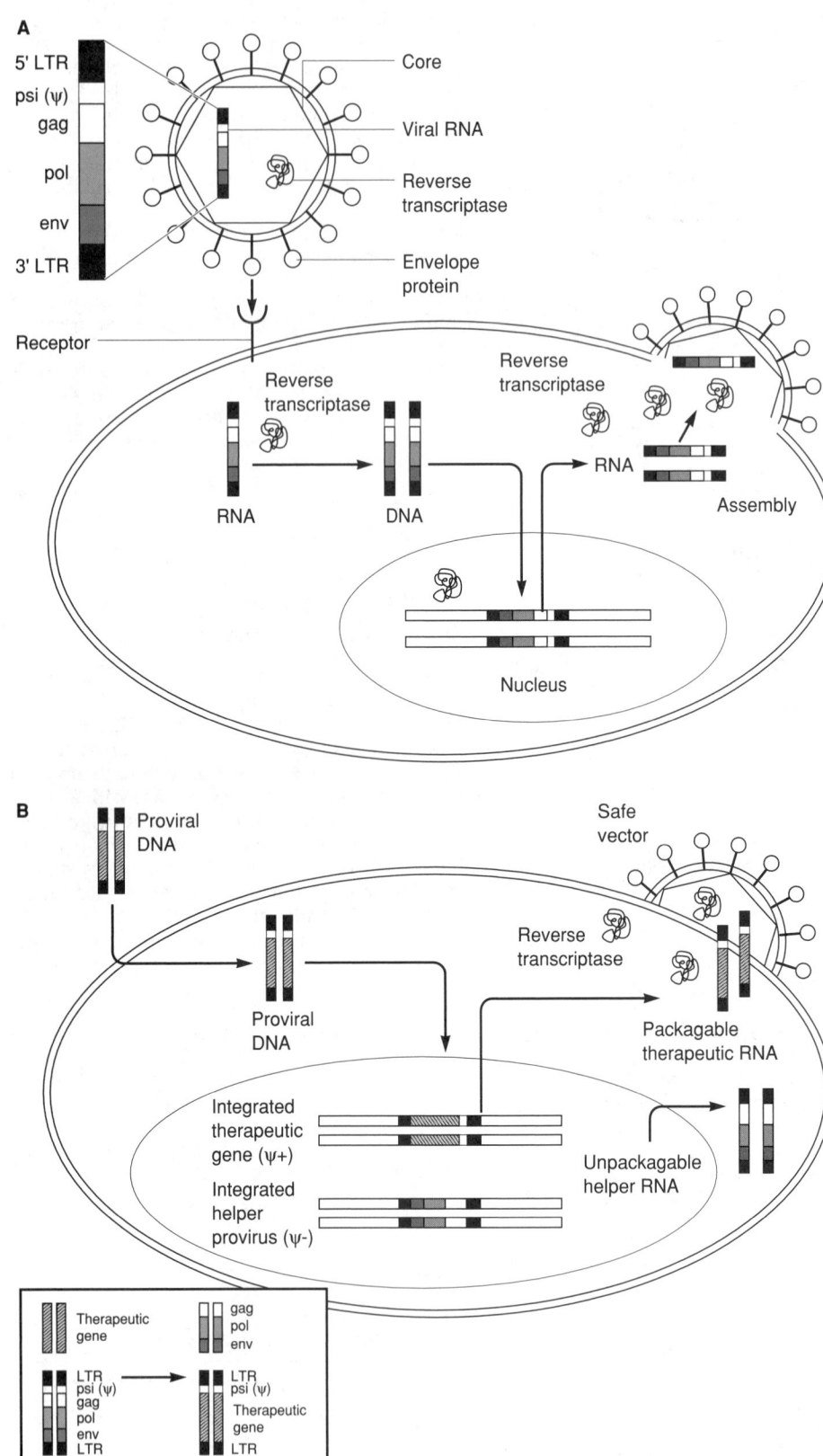

Figure 15-2. (*A*) Processes used in the construction of a retroviral vector. The schematic drawing represents the key features of a retroviral particle. Envelope (env) proteins are important in binding and uptake of the virus by the host cell. Viral reversed transcriptase allows conversion of viral RNA to a DNA provirus. Long terminal repeats (LTRs) are essential for viral integration into the host chromosome. The ψ sequence is necessary for packaging of RNA molecules into virions before budding from the host cell membrane. pol, reverse transcriptase; gag, core proteins.

(*B*) Steps in the life cycle of a retrovirus. The envelope glycoproteins bind to specific cell-surface proteins and allow fusion of the virus with the cell membrane, permitting entry of virion particles. Once in the cell, molecules of viral reverse transcriptase convert RNA to DNA. Proviral DNA integrates randomly into the genome of the proliferating host cell. Retroviral progeny are synthesized using host cell mechanisms. Packaging of infectious RNA requires ψ sequences.

(*C*) Steps in construction of therapeutic proviral DNA. Using standard DNA cloning techniques, one may substitute a therapeutic gene, along with desired promoters, enhancers, and selectable markers, for endogenous retroviral structural sequences, such as gag, pol, and env. By making the therapeutic DNA provirus ψ-positive, subsequent therapeutic RNA molecules can be selectively packaged. *(continues)*

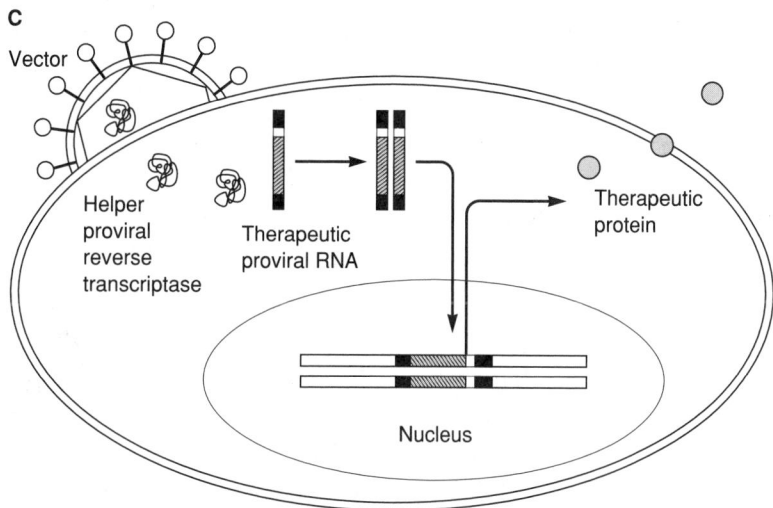

Figure 15-2. *(Continued).*

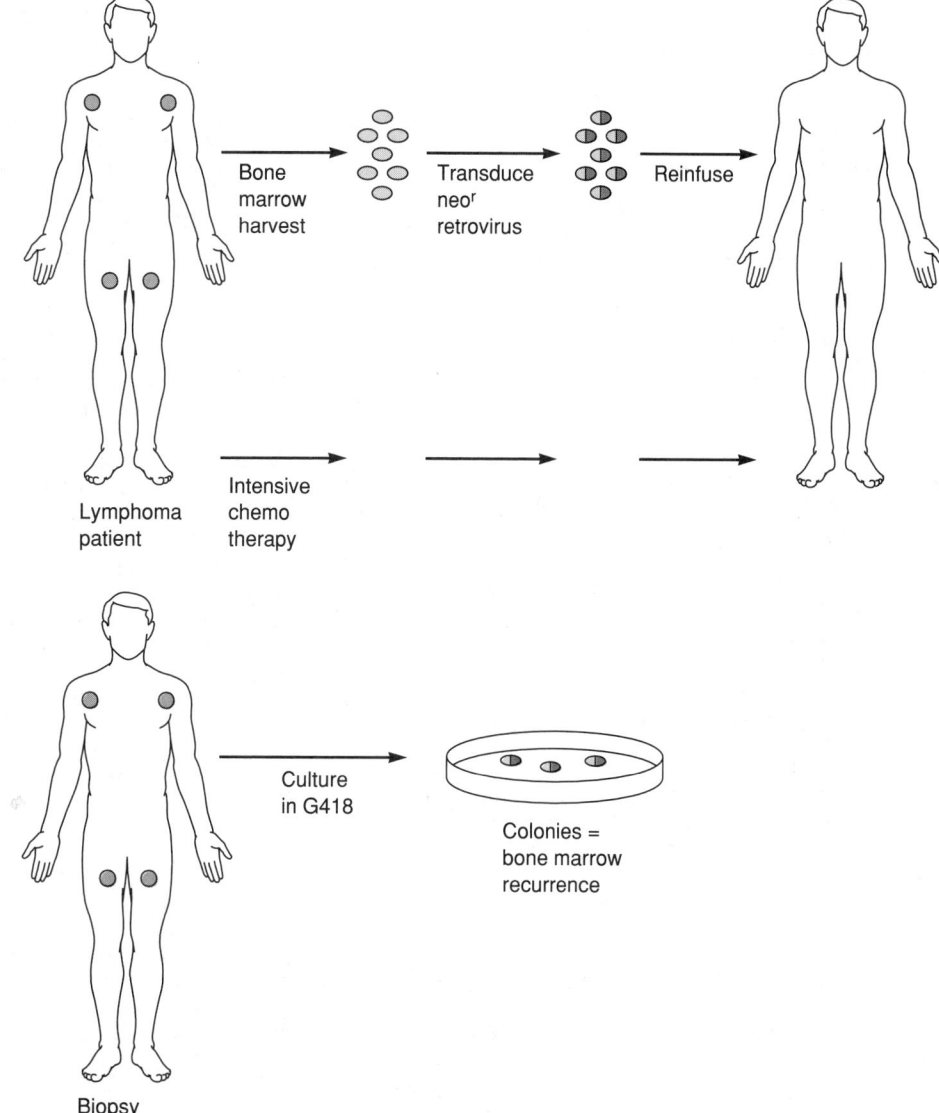

Figure 15-3. Use of a retroviral vector containing the neomycin resistance gene in marker studies for treatment of lymphoma patients. Presence of colonies later containing the neomycin resistance gene, surviving in the presence of the antibiotic G418, indicates bone marrow recurrence of the malignant cells.

Table 15-2. CANDIDATE CYTOKINES FOR CANCER-DIRECTED GENE THERAPY

Cytokine Gene	Action	Target Cells
IL-2	Growth factor Activation	T and B lymphocytes
IL-3	Growth factor	Stem cells Progenitor cells
IL-4	Growth factor Differentiation MHC class II expression	B and T lymphocytes (IgG1 and IgE) Macrophages
IL-6	Growth factor Differentiation	B and T lymphocytes Antibody-forming cells
IL-7	Growth factor Activation factor	Pre–B lymphocytes T lympyhocytes Macrophages Thymocytes
IL-12	Growth factor	Cytotoxic and natural killer cells T lymphocytes
Interferon-γ	MHC class I expression Immunoregulation B-cell differentiation Antiviral	Lymphocytes Monocytes
Tumor necrosis factor α	Inflammation Catabolism Cytokine production Adhesion molecule production	Fibroblasts Endothelium

Cytokine Gene Transfer

The genetic modification of tumor cells to secrete cytokines diminishes tumor growth and enhances host immune response in animals. Many cytokine genes have been used with different tumor models in preclinical trials. A recurring theme is that host cell response varies according to the cytokine used and the inherent immunogenicity of the native tumor.

Tumors modified to secrete cytokines are used to upregulate the host immune response against tumors. Because some cytokines have considerable toxicity when administered systemically, cytokine secretion of the tumor can theoretically attain maximal effects where it matters most while minimizing side effects. Interleukin (IL)-2 is one such cytokine (Fig. 15-4). TNFα, IFN , GM-CSF, and IL-12 are being tested in clinical trials involving patients with metastatic disease. A common objective in these trials is to enhance the immune system of the host against autologous tumors.

Gene Mutation-Directed Therapy

Probably the most mechanistic strategy to combat cancer involves manipulation of mutant genes responsible for unrestrained growth of tumors. The genes associated with carcinogenesis fall into two categories: protooncogenes and tumor suppressor genes (Table 15-3). *Protooncogenes* encode for proteins that participate in normal cellular proliferation. They can be altered to become oncogenes, the products of which allow unrestrained proliferation. *Tumor suppressor genes* encode proteins that inhibit cellular proliferation and promote cellular differentiation.

Oncogene mutations are dominant in that only one mutant allele is required for the development of a malignant phenotype. Tumor suppressor mutations are recessive—one normal allele maintains normal growth control and differentiation. There are exceptions to this pattern for both oncogenes and tumor suppressor genes. In the gene that encodes nuclear DNA binding protein *p53* the presence of mutant *p53* alleles acts as a dominant negative mutation. Normal protein must be present, and abnormal protein production must be suppressed (Fig. 15-5). The *ras* oncogene has highest mutation rate.

Many strategies for oncogene-directed cancer therapy involve the use of antisense oligodeoxynucleotides. Instead of engineering of a virus or other gene-delivery vehicle, a piece of DNA is inserted that is complementary to messenger RNA molecules. The antisense molecules bind to the sense mRNAs so that mRNA translation cannot occur (Fig. 15-6). If the bound mRNA escapes its antisense partner, translation proceeds. Antisense molecules are drugs that do not require virus-mediated gene transfer. The oligonucleotides can be made resistant to nuclease degradation.

Ribozymes are molecules that bind to mRNA, much like antisense molecules. However, ribozymes are catalytic and can cause structural modifications of mRNA, blocking transcription. The ability of ribozymes to catalyze post-transcriptional RNA modifications may be exploited in attempts to repair mutant RNA molecules and to revert them to the correct message.

Suicide Drug Therapy

Suicide drug therapy, originally used in the treatment of brain tumors, is based on selective introduction of the herpes simplex thymidine kinase (*HSVtk*) gene into tumor cells. Addition of ganciclovir leads to synthesis of toxic nucleotides, which are incorporated into newly synthesized DNA, causing cell death. *HSVtk*-ganciclovir therapy demonstrates a poorly understood phenomenon, the bystander effect, in which both transduced and nontransduced cells are killed when ganciclovir is added in vivo. The bystander effect can be advantageous, especially when technical limitations dictate that only a fraction of the tumor cells can be transduced. Human trials are being developed for mesothelioma, lymphoma, ovarian cancer, and hepatic metastases.

Cytosine deaminase is a suicide gene used to convert nontoxic 5-fluorocystine (5-FC) to 5-fluorouracil (5-FU). In vivo transduction of tumors with this gene has caused tumor regression and protection against wild-type tumor challenge.

In another approach, instead of selective targeting of tumor cells for suicide therapy, normal tissues are protected with the multidrug resistance gene (*MDR1*). The *MDR1* gene encodes P-glycoprotein, which exports a variety of chemotherapeutic agents from the cell, protecting the cells from destruction. Clinical trials have been approved for use of retroviruses expressing the MDR1 gene to target and, thus, protect bone marrow cells during therapy for breast and ovarian cancer.

Adenosine Deaminase Deficiency

Deficiency of adenosine deaminase (ADA) results in severe combined immunodeficiency. The first therapeutic human gene therapy trial involved retroviruses that expressed ADA. In 1990, a 4-year-old girl with severe combined immunodeficiency received infusions of autologous culture-expanded peripheral blood T lymphocytes. The T cells had been corrected in vitro by transduction of a retrovirus expressing the gene for ADA. Despite the need for repeated infusions, treatment was successful.

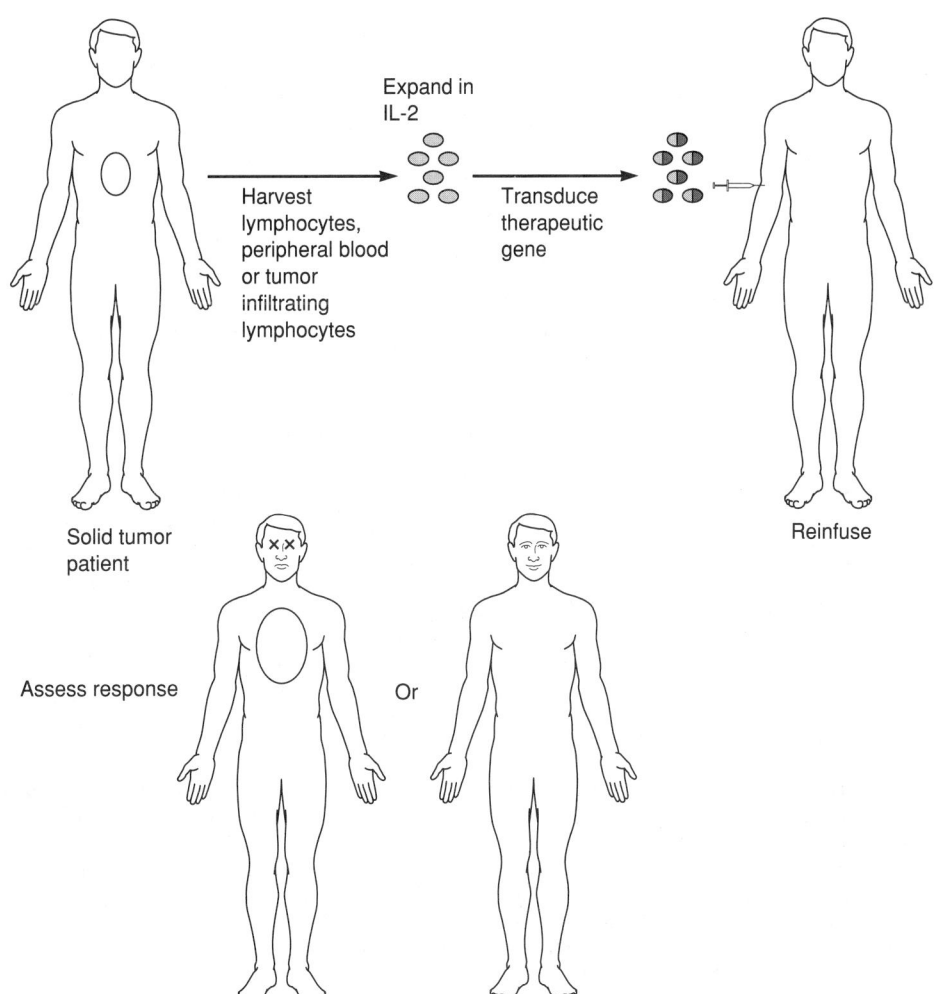

Figure 15-4. An example of the use of adoptive immunotherapy. Interleukin-2 (IL-2) and major histocompatibility complex antigen have been shown in animal models to augment native immune responses to solid organ tumors.

DISORDERS FOR WHICH GENE THERAPY IS PROPOSED

The Liver

A number of inborn errors of metabolism due to single-gene defects affect the liver or its secreted proteins (Table 15-4). Nonmetabolic diseases such as allograft rejection, cancer, and viral infection can be treated with liver-directed gene therapy.

DNA-Protein Complexes

Nonviral strategies are being developed to accomplish gene transfer in the liver along the receptor-mediated endocytosis pathway. Advantages include specific targeting of a defined cell population, physiologic cell entry, and the possibility of repetitive treatment with the therapeutic gene. Gene transfer by administration of DNA-protein complex is as efficient as transfer with viral vectors, but problems remain.

Ex Vivo Liver-Directed Gene Therapy

The choice in ex vivo therapy is to use autologous or allogeneic hepatocytes. Use of *autologous hepatocytes* does not require immunosuppression. However, a surgical procedure is needed to harvest cells. Only a small number of harvest procedures may be performed before the supply of cells is depleted. When *allogeneic hepatocytes* are used, and if rejection can be prevented, the recipient does not undergo surgical harvesting. Allogeneic cells provide a renewable resource for repeated treatment. Hepatocytes can be cryopreserved.

Although it is possible to isolate relatively pure fractions of hepatocytes and to establish primary cultures, the cells are difficult to maintain for long periods. Hepatocytes also begin to lose differentiated function within several days of isolation. Efficient transduction must be achieved in one short exposure to virus soon after the cells are isolated. Procedures have been developed for the transduction of

Table 15-3. ONCOGENES AND TUMOR SUPPRESSOR GENES AS TARGETS FOR GENE THERAPY

Gene	Designation	Function	Chromosome Location
Adenomatous polyposis coli	APC	Cytoskeletal	5q
Rous-associated sarcoma	K-*ras*-2	G protein	12p
Nuclear protein	*p53*	Cell cycle control	17p
Retinoblastoma	Rb	Cell cycle control	13q
Deleted in colon carcinoma	DCC	Cell adhesion	18q

p53 function: Dominant negative

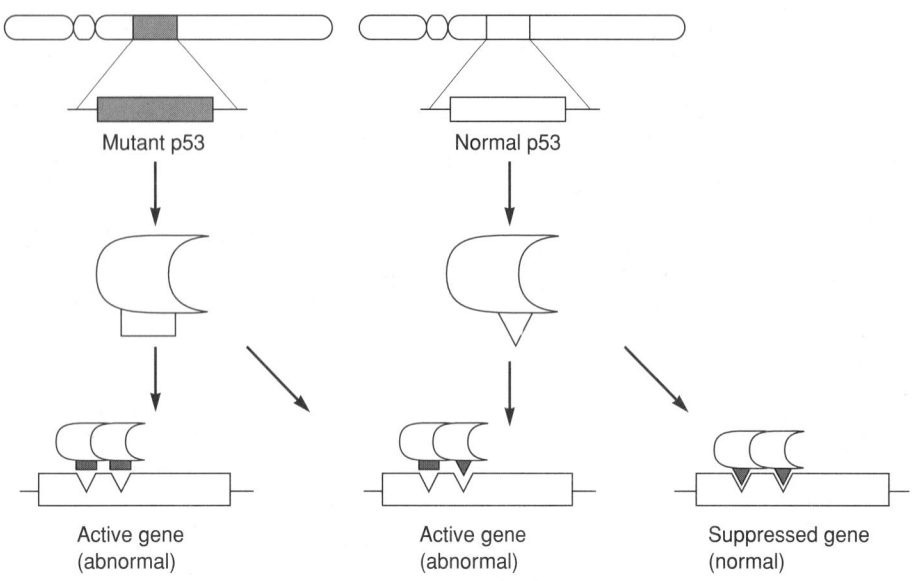

Active gene
(abnormal)

Active gene
(abnormal)

Suppressed gene
(normal)

Figure 15-5. The gene p53 functioning as a dominant negative mutation. The mutant p53 may form a heterodimer with normal p53. The formation of a heterodimer in this manner fails to suppress gene transcription appropriately. Formation of a normal homodimer suppresses transcription.

primary cultures of human hepatocytes with retroviral vectors.

Direct reinfusion of autologous human hepatocytes into a tributary of the portal venous system is the preferred approach to hepatocyte transplantation. Placing an indwelling catheter at the time of hepatocyte harvest allows readministration of autologous hepatocytes without another operation. The vessels can be studied with radiographs immediately before hepatocyte reinfusion to ensure that the vessel is open and that hepatopetal flow is present.

Complications of intraportal administration of autologous hepatocytes include portal vein thrombosis, portal hypertension with the development of ascites or variceal hemorrhage, infection, which may necessitate deferral of an urgently needed liver transplant, and complete thrombosis with organized clot adherent to the endothelium of the portal vein, which may also preclude liver transplantation.

Other strategies for the infusion of genetically altered hepatocytes into the portal vein may be appropriate in some patients. One approach, used in islet cell transplantation, is to cannulate the umbilical vein remnant in the falciform ligament. Although no clinical studies using hepatocytes have been performed, injection of highly purified pancreatic islets has been performed without evidence of portal vein thrombosis. Another approach to hepatocyte delivery is intrasplenic transplantation, which has been tried in animals. More than half of the cells originally transplanted into the spleen were engrafted into the liver, and function was demonstrated.

Familial Hypercholesterolemia

The molecular basis of familial hypercholesterolemia is a mutation in the gene that encodes the LDL receptor. People who inherit one abnormal allele have moderate elevations in plasma LDL and suffer premature coronary artery disease. Those with two abnormal LDL receptor alleles have severe hypercholesterolemia and life-threatening coronary artery disease. The hepatocyte is the preferred target cell for gene therapy for familial hypercholesterolemia (Fig. 15-7), because the liver modulates cholesterol homeostasis through metabolic functions expressed in the parenchymal cells.

Other disorders for which liver-based gene therapy is being studied include:

- Ornithine transcarbamylase (OTC) deficiency, an X-linked disorder related to disruption of the urea cycle

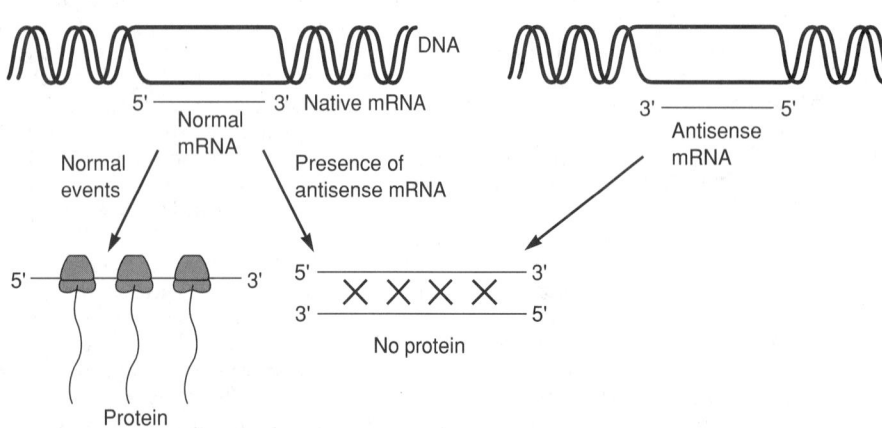

Figure 15-6. Diagrammatic representation of the use of antisense mRNA to block translation. The antisense mRNA is complementary to, and binds with, the targeted mRNA. Formation of a stable antisense mRNA-native mRNA complex prevents protein formation.

Table 15-4. GENETIC DISEASES THAT ARE POTENTIAL LIVER-DIRECTED EX VIVO GENE THERAPY CANDIDATES

Disease	Gene Defect
Familial hypercholesterolemia	Low-density lipoprotein receptor
Cystic fibrosis	Cystic fibrosis transmembrane conductance regulator
Neonatal hyperammonemia	Ornithine transcarbamylase
Hemophilia A	Factor VIII
Hemophilia B	Factor IX
Mucopolysaccharidosis type I	α-L-Iduronidase
Mucopolysaccharidosis type VII	β-glucuronidase
Crigler-Najjar syndrome type I	Uridine disphosphoglucuronate–bilirubin glucuronosyltransferase
Hereditary tyrosinemia type I	Fumarylacetoacetate hydrolase
Citrullinemia	Argininosuccinate synthetase

characterized by neonatal encephalopathy, hypothermia, apnea, and markedly elevated plasma ammonia levels in boys and men
- Crigler–Najjar syndrome type I, a rare, sometimes fatal neonatal kernicterus due to deficiency of the enzyme that catalyzes bilirubin
- α-1-Antitrypsin deficiency, which causes chronic obstructive pulmonary disease (COPD) and liver disease
- Hemophilia B

The Pancreas

Diabetes

Gene therapy for diabetes is based on the presumption that suitable genes can be identified as targets. Progress has been made in identifying the genetic contribution to insulin-dependent diabetes mellitus (IDDM). The finding of a major gene linkage with HLA on chromosome 6 fits with the known mechanism of IDDM-autoimmune destruction of insulin-producing pancreatic β-cells. The predominant phenotype in non–insulin-dependent diabetes mellitus (NIDDM) is obesity, arterial hypertension, dyslipidemia, and atherosclerotic coronary artery disease. NIDDM is inherited, but the mode of inheritance is not known. Some people with NIDDM of the young subtype may have glucokinase gene mutations, suggesting that ex vivo gene therapy to transfer the correct gene into islets may be an option. In the insulin receptor defect–insulin resistance syndromes, correcting the defect with gene transfer may involve most cells of the body, but especially skeletal muscle, fat, and the liver.

Islet Transplantation

Islet allografts help maintain normoglycemia without exogenous insulin therapy in immunosuppressed patients with diabetes. The research goal is early transplantation of islets to prevent diabetes-related complications and avoidance of immunosuppression. The autoimmune attack on autologous cells in patients with IDDM and rejection of allogeneic islets may be ameliorated by immunomodulation of the islet, the recipient, or both. In transgenic models of IDDM, antibody depletion has prevented diabetes. Research with these models suggests that it may be possible to prevent IDDM with immunoinhibitory cytokines.

Gene Transfer in Islets of Langerhans

Plasmid DNA has been used in vitro in transient transfection protocols to elucidate the mechanisms of transcriptional regulation of the insulin gene. Recombinant adenoviruses have been used to accomplish gene transfer into freshly isolated islets of Langerhans in rats. Basal levels of insulin release and glucose usage increased. The ability to engineer adenoviruses may allow investigation of regulatory enzymes in the pathway of glucose metabolism.

Cystic Fibrosis

Exocrine pancreatic insufficiency is present from birth in most patients with CF. Pathologic changes are caused by obstruction of ducts by abnormally thick, inspissated

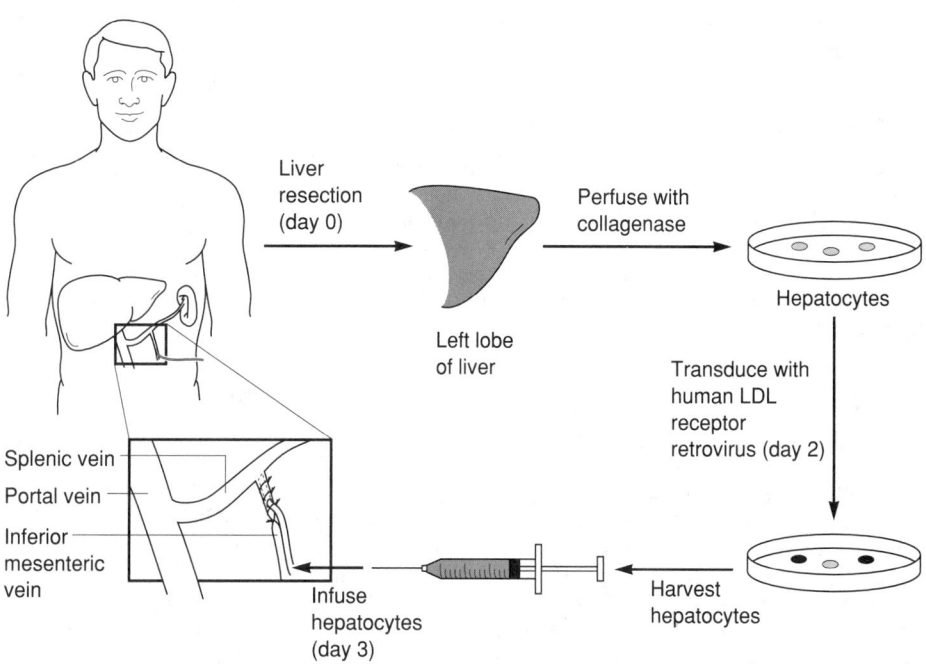

Figure 15-7. Strategy of ex vivo gene therapy for familial hypercholesterolemia. LDL, low-density lipoprotein.

Table 15-5. STRATEGIES FOR PERIPHERAL VASCULAR GENE THERAPY

Gene Product	Abbreviation	Action	Cell Type
Fibroblast growth factor	FGF	Induction of intimal hyperplasia	Smooth muscle cells
Platelet-derived growth factor	PDGF	Induction of intimal hyperplasia	Smooth muscle cells
Factor IX	FIX	Anticoagulation	Endothelial cells
Tissue plasminogen activator	tPa	Clot lysis	Endothelial cells
Herpes simplex virus thymidine kinase	HSVtk	Inhibition of intimal hyperplasia	Smooth muscle cells
Retinoblastoma protein	Rb	Inhibition of intimal hyperplasia	Smooth muscle cells
Vascular endothelial growth factor	VEGF	Arterial collateral development	Endothelial cells
Renin	—	Vascular smooth muscle growth	Smooth muscle cells
Angiotensin-converting enzyme	ACE	Vascular smooth muscle growth	Smooth muscle cells

secretions resulting in dilatation of secretory ducts and flattening of the cuboidal epithelium. There is widespread loss of acini and intraluminal calcifications, as seen with other types of chronic pancreatitis. The islets of Langerhans are preserved until late, but progressive scarring of the gland is associated with the development of diabetes. Pancreatic enzyme deficiency results in protein and fat malabsorption. Recombinant adenoviruses have been used to transduce genes that encode for pancreatic lipase as a way of treating pancreatic enzyme deficiency.

The Respiratory Tract

Adenoviruses

Recombinant adenoviruses represent important technology for in vivo gene therapy for pulmonary diseases. There are more than 40 human adenovirus serotypes, many of which are pathogenic in humans. Diseases caused by adenoviruses include hepatitis, conjunctivitis, upper respiratory tract infection, and diarrhea. Many episodes of the common cold are the result of adenovirus infections. Multiple exposures to adenoviruses throughout life result in the development of humoral immunity. The virus can be grown in large quantities and be highly purified. Administration of the virus in vivo has been associated with high-level gene expression in animals.

Gene therapy for cystic fibrosis is the paradigm for gene therapy in humans. Ex vivo gene therapy for cystic fibrosis uses recombinant retroviruses; in vivo gene therapy uses adenoviruses or cationic liposomes.

The Vascular System

Gene therapy should be useful for disease of the coronary arteries, aorta, and peripheral vessels. Target cells for atherosclerosis-mediated gene therapy include endothelial cells and smooth-muscle cells. A variety of genes have been proposed and have been used with success in vitro and in vivo in animals, although no human trials have yet been approved (Table 15-5).

Muscle

Uniform delivery of genes is important in gene therapy for muscle diseases. In inherited diseases such as muscular dystrophy, all muscle fibers must be treated to restore function, but delivery to muscles such as the diaphragm is critical to survival. There is interest in using myoblasts, muscle precursor cells, as factories for the production and secretion of serum proteins. Myoblasts can be isolated from adult skeletal muscle, cultured, transduced, and then returned to the host, where they fuse with existing muscle fibers. A myocyte cell line has been transduced with both human growth hormone and factor IX.

The Central Nervous System

The ability to manipulate the expression of genes in the mammalian brain leads to opportunities to treat neurologic disorders. DNA viruses have been used in most attempts at gene therapy for nonmalignant CNS disease. Herpes simplex type I (HSV I) has been used extensively because of its neurotropic host cell range. Like adenoviruses, recombinant HSV vectors retain functional viral genes, which may be cytotoxic or may reactivate preexisting latent virus in recipient cells. To circumvent these problems, defective HSV has been engineered to eliminate viral genes while retaining certain recognition sequences.

Adeno-associated virus (AAV) is a human parvovirus that can propagate as a lytic infection or integrate into the host genome as a provirus. It is used as a transduction vector for nerve tissue. Successful gene transfer has have been demonstrated in human erythroid cells and lymphocytes. AAV requires a helper virus, usually adenovirus, to initiate productive infection.

SUGGESTED READING

Blankenstein T, Qin Z, Uberla K, et al. Tumor suppression after tumor-cell targeted tumor necrosis factor gene transfer. J Exp Med 173:1047, 1991.

Brenner MK, Rill DR, Moen RC, et al. Gene marking to trace origin of relapse after bone marrow transplantation. Lancet 341:85, 1993.

Davies JL, Kawaguchi Y, Bennett ST, et al. A genome-wide search for human type 1 diabetes susceptibility genes. Nature 371:130, 1994.

Grossman M, Raper SE, Kozarsky K, et al. Successful ex vivo gene therapy directed to liver in a patient with familial hypercholesterolaemia. Nature 6:335, 1994.

Lindsten J, Pettersson U (eds). Etiology of Human Disease at the DNA Level. New York: Raven, 1991.

Ohno T, Gordon D, San H, et al. Gene therapy for vascular smooth muscle cell proliferation after arterial injury. Science 265:781, 1994.

Perales JC, Ferkol T, Beegen H, Ratnoff OD, Hanson RW. Gene transfer in vivo: Sustained expression and regulation of genes introduced into the liver by receptor-targeted uptake. Proc Natl Acad Sci 91:4086, 1994.

Sullenger BA, Cech TR. Ribozyme-mediated repair of defective mRNA by targeted trans-splicing. Nature 371:616, 1994.

Wagner E, Zatloukal K, Cotten M, et al. Coupling of adenovirus to transferrin-polylysine/DNA complexes greatly enhances receptor-mediated gene delivery and expression of transfected genes. Proc Natl Acad Sci 89:6099, 1992.

Weiss R, Teich N, Varmus, H Coffin J (eds). RNA Tumor Viruses. New York: Cold Spring Harbor Press, 1984.

ESSENTIALS OF SURGERY: SCIENTIFIC PRINCIPLES AND PRACTICE,
edited by Lazar J. Greenfield, Michael W. Mulholland, Keith T. Oldham, Gerald B. Zelenock,
and Keith D. Lillemoe. Lippincott–Raven Publishers, Philadelphia, © 1997.

CHAPTER 16

TRANSPLANTATION AND IMMUNOLOGY

JONATHAN S. BROMBERG, JEFFREY D. PUNCH, ROBERT M. MERION, MITCHELL L. HENRY, RONALD M. FERGUSON, DARRELL A. CAMPBELL, JR., JOHN M. HAM, JEREMIAH G. TURCOTTE, SARA J. SHUMWAY, R. MORTON BOLMAN III, LARRY R. KAISER, AND LAWRENCE ROSENBERG

TRANSPLANTATION IMMUNOLOGY

Initiation of the Immune Response

Initiation of the immune response involves: antigen recognition, direct recognition of antigen by immunoglobulin, recognition of antigen by the T-cell receptor in the context of the major histocompatibility complex (MHC; Table 16-1), antigen processing (Fig. 16-1), antigen presentation, and alloreactivity.

Clinical Immunosuppression

Immunosuppressive regimens for clinical transplantation are based on protocols with agents such as azathioprine and corticosteroids, or cyclosporine A (Table 16-2). Immunosuppression is induced with high doses of drugs to prevent rejection. The drugs are reduced rapidly in days to weeks to less toxic maintenance levels. Induction regimens rely on three or four drugs (azathioprine, corticosteroids, cyclosporine, antibodies), and maintenance regimens rely on two or three drugs (azathioprine, corticosteroids, cyclosporine). Therapy for first or mild rejections is usually high-dose "pulse" steroids. Therapy for steroid unresponsive, severe, or secondary rejections is antibodies, especially OKT3.

There are two main types of antibody preparations (Table 16-3). Polyclonal antibodies such as antilymphocyte (ALG) or antithymocyte globulin (ATG) are prepared by immunizing animals with human lymphocytes or lymphoid lines, bleeding the animals to obtain serum, and purifying whole immunoglobulin from serum. These preparations are directed primarily against many different antigens present on T cells (eg, CD2, CD3). They also recognize B-cell, monocyte, platelet, and granulocyte antigens. Polyclonal antibodies are used for induction but not for acute rejection.

They are associated with a number of side effects related to depletion of cell populations (leukopenia, thrombocytopenia) or allergic reactions related to host anti-immunoglobulin responses (urticaria, rash, pruritus). Monoclonal antibody (Orthoclone OKT3 [muromonab]) recognizes all T cells and interferes with their antigen recognition functions in the context of class I or class II MHC. OKT3 is used for induction of the immune response and management of rejection. It is first-line therapy for rejection or for rejection unresponsive to high-dose steroids or polyclonal antibodies.

Complications of Immunosuppression

Immunosuppressive drugs have numerous toxicities and adverse effects (Tables 16-2, 16-3). The complications include: infection, malignant neoplasia, squamous cell carcinoma, lymphoma, Karposi sarcoma, cervical carcinomas, atherosclerotic vascular disease, kidney damage, and graft-versus-host disease (GVHD).

Antigenicity and Immunity in Clinical Transplantation

Most laboratories use serologic, or antibody-based, techniques to type potential donors and recipients for HLA. The main loci typed are HLA-A, HLA-B, and HLA-DR. For a completely heterozygous person this results in six antigens typed (six-antigen match). Nucleic acid and polymerase chain reaction techniques are more accurate than serologically based techniques. They can be used to type for additional loci, which allows better matching.

An important test for graft compatibility is the crossmatch. This assay determines if there are preformed antibodies in the recipient's serum that react with antigens on the cell surface of the donor's lymphocytes (Fig. 16-2). A positive crossmatch means antibodies are present and hyperacute rejection would occur if the transplant were performed. Controls are always performed to exclude autoantibodies. Crossmatching is important for kidney, pancreas, lung, and heart allografting; hepatic allografts are resistant to hyperacute rejection.

Another test that reflects the presence of host anti-donor antibodies is the panel reactive antibody (PRA). Most patients on transplant waiting lists send serum samples to the transplant center on a regular basis. These sera are tested against a panel of typing cells of known HLA specificity by means of techniques identical to those for the crossmatch. The percentage of cells with which recipient serum reacts is determined, and this number is the PRA. Most healthy people have no

---

Table 16-1. **CLASS I AND CLASS II ANTIGENS: STRUCTURE AND FUNCTION**

Class I Antigens	Class II Antigens
STRUCTURE	
Encoded by HLA-A, -B, -C loci in humans	Encoded by HLA-D locus (DR, DP, DQ)
Single polymorphic heavy chain (45 kd)	Two chains α (29 kd) β (34 kd)
Associated with β_2-microglobulin (12 kd)	—
Five domains α_1, α_2, α_3 extracellular Transmembrane Cystoplasmic	Four domains α_1, α_2 or β_1, β_2 extracellular Transmembrane Cytoplasmic
Expressed on all nucleated cells	Expressed on B cells, antigen-presenting cells, and vascular endothelium
MAJOR FUNCTIONS	
Activator and target for cytotoxic T (CD8+) lymphocytes	Activator of helper T cells (CD4+) and stimulator in mixed lymphocyte reaction
Target for antibody-mediated rejection	Possible target for antibody-mediated rejection
Stimulate antibody response	Stimulator of antibody response (unknown significance)

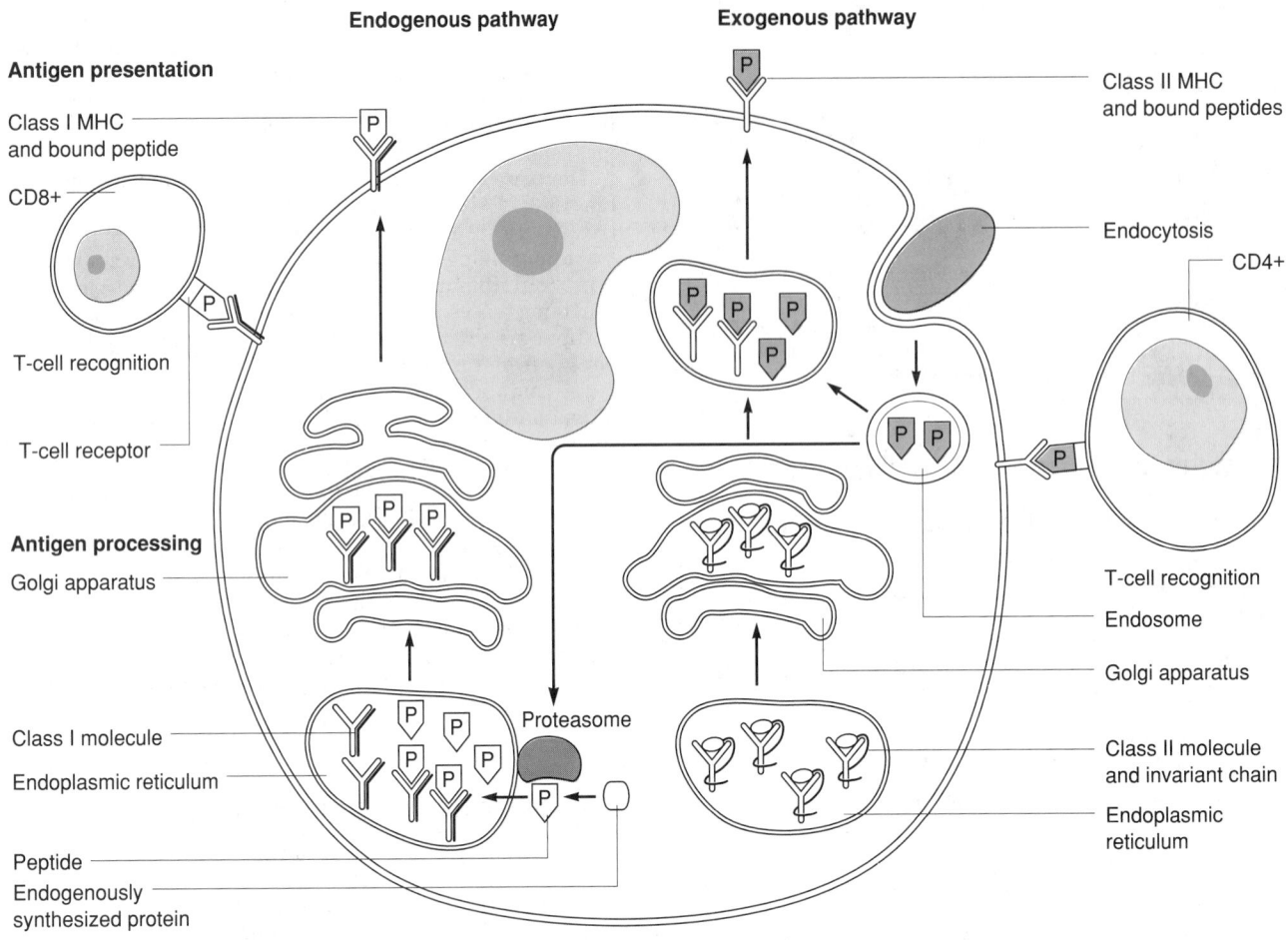

Figure 16-1. Antigen processing and presentation. Endogenously synthesized or intracellular proteins (eg, viral gene products) are degraded into peptides that are transported to the endoplasmic reticulum. These peptides bind to class I MHC molecules and are transported to the surface of the antigen-presenting cell. CD8+ T cells recognize the foreign peptide bound to class I MHC by way of the TCR complex. Exogenous antigen (eg, bacterial) is endocytosed and broken down into peptide fragments in endosomes. Class II molecules are transported to the endosome in association with the invariant chain, bind the peptide, and are delivered to the surface of the antigen-presenting cell, where they are recognized by CD4+ cells.

anti-HLA antibodies and have a low PRA. Patients who have undergone transfusion, are pregnant, have undergone earlier transplantation, or have an autoimmune disorder that induces many antibodies may have a high PRA. The presence of a very high PRA suggests a patient is likely to have a positive crossmatch.

A matching technique used in living related transplantation is the mixed lymphocyte culture (MLC) or mixed lymphocyte reaction (MLR). Lymphocytes are isolated from peripheral blood specimens from donor and recipient. The donor cells are irradiated to prevent mitosis, and the two cell populations are placed into culture together. Recipient cells recognize donor antigen in culture, are activated, and proliferate rapidly. After a few days of culture the amount of proliferation is quantitated by means of incorporation of radiolabeled nucleic acids into the cells. The amount or degree of proliferation compared with positive and negative controls is assumed to represent the potential for a host anti-donor response and risk for allograft rejection.

ORGAN PRESERVATION
Determination of Suitability for Cadaveric Organ Donation

An organ is considered acceptable for donation if the following general prerequisites are met:

- Establishment of a diagnosis of brain death
- Good health before the event that precipitated brain death
- Hemodynamic stability from the time of the event precipitating brain death until completion of organ procurement
- Informed consent from the donor's next of kin

An organ is unacceptable if one of the following is present: sepsis, viral infection, cancer, history of substance abuse, or specific organ dysfunction.

Brain Death

Any condition that causes overwhelming cerebral insult may be sufficient to cause brain death. These conditions

Table 16-2. CURRENTLY APPROVED IMMUNOSUPPRESSIVE AGENTS

Agent (Brand Name)	Mechanism of Action	Dosage	Monitoring	Clinical Uses	Adverse Effects
Azathioprine (Imuran)	Inhibits purine synthesis via active metabolites 6-thioinocinic acid (via conversion to 6-MP) and 6-thioguanine nucleotides; inhibits DNA and RNA synthesis; has greater effect on T cells than B cells	1–3 mg/kg/d IV or PO	Maintain WBCs >3000/μL	Part of regimens to lower doses of cyclosporine or prednisone	Myelosuppression (leukopenia, occasionally thrombocytopenia and megaloblastic anemia), hepatitis, cholestatis, hepatic vein thrombosis, pancreatitis dermatitis, alopecia, increased susceptibility to infections
Cytoxan	Alkylates DNA	0.5–1.5 mg/kg/d	Maintain WBCs >3000/μL	Substitution for azathioprine if adverse effects occur	Leukopenia, thrombocytopenia hemorrhagic cystitis, nausea, vomiting, increased susceptibility to infections
Glucocorticoids	Complex; affects T cells and macrophages; has little effect on antibody production by B cells. Steroid-receptor complex binds to DNA; alters transcription and translation of genes responsible for cytokine synthesis; blocks MLR and development of CTL; inhibits IL-1 and IL-6 synthesis	Prednisolone, 1–2 mg/kg/d induction; 0.1–0.2 mg/kg/d maintenance bid, qd, or qod dosing Prednisolone, 2 mg/kg/d for rejection; tapering schedule Solu-Medrol 5–15 mg/kg/d IV for rejection	No objective means to monitor; adjustment done by protocol; adverse effects	Foundation of most multidrug protocols; treatment of rejection	Cushingoid features (moon facies, acne, centripetal obesity, striae), hypertension, weight gain (increased appetite), hyperglycemia, osteoporosis, type II diabetes, poor wound healing, pancreatitis, peptic ulcer, colonic perforation, psychosis, increased susceptibility to infections
Cyclosporine (Sandimmune)	Binds to cyclophilin; blocks transcription of several early T-cell activation genes, including IL-2, IL-3, IL-4, and IFN-γ; inhibits IL-1 production by macrophages	8–10 mg/kg/d PO qd, bid, or tid or 2.5–3 mg/kg/d IV	Trough levels (usually 12 h); serum creatinine; mg/kg dose (protocol); biopsy (histologic evidence of cyclosporine toxicity)	Induction therapy with prednisolone or azathioprine in most multidrug regimens	Nephrotoxicity, hypertension, hyperkalemia, hyperuricemia and gout, gingival hypertrophy, hepatotoxicity, hirsutism, tremors, seizures, hyperglycemia, hemolytic uremic syndrome, increased susceptibility to infection
FK 506, Tacrolimus (Prograf)	Similar to cyclosporine (10–100 times more potent); binds to FKBP; blocks expression of IL-2 receptors on allostimulated T cells	0.15 mg/kg/d PO qd or bid or 0.075 mg/kg IV q 12 h	Trough levels; serum creatinine; dose mg/kg dose (protocol); adverse effects (neurologic)	Induction therapy with prednisone; treatment of rejection; maintenance without prednisolone	Nephrotoxicity, headache, weight loss, tremors, paresthesia, increased sensitivity to light, insomnia and mood changes, increased susceptibility to infections

MLR, mixed lymphocyte response; CTL, cytotoxic T lymphocytes.

Table 16-3. POLYCLONAL AND MONOCLONAL ANTIBODIES

Antibody	Source	Mechanism of Action	Dosage	Monitoring	Clinical Uses	Adverse Effects
ALG or ATG	Horse, goat, rabbit	Depletes T cells more than B cells as a result of complement-dependent lysis and opsonization	10–30 mg/kg/d IV qd over 6 h; must be given in central line	Peripheral T-cell levels; monitor for antihorse or antigoat antibody development; platelets; WBC count	Induction with azathioprine or prednisone as part of triple or quadruple therapy protocols; treatment of rejection with or without steroids	Fever, chills, leukopenia, thrombocytopenia, nausea, vomiting, diarrhea, arthralgia, headache, myalgia, rash, pruritus, urticaria, chest pain, phlebitis, rarely anaphylaxis or serum sickness
OKT3	Mouse	Reacts with CD3 recognition complex on T cells; blocks recognition of class I or II antigens; inhibits generation and function of effector T cells; opsonizes CD3+ cells; modulates CD3 antigen-recognition complex; renders T cells anergetic or kills them by apoptosis	2.5–10 mg/d IV over 30 min; can be given in peripheral vein	Peripheral CD3 levels; monitor for antimouse antibody development	Same as ALG, ATG	Usually with first dose: fever, chills, diarrhea, headache, nausea, vomiting dyspnea, wheezing, pulmonary edema, tachycardia, hypotension, aseptic meningitis, seizures, coma; markedly reduced with pretreatment with steroids, acetaminophen, indomethacin, and diphenhydramine hydrochloride

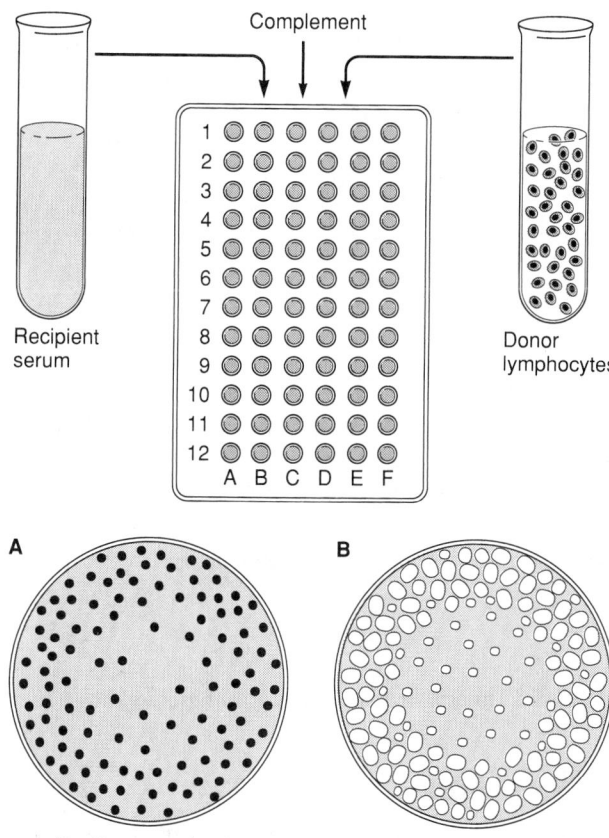

Figure 16-2. Lymphocytotoxicity crossmatch. Recipient serum is incubated with donor lymphocytes and complement in microtiter plates. If donor-specific lymphocytotoxic antibodies are present in the recipient serum, antibody binding results in complement fixation and lysis of the donor lymphocytes. This is detected by the addition of a dye that is taken up through the damaged cell membrane, and a positive crossmatch is noted (*A*). If no antibodies are present, cells remain viable and do not take up the dye (*B*). This is a negative crossmatch.

fall into the broad categories of subarachnoid hemorrhage, direct cerebral trauma, primary malignant tumor of the central nervous system, and other rare and miscellaneous entities. The following criteria indicate irreversible brain dysfunction: unreceptivity and unresponsivity, absence of spontaneous muscular movement, absence of reflexes, or a silent electroencephalogram (EEG).

Most hospitals have a brain death committee responsible for making uniform determinations of brain death according to locally established specific criteria. An example is as follows: 1) The presence of reversible causes of coma is excluded. Reversible causes of coma include sedation, hypothermia below 32.2°C, neuromuscular blockade, and shock. 2) Clinical criteria establishing the loss of all functions of the entire brain must be met. Such criteria include deep coma, absence of brain-stem function and absence of spontaneous respiration. A confirmatory diagnostic test must be performed.

Absence of brain-stem function can be documented with confirmation of the absence of pupillary light response, corneal reflex, oculocephalic reflex, oculovestibular reflex, and spontaneous respiration. The confirmatory test of choice is electrocerebral silence on an EEG. Four-vessel cerebral arteriography demonstrating cessation of blood flow to the brain may be performed within an hour of the clinical brain-death declaration.

Nuclear scintigraphic determination of cerebral blood flow provides definitive confirmation of brain death.

Request for Permission from Next of Kin

Organ donation is discussed at a time after and separate from informing the family of the patient's death. Although an organ donor card is an indication of the decedent's wishes, family consent is obtained before organ procurement. The hierarchy for permission from next of kin is as follows: spouse, adult son or daughter, either parent, adult brother or sister, guardian, any other person authorized to dispose of the body.

Donor-Organ Maintenance

Tissue Perfusion

Because most donors receive a minimum of fluids to prevent increased cerebral edema, an important step in donor-organ maintenance is prompt restoration of intravascular volume. This may necessitate 3 to 10 L of volume resuscitation. The dosage of pressor agents needed to support blood pressure can be progressively decreased as central venous pressure is raised to 10 to 12 cm H_2O. Crystalloid may be used, and lactated Ringer solution is often given because its slightly lower sodium concentration counteracts the sodium concentrating effects of diabetes insipidus. In the presence of severe hypernatremia, free water may be added. Colloid and blood are used to restore and maintain osmotic pressure and normovolemia. The hematocrit is kept at approximately 35% to replace traumatic losses and maintain oxygen-carrying capacity. Fluids are administered to achieve a urine output of at least 100 mL/h and a systolic arterial pressure of 90 to 120 mmHg. If diabetes insipidus is severe, exogenous vasopressin must be given.

Oxygenation and Ventilation

Arterial blood gases are checked regularly, and adjustments of the ventilator are made to optimize gas exchange and acidBbase balance. Oxygen supply must maintain arterial oxygen saturation >95% and mixed venous oxygen saturation >70%. Low levels of positive end-expiratory pressure may facilitate balanced oxygen supply and demand.

Inotropic Support

Most donors are hypovolemic at the time of brain death and are receiving inotropic support in lieu of volume to support their blood pressure. Dopamine hydrochloride is the most commonly used agent. The need for high doses of this drug indicates persistent hypovolemia, and restoration of normovolemia is almost always accompanied by a reduction in dopamine requirements. High doses of dopamine for long periods before organ procurement may be associated with increased rates of acute tubular necrosis and hepatic allograft failure. Cardiac procurement is often abandoned if high doses of inotropic support are needed, despite adequate volume status.

Prevention of Hypothermia

Thermoregulatory homeostatic mechanisms are destroyed when brain death occurs, and severe hypothermia may lead to ventricular arrhythmia and cardiac arrest. Warming blankets are used above and below the donor to keep body temperature >35°C, and exposure for examination or intervention is kept to a minimum. Intravenous fluids may be warmed before administration, and a heated humidifier circuit can be added to the ventilator.

Multiple-Organ Procurement

When brain death is declared, the decedent is identified as an organ donor, and permission is given by the next of kin, the logistics of organ procurement are arranged. The United Network for Organ Sharing (UNOS) is responsible for distribution of cadaveric donor organs throughout the United States. In each of 11 regions, organ procurement organizations (OPOs) maintain the list of potential recipients for their area. All potential recipients in the United States are entered into the UNOS computer system, and a point allocation system is used to determine in an OPO the recipient of a given organ. If a particular organ cannot be used by a recipient in the OPO, the next suitable recipient in the region is offered the organ. If no recipients in the UNOS region can be found, the organ is offered to any recipient in the United States. The only exception to these guidelines relates to renal transplant recipients who share six antigens with the donor. These kidneys are shared nationwide even if suitable local recipients are available.

Techniques of multiple organ procurement allow removal of the heart, lungs, kidneys, liver, and pancreas from a single donor for transplantation into six or more recipients. The steps in the procedure are as follows:

1. Incision
2. Exploration and inspection
3. Individual organ mobilization
4. In situ perfusion
5. Removal of organs
6. Closure of the incision
7. Processing, packaging, and transport to recipient centers

RENAL TRANSPLANTATION
Indications

The indication for renal transplantation is the presence of end-stage renal disease (Table 16-4). Contraindications are systemic malignant disease, active infection (including human immunodeficiency virus [HIV]), and inability to comprehend the procedure and follow-up requirements. An outline of the evaluation of a potential recipient is presented in Table 16-5.

Procedure

Nearly all transplanted kidneys (except in small children) are placed retroperitoneally in the iliac fossa. This provides proximity to blood vessels and the bladder, fixes

Table 16-4. CAUSES OF RENAL FAILURE IN RENAL TRANSPLANTATION

Congenital	Aplasia, obstructive uropathy
Hereditary	Alport syndrome, polycystic disease, tuberous sclerosis
Metabolic	Amyloidosis, cystinosis, nephrocalcinosis, oxalosis
Neoplasms	Renal cell carcinoma, Wilms tumor
Progressive	Diabetic nephropathy, chronic pyelonephritis, Goodpasture syndrome, hypertension, membranous glomerulonephritis, lupus nephritis, nephrotic syndrome, obstructive uropathies, scleroderma
Trauma	Vascular occlusion, parenchymal destruction

Table 16-5. PRETRANSPLANTATION WORKUP OF POTENTIAL RENAL RECIPIENTS

INITIAL WORKUP
History and physical examination
Laboratory analyses: serum electrolytes, calcium, magnesium, phosphorus, complete blood count, platelets, AST, APT, alkaline phosphatase, prothrombin time, partial thromboplastin time, viral serologies (including herpes simplex, cytomegalovirus, HIV, and hepatitis A, B, and C), urinalysis and urine culture, ABO and HLA typing, serum for frozen storage

ROUTINE EXAMINATIONS
Dental
Pap smear
Ophthalmologic (diabetic patients)
Psychosocial

SECONDARY WORKUP (BASED ON PRELIMINARY FINDINGS)
Cardiac: Stress ECG, stress MUGA, echo, coronary angiography
Gastrointestinal: upper and lower endoscopy, gallbladder echo
Genitourinary: voiding cystourethrogram, cystoscopy, retrograde ureterography
Pulmonary: arterial blood gases, pulmonary functions

the kidney anatomically, and does not violate the abdominal cavity.

Preservation

Simple cold storage may allow viability of a kidney up to 48 hours, and pulsatile preservation is effective up to 72 hours. The goals of each method are to maintain structural and metabolic integrity and to minimize reperfusion injury.

Immunosuppression

Cyclosporine has the following benefits over azathioprine: lower incidence of rejection episodes, lower incidence of infection (particularly cytomegalovirus [CMV]), lower cost associated with transplantation, and a shorter hospital stay and fewer readmissions.

The side effects of cyclosporine are nephrotoxicity, hypertension, and metabolic effects (including hyperuricemia, hyperkalemia, hypercholesterolemia, and hirsutism). Sequential therapy in which an ALG preparation, azathioprine, and prednisone are administered after transplantation and followed by cyclosporine avoids these complications.

Posttransplantation Care
Phase 1

The early phase is posttransplantation days 0 through 30. The goals of management are:

1) Prevention of death in the immediately postoperative period
2) Immediate function of the transplanted kidney
3) Baseline of stable renal function as close to normal as possible
4) Prevention of an early acute rejection episode

During the first week, a course of prophylactic ALG in conjunction with tapering doses of oral prednisone and azathioprine is often used. Cyclosporine is begun when serum creatinine is <2.5 mg/dL, usually by the 5th to 7th day after transplantation. At this time, ALG is discontinued, and the patient receives maintenance therapy with cyclosporine, prednisone, and azathioprine. This protocol meets the goals of achieving good immediate function and preventing early rejection.

Phase 2

The phase of acute rejection occurs in posttransplantation days 31 through 180. Two-thirds of recipients of first cadaveric renal grafts never have an acute rejection episode; some patients have only one rejection episode, and some have two or more. Acute rejection can be diagnosed and managed. Chronic rejection, slowly progressive loss of renal function, happens over months and occurs mostly among patients who have had a previous, successfully treated acute rejection episode. The treatment modalities commonly used are oral high-dose prednisone alone, oral prednisone with ALG, and oral prednisone with OKT3. The events of phase 2, although occurring in the first few months after transplantation, influence the long-term fate of an allografted kidney.

Phase 3

The quiescent phase is posttransplantation days 180 through 365. During this period few graft losses and few acute rejection episodes occur.

Phase 4

The chronic phase begins 1 year after transplantation and continues. Because most posttransplantation deaths are due to myocardial infarction and stroke, paying particular attention to the management of hypertension and lipid levels in these patients influences the prevention of cardiovascular complications.

Complications

Posttransplantation complications can be categorized as early or late. Most early complications are caused by infections, which range from simple wound infections to overwhelming bacterial or fungal sepsis. Other early problems include urologic complications, such as urine leaks associated with distal ureteral necrosis or bladder leaks or ureteral obstruction due to a lymphocele. Therapy for leaks is percutaneous ureteral drainage and stenting or Foley catheter drainage. Therapy for ureteral obstruction is drainage of the isolated retroperitoneal lymph collection into the abdominal cavity by making a peritoneal window. This allows decompression of the ureter and normalization of renal function.

The most important late complication is renal arterial stenosis. This condition may be heralded by uncontrolled hypertension and is diagnosed with renal transplant angiography. Percutaneous balloon angioplasty or surgical repair can be performed to correct the abnormality.

HEPATIC TRANSPLANTATION
Indications

Elective Transplantation for End-Stage Liver Disease

Rapidly deepening jaundice
Diuretic resistant ascites
Spontaneous hepatic encephalopathy
Recurrent sepsis (including spontaneous bacterial peritonitis)
Recurrent variceal hemorrhage
Prolongation of the prothrombin time to >8 seconds above control values in spite of vitamin K replacement
Severe fatigue

Emergency Transplantation

Fulminant hepatic failure (factor V level <20%) in which the patient's condition progresses to stage III (stuporous) or IV (unresponsive) coma

Contraindications

Inability to withstand the operation, usually for cardiovascular or pulmonary reasons
Recent intracranial hemorrhage or irreversible neurologic impairment
Active substance abuse
Intractable hypotension necessitating pressor support
Evidence of HIV infection
Ongoing bacterial infection
Extrahepatic malignant disease

Specific Indications

Primary biliary cirrhosis
Primary sclerosing cholangitis
Biliary atresia
Inherited metabolic disorders
Wilson's disease
α1-antitrypsin deficiency
Tyrosinemia
Type I glycogen storage disease
Fulminant hepatic failure
Budd-Chiari syndrome
Alcoholic liver disease
Primary liver tumors
Hepatitis B

Preoperative Assessment and Management

Urgent Transplantation

Assessment involves a neurologic examination with assessment of coma grade. Patients in grade IV coma (unresponsive) benefit from constant monitoring of intracranial pressure (ICP). An attempt is made to keep cerebral perfusion pressure (mean arterial blood pressure minus ICP) >60 mmHg. Therapy for low mean arterial blood pressure is pressors, and therapy for elevation of ICP is hyperventilation and mannitol. Severe elevations of ICP may cause brain death. Hemodynamic stability is assessed with monitoring of intravascular volume.

Expansion of intravascular volume may be limited by considerations about ICP, for which temporary inotropic support is needed. Acute renal failure is managed with continuous arteriovenous hemofiltration with or without dialysis, and this may be continued intraoperatively.

Because an acutely failing liver produces an acutely failing reticuloendothelial system, florid sepsis often occurs, and broad-spectrum antibiotics are needed. Pulmonary insufficiency is a common accompaniment of liver failure and is managed with intubation, high concentrations of inspired oxygen, and, if necessary, positive end-expiratory pressure.

Elective Transplantation

Under elective conditions, after a decision for hepatic transplantation is made, it is common to wait for several months for a suitable donor organ to become available. During this period, frequent examinations are performed so that rapid deterioration is recognized and managed. Therapy for encephalopathy is lactulose and protein restriction, for variceal hemorrhage is sclerotherapy, and for refractory ascites is large-volume paracentesis. Therapy for spontaneous bacterial peritonitis is hospital admission and antibiotics.

Hepatic Transplantation Procedure

Surgical Technique

A hepatic transplant operation has three and sometimes four phases:

1. Preliminary dissection and skeletonization of the recipient's diseased liver
2. Anhepatic phase, the period starting with devascularization of the recipient's liver and initiation of venovenous bypass and ending with revascularization of the newly implanted organ
3. The period after revascularization that includes biliary reconstruction and abdominal closure
4. Auxiliary liver transplantation (placement of the donor allograft in an heterotopic rather than orthotopic position,leaving the diseased liver in place)

Postoperative Complications

Primary Nonfunction

The clinical definition of primary nonfunction of hepatic allografts is as follows. The essential characteristics are: occurrence within 96 hours after the operation and patent portal vein and hepatic artery. Three of the following four characteristics are required for definition: bile output <20 mL in 12 hours, bilirubin level >10 or rising 5 mg/d or more, PT/PTT ratio of ≥1.5, and factors V and VIII <25% of normal.

Other Complications

Nonspecific cholestasis
Biliary leak or obstruction
Hemorrhage
Hepatic arterial thrombosis
Portal venous thrombosis
Vena caval thrombosis
Intraabdominal sepsis
Neurologic complications

Rejection and Immunosuppression

Acute Rejection

Acute, or cell-mediated, rejection is common but is blunted by means of antirejection therapy. Acute rejection usually occurs in the first 2 postoperative months. The diagnosis of cell-mediated rejection is made on clinical and histologic grounds (Table 16-6). Treatment ranges from full antirejection therapy to no therapy.

Chronic Rejection

Chronic rejection is characterized by a relentless immune attack on small bile ducts. The pattern is gradual biliary obstruction with elevation of alkaline phosphatase and bilirubin in the absence of abnormalities in large bile ducts. Small bile ducts are obliterated or completely absent. Retransplantation usually is needed.

Immunosuppression Induction and Maintenance

A common immunosuppressive protocol in hepatic transplantation consists of an initial 1 to 2 weeks course of ATG, high doses of prednisone with a rapid taper, azathioprine, and cyclosporine. Prophylactic administration of ATG starting the first posttransplantation day provides immunosuppression without nephrotoxicity. Cyclosporine, a nephrotoxic drug, can be added to the im-

---

Table 16-6. DIAGNOSIS OF HEPATIC ALLOGRAFT REJECTION

CLINICAL

Fever
Jaundice
Decrease in bile output
Change in consistency of bile

LABORATORY

Leukocytosis
Eosinophilia
Elevation of transaminases
Elevation of serum bilirubin
Elevation of prothrombin time

BIOPSY

Portal lymphocytosis
Endothelitis
Bile duct infiltration by cells, with duct injury

---

munosuppressive regimen when renal function is clearly improving, usually after 5 to 7 days. Because immunosuppression predisposes to infection, prophylactic antiviral and antibacterial drugs are administered. A typical regimen includes trimethoprim–sulfamethoxazone and acyclovir for the first postoperative month.

Management of Acute Rejection

When acute rejection is diagnosed, high doses of methylprednisolone are administered for 3 days. Steroid-resistant rejection is treated with OKT3.

CARDIAC TRANSPLANTATION

Indications

The primary indication for cardiac transplantation is end-stage heart disease in a patient who is not expected to survive more than 6 months to 1 year. Most candidates for cardiac transplantation are New York Heart Association class 3 or 4 as a result of cardiomyopathy. Other indications include congenital heart disease, valvular heart disease, viral cardiomyopathies, failed initial cardiac transplant, and familial and restrictive cardiomyopathies.

Preoperative Evaluation and Selection Criteria

The patient undergoes a complete history and physical examination. Any history or evidence of malignant disease or infection is pursued. Any other end-stage organ disease is a relative contraindication. All potential recipients must be nonsmokers who do not consume alcohol and are at an appropriate weight for their height and body build. Tests are performed (Table 16-7) to rule out the following contraindications to cardiac transplantation:

Age >65 years
History of malignant disease (not cured)
Ongoing infection, systemic disease, irreversible hepatic, pulmonary, or renal damage
Recent cerebrovascular or neurologic deficit
Pulmonary embolus within 6 weeks
Active ulcer or bleeding diathesis
Smoking, drinking, or recreational drug use
Poorly controlled diabetes mellitus
Pulmonary vascular resistance >6 to 8 Wood units (480 to 640 dynes/sec/cm5)
Psychologic instability or history of poor compliance

Table 16-7. PRETRANSPLANTATION TESTS AND EVALUATIONS

History and physical examination
Obstetric and gynecologic consultation for female patients, including Pap smear, herpes culture, and birth control counseling
Laboratory analyses
  Hematology: complete blood count, platelet count, coagulation battery, fibrinogen, factor V
  Chemistry: blood urea nitrogen, creatinine, electrolytes, calcium, PO_4, fasting, blood sugar, serum electrophoresis, cholesterol, triglycerides, amylase, SGOT, bilirubin, alkaline phosphatase, thyroid index, hepatitis profile, lipoprotein screen, creatinine clearance
  Microbiology: cytomegalovirus, Epstein-Barr virus, varicella-zoster, herpes simplex virus titers
  Immunology: ABO type and screen (this is double-checked), HLA-A, B, C, and DR typing and antileukocyte antibody screening, quantitative immunoglobulins, and human immunodeficiency virus (patient gives verbal consent)
Tests seen by nurse clinician, transplantation cardiologist, and transplantation cardiac surgeon)
  Chest radiograph, posteroanterior and lateral
  Bilateral mammogram for female patients
  Stool guaiac (three tests)
  12-lead electrocardiogram
  Cardiac catheterization, including pulmonary artery pressures and resistance
  MUGA scan; right and left ejection fractions or echo, or both
  Spine (thoracic, lumbar) and hip radiographs
  Pulmonary function tests, including lung volumes and DLCO
  Ventilation–perfusion lung scan
  Head CT scan without contrast
  Bone age for children
  Neuropsychologic evaluation
  Cardiopulmonary exercise test

Surgical Technique

The donor procurement team checks the donor's blood type, serologic tests, chest radiograph, and ECG. The recipient team does not anesthetize the patient until a report is received from the donor team that the donor heart looks functional. The diseases heart is not excised until the donor heart arrives in the operating room.

Immunosuppression Protocol

The triple-drug immunosuppression protocol is summarized in Table 16-8. Endomyocardial biopsy is obtained 7 to 10 days after transplantation. Rejection is treated with methylprednisolone. Lack of response to this regimen as suggested by biopsy findings is indication for use of ALG or ATG or OKT3.

Postoperative Care

Mechanical ventilation is gradually discontinued within 48 hours. Orogastric tubes are removed at the time of extubation. Isoproterenol is continued 72 hours postoperatively. Renal dose dopamine may be continued for 72 hours postoperatively to encourage brisk diuresis. A thermodilution pulmonary artery catheter is used almost routinely. Elevated pulmonary vascular resistance responds to perioperative prostaglandin or milronone administration. Some patients need atrial pacing as isoproterenol is discontinued. Calcium channel blockers are used to discontinue vasodilators.

Prophylactic antibiotics are discontinued when the chest tubes are removed, usually on the 2nd postoperative day. Oral intake is started after chest tube removal on the second postoperative day.

Endomyocardial biopsy is performed 7 to 10 days after transplantation, and pacing wires can be removed at that time. Preoperative recipient and donor titers are obtained for CMV, herpes simplex virus, varicella zoster virus, and Epstein–Barr virus. These titers are repeated before patient discharge. All patients receive trimethoprim-sulfamethoxazole. Pentamidine inhaler is given monthly to the few patients who are allergic to sulfa drugs. Acyclovir is given prophylactically to prevent viral infections and is continued as long as the patient does not have alterations in liver or renal function.

Rejection

The diagnosis of rejection is based on endomyocardial biopsies. Biopsies are performed 7 to 10 days after transplantation, then every 2 weeks for 3 months, then once a month for 6 months, then once every 3 months. After 2 years, biopsies are performed once a year.

PULMONARY TRANSPLANTATION

Unlike other solid organs, the lung has no systemic arterial supply that can be reconnected. Bronchial artery anatomy varies, and the size of bronchial arteries, even when they can be identified, precludes direct anastomosis.

Indications

The selection criteria for pulmonary transplant recipients are:

- End-stage disease resulting in a life expectancy <18 months
- No other systemic disease
- No clinically significant coronary artery disease
- No clinically significant psychiatric disorder
- No contraindication to immunosuppression
- Age ≤60 years (with some flexibility)
- Psychosocial support system

Donor Considerations

Unlike other solid organs for transplantation, potential donor lungs may be assessed with plain radiographs. Bronchoscopy provides a way to directly examine the potential

Table 16-8. IMMUNOSUPPRESSION PROTOCOL FOR CARDIAC TRANSPLANTATION

CYCLOSPORINE
Preoperative dose: 6–10 mg/kg PO
Maintenance dose: targeted to a 12-hour trough level of 200 ± 25 ng/mL by high-performance liquid chromatography during the first 6 months
After 6 months: trough level of 100 ± 25 ng/mL

AZATHIOPRINE
Preoperative dose: 2.5 mg/kg (round up to nearest 25 kg)
Maintenance dose: 2–2.5 mg/kg/d (titrated to keep WBCs ≥ 4000)

CORTICOSTEROIDS
Methylprednisolone, 500 mg IV, in operating room after release of aortic crossclamp, then 125 mg IV every 8 hours for three doses
Prednisone, 1 mg/kg/d starting on day 2 after transplantation, in divided doses, with tapering to 0.3 mg/kg/d by 3 months
0.15–0.10 mg/kg/d by the end of the first year

donor organs and to collect material for culture and Gram stain, the results of which may influence later care of the recipient. In no other organ is there the same risk for infection and, because of this, pulmonary infiltrate may preclude the use of a lung. A small infiltrate in one lung without evidence of purulent secretions may allow this lung to be used in double-lung transplantation. A pulmonary infiltrate does not necessarily preclude use of the contralateral lung for single lung transplant. The lungs of a particular donor may not be suitable when all other organs are acceptable. Because all brain-dead patients have endotracheal tubes and are on mechanical ventilation, it is likely that the airway is colonized with bacteria or that there is ongoing invasive infection. With pulmonary infection, there often is evidence of an infiltrate on the chest radiograph. Even with a clear chest radiograph, purulent secretions contraindicate use of the lungs for transplantation.

Problems with the lungs may begin at the time of the insult that has resulted in brain death because the patient may aspirate gastric contents. Signs of aspiration may not become evident on a chest radiograph for 24 to 48 hours, so bronchoscopy is performed before lungs are accepted for transplantation. Characteristic early bronchoscopic evidence of aspiration includes erythematous tracheobronchial mucosa, purulent secretions, and food particles. Pulmonary contusion due to blunt chest trauma may eliminate lungs from donor consideration, but minor-to-moderate contusion unilaterally may still allow use of the lungs in a bilateral lung recipient. It is often difficult to evaluate the extent of contusion at the time of donor retrieval because the interval from injury to determination of brain death and donation may be short. Although the detrimental effect of pulmonary contusion on gas exchange is usually transient, additional bleeding into the lung parenchyma can occur if cardiopulmonary bypass is needed for transplantation, as for a recipient with pulmonary hypertension.

Pulmonary edema may occur as a result of massive head injury and may be further complicated by donor management protocols. Renal transplantation teams try to ensure preservation of adequate urine output, so they infuse large volumes of crystalloid solution.

Cardiac transplantation teams use high doses of inotropic agents to maintain blood pressure, so they also administer large amounts of crystalloid solutions. Donor management must be coordinated to prevent "flooding" of the lungs, which are susceptible to edema after cerebral insult, if lungs are to be available for transplantation.

Size of donor lungs is less important when the recipient has emphysema, in which each hemithorax is very large, than with pulmonary fibrosis, in which the hemithorax is contracted. The important size consideration is a reasonable match between donor and recipient height.

Lung Preservation

The lung must be viable and must participate in gas exchange immediately after implantation. The protocol involves a flush technique with cold crystalloid solution and topical cooling by means of immersion. At the time of donor lung retrieval, just before crossclamping of the aorta, prostaglandin E1 is injected directly into the pulmonary artery to effect vasodilation of the pulmonary vascular bed. Vasodilation allows consistent distribution of the flush solution and consistent and rapid cooling. Prostaglandin E1 also may provide cytoprotection.

The maximal safe interval for the lung to be ischemic even when cooled is 6 hours. This time constraint places limits on the distance one may travel to procure lungs.

Transplantation Operation

Whether one lung or both lungs are replaced depends on recipient factors, including the cause of the end-stage lung disease and donor lung availability. Chronic infection, as in patients with cystic fibrosis, necessitates replacement of both lungs. Patients with pulmonary fibrosis do well with single-lung replacement. Single-lung transplantation is an acceptable operation for patients with emphysema and may be the operation of choice for patients older than 50 years.

Bilateral, sequential lung transplantation is performed for end-stage lung disease in which both lungs must be replaced and for pulmonary vascular disease. Patients with pulmonary hypertension undergo replacement of both lungs.

Other than procedures on patients with pulmonary hypertension, essentially all lung transplant procedures are performed without cardiopulmonary bypass. Lungs may be ischemic 7 to 9 hours and still actively participate in gas exchange.

Complications of Lung Transplantation

Intraoperative Complications
Technical problems with the vascular or bronchial anastomoses
Injury to the phrenic or recurrent laryngeal nerves
Myocardial infarction
Postoperative Complications
Infection of viral, bacterial, or fungal causes related to immunosuppression
Problems with airway healing
Intraabdominal complications

PANCREATIC TRANSPLANTATION

Pancreatic transplantation is performed to provide an endogenous source of insulin and other islet hormones. The ultimate goal is prevention, stabilization, or reversal of the degenerative complications of diabetes. Techniques for pancreatic transplantation are: polymer injection, enteric drainage, and bladder drainage.

Indications

Pancreatic transplantation can be applied to three categories of patients:

1. Patients with diabetes who have undergone successful renal transplantation
2. Patients with end-stage renal disease who need renal transplantation
3. Patients with nonuremic diabetes and other complications

The selection criteria for pancreatic transplantation are:

- IDDM, documented by an absence of circulating C peptide
- Age between 18 and 50 years
- Microalbuminuria with a creatinine clearance >60 mL/min (pancreas alone)
- Microalbuminuria with a creatinine clearance <60 mL/min (consider for simultaneous renal-pancreatic transplantation)
- Proteinuria with a projected requirement for dialysis or established end-stage diabetic nephropathy (consider for simultaneous renal-pancreatic transplantation)

- Autonomic neuropathy (not an independent inclusion criterion)
- Retinopathy (not an independent inclusion criterion)
- Labile diabetes and failure of medical management (may be an independent criterion for pancreatic transplantation alone)
- Sufficient cardiac reserve
- Psychosocial fitness
- Understanding of risks and benefits
- Absence of usual transplant recipient exclusion criteria

Simultaneous Renal and Pancreatic Transplantation

The advantages of simultaneous renalBpancreatic transplantation compared with the sequential procedure (renal followed by pancreatic) include: the recipient's need to accept only one set of donor antigens, ability to monitor rejection of the pancreas by identifying the well-recognized signs of renal allograft rejection, the immunosuppressive effect of uremia, transplantation in patients who have not been maintained on chronic immunosuppression, and one anesthetic exposure.

Pancreatic Transplantation Alone

Candidates for a pancreatic transplantation alone can be divided into two groups: those already possessing a renal allograft and those with no or only early diabetic nephropathy.

Procurement of a Pancreas

Donor Assessment

Most pancreatic transplantations are performed with organs from cadaveric donors. Absolute contraindications to cadaveric pancreatic organ donation include the presence of diabetes mellitus, chronic pancreatitis, and pancreatic damage due to trauma. Relative contraindications include a history of alcohol abuse and relapsing pancreatitis. Blood glucose and serum amylase levels are evaluated in cadaveric donors. The final decision concerning the suitability of the pancreas for transplantation is made during removal.

Organ Preservation

In situ perfusion techniques are used. A risk is thrombosis due to an intraglandular process that involves the pancreatic microvasculature. A low-pressure, low-volume flush to avoid intravascular damage to the gland is important.

Surgical Technique

An obstacle to pancreatic transplantation is that the organ comprises about 2 million endocrine islet cells randomly distributed in an organ that consists mainly of endocrine tissue.

Technical problems of transplanting endocrine tissue concern the exocrine part of the gland. Another problem is predisposition of the graft to vascular thrombosis. There are three options for managing exocrine secretions:

1. Maintain exocrine secretion by means of internal drainage of the exocrine pancreas by anastomosing the ductal system to the intestinal tract or urinary tract
2. Free drainage of pancreatic juice into the peritoneal cavity
3. Ablation of exocrine secretion by means of injection of a synthetic polymer that solidifies and blocks exocrine secretion

Perioperative Management

Immunosuppression—Induction and quadruple immunosuppression with ALG-ATG or OKT3, prednisone, cyclosporine, and azathioprine
Anticoagulation
Endocrine function—Glucose level returns to normal but may vary daily for 1 week after transplantation
Exocrine function—Serum amylase is measured (in the urine or intestinal drainage if diversion is performed). Octreotide administered to manage complications of continued exocrine secretion may interfere with absorption of cyclosporine

Complications

Postoperative complications of pancreatic transplantation are: Immunologic, including rejection and recurrence of diabetes; and Nonimmunologic, including thrombosis, bleeding, pancreatitis, anastomotic failure, sepsis, pancreatic ascites, pseudocyst, pancreatic fistula, intestinal obstruction, perforation (intestinal drainage), metabolic acidosis (bladder drainage), and urethritis, balanitis, cystitis (bladder drainage).

Late complications of pancreatic transplantation are nephropathy, neuropathy, and retinopathy.

Islet Transplantation

The objective of islet transplantation is the provision, early enough in the course of diabetes, of an effective islet cell mass that will function in a physiologic manner to prevent, stabilize, or reverse the secondary complications of diabetes. This technique is under investigation.

SUGGESTED READING

Almond PS, Matas A, Gillingham K, et al. Risk factors for chronic rejection in renal allograft recipients. Transplantation 1993; 55:752.

Belzer FO. Evaluation of preservation of the intra-abdominal organs. Transplant Proc 1993;25:2527.

Bergmeijer JH, Cransberg K, Nijman JM, Molenaar JC, Wolff ED, Provoost AP. Functional adaptation of en-bloc-transplanted pediatric kidneys into pediatric recipients. Transplantation 1994;58:623.

Clavien PA, Harvey RP, Strasberg SM. Preservation and reperfusion injuries in liver allografts. Transplantation 1992;53:957.

Davis RD, Pasque MK. Pulmonary transplantation. Ann Surg 1995;221:14.

Halloran PF, Broski AP, Batiuk TD, et al. The molecular immunology of acute rejection: an overview. Transplant Immunol 1993;1:3.

Momvaerts P, Arnoldi J, Russ, F, et al. Different roles of and T cells in immunity against an intracellular bacterial pathogen. Nature 1993;365:53.

Roth D, Fernandez JA, Babischkin S, et al. Detection of hepatitis C virus among cadaver organ donors: evidence for low transmission of disease. Ann Intern Med 1992;117:470.

Slaughter MS, Braunlin EA, Bolman RM III, et al. Pediatric cardiac transplantation: results of 2- and 5-year follow-up. J Heart Lung Transplant 1994;13:624.

Tesi RJ, Elkhammas EA, Henry ML, Ferguson RM. OKT3 for primary therapy of first rejection episode in kidney transplants. Transplantation 1993;55:1023.

TWO

SURGICAL PRACTICE

ESSENTIALS OF SURGERY: SCIENTIFIC PRINCIPLES AND PRACTICE,
edited by Lazar J. Greenfield, Michael W. Mulholland, Keith T. Oldham, Gerald B. Zelenock,
and Keith D. Lillemoe. Lippincott–Raven Publishers, Philadelphia, © 1997.

CHAPTER 17

HEAD AND NECK

JAMES P. NEIFELD

DIAGNOSTIC APPROACH

History

Important factors in the history include the site and duration of symptoms and exacerbating or ameliorating factors. Difficulty eating suggests a tumor of the oral cavity; hoarseness suggests laryngeal abnormality; and dysphagia suggests pharyngeal or cervical esophageal cancer.

Physical Examination

Intraoral examination requires use of a headlight. Dentures or other prostheses are removed from the patient's mouth, and all surfaces that can be reached by the examining finger are palpated. Palpation of the neck helps delineate the size, consistency, and extent of masses. Indirect laryngoscopy is used to view the vocal cords, supraglottic larynx, and piriform sinuses. A general physical examination is performed because cancers of the lung and breast and digestive, genital, and urinary tracts may present with neck masses.

Biopsy

If the results of physical examination are normal except for the head and neck, biopsy of the primary site is performed. Fine-needle aspiration biopsy is preferable to open biopsy to avoid contamination of tissue planes. If an experienced cytologist is not available, incisional biopsy of large masses or excisional biopsy of small masses may be performed after endoscopy has ruled out a tumor of the upper aerodigestive tract. *If the patient has a neck mass and an obvious cancer in the oral cavity, pharynx, or larynx, the mass in the neck should be assumed to be metastasis, and biopsy should not be performed.*

BENIGN LESIONS

Table 17-1 is a guide to benign lesions of the head and neck.

MALIGNANT LESIONS

Mucosal cancers are unusual in patients <40 years of age and are much more common in men than in women. A common predisposing factor is tobacco use, including chewing and pipe smoking in addition to cigarette smoking.

Staging

Clinical staging is mandatory. After the history, physical examination, indirect laryngoscopy, and panendoscopy, the lesion is staged according to the TNM system (Tables 17-2 and 17-3). *T* represents the size of the primary tumor; *N*, the size and extent of lymph node metastases; and *M*, distant disease. The staging of head and neck cancer is somewhat different from that of other cancers. It varies according to the primary site. For example, cancers of the oral cavity are staged according to size, whereas cancers of the larynx are staged according to involvement of one or both vocal cords, fixation of cords, and then deep extension. A complete description is given in Table 17-2.

Preoperative Evaluation

Preoperative evaluation includes routine laboratory tests and chest radiography. The evaluation is individualized to the site and size of the tumor. If a patient has dysphagia, a barium swallow examination may be indicated. Computed tomography (CT), magnetic resonance imaging (MRI), or other imaging techniques are indicated only for tumors that encroach on the base of the skull or are difficult to assess clinically. If a neck mass seems to involve the carotid artery, angiography is indicated.

Mucosal Cancers

Oral Cavity

Symptoms include difficulty eating, oral bleeding, a sore mouth, and substantial weight loss. Cancers of the oral cavity spread first to lymph nodes in the submental and submandibular areas and then to the midjugular chain.

Cancers of the Anterior Two-Thirds of the Tongue
Chronic, nonhealing ulcer
Cervical lymph node metastases in most patients
Excellent prognosis for small cancers
Poor prognosis once cervical lymph nodes become involved

Cancers of the Floor of the Mouth
Submandibular gland enlargement and pain, which may represent benign swelling rather than metastatic spread
Small tumors treated with surgery or radiation therapy
Large tumors and regional lymph nodes treated with surgery, usually radical neck dissection

Cancers of the Gingiva and Hard Palate
Uncommon sites of squamous cancers

Table 17-1. BENIGN LESIONS OF THE HEAD AND NECK

Lesion	Cause	Diagnosis and Treatment
TUMORS Lymphadenopathy	In children: viral infection, tonsillitis In adults: dental caries, mononucleosis, viral infection, sinusitis, tonsillitis, periodontal disease, skin disease Sinusitis Frontal Chronic maxillary Chronic ethmoid Peritonsillar abscesses Allergy, virus, bacteria, fungus (rare, seen in diabetic or immunosuppressed patients)	Biopsy Treatment of underlying disease
INFECTIONS Acute tonsillitis	Tonsillitis or pharyngitis, usually streptococcal Tumor or foreign-body perforation Pharyngeal infections Parapharyngeal Retropharyngeal	Antibiotics If no response: Opening and irrigation of sinus, possibly removal of infected mucosa Caldwell-Luc operation Ethmoidectomy High doses of penicillin if cellulitis is present Drainage, after tracheostomy if airway is compromised Incision and drainage if pus is present Tonsillectomy indicated because of recurrent nature of abscesses Penicillin
Salivary gland infections	Poor dental hygiene; salivary duct obstruction	Extraoral drainage Antibiotics Incision and drainage through posterior wall of pharynx Antibiotics Removal of obstruction If no response: excision of necrotic gland Tumor, infection, trauma
HEMORRHAGE Nasal Other sites	Malignant tumors: involvement of branch of carotid artery, tumor erosion into carotid artery, ulcerated tumor bed Epiglottitis Traumatic lesion Tumors	Anterior: pressure, topical vasoconstrictor, cautery Posterior: obstruction with Foley catheter balloon or nasal pack, possible ligation of internal maxillary artery, prophylactic antibiotics Tumor resection Ligation of carotid artery Packing of ulcerated tumor
UPPER AIRWAY OBSTRUCTION	Bacterial infection Trauma Tumor	Antibiotics, humidification of air, intubation if respiratory distress continues Emergency cricothyroidotomy in field Tracheostomy in emergency department *Oral intubation should not be attempted* Laryngoscopy in operating room with local anesthesia Tracheostomy if airway is narrow Laser treatment of tumor to open airway before definitive treatment of lesion

Treated with surgery
Spread to lymph nodes unusual

Cancers of the Buccal Mucosa
   Common in areas where tobacco and betel nuts are chewed
   Slow-growing, well-differentiated
   Low rate of lymph node metastasis

Verrucous Cancer
   Well-differentiated malignant tumor with benign-appearing histologic characteristics
   Rarely spreads to lymph nodes; commonly arises from buccal mucosa

Less responsive to radiation therapy than more invasive, less differentiated squamous cell carcinomas
Often treated with full-thickness resection of cheek; flap closure may be necessary

Cancers of the oral cavity are treated with wide resection. If the tumor is T2 or greater or is associated with clinically positive nodes, radical neck dissection is performed. Lymph node metastases are uncommon for small tumors but may occur in the presence of normal neck examinations when the primary tumor is T2 or greater. Survival rates for cancers of the hard palate are slightly lower than those for other cancers of the oral

Table 17-2. TNM CLASSIFICATION FOR STAGING OF CANCER OF THE HEAD AND NECK

PRIMARY TUMOR
Oral Cavity

TX   Primary tumor cannot be assessed
T0   No evidence of primary tumor
Tis   Carcinoma in situ
T1   Tumor 2 cm or less in greatest dimension
T2   Tumor more than 2 cm but not more than 4 cm in greatest dimension
T3   Tumor more than 4 cm in greatest dimension
T4   Tumor invades adjacent structures

Oropharynx

T1   Tumor 2 cm or less in greatest dimension
T2   Tumor more than 2 cm but not more than 4 cm in greatest dimension
T3   Tumor more than 4 cm in greatest dimension
T4   Tumor invades adjacent structures (eg, cortical bone, soft tissues of neck, deep [extrinsic] muscle of tongue)

Hypopharynx

T1   Tumor limited to one subsite of hypopharynx
T2   Tumor invades more than one subsite of hypopharynx or adjacent site, without fixation of hemilarynx
T3   Tumor invades more than one subsite of hypopharynx or adjacent site, with fixation of hemilarynx
T4   Tumor invades adjacent structures (eg, cartilage, soft tissues of neck)

Nasopharynx

T1   Tumor limited to one subsite of nasopharynx
T2   Tumor invades more than one subsite of nasopharynx
T3   Tumor invades nasal cavity or oropharynx
T4   Tumor invades skull or cranial nerve

Maxillary Sinus

T1   Tumor limited to antral mucosa, with no erosion or destruction of bone
T2   Tumor with erosion or destruction of infrastructure, including hard palate or middle nasal meatus
T3   Tumor invades any of following: skin of cheek, posterior wall of maxillary sinus, floor or medial wall of orbit, anterior ethmoid sinus
T4   Tumor invades orbital contents or any of the following: cribriform plate, posterior ethmoid or sphenoid sinuses, nasopharynx, soft palate, pterygomaxillary or temporal fossae, base of skull

Supraglottis

T1   Tumor limited to one subsite of supraglottis, with normal vocal cord mobility
T2   Tumor invades more than one subsite of supraglottis or glottis, with normal vocal cord mobility
T3   Tumor limited to laynrx, with vocal cord fixation, or invades postcricoid area, medial wall of piriform sinus, or preepiglottic tissues
T4   Tumor invades thyroid cartilage or extends to other tissues beyond larynx (eg, oropharynx, soft tissue of neck)

Glottis

T1   Tumor limited to vocal cord (may involve anterior or posterior commissures), with normal mobility
T1a   Tumor limited to one vocal cord
T1b   Tumor involves both vocal cords
T2   Tumor extends to supraglottis or subglottis or with impaired vocal cord mobility
T3   Tumor limited to larynx with vocal cord fixation
T4   Tumor invades thyroid cartilage or extends to other tissues beyond larynx (eg, oropharynx, soft tissues of neck)

Subglottis

T1   Tumor limited to subglottis
T2   Tumor extends to vocal cord, with normal or impaired mobility
T3   Tumor limited to larynx, with vocal cord fixation
T4   Tumor invades through cricoid or thyroid cartilage, or extends to other tissues beyond larynx (eg, oropharynx, soft tissues of neck)

REGIONAL LYMPH NODE INVOLVEMENT
NX   Regional lymph nodes cannot be assessed
N0   No regional lymph node metastasis
N1   Metastasis in single ipsilateral lymph node, 3 cm or less in greatest dimension
N2   Metastasis in single ipsilateral lymph node, more than 3 cm but not more than 6 cm in greatest dimension; or in multiple ipsilateral lymph nodes, none more than 6 cm in greatest dimension; or in bilateral or contralateral lymph nodes, none more than 6 cm in greatest dimension
N2a   Metastasis in single ipsilateral lymph node, more than 3 cm but not more than 6 cm in greatest dimension
N2b   Metastasis in multiple ipsilateral lymph nodes, none more than 6 cm in greatest dimension
N2c   Metastasis in bilateral or contralateral lymph nodes, none more than 6 cm in greatest dimension
N3   Metastasis in lymph node, more than 6 cm in greatest dimension

DISTANT METASTASIS
MX   Presence of distant metastasis cannot be assessed
M0   No distant metastasis
M1   Distant metastasis

Table 17-3. STAGING OF HEAD AND NECK CANCER

Stage	Stage Grouping
0	Tis, N0, M0
I	T1, N0, M0
II	T2, N0, M0
III	T3, N0, M0
	T1, N1, M0
	T2, N1, M0
	T3, N1, M0
IV	T4, N0–1, M0
	Any T, N2–3, M0
	Any T, any N, M1

cavity because of the difficulty in obtaining adequate margins.

Pharynx

Cancers from one of area of the nasopharynx may involve another area. The nasopharynx is the area above the soft palate. The oropharynx, the area between the upper portion of the epiglottis and the nasopharynx, includes the tonsils, soft palate, base of the tongue, and posterior pharyngeal wall. The hypopharynx, from the lower part of the epiglottis to the cervical esophagus, includes the piriform sinus area, the postcricoid area, and the inferior wall of the posterior pharynx.

Cancers of the Nasopharynx
Squamous-cell carcinoma, lymphoepithelioma, lymphoma
Nasal or eustachian tube obstruction, epistaxis, bloody rhinorrhea, decreased hearing
May present as lymph node metastases along the spinal accessory lymph node chain
Elevated levels of anti-Epstein–Barr virus antibodies
Treated with radiation therapy (preceded by chemotherapy for childhood and adolescent lymphoepitheliomas)

Cancers of the Oropharynx
Squamous-cell carcinomas that originate in the tonsil
Sore throat, ear pain, mass in the neck
Treated with radiation therapy or surgery

Cancers of the Hypopharynx
Early spread to lymph nodes
Treated with surgery (laryngectomy to obtain a margin around the tumor and ipsilateral radical neck dissection) and postoperative radiation therapy

Larynx

The larynx is divided into the supraglottis (epiglottis, aryepiglottic fold, and false vocal cords), glottis (true vocal cords), and subglottis (the area below the true vocal cords). Symptoms depend on where in the larynx the cancer arises.

Supraglottic Cancers
Hoarseness, difficulty swallowing, aspiration
Early spread to regional lymph nodes
Treated with radical neck dissection and laryngectomy
Spread to submental or submandibular lymph nodes, which must be removed during lymph node dissection
Radiation therapy after surgery

Cancers of the Glottis
Early presentation with hoarseness

Diagnosis with indirect and, if normal, direct laryngoscopy
Small cancers (T1 or T2) treated with radiation therapy and cordectomy for small recurrences after radiation therapy
Large cancers (T3 or T4) treated with surgery

Subglottic cancers
Hoarseness or dyspnea
Metastasis more common than with glottic cancers
Treated with laryngectomy and resection of lymph nodes in tracheoesophageal grooves

Paranasal Sinuses

Sinus cancers are unusual, and they are difficult to diagnose and treat. The symptoms are nasal stuffiness, epistaxis, a bulging cheek, nose, or forehead, or proptosis. Cancers that originate in the paranasal sinuses include squamous cell carcinomas and minor salivary gland cancers, especially adenoid cystic carcinomas (cylindromas). Lymphomas may also arise in these areas.

Treatment depends on the stage of the disease. Small cancers are treated with radiation therapy alone or with surgery. Surgery for maxillary sinus cancers includes maxillectomy. When resection cannot be performed, high-dose radiation therapy can be administered.

Salivary Gland Tumors

The major salivary glands are the parotid, submandibular (submaxillary), and sublingual glands. Thousands of minor salivary glands are present throughout the oral cavity, pharynx, and paranasal sinuses. The larger the salivary gland, the more likely the tumor is benign. The smaller the gland, the more likely it is malignant.

Benign Tumors
Benign Mixed Tumor
Epithelial and mesenchymal components
Wide variety of patterns
May rarely de-differentiate into a malignant tumor
Treated with excision with a margin of normal tissue in all directions around the tumor

Benign Parotid Tumor
Most common site is superficial lobe
Resected with superficial (or lateral) parotid lobectomy to avoid endangering the facial nerve
Recurrence rates high after enucleation or tumor spillage, which may necessitate another resection that includes the facial nerve
Postoperative radiation therapy effective in preventing recurrences or treating tumors with inadequate margins

Warthin tumors (papillary cystadenoma lymphomatosum)
Unusual, occur in men
Composed of lymphoid tissue that contains germinal centers
Treated with enucleation if diagnosis is made preoperatively; follow-up of contralateral gland required
Treated with parotid lobectomy if diagnosis is not made preoperatively
Other Benign Tumors
Diffuse enlargement of salivary gland: Sjögren syndrome, viral diseases such as mumps, ductal obstruction by sialolith
Cysts of parotid glands

Malignant Tumors

Malignant tumors of the salivary glands are uncommon. The most frequent site is the parotid gland.

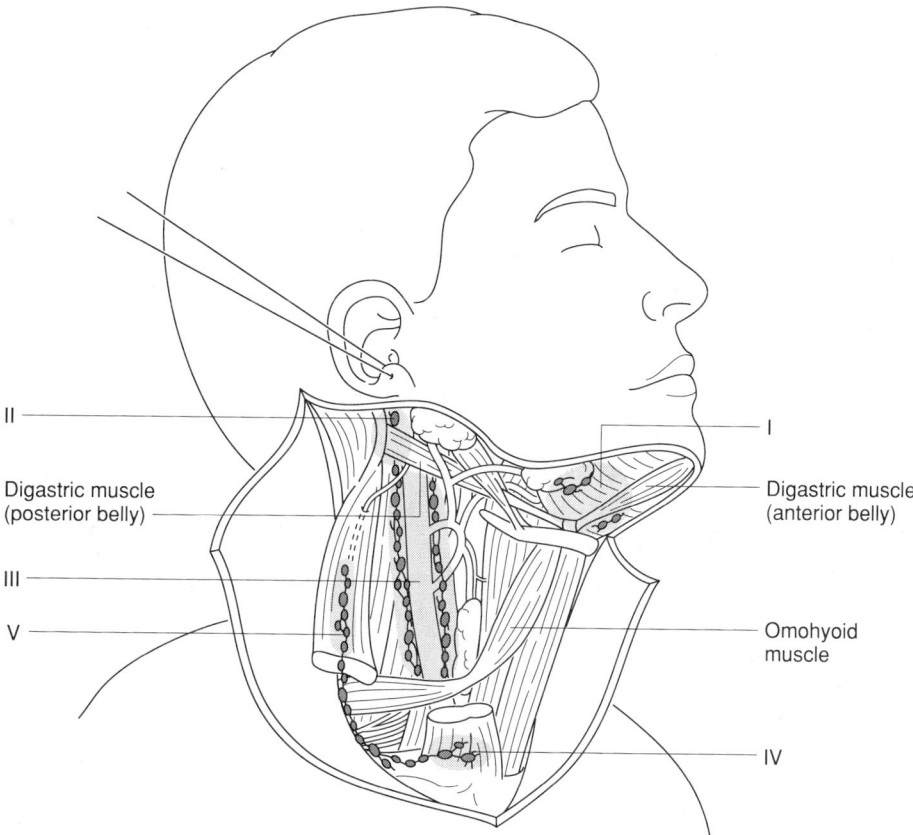

Figure 17-1. Lymphatic drainage of the head and neck. Level I includes the submental and submandibular lymph nodes. Level II includes the upper jugular chain (jugulodigastric) lymph nodes. Level III includes the middle jugular chain lymph nodes (those between the digastric muscle superiorly and the omohyoid muscle inferiorly). Level IV includes the lower jugular chain lymph nodes (below the omohyoid muscle). Level V includes the posterior triangle, or spinal accessory chain, lymph nodes.

Labels in figure: II — Digastric muscle (posterior belly) — III — V — I — Digastric muscle (anterior belly) — Omohyoid muscle — IV

Mucoepidermoid Cancer
   Contains both epidermoid cells and mucus-containing cells
   Treated with wide excision (low-grade tumors) or radical neck dissection (high-grade tumors)

Adenoid Cystic Carcinoma (Cylindroma)
   Slow-growing, spreads along nerve sheaths
   Extent of tumor difficult to determine; apparently wide excision may have positive margins
   Local disease treated with high-dose radiation therapy, but tumor usually spreads late in its course

Acinic Cell Carcinoma
   Low grade, slow spread
   Treated with local excision

Adenocarcinomas, Malignant Mixed Tumors
   Unusual
   Treated with wide excision; some surgeons advocate prophylactic radical neck dissection

Epidermoid Cancers
   Extremely rare, aggressive
   Treated with prophylactic radical neck dissection

Lymphomas and Sarcomas
   Treated as similar tumors elsewhere in the body

Other Tumors of the Head and Neck

Metastatic Tumor

Patients may present with metastatic tumor in a cervical lymph node but with no known primary site of tumor. These cancers are usually squamous cell epitheliomas. The primary site may be determined from the nodal metastasis (Fig. 17-1 and Table 17-4). If the evaluation for the primary site is unrevealing, radical neck dissection or radiation therapy may be used to treat the neck metastasis. The primary site becomes evident only about 25% of the time.

Soft-Tissue Sarcomas

Because of the proximity of vital structures, it is often difficult, if not impossible, to obtain a normal tissue plane in all directions around the tumor in the resection of tumors of the head and neck. Thus, many patients with soft-tissue sarcomas may undergo a resection with minimal or positive margins and should undergo postoperative ra-

Table 17-4. MOST COMMON PRIMARY SITES IN PATIENTS PRESENTING WITH NECK MASSES

Nodal Level	Primary Site
I	Anterior tongue Floor of mouth Anterior alveolar ridge
II	Oropharynx Nasophaynx
III	Hypopharynx Larynx Lateral tongue
IV	Usually subclavicular
V	Scalp Nasopharynx Parotid gland

diation therapy or brachytherapy or receive interstitial implants.

Melanoma

Melanomas are treated the same way as melanomas elsewhere in the body, except for melanomas that arise in the mucosa. Mucosal melanomas are rare, have a poor prognosis, and often present at an advanced stage. Adequate margins around a primary tumor may not be sufficient to prevent regional lymph node spread or systemic metastases. No adjuvant therapy has proved beneficial.

Hodgkin Disease

Patients with cervical masses, especially posterior masses, and no obvious malignant epithelial tumor are considered to have lymphoma. If the physical findings are unremarkable, fine-needle aspiration biopsy, open biopsy, or both are performed. Non-Hodgkin lymphoma arises in cervical lymph nodes less commonly than does Hodgkin disease.

Chromaffin Tumors

Tumors that arise from the chromaffin tissues (chemodectoma, paraganglioma) are rare. They usually originate in the carotid body or along the vagus nerve. Ninety percent are benign, but 10% are malignant and can spread hematogenously or to regional lymph nodes.

Vagal Paragangliomas

Vagal paragangliomas necessitate resection of the vagus nerve, resulting in paralysis of the recurrent laryngeal nerve. Histologic examination does not differentiate benign from malignant processes, and only the clinical behavior of the tumor can be used to determine if the tumor is malignant. The presence of regional lymph node metastases denotes a malignant tumor. No adjuvant therapy is known to be beneficial.

SURGICAL CONSIDERATIONS

Parotid Gland

Operations on the parotid gland are performed without paralyzing the patient. The facial nerve is preserved unless involved by tumor. Proximity to the nerve can be demonstrated during dissection by stimulating the main trunk or its branches.

The usual incision is preauricular, carried in front of the external auditory canal then curved anteriorly below the angle of the mandible. The digastric muscle is exposed, and the main trunk of the facial nerve is identified between the digastric muscle and the external auditory canal. The gland is retracted superiorly and anteriorly, and the nerve is traced distally. All branches of the nerve are identified and traced from proximal to distal until the superficial lobe is removed. Most malignant tumors in the deep lobe of the parotid gland require facial nerve resection followed by nerve grafting.

Submandibular Gland

Resection is usually performed through a submandibular incision carried through the subcutaneous tissue and platysma muscle. The ramus mandibularis branch of the seventh cranial nerve is identified. The lingual nerve, which is deep to the submandibular gland, is identified before division of the deep blood supply to the gland. The chorda tympani nerve, which arises from the lingual nerve, is divided during resection of the submandibular gland. Complications of removal of the submandibular gland include damage to the nerves resulting in loss of motor function or loss of taste.

Radical Neck Dissection

The incisions used for radical neck dissection (Fig. 17-2) depend on the experience of the surgeon, the site of the tumor, and whether a previous incision was made in the neck. If open biopsy was performed, the biopsy site is excised. Radical neck dissection removes the areolar tissue between the mandible superiorly, clavicle inferiorly, anterior border of the trapezius muscle posteriorly, midline in the upper neck, and strap muscles in the lower neck. Complications of radical neck dissection are presented in Table 17-5.

A classic radical neck dissection includes removal of the external and internal jugular veins, sternocleidomastoid and omohyoid muscles, spinal accessory nerve, and sensory nerves from C-2 through C-5 (Fig. 17-3). A modified radical neck dissection preserves the internal jugular vein, spinal accessory nerve, sternocleidomastoid muscle, and the submental and submandibular areas in tumors of the hypopharynx and larynx; dissects only certain areas of the neck; or enlarges the resection by removing the vagus nerve, hypoglossal nerve, carotid artery, or other structures that would be preserved.

Oral Cavity

A 1- to 2-cm margin is maintained around the tumor. This may necessitate resection of a segment of the mandible when bone is invaded by tumor.

A

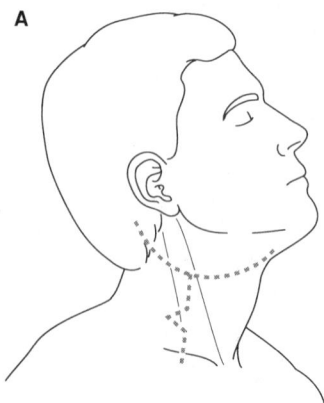

B

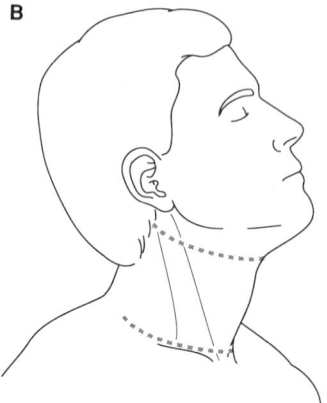

Figure 17-2. Frequently used incisions for radical neck dissection.

Table 17-5. COMPLICATIONS OF RADICAL NECK DISSECTION

Complication	Cause
Seroma	Drainage catheters removed too soon
Winged scapula and shoulder drop due to loss of support of the trapezius muscle	Resection of spinal accessory nerve
Involved side of neck flatter than other	Removal of sternocleidomastoid muscle
Division of hypoglossal nerve	Ligation of internal jugular vein at base of skull
Stroke	Resection of carotid artery

Larynx

Total laryngectomy is performed for advanced cancers of the larynx and for those that recur after irradiation. It can be performed in conjunction with a radical neck dissection. The lobe of the thyroid on the same side of the larynx as the tumor usually is removed. The parathyroid glands should not be resected during laryngectomy. Complications are presented in Table 17-6.

Pharynx

Tumors in the hypopharynx usually require laryngectomy to obtain an adequate margin. The resulting pharyngeal defect is often too large to close with local tissue, and rotation of outside tissue or use of free tissue transfer may be necessary. Pharyngeal tumors often involve the parapharyngeal and retropharyngeal lymph nodes. To remove potentially involved lymph nodes, pharyngectomy includes removal of all tissue to the prevertebral fascia.

Reconstruction

Pectoralis Major Musculocutaneous Flap
For defects in the pharynx, floor of mouth, and skin
Skin from the anterior chest wall, subcutaneous tissue, and pectoralis major muscle with underlying blood supply.

Trapezius Musculocutaneous Flap
For defects of the mandible, maxilla, and temporal bone
Can be rotated to higher areas than the pectoralis major flap cannot be used unless the transverse cervical artery and vein are preserved during radical neck dissection
Wing of the scapula can be used to provide a bone graft

Free Flaps
For skin defects, mucosal defects, or combined defects
Donor site depends on where graft is to be placed (Table 17-7)
Complications related to vascular anastomoses and venous congestion

Rehabilitation

Patients who have undergone resections of the head and neck require speech therapy; training to relearn swallowing; physical therapy; prosthodontic care for fitting a maxillary prosthesis, facial prosthesis, or dental restoration; plastic surgery; oral and neurosurgery; and occupational therapy.

ADJUVANT TREATMENT

Radiation Therapy
Purpose: To shrink tumors with microscopically involved margins or margins close to the tumor and to prevent metastatic cancer in the contralateral neck
Complications: Dry mouth, dysphagia, loss of taste, stricture, pharyngeal infection
Results: Seems to reduce local recurrence rates, but

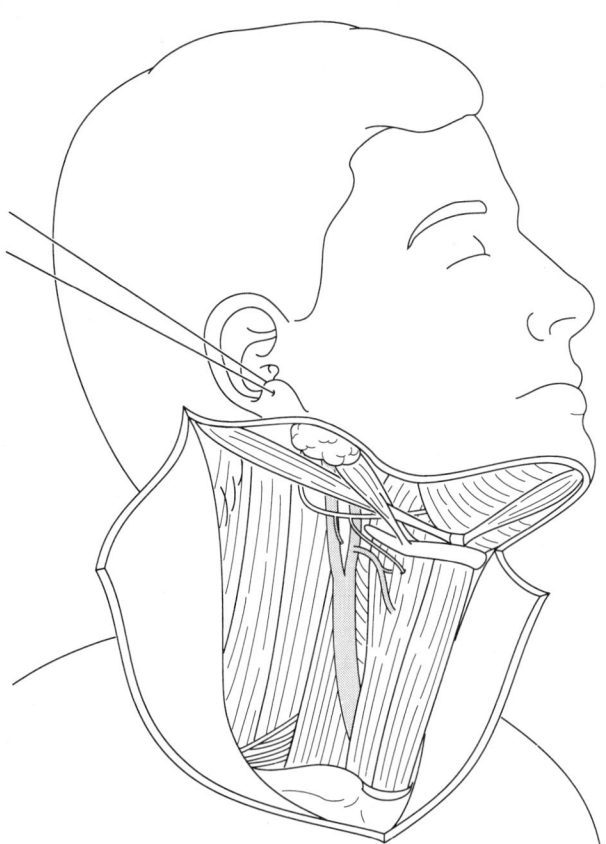

Figure 17-3. Schematic representation of operative field after radical neck dissection.

Table 17-6. COMPLICATIONS OF LARYNGECTOMY

Complication	Treatment
Breakdown of pharyngeal closure leading to wound infection and pharyngocutaneous fistula	Fistula: conservative care, sometimes surgical closure Neck infection: opening neck to facilitate drainage, frequent wound care
Hypoparathyroidism	Frequent measurement of serum calcium level for first 2–3 days after surgery
Pharyngeal stricture	Dilation with flexible dilators: sometimes revision of the closure
Tracheostomal stenosis	Enlargement of lumen with progressively larger tracheostomy tubes; largest tube left in place for months; if restenosis occurs, tracheostomal revision

Table 17-7. DONOR SITES OF FREE FLAPS

Defect	Flap
Circumferential pharyngeal defect	Free jejunal graft to replace section of pharynx resected
Skin or other soft-tissue defect	Radial forearm, latissimus dorsi muscle, circumflex iliac artery, or transverse rectus abdominis muscle (with epigastric vessels sutured to cervical vessels)

there has been no improvement in overall survival rate with surgery and radiation compared with surgery alone

Chemotherapy
Purpose: To shrink the tumor to enable radiation therapy or surgery to eradicate remaining tumor cells
Results: Randomized, prospective trials have not demonstrated better results with chemotherapy than with local therapy alone

Immunotherapy
Purpose: To produce a profound host response to the tumor, enabling the host to develop an immunity to the tumor cells
Results: Randomized, prospective trials have not demonstrated improvement in disease-free or overall survival rates

Intra-arterial Chemotherapy
Purpose: To shrink large, unresectable tumors by delivering high doses of chemotherapeutic agents directly to the tumor
Results: Randomized, prospective trials have not evaluated this expensive, time-consuming approach

Brachytherapy
Purpose: To deliver, through catheters left in the tumor bed, a high dose of radiation to the area in patients at high risk for local recurrence
Results: Has not been evaluated in randomized, prospective trials but appears promising because it can control local disease

METASTATIC DISEASE

Metastasis to the lung is frequent. When the mass is solitary, it may be difficult to determine if it is metastatic disease or primary lung cancer. The evaluation is identical to that of primary lung cancer. Chemotherapy is administered to patients with metastatic disease outside the confines of surgery or irradiation,. The response rates to single agents are low, and response durations are short. Combination chemotherapy has higher response rates, but response durations also are short.

SUGGESTED READING

Attie JN, Sciubba JJ. Tumors of major and minor salivary glands: clinical and pathologic features. Curr Probl Surg 1981;18:68.

Blot WJ, McLaughlin JK, Winn DM, et al. Smoking and drinking in relation to oral and pharyngeal cancer. Cancer Res 1988;48:3282.

Brachman DG. Molecular biology of head and neck cancer. Semin Oncol 1994;21:320.

Candela FC, Shah J, Jaques DP, Shah JP. Patterns of cervical node metastases from squamous carcinoma of the larynx. Arch Otolaryngol Head Neck Surg 1990;116:432.

Coleman JJ. Reconstruction of the pharynx after resection for cancer: a comparison of methods. Ann Surg 1989;209:554.

DeSanto LW, Beahrs OH. Modified and complete neck dissection in the treatment of squamous cell carcinoma of the head and neck. Surg Gynecol Obstet 1988;167:259.

Jacobs CD, Goffinet DR, Fee WE. Head and neck squamous cancers. Curr Probl Cancer 1990;14:1.

Ketcham AS, VanBuren JM. Tumors of the paranasal sinuses: a therapeutic challenge. Am J Surg 1985;150:406.

Spiro JD, Soo KC, Spiro RH. Squamous carcinoma of the nasal cavity and paranasal sinuses. Am J Surg 1989;158:328.

ESOPHAGUS

ESSENTIALS OF SURGERY: SCIENTIFIC PRINCIPLES AND PRACTICE,
edited by Lazar J. Greenfield, Michael W. Mulholland, Keith T. Oldham, Gerald B. Zelenock,
and Keith D. Lillemoe. Lippincott–Raven Publishers, Philadelphia, © 1997.

CHAPTER 18

ESOPHAGEAL ANATOMY AND PHYSIOLOGY AND GASTROESOPHAGEAL REFLUX

PETER F. CROOKES AND TOM R. DEMEESTER

ANATOMY

The esophagus is divided into cervical, thoracic, and abdominal portions. The *cervical esophagus* begins below the cricopharyngeus muscle at the level of C6 and extends to the lower border of T1, curving slightly to the left in its descent. The cervical esophagus abuts the trachea and posterior larynx.

The upper part of the *thoracic esophagus* is closely related to the posterior wall of the trachea. Above the level of the tracheal bifurcation, the esophagus is to the right of the descending aorta. At the tracheal bifurcation, it is behind the bifurcation and left main bronchus. Below the bifurcation the esophagus courses anteriorly and to the left to pass through the diaphragmatic hiatus.

The *abdominal esophagus* begins as the esophagus enters the abdomen through the diaphragmatic hiatus (Fig. 18-1, Fig. 18-2) and extends to the gastroesophageal (GE) junction and lower esophageal sphincter (LES).

Blood Vessels

The *inferior thyroid artery* provides the main blood supply to the cervical portion of the esophagus. The thoracic portion of the esophagus receives its blood supply from two to three *bronchial arteries* and *branches from the aorta*. The abdominal esophagus receives its blood supply from branches of the *left gastric artery* and *inferior phrenic arteries* (Fig. 18-3). Once the vessels enter the muscular wall of the esophagus, branching occurs at right angles to provide a longitudinal vascular plexus. This anatomic arrangement allows mobilization of the esophagus from the stomach to the aortic arch without ischemic injury.

A venous plexus in the submucosa collects capillary blood and delivers it to a periesophageal venous plexus. From this plexus, esophageal veins empty into the *inferior thyroid vein* proximally; into the *bronchial, azygos,* or *hemiazygos veins* in the thorax; and into the *left gastric vein* in the abdomen (Fig. 18-4).

Lymphatic Vessels

The lymphatic vessels of the esophagus form a submucosal network that drains into regional lymph nodes in the periesophageal connective tissue (Fig. 18-5). There is little barrier to longitudinal spread of cancer in the esophagus.

Nerves

The innervation of the cricopharyngeal sphincter and cervical portion of the esophagus is from the right and left recurrent laryngeal nerves, which originate from the vagus nerve. Vocal cord dysfunction, cricopharyngeal sphincter dysfunction, and motility problems of the cervical esophagus occur with surgical injury to these nerves. Branches from the left recurrent laryngeal nerve and from both vagus nerves innervate the upper thoracic esophagus. The esophageal plexus on the anterior and posterior walls of the esophagus innervates the lower esophagus. The esophageal plexus receives fibers from the thoracic sympathetic chain.

Efferent preganglionic sympathetic fibers that supply the esophagus originate from the fourth to sixth spinal cord segments and terminate in the cervical and thoracic sympathetic ganglions. Fibers from the superior cervical ganglion arrive at the pharyngeal plexus by way of vagal nerves. The postganglionic fibers reach the esophagus by branches from the cervical and thoracic sympathetic chain. The distal esophageal segments receive direct sympathetic fibers from the celiac ganglion.

Afferent visceral sensory pain fibers from the esophagus terminate without synapsing in the first four segments of the thoracic spinal cord, following both sympathetic and vagal pathways. Pain fibers from the heart travel these same pathways, explaining the similarity of symptoms in many esophageal and cardiac diseases.

INVESTIGATION OF STRUCTURAL ABNORMALITIES

Endoscopy

Endoscopy is the first diagnostic procedure performed in patients with symptoms of esophageal disease—*except when the chief symptom is dysphagia,* in which a barium swallow examination is performed first. Endoscopy allows visualization of a wide range of pathologic processes and can be used for therapeutic measures.

Esophageal landmarks are located in relation to the incisor teeth (Fig. 18-6). In adults, the tracheal bifurcation and indentation of the aortic arch are 24 to 26 cm from the incisor teeth. This landmark is helpful in localizing intraluminal lesions. The GE junction is best identified during insertion of the endoscope, before the scope is advanced into the stomach.

A *hiatal hernia* is present when the GE junction is >2 cm above the crura. *Barrett esophagus* is suggested when the squamocolumnar junction is more than 2 cm above the GE junction, but may be diagnosed if any specialized

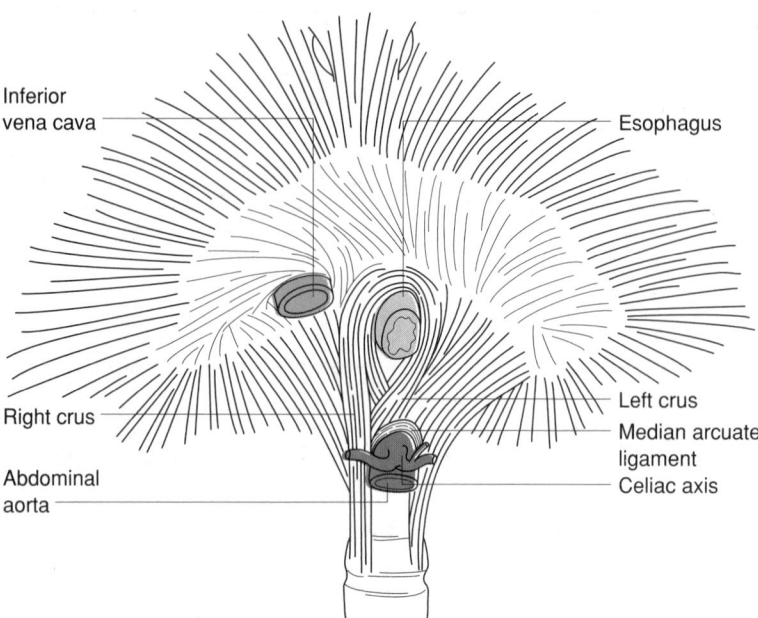

Inferior
vena cava

Esophagus

Right crus

Left crus

Median arcuate
ligament

Abdominal
aorta

Celiac axis

Figure 18-1. Diaphragm and esophageal hiatus seen from below.

epithelium (eg, intestinal type) is identified above the GE junction, regardless of the measured length of the columnar segment. *Esophagitis* is recognized by the presence of redness, linear erosions, or ulceration of the mucosa.

Radiography

Barium upper gastrointestinal radiographic studies complement endoscopy in providing both structural and functional information, especially when the entire examination is recorded on videotape. Three areas of esophageal narrowing are seen with both barium esophagography and endoscopy:

1. The cricopharyngeus muscle
2. The middle third of the esophagus at the level of the left main bronchus and aortic arch
3. The diaphragmatic hiatus

At a barium swallow examination, the pharyngoesophageal region is evaluated with the patient upright. Esophageal peristalsis is studied with the patient in the horizontal–prone–oblique position. Motility disorders characterized by disorganized activity with simultaneous contractions give rise to tertiary waves, often with a seg-

mented appearance to the barium column. This appearance is sometimes described as rosary beading or a corkscrew appearance. A hiatal hernia may be reducible at barium examination if the patient is upright.

Computed Tomography

Computed tomography (CT) is used to delineate the relation between esophageal lesions and adjacent structures, especially the trachea, left main bronchus, and aorta. The esophagus looks like a flattened hollow structure with a thin wall. A circular cross-sectional appearance with a fluid level is evidence of distal obstruction.

PHYSIOLOGY
Pharyngoesophageal Segment

When food is ready for swallowing, the tongue moves the bolus into the posterior oropharynx and forces it into the hypopharynx (Fig. 18-7A–D). As contact between the tongue and the hard palate moves posteriorly, the soft palate is elevated (Fig. 18-7C–H), closing the passage between the oro-and nasopharynx. This partitioning prevents

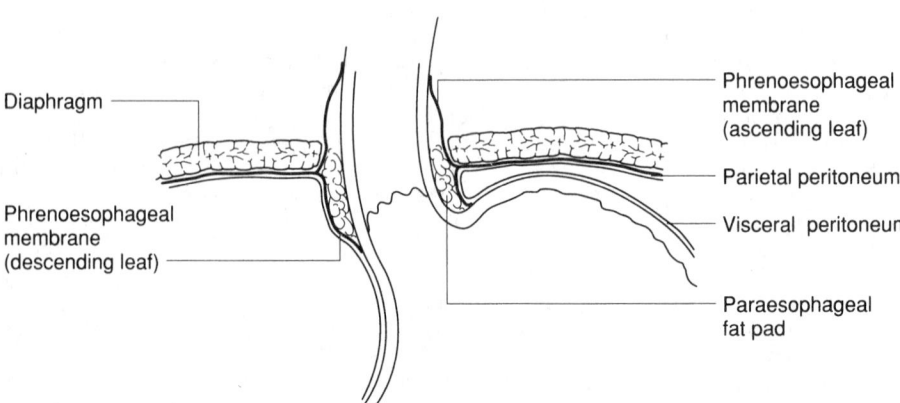

Diaphragm

Phrenoesophageal
membrane
(ascending leaf)

Parietal peritoneum

Visceral peritoneum

Phrenoesophageal
membrane
(descending leaf)

Paraesophageal
fat pad

Figure 18-2. Attachments of the phrenoesophageal membrane.

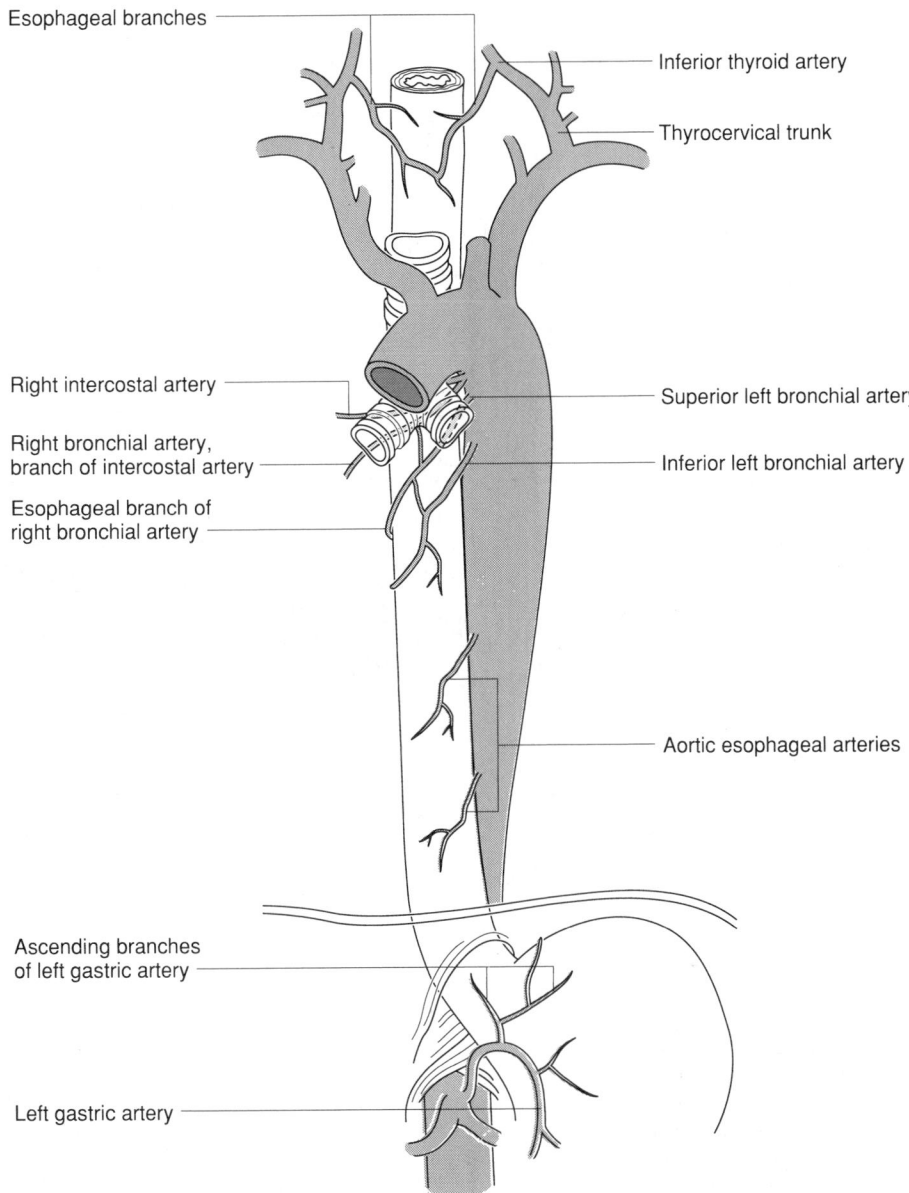

Figure 18-3. Arterial blood supply of the esophagus.

pressure generated in the oropharynx from being dissipated through the nose. During swallowing the hyoid bone moves upward and anteriorly, elevating the larynx and opening the retrolaryngeal space, bringing the epiglottis under the tongue (Fig. 18-7I–P). The backward tilt of the epiglottis covers the opening of the larynx to prevent aspiration.

Esophageal Body

The pressure gradient across the upper esophageal sphincter (UES) is accentuated by the subatmospheric environment of the cervical esophagus. Negative intraesophageal pressure increases until the food bolus reaches the midesophagus. Thereafter, bolus transport by peristalsis overcomes a pressure gradient and propels the bolus into the positive-pressure environment of the stomach.

To be effective, peristaltic contractions must be of sufficient amplitude to generate occlusion contraction and sufficiently organized for the wave of contraction to propel a food bolus aborally. Peristaltic defects fall into one of two categories:

1. Defects in organization of peristaltic waves are a neural phenomenon recognized by the presence of simultaneous waves on motility studies. They are typical of primary motility disorders, such as diffuse esophageal spasm.
2. Reduction of the power (amplitude) of peristalsis usually is due to muscle damage caused by severe reflux or replacement with fibrous tissue, as in scleroderma and other connective tissue diseases or severe reflux.

Lower Esophageal Sphincter

The LES provides a pressure barrier between esophagus and stomach. The sphincter normally remains closed to prevent reflux of gastric contents into the esophagus. The LES relaxes to allow food to enter or to allow air to exit during belching. The LES relaxes soon after initiation of a

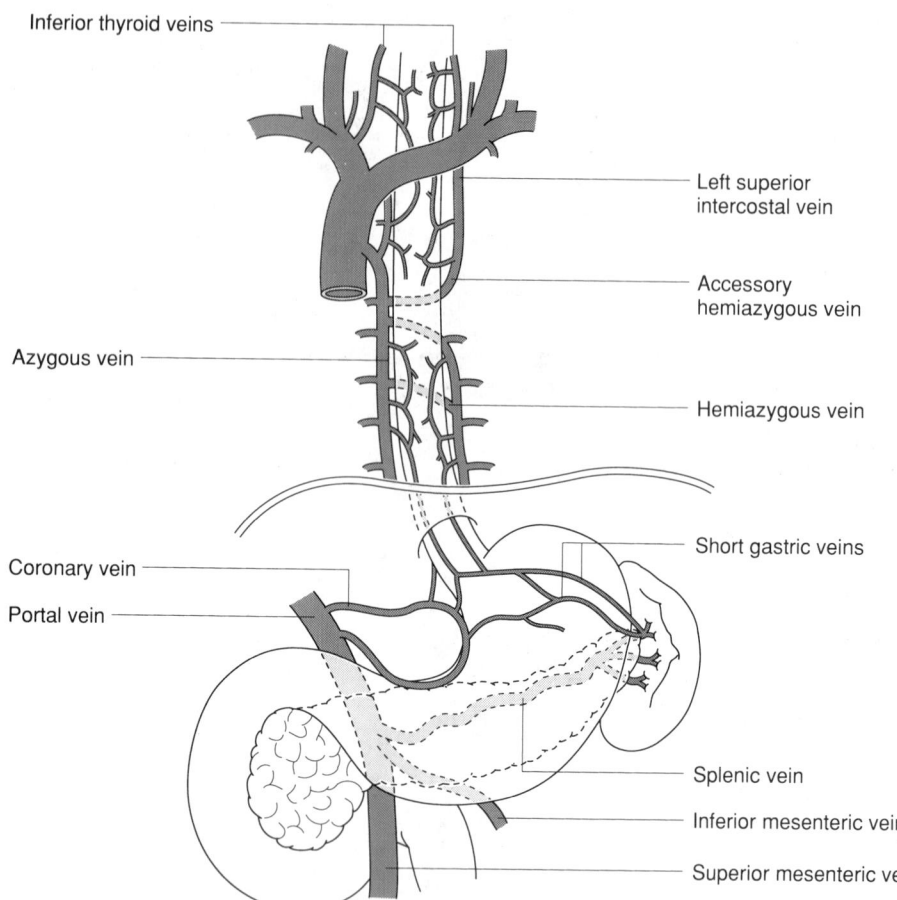

Figure 18-4. Venous drainage of the esophagus.

swallow. Relaxation of the LES is mediated by inhibitory neurons.

The Antireflux Barrier

Protection against reflux of gastric juice depends on the integrated effect of the LES, the esophageal body, and the gastric reservoir (Fig. 18-8). The competence of the LES is related to resting pressure, abdominal length of the LES, and overall length of the LES. A mechanically defective sphincter is not always associated with increased esophageal acid exposure because it may be compensated by the clearance function of the esophageal body. Abnormalities in the esophageal body and the stomach contribute to the development and progression of gastroesophageal reflux disease (GERD).

The role of the esophageal body in limiting acid reflux is related to its ability to clear the esophagus of acid. Clearance has two components: volume clearance, which requires peristalsis, and chemical clearance, which requires saliva. After a reflux episode, most of the acid is cleared by a peristaltic wave. Small residual amounts of acid on the mucosal surface are neutralized by saliva. Defective contractility and defective saliva production increase esophageal acid exposure. Clearance is aided by gravity and is impaired when a person is recumbent.

Abnormalities of the gastric reservoir that predispose to GE reflux include gastric dilatation, increased intragastric pressure, persistent gastric reservoir, and increased gastric acid secretion. The effect of gastric dilatation is to shorten the overall length of the LES, resulting in a decrease in

sphincter resistance to reflux. It most commonly results from aerophagia, which may itself be due to an unconscious increase in swallowing in an effort to improve esophageal clearance. Each swallow results in the propulsion of 1 to 2 cc of air into the stomach. This accounts for bloating. Increased intragastric pressure occurs because of loss of active relaxation as the stomach fills. A persistent gastric reservoir results from delay in gastric emptying. In a patient with a normal esophageal body and LES, the cause of excessive GE reflux is likely to be an abnormality in gastric function.

INVESTIGATION OF FUNCTIONAL ABNORMALITIES

Assessment of the contractility of the esophageal body and sphincters and measurement of esophageal acid exposure are the basis for therapy for most benign esophageal diseases.

Stationary Esophageal Manometry

A catheter containing pressure sensors is inserted into the esophagus and used to measure pressure in the esophageal body and sphincters at rest and in response to swallowing. It is indicated in the following situations:

- Nonobstructive dysphagia
- Noncardiac chest pain
- GERD

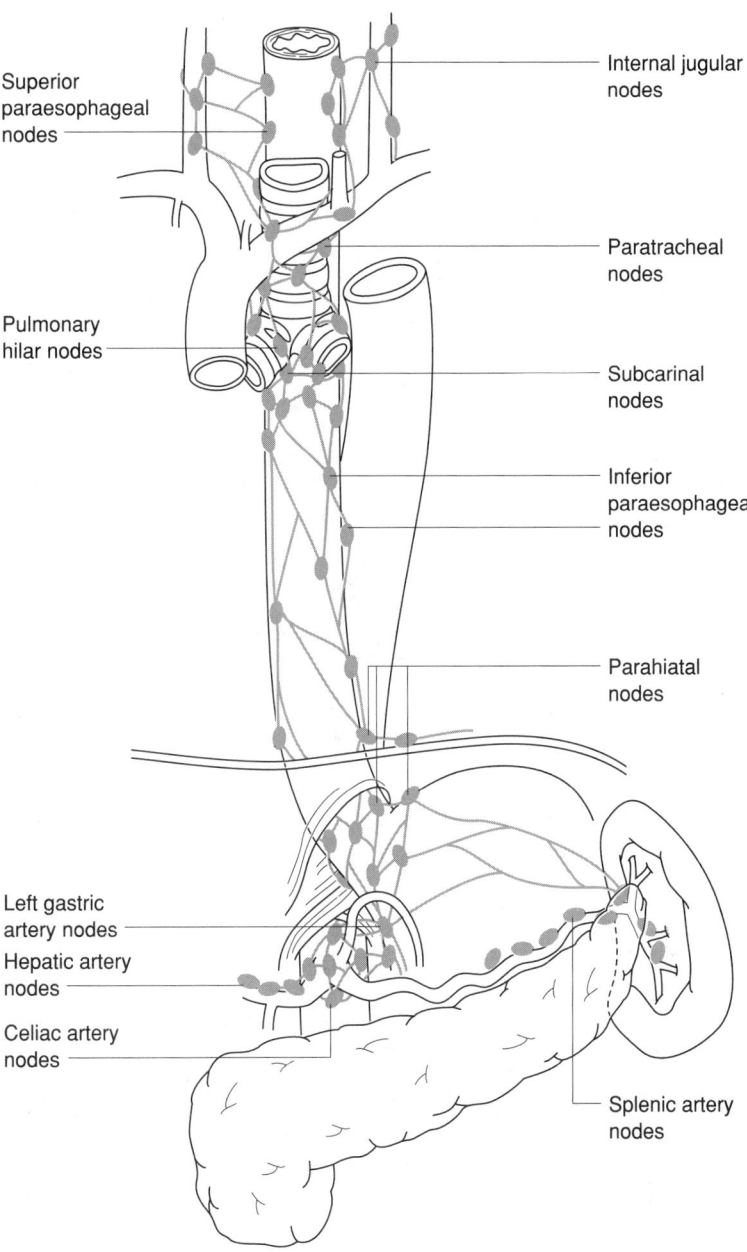

Figure 18-5. Lymphatic drainage of the esophagus.

- Placement of a pH electrode for 24-hour pH monitoring
- Postoperative manometry to assess success of an operation

A manometric study has the following four components:

1. Assessment of the LES (Fig. 18-9)
   - Resting pressure
   - Overall length of the sphincter
   - Abdominal length of the sphincter
2. Measurement of LES relaxation
3. Esophageal body manometry
4. Assessment of the UES

Measurement of Esophageal Acid Exposure: 24-hour pH Monitoring

Indications

Twenty-four-hour esophageal pH monitoring is measurement of esophageal acid exposure. It is the test used to confirm the diagnosis of GERD. It is indicated in any patient with symptoms suggestive of GERD, unless the symptoms are permanently abolished with a 12-week course of acid suppression therapy. The need for continued acid suppression is an indication for the pH monitoring. Monitoring is begun after the LES is located with manometry. An abnormal test is not proof of the presence of GERD. It is an indication for a search for the cause of excessive acid exposure.

Interpretation

Reflux episodes are defined as periods when esophageal pH is less than 4. Normal (physiologic) reflux occurs in the form of short, rapidly cleared postprandial episodes. Abnormal esophageal acid exposure is that which exceeds the 95th percentile for healthy people.

A few reflux episodes of long duration are more injurious than many brief episodes, even though the total acid exposure time may be similar. A scoring system integrates several features of the pH record into a single measurement of esophageal acid exposure (Table 18-1). Esophageal acid

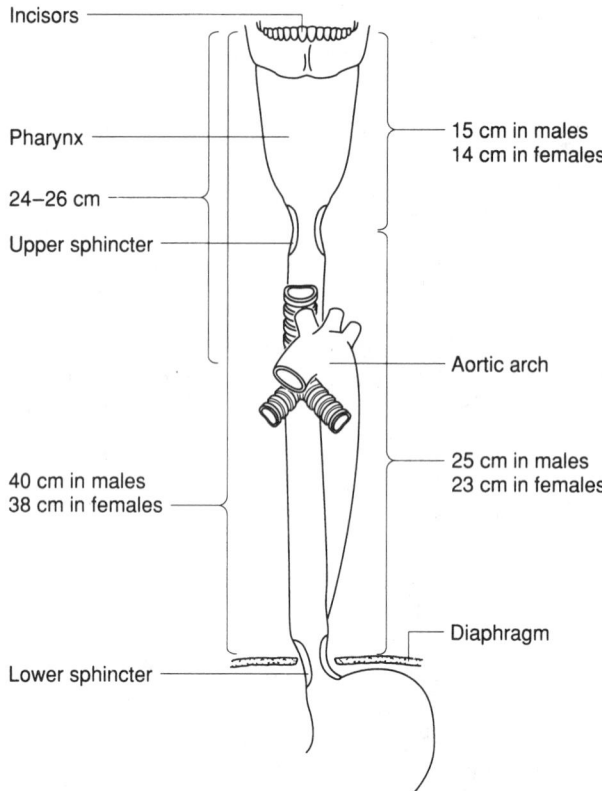

Incisors

Pharynx

24–26 cm

Upper sphincter

15 cm in males
14 cm in females

Aortic arch

25 cm in males
23 cm in females

40 cm in males
38 cm in females

Diaphragm

Lower sphincter

Figure 18-6. Important clinical endoscopic measurements of the esophagus in adults.

exposure quantifies the time the esophageal mucosa is exposed to gastric acid, gives a measurement of the ability of the esophagus to clear refluxed acid, and correlates esophageal acid exposure with symptoms.

Besides measurement of acid exposure, pH monitoring is used to detect excessive alkali in the esophagus (pH > 7). This is important because excess alkali may indicate that the refluxing gastric juice is mixed with duodenal content.

Other Tests for the Investigation of Esophageal Disease

- Dual esophageal pH monitoring
- Provocative testing
    Standard acid reflux test (SART)
    Bernstein test
    Edrophonium test
- Ambulatory 24-hour esophageal manometry
- Esophageal bile probe

Tests of Gastric Function

The function of the esophageal body and LES is affected by abnormalities in the stomach.

- Gastric emptying studies
- Ambulatory 24-hour gastric pH monitoring
- Gastric acid analysis
- Gastric bile probe
- Antroduodenal motility studies
- Cholescintigraphy

FUNCTIONAL DISORDERS OF THE ESOPHAGEAL BODY AND SPHINCTERS

Primary motor disorder implies the cause of the muscular defect is not known. *Secondary motor disorders* are the result of systemic diseases that affect the esophagus. The most common secondary motor disorder is hypoperistalsis associated with GERD, but the term usually refers to a systemic connective tissue or neuromuscular disease, such as scleroderma or polymyositis.

The five categories of primary motor disorders are achalasia, diffuse esophageal spasm, nutcracker esophagus, hypertensive LES, and nonspecific motor disorder, which is abnormal motor function that does not fall into one of the other categories.

Pharyngoesophageal Disorders

Disorders of the pharyngoesophageal phase of swallowing result from a discoordination of the neuromuscular events involved in chewing, initiation of swallowing, and propulsion of the material from the oropharynx to the cervical esophagus. The most common causes of pharyngoesophageal dysphagia are neuromuscular diseases, such as myasthenia gravis and Parkinson disease, and muscular diseases, such as myotonic dystrophy and polymyositis. Other important causes are structural lesions, including tumors, Zenker diverticula, and scarring of the tongue or pharynx from caustic injury, a surgical procedure, or radiation therapy.

Pathophysiology

All the aforementioned diseases disrupt one or more of the components of the pharyngeal mechanism (Fig. 18-10). In some patients with pharyngeal swallowing disorders, the UES relaxes at manometry, but there is radiographic evidence of diminished opening and increased pressure in the bolus. This intrabolus pressure, recognized as a small wave just before the pharyngeal wave, appears to reflect compliance of the pharyngoesophageal segment. It is elevated in the presence of muscle disease, indicating reduced compliance.

Investigation

An interview elicits a history of difficulty transferring food from the mouth to the pharynx. In neuromuscular diseases, dysphagia is often worse for liquids than for solids. Choking, repetitive pneumonia, nasal regurgitation, and hoarseness are prominent features. Examination in neuromuscular disorders may reveal a characteristic pattern of signs of the underlying disease. It is worthwhile watching the patient swallow during the consultation. Videoradiography, esophagoscopy, manometry with specially designed catheters, and 24-hour esophageal pH monitoring are used to identify the cause of pharyngoesophageal dysfunction.

Treatment

Medical treatment is drug treatment of the neurologic disease and work with a speech pathologist to improve swallowing.

Surgical treatment is cricomyotomy. The surgical options for Zenker diverticulum are excision or suspension. Suspension removes the risk of contamination of the operative site, the risk of breakdown of the closure site with fistula formation, and the risk of narrowing of the esophagus. With excision or suspension, recurrence is likely if cricomyotomy is not performed. It may be difficult to iden-

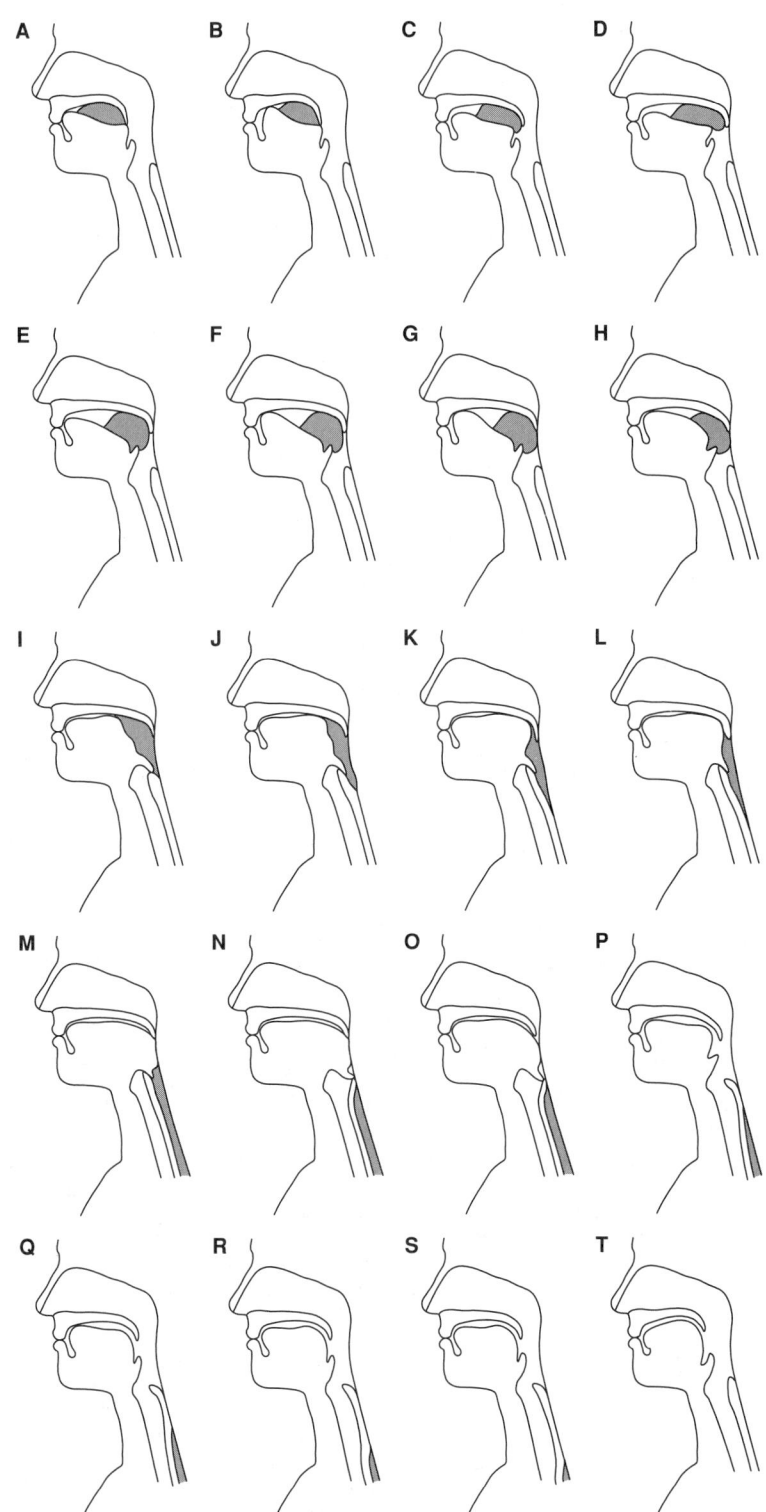

Figure 18-7. Sequence of events during the pharyngeal phase of swallowing, showing the action of the tongue coordinated with the movement of soft palate, larynx and epiglottis during a swallow. (Davenport HR. Physiology of the digestive tract, ed 5. Chicago, Yearbook, 1982:37)

tify the cricopharyngeus muscle if a diverticulum is not present. When local anesthesia is used, the patient is asked to swallow. This usually shows an area of persistent narrowing at the pharyngoesophageal junction. The myotomy is started in the easily identifiable cervical esophageal wall and extended cephalad 1 cm into the posterior pharyngeal muscle above the pharyngoesophageal junction.

In patients who do not benefit from reduction of outflow resistance and swallowing therapy, the only option is tube feeding through a percutaneous endoscopic gastrostomy.

Primary Motor Disorders of the Esophageal Body

Achalasia

Achalasia is characterized by failure of esophageal body peristalsis and incomplete relaxation of the LES. The causes appear to be neuronal degeneration in the myenteric plexus of the esophageal wall, which causes aperistalsis, and loss of activity of inhibitory neurons in the LES, which leads to incomplete sphincter relaxation.

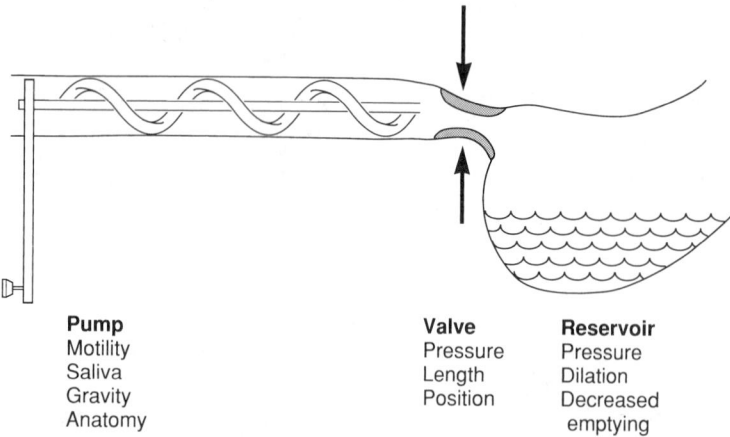

Pump	Valve	Reservoir
Motility	Pressure	Pressure
Saliva	Length	Dilation
Gravity	Position	Decreased
Anatomy		emptying
		Secretion

Figure 18-8. Mechanical model of the antireflux mechanism showing the esophageal body acting as a pump, the lower esophageal sphincter as a valve, and the stomach as a reservoir. (After DeMeester TR, Attwood SE. Gastroesophageal reflux disease, hiatus hernia, achalasia of the esophagus in spontaneous rupture. In: Schwartz SI, Ellis H. eds. Maingot's abdominal operations, vol 1, ed 9. Norwalk, CT, Appleton-Century-Crofts, 1989:514)

Diagnosis. The *symptoms and signs* of achalasia are:

- Dysphagia
- Regurgitation (Regurgitation must be differentiated from vomiting. Regurgitation occurs during or at the end of a meal, and the material tastes bland rather than sour or bitter.)
- Weight loss (late)
- Respiratory symptoms due to aspiration
- Long duration of symptoms before diagnosis
- Patient told symptoms are due to stress, may be taking antidepressive or anxiolytic medication
- Chest pain, sometimes unrelated to eating

The *radiographic* appearance of achalasia depends on the stage. In the early stages, the esophagus may appear normal, and patients may be falsely reassured. Esophageal dilatation develops, and an air fluid level may occur. Both these signs indicate outflow obstruction. Barium rarely enters the stomach; when a good view of the cardia is obtained, it has a narrow, tapering appearance. The late stage of achalasia is characterized by a tortuous, sigmoid esophagus, and an epiphrenic diverticulum may be present. The gastric air bubble may be absent because of inability to propel swallowed air into the stomach.

Endoscopy frequently reveals residual liquid or food in the esophagus. The narrowing at the lower end of the esophagus allows passage of the endoscope, usually with a characteristic "popping" sensation. When the patient has undergone previous treatment of achalasia, inflammation is likely to be caused by GE reflux.

Manometry is required to establish the diagnosis of achalasia. The manometric features (Fig. 18-11) are as follows. Not all patients have all four features.

1. Elevated LES pressure
2. Incomplete LES relaxation
3. Absence of esophageal body peristalsis
4. Positive intraesophageal body pressure

Treatment. Some patients show a short-lived symptomatic and manometric response to calcium channel blocking agents. However, definitive treatment of achalasia is balloon dilation or a surgical procedure.

Balloon dilation may be performed as an outpatient procedure and has minimal recovery time. It is less likely to be effective than surgical treatment and frequently must be repeated. The risk of perforation of the lower esophagus is high.

All surgical procedures are performed with a variant of the Heller myotomy in which the circular muscle of the lower esophagus is divided. The modified Heller myotomy is usually performed through a left thoracotomy in the seventh intercostal space. Four principles are important:

1. Adequate myotomy
2. Minimal hiatal disturbance
3. Antireflux protection without obstruction
4. Prevention of re-healing

If myotomy is performed through the abdomen, an antireflux procedure is added—either posterior or anterior hemifundoplication. A partial fundoplication is added to open transthoracic myotomy, but not to a thoracoscopic procedure. The enhanced view with thoracoscopy enables precise determination of the distal limit of the myotomy.

Diffuse Esophageal Spasm

Diffuse esophageal spasm is a primary motor disorder characterized by substernal chest pain, dysphagia or both. It produces a lesser degree of dysphagia, causes more chest pain, and has less effect on the patient's condition than does achalasia.

Diagnosis. *Radiographic* abnormalities such as segmental spasm with compartmentalization of the esophagus or formation of a diverticulum are the anatomic correlates of disordered motility function. The development of a diverticulum may temporarily alleviate dysphagia and replace it with postprandial pain and regurgitation of

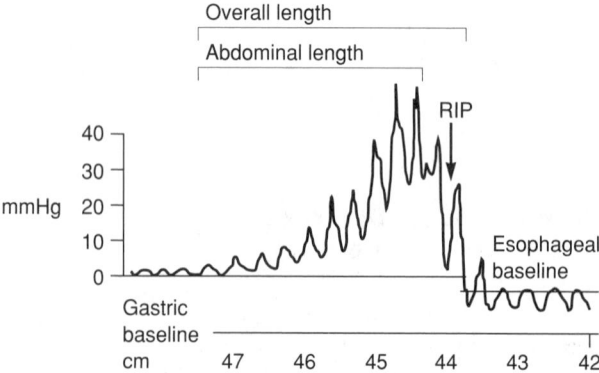

Figure 18-9. Manometric tracing as a transducer is pulled across the lower esophageal sphincter, showing the pressure, overall length, and abdominal length. RIP, respiratory inversion point.

Table 18-1. VALUES OF 24-HOUR ESOPHAGEAL pH MONITORING IN 50 HEALTHY ADULT VOLUNTEERS FOR pH LESS THAN 4.0

Measures	pH Values					
	Mean	SD	Median	Minimum	Maximum	95th Percentile
Total time pH <4 (%)	1.5	1.4	1.2	0.0	6.0	4.5
Upright time pH <4 (%)	2.2	2.3	1.6	0.0	9.3	8.4
Supine time pH <4 (%)	0.6	1.0	0.1	0.0	4.0	3.5
Episodes	19.0	12.8	16.0	2.0	56.0	46.9
Episodes ≥5 min	0.8	1.2	0.0	0.0	5.0	3.5
Longest episode (min)	6.7	7.9	4.0	0.0	46.0	19.8
Composite score	6.0	4.4	5.0	0.4	18.0	14.7

undigested food, suggesting achalasia. In patients with advanced disease, the radiographic appearance of tertiary contractions appears helical and is called *corkscrew esophagus* or *pseudodiverticulosis*.

Manometric abnormalities in diffuse esophageal spasm may be present over the total length of the smooth muscle portion of the esophageal body. The classic manometric finding is frequent simultaneous and repetitive esophageal contractions that may be of abnormally high amplitude or long duration. Key to the diagnosis of diffuse esophageal spasm is that the esophagus retains a degree of peristaltic ability. The LES in patients with diffuse esophageal spasm usually shows normal resting pressure and relaxation on deglutition. A hypertensive sphincter with poor relaxation may represent early achalasia.

Treatment. Symptom control is the only goal of treatment of diffuse esophageal spasm. Medical treatment is focused on abolishing strong simultaneous contraction with calcium channel blocking agents or long-acting nitrates.

Surgical treatment is myotomy of the esophageal body, which is not as strikingly successful as in achalasia and is considered only when medical treatment is ineffective. Myotomy of the esophageal body always is accompanied by myotomy of the LES (with partial fundoplication if an open procedure is performed) (Fig. 18-12).

Nutcracker Esophagus

Nutcracker esophagus is a manometric abnormality in which the amplitude of esophageal body peristalsis is greater than 2 standard deviations above normal. It is the most common primary motility disorder of the esophagus. The dominant symptom is central, crushing chest pain. The pain may have no relation to food ingestion and differs from angina in that it more frequently comes on at rest. Dysphagia or heartburn may be present but is overshadowed by the chest pain.

Diagnosis. Patients are usually referred from cardiologists with normal coronary angiograms and a request for esophageal motility testing. Barium radiography and endoscopy are not helpful. The pathognomic feature at *manometry* is the presence of prolonged high-amplitude waves. Many patients with noncardiac chest pain have increased esophageal acid exposure. It is important to identify these patients, because they respond well to fundoplication.

Treatment. Treatment of nutcracker esophagus is muscle-relaxing drugs (nitrates and calcium channel blockers). If features of diffuse esophageal spasm are identified at ambulatory manometry, myotomy is likely to be successful.

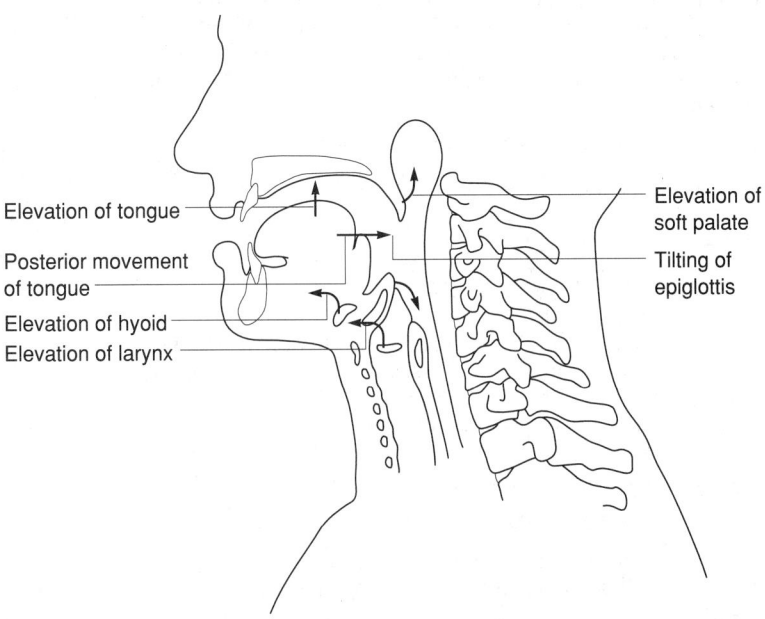

Figure 18-10. Sequence of events during the oropharyngeal phase of swallowing.

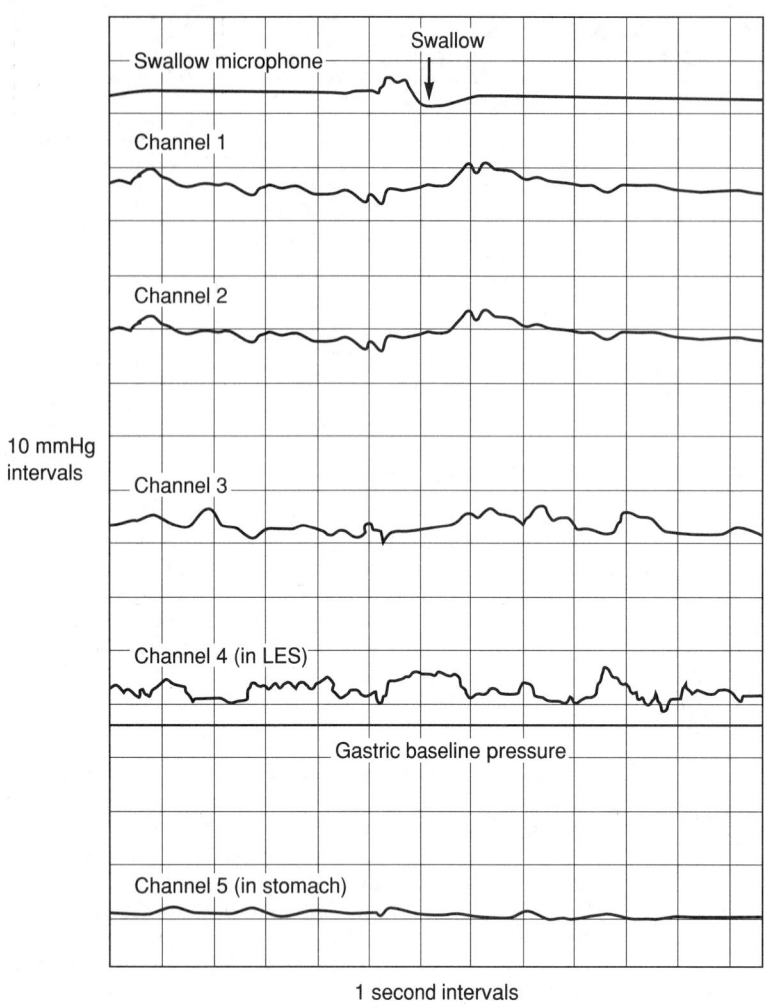

Figure 18-11. Manometric tracing in a patient with achalasia showing nonrelaxation of the lower esophageal sphincter and absent peristalsis.

Hypertension of the LES

This disorder is elevated basal pressure in the LES. Symptoms are chest pain and dysphagia. In about half of patients, LES relaxation, and esophageal body peristalsis are normal. The other half have motility disorders of the esophageal body; symptoms in these patients may be caused by prolonged postrelaxation contraction of the LES. Myotomy of the LES may be indicated for dysphagia in patients who do not respond to medical therapy or dilation.

Nonspecific Esophageal Motor Disorders

Many patients who report dysphagia or chest pain of noncardiac origin demonstrate a variety of esophageal contraction patterns at esophageal manometry that are clearly out of normal range but do not meet the criteria for a primary esophageal motility disorder. The importance of these abnormal contractions in chest pain or dysphagia is not clear. Surgery plays no role in the treatment of these disorders unless there is an associated diverticulum, in which case the diverticulum is suspended or resected, and distal myotomy across the LES is performed.

Secondary Motor Disorders of the Esophagus

Many connective tissue and neuromuscular diseases affect the esophageal body, but the most important is scleroderma. Most patients with this condition experience dysphagia. The loss of esophageal function is caused by replacement of the muscle of the lower esophagus and LES by fibrous tissue. The manometric finding is absence of LES pressure and severely impaired contraction amplitude in the smooth-muscle portion of the esophagus. The grossly defective LES allows superimposed reflux-induced injury, accelerating loss of function of the esophageal body. Many patients have a stricture. Antireflux surgery in this situation must involve a partial fundoplication, but some patients require esophageal replacement. Sometimes the situation is compounded by a severe delay in gastric emptying. Improvement is brought about with total gastrectomy and reconstruction.

GASTROESOPHAGEAL REFLUX DISEASE

GE reflux is a normal phenomenon. Most healthy people experience short episodes of reflux, usually after meals. GERD occurs when esophageal acid exposure exceeds that of a healthy population.

Pathophysiology

Increased esophageal acid exposure is caused by one of the following:

1. A mechanical defect in the LES
2. Inefficient esophageal clearance of refluxed gastric juice

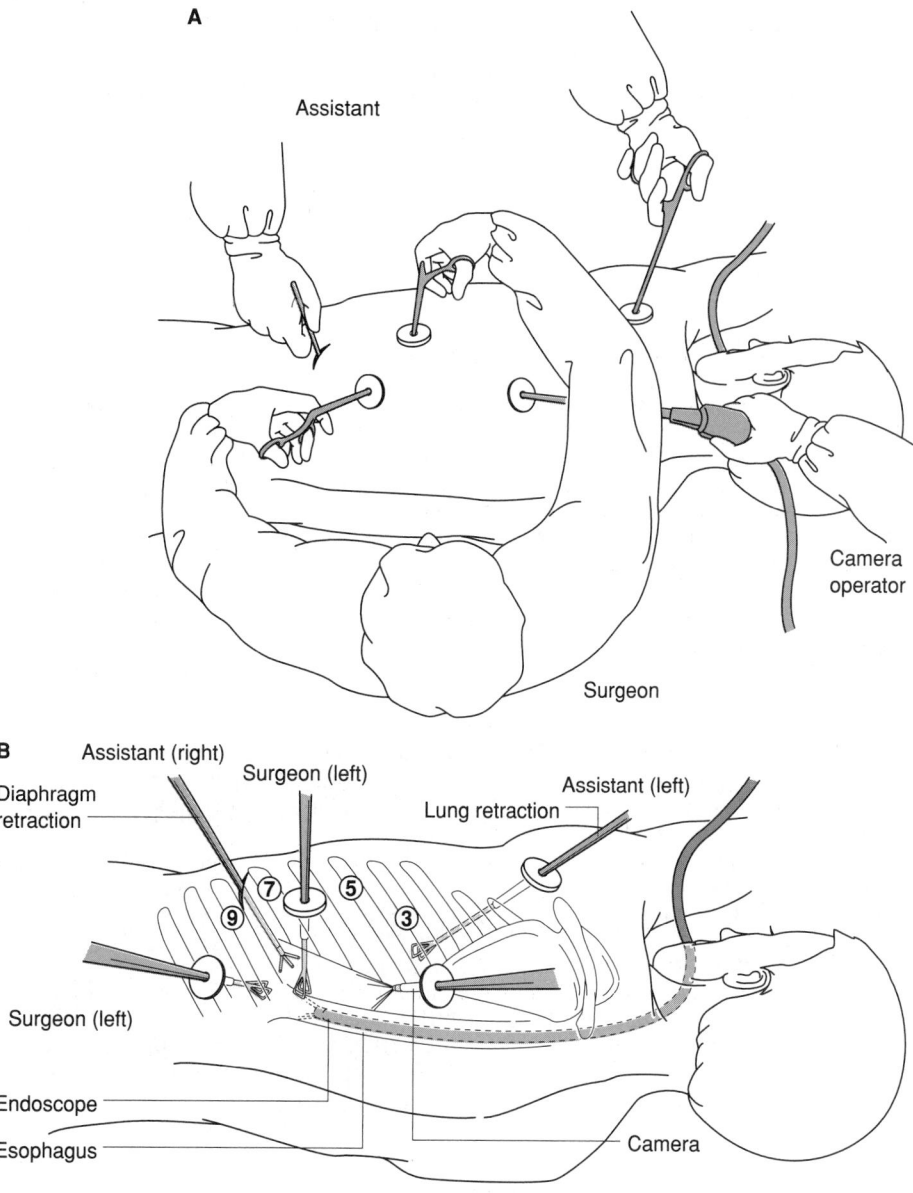

Figure 18-12. (*A*) Patient and surgeon positioning for thoracoscopic esophageal myotomy. (*B*) Trocar placement. Four 10-mm ports and a single 2- to 3-inch incision are used.

3. Abnormalities of the gastric reservoir that augment physiologic reflux

Complications of GERD include esophagitis, stricture, and Barrett esophagus. Esophagitis appears to develop as an isolated episode that does not return. In some patients with recurrent GERD, however, esophagitis becomes severe. The following factors are known to be associated with the development of complications:

1. Mechanical defects in the LES (Table 18-2)
2. Defects of esophageal clearance that prolong contact between refluxate and mucosa
3. Presence of a hiatal hernia
4. Alkali in the refluxed material

Clinical Features

Heartburn is the most common symptom of GERD. It occurs 30 to 60 minutes after meals. Heartburn exacerbated by lying flat or bending over suggests profound weakness of the LES. It may be associated with belching and *regurgi-*

tation of acid into the throat. Material regurgitated from the esophagus tastes bland and suggests a motor disorder. Material regurgitated from the stomach tastes bitter and suggests duodenogastric reflux.

If regurgitation is associated with *aspiration,* a variety of respiratory symptoms may occur. Sometimes the clinical features are those of asthma. A history of isolated episodes of pneumonia or frequent bouts of wheezing and coughing at night suggests GERD. Hoarseness may result from laryngeal irritation.

Dysphagia resulting from GERD is usually insidious. It results from a motility disorder caused by esophagitis, loss of esophageal compliance, or stricture formation. Patients usually localize dysphagia to the lower sternum, but cervical dysphagia is common in GERD. Heartburn often stops being a prominent symptom when a stricture has developed. The sudden development or rapid progression of dysphagia suggests a tumor.

Angina-like *chest pain,* sometimes called noncardiac chest pain, is frequently caused by GERD. Patients often report other classic symptoms of GERD, but the other symptoms are mild and overshadowed by the chest pain.

Table 18-2. COMPLICATIONS OF GASTROESOPHAGEAL REFLUX DISEASE
IN 150 CONSECUTIVE ADULT PATIENTS

Complication	Patients	Normal LES (%)	Defective LES (%)
None	59	58	42
Esophagitis	47	23*	77
Stricture	19	11	89
Barrett's esophagus	25	0	100

LES, lower esophageal sphincter.
* Grade of esophagitis more severe with defective LES.

Epigastric pain and *nausea* may be associated with GERD and are usually due to pathologic duodenogastric reflux or delayed gastric emptying. It is important to recognize these entities before recommending an antireflux procedure, because they may persist after the operation.

Bloating suggests gastric dilatation due to aerophagia or delayed gastric emptying.

Investigation

The initial examinations in patients with symptoms of GERD are *barium esophagography* and *upper gastrointestinal endoscopy*. In patients with GERD, these studies help identify a pathologic lesion only if a complication of the disease, such as esophagitis, stricture, or Barrett esophagus, or a potentially related condition, such as hiatal hernia, is present. The next step in investigation is *esophageal manometry* and *pH monitoring*.

Dual pH monitoring and chest radiography are helpful if there are respiratory symptoms. Gastric emptying tests, gastric acid analysis for hypersecretion, and esophageal and gastric bile probe monitoring may help elucidate gastric symptoms. Ambulatory esophageal motility studies may help define a disorder if stationary manometric findings are equivocal.

Complications of Gastroesophageal Reflux Disease

The complications of GERD are:

* Esophagitis
    Esophageal ulceration
    Esophageal stricture
    Barrett esophagus
    Short esophagus
* Respiratory symptoms caused by aspiration
* Nutritional failure

Surgical Treatment of Gastroesophageal Reflux Disease

The aim of surgical therapy is to help restore the patient to a life free of symptoms, without the need to take regular medications, and without undue social, dietary, or other restrictions. The indications for antireflux surgery are:

1. Demonstration of the presence of GERD with 24-hour pH monitoring
2. Symptoms or complications of GERD
3. Disease caused by a mechanically defective LES

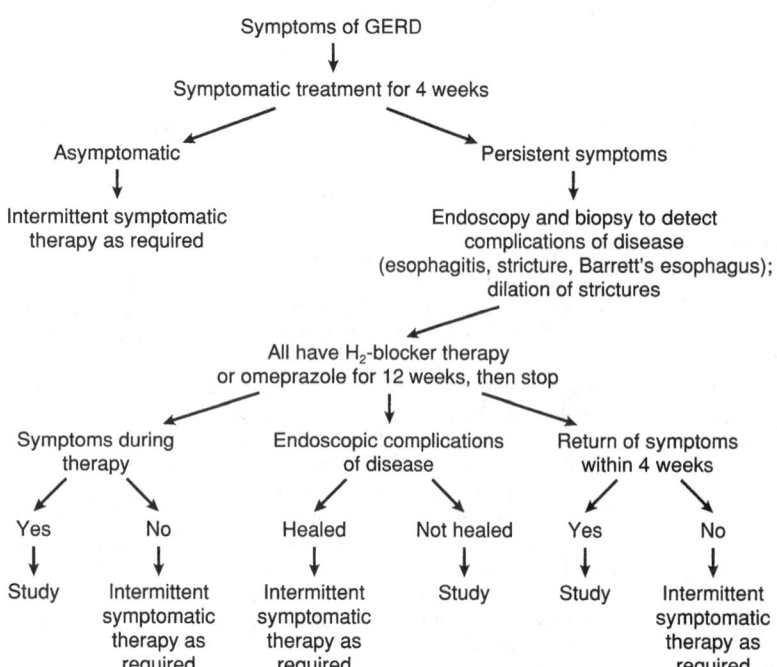

Figure 18-13. Algorithm for selecting patients with symptoms suggestive of gastroesophageal reflux disease (GERD) for further study.

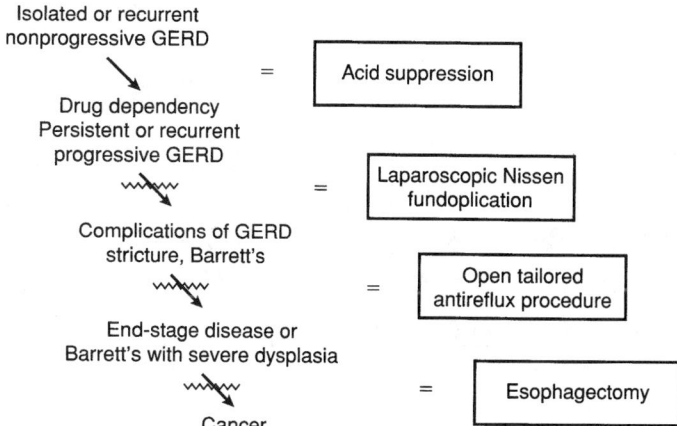

Figure 18-14. Conceptual scheme of the appropriate treatment at each stage of the spectrum of gastroesophageal reflux disease (GERD).

The algorithm in Figure 18-13 summarizes when patients are examined in the course of their disease to determine when surgical treatment is appropriate.

Principles of Antireflux Surgery

The therapy for GERD is summarized in Figure 18-14. Almost all antireflux operations involve plication of the esophagus with gastric fundus. The fundus is placed around the lower esophagus. The fundoplication must lie comfortably in the abdomen without tension, requiring only closure of the crura to maintain it there. The whole fundoplication may ride up into the chest if the crura are not closed or if there is tension on the fundoplication because of undetected esophageal shortening.

An antireflux barrier balances the risk of dysphagia against the risk of recurrent reflux. The Nissen fundoplication eliminates these problems. Partial fundoplications produce a lesser degree of resistance to outflow and are appropriate for patients with poor motility in the esophageal body. However, the long-term recurrence rate is higher than after a complete fundoplication.

Nissen Fundoplication

The elements of a transabdominal fundoplication are common to both laparoscopic and open procedures and include the following:

1. Crural dissection, identification and preservation of both vagi and the anterior hepatic branch
2. Circumferential dissection of the esophagus
3. Closure of the crura
4. Mobilization of the fundus by means of division of short gastric vessels
5. Construction of a short, loose fundoplication by enveloping the anterior and posterior walls of the fundus around the lower esophagus

Open Nissen fundoplication is easier than laparoscopic fundoplication when other complex procedures such as highly selective vagotomy or a bile diversion procedure are combined with the fundoplication.

Belsey Mark IV Repair

The techniques of the Belsey Mark IV and the transthoracic Nissen operations are similar, differing only in the construction of the gastric fundoplication.

Intraoperative Complications

The following complications can occur during antireflux operations:

- Splenic Injury
- Esophageal injury during hiatal dissection or during passage of the large bougie used to calibrate the fundoplication
- Hemorrhage that obscures the view during laparoscopic fundoplication—an indication for conversion to an open procedure
- Pneumothorax
- Inability to reduce the GE junction into the abdomen during abdominal fundoplication

SUGGESTED READING

Bechi P, Pucciani F, Baldini F, et al. Long-term ambulatory enterogastric reflux monitoring: Validation of a new fiberoptic technique. Dig Dis Sci 1993;38:1297.

Duranceau A. Pharyngeal and cricopharyngeal disorders. In: Pearson FG, ed. Esophageal Surgery. New York, Churchill Livingstone. 1995:389.

Kahrilas PJ, Dodds WJ, Hogan WJ. Effect of peristaltic dysfunction on esophageal volume clearance. Gastroenterology 1988; 94:73.

Peters JH, Heimbucher J, Kauer WKH, Incarbone R, Bremner CG, DeMeester TR. Clinical and physiologic comparison of laparoscopic and open Nissen fundoplication. J Am Coll Surg 1995;180:385.

Rothberg M, DeMeester TR. Surgical Anatomy of the Esophagus. In: Shields TW, General Thoracic Surgery, 3rd ed. Philadelphia, Lea & Febiger, 1989;79.

Sloan S, Rademaker AW, Kahrilas PJ. Determinants of gastroesophageal junction incompetence: Hiatal hernia, lower esophageal sphincter or both? Ann Intern Med 1992;117:977.

Stein HJ, Barlow AP, DeMeester TR, Hinder RA. Complications of gastroesophageal reflux disease: Role of the lower esophageal sphincter, esophageal acid and acid/alkaline exposure, and duodenogastric reflux. Ann Surg 1992;216:35.

Stein HJ, DeMeester TR, Eypasch EP, Klingman RP. Ambulatory 24-hour esophageal manometry in the evaluation of esophageal motor disorders and non-cardiac chest pain. Surgery 1991;110:753.

Stein HJ, DeMeester TR, Naspetti R, Jamieson J, Perry RE. Three-dimensional imaging of the lower esophageal sphincter in gastroesophageal reflux disease. Ann Surg 1991;214:374.

ESSENTIALS OF SURGERY: SCIENTIFIC PRINCIPLES AND PRACTICE,
edited by Lazar J. Greenfield, Michael W. Mulholland, Keith T. Oldham, Gerald B. Zelenock,
and Keith D. Lillemoe. Lippincott–Raven Publishers, Philadelphia, © 1997.

CHAPTER 19

TUMORS, INJURIES, AND MISCELLANEOUS CONDITIONS OF THE ESOPHAGUS

MARK B. ORRINGER

ESOPHAGEAL TUMORS

Almost all esophageal tumors are malignant. Benign tumors of the esophagus are extremely rare. They are classified into two main groups: epithelial (mucosal) and intramural (extramucosal). Even more rare are heterotopic collections of tissue within the esophageal wall. The diagnosis of an esophageal cyst usually can be made on the basis of its typical radiographic appearance.

Malignant Esophageal Tumors

Squamous Cell Carcinoma

The cause of esophageal carcinoma is unknown. It appears to be a result of prolonged exposure of the esophageal mucosa to noxious stimuli in patients who have a genetic predisposition to the disease. Alcohol, tobacco, zinc, nitrosamines, malnutrition, vitamin deficiencies, anemia, poor oral hygiene, dental caries, previous gastric operation, and chronic ingestion of hot foods or beverages are linked to the development of esophageal cancer. The most consistent risk factors are alcohol consumption and cigarette smoking.

The pathologic spectrum of esophageal carcinoma ranges from an early lesion (early carcinoma, superficial spreading carcinoma, intramucosal carcinoma, carcinoma in situ) limited to the mucosa to an advanced form in which the tumor penetrates the muscle layers of the esophagus or beyond. Most patients are 40 to 50 years of age. The tumor progresses to invasive squamous cell carcinoma over 2 to 4 years.

Early esophageal carcinoma is defined in terms of depth of tumor involvement—intraepithelial (carcinoma in situ), intramucosal (limited to the lamina propria), or submucosal. Advanced squamous cell carcinoma of the esophagus involves the muscular layers of the esophagus or beyond.

In the TNM classification for staging esophageal cancer (Table 19-1), the esophagus is divided into four main sections: 1) Cervical/lower border of the cricoid cartilage to the thoracic inlet, or 15-18 cm from the upper incisors; 2) Upper thoracic/thoracic inlet to the level of the carina, about 24 cm from the upper incisors; 3) Middle third/carina to half the distance to the esophagogastric junction, about 32 cm from the upper incisors; and 4) Lower/to the esophagogastric junction, about 40 cm from the upper incisors.

With this arbitrary division of the esophagus, 8% of squamous cell carcinomas occur in the cervical esophagus, 55% in the upper and midthoracic segments, and 37% in the lower thoracic segment. Esophageal carcinoma is notorious for its aggressive biologic behavior. It tends to

Table 19-1. TNM STAGING CLASSIFICATION FOR CANCER OF THE ESOPHAGUS

TNM DEFINITIONS

Primary Tumor

TX	Primary tumor cannot be assessed (cytologically positive tumor not evident endoscopically or radiographically)
T0	No evidence of primary tumor (eg, after treatment with radiation and chemotherapy)
Tis	Carcinoma in situ
T1	Tumor invades lamina propria or submucosa, but not beyond it
T2	Tumor invades muscularis propria
T3	Tumor invades adventitia
T4	Tumor invades adjacent structures (eg, aorta, tracheobronchial tree, vertebral bodies, pericardium)

Regional Lymph Node Involvement

NX	Regional nodes cannot be assessed
N0	No regional node metastasis
N1	Regional node metastasis

Distant Metastasis

MX	Presence of distant metastasis cannot be assessed
M0	No distant metastasis
M1	Distant metastasis

STAGE GROUPING

Stage 0	Tis, N0, M0
Stage I	T1, N0, M0
Stage IIA	T2, N0, M0
	T3, N0, M0
Stage IIB	T1, N1, M0
	T2, N1, M0
Stage III	T3, N1, M0
	T4, any N, M0
Stage IV	Any T, any N, M1

(Adapted from Beahrs OH, Henson DE, Hutter RVP, Kennedy BJ, eds. Manual for staging of cancer, ed 4. Philadelphia, JB Lippincott, 1992)

infiltrate locally, involve adjacent lymph nodes, and spread along the submucosal esophageal lymphatics.

Adenocarcinoma

Adenocarcinomas most often involve the distal third of the esophagus, have a peak prevalence in the sixth decade of life, and are three times more common among men than women. Esophageal adenocarcinoma has three possible origins: 1) Malignant degeneration of metaplastic columnar epithelium (Barrett mucosa), 2) Heterotopic islands of columnar epithelium, and 3) Esophageal submucosal glands.

The esophagus also may be involved in gastric carcinoma that grows cephalad. Severe gastroesophageal reflux (GER) is a factor in the development of a columnar epithelium-lined (Barrett) esophagus. Like squamous cell carcinoma, esophageal adenocarcinoma has an aggressive biologic behavior characterized by frequent transmural invasion and lymphatic spread.

Diagnosis

History and Physical Examination

Almost all patients with esophageal carcinoma have *dysphagia* as the primary presenting symptom. Dysphagia warrants barium swallow radiographic examination and endoscopic evaluation to rule out carcinoma. The combination of esophageal biopsy and brushings for cytologic evaluation establishes a diagnosis of carcinoma in almost all patients with malignant strictures.

The patient is asked to use one finger to localize on the chest or neck the point at which food lodges when swallowed. A patient with *mechanical* esophageal obstruction such as carcinoma localizes the consistent point of obstruction without difficulty. A patient with *neuromotor* obstruction may sense only slow, diffuse esophageal emptying in the retrosternal area.

Aside from weight loss, most patients with esophageal carcinoma have few objective findings at physical examination. Examination is performed to find cervical or supraclavicular lymph node metastases, abdominal masses, and liver nodularity. The finding of a hard, supraclavicular lymph node in a patient with an intrathoracic esophageal carcinoma warrants fine-needle aspiration biopsy. Documentation of metastatic disease establishes the presence of a stage IV tumor.

Laboratory Evaluation

Laboratory studies include complete blood count, blood urea nitrogen, and serum creatinine to assess hydration and liver function tests, including total protein and albumin levels to assess nutrition. Serum electrolytes, particularly potassium and calcium levels, are measured.

Imaging

A barium swallow examination is performed on all patients who describe dysphagia (Fig. 19-1). Computed tomography (CT) of the chest and upper abdomen is used for staging.

Bronchoscopy

Bronchoscopy is performed on patients with carcinoma of the upper- and middle-thirds of the esophagus to exclude invasion of the posterior membranous trachea or main-stem bronchi, which precludes esophagectomy.

Esophagoscopy

Esophagoscopy is the most important diagnostic tool. Vital staining of the esophageal mucosa is used to detect dysplastic esophageal lesions not obvious with direct endoscopic assessment. Endoscopic ultrasound is used to delineate mucosa, submucosa, and muscular layers of esophagus and adjacent tissue.

Premalignant Esophageal Lesions

Premalignant esophageal lesions include: chronic irritation of esophageal mucosa by noxious stimuli (alcohol, tobacco, hot foods and liquids); caustic esophageal strictures; Barrett esophagitis; reflux esophagitis; achalasia; Plummer–Vinson syndrome (Paterson–Kelly syndrome or sideropenic dysphagia); familial keratosis palmaris et plantaris (tylosis); and radiation esophagitis.

Management of Esophageal Cancer

Therapy for esophageal cancer is undertaken with the knowledge that for most patients local tumor invasion or distant metastatic disease precludes cure.

Radiation

Radiation therapy is used for palliation, in an attempt at cure, or as an adjunct to esophagectomy.

Intubation

A variety of endoesophageal tubes can be used to provide palliation to patients with esophageal carcinoma. Pulsion tubes are pushed through the tumor with the aid of

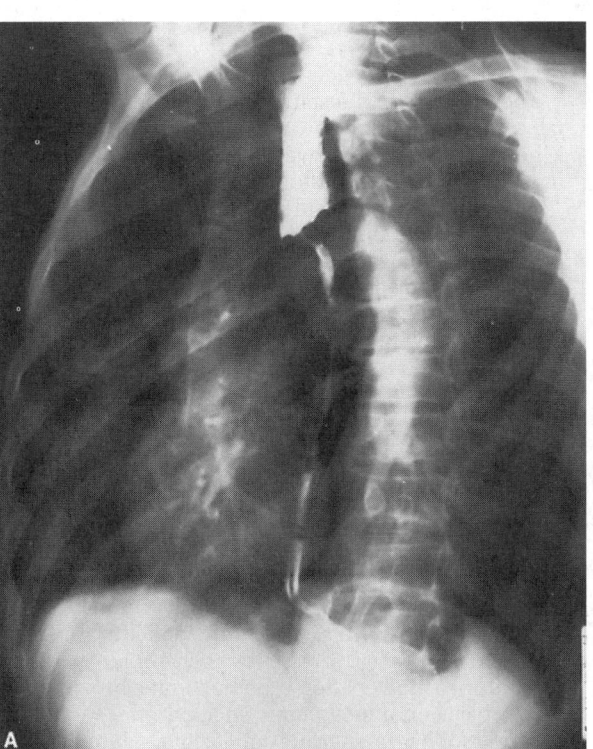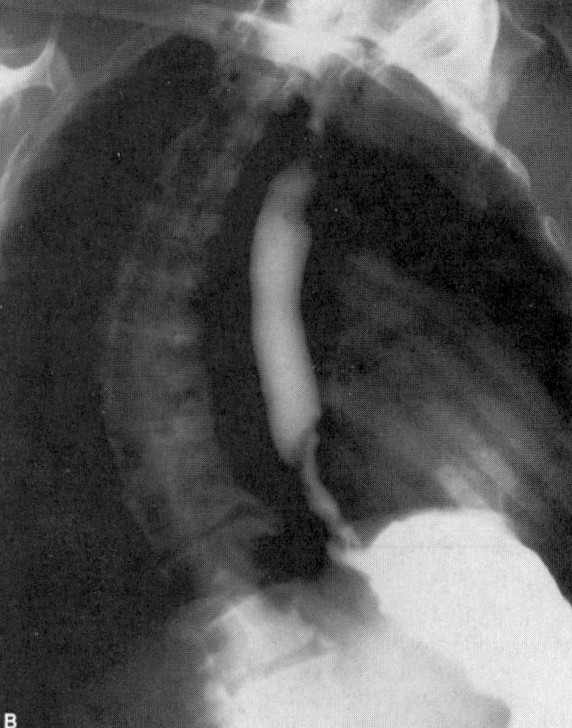

Figure 19-1. (*A*) Barium esophagogram showing an upper esophageal squamous cell carcinoma at the level of the aortic arch. Note the mucosal irregularity and shelf of tumor, which is characteristic of carcinoma. (*B*) Esophagogram showing a distal esophageal adenocarcinoma presenting as a characteristic apple-core constriction above the esophagogastric junction. (Orringer MB. Tumors of the esophagus. In: Sabiston DC Jr, ed. Textbook of surgery, ed 13. Philadelphia, WB Saunders, 1986:736)

an esophagoscope. Traction (pull-through) tubes are pulled into place by means of downward traction through a gastrotomy. This technique is reserved for patients with malignant tracheoesophageal fistulas. The tube is used to occlude the esophageal side of the fistula and allow oral alimentation.

Laser

Endoscopic laser fulguration of esophageal carcinoma can be used for temporary relief of esophageal obstruction if a tumor is unresectable.

Bypass

An internal bypass of unresectable esophageal carcinoma can be performed for palliation. Methods include substernal gastric or colonic bypass.

Resection

For most patients with localized esophageal carcinoma, resection is used for palliation of dysphagia.

Transhiatal Resection. Whenever possible, transhiatal esophagectomy without thoracotomy is performed to manage resectable esophageal carcinoma. Palpation through the diaphragmatic hiatus shows tumor invasion of the aorta or tracheobronchial tree. The entire intrathoracic esophagus is resected, the stomach is repositioned in the posterior mediastinum in the original esophageal bed, and the gastric fundus is anastomosed to the cervical esophagus above the level of the clavicles. The operation is performed through an upper-midline abdominal incision and a cervical incision. The mobilized stomach, based on the right gastric and right gastroepiploic vascular arcades, readily reaches above the level of the clavicles for a cervical anastomosis. Accessible cervical, intrathoracic, and intraabdominal lymph nodes are removed for staging, but en bloc resection of the esophagus and adjacent lymph node-bearing tissue is not performed.

Transthoracic Resection. The traditional operation for distal esophageal carcinoma is through a left thoracoabdominal incision. After the distal esophagus, proximal stomach, and adjacent lymph nodes are resected, an intrathoracic esophagogastric anastomosis is made. Tumors involving the midesophagus are resected through a thoracoabdominal or separate thoracic and abdominal incisions, and high intrathoracic esophagogastric anastomosis is performed. Pyloromyotomy or pyloroplasty is performed.

Radical Resection. Radical transthoracic esophagectomy with en bloc dissection of contiguous lymph node-bearing tissue is not much more effective than transhiatal esophagectomy without thoracotomy and without formal lymph node dissection. Stomach is used to replace the esophagus. Colonic interposition is used only when stomach is not available.

CERVICOTHORACIC ESOPHAGEAL CARCINOMA

Carcinoma that involves the cervicothoracic esophagus and adjacent larynx necessitates esophageal reconstruction after laryngopharyngectomy. Concomitant radical neck dissection may be needed. The pharynx and cervical esophagus may be replaced with skin tubes, rotated musculocutaneous flaps, or isolated, free jejunal grafts anastomosed to a cervical arterial blood supply.

Once the diagnosis of esophageal carcinoma is established, staging CT of the chest and abdomen is performed to rule out distant metastatic disease, which precludes even palliative resection. Fine-needle aspiration is used to confirm distant metastases suggested at CT. Esophagectomy is not performed on patients with proved pulmonary or hepatic metastases (stage IV disease). Patients with upper- or middle-third esophageal tumors need bronchoscopy to exclude tracheobronchial invasion that contraindicates resection. Brain and bone scans are obtained only when there are symptoms of metastases in these sites.

CAUSTIC INJURY

Caustic ingestion usually occurs among children <5 years of age who accidentally swallow caustic substances, or adults attempting suicide.

The most common caustic substances that cause esophageal injury are alkalis, acids, bleach, and detergents containing sodium tripolyphosphate. Ingestion of detergents and bleach causes only mild esophageal irritation, which heals without adverse sequelae. Acids and alkalis have devastating effects that range from acute multiorgan necrosis and perforation to chronic esophageal and gastric strictures. Alkalis produce liquefaction necrosis, which is almost always associated with deep tissue penetration. Acids usually cause coagulation necrosis, which limits the depth of injury.

The high viscosity of liquid *alkali* preparations, such as drain openers, prolongs contact between the substance and the mucous membranes and facilitates rapid transit into the stomach. Severe damage to the esophagus and stomach and adjacent organs, such as trachea, colon, small intestine, pancreas, and aorta, is common. Ingested *acid* passes through the esophagus, quickly producing gastric injury and sparing the esophagus, although extensive esophageal damage can occur.

Clinical Features

The clinical manifestations of caustic ingestion are related to the amount and character of the agent ingested. Mild pharyngeal, esophageal, or gastric burns may be almost completely asymptomatic.

Solid alkali (eg, crystal drain opener) burns the mouth, pharynx, and upper esophagus. The resulting severe pain causes immediate expectoration, so that little of the caustic agent is swallowed. These burns induce excessive salivation. At examination, the mucosa of the mouth and oropharynx shows white to gray-black patches. Patients may have hoarseness, stridor, aphonia, and dyspnea due to laryngotracheal edema or destruction.

Liquid alkali (eg, liquid drain opener) usually is swallowed quickly, producing minimal injury to the mouth and pharynx but severe damage to the esophagus, stomach, or both. Patients may have dysphagia, odynophagia, and aspiration. Severe retrosternal, back, or abdominal pain and signs of peritoneal irritation suggest mediastinitis or peritonitis due to esophageal or gastric perforation.

With *acid* ingestion, gastric injury is common, and signs and symptoms are localized to the abdomen.

When esophageal or gastric perforation results from caustic ingestion, patients demonstrate progressively severe sepsis and hypovolemic shock. In the absence of gastric or esophageal perforation, acute clinical manifestations resolve within several days. After this, chronic symptoms due to esophageal or gastric strictures begin. Strictures rarely form after ingestion of solid alkali. Patients who ingest liquid alkali, however, may have severe esophageal and severe gastric injury that results in stricture formation.

Immediate Diagnosis and Treatment

Initial management centers on stabilizing the patient's condition and assessing the severity of injury. *Vomiting must not be induced, and the patient must not be given anything to drink to dilute the fluid.* Hypovolemia is corrected with IV fluids. The patient undergoes observation for evidence of airway obstruction. Endotracheal intubation or tracheostomy may be needed if there is considerable laryngeal edema or actual laryngeal destruction. Broad-spectrum antibiotics are given once the diagnosis of esophageal injury is established.

Contrast-enhanced radiographic examination of the esophagus may provide important information about a caustic injury. Contrast esophagography with dilute barium is used to make the diagnosis of esophageal perforation. Identification of the site of perforation is crucial in planning intervention.

Management

Esophagogastroscopy is performed soon after admission to establish whether extensive esophageal injury has occurred and to grade the severity of the injury (Table 19-2).

After initial resuscitation and diagnostic evaluation, patients with caustic injuries undergo observation. Those with *first-degree* burns need no other therapy for 24 to 48 hours. Risk for esophageal stricture is low. Patients with *second-* or *third-degree* burns need prolonged observation for evidence of esophageal or gastric necrosis during the acute phase of the injury. Full-thickness necrosis of the esophagus, stomach, or other organs necessitates emergency resection.

Indications for immediate surgical exploration are: radiographic signs of free intraperitoneal air, mediastinal air, extravasation of contrast material from the stomach or esophagus, peritonitis, or abdominal or mediastinal sepsis; severe persistent back or retrosternal pain, which suggests mediastinitis; metabolic acidosis, which suggests visceral necrosis; and clinical evidence of peritonitis.

Patients with these findings who have swallowed a caustic *liquid* undergo abdominal surgical exploration. If during the operation esophageal resection is deemed necessary, a cervical incision can be added for transhiatal esophagectomy without thoracotomy. If esophageal or gastric resection is performed, alimentary continuity is not restored until after the patient has recovered from the acute insult and chronic stricture formation can be evaluated.

Some authors have advocated that all patients with second- or third-degree caustic injuries identified at endoscopy undergo immediate exploratory laparotomy. Patients with full-thickness injuries are treated by means of resection, usually esophagogastrectomy. Patients without full-thickness injuries undergo placement of a silicone stent, which is left in the esophagus for 3 weeks to prevent stricture formation.

Table 19-3. CAUSES OF ESOPHAGEAL PERFORATION

INSTRUMENTAL

Endoscopy
Dilation
Intubation
Sclerotherapy
Laser therapy

NONINSTRUMENTAL

Barogenic trauma
   Postemetic (Boerhaave syndrome)
   Blunt chest or abdominal trauma
   Other (eg, labor, convulsions, defecation)
Penetrating neck, chest, or abdominal trauma
Operative trauma
   Esophageal reconstruction (anastomotic disruption)
   Vagotomy, pulmonary resection, hiatal hernia repair,
      esophagomyotomy
Corrosive injuries (acid or alkali ingestion)
Erosion by adjacent infection
Swallowed foreign body

Chronic caustic esophageal strictures are dilated. This therapy is begun 6 to 8 weeks after the injury, when reepithelialization is complete, to minimize risk for esophageal perforation. If a caustic esophageal stricture is perforated during dilation, esophagectomy with visceral esophageal substitution is performed. Strictures that cannot be dilated and those that remain refractory to dilation after 6 to 12 months are managed by means of esophageal substitution. Stomach is used as the esophageal substitute unless the original injury has produced gastric scarring and contracture. In that case, colon is used.

ESOPHAGEAL PERFORATION

Esophageal perforation has a variety of causes (Table 19-3). Regardless of the cause, the pathophysiologic features and consequences are the same. Unless the perforation is contained by preexisting periesophageal fibrosis, saliva and gastric contents dissect into the fascial plains of the neck and mediastinum, and mediastinitis occurs. The presence of oral bacteria in these fluids initiates infection.

Diagnosis

Symptoms of esophageal perforation are pain (Table 19-4), difficulty swallowing, respiratory distress, and fever.

Pain or fever after esophageal instrumentation or operation is an indication for immediate contrast esophagogra-

Table 19-2. ENDOSCOPIC GRADING OF CAUSTIC ESOPHAGEAL INJURY

Severity of Injury	Endoscopic Findings
First-degree	Mucosal hyperemia and edema
Second-degree	Mucosal ulceration with vesicles and exudates; pseudomembrane formation
Third-degree	Deep ulceration with charring and eschar formation; severe edema obliterating the lumen

Table 19-4. SYMPTOMS AND SIGNS OF ESOPHAGEAL PERFORATION

Esophageal Segment Perforated	Symptom or Sign
Cervical or upper thoracic	Cervical or high retrosternal pain
Middle or distal	Anterior thoracic, posterior thoracic, interscapular, or epigastric pain
Upper thoracic	Signs of right pleural effusion
Distal esophagus	Signs of left pleural effusion

phy. When the diagnosis is considered, a water-soluble contrast agent is administered. If the study is normal, dilute barium is administered. If there is concern that perforation may have occurred during esophagoscopy, a chest radiograph may help to confirm the diagnosis. A normal chest radiograph, however, does not rule out esophageal perforation. Contrast-enhanced esophagography is performed to establish the diagnosis and determine the exact site of injury.

Management

Initial management of acute esophageal perforation focuses on decreasing bacterial and chemical contamination of the mediastinum and restoring intravascular volume losses. Oral intake is withheld, and the patient is instructed not to swallow saliva. Broad-spectrum IV antibiotics with activity against oral flora are administered. Nasogastric tube decompression of the stomach is instituted to minimize possible GER and further soiling of the mediastinum.

Nonsurgical Therapy

Although most esophageal perforations necessitate surgical intervention, some patients may undergo nonsurgical therapy that involves cessation of oral intake, administration of antibiotics, and IV hydration until the disruption heals or the small contained cavity begins to shrink. Nutrition is maintained through a nasogastric feeding tube, gastrostomy, jejunostomy, or IV hyperalimentation until oral intake can be resumed.

Criteria for nonsurgical therapy include the following:

Local, contained disruption without evidence of pleural contamination (hydrothorax or pneumothorax)
Walled-off extravasation in which contrast material drains back into the esophagus
Minimal or no symptoms
Minimal or no evidence of systemic infection (fever or leukocytosis)

The usual clinical settings in which such perforations are encountered are cervical esophageal tears caused by esophagoscopy; intramural dissection that occurs during dilation of a stricture or pneumatic dilation for achalasia; and asymptomatic esophageal anastomotic disruption discovered on a routine postoperative contrast examination.

Surgical Therapy

Cervical and Upper Thoracic Esophageal Perforations. Most cervical and upper thoracic perforations (to the level of the carina or the fourth thoracic vertebral body) are drained through the retroesophageal space. A well-drained cervical esophageal perforation usually heals spontaneously within several days. Insufflation of air into the esophagus through a nasogastric tube or small flexible esophagoscope may be used to identify the tear and allow direct closure if the tear is accessible. When a cervical esophageal perforation extends into the pleural cavity or lower mediastinum, transthoracic drainage is required.

Thoracoesophageal Perforations. The earlier an esophageal perforation is recognized and treated, the better is the likelihood of successful primary repair. Early esophageal perforations are those diagnosed within 24 hours of injury. Such perforations not associated with intrinsic esophageal disease are treated by means of primary repair of the tear combined with wide mediastinal drainage. Perforations of the lower third of the esophagus are approached through a left thoracotomy in the sixth or seventh interspace; more proximal thoracic esophageal tears are approached

through a right thoracotomy. Perforations of the intraabdominal esophagus not associated with pleural contamination are approached through the abdomen.

Primary repair is performed on perforations in an otherwise normal esophagus, regardless of the duration of the injury. The entire length of the mucosal injury is exposed by extending the muscle defect 1 to 2 cm beyond the extent of the mucosal tear. The defect is closed with staples. The stapled suture line is reinforced with adjacent muscle. The repair also can be reinforced with a pedicled flap of parietal pleura, anterior mediastinal fat, gastric fundus, or intercostal muscle.

After repair and drainage of the esophageal tear, a nasogastric tube is used to manage postoperative ileus, and nasogastric tube feedings can be instituted until oral intake is resumed. Once postoperative ileus has subsided, oral liquids may be resumed. A barium esophagogram is obtained 10 days after the repair to document the integrity of the esophagus; the chest tube is not removed until after this examination. If the repair is disrupted, the resulting esophagopleural cutaneous fistula heals spontaneously if external drainage through the chest tube is adequate and there is no distal esophageal obstruction.

Esophageal Perforation Associated with Intrinsic Disease. If perforation is associated with distal obstruction due to intrinsic esophageal disease, the obstruction must be relieved at the time of repair and drainage. Patients with intrinsic esophageal disease that cannot be managed conservatively undergo esophageal resection. Total thoracic esophagectomy eliminates the source of mediastinal and pleural contamination and allows cervical esophageal anastomosis.

If esophageal perforation is diagnosed promptly and mediastinal contamination is not excessive, immediate restoration of alimentary continuity can be achieved at the time of esophagectomy. This approach is used when the stomach is healthy and available for esophageal substitution and cervical esophagogastric anastomosis.

Patients with esophageal perforation due to caustic ingestion and those whose condition is unstable undergo esophagectomy with cervical esophagostomy, and reconstruction is performed later.

Late-Recognized Esophageal Perforation. The more time that passes between perforation and surgical treatment, the more inflamed are the tissues adjacent to the tear, and the greater is the risk for failure of primary suture repair. Every esophageal tear is inspected to ascertain if primary repair is feasible. Late-recognized esophageal perforations are managed in one of many ways: wide drainage alone, drainage and closure, drainage over a T tube, esophageal resection, exclusion and diversion, or nonsurgical management.

Most patients whose condition is stable can be treated with a feeding jejunostomy and a decompressing gastrostomy to prevent GER. Distal esophageal obstruction must be relieved, if necessary, by continuing dilations until the fistula closes. Well-drained esophagopleural cutaneous fistulas almost always heal spontaneously if there is no distal obstruction.

Late-recognized esophageal perforations can be closed. Chronic esophageal defects too large for direct closure without tension are closed with pedicled pleural flaps sutured around the edges of the defect.

INFECTIOUS ESOPHAGITIS

Chronic debilitation, immunosuppression, and prolonged use of antibiotics predispose to infectious esophagitis. *Candida albicans* is the most common organism. Other causes are other fungi, viruses (eg, human immunodeficiency virus), mycobacteria, and protozoa. Syphilis, tuberculosis, and Crohn disease of the esophagus are rare causes of infectious esophagitis.

DIVERTICULA

An esophageal diverticulum is an epithelium-lined mucosal pouch that protrudes from the esophageal lumen. Most esophageal diverticula are acquired. Esophageal diverticula may be classified according to location, extent of wall thickness that accompanies them, or presumed mechanism of formation:

Pharyngoesophageal (Zenker) diverticula occur at the junction of the pharynx and esophagus

Parabronchial (midesophageal) diverticula occur near the tracheal bifurcation

Epiphrenic (supradiaphragmatic) diverticula occur in the distal 10 cm of the esophagus

True diverticula contain all layers of normal esophageal wall (mucosa, submucosa, and muscle)

False diverticula consist of only mucosa and submucosa

Most esophageal diverticula are caused by elevated intraluminal pressure that forces the mucosa and submucosa to herniate through the esophageal musculature; these are false diverticula. Traction diverticula are caused by an external inflammatory reaction in adjacent mediastinal lymph nodes that adhere to the esophagus and pull the wall toward them as healing and contraction occur; these are true diverticula. Pharyngoesophageal and epiphrenic diverticula are pulsion diverticula associated with abnormal esophageal motility. Parabronchial diverticula are usually, but not always, of the traction variety and include all layers of the esophageal wall.

ACQUIRED TRACHEOESOPHAGEAL FISTULAS

Malignant Fistulas

Most acquired fistulas between the esophagus and the tracheobronchial tree are the result of malignant disease. Most patients die within 3 months of the onset of symptoms, and most of these die of aspiration pneumonia, not the malignant disease. The only therapy that may bring the patient some comfort is placement of an esophageal prosthesis.

Nonmalignant Fistulas

Only 10% of acquired fistulas between the esophagus and tracheobronchial tree are due to benign disease. These nonmalignant fistulas result from:

Erosion by contiguous infected subcarinal or mediastinal lymph nodes (tuberculosis, histoplasmosis, syphilis, actinomycosis)

Trauma (caustic injury, penetrating or blunt chest trauma, intubation, erosion of aspirated foreign body, dilation of esophageal stricture)

Late sequelae of chronic midesophageal traction diverticulum

Erosion by an endotracheal or tracheostomy tube cuff during prolonged ventilatory support.

Patients with tracheoesophageal fistulas have paroxysmal coughing while eating because swallowed food or liquid enters the tracheobronchial tree. Patients undergoing mechanical ventilation may have excessive tracheal secretions, difficulty with ventilation because of loss of inspired air into the gastrointestinal tract or out the mouth, or gastric distention. Regurgitation of gastric contents through the fistula and into the lungs may cause fulminant aspiration pneumonia.

The diagnosis of tracheoesophageal fistulas is established with contrast-enhanced esophagography. Bronchography may be used to delineate the site of the fistula and define diseased pulmonary parenchyma that may have to be resected during repair of the fistula. CT is used to define mediastinal adenopathy and to exclude the presence of a mediastinal tumor mass. Endoscopy is performed to exclude malignancy and to assess the size and location of the fistula. Biopsy specimens and brushings are taken from the tracheal and esophageal sides of the fistula for cytologic evaluation.

Benign acquired fistulas are identified and divided. The opening in the esophagus and the tracheal or bronchial defect are débrided and closed. Communication with a segment of lung may necessitate limited pulmonary resection. To prevent recurrence, viable adjacent tissue such as mediastinal fat may be interposed between the tracheobronchial and esophageal suture lines.

For patients undergoing mechanical ventilation, repair of the fistula is deferred until ventilation is discontinued. Initial management is removal of the nasogastric tube, if present, and replacement of the endotracheal or tracheostomy tube with a tube that has a large-volume, low-pressure cuff inflated below the fistula. The stomach is decompressed with a gastrostomy, and a feeding jejunostomy tube is inserted.

SUGGESTED READING

Castell DO, ed. The esophagus. Boston, Little, Brown, 1992.

Gudovsky LM, Koroleva NS, Biryukov YB, et al. Tracheoesophageal fistulas. Ann Thorac Surg 1993;55:868.

Mathiesen DJ, Grillo HC, Wain JC, Hilgenberg AD. Management of acquired nonmalignant tracheoesophageal fistula. Ann Thorac Surg 1991;52:759.

Orringer MB, Marshall B, Stirling MC. Transhiatal esophagectomy for benign and malignant disease. J Thorac Cardiovasc Surg 1993;105:265.

Orringer MB, Zuidema GD, eds. Shackelford's surgery of the alimentary tract, ed 4, vol 1. The esophagus. Philadelphia, WB Saunders, 1996.

Pearson FG, Deslauriers J, Ginsberg RJ, Hiebert CA, McKneally MF, Urschel HC Jr, eds. Esophageal surgery. New York, Churchill Livingstone, 1995.

Reed CE. Comparison of different treatments for unresectable esophageal cancer. World J Surg 1995;19:828.

Vandenplas Y, Helven R, Derop H, et al. Endoscopic obliteration of recurrent tracheoesophageal fistula. Dig Dis Sci 1993; 38:374.

White RI, Iannettoni MD, Orringer MB. Intrathoracic esophageal perforation: the merit of primary repair. J Thorac Cardiovasc Surg 1995;109:140.

Wright CD, Mathiesen DJ, Wain JC, et al. Reinforced primary repair of thoracic esophageal perforation. Ann Thorac Surg 1995; 60:245.

ESSENTIALS OF SURGERY: SCIENTIFIC PRINCIPLES AND PRACTICE,
edited by Lazar J. Greenfield, Michael W. Mulholland, Keith T. Oldham, Gerald B. Zelenock,
and Keith D. Lillemoe. Lippincott–Raven Publishers, Philadelphia, © 1997.

CHAPTER 20

ENDOSURGICAL PRINCIPLES

STEVE EUBANKS

Endosurgery entails operations performed with visualization provided through a telescope placed in a body space.

LAPAROSCOPY

Access

A needle (Veress needle) is placed into the peritoneal cavity through a small (<2 mm) skin incision by means of gradual advancement of the needle or a short, dartlike motion. Most insertions are safe and uneventful. However, intestinal injury, hemorrhage, exsanguination, and fatal air embolism can occur.

An alternative to use of a Veress needle is an open technique of trocar insertion. A 10 to 12 mm skin incision is made within the umbilicus or in the periumbilical area. Dissection of subcutaneous tissue is accomplished with sharp dissection or electrocauterization. The fascia is identified, grasped between clamps, and incised. The underlying peritoneum is elevated and incised under direct vision. The initial abdominal access port is then placed into the peritoneal cavity.

Complications can occur with either access method. Those associated with the open technique are generally limited to superficial bleeding or minimal injury to the intestine. Use of a Veress needle carries a small risk for serious intestinal injury. vascular trauma, and death.

After the establishment of pneumoperitoneum and placement of the first trocar, the laparoscopic telescope is placed into the abdominal cavity. All subsequent trocars enter the abdomen under direct visualization. The J maneuver is used for placement of secondary ports (Fig. 20-1).

Proper positioning of the trocars through the abdominal wall is crucial for a successful laparoscopic operation. *Triangulation* of the trocars allows convergence of the telescope and instrument tips on the target organ while minimizing extracorporeal interference between instruments (Fig. 20-2).

Three to five trocars are used to accomplish most laparoscopic operations. In adults the trocars are placed a minimum of 8 cm apart so that a wide range of extracorporeal manipulation is possible. Ideal placement of trocars and equipment allows the surgeon to squarely face the operative site and television monitor.

Physiology

Reduced tissue trauma and carbon dioxide (CO_2) pneumoperitoneum are two of the factors that account for the physiologic effects of laparoscopy. Reduced abdominal wall retraction, decreased manipulation of abdominal viscera, and lack of exposure of the viscera to room air during laparoscopy may be important secondary factors that contribute to improved gastrointestinal function compared with an open surgical procedure. Most physiologic effects of CO_2 pneumoperitoneum are detrimental; however, these generally are limited to the intraoperative period and are easily managed if anticipated. An optical cavity (or working space) is required for laparoscopy. This is most commonly produced by means of insufflation of CO_2 under pressure into the peritoneal cavity.

Alternatives to CO_2 include helium and argon. Inert gases potentially reduce many of the adverse hemodynamic and metabolic effects of CO_2 absorption. Alternative gases do not eliminate adverse effects related to elevations in abdominal pressure. CO_2 is preferred because it is inexpensive, readily available, rapidly absorbed and physiologically eliminated, and noncombustible.

The physiologic events that account for the hemodynamic effects of CO_2 insufflation are listed in Table 20-1.

Intraoperative physiologic effects of pneumoperitoneum on pulmonary function are undesirable, yet well-tolerated by most patients without serious existing pulmonary disease.

Postoperative ileus is not a problem with laparoscopy. Colonic electrical activity rapidly returns afterwards, and small-intestinal motility is preserved during laparoscopic cholecystectomy.

Laparoscopic surgical technique may avoid a maladaptive stress response by minimizing the systemic inflammatory response precipitated by multisystem trauma or severe infection that can lead to increased microvascular permeability, a hypermetabolic state, capillary thrombosis, and multiple-system organ failure.

Advantages and Disadvantages

Advantages of laparoscopy relative to laparotomy are: reduced pain, shorter hospital stay, fewer wound complications, and better cosmetic results. *Disadvantages* of laparoscopy are: negative physiologic effects of CO_2 pneumoperitoneum, technical challenges of operating with two-dimensional visualization on a television monitor, frustration and fatigue caused by working against the fulcrum of the abdominal wall and using long instruments, and the ability to view only surface anatomy (partially overcome with intraoperative ultrasonography). *Complications* of laparoscopy are: trocar injury to viscera or blood vessels, air embolism, trocar site hernia, and injury due to instrumentation.

Applications

The following procedures can be performed with laparoscopic technique: cholecystectomy, diagnosis of acute abdominal disorders, staging of malignant tumors, operations for gastroesophageal reflux disease, and appendectomy.

Laparoscopy is technically feasible but rarely performed for: colectomy, hernia repair, management of ulcer disease, splenectomy, adrenalectomy, and bypass procedures for malignant tumors of the pancreas. Procedures for which a laparoscopic approach is *not appropriate* are: pancreatoduodenectomy, resection of masses that necessitate a large incision for specimen removal, and major hepatic resections. Laparoscopic vascular procedures are under investigation.

THORACOSCOPY

Anesthesia Considerations

Most thoracoscopic operations are performed with general anesthesia with a dual-lumen endotracheal tube. This approach provides continuous airway control, allows single-lung ventilation, decreases risk for contralateral

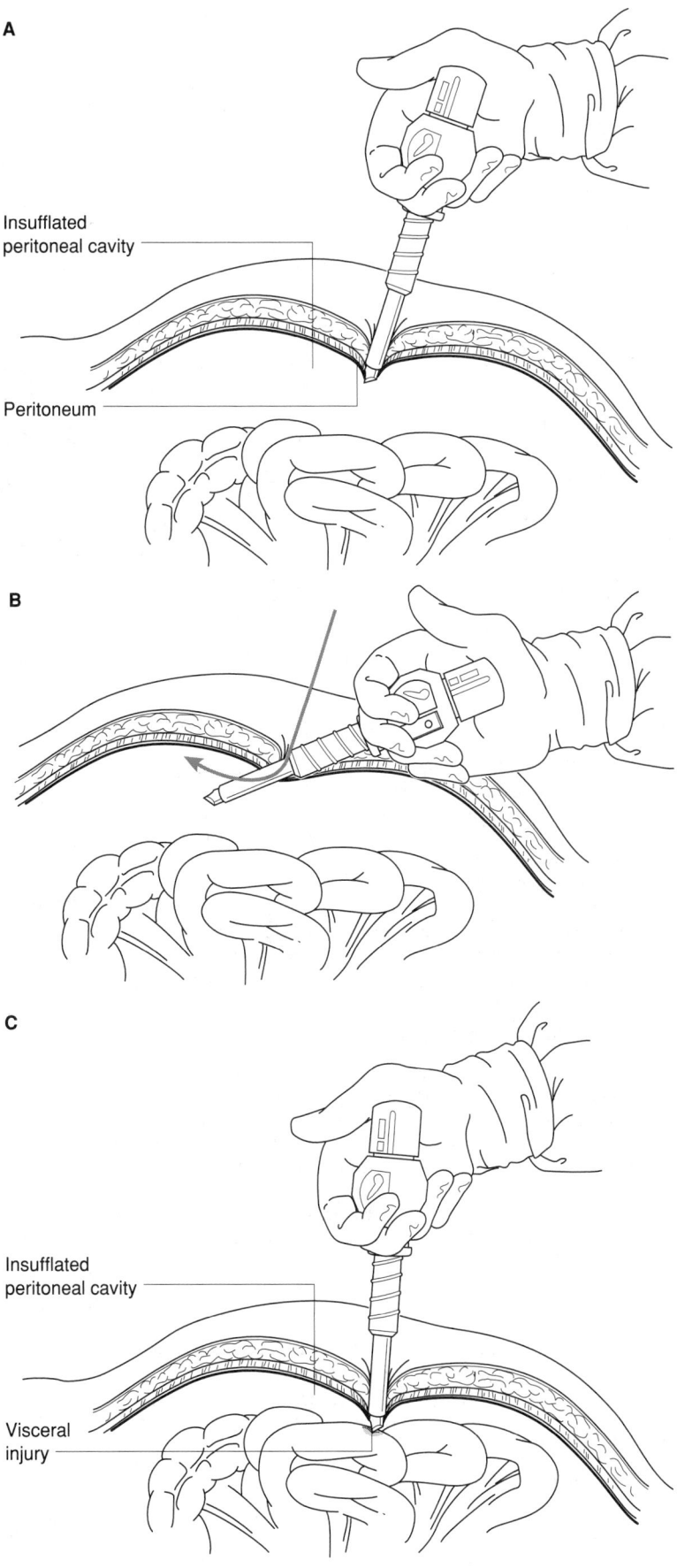

Figure 20-1. (*A*) A laparoscopic trocar is placed into the peritoneal cavity under direct vision after insufflation. (*B*) It can be placed safely using a J-maneuver as shown to direct the sharp tip tangentially away from the underlying viscera after penetration of the abdominal wall. This is done under visual control. (*C*) Laparoscopic port placement can lead to visceral injury if done without appropriate caution.

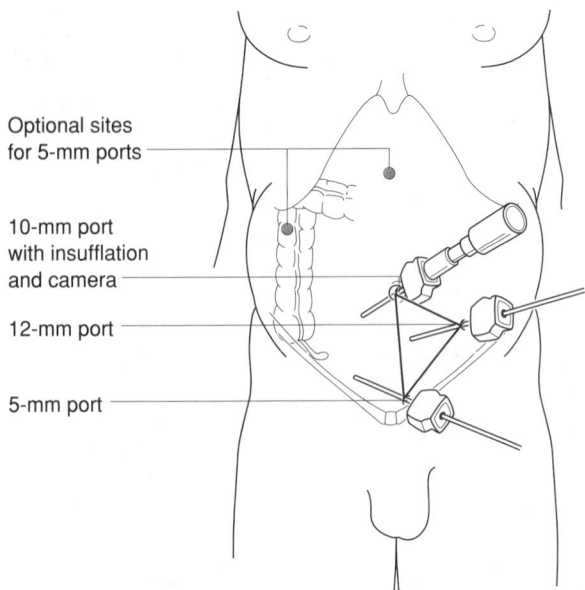

Figure 20-2. Trocar placement for a right colectomy. The general principle is to place the camera port so the surgeon's visual axis is parallel to the telescope, and to place the working ports so that the operative site is at the apex of an isosceles triangle.

lung contamination, and does not require patient cooperation.

Preoperative evaluation before elective thoracoscopy includes baseline arterial blood gases and pulmonary function studies to determine the patient's ability to tolerate single-lung ventilation. Preoperative pulmonary function is optimized by means of cessation of smoking, eradication of infection, chest physiotherapy, and treatment with bronchodilators and steroids if indicated. Most physiologic changes during thoracoscopy are the result of pneumothorax, single-lung ventilation, patient positioning, and the response to anesthesia.

Technical Considerations

The lateral decubitus position is routine for thoracoscopy. Access to the thoracic cavity is gained with a technique similar to placement of a chest tube. A 1 to 2 cm skin incision is placed on the lateral thorax. Electrocauterization is used to divide the subcutaneous tissues. A clamp is used to spread muscle fibers and is bluntly advanced through the parietal pleura. A fingertip is placed in the pleural space, and a 360° sweep is done to ensure that the lung is not at risk for injury.

Table 20-1. PHYSIOLOGIC EFFECTS OF PNEUMOPERITONEUM

Measurement	Effect
Mean arterial pressure	Increased
Systemic vascular resistance	Increased
Pulmonary vascular resistance	Increased
Heart rate	Increased
Central venous pressure	Increased
Venous return	Decreased
Cardiac output	Decreased
Cardiac index	Decreased

A thoracic cannula is placed over a blunt obturator and left in place throughout the procedure for instrument and telescope access to the pleural cavity. The skin incision must be immediately above the intercostal space selected for the procedure. Use of a skin incision removed from the intercostal space limits movement of the instruments.

The principle of *triangulation* is followed (Fig. 20-3). The target site is the apex of the triangle, and the telescope and cannulas provide points that converge on the target. The surgeon stands facing the surgical site with a television monitor directly in the line of sight. Cannulae are placed at sites that allow the surgeon and assistant to work parallel to the visual axis of the endoscope.

The optical cavity within which the surgeon operates is provided by collapse of the ipsilateral lung. The cavity is maintained by the fixed structure of the thoracic cage. Nonsealing cannulas are used for thoracoscopy because there rarely is a need to maintain a pressurized closed space. Additional instruments may be placed directly through thoracic wall incisions.

One to five cannulas are used for thoracoscopy. The sites are closed in layers after the cannulas are removed. A chest tube is placed in the pleural cavity through one cannula before inflation of the ipsilateral lung. The chest tube can be omitted if the procedure incurs minimal or no risk.

Advantages and Disadvantages

Advantages of thoracoscopy in relation to thoracotomy are: less pain, shorter hospital stay, faster return to normal activities, decreased tissue trauma, reduced cost, and better cosmetic results. *Disadvantages* of thoracoscopy are: loss of direct tactile feedback, difficulty of detection of deep parenchymal lesions, difficulty of technical maneuvers, such as suturing, anastomosis, ligation of blood vessels and loss of three-dimensional visualization.

Applications

Thoracoscopy can be used for the *diagnosis* of: pleural effusions, diffuse interstitial lung disease, isolated pulmonary infiltrates, solitary pulmonary nodules, mediastinal lymphadenopathy, neurogenic tumors, and mediastinal masses.

Thoracoscopy can be used in *therapy* for many diseases of the lung, pleura, mediastinum, and pericardium. The

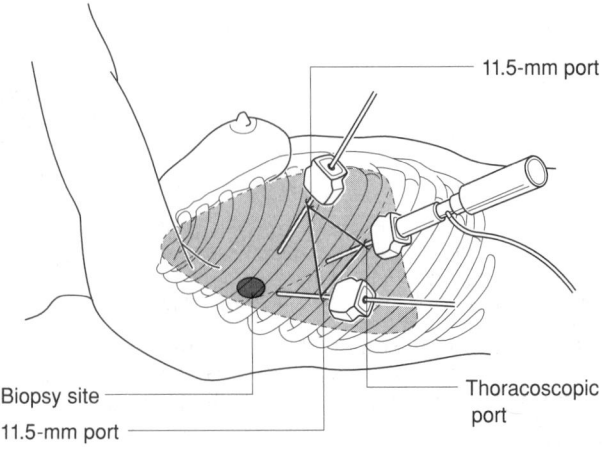

Figure 20-3. Example of thoracoscopic port placement. Positioning varies for individual need, but the principle of triangulation used for laparoscopic surgery is equally applicable in the thorax.

**Table 20-2. POTENTIAL COMPLICATIONS
OF THORACOSCOPIC
PULMONARY RESECTION**

Pneumothorax	Inadequate margin of resection
Persistent air leak	Lung injury
Hemorrhage	Intercostal neurovascular bundle injury
Air embolism	Equipment malfunction
Diaphragmatic perforation	Infection

(Modified from Mault JR, Harpole DH, Douglas JM. Thoracoscopic pulmonary resection. In: Pappas TN, Schwartz LB, Eubanks S, eds. Atlas of laparoscopic surgery. Philadelphia, Current Medicine, 1996;26:10)

limited cardiac applications include single-vessel coronary artery bypass grafting.

Conversion from a thoracoscopic procedure to thoracotomy is sometimes necessary to provide hemostasis, improve visibility, safely perform the procedure, or allow manual palpation.

The complications of thoracoscopic pulmonary resection are summarized in Table 20-2.

SUGGESTED READING

Arregui ME, Fitzgibbons RJ, Katkhouda M, McKernan JB, Reich H, eds. Principles of laparoscopic surgery: basic and advanced techniques. New York, Springer-Verlag, 1995.

DeCamp MM, Jaklitsch MT, Mentzer SJ, Harpole DH, Sugarbaker DJ. The safety and versatility of video-thoracoscopy: a prospective analysis of 895 cases. J Am Coll Surg 1995;181:113.

Farouck O, Saba A, Fath J, et al. Increases in intra-abdominal pressure affect pulmonary compliance. Arch Surg 1995; 130:544.

Pappas TN, Schwartz LB, Eubanks S, eds. Atlas of laparoscopic surgery. Philadelphia, Current Medicine, 1996.

Payne JH, Grininger LM, Izawam T, et al. Laparoscopic or open inguinal herniorrhaphy? A randomized prospective trial. Arch Surg 1994;129:973.

Peter H, DeMeester TR, eds. Minimally invasive surgery. St. Louis, Quality Medical, 1994.

Safran DB, Orlando R. Physiologic effects of pneumoperitoneum. Am J Surg 1994;167:281.

Schmieg RE, Schirmer BD, Combs MJ, Edwards M, Fariss A. Recovery of gastrointestinal motility after laparoscopic cholecystectomy. Surg Forum 1993;44:135.

Trokel MJ, Bessler M, Treat MR, Whelan RL, Nowygrod R. Preservation of immune response after laparoscopy. Surg Endosc 1994;8:1385.

ESSENTIALS OF SURGERY: SCIENTIFIC PRINCIPLES AND PRACTICE,
edited by Lazar J. Greenfield, Michael W. Mulholland, Keith T. Oldham, Gerald B. Zelenock,
and Keith D. Lillemoe. Lippincott–Raven Publishers, Philadelphia, © 1997.

CHAPTER 21

GASTRIC ANATOMY AND PHYSIOLOGY

MICHAEL W. MULHOLLAND

ANATOMY

Gross Anatomy

The stomach is composed of the cardia, which is just distal to the gastroesophageal junction; the fundus, above and to the left of the gastroesophageal junction; the corpus, between fundus and antrum; and the antrum, from corpus to pylorus (Fig. 21-1). The margin between corpus and antrum is not distinct. The pylorus is a thick ring of smooth muscle at the distal end of the stomach. The position of the stomach depends on the habitus of the person, the degree of gastric distention, and the position of the other abdominal organs. It is fixed only by the gastroesophageal junction and the retroperitoneal duodenum. The anterior surface of the stomach abuts the left hemidiaphragm, the left lobe and the anterior segment of the right lobe of the liver, and the anterior parietal surface of the abdominal wall. The posterior surface of the stomach abuts the left diaphragm; the left kidney and left adrenal gland; the neck, tail, and body of the pancreas; the aorta and celiac trunk; and the periaortic nerve plexuses. The greater curvature of the stomach abuts the transverse colon and transverse colonic mesentery. The left lateral portion of the stomach is in contact with the concavity of the spleen.

Blood Supply

The stomach is supplied by a number of major arteries and is protected by a large number of extramural and intramural collateral vessels. Gastric viability may be preserved after ligation of all but one primary artery. The rich network of vessels means that gastric hemorrhage cannot be controlled by the extramural ligation of gastric arteries. Most gastric blood flow is derived from the celiac trunk (Fig. 21-2). The lesser curvature is supplied by the right and left gastric arteries. The greater curvature is supplied by the short gastric and left gastroepiploic arteries and the right gastroepiploic artery.

Venous effluent from the stomach roughly parallels the arterial supply. The venous equivalent of the left gastric artery is the coronary vein.

Lymphatic Drainage

The lymphatic drainage of the stomach roughly parallels gastric venous return (Fig. 21-3). The lymphatic drainage, like the blood supply, has intramural ramifications and extramural communications. As a consequence, diseases that involve the gastric lymphatics often spread intramurally beyond the region of origin and to nodal groups far from the primary lymphatic zone.

Nerve Supply

The left and right vagus nerves descend parallel to the esophagus within the thorax before forming a periesophageal plexus between the tracheal bifurcation and the diaphragm. From this plexus, two vagal trunks coalesce before passing through the esophageal hiatus of the diaphragm (Fig. 21-4). The anterior vagus nerve supplies a hepatic division before innervating the liver and biliary tract. The remainder of the anterior vagal fibers run parallel to the lesser curvature of the stomach, branching to the anterior gastric wall. The posterior vagus nerve divides into the celiac branch, which passes to the celiac plexus, and a posterior gastric branch, which innervates the posterior gastric wall.

About 90% of the fibers in the vagal trunks are afferent, transmitting information from the gastrointestinal tract to the central nervous system. Only 10% of vagal nerve fibers are motor or secretory efferents. Acetylcholine is the neurotransmitter of primary vagal efferent neurons. The gastric sympathetic innervation is derived from spinal segments T-5 through T-10. Postsynaptic sympathetic nerve fibers enter the stomach with blood vessels. Afferent sympathetic fibers pass without synapse from the stomach to dorsal spinal roots. Pain of gastroduodenal origin is sensed through afferent fibers of sympathetic origin.

Microscopic Anatomy

The glandular portions of the stomach are lined by simple columnar epithelium composed of surface mucous cells. The luminal surface, at scanning electron microscopic examination, appears cobblestoned, interrupted at intervals by gastric pits. Opening into the gastric pits are one or more gastric glands.

Cardiac Glands

Cardiac glands occupy a narrow zone adjacent to the esophagus. They mark a transition from the stratified squamous epithelium of the esophagus to the simple columnar epithelium of the stomach. Cardiac glands contain mucous and undifferentiated and endocrine cells. The glands are usually branched and connect with short gastric pits. Secretion of mucus is the generally accepted function of the cardiac glands.

Oxyntic Glands

Oxyntic glands occupy the fundus and body of the stomach and contain the parietal cells, which are the sites of acid production. Oxyntic glands also contain chief cells, the site of gastric pepsinogen synthesis. Several oxyntic glands may empty into a single gastric pit.

Parietal Cells. Parietal cells contain intracellular canaliculi, a network of clefts that extend to the basal cytoplasm

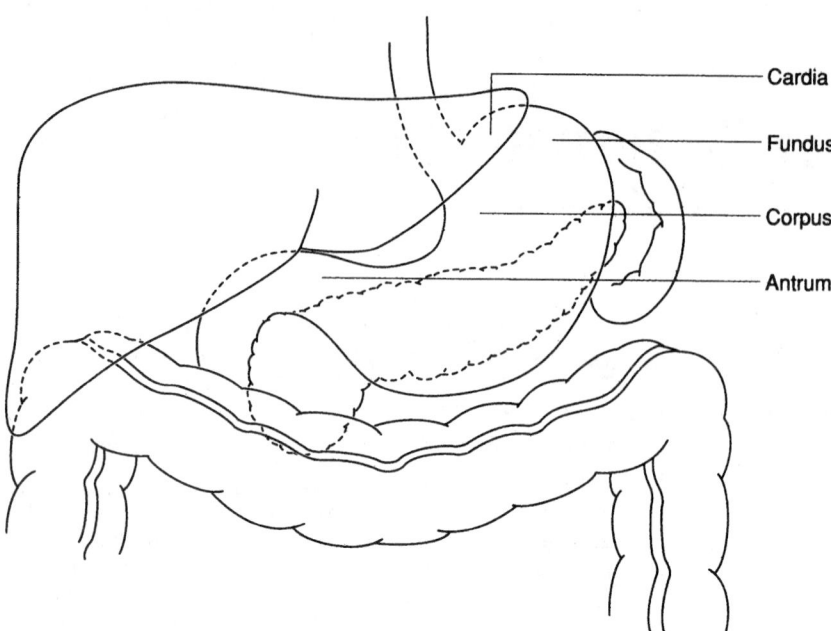

Figure 21-1. Topographic relations of the stomach.

and often encircle the nucleus, which is continuous with the lumen of the gland. The surface area provided by the intracellular secretory canaliculi is large, and is further enlarged by microvilli that line the canaliculi. In parietal cells not stimulated to secrete acid, the canaliculi are collapsed and inconspicuous. On stimulation, canalicular surface area increases and the intracellular clefts become prominent, producing an intracellular space that communicates with the gastric lumen, into which hydrogen ions are secreted in high concentration. Because the cytoplasm of parietal cells contains an abundance of large mitochon-

dria, the oxygen consumption of isolated parietal cells is about five times higher than that of gastric mucous cells. The cytoplasm also contains a small amount of rough endoplasmic reticulum, presumed to be the site of production of intrinsic factor.

Chief Cells. Chief cells synthesize and secrete pepsinogen. They are abundant in the bases of oxyntic glands. Chief cells have a morphology typical of protein-secreting exocrine cells. Rough endoplasmic reticulum is abundant within the cytoplasm and extends between secretory gran-

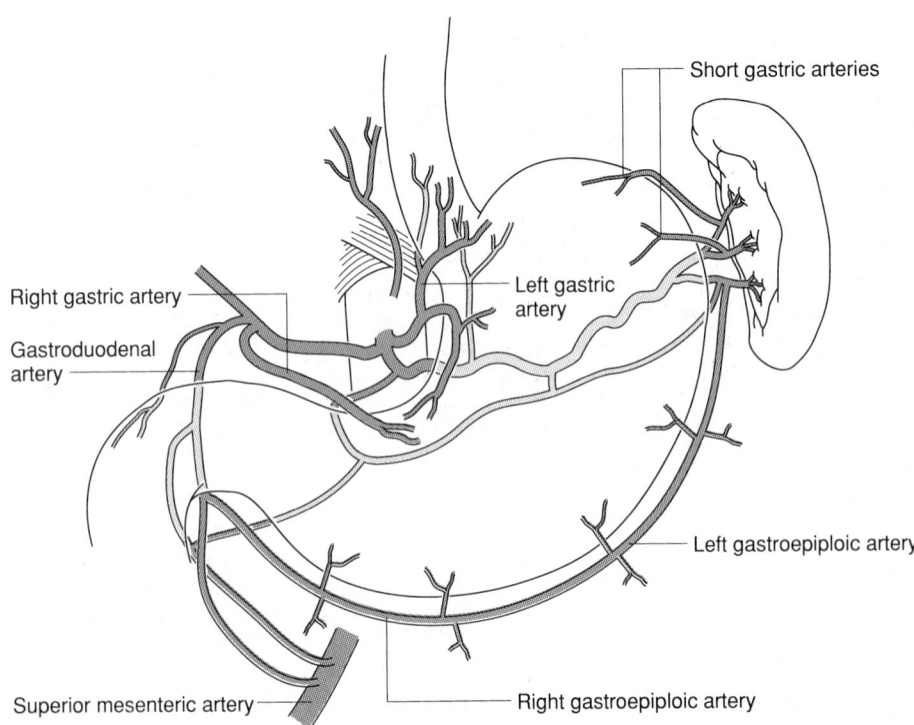

Figure 21-2. Arterial blood supply of the stomach.

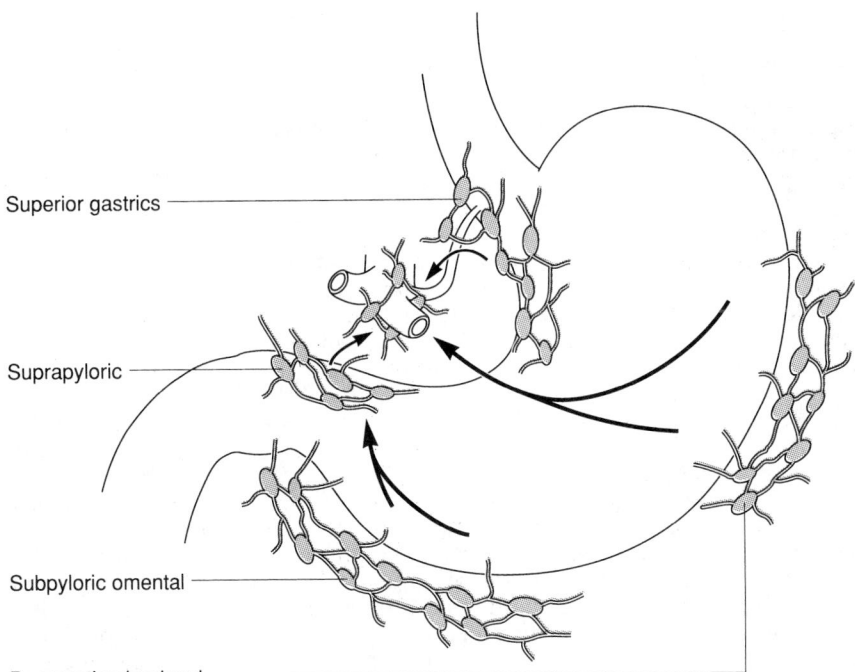

Figure 21-3. Lymphatic drainage of the stomach.

ules. Zymogen granules that contain pepsinogen are most concentrated within the apical cytoplasm. Pepsinogen is released by exocytosis from secretory granules at the apical surface of chief cells.

Antral Glands

Antral glands occupy the mucosa of the distal stomach and pyloric channel. The glands are relatively straight and often empty through deep gastric pits. Although most cells within the antral glands are mucus-secreting, gastrin cells are the distinctive feature of the mucosa in this area. Gastrin cells are pyramidal with a narrow area of luminal contact at the apex and a broad surface that overlies the lamina propria at the base. Gastrin cells are identified using immunocytochemical study by the presence of peptide. Granules 150 to 400 nm in diameter are the sites of gastrin storage and are most numerous in the basal cytoplasm. Gastrin is released by exocytotic fusion between secretory granule and plasma membrane.

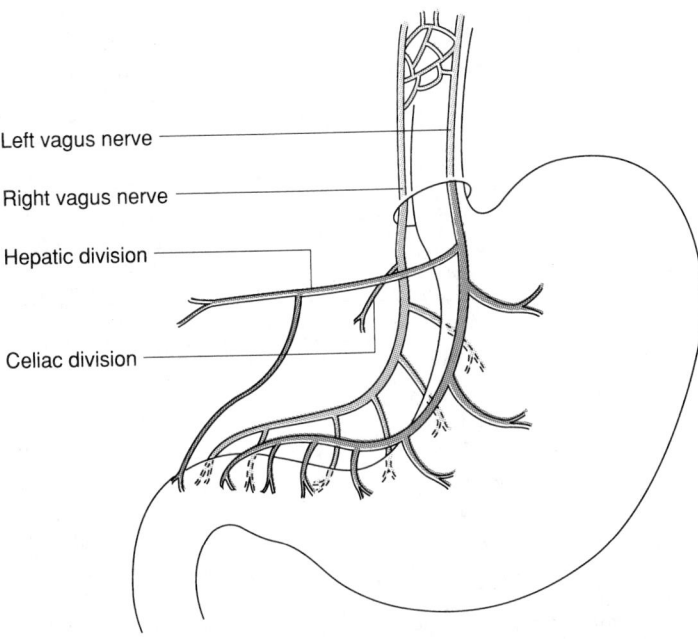

Figure 21-4. Vagal innervation of the stomach.

PHYSIOLOGY
Peptide Synthesis and Secretion

The stomach contains a number of biologically active peptides in nerves and mucosal endocrine cells. The two most important peptides are gastrin and somatostatin.

Gastrin

The most important stimulant of gastrin release is a meal. The most potent gastrin-releasing activities are triggered by the amino acids tryptophan and phenylalanine. Ingestion of fat and glucose does not cause gastrin release. Dietary amino acids are transported into gastrin cells, where decarboxylation enzymes convert the acids to amines, which promote gastrin release. Conditions that increase intracellular amine levels stimulate gastrin secretion, and those that prevent amino acids from entering gastrin cells inhibit gastrin release.

Gastrin release is inhibited when acidification of an ingested meal causes the intraluminal pH to fall to <3.0. Conversely, maintenance of intragastric pH >3.0 potentiates gastrin secretion after ingestion of protein or amino acids. Somatostatin has been implicated in the inhibited release of gastrin that occurs when luminal pH decreases. Release of mucosal somatostatin occurs with gastric acidification.

The vagus nerve appears to have both stimulatory and inhibitory effects on gastrin release. Hypergastrinemia after vagotomy suggests that inhibitory vagal effects on gastrin release exist. Vagal stimulation of gastrin release appears to be mediated by gastrin-releasing peptide, which acts as a neurotransmitter within the gastric wall. Adrenergic stimulation also appears to increase gastrin release.

Gastrin is important in the control of growth of the gastrointestinal mucosa. The acid-secreting oxyntic mucosa is sensitive to the trophic action of gastrin, but the mucous membranes of the duodenum, colon, and pancreatic parenchyma are also affected. The 17– and 34–amino acid forms of gastrin are equally potent in stimulating mucosal growth. Prolonged stimulation by high levels of gastrin, as in the Zollinger–Ellison syndrome, is associated with hypertrophy of the gastric mucosa. Small increases in circulating gastrin, such as those that follow vagotomy, do not cause mucosal hypertrophy.

Somatostatin

The most important gastric function of somatostatin appears to be regulation of acid secretion (circulating somatostatin) and gastrin release (locally released somatostatin). It decreases acid secretion and diminishes gastrin release. Concentrations of somatostatin capable of inhibiting acid secretion do so without altering serum gastrin levels, indicating a direct action on the acid-secreting fundic mucosa.

The presence of somatostatin where antral somatostatin cells contact antral gastrin cells, implies that somatostatin cells affect the function of gastrin cells through local release of the peptide. Somatostatin also may reach neighboring gastrin cells through diffusion or local blood flow. Cholinergic agents stimulate gastrin release and inhibit somatostatin release. Prostaglandin E_2, in contrast, inhibits gastrin release and stimulates somatostatin secretion.

Gastric Acid Secretion
Cellular Events

The basolateral membrane of parietal cells contains receptors for histamine, gastrin, and acetylcholine, the three most important stimulants of acid production. Histamine is released from mast-like cells within the lamina propria and diffuses to the mucosa; acetylcholine is released close

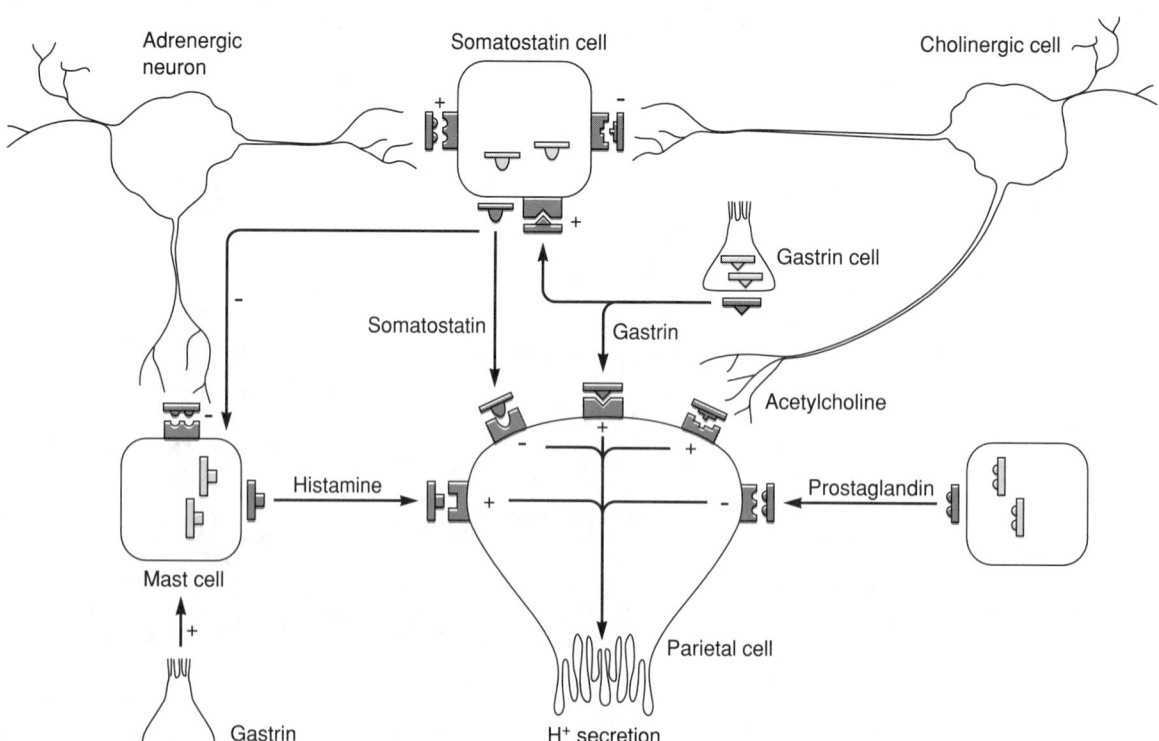

Figure 21-5. Interactions of cell types that affect parietal cell acid secretion.

to the parietal cells from cholinergic nerve terminals; and gastrin is delivered by the systemic circulation to the fundic mucosa from its source in the antrum and proximal duodenum (Fig. 21-5).

Histamine receptors in the gastric mucosa are classified as H2 receptors. Occupation of the histamine receptor activates a membrane-bound enzyme, adenylate cyclase (Fig. 21-6). Activated adenylate cyclase catalyzes conversion of intracellular adenosine triphosphate (ATP) to cyclic adenosine monophosphate (cAMP). Enhancement of cAMP production by histamine is closely linked to stimulation of parietal cell acid production. cAMP mediates histamine-stimulated acid production by activating protein kinases, which, in turn, catalyze protein phosphorylation. Acetylcholine and related cholinergic agonists activate parietal cells after binding to muscarinic receptors. The stimulatory effects of acetylcholine and its congeners can be abolished by atropine.

The transient increases in intracellular calcium produced by cholinergic stimulation of parietal cell function activate mechanisms that stimulate acid secretion. This intracellular calcium may modulate parietal cell function by means of protein phosphorylation or enzyme activation. The result of protein kinase C phosphorylation is parietal cell activation and hydrogen ion secretion.

Although histamine, acetylcholine, and gastrin occupy separate receptors on parietal cells, each secretagogue acts by means of a specialized ion transport system: the parietal cell proton pump. Membrane-bound protein is localized to the secretory canaliculus of the parietal cell. The proton pump concentrates hydrogen ions within the secretory canaliculus, and the hydrolysis

of ATP provides the energy for transport. For each H^+ ion transported to the luminal surface of the canalicular membrane, one K^+ ion is transported to the cytosolic surface. This cotransport requires that K^+ be continuously supplied to the luminal surface of the secretory membrane. This requirement is satisfied by conduction of K^+ across the canalicular membrane from intracellular stores. Chloride ions also enter the secretory canaliculus by diffusion. The transcellular exchange of H^+ for HCO_3^- ensures that the voluminous secretion of HCl at the luminal surface of the gastric mucosa is matched by equivalent delivery of base to submucosal capillaries.

Parietal cells contain membrane receptors that inhibit acid secretion. In histamine activation, the inhibitory effects appear to be mediated when somatostatin blocks production of cAMP. Parietal cells also contain receptors for prostaglandins, notably prostaglandin E_2 (PGE_2) an its derivatives. PGE_2 is a potent inhibitor of histamine-stimulated parietal cell activation, probably by a mechanism that inhibits formation of cAMP.

Gastric acid production can be blocked by receptor antagonists for each of the three primary stimulants—gastrin, acetylcholine, and histamine. Direct inhibition of acid production can be affected by derivatives of somatostatin or PGE_2. All forms of stimulated acid production can be blocked with agents that inhibit the parietal cell proton pump.

Regulation of Acid Secretion

Parietal cell activation and acid secretory response are greater when agonists are combined than when an agent is used alone. This increase in responsiveness is called

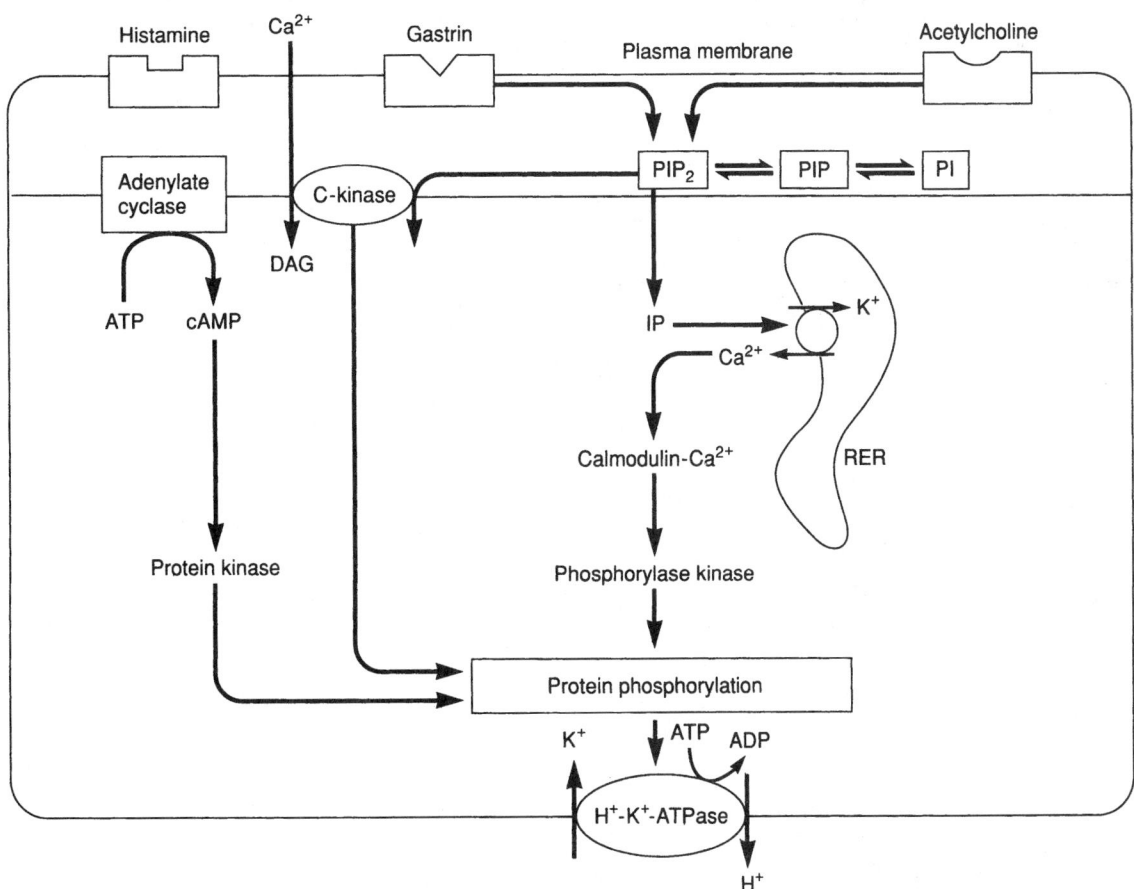

Figure 21-6. Cellular mechanisms controlling parietal cell acid secretion.

potentiation. Histamine strongly potentiates the acid secretory response to pentagastrin or to carbachol. Conversely, blockade of receptors to one stimulant decreases responsiveness to other agonists. For example, blockade of histamine receptors by agents such as cimetidine decreases responsiveness to pentagastrin even though gastrin receptors are not directly affected.

Humans secrete 2 to 5 mEq/h of HCl in the fasting state—basal acid secretion. Truncal vagotomy decreases basal acid secretion by about 85% and H2-receptor antagonists, by about 80%. Gastrin is not important in determining basal acid secretion.

Cephalic Phase. Acid secretion is stimulated with the thought, sight, or smell of food (Fig. 21-7). This cephalic phase of gastric acid secretion is mediated by the vagus nerve. Vagal discharge directs a cholinergic mechanism, and the cephalic phase of acid secretion can be inhibited by administration of atropine. Vagal discharge secondary to cephalic stimulation also inhibits the release of somatostatin.

Gastric Phase. The gastric phase of acid secretion begins when food enters the stomach. The presence of partially hydrolyzed food, gastric distention, and the buffering capability of food all stimulate acid secretion. Gastrin is the most important mediator of the gastric phase of acid secretion. The acid secretory rate after a mixed meal is 15 to 25 mEq/h. The meal response is less than the maximal response to exogenous stimulants because food causes the release of somatostatin and the initiation of other inhibitory responses.

Gastric acid secretion is inhibited by central nervous, gastric, and intestinal mechanisms. The vagus nerve stimulates and inhibits acid secretion and gastrin release. Vagotomy causes fasting and postprandial hypergastrinemia.

The most important and clearly established gastric inhibitory mechanism is suppression of gastrin release by exposure of the antral mucosa to acid. When luminal pH falls to 2.0, gastrin release stops. Acidification of the antrum increases somatostatin release and decreases gastrin secretion. Antral distention also inhibits acid secretion.

Intestinal Phase. Intestinal-phase inhibition of gastric acid secretion begins when digestive products enter the intestine. A large number of peptides have been proposed as mediators of the intestinal-phase effects, including secretin, somatostatin, peptide YY, gastric inhibitory peptide, and neurotensin.

Pepsin Secretion

Pepsins are proteolytic enzymes secreted by gastric chief cells. Once activated, pepsin is irreversibly denatured at pH 7.0 or greater. The most important function of pepsin is initiation of protein digestion. Intragastric protein hydrolysis by pepsin is incomplete, and the products of partial hydrolysis signal for gastrin and cholecystokinin release, which regulates digestion.

Secretion of Intrinsic Factor

Intrinsic factor, produced in the gastric mucosa, is necessary for absorption of cobalamin from the ileal mucosa. Intrinsic factor is synthesized and stored in the parietal cells. Intrinsic factor secretion, like acid secretion, is stimulated by histamine, acetylcholine, and gastrin. Unlike acid production, intrinsic factor secretion peaks soon after stimulation and returns to baseline. The amount of intrinsic factor secreted usually greatly exceeds the amount needed to bind and absorb available dietary cobalamin.

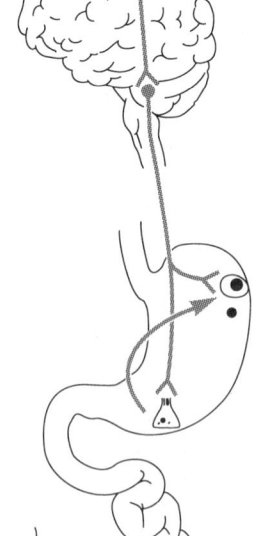

Stimulation
Cholinergic agonists
Prostaglandin inhibitors
GABAergic agonists
Gastrin
CCK-8
TRH
Somatostatin

Inhibition
Cholinergic antagonists
Andrenergic agonists
Prostaglandins
Seratonin
Bombesin
Opiod peptides
Calcitonin
Calcitonin gene–related peptide

Acetylcholine
Histamine
Gastrin

Somatostatin
Prostaglandins

Entero-oxyntin

Neurotensin
Secretin
Somatostatin
PeptideYY
Gastric inhibitory peptide

Figure 21-7. Regulation of acid secretion in vivo.

Production of Gastric Bicarbonate

The gastric mucosa secretes HCO_3^- in addition to acid. The surface mucous cells that face the gastric lumen are presumed to be responsible for HCO_3^- production. HCO_3^- transport appears to protect the mucosa against damage from luminal acid. H^+ ions diffusing from luminal fluids toward the gastric mucosa appear to be neutralized by HCO_3^- secreted close to the surface. This allows a pH near 7.0 to be maintained at the mucosal surface, even if the total amount of HCl secreted greatly exceeds gastric HCO_3^- production. Drugs or chemicals that inhibit bicarbonate secretion acidify the mucosal surface.

Gastric Blood Flow

Because the gastric mucosa has high metabolic activity, control of mucosal blood flow is important. Perfusion abnormalities appear to promote development of mucosal lesions during periods of stress. Mucosal blood flow is regulated by neural, hormonal, and locally active influences.

Postganglionic sympathetic fibers innervate small mucosal arteries. Mucosal capillaries do not receive adrenergic innervation. Electrical stimulation of sympathetic nerves that supply the stomach decreases total gastric blood flow, decreases flow within celiac and gastroepiploic vessels, and diminishes blood flow to the mucosa. Stimulation of the vagus nerve is followed by a prompt increase in blood flow, suggesting a dilatory effect of parasympathetic nerves. The finding that vagotomy is accompanied by modest decreases in total gastric and mucosal blood flow is consistent with this concept. The effects of vagal stimulation on mucosal blood flow are complicated by accompanying increases in acid secretion. Almost all stimuli that increase acid production also increase blood flow.

Gastrointestinal peptide hormones affect gastric blood flow because they increase or decrease acid secretion. Gastrin, because it is a potent stimulant of acid secretion, also increases mucosal blood flow. PGE increases gastric blood flow at doses that decrease acid secretion.

Gastric Motility

Gastric Smooth Muscle

The stomach has two functional regions—the proximal third and the distal two-thirds. These areas are distinct in smooth-muscle anatomy, electrical activity, and contrac-tile function. The regions do not correspond to the anatomic divisions of fundus, corpus, and antrum.

The proximal stomach has three layers of gastric smooth muscle—an outer longitudinal layer, a middle circular layer, and an inner oblique layer. In the distal stomach, the longitudinal layer is clearly defined, and the inner oblique layer is not distinct. The gastric smooth muscle ends at the pylorus (Fig. 21-8). The smooth muscle of the proximal stomach is electrically stable, whereas the smooth muscle of the distal stomach demonstrates spontaneous, repeated electrical discharges. Peristalsis occurs in the distal but not in the proximal stomach.

Coordination of Contraction

Vagally mediated reflexes influence intragastric pressure, presumably by affecting the contractile activity of the smooth muscle of the proximal stomach. When a meal is ingested, the increasing gastric volume is accommodated by receptive relaxation of the proximal stomach with little increase in intragastric pressure. Relaxation of the proximal stomach allows it to store ingested food in the immediately postprandial period. Gastric accommodation due to receptive relaxation is lost after truncal or proximal gastric vagotomy.

After a meal has been ingested, proximal contractile activity increases, and alterations in proximal gastric tone cause the compressive movement of gastric content from the fundus to the antrum. Food that enters the distal stomach is propelled by peristalsis toward the pylorus. The pylorus closes 2 to 3 seconds before the antrum contracts, allowing a small bolus of liquid and suspended food particles to pass through the pylorus while the main mass of gastric content is pushed back into the antrum. The churning that results mixes ingested food particles, gastric acid, and pepsin. Solid food particles do not ordinarily pass through the pylorus unless they are no larger than 1 mm in diameter.

Liquid emptying occurs more quickly than solid emptying. The actions of the proximal stomach in liquid emptying are regulated by the sieve-like action of the antropyloric segment and are modified by the nutrient composition of the ingested meal. The distal gastric segment appears to control solid emptying through grinding and peristalsis. This concept of the two-component stomach is useful in treating patients who have undergone gastric operations. Patients who undergo proximal gastric vagotomy exhibit accelerated emptying of liquids but have normal solid emptying. Because receptive relaxation is

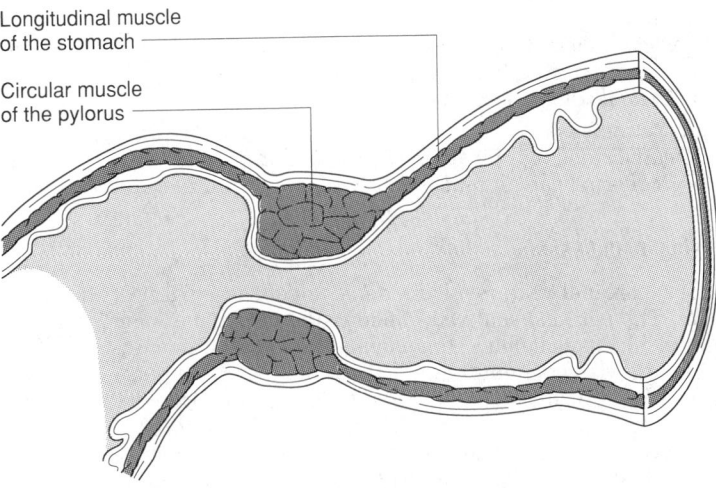

Figure 21-8. Cross-sectional anatomy of pyloric sphincter.

lost, denervation of the proximal stomach appears to increase intragastric pressure and accelerate liquid emptying while leaving the distal stomach unaffected. Vagal denervation of the antrum interrupts gastric emptying of solids to a greater degree than that of liquids.

SUGGESTED READING

Andrews PC, Dixon JE. Biosynthesis and processing of the somatostatin family of peptide hormones. Scand J Gastroenterol 1986;21(Suppl):22.

Chew CS, Nakamura K, Ljungstrom M. Calcium signaling mechanisms in the gastric parietal cell. Yale J Biol Med 1992;65:561.

Debas HT, Mulholland MW. Drug therapy in peptic ulcer disease. Curr Probl Surg 1989;26:1.

DelValle J, Wang, L, Gantz, I, Yamada T. Characterization of H2 histamine receptor: linkage to both adenylate cyclase and [Ca^{2+}]i signaling systems. Am J Physiol 1992;263:G967.

Malinowski D, Sachs G, Cuppoletti J. Gastric H$^+$ secretion: histamine (cAMP-mediated) activation of protein phosphorylation. Biochim Biophys Acta 1988;972:95.

Mulholland MW, Debas HT. Physiology and pathophysiology of gastrin: a review. Surgery 1988;103:135.

Prinz C, Kajimura M, Scott D, et al. Acid secretion and the H, K, and ATPase of stomach. Yale J Biol Med 1992;65:577

Schubert ML, Jong NJ, Makhlouf GM. Bombesin/GRP-stimulated somatostatin secretion is mediated by gastrin in the antrum and by intrinsic neurons in the fundus. Am J Physiol 1991; 261:G885.

ESSENTIALS OF SURGERY: SCIENTIFIC PRINCIPLES AND PRACTICE, edited by Lazar J. Greenfield, Michael W. Mulholland, Keith T. Oldham, Gerald B. Zelenock, and Keith D. Lillemoe. Lippincott–Raven Publishers, Philadelphia, © 1997.

CHAPTER 22

DUODENAL ULCER

MICHAEL W. MULHOLLAND

The pathogenesis of duodenal ulcers is usually attributed to one of the following factors:

Acid secretion
- Increased acid secretory capacity
- Increased basal acid secretion
- Increased pentagastrin-stimulated output
- Increased meal response

Abnormal gastric emptying

Environment
- Cigarette smoking
- Use of nonsteroidal antiinflammatory drugs
- *Helicobacter* infection

Mucosal defense

Decreased duodenal bicarbonate production
- Decreased gastric mucosal prostaglandin production

DIAGNOSIS

The cardinal feature of duodenal ulcers is epigastric pain. The pain is usually confined to the upper abdomen and is burning, stabbing, or gnawing. Referred pain is uncommon. Many patients report pain on arising in the morning and that ingestion of food or antacids usually provides prompt relief. There are few abnormal physical findings.

The differential diagnosis of duodenal ulcer includes nonulcerative dyspepsia, gastric neoplasia, cholelithiasis and related diseases of the biliary system, and inflammatory and neoplastic disorders of the pancreas. If a patient has dyspepsia, the differential diagnoses are peptic ulcer and gastric cancer.

Endoscopy

Evaluation for peptic ulcers usually involves either a barium contrast radiographic examination of the stomach and duodenum or endoscopy. Endoscopy eliminates the need for radiation, is safe, is preferred by elderly patients, and allows biopsy of the esophagus, stomach, and duodenum. Endoscopy, however, does have a morbidity of about 1 complication per 5000 examinations and is more expensive than radiography.

Duodenal ulcers are characterized by lesions that erode the intestinal wall. Endoscopy shows sharply demarcated edges of the lesions and an exposed submucosa. The base of the ulcer is often clean and smooth, although acute ulcers and those with recent hemorrhage may demonstrate eschar or adherent exudate. Surrounding mucosal inflammation is common. The most frequent site of peptic ulcers is the first portion of the duodenum. Ulcers of the third or fourth portions of the duodenum are unusual and suggest an underlying gastrinoma. Ulcers within the pyloric channel or in the prepyloric area are similar in endoscopic appearance to duodenal ulcers and have clinical features similar to those of duodenal ulcers.

Diagnostic Imaging

Barium meal radiographs demonstrate retention of contrast material in the ulcer. When viewed in profile, the ulcer may appear to project beyond the level of the duodenal mucosa. Distortion of the duodenal bulb by spasm or cicatrization is a secondary sign of current or previous ulcers.

Histologic Evaluation

Duodenal ulcers are characterized by chronicity and invasiveness. Chronic injury is suggested by surrounding fibrosis. Collagen is deposited within the submucosa during each round of ulcer relapse and healing. The adjacent mucosa often bears evidence of chronic injury with infiltration of acute and chronic inflammatory cells. Gastric metaplasia, in which the duodenum exhibits histologic features of gastric mucosa, is common in the surrounding, nonulcerated mucosa. The ulcer may invade a variable distance through the wall of the duodenum, including the full thickness of the intestine in instances of perforation.

DRUG TREATMENT

There are several potential sites of action for drugs that inhibit acid secretion (Fig. 22-1). Receptor antagonists for histamine, gastrin, or acetylcholine; antagonists of the parietal cell proton pump; and antagonists of agents that supplement or restore mucosal defenses are used to treat uncomplicated ulcer disease. Surgeons who treat patients with duodenal ulcers should be aware of the uses and limits of drug therapy (Table 22-1).

Histamine–Receptor Antagonists

Histamine, released into the intestinal fluid by cells within the fundic mucosa, diffuses to the mucosal parietal cells. It stimulates acid production by occupying a membrane-bound receptor and activating parietal cell adenylate cyclase. Blockade of histamine receptors inhibits

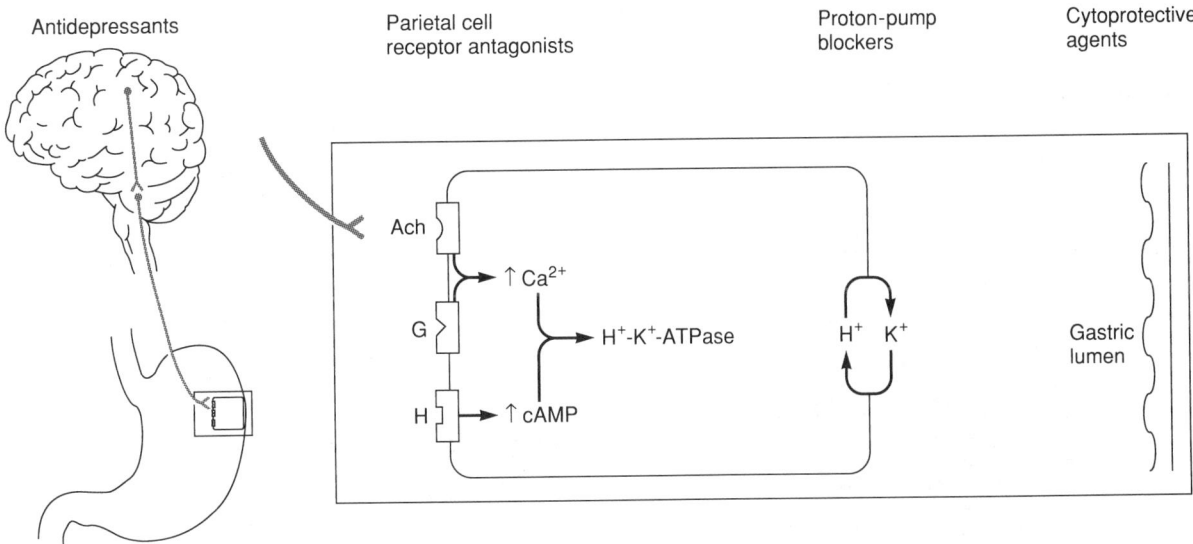

Figure 22-1. Overview of the sites of action of drugs with antiulcer activities.

most forms of stimulated acid secretion. Cimetidine, ranitidine, famotidine, and newer H_2-receptor antagonists bind competitively to parietal cell H_2-receptors to produce reversible inhibition of acid secretion.

Anticholinergic Drugs

Anticholinergic drugs block acid secretion by occupying muscarinic receptors for acetylcholine. Although most antimuscarinic agents inhibit acid secretion, nonselective anticholinergic drugs like atropine have unpleasant side effects, such as dry mouth, blurred vision, and urinary retention. For atropine, these limiting side effects occur at doses lower than necessary to inhibit acid secretion. "Selective" anticholinergic agents interact specifically with muscarinic receptors on postganglionic nerves of the stomach while having less effect on receptors on parietal cells and muscle cells of pupil, bladder, and heart. Pirenzepine inhibits vagally stimulated acid secretion and has minimal undesirable visual, urinary, or cardiac effects.

Proton Pump Blockers

Acid secretion by the parietal cells is caused by the transport of hydrogen ions from the parietal cell cytoplasm to secretory canaliculi in exchange for potassium. Because

the proton pump is present only in gastric mucosa, its blockade has a minimal effect on nongastric functions.

Omeprazole is one of a family of compounds that selectively block the parietal cell proton pump. Omeprazole accelerates the healing of ulcers and provides symptomatic relief. Direct comparisons with H_2-receptor antagonists favor omeprazole in terms of pain relief and in the rate of ulcer healing. Omeprazole is not used for long-term maintenance therapy because of concerns about chronic hypergastrinemia, hyperplasia of the enterochromaffin-like cells, and bacterial overgrowth in the achlorhydric stomach. Peptic ulcers recur in a large number of patients after cessation of omeprazole therapy.

When long-term omeprazole therapy is necessary, dosage should be adjusted to achieve an acid production of approximately 10 mEq/h in the hour before the next dose. Continuous anacidity may be deleterious and is not necessary to achieve ulcer healing.

Sucralfate

Sucralfate is the aluminum salt of sulfated sucrose. In the acidic environment of the stomach, sucralfate polymerizes, becoming viscous, and adheres to the gastroduodenal mucosa. Coating of the ulcer base by the polymer provides a protective barrier, binding bile salts and inhibiting the

Table 22-1. PHARMACOLOGIC PARAMETERS OF COMMONLY USED ANTIULCER DRUGS

Agent	Ulcer Therapy (Daily Dose)	Bioavailability (%)	Major Route of Excretion	Most Frequent Side Effects	Important Drug Interactions
Cimetidine	800–1200 mg	70	Renal	Neuropsychiatric effects, endocrine disorders	Hepatically metabolized drugs
Ranitidine	300–400 mg	70	Renal	Neuropsychiatric effects	Warfarin
Famotidine	40 mg	70	Renal	Nonspecific	
Prenzepine	100–150 mg	25	Feces	Dry mouth	
Omeprazole	20–30 mg	40–50	Renal	Nonspecific	
Sucralfate	4 g	Unabsorbed	Unabsorbed	Constipation	
Microprostol	800 μg	—	Tissue metabolism	Diarrhea	

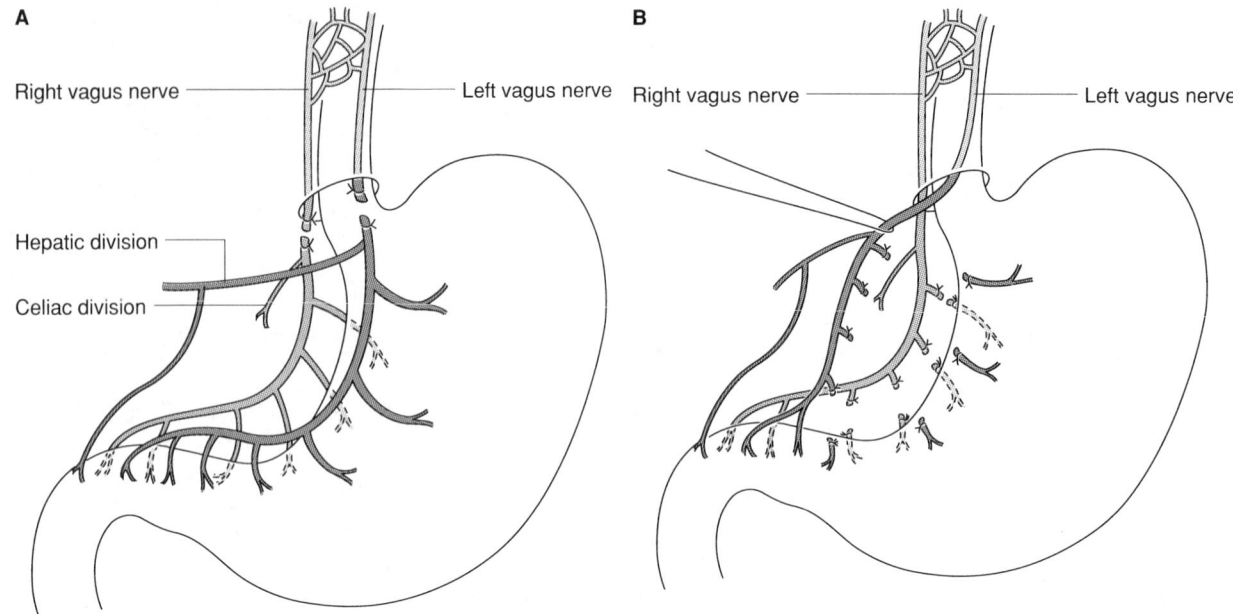

Figure 22-2. Truncal vagotomy and proximal gastric vagotomy. (*A*) With truncal vagotomy, both nerve trunks are divided at the level of the diaphragmatic hiatus. (*B*) Proximal gastric vagotomy involves division of the vagal fibers that supply the gastric fundus. Branches to the antropyloric region of the stomach are not transected, and the hepatic and celiac divisions of the vagus nerves remain intact.

action of pepsin. Sucralfate stimulates production of mucus, increases mucosal production of prostaglandin E_2, increases bicarbonate secretion, binds epidermal growth factor and may protect the mitogen from acid degradation, and stimulates epithelial proliferation at the ulcer margin. The drug has almost no buffering capability. Virtually no systemic absorption occurs. Because of this property, sucralfate is recommended for pregnant women.

Sucralfate promotes healing of acute duodenal ulcers. When the drug is administered at a dose of 1 g four times a day, >80% of ulcers heal within 6 weeks, a rate roughly equivalent to that achieved with H_2-receptor antagonists. Pain is relieved less quickly with sucralfate than with antisecretory drugs. The side effects of sucralfate are infrequent and mild; constipation is the most frequent. The lack of systemic absorption and the low incidence of side effects make sucralfate attractive for long-term maintenance therapy.

Prostaglandin Analogues

Prostaglandins are 20-carbon oxygenated fatty acids synthesized from fatty acids through the action of cyclooxygenase. They are cytoprotective and, at higher doses, also have an antisecretory action. Antisecretory doses are required to heal ulcers.

Misoprostol, the most widely used prostaglandin analogue, heals duodenal ulcers in > 60% of patients after 4 weeks of treatment when administered in 200-mg doses four times a day. Misoprostol and H_2-receptor antagonists have comparable efficacy in healing acute duodenal ulcers.

The worst side effect of prostaglandin derivatives is diarrhea. In most patients, diarrhea stops even though drug administration is continued. Uterine bleeding has been reported in some women who take the drug, which also may be an abortifacient.

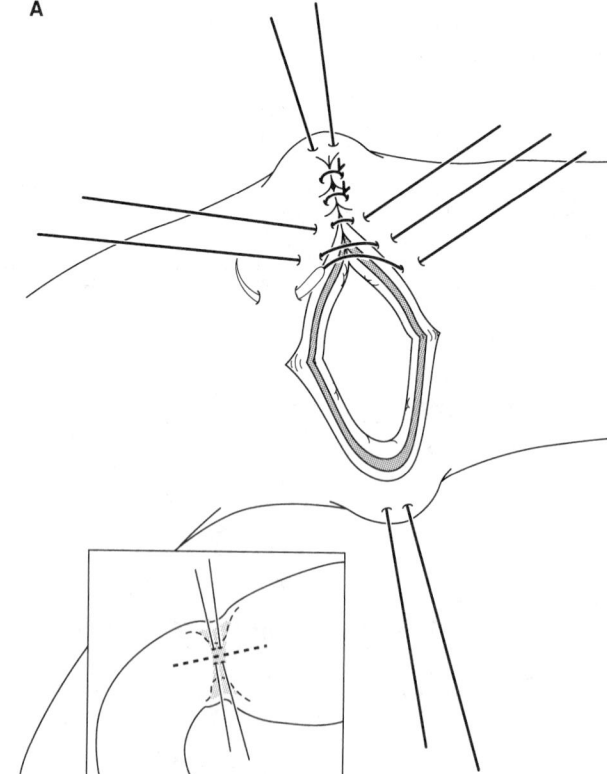

Figure 22-3. Pyloroplasty formation. A Heineke-Mikulicz pyloroplasty (*A*) involves a longitudinal incision of the pyloric sphincter followed by a transverse closure. The Finney pyloroplasty (*B*) is performed as a gastroduodenostomy with division of the pylorus. The Jaboulay pyloroplasty (*C*) differs from the Finney procedure in that the pylorus is not transected. *(continues)*

Antacids

Compounds that effectively suppress acid production have greatly reduced the need for antacids in the treatment of acute ulcers. Properly used, however, antacids can be effective in healing ulcers. Intensive treatment with antacids (30 mL of liquid antacid seven times a day, providing about 1000 mEq of buffer) heals ulcers in 78% of patients within 4 weeks. In spite of this high rate of healing, the large and frequent doses are unacceptable to many patients, and many patients experience diarrhea during such a regimen. More palatable alternatives include low-dose antacid therapy (<200 mmol/day) and the use of antacids as supplements to other acid-suppressive agents.

Antimicrobial Therapy

The realization that *Helicobacter pylori* infection is important in ulcer pathogenesis led to the development of antimicrobial therapy for ulcers. Single-, double-, and triple-agent regimens have been used. Triple therapy with bismuth (colloidal bismuth subsalicylate or colloidal bismuth subcitrate), metronidazole, and tetracycline or amoxicillin eradicates *H pylori* in 90% of patients. Inclusion of an H_2-receptor antagonist or omeprazole appears to increase the efficacy of antimicrobial therapy. Antimicrobial therapy is recommended for peptic ulcer disease resistant to conventional therapy, including relapses during maintenance therapy and ulcers that do not heal with H_2-receptor antagonist or omeprazole therapy.

SURGICAL TREATMENT

Surgical intervention is reserved for the treatment of complicated ulcer disease. Four complications are the classic indications for peptic ulcer operations—intractability, hemorrhage, perforation, and obstruction. The goals of surgical therapy are as follows:

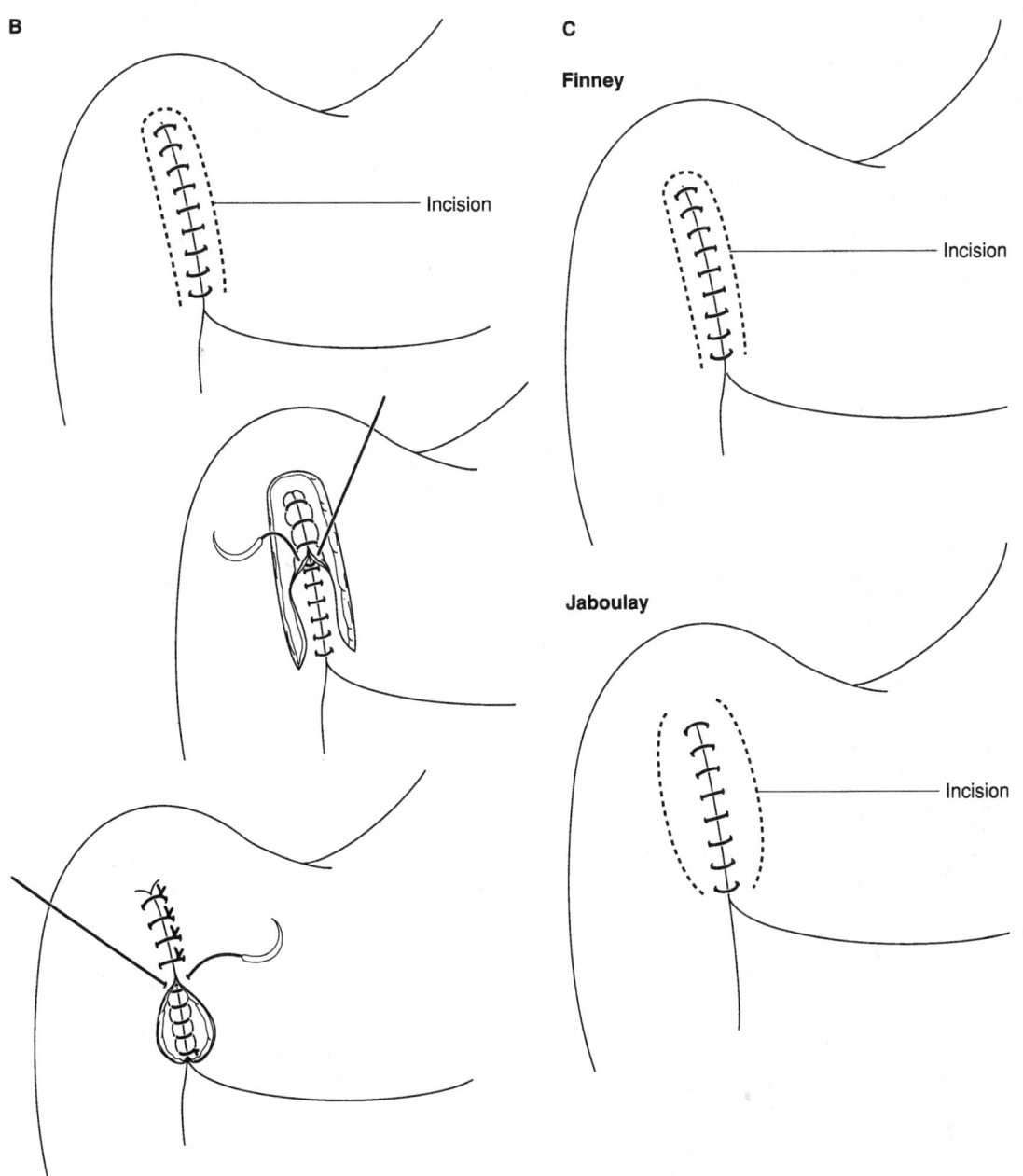

Figure 22-3. (Continued)

1. To alter the ulcer diathesis to achieve ulcer healing and minimize the risk of recurrence
2. To treat coexisting anatomic complications, such as pyloric stenosis or perforation
3. To protect the patient from chronic side effects

Surgical Procedures

Three procedures—truncal vagotomy and drainage, truncal vagotomy and antrectomy, and proximal gastric vagotomy—are the operations most widely used to treat peptic ulcers. Division of both vagal trunks at the esophageal hiatus—truncal vagotomy—denervates the acid-producing fundic mucosa and the remaining vagally supplied viscera (Fig. 22-2).

Truncal Vagotomy with Pyloroplasty

Because denervation impedes normal pyloric contraction and may impair gastric emptying, truncal vagotomy must be combined with a procedure to eliminate function of the pyloric sphincter. Gastric drainage is assured by a pyloroplasty (Fig. 22-3).

Truncal Vagotomy with Antrectomy

Truncal vagotomy may be combined with resection of the gastric antrum to effect further reduction in acid secretion, presumably by removing antral sources of gastrin. The limits of antral resection are usually defined by external landmarks, rather than the histologic transition from fundic to antral mucosa. The stomach is divided proximally along a line from a point above the incisura angularis to a point along the greater curvature midway from the pylorus to the gastroesophageal junction. Restoration of gastrointestinal (GI) continuity by a gastroduodenostomy is called a Billroth I reconstruction. A Billroth II procedure uses a gastrojejunostomy (Fig 22-4).

Proximal Gastric Vagotomy

Proximal gastric vagotomy (PGV) differs from truncal vagotomy in that only the nerve fibers to the acid-secreting fundic mucosa are divided. Vagal nerve fibers to the antrum and pylorus are left intact, and the hepatic and celiac divisions are not transected. Denervation begins about 5 cm from the pylorus and extends proximally along the lesser curvature. In PGV, the distal esophagus is skeletonized for 5 to 7 cm to divide any vagal fibers to the fundus running intramurally within the esophagus. The operation also has been called parietal cell vagotomy.

Physiologic Consequences of Surgical Therapy

Division of efferent vagal fibers affects acid secretion by reducing cholinergic stimulation of parietal cells. Vagotomy also diminishes parietal cell responsiveness to gastrin and histamine. Basal acid secretion is reduced by about 80% in the immediate postoperative period. Basal acid secretion increases slightly within months of the operation but remains unchanged thereafter. The maximal acid output (MAO) in response to exogenously administered stimulants, such as pentagastrin, is reduced by about 70% soon after the operation. After 1 year, pentagastrin-stimulated MAO rebounds to 50% of prevagotomy values but remains at this level. Acid secretion due to endogenous stimulation by a liquid meal is reduced 60% to 70% relative to normal values. The acid-reducing properties of PGV and truncal vagotomy are roughly equivalent (Table 22-2).

Truncal vagotomy and PGV both cause postoperative hypergastrinemia. Fasting gastrin values are elevated to

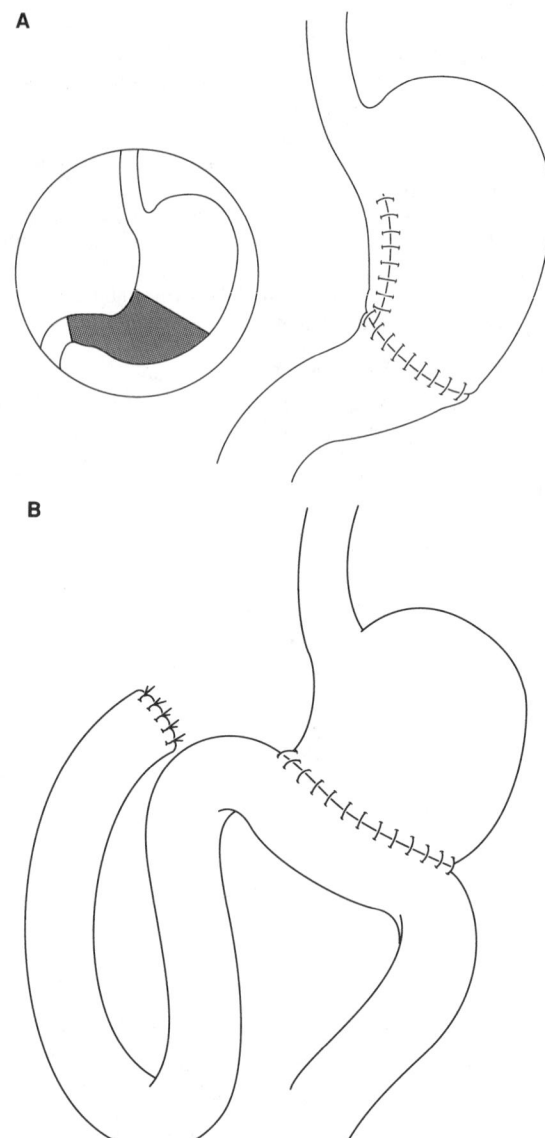

Figure 22-4. Antrectomy involves resection of the distal stomach (*blue area in inset*). Restoration of gastrointestinal continuity may be accomplished as a Billroth I gastroduodenostomy (*A*) or Billroth II gastrojejunostomy (*B*) reconstruction.

about twice preoperative levels, and the postprandial response is exaggerated. Immediately after vagotomy, hypergastrinemia appears to be caused by a decrease in luminal acid with loss of feedback inhibition of gastrin release. Chronic hypergastrinemia is caused by gastrin cell hyperplasia and loss of inhibitory feedback. When antrectomy is added to vagotomy, circulating gastrin levels decrease, basal gastrin levels are reduced by about half, and postprandial gastrin levels by about two-thirds.

PGV denervation abolishes vagally mediated receptive relaxation. When food is ingested, the increase in intragastric pressure is greater and the gastroduodenal pressure gradient is higher than in normal GI tracts. As a result, emptying of liquids, which depends on the gastroduodenal pressure gradient, is accelerated after PGV. Emptying of solids, however, is nearly normal because nerve fibers to the antrum and pylorus are retained, preserving the ability of the distal stomach to mix and grind solid food.

Table 22-2. PHYSIOLOGIC ALTERATIONS CAUSED BY TRUNCAL VAGOTOMY

GASTRIC EFFECTS

Decreased basal acid output
  Reduced cholinergic input to parietal cells
Decreased stimulated maximal acid output
  Diminished sensitivity to histamine gastrin
  Decreased meal-induced acid secretion
Increased fasting and postprandial gastrin
Gastrin cell hyperplasia
Accelerated liquid emptying
Altered emptying of solids

NONGASTRIC EFFECTS

Decreased pancreatic exocrine secretion
  Decreased pancreatic enzymes and bicarbonate
Decreased postprandial bile flow
Increased gallbladder volumes
Diminished release of vagally mediated peptide hormones

Truncal vagotomy affects the motor activities of both proximal and distal stomach. Solid and liquid emptying rates are usually increased when truncal vagotomy is accompanied by pyloroplasty.

Truncal vagotomy affects a number of other GI functions. These extragastric alterations in digestive function usually are subclinical. PGV, in which the vagal innervation to nongastric viscera is preserved, produces fewer physiologic alterations than truncal vagotomy.

TREATMENT OF COMPLICATED ULCER DISEASE

Intractability

Most patients believe the most important aspect of ulcer treatment is pain relief. Pain relief, however, should not be equated with complete healing of ulcers. Intractability, therefore, is defined as mucosal damage refractory to drug treatment. Ulcers are considered intractable if they meet any of the following criteria:

1. The ulcer persists >3 months despite active drug therapy
2. The ulcer recurs within 1 year after initial healing despite maintenance therapy
3. The ulcer disease is characterized by cycles of prolonged activity with brief remissions

Intractability is an indication for surgical therapy. With agents such as omeprazole, pain relief can be achieved by as many as 90% of patients within 2 weeks of beginning therapy; so pain is infrequently a motive for surgical intervention.

Intractable ulcers are treated with PGV. Permanent symptoms of dumping are rare after PGV, and reoperation is rarely needed for symptoms that result from the operation. The low incidence of postoperative symptoms is obtained at the cost of a high ulcer recurrence rate, about 10%. This rate is similar to that after truncal vagotomy and drainage, but considerably higher than that after truncal vagotomy and antrectomy.

Hemorrhage

Hemorrhage is the leading cause of death due to peptic ulcer. The incidence of hemorrhage has not changed since the introduction of H2-receptor antagonists. Most hemorrhage occurs during the initial episode of ulceration or during a relapse. Patients who have had hemorrhages have a high risk of rebleeding. Patients with recurrent hemorrhage and elderly patients are at greatest risk of dying, and these two groups should be resuscitated vigorously, examined promptly, and treated aggressively.

Upper GI endoscopy is the initial diagnostic test when there is evidence of hemorrhage from a duodenal ulcer. An ulcer should be accepted as the bleeding source only if it has one of the following endoscopic signs of active or recurrent hemorrhage:

Signs of Active Hemorrhage
- Arterial jet
- Active oozing
- Oozing beneath an adherent clot

Signs of Recurrent Hemorrhage
- Adherent clot without oozing
- Adherent slough within the ulcer base
- Visible vessel within the ulcer

The ability of these findings to predict recurrent hemorrhage is controversial, so these signs cannot be used alone as indications for an operation. They are warnings that aggressive therapy is needed, and close follow-up therapy is mandatory.

Endoscopic Therapy

The ability to visualize bleeding duodenal ulcers with endoscopy has led to attempts to treat hemorrhage endoscopically. The most established method is thermal coagulation. An NIH Consensus Development Conference has recommended endoscopic hemostatic therapy for patients >60 years with hemodynamic instability, the need for continual transfusions, red stool or hematemesis, and a serious comorbid condition. Failure of endoscopic hemostasis is usually due to scarring, rapid active bleeding, or an adherent clot.

Surgical Therapy

Surgical intervention is appropriate for massive hemorrhage that causes shock, prolonged blood loss that necessitates continual transfusions, recurrent bleeding during medical therapy or after endoscopic therapy, and recurrent hemorrhage that necessitates hospitalization. Surgical therapy consists of duodenotomy with direct ligation of the bleeding vessel within the ulcer base, followed by a procedure to effect a permanent reduction in acid production, such as truncal vagotomy with pyloroplasty or truncal vagotomy and antrectomy.

Perforation

Perforation of a duodenal ulcer is usually accompanied by sudden and severe epigastric pain. The pain, caused when highly caustic gastric secretions spill onto the peritoneum, rapidly reaches peak intensity and remains constant. Radiation to the right scapular region is common. Pain may be sensed in the lower abdomen if gastric contents travel caudally through the paracolic gutter. Peritoneal irritation is usually intense, and most patients avoid movement to minimize discomfort.

Physical examination reveals a low-grade fever, diminished bowel sounds, and rigid abdominal muscles. Upright abdominal radiographs may reveal pneumoperitoneum. Upper GI contrast studies performed with water-soluble contrast material may be helpful if a pneumoperitoneum is not demonstrated but there is still evidence of perforation.

Perforation is usually an indication for operation. Laparotomy allows the opportunity to relieve intraperitoneal contamination and to permanently reduce acid production.

About two-thirds of patients with perforation have chronic symptoms and are at risk for recurrent disease. These patients should consider a definitive antiulcer operation if there is evidence of chronic ulcer, there has been no preoperative shock, there is no life-threatening illness, and the perforation has been present < 48 hours. If these criteria are not met, simple omental patching of the perforation with peritoneal débridement is usually safer than a definitive antiulcer operation. The antiulcer operation can be performed later.

Patients without antecedent symptoms also may be at risk for recurrent ulcers. After a recurrent ulcer is present for 5 to 6 years, the recurrence rates of acute perforation are similar to those of chronic disease. A definitive antiulcer operation should, therefore, be considered for patients with perforated acute ulcers.

PGV with patch closure of the perforation has been shown to be safe and effective in preventing ulcer relapse. Incorporation of the perforation as part of a pyloroplasty or resection of the site of perforation during antrectomy also may be combined with truncal vagotomy.

Obstruction

Gastric outlet obstruction may be acute or chronic in patients with duodenal ulcers. Acute obstruction is caused by edema and inflammation associated with ulcers in the pyloric channel and the first portion of the duodenum. Pyloric obstruction is suggested by recurrent vomiting, dehydration, and hypochloremic alkalosis due to loss of gastric secretions. Acute obstruction is treated by intravenous administration of antisecretory agents. It usually resolves within 72 hours. Repeated episodes of ulceration and healing may lead to pyloric scarring and fixed stenosis with chronic gastric outlet obstruction.

Upper GI endoscopy is used to confirm the nature of the obstruction and to exclude neoplasia. Endoscopic hydrostatic balloon dilation of the pyloric stenosis may be attempted at this time. Only about 40% of patients, however, have improvement that lasts longer than 3 months after dilation. Recurrent stenosis appears to be caused by scarring within the pyloric channel.

The surgical treatment of gastric outlet obstruction should address the underlying ulcer disease and relieve the anatomic abnormality. Truncal vagotomy with antrectomy or truncal vagotomy with drainage is performed.

SUGGESTED READING

Ateshkadi A, Iam NP, Johnson CA. Helicobacter pylori and peptic ulcer disease. Clin Pharmacol 1993;12:34.

Glise H. Epidemiology in peptic ulcer disease: current status and future aspects. Scand J Gastroenterol 1990;25(suppl) 175:13.

Goh P, Tekant Y. Endoscopic hemostasis of bleeding peptic ulcers. Dig Dis 1993;11:216.

Labenz J, Gyenes E, Ruhl GH, Borsch G. Amoxicillin plus omeprazole versus triple therapy for eradication of Helicobacter pylori in duodenal ulcer disease; a prospective, randomized, controlled study. Gut 1993;34:1167.

Lamers CBHW, Bijlstra AM, Harris AG. Ocreotide, a long-acting somatostatin analog, in the management of postoperative dumping syndrome. Dig Dis Sci 1993;38:359.

Massoomi F, Savage J, Destache CJ. Omeprazole: a comprehensive review. Pharmacotherapy 1993;13:46.

Netchvolodoff CV. Refractory peptic lesions. Postgrad Med 1993;93:143.

Soll A. Pathogenesis of peptic ulcer and implications for therapy. N Engl J Med 1990; 32:909.

ESSENTIALS OF SURGERY: SCIENTIFIC PRINCIPLES AND PRACTICE, edited by Lazar J. Greenfield, Michael W. Mulholland, Keith T. Oldham, Gerald B. Zelenock, and Keith D. Lillemoe. Lippincott–Raven Publishers, Philadelphia, © 1997.

CHAPTER 23

STRESS ULCER AND GASTRIC ULCER

GORDON L. KAUFFMAN, JR., AND ROBERT L. CONTER

GASTRIC MUCOSAL DEFENSE

Stress gastritis and gastric ulcers originate with damage to the surface epithelium caused by alterations or defects in mucosal defense factors. Gastric mucosal barrier function is compromised by the presence in the gastric lumen of substances, such as acetylsalicylic acid (ASA), bile acids, ethanol, or lysolecithin, that allow protons to diffuse from lumen to mucosa. When the protons flow into the mucosa, sodium, water, glucose, and protein move from mucosa to lumen. With the change in permeability, histamine is released into the mucosa, enhancing blood flow. The result is mucosal damage with gross hemorrhage.

STRESS GASTRITIS

The causes of stress gastritis are well-defined. Acute stress gastritis occurs after physical trauma, shock, sepsis, hemorrhage, respiratory failure, severe burns (Curling ulcer), or central nervous system disease (Cushing ulcer). Predisposing factors are listed in Table 23-1. Increased gastric acid secretion is probably not the cause of stress gastritis, but acid must be present in the lumen for this form of gastritis to occur.

Definition of Lesions

Early Lesions

Occur within 24 hours of the precipitating event
Begin in the proximal stomach, only rarely occur in the antrum

Table 23-1. PREDISPOSING FACTORS FOR STRESS GASTRITIS

GASTRIC CONDITIONS

Luminal acid secretion
Mucosal permeability
Mucosal blood flow
Mucus and bicarbonate production
Epithelial cell renewal
Endogenous prostaglandins
Systemic acid–base status

CLINICAL CONDITIONS

Multiple trauma
Hypotension
Sepsis
Adult respiratory distress syndrome
Major burn
Oliguric renal failure
Hepatic dysfunction
Prolonged surgical procedures
Massive transfusion requirements
Extended intensive care stay

Multiple, shallow, discrete (1 to 2 mm) areas of erythema with focal hemorrhage or an adherent clot

Frank bleeding only after the gastric mucosa has eroded into the submucosa

Central area of pallor sometimes surrounded by erythema rather than intramucosal bleeding, suggesting ischemia and reperfusion

No fibrosis or scarring

Histologic features

Wedged-shaped mucosal hemorrhages with coagulation necrosis of the superficial mucosal cells

Surface epithelium may be intact, and scattered leukocytes may be present within lamina propria (nonaggressive form)

Pronounced inflammatory cellular infiltrate and coagulation necrosis may be present (aggressive form)

Late Lesions

Present 24 to 72 hours after injury

Tissue reaction, organization around a clot, or inflammatory exudate

Appearance identical to that of regenerating mucosa around a healing gastric ulcer

Histologic features

Hemorrhage, inflammatory cell infiltration, and coagulation necrosis extending into muscularis mucosae

Presentation and Diagnosis

Hemorrhaging usually begins 3 to 10 days after the precipitating event. Painless upper GI bleeding may be the only clinical sign, presenting as only a few flecks of blood in the nasogastric tube or an unexplained drop in hematocrit. The bleeding is slow and intermittent, but it can be rapid, heralded by hypotension and hematemesis. Guaiac-positive stools are usually found early.

Esophagogastroduodenoscopy confirms the diagnosis and differentiates stress erosion from other sources of upper GI hemorrhage. If endoscopy is not diagnostic, visceral angiography through selective catheterization of the left gastric or splenic vessels may identify the vessel supplying the bleeding site. Barium radiographs are of little value. They also interfere with the interpretation of arteriograms.

Medical Treatment

Hypovolemic shock is corrected with whole blood replacement. Clotting abnormalities are corrected with fresh-frozen plasma, platelets, or both. The source of sepsis is identified, and antibiotics accompany surgical drainage of the septic focus. Initial efforts to control gastric hemorrhage include gastric saline lavage and nasogastric decompression.

Once acute bleeding has stopped, the pH of gastric fluid is kept >5.0 with antacids, H_2-receptor antagonists, omeprazole, or combination therapy. Antacids and H_2-receptor blocking agents are ineffective in the presence of active GI bleeding, so they are not used for definitive therapy. Because of the high mortality associated with active hemorrhage from acute lesions, patients at high risk for stress gastritis are given prophylactic treatment (Table 23-2).

An angiographic technique can be tried to control acute bleeding. In selective angiographic catheterization of the gastric vessels, vasopressin is infused into the splanchnic circulation via the left gastric artery. Another technique, transcatheter embolization with gelatin foam, metal coils, or autologous blood clot, is probably not feasible because

Table 23-2. MEDICAL PROPHYLAXIS FOR STRESS GASTRITIS

Agent	Efficacy (%)
Antacid	>96
H_2 antagonists	>97
Sucralfate	96–100
Prostaglandins	<50

of the extensive plexus of submucosal arteries in the stomach.

Surgical Therapy

Ten percent to 20% of acute stress ulcers continue to bleed, or bleeding recurs despite aggressive medical therapy. A definitive operation controls bleeding and carries the lowest possible mortality and rate of recurrent hemorrhage. The following procedures fulfill these requirements: vagotomy and drainage, vagotomy and antrectomy, vagotomy and subtotal gastrectomy, total gastric resection, gastric devascularization, or vagotomy and pyloroplasty with oversewing of isolated, actively bleeding erosions. Vagotomy with partial gastrectomy or gastric devascularization may be appropriate for patients with diffuse mucosal bleeding. For patients with massive, life-threatening hemorrhage, total gastrectomy may be the only choice.

GASTRIC ULCER

Definition of Lesion

It is often impossible to differentiate between gastric carcinoma and benign gastric ulcer based solely upon symptoms. A classic gastric ulcer is a circular area devoid of mucosa, has a fibrous base, and is lined by granulation tissue.

Barium Radiographic Signs of Benign Ulcer
- A radiolucent line, usually about 1 mm wide, that partially or completely traverses the orifice of an ulcer
- Mucosal folds that radiate to the edge of the ulcer crater
- Spasm of gastric circular muscles on the gastric wall opposite the ulcer

Barium Radiographic Signs of Malignant Tumor
- Demonstration of a tumor in the vicinity of the ulcer or a mass with central ulceration
- Abnormal mucosal folds near the base of the crater or folds that are interrupted near the ulcer
- A nodular or irregularly shaped ulcer base

Some patients with gastric carcinoma do not have obvious ulcers on radiographs but present with a nondistensible stomach indicative of diffusely spreading carcinoma (linitis plastica).

Endoscopic Identification

Upper GI endoscopy is used to diagnose gastric ulcers. Benign ulcers can de differentiated from malignant ulcers with examination of the ulcer base, the margin of the crater, the relation of the margin to the surrounding mucosal folds, and the size of the ulcer. Ulcers <1 cm in diameter are associated with only a 5% risk for malignancy.

- Endoscopic Features of Benign Gastric Ulcers

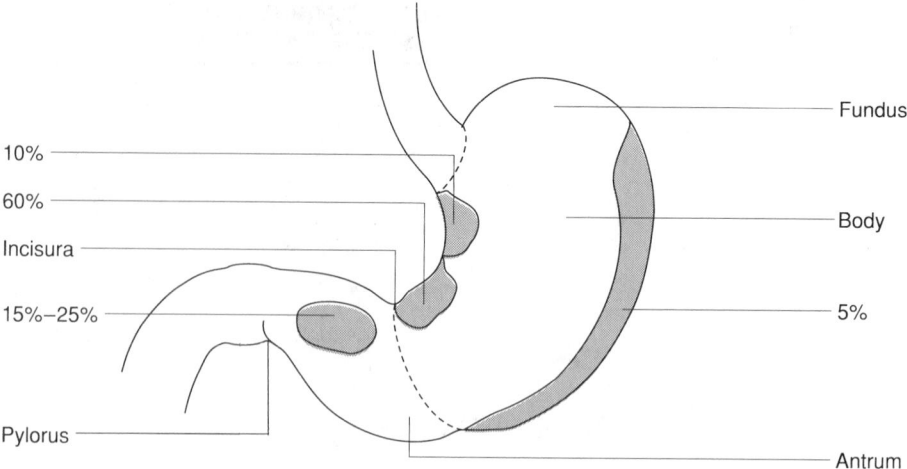

Figure 23-1. Location of gastric ulcers.

- Base—smooth, flat, covered by a gray-to-white fibrinous exudate
- Crater—round or oval, but may be linear
- Margin—slightly raised, erythematous, smooth
- Mucosal folds—symmetric and taper smoothly to the edge of the ulcer

Histologic Appearance

A gastric ulcer extends through the muscularis mucosae. Healing depends on the migration of adjacent mucosal cells to cover the defect. Histologic appearance varies. Active ulcers have four histologic zones:

1. The base of the ulcer, which is covered with a thin layer of fibrinous material
2. A region of intense cellular (neutrophil) infiltrate immediately under the base
3. A region of active granulation tissue characterized by a mononuclear leukocytic infiltrate
4. A region of fibrous or collagenous scar in the deepest tissue

Location

Gastric ulcers can occur anywhere in the stomach, although they usually occur on the lesser curvature near the incisura angularis (Fig. 23-1). Most ulcers on the greater curvature prove to be benign. Gastric ulcers are classified by location and gastric acid secretory status (Table 23-3; Figs. 23-2 through 23-5).

Incidence

The incidence of gastric ulcer varies widely throughout the world. In the United States, gastric ulcer is more common in men and elderly people than women and young people. Gastric ulcers rarely develop before the age of 40 years; the peak incidence is 55 to 65 years. Predisposing factors are listed in Table 23-4.

Associated Factors

Acid and Pepsin Secretion

The role of acid and pepsin secretion in the pathogenesis of gastric ulcer is not clear. Although the presence of acid is essential to the production of gastric ulcer, the amount secreted is not important. Pepsin secretion usually parallels acid secretion. The luminal concentration of pepsin may be elevated in patients with gastric ulcers.

Gastric Motility

Alterations in gastric motility may contribute to the formation of gastric ulcers. Gastric stasis with antral food retention may cause increased gastrin release and acid secretion. Delayed gastric emptying may prevent clearing of refluxed duodenal contents. Other motility defects include an incompetent pyloric sphincter mechanism, presence of prominent muscle bands near the incisura, alterations in the migrating motor complex, prolonged high-amplitude gastric contractions, and chronic mesenteric ischemia with resultant gastroparesis.

Gastritis

Chronic superficial and atrophic gastritis are associated with gastric ulcer. It is not known whether the ulcer or the gastritis occurs first. The greater the extent of gastritis, the more proximal is the ulcer.

Infection

A direct cause-and-effect relationship between peptic ulcer disease and Helicobacter pylori colonization has not been established, but circumstantial evidence is convincing. *H pylori* is present in most patients with gastric or duodenal ulcers. Colonization with *H. pylori* is confirmed at histologic evaluation of endoscopically obtained biopsy

Table 23-3. CLASSIFICATION OF GASTRIC ULCERS

Type	Location	Acid Secretory Status
I	Gastric body, usually lesser curvature	Low
II	Gastric body, in association with duodenal ucler	High
III	Prepyloric region	High
IV	High on lesser curvature	High
V	Anywhere in stomach	*

* Result of chronic ingestion of ASA or nonsteroidal anti-inflammatory drugs (NSAIDs).

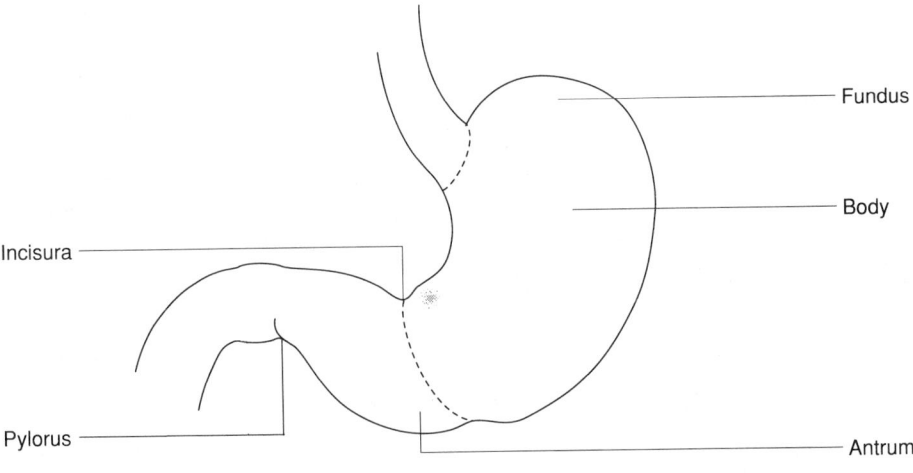

Type I Gastric Ulcer
Gastric body usually lesser curvature
Normal or low acid secretion
Hemorrhage infrequent, penetration common
Blood group A

Figure 23-2. Location of type I gastric ulcer with associated conditions.

specimens or with a culture, the former having a greater sensitivity and specificity. Another technique is the urea breath test. Enzyme-linked immunosorbent assay (ELISA) is the most frequently used serologic test. Antimicrobial therapy reduces recurrence rates of gastric ulcers in patients whose antrum is colonized by *H pylori*.

Intraarterial Chemotherapy

Gastric and duodenal ulcers occur in some patients who receive hepatic arterial infusion chemotherapy, usually 5-fluorouracil as a single agent or in combination with cisplatin, doxorubicin, and mitomycin C. These chemotherapeutic agents may have a direct toxic effect on the nutrient side of the gastric mucosa, because symptoms improve when chemotherapy is suspended.

Natural History

Gastric ulcers have recurrent cycles of healing and relapse. Ulcers that recur usually do so in the area of the initial ulcer. In addition to causing pain, gastric ulcers may bleed, obstruct, or perforate. Perforation is the most frequent complication. Most perforations occur along the anterior or anterosuperior aspect of the lesser curvature. The older the patient, the higher is the perforation, the larger is the ulcer, and the greater are the associated morbidity and mortality.

Hemorrhaging from gastric ulcers occurs in older patients, is less likely to stop, and carries a higher morbidity and mortality than bleeding from duodenal ulcers. Hemorrhage occurs most frequently with types II and III ulcers, but patients with type IV ulcers may present with massive, life-threatening hemorrhage.

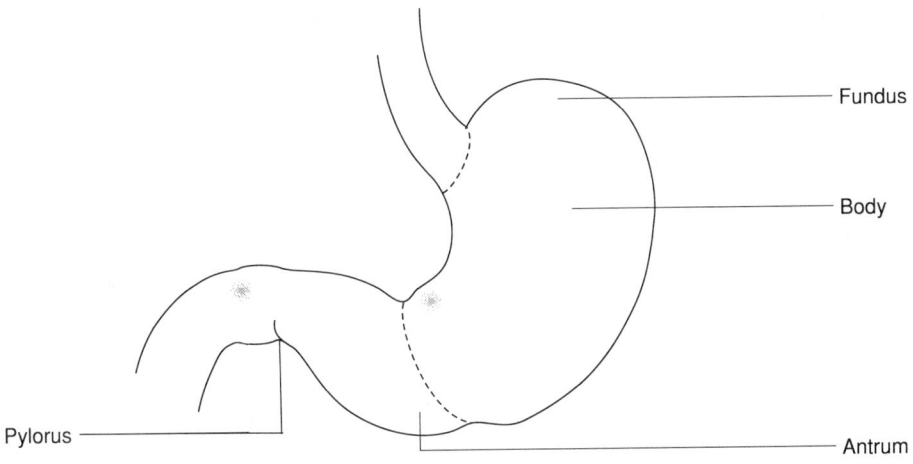

Type II Gastric Ulcer
Gastric body and duodenal ulcer
Hypersecretion of acid
Hemorrhage, obstruction, and perforation frequent
Blood group O

Figure 23-3. Location of type II gastric ulcer with associated conditions.

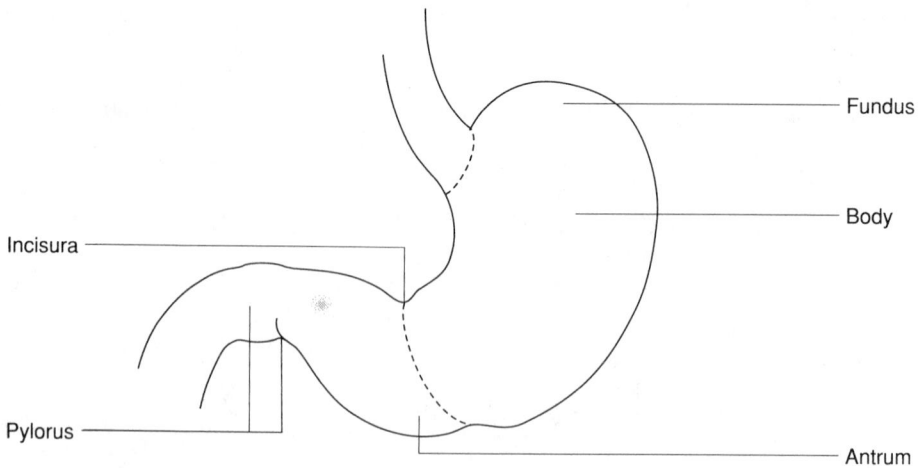

Type III Gastric Ulcer
Prepyloric
Hypersecretor of acid
Hemorrhage and perforation frequent
Blood group O

Figure 23-4. Location of type III gastric ulcer with associated conditions.

Gastric outlet obstruction is most common in patients with a type II or III gastric ulcer. Benign obstruction must be differentiated from antral carcinoma. Type I ulcers may interfere with gastric motility but usually do not cause obstruction.

Presentation

The symptoms of chronic gastric ulcer include gnawing, dull, or burning abdominal pain localized to the midline or the left upper quadrant. Pain may be aggravated or precipitated by the ingestion of food. Other reported symptoms of gastric ulcer include nausea, vomiting, anorexia, and weight loss. Patients may not eat because they fear postprandial symptoms. Physical examination may show epigastric tenderness. Laboratory studies usually are normal.

Acute gastric ulcers may present with either hemorrhage or perforation. It is unusual for an acute ulcer to present with obstruction. Asymptomatic or silent ulcers may be discovered in elderly patients with no history of ulcer disease; these ulcers may be severe and life-threatening in patients taking NSAIDs.

Diagnosis

History and physical examination may be of limited value in differentiating gastric from duodenal ulcers. The two principal means of diagnosing gastric ulcers are upper GI radiography and fiberoptic endoscopy. Ninety percent

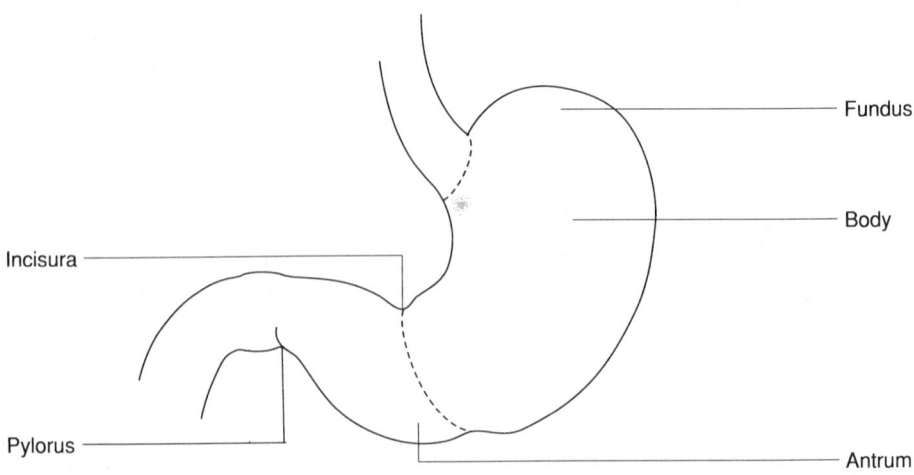

Type IV Gastric Ulcer
High on lesser curvature
Low acid secretion
Hemorrhage common, penetration frequent
Blood group O

Figure 23-5. Location of type IV gastric ulcer with associated conditions.

Table 23-4. PREDISPOSING FACTORS FOR GASTRIC ULCER

GASTRIC CONDITIONS
Acid and pepsin
Gastric stasis
Coexisting duodenal ulcer
Duodenogastric reflux
Gastritis
Infection with *Helicobacter pylori*

CLINICAL CONDITIONS
Chronic alcohol use
Nonsteroidal antiinflammatory drugs
Smoking
Long-term corticosteroid therapy
Infection
Intraarterial chemotherapy

of gastric ulcers are diagnosed accurately with contrast radiography. About 5% of ulcers that benign appear on radiographs are malignant.

Gastroscopy is the most reliable method of diagnosing a gastric ulcer. Clinical features that prompt early endoscopic evaluation include weight loss, symptoms of gastric outlet obstruction, a palpable abdominal mass, guaiac-positive stools, and blood-loss anemia. Endoscopic features that suggest a malignant lesion include an exophytic mass, abnormal or disrupted mucosal folds, a necrotic ulcer crater, bleeding from the edge of the ulcer crater, a stepwise depression of the ulcer edge, heaped-up margins, or small extensions of the ulcer that blur a portion of the ulcer wall. If biopsies do not demonstrate malignant cells but the endoscopic appearance suggests a carcinoma under the ulcer, endoscopy is repeated to obtain deeper biopsy specimens.

Medical Therapy

Medical therapy for gastric ulcer is summarized in Table 23-5.

Antacids

The larger the gastric ulcer, the longer are antacids required for healing. The frequent dosing and unpleasant side effects, such as diarrhea, constipation, and alkalosis, associated with prolonged antacid use may decrease patient compliance.

Histamine-Receptor Antagonists

H_2-receptor antagonists are the most commonly prescribed antisecretory drugs used to treat benign gastric ulcers. The five H_2-receptor antagonists—cimetidine, ranitidine, famotidine, nizatidine, and roxatidine—appear to be equally effective in healing. Gastric ulcer healing rates are >80% after 8 weeks of therapy with these agents.

Omeprazole

Omeprazole appears to produce rapid symptomatic relief and healing and promotes healing of gastric ulcers in patients who continue to use NSAIDs.

Anticholinergics

Pirenzepine and telenzepine block acid secretion to a greater extent than they inhibit cardiac, smooth muscle, and salivary gland function. The efficacy of pirenzepine approximates that of the H_2-receptor antagonists in gastric ulcer healing. Although healing rates are lower than for duodenal ulcers, these drugs appear to be as effective as cimetidine in the treatment of gastric ulcers.

Sucralfate

Sucralfate heals gastric ulcers as effectively as cimetidine.

Prostaglandins

Prostaglandins A, E, and I are produced by the gastric and duodenal mucosa. In addition to their antisecretory effects, they protect the mucosa. Prostaglandin analogues include rioprostil, enprostil, arbaprostil, enisoprost, and trimoprostil. Prostaglandins are as effective as H_2-receptor antagonists for healing gastric ulcers.

Dietary Considerations

Dietary restrictions do not appear to enhance the healing rate of gastric ulcers. Patients are advised to avoid alcoholic beverages, chocolate, and fatty meals, which tend to decrease lower esophageal sphincter pressure and promote reflux of gastric acid into the esophagus. Patients are advised to stop smoking, not only because smoking decreases esophageal sphincter tone but also because it is associated with failure of medical therapy for gastric ulcer.

Treatment of *Helicobacter pylori* Infection

If *H. pylori* colonization is present, a triple-therapy regimen of bismuth subsalicylate, tetracycline, and metronidazole accompanies antisecretory therapy. Amoxicillin can be substituted for tetracycline or metronidazole with only a slight reduction in efficacy. Another regimen is ranitidine, metronidazole, and amoxycillin. The eradication rate is >90%; the ulcer recurrence rate after discontinuation of this therapy is 20%.

Treatment of NSAID-induced Mucosal Injury

The treatment of ulcers in patients taking NSAIDs is complicated because many of these ulcers are clinically silent and may not respond to standard therapy. The ideal medical therapy for NSAID-induced gastric mucosal injury is not clearly established, although synthetic prostaglandins appear to have a role in prevention and treatment. If possible, NSAIDs are discontinued, and the lesions heal rapidly once the agent is withdrawn. If NSAIDs cannot be discontinued, omeprazole or a synthetic prostaglandin is prescribed.

Table 23-5. MEDICAL TREATMENT OF GASTRIC ULCER

Agent	Mechanism of Action
Antacids	Neutralize gastric acidity and decrease activity of pepsin
H_2 antagonists	Block parietal cell H_2 receptor
Omeprazole	Inhibits H^+-K^+-ATPase pump
Anticholinergics	Block specific M_1 (muscarinic) receptor blocker in stomach wall
Sucralfate	Complexes with pepsin and bile salts and binds to proteins in mucosa
Prostaglandins	Inhibit acid secretion, increase endogenous mucosal defense

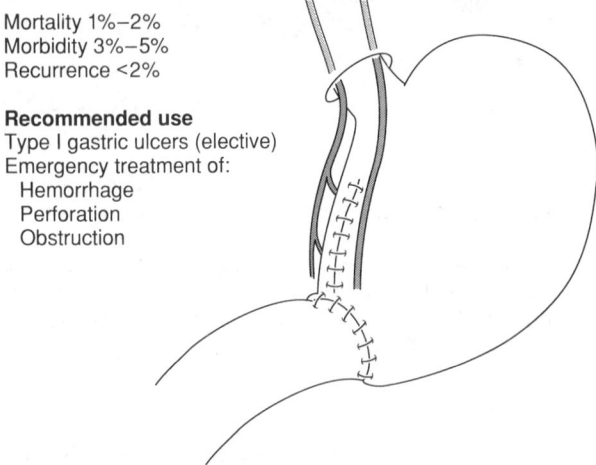

Mortality 1%–2%
Morbidity 3%–5%
Recurrence <2%

Recommended use
Type I gastric ulcers (elective)
Emergency treatment of:
  Hemorrhage
  Perforation
  Obstruction

Figure 23-6. Distal gastrectomy (without vagotomy), with associated morbidity, mortality, and recurrence rates, as well as indications.

Surgical Therapy

Surgical intervention allows for total excision of the ulcer for histologic evaluation and reduces gastric secretion.

- Indications
- Failure of a newly diagnosed ulcer to heal completely within 12 weeks of initiation of medical therapy
- Failure of a recurrent ulcer to respond to medical therapy or recurrence after two successful courses of initial treatment
- Inability to exclude malignant disease

Surgical Treatment of Type I Gastric Ulcers

Type I benign gastric ulcers are treated with elective distal gastrectomy with gastroduodenal (Billroth I) anastomosis (Fig. 23-6). Gastrojejunostomy (Billroth II) is an acceptable alternative, although this reconstruction is less physiological. The ulcer is included in the antrectomy specimen. Another operation for type I gastric ulcer is proximal gastric vagotomy (PGV) (highly selective or parietal cell vagotomy) with excision of the ulcer. Depending on the size of the ulcer and the degree of surrounding inflammation, excision of the ulcer may not be technically feasible.

Surgical Treatment of Type II Gastric Ulcers

Antrectomy that includes the gastric ulcer and truncal vagotomy are performed because the procedure reduces acid secretion and removes the gastric mucosa at risk for ulcer and the ulcer itself. Gastroduodenal reconstruction is performed. The type of reconstruction—gastroduodenostomy or gastrojejunostomy—depends on how badly the duodenum is inflamed. An alternative is truncal vagotomy and drainage alone. A third option is vagotomy and pyloroplasty.

Surgical Treatment of Type III Gastric Ulcers

Type III gastric ulcers are treated with vagotomy and antrectomy that includes the ulcer.

Surgical Treatment of Type IV Gastric Ulcers

Type IV ulcers are difficult to treat. The choice of operation depends on the size of the ulcer, the distance from the gastroesophageal junction, and the degree of surrounding inflammation. Whenever possible, the juxtaesophageal ul-

cer is excised. The most aggressive technique is a generous distal gastrectomy that includes a small portion of the esophageal wall and ulcer with a Roux-en-Y esophagogastrojejunostomy to restore continuity. A less aggressive procedure for type IV ulcers 2 to 5 cm from the gastroesophageal junction is distal gastric resection extended vertically to include the lesser curvature with the ulcer. After resection, intestinal continuity is restored with an end-to-end gastroduodenostomy.

Another approach is a transgastric approach to the juxtaesophageal gastric ulcer. The procedure requires an 8-cm gastrotomy over the anterior gastric wall parallel to and just below the esophagus. The left gastric vessels are ligated close to the stomach, and a generous wedge resection of the anterior and posterior walls of the lesser curvature is completed to include the ulcer. The defect is closed transversely, and a pyloroplasty is performed.

Surgical Treatment of Type V Gastric Ulcers

If a suspected type V ulcer does not heal rapidly with cessation of the offending agent and antisecretory therapy, the patient may have a malignant tumor. Except for perforation or unrelenting hemorrhage, chemically induced ulcers are not treated surgically.

Surgical Treatment of Complications of Gastric Ulcer

Hemorrhage and perforation are emergencies. Gastric outlet obstruction is treated with preoperative gastric decompression for several days, correction of fluid and electrolyte imbalance, and endoscopy with biopsies before surgical intervention. Definitive treatment of all complications corrects the emergency condition and prevents recurrent ulcers. Antrectomy that includes the ulcer and gastroduodenostomy meets this goal. For patients with life-threatening hemorrhage whose condition is unstable, vagotomy and pyloroplasty with suture ligation of the ulcer is an acceptable but less effective alternative. Multiple biopsy specimens are obtained to exclude the presence of malignant disease. For patients at extremely high risk, alternative procedures include vagotomy with excision of the ulcer or biopsy with simple closure of a perforated ulcer with an omental patch. Care must be taken to avoid gastric outlet obstruction at the site of the closure.

Although most instances of obstruction by a gastric ulcer can be treated with antrectomy and gastroduodenostomy, scarring may be so severe as to preclude safe anastomosis. If resection is performed but gastroduodenostomy is deemed risky, gastrojejunostomy is undertaken.

SUGGESTED READING

Craham DY, Smith JL. Gastroduodenal complications of chronic NSAID therapy. Am J Gastroenterol 1988;83:1081.

Emas S, Grupcev G, Eriksson B. Ten-year follow-up of a prospective, randomized trial of selective proximal vagotomy with ulcer excision and partial gastrectomy with gastroduodenostomy for treating corporal gastric ulcer. Am J Surg 1994; 167:596.

Forbes GM, Glaser ME, Cullins DJE. Duodenal ulcer treated with Helicobacter pylori eradication: seven year follow-up. Lancet 1994;343:258.

Herting RL, Nissen CH. Overview of misoprostil clinical experience. Dig Dis Sci 1986;31(Suppl):47S.

Marrone GO, Silen W. Pathogenesis, diagnosis and treatment of acute mucosal lesions. Clin Gastroenterol 1984;13:635.

Tryba N, Zeuvonou F, Torok M, et al. Prevention of acute stress bleeding with sucralfate, antacids or cimetidine: a controlled study with pirenzepine as a basic medication. Am J Med 1985;79(Suppl):21.

Walan A, Baclar JP, Classen M, et al. Effect of omeprazole and ranitidine on ulcer healing and relapse rates in patients with benign gastric ulcer. N Engl J Med 1989;320:69.

Zinner MJ, Zuidema GD, Smith PL, et al. The prevention of upper gastrointestinal tract bleeding in patients in an intensive care unit. Surg Gynecol Obstet 1981;153:214.

ESSENTIALS OF SURGERY: SCIENTIFIC PRINCIPLES AND PRACTICE, edited by Lazar J. Greenfield, Michael W. Mulholland, Keith T. Oldham, Gerald B. Zelenock, and Keith D. Lillemoe. Lippincott–Raven Publishers, Philadelphia, © 1997.

CHAPTER 24
MORBID OBESITY

HARVEY J. SUGERMAN

Morbid obesity is the degree of overweight clearly associated with increased disability and mortality (Fig. 24-1). Severe obesity (>100 lb. above ideal weight) is estimated to affect 4.9% (2.8 million) of men and 7.2% (4.5 million) of women in the United States. The causes of morbid obesity are unknown but probably include genetic factors, abnormalities of neural or humoral transmitters to the hypothalamic hunger or satiety centers, dysfunction of the hypothalamic centers themselves, and psychologically induced oral dependency drives. Morbidly obese adults have been found to have a lower basal energy expenditure than people of normal weight.

The large number of problems that cause morbid obesity are listed in Table 24-1. Many morbidly obese people suffer from severe psychologic and social disability. Premature death is common.

CENTRAL VERSUS PERIPHERAL OBESITY

Central obesity, in which excess fat is carried at the waist, is associated with a greater morbidity than peripheral obesity, in which excess fat is carried on the hips, thighs, and buttocks. This increased morbidity is caused by the increased metabolism of visceral fat, which leads to increased blood glucose levels, hyperglycemia, increased insulin secretion, insulin-induced sodium reabsorption, which leads to hypertension, and increased fatty acid and cholesterol turnover with an increased risk of atherosclerosis and gallstones. Another complication of central obesity is increased intra-abdominal pressure, which may cause venous stasis disease, gastroesophageal reflux, stress and urge urinary incontinence, obesity hypoventilation syndrome, nephrotic syndrome, incisional and inguinal hernia, and elevated pleural pressures, which can markedly increase pulmonary artery and pulmonary capillary wedge pressures, which may cause pseudotumor cerebri.

DIETARY MANAGEMENT OF MORBID OBESITY

Dietary programs for weight reduction include hospital-supervised programs, psychiatric behavior-modification programs, commercial organizations, commercial diets, protein-sparing fast programs, and diet pills provided by unscrupulous physicians. No dietary approach has achieved uniform, long-term success for morbidly obese people. Although many people can lose weight through

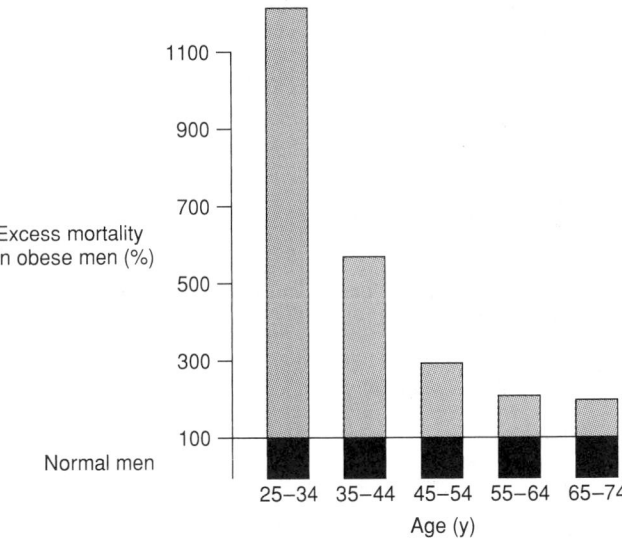

Figure 24-1. Percentage of excess probability of dying among morbidly obese men as computed for decades relative to mortality of US men as a whole. (After Drenick EJ, Bale GS, Seltter F, et al. Excessive mortality and causes of death in morbidly obese men. JAMA 1980;243:443)

dietary manipulation, almost 95% of morbidly obese people regain the weight they lose.

SURGICAL MANAGEMENT OF MORBID OBESITY
Surgical Eligibility

Patients are considered eligible for surgical treatment of obesity if they have a body mass index (BMI; weight [kg]/height [cm]^2) of ≥40 without comorbidity or a BMI of ≥35 with comorbidity (eg, diabetes, respiratory insufficiency, pseudotumor cerebri).

Jejunoileal Bypass

Because of the high complication rate, standard jejunoileal bypass should no longer be performed. Some surgeons believe that patients who have undergone the procedure should have jejunoileal bypasses reversed. If medical problems are severe (ie, progressive liver or renal dysfunction), a jejunoileal bypass can be reversed. Because these patients regain their lost weight, conversion to a gastric procedure for obesity may be considered unless the patient is too ill (ie, severe cirrhosis with portal hypertension).

Gastric Procedures for Morbid Obesity

Gastric operations are associated with weight loss comparable to jejunoileal bypass, and with less of a complication rate.

Gastroplasty

In gastroplasty, the stomach is stapled so that a small opening allows normal passage of food into the distal stomach and duodenum. Gastroplasties have been performed with either horizontal or vertical placement of the staples. Horizontal gastroplasty usually requires ligation and division of the short gastric vessels between the stomach and

Table 24-1. MORBIDITY ASSOCIATED WITH OBESITY

Cardiac dysfunction
   Cardiomegaly and impaired left ventricular function
   High cardiac output and low systemic vascular resistance
   Left ventricular hypertrophy and failure
   Coronary atherosclerosis
   Angina or myocardial infarction
   Hypoxemic pulmonary artery vasoconstriction, which may lead to
      right-sided heart failure
   Prolonged sinus arrest, premature ventricular contractions, and
      sudden death due to sleep apnea syndrome
Pulmonary dysfunction
   Obesity hypoventilation syndrome
   Obstructive sleep apnea syndrome
   A combination of the two (Pickwickian syndrome)
Non–insulin-dependent diabetes mellitus (Adult-onset, Type II)
   venous stasis disease
   Deep venous thrombosis
   Pulmonary embolism
   Stasis ulcers
Degenerative joint disease
Other conditions
   Gastroesophageal reflux
   Stress overflow urinary incontinence
Pseudotumor cerebri (benign intracranial hypertension)
Sexual dysfunction, infertility, hirsutism, ovarian cysts,
   hypermenorrhea, endometrial carcinoma.

spleen and carries the risk of devascularization of the gastric pouch or splenic injury. Horizontal gastroplasties include a single application of a 90-mm stapling device, without suture reinforcement of the opening between upper and lower gastric pouches, or a double application of staples with either a central or lateral polypropylene-reinforced stoma.

Vertical banded gastroplasty (VBGP) is a procedure in which a stapled opening is made in the stomach 5 cm from the cardioesophageal junction (Fig. 24-2). Two applications of a 90-mm stapling device are made between this opening and the angle of His, and a 1.5-cm by 5-cm strip of polypropylene mesh is wrapped around the stoma on the lesser curvature and sutured to itself, but not to the stomach. Erosion of the mesh into the stomach is an unusual complication of this procedure. Pouch enlarge-ment is much less likely to occur with a vertical staple line in the thicker, more muscular part of the stomach than in horizontal gastroplasty, and the stomal diameter is fixed with the mesh band. Vertical silicone-ring gastroplasty is a similar procedure (Fig. 24-3) in which a vertical staple line and silicone tubing reinforce the stoma. Weight loss with vertical silicone ring gastroplasty appears to be similar to that with VBGP. Use of the four-row parallel bariatric stapler has been associated with a 35% rate of staple-line disruption, leading to failure of the operative procedure. Some surgeons now recommend transecting the stomach.

Gastric Bypass

In gastric bypass the staples can be placed in a vertical or a horizontal direction. Vertical stapling is preferred because there is less risk of devascularization of the gastric pouch or splenic injury. Because of the high incidence of staple-line disruption, some surgeons recommend transecting the stomach for patients undergoing gastric bypass. However, with three superimposed applications of a 90-mm stapler, the incidence of staple-line disruption is <2%. The gastrojejunostomy used to drain the gastric pouch can be a loop, a loop with a jejunojejunostomy constructed below the gastrojejunostomy, or a Roux-en-Y limb. The latter two techniques prevent bile reflux into the gastric pouch. The length of the Roux-en-Y jejunal limb is usually 45 cm. Patients with a BMI of ≥50 have better weight loss with a 150-cm Roux limb (long-limb gastric bypass). The gastric pouch should be small (1 to 30 mL) and the stoma restricted to 1 cm (Fig. 24-4). The small gastric pouch has a limited volume of acid secretion and is associated with a low incidence of marginal ulcer in the absence of vagotomy.

Gastroplasty Versus Gastric Bypass

Roux-en-Y gastric bypass allows better weight loss than VBGP (Fig. 24-5). VBGP may be associated with severe gastroesophageal reflux, which resolves after the VGBP is converted to a gastric bypass. Patients who undergo gastric bypass have a higher incidence of stomal ulcer, stomal stenosis, vitamin B_{12} deficiency, and, in menstruating women, iron-deficiency anemia than do patients who have undergone gastroplasty. Gastric bypass, however, is more effective than VBGP in correcting glucose intolerance in patients without overt non–insulin-dependent diabetes mellitus.

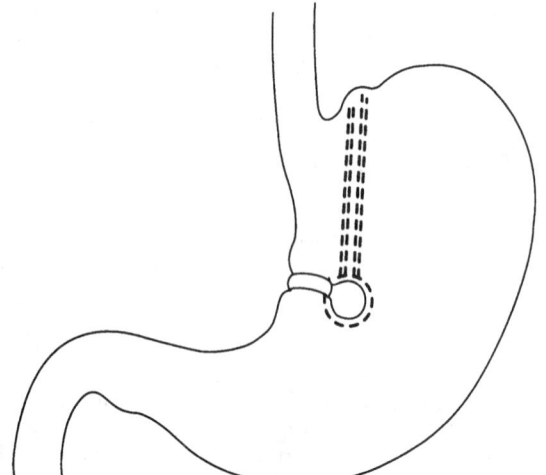

Figure 24-2. Vertical banded gastroplasty.

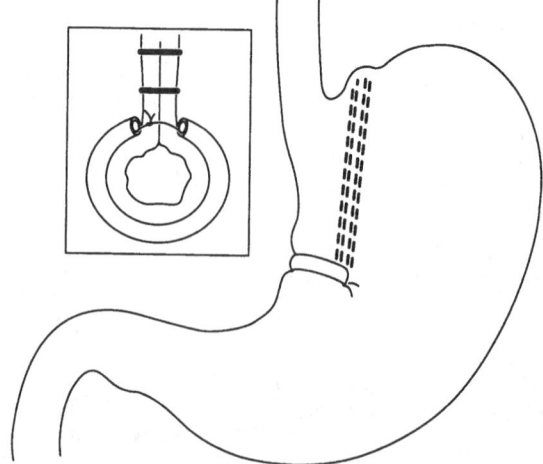

Figure 24-3. Vertical Silastic ring gastroplasty.

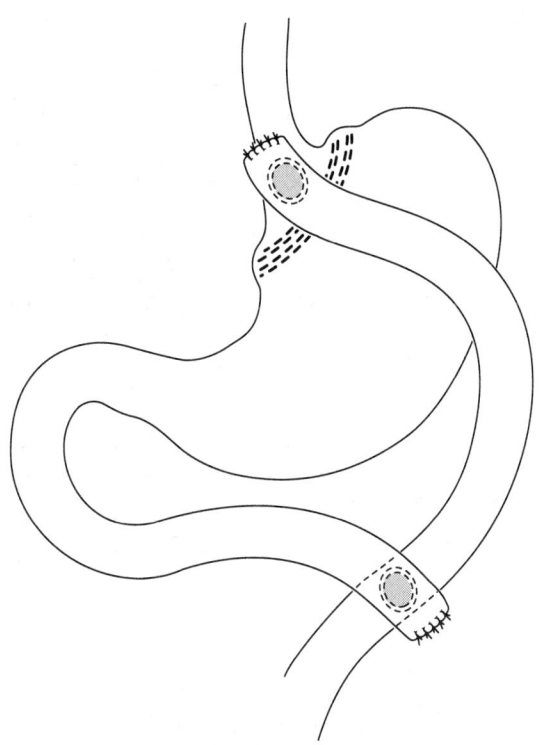

Figure 24-4. Proximal Roux-en-Y gastric bypass.

About 10% to 15% of patients who undergo gastric bypass regain lost weight or do not achieve acceptable weight loss. Although regained weight may be a result of expansion of either the stoma or the pouch, this finding is not observed in most patients. The cause of failure appears to be excessive, constant nibbling on foods with high caloric density.

Complications of Gastric Operations for Morbid Obesity

Leak

The worst complication of gastric surgery for morbid obesity is a postoperative gastric leak that leads to peritonitis. After gastroplasty, this leakage can occur at the staple line, from the proximal gastric pouch, or from the distal stomach. The most dangerous aspect of a gastric leak is difficulty recognizing the symptoms of peritonitis. By the third day after surgery, patients should have little pain. Worsening postoperative pain and pain in the back or the left shoulder (consistent with inflammation of the left hemidiaphragm), urinary frequency, or rectal tenesmus (implying pelvic irritation) is evidence of a leak. Tachycardia, tachypnea, fever, and leukocytosis are usually present. A leak can usually be confirmed with an emergency upper gastrointestinal radiographic series using water-soluble contrast material. If a leak is noted, or if the radiograph is normal but suspicion is high, urgent exploration of the abdomen is necessary. An attempt should be made to repair the leak. A large sump drain should be placed nearby, because the repair frequently breaks down. This leads to a controlled fistula, which usually heals with total parenteral nutrition or a distal feeding jejunostomy.

Necrosis

Necrosis of the distal stomach due to dilatation can occur after a gastric bypass as a result of afferent limb obstruction of a loop gastrojejunostomy or obstruction at

the jejunojejunostomy of a Roux-en-Y procedure. This complication is usually heralded by frequent hiccoughs and can be diagnosed by visualization of a large gastric bubble on a plain abdominal radiograph. Impending gastric necrosis necessitates urgent percutaneous or surgical decompression.

In patients who have had a jejunoileal bypass converted to a gastric bypass or patients with extensive adhesions from previous abdominal operations, a gastrostomy tube should be inserted prophylactically for decompression. The gastrostomy tube also can be used for feeding until the patient's oral intake allows weight stabilization. A gastrostomy can be used to feed patients with leaks from the proximal gastric pouch.

Ulcer

A marginal ulcer develops in about 10% of patients who undergo gastric bypass. These ulcers usually respond to acid suppression therapy (H_2 receptor blocker or omeprazole) or sucralfate.

Stenosis

Stomal stenosis may develop after Roux-en-Y gastric bypass or VBGP. Outpatient endoscopic balloon stomal dilation should be attempted and is usually successful in patients who have undergone gastric bypass. It is effective in only half of stenoses in patients who have undergone VBGP.

Gallstones

Rapid weight loss after either VBGP or gastric bypass is associated with a high incidence of gallstone formation. Ten to twenty percent of patients need cholecystectomy for acute biliary colic or cholecystitis within 3 to 5 years after obesity surgery. Some surgeons recommend routine prophylactic cholecystectomy at the time of the obesity operation; others perform cholecystectomy only when there is sonographic evidence of gallstones or biliary sludge. Prophylactic administration of ursodeoxycholic acid, 300 mg by mouth twice a day, reduces the risk of gallstone formation when given for 6 months after gastric bypass. There is a low risk of additional gallstone formation over the 6 months after the medication has been discontinued.

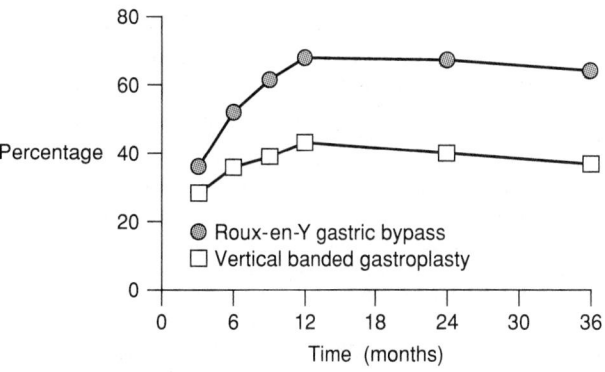

Figure 24-5. Percentage loss of excess weight over 3 years after Roux-en-Y gastric bypass compared with vertical banded gastroplasty. (After Sugerman HJ, Starkey J, Birkenhauer R. A randomized prospective trial of gastric bypass versus vertical banded gastroplasty for morbid obesity and their effects on sweets versus non-sweets eaters. Ann Surg 1987;205:613)

Polyneuropathy

A rare syndrome of polyneuropathy has been noted after gastric operations for morbid obesity. It occurs in association with intractable vomiting and severe protein–calorie malnutrition. Acute thiamine deficiency has been thought to be responsible for this condition.

Vitamin B$_{12}$ Deficiency

Vitamin B$_{12}$ deficiency has been observed after gastric bypass. It mandates long-term follow-up with annual measurement of vitamin B$_{12}$ level. Deficiency of vitamin B$_{12}$ is probably due to decreased acid digestion of vitamin B$_{12}$ from food with subsequent failure of coupling to intrinsic factor.

Anemia

Iron-deficiency anemia can occur in menstruating women after gastric bypass. It can be refractory to supplemental ferrous sulfate, because iron absorption requires acid and takes place primarily in the duodenum and upper jejunum. Iron-dextran injections may be necessary. All women should take two (325 mg/d) iron sulfate tablets by mouth after gastric bypass as long as they continue to menstruate.

Other Complications

Other complications, which can occur with any type of operation on obese patients, include wound infection, wound dehiscence, incisional hernia, venous thrombosis, and pulmonary embolism. The incidence of lower-leg venous thrombosis and pulmonary embolism can be reduced with the use of intermittent venous compression boots. Early ambulation is important. Pulmonary embolism is a frequent fatal complication in patients with heart failure associated with hypoxemic pulmonary hypertension and a mean pulmonary artery pressure greater than 40 mmHg. It has been recommended that a vena caval filter be placed in these patients prophylactically at the time of obesity surgery. The operative mortality after gastric surgery for obesity is about 0.5%.

OVERVIEW OF GASTRIC SURGERY FOR MORBID OBESITY

Selectively applied gastric procedures for morbid obesity can yield satisfactory weight reduction, with the average loss of one-half to two-thirds of excess weight within 1 to 1.5 years. Weight becomes stable at this level in most patients, as caloric intake meets caloric expenditure. Patients must be followed carefully to ensure adequate levels of protein, vitamins, and other micronutrients.

Weight loss completely corrects insulin-dependent diabetes in almost all patients, hypertension in 80%, and headaches associated with cerebrospinal fluid pressure elevation in pseudotumor cerebri. Obstructive sleep apnea syndrome resolves with weight loss. The hypoxemia and hypercarbia seen in the obesity hypoventilation syndrome return toward normal with weight loss. Elevated pulmonary artery and pulmonary capillary wedge pressures also improve after weight loss with correction of abnormal arterial blood gases. Loss of weight usually corrects sex hormone abnormalities in women, allows healing of chronic venous stasis ulcers associated with venous insufficiency, prevents reflux esophagitis, relieves stress overflow urinary incontinence, and improves low-back and joint-related pain. Weight loss may allow total joint replacement with artificial joints. Patient self-image is often markedly improved after gastric surgery for obesity.

SUGGESTED READING

Bjorntorp P. Abdominal obesity and the metabolic syndrome. Ann Med 1992;24:465.

Brolin RE, Kenler HA, Gorman JH, Cody RP. Long-limb gastric bypass in the superobese: a prospective randomized study. Ann Surg 1992;215:387.

Hocking MP, Duerson MC, O'Leary JP, Woodward EF. Jejunoileal bypass for morbid obesity: late follow-up in 100 cases. N Engl J Med 1983;308:995.

National Institutes of Health Technology Assessment Panel. Methods for voluntary weight loss and control. Ann Intern Med 1992;116:942.

Ravussin E, Lillioja S, Knowler WC, et al. Reduced rate of energy expenditure as a risk factor for body-weight gain. N Engl J Med 1988;318:467.

Roberts SB, Savage J, Coward WA, et al. Energy expenditure and intake in infants born to lean and overweight mothers. N Engl J Med 1988;318:461.

Stunkard AJ, Harris JR, Pedersen NL, McClearn GE. The body-mass index of twins who have been reared apart. N Engl J Med 1990;322:1483.

Sugerman JH, Wolper JL. Failed gastroplasty for morbid obesity: revised gastroplasty versus Roux-en-Y gastric bypass. Am J Surg 1984;148:331.

ESSENTIALS OF SURGERY: SCIENTIFIC PRINCIPLES AND PRACTICE, edited by Lazar J. Greenfield, Michael W. Mulholland, Keith T. Oldham, Gerald B. Zelenock, and Keith D. Lillemoe. Lippincott–Raven Publishers, Philadelphia, © 1997.

CHAPTER 25

GASTRIC NEOPLASMS

MICHAEL W. MULHOLLAND

ADENOCARCINOMA

Epidemiology

Gastric cancer is one of the ten most common causes of cancer-related death in the United States (Fig. 25-1). The worldwide incidence and death rate for gastric cancer vary markedly. In Japan, the disease accounts for about 50% of cancer-related deaths among men and 40% of cancer deaths among women. Exposure to environmental carcinogens, probably in the diet, appears to account for the high frequency of disease. Although nitrites in the diet appear to have a role in gastric carcinogenesis, specific dietary constituents that promote tumor formation have not been identified. It appears that exposure to *Helicobacter pylori* has a role in the development of gastric carcinoma.

Premalignant Lesions

Gastric Polyps

The risk for gastric cancer is greater in stomachs that harbor polyps. This risk is related most closely to polyp histology, size, and number. In terms of malignant potential, gastric polyps may be divided into two broad categories—hyperplastic polyps and adenomatous polyps.

Hyperplastic Polyps

Hyperplastic polyps occur in 0.5 to 1% of the general population and account for 70% to 80% of all gastric polyps. Hyperplastic polyps contain an overgrowth of gastric epithelium that appears normal at histologic examination.

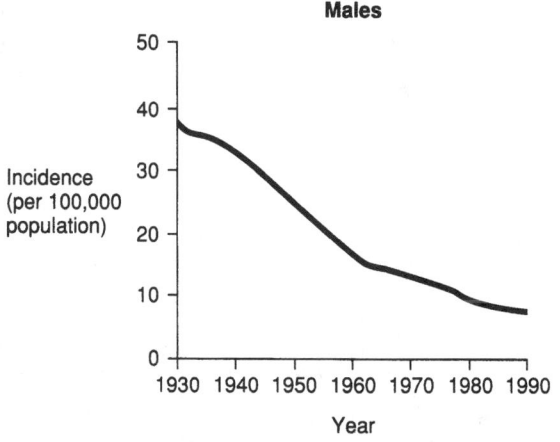

Males

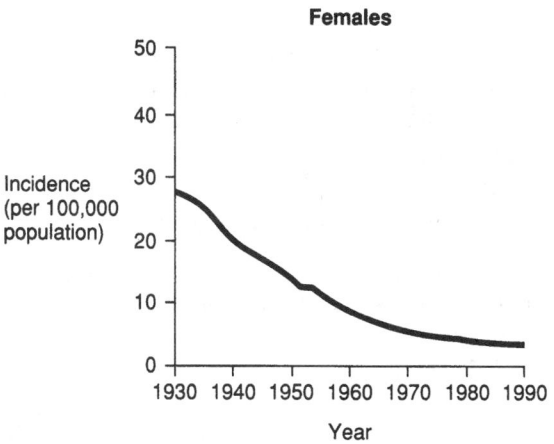

Females

Figure 25-1. Incidence of gastric cancer deaths in the United States.

Atypia is rare. Hyperplastic gastric polyps are considered to have no neoplastic potential.

Most hyperplastic polyps are asymptomatic. Dyspepsia and vague epigastric discomfort are the most common symptoms, although coexistent gastroduodenal disease is also frequently identified. Complications are unusual, and gastrointestinal hemorrhage occurs <20% of the time. When hyperplastic polyps are discovered, endoscopic removal for histologic examination is sufficient treatment.

Adenomatous Polyps

Adenomatous polyps carry a risk for carcinoma of 10% to 20%; the risk is greatest for polyps >2 cm in diameter. Mucosal atypia is frequent, and mitotic figures are more common than in hyperplastic polyps. Dysplasia and carcinoma in situ may develop in adenomatous polyps. Multiple adenomatous polyps increase the risk for cancer. Symptoms are similar to those of hyperplastic polyps. Endoscopic removal is indicated for pedunculated lesions and is sufficient if the polyp is completely removed and shows no evidence of invasive cancer on histologic examination. Operative excision is recommended for sessile lesions >2 cm, for polyps with biopsy-proved invasive carcinoma, and for polyps complicated by pain or bleeding. After removal, endoscopic surveillance of the gastric mucosa is indicated.

Gastritis

The incidence of both gastric cancer and atrophic gastritis increases with age. Chronic gastritis is frequently associated with intestinal metaplasia and mucosal dysplasia;

these histologic features are often observed in mucosa adjacent to gastric cancer. Gastritis is frequently progressive and severe in the gastric mucosa of patients with cancer.

***Helicobacter pylori* Infestation.** *H. pylori* chronic gastritis has been postulated to cause gastric cancer, but the evidence is considerably weaker than evidence linking the organism to benign ulceration. A higher than expected prevalence of *H. pylori* infestation has been reported in regions of the world with high cancer rates. In developed nations, however, the frequency of *H. pylori* infestation among patients with gastric adenocarcinoma is similar to the incidence in age-matched controls. The reduction in gastric cancer in developed countries may be due to a reduction in *H. pylori* infestation because of improved nutrition and hygiene.

Pernicious Anemia. The incidence of malignant gastric tumors seems to be high among patients with chronic gastritis associated with pernicious anemia. The disease is characterized by fundic mucosal atrophy, loss of parietal and chief cells, hypochlorhydria, and hypergastrinemia. The increased risk warrants aggressive investigation of new symptoms in patients with long-standing pernicious anemia, but it is not high enough to justify repeated endoscopic examinations. There is no evidence that antral gastritis, frequently observed in patients with peptic ulcers, has any malignant potential.

Intestinal Metaplasia. Intestinal metaplasia, the presence of intestinal glands within the gastric mucosa, is associated with both gastritis and gastric cancer. The evolution from metaplasia to dysplasia to carcinoma to invasive cancer has been demonstrated in other organs, but no direct evidence can be provided for this progression in gastric cancer.

Previous Gastric Operations

Gastric cancer may be more likely to develop in patients who have undergone partial gastrectomy than in those who have not. The true risk for gastric neoplasia, however, appears to be overestimated.

Clinical Features

The symptoms of gastric cancer may mimic those of a number of nonneoplastic gastroduodenal diseases (Fig. 25-2; Table 25-1). Most patients with early gastric cancer have normal physical examinations. Guaiac-positive stool is noted in one-third of patients. Abnormal physical findings usually reflect advanced disease. Cachexia, abdominal mass, hepatomegaly, and supraclavicular adenopathy usually indicate metastasis. No simple laboratory tests are specific for gastric neoplasms.

Diagnosis and Screening

Endoscopy

Fiberoptic endoscopy is the definitive diagnostic method when gastric neoplasia is suspected. The findings are as follows:

Early Cancer
- Polypoid lesion
- Flat plaque-like lesion, or
- Shallow ulcer

Advanced Cancer
- Ulcerated lesion
- Irregular border, beaded because of infiltrating cancer cells
- Necrotic, shaggy base
- Ulcer that appears to arise from underlying mass

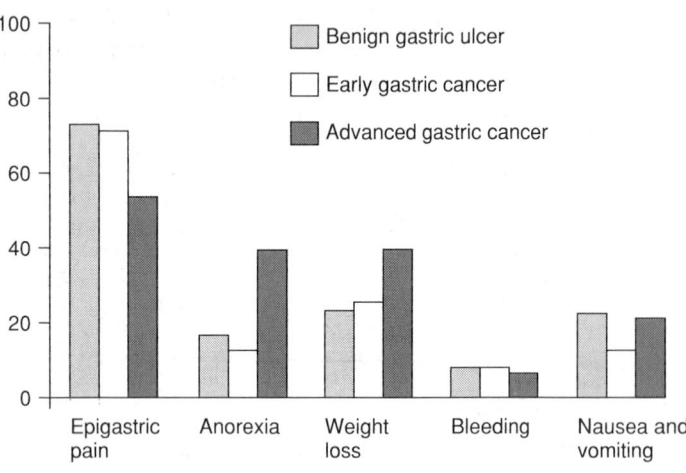

Figure 25-2. Clinical symptom frequency in benign gastric ulcer, early gastric cancer, and advanced gastric cancer. (After Meyer WC, Damiano RJ, Postlethwait RW, Rotolo FS. Adenocarcinoma of the stomach: changing patterns over the past four decades. Ann Surg 1987;205:18)

Benign gastric ulcers can be differentiated from malignant gastric ulcers only with gastric biopsy. The accuracy of diagnosis can exceed 95% if several biopsy specimens are obtained. Diagnostic accuracy can be enhanced with direct brush cytology.

The ability to diagnose gastric adenocarcinoma at endoscopy has prompted screening programs for populations at high risk. Because the incidence of gastric cancer is relatively low in the United States and Canada, mass screening is not performed.

Radiography

Single-contrast barium examinations have a diagnostic accuracy of 80%. This diagnostic yield increases to about 90% when double-contrast (air and barium) is used. Typical findings include ulceration, a gastric mass, loss of mucosal detail, and distortion of the gastric silhouette (Fig. 25-3).

Computed Tomography

Computed tomography (CT) is used as a primary diagnostic method and to assess extragastric spread. When performed with intraluminal contrast, CT can demonstrate infiltration of the gastric wall by tumor, gastric ulcer, and hepatic metastasis (Fig. 25-4). The technique is not reliable in depicting invasion of adjacent organs or the presence of lymphatic metastases. Because of these limitations, CT is not a reliable staging method and usually does not eliminate the need for laparotomy.

Endoscopic Ultrasonography

Endoscopic ultrasonography shows that the gastric wall is a five-layered structure with alternating hyperechoic and hypoechoic layers. The examination allows the examiner to differentiate gastric submucosal lesions from compression by adjacent organs or disease processes.

Benign Lesions

Benign leiomyomas appear as round, hypoechoic masses with smooth margins, usually contiguous with muscularis propria. Malignant transformation is suggested by a diameter of >3 cm, irregular margins, destruction of normal layers of the gastric wall, and hypoechoic foci caused by necrosis.

Gastric Cancer

The gastric wall thickens when it is infiltrated by tumor. Ultrasound allows accurate measurement of the depth of gastric cancer invasion. Early gastric cancer, confined to

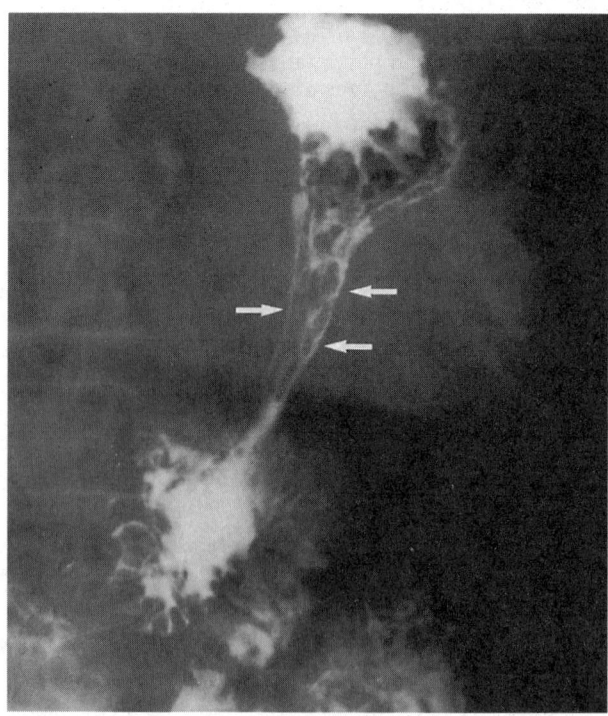

Figure 25-3. Barium contrast radiograph demonstrating extensive involvement of the gastric body by infiltrating adenocarcinoma (linitis plastica). The gastric silhouette is narrowed (*arrows*), and the stomach is nondistensible.

Table 25-1. COMMON SYMPTOMS AND PHYSICAL FINDINGS IN GASTRIC CANCER

Symptoms	Physical Findings
Weight loss	Guaiac-positive stool
Pain	Cachexia
Nausea and vomiting	Abdominal mass
Anorexia	Abdominal tenderness
Dysphagia	Hepatomegaly
Melena	—

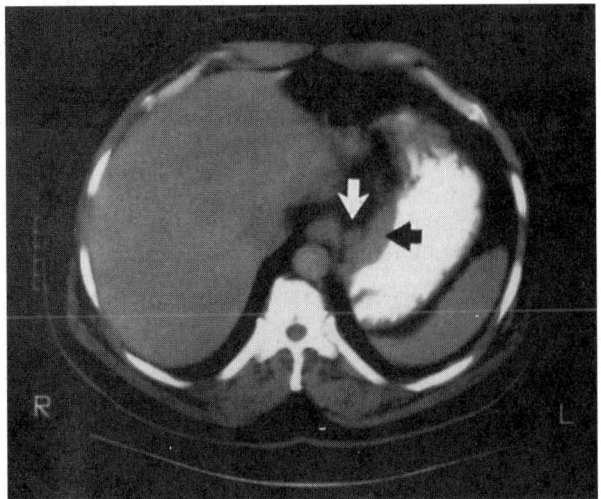

Figure 25-4. CT scan demonstrating mass along lesser curvature of the stomach (*black arrow*) and associated lymph node enlargement (*white arrow*).

the mucosa and submucosa, can be differentiated from advanced cancer in >90% of examinations. Gastric adenocarcinoma can be differentiated from gastric lymphoma on the basis of ultrasonographic characteristics. Scirrhous carcinoma demonstrates preservation of the normal five-layer structure with hypoechoic thickening of the 3rd and 4th layers. With lymphoma, there is diffuse thickening of the gastric wall and blurring of the layered pattern. Endoscopic ultrasonography is not helpful in the nodal staging of gastric cancer. Evaluation for hepatic and distant metastasis requires CT.

Pathology

Gastric adenocarcinoma occurs in two histologic subtypes—intestinal and diffuse (Table 25-2).

Gastric adenocarcinomas demonstrate a number of chromosomal and genetic abnormalities. Cytometric analysis reveals that gastric tumors with a large fraction of aneuploid cells (with a greater than normal amount of nuclear DNA) tend to be highly infiltrative and have a poor prognosis. Chromosomal abnormalities are frequent in gastric adenocarcinomas.

Many gastric adenocarcinomas demonstrate increased expression of the K-*ras* protooncogene and tumor growth

factor a (TGF-α). Increased expression correlates with advanced stage, grade, depth of invasion, lymphatic metastasis, and bad prognosis. Mutations of the p53 tumor suppressor gene are found in a high proportion of gastric cancers. Overexpression of the receptor for epidermal growth factor is noted consistently.

In the United States, gastric adenocarcinomas occur with equal frequency in the proximal and distal regions of the stomach. About 40% of tumors involve the proximal stomach (the esophagogastric junction and fundus), and an equal percentage arise in the antrum. In 15% of patients, the stomach is diffusely involved at the time of diagnosis. Proximal involvement is more common in elderly patients. The proportion of tumors involving the proximal stomach has increased dramatically. The prognosis is not good for tumors that originate in the proximal stomach or for those with diffuse involvement of the stomach.

The gastric cancer staging format used by the American Joint Commission is presented in Table 25-3. The staging system is oriented toward surgical and pathologic examinations but accurately reflects prognosis (Fig. 25-5). Staging data illustrate the high frequency with which lymph node metastases are present at the time of diagnosis in the United States and the severe impact of this lymphatic involvement on survival. Even early gastric cancers have a 15% prevalence of nodal metastasis.

Curative Treatment

Surgical resection is the only hope for cure of gastric cancer, and advanced stage of disease at the time of diagnosis precludes curative resection for most patients. The surgical objectives in gastric cancer therefore are the following:

1. To maximize chances for cure in patients with localized tumor
2. To provide effective and safe palliation to patients with advanced malignant disease

Table 25-2. SUBTYPES OF GASTRIC ADENOCARCINOMA

Intestinal	Diffuse
Cells form glands	No gland formation
Associated with chronic mucosal atrophy, chronic gastritis, intestinal metaplasia, dysplasia	Infiltrates tissues as a sheet of loosely adherent cells
Blood-borne metastases	Lymphatic invasion
More frequent in populations at high risk gastric cancer (Japan, China)	More frequent in populations with a low incidence of gastric cancer (United States)
More frequent in men and older patients	More frequent in women and younger patients
	Less favorable prognosis

Table 25-3. TNM CLASSIFICATION FOR STAGING OF GASTRIC CANCER

TNM DEFINITIONS
Primary Tumor
T1 Tumor confined to the mucosa
T2 Tumor involves the mucosa and submucosa, and extends to but does not penetrate serosa
T3 Tumor penetrates serosa with or without invasion of adjacent structures
T4 Diffuse involvement on gastric wall without obvious boundaries (linitis plastica)

Regional Lymph Node Involvement
N0 No nodal metastasis
N1 Metastasis to perigastric lymph nodes in immediate vicinity of tumor
N2 Metastasis to lymph nodes distant from primary tumor or along both curvatures of the stomach

Distant Metastasis
M0 No distant metastasis
M1 Metastasis beyond regional lymph nodes

STAGE GROUPING
Stage I   T1, N0, M0
Stage II   T2–3, N0, M0
Stage III T1–3, N1–3, M0
Stage IV   Tumor unresectable or metastatic

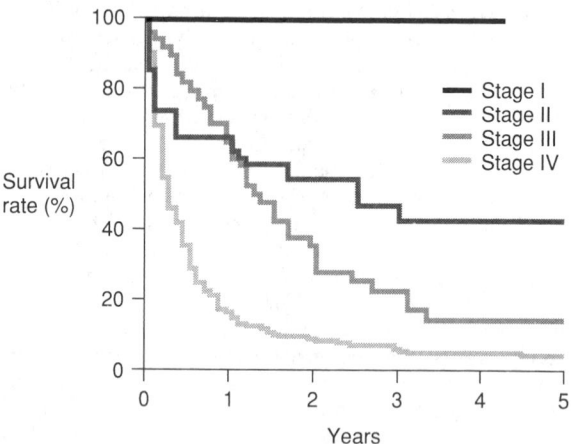

Figure 25-5. Survival rate of gastric cancer by stage.

Evolution of the surgical approach to gastric adenocarcinoma has focused on the following five issues:

1. The extent of gastric resection needed for potentially curable lesions
2. The role of perigastric lymphadenectomy
3. The adequacy of proximal and distal resection margins
4. The role of splenectomy
5. The implications of involvement of adjacent organs

Radical operations increase operative morbidity but do not improve survival. For early lesions (N0–1, M0) of the antrum or middle stomach, distal subtotal gastrectomy including 80% of the stomach provides a satisfactory 5-year survival rate without an increase in operative morbidity. Proximal gastric lesions or larger lesions of the mid-stomach may require total gastrectomy or esophagogastrectomy to encompass the tumor. Regardless of the extent of gastric resection, patients with more advanced tumors fare poorly because of the increased likelihood of lymphatic and hematogenous spread.

The extent of gastric resection is determined, in part, by the need to obtain a resection margin free of microscopic disease. Microscopic involvement of the resection margin by tumor cells is associated with poor prognosis. Gastric cancer demonstrates extensive intramural spread. The propensity for intramural metastasis is related, in part, to the extensive anastomosing capillary and lymphatic network within the wall of the stomach. A line of resection 6 cm from the tumor mass is necessary to ensure a low rate of anastomotic recurrence.

The value of extended lymphadenectomy in the treatment of gastric adenocarcinoma is controversial. Because the benefits of extended lymphadenectomy accrue only to patients with local or regional disease, intraoperative staging must be undertaken to exclude patients with spread to liver, peritoneum, or serosa of the stomach. Resections are characterized as follows:

R1—resection of stomach, omentum, and perigastric lymph nodes
R2—resection of stomach and omentum and en bloc removal of the superior leaf of the transverse mesocolon, the pancreatic capsule, and lymph nodes along the branches of the celiac artery and in the infraduodenal and supraduodenal areas
R3—resection of the foregoing structures, the spleen, the tail of the pancreas, and the lymph nodes along the aorta and esophagus

Histologically positive lymph nodes are frequently present in the splenic hilum and along the splenic artery. Routine splenectomy is performed in some centers, but prophylactic splenectomy has not been demonstrated to improve outcome. Likewise, resection of the tail or body of the pancreas has not been demonstrated to improve survival. Resection of adjacent organs may be required for local control if direct invasion has occurred. In this circumstance, operative morbidity is increased, and long-term survival is rare.

Palliative Treatment

When preoperative evaluation demonstrates disseminated disease, palliation of symptoms becomes a primary consideration. Palliation does not always require surgical intervention. Endoscopic laser fulguration can be used to treat obstruction, bleeding, and dysphagia. Successful laser treatment requires adequate visualization and is hampered by circumferential tumor growth that impedes passage of the endoscope, by sharp angulation of the esophagogastric junction, and by lesions >6 cm in length.

Surgical palliation, usually in the form of gastric resection, may be considered for patient comfort if laparotomy can be performed with acceptable morbidity and mortality. No prospective studies have proved that palliative resection prolongs survival. Nonetheless, resection appears to relieve symptoms, particularly dysphagia. Bypass of obstructing distal gastric lesions without resection provides relief to less than half of patients, and the mean survival period is <6 months. For proximal obstructing lesions, total gastrectomy with Roux-en-Y esophagojejunal reconstruction may be necessary. An operative mortality of <5% has been reported. The mean survival period after palliative gastric resection is about 9 months. For nonresectable gastric adenocarcinomas, when dysphagia is present, radiation therapy may have a palliative role.

Chemotherapy

Chemotherapy has limited use in the treatment of disseminated gastric adenocarcinoma. The drugs most commonly used are 5-fluorouracil (5FU), mitomycin C, and doxorubicin. The rate of partial response to single-agent therapy is rarely >25% to 30%, and complete responses have not occurred. Because long-term survival can only be expected in patients who have a complete response, single-drug approaches have had no impact on survival rates. FAM (the combination of 5FU, doxorubicin, and mitomycin C for the treatment of advanced gastric cancer, has an overall partial response rate of about 33%. The combination of 5FU, doxorubicin, and cisplatin has been associated with complete responses in 12% of patients. Increases in mean survival rates with multiple-agent chemotherapy have not been proved.

The addition of radiation therapy to chemotherapy has modest benefit. Single-agent adjuvant chemotherapy after potentially curative surgery for gastric adenocarcinoma has not been proved to be beneficial. No definitive data are available to suggest that multiple-agent adjuvant combinations based on 5FU are more effective than single agents, although several trials indicate that benefit may exist.

GASTRIC LYMPHOMA
Clinical Features

The stomach is the site of more than half of gastrointestinal lymphomas and is the organ most commonly involved in extranodal lymphomas. Non-Hodgkin lymphomas ac-

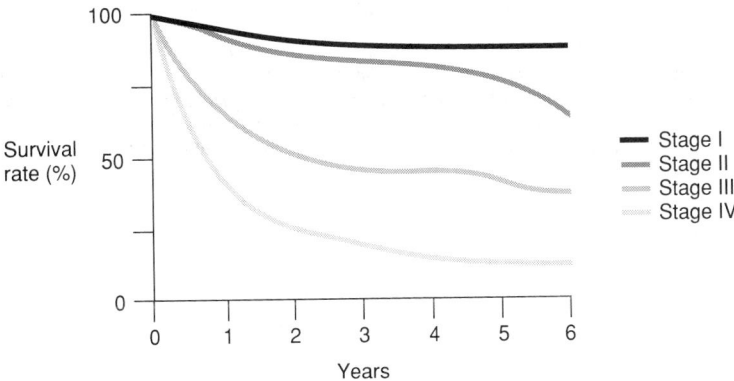

Figure 25-6. Survival of gastric lymphoma by stage.

count for about 5% of malignant gastric tumors. Patients are considered to have primary gastric lymphoma if initial symptoms are gastric and the stomach is exclusively or predominantly involved with the tumor. Patients who do not fulfill these criteria are considered to have secondary gastric involvement from systemic lymphoma.

The peak incidence of gastric lymphoma is in the sixth and seventh decades of life. Symptoms are indistinguishable from those of gastric adenocarcinoma. Epigastric pain, weight loss, anorexia, nausea, and vomiting are common. Although gross bleeding is uncommon, occult hemorrhage and anemia are observed in more than half of patients.

Diagnosis

Radiographic findings are similar to those for adenocarcinoma. Endoscopic biopsy, combined with endoscopic brush cytology and ultrasonography, provides the diagnosis 90% of the time. Submucosal growth without ulceration of the overlying mucosa may occasionally render endoscopic biopsy nondiagnostic. When gastric lymphoma is first diagnosed by endoscopic means, evidence of systemic disease should be sought. CT of chest and abdomen (to detect lymphadenopathy), bone marrow biopsy, and biopsy of enlarged peripheral lymph nodes may be appropriate. A commonly used staging system is as follows:

* Stage I—tumor confined to stomach
* Stage II—tumor with spread to perigastric lymph nodes
* Stage III—nodal involvement beyond perigastric lymph nodes (eg, paraaortic nodes)
* Stage IV—tumor spread to other organs in the abdomen (spleen, liver)

Treatment

A multimodality treatment program with gastrectomy as the first step is used to treat primary gastric lymphomas. This approach has the following advantages:

Accurate histologic evaluation
Cure of localized tumor
Elimination of the risk of life-threatening hemorrhage or perforation

The role of resection in the treatment of gastric lymphoma is controversial, and increasing numbers of patients are treated with chemoradiation therapy alone. The risk of hemorrhage or perforation is probably overstated. The use of endoscopic ultrasonography to detect full-thickness

involvement of the gastric wall may identify patients at risk for perforation.

If gastrectomy is performed before chemotherapy or radiation therapy, extended radical resections are not indicated. Unlike in adenocarcinoma, microscopically positive resection margins do not predict local recurrence in cases of lymphoma when radiation therapy is administered postoperatively. The postoperative mortality is 0% to 5%. In a small number of patients with stage I disease, surgery may be considered curative and no further therapy is required. Postoperative radiation to the gastrectomy bed appears to improve local and regional control.

In >30% of patients with stage II disease who undergo apparently adequate surgery and radiation therapy, the cancer recurs outside the treatment field. Patients with stage II primary gastric lymphoma should, therefore, be considered to have systemic disease and to require systemic therapy in addition to surgery or radiation therapy. Chemotherapy, either primarily or as postoperative adjuvant therapy, is appropriate. Survival from gastric lymphoma is linked to stage at diagnosis (Fig. 25-6).

GASTRIC CARCINOIDS

Gastric carcinoid tumors are extremely rare. Most small gastric carcinoids are asymptomatic. Large tumors may cause ulceration of the overlying mucosa. Because of the potential for invasion, curative resection is attempted. Patients with pernicious anemia appear to be at high risk for gastric carcinoids.

GASTRIC SARCOMAS

Sarcomas constitute approximately 3% of malignant gastric tumors. Leiomyosarcomas are predominant, and angiosarcomas and fibrosarcomas are rare. Intraperitoneal sarcomatosis is frequent, as is local recurrence after resection. Metastasis occurs by the hematogenous route, so hepatic involvement is common. En bloc resection of the tumor and involved structures is the treatment of choice.

SUGGESTED READING

Bozzetti F, Audisio RA, Giardini R, Gennari L. Role of surgery in patients with primary non-Hodgkin's lymphoma of the stomach: an old problem revisited. Br J Surg 1993; 80:1101.

Findlay M, Cunningham D. Chemotherapy of carcinoma of the stomach. Cancer Treat Rev 1993;19:29.

Harju E. Gastric polyposis and malignancy. Br J Surg 1986; 73:532.

Nicholson DA, Shorvon PJ. Review article: endoscopic ultrasound of the stomach. Br J Surg 1993;66:487.

Robertson CS, Chung SCS, Woods SDS, et al. A prospective randomized trial comparing R_1 subtotal gastrectomy with R_3 gastrectomy for antral cancer. Ann Surg 1994;250: 176.

Silverberg E, Boring CC, Squires TS. Cancer statistics, 1990. CA 1990;40:9.

Veldhuyzen, van Zanten, Sherman PM. *Helicobacter pylori* infection as a cause of gastritis, duodenal ulcer, gastric cancer and nonulcer dyspepsia: a systematic overview. Can Med Assoc J 1994;150:177.

Wyatt JI. Gastritis and its relation to gastric carcinogenesis. Semin Diagn Pathol 1991;8:137.

SMALL INTESTINE

ESSENTIALS OF SURGERY: SCIENTIFIC PRINCIPLES AND PRACTICE,
edited by Lazar J. Greenfield, Michael W. Mulholland, Keith T. Oldham, Gerald B. Zelenock,
and Keith D. Lillemoe. Lippincott–Raven Publishers, Philadelphia, © 1997.

CHAPTER 26

ANATOMY AND PHYSIOLOGY OF THE SMALL INTESTINE

WALTER A. KOLTUN AND THEODORE N. PAPPAS

GROSS ANATOMY

Duodenum

The duodenum extends 20 to 30 cm from the pyloric sphincter to the ligament of Treitz, where the jejunum begins. It is divided into four parts—the cap (bulb) and the second (descending), third (transverse), and fourth (ascending) portions. The blood supply is illustrated in Figure 26-1.

Duodenal Cap

The duodenal cap is a triangular structure 5 cm long that projects slightly cephalad from the pylorus. It overlies the common bile duct and is the anchor point for the hepatoduodenal ligament. The cap is the site of >90% of duodenal ulcers. The posterior wall of the duodenal cap is adjacent to the head of the pancreas. Posterior penetrating ulcers in this area erode into the pancreas and the underlying gastroduodenal artery.

Second Portion

The second (descending) portion of the duodenum courses about 10 cm posteriorly and caudally from the duodenal cap to the level of the first lumbar vertebra. It is attached to the head of the pancreas and becomes a retroperitoneal structure as it courses posteriorly. In this retroperitoneal position, the duodenum overlies the Gerota fascia and the inferior vena cava. At the junction between the duodenal cap and descending portion is the foramen of Winslow, posterior to the hepatoduodenal ligament. The hepatic flexure of the colon is draped on the anterior surface of the second portion of the duodenum.

Endoscopic examination of this portion of the duodenum shows valvulae conniventes, which are concentric mucosal folds 1 to 2 mm thick and 2 to 4 mm high separated by 2 to 4 mm of flat, smooth mucosa. The diameter of the second portion of the duodenum varies from 3 to 5 cm. The ampulla of Vater is a hooded fold that marks the confluence of the common bile duct and the main pancreatic duct (duct of Wirsung). It enters the midpoint of the second portion of the duodenum surrounded by the sphincter of Oddi. In 50% to 60% of patients, an accessory pancreatic duct (the duct of Santorini) enters the duodenum proximal to the ampulla of Vater.

Third and Fourth Portions

The third (transverse) portion of the duodenum is almost entirely retroperitoneal. It is attached to the uncinate process of the pancreas and extends from the second portion of the duodenum to the level of the third lumbar vertebra directly over the aorta. The third portion of the duodenum is wedged between the superior mesenteric artery (SMA) and the aorta. The transition between the third and fourth portions of the duodenum is the acute angle made by these two arteries.

The fourth (ascending) portion of the duodenum passes superiorly and obliquely to reach the ligament of Treitz. The ligament of Treitz consists of a slip of muscle that extends downward from the right crus of the diaphragm and a fibromuscular band that passes from the duodenum toward the celiac axis. At the ligament, the jejunum passes directly forward and inferiorly and is no longer attached to the retroperitoneum.

Jejunum and Ileum

The jejunum extends about 100 cm from the ligament of Treitz to the arbitrary point at which the ileum begins. The ileum extends 100-150 cm from its junction with the jejunum to the ileocecal valve. The jejunum is the widest portion of the small intestine, which narrows from the jejunum to the ileocecal valve.

In contrast to the approximately 250 cm of jejunum and ileum, the small-intestinal mesentery has a base of only about 15 cm. The mesentery extends from the ligament of Treitz, left of the midline, near the second lumbar vertebra across the midline on a tangent toward the right lower quadrant. The mesentery tethers the small intestine, preventing kinking of its blood supply. The mesentery contains a large supply of lymphatic vessels and fat.

The mucosal surface of the jejunum is characterized by smooth surfaces interrupted by valvulae conniventes. These folds are tall and numerous in the jejunum but short and infrequent in the distal ileum.

The blood supply of the jejunum and the ileum originates from the SMA. The first jejunal branch of the mesenteric artery is at the point where the SMA crosses the duodenum. After this point, several jejunal and ileal branches arise from the SMA. The SMA accompanies the length of the distal small intestine as a marginal artery before anastomosing with the ileal branch of the ileocolic artery. The arterial supplies of the jejunum and the ileum have different structures (Fig. 26-2).

HISTOLOGY OF THE SMALL INTESTINE

The wall of the small intestine is made up of mucosa, submucosa, muscle, and serosa. The serosa, or outer coat, is incomplete where the duodenum is a retroperitoneal

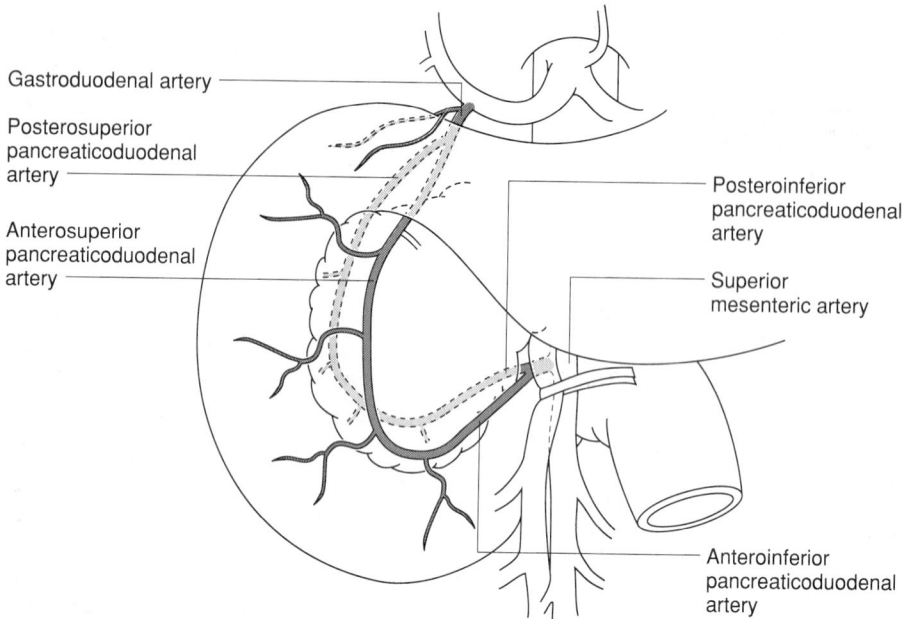

Gastroduodenal artery

Posterosuperior pancreaticoduodenal artery

Anterosuperior pancreaticoduodenal artery

Posteroinferior pancreaticoduodenal artery

Superior mesenteric artery

Anteroinferior pancreaticoduodenal artery

Figure 26-1. Arterial supply to the duodenum.

structure, but it completely surrounds the jejunum and ileum.

Mucosa

The mucosa, or inner lining, is responsible for absorption and secretion. Multiple villi increase the surface area of the mucosa (Fig. 26-3). The mucosa has both exocrine and endocrine functions.

Most of the columnar cells of the villi are *absorptive cells.* The absorptive cells at the apex of the villi contain microvilli, which appear to bind substances for absorption. The absorptive cells also contain lysosomes, which hold hydrolytic digestive enzymes. Absorptive cells have abundant mitochondria, a Golgi complex, granular endoplasmic reticulum, and a basal nucleus.

Goblet cells, exocrine secretory cells in the absorptive epithelium, secrete mucin which lubricates the surface of the epithelium. *Paneth cells,* at the base of the villi in the crypts of LieberkÅhn, contain secretory granules, which contain lysosomal enzymes. *Theliolymphocytes,* T-cell lymphocytes distributed among absorptive cells in the mucosa, have both suppressor and cytolytic activity.

APUD cells (amine precursor uptake and decarboxylation) are dispersed throughout the mucosa of the small intestine. These endocrine cells produce hormones, neuropeptides, and paracrine agents. The most well-known of these cells are the enterochromaffin cells, which occupy the basal portion of the crypts and are thought to secrete 5-hydroxytryptamine. The areas of the small intestine have varying concentrations of neuroendocrine cells (Fig. 26-4).

Submucosa

The submucosa, the layer just beneath the mucosa, has a rich network of blood vessels, lymphatics, and nerves. *Brunner glands* in the submucosa of the duodenum and upper jejunum are connected to the crypts of LieberkÅhn by small ducts, which empty into the lumen of the small intestine. Brunner glands produce an alkaline solution that appears to protect the duodenal mucosa. *Peyer patches* in the submucosa, predominantly in the ileum, consist of dense lymphatic tissue. A large number of lymphocytes usually surround these patches.

Muscle

The small intestine has two muscular layers—an inner circular layer and an outer longitudinal layer. These layers are responsible for intestinal motility. Within the muscular layers are the myenteric plexus of Auerbach and a plexus of ganglia for nonmyelinated nerve fibers.

SMALL-INTESTINAL HORMONES, NEUROTRANSMITTERS, AND PARACRINE SUBSTANCES

Cholecystokinin (CCK)

A peptide, neurotransmitter, and true hormone present in high concentrations in both brain and intestine. Released from the mucosa of the duodenum and jejunum in response to the presence of fats and proteins. After release, the gallbladder contracts and the sphincter of Oddi relaxes, emptying bile into the duodenum. Works with secretin to stimulate pancreatic exocrine secretion.

Secretin

A peptide and true hormone present in the duodenum and jejunum. Released in response to acid in the duodenum when luminal pH falls to <4.5. It stimulates pancreatic secretion.

Somatostatin

A peptide present in multiple areas of the central nervous system, peripheral nervous system, and intestine. Released during a meal and regulates the release of gastric acid and gastrin. Appears to be a neurotransmitter and paracrine agent in the pancreatic islets and in the mucosa of the stomach.

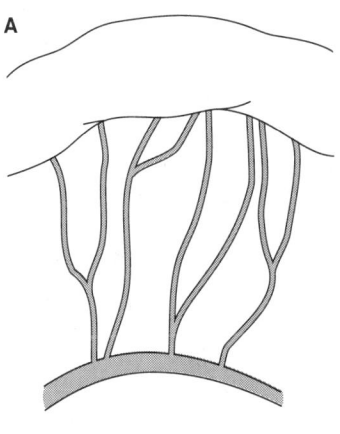

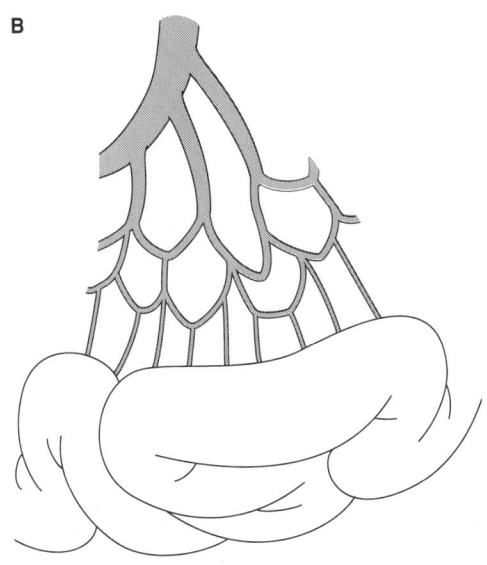

Figure 26-2. Contrasting vasa recta of jejunum (*A*) and ileum (*B*).

Gastric Inhibitory Polypeptide

A peptide present in highest concentration in the mucosa of the duodenum and jejunum. Appears to be a true hormone. May regulate insulin release by augmenting the insulin response to an orally ingested meal.

Motilin

A peptide localized in enterochromaffin cells of the mucosa of the upper small intestine. Released during the fasting state; increased levels correspond with the onset of the migrating motor complex (MMC).

Neurotensin

A neurotransmitter in the central nervous system and intestine, mainly the ileal mucosa. Released in greatest quantity in response to fats but also released in the presence of carbohydrates and protein.

Glucagon

A peptide that functions in opposition to insulin to promote glycogenolysis, lipolysis, gluconeogenesis, and ketogenesis.

Peptide YY

A peptide present predominantly in the mucosa of the terminal ileum and right colon. Released in response to mixed meals and fats. Inhibits acid secretion.

IMMUNOLOGY OF THE SMALL INTESTINE

Both immunologic and nonimmunologic processes provide protection from the entry of noxious materials while allowing the intestine to absorb needed nutrients. Nonimmunologic defense mechanisms include the following:

- Gastric acidity and enteric proteolytic enzymes (including lysozymes), which degrade harmful toxins and organisms
- Mucin production, which coats and protects the epithelium and inhibits the growth of bacteria
- Peristalsis, which can remove and cleanse the intestine of macromolecules, microbes, and parasites
- Rapid epithelium turnover, which tends to dilute and exclude antigens attempting entry at the surface
- Competitive inhibition between endogenous and pathologic bacteria

Gut-associated lymphoid tissue is an important component of the immune system. It is made up of aggregated (Peyer patches, lymphoid follicles, mesenteric lymph nodes) and nonaggregated (luminal, intraepithelial, and lamina propria leukocytes) cellular components.

Secretory Immune System

The most important immunoglobulin of the intestinal immune system is IgA. It binds the threatening antigen while resisting enzymatic degradation by intestinal enzymes. The binding of antigen to IgA stimulates protective mucus secretion and prevents the uptake of viruses and bacteria by promoting contact and entrapment within the epithelial mucous layer. Bacteria can be immobilized by IgA attachment to pili or fimbriae, leading to impaired cellular division and enhanced degradation by luminal enzymes. Secretory IgA can bind to macromolecules and toxins, altering their biologic activity and impeding transmucosal entry.

Migratory Pathways and Gastrointestinal Immunoresponsiveness

The migratory path of enteric lymphocytes begins with exposure to antigen within the intestinal lumen. Small amounts of antigen are sampled by the M cells and presented to the underlying antigen- processing cells, which then stimulate the IgA-bearing lymphocytes in the Peyer patches (Fig. 26-5). In the Peyer patches, stimulated cells leave via the lymphatics, populate mesenteric lymph nodes, and drain through the thoracic duct into the systemic circulation. They then migrate to the lamina propria or other tissues such as the mammary or salivary glands, cervix, and lungs. At these sites, final maturation takes place, and antigen-specific IgA production occurs.

SMALL-INTESTINAL MOTILITY

The motility of the small intestine enables digestion and absorption. Motile contractions promote contact of ingested material with enzymes, chyme, and intestinal mucosa, and deliver food to portions of the intestine where

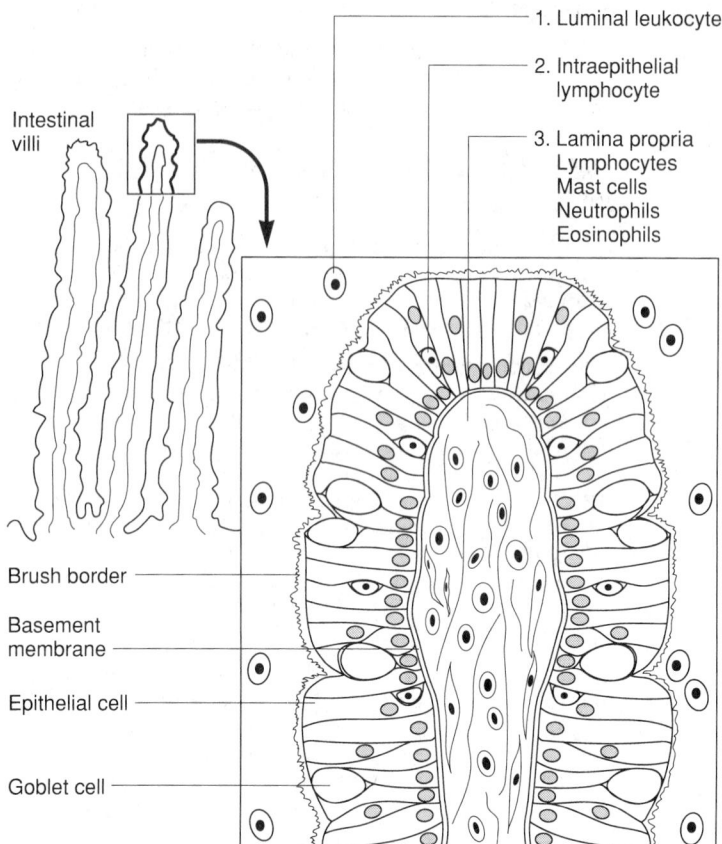

Intestinal villi

1. Luminal leukocyte

2. Intraepithelial lymphocyte

3. Lamina propria
   Lymphocytes
   Mast cells
   Neutrophils
   Eosinophils

Brush border

Basement membrane

Epithelial cell

Goblet cell

Figure 26-3. Small intestinal villus with associated immunologic cells.

specialized absorptive functions take place. Motility participates in enteric defense by evacuating offending ingested material such as toxins and bacteria. Decreased intestinal motility can lead to stasis and bacterial overgrowth, which compromise absorption and nutrition. Mechanical contraction is correlated with myoelectric activity.

Intrinsic Electrical Activity

The smooth-muscle cells of the intestine have a resting membrane potential of 40 to 50 mV, which varies in a cyclic manner by 5 to 15 mV. This variation results in phasic depolarization, referred to as slow waves, basic electrical rhythm, pacemaker potential, or electrical control activity. In the duodenum slow-wave frequency is 11 to 12 cycles/min; in the ileum it is 8 to 9 cycles/min. The proximal high frequencies cause more contractions, propelling intestinal contents aborally.

Slow waves do not cause muscular contractions by themselves. Spike, or action, potentials represent a rapid change in membrane potentials. When they occur repetitively during slow-wave depolarization, spike potentials cause smooth muscle to contract. Unlike slow waves, spike potentials conduct only over a short distance, causing discrete ring-like contractions of the intestine. Also, unlike slow waves, spike potentials are not constantly present. Only when the two are superimposed does the intestine contract.

The nerves within the myenteric nerve plexus of the intestinal wall have efferent, afferent, and intrinsic reflex functions, which produce various patterns of depolarization on stimulation. One such pattern results in the peristaltic reflex—contractions above and relaxation below a site of small-intestinal distention. Acetylcholine is the probable neurotransmitter of excitatory neurons. Adenosine triphosphate (ATP), vasoactive intestinal peptide, somatostatin, serotonin, and substance P all may be neurotransmitters of inhibitory neurons.

Interdigestive Motility Pattern

During the fasting state, spike bursts and muscular contractions migrate from duodenum to terminal ileum in a cyclic pattern known as the interdigestive myoelectric complex or migrating motor complex (MMC). This complex is divided into four phases:

Phase I—quiescence, no spikes or contractions
Phase II—accelerating irregular spiking activity
Phase III—activity front, a series of high-amplitude, rapid spikes corresponding to strong, rhythmic intestinal contractions
Phase IV—subsiding activity

The cycle lasts 90 to 120 minutes. The MMC is interrupted and replaced by rapid spiking activity (similar to phase II) when the intestine receives a food bolus. The duration of the interruption depends on the volume and nature of the food; fats cause the longest duration of rapid spiking.

The function of the MMC is not clear. It periodically sweeps residual luminal contents, bacteria, desquamated cells, and other debris out of the small intestine, preventing bacterial overgrowth. Intestinal function varies during the four phases. Absorption is greatest during phase I and poorest in phase III; transit is most rapid in phase III.

Disruption of the MMC by feeding is at least partially

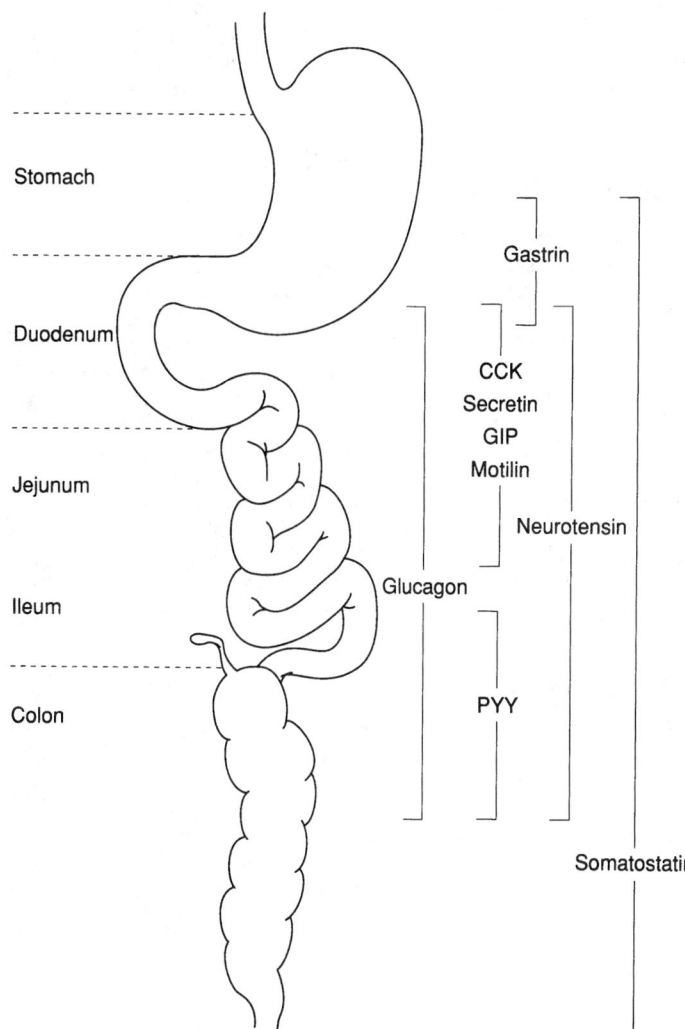

Figure 26-4. Distribution of peptide hormones within the gastrointestinal tract.

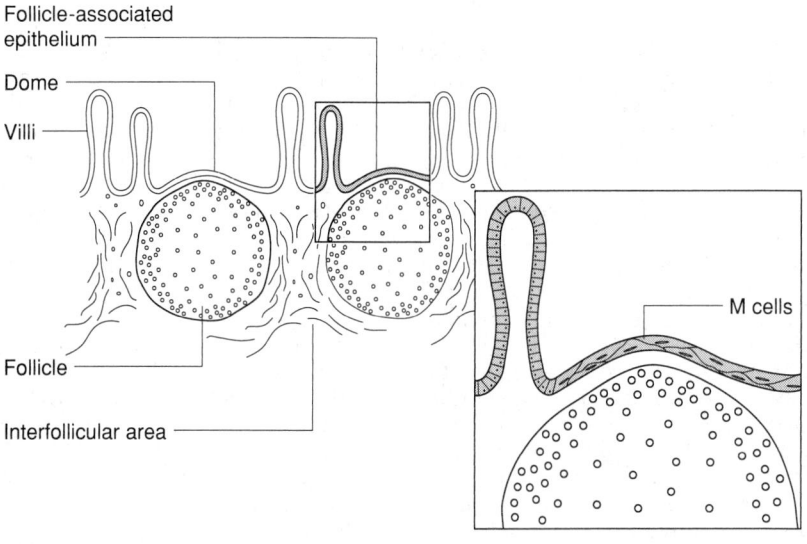

Figure 26-5. Epithelial anatomy in the area of Peyer patches.

hormonally mediated. The MMC can be disrupted by the sight or smell of food but not by parenteral nutrition. Orally consumed fats are much more effective at interrupting the MMC than equicaloric amounts of carbohydrate or protein.

SMALL-INTESTINAL DIGESTION AND ABSORPTION

The function of the GI tract is digestion and absorption of food for the continued growth and survival of the organism. The small intestine plays the largest role in absorption, which begins in the duodenum. Chyme stimulates the release of secretin and CCK from the duodenal mucosa, which aids in digestion by promoting pancreatic secretion and gallbladder emptying.

The jejunum is the site of maximum absorption of all ingested material except for vitamin B_{12} (cobalamin). Besides being the site of transport processes, the jejunal mucosa contains numerous large intercellular pores that allow rapid passive transfer of solutes and water. The ileum is less permeable and makes greater use of active-transport mechanisms, such as specific receptors for vitamin B_{12} and bile salts.

Absorption of Water

About 1 to 1.5 L of water is ingested each day. Another 5 to 10 L is secreted by the GI tract. About 80% of this fluid is reabsorbed by the small intestine. Net water movement into or out of the intestinal lumen is determined by the tonicity of the enteric material. When a meal is ingested, a hypotonic solution of chyme is deposited in the upper small intestine. Water rapidly leaves the lumen through the large intercellular pores in the jejunum, bringing enteric contents closer to isotonicity. Of the original 6 to 11 L of water that enters the duodenum in 24 hours, <1 L is delivered to the colon.

Absorption of Electrolytes

The four basic mechanisms of sodium absorption are: (1) simple electrogenic absorption; (2) non–electrolyte-stimulated absorption; (3) neutral absorption; and (4) solvent drag. The first three depend on the $Na^+\phi K^+\phi ATPase$ pump in the basolateral cell membrane. This process extrudes three Na^+ ions from the cell for every two K^+ ions that enter, using energy generated by hydrolysis of ATP.

Sodium

Absorption of sodium is an electrochemical process that causes sodium to leave the electrically neutral, high-sodium concentration of the intestinal lumen to enter the negatively charged, low-sodium concentration of the cell interior. Non–electrolyte-stimulated sodium absorption involves the absorption of sodium with an organic solute, such as glucose, and is mediated by a specific carrier molecule in the apical membrane. Neutral sodium chloride absorption couples sodium and chloride transport.

A large portion of sodium absorption, especially in the jejunum, where intercellular junctions are large and osmotic forces great, depends on the phenomenon of solvent drag. When osmotic forces generate rapid movement of water from the intestinal lumen through intercellular tight junctions into the interstitium, the friction between the water and the dissolved electrolytes drags sodium ions along with the movement of water.

Although the intestine has a high bidirectional sodium flux, it is highly sodium-preserving. Of the 250 to 300 mEq/d of sodium consumed by the average adult, >95% is absorbed; <5 mEq/d is excreted in the stool.

Chloride

Active sodium chloride cotransport predominates in the ileum. Passive diffusion of chloride can occur through paracellular spaces because the interstitium is slightly electrically positive in relation to the intestinal lumen. A large portion of chloride transport is reabsorption of chloride ion secreted as hydrochloric acid by the stomach.

Bicarbonate

Bicarbonate absorption in the jejunum involves the formation of carbon dioxide in the intestinal lumen from bicarbonate ion and secreted hydrogen ion. This process generates a high partial pressure of carbon dioxide in the lumen, causing the carbon dioxide to diffuse back into the cell and re-form bicarbonate and hydrogen ion by way of carbonic anhydrase. Bicarbonate diffuses into the blood, whereas hydrogen ion is resecreted, partly in exchange for sodium. In the ileum and duodenum, bicarbonate is actively secreted in exchange for chloride and assists in the neutralization of stomach acid and the generation of alkaline succus entericus.

Potassium

Potassium absorption is largely passive, taking place through the intercellular pores in the jejunum where concentration gradients are greatest.

Calcium

The acidic environment of the stomach assists in calcium absorption by solubilizing ingested nonionic calcium carbonate salts. The intestine absorbs 40% of the calcium to which it is exposed, all in the duodenum and jejunum. At high concentrations, the active-transport process is saturated, and passive absorptive diffusion of calcium occurs. At low concentrations, calcium absorption involves the capture of calcium by calcium-binding protein facilitated by active transport across the apical membrane into the cell, and active transport out of the cell at the basolateral surface by means of a Ca^{++}-ATPase pump. This process is regulated by parathyroid hormone (PTH). PTH is released in low-calcium states and promotes the conversion of vitamin D to its active form. The active form increases the synthesis of calcium-binding protein, increasing absorption of calcium.

Iron

Most dietary iron comes from ingested meat as myoglobin and hemoglobin, and is absorbed in the duodenum and proximal jejunum. There are separate transport mechanisms for complexed iron (heme), which is most rapidly absorbed, and inorganic iron, which is absorbed in the ferrous (Fe^{++}) form. Dietary ascorbic acid aids in iron absorption by reducing ferric (Fe^{+++}) ion to the more absorbable ferrous form. Within the cell, enzyme mechanisms liberate ferrous ion from the heme moiety. The ferrous iron can then be complexed with apoferritin to form ferritin, an intracellular storage form of iron. Alternatively, ferrous iron can be extruded from the serosal surface of the cell by a carrier protein, and then delivered to other tissues complexed with transferrin, a plasma transport protein.

Carbohydrate Digestion and Absorption

A typical adult in the western world consumes about 400 g/d of carbohydrate in the form of starch (about 60%), sucrose (30%), and lactose (10%), yielding about 1600 kcal

(4 kcal/g) of energy. Starch digestion is usually complete by the time the carbohydrate load reaches the distal duodenum. The oligosaccharides that result, along with sucrose and lactose, are then presented to the brush border of the jejunum to complete digestion and absorption. In the brush border, enzymes catalyze the hydrolysis of these sugars into glucose, galactose, and fructose. These monosaccharides are then absorbed into the cell. Glucose and galactose compete for the same carrier mechanism and require sodium for transport across the cell membrane. The sugar then exits the cell at the basolateral surface. Absorption of fructose does not require sodium.

Dietary fiber is nondigestible carbohydrate, such as cellulose. High-fiber diets retain water within the intestinal lumen and shorten intestinal transit time. Dietary fiber can adsorb organic materials such as bile salts and lipids, and inorganic minerals such as zinc, calcium, magnesium, and iron.

Protein Digestion and Absorption

The hydrolysis of protein into its constituent amino acids starts in the stomach with the secretion and activation of pepsinogen into pepsin. In the duodenum, peptidases from the pancreas break the protein molecules into peptide chains. About 30% of protein is digested to free amino acids, and the remainder to oligopeptides of two to six amino acids. Hydrolysis of the latter occurs either at the brush border or within the cellular cytoplasm. In the apical cells, membrane transport mechanisms transfer dipeptides or tripeptides into the cytosol, where specific peptidases further hydrolyze the peptides to their component amino acids. Larger peptides are first enzymatically cleaved in the brush border and then absorbed as either dipeptides, tripeptides, or free amino acids.

There are at least four different amino-acid transport mechanisms, each based on the electrochemical characteristics of the amino acid to be transported—neutral, dibasic, acidic (or dicarboxylic), and imino. Energy for transport is derived from cotransport of sodium and, ultimately, from the Na^+-K^+-ATPase pump. The absorption of dipeptides and tripeptides is more rapid than that of single amino acids and accounts for the largest part of protein absorption. These transport processes use sodium- and energy-dependent carrier mechanisms. After digestion within the cell, free amino acids diffuse into the portal circulation.

Fat Digestion and Absorption

The average western diet contains 60 to 100 g of fat, 90% in the form of triglycerides and the remainder in the form of cholesterol, phospholipids, and fat-soluble vitamins. Fat digestion and absorption begin with triglyceride digestion in the intestinal lumen. Lipase, a pancreatic enzyme, cleaves the fatty moieties, yielding two fatty acids and a monoglyceride (a fatty acid esterified to glycerol). The secretion of lipase (and its necessary cofactor, colipase) from the pancreas, is stimulated by CCK, which is secreted by the duodenal mucosa in response to the presence of fatty acids in the duodenum.

After lipolysis, the free fatty acids and monoglycerides are solubilized in the aqueous contents of the intestine by forming bile micelles, which are aggregations of bile salts and fatty acids. The micelles traverse the water layer next to the brush border and approximate themselves and their component molecules to the mucosal cell for absorption. Absorption of micelle contents occurs by dissolution within the lipid bilayer of the mucosal cell. This process does not require energy and is rapid. Once within the cell, fatty acids are transferred to the endoplasmic reticulum by means of fatty acid-binding protein. In the endoplasmic reticulum, triglycerides are resynthesized, and a chylomicron is formed. Chylomicrons are large particles that consist of 90% triglyceride and 10% phospholipid, cholesterol, and protein. After exocytosis, chylomicrons enter the lymphatics through the terminal villus lacteal.

Very low-density lipoproteins, particles that have a high cholesterol-to-triglyceride ratio, manufactured by the mucosal cells, seem to be the most important route of entry into the bloodstream for dietary cholesterol.

Long-chain fatty acids are largely absorbed by the foregoing process and eventually enter the bloodstream through the thoracic duct. Short-chain fatty acids (fewer than 8 carbon atoms) are water-soluble and enter and exit enterocytes by simple diffusion without the need for bile micelles or chylomicrons. They are removed in the portal circulation without entering the lymphatics. Medium-chain triglycerides (6 to 14 carbon atoms) are absorbed and removed from the intestine by simple diffusion and the absorptive process used by long-chain fatty acids.

Absorption of Bile Salts

Eighty to ninety percent of secreted bile salts in the micelles are reabsorbed and returned to the liver through the portal circulation. In the liver, bile salts are resecreted and stored in the gallbladder in preparation for the next meal. Passive absorption of bile occurs along the entire length of the small intestine and depends on the lipid solubility of the bile salt. As much as 50% of bile is passively absorbed. Active absorption of bile occurs only in the terminal ileum, probably through a sodium-linked cotransport system. A small amount of bile escapes into the colon, where it is deconjugated by bacteria, promoting lipid solubility and further passive absorption. Compromise of fat absorption can decrease bile absorption by stabilizing the bile micelles.

Vitamin Absorption

Fat-soluble vitamins (A, D, E, and K) are principally absorbed by micelles along with fats and exit the mucosal cells in chylomicrons to enter the lymph. Water-soluble vitamins are absorbed in the ileum and jejunum. Vitamins C (ascorbic acid), B_1 (thiamine), B_{12} (cobalamin), and niacin use active-transport mechanisms linked to sodium cotransport. Folic acid and vitamin B_2 (riboflavin) are absorbed by facilitated diffusion. Pyridoxine (B_6) is absorbed by simple diffusion.

Glutamine and Ammonia Metabolism

Glutamine is the most abundant amino acid in the blood and is the most important respiratory fuel of the enterocyte. This amino acid is important in total body nitrogen and ammonia metabolism. Ammonia is part of all amino acids, proteins, and nucleic acids, yet is relatively toxic when free in the blood. Glutamine detoxifies ammonia in peripheral tissues such as muscle. Twenty to thirty percent of circulating plasma glutamine is taken up by the small intestine and accounts for approximately half of the ammonia generated by the intestine. The remaining ammonia is largely the product of colonic bacterial metabolism. Surgical patients who receive glutamine-supplemented hyperalimentation solutions show improved nitrogen balance and protein metabolism. Most standard hyperalimentation solutions do not contain glutamine, however, because of its short shelf-life and its potential for ammonia toxicity. This problem can be circumvented by the use of glutamine dipeptides, or the addition of glutamine at the time of administration of hyperalimentation solutions. Early resumption of enteral feeding, however, provides the safest and most effective way to maintain a healthy intestinal mucosa.

SUGGESTED READING

Cohen S, Snape WJ. Movement of the small and large intestine. In: Sleisenger MH, Fordtran JS, eds. Gastrointestinal disease: pathophysiology, diagnosis, management, ed 4, vol 2. Philadelphia, Saunders, 1989:1088.
Davenport HW. Physiology of the digestive tract, ed 5. Chicago, Year Book, 1982.
Faucett DW. A textbook of histology, ed 11. Philadelphia, Saunders, 1986:641.
Granger DN, Barrowman JA, Kuietys PR. Clinical gastrointestinal physiology. Philadelphia, Saunders, 1985.
Hanaver SB, Kraft SC. Intestinal immunology. In: Berk JE, ed. Bockus gastroenterology, ed 4, vol 3. Philadelphia, Saunders, 1985:1607.
Kagnoff MF. Immunology of the digestive system. In: Johnson LR, ed. Physiology of the gastrointestinal tract, ed 2. New York, Raven, 1987:1699.
Souba WW. The gut as a nitrogen-processing organ in the metabolic response to critical illness. Nutr Support Serv 1988; 8:15.
Weisbrodt NW. Motility of the small intestine. In: Johnson LR, ed. Physiology of the gastrointestinal tract, ed 2. New York, Raven, 1987:631.

ESSENTIALS OF SURGERY: SCIENTIFIC PRINCIPLES AND PRACTICE, edited by Lazar J. Greenfield, Michael W. Mulholland, Keith T. Oldham, Gerald B. Zelenock, and Keith D. Lillemoe. Lippincott–Raven Publishers, Philadelphia, © 1997.

CHAPTER 27

ILEUS AND BOWEL OBSTRUCTION

DAVID I. SOYBEL

Mechanical obstruction means that luminal contents cannot pass through the intestinal tube because the lumen is blocked. In neurogenic or functional obstruction, luminal contents do not pass because of disturbances in intestinal motility that prevent peristalsis. Functional obstruction is also called ileus.

MECHANICAL OBSTRUCTION

In simple mechanical obstruction the intestinal lumen is partially or completely occluded without compromise of intestinal blood flow. Simple obstruction may be complete (the lumen is totally occluded (Fig. 27-1)), or incomplete (the lumen is narrowed but allows distal passage of some fluid and air). In strangulation, blood flow to the obstructed segment is compromised, and tissue necrosis and gangrene are imminent. Obstruction is classified according to cause and location of the obstructing lesion (Table 27-1).

Open-loop obstruction occurs when intestinal flow is blocked but proximal decompression is possible by means of vomiting. Closed-loop obstruction occurs when inflow to and outflow from the loop of intestine are blocked (Fig. 27-2). Gas and secretions accumulate in the loop without a means of decompression. Examples of closed-loop ob-

struction include torsion of a loop of small intestine around an adhesive band, incarceration of intestine in a hernia, volvulus of the cecum or colon, or obstructing carcinoma of the colon with a competent ileocecal valve.

Pathophysiologic Features

Local Effects

When a loop of intestine becomes obstructed, intestinal gas and fluid accumulate. The rate at which symptoms and complications develop depends on luminal volume, bacterial proliferation, and alterations in motility and perfusion.

Intestinal Gas

In the setting of acute pain and anxiety, patients with intestinal obstruction may swallow excessive amounts of air. Distal passage of swallowed air is prevented with nasogastric suction.

Intestinal Flora

Normal digestive function depends on the resident bacterial population. Maintenance of this flora depends on intact motor activity of the intestines and interactions among the bacterial species present. This balance is disturbed by antibiotic therapy or surgical procedures that result in stasis within intestinal segments.

Intestinal Fluid

Fluid accumulates in the lumen in the presence of intestinal obstruction. Elevation of luminal pressure >20 cm H_2O inhibits absorption and stimulates secretion of salt and water into the lumen proximal to an obstruction.

Intestinal Blood Flow

In response to heightened luminal pressure, total blood flow to the intestinal wall may increase. Enzymatic breakdown of stagnant intestinal contents leads to increased osmolarity of luminal contents. The simultaneous changes in hydrostatic and osmotic pressures on the blood and lumen sides of the mucosa favor flow of extracellular fluid into the lumen. Blood flow is compromised as luminal pressure increases, bacteria invade, and inflammation leads to edema within the intestinal wall.

Intestinal Motility

Obstruction of the intestinal lumen does not simply block distal passage of luminal contents. Accumulation of fluid and gas in the obstructed lumen elicits changes in myoelectrical function proximal and distal to the obstructed segment. In response to this distention, the obstructed segment may dilate, a process known as receptive relaxation. Such changes ensure that, despite accumulation of air and fluid, intraluminal pressures do not rise easily to the point of compromising blood flow to the intestinal mucosa.

Complications of Intestinal Obstruction

Closed-Loop Obstruction

The complications of closed-loop obstructions evolve rapidly. The reasons for this rapid evolution are best understood by considering the simplest and most common form of closed-loop obstruction: appendicitis.

When a fecalith obstructs the blind-ended appendix, secretion of mucus and enhanced peristalsis represent an initial attempt to clear the blockage. Intense, crampy ab-

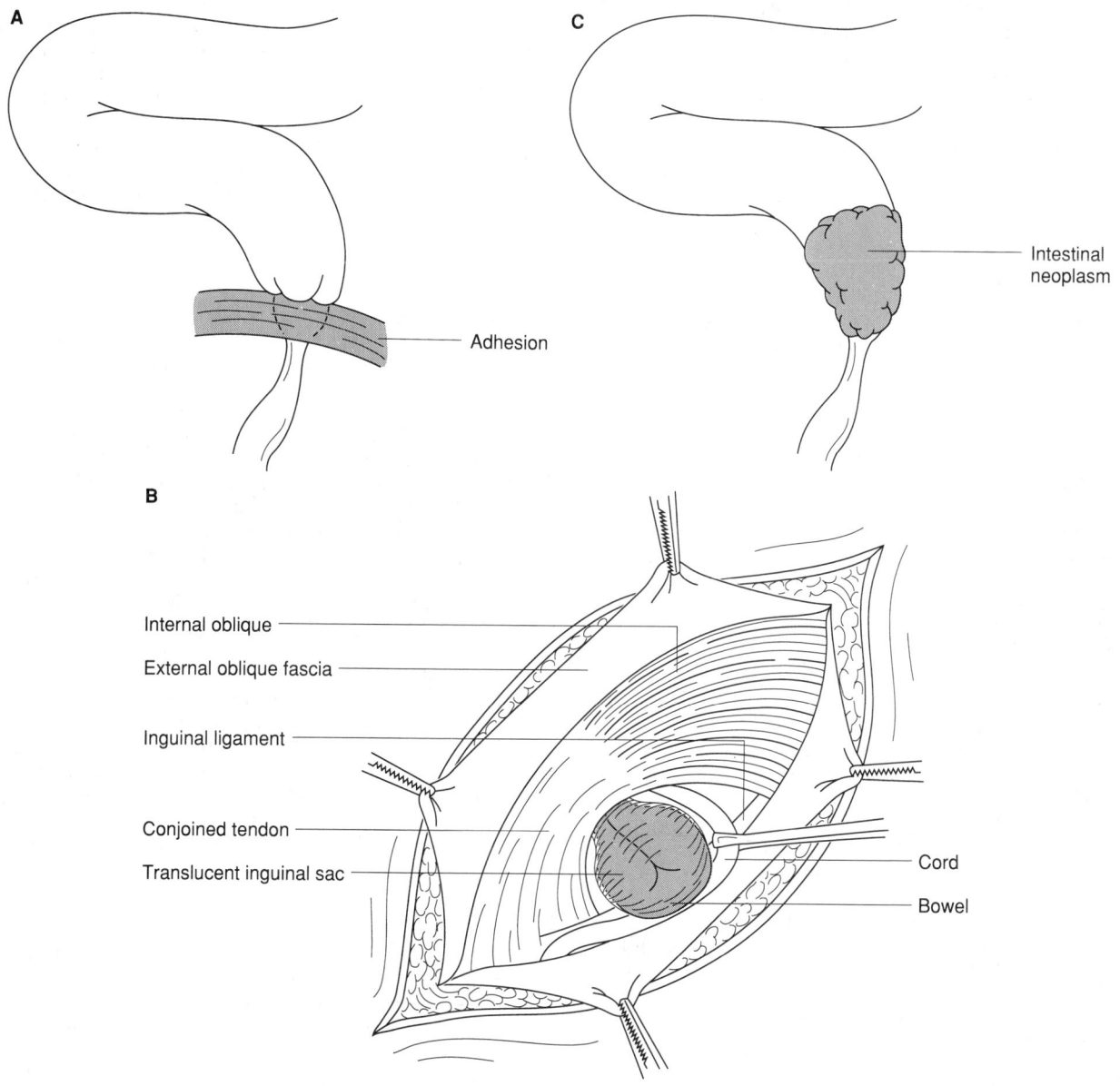

Figure 27-1. Schematic illustration of different forms of simple mechanical obstruction. Simple obstruction is most often due to adhesion (*A*), groin hernia (*B*), or neoplasm (*C*). The hernia can act as a tourniquet, causing a closed-loop obstruction and strangulation.

dominal pain focused at the umbilicus results. Nausea and vomiting occur in response to hyperperistalsis and stretching of the mesentery. Over the next 8 to 18 hour, continued secretion of mucus leads to high intraluminal pressure, stasis, bacterial overgrowth, and mucosal disruption. When luminal pressure exceeds mural venous pressure and capillary perfusion pressure, inflammatory cells are recruited from surrounding peritoneal structures. This sequence leads to intense inflammation, release of exudate in the area of the appendix, and the localization of pain from the umbilicus to the area of peritoneum nearest the inflamed appendix.

Peritoneal findings (localized tenderness, involuntary guarding, rebound or referred tenderness) and fever appear. Twenty to 24 hours into the illness, the blood supply of the appendix is compromised. Gangrene and perforation follow, and if not contained by surrounding structures,

free perforation leads to peritonitis. Toxins from necrotic tissue and bacterial overgrowth are released into the systemic circulation, and shock occurs. Torsion of a loop of small intestine around an adhesive band or inside a hernia leads to a similar sequence of events. Torsion of the large intestine is usually accompanied by massive distention of the loop by air and feces.

Open Loop Obstruction

Complications of open-loop obstruction do not evolve rapidly. Open-loop obstruction in the proximal jejunum (high obstruction) can be decompressed with vomiting. The obstruction is characterized by loss of gastric, pancreatic, and biliary secretions with resulting electrolyte disturbances. Obstruction of the distal ileum (low obstruction) may lead only to slowly progressive distention of the small intestine, with accommodation by intestinal myo-

Table 27-1. CLASSIFICATION OF ADULT MECHANICAL INTESTINAL OBSTRUCTIONS

INTRALUMINAL	EXTRINSIC
Foreign bodies	Adhesions
Barium inspissation (colon)	Congenital
Bezoar	Ladd or Meckel's
Inspissated feces	bands
Gallstone	Postoperative
Meconium (cystic fibrosis)	Postinflammatory
Parasites	Hernias
Other (eg, swallowed objects,	External
enteroliths)	Internal
Intussusception	Volvulvus
Polypoid, exophytic lesions	External mass effect
INTRAMURAL	Abscess
	Annular pancreas
Congenital	Carcinomatosis
Atresia, stricture, or stenosis	Endometriosis
Web	Pregnancy
Intestinal duplication	Pancreatic pseudocyst
Meckel's diverticulum	
Inflammatory process	
Crohn's disease	
Diverticulitis	
Chronic intestinal ischemia or	
postischemic stricture	
Radiation enteritis	
Medication induced (nonsteroidal	
antiinflammatories, postassium	
chloride tablets)	
Neoplasms	
Primary bowel (malignant or benign)	
Secondary (metastases, especially	
melanoma)	
Traumatic	
Intramural hematoma of duodenum	

electrical function and minor alterations in fluid and electrolyte balances. Open-loop obstruction from midjejunum to midileum (intermediate obstruction) is often characterized by events similar to those of closed-loop obstruction or combinations of the events of high and low obstruction (Table 27-2).

Clinical Presentation

The following questions must be addressed expeditiously:

1. Is pain out of proportion to the physical findings?
2. How rapidly are the symptoms and signs evolving (minutes, hours)?
3. Is the patient experiencing dehydration and serum electrolyte and pH imbalances?
4. Is the obstruction complete or incomplete?
5. Is there a possibility of strangulation?

The presentation of small-intestinal obstruction depends on level of obstruction, open- or closed-loop nature, and interval since onset of symptoms. Pain, vomiting, obstipation, and distention are present in variable degrees. Vomiting and acute fluid and electrolyte imbalances are sometimes prominent. Elderly patients are prone to dehydration.

Diagnosis

Plain abdominal radiographs and laboratory studies are used to confirm the diagnosis of obstruction and determine the extent of physiologic impairment. The patient's history

and the clinical course in the first few hours of observation are evaluated to determine the likelihood of strangulation. Key factors in the history and clinical examination include: (1) previous abdominal operation; (2) quality of pain (colicky and intermittent as opposed to steady); (3) abdominal distention; and (4) hyperactivity of bowel sounds. Contrast radiography or computed tomography (CT) are used only when symptoms are not evolving rapidly or when identification of the underlying lesion might alter surgical strategy.

Treatment

Initial treatment of all patients with suspected intestinal obstruction includes restriction of oral intake and IV administration of fluids. Restoration of fluid and electrolyte balance necessitates frequent assessment of serum electrolyte levels and pH. In the presence of rapidly evolving obstruction or in patients with marked dehydration, an indwelling urinary catheter is placed to monitor urine output. Invasive hemodynamic monitoring (eg, with a Swan–Ganz catheter) may be necessary to monitor the response to fluid resuscitation in patients with underlying cardiac, pulmonary, or renal insufficiency. Nasogastric decompression is indicated in all but the most mild cases of obstruction. The nasogastric tube prevents distal passage of swallowed air and minimizes the discomfort of reflux of intestinal content.

Perioperative administration of antibiotics reduces risk for wound infection and abdominal sepsis in patients undergoing operations to relieve intestinal obstruction. Only when the decision has been made to proceed with an operation are antibiotics administered. Giving antibiotics to patients who are being observed can obscure the underlying process and delay therapy.

Abdominal exploration is performed when the diagnosis

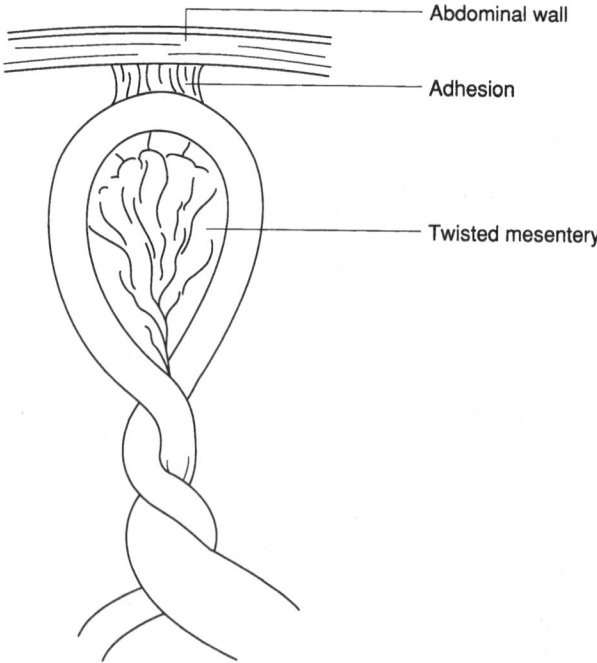

Figure 27-2. Schematic illustration of a closed-loop obstruction. The small intestine twists around its mesentery, compromising inflow and outflow of luminal contents from the loop. Also, the vascular supply to the loop may be compromised because of the twisting of the mesentery. The risk of strangulation is high.

Table 27-2. SYMPTOMS AND SIGNS OF BOWEL OBSTRUCTION

Symptom or Sign	Proximal Small Bowel (Open Loop)	Distal Small Bowel (Open Loop)	Small Bowel (Closed Loop)	Colon and Rectum
Pain	Intermittent, intense, colicky; often relieved by vomiting	Intermittent to constant	Progressive, intermittent to constant; rapidly worsens	Continuous
Vomiting	Large volumes, bilious and frequent	Low volume and frequency; progressively feculent with time	May be prominent (reflex)	Intermittent, not prominent; feculent when present
Tenderness	Epigastric or periumbilical; quite mild unless strangulation is present	Diffuse and progressive	Diffuse, progressive	Diffuse
Distention	Absent	Moderate to marked	Often absent	Marked
Obstipation	May not be present	Present	May not be present	Present

(Adapted from Schuffler MD, Sinanan MN. Intestinal obstruction and pseudo-obstruction. In: Sleisenger MH, Fordtran JS, eds. Gastrointestinal disease, ed 5. Philadelphia, WB Saunders, 1993:898)

of intestinal obstruction is likely or certain, and when resuscitation has been completed. The indications are as follows:

Rapidly progressing abdominal pain or distention, with or without peritoneal findings

Peritoneal findings, fever, diminished urine output, leukocytosis, hyperamylasemia, metabolic acidosis

Failure of signs and symptoms of obstruction to resolve over 24-48 hour, even in the absence of peritoneal findings

Once a diagnosis of complete obstruction is made, an operation is performed without delay. It is reasonable to observe the patient when the diagnosis is uncertain or if the obstruction is incomplete.

Types of Intestinal Obstruction

Adhesions

Operations on the lower part of the abdomen, such as appendectomy, hysterectomy, and abdominoperineal resection, often are complicated by adhesive obstruction. Adhesions can form after any abdominal procedure, however, including cholecystectomy, gastrectomy, and vascular procedures. Mechanisms of adhesion formation include foreign body reaction to talc, starch, lint, intestinal content, or suture; intussusception; hernia; abscess; or technical error. The most reasonable approach to reducing adhesion formation includes meticulous attention to hemostasis, gentle surgical technique, and removal of foreign material from the peritoneal cavity. The use of monofilament sutures for fascial closure and avoidance of closure of the peritoneum as a separate layer, reduce the likelihood of formation of adhesions between viscera and abdominal wall.

Acute symptoms denote complete obstruction, which must be treated immediately. Delays in recognition and operative intervention can be fatal. Loss of bowel sounds after a short period of normal or increased activity is a sign of ischemia.

Most postoperative adhesions are treated as partial intestinal obstruction. Nasogastric suction and IV fluids usually relieve symptoms within a few days (Fig. 27-3). When the clinical course does not call for early surgical intervention, nonsurgical therapy may be tried for 10 to 14 days.

Hernia

When herniation causes obstruction, the patient is quickly resuscitated and taken to the operating room. The hernia is reduced and the viability of the intestine assessed. If viable, the intestine is left alone; if not, it is resected. The hernial defect is repaired.

Gallstone Ileus

As a result of intense inflammation surrounding a gallstone, a fistula may develop between the biliary tree and the small or large intestine. Patients usually are elderly and present with intermittent symptoms over several days, as the stone tumbles toward the ileum. The classic findings on plain radiographs include intestinal obstruction, a stone outside the right upper quadrant, and air in the biliary tree.

Treatment is removal of the stone and resection of the obstructed segment of intestine if there is evidence of tissue necrosis. The entire intestine is searched to exclude the presence of additional gallstones. Cholecystectomy is not performed at the initial operation. The risk for recurrent gallstone ileus is 5% to 10%. Recurrences usually take place within 30 days of the initial episode and are usually caused by stones in the small intestine that were missed at the original operation.

Intussusception

Intussusception occurs when one segment of intestine telescopes into an adjacent segment, causing obstruction and ischemic injury. The obstruction may become complete, particularly if inflammation and necrosis occur. Tumors, benign or malignant, cause most cases of intussusception. Intussusception may be a postoperative complication related to the suture line, adhesions, or the presence or withdrawal of an intestinal tube. Perioperative intussusception frequently subsides without intervention.

The radiographic features of intussusception are not specific. Plain films reveal evidence of partial or complete obstruction. Sometimes a sausage-shaped area of soft-tissue opacity is outlined by two strips of air. Sonography may be useful in diagnosis, but the mainstay is contrast radiography (Fig. 27-4). Because of the relation between tumors and intussusception, surgical treatment is recommended. Reduction with hydrostatic pressure is the standard of care in children; it should not be attempted in adults.

Crohn's Disease

Intestinal obstruction is the most frequent indication for surgical intervention in Crohn's disease. Obstruction occurs under two sets of circumstances:

1. Acute episodes of the disease. The lumen may be narrowed by a reversible inflammatory process. The

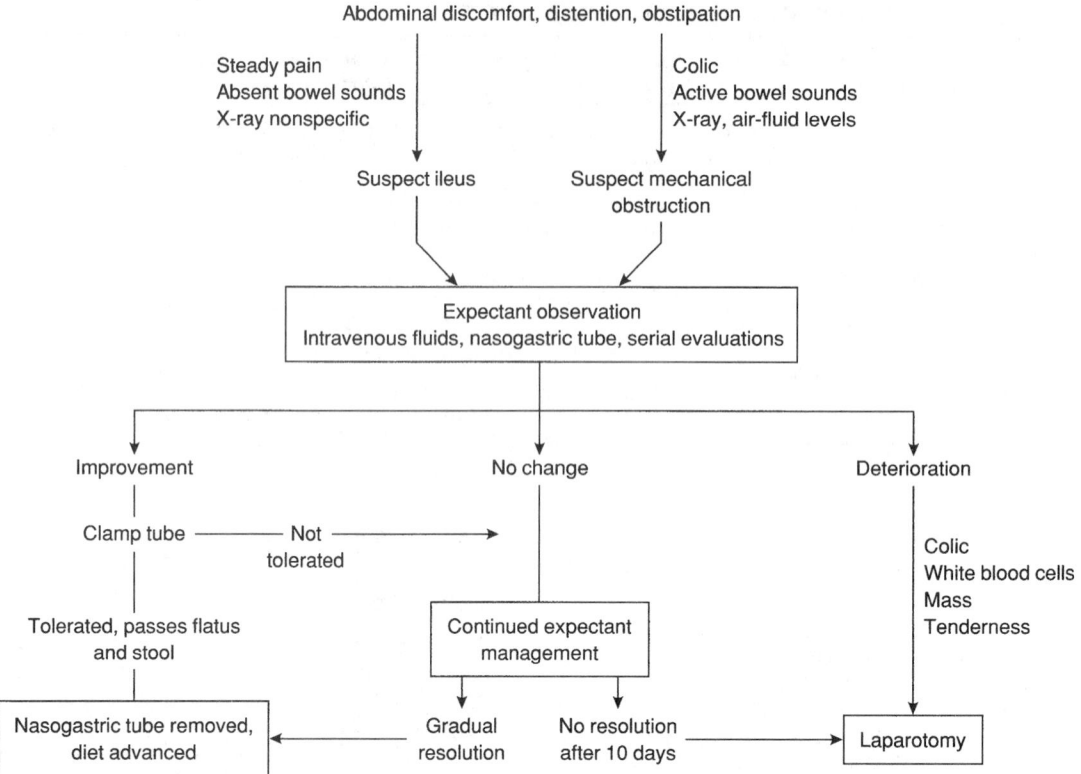

Abdominal discomfort, distention, obstipation

Steady pain
Absent bowel sounds
X-ray nonspecific

Colic
Active bowel sounds
X-ray, air-fluid levels

Suspect ileus

Suspect mechanical obstruction

Expectant observation
Intravenous fluids, nasogastric tube, serial evaluations

Improvement

No change

Deterioration

Clamp tube — Not tolerated

Colic
White blood cells
Mass
Tenderness

Tolerated, passes flatus and stool

Continued expectant management

Nasogastric tube removed, diet advanced

Gradual resolution

No resolution after 10 days

Laparotomy

Figure 27-3. An approach to postoperative intestinal obstruction. (Adapted from Welch JP. Bowel obstruction: differential diagnosis and clinical management. Philadelphia, WB. Saunders, 1989)

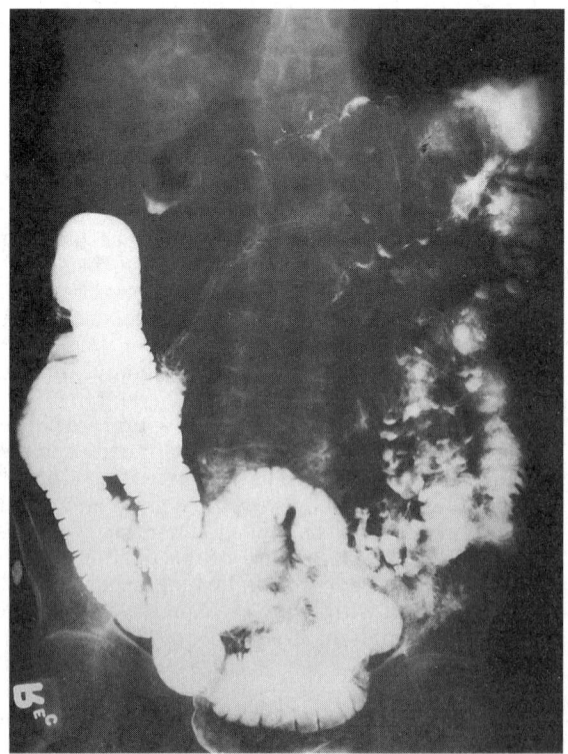

Figure 27-4. Barium enema showing intussusception of ileum (*arrows*) into ascending colon shortly after a cecectomy for tumor with ileal to ascending colon anastomosis. (Courtesy of John Braver, MD, Department of Radiology, Brigham and Women's Hospital, Harvard Medical School, Boston)

result is open-loop obstruction that may respond to IV hydration, nasogastric decompression, and therapy with corticosteroids or other anti-inflammatory drugs

2. Chronic strictures that do not respond to conservative measures. Affected intestine may not dilate proximal to the obstruction, and a small perforation develops that may not be large enough to show free air on a radiograph. Once the diagnosis is made, operative therapy is not delayed

A CT scan may help differentiate the two types of obstruction.

Malignant Obstruction

Obstruction can complicate malignant disease of the small and large intestine. Most often, a primary lesion such as an adenocarcinoma or lymphoma enlarges until the intestinal lumen is blocked. The lesion then causes symptoms and signs associated with the level of obstruction.

A second setting involves evidence of intestinal obstruction after a cancer operation. The likelihood that the obstruction is due to recurrent disease is related to (1) the origin of the primary tumor, (2) the stage of the primary tumor, and (3) whether the original operation was curative or palliative. Gastric and pancreatic carcinomas often present with, or are complicated by, peritoneal carcinomatosis and obstruction. Obstruction after resection of carcinoma of the colon and rectum is usually due to adhesions, and not recurrence of the malignant tumor. Even if obstruction is due to unresectable disease, palliation can be achieved with bypass or enterostomy (Fig. 27-5).

Volvulus

Volvulus occurs when a loop of intestine is twisted more than 180° about the axis of its mesentery. The most common site is the sigmoid colon. Volvulus is a form of closed-

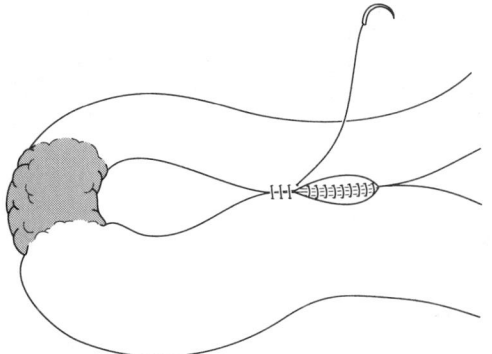

Figure 27-5. Significant palliation can be achieved in a patient with obstructing, but unresectable, malignancy. Enteroenterostomy is performed to bypass the obstructing segment.

loop obstruction. Volvulus of any segment of the colon is associated with abdominal distention and, usually, severe abdominal pain. The most common radiographic feature is a bent-inner-tube appearance of the sigmoid.

Treatment is with endoscopic decompression. A flexible sigmoidoscope is advanced into the rectum until a rush of air and feces indicates that torsion has been relieved. A rectal tube is advanced into the loop as a stent to prevent retorsion. Gangrene does not usually develop if treatment is prompt. After endoscopic decompression, volvulus is likely to recur if sigmoid resection is not performed. Sigmoid resection should be performed if the patient is fit for surgical therapy. If the patient presents with peritoneal findings, sepsis, and shock, rapid resuscitation followed by urgent resection and colostomy is warranted. Volvulus other than sigmoid volvulus usually cannot be relieved without an operation. Fixation of the twisted segment is a less satisfactory solution than resection of the involved segment.

Radiation Enteritis

Radiation injury elicits vasculitis and fibrosis that lead to chronic, recurrent low-grade partial obstruction of the small intestine and to strictures and bleeding in the colon and rectum. Surgical treatment is indicated for incapacitating symptoms but is risky. Attempts to suture scarred loops can result in chronic inflammation and formation of interloop abscesses and fistulas. The incidence of suture-line leak is high.

The Role of Laparoscopic Surgery in Intestinal Obstruction

Laparoscopic approaches to intestinal obstruction include lysis of adhesions, enterolithotomy for gallstone ileus, and fixation of volvulus segments. Laparoscopic approaches to all forms of abdominal surgery have been advocated as a way of reducing formation of adhesions and, thus, of reducing long-term risk for adhesive intestinal obstruction. This benefit has not been documented. In anecdotal reports, intestinal obstruction is mentioned as a complication of laparoscopic procedures. Causes of obstruction include Richter hernias due to entrapment of intestine in trocar entry sites, and unrecognized internal or abdominal-wall hernias. The incidence of complications should diminish with improvements in trocar design and operator experience.

ILEUS AND PSEUDOOBSTRUCTION
Ileus

Ileus reflects underlying alterations in motility of the GI tract that lead to functional obstruction. Ileus is the interval between an abdominal operation and the return of flatus and bowel movements. The factors implicated in the development and persistence of ileus are listed in Table 27-3.

The distinction between normal postoperative ileus and paralytic ileus is based on time elapsed since the operation and clinical circumstances. For example, after elective cholecystectomy, normal postoperative ileus lasts 48 hours. After low anterior resection of the colon, it may last 3 to 5 days. The absence of bowel sounds, flatus, or bowel movements beyond the expected period indicates delayed resolution, or paralytic ileus.

Diagnosis

When postoperative ileus extends beyond the expected period, plain radiographs of the abdomen reveal gas in segments of both small and large intestine. The patient may experience discomfort and distention as swallowed air fills loops that do not have effective peristalsis. Contrast radiography or CT is helpful in differentiating early postoperative obstruction and ileus. CT may be useful if abdominal abnormalities such as an abscess are suspected. Flow of contrast material to the large intestine excludes the diagnosis of complete obstruction but not of partial obstruction.

Treatment

Measures to prevent prolongation of ileus include: (1) meticulous technique in the operating room; (2) limiting use of narcotics for analgesia; (3) correction of electrolyte or metabolic imbalances; and (4) early recognition of septic complications.

Pseudoobstruction

Acute pseudoobstruction, also known as Ogilvie syndrome, is paralytic ileus of the large intestine. It is characterized by rapidly progressive abdominal distention, often without pain. Although the distention is not caused by mechanical obstruction, the intestinal wall, particularly

Table 27-3. POTENTIAL CONTRIBUTIONS TO PROLONGED ILEUS

NEUROGENIC	PHARMACOLOGIC
Spinal cord lesions or injury	Anticholinergics
Retroperitoneal process, hematoma, tumor	Opiates
Ureteral colic	Autonomic blockers
	Antihistamines
METABOLIC	Psychotropics
Hypokalemia	Phenothiazines
Uremia	Haloperidol
Ca^{2+}, Mg^{2+} imbalance	Tricyclic antidepressants
Hypothyroidism	Clonidine
Diabetic coma or ketoacidosis	Vincristine
	INFECTIOUS
	Systemic sepsis
	Pneumonia
	Peritonitis
	Herpes zoster
	Tetanus
	Bacterial overgrowth of bowel

of the cecum, can become so distended its blood supply is compromised. Gangrene, perforation, peritonitis, and shock follow. Risk factors include severe blunt trauma, orthopedic trauma or procedures, acute cardiac disease or a coronary bypass operation, acute neurologic disease or a neurosurgical procedure, and acute metabolic derangements.

Diagnosis

Plain radiographs of the abdomen reveal air in the small intestine and distention of discrete segments of colon (cecum or transverse colon) or the entire abdominal portion of the colon. When intestinal necrosis is not a concern, a radiographic enema examination with water-soluble contrast material can depict the nonmechanical nature of the dilatation. Colonoscopy may be therapeutic as well as diagnostic. Features of ischemia include localized tenderness, leukocytosis, metabolic acidosis, evidence of sepsis, and a rapidly deteriorating clinical course.

Treatment

Initial management of pseudoobstruction is resuscitation and correction of metabolic or electrolyte imbalances. A nasogastric tube is helpful if the patient is vomiting, and it prevents swallowed air from passing distally. Intestinal ischemia is an indication for surgical treatment. If intestinal necrosis is found, the affected segment is resected and an ileostomy or colostomy is established. If the intestine is viable, a cecostomy is placed to vent the colon and prevent distention.

If distention is painless and the patient shows no signs of toxicity or small-intestinal ischemia, expectant management is successful about 50% of the time. If the distention worsens so that the cecal diameter increases beyond 10 to 12 cm, or if distention persists for more than 48 hours, colonoscopy is recommended.

Endoscopic decompression may be successful, but colonic distention is likely to recur. Rectal tubes are ineffective in the treatment of distention of the proximal colon.

SUGGESTED READING

Cullen JJ, Eagon JC, Kelly KA. Gastrointestinal peptide hormones during postoperative ileus. Dig Dis Sci 1994;39:1179.

Eskelinen M, Ikonen J, Liponen P. Contributions of history-taking, physical examination, and computer assistance to diagnose small bowel obstruction: A prospective study of 1333 patients with acute abdominal pain. Scand J Gastroenterol 1994;29: 715.

Frager D, Medwid SW, Baer JW, Mollinelli B, Friedman M. CT of small bowel obstruction: Value in establishing the diagnosis and determining the degree and cause. Am J Roentgenol 1994;162:37.

Frank JW, Sarr MG, Camilleri M. Use of gastroduodenal motility to differentiate mechanical and functional intestinal obstruction: An analysis of clinical outcome. Am J Gastroenterol 1994;89:339.

Frantzides CT, Cowles V, Salaymeh B. Morphine effects on human colonic myoelectric activity in the post-operative period. Am J Surg 1992;163:144.

Garcia-Caballero M, Vara-Thorbeck C. The evolution of postoperative ileus after laparoscopic cholecystectomy: A comparative study with conventional cholecystectomy. Surg Endosc 1993;7:416.

Ogata M, Imai S, Hosotani R, Aoyama H, Hayashi M, Ishikawa T. Abdominal ultrasonography for the diagnosis of strangulation in small bowel obstruction. Br J Surg 1994;81:421.

O'Leary DP, Coakley JB. The influence of suturing and sepsis on the development of post-operative peritoneal adhesions. Ann R Coll Surg Engl 1992;74:134.

Reisner RM, Cohen JR. Gallstone ileus: A review of 1001 reported cases. Am Surg 1994;60:441.

Serror D, Feigin E, Szold A, et al. How conservatively can post-operative small bowel obstruction be treated? Am J Surg 1993;165:121.

ESSENTIALS OF SURGERY: SCIENTIFIC PRINCIPLES AND PRACTICE, edited by Lazar J. Greenfield, Michael W. Mulholland, Keith T. Oldham, Gerald B. Zelenock, and Keith D. Lillemoe. Lippincott–Raven Publishers, Philadelphia, © 1997.

CHAPTER 28
CROHN'S DISEASE
WOLFGANG H. SCHRAUT AND DAVID S. MEDICH

Crohn's disease is an incurable chronic inflammatory disorder of the alimentary tract. The terminal ileum and proximal colon are affected most often, but any portion from mouth to anus can be involved. Involvement of extraintestinal tissues (joints, skin, eyes) is common, indicating that Crohn's disease is a systemic disorder, not a localized intestinal disease. The disease course is characterized by histopathologic and physiologic changes and signs and symptoms that wax and wane. The cause and pathogenesis are not known.

ETIOLOGIC THEORIES

The two following etiologic hypotheses have evolved:

1. The infectious theory. An unidentified microbe or agent causes the disease, and the immune system responds appropriately to the invasion.
2. The immunologic theory. The immune system reacts inappropriately to antigenic challenge.

Proposed infectious causes are as follows:

- Bacterial infection, most notably with Mycobacterium spp
- The presence of abnormal qualitative and quantitative microflora in the small intestine, most likely the result of inflammation and fecal stagnation
- Viral infection
- Proposed immunogenetic causes are as follows:
- Genetic predisposition
- Aberrations in the mechanisms of the intestinal mucosal immune system (Figs. 28-1, 28-2).

Pathologic Features

Crohn's disease may be rapidly progressive or may run an indolent course with intermittent episodes of exacerbation. The acute, active phase is marked by aphthous mucosal ulcers, lymphoid aggregates, granulomas, and transmural chronic inflammation with fissures and fistulas. The quiescent, healing phase is characterized by fibrosis with stricture formation and chronic ulcers. The granulomatous inflammatory process may involve other tissues and organs.

Macroscopic Appearance

Segments of intestine involved in Crohn's disease are rigid and thickened as a result of fibrosis and inflammatory edema that narrow the intestinal lumen. Mesenteric fat

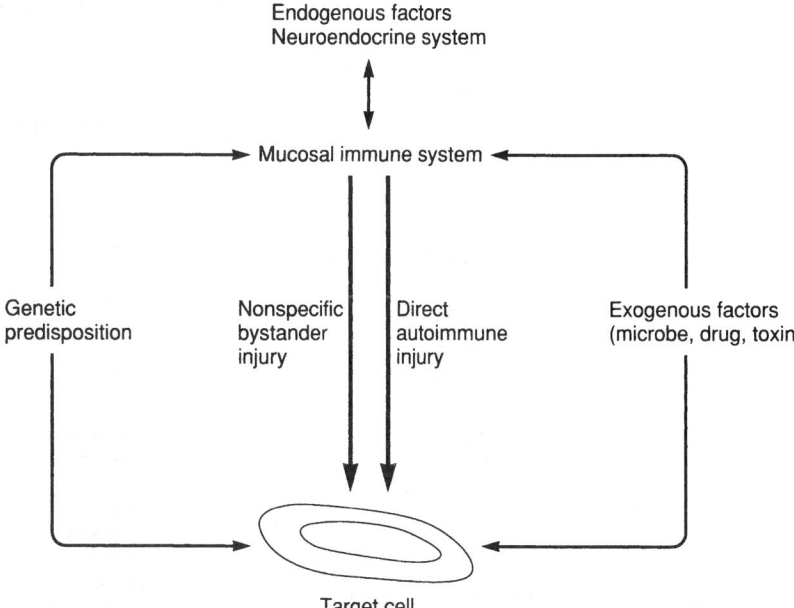

Figure 28-1. Overview of the elements that may contribute to the pathogenesis of inflammatory bowel disease. (After Shanahan F, Targan S. Immunology of inflammatory bowel disease. In: Shaffer E, Thomson ABR, eds. Modern concepts in gastroenterology, vol 2. New York, Plenum, 1989:293)

reaches over the antimesenteric intestinal wall. The serosa may be granular and dulled by exudate. The mesentery is foreshortened, thickened, and edematous and contains enlarged, inflamed mesenteric lymph nodes. The inflammatory process may extend into adjacent tissues and structures, causing fistulas, abscesses, and sinus tracks. Inflammation and fibrosis often distort normal anatomic boundaries, causing ureteral deviation and obstruction or intestinal obstruction with matting-together of involved and uninvolved loops of intestine. Fistulous communications may occur between the diseased intestine and any intraabdominal or extraabdominal structure or organ. Opening a segment of intestine affected by Crohn's disease reveals a thick wall, a narrow lumen, longitudinal ulcerations, cobblestoning, aphthoid ulcers, and dilatation of proximal uninvolved intestine.

Microscopic Features

The pathologic changes of Crohn's disease begin with focal accumulation of inflammatory cells adjacent to a crypt. Localization at the crypt leads to aphthoid ulcers, fissure-like ulcers, and crypt abscesses. Granulomas are localized, well-formed aggregates of epithelioid histiocyte surrounded by lymphocytes and giant cells. Caseation is absent. Fistulas and sinus tracks develop from confluent crypt abscesses and transmural inflammation. Transmural inflammation is characterized by lymphoid aggregates in a widened submucosa and similar accumulations external to the muscularis propria. Transmural inflammation is accompanied by serositis that causes adherence to other loops of intestine or adjacent organs.

Epithelial cell injury with necrosis is not the initial event but evolves as the inflammatory process matures. Often the overlying mucosa is edematous only while the submucosal compartment is edematous and infiltrated with lymphoid and inflammatory cells. A mature inflammatory lesion contains lymphocytes (more T cells than B cells), macrophages, and neutrophils. T cells are both suppressor and helper cells. B cells producing IgG are more common than in normal intestine. The most common B cells are IgA-positive plasma cells.

Differentiation between Crohn's disease of the colon and

ulcerative colitis is difficult. Ulcerative colitis is a mucosal disease that begins at the rectum and is contiguous, whereas Crohn's colitis may involve all layers of the intestinal wall and is often discontinuous (Table 28-1).

Clinical Features

The location of Crohn's disease in the GI tract determines the clinical features, the nature of complications, the surgical procedure, and the prognosis. Three categories of disease are recognized—ileocolic, small-intestinal, and colonic (Table 28-2). Classification according to histopathologic and pathophysiologic criteria is as follows:

1. Stenosing, fibrosing, stricturing Crohn's disease that necessitates and is amenable to surgical therapy
2. Fistulizing, abscess-forming disease treated with medical and surgical therapy
3. Aggressive, inflammatory disease treated with anti-inflammatory agents and immunosuppressive therapy

Crohn's disease usually arises between 15 and 35 years of age. In most patients, the clinical signs and symptoms center on the triad of abdominal pain, diarrhea, and weight loss. These signs and symptoms have an insidious, gradual onset. Symptoms usually last for 2 to 3 years before the diagnosis is confirmed. The diagnosis is usually made during an acute exacerbation. Sometimes extraintestinal manifestations are the initial clinical presentation (Table 28-3).

Abdominal pain is due to partial obstruction and is worsened by oral intake. Pain is often accompanied by a tender mass in the right lower abdominal quadrant and by febrile episodes. Signs and symptoms may mimic acute appendicitis and often precipitate abdominal exploration to establish the diagnosis. A common manifestation of Crohn's disease is perianal disease, including anal fistulas with extension to adjacent organs and regions, fissures, and perirectal abscesses.

The clinical manifestations of Crohn's disease in children are similar to those in adults. The most disconcerting aspect is growth failure and retardation of sexual development.

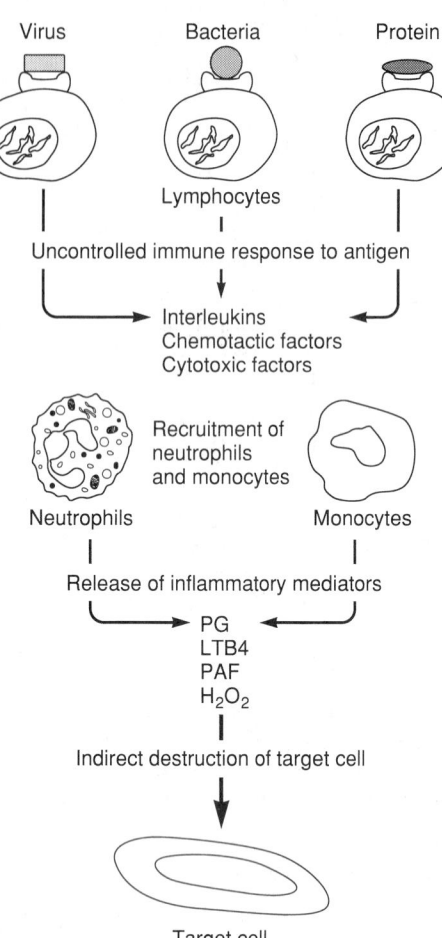

Figure 28-2. Mucosal immune effector mechanisms that have been proposed as possible mediators of a direct specific attack against the putative target cell in inflammatory bowel disease. These may be generated in response to either an alteration in the target cell or an external agent, or they may arise from a breakdown in mucosal immune tolerance to normal host epithelial cells. PG, prostaglandin; PAF, platelet-activating factor. (After Shanahan F, Targan S. Immunology of inflammatory bowel disease. In: Shaffer E, Thomson ABR, eds. Modern concepts in gastroenterology, vol 2. New York, Plenum, 1989:293)

COMPLICATIONS

Crohn's disease is associated with the following complications:

- Small-intestinal obstruction
- Fistula formation (Table 28-4)
- Intraabdominal abscesses
- Toxic megacolon or toxic dilatation of the ileum Perianal or anorectal disease
- Free perforation with peritonitis Carcinoma of the small or large intestine.

DIAGNOSIS

History and Physical Examination

The history reveals intermittent episodes of abdominal pain, diarrhea, and weight loss. Examination frequently discloses pallor and signs of undernutrition and malabsorption. The abdominal examination may disclose altered bowel sounds, distention, an inflammatory mass or ab-

Table 28-1. HISTOPATHOLOGIC DIFFERENTIATION OF CROHN'S COLITIS AND ULCERATIVE COLITIS

Crohn's Colitis	Ulcerative Colitis
MACROSCOPIC	
Transmural involvement	Disease confined to mucosa except in toxic dilation
Segmental disease, fistulas	Rectum always involved
Thickened wall with "creeping fat"	Normal thickness of bowel wall
Occasional pseudopolyps	Pseudopolyps
Small bowel may be involved	Small bowel not involved (except as backwash ileitis)
Perianal disease common	Perianal disease less common
MICROSCOPIC	
Transmural inflammation and fibrosis	Inflammation of mucosa and submucosa
Crypt abscesses less common	Crypt abscesses common
Cobblestoning	Pseudopolyps
Narrow, deeply penetrating ulcers	Shallow, wide ulcers
Fissures, fistulas	
Granuloma common	Granuloma rare
Mucus secretion increased	Mucus secretion decreased

scess, tenderness, or fistulas. Examination of the perineum and anorectum may demonstrate tender, ulcerated anal tags, eccentrically located fissures, fistulas, abscesses, rectal ulcers, and strictures.

Laboratory Findings

There is no specific test for Crohn's disease. Anemia, leukocytosis, and hypoproteinemia are common.

Endoscopic Examination

Colonoscopy is used to determine the extent of disease, to confirm radiographic abnormalities, and to perform biopsies of abnormal areas. Most patients have erythema and

Table 28-2. CLINICAL FEATURES OF CROHN'S DISEASE

Disease Manifestations	Site of Disease (%)		
	Small Intestine Only	Small Intestine and Colon	Colon Only
Diarrhea	87	92	88
Abdominal pain	78	79	74
Hematochezia	10	22	46
Intestinal obstruction	34	44	17
Fissures and fistulas			
Anal, perirectal	22	50	51
Internal, cutaneous	18	34	13
Systemic manifestations			
Arthritis, arthralgia	18	19	27
Iritis, uveitis	3	4	7
Liver disease	3	5	5
Skin lesions	3		8

(Donaldson RM Jr. Small and large intestine in Crohn's disease. In: Sleisinger MH, Fordtran JS, eds. Gastrointestinal disease, ed 4. Philadelphia, WB Saunders, 1989:1336)

Table 28-3. EXTRAINTESTINAL MANIFESTATIONS OF CROHN'S DISEASE

SKIN
Pyoderma gangrenosum
Erythema nodosum multiforme
Vasculitis
Aphthous stomatitis

EYES
Conjunctivitis
Iritis
Iridocyclitis, episcleritis
Uveitis
Vasculitis

JOINTS
Arthritis
Ankylosing spondylitis
Hypertrophic osteoarthropathy

LIVER
Sclerosing cholangitis
Pericholangitis (rare)
Granulomatous hepatitis (rare)

Table 28-5. COLONOSCOPIC MUCOSAL FEATURES AND THEIR DIAGNOSTIC SPECIFICITY IN INFLAMMATORY BOWEL DISEASE*

Lesion	Ulcerative Colitis	Crohn's Disease
INFLAMMATION		
Distribution		
Colon		
Contiguous	+++	+
Symmetric	+++	+
Rectum	+++	+
Friability	+++	+
Topography		
Granularity	+++	+
Cobblestoned	+	+++
ULCERATION		
Location		
Overt colitis	+++	+
Ileum	0	++++
Discrete lesion	+	+++
Features		
Size > 1 cm	+	+++
Deep	+	++
Linear	+	+++
Aphthoid	0	++++
BRIDGING	+	++

* Specificity index range of 0 (not seen) to ++++ (diagnostic).
(Hogan WJ, Hensley GT, Geenen JE. Endoscopic evaluation of inflammatory bowel disease. Med Clin North Am 1980;64:1084)

edema as a result of chronic diarrhea. The colonoscopic features are listed in Table 28-5.

Diagnostic Imaging

Contrast radiography of the GI tract is essential for differential diagnosis (Table 28-6) and delineation of the extent and severity of disease (Table 28-7). Radiographic examination is indicated to prepare for surgical therapy, for patients who require a change in medical management, and for patients with recurrent symptoms after surgical resection. Computed tomography (CT) delineates masses and abscesses, and endoscopic retrograde cholangiopancreatography (ERCP) is used to diagnose hepatobiliary involvement (sclerosing cholangitis).

MANAGEMENT

Management of Crohn's disease includes supportive medical therapy for acute exacerbations and surgical therapy for complications of long-standing intestinal inflammation. Disease-specific treatment does not exist. Emphasis is on alleviation of symptoms, nutritional support, and suppression of the inflammatory process.

Treatment of Symptoms

Abdominal Pain

Opiates and other analgesics are used with great caution. These agents decrease intestinal motility and increase the risk of ileus and obstruction. Antispasmodics may be used

to decrease postprandial hypermotility, but inhibition of peristalsis leading to ileus or toxic dilatation must be recognized and avoided.

Diarrhea

Opiates and opiate derivatives provide some diminution of symptoms. Codeine, diphenoxylate, and loperamide are the commonly used agents. They are most effective in patients whose diarrhea is caused by chronic active disease or intestinal resection. Use of these drugs during severe, acute flares may cause toxic megacolon, dilatation, and obstruction.

Cholestyramine is effective for bile–salt-induced diarrhea due to ileal disease or resection. Dietary restriction of fats is effective for steatorrhea. In refractory cases of diarrhea, administration of octreotide, a synthetic analog of somatostatin, may be considered.

Nutritional Therapy

An association between diet and etiologic factors has not been documented, nor does direct evidence suggest that diet alters disease activity. Many patients report fewer

Table 28-4. TYPES OF FISTULAS IN CROHN'S DISEASE

Type	Occurrence (%)
Enteroenteric	>20
Enterocutaneous	>20
Enterovesical, enteroureteral, enterourethral, ileosigmoid	2–6
Duodenoenteric	1–2
Enterorectal	1–2
Enterovaginal	3–5

Table 28-6. RADIOLOGIC FINDINGS IN INFLAMMATORY BOWEL DISEASE

Crohn's Disease	Ulcerative Colitis
Segmental involvement	Contiguous involvement
Skip lesions	Rectum always involved
Cobblestoning	Pseudopolyps
Pseudodiverticula	Loss of haustral markings
Strictures	Strictures (cancer)
Toxic dilation rare	Toxic megacolon
Longitudinal ulcers	
Transverse fissures	
Intramural fistulas	

Table 28-7. DIFFERENTIAL DIAGNOSIS OF CROHN'S DISEASE

INFECTIOUS CONDITIONS	OTHER CONDITIONS
Yersinia infection	Ulcerative colitis
Salmonellosis, shigellosis	Radiation enteritis
Campylobacter enteritis	Ischemic colitis
Tuberculosis	Irritable bowel disease
Pseudomembranous colitis	Diverticulitis
(*Clostridium difficile*)	Appendicitis
Staphylococcal enteritis	Behçet syndrome
Viral enteritis (lymphogranuloma	Sprue
venereum)	Sarcoidosis
Fungal Infections	**NEOPLASIA**
Histoplasmosis	Lymphoma
Candidiasis	Adenocarcinoma
	Polyposis syndromes
Protozoal Infections	
Amebiasis	
Lambliasis	
Giardiasis	
Schistosomiasis	

symptoms after an exclusion diet based on personal experience, but this practice can lead to food avoidance and severe malnutrition.

Nutritional support of malnourished patients with Crohn's disease increases body weight, visceral protein status, and nitrogen balance. Bowel rest with total parenteral nutrition (TPN) or enteral elemental diets has been used to treat acute disease, both as supportive and as primary therapy.

Drug Therapy

Drugs being evaluated for the treatment of Crohn's disease include corticosteroids, sulfasalazine (5-ASA), broad-spectrum antibiotics such as metronidazole, and immunosuppressive agents such as azathioprine and its active metabolite, 6-mercaptopurine, methotrexate, and cyclosporine (Fig 28-3).

Surgical Therapy

Surgical therapy is palliative, not curative. It is reserved for complications of the disease. Intestinal resection in patients with uncomplicated disease is justified only in unusual circumstances. Surgical intervention also is indicated when medical therapy has failed and the patient's condition is chronically debilitated because of the disease.

Preoperative Preparation

Preoperative intestinal preparation is with enemas, a clear liquid diet, and oral electrolyte catharsis. If the patient has a stenotic lesion in the intestinal tract and complete or partial small-intestinal obstruction, oral intestinal preparation is undertaken cautiously and may not be possible. Prophylactic parenteral antibiotics are administered perioperatively. Antibiotic coverage is continued postoperatively beyond the usual two doses only when there is obvious sepsis.

Surgical Technique

Abdominal exploration must be complete and nearly always requires division of all adhesions. The site of disease or recurrence is assessed, and the length of the uninvolved proximal small intestine is estimated. A meticulous search

for skip lesions is undertaken. The colon is inspected for the presence or absence of Crohn's colitis.

The proposed sites of intestinal transection are identified; these are adjacent to the clinically obvious limits of involvement. The lines of resection are conservative. They are only a few centimeters proximal and distal to the site of visible changes of Crohn's disease—narrowing of the intestinal lumen, thickening of the intestinal wall, serositis, tortuosity of the serosal vessels, creeping fat over the intestinal surface, and thickening of the mesenteric margins of the intestine.

The site of intestinal transection is cleared of mesenteric tissue for about 1 cm. Microscopic evidence of Crohn's disease at the resection margins does not compromise safe anastomosis. Frozen-section examination of resection margins is not necessary. After anastomosis, the mesenteric rent is closed, the peritoneal cavity is irrigated, the retroperitoneum is inspected for possible sites of bleeding, and the incision is closed in layers. In a large number of patients, especially those undergoing reoperation, extensive mesenteric foreshortening with dense adherence of the diseased intestine to the retroperitoneum may be encountered in the region of the upper ureter, pancreas, and third and fourth portions of the duodenum. In this situation, the risk of pancreatic, duodenal, and ureteral injury is high. There also is risk for intraoperative hemorrhage if the foreshortened mesentery, which always contains enlarged and engorged mesenteric arteries and veins, is injured or torn.

Management of Fistulas and Abscesses

As soon as the extent of a fistula track and its communication with abdominal organs is determined, surgical correction is planned. The surgical procedure is undertaken when the fistula tracks are as clean as possible, when active inflammatory processes are under control, and when the patient is in good nutritional condition and has undergone intestinal preparation. Enteroenteric fistulas, ileosigmoid fistulas, and low-output enterocutaneous fistulas are not repaired if the fistula track is well established and does not cause bleeding or febrile episodes and does not interfere with the patient's well-being.

If a retroperitoneal fistula track is encountered during mobilization of the diseased segment of intestine, the diseased intestine is removed and the fistula track is transected. When a fistula track is encountered or an abscess is opened, the contents are evacuated with suction, and all necrotic tissue is excised. Care is taken to avoid injury to the right ureter, the third and fourth portions of duodenum, and the inferior vena cava and superior mesenteric vein.

In patients with duodenal fistulas, the duodenum is mobilized completely to allow excision of the margins of the duodenal fistula and closure of the defect. If the fistulous communication between the diseased intestine and duodenum involves the mesenteric side of the duodenum, adjacent pancreatitis is always present to some degree. Fistulous communication between the intestine and the pancreatic ductal system is possible. This defect can be repaired with ileocolonic resection of the involved intestine supplemented with a Roux-en-Y pancreatojejunostomy or distal pancreatectomy.

Intestinal preparation of patients with enterocutaneous fistulas is best achieved with TPN. The fistula tracks are cleared of fecal material, and the skin opening is allowed to heal as much as possible. The intestine that contains the fistula is separated from surrounding loops of uninvolved intestine and resected. The fistula track is transected where it penetrates the abdominal wall. Spillage of purulent and fecal material usually is minimal. The track through the

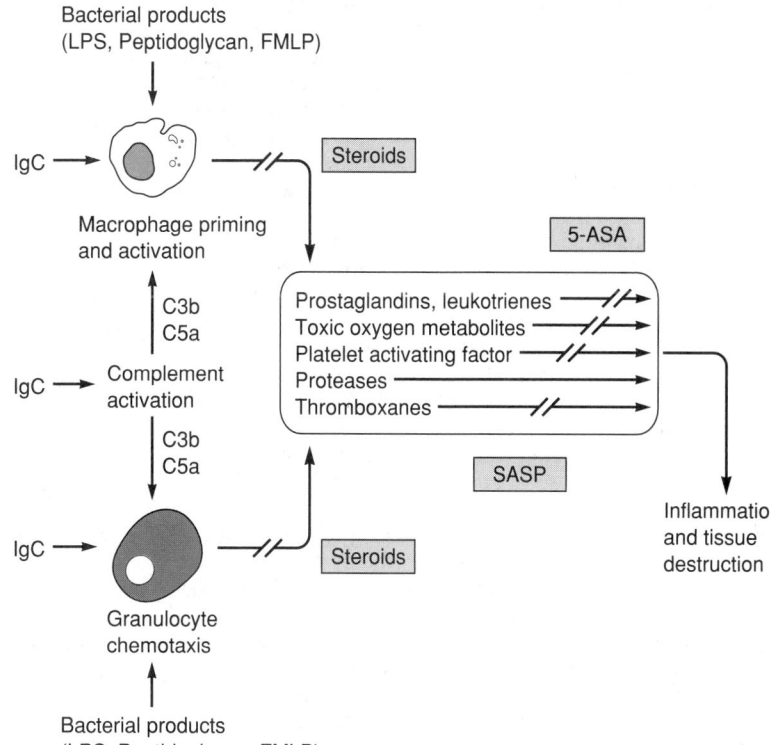

Figure 28-3. Mechanisms of tissue injury in inflammatory bowel disease. The events that initiate inflammatory bowel disease are largely undefined but involve activation of cells and initiation of the inflammatory cascade. Antibiotics may reduce the antigen load; steroids and immunosuppressive drugs block immunologic processes at various sites; 5-ASA compounds have inhibitory effects at multiple sites of the immune system. LPS, lipopolysarcharide; FMLP, formyl-methionyl-leucyl-phenylalanine; SASP, sulfasalazine. (After Hanauer SB. Highlights of controversies in IDB workshop. IBD Chronicle 1993;1:7)

abdominal wall is vigorously débrided, and the fistula opening at the skin level is excised.

Fistulas with the sigmoid colon, bladder, or any abdominal organ not primarily involved with Crohn's disease all are treated the same way. The opening in the nondiseased organ is cleared and closed in layers. An ileosigmoid fistula is treated by means of resection of the diseased small intestine and wedge resection of the sigmoid or by means of simple closure of the colonic defect. A fistula that coexists with an inflammatory mass or abscess and leads to partial or complete intestinal obstruction is a frequent reason for a primary surgical procedure and is equally often an indication for reoperation. The development of an enteric fistula, whether it communicates with another abdominal structure or with the skin, almost always is associated with an inflammatory mass. The mass consists of inflamed mesentery that contains markedly enlarged lymph nodes, loops of diseased and nondiseased intestine, and the parietal peritoneum. Often there is purulent material within the interstices of the inflammatory mass, and at times there is a frank abscess.

Percutaneous drainage of abscesses under sonographic or CT guidance is not always suitable for patients with Crohn's disease, because multiple loops of diseased and nondiseased intestine are transgressed. Resection with drainage is safer than percutaneous drainage. Temporary closure of an enterocutaneous or enteroenteric fistula can sometimes be achieved with TPN and bowel rest. A lasting closure is possible only with resection of the diseased intestine from which the fistula arises.

Stricture

Patients with recurrent Crohn's disease may have multiple strictures of the small intestine, which cause symptoms of partial obstruction and weight loss. Resection of multiple strictures may result in short-bowel syndrome and is, therefore, avoided. For short strictures, strictureplasty is an excellent alternative to resection.

Strictureplasty is achieved with a longitudinal incision across the short stenotic segment into the prestenotic and poststenotic intestine. For strictureplasty, the longitudinal enterotomy is converted into a transverse closure. Recurrence rates are not substantially increased after strictureplasty, even though inflamed intestinal tissue is left in situ. Resection and strictureplasty are complementary techniques and not used in lieu of each other. Inflammatory changes at the margin of resection are acceptable and are compatible with a safe anastomosis. Consequently, frozen-section histologic evaluation of the margins of resection is not necessary.

Colonic Crohn's Disease

Most patients with Crohn's disease have inflammatory changes limited to the colon or have marked colonic involvement. Although disease in the colon is often segmental, colonic recurrences are frequent after limited segmental resection. In patients with diffuse disease of the colon and rectum, proctocolectomy with ileostomy is the treatment of choice. If the disease is less extensive and the rectum is spared, limited resection with anastomosis is an acceptable approach. Because recurrence is inevitable, reoperations are common. Placement of the abdominal incision must take into account the likelihood of future intestinal stomas.

Perianal Disease

Two types of perianal lesions occur in Crohn's disease:

- Primary lesions specific to Crohn's disease (eg, anal fissure, ulcerated hemorrhoidal tissues, cavitating intrarectal ulcer), often accompanied by active disease in the proximal GI tract.
- Secondary nonspecific lesions (eg, subcutaneous fistulas, ulcerated external and internal hemorrhoids, anal stricture, and deep perianal abscesses and fistulas)

A conservative surgical approach to these lesions is prudent. Many patients with indolent anal fistulas can live comfortably for years. The development of an abscess, however, necessitates drainage. In the presence of active proximal Crohn's disease and a concomitant flare of perianal disease, both entities must be treated. In the absence of Crohn's proctitis and during quiescence of proximal intestinal disease, an uncomplicated fistula track may be treated with standard surgical procedures.

An anorectovaginal fistula can be treated with a rectal advancement flap. Standard operations are impossible because of the transsphincteric nature of multiple interconnected fistula tracks. A combination of partial excision, fistulotomy, and placement of drains may provide drainage and maturation of the fistula tracks without leading to complete destruction of the sphincter mechanism. Patients with perianal disease in direct continuity with active rectal disease may undergo proctectomy. Fecal diversion with a proximal colostomy does not improve healing but may provide relief of symptoms.

Extensive perineal sepsis complicating ischiorectal abscesses, rectocutaneous fistulas, or rectovaginal fistulas may involve the entire perineum and groin as a manifestation of Crohn's proctocolitis. In these patients, the perineum and the rectal sphincter are usually destroyed, and the rectum is extensively diseased. Proctocolectomy, performed in two stages, may be necessary. At the first operation, the entire abdominal colon is resected with the upper two-thirds of the rectum. An end ileostomy is constructed, and the rectum is closed. At the end of the first operation, the abscesses are drained and the fistula tracks are opened. Once suppuration has subsided, the rectum is resected with a perineal approach, residual fistula tracks are excised, and vaginal defects are repaired. Extensive destruction of the posterior vaginal wall occasionally requires the use of a musculocutaneous flap for repair. Some patients have a persistent nonhealing perineal wound.

Some persistent wounds are minor cutaneous sinuses, whereas others are large, infected cavities that destroy the perineum and adjacent tissue. Surgical treatment is excision of the fibrous wall of the cavity that also may include the coccyx and portions of the sacrum. The wound is left open and heals by secondary intention in most instances.

SUGGESTED READING

Allan RN, Keighly MRB, Alexander-Williams J, Hawkins C, eds. Inflammatory bowel disease. Edinburgh, Churchill Livingstone, 1983.

Cottone M, Rosselli M, Orlando A, et al. Smoking habits and recurrence in Crohn's's disease. Gastroenterology 1994;106:643 Crohn's BB, Ginsberg L, Oppenheimer GD. Regional ileitis: A pathological and clinical entity. JAMA 1932;99:1323.

Hanauer SB. Evolving medical therapies for inflammatory bowel disease. Prog Inflamm Bowel Dis 1994;15.

Kirsner JB, Shorter RG, eds. Inflammatory bowel disease. Philadelphia, Lea & Febiger, 1988.

Kornbluth A, George J, Sachar D. Immunosuppressive drugs in Crohn's's disease. Gastroenterologist 1994;2:239.

McLeod RS, Wolff BG, Steinhart H, et al. Delayed recurrence following surgery for Crohn's's disease. Gastroenterology 1994; 106:A733.

Rutgeerts P, Geboes K, Van Trappen G, et al. Predictability of the postoperative course of Crohn's's disease. Gastroenterology 1990;99:956.

Strober W, James S. The immunologic basis of inflammatory bowel disease. J Clin Immunol 1986;6:415.

Thayer WR, Coutu JA, Chiodini RJ, Van Kruiningen HJ, Merkal RS. Possible roll of mycobacteria in inflammatory bowel disease. II. Mycobacteria antibodies in Crohn's's disease. Dig Dis Sci 1984;29:1080.

ESSENTIALS OF SURGERY: SCIENTIFIC PRINCIPLES AND PRACTICE, edited by Lazar J. Greenfield, Michael W. Mulholland, Keith T. Oldham, Gerald B. Zelenock, and Keith-D. Lillemoe. Lippincott–Raven Publishers, Philadelphia, © 1997.

CHAPTER 29
SMALL-INTESTINAL NEOPLASMS

MICHAEL G. SARR AND MICHEL M. MURR

Neoplasms of the small intestine are unusual, especially considering the great length of the organ. Benign lesions are more frequent than malignant tumors.

CLINICAL PRESENTATION

Most benign tumors remain asymptomatic. Malignant neoplasms eventually produce symptoms that vary according to site and size of the tumor, location and spread within the intestinal wall, and degree of necrosis and ulceration. The clinical features are presented in Table 29-1.

DIAGNOSIS

Symptoms are often overlooked by patients and physicians. Preoperative diagnosis always requires the use of an imaging technique, but surgical exploration usually is the definitive procedure in establishing the diagnosis.

Plain abdominal radiographs may show signs of intestinal obstruction but otherwise are nonspecific. Upper gastrointestinal (GI) barium radiographs with small-intestinal follow-through show a filling defect, mass lesion, or evidence of intussusception. A more sensitive technique is enteroclysis, in which barium contrast material is introduced directly into the proximal jejunum with an orojejunal tube. Computed tomography (CT), ultrasonography, and magnetic resonance imaging (MRI) may aid in preoperative staging by showing extraluminal extent and the presence of nodal or liver metastases. Angiography has no role in screening or staging. It may have clinical value in the diagnosis and localization of neoplasms of vascular origin or carcinoid tumors that have a severe perivascular sclerosing reaction.

Table 29-1. CLINICAL PRESENTATION OF SMALL INTESTINAL NEOPLASMS

Findings	Occurrence (%)
BENIGN NEOPLASMS	
No symptoms	>50
Abdominal pain*	25
Intestinal obstruction	20
Hemorrhage	10
MALIGNANT NEOPLASMS	
Weight loss	90–100
Abdominal pain*	80
Intestinal obstruction	30
Abdominal mass	15
Perforation	10
Jaundice (periampullary neoplasms)	1–2

* Usually related to intermittent or incomplete mechanical obstruction

Endoscopy can help detect duodenal neoplasms. Extended upper endoscopy or Sunde-type enteroscopy allows examination of most of the intestinal lumen. Extended colonoscopy allows examination of the distal 10 to 30 cm of the small intestine.

BENIGN NEOPLASMS

Benign tumors originate from epithelium or mesenchyme. The common lesions are leiomyomas, adenomas, and lipomas (Table 29-2).

Leiomyomas

Leiomyomas occur most frequently in the jejunum as single, firm, grayish-white lesions composed of well-differentiated smooth-muscle cells without mitoses. On radiographs, an ovoid, intraluminal filling defect with an intact overlying mucosa is highly suggestive of leiomyoma. Most leiomyomas grow extraluminally and may become quite large, even palpable, before being recognized. The lesion eventually outgrows its highly vascular blood supply, leading to central necrosis, ulceration, and intraluminal bleeding. Differentiation between large leiomyomas and their malignant counterparts, leiomyosarcomas, is difficult, even after pathologic review. Leiomyomas are treated with segmental resection.

Adenomas

Tubular Adenomas
Occur most commonly in the duodenum
Asymptomatic but sometimes may bleed or cause obstruction
Treatment
  Simple endoscopic polypectomy
  Enterotomy or segmental intestinal resection if in the jejunum or ileum
Villous Adenomas
Occur most commonly in the duodenum, especially the periampullary region
Potentially malignant
May present with occult bleeding, gastric outlet obstruction, or biliary obstruction
Diagnosis confirmed with endoscopic biopsy, which does not ensure absence of malignancy
Treatment
  Endoscopic polypectomy when no invasive carcinoma can be found in the polypectomy specimen
  Local surgical resection for large sessile lesions

Table 29-2. RELATIVE INCIDENCE OF BENIGN NEOPLASMS OF THE SMALL INTESTINE

Type	Occurrence (%)
Leiomyomas	18
Lipomas	15
Adenomas	15
Polyps (polyposis, Peutz-Jeghers)	15
Hemangiomas	13
Fibromas	10
Neurogenic tumors	7
Lymphangiomas	3
Myxomas	2
Other tumors	2

Extensive resection for invasive carcinoma, often involving pancreatoduodenectomy for periampullary lesions
Brunner gland adenomas
Hyperplasia of exocrine glands of proximal duodenal mucosa
Present as polypoid lesions of first portion of duodenum
Symptoms unusual; bleeding or obstructive symptoms may occur
Treatment
  Simple local resection, either with endoscopy or, rarely, submucosal excision through a duodenotomy

Lipomas

Lipomas are found most commonly in the ileum and the duodenum. They originate from submucosal adipose tissue or mesenteric fat. The lesions are extraluminal. CT can help define the density of the lesion and thus confirm the diagnosis. Because lipomas have no malignant potential, they are excised only if the tumor is symptomatic.

Peutz–Jeghers Syndrome

Peutz–Jeghers syndrome is an inherited syndrome of mucocutaneous melanotic pigmentation and multiple GI polyps. The polyps are actually hamartomas, and occur primarily in the jejunum and ileum. Peutz–Jeghers lesions most often present as intermittent intussusception. Occult hemorrhage occurs but infrequently. Because patients with this syndrome have a high incidence of extraintestinal malignant tumors, aggressive diagnostic evaluation and follow-up care are necessary. Because the lesions are widespread, extensive resection is not justified, and treatment is limited to the segment producing the complications.

Hemangiomas

Hemangiomas vary in size, from pinpoint lesions to large cavernous forms, which are unusual. These lesions cause occult or recurrent acute GI bleeding. The diagnosis is difficult but is possible with angiography or endoscopy. Many hemangiomas are found during exploration for GI bleeding of unknown causation. Small tumors are destroyed by electocauterization or laser therapy. Large lesions may require segmental resection. Multiple lesions may be confined to the proximal small intestine, and can be treated with extensive small-intestinal resection to prevent the need for frequent blood transfusions.

Endometriosis

Endometriosis is the presence of benign endometrial tissue in areas other than the uterus. Endometriosis of the small intestine appears as puckered, bluish-red nodules, most commonly in the serosa of the ileum. The adjacent small intestine is often scarred, thickened, and adherent in reaction to the cyclic hormonal responses of the endometrioma. Endometriosis of the small intestine usually is found incidentally at celiotomy or laparoscopy. A biopsy excludes metastatic malignant growth. Treatment is noninterventional unless mechanical obstruction has occurred. Hormonal therapy may alter the behavior of the endometriosis, preventing further GI complications.

MALIGNANT NEOPLASMS

Malignant neoplasms of the small intestine include adenocarcinoma, leiomyosarcoma, lymphoma, and carcinoid tumors. Metastasis from tumors of other parts of the body may mimic primary GI tumors. Most malignant tumors of the small intestine occur in the fifth or sixth decade of life, slightly more often in men than in women. The relative frequency of malignant small-intestinal tumors is shown in Table 29-3.

Adenocarcinoma

Given the difference in lengths of duodenum, jejunum, and ileum, the duodenal epithelium shows a great propensity toward malignant transformation (Fig. 29-1).

Origin

Adenocarcinomas originate in the epithelial cells of the small-intestinal mucosa. Previously benign periampullary villous adenomas can undergo malignant transformation to adenocarcinoma, but the polyp-to-cancer sequence is not well established. In Peutz–Jeghers syndrome, hereditary factors may effect malignant transformation. The chronic inflammatory changes of Crohn's disease may lead to adenocarcinoma, especially in the ileum.

Presentation and Diagnosis

The presentation of adenocarcinoma varies with the location of the tumor. The following clinical features may be present:

All Locations
Weight loss and abdominal pain
Duodenum
Intermittent jaundice
Hematochezia
Jejunum and ileum
Slowly progressive intestinal obstruction
Apple-core defect on GI barium-enema radiograph
Blood loss, usually occult

A palpable mass or perforation is unusual. Duodenal tumors can be detected with endoscopy but jejunoileal adenocarcinomas cannot. Distal lesions often are detected during surgical exploration for small-intestinal obstruction of unknown causation. Dilatation of the intrapancreatic portion of the common bile duct on CT or ultrasonographic scans may be evidence of duodenal or ampullary adenocarcinoma.

Treatment

Surgical treatment of adenocarcinoma requires wide segmental resection, including the draining nodal system. Most duodenal adenocarcinomas require pancreatoduodenectomy (Whipple resection) to incorporate the draining nodal basin. Small lesions in the first portion of the duodenum and tumors in the fourth portion of the duodenum sometimes are removed by segmental resection. Unresectable duodenal cancers that cause intestinal obstruction can be palliated with gastrojejunostomy, unless the tumor

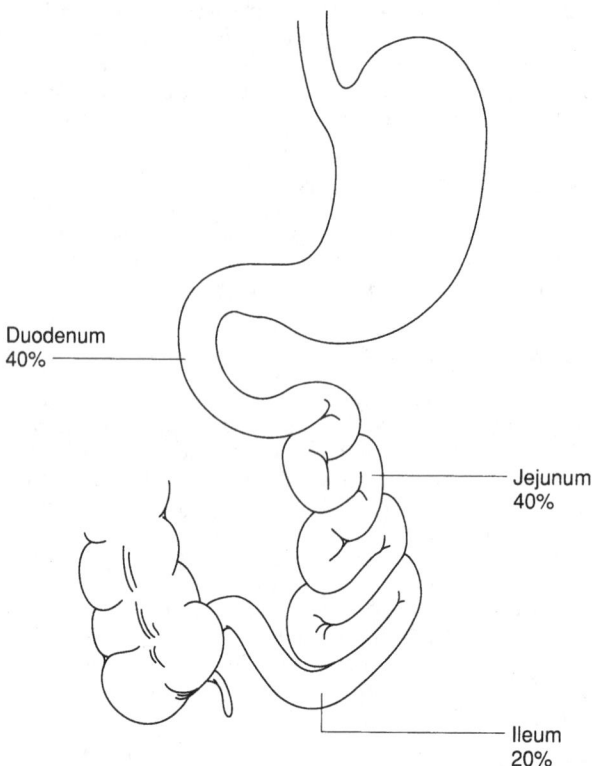

Figure 29-1. The duodenal mucosa has a substantially greater propensity for development of adenocarcinoma, especially considering its shorter length compared with the jejunum and ileum.

causes bleeding. If bleeding occurs, endoscopic laser photocoagulation may provide short-lived benefit.

Jejunoileal adenocarcinomas are removed by segmental resection. The proximal extent of the mesenteric lymphadenectomy is limited by the superior mesenteric artery. Distal ileal lesions are best managed with right hemicolectomy that includes the draining lymph nodes. Adenocarcinomas in the mid-portion of the small intestine may be treated with laparoscopy-assisted resection. Laparoscopic examination of the small intestine reveals the involved segment. If the segment is mobile, an incision can be made over the mass just large enough to allow the segment to be exteriorized, and an extra-abdominal resection can be performed.

Chemotherapy and Radiation Therapy

Response to 5-fluorouracil (5-FU) alone is poor, and experience with other agents is limited. These tumors are radioresistant.

Leiomyosarcoma

Origin

Leiomyosarcomas originate in the tunica muscularis or the muscularis mucosae of the small intestine. They can be difficult to differentiate from leiomyomas. Leiomyosarcomas have more than two mitoses per high-power microscopic field, concomitant cellularity, and nuclear atypia; they are larger than leiomyomas, and are accompanied by necrosis. About 20% of leiomyosarcomas are epithelioid leiomyosarcomas, characterized by bizarre pleiomorphic cells; these epithelioid lesions appear to have a better prognosis than other leiomyosarcomas. Leiomyosarcomas occur most commonly in the jejunum and ileum.

Table 29-3. RELATIVE FREQUENCY OF MALIGNANT TUMORS OF THE SMALL INTESTINE

Type	Occurrence (%)
Adenocarcinoma	30–50
Leiomyosarcoma	10–20
Lymphoma	10–15
Carcinoid tumors	30–50

Presentation and Diagnosis

Leiomyosarcomas tend to grow outside the lumen and obstruct the small intestine only late in their course. They often become quite large before causing symptoms that warrant investigation. The following clinical features may be present:

- Abdominal pain and weight loss
- Hemorrhage when ischemia within the tumor causes necrosis
- Acute abdomen due to intestinal perforation
- Intestinal obstruction
- Palpable abdominal mass

On radiographs, a barium-filled cavity indicative of central necrosis suggests the diagnosis. CT may reveal a large, bulky, extraluminal mass with central necrosis and sometimes calcification. Angiography may depict a vascular mass. Celiotomy usually is required for diagnosis and treatment.

Treatment

Surgical treatment requires a wide, en bloc segmental resection that includes the associated mesentery. Extended lymphadenectomy is not indicated because leiomyosarcomas spread by the hematogenous route. Most resections of duodenal lesions involve a pancreatoduodenectomy because of the large tumor size. Palliative bypass may be indicated.

Chemotherapy and Radiation Therapy

Chemotherapy is of no benefit; palliation is of short duration, and side effects are common. Leiomyosarcomas are radioresistant.

Lymphoma

Lymphomas occur as primary local neoplasms without concurrent peripheral lymphadenopathy or splenomegaly or as secondary neoplasms that present as part of a systemic disseminated lymphoma. Although primary GI lymphomas are the most common form of extranodal lymphomas, they account for only 5% of all lymphomas. Small-intestinal lymphomas most commonly occur during the fifth and sixth decades of life, mostly in men. The lesions may be multifocal. Conditions such as celiac disease, Crohn's disease, and immunodeficiency syndromes, including pharmacologic immunosuppression, increase the risk for extranodal GI lymphomas.

Origin

Lymphomas arise from the lymphoid tissue within the wall of the small intestine. They predominate in the ileum, where the greatest concentration of GI lymphoid tissue occurs. Almost all primary small-intestinal lymphomas are non-Hodgkin, B-cell lymphomas. They exhibit immunohistochemical characteristics similar to those of lymphomas in other parts of the body. Most small-intestinal lymphomas are intermediate or high-grade tumors with large-cell or immunoblastic features that have a diffuse rather than nodular growth pattern. Clinicopathologic staging is not standardized; one system is presented in Table 29-4.

Presentation and Diagnosis

The clinical features of lymphomas are as follows:

- Fatigue and weight loss
- Abdominal pain
- Acute abdomen with perforation, obstruction, intussusception, or hemorrhage

Table 29-4. MODIFIED ANN ARBOR CLASSIFICATION OF PRIMARY NON-HODGKIN GASTROINTESTINAL LYMPHOMA

Stage	Description
IE	Tumor confined to small intestine
IIE	Spread to regional lymph nodes
IIIE	Spread to nonresectable nodal involvement beyond regional nodes
IVE	Spread to other organs within or beyond abdomen

- Abdominal mass
- Malabsorption

The diagnosis of small-intestinal lymphoma is usually made on the basis of findings at GI contrast studies that suggest submucosal nodules, mucosal ulcerations, or diffuse, coarse mucosal folds. Other findings may include fixation of involved loops of intestine or, sometimes, aneurysmal dilatation of the involved segment due to ulceration and necrosis of the tumor mass. CT can help in diagnosis and staging by showing the presence of bulky mesenteric nodes in association with diffuse thickening of the intestinal wall or a large tumor mass. Peroral or endoscopic biopsies are not helpful because most lymphomas occur in the distal small intestine.

Intestinal lymphomas are associated with several malabsorptive conditions. Clinical deterioration in a patient with previously controlled celiac disease suggests the diagnosis of lymphoma and may require celiotomy for confirmation. Lymphoma appears to be associated with Crohn's disease and dermatitis herpetiformis. Disorders of immunologic function sometimes are associated with extranodal intestinal lymphoma.

Treatment

Intestinal lymphoma necessitates surgical intervention for diagnosis, staging, relief of obstruction and perforation, and resection or debulking. Because intraoperative staging affects postoperative management, liver biopsy and sampling of the para-aortic and mesenteric nodes outside the field of resection are performed. Localized tumors are resected wide, en bloc lymphadenectomy. Widespread or multicentric intestinal lymphomas are impossible to resect. Debulking is performed if the patient's overall health will not be jeopardized by removal of an excessive length of intestine.

Chemotherapy and Radiation Therapy

Most stage IE and IIE lymphomas are treated with chemotherapy and radiation therapy, under the assumption that lymphoma is a systemic disease that requires adjuvant systemic therapy. When surgical management has been directed at palliation or debulking or when disease is in stage IIIE or IVE, localized radiation therapy with combination cytotoxic chemotherapy is usually given.

Mediterranean Lymphoma

Mediterranean lymphoma, or immunoproliferative small-intestinal disease, is a variant of primary intestinal lymphoma. It is most commonly found in lower socioeconomic populations in underdeveloped countries. The disease primarily affects young adults, has a male predominance. It presents with weight loss, intestinal cramps, diarrhea, steatorrhea, and clubbing of the fingers. Death is caused by progressive malnutrition or transformation to disseminated, aggressive lymphoma. Chemotherapy and radiation therapy sometimes are successful, but administration of a full-dose regimen is limited by malnutrition and malabsorption.

Post-transplant Lymphoproliferative Disease

Immunocompromised transplant recipients are at high risk for extranodal lymphoma. Post-transplant lymphoproliferative disease presents with intestinal bleeding and perforation. The mortality is high, and all modalities of treatment are used, including wide resection, chemotherapy or radiation therapy or both, and most important, reduction in the dosages of immunosuppressive drugs.

Carcinoid Tumors

Carcinoid tumors originate from cells of the APUD (amine precursor uptake and decarboxylation) system. Carcinoid is a misnomer because although they are populations of innocuous-appearing cells with uniform nuclei and few mitoses, these tumors are true malignant neoplasms. After the appendix, which harbors 85% of all carcinoids, the small intestine is the most common site of origin (Fig 29-2). The peak prevalence is in the sixth decade, but the age range is broader than for other malignant tumors of the small intestine (ie, 20 to 80 years).

Presentation and Diagnosis

As with other small-intestinal tumors, symptoms are nondescript. The clinical features are as follows:

- Carcinoid syndrome
- Anorexia, weight loss, and fatigue
- A desmoplastic reaction in which the mesentery becomes shortened, thickened, and fixed, kinking and angulating the intestinal loops, and producing symptoms of distal partial intestinal obstruction
- Abdominal pain
- Intestinal ischemia or infarction due to vascular thickening and sclerosis accompanying the desmoplastic reaction

It is difficult to differentiate carcinoid tumors from inflammatory processes such as Crohn's disease. On contrast-enhanced GI radiographs, carcinoids show tethering and pleating of ileal folds with abrupt demarcation between stenotic tumor-involved ileum and normal adjacent intestine. Submucosal nodules are sometimes present. The primary tumor may not be evident. CT may suggest carcinoid disease, not by showing the primary tumor but by demonstrating nodal metastases within the mesentery or multiple hepatic nodules. Endoscopy is of little use in the diagnosis of small-intestinal carcinoid tumors.

Treatment

In the absence of the carcinoid syndrome, surgical management of primary small-intestinal carcinoid tumors involves wide en bloc resection of as much of the nodal drainage pathways as possible. Most distal ileal carcinoids are treated with right hemicolectomy. Proximal tumors are treated with wedge-shaped segmental resection that includes the mesentery. A diligent search is made for other primary carcinoids of the small intestine and for malignant neoplasms of other organs.

Carcinoid Syndrome

Carcinoid syndrome manifests as late-stage disease with a large bulk of tumor deposits in the liver. The prominent feature is intermittent flushing with diarrhea, which may be provoked by foods, alcohol, or emotional or physical

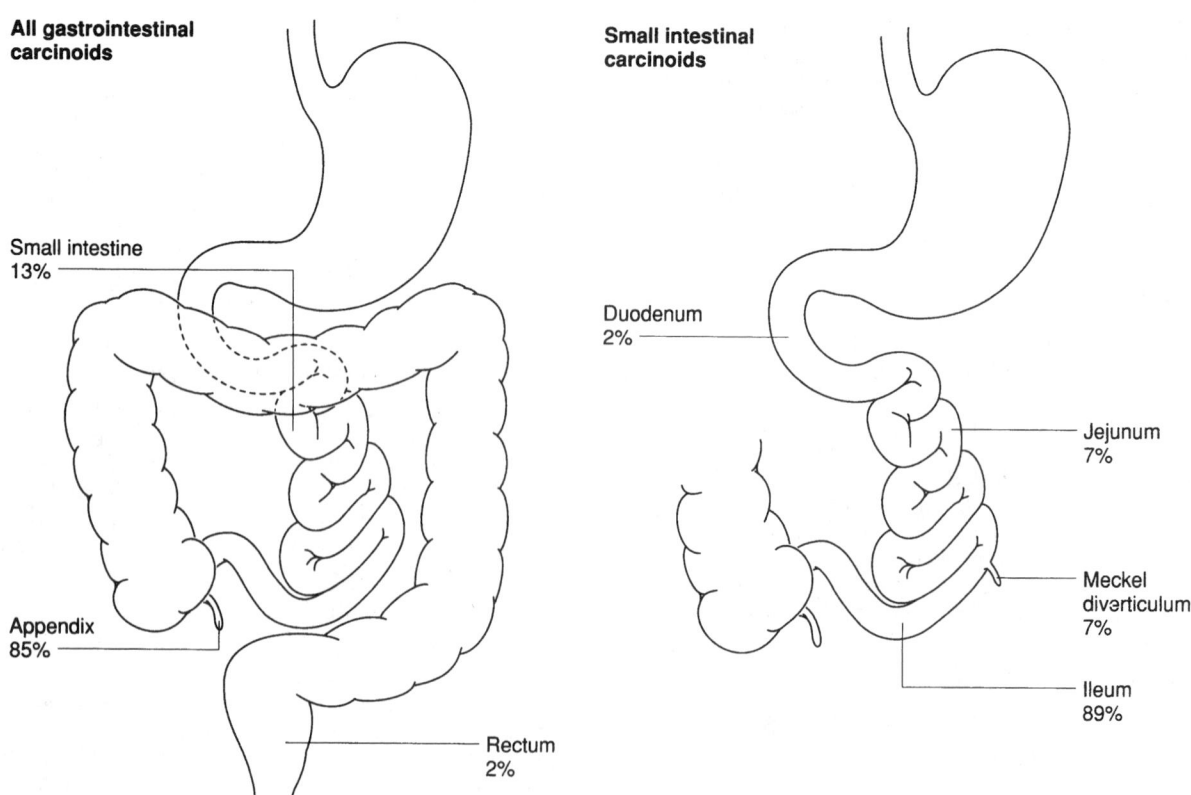

All gastrointestinal carcinoids

Small intestine 13%

Appendix 85%

Rectum 2%

Small intestinal carcinoids

Duodenum 2%

Jejunum 7%

Meckel diverticulum 7%

Ileum 89%

Figure 29-2. Relative incidence of gastrointestinal carcinoid tumors.

stress, including induction of anesthesia. Heart failure is unusual at presentation but can develop later in the clinical course. Carcinoid crisis is a life-threatening reaction that includes intense, persistent, generalized flushing, severe diarrhea, and central nervous system symptoms that range from mild light-headedness and vertigo to somnolence or coma. Associated cardiovascular abnormalities may include tachycardia, arrhythmias, and hyper- or hypotension. Carcinoid crisis requires active and aggressive pharmacologic intervention.

The vasomotor sequelae of carcinoid syndrome are probably related to the effects of several vasoactive substances acting in concert, most likely serotonin and bradykinin. The clinical diagnosis of carcinoid syndrome is confirmed by increased levels of 5-hydroxyindoleacetic acid (5-HIAA), a metabolite of serotonin. Normal 24-hour urinary 5-HIAA level is less than 9 mg.

Treatment of the carcinoid syndrome is directed at relief of the symptoms. The most effective treatment is pharmacologic, usually with octreotide, the synthetic analogue of somatostatin. Somatostatin or octreotide is used when patients with the carcinoid syndrome are exposed to stressful situations, such as an operation or courses of intense chemotherapy. It can be life-saving in patients in carcinoid crisis.

Chemotherapy and Radiation Therapy

Chemotherapy for metastatic carcinoids is of little benefit. The most effective agents include doxorubicin, 5-FU, and streptozocin, as single- or multiple-drug regimens. Radiation therapy is of essentially no benefit.

Metastatic Tumors

The small intestine may be the site of metastatic spread by direct extension through peritoneal seeding from other intraperitoneal organs. Less commonly, hematogenous spread may occur from another primary neoplasm. Pain and obstruction are the most common symptoms. The prognosis is poor because this clinical situation represents distant metastatic disease. Metastatic foci of malignant melanoma, when symptomatic, are best diagnosed with a radiographic contrast study. If intestinal metastases are symptomatic, or if they represent the only site of known metastasis, aggressive resection may be warranted.

SUGGESTED READING

Amer MH, El-Akkad S. Gastrointestinal lymphoma in adults: clinical features and management of 300 cases. Gastroenterology 1994;106:846.

Ashley SW, Wells SA Jr. Tumors of the small intestine. Semin Oncol 1988;15:116.

Bjorck KJ, Davis CG, Nagorney DM, Mucha P Jr. Duodenal villus tumors. Arch Surg 1990;125:961.

Godwin JD II. Carcinoid tumors: an analysis of 2837 cases. Cancer 1975;36:560.

Licht JD, Weissman LB, Antman K. Gastrointestinal sarcomas. Semin Oncol 1988;15:181.

Moertel CG. An odyssey in the land of small tumors. J Clin Oncol 1987;5:1503.

Morgan BK, Compton C, Talbert M, Gallagher WJ, Wood WC. Benign smooth muscle tumors of the gastrointestinal tract: a 24-year experience. Ann Surg 1990;211:63.

Prystowsky JB, Stryker SJ, Ujiki GT, Poticha SM. Gastrointestinal endometriosis: incidence and indications for resection. Arch Surg 1988;123:855.

PANCREAS

ESSENTIALS OF SURGERY: SCIENTIFIC PRINCIPLES AND PRACTICE,
edited by Lazar J. Greenfield, Michael W. Mulholland, Keith T. Oldham, Gerald B. Zelenock,
and Keith D. Lillemoe. Lippincott–Raven Publishers, Philadelphia, © 1997.

CHAPTER 30

PANCREATIC ANATOMY AND PHYSIOLOGY

DANA K. ANDERSEN AND F. CHARLES BRUNICARDI

ANATOMY

The pancreas lies behind the posterior peritoneal membrane at the level of the second lumbar vertebra. It weighs 75 to 100 g and is 15 to 20 cm long. The pancreas has three regions—the head, the neck, and the body and tail.

Relations to Other Structures

The pancreas is almost entirely retroperitoneal and lies close to a number of organs (Fig. 30-1).

Head

The head of the pancreas fits closely into the curve of the duodenum and lies to the right of the superior mesenteric vessels. The anterior aspect of the head is crossed by the root of the transverse mesocolon and lies anterior and adjacent to the vena cava, the renal veins, and the right renal artery. The uncinate process, which is part of the head, wraps around and extends posteriorly to the superior mesenteric vessels. The common bile duct descends in the posterior surface of the head to join the main pancreatic duct at the ampulla of Vater.

Neck

The neck of the pancreas lies over the superior mesenteric vessels and is differentiated from the head by a notch that contains the superior mesenteric vessels.

Body

The body of the pancreas begins to the left of the neck. Its anterior surface is covered with peritoneum, which forms the posterior floor of the lesser sac. The transverse mesocolon attaches to the inferior margin. The body lies behind the posterior wall of the stomach and overlies the aorta at the origin of the superior mesenteric artery.

Tail

The tail is the small portion of the pancreas, and is anterior to the left kidney. The tail lies close to the spleen, the left colic flexure, and the splenorenal ligament, making it susceptible to injury during splenectomy.

Pancreatic Ducts

The main pancreatic duct, or duct of Wirsung, runs the length of the pancreas and joins the common bile duct to empty into the duodenum at the ampulla of Vater. The duct is usually in the center of the pancreas but sometimes is near the posterior or anterior surface. The pancreatic duct is 2 to 3.5 mm in diameter and contains 20 secondary branches, which drain the tail, body, and uncinate process.

The drainage of the lesser duct, or duct of Santorini, is variable. The lesser duct usually drains the superior portion of the head of the pancreas. It empties into the second portion of the duodenum through the lesser papilla, located 2 cm proximal to the ampulla of Vater.

The main pancreatic duct joins with the common bile duct and empties at the ampulla of Vater. The surrounding sphincter of Oddi, which is regulated by neural and hormonal factors, controls pancreatic and biliary secretions into the duodenal lumen. This sphincter prevents reflux of duodenal contents into the ducts and may prevent reflux of bile into the pancreatic duct because of the difference in pancreatic and biliary ductular pressures.

Arterial Supply

The celiac and superior mesenteric arteries supply blood to the pancreas through their main branches (Fig. 30-2).

Head

In the head of the pancreas, arcades in the anterior and posterior surfaces collateralize. These arcades originate from branches of the gastroduodenal and the superior mesenteric arteries. Just distal to the first portion of the duodenum, the gastroduodenal artery becomes the superior pancreatoduodenal artery, which divides into anterior and posterior branches. The inferior pancreatoduodenal artery is the first branch of the superior mesenteric artery, and divides into anterior and posterior branches. The anterosuperior pancreatoduodenal artery lies in the anterior portion of the head of the pancreas and collateralizes with the anteroinferior pancreatoduodenal artery. The posterosuperior pancreatoduodenal artery crosses the common bile duct and forms the posterior arcade with the posteroinferior pancreatoduodenal artery. These arcades supply the head of the pancreas and the second and third portions of the duodenum. Because the duodenum and head of the pancreas share a vascular supply, the two structures must be resected together. In some people, the common hepatic, right hepatic, or gastroduodenal artery may originate from the superior mesenteric artery.

Body and Tail

The body and tail of the pancreas are supplied by the splenic artery. The splenic artery originates from the celiac trunk and courses along the superior surface of the pancreas to the spleen. Approximately 10 branches of the splenic artery supply the body and tail of the pancreas. Three of the larger branches are (1) the dorsal pancreatic

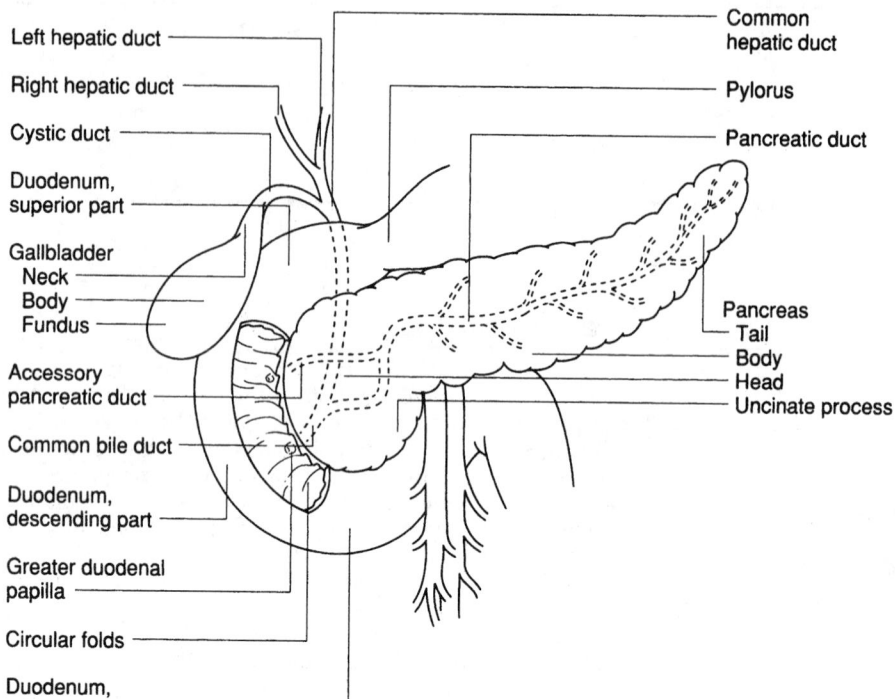

Left hepatic duct

Right hepatic duct

Cystic duct

Duodenum, superior part

Gallbladder
  Neck
  Body
  Fundus

Accessory pancreatic duct

Common bile duct

Duodenum, descending part

Greater duodenal papilla

Circular folds

Duodenum, inferior part

Common hepatic duct

Pylorus

Pancreatic duct

Pancreas
  Tail
  Body
  Head
  Uncinate process

Figure 30-1. Relation of the pancreas to the duodenum and extrahepatic biliary system. (After Woodburne RT. Essentials of human anatomy. New York, Oxford University Press, 1973)

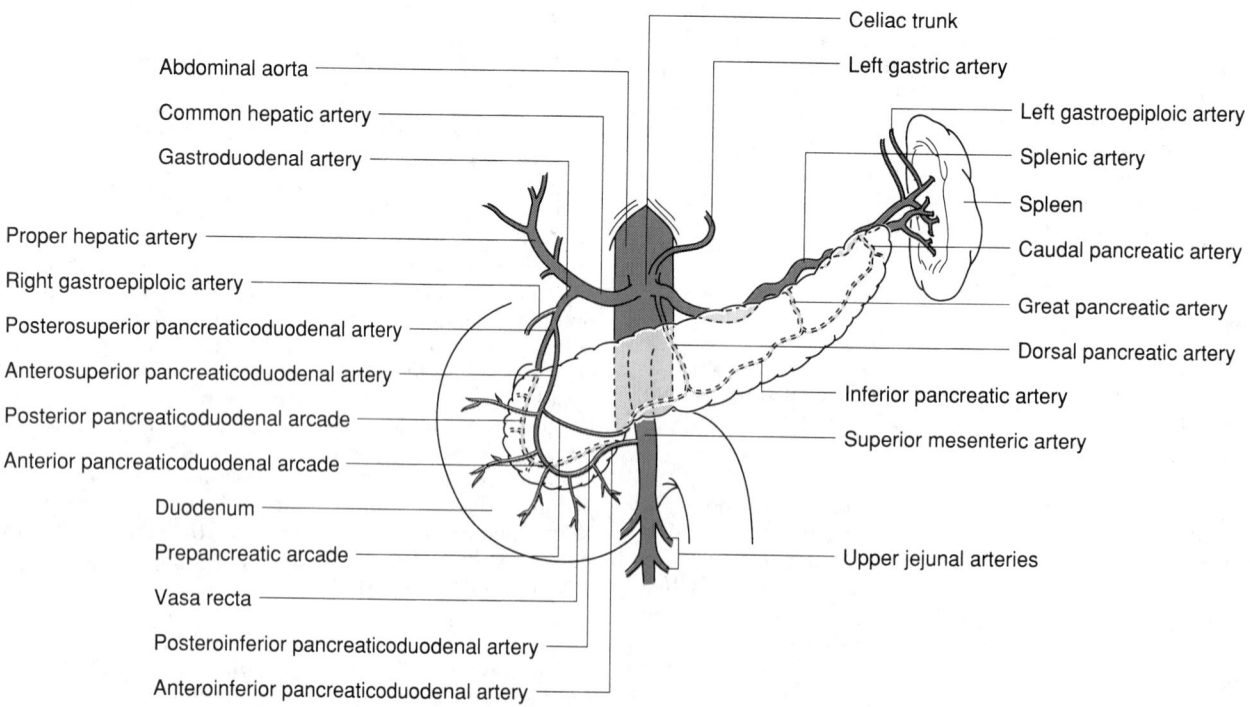

Abdominal aorta

Common hepatic artery

Gastroduodenal artery

Proper hepatic artery

Right gastroepiploic artery

Posterosuperior pancreaticoduodenal artery

Anterosuperior pancreaticoduodenal artery

Posterior pancreaticoduodenal arcade

Anterior pancreaticoduodenal arcade

Duodenum

Prepancreatic arcade

Vasa recta

Posteroinferior pancreaticoduodenal artery

Anteroinferior pancreaticoduodenal artery

Celiac trunk

Left gastric artery

Left gastroepiploic artery

Splenic artery

Spleen

Caudal pancreatic artery

Great pancreatic artery

Dorsal pancreatic artery

Inferior pancreatic artery

Superior mesenteric artery

Upper jejunal arteries

Figure 30-2. Arterial supply to the pancreas. (After Woodburne RT. Essentials of human anatomy. New York, Oxford University Press, 1973)

artery, which lies close to the celiac trunk; (2) the great pancreatic artery, which supplies the mid-portion of the body; (3) and the caudal pancreatic artery, which supplies the tail. These three arteries form channels that course the length of the pancreas and collateralize with the inferior pancreatoduodenal artery, which originates from the superior mesenteric artery.

Venous Drainage

The venous drainage of the pancreas and duodenum follows the arterial supply (Fig. 30-3). The veins are usually superficial to the arteries, and there is a similar frequency of anomalies. The anterior and posterior venous arcades drain the pancreatic head, and the splenic vein drains the body and tail. All venous effluent from the pancreas drains into the portal vein. The main areas of venous drainage are the suprapancreatic portal vein, the retropancreatic portal vein, the splenic veins, and the infrapancreatic superior mesenteric vein. The anterior and posterior venous arcades in the head of the pancreas drain directly into the suprapancreatic portal vein. The anteroinferior pancreatoduodenal arcades drain with the right gastroepiploic vein to form a common venous trunk with the right colic vein. This gastrocolic trunk enters the superior mesenteric vein at the inferior border of the neck of the pancreas. The posteroinferior venous arcade empties directly into the superior mesenteric vein. Because the veins of the pancreatic head drain laterally into the superior mesenteric and portal veins, it is safe to dissect the neck of the pancreas directly anterior to the portal vein during pancreatoduodenectomy.

Three venous branches drain the body and tail of the pancreas. These are (1) the inferior pancreatic vein, (2) the caudal pancreatic vein, and (3) the great pancreatic vein. All three branches drain into the splenic vein. The inferior mesenteric vein courses behind the pancreas and joins with the splenic vein or directly with the superior mesenteric vein.

Lymphatic Drainage

The lymphatic drainage of the pancreas is abundant and diffuse and most likely is responsible for the high incidence of metastases associated with pancreatic cancer (Fig. 30-4). Lymphatic vessels of the pancreatic head and duodenum drain into the celiac and superior mesenteric lymph nodes, constituting the predominant drainage. The anterior lymphatic vessels drain into the peripyloric nodes,

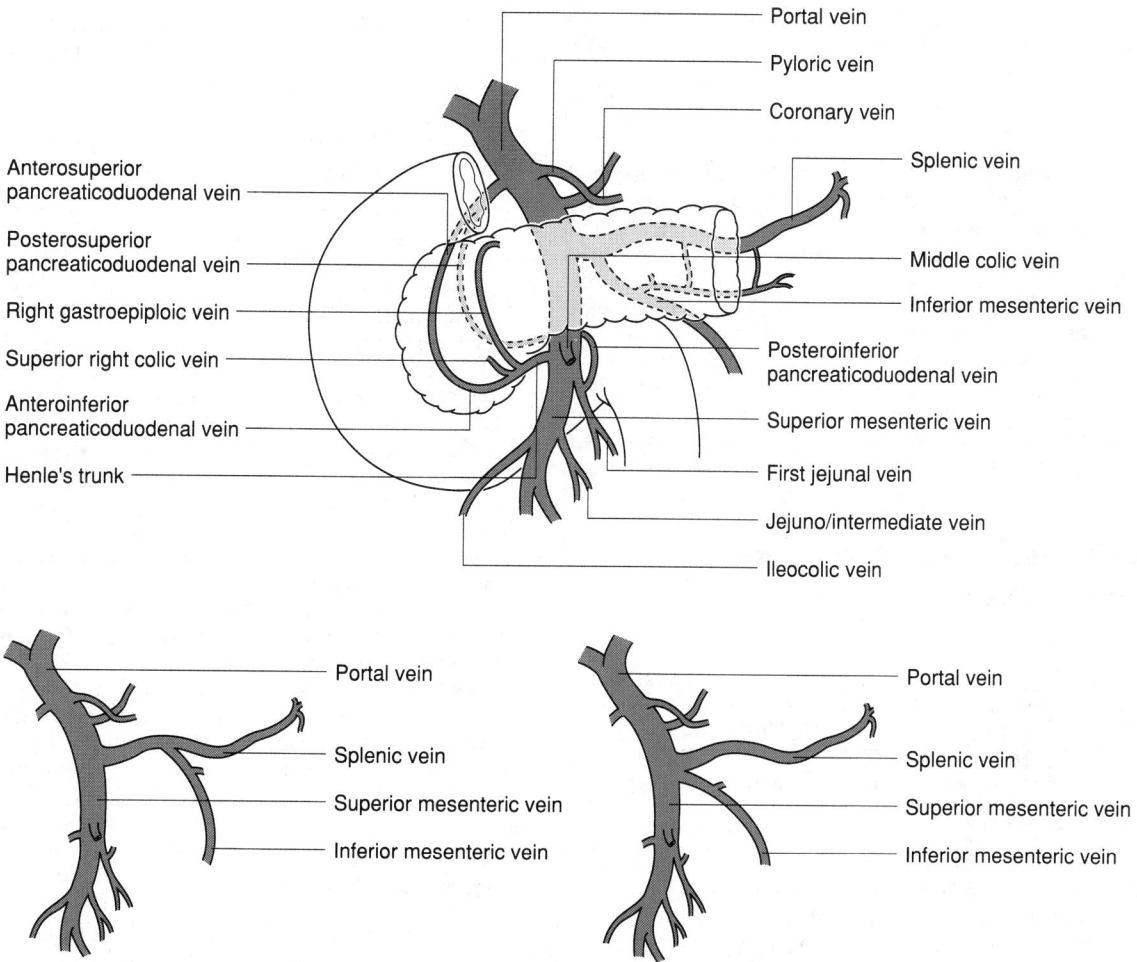

Figure 30-3. Venous drainage of pancreas. Variations in the relation of the portal, splenic, superior mesenteric, and inferior mesenteric veins are shown at the bottom. (After Mackie CR, Moossa AR: Surgical anatomy of the pancreas. In: Moossa AR, ed. Tumors of the pancreas. Baltimore, Williams & Wilkins, 1980)

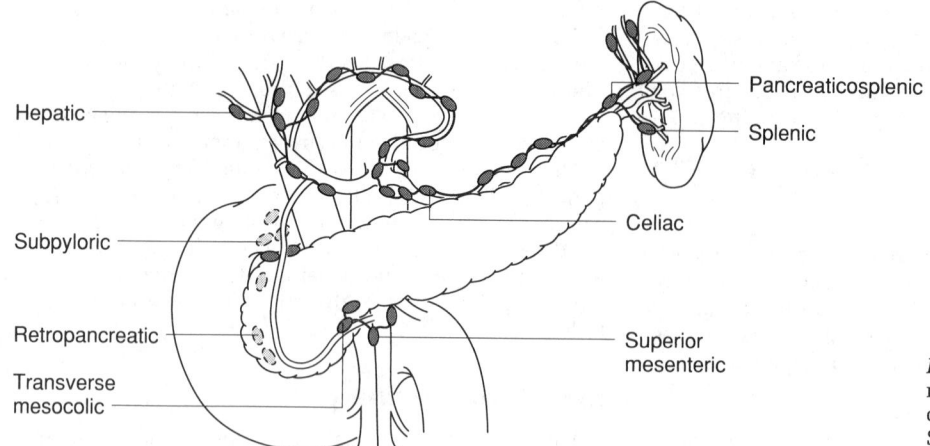

Hepatic

Subpyloric

Retropancreatic

Transverse
mesocolic

Pancreaticosplenic

Splenic

Celiac

Superior
mesenteric

Figure 30-4. Lymph node groups receiving drainage from the pancreas. (After Mackie CR, Moossa AR. Surgical anatomy of the pancreas. In: Moossa AR, ed. Tumors of the pancreas. Baltimore, Williams & Wilkins, 1980)

and the lymphatic vessels of the tail and body drain into the pancreatosplenic nodes along the splenic vessels. The absence of a peritoneal barrier on the posterior surface of the pancreas allows direct communication between the intrapancreatic lymphatic vessels and the retroperitoneal tissues. This anatomic feature probably contributes to the high incidence of recurrence after resections of pancreatic cancer.

Innervation

The exocrine and endocrine secretions of the pancreas are regulated by sympathetic fibers from the splanchnic nerves, parasympathetic fibers from the vagus nerve, and peptidergic neurons, which secrete amines and peptides (Fig. 30-5). Parasympathetic fibers stimulate both exocrine and endocrine secretion, whereas sympathetic fibers have a predominantly inhibitory effect. The peptidergic neurons secrete hormones such as somatostatin, vasoactive intestinal peptide (VIP), calcitonin gene-related peptide (CGRP), and galanin. The pancreas has a rich afferent sensory fiber network, which probably contributes to the intrinsic pancreatic pain associated with pancreatic cancer and chronic pancreatitis.

STRUCTURE AND HISTOLOGY
Exocrine Structure

Acinar Cells

The acinar cells secrete the enzymes responsible for digestion. Twenty to 40 acinar cells form an acinus. Centroacinar cells are responsible for fluid and electrolyte secretion by the pancreas. These cells contain enzymes necessary for bicarbonate and electrolyte transport.

Ductular Network

A network of conduits carries exocrine secretions into the duodenum. The acinus drains into small intercollated ducts. Several small intercollated ducts join to form an interlobular duct. The interlobular ducts contribute to fluid and electrolyte secretion. The interlobular ducts form secondary ducts that empty into the main pancreatic duct. The ductular network is progressively destroyed with recurrent episodes of pancreatitis, contributing, in part, to exocrine insufficiency and pain.

HISTOLOGY
Endocrine Structure

Within the pancreas are small nests of cells that secrete hormones that control glucose homeostasis. These islets of Langerhans constitute 2% of the pancreatic mass. The islets contain an average of 3000 cells of the following types:

- Alpha (A), which secrete glucagon
- Beta (B), which secrete insulin
- Delta (D), which secrete somatostatin
- PP or F, which secrete pancreatic polypeptide

The B cells are located in the center of the islet and constitute 70% of islet mass. The PP, A, and D cells are located at the periphery of the islet. D cells sometimes are present in the core of islets. Islet cells may secrete more than one hormone. For example, in addition to insulin, B cells secrete amylin, which may regulate glucose metabolism.

The cellular composition of the islets varies throughout the pancreas. Islets in the uncinate process are rich in PP cells and poor in A cells. Islets in the body and tail are rich in A cells and poor in PP cells. B cells and D cells are evenly distributed throughout the pancreas. The physiologic significance of this distribution remains unknown. Certain operations may remove certain islet populations. For example, pancreatoduodenectomy removes 95% of the functioning PP cell mass, which may contribute to glucose intolerance.

Islets contain small numbers of cells that secrete hormones such as VIP, serotonin, and pancreastatin. The islets also secrete numerous neuropeptides such as CGRP, neuropeptide Y, bombesin, and somatostatin, which probably have local regulatory effects on endocrine and exocrine secretion. Islet cells are physiochemically distinct and are related to other neuroendocrine cells derived from the neural crest of the embryo. These groups of cells are capable of amine precursor uptake and decarboxylation and may give rise to APUDomas.

Intravascular Pattern

The islets comprise 2% of pancreatic tissue but receive 20 to 30% of pancreatic arteriolar flow. The distribution of blood flow can change after a meal. Two microvascular patterns within the islets have been proposed:

1. The arteriole of the islet penetrates the islet and perfuses the center, where the B cells are located. The

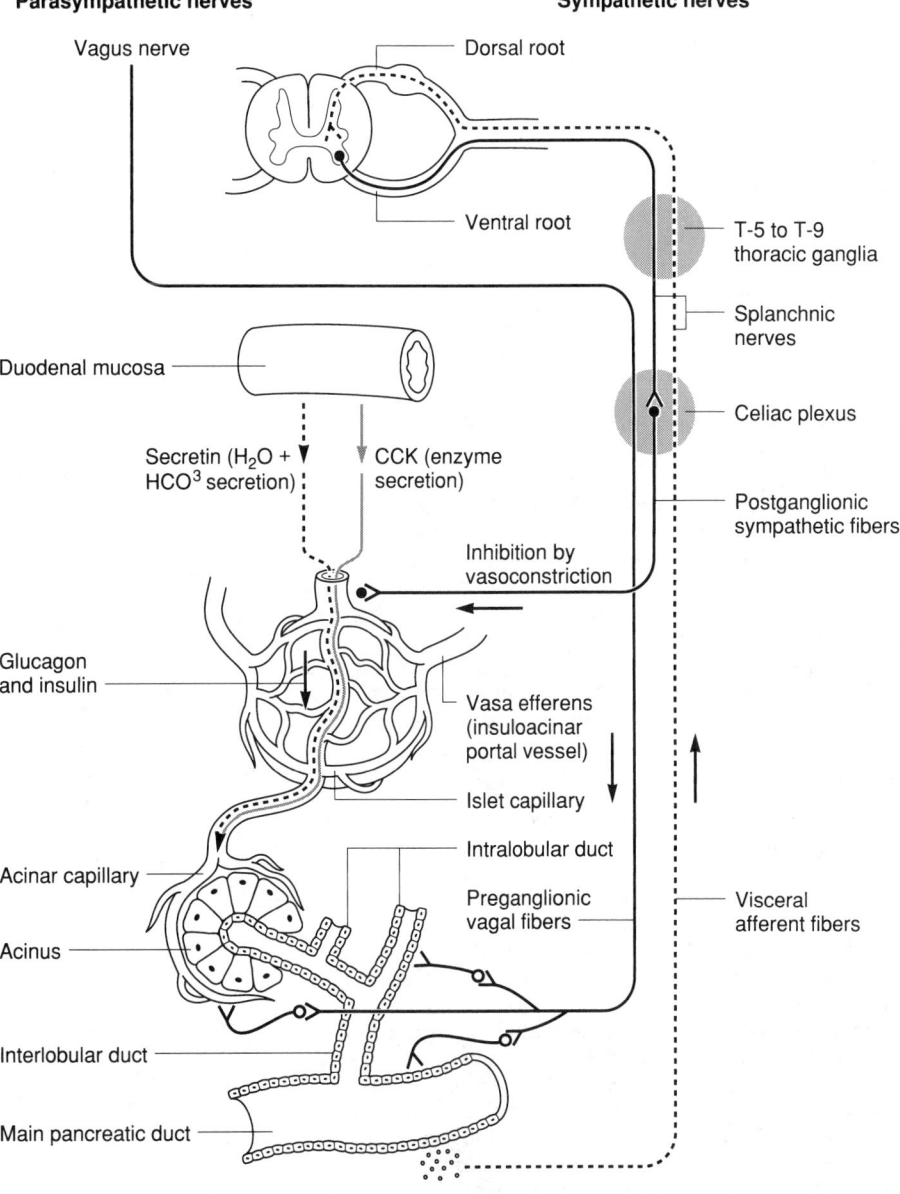

Parasympathetic nerves

Sympathetic nerves

Figure 30-5. Schematic diagram of the neurohormonal control of the exocrine cells. Visceral receptors line the ductule system and carry the sensation of pain to the spinal cord. Sympathetic fibers first synapse in the celiac plexus after traveling through the thoracic ganglia and the splanchnic nerves. Postganglionic fibers then synapse on intrapancreatic arterioles. Parasympathetic preganglionic fibers travel through the celiac plexus after leaving the vagus nerves and course with vessels and ducts to synapse on postganglionic fibers near acinar cells, islet cells, and the smooth muscle of major ducts. Stimulation of these parasympathetic fibers results in an immediate release of pancreatic enzymes. Secretin and CCK first enter the pancreas through the capillary network of the islet cells, then enter the separate capillary network of the acinar tissue through the insuloacinar portal vessels. Glucagon, somatostatin, pancreatic polypeptide, and insulin from the islet cells reach the acinar tissue immediately after release. In this way, the islet cells can influence the acinar tissue responses to CCK and secretin. (After Tompkins RK, Traverso LW. The exocrine cells. In: Keynes WM, Keith RG, eds. The pancreas. New York, Appleton-Century-Crofts, 1981)

blood then flows toward the periphery, or mantle, of the islet, where the non-B cells are located. This process allows high concentrations of insulin to modulate secretion of non-B cells through paracrine action.

2. The arteriole perfuses the mantle, then the core. The collecting vessels that drain the islets then perfuse the acinar tissue. The perfusion of acinar tissue with venous blood from the islet—the insuloacinar portal system—allows endocrine regulation of the exocrine pancreas. This regulation is performed by insulin, but other islet hormones, such as PP and somatostatin, also influence exocrine secretion. Much of the acinar tissue is perfused directly by pancreatic arterial blood that bypasses the endocrine tissue.

PHYSIOLOGY
Exocrine Function

The pancreas secretes 500 to 800 mL/d of an alkaline fluid (or juice) that contains digestive enzymes. The alkaline pH is caused by secreted bicarbonate, which neutral-

izes gastric acid and regulates the pH of the intestine, where the enzymes digest carbohydrates, proteins, and fats. Pancreatic fluid is colorless, odorless, and isosmotic. It contains 0.2% protein, mostly enzymes such as amylase, lipase, and trypsinogen.

Bicarbonate Secretion

The centroacinar cells and ductular epithelium secrete fluid that contains 20 mmol/L bicarbonate in the basal state and as much as 150 mmol/L under maximal stimulation. pH is 7.6 to 9.0. The fluid carries inactive proteolytic enzymes to the duodenal lumen. Sodium and potassium concentrations are constant and equal those of plasma. Chloride secretion varies inversely with bicarbonate secretion; the sum of these two cations remains constant and equal to that of plasma. Secretin, the main stimulant of bicarbonate secretion, is released from the duodenal mucosa when duodenal luminal pH is <3.0. Cholecystokinin (CCK) weakly stimulates bicarbonate secretion, but it potentiates secretin-stimulated bicarbonate secretion. Gastrin and acetylcholine also are weak stimulants of bicarbonate secretion. Bicarbonate secretion is inhibited by atropine, and is reduced 50% with truncal vagotomy.

Enzyme Secretion

The acinar cells secrete isozymes that fall into three enzyme groups—amylases, lipases, and proteases. The enzymes are not secreted in a fixed ratio, and specific nutrient stimulants may increase one enzyme over another. Dietary alterations also change the relative amounts of amylase, lipases, and proteases secreted. When enzyme secretion is absent or impaired, malabsorption or incomplete digestion occurs, resulting in fecal loss of fat and protein.

Enzyme secretion is regulated through hormonal and neural factors. The enteric hormone CCK is the predominant regulator and stimulates acinar cells through specific membrane-bound receptors. The intracellular effectors, or second messengers, are calcium and diacylglycerol. Acetylcholine strongly stimulates acinar cells when released from postganglionic fibers of the pancreatic plexus and with CCK potentiates enzyme secretion. Secretin and VIP weakly stimulate acinar cell secretion and potentiate the effect of CCK on the acinar cells. Acinar cell secretion is influenced by islet hormones through the insuloacinar portal system. The enzymes are synthesized in the endoplasmic reticulum of the acinar cells and packaged in zymogen granules. The enzymes are released from the apical portion of the acinar cells into the lumen of the acinus, and are transported into the duodenal lumen, where they are activated.

Enzyme Groups

Through secretion of three classes of enzymes, the pancreas regulates digestion of fats, carbohydrates, and proteins.

Amylase hydrolyzes starch and glycogen to glucose, maltose, maltotriose, and dextrins.

Lipases emulsify and hydrolyze fat in the presence of bile salts. They hydrolyze insoluble esters of glycerol, alcohol esters, and water-soluble esters.

The proteolytic enzymes are essential for protein digestion. These enzymes are secreted as proenzymes and require activation for proteolytic activity. The proenzymes of trypsin and chymotrypsin are trypsinogen and chymotrypsinogen. They are activated by a duodenal enzyme, enterokinase, which converts trypsinogen to trypsin. Trypsinogen can also be activated by a decrease in pH to <7.0.

Endocrine Function

Insulin Synthesis, Secretion and Action

Insulin is a 56−amino acid polypeptide synthesized in the B cells of the islets of Langerhans. The B cells are destroyed in insulin-dependent diabetes mellitus (IDDM; type 1), resulting in insulin deficiency.

Insulin is secreted in two phases. The first phase is a burst of stored insulin that lasts 4to6 min. The second phase is sustained secretion attributed to ongoing synthesis of insulin. Secretion of insulin is regulated by nutrient, neural, and hormonal factors. Glucose is the predominant nutrient regulator. Additional nutrient regulators are amino acids, such as arginine, lysine, and leucine, and free fatty acids. Hormones that stimulate insulin secretion include glucagon, gastric inhibitory polypeptide (GIP), and CCK. Hormones that inhibit insulin secretion are somatostatin, amylin, and pancreastatin.

Glucagon Synthesis, Secretion and Action

Glucagon is a single-chain, 29−amino acid polypeptide secreted by the A cells of the islets. It promotes hepatic glycogenolysis. Other forms of glucagon released from the gastrointestinal tract include gastric glucagon, enteroglucagon, and glucagon-like peptides. Their physiologic role is not clear.

Pancreatic glucagon secretion is controlled by neural, hormonal, and nutrient factors. Glucose is the primary regulator and suppresses glucagon secretion. Glucagon and insulin respond in a reciprocal manner to changes in glucose concentrations; therefore, glucagon is considered a counterregulatory hormone to insulin—the two hormones work together to maintain basal glucose levels. Exaggerated or excess glucagon secretion may contribute to hyperglycemia, whereas a failure of glucagon secretion or absence of glucagon-rich portions of the pancreas may contribute to profound hypoglycemia. Glucagon is stimulated by the amino acids arginine and alanine. Insulin and somatostatin have a potent suppressive effect on glucagon secretion and may regulate glucagon secretion through paracrine effects within the islet.

Somatostatin Synthesis, Secretion and Action

Somatostatin is a 14−amino acid polypeptide that inhibits the release of almost all peptide hormones and inhibits gastric, pancreatic, and biliary secretion. It is present in the D cells of islets. The role of the hormone in the pancreas is not clear. Somatostatin has been found in the neurons of islets, and may act as an inhibitory neuropeptide. Because of its potent inhibitory effect, the peptide has been used to treat both endocrine and exocrine disorders.

Pancreatic Polypeptide Synthesis, Secretion and Action

PP is a 36−amino acid peptide secreted by the F cells of the islet. F cells are located predominantly in the uncinate process and represent 5 to 15% of the islet cell mass. The role of PP is not clear. PP has been shown to inhibit exocrine secretion as well as choleresis and gallbladder emptying. Release of PP is regulated predominantly by cholinergic innervation. The rise in PP levels after a meal is ablated by vagotomy and can be used as a marker of completeness of vagotomy. Circulating PP levels are increased in diabetes and in normal aging because of increased secretion. PP may be involved in glucose homeostasis, and PP deficiency after chronic pancreatitis or pancreatoduodenectomy may contribute to glucose intolerance, linking PP deficiency to pancreatogenic diabetes.

Other Peptide Products

Neuropeptides, such as VIP, galanin, and serotonin, may have a role in regulation of islet-cell secretion. Amylin is a 36−amino acid polypeptide secreted by the B cells. It inhibits insulin secretion and peripheral insulin uptake and has been implicated in the development of non−insulin-dependent diabetes mellitus (NIDDM; type 2). Pancreastatin is a derivative of chromogranin A, and has been shown to inhibit insulin secretion. Its role is not known.

Intraislet Regulation of Hormone Secretion

Because exogenous infusions of insulin, glucagon, and somatostatin affect islet hormone secretion, paracrine regulation of islet hormone secretion has been an area of intense investigation. Blood flow in islets is centripetal, that is, a central artery penetrates into the islet and perfuses the centrally located B-cell mass. The blood then flows outward toward the A, D, and F cells, allowing a paracrine cascade. By using antibodies specific for each hormone, researchers have demonstrated that insulin secretion within islets regulates secretion of glucagon and somatostatin. This observation suggests that the suppression of glucagon during hyperglycemia is regulated not by glucose

Table 30-1. CHARACTERISTIC RESULTS OF SECRETIN TESTING: FLOW, BICARBONATE, AND ENZYME CHANGES OBSERVED IN PATIENTS WITH VARIOUS PANCREATIC AND OTHER DISORDERS

Disorder	Pattern	Flow Rate	Maximum Bicarbonate Concentration	Enzyme Secretion
End-stage pancreatitis, advanced pancreatic cancer	Total insufficiency	Decreased	Decreased	Decreased
Chronic pancreatitis	Qualitative insufficiency	Normal	Decreased	Normal
Pancreatic cancer	Quantitative insufficiency	Decreased	Normal	Normal
Malnutrition*	Isolated enzyme deficiency	Normal	Normal	Decreased
Hemochromatosis, Zollinger-Ellison syndrome, various cirrhoses	Hypersecretion	Increased	Normal	Normal

* Sprue, ulcerative colitis, and regional enteritis
(Dreiling DA, Wolfson P. New insights into pancreatic disease revealed by the secretin test. In: Berk JE, ed. Developments in digestive diseases, vol 2. Philadelphia, Lea & Febiger, 1979:155)

but by an increase in insulin secretion. It has been demonstrated that intraislet somatostatin regulates insulin secretion. The physiologic importance of the paracrine cascade is not known.

TESTS OF PANCREATIC FUNCTION

Exocrine Function

Secretin Test

The standard test of exocrine pancreatic function. Before and after administration of secretin, duodenal fluid is analyzed for total volume, bicarbonate output, and enzyme secretion. The test is positive when abnormal values indicate exocrine pancreatic insufficiency (Table 30-1).

Fecal Fat Test

Used to differentiate pancreatic dysfunction and malabsorption due to enteric disease. Steatorrhea due to pancreatic disease is the result of lipase deficiency; fecal fat content increases.

Dimethadione Test

Used to assess exocrine function. After administration of tridione, the secretin test is performed. Duodenal output of dimethadione correlates with exocrine function; it is impaired in patients with exocrine insufficiency.

Lundh Test

Used to measure pancreatic enzyme secretion in response to a meal of carbohydrate, fat, and protein. The test is abnormal in patients with chronic pancreatitis and diminished pancreatic reserve.

Triolein Breath Test

A noninvasive test of exocrine insufficiency. Radiolabeled triglycerides are given orally, and the metabolite, $^{14}CO_2$, is measured in the breath. Patients with disorders of fat digestion or absorption exhale only a small amount of the ^{14}C-triolein dose.

PABA Test

A noninvasive test of pancreatic insufficiency. N-benzoyl-L-tyrosyl-paraaminobenzoic acid (BT-PABA) is cleaved by chymotrypsin to form PABA. PABA is excreted in the urine after being absorbed from the small intestine. BT-PABA is administered, and urine is collected. Patients with chronic pancreatitis excrete <60% of the ingested BT-PABA.

Test Meal PP Response

Allows confirmation of suspected pancreatic disease based on plasma levels of PP (Table 30-2).

Endocrine Function

Oral Glucose Tolerance Test (OGTT)

An indirect assessment of the insulin response to an oral glucose load. Used to confirm the diagnosis of diabetes (Table 30-3). Caution must be used in the interpretation of OGTT results, because the test measures glucose profile and not actual insulin response.

IV Glucose Tolerance Test

Reflects the pancreatic endocrine response to glucose. Used to measure the disappearance of plasma glucose after administration of a glucose bolus, indirectly reflecting insulin secretion and action. Eliminates gastrointestinal influences of glucose metabolism that occur with the OGTT. IVGTT response decreases with age, so results are evaluated with age-adjusted criteria.

Table 30-2. DIFFERENTIAL DIAGNOSIS OF INTESTINAL AND PANCREATIC STEATORRHEA

Parameter	Intestinal Steatorrhea	Pancreatitis
Fecal fat	<20 g monoglycerides and diglycerides; soapy consistency	>20 g triglycerides; oily seepage
D-Xylose	Low	Normal
Secretin test	Normal	Abnormal
Small bowel series	Abnormal	Normal
Small bowel biopsy	Abnormal	Normal
Lundh meal	Normal	Abnormal
PABA test	Normal	Abnormal
PP response to test meal	Normal	Low
Vitamin B_{12} and folate	Low	Normal
Treatment with pancreatic enzymes	No change	Improvement

(Modified from Brandt LJ. Gastrointestinal disorders of the elderly. New York, Raven Press, 1984:470)

Table 30-3. INTERPRETATION OF ORAL GLUCOSE TOLERANCE TEST RESULTS

Interpretation	Fasting Glucose Value (mg/dL)		Intermediate Glucose Value (mg/dL)		2-Hour Glucose Value (mg/dL)
Normal	<115	and	All values < 200	and	<140
Impaired glucose tolerance	<140	and	Any value ≥ 200	and	140–199
Diabetic	≥140		(Glucose tolerance test		
	or		not necessary)		
	<140	and	Any value ≥200	and	≥200
Nondiagnostic	Any combination of glucose values that does not fit into another category				

(Modified from National Diabetes Data Group. Classification and diagnosis of diabetes mellitus and other categories of glucose intolerance. Diabetes 1979;28:1039)

IV Arginine Test

Used to diagnose hormone-secreting tumors. Arginine stimulates secretion of islet hormones.

Tolbutamide Response Test

Used to detect hormone-secreting tumors. Tolbutamide stimulates insulin secretion.

SUGGESTED READING

Ahren B, Taborsky GJ Jr, Porte D Jr. Neuropeptidergic versus cholinergic and adrenergic regulation of islet hormone secretion. Diabetologia 1986;29:827.

Bell GI, Kayano T, Buse JB, et al. Molecular biology of mammalian glucose transporters. Diabetes Care 1990;13:198.

Havel PJ, Taborsky GJ Jr. The contribution of the autonomic nervous system to changes in glucagon and insulin secretion during hypoglycemic stress. Endocr Rev 1989;10:332.

Jansson L, Hellerstrom C. Glucose-induced changes in pancreatic islet blood flow mediated by central nervous system. Am J Physiol 1986;25:E644.

Kennedy FP. Pathophysiology of pancreatic polypeptide secretion in human diabetes mellitus. Diabetes Nutr Metab 1990;2:155.

Kleinman R, Gingerich R, Wong H, et al. The use of the Fab fragment for immunoneutralization of somatostatin in the isolated perfused pancreas. Am J Surg 1994;167:114.

Liu Y, Guth PH, Kaneko K, et al. Dynamic in vivo observation of rat islet microcirculation. Pancreas 1993;8:15.

Murakami T, Fujita T, Ohtsuka A, et al. The insulino-acinar portal and insulino-venous drainage systems in the pancreas of the mouse, dog, monkey and certain other animals: a scanning electron microscopic study of corrosion casts. Arch Histol Cytol 1993;56:127.

Opara EC, Atwater I, Go VLM. Characterization and control of pulsatile secretion of insulin and glucagon. Pancreas 1988;3:484.

ESSENTIALS OF SURGERY: SCIENTIFIC PRINCIPLES AND PRACTICE, edited by Lazar J. Greenfield, Michael W. Mulholland, Keith T. Oldham, Gerald B. Zelenock, and Keith D. Lillemoe. Lippincott–Raven Publishers, Philadelphia, © 1997.

CHAPTER 31

ACUTE PANCREATITIS
KAREN S. GUICE

Acute pancreatitis is a complex disorder of the exocrine pancreas characterized by acute acinar cell injury and regional and systemic inflammatory responses. Because the pathogenic mechanisms are unclear, specific treatment is not available. Empiric supportive care is the standard. Clinical outcome has improved only to the extent that critical care has improved.

PATHOLOGY

Acute pancreatitis is characterized by alterations in acinar cell structure and function and by an acute regional and systemic inflammatory responses. The pancreas enlarges and becomes edematous with small areas of focal necrosis that involve the pancreas and areas of adjacent retroperitoneal fat. Although pancreatitis usually is reversible, frank pancreatic necrosis develops in some patients and may lead to irreversible regional injury or multiple-system organ failure (MSOF). Histologic characteristics of advanced disease include extensive acinar cell necrosis, interstitial microabscess formation, extensive peripancreatic fat necrosis, microvascular thrombosis, and local hemorrhage.

PATHOPHYSIOLOGY

A variety of substances normally present in pancreatic tissue and secretions and in plasma protect against premature or inappropriate activation of digestive enzymes. Although the specific mechanisms are not known, the normal secretory sequence appears to be disrupted in acute pancreatitis. Once initiated, protease release perpetuates acinar cell injury and initiates a regional acute inflammatory response, generating additional injury.

The endogenous inflammatory system participates early in the development of acute pancreatitis. Both humoral factors and cellular elements appear to be involved. Complement is activated, histamine is released, and bradykinin is generated. Cytokines also appear to have a role.

Systemic Consequences

In addition to localized inflammation, acute pancreatitis involves a systemic inflammatory response, which may lead to MSOF. A common event appears to be microvascular endothelial cell injury in diverse target organs. Pancreatitis-induced/dependent microvascular lung injury is one such example. This process may explain the frequent pulmonary symptoms and the occasional case of acute respiratory distress syndrome (ARDS) in patients with acute pancreatitis.

The role of the microcirculation in the development of acute pancreatitis is poorly understood. Increased permeability, microvascular thrombosis, or obstruction by leukoaggregates may lead to local or regional tissue hypoxia. Diminished microvascular blood flow may initiate acute pancreatitis. Hypoxic acinar cell injury appears to be associated with cardiopulmonary bypass, thromboembolic disease, and myocardial infarction.

Complications

Complications of acute pancreatitis are as follows:

Early
  Shock
  Multiple-system organ failure
  Encephalopathy
  Coagulopathy
  Sepsis
  Hypocalcemia
Late
  Pseudocyst
  Diabetes
  Abscess

INCIDENCE

The incidence of acute pancreatitis is estimated to be 0.14 to 1.3%. Incidence is difficult to determine because patients with mild pancreatitis may not seek medical care and because diagnostic criteria vary among institutions. Variations among populations depend on social factors, such as ethanol use and on environmental and hereditary determinants, such as the incidence of gallstones.

Acute pancreatitis may occur at any age but is most common in adults 30 to 70 years of age. In general, patients with gallstone-induced pancreatitis are older (40 to 60 years), whereas those with alcohol-associated pancreatitis are younger (30 to 40 years). Sex distribution depends on the cause of the disease. Women more frequently have gallstone-associated pancreatitis; men more frequently have pancreatitis associated with alcohol use.

The mortality for acute pancreatitis is 6% to 20.5%. Acute hemorrhagic or necrotizing pancreatitis has a mortality of 50% or more. Necrotizing pancreatitis occurs in 5% to 10% of patients.

CLINICAL ASSOCIATIONS

Clinical associations with acute pancreatitis occur in three categories—biliary stones, ethanol ingestion, and other conditions. The distribution of causes reflects the patient population (Table 31-1).

Because the distal common bile duct and pancreatic duct have a common channel, pancreatic ductal hypertension may occur when a gallstone obstructs the ampulla of Vater. If transient obstruction causes edema and ampullary dysfunction, reflux of bile or duodenal contents into the pancreatic duct may initiate acute pancreatitis. Choledocholithiasis is not always found, because the stone usually passes before the patient seeks care. When stools are screened, gallstones are found in almost all patients within 10 days of the onset of disease.

Ethanol use is the most common cause of acute pancreatitis in the United States. Ethanol ingestion usually leads to pancreatic ductal hypertension.

Other Conditions

  Trauma
  Surgical
  During ERCP
  Accidental trauma, blunt or penetrating
  Obstruction, other than gallstone
  Tumors of pancreas, duodenum, or bile duct
  Duodenal obstruction
  Pancreas divisum
  Infection (Table 31-2)
  Hyperlipidemia
  Hyperparathyroidism
  Vascular disease
  Immunologic factors
  Pregnancy
  Drugs
  Steroids
  Estrogen
  Corticosteroids
  Diuretics
  Furosemide
  Thiazides
  Ethacrynic acid
  Diazoxide
  Calcium
  Warfarin
  Cimetidine
  Quinidine
  Phenformin
  Azathioprine
  Mercuric chloride
  Paracetamol
  Sulfonamides
  Tetracyclines
  L-asparaginase
  Methyldopa
  Clonidine

PRESENTATION

The cardinal clinical symptom of acute pancreatitis is visceral epigastric pain that radiates to the back. The pain may be similar to that of acute peritonitis and may mimic that of a perforated viscus, or it may be minimal. Other common signs and symptoms are nonspecific (Table 31-3).

The clinical signs of complex disease or necrotizing pancreatitis are jaundice and hypotension. Retroperitoneal hemorrhage associated with pancreatic necrosis may become apparent as blood dissects into the subcutaneous tissues, producing blue discoloration of the flanks (Grey Turner sign), the umbilicus (Cullen sign), or the inguinal ligament (Fox sign).

The clinical course of acute pancreatitis is extremely variable. One patient may have minimal symptoms, few signs, and only mild hyperamylasemia, require little or no treatment, and have few, if any, complications. Another patient may experience fulminant pancreatic necrosis, hemorrhage, MSOF, or death.

Several grading systems are used to estimate risks and outcomes on the basis of presenting clinical features. The

Table 31-1. CLINICAL ASSOCIATIONS WITH ACUTE PANCREATITIS FROM COLLECTED REVIEWS AROUND THE WORLD

Country	Patients	Cause (%)			
		Biliary Stones	Ethanol	Idiopathic	Other
United States	7147	28	53	8	11
Great Britain	1539	52	7	34	7
Germany	279	51	22	24	3
France	294	34	33	—	—
Sweden	207	48	21	15	16
Denmark	163	33	42	21	4
India	42	17	23	31	29
Hong Kong	483	41	10	39	10

Ranson criteria are widely adopted. A patient with three or more of the following findings has a 30% chance of death.

RANSON GRAVE PROGNOSTIC SIGNS ASSOCIATED WITH ACUTE PANCREATITIS

At admission
  Age >55 years
  White blood cell count >16,000/mL
  Glucose level >200 mg/dL
  Lactate dehydrogenase level >350 IU/L
  Aspartate aminotransferase (formerly SGOT) value >250 IU/L

After 48 hours
  Hematocrit decrease of 10%
  Blood urea nitrogen increase of 5 mg/dL
  Ca^2-level <8 mg/dL
  P_aO_2 <60 mmHg
  Base deficit value >4 mEq/L
  Fluid sequestration >6 L

DIAGNOSIS

The diagnosis of acute pancreatitis based on the physical finding of epigastric abdominal pain and tenderness and the laboratory finding of hyperamylasemia.

Imaging

Although diffuse ileus and a solitary left upper abdominal sentinel loop are classic findings on plain abdominal radiographs, neither is specific for acute pancreatitis. About one-third of patients with acute pancreatitis have abnormal chest radiographs at the time of diagnosis. Barium studies of the GI tract are seldom helpful in the evaluation of simple acute pancreatitis.

Ultrasonography (US) is a readily available, rapid, and noninvasive means of imaging the pancreas. In simple acute pancreatitis, an enlarged, anechoic gland is seen. US examination yields information about cholelithiasis, choledocholithiasis, and the status of the intrahepatic and extrahepatic biliary ducts. US is valuable for evaluating peripancreatic fluid collections and pancreatic pseudocysts.

Computed tomography (CT) has capabilities similar to those of US, although the sensitivity for detecting cholelithiasis is lower. Contrast enhancement in the duodenum and small intestine is necessary. Dynamic CT with simultaneous IV contrast enhancement provides valuable information about regional pancreatic perfusion and may allow estimation of the extent of pancreatic necrosis. Either CT- or US-guided diagnostic needle aspiration allows access to peripancreatic or pancreatic fluid collections for diagnostic sampling, therapeutic drainage, and collection of culture specimens.

The role of endoscopic retrograde cholangiopancreatography (ERCP) to evaluate acute pancreatitis is limited be-

Table 31-2. INFECTIOUS CAUSES LINKED TO THE DEVELOPMENT OF ACUTE PANCREATITIS

Viral	Bacterial	Fungal	Parasitic
Mumps	*Staphylococcus* sp	Aspergillosis	*Ascaris lumbricoides*
Coxsackie B	*Escherichia coli*	Actinomycosis	*Opisthorchis sinensis*
Enterovirus	*Enterococcus* sp		*Echinococcus granulosus*
Epstein-Barr virus	*Enterobacter* sp		*Giardiasis lamblia*
Cytomegalovirus	*Proteus* sp		*Plasmodium falciparum*
Hepatitis B	*Pseudomonas aeruginosa*		
Hepatitis A	Spirochetes		
Hepatitis C	*Corynebacterium diphtheriae*		
	Legionnella spiro		
	Yersinia sp		
	Campylobacter sp		
	Salmonella typhimurium		
	Mycobacteria sp		
	Mycoplasma sp		

Table 31-3. COMMON SIGNS AND SYMPTOMS OF UNCOMPLICATED ACUTE EDEMATOUS PANCREATITIS

Sign or Symptom	Frequency (%)
Abdominal pain	85–100
Nausea and vomiting	54–92
Anorexia	83
Fever	12–80
Abdominal mass	6–20
Ileus	50–80

cause of the high risk for exacerbation of existing inflammation. It is used to delineate the structure of the pancreatic ducts.

Biochemical Markers

Characteristic but nonspecific biochemical features associated with acute pancreatitis are summarized in Table 31-4.

One of the pathophysiologic events in pancreatitis is release of amylase from acinar cells into the pancreatic microcirculation. The laboratory finding of hyperamylasemia in a patient with signs and symptoms of acute pancreatitis usually confirms the diagnosis. However, the clinician must be aware of the following:

- In pancreatitis due to a discrete event, such as transient pancreatic duct obstruction with a gallstone, serum amylase rises once and clears rapidly, usually within hours. Because patients usually do not seek care immediately, the peak may have passed, and serum amylase level may be normal.
- In necrotizing or chronic pancreatitis, the acinar cell population may be damaged or destroyed, reducing amylase output. Serum amylase level may be normal or minimally elevated.
- Nonpancreatic sources of amylase exist, so hyperamylasemia may be caused by another disease. The salivary glands, fallopian tubes, and small intestine are sources of amylase.

Lipase and other acinar cell products (eg, immunoreactive trypsin, chymotrypsin, elastase, ribonuclease, and phospholipase A2) may be detected in plasma after the onset of acute pancreatitis. Measurement of these substances has not proved more reliable than measurement of amylase. Plasma levels of methemalbumin also may be elevated in acute pancreatitis.

TREATMENT

The closest approximation to specific therapy for acute pancreatitis is surgical relief of pancreatic ductal obstruction or elimination of stimuli, such as alcohol. Otherwise treatment is general supportive care.

Medical Therapy

Fluid Resuscitation

Regional retroperitoneal inflammation and systemic microvascular injury contribute to loss of intravascular plasma volume. Hypovolemia may be mild or profound to the point of shock. More than half of patients with acute pancreatitis have evidence of inadequate end-organ perfusion. Resuscitation requires IV administration of large vol-

umes of isotonic crystalloid solution and use of invasive hemodynamic monitoring devices.

Hypovolemia almost invariably causes renal dysfunction in patients with acute pancreatitis. Renal function must be evaluated with biochemical tests, and urine output must be monitored during acute resuscitation. Early recognition of oliguria or azotemia allows correction.

Blood Gases

Pulmonary dysfunction occurs in two-thirds of patients with acute pancreatitis. Most patients have transient hypoxemia, defined as $P_aO_2 <70$ mmHg. Monitoring of pulmonary gas exchange with periodic measurement of arterial blood gases is standard in all patients with acute pancreatitis. Continuous transcutaneous monitoring of capillary hemoglobin saturation or measurement of mixed venous saturation is appropriate if there is evidence of ARDS.

Nutritional Support

Acute pancreatitis has many of the hemodynamic and metabolic characteristics of sepsis. Glucose production is exaggerated, insulin resistance and pancreatic endocrine insufficiency may develop, and protein catabolism is marked. It is appropriate to begin nutritional support immediately after acute resuscitation because of the unpredictable return of intestinal function and the extraordinary metabolic requirements. The choice of route—parenteral or enteral—is less important than the need to provide adequate calories and to establish positive nitrogen balance.

Antibiotics

Antibiotic therapy is reserved for specific infectious complications, such as pneumonia or pancreatic abscess.

Correction of Metabolic Imbalance

Hypokalemia, hypocalcemia, hemorrhage, and consumptive coagulopathy are treated with appropriate replacement products, such as potassium chloride, IV calcium gluconate or chloride, RBCs, and fresh-frozen plasma. Hyperglycemia and glycosuria are manifestations of altered carbohydrate metabolism. Hyperglycemia is usually transient. Permanent residual diabetes mellitus is infrequent.

Table 31-4. BIOCHEMICAL FEATURES OF ACUTE PANCREATITIS

INCREASED

Hematocrit, hemoglobin (hemoconcentration)
White blood cell count
Blood urea nitrogen
Creatinine
Bilirubin
Lipid, triglyceride levels
Glucose
Alkaline phosphatase
SGOT, SGPT

DECREASED

Hematocrit, hemoglobin (hemorrhage)
Calcium
Magnesium
PaO_2

OTHER

Respiratory alkalosis (early)
Metabolic alkalosis (early)
Consumptive coagulopathy
Metabolic acidosis (late)
Respiratory acidosis (late)

Treatment of acute illness is titrated administration of exogenous glucose and insulin to maintain euglycemia.

Monitoring for Encephalopathy

Some patients with acute pancreatitis have evidence of encephalopathy. Symptoms include disorientation, confusion, delirium, delusions, or hallucinations. Transient acute psychosis also occurs. Because ethanol ingestion and withdrawal also produce these symptoms, it is often difficult to determine the cause. Cerebral edema, hemorrhage, and focal necrosis, presumably due to alterations in microvascular blood flow, also may occur. Treatment is nonspecific and supportive.

Anticoagulants

Coagulation disorders, such as microvascular thrombosis and disseminated intravascular coagulopathy (DIC), are common in acute pancreatitis. DIC occurs early unless it is a complication of late sepsis. Hyperfibrinogenemia and increased platelet counts occur late, suggesting enhanced thrombotic potential. Use of heparin, low–molecular-weight dextran, and fibrinolytic agents therapy to prevent the development of acute hemorrhagic pancreatitis is being investigated.

Calcium Replacement

Hypocalcemia frequently accompanies acute pancreatitis. It appears that large quantities of calcium are bound in the tissues during peripancreatic fat saponification. Other factors, such as changes in plasma levels of parathyroid hormone, glucagon, and calcitonin, may contribute. Unattended, hypocalcemia may progress to tetany. Monitoring of serum calcium level is standard during acute illness. Treatment is IV calcium replacement.

Surgical Treatment

Surgical therapy for acute pancreatitis is reserved for complications and for correction of anatomic defects. Acute pancreatitis may be indistinguishable from perforated duodenal ulcer, acute appendicitis, and ruptured abdominal aortic aneurysm. Correct diagnosis is crucial. It is important to avoid biopsy, resection, or other high-risk nontherapeutic procedures.

Endoscopic Sphincterotomy

Endoscopic sphincterotomy is the initial therapeutic procedure for relief of biliary ductal obstruction when acute pancreatitis is associated with choledocholithiasis. The procedure decompresses the ampulla of Vater and disimpacts the gallstone.

Cholecystectomy

More common than a blocked common bile duct is simple cholelithiasis associated with an episode of acute pancreatitis, which usually resolves without surgical treatment. However, biliary pancreatitis usually recurs within 6 weeks, so cholecystectomy is performed as soon as the acute pancreatitis resolves.

Anatomic Repair

Correctable lesions that cause acute pancreatitis include pancreas divisum, choledochal cysts, and pancreatic ductal obstruction related to tumor, stricture, or injury. Surgical therapy for obstruction is directed at achieving pancreatic ductal drainage by means of diversion into the jejunum for benign obstructions or by means of tumor resection. Pancreas divisum is treated with transduodenal sphincteroplasty. A choledochal cyst is marsupialized into the duodenum.

Surgical Management of Necrotizing Pancreatitis

When pancreatitis does not resolve spontaneously, infected and uninfected areas of pancreatic necrosis must be differentiated. This is done with needle aspiration of peripancreatic fluid collections under CT or US guidance. The presence of an infected sequestrum mandates surgical exploration, debridement of devitalized tissue, and external drainage. Antibiotic coverage is dictated by intraoperative cultures or examination of aspirates of necrotic tissue. Several debridements are required, usually every 24 to 48 hours, until the necrotic tissue is replaced with a granulating wound.

Peritoneal Drainage

Results with open and closed systems are comparable as long as colonized or infected devitalized tissue is not left in a closed abdominal cavity. If areas of pancreatic necrosis are not infected, surgical intervention may be deferred unless clinical evidence of deterioration develops.

PANCREATIC PSEUDOCYSTS

Pancreatic pseudocysts are fluid-filled cystic structures without a true epithelial lining. The wall of a pseudocyst is composed of displaced adjacent viscera (stomach, small intestine, or colon) and a fibrous capsule that bears evidence of acute and chronic inflammation. The fluid in the cavity is serous and contains pancreatic secretions, albumin, and inflammatory cells. Bacteria are cultured in about 35% of pseudocysts.

Pancreatic pseudocysts usually present with persistent visceral pain or ileus after an episode of acute pancreatitis. Fever, leukocytosis, and a palpable epigastric mass are common, nausea and vomiting less so. Jaundice suggests common bile duct obstruction. Most pseudocysts are located in the head of the pancreas, but they dissect almost anywhere in the retroperitoneal space or mediastinum.

If the patient has no symptoms and a pseudocyst is small (<5.0 cm), treatment is observation; many of these pseudocysts resolve in a few weeks. If the pseudocyst is large (>5 cm), the patient has chronic alcoholic pancreatitis, and the pseudocyst cavity is multilocular or debris-filled, ERCP is performed. If ERCP shows a pancreatic duct communicating with a pseudocyst, an operation usually is necessary.

If no ductal communication is demonstrated at ERCP, percutaneous drainage may be attempted. Results of pseudocyst drainage are summarized in Table 31-5. Before an open surgical drainage procedure is performed, a waiting period of at least 6 weeks is allowed for the pseudocyst to resolve or for the wall to develop a thick fibrous capsule. Wall thickness is estimated with US or CT. Pancreatic resection has the lowest recurrence rate, but is performed only if the pseudocyst is in the tail of the pancreas.

PANCREATIC ABSCESS

Pancreatic abscesses are usually caused by an infected pancreatic pseudocyst or necrotizing pancreatitis. The signs are persistent fever, leukocytosis, and a palpable abdominal mass. Bacteremia and systemic toxicity are late clinical features. At imaging, debris within a cyst suggests an abscess. Percutaneous aspiration with positive cultures is the definitive preoperative test. Treatment is wide surgical debridement of all infected and devitalized tissue, external drainage, and antibiotics.

Table 31-5. RESULTS OF PSEUDOCYST DRAINAGE PROCEDURES

Type	Complication Rate (%)	Recurrence Rate (%)	Mortality Rate (%)
Percutaneous aspiration	0	63	0
Percutaneous catheter	16	8	3
Surgical external drainage	35	20–25	7–27
Surgical internal drainage	25–35	5–9	3–9

SUGGESTED READING

Grewal HP, El Din AM, Gaber L, Kotb M, Gaber AO. Amelioration of the physiologic and biochemical changes of acute pancreatitis using an anti-TNF-polyclonal antibody. Am J Surg 1994;167:214.

Howard JM, Jordan GL Jr, Reber HA, eds. Surgical diseases of the pancreas. Philadelphia, Lea & Febiger, 1987.

Huibregtse K, Smits ME. Endoscopic management of diseases of the pancreas. Am J Gastroenterol 1994;8:S66.

McKay C, Gallagher G, Baxter JN, Imrie CW. Systemic complications in acute pancreatitis are associated with increased monocyte cytokine release. Gut 1994;35:A575.

Norman J, Franz M, Fabri PJ, Gower WR. Decreased severity of experimental acute pancreatitis by pre or post treatment with interleukin-1 receptor antagonist. Gastroenterology 1994; 106:A311.

Poston GJ, Williamson RCN. Surgical management of acute pancreatitis. Br J Surg 1990;77:5.

Ranson JHC. Etiological and prognostic factors in human acute pancreatitis: a review. Am J Gastroenterol 1982;77:633.

Rinderknecht H. Activation of pancreatic zymogens: Normal activation, premature intrapancreatic activation, protective mechanisms against inappropriate activation. Dig Dis Sci 1986;31:314.

Steer ML, Meldolesi J. The cell biology of experimental pancreatitis. N Engl J Med 1987;316:144.

ESSENTIALS OF SURGERY: SCIENTIFIC PRINCIPLES AND PRACTICE, edited by Lazar J. Greenfield, Michael W. Mulholland, Keith T. Oldham, Gerald B. Zelenock, and Keith D. Lillemoe. Lippincott–Raven Publishers, Philadelphia, © 1997.

CHAPTER 32

CHRONIC PANCREATITIS

MICHAEL W. MULHOLLAND

Chronic pancreatitis is progressive and permanent fibrosis of the pancreatic exocrine parenchyma, often accompanied by endocrine dysfunction.

ETIOLOGY

The following are etiologic factors in the development of chronic pancreatitis:

- Alcohol consumption
- Heredity
- Hyperparathyroidism
- Tropical pancreatitis—a nutritional disease in tropical Africa and Southeast Asia
- Obstruction of the main pancreatic duct
- Idiopathic causes

PATHOGENESIS

The initial lesion in chronic pancreatitis appears to be acinar cell injury. A characteristic of early alcoholic chronic pancreatitis is a patchy distribution of normal acinar tissue among abnormal lobules. Microscopic examination shows irregular dilatation of ductules, loss of ductal epithelium and acinar tissue, localized obstruction, and formation of small intraparenchymal cysts. Abnormal pancreatic protein and calcium secretion causes precipitated proteinaceous material to collect in intercalated and canalicular ducts. As the disease progresses, these protein plugs cause increasing ductal obstruction. Infiltration of the interstitium by inflammatory cells is followed by deposition of fibrous tissue within and between lobules. In advanced stages, exocrine tissue is replaced by fibrosis. Endocrine islets survive in isolated nests among broad areas of scar tissue.

CLINICAL PRESENTATION

Pain

Pain is the predominant symptom of chronic pancreatitis. The pain is usually localized to the epigastrium and radiates to the back in the region of the upper lumbar vertebrae. The pain is dull rather than sharp, and constant rather than intermittent or colicky. The discomfort sometimes is alleviated by bending forward, and is worsened by lying supine. Ingestion of food or alcohol exacerbates the pain in many patients. Most patients experience pain everyday, but some have an attack of pain followed by several pain-free days and another episode of pain.

The mechanisms responsible for causing pain in chronic pancreatitis are not known. Possibilities are:

- Inflammation
- Damage to intrapancreatic nerves
- Increased pancreatic interstitial and intraductal pressure
- Associated conditions, such as pseudocysts, bile duct stenosis, and duodenal obstruction

Malabsorption and Weight Loss

Malabsorption occurs when most of the exocrine tissue is lost. Steatorrhea occurs when lipase secretion falls to <5% to 10% of normal. Bulky, oily bowel movements and abdominal bloating are common symptoms. Weight loss nearly always occurs. Syndromes associated with deficiencies of fat-soluble vitamins are coagulopathy (vitamin K), osteomalacia (vitamin D), neuropathy (vitamin E), night blindness (vitamin A), and dermatitis (essential fatty acids).

Coincident with a reduction in enzyme production, is a decrease in pancreatic bicarbonate secretion. As a result, postprandial duodenal pH may be decreased for prolonged periods. If duodenal pH is <4, acid denaturation of pancreatic enzymes may exacerbate malabsorption. Postprandial abdominal pain is common in patients with chronic pancreatitis, and the fear of this pain may lead to a further reduction in food intake.

Endocrine Insufficiency

Altered insulin secretion occurs in almost all patients with chronic pancreatitis, abnormal glucose tolerance in most, and overt diabetes in a large number. These deficits are progressive. The long-term complications of pancreatic diabetes are not known, in part because many patients with chronic pancreatitis do not live long enough to participate in follow-up studies.

DIAGNOSIS
Laboratory Tests

Routine tests of blood or serum are not helpful in the diagnosis of chronic pancreatitis.

Tests of Pancreatic Exocrine Function

Direct measurement of exocrine function requires collection of pancreatic secretions by means of direct cannulation of the pancreatic duct. Indirect tests of pancreatic function measure absorption of a nutrient that requires pancreatic digestion. Neither type of test detects early disease.

Diagnostic Imaging

The simplest way to confirm chronic pancreatitis is a plain abdominal radiograph that demonstrates calcification of the pancreas.

Ultrasound (US) is useful in the initial evaluation of suspected chronic pancreatitis. Supportive findings are atrophy of the gland, hypoechoic areas, dilatation of the pancreatic duct to >4 mm, and associated cystic lesions. US examination of the pancreas may sometimes be compromised by overlying intestinal gas.

Computed tomographic (CT) findings are glandular atrophy, irregularity of the pancreatic outline, calcification, and ductal dilatation. Small cystic lesions are well demonstrated with CT.

Endoscopic retrograde cholangiopancreatography (ERCP) is the most sensitive and reliable method for diagnosing chronic pancreatitis. In earliest chronic pancreatitis, ductal changes are limited to secondary and tertiary ducts that show irregular dilatation. In moderate disease, the main pancreatic duct may be dilated with alternating areas of stenosis. In advanced chronic pancreatitis, marked ductal changes may form a chain-of-lakes appearance. ERCP is useful in demonstrating anatomic abnormalities, such as common bile duct stenosis or pancreatic pseudocyst.

TREATMENT OF COMPLICATIONS
Pain

Abstinence

Management of pain in patients with chronic pancreatitis begins with abstinence from alcohol. With elimination of alcohol, most patients experience a decrease in pain, although most do not become pain-free. Because alcohol is a secretagogue for pancreatic enzymes, pain relief is more likely in patients who retain some exocrine function.

Enzyme Replacement

Patients with chronic pancreatitis appear to experience continuous hormonal or neural stimulation to secrete digestive enzymes (Fig. 32-1). The increased stimulatory signals are presumed to cause or exacerbate pain. If this theory is correct, effective delivery of pancreatic enzymes to the duodenum should reduce chronic stimulation, decrease ductal pressure, and relieve pain. This therapy is under investigation.

Endoscopic Therapy

The use of endoprostheses or stents placed in the pancreatic duct under endoscopic guidance is associated with a risk of pancreatic ductal injury and fibrosis. For this reason, stents are used only for short periods to identify patients most likely to benefit from surgical drainage. The role of endoscopic removal of pancreatic ductal stones is under investigation. Stones fragmented with extracorporeal shock wave lithotripsy are extracted after sphincterotomy of the pancreatic duct. When stones are cleared, half

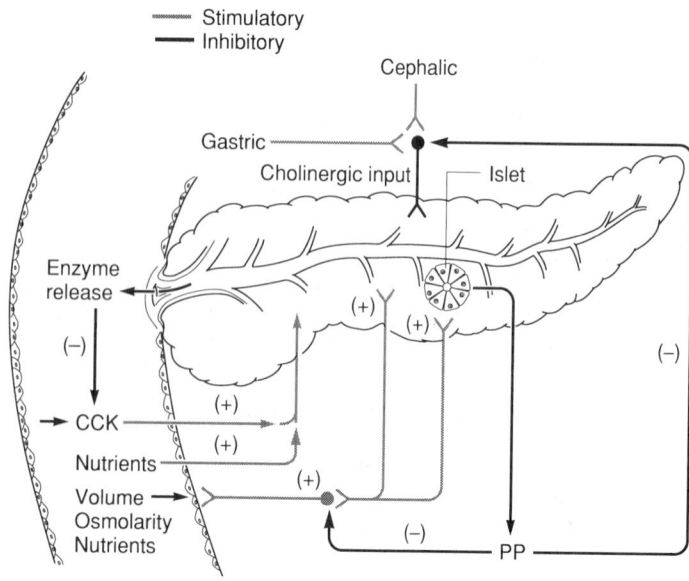

Figure 32-1. Schematic diagram of stimulatory and inhibitory influences on pancreatic exocrine secretion. CCK, cholecystokinin; PP, pancreatic polypeptide.

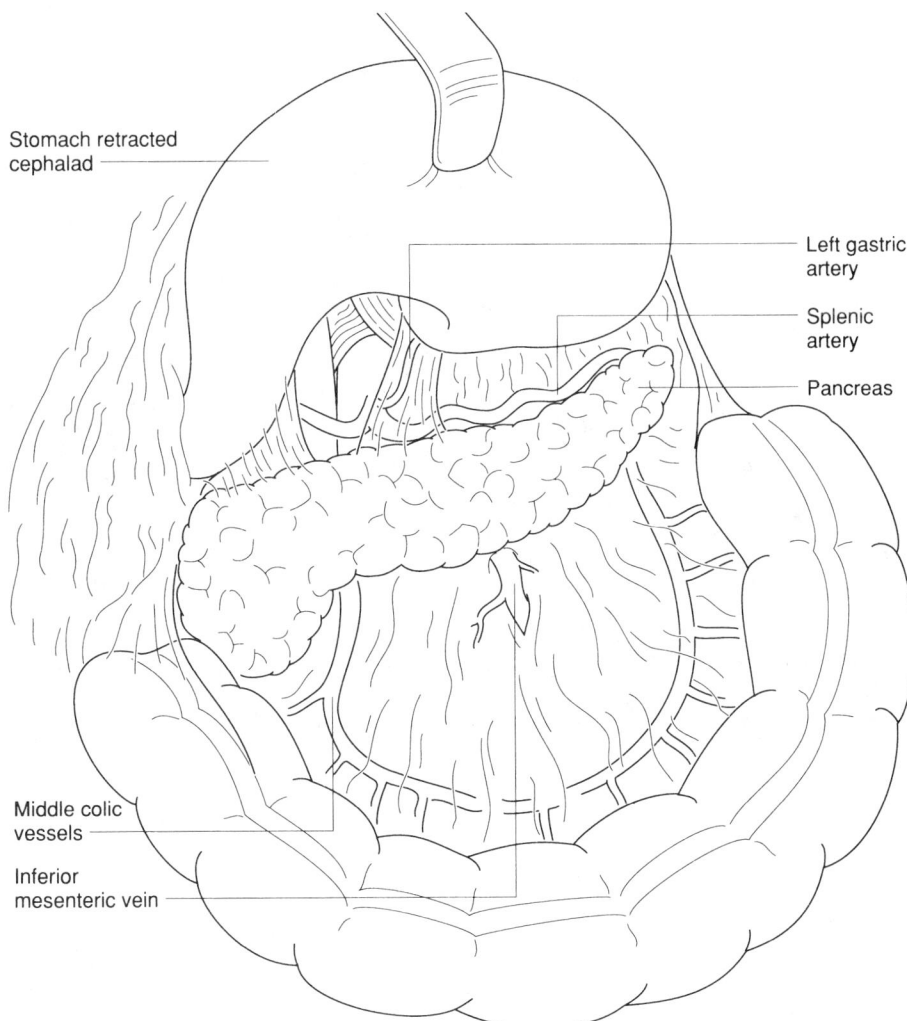

Figure 32-2. Exposure of the anterior surface of the pancreas through the lesser sac.

of patients experience long-term improvement in pancreatic pain.

Analgesics

Analgesics are the mainstay for nonsurgical treatment of pain in chronic pancreatitis. Nonnarcotic analgesics are used first. Eventually, most patients with chronic pancreatitis require narcotics.

Surgical Treatment

Intractable pain is the most frequent indication for surgical treatment of chronic pancreatitis. An operation is considered when pain is severe enough to interfere with the quality of life, to interfere with nutrition, or to cause narcotic addiction.

Pancreatojejunostomy. If the pancreatic ducts are dilated to >8 mm, ductal decompression with pancreatojejunostomy (Puestow procedure) is used for relief of pain (Figs. 32-2 through 32-4). This operation does not remove pancreatic tissue and does not cause diabetes or worsen exocrine deficits. However, neither does it improve malabsorption, although secretions empty freely through the pancreatojejunostomy into the small intestine. Fibrotic replacement of pancreatic tissue usually continues postoperatively, although an operation may slow this process.

Most patients experience complete or substantial improvement in pain soon after pancreatojejunostomy. Recurrent or

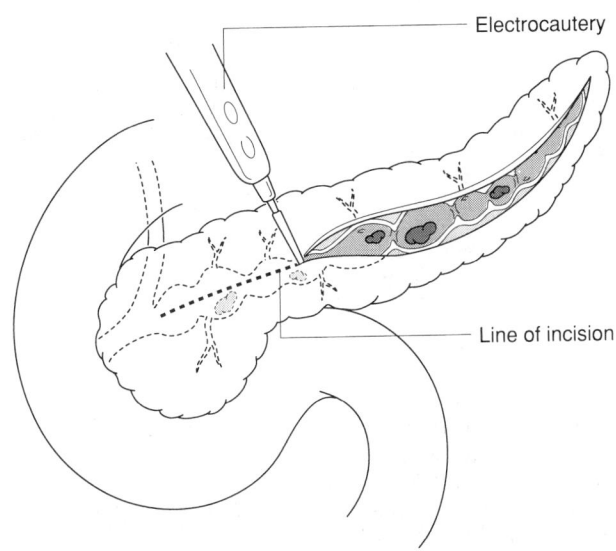

Figure 32-3. Longitudinal incision of the main pancreatic duct preparatory to performing lateral pancreaticojejunostomy.

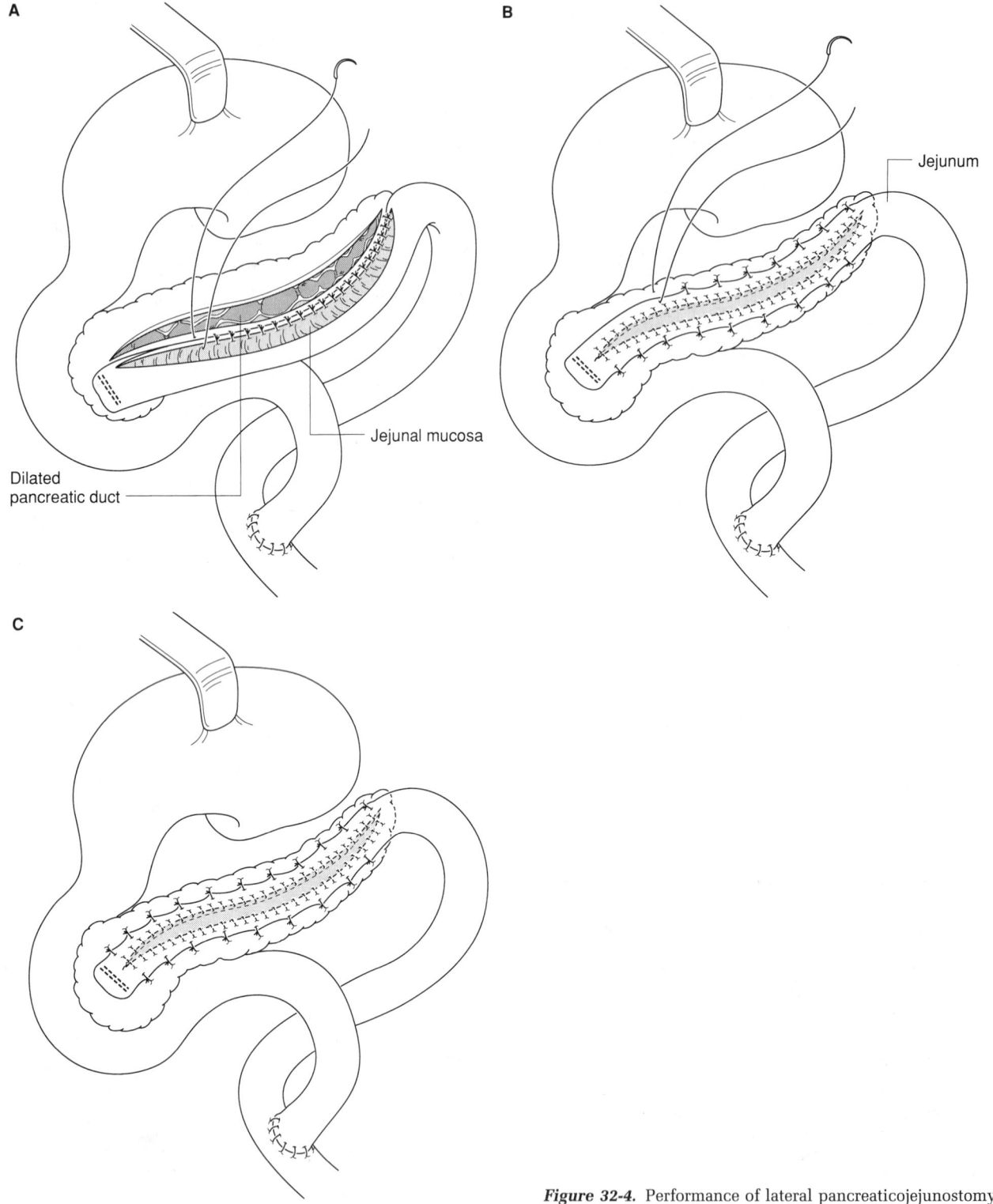

A

Dilated
pancreatic duct

Jejunal mucosa

B

Jejunum

C

Figure 32-4. Performance of lateral pancreaticojejunostomy.

persistent pain after pancreatojejunostomy requires reevaluation to exclude another disease, such as pancreatic carcinoma, peptic ulcer, calculous biliary disease, or bile duct stricture. If another disease is excluded, patency of the pancreatojejunal anastomosis must be assured with ERCP.

Pancreatic Resection. Pancreatic drainage is not feasible when pancreatic ducts are small or normal in diameter.

Pancreatic resection is considered when patients have small ducts, when the disease involves one portion of the gland and the rest of the gland is nearly normal, or after failed pancreatojejunostomy. The rationale for pancreatic resection is that pain and risk of complications are reduced with removal of the diseased portion of the gland.

Distal pancreatectomy may be performed when pathologic changes are confined to the tail or body of the pancreas. The proportion of pancreatic tissue resected is determined by the point of transection. For example, about half of the pancreatic mass is removed when the gland is divided at the level of the superior mesenteric vessels; a 95% pancreatectomy leaves only a thin rim of pancreatic tissue within the duodenal C loop (Fig. 32-5). Pancreatic resection always reduces the amount of residual functioning endocrine and exocrine tissue. Postoperative diabetes occurs with a frequency proportional to the degree of pancreatic resection and contributes substantially to late mortality after extended resection. Immediate pain relief occurs in most patients after distal pancreatectomy.

Resection of the pancreatic head by means of pancreatoduodenectomy (Whipple operation) is performed in some patients (Fig. 32-6). Indications for pancreatoduodenectomy are:

- A chronic inflammatory mass that involves primarily the head of the gland and the uncinate process
- A chronic inflammatory mass in the head of the pancreas associated with duodenal stenosis
- Multiple pseudocysts confined to the head of the pancreas
- Failure of pancreatojejunostomy due to inadequate drainage of the uncinate process.

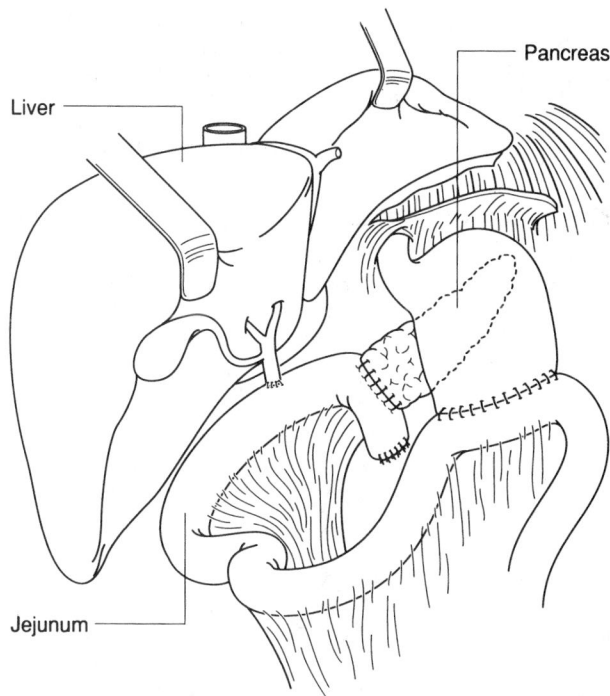

Figure 32-6. Reconstruction after standard pancreaticoduodenectomy.

A modified pancreatoduodenectomy with preservation of the gastric antrum and pylorus also can be performed (Fig. 32-7).

Malabsorption

Treatment of pancreatic insufficiency begins with the administration of sufficient enzyme tablets to abolish azotorrhea and to reduce steatorrhea to tolerable levels. This

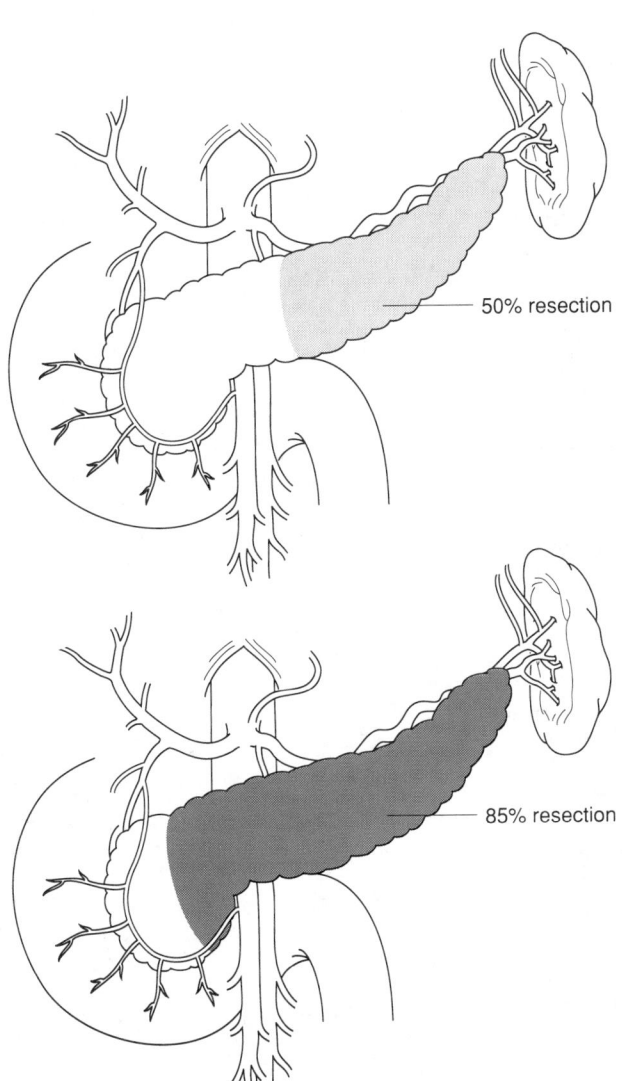

Figure 32-5. Points of parenchymal transection for 50% and 85% distal pancreatectomies.

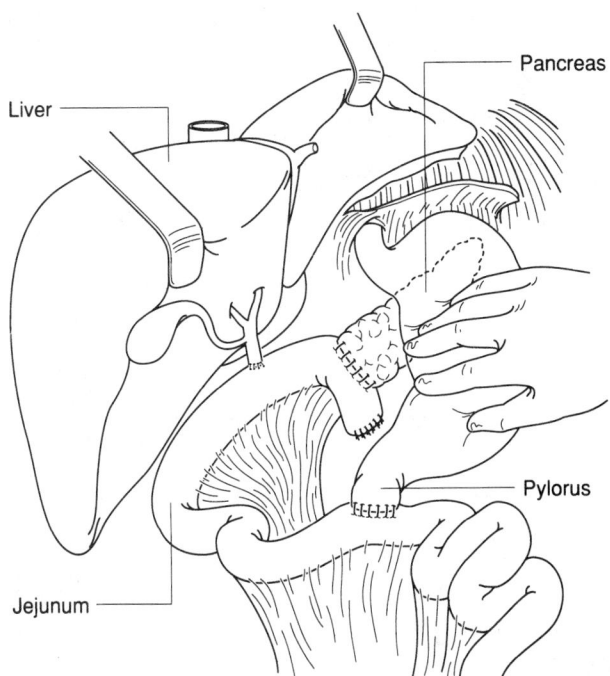

Figure 32-7. Reconstruction after pylorus-preserving pancreaticoduodenectomy.

often means ingestion of several tablets with each meal. If symptoms persist, the number of tablets is increased or the fat content of meals is decreased. H_2-receptor antagonists may be added for patients resistant to these measures. If steatorrhea persists, a search is performed for other contributing causes (bacterial overgrowth, ileal disease).

Biliary Complications

Complications that involve the common bile duct occur in chronic pancreatitis because of the association between the bile duct and the head of the pancreas. The fibrosis associated with chronic pancreatitis encases and compresses the common bile duct.

Common bile duct stenosis is a common complication. Cholangiography is performed by the transhepatic or retrograde endoscopic route. Because patients with chronic pancreatitis with common bile duct disease frequently require treatment of concurrent pancreatic disease, examination of both systems is best accomplished with ERCP. Bile duct fibrosis results in long, gradually tapering strictures that conform to the intrapancreatic duct. Malignant strictures usually result in abrupt termination of the biliary duct. The proximal suprapancreatic portion is variably dilated.

The most serious sequelae of unrelieved biliary obstruction are cholangitis and biliary cirrhosis. The degree of biliary obstruction at cholangiography does not correlate

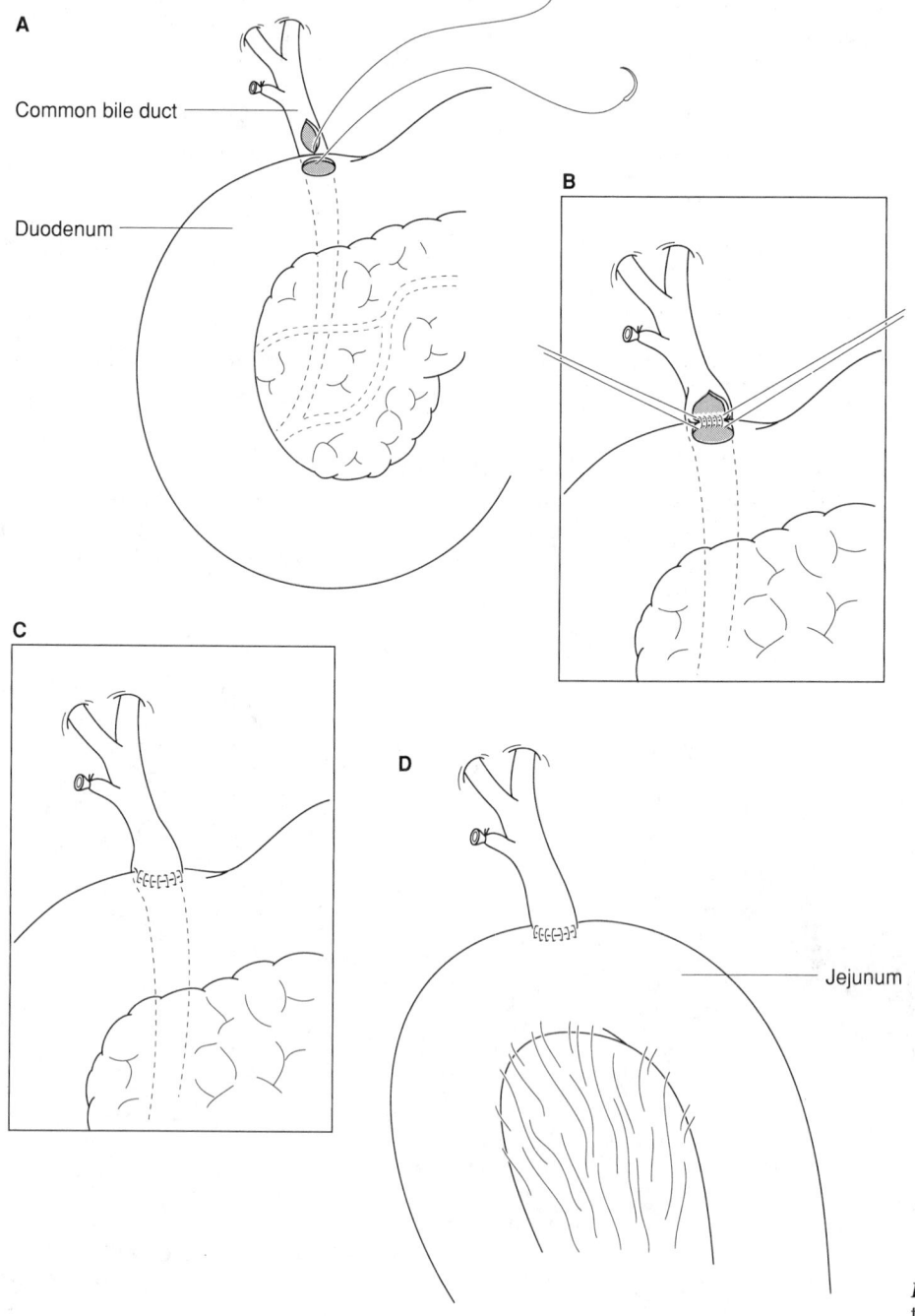

Figure 32-8. Operative construction of choledochoduodenostomy (*A* through *C*) and choledochojejunostomy (*D*).

with the severity of pancreatic disease, histologic findings in the liver, or biochemical abnormalities. Therapeutic decisions are based on clinical factors rather than radiologic criteria. Persistent elevation of serum alkaline phosphatase level is probably the best predictor of progressive biliary stenosis.

Patients with stricture of the common bile duct associated with chronic pancreatitis undergo surgical intervention for treatment of symptoms or prevention of biliary cirrhosis. Indications for surgical intervention are the following:

- Persistent jaundice
- Cholangitis
- Liver biopsy evidence of biliary cirrhosis
- Inability to exclude pancreatic cancer
- Progressive stricture supported by radiologic evidence of progressive dilatation of extrahepatic and intrahepatic bile ducts
- Persistent elevation of alkaline phosphatase at more than three times normal.

Intrapancreatic strictures of the common bile duct are treated with choledochoduodenostomy or choledochojejunostomy (Fig. 32-8). Complications of chronic pancreatitis include pancreatic pseudocyst, pancreatic ascites, and splenic vein thrombosis.

SUGGESTED READING

Cremer M, Deviere J, Delhaye M, et al. Stenting in severe chronic pancreatitis: results of medium-term follow-up in seventy-six patients. Endoscopy 1991;23:171.

Ebbohoj N, Borly L, Madsen P, Svendsen LB. Pancreatic tissue pressure and pain in chronic pancreatitis. Pancreas 1986; 1:556.

Folsch UR. Feedback regulation of pancreatic exocrine secretion in animals and man. Eur J Clin Invest 1990;20:S40.

Frey CF, Suzuki M, Isaji S. Treatment of chronic pancreatitis complicated by obstruction of the common bile duct or duodenum. World J Surg 1990;14:59.

Geenen JE, Rolny P. Endoscopic therapy of acute and chronic pancreatitis. Endoscopy 1991;37:377.

Huibregtse K, Schneider B, Vrij AA, Tytgat GN. Endoscopic pancreatic drainage in chronic pancreatitis. Gastrointest Endosc 1988;34:9.

Ihse I, Borch K, Larsson J. Chronic pancreatitis: results of operations for relief of pain. World J Surg 1990;14:53.

Levy P, Milan C, Pignon JP, et al. Mortality factors associated with chronic pancreatitis: unidimensional and multidimensional analysis of a medical–surgical series of 240 patients. Gastroenterology 1989;96:1165.

Nealon WH, Thompson JC. Progressive loss of pancreatic function in chronic pancreatitis is delayed by main pancreatic duct decompression: a longitudinal prospective analysis of the modified Puestow procedure. Ann Surg 1993;217:458.

Roberts IM. Enzyme therapy for malabsorption in exocrine pancreatic insufficiency. Pancreas 1989;4:496.

Sidhu SS, Tandon RK. The pathogenesis of chronic pancreatitis. Postgrad Med J 1995;71:67.

Steer ML, Waxman I, Freedman S. Chronic pancreatitis. N Engl J Med 1995;332:1482.

ESSENTIALS OF SURGERY: SCIENTIFIC PRINCIPLES AND PRACTICE, edited by Lazar J. Greenfield, Michael W. Mulholland, Keith T. Oldham, Gerald B. Zelenock, and Keith D. Lillemoe. Lippincott–Raven Publishers, Philadelphia, © 1997.

CHAPTER 33

NEOPLASMS OF THE EXOCRINE PANCREAS

RICHARD H. BELL, JR.

Ductal adenocarcinoma of the pancreas is the fifth most common cause of cancer death in the United States. It is, for the most part, recalcitrant to treatment.

EPIDEMIOLOGY AND ETIOLOGY

Adenocarcinoma of the pancreas most commonly develops in the seventh decade of life. The cause is not known. Possible etiologic environmental factors include:

- Cigarette smoking
- High consumption of dietary fat. This does not mean that fatty foods contain carcinogens; it is more likely that fats promote the effects of carcinogens derived from other sources
- Alcohol consumption does not appear to be a risk factor

Possible etiologic host factors include:

- Chronic pancreatitis
- Gastric resection
- Cholecystectomy, in women
- Family history, rare autosomal dominant syndromes. People with long-standing diabetes do not appear to be at increased risk for pancreatic cancer. In most patients, diabetes manifests at about the same time as the pancreatic neoplasm, and the onset of diabetes may be an early sign of pancreatic cancer.

PATHOLOGY

Although ductal epithelial cells are <5% of pancreatic mass, they appear to be the cell of origin of most pancreatic carcinomas (Table 33-1). The typical microscopic appearance of a ductal pancreatic tumor is large and small glands lined by cuboidal or columnar epithelium that produce variable amounts of mucin. The glands are embedded in a dense fibrous matrix, which is why the tumors are hard. The degree of differentiation of ductal carcinoma varies. Poorly differentiated tumors demonstrate less gland formation and mucus production and more epithelial anaplasia.

Most patients with pancreatic cancer have chronic obstructive pancreatitis with ductal dilatation, atrophy and fibrosis of the acinar parenchyma, and varying degrees of chronic lymphocytic infiltration. Some patients have histologic evidence of superimposed acute pancreatitis with a polymorphonuclear cell infiltrate. Pseudocysts are rare.

Ductal carcinoma of the pancreas probably begins with ductal hyperplasia followed by atypical hyperplasia, carcinoma in situ, and invasive carcinoma. Interpretation of preneoplastic changes in the pancreas is difficult because obstructive pancreatitis can lead to hyperplastic changes near carcinomas, and intraductal spread of carcinoma can mimic multifocal atypia.

Table 33-1. HISTOLOGIC CLASSIFICATION OF 645 CASES OF PRIMARY, NONENDOCRINE CANCER OF THE PANCREAS

Classification	Number
DUCT (DUCTULAR) CELL ORIGIN	572 (89%)
Duct cell adenocarcinoma	494
Giant cell carcinoma	27
Giant cell carcinoma (osteoid)	1
Adenosquamous carcinoma	20
Microadenocarcinoma	16
Mucinous (colloid) carcinoma	9
Cystadenocarcinoma (mucinous)	5
ACINAR CELL ORIGIN	8 (1%)
Acinar cell carcinoma	7
Cystadenocarcinoma (acinar cell)	1
UNCERTAIN HISTOGENESIS	61 (9%)
Pancreaticoblastoma	1
Papillary and cystic neoplasm	1
Mixed type—duct and islet cells	1
Unclassified	58
CONNECTIVE TISSUE ORIGIN	4 (1%)
TOTAL	645 (100%)

(Adapted from Cubilla AL, Fitzgerald PJ. Cancer [non-endocrine] of the pancreas: a suggested classification. In: Fitzgerald PJ. Morrison AB, eds. The pancreas. Baltimore, Williams & Wilkins, 1980:83)

Site of Ductal Adenocarcinoma

Sixty percent to 70% of pancreatic ductal adenocarcinomas occur in the head of the gland; about 15% occur in the body of the gland; 10% in the tail; and 5% to 15% are diffuse.

Local Extension

Extension beyond the pancreas is the rule rather than the exception in ductal carcinoma of the pancreas. The bile duct and the first or second portion of the duodenum are invaded early. Most pancreatic cancers involve early invasion of the retroperitoneum, either directly or along autonomic nerves of the celiac plexus. Perineural invasion is almost always present. In about one-half of patients, the walls of the portal or superior mesenteric veins are invaded; complete transmural invasion leads to thrombosis. Carcinoma of the body and tail may invade the splenic vein with thrombosis and gastric varices. Other sites of local invasion are the superior mesenteric and splenic arteries, transverse mesocolon, stomach, kidneys, and left adrenal gland.

Metastatic Disease

The common sites of metastatic spread of carcinoma of the pancreas are regional and juxtaregional lymph nodes and liver (Table 33-2). Lymphatic spread usually precedes hematogenous spread. Although lymph node involvement is not a contraindication to resection, the involved nodes must be included in the resection (Fig. 33-1).

Staging of Pancreatic Cancer

Table 33-3 shows a staging system oriented toward surgical resectability.

DIAGNOSIS

The vague early symptoms of pancreatic cancer are often minimized by both patient and physician, causing a delay in diagnosis. It is usually not until jaundice or extreme weight loss occurs that the diagnosis is made. By this time, the pancreatic tumor is large and has grown beyond the confines of the pancreas.

Clinical Symptoms and Signs

The presenting symptoms and signs of pancreatic cancer are listed in Tables 33-4 and 33-5.

Weight Loss

Average loss is 10 kg. Unexplained weight loss should prompt a search for a malignant tumor. In older adults, it is appropriate to perform computed tomography (CT) of the abdomen for this indication alone. Other digestive symptoms include nausea, vomiting, and constipation.

Jaundice

In people older than 60 years, the combination of jaundice and weight loss usually means carcinoma of the pancreas or periampullary region. The diagnosis requires imaging studies for confirmation. Jaundice is associated with dark urine and light stools. Pruritus sometimes is present.

When bilirubin levels are only minimally elevated, icterus may be confined to the sclera, but most patients have cutaneous changes by the time of presentation. Hepatomegaly usually reflects congestion due to biliary obstruction, and does not imply the presence of metastatic disease unless the liver is nodular or hard. The obstructed gallbladder is palpable in about one-fourth of patients with pancreatic cancer. In most patients, the tumor itself is not palpable.

Pain

Pain is usually perceived in the epigastrium but can occur in any part of the abdomen and may radiate to the back. In older adults, persistent, unexplained abdominal pain merits CT evaluation. Most patients with pancreatic cancer eventually experience moderate to severe pain, especially with tumors of the body and tail, probably because of invasion of the celiac plexus.

Table 33-2. SITES OF METASTASIS IN PANCREATIC CANCER

Site of Metastasis	Head (n = 106)	Body and Tail (n = 34)	Head, Body, and Tail (n = 24)
Regional lymph nodes	85	34	24
Juxtaregional lymph nodes	52	25	18
Liver	80	28	21
Stomach	15	7	13
Peritoneum	23	17	11
Lungs	28	8	7
Pleura	29	13	6
Pericardium	3	2	1
Colon	3	4	4
Spleen	6	11	4
Adrenal glands	15	9	5
Bones	13	5	3
Kidneys	9	7	6
Skin	1	1	2
No metastases	15	1	0

(Adapted from Kloppel G. Pancreatic, non-endocrine tumors. In: Kloppel G, Heitz PU, eds. Pancreatic pathology. New York, Churchill Livingstone, 1984:96)

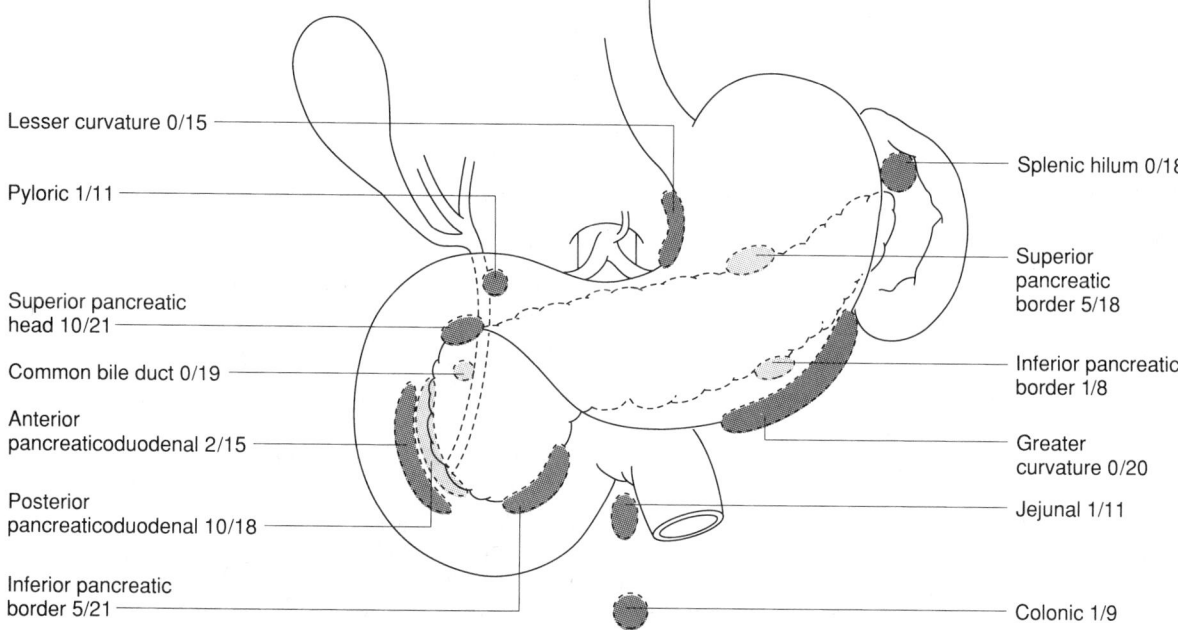

Figure 33-1. Lymph node involvement in duct cell carcinoma of the head of the pancreas in patients undergoing "curative" resection, most of whom were treated by total or regional pancreat-ectomy. The denominator indicates the number of patients in whom lymph nodes of that group were found, and the numerator indicates the number of patients in whom lymph nodes contained microscopically verified cancer. (After Cubilla AL, Fitzgerald PJ. Surgical pathology aspects of cancer of the ampulla-head-of-pancreas region. In: Fitzgerald PJ, Morrison AB, eds. The pancreas. Baltimore, Williams & Wilkins, 1980;72)

Table 33-3. TNM CLASSIFICATION FOR STAGING OF CANCER OF THE PANCREAS

TNM DEFINITIONS

Primary Tumor

T1 No direct extension of the primary tumor beyond the pancreas
T2 Limited direct extension (to duodenum, bile ducts, or stomach), still possibly permitting tumor resection
T3 Further direct extension, incompatible with surgical resection
TX Direct extension not assessed or not recorded

Regional Lymph Node Involvement

N0 Regional nodes not involved
N1 Regional nodes involved
NX Regional node involvement not assessed or not recorded

Distant Metastasis

M0 No distant metastasis
M1 Distant metastatic involvement
MX Distant metastatic involvement not assessed or not recorded

STAGE GROUPING

Stage I   T1, T2, N0, M0—No or limited direct extension to adjacent viscera, with no regional node extension and absence of distant metastases. Limited direct extension defined as involvement of organs adjacent to the pancreas that could be removed en bloc with the pancreas if a curative resection were attempted.
Stage II T3, N0, M0—Further direct extension of tumor into adjacent viscera, with no lymph node involvement and no distant metastases, which precluded surgical resection.
Stage III T1–3, N1, M0—Regional node metastases without clinical evidence of distant metastases.
Stage IV T1–3, N0–1, M1—Distant metastatic disease in liver or other sites.

(Adapted from Pollard HJ, et al. Staging of cancer of the pancreas. Cancer of the Pancreas Task Force. Cancer 1981;47:1631)

Other Signs

Ascites is present in some patients. With large tumors there may be gross or occult blood in the stool due to invasion of the duodenum, stomach, or colon.

Laboratory Investigation

Routine Tests

Routine laboratory determinations add little to the diagnosis of pancreatic cancer other than reinforcing the suspicion of extrahepatic biliary obstruction. The findings are as follows:

- Elevated bilirubin, particularly the conjugated fraction
- Elevated alkaline phosphatase
- Elevated transaminases
- Prolonged prothrombin time
- Mildly elevated serum amylase

Serum Markers

Considerable effort has been expended to find serum markers of pancreatic cancer. Mucins, CA 19-9, and the c-K-ras oncogene are being evaluated.

Diagnostic Imaging

Ultrasonography

Transcutaneous ultrasonography (US) is the first test in the evaluation of jaundice. The presence of a dilated common bile duct or intrahepatic bile ducts is diagnostic of extrahepatic biliary obstruction. This finding directs the physician to search for the cause of the obstruction. If the bile ducts are not dilated, mechanical obstruction is unlikely. US is also the best test to determine if gallstones

Table 33-4. SYMPTOMS OF PANCREATIC CANCER

Symptom	Patients (%)
HEAD	
Weight loss	92
Jaundice	82
Pain	72
Anorexia	64
Dark urine	63
Light stools	62
Nausea	45
Vomiting	37
Weakness	35
Pruritus	24
Diarrhea	18
Melena	12
Constipation	11
Fever	11
Hematemesis	8
BODY AND TAIL	
Weight loss	100
Pain	87
Weakness	43
Nausea	43
Vomiting	37
Anorexia	33
Constipation	27
Hematemesis	17
Melena	17
Jaundice	7
Fever	7
Diarrhea	3

(Adapted from Howard JM, Jordan GL Jr. Cancer of the pancreas. Curr Probl Cancer 1977;2:5)

are present. If US shows gallstones and no evidence of a pancreatic mass, the next step is endoscopic retrograde cholangiopancreatography (ERCP) to document common duct stones. If no gallbladder stones are detected with US, choledocholithiasis is unlikely, and a pancreatic or periampullary tumor or chronic pancreatitis is the likely cause of the obstruction. CT is the next examination. For patients who may have pancreatic cancer but do not have jaundice (ie, they have weight loss only), US is not appropriate, and CT is performed first.

Computed Tomography

CT is the single most useful diagnostic examination. It depicts the tumor mass and provides information about the extent of the tumor. CT scans may not depict tumors <2 cm. In such cases, the findings may be limited to pancreatic or bile duct dilatation. Such findings are highly suggestive of malignant pancreatic tumor and are further evaluated, ordinarily with ERCP. Dynamic CT, in which high-speed scans are obtained during rapid IV administration of iodinated contrast material, and three-dimensional reconstruction from spiral scans, provide information about vascular invasion.

Fine-needle Aspiration Biopsy With CT or US Guidance

A needle is passed into the pancreatic mass, and a cytologic examination is performed on aspirated cells. The technique is useful to differentiate chronic pancreatitis and pancreatic cancer and to provide a tissue diagnosis in patients with advanced disease who are not considered candidates for palliative or curative surgical therapy.

ERCP

ERCP is indicated to solve the following problems in the diagnosis of pancreatic cancer:

- There is CT evidence of bile duct or pancreatic duct obstruction but there is no mass
- Differentiation between chronic pancreatitis and pancreatic cancer is difficult
- Cholelithiasis and bile duct obstruction without a pancreatic mass are depicted with US

Findings at ERCP that suggest pancreatic cancer are as follows:

- Irregular narrowing of the pancreatic duct
- Displacement of the main pancreatic duct
- Destruction or displacement of side branches of the duct
- Pooling of contrast material in necrotic areas of tumor
- Irregular stenosis and proximal dilatation of the bile duct.

Chronic pancreatitis is characterized by multiple or long stenoses of the pancreatic duct. Pancreatic cancer causes abrupt focal interruption of the duct.

Upper Gastrointestinal Endoscopy

Upper GI endoscopy is used to find tumors of the ampulla of Vater or duodenum, which have a considerably better prognosis than pancreatic cancers. It may be possible to obtain a tissue diagnosis of pancreatic cancer if the duodenum is invaded. Upper GI endoscopy makes it possible to estimate the degree of duodenal obstruction in pancreatic cancer.

Endoscopic Ultrasonography

Endoscopic US appears to be more sensitive than transcutaneous US or CT in detection of tumors <2.5 cm in diameter. Pancreatic carcinomas appear as hypoechoic areas in the pancreatic substance. Endoscopic US is useful in the evaluation of vascular invasion.

CURATIVE TREATMENT
Surgical Therapy

Surgical resection is the only potentially curative therapy for pancreatic cancer. Unfortunately, few patients are actually cured of the disease. There have been some mildly encouraging improvements in surgical therapy for pancre-

Table 33-5. SIGNS OF PANCREATIC CANCER

Sign	Patients (%)
HEAD	
Jaundice	87
Palpable liver	83
Palpable gallbladder	29
Tenderness	26
Ascites	14
Abdominal mass	13
BODY AND TAIL	
Palpable liver	33
Tenderness	27
Abdominal mass	23
Ascites	20
Jaundice	13

(Adapted from Howard JM, Jordan GL Jr. Cancer of the pancreas. Curr Probl Cancer 1977;2:5)

atic cancer, and results may be improved by combining chemotherapy and radiation therapy with surgical therapy. Most resectable carcinomas of the pancreas are located in the head of the gland, probably because the onset of jaundice prompts diagnosis sooner than with tumors of the body or tail.

Pancreatoduodenectomy

The steps in pancreatoduodenectomy are as follows:

- Upper abdominal incision
- Inspection of the entire peritoneal cavity for evidence of metastatic disease, especially the liver, omentum, peritoneal surfaces, and subdiaphragmatic periaortic lymph nodes
- If findings are normal, mobilization of pancreas by reflecting hepatic flexure of the colon downward and mobilizing the head of the pancreas from the retroperitoneum
- Palpation for tumor, which is harder than the rest of the pancreas and surrounding tissues
- If the tumor mass can be palpated, fine-needle aspiration for cytologic examination
- While cytologic examination is being performed, opening of lesser sac through gastrocolic omentum
- Inspection of body and tail of the pancreas to determine extent of tumor involvement
- Examination of lymph nodes along the superior and inferior body of the pancreas and around the celiac axis
- Biopsy of enlarged nodes
- Frozen-section examination—extrapancreatic tumor is a contraindication to resection
- If there is no evidence of lymphadenopathy, dissection between anterior surface of the portal vein and posterior surface of the neck of the pancreas
- Establishment of communication, inferior to superior, behind the neck of the pancreas and the portal vein. The presence of hard tissue and an inability to establish a communication imply invasion of the anterior surface of the portal vein. The tumor is unresectable with conventional methods.
- If the anterior surface of the portal vein is free and the decision is to proceed with resection, division of the antrum of the stomach
- Division of right gastric and gastroduodenal arteries between ligatures
- Removal of gallbladder, division of common hepatic duct, and freeing of distal duct to the level of the upper edge of the duodenum
- Division of jejunum about 15 cm distal to the ligament of Treitz, in a location with sufficient mobility to allow the distal end of the jejunum to reach into the right-upper quadrant
- Incision of ligament of Treitz and division of mesentery of proximal jejunum
- Division of the neck of the pancreas over the portal vein
- Ligation and division of the branches of the portal vein that emanate from the head of the pancreas
- Dissection of the uncinate process from beneath the portal vein. The inferior pancreatoduodenal branch of the superior mesenteric artery supplies the uncinate process and is ligated in the course of this dissection.
- Removal of the resected specimen

Reconstruction, which requires three anastomoses:

1. The pancreatic remnant to the free end of the jejunum
2. The bile duct to the side of the jejunum
3. The stomach to the side of jejunum downstream from the other anastomoses.

Conventional pancreatoduodenectomy can be modified to allow preservation of the antrum and pylorus of the stomach. The proximal duodenum is transected just distal to the pylorus and is anastomosed end-to-side to the jejunum. After this operation, emptying of liquids and solids from the stomach seems to be better than after conventional pancreatoduodenectomy, and patients seem to regain weight more easily. A disadvantage of pylorus preservation is that return of gastric emptying in the immediately postoperative period seems to take longer than after the conventional operation.

Complications

- Disruption of the anastomosis
- Upper GI hemorrhage
- Marginal ulceration
- Biliary fistulas
- Delayed gastric emptying

Results. The results of conventional pancreatoduodenectomy are discouraging. Most known cures of pancreatic cancer have been achieved with pancreatoduodenectomy. However, relatively few patients who undergo pancreatoduodenectomy are alive and free of disease 5 years after the operation.

Causes of local failure:

- Inadequate tumor margins because of proximity to vital structures (portal vein, superior mesenteric artery)
- Failure to identify and resect regional lymphatic disease
- Unresected direct retroperitoneal extension
- Unrecognized extension of disease into the remaining pancreas

Causes of systemic failure

- Micrometastases unrecognized and untreated at operation
- Spread of recurrent locoregional disease

Extended Radical Pancreatectomy

Because of the high incidence of direct retroperitoneal invasion and regional lymph node metastasis, it has been argued that the scope of resection for pancreatic cancer be enlarged to include a radical regional lymphadenectomy and resection of areas of retroperitoneal invasion. The operation has the following features:

- Extension of the pancreatic resection from the neck to the middle of the body of the pancreas
- Segmental resection and re-anastomosis of the portal vein, if necessary, to achieve tumor-free margins
- Extensive lymphadenectomy to include the peripancreatic and celiac nodes
- Resection of retroperitoneal tissue, particularly in the right perinephric area and celiac plexus

Results. Results of extended radical pancreatectomy are inconsistent. They range from no improvement and a high operative morbidity and mortality to high 5-year survival rates and low operative mortality. Survival rates may improve with the combination of radical pancreatectomy and intraoperative radiation therapy.

Intraoperative Radiation Therapy

Intraoperative radiation therapy (IORT) allows a full therapeutic dose of radiation to be delivered directly to the operative bed at the time of surgical resection. The advantage is that therapy can be delivered to areas where tumor margins may be inadequate, to local lymphatics, and to areas where tumor cells may have been spilled during resection. Radiation doses to surrounding normal areas are minimized. The use of IORT as an adjuvant to surgical resection has been limited, and insufficient information exists to judge its value.

Postoperative or Preoperative Adjuvant Chemotherapy and Radiation Therapy

Postoperative

The use of 5-fluorouracil (5-FU) and external beam radiation therapy after resection appears to provide a therapeutic benefit. Patients experience leukopenia, mucositis, and diarrhea, but there are no life-threatening complications. Because of the efficacy and low toxicity, this therapy is advised for patients who undergo successful resection of ductal carcinoma of the pancreas.

Preoperative

For many patients, radiation therapy is delayed while they recover from their operations. The ability to palliate jaundice with endoscopic techniques has allowed patients with apparently resectable tumors to undergo preoperative treatment with 5-FU and radiation therapy, which nearly all patients are able to complete. Tumors are restaged after completion of the therapy. If no distant metastases are evident at restaging, laparotomy is performed. Preoperative chemoradiation therapy appears to be effective in preventing local recurrence, and increases median survival to about 2 years, results similar to those with postoperative adjuvant therapy.

PALLIATIVE TREATMENT OF PANCREATIC CARCINOMA

Palliative Treatment of Symptoms

Jaundice

If mild, jaundice may not require therapy. The natural progression in most patients is deepening jaundice with hepatocellular failure and coagulation abnormalities. Extrahepatic biliary obstruction contributes to anorexia and digestive symptoms. Pruritus is justification for relief of bile duct stasis. When patients undergo exploration for resection but unresectable disease is found, biliary bypass is routine. The jejunum rather than the duodenum is used as a conduit because duodenal obstruction may occur as the tumor advances.

Although endoscopic decompression of the bile duct can be performed in most patients, the stents are not as durable as a surgical bypass. Biliary sepsis and recurrent jaundice develop more often in patients with stents than in those who undergo surgical bypass; surgical bypass, however, has a high morbidity and mortality. Nonsurgical methods are best for patients with severe symptoms (eg, pruritus) but with advanced disease. Surgical bypass is reserved for patients with a life expectancy of at least 3 months.

Vomiting and Duodenal Obstruction

Duodenal invasion is present at the time of diagnosis in about one-fourth of patients with pancreatic cancer. About one-third of patients experience nausea and vomiting. Although it is not always possible to detect duodenal nar-

rowing, many patients have motor abnormalities of the duodenum caused by tumor involvement. The role of prophylactic gastroenterostomy is controversial. Gastroenterostomy at biliary bypass does not appear to add to overall operative mortality, and gastroenterostomy avoids a second operation. However, some patients experience prolonged delays in gastric emptying after gastroenterostomy, defeating the purpose of palliation.

Pain

Abdominal pain may be mild and manageable with oral medication, but most patients experience moderate to severe pain, probably due to invasion of retroperitoneal nerve trunks. Percutaneous chemical celiac plexus blockade in patients with advanced pancreatic cancer can relieve pain. The most common complication is transient orthostatic hypotension, which lasts a few days. Alcohol ablation of the celiac plexus during biliary and gastric bypass also effectively controls pain.

Palliative Antineoplastic Therapy

5-Fluorouracil and External Beam Radiation Therapy

The combination of 5-FU and external beam radiation therapy results in prolonged survival of patients with unresectable pancreatic cancer. Although the toxicity of the regimen is mild, a small percentage of patients have severe thrombocytopenia or leukopenia. Nausea and vomiting are common. Because of toxic side effects, it may be inappropriate to recommend therapy to patients with widespread and extensive metastatic disease.

Intraoperative Radiation Therapy

Most researchers evaluating IORT believe it has been effective in the amelioration of pain, but evidence suggests that IORT has little advantage over external beam therapy in terms of tumor control.

SUGGESTED READING

Brown DL, Bulley CK, Quiel EL. Neurolytic celiac plexus block for pancreatic cancer pain. Anesth Analg 1987;66:869.

Fortner JG. Regional pancreatectomy for cancer of the pancreas, ampulla, and other related sites: tumor staging and results. Ann Surg 1984;199:418.

Gudjonnson B. Cancer of the pancreas: 50 years of surgery. Cancer 1987;60:2284.

Ishikawa O, Ohhigashi H, Sasaki Y, et al. Practical usefulness of lymphatic and connective tissue clearance for the carcinoma of the pancreas head. Ann Surg 1988;208:215.

Johnstone PA, Sindelar WF. Patterns of disease recurrence following definitive therapy of adenocarcinoma of the pancreas using surgery and adjuvant radiotherapy: correlations of a clinical trial. Int J Radiat Oncol Biol Phys 1993;27:831.

Kalser MH, Ellenberg SS. Pancreatic cancer: adjuvant combined radiation and chemotherapy following curative resection. Arch Surg 1985;120:899.

Manabe T, Ohshio G, Baba N, et al. Radical pancreatectomy for ductal cell carcinoma of the head of the pancreas. Cancer 1989;64:1132.

Nitecki SS, Sarr MG, Colby TV, van Heerden JA. Long-term survival after resection for ductal adenocarcinoma of the pancreas. Ann Surg 1995;221:59.

Traverso LW, Longmire WP Jr. Preservation of the pylorus in pancreatoduodenectomy. Surg Gynecol Obstet 1978;146:959.

ESSENTIALS OF SURGERY: SCIENTIFIC PRINCIPLES AND PRACTICE,
edited by Lazar J. Greenfield, Michael W. Mulholland, Keith T. Oldham, Gerald B. Zelenock,
and Keith D. Lillemoe. Lippincott–Raven Publishers, Philadelphia, © 1997.

CHAPTER 34

NEOPLASMS OF THE ENDOCRINE PANCREAS

CHARLES J. YEO

Neoplasms of the endocrine pancreas are rare. The annual clinical incidence is five cases per one million person–years. According to autopsy reports, however, the prevalence is one per hundred autopsies.

Cells of the pancreatic islets are presumed to originate from neural crest cells. Cells of this origin are called *APUD cells,* indicating they have a high content of *a*mine, have the capacity for amine *p*recursor *u*ptake, and contain an amino acid *d*ecarboxylase. A generalized derangement of the APUD system may cause abnormalities of multiple endocrine cells, as in the multiple endocrine neoplasia (MEN) syndromes.

Neoplasms of the endocrine pancreas are functional or nonfunctional. *Functional* tumors elaborate one or more hormonal products into the blood, leading to a recognizable clinical syndrome. most pancreatic endocrine neoplasms are functional (Table 34-1). *Nonfunctional* endocrine tumors of the pancreas are associated with normal serum hormone levels and have no recognizable clinical syndrome.

Histologic findings do not predict the biologic behavior or the endocrine manifestations of these neoplasms. Immunofluorescence techniques and the peroxidase–antiperoxidase test allow demonstration of specific hormones within neoplastic cells. Malignancy is identified on the basis of presence of local invasion, spread to regional lymph nodes, or existence of hepatic or distant metastases.

Three principles apply to the diagnosis of functional neoplasms of the endocrine pancreas:

1. Recognition of the abnormal physiologic condition or characteristic syndrome
2. Detection of hormone elevations in serum with radioimmunoassay
3. Localization and staging of the tumor in preparation for possible surgical intervention.

LOCALIZATION AND STAGING
Diagnostic Imaging
Computed Tomography

The initial imaging technique for localization of a pancreatic endocrine neoplasm is dynamic abdominal CT with IV and oral administration of contrast material. CT also is used to detect peripancreatic lymph node enlargement and the presence of hepatic metastases.

Angiography

If CT does not depict the primary tumor, visceral angiography is performed that focuses on the arterial supply to the pancreas and peripancreatic region.

Endoscopic Ultrasonography

Endoscopic ultrasonography (US) is more sensitive than the combination of CT and visceral angiography.

Somatostatin Receptor Imaging

Whole-body radionuclide scanning with iodine-labeled tyrosine^3-octreotide or indium-labeled pentetreotide, an octreotide analog, relies on the presence of somatostatin receptors on many islet cell tumors. These modalities are used to identify primary tumors and hepatic and extrahepatic metastases.

Selective Transhepatic Portal Venous Hormone Sampling

Selective transhepatic portal venous hormone sampling is an invasive technique that demonstrates an increase in hormone concentration where the tumor drains its hormonal product into the portal venous system. The results of sampling are used to define the region of the pancreas (or duodenum with gastrinoma) that harbors the occult tumor.

Selective Arterial Secretin Stimulation Test

This test combines selective arterial injection of secretin with hepatic venous sampling for gastrin. It takes advantage of the biology of gastrinoma in that gastrinoma cells respond to secretin with the release of gastrin. Secretin is administered by means of serial injection through an arterial catheter into at least three sites: the splenic, gastroduodenal, and inferior pancreatoduodenal arteries. Samples are drawn from a hepatic vein catheter before and immediately after the injections. The arterial supply to the occult

Table 34-1. **CLASSIFICATION OF FUNCTIONAL PANCREATIC ENDOCRINE TUMORS**

Tumor (Syndrome)	Clinical Features	Extrapancreatic Location	Malignancy Rate
Insulinoma	Hypoglycemia	Rare	10%
Gastrinoma (Zollinger-Ellison)	Peptic ulcer Diarrhea	Frequent	50%
VIPoma (Verner-Morrison; watery diarrhea, hypokalemia, achlorhydria or hypochloride; pancreatic cholera)	Watery diarrhea Hypokalemia Achlorhydria	10%	Most
Glucagonoma	Hyperglycemia Dermatitis	Rare	Most
Somatostatinoma	Hyperglycemia Steatorrhea Gallstones	Rare	Most

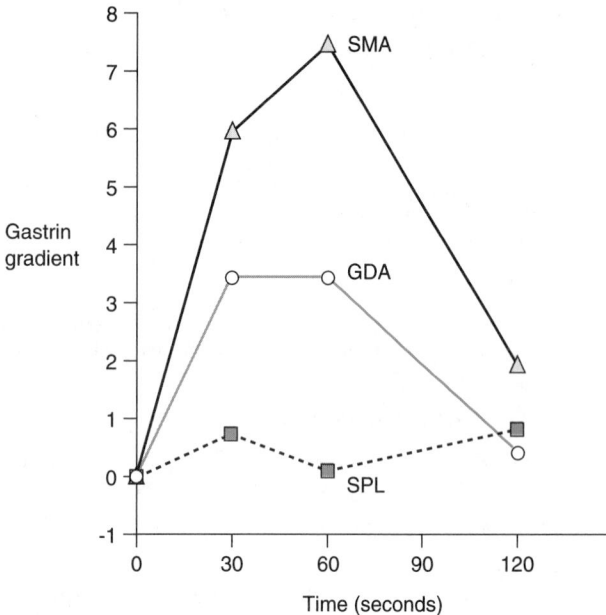

Figure 34-1. Graphic depiction of the results of a selective arterial secretin stimulation test in a patient with gastrinoma. The Y axis plots the rise in hepatic vein gastrin concentration (gastrin gradient) compared with basal values plotted on the X axis: 1 = 100% rise; 2 = 200% rise; and so forth. A rise in the hepatic vein gastrin concentration is observed following superior mesenteric artery (SMA) and gastroduodenal artery (GDA) secretin injections, localizing the neoplasm to the head of the pancreas or duodenum. SPL, splenic artery. (After Thom AK, Norton JA, Doppman JL, et al. Prospective study of the use of intraarterial secretin injection and portal venous sampling to localize duodenal gastrinomas. Surgery 1992;112:1002)

gastrinoma is determined on the basis of which selective secretin injection is followed by an increase in hepatic vein gastrin concentration (Fig. 34-1). The results localize the region of the gastrinoma—the duodenum and head of the pancreas or the body or tail of the pancreas.

SURGICAL EXPLORATION

The goals of surgical therapy for pancreatic endocrine neoplasms are: (1) control of symptoms caused by hormone excess; (2) resection of maximal tumor mass; and (3) preservation of maximal pancreatic parenchyma.

Surgical exploration proceeds as follows:

- Exposure of the body and tail of the pancreas with division of the gastrocolic ligament
- Elevation of the body and tail out of the retroperitoneum with division of the inferior retroperitoneal attachments
- Elevation of the second portion of the duodenum out of the retroperitoneum with a Kocher maneuver
- Bimanual palpation of the pancreatic head and uncinate process
- Assessment of the liver for evidence of metastatic disease
- Evaluation of possible extrapancreatic sites of tumor—duodenum, splenic hilum, small intestine and its mesentery, peripancreatic lymph nodes, and reproductive tract in women

Real-time US can assist in tumor identification.

TYPES OF TUMORS

Insulinoma

Insulinoma is the most common neoplasm of the endocrine pancreas. It is associated with the Whipple triad:

1. Symptoms of hypoglycemia during fasting
2. Hypoglycemia with serum glucose <50 mg/dL
3. Relief of hypoglycemic symptoms after administration of exogenous glucose.

Autonomous insulin secretion from the tumor causes the hypoglycemia of insulinoma (Table 34-2).

A common mistake made in the diagnosis of insulinoma is to begin with an oral glucose tolerance test. Instead, insulinoma is most reliably diagnosed with a monitored-fast study. Additional support for the diagnosis of insulinoma comes from calculation of the insulin-to-glucose ratio (I:G ratio) at different times during the monitored fast. Healthy people have I:G ratios <0.3, whereas patients with insulinoma have I:G ratios >0.4 after a prolonged fast.

The possibility of surreptitious administration of insulin or oral hypoglycemic agents must be considered in the diagnosis of insulinoma. C peptide and proinsulin levels are not elevated in patients who self-administer insulin. Patients who self-administer bovine or porcine insulin may have anti-insulin antibodies in the blood. The presence of oral hypoglycemic agents is assessed with conventional toxicologic screening.

After the diagnosis of insulinoma is confirmed with biochemical analysis, localization and staging studies are performed—abdominal CT, endoscopic US, and visceral angiography.

The treatment of insulinoma is surgical. Almost all patients have benign solitary adenomas. The few patients with MEN-1 may have multiple insulinomas. In about 10% of patients, insulinoma is metastatic to peripancreatic lymph nodes or the liver.

During surgical exploration, the pancreas is assessed with operative palpation and intraoperative real-time US, to allow evaluation of the entire pancreas and a search for the site of the primary tumor. Small, benign insulinomas not close to the main pancreatic duct may be removed with enucleation, regardless of location within the gland (Fig. 34-2). Insulinomas in the body and tail of the pancreas, those >2 cm in diameter, and those close to the pancreatic duct are excised with distal pancreatectomy. Large insulinomas deep in the head or uncinate process may not be amenable to local excision, and may require pancreatoduodenectomy.

Some patients may undergo exploration for insulinoma without preoperative tumor localization, and no tumor is identified with visualization, palpation, or real-time US. This situation presents a management problem. The fa-

Table 34-2. INSULINOMA

Parameter	Description
Symptoms	
Neuroglycopenia causes	Confusion, personality change, coma
Catecholamine surge causes	Trembling, diaphoresis, tachycardia
Diagnostic tests	Monitored fast
	Insulin/glucose ratio
	C-peptide and proinsulin blood levels
Anatomic localization	Evenly distributed throughout pancreas

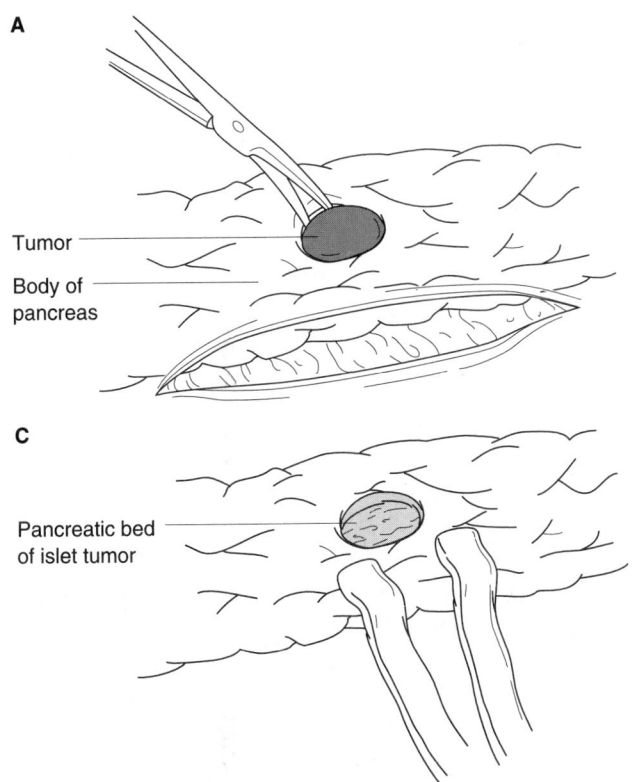

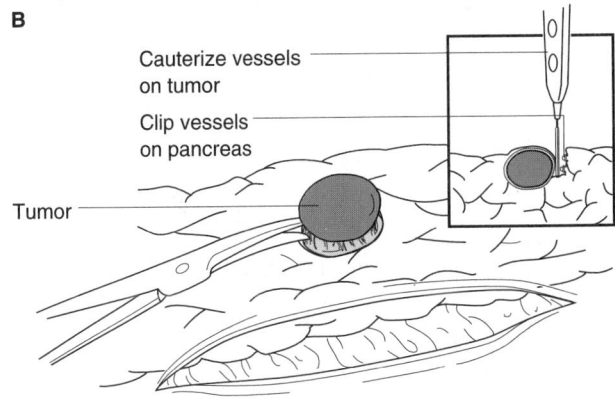

Figure 34-2. The technique used for enucleation of a benign pancreatic endocrine neoplasm, using the scissors (*A*) or electrocautery (*B*). (*C*) After enucleation, the site of neoplasm excision is drained. (After Cameron JL. Atlas of surgery, vol 1. Philadelphia, BC Decker/Mosby–Year Book, 1990:441)

vored option is to defer blind resection and perform postoperative selective transhepatic portal venous insulin sampling to allow tumor localization and directed surgical excision at a second operation.

About 10% of insulinomas are malignant, usually with evidence of lymph node or hepatic metastases. Resection of the primary tumor and accessible metastases reduces hypoglycemic symptoms, which can threaten long-term survival. In patients with unresectable insulinoma, dietary therapy that includes judicious spacing of carbohydrate-rich meals and night-time snacks may help minimize hypoglycemic episodes. Medications such as diazoxide and octreotide are used to inhibit insulin release and raise serum glucose level. Chemotherapeutic agents that have some efficacy against malignant insulinoma include streptozocin, dacarbazine (DTIC), doxorubicin, and 5-fluorouracil (5-FU). The highest response rates to chemotherapy occur with combination therapy.

Gastrinoma (Zollinger–Ellison Syndrome)

Zollinger–Ellison syndrome is the association between severe peptic ulcer disease and pancreatic endocrine tumors. Seventy-five percent of gastrinomas occur sporadi-

cally, whereas 25% are associated with MEN-1. The presenting clinical symptoms of gastrinoma are a direct result of circulating hypergastrinemia (Table 34-3).

Laboratory Diagnosis

Serum gastrin measurement is used to screen for gastrinoma (Table 34-4). In most patients with gastrinoma, the fasting serum gastrin level is elevated to more than 200 pg/mL. Gastrin values >1000 pg/mL are virtually diagnostic of gastrinoma, particularly when they are accompanied by hyperchlorhydria or well-established ulcer disease. However, fasting hypergastrinemia alone is not sufficient for the diagnosis of gastrinoma, because hypergastrinemia can exist in other pathophysiologic states.

Gastric acid analysis is important in the diagnosis of gastrinoma. It can differentiate ulcerogenic (high gastric acid) hypergastrinemia and nonulcerogenic (low gastric acid) hypergastrinemia. For accurate gastric acid analysis,

Table 34-3. GASTRINOMA

Parameter	Description
Symptoms	Peptic ulcer disease Diarrhea Esophagitis
Diagnostic tests	Serum gastrin measurement Gastric acid analysis Secretin stimulation test
Anatomic localization	Duodenum and head of pancreas (gastrinoma triangle)

Table 34-4. DISEASE STATES ASSOCIATED WITH HYPERGASTRINEMIA

NONULCEROGENIC CAUSES (NORMAL TO LOW ACID SECRETION)
Atrophic gastritis
Pernicious anemia
Previous vagotomy
Renal failure
Short-gut syndrome

ULCEROGENIC CAUSES (EXCESS ACID SECRETION)
Antral G-cell hyperplasia or hyperfunction
Gastric outlet obstruction
Retained excluded antrum
Zollinger-Ellison syndrome

patients must stop taking antisecretory medications, such as histamine H_2 antagonists or omeprazole. The diagnosis of gastrinoma is made with a basal acid output (BAO) >15 mEq/h in patients who have never had an operation, a BAO >5 mEq/h in patients with previous vagotomy or antiulcer operation, or a basal-to-maximal acid output ratio (BAO/MAO) >0.6.

After documentation that hypergastrinemia is associated with excessive acid secretion, provocative testing with secretin is performed to differentiate gastrinoma, antral G cell hyperplasia or hyperfunction, and other causes of ulcerogenic hypergastrinemia. The secretin stimulation test is performed after the patient has fasted. An increase in gastrin level to >200 pg/mL above basal level supports the diagnosis of gastrinoma (Fig 34-3).

Management

After biochemical confirmation of the diagnosis of gastrinoma, management is as follows:

1. Gastric acid hypersecretion is controlled with omeprazole.
2. After initiation of omeprazole therapy, imaging studies are performed to localize the primary tumor and assess for metastatic disease.

If the localization and staging studies indicate *unresectable hepatic metastases,* percutaneous or laparoscopically directed liver biopsy is performed for histologic verification. If unresectable gastrinoma is confirmed, open surgical exploration is not performed, and the patient undergoes long-term omeprazole therapy. Almost all patients are rendered achlorrhydric with appropriate doses of omeprazole. Patients who do not take appropriate doses of omeprazole and who have complications related to ulcer diathesis may need total gastrectomy, which removes the parietal cell mass.

In most patients, *unresectable disease is not identified* at staging studies, and patients undergo surgical exploration with curative intent. The entire abdomen is assessed for areas of extrapancreatic and extraduodenal gastrinoma. Most gastrinomas are located to the right of the superior mesenteric vessels (Fig. 34-4) within the head of the pancreas or the duodenum—the gastrinoma triangle. Intraoperative US assists in tumor localization. Intraoperative upper GI endoscopy may be helpful because it allows transillumination of the duodenal wall and identification of small duodenal gastrinomas. Any suspicious peripancreatic lymph nodes are excised, and a frozen-section histologic examination is performed. Primary tumors within the substance of the pancreas <2 cm in diameter and well encapsulated may be enucleated. Pancreatic tumors without defined capsules or situated deep in the pancreatic parenchyma may require partial pancreatic resection—either distal pancreatectomy or pancreatoduodenectomy.

If there is *no identifiable pancreatic or duodenal tumor,* a longitudinal duodenotomy may be performed at the level of the second portion of the duodenum to allow eversion of the duodenum in a search for duodenal microgastrinomas. Primary gastrinomas within the duodenal wall are resected locally, with primary closure of the duodenal defect. In a small percentage of patients, gastrinoma may be found only in peripancreatic lymph nodes. Resection of these apparent lymph-node primary gastrinomas is associated with long-term eugastrinemia and biochemical cure in as many as 50% of patients.

If localization studies, such as portal venous gastrin sampling or the selective arterial secretin stimulation test, identify the tumor as within the *gastrinoma triangle, but no tumor is found at laparotomy,* the surgical options are as follows:

1. Parietal cell vagotomy to reduce dosages of antisecretory drugs. It is not well established that this operation decreases dose requirements. The operation also leaves behind potentially resectable gastrinoma.
2. Total gastrectomy. Omeprazole has drastically reduced the need for total gastrectomy. The operation is sometimes performed on patients whose tumors cannot be localized or if the patient will not take adequate doses of omeprazole. Total gastrectomy leaves the primary tumor behind, with the potential for subsequent tumor growth and metastases.
3. Blind pancreatoduodenectomy. This operation is performed on patients with clear-cut biochemical documentation of hypergastrinemia, hyperchlorhydria, and tumor localization within the gastrinoma trian-

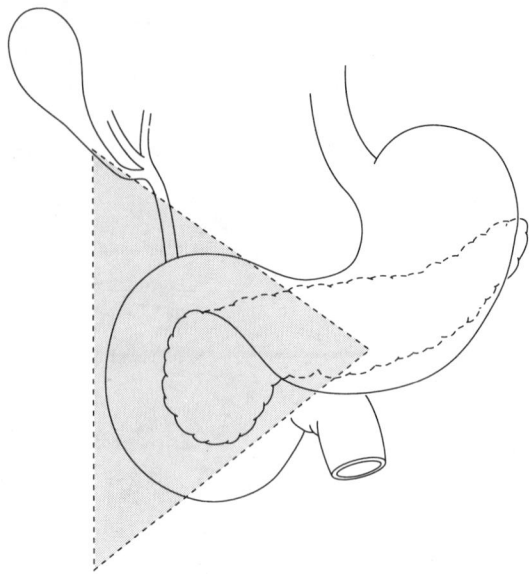

Figure 34-4. Most gastrinomas are found within the gastrinoma triangle. (After Stabile BE, Morrow DJ, Passaro E. The gastrinoma triangle: operative implications. Am J Surg 1984;147:26)

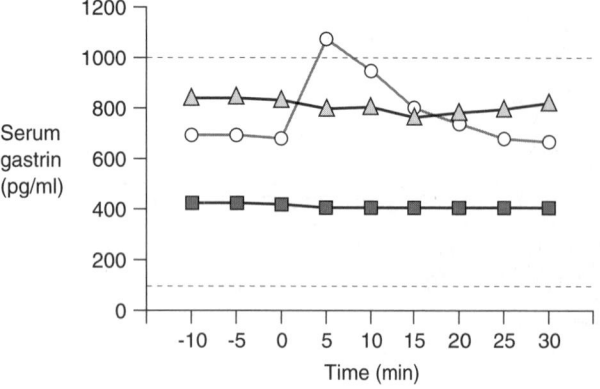

Figure 34-3. Results of intravenous secretin stimulation tests in patients with atrophic gastritis (*triangles*), gastric outlet obstruction (*squares*), and gastrinoma (*circles*). A positive test, consistent with the presence of gastrinoma, is indicated by an increase over basal serum gastrin levels of at least 200 pg/mL. (After Wolfe MM, Jensen RT. Zollinger-Ellison syndrome: current concepts in diagnosis and management. N Engl J Med 1987;317:1200)

Table 34-5. VERNER-MORRISON SYNDROME: DIFFERENTIAL DIAGNOSIS

Entity	Workup
Villous adenoma	Lower GI endoscopy
Laxative abuse	Stool examination for phenolphthalein
Celiac disease	Fecal fat measurement
	D-Xylose tolerance test
	Small bowel biopsy
Parasitic and infectious diseases	Stool culture
	Ovum and parasite analysis
	Clostridium difficile toxin assay
Inflammatory bowel disease	Lower GI endoscopy
	Upper GI and small bowel series
Carcinoid syndrome	Urinary 5'-HIAA
	Upper GI and small bowel series
	Abdominal CT scan
	Serum serotonin measurement
Gastrinoma	Serum gastrin measurement
	Gastric acid analysis
	Secretin stimulation test

gle. In a small number of patients, such blind resections have yielded pathologically verified primary gastrinomas within the duodenal wall or the head of the pancreas that were not apparent at laparotomy. Conventional pancreatoduodenectomy is performed because duodenal gastrinomas may originate close to the pylorus and be left behind with pylorus-sparing pancreatoduodenectomy. A small number of patients are rendered eugastrinemic with blind resection.

The following modalities are used to treat metastatic gastrinoma (none has improved the survival rate):

- Chemotherapy
- Hormonal therapy with octreotide
- Aggressive resection and palliative debulking of metastatic gastrinoma
- Hepatic transplantation, hepatic artery embolization, and interferon therapy for gastrinoma metastatic to the liver

Management of *gastrinoma associated with MEN-1* is difficult. Omeprazole is used to control gastric acid hypersecretion. Surgical treatment of hypercalcemia due to parathyroid hyperplasia precedes any surgical treatment of hypergastrinemia. MEN-1 gastrinoma involves multiple pancreatic or duodenal neoplasms, and preoperative and intraoperative localization techniques are needed to guide resection. In some patients, hypergastrinemia associated with MEN-1 gastrinoma is corrected with surgical resection.

VIPoma

The active agent in VIPoma is vasoactive intestinal polypeptide (VIP). VIPoma is also called Verner–Morrison syndrome, WDHA syndrome (watery diarrhea, hypokalemia, and either achlorhydria or hypochlorhydria), and pancreatic cholera syndrome. Symptoms and signs are summarized in Table 34-5. The diagnosis of VIPoma is made after other more common causes of diarrhea are excluded. Some patients have elevations of other mediators, such as peptide histidine–isoleucine (PHI) or prostaglandins. Because VIP secretion may be episodic in patients with VIPoma, several fasting VIP levels are measured—one low VIP level does not rule out the syndrome.

After elevated VIP levels are documented, tumor local-

Table 34-6. GLUCAGONOMA

Parameter	Description
Symptoms	Dermatitis manifested as necrolytic migratory erythema
	Stomatitis
	Weight loss
Diagnostic tests	Hyperglycemia
	Hypoproteinemia
	Serum glucagon measurement
	Serum amino acid profile
Anatomic localization	Most in body or tail of pancrreas

ization and staging begin with dynamic abdominal CT with IV and oral contrast enhancement. Because 10% of patients with VIPoma may have extrapancreatic tumors in the retroperitoneum or thorax, thoracic CT is indicated if abdominal CT does not depict a tumor. Visceral angiography and portal venous hormone sampling are not necessary in most patients.

Preparation for surgical exploration includes correction of fluid and electrolyte losses with vigorous IV fluid and electrolyte replacement. Parenteral administration of octreotide reduces circulating VIP levels, decreasing the volume of diarrhea.

Surgical excision of VIPoma is appropriate in all patients. Most VIPomas occur in the distal pancreas, where they are amenable to resection with distal pancreatectomy. If no tumor is found in the pancreas, exploration of the retroperitoneum is performed to include both adrenal glands. Metastatic disease to lymph nodes and the liver occurs in 50% of patients. In the presence of metastatic disease, palliative debulking is indicated.

In patients with recurrent or unresectable VIPoma, octreotide therapy reduces circulating VIP levels and controls diarrhea. Some patients have had partial responses to streptozocin, combination chemotherapy, and interferon.

Glucagonoma

The findings in patients with glucagonoma are summarized in Table 34-6. The cardinal finding is severe dermatitis. The diagnosis is suggested by clinical presentation and biopsy of the skin lesions. It is secured with documentation of elevated fasting levels of serum glucagon.

After biochemical documentation of hyperglucagonemia, localization and staging are performed with dynamic contrast-enhanced abdominal CT. Because the tumors are usually large and solitary, CT localizes the tumor in most patients.

Before surgical exploration, malnutrition must be managed. Total parenteral nutrition (TPN) is used to improve

Table 34-7. SOMATOSTATINOMA

Parameter	Description
Symptoms	Steatorrhea
	Right upper quadrant pain
Diagnostic tests	Hyperglycemia
	Hypochlorhydria
	Gallstones
	Serum somatostatin level
Anatomic localization	Most in head or uncinate process of pancreas

Table 34-8. RARE FUNCTIONAL PANCREATIC ENDOCRINE NEOPLASMS

Tumor	Hormone/Candidate	Features
Calcitoninoma	Calcitonin	Secretory diarrhea
Parathyrinoma	PTH-related protein	Hypercalcemia
		Bone pain
		Normal serum PTH
GRFoma	Growth hormone releasing factor	Acromegaly
ACTHoma	Adrenocorticotropic hormone	Cushing syndrome
Neurotensinoma	Neurotensin	Tachycardia
		Hypotension
		Malabsorption

PTH, parathyroid hormone.

the catabolic state caused by hyperglucagonemia, reverse malnutrition, and improve the dermatitis. Octreotide reduces circulating glucagon levels and improves response to TPN.

Most glucagonomas occur in the body and tail of the pancreas. Because these tumors are large and bulky, surgical resection is performed with distal pancreatectomy. Metastases are found in most patients, and debulking of the lesions is considered.

Patients with incurable or recurrent glucagonoma have low response rates to chemotherapeutic agents, such as streptozocin and dacarbazine. Octreotide reduces elevated glucagon levels and controls the hyperglycemia and dermatitis associated with incurable glucagonoma.

Somatostatinoma

The clinical features of the somatostatinoma syndrome are summarized in Table 34-7. A high fasting plasma somatostatin level confirms the diagnosis. Most somatostatinomas occur in the head of the pancreas and periampullary region. The most useful study for localization and staging is abdominal CT.

Preoperative management of somatostatinoma is treatment of hyperglycemia and malnutrition. Resection for cure is not common because most patients have metastatic disease. Resection of the primary tumor and debulking of hepatic metastases are indicated. Cholecystectomy is indicated, even in the absence of documented gallstones, because of concern about the development of cholelithiasis with persistently elevated somatostatin levels.

Nonfunctional Islet Cell Tumors

Approximately one-third of patients with neoplasms of the endocrine pancreas have no defined clinical syndrome, and serum insulin, gastrin, VIP, glucagon and somatostatin levels are not elevated. These patients are considered to have nonfunctional endocrine neoplasms (Table 34-8). The

one hormone that may be elevated in the serum is pancreatic polypeptide (PP). PP appears to be a marker for some pancreatic endocrine tumors without being the mediator of any specific PP-related clinical syndrome.

Nonfunctional endocrine neoplasms present with clinical manifestations, such as abdominal pain, weight loss, and jaundice, which result from space-occupying lesions in the pancreas. These clinical manifestations are similar to those of ductal adenocarcinoma of the exocrine pancreas. Nonfunctional tumors may occur in the head, neck, or uncinate process of the pancreas. The malignancy rate is 50% to 90%. Nonfunctional tumors grow in a more indolent way than ductal adenocarcinoma, and are associated with longer survival periods.

Localization and staging studies are similar to those for ductal adenocarcinoma. Abdominal CT is used for evaluation of the primary tumor and to assess for hepatic metastases. Preoperative cholangiography may be indicated for jaundice.

Most nonfunctional neoplasms are >2 cm in diameter and cannot be excised. Tumors in the head, neck, or uncinate process are resected with pancreatoduodenectomy. Tumors that originate in the body or tail are treated with distal pancreatectomy. Patients with unresectable tumors in the head of the pancreas undergo surgical palliation of obstructive jaundice and gastric outlet obstruction with bilioenteric and gastroenteric bypass, respectively. Some patients with unresectable disease may respond to combination chemotherapy.

SUGGESTED READING

Chiarugi M, Pucciarelli M, Goletti O, et al. Outcome of surgical treatment for extrapancreatic gastrinomas. Surg Gynecol Obstet 1993;177:153.

Farley DR, van Heerden JA, Grant CS, Thompson GB. Extrapancreatic gastrinomas: surgical experience. Arch Surg 1994;129:506.

Fedorak IJ, Ko TC, Gordon D, Flisak M, Prinz RA. Localization of islet cell tumors of the pancreas: a review of current techniques. Surgery 1993;113:242.

Fraker DL, Norton JA, Alexander HR, et al. Surgery in Zollinger-Ellison syndrome alters the natural history of gastrinoma. Ann Surg 1994;220:320.

Menegaux F, Schmitt G, Mercadier M, Chigott JP. Pancreatic insulinomas. Am J Surg 1993;165:243.

Modlin IM, Lewis JJ, Ahlman H, et al. Management of unresectable malignant endocrine tumors of the pancreas. Surg Gynecol Obstet 1993;176:507.

Sugg SL, Norton JA, Fraker DL, et al. A prospective study of intraoperative methods to diagnose and resect duodenal gastrinomas. Ann Surg 1993;218:138.

Udelsman R, Yeo CJ, Hruban RH, et al. Pancreaticoduodenectomy for selected pancreatic endocrine tumors. Surg Gynecol Obstet 1993;177:269.

White TJ, Edney JA, Thompson JS, et al. Is there a prognostic difference between functional and nonfunctional islet cell tumors? Am J Surg 1994;168:627.

LIVER AND PORTAL VENOUS SYSTEM

ESSENTIALS OF SURGERY: SCIENTIFIC PRINCIPLES AND PRACTICE,
edited by Lazar J. Greenfield, Michael W. Mulholland, Keith T. Oldham, Gerald B. Zelenock,
and Keith D. Lillemoe. Lippincott–Raven Publishers, Philadelphia, © 1997.

CHAPTER 35

HEPATOBILIARY ANATOMY

DAVID R. BYRD

Several anatomic features pose obstacles to operations on the liver:

- The liver is prone to fracture and bleeding with manipulation
- A dual efferent blood supply is intertwined with delicate afferent biliary ducts in a crowded hepatic hilum
- The three hepatic veins empty directly into the inferior vena cava posterior to the liver and are obscured unless extensive retrohepatic dissection is performed

TOPOGRAPHIC ANATOMY AND RELATIONSHIPS TO PERIHEPATIC STRUCTURES

The liver occupies the right upper quadrant of the abdomen. It extends vertically on the right side from the undersurface of the right hemidiaphragm to the anterior costal margin. It extends horizontally on the left midclavicular line at the superior pole of the spleen.

The anterior surface of the liver is covered by peritoneum that extends to the anterior abdominal wall in the midline from the ligamentum teres, or round ligament (the obliterated umbilical vessels), and the falciform ligament, an obliquely oriented fusion of peritoneum. In the posterior aspect of the liver, the investing peritoneum is contiguous with the peritoneum of the diaphragm at the coronary and triangular attachments, leaving a rhomboid retroperitoneal area not covered by peritoneum (Fig. 35-1). The Glisson capsule is a thin, fibrous covering that envelopes the entire liver deep to the peritoneum and sends thin fibrous septa into the hepatic parenchyma.

The liver can be surgically separated from adjacent organs and structures through division of areolar tissue planes. Neoplasms or inflammatory conditions of the liver or surrounding structures may obliterate these tissue planes. In the superior and anterior aspects, the diaphragm or abdominal wall may be invaded by cancer or abscess. In the posterior aspect, neoplasms of the right adrenal gland or superior pole of the right kidney may adhere to the right hepatic lobe. In the inferior aspect, the gallbladder, duodenum, hepatic flexure of the colon, or periportal lymph nodes may be inseparable from the liver edge. On the left side, cancer of the stomach or gastroesophageal junction may invade the left hepatic lobe.

MORPHOLOGIC AND FUNCTIONAL ANATOMY

The original morphologic division of the liver into right and left lobes separated by the falciform ligament has been replaced with functional division into eight segments,

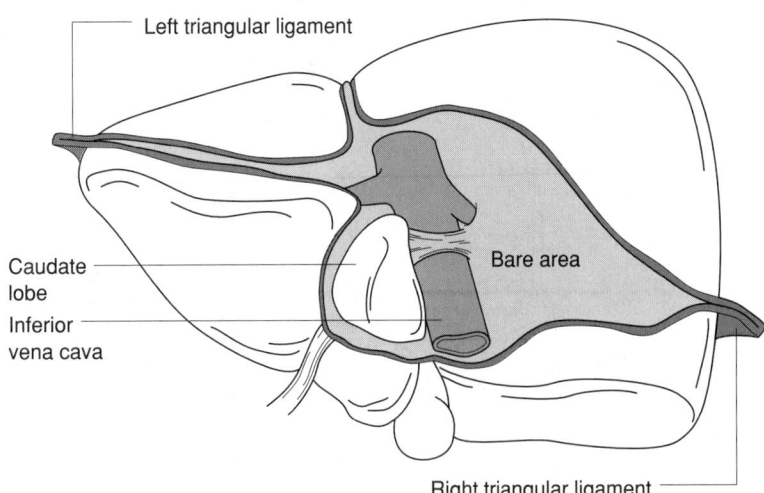

Figure 35-1. Posterior view of liver, showing the level of peritoneal reflections.

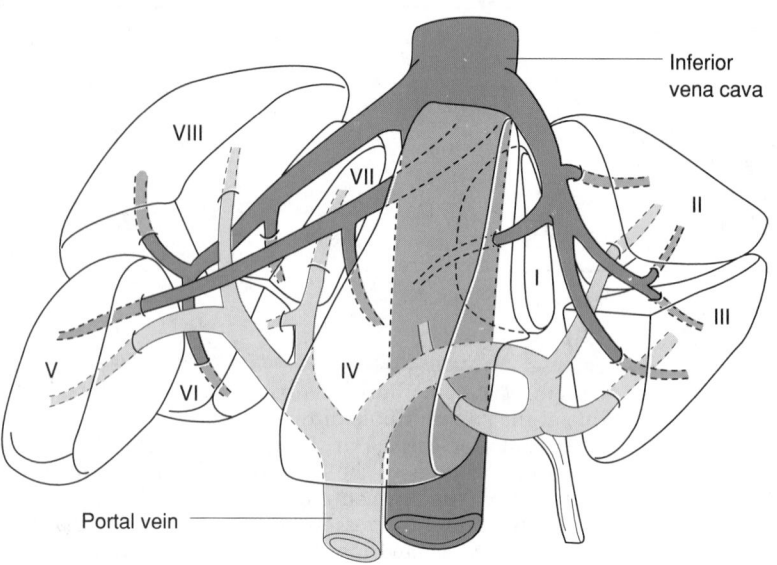

Figure 35-2. Functional division of the liver and the liver segments according to Couinaud's nomenclature.

based on hepatic venous drainage and portal pedicles (branches of the hepatic artery, portal vein, and bile duct; Fig. 35-2).

Enumeration of the segments begins left to right, beginning with segment I, the caudate lobe. The left lateral sector (lobe) consists of a superior segment II and an inferior segment III (left lateral segment in old terminology). The left vertical incisura separates the left lateral sector from segment IV, which comprises a superior segment IVa and an inferior segment IVb (quadrate lobe or medial segment of the left lobe). The main incisura separates the right and left lobes. The right vertical incisura divides the right lobe into an anteromedial sector and a posterolateral sector. The anteromedial sector comprises inferior segment V and a superior segment VIII. The posterolateral sector comprises inferior segment VI and superior segment VII.

THE HEPATIC VEINS

Three major hepatic veins carry blood from the central veins of the hepatic substance to the inferior vena cava (IVC). The left hepatic vein drains segments II, III, and IV.

The middle hepatic vein drains a portion of segment IV and anterior segments V and VIII. The right hepatic vein drains posterior segments VI and VII and a portion of the anterior segments.

Branches of the hepatic veins drain obliquely from inferior to superior and posterior within the hepatic parenchyma. In two-thirds of people, a single large right hepatic vein joins the right anterior wall of the IVC and a middle and left hepatic vein converge 1–2 cm from the IVC and enter the left anterior wall of the IVC as a single vessel adjacent to the confluence of the right hepatic vein and IVC (Fig. 35-3). In one-third of people, each major hepatic vein joins the IVC as a separate trunk at the same horizontal level. In some people, one or more of the hepatic veins has a short extraparenchymal segment at the confluence with the IVC. More frequently, the entire length of the hepatic veins is intraparenchymal, which may preclude early, safe hepatic venous isolation during hepatic resection. These veins have a fragile, thin wall, and surgical injury may cause rapid hemorrhage, that is difficult to isolate and control.

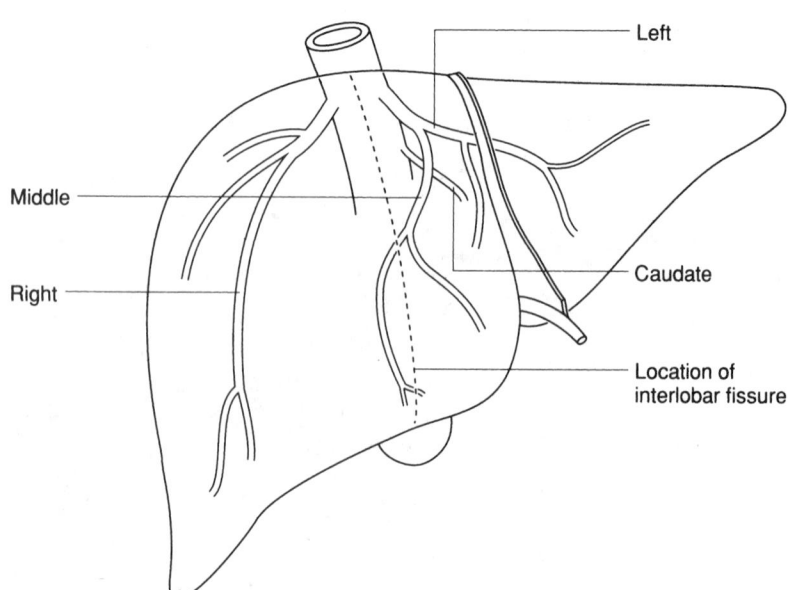

Figure 35-3. Three major hepatic veins drain the liver. The caudate segment of the liver usually drains directly into the inferior vena cava.

Venous drainage of the caudate lobe is through multiple short posterior veins, which empty directly into the IVC. Several posterior accessory veins drain the medial aspect of the right lobe and empty directly into the right anterior surface of the IVC. Identification of these accessory veins is essential during right hepatic lobectomy, caudate lobe resection, and right adrenalectomy.

HEPATIC PORTAL SYSTEM

The origin of the main hepatic portal vein is posterior to the neck of the pancreas at the confluence of the superior mesenteric and splenic veins. Here the portal vein receives the pyloric and coronary veins. The portal vein then courses cephalad and slightly obliquely to form the posterior-most structure within the hepatoduodenal ligament (portal triad), which is invested by leaves of the lesser omentum.

The hepatic hilum posterior to the hepatic duct and hepatic arterial bifurcation contains an extrahepatic portal bifurcation into a short oblique right portal vein and a longer and more transverse left portal vein (Fig. 35-4). These branches become intraparenchymal and invested with the bile duct and hepatic arterial branches by extensions of the Glisson capsule. One or two small posterior branches originate from both the right and left portal veins, providing a dual blood supply to the caudate lobe. The left portal vein courses anteriorly in the pars umbilicus to give off a medial branch or branches to segment IV (quadrate lobe) and lateral branches to the left lateral sector.

The left portal vein subdivides into a superior branch to segment II and an inferior branch to segment III. The right portal vein branches within 1 to 2 cm of the main portal bifurcation into an anterior division, which sends an inferior branch to segment V and a superior branch to segment VIII, and a posterior division, which sends an inferior branch to segment VI and a superior branch to segment VII.

THE HEPATIC ARTERIES

There is considerable variability in the origin and course of the right and left hepatic arteries. The most common finding is a transverse common hepatic artery from the celiac trunk, which gives off the gastroduodenal, right gastric, and supraduodenal arteries and courses obliquely in

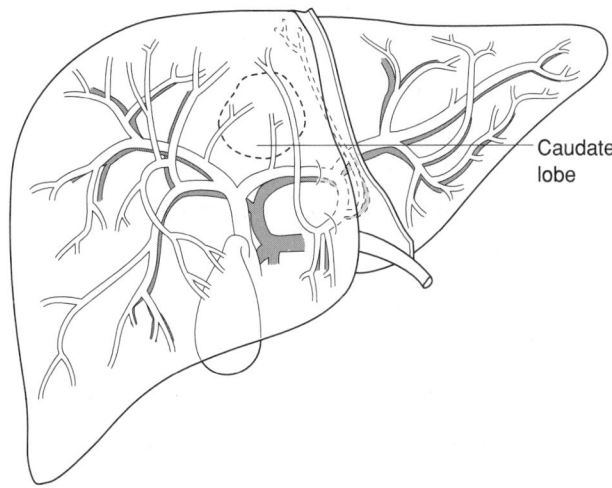

Figure 35-5. Intrahepatic divisions of bile ducts and hepatic arteries. Arterial and ductal supplies to liver parenchyma run in parallel.

the left anterior aspect of the hepatoduodenal ligament as the proper hepatic artery. Distal to the point at which the cystic artery branches to the gallbladder, there is a fairly low trifurcation into single right, middle, and left hepatic arteries. Within the hepatic parenchyma, the hepatic arterial branches course closely with bile duct branches and fairly closely with portal venous branches, invested by the Glisson capsule, to supply portal pedicle branches to each hepatic segment (Fig. 35-5).

Knowledge of the variations in the hepatic arteries (Table 35-1) is important because unintentional division may occur during gastric, pancreatic, and hepatobiliary procedures. One variation is that the middle hepatic artery originates from either the right or left hepatic artery distal to a bifurcation of the proper hepatic artery. This pattern is found 55% of the time. In another variation, a replaced or accessory left hepatic artery originates from the left gastric artery and courses transversely in the lesser omentum. With nearly equal frequency, a replaced or accessory right hepatic artery from the superior mesenteric artery near its origin may course posteriorly or through the head of the pancreas and obliquely along the right posterior border of the hepatoduodenal ligament.

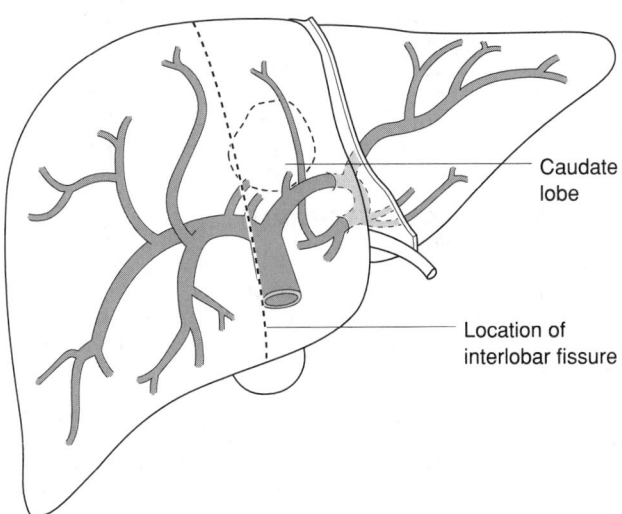

Figure 35-4. Intrahepatic divisions of the portal vein.

Table 35-1. HEPATIC ARTERIAL VARIATIONS

Variation (order in which arteries originate from proper hepatic artery)	Frequency (%)
Right, left middle	55
Right, middle replaced left (off left gastric)	10
Left, middle replaced right (off superior mesenteric)	11
Middle, replaced right and left	1
Right, left, middle, accessory left	8
Right, left, middle, accessory right	7
Right, left, middle, accessory right and left	2
Combined replaced right, accessory left or replaced left, accessory right	2
No celiac trunk, common hepatic origin off superior mesenteric	2
No celiac trunk, common hepatic origin off left gastric	0.5

(From Michels NA. Newer anatomy of the liver and its variant blood supply and collateral circulation. Am J Surg 1966;112:337).

IMAGING EVALUATION OF HEPATIC ANATOMY

Ultrasonography

US is used to:

- Identify lesions within the hepatic parenchyma
- Describe the consistency and homogeneity of the liver (fatty or cirrhotic)
- Identify dilatation of the biliary tree and the presence of abnormalities or stones within the gallbladder

At intraoperative US probes with horizontal or vertical orientation and different depths of resolution are placed directly on the surface of the liver. Beginning superiorly at the IVC, the confluence and course of each of the hepatic veins is delineated. More inferiorly, the main right and left portal pedicles course transversely in the transverse incisura. The left portal pedicle courses anteriorly as the pars umbilicus in the ligamentum teres. Portal and hepatic veins are easily differentiated because of the hyperechoic extensions of the Glisson capsule that surround the portal veins. Flattening of a circular mass with external compression with a US probe differentiates a blood vessel and a solid mass.

Computed Tomography

Not all of the abdomen and pelvis can be imaged with US. Some intra-abdominal regions are distorted because of the presence of air in the stomach, small intestine, or colon. CT is used to screen for hepatic and other abdominal or retroperitoneal lesions.

Resolution of hepatic lesions is enhanced with the combination of visceral angiography and CT, known as CT arterioportography (CTAP). Most primary or secondary hepatic lesions are supplied by branches of the hepatic artery. CT performed immediately after injection of contrast material into the common hepatic artery (CT arteriography) may depict small hepatic lesions, which usually show increased attenuation relative to the surrounding hepatic parenchyma. CT portography involves direct injection of contrast material into the splenic or superior mesenteric arteries and CT during the portal venous phase of injection. Hepatic lesions supplied by the hepatic artery appear as discrete lesions of low attenuation, surrounded by normal hepatic parenchyma, enhanced with portal venous contrast material. Depiction of anatomic relations between hepatic lesions and portal structures aids in preoperative planning and determination of the feasibility of surgical resection.

Double helical (spiral) CT allows total hepatic imaging in both the arterial and arteriovenous phases after one rapid IV bolus injection of contrast material during one breath hold. It is possible to visualize the portal structures and hepatic veins on one scan that provides high resolution of small hepatic lesions. Three-dimensional reconstructions in different planes can be used to delineate hepatic parenchyma and arteries.

Magnetic Resonance Imaging

Magnetic resonance imaging (MRI) of the liver has results similar to those of CT, but the results are not good enough to justify the increased cost of employing this modality. MRI does not provide optimal images of the intestine or retroperitoneum.

Positron Emission Tomography

Total body imaging with positron emission tomography (PET) increases resolution of primary and secondary hepatic tumors by taking advantage of the fact that glucose has an increased metabolism in neoplasms. With IV injection of radiolabeled glucose before scanning, areas of increased uptake are depicted in the liver and areas outside the liver, such as the primary tumor basin, regional nodes, or distant sites, such as the lung.

HEPATIC RESECTION

Preoperative Evaluation of Hepatic Reserve

Liver function tests that measure synthetic ability (albumin and prothrombin time), bile excretory function (total bilirubin and alkaline phosphatase), and prognostic scores (Child–Pugh score) are helpful only in determining the presence of hepatic dysfunction before surgical intervention. More sophisticated dynamic tests include the following, but none of these techniques is universally accepted or reliable:

- Measurement of hepatic perfusion by the clearance of galactose or organic anionic dyes, such as indocyanine green and sulfobromophthalein
- Tests of microsomal function, such as the aminopyrine breath test, caffeine clearance, or lidocaine clearance
- Measurement of mitochondrial oxidative metabolism of the liver with the ketone body ratio or redox tolerance index

The guidelines for hepatic resection are as follows:

- In a liver without evidence of hepatitis or cirrhosis, resection of 75% to 80% of liver volume is safe.
- In a cirrhotic liver, wedge resection or segmental resection may be safe under some circumstances.
- Full lobar resection in a cirrhotic liver is performed only in special circumstances and by experienced hepatic surgeons.

Correlation of CT Findings With Segmental Anatomy

Preoperative CT is used to determine the location of hepatic lesions and to estimate the extent of resection needed to remove all disease. One can define each sector of the liver by noting the location and course of the major hepatic veins that separate each sector. Segments within each sector are identified on the basis of superior or inferior location, relative to the main portal structures within the transverse incisura. Some lesions may straddle two or more segments, and bisegmentectomy may be feasible.

Oncologic Considerations in Hepatic Resection

The goals of surgical management of primary or secondary neoplasms of the liver must be delineated before any attempt at resection. The following questions must be answered:

- What is the diagnosis?
- What is the biology of the tumor in this patient?
- Is the goal of resection curative or palliative?
- Has other distant disease been excluded with a reasonable number of preoperative tests?
- What is the comorbid status of the patient?

• What other treatments are effective, and what is the optimal sequence of these treatments?

Intraoperative Assessment

The incision most commonly used for hepatic resection is an extended right subcostal incision with vertical or intercostal extension, if necessary. A generous vertical incision is sometimes used for left-sided resection; a right thoracoabdominal incision may be used for right-sided resection. A self-retaining costal-margin retractor provides access to the entire subdiaphragmatic surface, and may be combined with self-retaining ringed retractors to keep the stomach, colon, and small intestine from the operative field.

Complete mobilization of the liver may be required for major resection and for intraoperative US. After detachment of the hepatic flexure of the colon and ligation and division of the falciform ligament, the left and right triangular ligaments are sharply divided to fully mobilize the liver. During division of the left triangular ligament, care must be taken to avoid injury to the spleen, the left phrenic vein, the left hepatic vein, and the IVC. During division of the right triangular ligament, care must be taken to avoid injury to the right hemidiaphragm, the right adrenal gland and adrenal vein, the right phrenic vein, several moderate-sized accessory right hepatic veins that drain into the right lateral wall of the IVC, the main right hepatic vein, and the IVC. After mobilization, digital and bimanual palpation and intraoperative US are performed.

Two of the three vertical incisurae usually can be identified: the left lateral incisura courses immediately to the left of the umbilical fissure, and the main incisura courses from the gallbladder fossa anteriorly to the IVC posteriorly. The right vertical incisura is not reliably identified on the basis of external landmarks. It begins at the anterior border of the liver halfway between the right angle of the liver and the right side of the gallbladder bed and courses vertically three finger-breadths anterior and parallel to the right lateral edge of the liver.

The porta hepatis is dissected to allow identification of the main bifurcations of the hepatic artery, bile duct, and portal vein. This allows ligation of unilateral branches of each of these structures during hepatic lobectomy but before parenchymal dissection. Ligation delineates the surface line of devascularization and eliminates the portal contribution of blood loss during parenchymal dissection. This technique requires tedious dissection, which may take a considerable amount of time to complete. An alternative is to leave the main portal structures undisturbed and ligate branches to a given lobe during parenchymal transection. Hemorrhage can be minimized with intermittent portal inflow occlusion by means of clamping or compression of the portal triad (Pringle maneuver). Greater exposure of the superior aspect of the hepatic hilum and exposure of a high or intraparenchymal bifurcation of a portal structure may be aided with exposure of the hilar plate (Fig. 35-6) and transverse division of the Glisson capsule at the inferior-most border of segment IV (the quadrate lobe).

There has been considerable debate over early versus late isolation and ligation of a given hepatic vein during lobectomy because the extraparenchymal component of the hepatic vein may be short or absent. Because hemorrhage in this location may be difficult to expose and control, a safe strategy is to avoid early isolation of a hepatic vein or attempt isolation only if a considerable length of vein is found when the triangular ligament is mobilized.

Major Lobectomy

Major lobectomy or hemihepatectomy includes segments V, VI, VII, and VIII (right hepatic lobectomy) or resection of segments II, III, and IV (left hepatic lobectomy). Extended resection of each major lobe includes segments IV (right trisegmentectomy) through VIII, or segments II, III, IV, and anterior segments V and VIII (left trisegmentectomy). The caudate lobe may be included in major resection, but care must be taken to preserve portal pedicle branches to this lobe if it is to be saved. A cholecystectomy is included in all hepatic resections.

The steps in all major resections are similar. They adhere to the principles of optimal operative exposure and control of vascular inflow and outflow. In some operations, the vena cava must be controlled. The infrahepatic vena cava is encircled superior to the junction of the renal veins. The

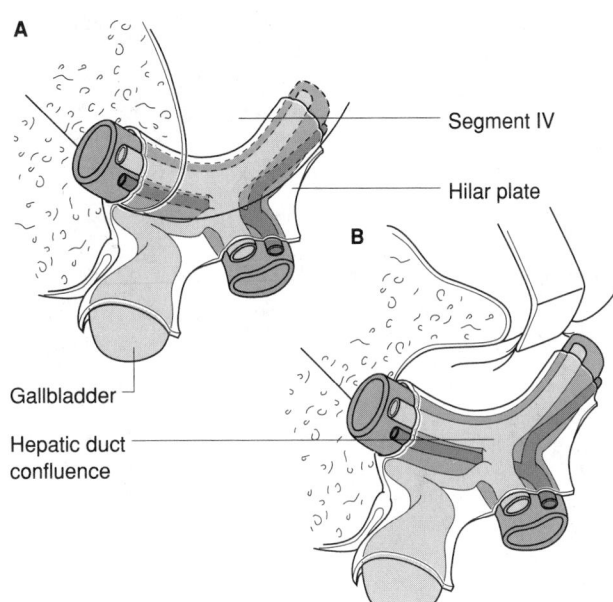

Figure 35-6. (*A*) Relation between the posterior aspect of the quadrate lobe and the biliary confluence. The connective tissue surrounding the bile ducts and vascular structures fuses with the Glisson capsule to form the hilar plate. (*B*) The biliary duct confluence and left hepatic duct can be exposed by incising the Glisson capsule and retracting the quadrate lobe upward.

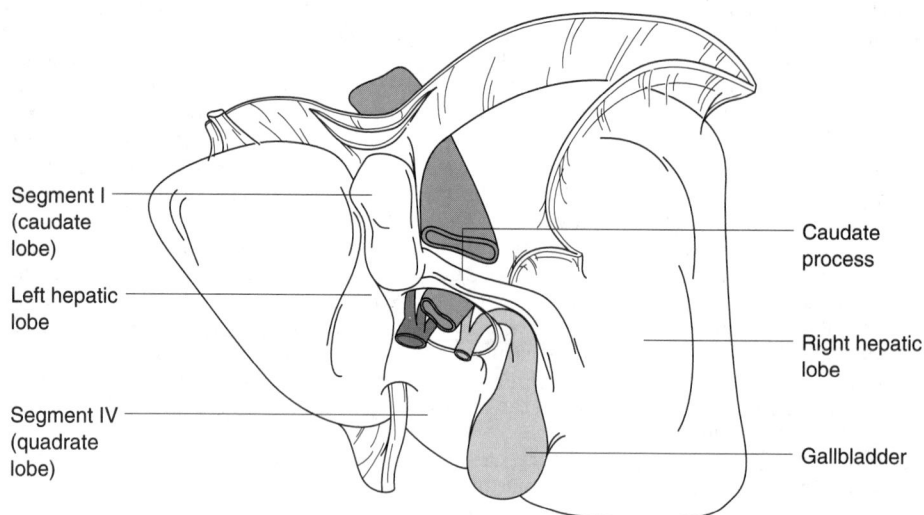

Segment I
(caudate
lobe)

Left hepatic
lobe

Segment IV
(quadrate
lobe)

Caudate
process

Right hepatic
lobe

Gallbladder

Figure 35-7. Inferior aspect of the liver, demonstrating relation of the caudate lobe to other hepatic structures.

suprahepatic vena cava is encircled just inferior to the diaphragm or within the pericardium. Preparation for the Pringle maneuver is to encircle the main portal vein and proper hepatic artery with umbilical-tape tourniquets or a noncrushing vascular clamp.

One begins division of the hepatic parenchyma by scoring the Glisson capsule with cautery or knife. The hepatic substance is divided by means of blunt dissection with a finger, the blunt end of an instrument or suction tip, or an ultrasonic

desiccator. Blood vessels and bile ducts are cauterized, sutured, or clipped in rapid succession from anterior to posterior. Constant evaluation of the direction of transection prevents unintentional division of vital vessels in adjacent segments. If temporary portal inflow occlusion is used, 10 to 20 minutes intervals of unclamping every 3 to 5 minutes to re-establish blood flow is recommended.

The hepatic veins are encountered in the hepatic substance near the vena cava and are clamped and suture-

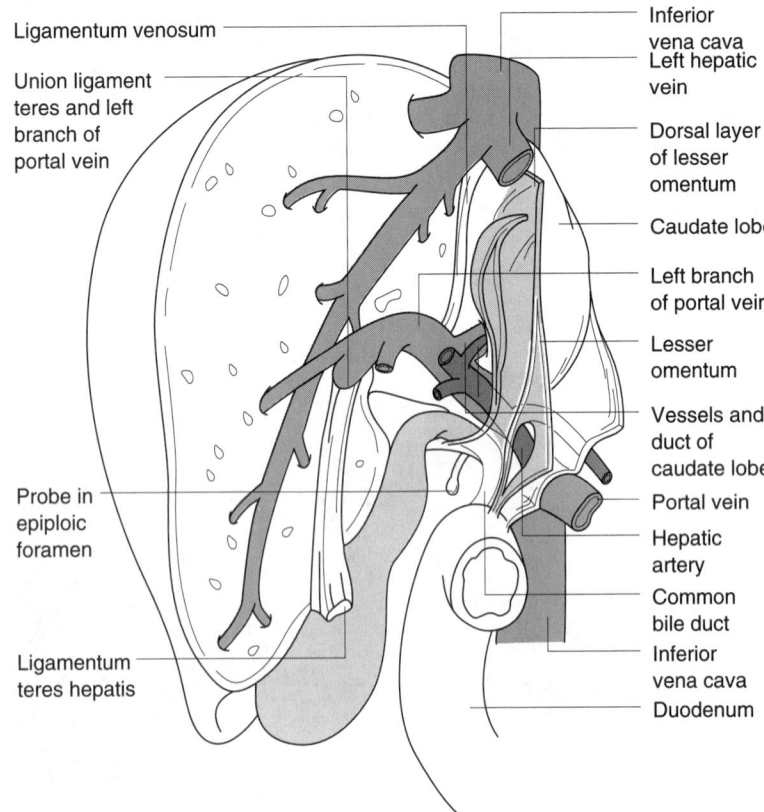

Ligamentum venosum

Union ligament teres and left branch of portal vein

Probe in epiploic foramen

Ligamentum teres hepatis

Inferior vena cava
Left hepatic vein

Dorsal layer of lesser omentum

Caudate lobe

Left branch of portal vein

Lesser omentum

Vessels and duct of caudate lobe

Portal vein

Hepatic artery

Common bile duct

Inferior vena cava

Duodenum

Figure 35-8. Relation of caudate lobe to right and left hepatic lobes and to structures in hepatic hilum.

ligated to complete the resection. The raw hepatic surface is inspected for bleeding and bile leaks, which may be controlled with suture ligation, argon beam coagulation, or use of fibrin glue. The greater omentum may be used to buttress the transected liver edge. Perihepatic closed-suction drains often are placed to monitor for unrecognized postoperative bile leaks.

Segmental Resection

Segmental, bisegmental, and subsegmental or nonanatomic partial resection focuses on maximizing functional reserve without compromising safety.

The caudate lobe (segment I) has several features that are important to consider before and during resection. This segment can be thought of as a separate, smaller liver. Although segment I receives its afferent blood supply from both the right and left portal pedicles, which originate just distal to the main portal bifurcation, the only parenchymal attachment to the remainder of the liver is the thin caudate process, which extends from the posterior aspect of the right lobe (Fig. 35-7). The anterior surface of segment I is separated from the left lobe by the extension of the lesser omentum known as the ligamentum venosum (Fig. 35-8). There is a completely different route of hepatic venous drainage through multiple short veins that pass directly posteriorly into the left and anterior surface of the vena cava. It is often unnecessary to remove this segment during hemihepatectomy unless the blood supply is compromised or there are oncologic reasons to remove it. Isolated resection of segment I can be performed to treat solitary lesions in this segment.

SUGGESTED READING

Adson MA, Beart RW. Elective hepatic resections. Surg Clin North Am 1977;57:339.

Bismuth H, Houssin D, Castaing D. Major and minor segmentectomies "réglées" in liver surgery. World J Surg 1982;6:10.

Cantlie J. On a new arrangement of the right and left lobes of the liver. J Anat 1897;32:4.

Goldsmith NA, Woodburne RT. The surgical anatomy pertaining to liver resections. Surg Gynecol Obstet 1975;105:310.

Healey JE Jr. Clinical anatomic aspects of radical hepatic surgery. J Int Coll Surg 1954;22:542.

McIndoe AH, Counseller VS. The bilaterality of the liver. Arch Surg 1927;15:589.

Yanaga K, Matsumata T, Hayashi H, Shimada M, Urata K, Sugimachi K. Isolated hepatic caudate lobectomy. Surgery 1994;115:757.

ESSENTIALS OF SURGERY: SCIENTIFIC PRINCIPLES AND PRACTICE, edited by Lazar J. Greenfield, Michael W. Mulholland, Keith T. Oldham, Gerald B. Zelenock, and Keith D. Lillemoe. Lippincott–Raven Publishers, Philadelphia, © 1997.

CHAPTER 36
HEPATIC PHYSIOLOGY
STEVEN E. RAPER

HISTOLOGIC ORGANIZATION OF THE LIVER

The free surface of the liver is lined with a single layer of mesothelial cells. Beneath this layer is the Glisson capsule, which is composed of collagen bundles, fibroblasts, and small blood vessels. At the hepatic hilus, the capsule joins with dense connective tissue inside the liver. In the lobules, the connective tissue is replaced with a loosely organized reticular network.

The smallest functional unit of the liver is the acinus—a small mass of hepatic parenchyma. The apices of the acinus are the terminal hepatic venules. The axis is the terminal branches of the portal vein, hepatic arteriole, and bile ductule. The hepatocytes near the portal structures are the first to receive nutrients, the first to regenerate, and the last to die. Cells near the terminal hepatic venules receive blood of poorest quality and lack resistance to toxic injury.

PARENCHYMAL CELL ULTRASTRUCTURE
Plasma Membrane

The plasma membrane consists of a phospholipid bilayer in which hydrophobic fatty acid tails are oriented to the interior membrane and hydrophilic phospholipid heads are oriented to the exterior membrane. Within this phospholipid bilayer are proteins, often complexed with sugar molecules (glycoproteins), with structural or metabolic functions.

The cell membrane allows lipid-soluble molecules to enter the cell by simple diffusion. Polar molecules enter cells via membrane transport proteins.

Passive transport occurs by simple or facilitated diffusion. Channel proteins allow molecules to diffuse into cells without binding; carrier proteins first bind the solute and allow it to be transported into the cell. Active transport requires an energy source, usually adenosine triphosphate (ATP), to transport molecules against a thermodynamically unfavorable electrochemical or concentration gradient.

The plasma membrane regions are characterized by function:

- Sinusoidal membrane—allows active bidirectional transport of proteins, water, and organic and inorganic solutes
- Basolateral membrane—contains structural proteins that allow attachment and communication between cells
- Bile canalicular membrane—appears to be responsible for canalicular shape and bile formation

The plasma membrane is the site of endocytosis, the process by which hepatocytes take up extracellular fluids and macromolecules.

Cell Surface Receptors

The sinusoidal membrane is studded with receptors, large glycoprotein molecules that span the plasma membrane lipid bilayer (Table 36-1). Besides undergoing receptor binding and internalization at the plasma membrane, ligands may follow a number of intracellular pathways. Molecular sorting occurs in the intracellular compartments that process receptor-bound proteins, in effect, targeting proteins to various intracellular destinations. Some cell surface receptors initiate a cascade of intracellular events by generating intracellular second messengers. Such second messengers include cyclic adenosine monophosphate (cAMP), inositol triphosphate, and diacylglycerol (Fig. 36-1).

Mitochondria

Liver mitochondria are self-replicating organelles that contain an independent complement of DNA. The outer membrane is freely permeable. The inner membrane con-

Table 36-1. KNOWN HEPATIC RECEPTORS, LIGAND SPECIFICITY, AND FUNCTION

Receptor	Ligand	Function
Asialoglycoprotein	Desialylated proteins with exposed terminal galactose residues	Targeting of senescent proteins to lysomes for degradation
Chylomicron remnant	Lipoproteins containing apolipoprotein B-48	Triglyceride and cholesterol metabolism
Epidermal growth factor	Epidermal growth factor; transforming growth factor α	Hepatic growth
Growth hormone	Growth hormone	Hepatotrophic factor
Immunoglobulin A (IgA)	Polymeric IgA	Secretory component formation; intestinal immunity
Insulin	Insulin	Hepatotrophic factor; glycogenesis
Insulin-like growth factor 1 (IGF-1)	IGF-1 Lysosomal enzymes	Hepatotrophic factor; lysosomal enzyme processing
Low-density lipoprotein	Lipoproteins containing apolipoprotein B-100 or E	Triglyceride and cholesterol metabolism
Transferrin	Transferrin–iron complexes	Iron uptake and storage

tains the enzymes of the electron transport chain and ATP synthetase. The primary role of mitochondria is to generate large amounts of ATP through the citric acid cycle and oxidative phosphorylation.

Endoplasmic Reticulum and Golgi Complex

The smooth ER, rough ER, and Golgi complex compose the liver microsomal fraction. The liver microsomes participate in (1) synthesis of albumin, fibrinogen, and other proteins destined for export to the plasma; (2) synthesis of cholesterol and bile salts; (3) glucuronidation of bilirubin, drugs, and steroids; (4) esterification of free fatty acids to triglycerides; and (5) glycogenolysis.

The Nucleus

The nucleus is separated from the cytoplasm by an envelope that consists of an inner and an outer membrane. All the chromosomal DNA is packed into chromatin fibers in association with DNA-binding proteins called histones. Ribosomes are synthesized in the nucleolus to aid in protein synthesis. The cytoplasm and nucleus communicate through nuclear pores.

HEPATIC BLOOD FLOW
Control of Hepatic Blood Flow

Total hepatic blood flow is 100 to 130 mL/min/kg. About two-thirds of total hepatic flow is derived from the portal vein and one-third from the hepatic artery. Both intrinsic and extrinsic mechanisms of flow regulation operate in the hepatic artery. Intrinsic flow regulation occurs through arterial autoregulation based on the local concentration of adenosine surrounding the hepatic arteriole and portal venule. An increase in portal venous flow increases washout of adenosine and hepatic arteriolar constriction. If portal venous flow is reduced, local concentrations of adenosine increase, and the hepatic arterioles dilate, leading to a compensatory increase in hepatic arterial flow and maintaining a constant total hepatic blood flow.

Both humoral and neural mechanisms may play a role in extrinsic flow regulation. The hepatic artery does not constrict after meals, despite marked increases in portal flow. Possible humoral mediators of extrinsic regulation include gastrin, glucagon, secretin, and bile salts. The hepatic artery is densely innervated by sympathetic nerves, which are known to cause vasoconstriction mediated by α-adrenergic receptors. The liver is a physiologic blood reservoir, about 25% to 30% of its volume being blood. In acute blood loss, as much as 30%, or 300 mL, of hepatic blood volume can be released into the systemic circulation without an adverse effect on liver function. In systemic volume overload, however, as much as 1 L of extra blood may be stored in the liver before passive congestion and liver injury occur.

Blood-cleansing Function

Hepatic sinusoids are lined with endothelium punctuated with pores that allow proteins as large as albumin to diffuse out of the vascular tree and into proximity with

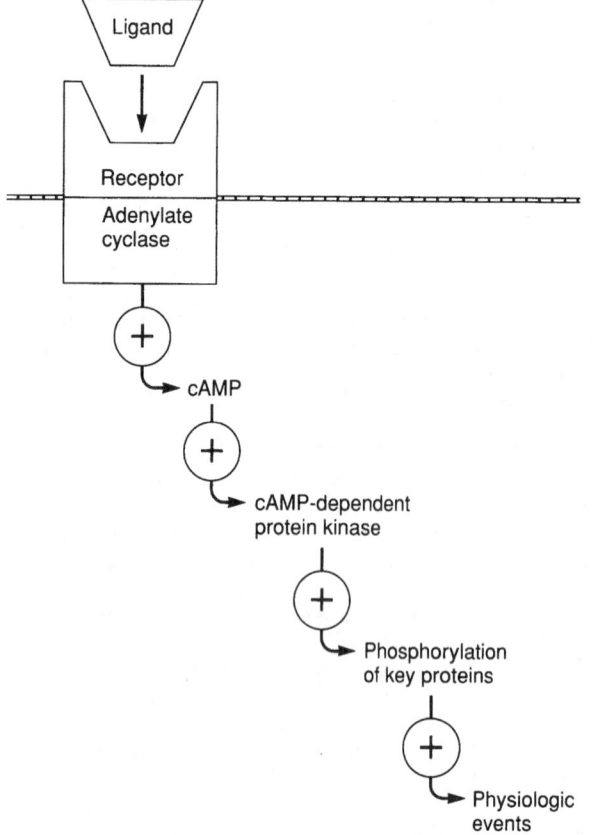

Figure 36-1. Role of cyclic adenosine monophosphate (cAMP)–dependent protein kinase in signal transduction. A single ligand–receptor interaction at the membrane is amplified many times by the stimulation of adenyl cyclase.

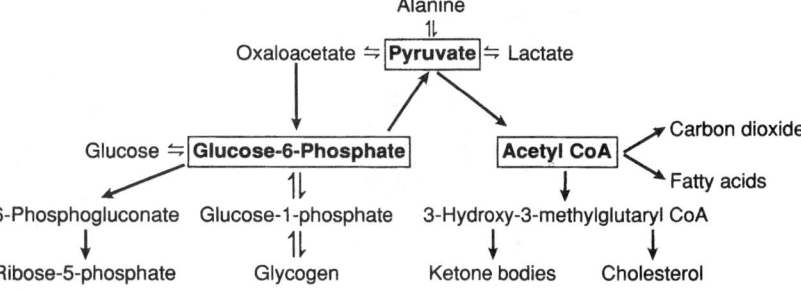

Figure 36-2. A summation of the key regulatory molecules the liver uses to perform its diverse metabolic duties. Essentially, any compound found in the body can be synthesized in the liver from glucose-6-phosphate, acetyl CoA, or pyruvate. The inability of mammalian liver to convert acetyl CoA to pyruvate means that fats cannot be converted to carbohydrates.

hepatocytes. Because sinusoidal pressure is low, proteins can diffuse back into the blood vessels. Much of the extravasated protein enters the lymphatics, so hepatic lymph contains as much protein as plasma. The extreme permeability of the liver allows rapid exchange of a diverse number of nutrients, hormones, and environmental agents between blood and hepatocyte. The liver is a filter for particulate debris, which enters the portal circulation through intestinal capillaries. Particles such as bacteria are ingested by the Kupffer cells that line the hepatic sinusoidal endothelium. After particulate matter is internalized, degradative enzymes neutralize the threat to the host.

HEPATIC METABOLISM

Metabolic processes in the liver are essential for the production of fuel substrates for other organs. The liver regulates intestinally absorbed nutrients for tissue consumption or storage. It accomplishes this task by synthesizing three key metabolites—glucose-6-phosphate (G6P), pyruvate, and acetyl coenzyme A (CoA) (Fig. 36-2). Each of these molecules is modified by the liver to allow an almost limitless number of metabolic processes. G6P is stored as glycogen or converted into glucose, pyruvate, or ribose-5-phosphate (a nucleotide precursor). Pyruvate is converted into lactate, alanine (and other amino acids), and acetyl CoA, or it enters the tricarboxylic acid cycle. Acetyl CoA is converted to 3-hydroxy-3-methylglutaryl CoA (HMG-CoA), a cholesterol and ketone body precursor, or citrate (for fatty acid and triglyceride synthesis), or it is degraded to carbon dioxide and water for energy. Glucose produced by the dephosphorylation of G6P rapidly diffuses out of the cell and is taken up by the brain, muscle, and other organs. Hepatic glycolysis is used primarily for production of intermediates of metabolism, and not for energy.

CARBOHYDRATE METABOLISM

The products of intestinal carbohydrate digestion are glucose (80%) and fructose and galactose (20%). Fructose and galactose are rapidly converted to glucose, which the body uses for transport and uptake of carbohydrate by cells. The liver takes up as much as 100 g/day of glucose and converts it into glycogen (glycogenesis). The liver releases glucose into the blood by glycogenolysis, the breakdown of glycogen, or by gluconeogenesis, the formation of new glucose from substrates such as alanine, lactate, glycerol, and dietary amino acids.

Glycogen Storage and Metabolism

The first step in glycogen storage is the transport of glucose through the hepatocyte plasma membrane. About 90% of portal venous glucose is removed from the blood by liver cells by carrier-facilitated diffusion.

Glycogenesis and Glyconeolysis

In the hepatocyte, glucose and ATP are converted by the enzyme glucokinase to G6P, the first intermediate in the synthesis of glycogen (Fig. 36-3). Glycogenolysis does not occur by simple reversal of glycogenesis. Each succeeding glucose on a glycogen chain is released by glycogen phosphorylase (Fig. 36-4). Eventually, G6P is re-formed. G6P cannot exit the cells, and must be converted back to glucose. This reaction is catalyzed by G6Pase, which is present only in hepatocytes and renal and intestinal epithelial cells. Brain and muscle cells do not contain the phosphatase enzyme. This lack of G6Pase ensures a ready supply of glucose for the energy needs of brain and muscle. The liver does not use glucose as a primary fuel source but as a precursor for other molecules.

Glycolysis

Glycolysis converts glucose to two molecules of pyruvate (Fig. 36-5). Glycolysis occurs in the cytoplasm, and the citric acid cycle occurs in the mitochondria (Fig. 36-6). During times of glucose excess, as in the fed state, the liver may use glycolysis to generate energy in the form of ATP, but the oxidation of ketoacids is preferred.

Phosphogluconate Pathway

When glucose enters the liver, glycogen is formed until hepatic glycogen capacity is reached. The liver converts excess glucose to fat by means of the phosphogluconate pathway.

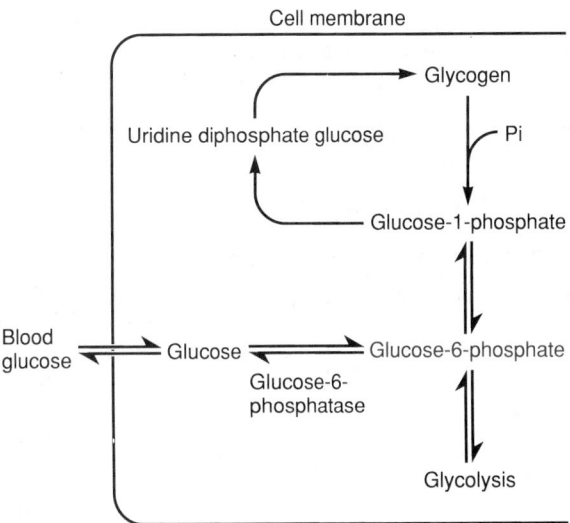

Figure 36-3. The chemical reactions of glycogenesis and glycolysis. Glucose-6-phosphatase allows hepatic glucose to be transported out of the hepatocyte for use in other tissues. Glucose-6-phosphate has a central role in carbohydrate metabolism.

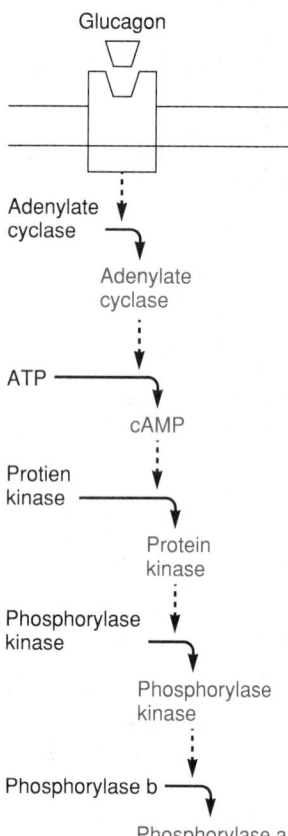

Figure 36-4. Glucagon-stimulated enzyme cascade responsible for control of glycogen metabolism. Inactive forms are shown in black, active forms in blue.

Gluconeogenesis

When glycogen stores are depleted, the liver synthesizes new glucose by means of gluconeogenesis. About 60% of the naturally occurring amino acids, in addition to glycerol, and lactate can be used as a substrate for glucose production. Alanine is the amino acid easiest to convert into glucose. Simple deamination allows conversion to pyruvic acid, which is converted to glucose. Other amino acids are converted to sugars and enter the phosphogluconate pathway. Gluconeogenesis is enhanced by fasting, critical illness, and periods of anaerobic metabolism. Active skeletal muscle and erythrocytes form large quantities of lactate, which the liver converts to glucose.

LIPID METABOLISM

Lipid Transport Into Liver

After absorption into the small-intestinal cells, triglycerides are re-formed and aggregate into chylomicrons, which enter the bloodstream in lymph. Chylomicrons are removed from the blood by the liver and adipose tissue. The capillary surface of the liver contains large amounts of lipoprotein lipase, which hydrolyzes triglycerides into fatty acids and glycerol. The fatty acids diffuse into the hepatocytes for further metabolism.

Fatty Acid Metabolism

Most fatty acids in plasma are long-chain acids. Because long-chain fatty acids are not readily absorbed by the intestinal mucosa, they must first be incorporated into chylomi-

crons. Short-chain and medium-chain fatty acids are absorbed directly into the portal circulation and are avidly taken up by hepatocytes. Free fatty acids in the circulation are noncovalently bound to albumin and are transferred to the hepatocyte cytosol by fatty acid-binding proteins (FABP). Most free fatty acids are catabolized for energy by cardiac and skeletal muscle. Structural elements of all tissues contain large amounts of unsaturated fats, and the liver produces these unsaturated fatty acids. Fatty acid CoA esters are synthesized in the cytosol after hepatic uptake. These fatty acid CoA esters may be converted into triglyceride, transported into mitochondria for the production of acetyl CoA and ATP, or stored in the liver as triglycerides (Fig. 36-7). The mitochondrial hydrolysis of fatty acids is a source of large quantities of ATP.

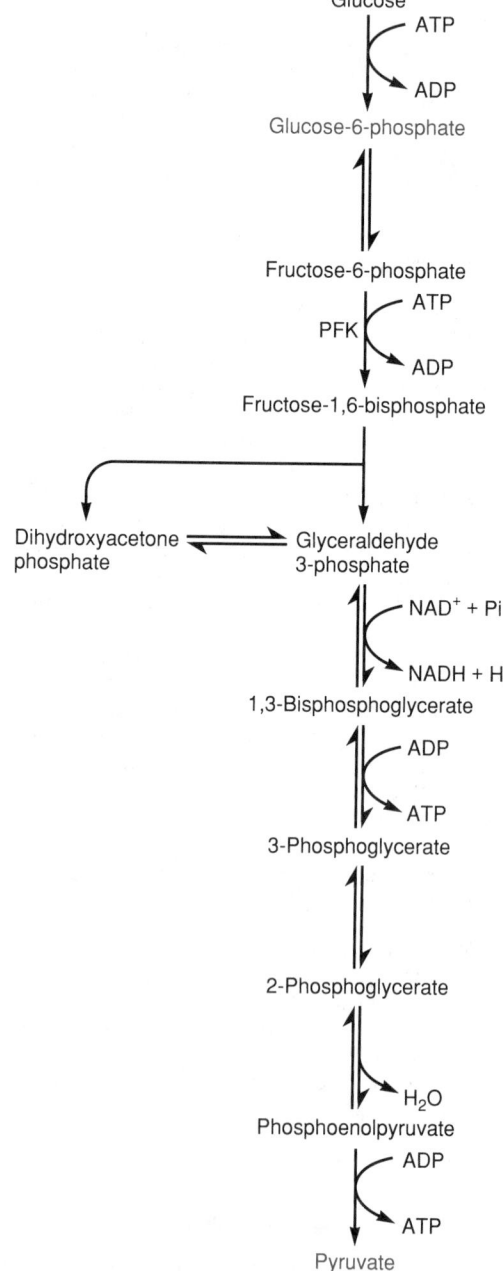

Figure 36-5. The glycolytic pathway. There is a net gain of two ATP molecules per glucose molecule. Phosphofructokinase (PFK) is the key regulatory enzyme in this pathway.

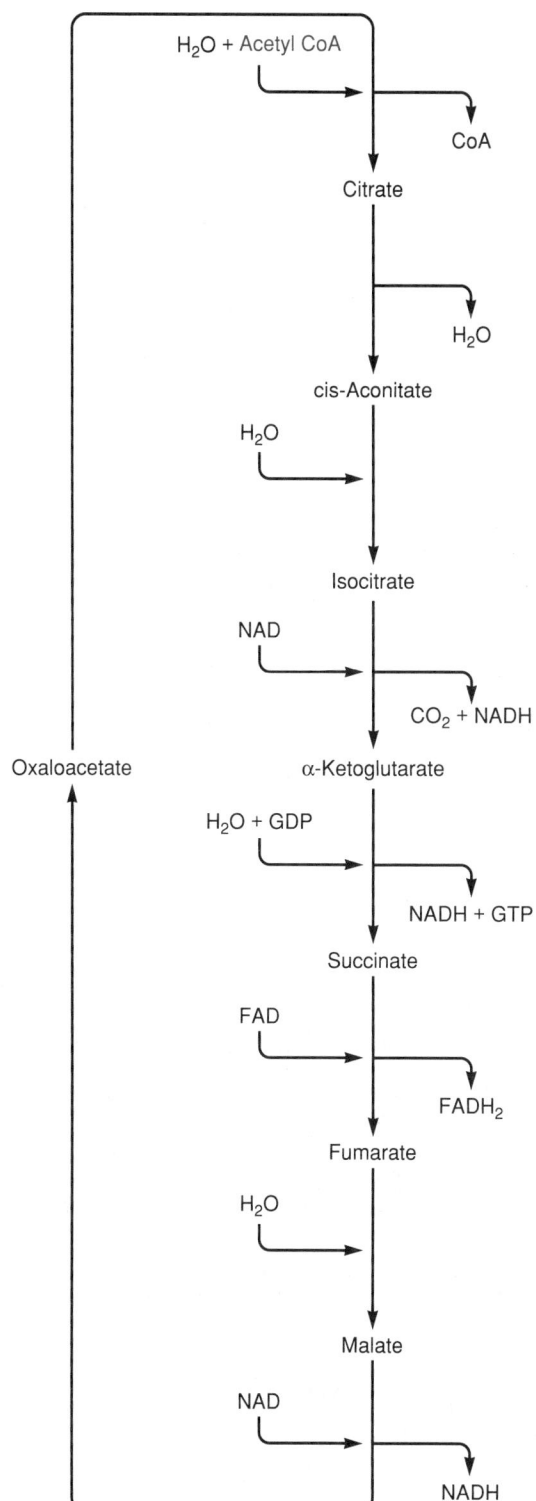

Figure 36-6. The citric acid cycle. NADH and FADH$_2$, formed in the citric acid cycle, are subsequently oxidized in mitochondria by means of the electron transport chain to generate ATP. Acetyl CoA plays a key role.

Cholesterol Metabolism

Cholesterol is an important regulator of membrane fluidity and is a substrate for synthesis of bile acids and steroid hormones. Cholesterol is available by dietary intake or by synthesis. About 90% of new cholesterol is synthesized in the liver from its precursor, acetyl CoA. Dietary cholesterol intake suppresses synthesis. Newly synthesized hepatic cholesterol is used primarily for bile acid synthesis for intestinal absorption of dietary fats.

Phospholipids

Three classes of phospholipid are synthesized by the liver—lecithins, cephalins, and sphingomyelins. The main role of phospholipids of all types is to form plasma and organelle membranes. Phospholipids are essential for reducing surface tension between membranes and surrounding fluids. Phosphatidylcholine, a lecithin, is the most important biliary phospholipid. It promotes the secretion of free cholesterol into bile. Thromboplastin, a cephalin, is needed to initiate the clotting cascade. Sphingomyelins are necessary for the formation of the myelin nerve sheath.

PROTEIN METABOLISM

Amino Acid Transport and Storage

Almost all the end products of dietary protein digestion are amino acids, which are absorbed by the enterocytes into the portal circulation. Amino acids are taken up by hepatocytes by one of the active transport mechanisms. Amino acids are not stored in the liver but are used rapidly to produce plasma proteins, purines, heme proteins, and hormones. The ammonia formed in deamination of amino acids is detoxified by one of two routes. The most important pathway is the conversion of ammonia to urea by enzymes of the Krebs-Henseleit cycle, present only in the liver (Fig. 36-8). A second pathway is deamination of L-glutamine by the kidney, in which ammonia is excreted into the urine.

Formation of Plasma Proteins

Essentially all albumin, fibrinogen, and apolipoproteins are derived from the liver, which adds as much as 50 g of protein to the plasma per day. Seventy-five percent of protein synthesized in the liver is exported in plasma. Most newly synthesized proteins are not stored in the liver. The rate of protein synthesis is determined by the intracellular levels of amino acids (Table 36-2). Albumin, a single-chain polypeptide of 584 amino acids, binds with a variety of smaller molecules. Albumin does not contain terminal galactose residues and is not rapidly cleared. As a result, the half-life of albumin in plasma is 19 days. This long half-life makes albumin an insensitive indicator of hepatic synthetic function. Many proteins are modified after being synthesized in the rough ER of the liver. Glycosylation, addition of carbohydrate moieties, allows some proteins to bind with receptors for hepatic uptake and processing. Desialation, removal of sialic acid residues from glycoproteins, is important in the clearance of senescent proteins from the plasma.

Protein Uptake and Degradation

Asialoglycoproteins (ASGPs) are proteins from which sialic acid residues have been removed by tissue neuraminidases. Terminal galactose residues are exposed that are recognized by the ASGP receptor, allowing hepatic

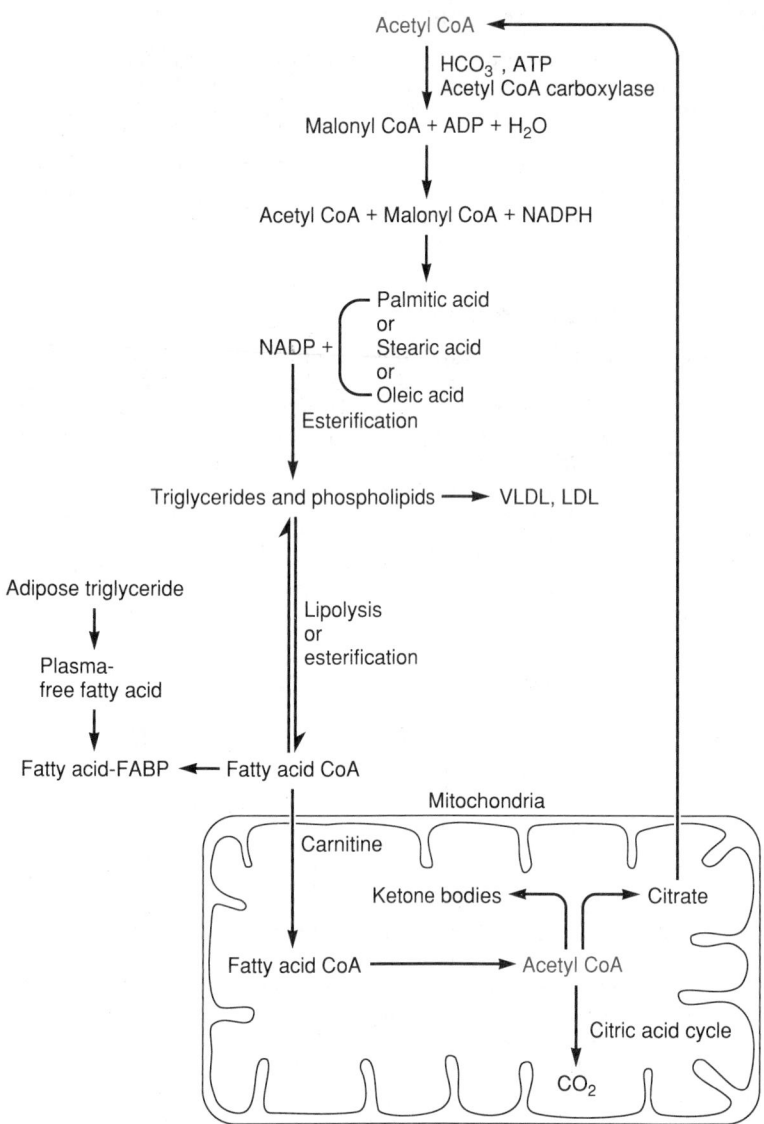

Figure 36-7. Diagram of hepatic fatty acid metabolism. Both dietary and newly synthesized fatty acids are esterified and subsequently degraded in the mitochondria for energy.

receptor-mediated endocytosis. Protein degradation occurs primarily in lysosomes, which contain more than 20 nonselective hydrolytic enzymes.

HEME AND PORPHYRIN METABOLISM

Heme is formed from glycine and succinate. It is the functional iron-containing center of hemoglobin, myoglobin, cytochromes, catalases, and peroxidases. From glycine and succinate precursors, α-aminolevulinic acid (α-ALA) is synthesized by ALA synthase. The porphyrinogens are intermediates in the pathway from α-ALA to heme, and porphyrins are oxidized forms of porphyrinogen. Inherited enzyme defects in the heme synthetic pathway lead to porphyria, the overproduction of porphyrinogens. Porphyria is caused by heavy-metal intoxication, excessive estrogen, alcohol ingestion, or exposure to chlorinated hydrocarbons. Bilirubin IX α, the predominant heme degradation product, is derived mostly from hemoglobin. Heme oxygenase, present in the reticuloendothelial system, aids in this conversion. Heme oxygenase is present in the ER

and requires the reduced form of nicotinamide-adenine dinucleotide phosphate (NADPH) as a cofactor.

METAL METABOLISM

Iron

Iron uptake in liver cells appears to occur by two processes: (1) receptor-mediated endocytosis of iron–transferrin complexes and (2) facilitated diffusion across the plasma membrane. Transferrin is synthesized in the liver and has plasma membrane receptors on a number of different tissues. After endocytosis, the transferrin and iron dissociate, and the transferrin and transferrin receptor return to the cell surface for recycling, and iron is internalized by carrier-mediated diffusion. After it is internalized, iron is stored and complexed to apoferritin. The iron-apoferritin complex is called *ferritin* and is responsible for iron storage. It is essential that iron be stored in a protein-bound form, because free iron catalyzes free radical formation, which leads to cell injury.

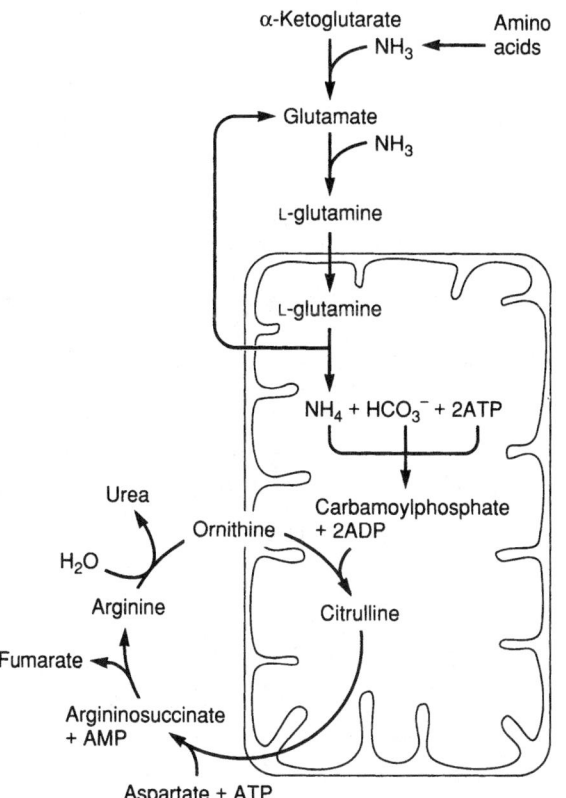

Figure 36-8. The urea cycle. Ammonia entering the urea cycle is derived from protein and amino acid degradation in tissues (endogenous) and colonic lumen (exogenous).

Copper

Copper is transported to the liver bound to albumin or histidine, and enters the hepatocytes by facilitated diffusion. Inside the cell, copper binds to several proteins for storage or as a necessary enzyme cofactor. Ceruloplasmin is a liver-derived protein that binds hepatic copper for transport to other tissues.

Other Metals

Zinc is taken up by, and competes for, the same binding sites as copper. In hepatocytes, zinc binds to metallothionein and is excreted into bile. Metals present in trace amounts are lead, cadmium, selenium, mercury, and nickel. These metals are usually bound to metallothionein or glutathione. Metal intoxication is associated with free radical formation and liver injury.

VITAMIN METABOLISM

The liver metabolizes the fat-soluble vitamins A, D, and K. Hepatic bile salt secretion is necessary for solubilization and absorption of dietary fat-soluble vitamins from the intestine. The liver stores large amounts of fat-soluble vitamins and synthesizes transport proteins for the vitamins. Vitamin A is stored only in the liver; excessive ingestion of vitamin A may cause liver injury. Retinol-binding protein, synthesized by the liver, is responsible for the plasma transport of vitamin A. Vitamin D must undergo metabolism in the liver to produce 25-hydroxyvitamin D, a necessary step in the conversion from dietary to biologically active vitamin D. Vitamin D undergoes biliary secretion, intestinal absorption, and hepatic uptake or enterohepatic

Table 36-2. MAJOR PROTEINS SYNTHESIZED BY THE LIVER

Broad Category	Protein	Molecular Weight	Function
Transport proteins	Albumin	66,000	Multiple
	Transferrin	57,000	Transports iron
	Hemopexin	80,000	Transports heme to liver
	Ceruloplasmin	132,000	Transports copper
	Haptoglobin	90,000	Transports free hemoglobin
	Thyroxine-binding globulin	55,000	Transports thyroid hormone
	Thyroxine-binding prealbumin	50,000	Transports thyroid hormone
	Testosterone-estradiol–binding globulin	90,000	Facilitates testosterone action
	Retinol-binding protein	21,000	Transports vitamin A
	Vitamin D–binding protein	52,000	Transports vitamin D
Coagulation proteins	Fibrinogen (factor I)	340,000	Forms fibrin
	Prothrombin (factor II)	73,000	Converts fibrinogen to fibrin
	Factors V, VII, IX, X, XI, XII	50,000–75,000	Extrinsic and intrinsic pathway
	Plasminogen	90,000	Forms plasmin
	α_2-antiplasmin	70,000	Inhibits plasmin
	Antithrombin III	60,000	Protease inhibitor
	Protein S	50,000	Protein C cofactor
	Protein C	55,000	Anticoagulant
Acute-phase reactants	α_2-macroglobulin	720,000	Binds endopeptidases
	α_1-antitrypsin	54,000	Inhibits serine proteases
	C-reactive protein	105,000	Modifies inflammation
	Orosomucoid	40,000	Unknown
Lipoprotein metabolism	Apolipoprotein AI, AII	17,000–30,000	LCAT cofactors
	Apolipoprotein CI, CII, CIII	6000–10,000	Inhibit binding to liver
	Apolipoprotein E	34,000	Receptor recognition
	Apo B100	510,000	VLDL synthesis and secretion
	LCAT	—	Cholesterol synthesis in blood

LCAT, lecithin–cholesterol acetyl transferase; VLDL, very-low-density lipoprotein.

circulation. Vitamin D-binding globulin is synthesized in the liver and aids in the transport of all forms of vitamin D. Vitamin K_1 is ingested with food; vitamin K_2 is a product of bacterial action in the intestinal lumen. Vitamin K is required for hepatic synthesis of biologically active coagulation factors II, VII, IX, and X. Of the water-soluble vitamins, only vitamin B_{12} is stored to an appreciable extent in the liver.

BILE FORMATION

Composition and Secretion

The liver secretes about 1.5 L of bile a day. Eighty percent of this volume is secreted by the hepatocytes (canalicular bile), and 20% is secreted by the bile duct epithelial cells (ductular bile). Bile acids are the main determinant of bile production.

Bile Acid Metabolism

Primary bile acids—cholic acid and chenodeoxycholic acid—are synthesized from cholesterol in the liver. Secondary bile acids— deoxycholic acid and lithocholic acid—are formed in the intestinal lumen by bacterial dehydroxylation. Essentially all the primary and secondary bile acids are conjugated with the amino acids glycine or taurine. Conjugated bile acids form micelles, which facilitate lipid digestion and absorption from the small intestine.

Biliary Lecithin and Cholesterol Secretion

The main biliary phospholipid is lecithin. Lecithin has two main purposes in bile: (1) to solubilize free biliary cholesterol and (2) to emulsify dietary fats in the intestine. Free cholesterol is not soluble in water or simple micelles of bile acids but is readily solubilized in mixed micelles of both bile acids and lecithin.

Biliary Proteins

Proteins constitute about 5% of the total biliary solute. Intact proteins in bile appear to help in intestinal immunity and in the prevention of gallstone nucleation. Some proteins are degraded in lysosomes before biliary excretion. This mechanism eliminates senescent plasma proteins.

HEPATIC BIOTRANSFORMATION

Biotransformation is the intracellular metabolism of endogenous organic compounds (eg, heme proteins and steroid hormones) and exogenous compounds (eg, drugs and environmental compounds). The liver contains enzyme systems that expose functional groups such as hydroxyl ions or alter the size and solubility of organic and inorganic compounds by conjugation with small polar molecules. The liver converts hydrophobic, potentially toxic compounds, into hydrophilic conjugates, which are excreted into bile or urine. Four enzyme families are responsible for hepatic biotransformation—the cytochromes P-450, the uridine diphosphate-glucuronyl (UDP-glucuronyl) transferases, the glutathione S-transferases, and the sulfotransferases.

SUGGESTED READING

Casanova JE, Breitfeld PP, Ross SA, Mostov KE. Phosphorylation of the polymeric immunoglobulin receptor required for its efficient transcytosis. Science 1990;248:742.
Geuze HJ, Van der Donk HA, Simmons CF, et al. Receptor mediated endocytosis in liver parenchymal cells. Int Rev Exp Pathol 1986;29:113.
Havel RJ, Hamilton RL. Hepatocytic lipoprotein receptors and intracellular lipoprotein catabolism. Hepatology 1988;8:1689.
Hoffman AF. Chemistry and enterohepatic circulation of bile acids. Hepatology 1984;4(Suppl 5):4.
LaRusso NF. Proteins in bile: how they get there and what they do. Am J Physiol 1984;247:G199.
Lautt WW, Legare DJ, Ezzat WR. Quantitation of the hepatic arterial buffer response to graded changes in portal blood flow. Gastroenterology 1990;98:1024.
Styrer L. Pentose phosphate pathway and gluconeogenesis. In: Styrer L, ed. Biochemistry, ed 3. New York, Freeman, 1988: 427.
Wu CH, Wu GY. Targeting genes: delivery and persistent expression of a foreign gene driven by mammalian regulatory elements in vivo. J Biol Chem 1989;264:1698.

ESSENTIALS OF SURGERY: SCIENTIFIC PRINCIPLES AND PRACTICE, edited by Lazar J. Greenfield, Michael W. Mulholland, Keith T. Oldham, Gerald B. Zelenock, and Keith D. Lillemoe. Lippincott–Raven Publishers, Philadelphia, © 1997.

CHAPTER 37

HEPATIC INFECTION AND ACUTE HEPATIC FAILURE

MICHAEL R. LUCEY

VIRAL HEPATITIS

Five viruses cause acute viral hepatitis (Table 37-1).

Hepatitis A

Humans appear to be the only host for hepatitis A virus (HAV) infection. The principal mode of transmission of HAV infection is fecal–oral, although parenteral transmission is possible. The incubation period is usually about 28 days.

Clinical Features

An anicteric prodrome that lasts 2 days to 3 weeks consists of malaise, arthralgia, myalgia, anorexia, loss of taste for food, possibly coryza, headache, photophobia, fever, pharyngitis, dark urine, pale stools, and, sometimes, epigastric or right-upper-quadrant pain accompanied by diarrhea. The prodrome subsides with the onset of jaundice. The liver may be enlarged and slightly tender. Spider angiomata may appear. Jaundice persists 1 to 6 weeks. Lassitude may last for months.

Fecal shedding of HAV usually continues 7 to 10 days after the onset of jaundice. Serum transaminases usually are elevated. Serum anti-HAV IgM is usually detectable when jaundice appears, and strongly indicates the diagnosis. Elevated titers of anti-HAV IgM may persist for months. The IgG fraction of anti-HAV rises as jaundice subsides and persists for years.

Liver biopsy is rarely required to make the diagnosis, but if performed, it demonstrates periportal and lobular infiltration by lymphocytes and macrophages associated

Table 37-1. CHARACTERISTIC OF VIRUSES

Virus	Genus	Genome	Genome Length (kb)	Mode of Transmission	Incubation* (d) Mean	Range	Acute Hepatitis	Consequences of Infection Fulminant Hepatic Failure	Chronic Hepatitis	Hepatoma	Posttransplantation Infection Recipient to Allograft	New Acquisition
Hepatitis A	Picornavirus	RNA	7.5	Fecal–oral Parenteral	28	15–50	Yes	Yes	No	No	No	No
Hepatitis B	Hepadnavirus	DNA	3.2	Parenteral Venereal ? Fecal–oral	84	28–160	Yes	Yes	Yes	Yes	Yes	Yes
Hepatitis C	Flavivirus	RNA	10.2	Parenteral ? Venereal ? Fecal–oral	56	14–160	Yes	Probable	Yes	Yes	Yes	Yes
Hepatitis D	Viroid	RNA	1.67	Parenteral	—	—	Yes	Yes	Yes	No	Yes	Uncertain
Hepatitis E	Probably calicivirus	RNA	7.6	Fecal–oral	40	22–60	Yes	Yes†	No	No	Uncertain	No

* Time from exposure to clinical hepatitis.
† Especially in pregnant women in third trimester.

with parenchymal injury. Hepatocellular injury is characterized by balloon degeneration of hepatocytes, acidophil bodies, and hepatocyte dropout. These changes lead to loss of the normal hepatic lobular architecture.

Serious consequences of HAV infection are uncommon. Some patients who have recovered from a typical HAV infection have a relapse 7 to 10 weeks after the initial recovery, but no chronic carrier state for HAV has been identified, nor does HAV cause chronic active hepatitis or cirrhosis.

Treatment

HAV infection is treated with simple nursing care, adequate nutrition, and attention to hygiene after defecation. A formalin-inactivated HAV vaccine induces an immune response after one or two doses. Vaccination is recommended for travelers to endemic areas and for people, such as sewage workers, whose occupation places them at high risk of exposure to HAV. Passive prophylaxis with intramuscular injection of immune globulin is recommended for people at risk, such as household contacts of a person with hepatitis A and employees of day care centers in which children or employees have acute hepatitis A.

Hepatitis B

Hepatitis B virus (HBV) infection is spread by the parenteral route and by intimate personal contact. The onset of acute hepatitis B is insidious. The incubation period is about 8 weeks.

Clinical Features

Many cases of hepatitis B are asymptomatic and recognized only at serologic screening during an outbreak. A diagnosis of previous acute HBV infection often is made in a patient with newly diagnosed chronic hepatitis B. The first serum indicator of HBV infection is the presence of hepatitis B surface antigen (HBsAg), which may precede the onset of jaundice. Acute HBV infection is accompanied by the serum and liver markers of viral replication—serum HBV DNA, serum HBV DNA polymerase, serum HBeAg, liver HBV DNA, and liver HBcAg. With the onset of clinical hepatitis, serum anti-HBc IgM becomes detectable. When HBV infection is self-limited and does not progress to chronic hepatitis, anti-HBc IgM does not persist for more than 6 months after acquisition of HBV. Thus, serum anti-HBc IgM is used to differentiate acute and chronic hepatitis B.

Most patients experience subclinical HBV infection with complete recovery. About 25% experience clinical jaundice, which resolves without development of the carrier state.

Chronic HBV exists in two related forms. Most patients have a benign carrier state. These patients produce an excess of HBsAg in the liver but do not have evidence of ongoing liver injury or of active viral replication. The other HBV carriers have evidence of ongoing active viral replication and clinical features of chronic active hepatitis.

Histologic examination in benign chronic hepatitis shows hepatocytes with a ground-glass appearance due to an excess of cytoplasmic HBsAg proteins. There may be no inflammation, or inflammation may be confined only to the portal triad without evidence of liver injury. Chronic hepatitis with progressive liver injury usually shows serum markers of active viral replication, ongoing liver injury, and a histologic pattern of active inflammation. Chronic replicative hepatitis B can progress to cirrhosis.

Patients with chronic hepatitis B sometimes spontaneously become benign chronic carriers. This seroconversion is often accompanied by an acute exacerbation of hepatitis with a typical viral syndrome and elevated levels of transaminases. A similar phenomenon is observed when seroconversion is induced by interferon therapy.

Hepatoma is a consequence of chronic hepatitis B; it occurs 10 to 20 years after HBV infection. The risk factors are male sex, cirrhosis, viral infection with HBV or HCV, inherited disorders such as hemochromatosis or tyrosinemia, and environmental exposure to the procarcinogen aflatoxin.

Treatment

The best way to treat hepatitis B is to prevent it with vaccination, passive prophylaxis with HB immunoglobulin (HBIG), and use of condoms. No treatment ameliorates acute hepatitis B or prevents its progression to chronic infection. Patients with HBV-induced fulminant hepatic failure may require liver transplantation.

Hepatitis C

The most common identifiable sources of hepatitis C virus (HCV, formerly called non-A non-B hepatitis) infection in the United States are transfusion of blood or blood-derived products and illicit use of IV drugs. The incubation period is 5 to 10 weeks.

Clinical Features

Posttransfusion hepatitis C leads to chronic hepatitis and cirrhosis. The initial elevated ALT level may be associated with little or no clinical disturbance. Viral replication coincides with this initial episode of hepatitis. Anti-HC antibody does not appear until 18 weeks after the initial posttransfusion hepatic illness. In some people, acute hepatitis C does not progress to chronic infection, and anti-HCV antibody may appear in serum.

Chronic HCV infection is characterized by an indolent clinical syndrome in which transaminase levels fluctuate. During this time, viral replication is usually detectable with polymerase chain reaction (PCR) amplification of HCV in serum. However, a negative HCV PCR in a previously positive person does not necessarily mean the patient no longer has HCV infection. Patients can harbor HCV for many years without ill effects, except fluctuating mild elevations in liver enzyme levels.

Biopsy of a liver affected by hepatitis C shows appearances ranging from normal, through slight or aggressive hepatitis, to frank cirrhosis. Histologic features of chronic hepatitis C include a lymphocytic infiltrate in the portal triad, bile duct injury, acidophil bodies, and macrovesicular fat deposition.

Hepatitis C does not appear to alter life expectancy, at least in the first 15 years of infection. Once cirrhosis and end-stage liver disease develop, however, the clinical syndrome cannot be differentiated from other forms of chronic liver failure.

Treatment

Interferon α is the only FDA-approved therapy for chronic HCV infection. Early administration of interferon in acute HCV may reduce the risk of progression to chronic HCV. The biochemical response is usually transient, however, and enzyme levels increase either during therapy or after interferon is stopped. People infected with HCV are advised to abstain from alcohol. Liver transplantation is used to treat incapacitating liver failure due to chronic hepatitis C, even though HCV usually infects the allograft.

Hepatitis D

Humans appear to be the only host of hepatitis D virus (HDV, formerly called hepatitis). The incubation period is 4 to 20 weeks.

HDV requires simultaneous infection with HBV to complete its life cycle. HDV infection acquired simultaneously with HBV infection is called *coinfection.* HDV infection in a host with prior HBV infection is called *superinfection.*

Clinical Features

Coinfection is a mild transient clinical phenomenon sometimes recognizable only by detection of anti-hepatitis B core antibody (HBcAb) IgM and anti-HD IgM. There may be a biphasic pattern of elevated transaminases. The first peak corresponds to acute HBV replication, and the second to acute HDV replication. A common cause of coinfection is abuse of IV drugs. Patients with acute coinfection usually do not become chronic carriers of HDV. Chronic hepatitis with progression to cirrhosis is one consequence of HDV infection.

Treatment

Interferon α is used to treat chronic HDV infection. Recrudescence of both HDV and HBV after interferon is discontinued is common. HDV and HBV coinfection can recur after liver transplantation.

Hepatitis E

Hepatitis E (formerly called epidemic waterborne non-A non-B hepatitis) is associated with fecal contamination of drinking water. The incubation period is 40 days.

Clinical Features

Transient cholestatic jaundice develops, and the patient recovers without chronic sequelae. An important exception is HEV infection in pregnant women. Fulminant hepatic failure due to hepatitis E is common in the third trimester.

Treatment

The provision of clean water and means for hygienic disposal of excreta are goals to control HEV infection.

PYOGENIC HEPATIC ABSCESS

Pyogenic hepatic abscesses are caused by benign or malignant biliary obstruction accompanied by cholangitis; extrahepatic abdominal sepsis; trauma to, or operations on, the right-upper quadrant; and hepatic arterial occlusion after a liver transplant or intra-arterial chemotherapy or injection of ethanol for hepatoma. Pyogenic hepatic abscess after intraabdominal sepsis is probably caused by hematogenous spread through the portal bloodstream. Abscesses due to hematogenous transmission are usually unifocal, whereas those due to biliary obstruction are usually multifocal. Metastatic cancer in the liver, diabetes mellitus, and alcoholism are predisposing factors.

The organisms that predominate in pyogenic hepatic abscesses are gram-negative aerobic rods, streptococci, and anaerobes, including *Bacteroides fragilis.* Pyogenic hepatic abscesses occur with equal frequency in men and women. The median age at presentation is 40 to 49 years. About 15% of patients die, usually of uncontrolled sepsis.

Diagnosis

Pyogenic hepatic abscess presents with fever, chills, abdominal pain, and weight loss. Forty percent of patients have abdominal tenderness. Overt jaundice is present in 20%. Almost all patients have polymorphonuclear leukocytosis and nonspecific abnormalities in biochemical tests, including elevated alkaline phosphatase and transaminase levels and hypoalbuminemia.

The differential diagnosis of pyogenic hepatic abscess includes ascending cholangitis, amebic hepatic abscess, and sepsis elsewhere in the body associated with hepatic dysfunction. About 40% of patients have abnormal chest radiographs, including atelectasis, pulmonary infiltrate, or elevated right hemidiaphragm.

Pyogenic hepatic abscess is detected with real-time ultrasonography (US), computed tomography (CT), radionuclide imaging, and contrast-enhanced magnetic resonance imaging (MRI). CT, especially with IV contrast, is as sensitive as US. Imaging does not differentiate pyogenic and amebic abscesses.

Once a hepatic abscess is detected with US or CT, diagnostic percutaneous aspiration is performed, unless there are clear indications that the abscess is amebic. Diagnostic aspiration allows identification of the causative organism, even after antibiotics are started. The antibiotic regimen can be modified on the basis of culture results.

Treatment

Most pyogenic hepatic abscesses are treated with antibiotics and drainage. Antibiotic therapy alone may be advisable for patients in whom drainage is considered hazardous or patients with multiple small abscesses. Percutaneous drainage with US or CT guidance sometimes is sufficient to evacuate pus. Surgical exploration is advised for patients in unstable condition who have signs of continued sepsis despite nonsurgical treatment, or patients in stable condition in whom fever persists for >2 weeks after percutaneous catheter drainage and institution of appropriate antibiotics.

AMEBIC HEPATIC ABSCESS

Entamoeba histolytica is the only ameba that causes tissue invasion in humans. Risk factors are spending time in a high-risk area and alcoholism. Homosexual men are at risk because they have a high frequency of intestinal carriage of E. histolytica.

Diagnosis

The duration of illness at presentation of amebic hepatic abscess varies. An acute form with symptoms for <2 weeks can be differentiated from a chronic form. About half of patients with amebic abscesses have abnormalities in the right lung (atelectasis, infiltrate, effusion, or elevated hemidiaphragm). Moderate elevation in serum aminotransferases and alkaline phosphatase levels are common. Liver US is followed by CT. Imaging does not differentiate amebic and pyogenic abscesses. Serologic tests positive for E. histolytica confirm the diagnosis of amebic hepatic abscess.

Treatment

Amebic hepatic abscesses are treated with metronidazole. Chloroquine phosphate may be added for acutely illness. Alternatives include dehydroemetrine, iodoquinol, and emetine.

Most uncomplicated amebic hepatic abscesses do not require aspiration. Superinfection of an amebic abscess is a complication of invasive aspiration procedures or abscess rupture. Therapeutic aspiration is performed to exclude pyogenic abscess in patients who do not respond to metronidazole or chloroquine and in patients with large leftlobe amebic abscesses, which may rupture into the pericardium.

HYDATID DISEASE OF THE LIVER

Echinococcosis is caused by infestation with the tapeworms. Humans are intermediate hosts and acquire echinococcal eggs by ingesting contaminated food. An egg digested in the duodenum yields an embryo that travels through the portal bloodstream to the liver and lodges there, developing into a hydatid cyst.

Diagnosis

The only clinical finding of hepatic hydatid cyst is a palpable hepatic mass. Because the cysts grow slowly, there is usually a protracted asymptomatic stage. Symptoms, when they occur, are due to increases in cyst size, which leads to abdominal pain, biliary obstruction and jaundice, and, rarely, portal hypertension.

Routine laboratory tests in patients with hydatid cysts may be normal or nonspecifically abnormal, such as showing features of obstructive jaundice. Serologic tests are specific and sensitive. Although routine chest or abdominal radiographs may show a mass, sometimes with a calcific rim, US and CT are the favored means of imaging. The presence of calcification and daughter cysts within the parent cyst suggests echinococcosis.

Treatment

Percutaneous needling of hydatid cysts is unwise. The cyst fluid is under pressure, and needling may rupture the cyst, causing anaphylaxis or intraperitoneal seeding. Serologic testing should precede needling of any mass that may be a hydatid cyst.

The treatment of hydatid cysts is surgical. The aim is to remove the cyst or cysts without dissemination of the organism. At operation, the cyst is drained of fluid through a cannula, after the operative field is protected from fluid leakage. If the aspirate is clear, ethyl alcohol or 20% sterile saline solution is injected into the cyst to kill any adherent scoleces. If the cyst fluid is bilious, solution is not injected to avoid infusion of irritant solution into the biliary tree. The cyst contents and pericystic wall are removed with careful dissection. Often the surgical procedure is preceded by albendazole therapy to eradicate viable scoleces and reduce the risk of dissemination during the operation.

SCHISTOSOMAL HEPATIC DISEASE
Diagnosis

Acute schistosomiasis occurs soon after cercariae enter the human host by penetrating the skin. An early manifestation is an irritating maculopapular rash that lasts several days. After an incubation period of 1 to 2 months, a syndrome of lassitude, anorexia, and GI upset with intermittent fever, chills, sweating, headache, diarrhea, muscle aches, or bronchospasm develops. Clinical examination reveals hepatomegaly, moderate splenomegaly, and generalized lymphadenopathy. Sigmoidoscopy shows a red edematous mucosa with fine granulation, petechiae, and ulcers. The diagnosis is established with demonstration of ova in stool or within the submucosa of the rectum.

Chronic schistosomiasis is usually asymptomatic until variceal hemorrhage occurs. Hepatosplenomegaly is progressive. The typical manifestations of chronic liver insufficiency (jaundice, spider angiomata, palmar erythema, gynecomastia) are unusual. Laboratory features of chronic schistosomiasis include eosinophilia, hypoalbuminemia, hypergammaglobulinemia, and elevated serum alkaline phosphatase. Serum transaminases are normal. Inspection of feces for ova is the most reliable diagnostic test.

Treatment

Schistosomiasis is treated with praziquantel. Bleeding esophageal varices are managed with variceal sclerotherapy.

ACUTE HEPATIC FAILURE

Hepatic failure is caused by acute necrosis of a large number of hepatocytes. Fulminant hepatic failure is the development of acute hepatic encephalopathy within 8 weeks of the onset of symptomatic hepatocellular disease in a previously healthy person. The causes of fulminant hepatic failure are listed in Table 37-2. Submassive hepatic necrosis is the development of acute hepatic encephalopathy 8 to 24 weeks after the onset of symptomatic hepatocellular disease.

About 2000 cases of acute hepatic failure occur in the United States each year; 80% of patients die. Outcome is determined by the course of encephalopathy (Table 37-3). Cerebral edema, which leads to increased intracran-

Table 37-2. CAUSES OF FULMINANT HEPATIC FAILURE

VIRAL INFECTION
Hepatitis A
Hepatitis B
Hepatitis D
Other viruses (less common)
  Cytomegalovirus
  Epstein-Barr
  Varicella
  Herpes

POISONS, CHEMICALS, AND DRUGS
Amanita phalloides
Acetaminophen
Tetracycline
Phosphorus
Halogenated volatile anesthetics (especially halothane)
Isomazid
Methyldopa
Valproate
Monoamine oxidase inhibitors

ISCHEMIA AND HYPOXIA
Hepatic vascular occlusion
Acute circulatory stroke
Heat stroke
Gram-negative sepsis

MISCELLANEOUS
Acute fatty liver of pregnancy
Reyes syndrome
Wilson disease
Hodgkin and other lymphomas
Hereditary fructose intolerance
Galactosemia, tyrosinemia
Idiopathic (also called non-A non-B)

ial pressure (ICP), may cause permanent cerebral injury or death. Fulminant hepatic failure and submassive hepatic necrosis are always accompanied by severe coagulopathy.

Medical Management

- Transfer to the ICU of a liver transplant center
- Diagnosis with tests for anti-HBc antibody IgM, HBsAg, anti-HAV IgM, cytomegalovirus (CMV), Epstein–Barr virus (EBV), herpes simplex virus (HSV), and varicella–zoster virus (VZV) antibodies, serum ceruloplasmin, toxins, and examination of the eyes for corneal rings.
- N-acetyl cysteine for patients who have ingested acetaminophen
- Avoidance of renal failure (aminoglycosides, radiographic dye, and other nephrotoxic agents are used with caution)
- Regulation of hypoglycemia, hypokalemia, and acidosis
- Correction of coagulopathy with fresh frozen plasma
- Management of hypotension with assisted ventilation
- Monitoring for sepsis with daily cultures of blood, urine, and other body fluids
- Management of cerebral edema with mannitol and ICP monitoring

Surgical Treatment

Liver transplantation is a life-saving procedure for patients with hepatic failure or submassive hepatic necrosis that does not respond to medical management. The most important indicators that a liver transplant is needed are the level of encephalopathy and the trend of change in encephalopathy. Because of difficulty procuring a donor organ, human heterotopic transplants, extracorporeal perfusion through human or pig livers or artificial hepatocyte perfusion devices, and xenografts may be used to sustain the patient until spontaneous recovery occurs or a suitable organ is found.

HEPATIC INFECTIONS ASSOCIATED WITH HIV OR AIDS

Patients with asymptomatic human immunodeficiency virus (HIV) infection may have abnormal liver chemistry tests. Liver disturbances in these patients may have any of the causes of noninfectious liver disease. Many patients with asymptomatic positive evidence of HIV antibody have markers of exposure to HBV and HDV. HCV antibodies are common in people with hemophilia. Diagnosis and management of abnormal liver tests in people who are HIV Ab-positive without AIDS are the same as for anyone who has abnormal liver tests.

Many patients with AIDS carry markers for exposure to viral hepatitis. AIDS also may be accompanied by opportunistic infections that localize to the liver. These include infection with *Mycobacterium avium-intracellulare, M. tuberculosis,* CMV, EBV, HSV, and fungal infections. These infections present with fever, hepatomegaly, and abnormal liver chemistries. Jaundice is unusual. The presence of opportunistic viral bacterial or fungal infections in AIDS is usually a manifestation of disseminated infection in patients with advanced disease.

Therapy for hepatic infection in the presence of HIV infection requires changing the underlying process of immunodeficiency. There is no effective therapy for *M. avium-intracellulare* infection. *M. tuberculosis* infection is treated with antituberculosis chemotherapy. CMV hepatitis in AIDS may respond to ganciclovir. Therapy for hepatic fungal infection is amphotericin B and fluconazole.

Table 37-3. PROGNOSTIC CRITERIA FOR PREDICTING REQUIRED LIVER TRANSPLANTATION IN PATIENTS WITH FULMINANT HEPATIC FAILURE

Cause of Liver Failure	Criteria
Acetaminophen toxicity	pH <7.3 (irrespective of grade of encephalopathy) *or* Prothrombin time >100 s and serum creatinine >3.4 mg/dL (300 µmol/L) in patients with grade III or IV encephalopathy
All other causes	Prothrombin time >100 s (irrespective of grade encephalopathy) *or* Any three of the following variables (irrespective of grade of encephalopathy): Age <10 years or >40 years; Liver failure due to halothane or other drug idiosyncrasy or idiopathic hepatitis; Duration of jaundice prior to encephalopathy >7 d; Prothrombin time >50 s; Serum bilirubin >17.5 mg/dL (300 µmol/L)

(Adapted from O'Grady JG, Alexander GJM, Hayllar KM, Williams R. Early indicators of prognosis in fulminant hepatic failure. Gastroenterology 1989;97:439)

HEPATIC INFECTIONS IN IMMUNOSUPPRESSED HOSTS

Systemic infections that affect the liver and other tissues in immunosuppressed patients include infections with *M. tuberculosis*, CMV, VZV, and *Candida albicans*.

When a patient with chronic HBV receives an orthotopic liver graft, infection of the grafted liver with HBV is almost invariable and often causes liver injury. Frequent administration of exogenous anti-HBsAg may reduce the frequency and severity of recurrent HBV infection in the allograft. HDV infection recurs in the grafted liver but may not have a severe course. HCV infection commonly recurs in a grafted liver. CMV infection of a liver graft is rarely disseminated and often resolves without treatment, but ganciclovir is effective if treatment is needed.

Hepatitis B in recipients of renal grafts usually represents HBV infection acquired before transplantation. HCV infection may occur in renal transplants. CMV hepatitis in renal graft recipients is probably part of a disseminated CMV infection.

SUGGESTED READING

Farci P, Mandas A, Coiana A, et al. Treatment of chronic hepatitis D with interferon alpha-2a. N Engl J Med 1994;330:88.

Innes BL, Snitbhan R, Kunasol P, et al. Protection against hepatitis A by an inactivated vaccine. JAMA 1994;271:1328.

Jones EA, Schafer DF. Fulminant hepatic failure. In: Zakin D, Boyer TWB, eds. Hepatology: a textbook of liver disease, ed 2. Philadelphia, WB Saunders, 1990.

Krawczynski K. Hepatitis E. Hepatology 1993;17:932.

Lau JYN, Wright TL. Molecular virology and pathogenesis of hepatitis B. Lancet 1993;342:1335.

Samuel D, Muller R, Alexander G, et al. Liver transplantation in European patients with the hepatitis B surface antigen. N Engl J Med 1993;329:1842.

Schneiderman DJ, Arenson DM, Cello JP, Margaretten W, Weber TE. Hepatic disease in patients with the acquired immune deficiency syndrome (AIDS). Hepatology 1987;7:925.

Takahashi M, Yamada G, Miyamoto R, Doi T, Endo H, Tsuji T. Natural course of chronic hepatitis C. Am J Gastroenterol 1993;88:240.

ESSENTIALS OF SURGERY: SCIENTIFIC PRINCIPLES AND PRACTICE, edited by Lazar J. Greenfield, Michael W. Mulholland, Keith T. Oldham, Gerald B. Zelenock, and Keith D. Lillemoe. Lippincott–Raven Publishers, Philadelphia, © 1997.

CHAPTER 38

CIRRHOSIS AND PORTAL HYPERTENSION

FREDERIC E. ECKHAUSER AND JEREMIAH G. TURCOTTE

CIRRHOSIS

Cirrhosis is necrosis, regeneration, and scarring of the liver. The disease is classified according to morphologic, histologic, and etiologic criteria (Table 38-1). Etiologic factors include alcohol consumption (Table 38-2), viral hepatitis, toxins, chronic biliary obstruction, genetically transmitted metabolic disorders, and possibly malnutrition.

Table 38-1. CLASSIFICATION OF CIRRHOSIS

MORPHOLOGIC	ETIOLOGIC
Macronodular	Alcohol
Micronodular	Viral hepatitis
Mixed	Biliary obstruction
	Primary
HISTOLOGIC	Secondary
Portal	Venoocclusive
Postnecrotic	Hemochromatosis
Posthepatitic	Wilson disease
Primary obstructive	Autoimmune
Primary	Syphilis
Secondary	Drugs and toxins
Venoocclusive	α_1-Antitrypsin deficiency
	Cystic fibrosis
	Glycogen storage disease
	Other metabolic diseases
	Sarcoidosis
	Copper
	Small bowel bypass
	Idiopathic

(Modified from Conn HO, Atterbury CE. Cirrhosis. In: Schiff L, Schiff ER, eds. Diseases of the liver, ed 6. Philadelphia, JB Lippincott, 1987:726)

Pathogenesis

The normal hepatic response to necrosis is an attempt at regeneration, which may be impaired in several ways (Fig. 38-1). Fibrogenesis occurs in the nonregenerating areas of necrosis, producing scars. As attempts at restoration continue, fibrotic zones connect to produce septa, which surround the residual parenchyma. Proliferation of residual parenchyma is limited by the enveloping scars, producing nodular areas. The process of destruction, scarring, and nodularity distorts the vascular architecture. Venous obstruction causes portal hypertension and formation of intrahepatic arterioportal and portohepatic venous shunts that impair sinusoidal perfusion and hepatocyte function.

Clinical Features

Latent (Compensated) Cirrhosis

Latent cirrhosis may be discovered during a routine physical examination for nondescript symptoms, such as fatigue, anorexia, and weight loss. Physical findings include palmar erythema, spider angiomata, Dupuytren contractures, and hepatosplenomegaly. Ascites and dilated abdominal wall veins indicate portal hypertension.

Biochemical studies may be normal or abnormal. Subtle changes in serum transaminases, hypoalbuminemia, and hyperglobulinemia may be the earliest biochemical clues. The diagnosis is made only with liver biopsy. Patients with compensated cirrhosis usually remain free of symptoms for many years, but eventually most have complications related to hepatic failure or portal hypertension (variceal bleeding, ascites, or encephalopathy).

Active (Decompensated) Cirrhosis

Patients have failing general health, muscle wasting, jaundice, and ascites, with or without peripheral edema. Precipitating factors include exposure to hepatotoxins such as alcohol, drugs, and anesthetic agents; GI bleeding; electrolyte imbalances; and intercurrent infections. Unexplained fever or sepsis may be due to spontaneous bacterial peritonitis or altered hepatic reticuloendothelial function and intrahepatic portosystemic shunting. Mental aberra-

Table 38-2. EFFECTS OF ALCOHOL ON LIVER CELL FUNCTION

Disorganizes the lipid portion of cell membranes, leading to adaptive changes in their composition
Alters capacity of cells to cope with environmental toxins
  Biotransformation to create toxic intermediates
  Interference with normal detoxifying mechanisms
  Increased synthesis of endogenous toxins
Oxidation of alcohol produces acetaldehyde, a toxic and reactive intermediate
Inhibits protein export from liver
Modifies hepatic protein synthesis in fasted animals
Alters structure and function (energy production) of mitochondria
Alters metabolism of cofactors essential for enzyme activity (pyridoxine, folate, choline, vitamin E)
Alters oxidation reduction potential of liver cell

(Modified from Zakim D, Boyer TD. Hepatology: a textbook of liver disease. Philadelphia, WB Saunders, 1982:759)

tions, a flapping tremor, and fetor hepaticus may be present in patients with severe decompensation. Jaundice is common, and its intensity correlates roughly with the severity of hepatic dysfunction.

Abnormal laboratory findings include elevated levels of serum bilirubin, alkaline phosphatase, and γ-globulin. Anemia is a frequent finding. Hypersplenism may cause leukopenia or thrombocytopenia. Prothrombin time is prolonged and may be unresponsive to parenteral vitamin K.

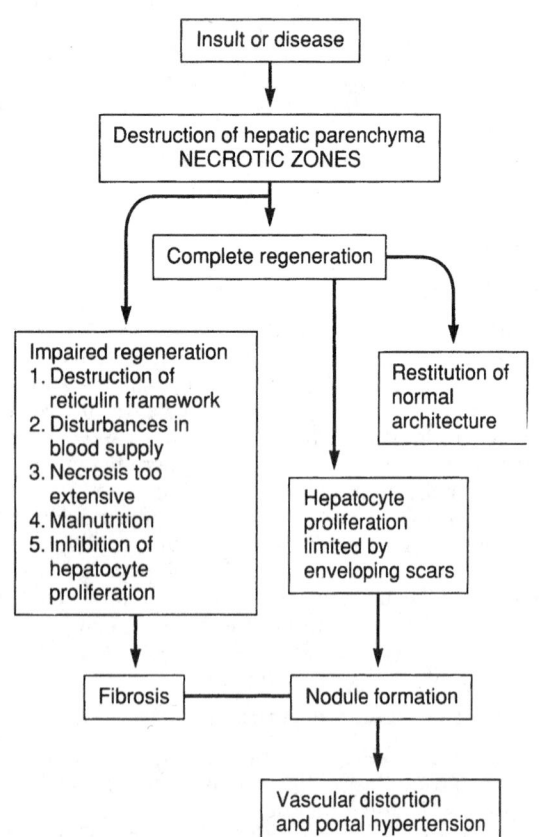

Figure 38-1. The evolution of cirrhosis. Fibrosis occurs in nonregenerative necrotic areas, producing scars. The pattern of nodularity and scars reflects the type of response to injury (eg, uniform versus nonuniform necrosis) and the extent of injury.

Systemic Manifestations of Chronic Liver Disease

Hepatic failure affects virtually every organ system in the body. It may occur as a rapidly progressive lesion in the absence of preexisting liver disease or as a terminal event in patients with chronic active hepatitis or end-stage cirrhosis.

Cardiorespiratory Manifestations

Table 38-3 summarizes the cardiorespiratory abnormalities observed in patients with cirrhosis. Patients with progressive hepatic decompensation often have an unbalanced hyperdynamic state similar to that seen in sepsis. Findings include an increase in mixed venous oxygen saturation, a decrease in the arteriovenous oxygen gradient, and metabolic acidosis. These changes are consistent with arteriovenous shunting and diversion of blood away from nutrient capillary beds. Patients in this decompensated state frequently exhibit altered cardiovascular reactivity with decreased responsiveness to administration of exogenous norepinephrine.

Pulmonary Manifestations

The pulmonary manifestations of cirrhosis include dyspnea, cyanosis, clubbing, and arterial oxygen desaturation. Abdominal distention due to ascites may produce areas of pulmonary collapse and alter the ventilation–perfusion ratio.

Renal Manifestations

Renal manifestations of hepatic failure include impaired sodium handling, impaired water excretion, and progressive, oliguric renal failure (hepatorenal syndrome). These patients exhibit renal function abnormalities different from those of acute renal failure, but often indistinguishable from those of prerenal azotemia. Therapy is discontinuation of diuretics and other drugs that may impair renal function, provision of satisfactory intravascular volume, and treatment of septicemia.

Endocrine Function (Disorders of Glucose Homeostasis)

Under normal fasting conditions, hepatic glucose production is necessary to supply glucose as an energy source for obligate glucose-metabolizing tissues, such as red blood cells (RBCs) and the central nervous system. Glucose intolerance is seen in patients with chronic forms of cirrhosis, hemochromatosis, and acute hepatitis. Growth hormone also is implicated in the glucose intolerance of chronic liver disease.

Table 38-3. CARDIORESPIRATORY ABNORMALITIES IN CIRRHOSIS

Abnormality	Pathophysiology
↓ Arterial P_{O_2}	Portopulmonary and intrapulmonary shunts
↓ Arteriovenous O_2 difference	Arteriolar and capillary shunts
↓ Peripheral resistance	Systemic-splanchnic arteriovenous shunts
↑ Cardiac output	Low peripheral resistance
↑ Plasma volume	Increased whole body sodium and water secondary to hyperaldosteronism
	Low peripheral resistance

Neuropsychiatric Manifestations

Hepatic encephalopathy is related to impaired hepatic extraction and metabolism of neuroactive metabolites that cause neural inhibition. Patients present with variable obtundation and mental confusion. Progression of encephalopathy is characterized by the development of asterixis (a coarse, flapping hand tremor elicited by asking the patient to hyperextend the wrist) and fetor hepaticus (a breath odor probably related to pulmonary excretion of mercaptans). Laboratory studies are nonspecific and reflect only the presence of advanced liver disease. EEG abnormalities are nonspecific. Treatment is outlined in Table 38-4.

PORTAL HYPERTENSION

Anatomy

The three major splanchnic veins are the hepatic portal vein and its two major tributaries, the superior mesenteric and splenic veins. Variations in the confluence of the splenic vein and superior mesenteric vein preclude some portosystemic shunts.

Physiology

Portosystemic Collaterals and the Hyperdynamic State

An increase in portal pressure leads to spontaneous development of portosystemic collateral vessels in an attempt to decompress the portal system. These collateral vessels increase venous return to the heart and increase cardiac output (Fig. 38-2). With portal vein stenosis, increases in blood flow occur in all segments of the GI tract, muscle, and kidney, primarily as a result of precapillary vasodilatation. Peripheral vasodilatation leads to increased venous return, decreased systemic vascular resistance, and increased cardiac output. Arteriovenous connections in the gastric submucosa may cause portal hypertensive gastropathy.

Table 38-4. TREATMENT OF HEPATIC ENCEPHALOPATHY

Identify precipitating factors
    Disordered carbohydrate metabolism
    Narcotics
    Infection
    Hypotension
    Hypoxia
    Excess exogenous protein
    Gastrointestinal bleeding
    Electrolyte abnormalities
    Alkalosis
Supportive therapy
    Eliminate dietary nitrogen
    Purge gastrointestinal tract to remove blood and other
      nitrogenous compounds
    Nonabsorbable antibiotics (neomycin or metronidazole)
    Lactulose or lactilol
Dopamine receptor agonists
    L-Dopa and bromocriptine*
Branched-chain amino acids†
Temporary liver support
Orthotopic liver transplantation

---

* Arousal effect in selected patients may be due to enhanced renal function.

† High cost and equivocal benefits of intravenous amino acid mixtures make it difficult to justify routine use.

Changes in Blood Volume and Hepatic Resistance

Plasma volume is increased in patients with cirrhotic and noncirrhotic portal hypertension and in patients with cirrhosis with acute variceal hemorrhage. In a vessel at the limits of compliance, such as an esophageal varix, a small increase in volume causes a large increase in wall tension that results in rupture. Injudicious volume overexpansion may precipitate variceal bleeding.

Extrinsic neurohumoral mechanisms exist to control resistance of the hepatic vasculature. The following endogenous compounds modulate hepatic resistance:

Agents That Increase Splanchnic Flow

Bile acids
Bradykinin
Cholecystokinin
Epinephrine
Gastrin
Glucagon
Histamine
Neurotensin
Prostaglandins PGI_2, PGE_1, PGA_1, and PGA_2
Vasoactive intestinal peptide (VIP; in high doses)

Agents That Decrease Splanchnic Flow

Epinephrine (in high doses)
Norepinephrine
Prostaglandins PGF_{2a} and PGD_2
Thromboxane B_2
Somatostatin
VIP (in low doses)

Pathophysiology of Variceal Hemorrhage

Portal and Variceal Pressure

Measurement of portal pressure is used to estimate risk for variceal hemorrhage and response to therapy. It is presumed that portal pressure is directly proportional to variceal pressure.

Variceal Size and Appearance

Size of varices alone is not predictive of variceal hemorrhage. Signs associated with impending rupture are listed in Table 38-5.

Ascites

Pathophysiology

Scarring and regeneration that distort the intrahepatic vascular architecture elevate hepatic sinusoidal and intestinal capillary pressures. These factors contribute to transudation of fluid into the peritoneal cavity. Ascitic fluid is a mixture of hepatic and splanchnic lymph.

The pathogenesis of ascites in cirrhosis has not been fully elucidated. Theories are contraction or expansion of plasma volume that lead to stimulation or suppression of the renin-angiotensin-aldosterone system.

Clinical Features

Ascites may develop abruptly or slowly over several months. The onset of ascites usually indicates the presence of advanced liver disease. Rapid-onset ascites is usually related to a precipitating event, such as upper GI hemorrhage, excessive diuretic therapy with dehydration, electrolyte imbalance, exposure to hepatotoxins, or growth of

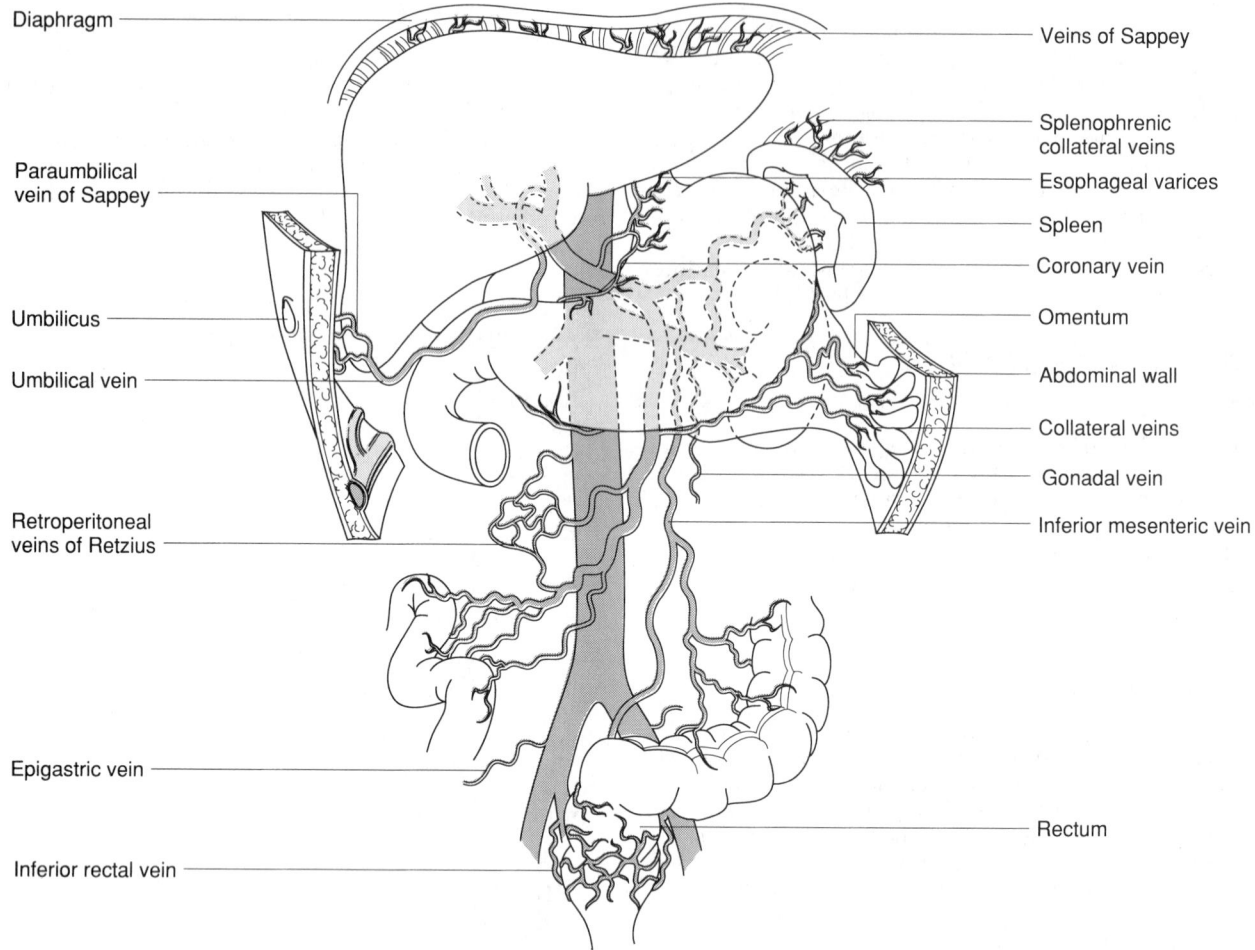

Figure 38-2. Potential venous collaterals that develop with portal hypertension. The veins of Sappey drain portal blood through the bare areas of the diaphragm and through paraumbilical vein collaterals to the umbilicus. The veins of Retzius form in the retroperitoneum and shunt portal blood from the bowel and other organs to the vena cava.

a cirrhosis-associated hepatic tumor. The short-term prognosis is good if the underlying cause can be corrected.

Patients with cirrhosis and ascites exhibit the following physical findings:

Peripheral muscle wasting
Conspicuous abdominal distention
Umbilical and inguinal hernias

Recanalization of the umbilical vein with distention of periumbilical collaterals to form a caput medusa
A thrill and a bruit over the epigastrium
Pleural effusion (10% of patients)
Peripheral edema of the lower extremities

Diagnosis

Diagnostic paracentesis is performed to confirm the cause of ascites. The abdominal wall is examined with Doppler ultrasound (US) to identify sites of high flow, indicating the presence of nearby dilated collaterals or epigastric vessels.

Cirrhotic ascitic fluid is usually straw-colored, clear, or greenish. Blood-staining indicates a malignant tumor. To help differentiate the causes of ascites (Table 38-6), an aliquot of ascitic fluid is evaluated for protein, RBC count, white blood cell (WBC) count and differential, amylase, pH, glucose, and culture and sensitivity.

Complications

Spontaneous bacterial peritonitis (SBP) is the presence of infected ascitic fluid without a demonstrated site of infection. SBP appears to be caused by translocation of bacteria through the intestinal wall (Table 38-7). SBP must be differentiated from other causes of peritonitis (Table 38-8).

Umbilical and other abdominal wall hernias result from

Table 38-5. ENDOSCOPIC SIGNS THAT CORRELATE WITH RISK OF VARICEAL RUPTURE

Category	Subcategory
Basic color	White varices
	Blue varices
Signs	Red color sign
	Red wale marking
	Cherry red spot
	Hematocystic spot
	Diffuse redness
Form	Linear
	Tortuous
	Large

(Japanese Research Society for Portal Hypertension)

Table 38-6. DIFFERENTIAL DIAGNOSIS OF ASCITES

PORTAL HYPERTENSION

Cirrhosis and other intrahepatic diseases
Hepatic congestion
    Congestive heart failure
    Constrictive pericarditis
    Inferior vena cava obstruction
    Budd-Chiari syndrome
Portal vein occlusion

HYPOALBUMINEMIA

Nephrotic syndrome
Protein-losing enteropathy
Malnutrition

MISCELLANEOUS DISORDERS

Myxedema
Ovarian disease (Meig syndrome, struma ovarii)
Peritoneal carcinomatosis
Pancreatic ascites
End-stage renal disease
Chylous ascites
Bile ascites
Urine ascites

(Sleisenger MH, Fordtran JS. Gastrointestinal disease: pathophysiology, diagnosis and management, ed 4. Philadelphia, WB Saunders, 1989:433)

increased intraabdominal pressure and wasting of abdominal wall muscles.

Therapy

Ascites unresponsive to medical therapy is usually a manifestation of end-stage liver disease. The most expedient treatment is orthotopic hepatic transplantation. This solution is not feasible for many patients, so therapy involves:

- Sodium and fluid restriction
- Diuretics
- Therapeutic paracentesis
- Surgical implantation of a peritoneovenous shunt or a transjugular intrahepatic portosystemic shunt (TIPS)

Budd–Chiari Syndrome and Venoocclusive Disease

Budd–Chiari syndrome is obstruction of venous outflow from the liver due to endophlebitis obliterans and occlusion of the hepatic veins or suprahepatic inferior vena cava

Table 38-7. BACTERIOLOGY OF SPONTANEOUS BACTERIAL PERITONITIS

Organisms	Percentage of Total
Escherichia coli	40
Pneumococci	15
Streptococci	14
Klebsiella	7
Pseudomonas	3
Proteus	3
Staphylococci	3
Anaerobes	5
Other	20
Multiple isolates	10

(Adapted from Targan S, Chow A, Gluze L. Role of anaerobic bacteria in spontaneous peritonitis of cirrhosis. Am J Med 1977;62:397)

Table 38-8. DIFFERENTIAL DIAGNOSIS OF SPONTANEOUS BACTERIAL PERITONITIS AS DISTINGUISHED FROM NONSPONTANEOUS BACTERIAL PERITONITIS

Feature	Spontaneous	Nonspontaneous
History of GI disease	Usually negative	Often positive
Abdominal examination	Positive rebound	Pain, rigidity
Pneumoperitoneum	Absent	Often present
Appearance of fluid	Frequently clear	Cloudy to purulent
Ascites fluid pH	7.0–7.4	6.5–7.3
Ascites fluid glucose	Same as blood	Lower than blood
Species of bacteria	Single	Multiple
Anaerobes	Rare	Common
Blood in ascites fluid	Rare	Common

(Adapted from Schiff L, Schiff ER. Diseases of the liver, ed 6. Philadelphia, JB Lippincott, 1987:83)

from thrombosis or obstructing webs. The causes vary (Table 38-9).

Clinical Features

    Right-upper-quadrant pain
    Hepatomegaly
    Ascites
    Fulminant hepatic failure (small percentage of patients)
    Slowly progressive disease
    Peripheral muscle wasting

Diagnosis

Figure 38-3 is an algorithm for the management of Budd–Chiari syndrome. Routine determinations of liver function, including serum aminotransferases, and alkaline phosphatase are only moderately abnormal. Technetium colloid hepatic scintiscans show diffuse, nonhomogeneous uptake in the periphery of the liver with pronounced central concentration over the caudate lobe. Vena caval and

Table 38-9. ETIOLOGIC FACTORS IN BUDD-CHIARI SYNDROME

Idiopathic
Hematologic disorders
    Polycythemia vera
    Paroxysmal nocturnal hemoglobinuria
    Myeloproliferative disorders
    Antithrombin ill deficiency
    Circulating lupus anticoagulants
Oral contraceptives
Pregnancy and postpartum
Tumors
    Hepatocellular carcinoma
    Renal cell carcinoma
    Adrenal carcinoma
    Leiomyosarcoma of the inferior vena cava
Vena caval webs
Infections
    Amebic abscess
    Aspergillosis
    Hydatid cyst
Phlebitis
Trauma
Venocclusive disease

(Adapted from Maddrey WS. Hepatic vein thrombosis [Budd-Chiari syndrome]. Hepatology 1984;4:44S)

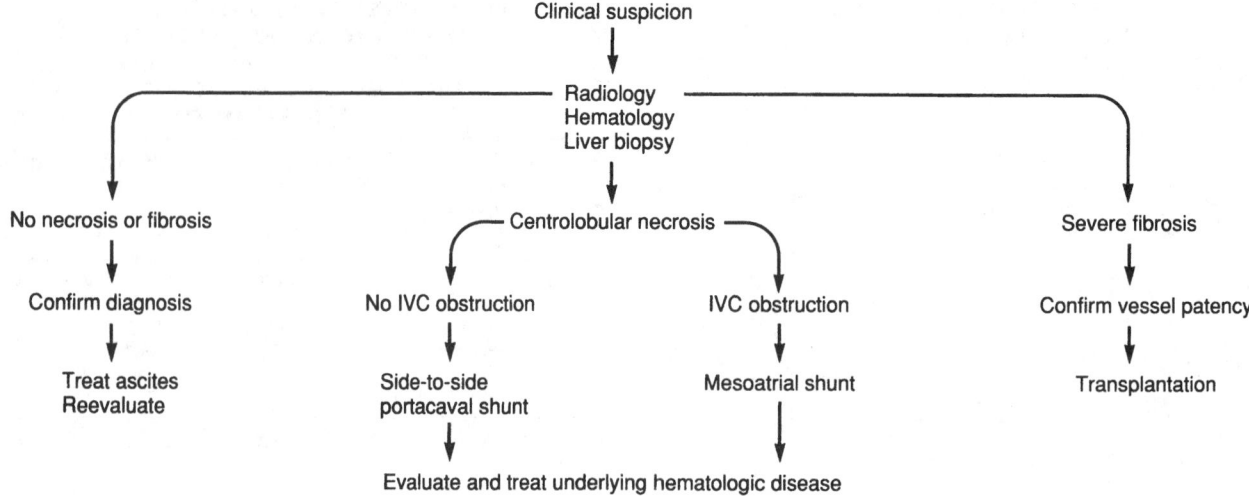

Figure 38-3. Algorithm for treating patients with Budd-Chiari syndrome. IVC, inferior vena cava. (After Henderson JM, Warren WD, Millikan WJ, et al. Surgical options: hematologic evaluation and pathologic changes in Budd-Chiari syndrome. Am J Surg 1990;1959:41)

hepatic vein catheterization is the standard for establishing the diagnosis. Liver biopsy is performed whenever possible. Features include centrilobular congestion, sinusoidal dilatation, cell dropout in the absence of a marked inflammatory response, and fibrosis.

Treatment

Intensive medical treatment with diuretics and anticoagulants may relieve symptoms but does not appear to confer survival benefit. Peritoneovenous shunts relieve ascites but do not decompress the liver or halt the progression of liver injury. Effective surgical approaches to Budd–Chiari syndrome are construction of a portosystemic shunt, resection of membranous webs, and orthotopic hepatic transplantation.

Differential Diagnosis of Portal Hypertension

The causes of portal hypertension are disorders that increase resistance or disorders that increase flow (Table 38-10).

Therapy for Gastroesophageal Variceal Hemorrhage

The choice of elective therapy for gastroesophageal variceal hemorrhage depends on:

*   The natural history of the disease causing the portal hypertension
*   Residual hepatic function
*   The presence of associated disease
*   Continuing drug or alcohol abuse
*   The patency of the splanchnic veins
*   The location of the varices causing the bleeding

Laboratory and clinical factors used to categorize portal hypertension are presented in Table 38-11.

By far, the most common location of bleeding varices is the esophagus, followed by the stomach, duodenum, ileum, bladder, and colostomy or ileostomy stomas.

Most patients with bleeding varices who have good or moderate hepatic function undergo a trial of serial sclerotherapy. If sclerotherapy fails or is not feasible, a portosys-temic shunt is considered. Decompression with a portosystemic shunt is the most feasible therapy for bleeding varices distal to the esophagus and for portal hypertensive gastropathy. Patients with poor liver function or with rapidly progressive liver disease undergo hepatic transplantation.

Medical Management

Drugs used to treat gastroesophageal variceal hemorrhage are vasopressin, somatostatin, and propranolol. Balloon tamponade is used to treat acute variceal hemorrhage unresponsive to drugs or sclerotherapy.

Endoscopic Sclerotherapy

The goal of sclerotherapy is to obliterate the variceal lumen or induce sclerosis of the submucosa, where varices usually originate (Fig. 38-4). A substance, usually sodium morrhuate, is injected directly into a varix (intravariceal) or into the submucosa between varices (paravariceal). The goal of paravariceal injection is to eradicate the submucosal space and compress the varices. Such an approach may take several days to be effective and is not suitable for controlling acute hemorrhage.

Complications of sclerotherapy are:

Transient substernal chest pain

*   Dysphagia
*   Stricture
*   Ulceration
*   Esophageal perforation
*   Cardiac arrest, coronary spasm and tamponade
*   Asymptomatic pleural effusions, aspiration pneumonia, ARDS
*   Bacteremia, perinephric abscess, brain abscess, endocarditis

Endoscopic Variceal Ligation

In endoscopic variceal ligation (EVL) suction and O rings are used to arrest bleeding or achieve complete variceal obliteration (Fig. 38-5). EVL produces superficial mucosal ulcerations that epithelialize and heal within 21 days.

Table 38-10. COMMON CAUSES OF PORTAL HYPERTENSION

DISORDERS THAT PRIMARILY INCREASE RESISTANCE TO FLOW

Prehepatic

Congenital atresia
Extrinsic compression
Portal, superior mesenteric, or splenic vein thrombosis

Hepatic

CIRRHOSIS

α_1-Antitrypsin deficiency
Cryptogenic cirrhosis
Cystic fibrosis
Hemochromatosis
Nutritional (alcoholic)
Posthepatic
Wilson disease

CONGENITAL HEPATITIC FIBROSIS

Focal regenerative hyperplasia
Hepatic venoocclusive disease
Idiopathic
Metastatic carcinoma
Sarcoidosis
Schistosomiasis
Toxin and drug injuries

ACUTE DISEASE

Acute fatty liver
Alcoholic hepatitis
Fulminant hepatic failure

Posthepatic

Budd-Chiari syndrome
Chronic heart failure
Constrictive pericarditis
Vena caval webs

DISORDERS THAT PRIMARILY INCREASE FLOW

Arterioportal Fistula

Hepatocellular carcinoma
Mesenteric arteriosclerotic or aneurysmal vascular disease
Osler-Weber-Rendu syndrome

Splenomegaly

Transjugular Intrahepatic Portosystemic Shunt

TIPS is used to treat protracted bleeding with hemodynamic instability, progressive coagulopathy, and visceral hypoperfusion. It is easier to perform and is safer than a portosystemic shunt. The procedure is as follows:

- Cannulation of the suprahepatic inferior vena cava and hepatic veins with an angiography catheter introduced through the jugular vein
- Replacement of the angiography catheter with a specialized instrument advanced under fluoroscopic guidance through the hepatic parenchyma to establish a track between branches of the hepatic and portal veins
- Positioning of an angioplasty balloon catheter across the parenchymal track and inflation of the balloon
- Withdrawal of the balloon catheter and insertion of a delivery catheter that contains a metal stent
- Deployment of the stent to cover the entire parenchymal track and to extend several millimeters into the lumen of the hepatic and portal veins

- Radiographic confirmation of stent placement and measurement of pressure across the stent to ensure portal decompression
- If portal decompression is suboptimal, dilation of the stent with an angiographic balloon or a second stent

Complications of TIPS include encephalopathy and stenosis or occlusion of the stent. Encephalopathy is managed with dietary protein restriction and lactulose. All patients with TIPS are examined with duplex US at intervals to assess shunt patency and flow. Equivocal results prompt angiographic evaluation.

Portosystemic Shunts

Portosystemic shunts may be categorized according to their hemodynamic characteristics:

Nonselective Shunts
End-to-side portacaval shunt—diverts all portal blood around the liver (Fig. 38-6)
Lateral shunt—diverts all or some portal blood
   Side-to-side portacaval
   Interposition portacaval
   Marion–Clatworthy cavomesal
   Central splenorenal
Selective Shunts
Distal splenorenal shunt
Small-diameter portacaval shunt
Small-diameter mesocaval shunt

Preoperative and Postoperative Care

Fluid. Sodium and water replacement are restricted preoperatively and postoperatively, especially if ascites is present. Third-space losses are replaced conservatively with crystalloid in the early postoperative phase. After third-space fluid sequestration is replaced, little or no additional sodium is administered. The patients receive sufficient sodium because most drugs are in the form of a sodium salt and all blood products contain large quantities of sodium. Potassium is monitored and replaced.

Cardiorespiratory Function. Arterial oxygen pressure is low, cardiac output high, peripheral resistance low, and plasma volume expanded (Table 38-12). The baseline values for blood gas and Swan-Ganz pressure and cardiac output determinations may vary substantially from normal ranges.

Table 38-11. CHILD-TURCOTTE HEPATIC RISK CLASSIFICATION*

Parameter	Category		
	A	B	C
Bilirubin (mg/dL)	<2	2–3	>3
Albumin (g/dL)	>3.5	3–3.5	<3
Ascites	None	Treatable	Refractory
Encephalopathy	None	Minimal	Severe
Nutrition (muscle mass)	Normal	Fair	Poor

* This system correlates with operative mortality and long-term prognosis after construction of portosystemic shunts and has been used to estimate hepatic reserve and prognosis in many other clinical settings. Five variables are included because no single test reliably estimates operative mortality or long-term prognosis. Some judgment is needed in applying this system, because patients' laboratory studies or clinical status frequently overlap into more than one risk category.

(Wantz GE, Payne MA. Experience with portacaval shunt for portal hypertension. N Engl J Med 1961;265:721.)

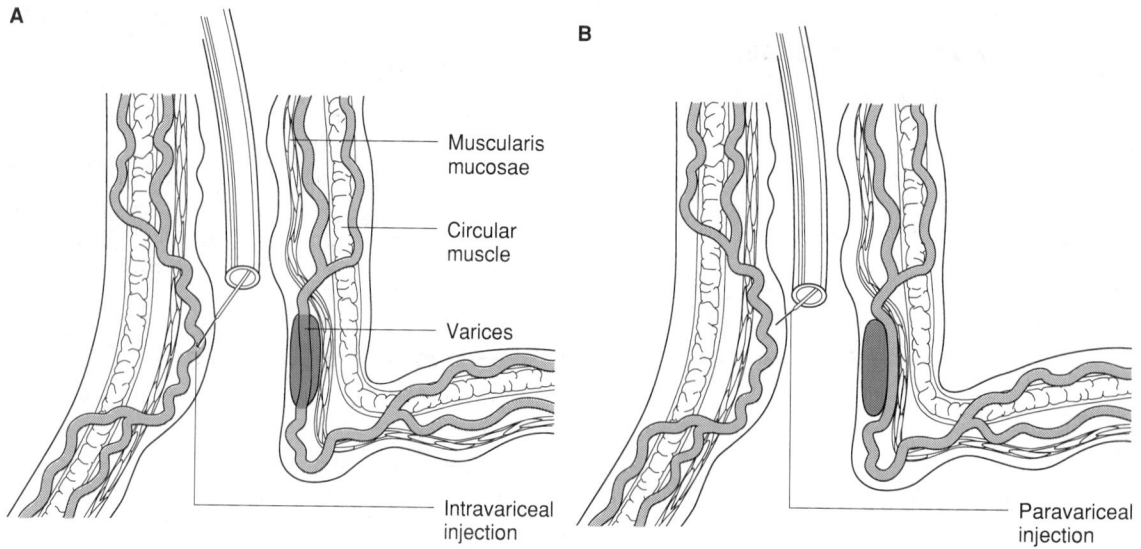

Figure 38-4. Techniques of intravariceal (*A*) and paravariceal (*B*) injection of esophageal varices.

These baseline deviations from normal are corrected when severe and are taken into account in interpretation of blood gas and pulmonary artery tests, both before and after the operation.

Coagulation Abnormalities. If secondary hypersplenism is present, platelet, WBC, and RBC counts may be low. Replacement with fresh frozen plasma, platelets, and cryoprecipitate (factor VIII) is almost always needed intraoperatively, and is continued postoperatively until the coagulation status has stabilized and all bleeding has halted.

Nutrition. As much as twice normal caloric intake may be needed to achieve caloric balance. Most patients tolerate IV hyperalimentation if excessive amounts of protein or amino acids are not infused. Early enteral feeding is desirable to avoid infection due to translocation of bacteria from the GI tract. Vitamin supplementation, especially A, D, K,

and B, is recommended. Magnesium, zinc, calcium, and phosphorous are monitored and replaced, if needed.

Devascularization and Transection Procedures

Nonshunting procedures to treat gastroesophageal hemorrhage range from simple transection or stapling of the esophagus or proximal stomach to extensive esophagogas-

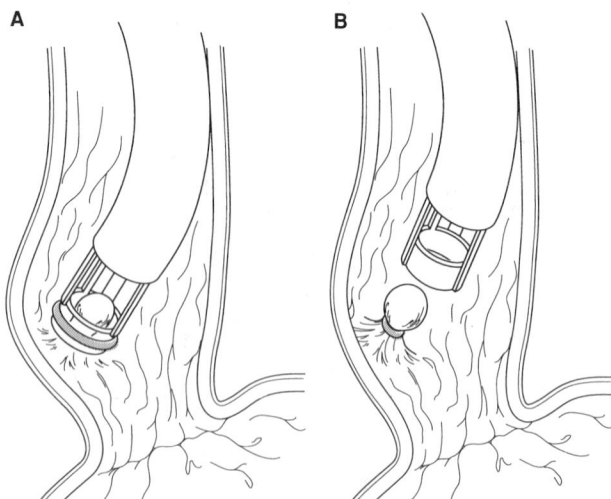

Figure 38-5. Endoscopic ligation of esophageal varices. The device for ligation is based on the standard Barron-type ligater used in the treatment of anal hemorrhoids. The esophageal varix is drawn up into the ligating device with suction (*A*), and the base of the varix is ligated with an O-ring (*B*). Up to six varices can be treated at a single session.

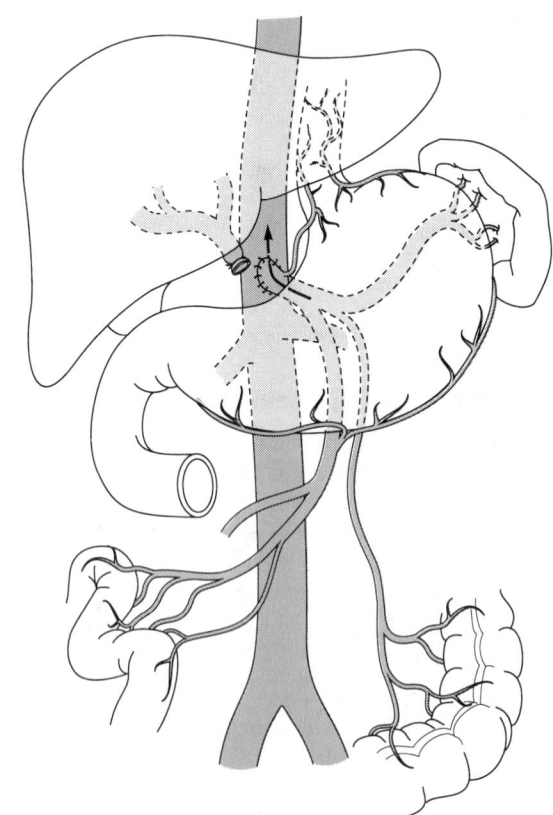

Figure 38-6. End-to-side portocaval shunt. This shunt is also referred to as an Eck fistula. The portal vein is divided. The hepatic limb of the portal vein is ligated. The splanchnic end of the portal vein is anastomosed end to side of the vena cava. All portal blood is necessarily diverted into the cava, and the hepatic limb of the portal vein cannot serve as an outflow track.

Table 38-12. CARDIORESPIRATORY PHYSIOLOGY IN PATIENTS WITH HEPATIC CIRRHOSIS

Abnormality	Pathophysiology	Physical Signs
P_{O_2} and oxyhemoglobin saturation decreased	Portopulmonary and intrapulmonary shunts	Cyanosis, clubbing of fingers
Arteriovenous oxygen difference decreased	Arteriolar or capillary shunts	Palmer erythema, spider telangiectasia
Peripheral resistance decreased	Systemic and splanchnic arteriovenous shunts	Tendency to hypotension, hypertension unusual, widened pulse pressure
Cardiac output increased	Low peripheral resistance, expanded plasma volume	Systolic ejection murmur, short occlusion time, rapid pulse
Plasma volume increased	Increased total body sodium and water, secondary aldosteronism	Edema, ascites, high-output cardiac failure if severe

tric devascularization and splenectomy. Transection of the esophagus or stomach interrupts the submucosal and intermuscular venous collateral vessels. Splenectomy eliminates the splenic component of portal blood flow, which may temporarily lower portal pressure.

Most esophageal and gastric transection procedures are performed with stapling devices. Perioperative complications include leaks due to faulty technique, ischemia, and stenosis of the anastomosis. Late complications of esophageal transection are stricture formation and recurrence of variceal bleeding.

The role of devascularization and transection procedures is not clear. Some surgeons believe these operations can be performed on patients at good risk in whom sclerotherapy is not feasible or has failed, especially patients in whom the portal, splenic, or superior mesenteric veins are thrombosed, precluding construction of a conventional shunt.

SUGGESTED READING

Benner KG, Sahagun G, Saxon R, Barton RE, et al. Selection of patients undergoing transjugular intrahepatic portosystemic shunting for refractory ascites. Hepatology 1994;20:69A.

Conn HO. Transjugular intrahepatic portal-systemic shunt: the state of the art. Hepatology 1993;17:148.

Gimson AE, Ramage JK, Panos MZ, et al. Randomized trial of variceal band ligation versus injection sclerotherapy for bleeding esophageal varices. Lancet 1993;342:391.

Hashizume M, Ohta M, Ueno K, et al. Endoscopic ligation of esophageal varices compared with injection sclerotherapy: a prospective, randomized trial. Gastrointest Endosc 1993; 39:123.

Hillaire S, Labianca M, Borgonovo G, et al. Peritoneovenous shunting of intractable ascites in patients with cirrhosis: improving results and predictive factors of failure. Surgery 1993;113:373.

Lebrec D, Giuily N, Hadeneque A, et al. Transjugular intrahepatic portosystemic shunt vs. paracentesis for refractory ascites: results of a randomized trial. Hepatology 1994;20:417A.

Pomier-Layragues G, Legault L, Roy L, et al. TIPS for treatment of refractory ascites: a pilot study. Hepatology 1993;18:187A.

Ring EJ, Lake JR, Roberts JP. Using transjugular intrahepatic portosystemic shunts to control variceal bleeding before liver transplantation. Ann Intern Med 1992;16:304.

Stiegmann GV, Goff JS, Michaletz-Onody PA, et al. Endoscopic sclerotherapy compared to endoscopic ligation for bleeding esophageal varices. N Engl J Med 1992;326:1527.

ESSENTIALS OF SURGERY: SCIENTIFIC PRINCIPLES AND PRACTICE, edited by Lazar J. Greenfield, Michael W. Mulholland, Keith T. Oldham, Gerald B. Zelenock, and Keith D. Lillemoe. Lippincott–Raven Publishers, Philadelphia, © 1997.

CHAPTER 39

HEPATIC NEOPLASMS

JOHN B. HANKS AND W. SCOTT ARNOLD

BENIGN LIVER DISEASE

Benign Solid Tumors

Hepatocellular Adenoma

More than 90% of adenomas occur in women 20 to 40 years of age, most of whom have used oral contraceptives. Adenomas also may occur in patients who take conjugated estrogens and in those with estrogen-producing tumors. The risk of hepatic adenoma appears to be related to the dosage and duration of use of estrogens. Adenoma also is associated with glycogen storage disease type 1 and use of anabolic steroids.

Histologic examination of hepatocellular adenoma shows benign, normal-appearing well-circumscribed hepatocytes that can be differentiated from normal parenchyma by a lack of bile duct architecture. Adenomas are not considered premalignant.

Symptoms of hepatocellular adenoma are abdominal pain and acute signs and symptoms, due to bleeding or rupture with intraperitoneal hemorrhage. Hepatomegaly or an upper abdominal mass is a common finding.

Laboratory tests are normal unless there has been bleeding.

Computed tomography (CT) is the most useful preliminary imaging study and often reveals areas of hemorrhage and necrosis. Angiography may add to CT findings by depicting a hypervascular tumor with a peripheral blood supply. ^{99m}Tc sulfur colloid scans show a cold spot, differentiating adenoma and focal nodular hyperplasia (FNH) but not other solid masses.

Treatment for patients with an acute abdomen and shock is emergency resection. Asymptomatic, or less acutely symptomatic, tumors also are treated with resection because the tumor tends to bleed and there is a small risk of coexistent malignant disease. Oral contraceptives are discontinued. If resection is too hazardous, conservative management is discontinuation of oral contraceptives and avoidance of pregnancy. Pregnancy is not associated with an increased incidence of adenoma, but it is associated with tumor growth, symptoms, and an increased tendency for the tumors to rupture.

Focal Nodular Hyperplasia

FNH predominantly affects young women, but it is also found in men and children. There is no clear relation between use of oral contraceptives and the development of FNH. FNH usually is asymptomatic and does not bleed or undergo malignant change. The lesion is usually an incidental finding. Patients who do have symptoms report abdominal discomfort. A few patients have hepatomegaly, a mass, or tenderness. Bleeding is rare.

Unlike adenomas, lesions of FNH are lobulated. Large lesions also have a central stellate scar. The histologic appearance of FNH is normal-appearing hepatocytes, bile ducts, and Kupffer cells.

Laboratory tests are normal in patients with FNH.

Imaging with CT, magnetic resonance imaging (MRI), and ultrasound (US) is sensitive for FNH, but frequently is nonspecific. Angiograms show a hypervascular mass similar to adenoma. Radionuclide imaging can be useful. FNH is the only lesion that contains Kupffer cells and, therefore, appears isodense rather than as a defect.

Treatment of asymptomatic disease is conservative when the diagnosis is clear. If there is any doubt about the diagnosis, an excisional biopsy is performed for small, easily removed lesions. An incisional or percutaneous core biopsy may be performed for large or inaccessible lesions. Therapy for symptomatic disease is individualized; the risk of removal of a large mass is greater than the risk of observation.

Bile Duct Hamartomas and Adenomas

Bile duct hamartoma and *bile duct adenoma* are two separate entities. Hamartomas are more common than adenomas. Both are small, incidental findings that are important because they are confused with metastatic or primary malignant tumors.

Benign Vascular Lesions

Cavernous hemangiomas of the liver are the most common benign hepatic tumor. They are the second most common hepatic tumor, exceeded only by metastases. The lesions occur in all age groups and more commonly in women and girls. Hemangiomas are not premalignant. The etiologic factors have not been defined. *Capillary* hemangiomas rarely occur in the liver and are of minimal clinical significance.

The histologic appearance of cavernous hemangiomas is cystically dilated, endothelium-lined vascular spaces.

Patients with symptoms usually have large masses. Symptoms include vague right-upper-quadrant discomfort, pain, fullness, early satiety, and sometimes nausea, vomiting, and fever. Physical examination may show hepatomegaly, mass, or bruit. Complications are rare but include obstructive jaundice, gastric outlet obstruction, and consumptive coagulopathy initiated by thrombosis within large hemangiomas. Spontaneous rupture or hemorrhage is infrequent.

Laboratory findings are normal in patients with hemangioma.

The most useful imaging studies are MRI, CT, and tagged red blood cell (RBC) scanning. These tests have largely replaced angiography. CT scans often have a characteristic enhancement pattern. Gadolinium-enhanced MRI is sensitive and specific in the diagnosis of hemangioma and has better resolution than tagged RBC scan. Fine-needle aspiration (FNA) biopsy of suspected hemangiomas is avoided if the diagnosis is secure with less-invasive procedures. A

common clinical problem is differentiating incidentally discovered hemangioma and malignant tumor. If the CT appearance is compatible with hemangioma, a tagged RBC scan or MRI is used to confirm the diagnosis.

Because of the benign natural history of hemangioma and its low risk of rupture, treatment is observation if there are no symptoms, especially for lesions <4 cm in diameter. Surgical excision is the only effective treatment of symptomatic masses, and is performed if the lesion is localized and accessible.

Benign Cystic Diseases

Congenital Hepatic Cysts

The pathogenesis of congenital hepatic cysts is unclear; they most likely occur when intralobular bile ducts fail to fuse with interlobular bile ducts because of dysgenesis, stenosis, or obstruction. Another theory is that the cysts are caused by congenital lymphatic obstruction.

Solitary Cysts. Solitary cysts are somewhat more common in women than in men and occur most frequently in the right lobe. They are more often multilocular than unilocular. There is no apparent genetic transmissibility or association with renal cysts.

Most congenital solitary cysts are asymptomatic. Symptoms if they occur include vague right-upper-quadrant discomfort or pain, a sensation of epigastric fullness or heaviness, early satiety, and nausea and vomiting from pressure of the cyst on adjacent viscera. Hepatomegaly or a palpable mass may occur; respiratory symptoms occur if the cyst is large. Complications are rare but include hemorrhage into the cyst, secondary bacterial infection, torsion (if pedunculated), and obstructive jaundice from compression of extrahepatic ducts.

The histologic appearance is cuboidal epithelium resembling bile duct epithelium. The cyst is filled with fluid that can be clear, mucoid, bloody, or bilious.

In the absence of complications, laboratory tests are normal.

If the patient has no symptoms, the cyst was discovered incidentally, and there is no evidence of infection or malignancy, treatment is observation. Indications for surgical intervention include symptoms, rupture, hemorrhage, and infection. A symptomatic, uninfected simple cyst is treated with excision. Large cysts are unroofed with free peritoneal drainage, unless there is a history of hemorrhage or evidence of biliary communication. If the cyst communicates with the biliary system, the leak may be oversewn or the cyst drained by means of Roux-en-Y cystojejunostomy. Infected cysts are drained externally and resected later or marsupialized.

Polycystic Disease. Polycystic liver disease is associated with polycystic kidney disease. Hepatic polycystic disease is most often bilobar and may be microscopic or large. The cysts usually contain clear fluid. Hepatic cysts in infantile disease may be an incidental finding during evaluation for renal symptoms or may present as congenital hepatic fibrosis. Adult polycystic liver disease is frequently asymptomatic and may be discovered during an evaluation of renal symptoms. Symptomatic cysts cause disturbances similar to those of solitary cysts.

Treatment is reserved for patients with symptoms or complications and consists of unroofing or excision of accessible cysts or fenestration to drain deep cysts into superficial cysts. Extensive unresectable disease is treated with liver transplantation.

Acquired Hepatic Cysts

Traumatic

Traumatic hepatic cysts are false cysts (they have no true epithelial lining) that result from a resolved subcapsular or intraparenchymal hematoma. Other than lack of a capsule, a history of trauma, and a fibrotic wall that contains hemosiderin, these cysts are similar to solitary congenital cysts and are treated in a similar conservative way.

Neoplastic

Neoplastic cysts of the liver can be primary biliary cystadenomas or cystadenocarcinomas but more commonly are metastases from cystic primary tumors such as pancreatic or ovarian carcinoma. These cysts also may represent cystic degeneration of a solid primary tumor or metastasis.

MALIGNANT PRIMARY HEPATIC TUMORS

In North America and western Europe, most malignant tumors of the liver are metastases. Primary liver cancer is more common in the rest of the world.

Hepatocellular Carcinoma

Epidemiology, Etiology, and Pathogenesis

Hepatocellular carcinoma (HCC) has three well-known epidemiologic associations—hepatitis B virus (HBV) infection, cirrhosis, and hepatotoxins, especially aflatoxin B1. Other risk factors for HCC include type 1 glycogen storage disease, α_1-antitrypsin deficiency, hemochromatosis, tyrosinemia, and use of androgens. HCC is more common among men.

Pathology

HCC may be a unifocal, multifocal, or infiltrative mass. It may be difficult to differentiate well-differentiated HCC and normal liver or adenoma. Poorly differentiated HCC may appear as giant cells, small cells, or spindle cells (mimicking a sarcoma). The clear-cell type and any HCC with a lymphocytic infiltrate have better prognoses than other types. There is no premalignant lesion, although well-differentiated cellular atypia may resemble hepatic adenoma.

Cellular components of HCC may have sex steroid receptors, and these receptors may have implications for hormonal therapy. The tumors frequently stain positive for α-fetoprotein (AFP), α_1-antitrypsin, and sometimes carcinoembryonic antigen (CEA).

The fibrolamellar variant of HCC has a good prognosis. Fibrolamellar tumors are usually associated with normal AFP levels and are infrequently associated with HBV or cirrhosis. The tumor is composed of polygonal cells that grow in nests or cords separated by fibrous stroma. Because of the good prognosis, surgical resection is more feasible than with other tumors.

Clinical Presentation

Symptoms of HCC often are masked by hepatitis or cirrhosis, and the only sign may be sudden clinical deterioration. The signs and symptoms are:

- Painful hepatomegaly, with or without nodular enlargement
- Right-upper-quadrant pain
- Palpable mass
- Weight loss, anorexia, and malaise
- Fever
- Splenomegaly, varices, ascites
- Severe, sudden abdominal pain that indicates hemorrhage into the mass
- Intraperitoneal bleeding (10% of patients)
- Jaundice, rarely due to biliary obstruction
- Anemia
- Paraneoplastic syndromes—erythrocytosis, dysfibrinogenemia, hypoglycemia, hypercalcemia, hypertension (from angiotensin production), and diarrhea (from vasoactive intestinal peptide or gastrin production)

Diagnosis

Abdominal CT is the most commonly used radiologic study in the evaluation of HCC. It yields good anatomic resolution and can depict extrahepatic disease. Percutaneous FNA or core biopsy can be used for tissue diagnosis. Chest radiography and cytologic examination of ascitic fluid are performed to rule out metastatic disease. Liver enzyme tests may be abnormal, but are nonspecific, often reflecting underlying liver disease. Levels of serum AFP correlate with tumor size. Laparotomy is the best method for determining extrahepatic spread of disease. Intraoperative US is used to guide resection.

Staging

Table 39-1 shows the TNM staging system for HCC.

Screening Recommendations

If HCC is to be found at a small, asymptomatic, and surgically curable stage, a screening program is necessary. Table 39-2 shows one proposed screening regimen.

Natural History

HCC has a tendency for local and vascular invasion. Untreated patients survive only 3 to 4 months after diagnosis. The tumor metastasizes mainly to the lung but also to the regional nodes, adrenal glands, bone, kidney, heart, pancreas, and central nervous system. Direct extension of the tumor through the portal or hepatic venous system may occur.

Cholangiocarcinoma

Cholangiocarcinoma is a malignant tumor of the bile duct epithelium and may have either intrahepatic or extrahepatic location. Cholangiocarcinomas are associated with clonorchiasis, ulcerative colitis, hemochromatosis, chronic cholangitis, and choledochoceles. Intrahepatic cholangiocarcinoma is much less common than extrahepatic cholangiocarcinoma. Intrahepatic cholangiocarcinoma is usually discovered at evaluation of a liver mass.

Primary Hepatic Sarcomas

Primary hepatic sarcomas are rare. The most common is angiosarcoma, which is associated with the following carcinogens: vinyl chloride monomer, a volatile chemical used in the plastics industry; Thorotrast, a radiographic contrast medium used between 1928 and 1950; and arsenic. Exposure to androgens such as methyltestosterone also is a risk factor. There is a long latent period between exposure and development of malignancy. The tumor is highly malignant, has high metastatic potential, is locally invasive, and is rapidly fatal.

Epithelioid hemangioendothelioma, an intermediate-grade sarcoma that is the malignant counterpart of pediatric hemangioendothelioma. The tumor is regarded as malignant and treated as such. Although sarcomas are usually primary, they may be metastatic. Examination of the retro-

Table 39-1. TNM CLASSIFICATION FOR STAGING OF LIVER TUMORS

TNM DEFINITIONS
Primary Tumor

TX   Primary tumor cannot be assessed
T0   No evidence of primary tumor
T1   Solitary tumor 2 cm or less in greatest dimension without vascular invasion
T2   Solitary tumor 2 cm or less in greatest dimension with vascular invasion, or
     Multiple tumors limited to one lobe, none more than 2 cm in greatest dimension, without vascular invasion, or
     A solitary tumor more than 2 cm in greatest dimension without vascular invasion
T3   Solitary tumor more than 2 cm in greatest dimension with vascular invasion, or
     Multiple tumors limited to one lobe, none more than 2 cm in greatest dimension, with vascular invasion, or
     Multiple tumors limited to one lobe, any more than 2 cm in greatest dimension, with or without vascular invasion
T4   Multiple tumors in more than one lobe, or tumor involves a major branch of portal or hepatic veins

Lymph Node Involvement

NX   Regional lymph nodes cannot be assessed
N0   No regional lymph node metastasis
N1   Regional lymph node metastasis

Distant Metastasis

MX   Presence of distant metastasis cannot be assessed
M0   No distant metastasis
M1   Distant metastasis

STAGE GROUPING

Stage I   T1, N0, M0
Stage II   T2, N0, M0
Stage III   T1, N1, M0
            T2, N1, M0
            T3, N0, M0
            T3, N0, M0
Stage IVA   T4, any N, M0
Stage IVB   Any T, any N, M1

(Union Internationale Contra le Cancer)

peritoneum is performed to exclude metastatic spread to the liver.

Therapeutic Options for Malignant Primary Hepatic Tumors

Curative Therapy

Surgical resection offers the only chance for cure of primary hepatic malignant tumors. Unfortunately, only a few tumors are resectable, usually because of cirrhosis, extensive involvement of structures at the porta hepatis, and metastasis.

Small tumors are removed with wedge resection or segmentectomy; large tumors require lobectomy. The operation is often aided by intraoperative US. Most patients who undergo resection have recurrences. The recurrence usually is local—at the margin of resection or within the parenchyma of the residual lobe. For tumors >4 cm, a tumor-free margin of >1 cm is required to limit recurrence.

Palliative hepatic artery embolization may be performed for unresectable HCC but is subject to the constraints of decreased hepatic reserve. When resection is not possible, chemotherapy, immunotherapy, and transplantation are alternatives.

Transplantation

Orthotopic liver transplantation is performed for severe hepatic dysfunction, large or centrally located tumors, or bilobar tumors. Extrahepatic disease, including lymph node involvement, is a contraindication to resection or transplantation. Patients with tumors >5 cm in diameter that are not encapsulated or associated with vascular invasion undergo neoadjuvant or adjuvant multimodality therapy.

Palliative Therapy

Chemotherapy. Doxorubicin is the recommended agent. 5-Fluorouracil, FUDR, cisplatin, and mitomycin are under investigation for use in regional chemotherapy, which involves surgical or percutaneous placement of a hepatic arterial catheter and a continuous infusion pump. Despite tumor response, systemic or regional chemotherapy does not increase survival rate.

Ischemic Therapy. Hepatic artery *ligation*, alone or in combination with regional chemotherapy, is ineffective for primary liver cancer. It has a high complication rate, and often cannot be used in patients with cirrhosis. Hepatic artery *embolization* does have palliative benefit, especially in combination with regionally delivered doxorubicin or cisplatin. Both procedures can be used for control of tumor rupture.

Radiation Therapy. Radiation therapy for primary liver cancer is limited by dose-related hepatitis, which occurs after 2500 to 3000 cGy. It is useful for acute palliation. When used in combination with systemic chemotherapy, radiation therapy may be equivalent or superior to intra-arterial chemotherapy.

METASTATIC LIVER DISEASE

Biology of Hepatic Metastases

The liver is a frequent site of metastatic deposits because of its dual blood supply (75% from the portal vein, 25% from the hepatic artery) and histologic filtering structure. Liver metastases from tumors that do not drain into the portal vein (eg, breast, lung, melanoma) are not resected because of the probability of systemic metastasis. Only colorectal, pancreatic, and carcinoid tumors are likely to have liver-only metastases. Only colorectal cancer has been extensively studied.

Table 39-2. SCREENING FOR HEPATOCELLULAR CARCINOMA

Risk Category	Characteristics	Screening Regimen
High	Replicative HBV infection or cirrhosis Male, nonwhite	AFP measurement every 3–4 mo US examination every 4–6 mo
Moderate	Childhood HBV infection Nonreplicative HBV infection	AFP every 3–4 mo
	Adult HBV infection Female, white	Annual US examination
Low	No HBV infection or cirrhosis	Screening not justified as cost effective After operation, patients undergo regular AFP determinations and US examinations as for high risk

Natural History of Metastatic Colorectal Cancer

Metastases are most commonly asymptomatic and are discovered at biochemical and radiologic evaluation. They are found during primary cancer resection in 8 to 30% of patients. If present, symptoms and signs include malaise, fever, weight loss, right-upper-quadrant pain or fullness, a palpable mass, and occasionally ascites or splenomegaly. Jaundice is infrequent and may be due to metastatic obstruction of the biliary tract, or it may occur late as a result of loss of parenchyma and cholestasis. Most primary colorectal tumors recur after resection. Twenty percent of the patients in whom disease recurs have only hepatic metastases. These tumors are curable with surgical treatment.

Evaluation

No laboratory test is specific or sensitive enough to be used exclusively for the detection of hepatic metastases. The most useful tests are CEA determination (for colorectal metastases), alkaline phosphatase, aspartate aminotransferase, γ-glutamyltransferase, lactate dehydrogenase, and 5'-nucleotidase (Table 39-3). Although conventional laboratory tests such as CEA are helpful, levels frequently are not elevated until disease is extensive; therefore, these tests are not used alone for evaluation of metastatic disease. Preoperative evaluation is often performed with CT, US, and angiography to define vascular anatomy. A patient with suspected colorectal metastases after previous resection undergoes colonic evaluation.

Surgical Treatment

Preoperative evaluation of hepatic metastases determines resectability and identifies favorable prognostic factors.

Prognostic Factors

Extrahepatic Disease.   Extrahepatic disease is a contraindication to surgical intervention.

Margin of Resection.   Inability to obtain margins of resection >1 cm is a contraindication to resection.

Number of Metastases.   Four or more metastases is a contraindication to resection if there are other negative prognostic factors.

Size of Metastases.   Size of metastases is a factor only because large metastases necessitate large hepatic resection. Large metastases may preclude adequate margins and indicate an increased likelihood of micrometastases.

Intrahepatic Distribution.   Bilobar metastases amenable to a parenchyma-sparing resection with adequate margins are not a contraindication to surgical treatment.

Type of Resection.   Anatomic resections appear to confer an advantage over wedge resections, probably because of better ability to obtain margins.

Stage.   Patients with Dukes C tumors have a high incidence of extrahepatic recurrence despite complete resection of the primary and hepatic metastases.

Age and Sex.   Patient age and sex are not prognostic factors.

Surgical Options

The best technique allows the best margins with sparing of liver mass. The surgical options are:

- Nonanatomic wedge resection for peripherally located lesions
- Anatomic segmentectomy, which allows good margins and sparing of uninvolved parenchyma
- Lobectomy or trisegmentectomy

Repeat hepatic resection can be performed for recurrent colorectal metastases. About 80% of patients have recurrence after resection of colorectal liver metastases; 65% have liver involvement. When patients with inadequate resection margins are excluded, the liver-only recurrence rate is reduced. Thus, most patients with recurrence after adequate resection have disease spread beyond the liver at the time of hepatic resection, and recurrence is likely because of missed occult metastases.

Palliative Therapy

Palliative options for patients with unresectable metastases are limited to systemic or regional chemotherapy, hepatic artery ligation, cryosurgery, percutaneous ethanol in-

---

Table 39-3. LABORATORY EVALUATION IN PATIENTS WITH SUSPECTED HEPATIC METASTASES

Test	Results	Description
CEA		
CEA alone	86% sensitivity	CEA is used in the detection of colorectal cancer and its metastatic spread. Although not specific for colorectal cancer, serial CEA levels are sensitive for disease recurrence in patients with colorectal cancer.
CEA & LDH together	87% sensitivity	
	47% specificity	
AP		
AP	77% sensitivity	AP is an enzyme with distribution in the liver, bile duct, bone, placenta, kidney, and WBCs. Like GGT and 5'-nucleotidase, it is elevated in cases of biliary obstruction or infiltrating diseases more than with hepatocellular injury.
AP with positive CEA	88% sensitivity	
	12% false-positive	
GGT	97% sensitivity	GGT is found in the liver, kidney, pancreas, heart, brain, and spleen. It has been most consistently sensitive, alone and in combination with AP, in hepatic metastatic disease.
5'-NUCLEOTIDASE	65% sensitivity	Despite a wide tissue distribution, increased serum levels occur only with hepatobiliary disease. Its values correlate closely with AP and GGT. Compared with AP, GGT, and SGOT, it had the lowest false-positive rate and best positive predictive value.

AP, alkaline phosphatase; CEA, carcinoembryonic antigen; GGT, γ-glutamyltransferase; LDH, lactate dehydrogenase; WBCs, white blood cells.

jection, chemoembolization, immunotherapy, or radiation therapy.

SUGGESTED READING

Doty JE, Tompkins RK. Management of cystic diseases of the liver. Surg Clin North Am 1989;69:285.

Ekberg H, Tranberg KG, Anderson R, et al. Patterns of recurrence in liver resection for colorectal secondaries. World J Surg 1987;11:541.

Farmer DG, Rosove MH, Shaked A, et al. Current treatment modalities for hepatocellular carcinoma. Ann Surg 1994;219:236.

Ferrucci JT. Liver tumor imaging. Cancer 1991;67:1189.

Johnson PJ. Hepatic virsuses, cirrhosis, and liver cancer. J Surg Oncol (Suppl) 1993;3:28.

Nelson RC, Chezmar JL. Diagnostic approach to hepatic hemangiomas. Radiology 1990;176:11.

Nichols FC, van Heerden JA, Weiland LH. Benign liver tumors. Surg Clin North Am 1989;69:297.

Saenz NC, Cady B, McDermott WV, Steele GO. Experience with colorectal cancer metastatic to the liver. Surg Clin North Am 1989;69:361.

Soyer P, Levesque M, Elias D, et al. Dectection of liver metastases from colorectal cancer: comparison of intraoperative ultrasound and CT during arterial portography. Radiology, 1992;183:541.

Yoshida Y, Kanematsu T, Matsumata T, et al. Surgical margins and recurrence after resection of hepatocellular carcinoma in patients with cirrhosis: further evaluation of limited hepatic resection. Ann Surg 1989;209:297.

GALLBLADDER AND BILIARY TRACT

ESSENTIALS OF SURGERY: SCIENTIFIC PRINCIPLES AND PRACTICE,
edited by Lazar J. Greenfield, Michael W. Mulholland, Keith T. Oldham, Gerald B. Zelenock,
and Keith D. Lillemoe. Lippincott–Raven Publishers, Philadelphia, © 1997.

CHAPTER 40

BILIARY ANATOMY AND PHYSIOLOGY

NATHANIEL J. SOPER

ANATOMY
Gallbladder

The gallbladder is a pear-shaped organ bound to a fossa on the right inferior surface of the liver by connective tissue and vessels. It is 7 to 10 cm long, with an average volume of about 30 mL. With marked distention or acute obstruction, the gallbladder may contain as much as 300 mL of fluid.

The gallbladder lies among the right, left, and quadrate hepatic lobes, or between hepatic segments IV and V (Fig. 40-1). The gallbladder sometimes has a complete peritoneal covering and true mesentery, which predispose the organ to torsion. The fundus and inferior surface of the gallbladder are covered with peritoneum reflected from the liver.

The gallbladder has four areas—the fundus, body, infundibulum, and neck (Fig. 40-2). The *fundus* of the gallbladder originates at the anterior border of the liver and duodenum or transverse colon. The fundus usually projects 1–2 cm below the edge of the liver and contacts the anterior abdominal wall near the lateral border of the right rectus muscle. The *body* of the gallbladder extends from the fundus into the tapered portion, or *neck,* which curves backward and upward toward the transverse fissure of the liver and terminates in the cystic duct. The neck usually has a gentle curve, the convexity of which may be enlarged to form the *infundibulum,* or Hartmann pouch. The neck occupies the deepest part of the gallbladder fossa and lies in the free portion of the hepatoduodenal ligament (Fig. 40-1). The cystic duct lumen contains a thin mucosal septum, the spiral valve (Fig. 40-2), which may make catheterization of the cystic duct difficult but does not have true valvular function.

Blood Vessels, Nerves and Lymphatic Vessels
Arteries

The arteries of the gallbladder are derived from the cystic branch of the hepatic artery. The cystic artery arises from the right hepatic artery 95% of the time, but it may arise from the left hepatic, common hepatic, gastroduodenal, or superior mesenteric arteries (Fig. 40-3). Double cystic arteries are present 8% of the time and an accessory cystic artery 12% of the time.

The course of the cystic artery varies, but the artery almost always is situated in the hepatocystic triangle—the area bounded by the cystic duct, common hepatic duct, and liver margin. From its origin, the cystic artery usually crosses behind the hepatic duct, but sometimes is anterior to the duct. The cystic artery courses to the neck of the gallbladder, where it divides into anterior and posterior divisions that supply the corresponding areas of the gallbladder. When the cystic artery originates from the right hepatic artery, its course from its origin to the gallbladder is usually parallel and medial to the cystic duct. A cystic artery that originates from the right hepatic artery or the common hepatic artery may lie close to the common hepatic duct, which may be injured when the artery is clamped or ligated. When the cystic artery originates from the right hepatic artery close to the liver, the artery is related only to the upper part of the cystic duct (Fig. 40-4).

Veins

The cystic veins empty into the right branch of the portal vein and directly into the liver.

Lymphatic Vessels

Gallbladder lymphatic vessels drain into nodes at the neck of the gallbladder. Often, a visibly enlarged lymph node (cystic artery node or sentinel node) overlies the insertion of the cystic artery into the gallbladder wall.

Nerves

The nerves of the gallbladder are branches of the vagus and sympathetic nerves, which pass through the celiac plexus. The left (anterior) vagal trunk branches into hepatic and gastric components. The hepatic branch supplies fibers to the gallbladder, bile ducts, and liver. In addition to cholinergic fibers, the vagi have numerous fibers that contain peptides, such as substance P, somatostatin, enkephalins, and vasoactive intestinal polypeptide (VIP). Sympathetic innervation comes from the 7th to 10th thoracic segments and passes through the splanchnic ganglion to the celiac ganglion. Most of the postganglionic fibers that innervate the gallbladder, bile ducts, and liver pass through the celiac ganglion. Afferent nerve fibers from the liver, gallbladder, and bile ducts pass via sympathetic afferent fibers through the splanchnic nerves and mediate the pain of biliary colic.

Extrahepatic Biliary Ducts
Common Hepatic Duct

The left hepatic duct usually has a longer extrahepatic course than does the right hepatic duct. The common hepatic duct is formed by the union of the right and left

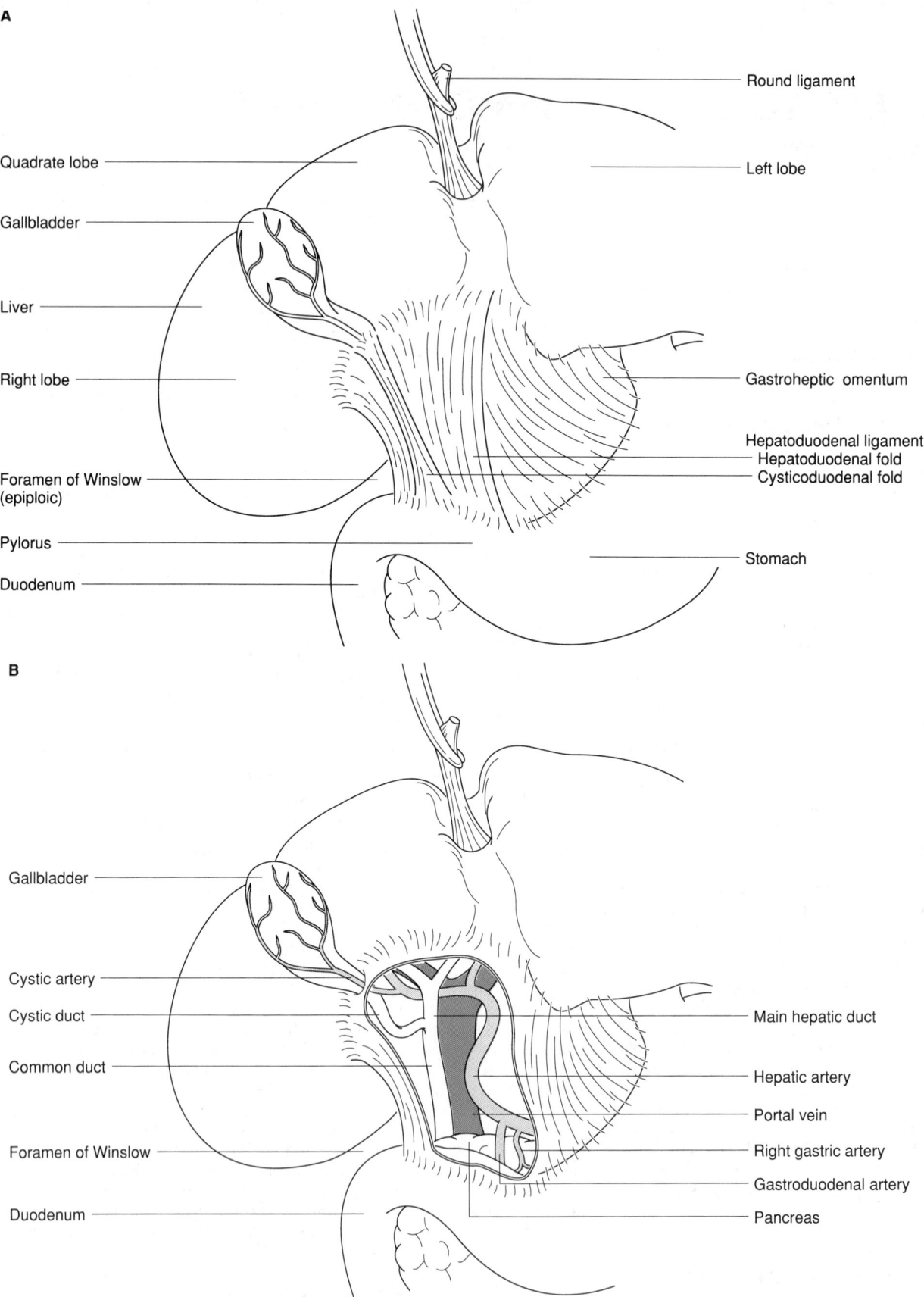

A

Round ligament

Quadrate lobe

Left lobe

Gallbladder

Liver

Right lobe

Gastroheptic omentum

Hepatoduodenal ligament
Hepatoduodenal fold
Cysticoduodenal fold

Foramen of Winslow
(epiploic)

Pylorus

Stomach

Duodenum

B

Gallbladder

Cystic artery

Cystic duct

Main hepatic duct

Common duct

Hepatic artery

Portal vein

Foramen of Winslow

Right gastric artery

Gastroduodenal artery

Duodenum

Pancreas

Figure 40-1. Anatomic relations of structures within the hepatoduodenal ligament.

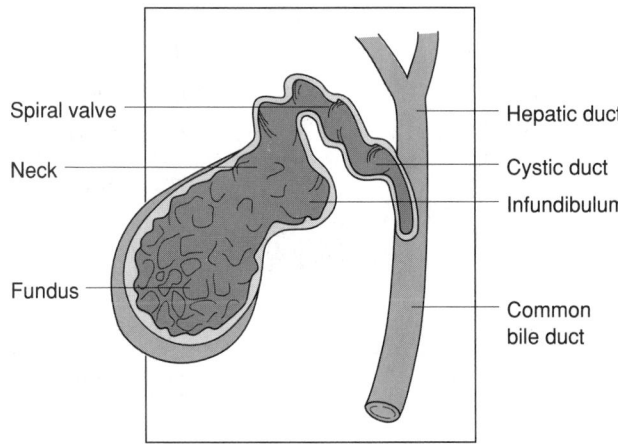

Figure 40-2. Cross section of the gallbladder and cystic duct.

Labels: Spiral valve, Neck, Fundus, Hepatic duct, Cystic duct, Infundibulum, Common bile duct

hepatic ducts close to their emergence from the liver (Fig. 40-5). This "normal" configuration occurs only one-third of the time. The common hepatic duct is 1 to 2.5 cm long and has a diameter of about 4 mm. The duct passes downward in the superior and lateral portion of the hepatoduodenal ligament and lies in front of the portal vein and to the right of the hepatic artery. The common hepatic duct unites with the cystic duct to form the common bile duct. An accessory right hepatic duct is present 5% of the time.

Cystic Duct

The cystic duct is 0.5 to 4 cm long, begins at the neck of the gallbladder, and courses slightly to the left. The cystic duct passes downward, backward, and to the left in the hepatoduodenal ligament and usually unites with the main hepatic duct at an acute angle. The cystic duct usually lies to the right of the hepatic artery (Fig. 40-6) and portal vein. Its course and mode of insertion into the common duct are highly variable. The cystic duct may be extremely short or run behind or parallel to the main hepatic duct and, after a spiral course, empty into the posterior or left side of the hepatic duct.

Common Bile Duct

The common bile duct is formed by union of the common hepatic and cystic ducts. The common bile duct is 7 to 9 cm long, depending on the site of union of the cystic and main hepatic ducts. Normal internal diameter is about 5 mm. However, the duct may be quite narrow or dilate to enormous dimensions when obstructed.

The supraduodenal portion of the common bile duct passes downward and backward in the hepatoduodenal ligament in front of the epiploic foramen (foramen of Winslow) anterior and to the right of the portal vein. The hepatic artery and its gastroduodenal branch lie to the left of the supraduodenal portion of the duct. The retroduodenal portion lies behind and adherent to the first part of the duodenum, lateral to the portal vein, and in front of the vena cava. The pancreatic portion extends from the lower border of the first part of the duodenum to the point on the posteromedial wall of the second or descending part of the duodenum where the duct penetrates the intestine. This portion of the duct is either surrounded by the pancreas or runs in a groove in the posterior surface of the pancreas.

The intramural portion of the common bile duct runs obliquely downward and laterally within the wall of the duodenum for 1 to 2 cm. It opens on a papilla of mucous membrane about 10 cm from the pylorus. The junction of

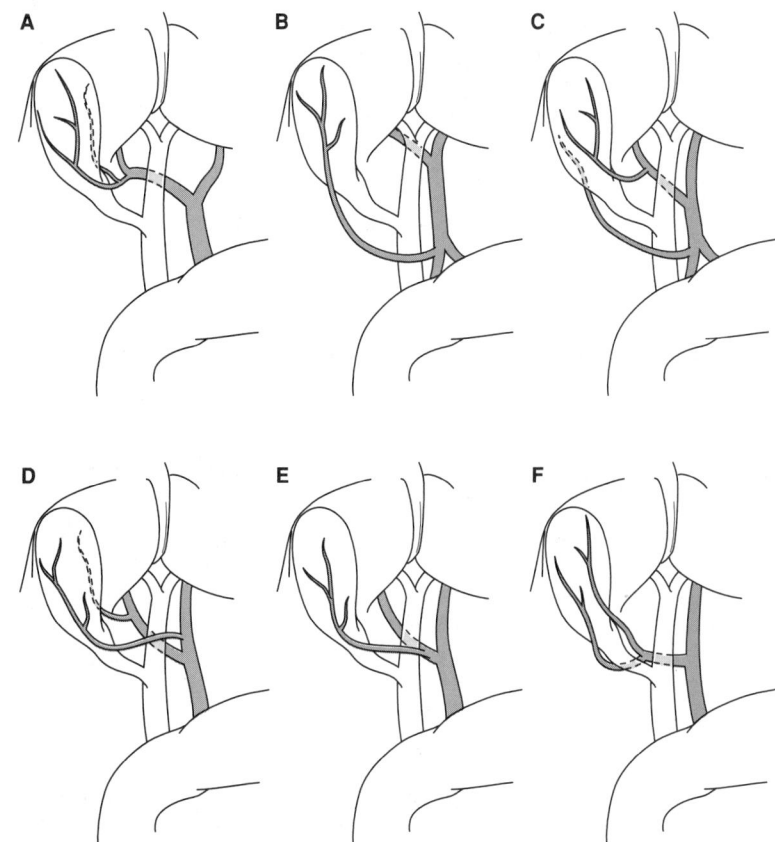

Figure 40-3. Normal and anomalous arterial supply to the gallbladder.

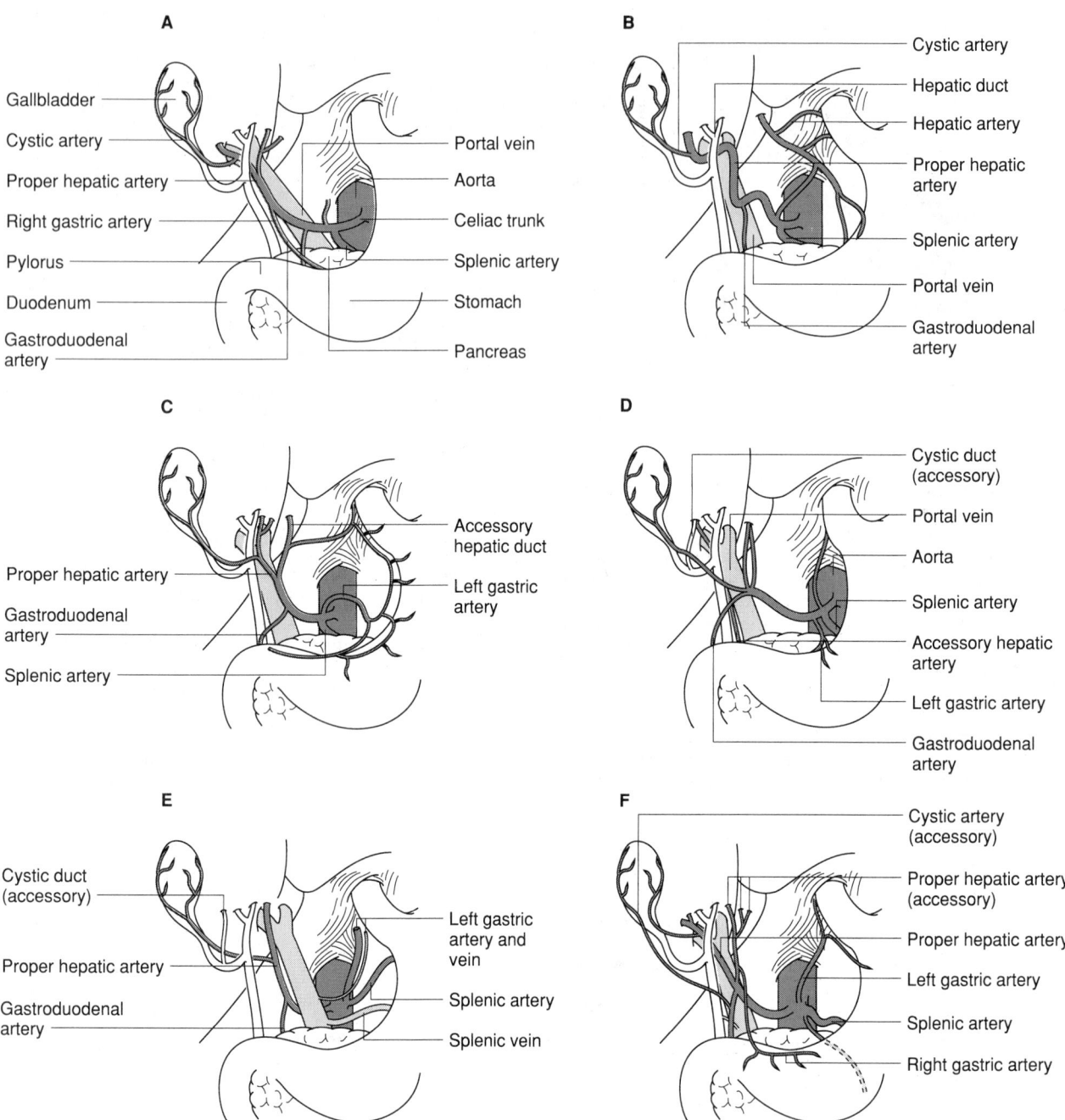

A

Gallbladder
Cystic artery
Proper hepatic artery
Right gastric artery
Pylorus
Duodenum
Gastroduodenal artery

Portal vein
Aorta
Celiac trunk
Splenic artery
Stomach
Pancreas

B

Cystic artery
Hepatic duct
Hepatic artery
Proper hepatic artery
Splenic artery
Portal vein
Gastroduodenal artery

C

Proper hepatic artery
Gastroduodenal artery
Splenic artery

Accessory hepatic duct
Left gastric artery

D

Cystic duct (accessory)
Portal vein
Aorta
Splenic artery
Accessory hepatic artery
Left gastric artery
Gastroduodenal artery

E

Cystic duct (accessory)
Proper hepatic artery
Gastroduodenal artery

Left gastric artery and vein
Splenic artery
Splenic vein

F

Cystic artery (accessory)
Proper hepatic artery (accessory)
Proper hepatic artery
Left gastric artery
Splenic artery
Right gastric artery

Figure 40-4. Variations in relations among the hepatic artery, portal vein, and bile ducts.

the terminal common bile duct and pancreatic duct at the papilla takes one of three configurations:

- the bile duct and pancreatic ducts have a common channel
- the common channel is nonexistent
- the two ducts enter the duodenum through separate openings

Blood Vessels and Nerves

Arteries

The arteries to the extrahepatic biliary ducts anastomose freely within the duct walls. The arterial supply is derived from the gastroduodenal and right hepatic arteries. Two

trunks run along the medial and lateral walls of the common duct.

Veins

The anterior surface of the common bile duct is covered by a plexus of thin-walled veins from which troublesome bleeding may occur while the duct is being exposed. These veins usually can be pushed aside.

Nerves

The nerve supply to the common bile duct and sphincter of Oddi is the same as for the gallbladder. The density of neural fibers and ganglia increases near the sphincter of Oddi and includes several ganglionated plexuses connected to those of the gallbladder and duodenum.

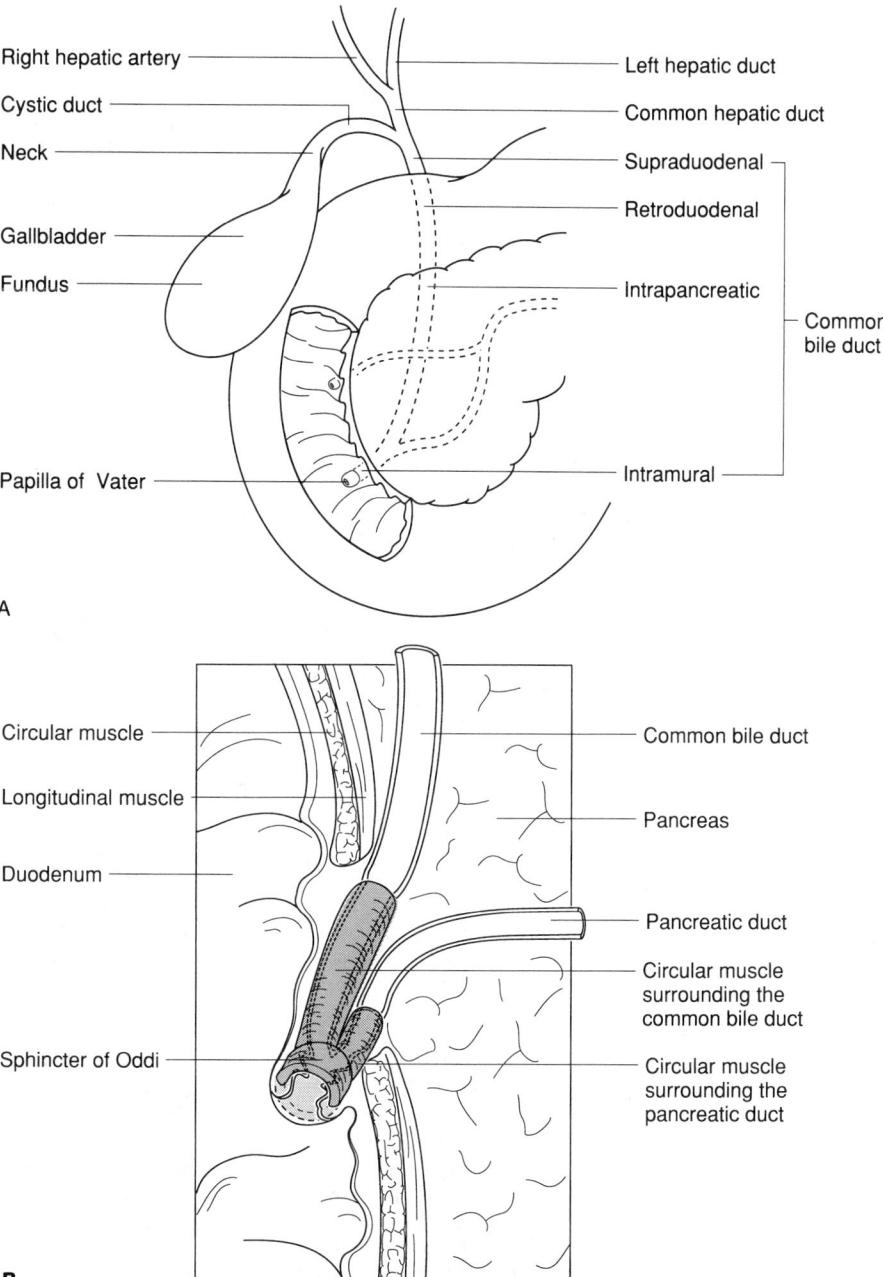

Figure 40-5. (*A*) Anatomic divisions of the gallbladder and the bile ducts. (*B*) Cross section of the sphincter of Oddi.

HISTOLOGY AND ULTRASTRUCTURE

Gallbladder

The gallbladder wall consists of five layers. From innermost to outermost they are:

- Epithelium
- Lamina propria
- Smooth muscle
- Perimuscular subserosal connective tissue
- Serosa

The gallbladder contains no muscularis mucosae or submucosa. Most cells in the mucosa are columnar cells, the main function of which is absorption. The cells are aligned in one row and have slightly eosinophilic cytoplasm, apical vacuoles, and basal or central nuclei.

The ultrastructure of the columnar cells features apical microvilli with filamentous rootlets. Vesicles in these cells originate from the intervillous cell membrane. The lateral membranes between cells are connected by junctional complexes that have complex interdigitations near the base. The intercellular spaces vary in size with the absorptive activity of the mucosa; spaces are distended during water transport, but otherwise are collapsed. The cytoplasmic structures consist of endoplasmic reticula, Golgi complexes, lysosomes, glycogen, mitochondria, mucous granules, and vesicles. The nucleus is rounded and sometimes contains a small nucleolus. The histologic features of the mucosa are different in different parts of the gallbladder. For example, the epithelial cells in the neck are tubuloalveolar and consist of cuboidal or low columnar cells with clear cytoplasm and basal nuclei.

The lamina propria contains nerve fibers, blood vessels, lymphatic vessels, elastic fibers, loose connective tissue,

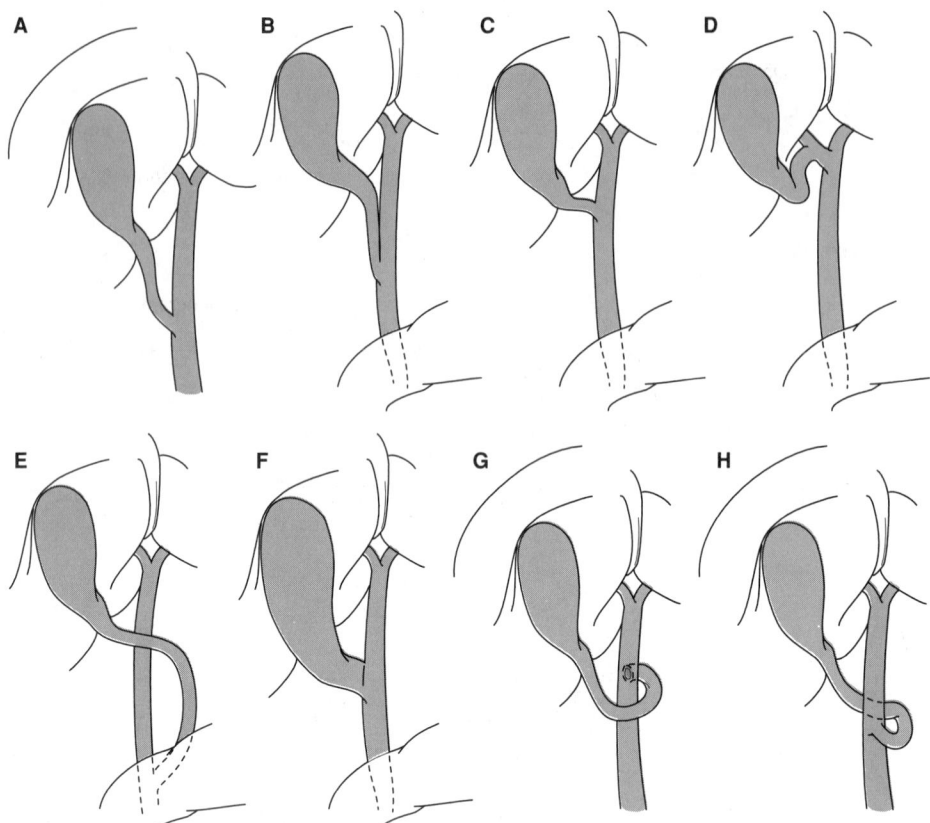

Figure 40-6. Variations in cystic duct anatomy.

and occasional mast cells and macrophages. The muscle layer is a loose arrangement of circular, longitudinal, and oblique fibers without well-developed layers. Ganglia are present between smooth-muscle bundles. The subserosa comprises a loose arrangement of fibroblasts, elastic and collagen fibers, vessels, nerves, lymphatics, and adipocytes.

Rokitansky-Aschoff sinuses are invaginations of epithelium into the lamina propria, muscle, and subserosal connective tissue. These sinuses are present in about 40% of normal gallbladders and are present in abundance in almost all inflamed gallbladders. Ducts of Luschka are tiny bile ducts that drain directly from the liver into the body of the gallbladder. They occur in about 10% of normal gallbladders, and have no relation to the Rokitansky–Aschoff sinuses or to cholecystitis, but may lead to a bile leak after otherwise-uncomplicated cholecystectomy.

Cystic Duct

The epithelium of the cystic duct is similar to that of the gallbladder. At the origin of the cystic duct is the spiral valve of Heister, which consists of bundles of transversely oriented smooth muscle that are thought to have a small role in filling and emptying of the gallbladder.

Extrahepatic Bile Ducts

The extrahepatic bile ducts are composed of columnar mucosa surrounded by a layer of connective tissue. The surface is flat, and the cells have basal nuclei and a small nucleolus. The mucosa of the most distal segment of a bile duct contains mucus-secreting glands and forms longitudinal folds called *mucosal valvules.* The lamina propria consists of collagen, elastic fibers, and vessels. There are a few

lymphocytes, and pancreatic acini and ducts are present in the wall of the intrapancreatic portion of the distal common bile duct.

The bile duct wall is fibromuscular with smooth muscle cells scattered throughout. Muscle fibers in the bile ducts are sparse and discontinuous. Those that are present are usually longitudinal, although there are occasional circular fibers. The distal common bile duct has a more substantial muscle layer in the intraduodenal portion of the duct, which becomes prominent at the sphincter of Oddi, where distinct bundles of longitudinal and circular fibers are situated.

PHYSIOLOGY

Motor Function

As bile is secreted from the liver, it flows through the hepatic ducts into the common hepatic duct and continues through the common bile duct into the duodenum. When the sphincter of Oddi is intact and contracted, bile is directed into the gallbladder, where it is concentrated and stored (Fig. 40-7).

In the *postprandial* state, about 70% of hepatic bile flows into the gallbladder before reaching the duodenum and entering the enterohepatic cycle. Patterns of gallbladder storage and emptying depend on a pressure gradient between the bile ducts and the gallbladder produced by contraction of the sphincter of Oddi. Peptide hormones and neural factors influence this gradient.

During the *interdigestive* phase, 90% of bile from the liver enters the gallbladder, and only a small fraction of gallbladder bile enters the duodenum. Like a bellows, the gallbladder empties small volumes of bile into the duodenum, but there is a net gain in volume of gallbladder bile.

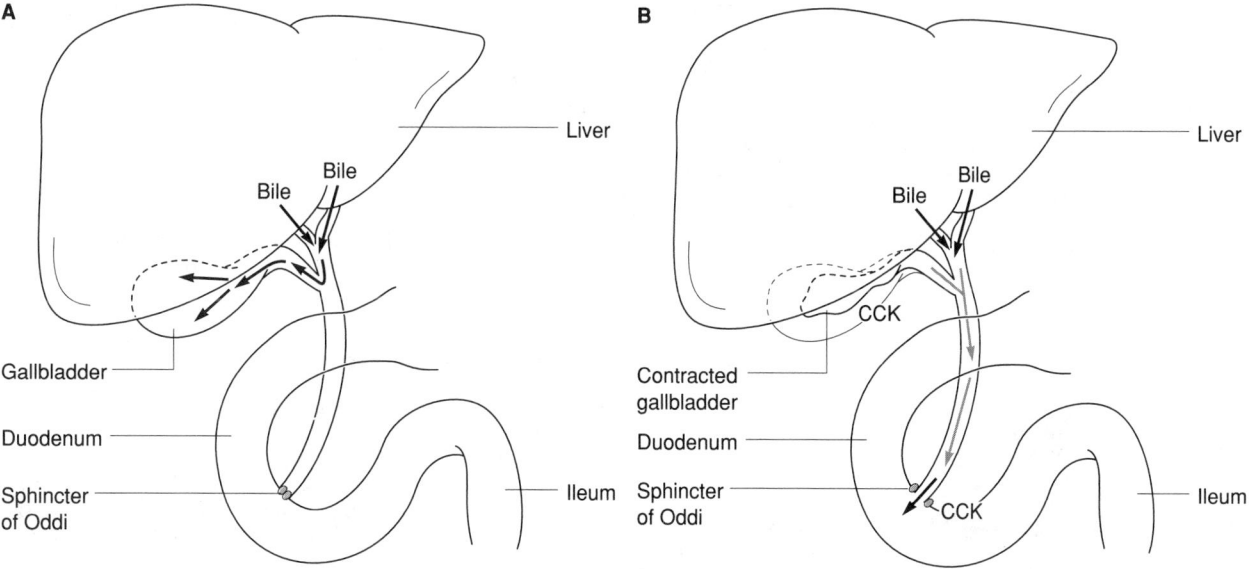

Figure 40-7. Effect of CCK on gallbladder and sphincter of Oddi.

After a meal, the gallbladder empties by means of steady tonic contraction that appears to be due to release of endogenous cholecystokinin (CCK) from the mucosa of the small intestine.

The importance of these gallbladder motor events is not clear. They have been used to explain cholesterol nucleation and gallstone formation. The bellows action of the gallbladder may reduce the vesicular phase (liquid crystals that cause stone formation) and increase the micellar phase of bile storage. Periodic emptying during the interdigestive phase would remove the less-dense vesicles, and alterations in the normal motor function would increase the risk of cholesterol stone formation.

Sphincter of Oddi Function

The sphincter of Oddi (Fig. 40-5B) is 4 to 6 mm long. The basal resting pressure in the sphincter is about 13 mmHg above duodenal pressure. The sphincter exhibits phasic contractions with a frequency of four per minute and a duration of 8 seconds. Pressure increases dramatically with phasic contractions, which have an amplitude of 120 to 140 mmHg. The sphincter relaxes with CCK stimulation, leading to diminished amplitude of phasic contractions and reduced basal pressure, allowing increased passive flow of bile into the duodenum. Parasympathetic stimulation also causes intermittent relaxation of the sphincter, and sympathetic splanchnic stimulation causes increased pressure.

Neurohormonal Regulation

The extrinsic nerves of the gallbladder consist of sympathetic fibers from the celiac ganglion and parasympathetic fibers from the vagus nerve. The sympathetic fibers innervate the smooth muscle of the blood vessels and the nonadrenergic cells of the intramural neural plexuses, but they do not contact epithelial cells. The parasympathetic fibers are situated in the ganglia of the lamina propria. The intrinsic nerves consist of cholinergic and peptidergic fibers, which occur in all layers of the gallbladder and terminate close to smooth muscle cells, basement membrane of the epithelial cells, and blood vessels. Cholinergic and CCK-containing nerves contract the gallbladder, and VIP-positive nerves inhibit gallbladder contraction and dilate the gallbladder.

Gallbladder motility is an interactive process that involves direct neural control, neural stimulation with the release of adrenergic and cholinergic substances, neural stimulation with the release of peptides, and the direct effect of hormones and peptides on smooth muscle. Adrenergic stimulation usually causes relaxation because most α-adrenergic receptors are inhibitory. Selective stimulation of excitatory α-adrenergic receptors causes contraction. Sympathetic stimulation also causes increased net water absorption, probably through an α-adrenergic mechanism. The pylorocholecystic reflex is a cholinergic mechanism in which the gallbladder contracts in response to antral distention. CCK works directly on smooth muscle fibers, or the response is mediated through cholinergic nerves.

Afferent fibers transmit the sensation of biliary discomfort to the right-upper quadrant and to the right side of the back by way of the splanchnic system. The cause of biliary colic appears to be increased pressure in the gallbladder due to transient gallstone obstruction of outflow of bile from the gallbladder.

Hormonal and peptidergic receptors are located on the

Table 40-1. COMPARISON OF HEPATIC AND GALLBLADDER BILE

	Hepatic Bile	Gallbladder Bile
Na (mEq/L)	140–159	220–340
K (mEq/L)	4–5	6–14
Ca (mEq/L)	2–5	5–32
Cl (mEq/L)	62–112	1–10
Bile salts (mEq/L)	3–55	290–340
Cholesterol (mg/dL)	60–70	350–930
Pigment (mg/dL)	50–170	
pH	7.2–7.7	5.6–7.4

(Davenport HW. Physiology of the digestive tract, ed 4. Chicago, Year Book, 1977)

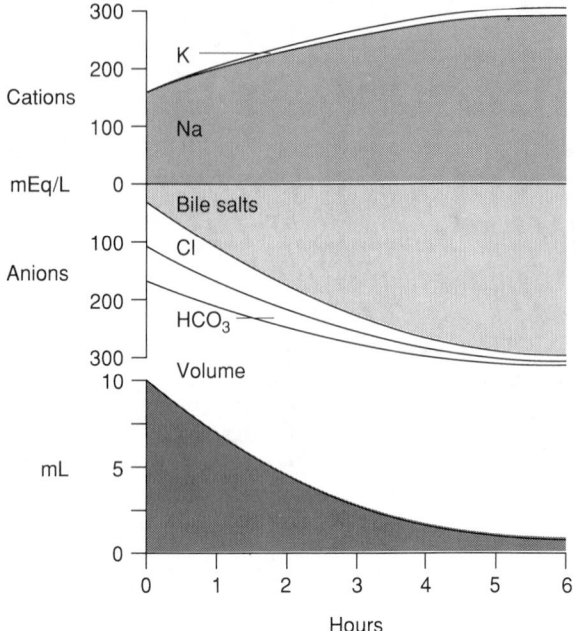

Figure 40-8. Changes in the volume and concentration of hepatic bile (*left*) to gallbladder bile (*right*).

smooth muscle, blood vessels, nerves, and epithelium of the gallbladder. CCK stimulates gallbladder contraction (Fig. 40-7). CCK is localized in epithelial cells of the small intestine; the highest concentration is in the duodenum. It is released into the blood stream by acid, fat, and amino acids in the duodenum. Intraduodenal bile inhibits the release of CCK.

CCK has a plasma half-life of 2.5 minutes and is metabolized by both the liver and the kidney. The degree of gallbladder contraction is related to the plasma concentration of CCK. CCK acts directly on smooth muscle receptors of the gallbladder; optimal binding occurs at a pH of 5.5 and requires the presence of magnesium. CCK-stimulated gallbladder muscle contraction is calcium-dependent and is mediated by cholinergic vagal neurons. Gallbladder response to CCK stimulation decreases after vagotomy or cholinergic blockade.

VIP inhibits contraction and causes gallbladder relaxation. Somatostatin inhibits gallbladder contraction mediated by CCK or vagal stimulation. Patients with somatostatinomas and those being treated with somatostatin analogs have a high incidence of gallstones, presumably because of the inhibitory effect of somatostatin on gallbladder emptying. The effect of other hormones on gallbladder motor activity is unclear.

Gallbladder afferent innervation is mediated by capsaicin-sensitive neurons. These neurons contain a number of neuropeptides, including substance P, neurokinin A, and calcitonin gene-related peptide.

MOTOR DYSFUNCTION

Gallbladder Dyskinesia

Motility abnormalities of the gallbladder and cystic duct present with symptoms that suggest gallstones. The most common presentation of gallbladder motility disorders—chronic acalculous cholecystitis or gallbladder dyskinesia—is recurrent biliary-type pain. However, examinations of the biliary tree with ultrasonography (US) or endoscopic retrograde cholangiopancreatography (ERCP) show no evidence of gallstones or other anatomic abnormalities.

The most specific test for diagnosing gallbladder dyskinesia is CCK-enhanced *cholescintigraphy* with assessment of gallbladder ejection fraction. A number of factors may lead to decreased gallbladder contraction, such as a primary abnormality of gallbladder muscle, motor dysfunction due to chronic inflammation or lithogenic bile, suboptimal hormonal or neural stimulation, or circulation of an inhibiting substance.

Sphincter of Oddi Dysfunction

Abnormalities of the sphincter of Oddi may cause symptoms suggestive of diseases of the biliary tree or of the pancreas. Sphincter of Oddi dysfunction may occur de novo or lead to symptoms after cholecystectomy. *Manometry* of the sphincter of Oddi may be performed at ERCP to characterize basal pressure, the amplitude and frequency of contractions, and the direction of propagation of contractile waves. Stenosis of the sphincter of Oddi is characterized by elevated basal pressure (>40 mmHg), whereas

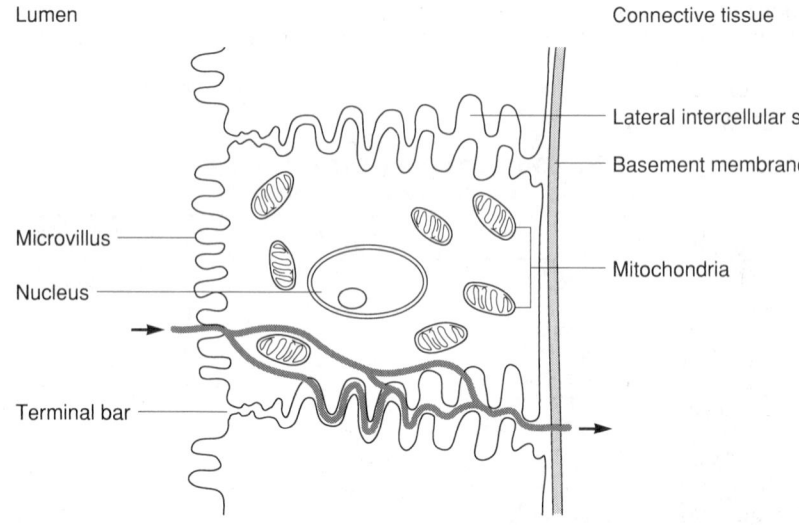

Figure 40-9. Cellular mechanisms of gallbladder mucosal absorption. The arrows indicate the route of water flow across the cell membrane and into the intercellular spaces. NaCl is pumped into the intercellular space, resulting in a hypertonic environment. As water enters, the space distends, and an isotonic solution enters the connective tissue space.

dyskinesia is characterized by abnormalities of the other manometric values.

Absorption

The gallbladder mucosa rapidly absorbs water and solutes from bile and concentrates the solute components. The changes in concentration of solute components from hepatic bile to gallbladder bile are shown in Table 40-1 and Figure 40-8. In *passive absorption,* sodium and chloride enter the gallbladder epithelial cells along electrochemical gradients. This results in an osmotic gradient, and water flows into the cell. In *active transport,* intracellular sodium is extruded across the basolateral membrane into the lateral intercellular spaces. The active transport of sodium against an electrochemical gradient is assisted by the Na^+-K^+-ATPase pump. The transport of electrolytes and fluid along the lateral intercellular spaces appears to be an important site for absorption (Fig. 40-9).

Secretion

Secretion occurs by means of inhibition of net ion and fluid absorption or stimulation of a bicarbonate secretory mechanism. The mechanism of gallbladder secretion is not understood. It may be related to elevations of cAMP or exposure to prostaglandins and possibly peptides such as VIP and secretin. The gallbladder epithelium secretes mucin and nonmucin glycoproteins, which may be important in the formation of gallstones. In experimental cholecystitis, substances such as morphine, loperamide, and enkephalin inhibit gallbladder secretion, which may contribute to the relief of symptoms that occurs with opiate treatment.

SUGGESTED READING

Dodds WJ. Biliary tract motility and its relationship to clinical disorders. AJR 1990;155:247.

Fisher RS, Rock E, Levin G, Malmud L. Effects of somatostatin on gallbladder emptying. Gastroenterology 1987;92:885.

Frierson JF Jr. The gross anatomy and histology of the gallbladder, extrahepatic bile ducts, vaterian system and minor papilla. Am J Surg Pathol 1989;13:146.

Geenen JE, Hogen WJ, Dodds WJ, Toouli J, Venu RP. The efficacy of endoscopic sphincterotomy in post-cholecystectomy patients with Sphincter of Oddi dysfunction. N Engl J Med 1989;320:82.

Gilloteaux J, Pomerants B, Kelly TR. Human gallbladder mucosa ultrastructure: evidence of intraepithelial nerve structures. Am J Anat 1989;184:321.

Lanzini A, Northfield TC. Assessment of the motor functions of the gallbladder. J Hepatol 1989;9:383.

Lipsett PA, Hildreth J, Kaufman HS, Lillemoe KD, Pitt HA. Human gallstones contain pronucleating non-mucin glycoproteins that are immunoglobulins. Ann Surg 1994;219:25.

Lundgren O, Svanvik J, Jivegard L. Enteric nervous system. II. Physiology and pathophysiology of the gallbladder. Dig Dis Sci 1989;34:284.

Sorensen MK, Fancher S, Lang MP, Eidt JF, Broadwater JR. Abnormal gallbladder nuclear ejection fraction predicts success of cholecystectomy in patients with biliary dyskinesia. Am J Surg 1993;166:670.

Toouli J. Biliary tract. In: Kumar D, Wingate D, eds. An illustrated guide to gastrointestinal motility, 2nd ed. Edinburgh, Churchill Livingstone, 1993;393–409.

ESSENTIALS OF SURGERY: SCIENTIFIC PRINCIPLES AND PRACTICE, edited by Lazar J. Greenfield, Michael W. Mulholland, Keith T. Oldham, Gerald B. Zelenock, and Keith D. Lillemoe. Lippincott–Raven Publishers, Philadelphia, © 1997.

CHAPTER 41

CALCULOUS BILIARY DISEASE

DAN I.N. GIURGIU AND JOEL J. ROSLYN

Calculi occur in the gallbladder, extrahepatic biliary tract, or the intrahepatic ductal system. They may be single or multiple and vary in color, size, shape, and configuration. There are three types of gallstones—cholesterol, pigment, and mixed cholesterol and pigment stones.

EPIDEMIOLOGIC FACTORS

- Age (Table 41-1)
- Hereditary and ethnicity (the incidence of gallstones in ethnic groups varies in different geographic areas, so environment and diet may be as important as hereditary)
- Sex and hormones
    Gallstone disease is more common in women than in men. After the seventh or eighth decade of life, however, the incidence in men and women is the same
    During the second and third trimesters of pregnancy, the rate of gallbladder emptying and the percentage of initial volume emptied decrease
- Obesity
- Diabetes
- Cirrhosis
- Vagotomy
- Total parenteral nutrition (TPN)

CHOLESTEROL GALLSTONES

The following factors are implicated in gallstone formation (Figs. 41-1, 41-2):

- Cholesterol solubilization
- Cholesterol saturation
- Nucleation and mucous secretion
- Gallbladder stasis
- Increase in biliary calcium concentration

Table 41-1. GALLBLADDER DISEASE PREVALENCE BY AGE GROUP

Age (yr)	Percentage With Stones	
	Female	Male
10–39	5.0	1.5
40–49	12.0	4.4
50–59	15.8	6.2
60–69	25.4	9.9
70–79	28.9	15.2
80–89	30.9	17.9
90+	35.4	24.4

(Modified from Bateson MC. Gallbladder disease and cholecystectomy rates are independently variable. Lancet 1984;2:621)

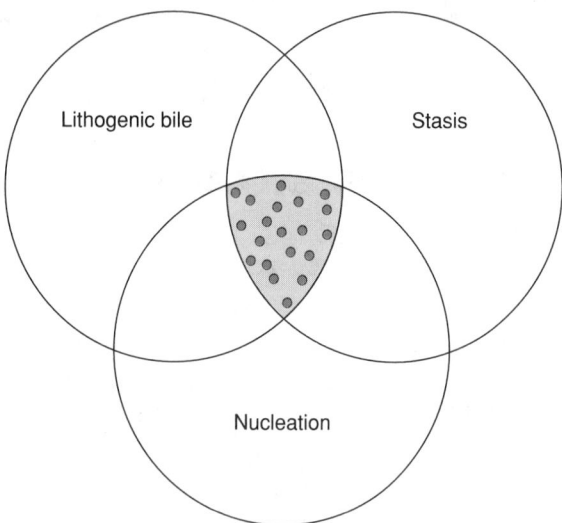

Figure 41-1. Gallstone pathogenesis is a multifactorial process that results from stasis of bile in the gallbladder in combination with a nucleation defect, all in the presence of cholesterol-saturated bile.

- Altered gallbladder absorption of sodium, water, and calcium
- Changes in biliary prostaglandin synthesis

PIGMENT GALLSTONES

Pigment stones are the most common type of gallbladder calculi worldwide. Cholesterol calculi account for most gallstones in the United States. The mechanism by which pigment gallstones form is not clear. The final pathway is altered solubilization of unconjugated bilirubin with precipitation of calcium bilirubinate and insoluble salts.

Classification

Pigment gallstones are characterized by their high concentration of bilirubin and their low cholesterol content. Most pigment gallstones are mixed stones and contain calcium bilirubinate as the main component. *Black* stones occur in patients with hemolytic disorders or cirrhosis. These stones are tarry, almost always occur in the gallbladder, and are believed to be caused by alterations in biliary metabolism. *Brown* stones are similar in composition to primary common bile duct stones, may be located throughout the intrahepatic or extrahepatic biliary tract, and are associated with infection.

Pathogenesis

Important factors in the pathogenesis of pigment gallstones are:

- Infection—free unconjugated bilirubin, produced by bacterial deconjugation, combines with calcium in bile to produce a calcium bilirubinate matrix
- In patients with hemolytic disorders, presentation of excessive loads of bilirubin to the liver for excretion
- In patients with cirrhosis
  Hypersplenism, which leads to increased hemolysis
  Impaired hepatic conjugation of bilirubin
- Biliary secretion of endogenously synthesized β-glucuronidase

- Changes in bile acid composition that decrease calcium solubility
- Bile stasis
- Sepsis

GALLSTONE DISEASE

Asymptomatic Stones

Half of patients with gallstones experience no symptoms. The gallstones are benign, and prophylactic management rarely is needed. Early cholecystectomy is considered for patients with asymptomatic gallstones who are at risk for complications of gallstone disease—acute cholecystitis, choledocholithiasis, and gallstone pancreatitis.

Diagnosis

The following examinations are performed:

- Oral cholecystography
- Abdominal ultrasonography (US)
- Hepatobiliary scintigraphy
- Duodenal drainage studies with examination of bile for cholesterol crystals and cholecystokinin (CCK) cholecystography

Clinical Features

Nonspecific Symptoms

Patients with cholelithiasis describe vague, poorly localized abdominal discomfort, often after meals. The discomfort usually is localized in the right-upper quadrant, although a large number of patients report midepigastric pain. Other symptoms are flatulence, eructation, and heartburn.

Biliary Colic

Biliary colic results from the presence of an impacted stone in the cystic duct or Hartmann pouch or from passage of a stone through the duct. Biliary colic is characterized by a rapid increase in intensity of pain, a plateau of discomfort that lasts for several hours, and a gradual decrease in intensity. The pain is felt in the right-upper quadrant or midepigastrium. The back discomfort felt by patients with biliary colic usually occurs in the inferomedial aspect of the right scapula, although pain sometimes is felt in the right shoulder. Episodes of biliary colic occur after meals and often are accompanied by nausea and emesis. These

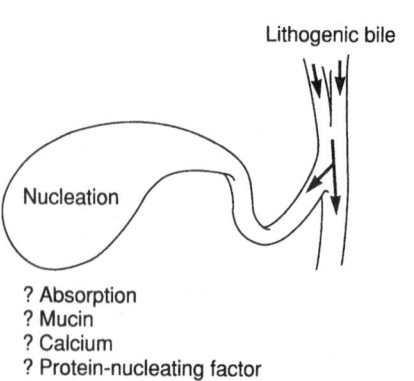

Figure 41-2. Proposed events that occur during cholesterol gallstone formation. A relation can be seen between hepatic metabolism and altered gallbladder physiology.

attacks often are precipitated by fatty meals, although most foods can cause gallbladder contraction and pain.

Acute Cholecystitis

The clinical manifestations of biliary colic and acute cholecystitis overlap, and differentiation is difficult. As in biliary colic, the initiating factor in acute cholecystitis is impaction of a stone in the cystic duct or pouch of Hartmann (Fig. 41-3).

The onset and character of pain of acute cholecystitis are similar to those of biliary colic. The pain of acute cholecystitis, however, persists and may be unremitting for several days. Progression of inflammation causes gallbladder distention, which leads to inflammation of the contiguous parietal peritoneum and causes right-upper-quadrant pain. This change in the pattern of symptoms reflects the shift from visceral to parietal pain. Many patients experience anorexia, nausea, or vomiting. As a result of peritoneal irritation, the patient is most comfortable lying still and is reluctant to move. The classic physical finding of acute cholecystitis is a positive Murphy sign—inspiratory arrest during deep palpation in the right-upper quadrant. Mild jaundice may be present, and is due to contiguous inflammation rather than bile duct obstruction.

Laboratory data are helpful but nonspecific. Most patients with uncomplicated acute cholecystitis have mild leukocytosis.

Most instances of acute cholecystitis are self-limiting because the stone frequently dislodges and patency of the cystic duct is restored. Symptoms abate in 3 to 4 days. If cystic duct obstruction is maintained because the stone stays in the lumen or the pouch of Hartmann, the disease may be ongoing. As many as 10% of these patients experience a complication of cholecystitis—gangrene, empyema, perforation, or cholangitis.

Most bacteria cultured from patients with acute cholecystitis are of enteric origin, the most common being *Escherichia coli. Enterobacter* sp. and *Klebsiella* sp. also are found. Sepsis often occurs after cholecystectomy, especially when the operation is performed for acute cholecystitis. Sepsis is prevented with judicious use of antimicrobial agents.

MANAGEMENT OF GALLSTONES

Cholecystectomy

Laparoscopic cholecystectomy (LC) has supplanted open cholecystectomy (OC) in the management of calculous biliary disease. The advantages of LC over OC are reduced hospital stay, earlier return to normal activity, less

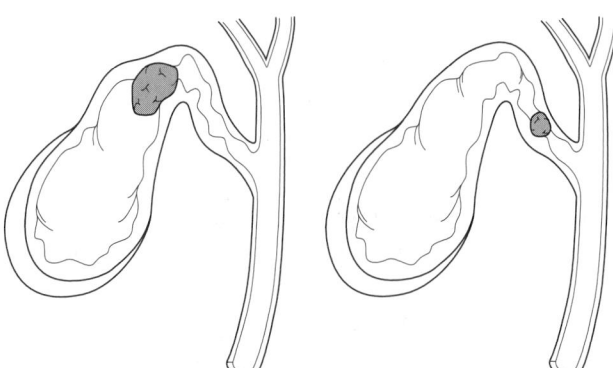

Figure 41-3. Acute cholecystitis occurs when a stone becomes lodged in the cystic duct or Hartmann pouch.

pain, and less scarring. The steps in LC are illustrated in Figure 41-4.

The indication for LC and OC is the same—the presence of symptomatic gallstones. *Contraindications* to LC are:

- Inadequate training or equipment
- High risk of general anesthesia
- Uncorrected coagulopathy
- Peritonitis
- Suspected gallbladder carcinoma

Patients with acute cholecystitis, morbid obesity, previous upper-abdominal operations, or cirrhosis and portal hypertension and pregnant may not be able to undergo LC, depending on the clinical circumstances.

Injury to the bile ducts occurs in a small number of patients during LC (Table 41-2) and is most likely to occur early in a surgeon's experience with LC. Trainees must be supervised closely by an experienced laparoscopic surgeon.

Medical Dissolution

Only cholesterol gallstones are treated with medical dissolution. Chenodeoxycholic acid (CDCA) is the pharmacologic agent used. Problems with the use of CDCA are:

- The need for at least 9 months of intense therapy, and probably lifetime maintenance therapy to prevent recurrence of stones
- The need to limit dietary cholesterol, especially in obese patients
- Toxicity and side effects
- High cost

Ursodeoxycholic acid (UDCA) may be a safer and more effective drug for gallstone dissolution than CDCA.

Only about 10% of patients in the United States with gallstones are candidates for medical dissolution therapy. The indications for the use of CDCA and UDCA are limited, especially since the introduction of LC.

Contact Dissolution

Percutaneous transhepatic cholecystolitholysis (direct contact dissolution) can be used to treat symptomatic cholesterol gallstones. The procedure involves percutaneous placement of a catheter through the liver and into the gallbladder and rapidly alternating infusion and aspiration of an agent, usually methyl tert-butyl ether (MTBE), that dissolves cholesterol (Fig. 41-5). The procedure is performed with local analgesia and fluoroscopic or US guidance.

Candidates for MTBE dissolution are patients at high risk with symptomatic stones and those who refuse an operation. For this modality to be effective, stones must be composed of cholesterol, and a patent cystic duct must be demonstrated with oral cholecystography or biliary scintigraphy. Side effects are transient abdominal pain, nausea, emesis, duodenitis, sedation, and complications of catheter placement.

Biliary Lithotripsy

The selection criteria for biliary lithotripsy are:

- History of biliary tract pain
- One to three radiolucent gallbladder stones <30 mm in diameter
- Gallbladder function demonstrated with oral cholecystography

Contraindications to biliary lithotripsy are:

- More than three stones
- Large or calcified stones

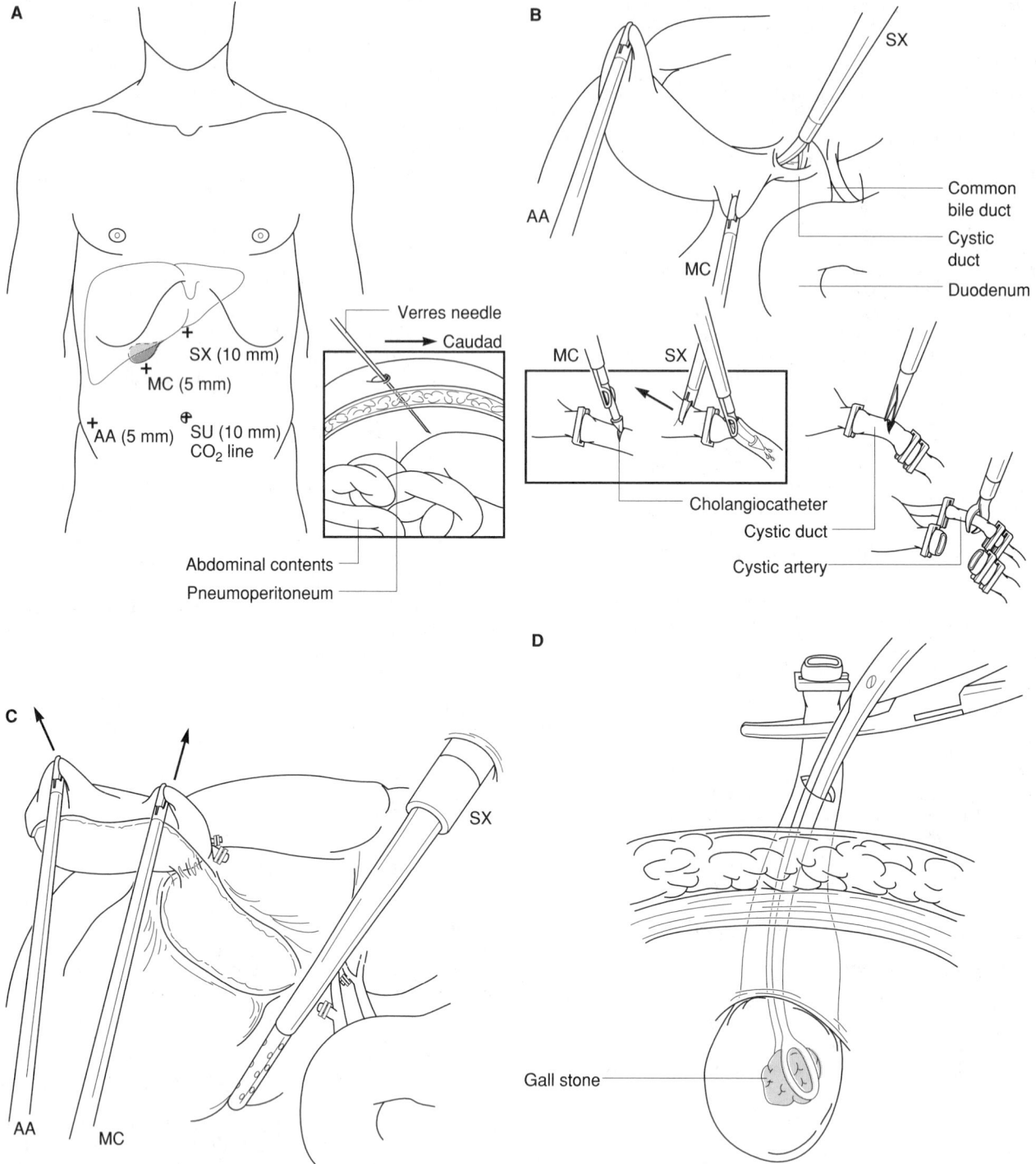

Figure 41-4. (*A*) Laparoscopic cholecystectomy is performed in a series of steps designed to create a pneumoperitoneum and provide exposure. (*B*) Careful identification of ductal and vascular anatomy. (*C*) Dissection of the gallbladder. (*D*) Extraction.

- A nonfunctioning gallbladder
- Complications of gallstone disease, such as cholecystitis, cholangitis, jaundice, or pancreatitis

CHOLECYSTITIS IN SPECIFIC CLINICAL SETTINGS

Acalculous Cholecystitis

Acalculous cholecystitis is an unusual but potentially lethal condition. It is a postoperative complication, but it also occurs after trauma or burns. A combination of bile stasis (due to ampullary spasm caused by narcotics, prolonged fasting, or edema) and increased bile viscosity (due to dehydration and multiple transfusions) changes the concentration of biliary lipids and other luminal factors, leading to irritation and inflammation of the gallbladder mucosa.

Patients usually have multiple medical and surgical problems, and the diagnosis may be delayed. Early diagnosis, by means of liberal use of US, and prompt surgical treatment may reduce the high mortality of this disease. If cholecystectomy is contraindicated because the patient is

Table 41-2. COMPLICATIONS OF LAPAROSCOPIC CHOLECYSTECTOMY*

Complication	No. of Patients	Percentage
Bile duct injury	459	0.6
Vascular injury	193	0.25
Intestinal injury	109	0.14
Mortality	33	0.04

*N = 77,604 patients
(Modified from Deziel DJ, Millikan KW, Economou SG, et al. Complications of laparoscopic cholecystectomy: A national survey of 4,292 hospitals and an analysis of 77,604 cases. Am J Surg 1993;165:9.)

in unstable condition, cholecystostomy, percutaneous or with a minilaparotomy, is performed.

Diabetes

Diabetes is not a risk factor for severe biliary tract disease. Care is the same as for any patient with cholecystitis.

Advanced Age

Gallstone disease is more severe in elderly than in younger patients. Elderly patients have an increased incidence of choledocholithiasis, emphysematous cholecystitis, perforation of the gallbladder, and sepsis, probably as the result of delayed diagnosis. Elderly patients undergo elective cholecystectomy with minimal morbidity and mortality. The extremely high mortality for emergency cholecystectomy in the elderly warrants early treatment of symptomatic gallstone disease. Elderly patients with acute cholecystitis are best treated with timely diagnosis, early stabilization, and semiurgent cholecystectomy.

Cirrhosis

Difficulties in patients with cirrhosis who undergo cholecystectomy are caused by portal hypertension, thrombocytopenia due to hypersplenism, and coagulopathy. Cholecystectomy is undertaken only for symptomatic disease or complications such as acute cholecystitis, perforation, fistula formation, or empyema of the gallbladder. Because most bleeding during cholecystectomy in patients with cirrhosis results from attempts at complete removal of the gallbladder from its hepatic bed, the posterior wall of the gallbladder may be left in situ and the remaining mucosa cauterized.

TPN-Induced Gallbladder Disease

Patients who undergo long-term TPN (both children and adults) have a high incidence of asymptomatic and symptomatic gallstone disease. Cholecystectomy is indicated when stones first appear. Cholecystectomy also is considered for patients without stones who are to undergo long-term TPN and who are undergoing laparotomy for other reasons.

COMPLICATIONS OF CHOLECYSTITIS

Hydrops

Obstruction of the cystic duct by an impacted stone can result in hydrops, in which the gallbladder is filled with a clear or whitish mucoid material. The gallbladder enlarges,

and patients experience signs and symptoms of acute cholecystitis, although sometimes the only finding is a mass in the right-upper quadrant. Cholecystectomy is performed.

Emphysematous Cholecystitis

Emphysematous cholecystitis is an unusual but lethal complication of cholecystitis. It is manifested by the radiographic demonstration of gas in the gallbladder lumen or wall. The gas is produced by bacteria. The organism most often cultured is *Clostridium perfringens*, sometimes mixed with *E. coli* and *Klebsiella* sp. The clinical course is rapid onset with severe abdominal pain, nausea and vomiting, and severe sepsis. Gangrene and perforation of the gallbladder are common sequelae. Emergency cholecystectomy is warranted.

Empyema

The pathogenesis of empyema is similar to that of acute uncomplicated cholecystitis. The only difference is that empyema is characterized by the presence of pus in the gallbladder lumen. Patients are often in toxic condition. Emergency cholecystectomy is required.

Gallbladder Perforation

Perforation of the gallbladder sometimes accompanies acute cholecystitis. It is classified as follows:

Type 1—Acute free perforation with bile-stained peritoneal fluid
Type 2—Subacute perforation with pericholecystic or right-upper-quadrant abscess formation
Type 3—Chronic perforation with formation of cholecystoenteric or cholecystocutaneous fistulas

Type 1 and 2 perforations are associated with vascular, metabolic, and other disorders. Computed tomography (CT) is better than US in the detection of abscesses and free fluid that accompany type 1 or 2 perforation. Barium upper GI radiographic examinations help define fistulous communication between stomach, duodenum, and gallbladder. Clinical suspicion of type 1 perforation warrants prompt treatment with fluid resuscitation, nasogastric decompression, IV broad-spectrum antibiotics, and laparotomy.

Type 3 is the most common type of gallbladder perforation. Depending on the size of the fistula, a gallstone may pass through the track. In most patients, the stone passes

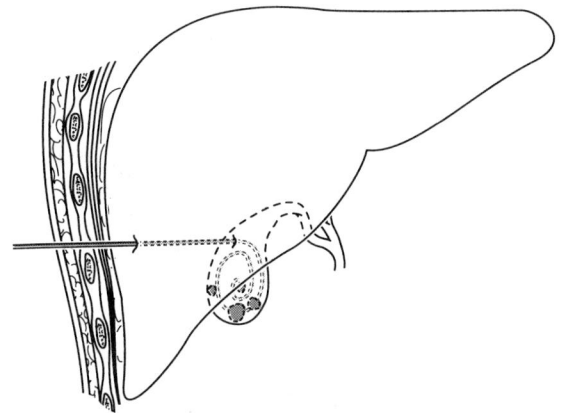

Figure 41-5. Schematic demonstration of the technique of percutaneous placement of pigtail catheter into the gallbladder. Methyl tert-butyl ether is infused and aspirated through the catheter.

through the intestine without symptoms. Stones >2 cm in diameter, however, may lodge in the GI tract and cause mechanical small-intestinal obstruction (gallstone ileus).

Patients with gallstone ileus are treated with aggressive fluid resuscitation, broad-spectrum antibiotics, and early laparotomy. The diagnosis usually is made at the time of laparotomy when a gallstone is palpated at the site of obstruction. The primary goals at laparotomy are correction of the obstruction and removal of the stone.

CHOLEDOCHOLITHIASIS

Primary, or recurrent, common duct stones form outside the gallbladder in the intrahepatic or extrahepatic bile ducts. Primary stones form as a result of biliary stasis and biliary

infection. Removing a stone without correcting the underlying abnormality may predispose to stone recurrence. *Secondary,* or retained, stones form in the gallbladder and pass into the choledochus through the cystic duct or sometimes through a cholecystocholedochal fistula. These stones are removed without biliary bypass or drainage.

Primary bile duct stones are always pigment stones. Primary stones are earthy, soft, brown, easily crushable, and conform to the shape of the duct. The following factors are implicated in the pathogenesis of primary choledocholithiasis:

- Ampullary stenosis and ductal dilatation
- Aberrant sphincter of Oddi motility

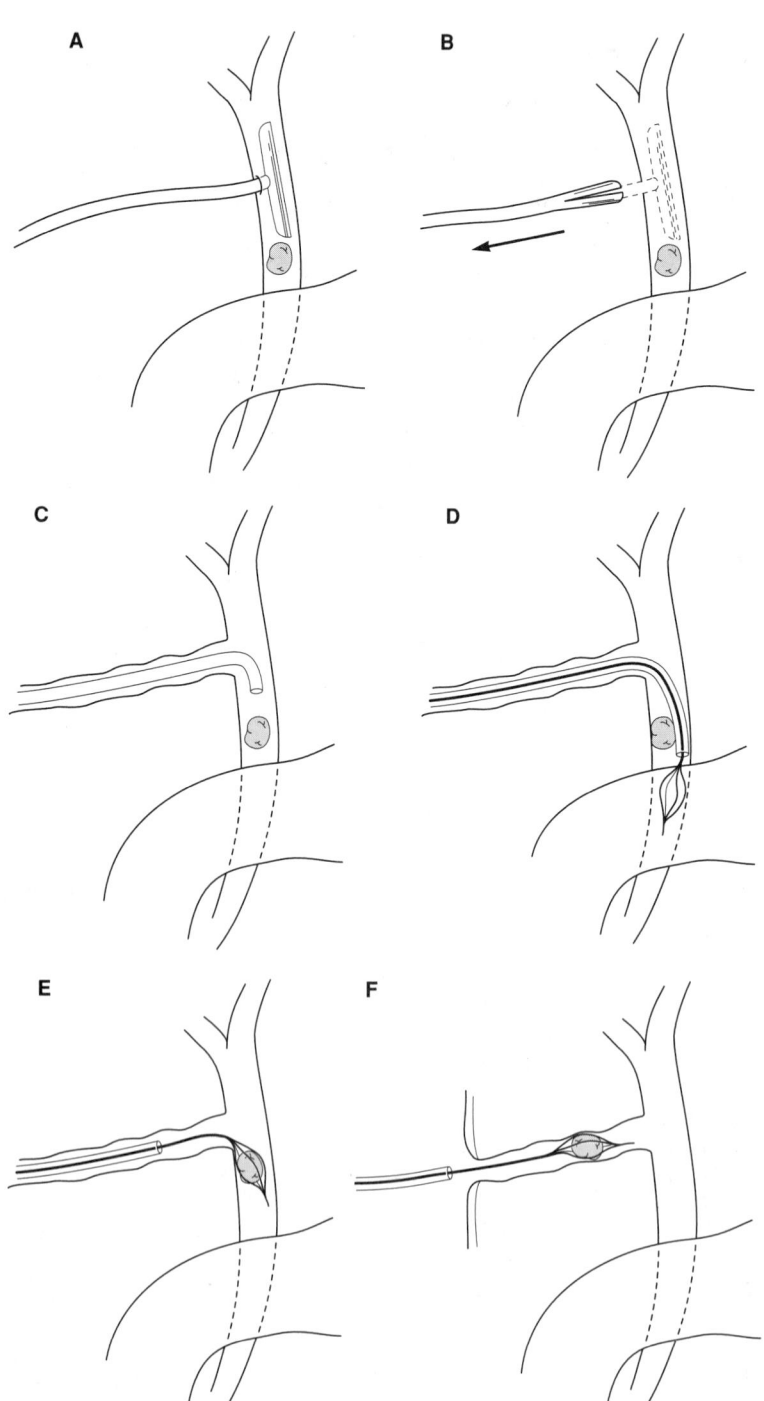

Figure 41-6. Illustration of Burhenne technique with placement of basket down matured tract and stone extraction.

- The presence of paravaterian diverticula of the duodenum
- The presence of bacteria
  - Aerobes—*E. coli* and *Klebsiella pneumoniae*
  - Anaerobes—*Bacteroides* sp. and *Clostridium* sp.

The bacteriologic profile reflects an ascending route of infection from the small intestine.

Clinical Evaluation and Diagnosis

Stones may be present for years in the bile duct without causing problems and may come to the attention of both patient and physician only when common duct obstruction occurs. When obstruction is sudden and complete, the patient experiences biliary colic; bacteremia with chills, fever, leukocytosis; and jaundice. When stones in the bile duct are not impacted, the manifestations may be pruritus, with or without jaundice, transient elevation of alkaline phosphatase, and episodic abdominal or back discomfort.

Common duct obstruction due to stone disease, as opposed to malignant stricture, is characterized by incomplete obstruction, low levels of hyperbilirubinemia, and fluctuating pain and jaundice. Pain is midepigastric and radiates to the back.

Laboratory Evaluation

In the absence of clinically significant obstruction, liver function tests may be normal. Increases in serum alkaline phosphatase are the most sensitive indicator of ductal obstruction, because this enzyme is released from the biliary ductal epithelium.

Diagnostic Imaging

US is used to identify biliary dilatation. CT provides comparable information and may depict masses, such as tumors in the distal bile duct, periampullary region, or head of the pancreas. In patients with primary common duct stones or patients in whom the cause of obstruction is not known, percutaneous transhepatic cholangiography (PTC) or endoscopic retrograde cholangiopancreatography (ERCP) is helpful to define the intrahepatic and extrahepatic biliary tree and localize anatomic abnormalities. In patients who may have primary common duct stones, ERCP allows visualization of the ampulla and periampullary region and therapeutic intervention if sphincterotomy is indicated and feasible.

Clinical Syndromes

Common Bile Duct Stones Found During Cholecystectomy

Complete stone removal is the goal when common duct stones are identified during cholecystectomy. The first step is dissection of the duct. A Kocher maneuver and choledochotomy facilitate stone extraction with a forceps, irrigation, or milking of the duct. Choledochoscopy aids visualization of stones and stone removal with endoscopic grasping forceps, baskets, or biliary balloons. Completion

choledochoscopy is performed to confirm that the duct has been cleared of stones and debris.

Common bile duct stones discovered during LC often necessitate conversion to OC for common duct exploration. Alternatives are:

- Trancystic dilatation and exploration with stone removal
- Laparoscopic choledochotomy
- Completion of LC and postoperative ERCP, sphincterotomy, and stone removal

Secondary (Retained) Common Bile Duct Stones

Reoperation can be used to treat secondary common bile duct stones, but the following are alternatives.

Radiologic extraction (Burhenne technique) is performed when a T tube is in place. Six to 8 weeks after the operation, the T tube is removed and a basket is passed down the T-tube track. The basket is manipulated under fluoroscopic guidance, and stones are removed (Fig. 41-6).

Endoscopic sphincterotomy provides access to the common bile duct when a T tube is not in place.

Primary (Recurrent) Common Bile Duct Stones

The goals of management of primary common bile duct stones are removal of stones and prevention of recurrence. Because many patients have multiple stones in both the choledochus and intrahepatic ducts, complete removal may not be feasible. The goal is to facilitate passage of stones into the small intestine to reduce the likelihood of cholangitis, jaundice, or pancreatitis.

The surgical options for primary common duct stones are:

- Transduodenal sphincteroplasty
- Side-to-side choledochoduodenostomy
- Roux-en-Y choledochojejunostomy

The presence of primary common duct stones is absolute indication for drainage of the biliary tree by means of choledochoduodenostomy, choledochojejunostomy, or transduodenal sphincteroplasty.

Alternatives to surgical treatment are endoscopic sphincterotomy (papillotomy), US fragmentation, and electrohydraulic laser lithotripsy. Because they are pigment stones, primary common duct stones cannot be treated with dissolution agents.

SUGGESTED READING

Burnett D, Ertan A, Jones R, et al. Use of external shockwave lithotripsy and adjuvant ursodiol for treatment of radiolucent gallstones: a national multicenter study. Dig Dis Sci 1989; 34:1011.

Deziel DJ, Millikan KW, Economou SG, et al. Complications of laparoscopic cholecystectomy: a national survey of 4,292 hospitals and an analysis of 77,604 cases. Am J Surg 1992;165:9.

Roslyn JJ, Binns GS, Hughes EF, et al. Open cholecystectomy: a contemporary analysis of 42,474 patients. Ann Surg 1993; 218:129.

Thistle JL, May GR, Bender CE, et al. Dissolution of cholesterol gallbladder stones by methyl tert-butyl ether administered by percutaneous transhepatic catheter. N Engl J Med 1989; 320:633.

ESSENTIALS OF SURGERY: SCIENTIFIC PRINCIPLES AND PRACTICE,
edited by Lazar J. Greenfield, Michael W. Mulholland, Keith T. Oldham, Gerald B. Zelenock,
and Keith D. Lillemoe. Lippincott–Raven Publishers, Philadelphia, © 1997.

CHAPTER 42

BILIARY NEOPLASMS

DAVID L. NAHRWOLD AND LILLIAN G. DAWES

GALLBLADDER CANCER

The incidence of gallbladder cancer is 2.5 cases per 100,000 population. About 6500 people die of gallbladder cancer each year. The disease is more common in women than men. The mean age at diagnosis is 65 years.

Gallbladder cancer is associated with gallstones. Large gallstones, probably because they are present in the gallbladder a long time, irritate the gallbladder wall, predisposing to the development of carcinoma.

The low incidence of gallbladder cancer does not warrant routine cholecystectomy in all patients with gallstones. There are exceptions, however. Calcification of the wall of the gallbladder, so-called porcelain gallbladder, is associated with a high incidence of gallbladder cancer. The presence of a porcelain gallbladder, therefore, should alert the physician to the high probability of malignancy, and a cholecystectomy should be performed unless contraindicated for other reasons .

Pathology

Most gallbladder cancers are well-differentiated adenocarcinomas. Adenocarcinomas of the gallbladder are papillary, serous, colloid, or glandular. A small percentage of gallbladder cancers are squamous cell in origin. The rest are anaplastic neoplasms.

The spread of gallbladder cancer follows the lymphatic and venous drainage of the organ. Venous drainage is into the venules that drain directly into the liver. The most common mode of spread of gallbladder cancer is direct extension into the liver, particularly liver segments IV and V. The lymphatic drainage of the gallbladder is to the cystic duct lymph node, to periportal lymph nodes, and then to celiac and superior mesenteric lymph nodes. Spread to the cystic lymph node and other periportal lymph nodes is of diagnostic significance. These tumors also can spread into and around the cystic duct and may extend into the common bile duct, causing biliary obstruction. Thus, the first clinical symptom encountered is often jaundice (Fig. 42-1). Besides direct extension and lymphatic spread of tumor, distant metastasis is possible but not common.

The staging system takes into consideration the lymphatic and venous drainage of the gallbladder. This system is used to describe the extent of gallbladder carcinoma and is of prognostic value (Table 42-1). A TNM classification also can be used to describe the extent of gallbladder cancer (Table 42-2).

Diagnosis

The signs and symptoms of gallbladder cancer are similar to those of gallstones—right-upper-quadrant pain, discomfort, and dyspepsia. Patients with gallbladder cancer frequently have advanced disease and present with nonspecific malaise, weight loss and anorexia, or obstructive jaundice. In the later stages of the disease, some patients present with a mass in the right-upper quadrant.

Tumor invasion of the cystic duct causing obstruction can result in the development of acute cholecystitis. Jaundice occurs when the tumor extends into the common bile duct. The diagnosis often is not made preoperatively but is made at laparotomy for jaundice or acute cholecystitis. Tumors with the best prognosis are those found incidentally at cholecystectomy for symptomatic gallstone disease. This emphasizes the importance of opening all gallbladders at cholecystectomy so that any suspicious lesions can be subjected to histologic examination.

Treatment
Surgical Therapy

When gallbladder cancer is limited to the mucosa and submucosa, cholecystectomy is adequate treatment and has a good prognosis. When the cancer involves the deeper layers of the gallbladder wall, the prognosis is grim.

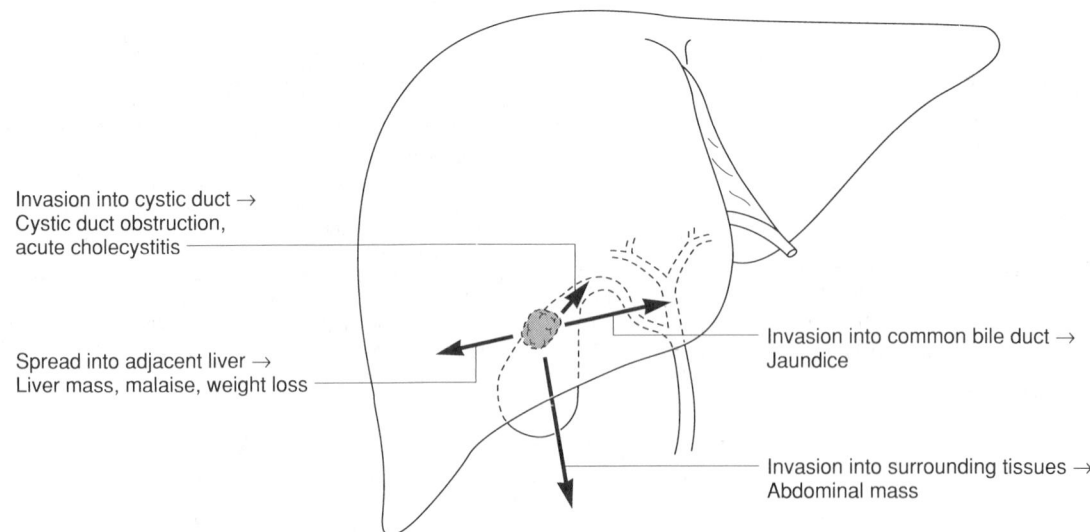

Figure 42-1. Tumor spread and presenting signs in gallbladder cancer. Gallbladder cancer commonly spreads by direct extension into surrounding tissues. This tumor extension results in the clinical presentations of jaundice, acute cholecystitis, abdominal mass, and weight loss.

Table 42-1. STAGING SYSTEM FOR GALLBLADDER CANCER

Stage	Extent of Tumor
I	Mucosa only
II	Muscularis and mucosa
III	Subserosa, muscularis, and mucosa
IV	Cystic lymph node involvement and layers of the gallbladder wall
V	Distant spread

Table 42-2. TNM CLASSIFICATION FOR STAGING OF CANCER OF THE GALLBLADDER

Stage	Stage Grouping
I	T1, N0, M0
II	T2, N0, M0
III	T1, T2 or T3, N0 or N1, M0
IVA	T4, N0 or N1, M0
IVB	Any T, N2, M0 or any T, any N, M1

To improve survival rates, and considering the lymphatic and venous drainage of the gallbladder, gallbladder cancer is treated with cholecystectomy and wide resection of the liver around the gallbladder bed (liver segments IV and V) and regional lymphadenectomy. This procedure— *radical cholecystectomy* or *extended cholecystectomy*— may involve resection of the adjacent bile duct. Some surgeons perform a more radical operation that includes hepatic resection, bile duct resection, and sometimes a pancreatoduodenectomy. This procedure may increase survival time, but it has a high mortality. Given improved surgical technique and improved perioperative care, hepatic lobectomy or pancreatoduodenectomy or both may be indicated.

Patients with invasive but resectable disease undergo wedge resection of the liver with a 2- to 3-cm margin around the gallbladder with cholecystectomy and lymph node dissection. The lymph node dissection includes all lymph nodes and surrounding areolar tissue from the bifurcation of the common hepatic ducts to the distal common bile duct, as well as the lymph nodes along the hepatic artery up to the celiac axis (Fig 42-2). If the gallbladder cancer is near the cystic duct or the bile duct is involved with tumor, bile duct resection and extended cholecystectomy are warranted.

Palliative Treatment

For stage V disease, treatment is palliation. Because patients with disease in this stage frequently present with obstructive jaundice, a goal of treatment is relief of jaundice and its attendant symptoms, such as pruritus and cholangitis. Percutaneous, endoscopic, or surgical drainage of the biliary tree is performed. A biliary–enteric anastomosis (anastomosis of a loop of intestine to the biliary ducts proximal to the obstruction) can be performed for palliation when the diagnosis is made during an operation. When both the diagnosis and unresectability of the tumor are determined before an operation, drainage of the biliary tree for palliation may be performed by means of stent placement, either with endoscopy or by the transhepatic route.

Radiation and Chemotherapy

No radiation or chemotherapy regimen provides a good response. Further investigation is needed to determine the exact roles of chemotherapy and radiation in the treatment of gallbladder carcinoma.

Laparoscopy

Laparoscopic removal of gallbladder cancer is not recommended. Tumor implantation occurs at the trocar sites, and laparoscopic manipulation of the tumor may lead to tumor dissemination. If gallbladder cancer is suspected, open cholecystectomy with exploration is warranted. Staging laparoscopy may be appropriate before an open operation if metastatic disease is suspected.

Prognosis

The prognosis of gallbladder cancer is poor; the average survival time is 6 months. Less than 5% of patients survive 5 years, because 90% of patients with gallbladder cancer present with stage V disease.

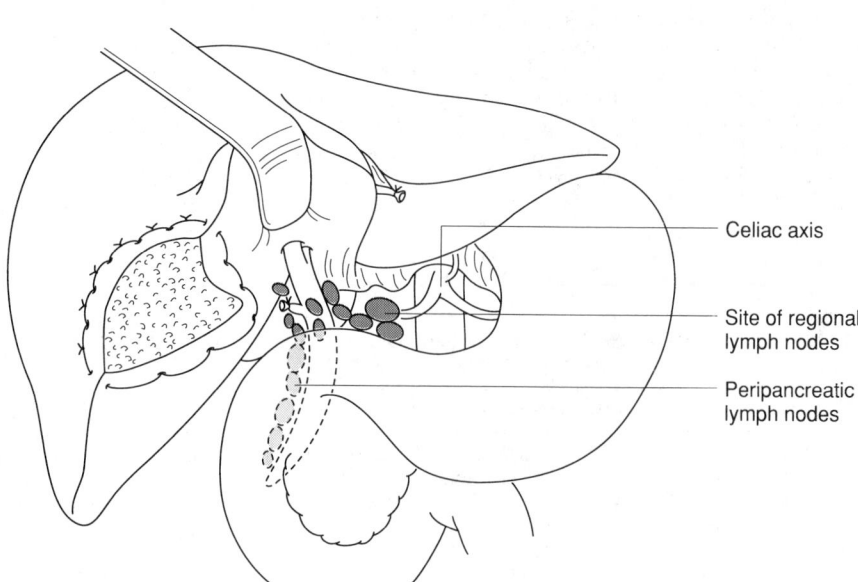

Figure 42-2. Treatment for invasive gallbladder cancer is cholecystectomy and a wedge resection of the liver along with a regional lymphadenectomy. The wedge resection of the liver is illustrated along with the lymph node regions that drain the gallbladder and that should be removed during operation for gallbladder cancer.

Celiac axis

Site of regional lymph nodes

Peripancreatic lymph nodes

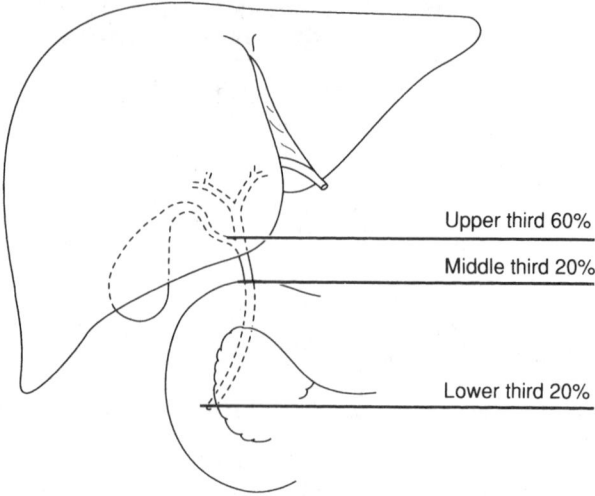

Figure 42-3. Distribution of bile duct cancers.

CARCINOMA OF THE BILE DUCTS
Incidence

Cancer of the bile ducts is less common than gallbladder carcinoma. Unlike gallbladder cancer, bile duct cancer is more frequent in men than women. The mean age at diagnosis is 50 to 70 years. The following conditions are associated with bile duct cancer:

- Gallstones (the association is not as striking as with gallbladder cancer)
- Biliary tract infection
- *Opisthorchis sinensis* infestation
- Chronic carriage of typhoid
- Congenital hepatic fibrosis
- Choledochal cysts
- Ulcerative colitis

Staging

Bile duct cancer is classified according to its location within the ductal system. The tumors are divided into three locations: upper-third (Klatskin tumors), middle-third, and lower-third (Fig. 42-3). The most common location is the upper-third, at the confluence of the hepatic ducts. Middle-third tumors are located between the cystic duct and the upper border of the duodenum. Lower-third lesions are located between the upper border of the duodenum and up to, but not including, the ampulla of Vater. Bile duct cancer can be staged with the TNM system (Table 42-3).

Clinical Findings

Bile duct cancers spread by direct extension. Because the bile ducts are close to the branches of the portal veins and hepatic arteries, these tumors are often unresectable because of vascular invasion, especially when they are located near the bifurcation of the hepatic duct. The symptoms are as follows:

Early
Jaundice
Abdominal pain
Cholangitis
Late
Anorexia and weight loss
Pruritus
Anemia

Diagnosis

Diagnosis is most often made during evaluation of jaundice. Elevated alkaline phosphatase levels may be the only laboratory finding.

Ultrasound (US) examination demonstrates intrahepatic ductal dilatation and, depending on the site of the tumor, variable degrees of common bile duct dilatation. US or computed tomography (CT) demonstrates intrahepatic biliary obstruction but rarely the tumor itself.

When biliary obstruction is present, visualization of the biliary tree is required with percutaneous transhepatic cholangiography (PTC) or endoscopic retrograde cholangiopancreatography (ERCP). PTC is used for proximal lesions because ERCP may not depict the proximal portion of the biliary tree. For distal lesions, however, ERCP provides the opportunity to obtain brushings for cytologic diagnosis and decreases the risk for bile leak because liver puncture is avoided.

Selective celiac angiography helps identify tumor involvement with major adjacent blood vessels, such as the portal veins, to aid in determination of surgical resectability.

Surgical Therapy

Tumors of the Middle- and Lower-Thirds of the Bile Duct

Resection of the bile duct tumor with reanastomosis is performed when possible. This approach may be possible for small carcinomas of the middle-third of the bile duct. For large lesions, reconstruction with a biliary–enteric anastomosis, usually a choledochojejunostomy, is required. For lower-third lesions, a Whipple procedure (pancreatoduodenectomy) is necessary. Middle- and lower-

---

Table 42-3. ADVANTAGES AND DISADVANTAGES OF ENDOSCOPIC AND TRANSHEPATIC STENTING

	Endoprosthesis	External Stents
Placement	With endoscopic retrograde cholangiopancreatography and sphincterotomy	Percutaneous transhepatic approach
Electrolyte balance	No loss of fluid and electrolytes	External loss of fluid and electrolytes
Incidence of cholangitis	Less cholangitis and infection	Permits entry of bacteria from external sources
Care and comfort	Better patient comfort	Requires daily care
Access	Does not permit easy access	Easily exchanged; permits cholangiographic follow-up and placement of intracavitary radiotherapy

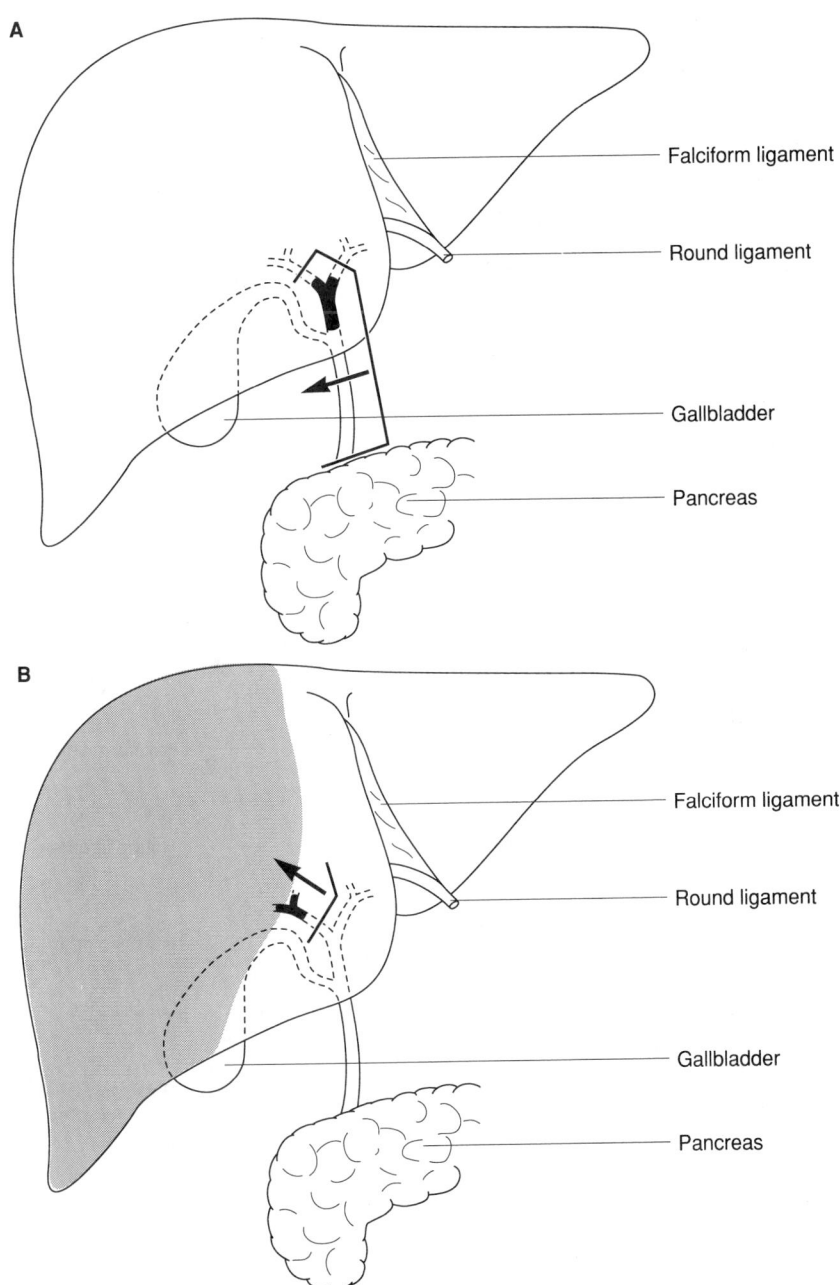

Figure 42-4. Surgical resection of hilar bile duct tumors in different locations. (*A*) Resection limited to extrahepatic bile ducts. (*B*) Resection of right bile duct with concomitant right hepatic lobectomy (*blue area*). (*C*) Resection of ductal bifurcation combined with right hepatic trisegmentectomy (*blue area*). (*D*) Resection of left bile duct with concomitant left hepatic lobectomy (*blue area*). (*E*) Resection of duct bifurcation with left hepatic lobectomy (*blue area*).

third lesions have better prognoses than tumors in the hilum.

Hilar Tumors

Most hilar tumors are unresectable at diagnosis. Unless contraindicated for other reasons, surgical exploration is performed in all patients whose tumors may be resectable. Hepatic lobectomy is indicated for cure. Resection may include extended right hepatic lobectomy for lesions extending along the right hepatic ducts into the liver or invading the vascular supply to the right lobe. A left hepatic lobectomy or extended left hepatic lobectomy is performed for lesions extending into the left lobe of the liver (Fig. 42-4).

Regardless of the surgical therapy, stenting of the biliary anastomosis is important because postoperative strictures and recurrent tumor are common. Presence of a stent facilitates follow-up cholangiography and dilatation if strictures occur.

Aggressive surgical therapy with vascular reconstruction has been proposed to improve the dismal prognosis of extensive disease. Hepatic transplantation has been performed for these tumors, but the cancer recurrence rate is high, so hepatic transplantation is not recommended treatment.

Determination of Resectability. Hilar bile duct tumors are considered unresectable if there is (1) metastatic disease, growth into surrounding structures, or peritoneal metastasis; (2) extensive vascular invasion, that is, tumor invading the main portal vein or involving both right and left portal veins or right and left hepatic arteries; or (3) tumor within the second-order biliary radicles of both hepatic lobes.

CT helps delineate the extent of local invasion.

If cholangiograms show extension of tumor into both the right and left biliary ducts beyond the secondary biliary radicles, the tumor is unresectable.

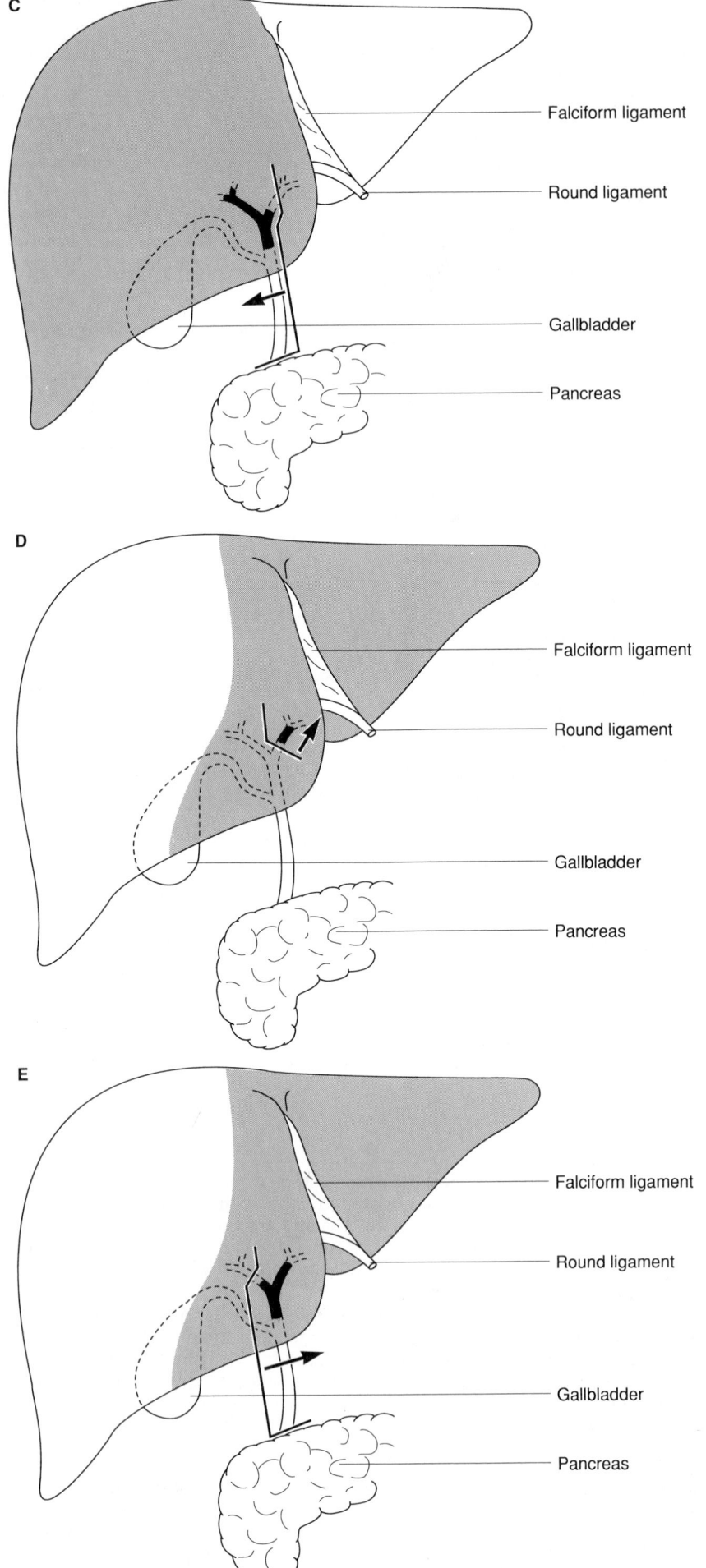

Figure 42-4. *(Continued)*

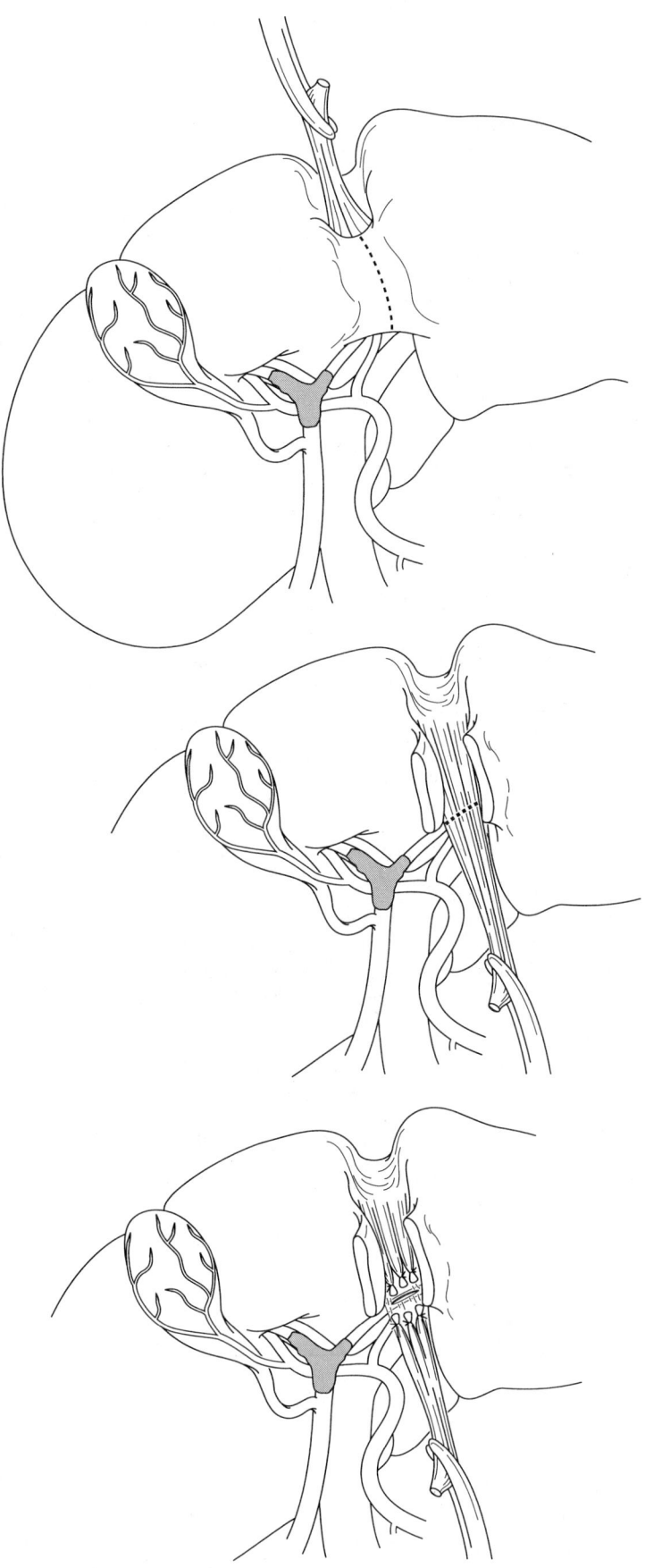

Figure 42-5. Surgical approach to biliary drainage for the left ductal system, illustrating round ligament approach to the left hepatic duct.

Angiography aids in determination of the extent of vascular involvement.

Surgical exploration is considered for all patients at good risk whose tumors may be resectable.

Surgical Treatment of Unresectable Tumors. Unresectable tumors are treated with surgical decompression of the biliary tree. Some approaches are as follows:

- The bridge of tissue just beneath the ligamentum teres is opened to expose the dilated left hepatic duct. An anastomosis is made with a loop or Roux-en-Y limb of jejunum (Fig. 42-5).
- The right hepatic ductal system is approached from beneath the gallbladder bed, and a right hepatojejunostomy is performed.
- A U-tube stent is placed through the abdominal wall, through the liver, across the tumor, out the bile duct, and through the abdominal wall. Because of problems with leakage around the exit site from the common bile duct, a Roux-en-Y limb of jejunum sometimes is used as a conduit for this tube from the common duct to the abdominal wall.

Nonsurgical Palliative Stenting

Nonsurgical percutaneous or endoscopic stenting can be used to improve palliation of extensive unresectable bile duct cancer. Stents are placed across an obstructing, unresectable bile duct cancer, either at ERCP or with a percutaneous transhepatic approach.

Endoprostheses improve patient comfort, avoid loss of electrolytes, and a reduce the incidence of cholangitis and infection. The disadvantages are that endoprostheses are difficult to place in proximal bile duct lesions and they do not provide easy access for changing catheters or repeat cholangiography. For proximal ductal lesions, the transhepatic approach is preferred.

With external catheters, iridium (^{192}Ir) wires are placed for administration of intracavitary radiation therapy. Because percutaneous drains are used for palliation, drainage of one ductal system may be sufficient to relieve jaundice or pruritus or to treat cholangitis. Bilateral stent placement may be necessary to control biliary infection if an undrained segment is infected.

The complications of use of palliative percutaneous or endoscopic stents are cholangitis, bleeding, bile leakage, and recurrent obstruction due to catheter occlusion. The 30-day mortality for percutaneous or endoscopic stenting is 15% to 33%. This high mortality may reflect the advanced stage of disease at stenting. Surgical bypass also carries a high mortality.

Patients with bile duct tumors who have metastatic or unresectable disease should undergo percutaneous or endoscopic stenting to avoid the complications and discomfort of surgical intervention. If tumors are explored for resectability and are found to be unresectable, one of the surgical drainage or stenting procedures should be performed, if possible. Patients with surgical bypass for palliation have a lower incidence of cholangitis and may have improved quality of life and survival.

Adjuvant Therapy

Treatment with postoperative radiation therapy—external beam radiation, intraoperative radiation, or local radiation with a ^{192}Ir wire—may reduce recurrence rates and prolong survival in patients with surgically resected tumors. Various chemotherapeutic regimens have been tried, but no effective treatment of bile duct cancer has been developed.

SUGGESTED READING

Cameron JL, Pitt HA, Zinner MJ, Kaufman SL, Coleman J. Management of proximal cholangiocarcinomas by surgical resection and radiotherapy. Am J Surg 1990;159:91.

Clair DG, Lautz DB, Brooks DC. Rapid development of umbilical metastases after laparoscopic cholecystectomy for unsuspected gallbladder carcinoma. Surgery 1993;113:355.

Donahue JH, Nagorney DM, Grand CS, Tsushima K. Carcinoma of the gallbladder: Does radical resection improve outcome? Arch Surg 1990;125:237.

Nakamura S, Mishiyama R, Yokoi Y, et al. Hepatopancreatoduodenectomy for advanced gallbladder carcinoma. Arch Surg 1994;129:625.

Ottow RT, August DA, Sugarbaker PH. Treatment of proximal biliary tract carcinoma: overview of techniques and results. Surgery 1985;97:251.

Piehler JM, Crichlow RW. Primary cancer of the gallbladder: a collective review. Surg Gynecol Obstet 1978;147:929.

Pinson CW, Rossi RL. Extended right hepatic lobectomy, left hepatic lobectomy and skeletonization resection for proximal bile duct cancer. World J Surg 1988;12:52.

Silk YN, Douglass HO, Nava HR, Driscoll DL, Tartarian G. Carcinoma of the gallbladder: the Roswell Park experience. Ann Surg 1989;210:751.

Terblanche J, Kahn D, Bornman PC, Werner D. The role of U-tube palliative treatment in the high bile duct carcinoma. Surgery 1988;103:624.

Tompkins RK. Treatment and prognosis in bile duct cancer. World J Surg 1988;12:109.

ESSENTIALS OF SURGERY: SCIENTIFIC PRINCIPLES AND PRACTICE, edited by Lazar J. Greenfield, Michael W. Mulholland, Keith T. Oldham, Gerald B. Zelenock, and Keith D. Lillemoe. Lippincott–Raven Publishers, Philadelphia, © 1997.

CHAPTER 43

BILIARY STRICTURES AND SCLEROSING CHOLANGITIS

KEITH D. LILLEMOE

Benign bile duct strictures have numerous causes:

Postoperative strictures
Injury at primary biliary operation
   Laparoscopic cholecystectomy
   Open cholecystectomy
   Common bile duct exploration
Injury at other operative procedures
   Gastrectomy
   Hepatic resection
   Portacaval shunt
Stricture of a biliary–enteric anastomosis
Blunt or penetrating trauma
Strictures due to inflammatory conditions
Chronic pancreatitis
Cholelithiasis and choledocholithiasis
Primary sclerosing cholangitis
Stenosis of the sphincter of Oddi
Duodenal ulcer
Crohn's disease
Viral infection
Toxic drugs

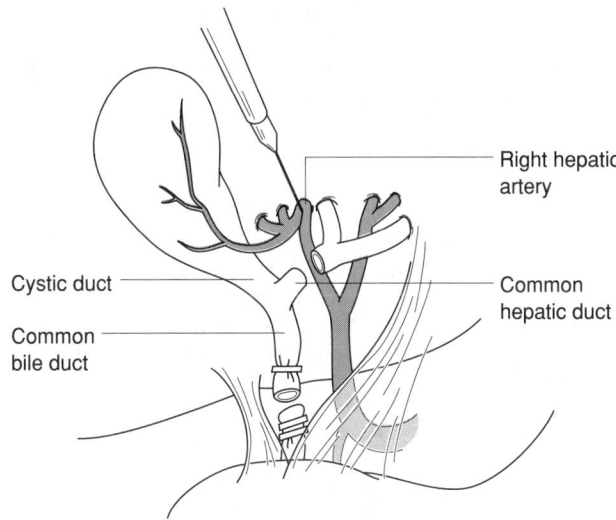

Figure 43-1. Classic laparoscopic bile duct injury. The common bile duct is mistaken for the cystic duct and transected. A variable extent of the extra-hepatic biliary tree is resected with the gallbladder. The right hepatic artery, in background, is also often injured. (After Branum G, Schmidt C, Baile J, et al. Management of major biliary complications after laparoscopic cholecystectomy. Ann Surg 1993;217:532)

POSTOPERATIVE BILE DUCT STRICTURES

Pathogenesis

Most benign bile duct strictures result from operations in or near the right-upper quadrant. More than 80% of strictures occur after injury to the bile ducts during cholecystectomy.

Biliary Operations

The incidence of bile duct injury is higher during laparoscopic than during open cholecystectomy. Associated factors include:

- Technical difficulties such as acute or chronic inflammation, obesity, inadequate surgical exposure, and failure to identify structures before clamping, ligation, or division
- Bleeding from the cystic or hepatic arteries
- Overly generous application of ligation clips to poorly visualized areas in the hilum
- Failure to recognize congenital anatomic anomalies of the bile ducts, such as insertion of the right hepatic duct into the cystic duct or a long common wall between the cystic duct and the common bile duct
- During laparoscopic cholecystectomy, distortion of the surgeon's perspective in which the common bile duct is mistaken for the cystic duct and clipped and divided (Fig. 43-1)
- Surgeon's lack of experience with laparoscopic cholecystectomy
- Unnecessary dissection around the bile duct during cholecystectomy or bile duct anastomosis resulting in division of, or injury to, the arteries of the bile duct (Fig. 43-2)
- Local inflammatory response in adjacent tissue associated with bile leakage, which leads to fibrosis and scarring

Other Operations

The most common situation resulting in bile duct injury during *gastrectomy* is dissection of the pyloric region and the first portion of the duodenum in the presence of inflammation from peptic ulcer disease. The injury occurs during mobilization of the duodenum for Billroth I gastroduodenostomy or for closure of the duodenal stump.

Biliary injury during *liver resection* is most likely to occur during dissection of the hepatic hilum.

Biliary Anastomoses

Strictures occur at biliary–enteric anastomoses performed for reconstruction after resection for benign or malignant disease of the pancreatobiliary system and at

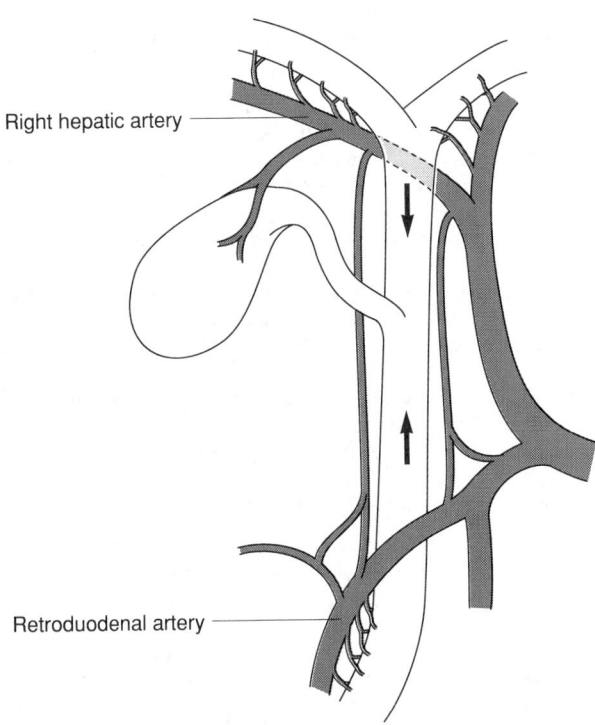

Figure 43-2. Diagrammatic view of the blood supply of the human bile duct. The blood supply to the bile ducts in the hilum of the liver (*above*) and to the intrapancreatic bile duct (*below*) from adjacent arteries is profuse. The supraduodenal bile duct blood supply is axial and tenuous, with 60% from below and 38% from above. The small main axial vessels (3- and 9-o'clock arteries) are vulnerable and easily damaged. (After Terblanche J, Allison HF, Northover JMA. An ischemic basis for biliary strictures. Surgery 1983;94:52)

end-to-end bile duct anastomoses performed for hepatic transplantation or repair of traumatic injury. Ischemia of the anastomosis due to excessive skeletonization of the duct appears to be an important factor in many such strictures.

Stricture Recurrence

Factors associated with recurrent bile duct stricture are:

- Location of the stricture: strictures high in the biliary tree appear to have a rate of recurrence
- Length of follow-up period: long-term follow-up evaluation of bile duct anastomoses is important because strictures can develop years after the original anastomosis
- Influence of previous operations: previous attempts at repair are associated with a high rate of stricture recurrence
- Type of operation: procedures other than choledochojejunostomy or hepaticojejunostomy have a high rate of stricture recurrence
- Use and duration of postoperative stenting: a longer period of stenting appears to be beneficial

Clinical Presentation

Most benign postoperative bile duct strictures present soon after the initial operation. After open cholecystectomy, only about 10% of postoperative strictures are suspected within the first week, but nearly 70% are diagnosed within the first 6 months and >80% within 1 year of the operation. During laparoscopic cholecystectomy, the injury may be recognized during the procedure or, more commonly, in the early postoperative period.

Postoperative bile duct strictures that occur within *days to weeks* of the initial operation usually present in one of two ways:

1. Progressive elevation of liver function tests, particularly total bilirubin and alkaline phosphatase levels. These changes often are seen as early as the second or third postoperative day.
2. Leakage of bile from an injured bile duct. This mode of presentation appears to be more common after laparoscopic cholecystectomy. Bilious drainage from surgically placed drains or through the wound after cholecystectomy is abnormal and represents biliary injury. In patients without drains, or from whom drains have been removed, the bile may leak freely into the peritoneal cavity, or it may collect in loculi. Free accumulation of bile in the peritoneal cavity results in biliary ascites or bile peritonitis. A loculated bile collection may result in a sterile biloma or an infected subhepatic or subdiaphragmatic abscess.

Patients with postoperative bile duct strictures that present *months to years* after the initial operation frequently have evidence of cholangitis, which is often mild and responds to antibiotic therapy. Repetitive episodes usually occur before the definitive diagnosis. Less commonly, patients may present with painless jaundice and no evidence of sepsis. Patients with markedly delayed diagnoses may present with advanced biliary cirrhosis and its complications.

Laboratory Investigation

- Serum bilirubin level may fluctuate
- Serum alkaline phosphatase is usually elevated
- Serum transaminase levels may be normal or minimally elevated, except during episodes of cholangitis

- If advanced liver disease exists, hepatic synthetic function may be impaired with lowered serum albumin and a prolongation of prothrombin time
- Serum electrolytes and complete blood count are normal, unless there is associated biliary sepsis

Diagnostic Imaging

In patients with strictures in the early postoperative period with evidence of a bile leak or biliary sepsis, ultrasonography (US) and computed tomography (CT) are useful to rule out the presence of intra-abdominal collections that might require drainage. Months to years after the initial operation, both studies help confirm biliary obstruction by demonstrating a dilated biliary tree. CT is useful in identification of the level of obstruction of the extrahepatic bile duct.

In patients who may have early postoperative bile duct injury, a radionuclide biliary scan helps confirm bile leakage.

In patients with postoperative external bile fistulas, injection of water-soluble contrast medium through the drainage tract (sinography) often defines the site of leakage and the anatomy of the biliary tree. Sinography also depicts intraabdominal collections and facilitates nonoperative drainage.

The standard for evaluation of bile duct strictures is cholangiography. Percutaneous transhepatic cholangiography (PTC) is generally more valuable than endoscopic retrograde cholangiography (ERC), because PTC helps define the anatomy of the proximal biliary tree to be used in surgical reconstruction. Percutaneous transhepatic catheters, which are useful for decompression of the biliary system to treat or prevent cholangitis, can be placed after PTC. These catheters may be helpful in surgical reconstruction, and they provide access to the biliary tree for nonsurgical dilation.

ERC is less useful than PTC because discontinuity of the extrahepatic bile duct usually prevents adequate filling of the proximal biliary tree. ERC may demonstrate a normal-sized distal bile duct up to the site of the stricture without depicting the proximal biliary system. This finding is frequent with injury during laparoscopic cholecystectomy when the distal bile duct is clipped and divided.

Preoperative Care

Early Strictures

Strictures that present soon after an operation may be associated with sepsis due to cholangitis or intraabdominal bile collections. Sepsis must be controlled with broad-spectrum parenteral antibiotics, percutaneous biliary drainage, and percutaneous or operative drainage of biliary leaks. Once sepsis is controlled, there is no hurry to perform surgical reconstruction of the bile duct stricture. The combination of proximal biliary decompression and external drainage allows most biliary fistulas to be controlled or even closed. The patient can be discharged home to allow several months to elapse for resolution of the inflammation in the periportal region and recovery of overall health status.

Late Strictures

Symptoms of cholangitis may necessitate urgent cholangiography and biliary decompression. Biliary drainage is best accomplished with the transhepatic method, although endoscopic stent placement can be successful. Parenteral antibiotics and biliary drainage are continued until sepsis is controlled. If patients present with jaundice but without cholangitis, cholangiography is performed to define the anatomy.

Surgical Management

The goal of surgical management of bile duct stricture is establishment of bile flow into the proximal gastrointestinal tract in a manner that prevents cholangitis, sludge or stone formation, stricture recurrence, and biliary cirrhosis. This goal is met with a tension-free anastomosis between healthy tissues. Surgical techniques for primary repair of bile duct strictures include end-to-end repair, Roux-en-Y hepaticojejunostomy or choledochojejunostomy, choledochoduodenostomy, and mucosal grafting.

Immediate Repair of Intraoperative Bile Duct Injury

Recognition of a bile duct injury is uncommon during open or laparoscopic cholecystectomy. If bile leakage or atypical anatomy is encountered during laparoscopic cholecystectomy, early conversion to an open operation and prompt cholangiography are imperative. If a segmental or accessory duct <3 mm in diameter is injured, and cholangiography demonstrates segmental or subsegmental drainage of the injured ductal system, simple ligation of the injured duct is adequate. If the injured duct is ≥4 mm in size, however, it is likely to drain multiple hepatic segments or the entire right or left lobe and, thus, requires surgical repair.

If the injury involves the common hepatic duct or the common bile duct, repair is performed at the time of injury. The aims of repair are to maintain duct length, to avoid sacrificing tissue, and to effect a repair that does not allow postoperative bile leakage. Therefore, all repairs at the initial operation involve external drainage. If the injured segment of bile duct is <1 cm long, and the two ends can be apposed without tension, an end-to-end anastomosis is performed and a T tube is placed through a separate choledochotomy above or below the anastomosis. Generous mobilization of the duodenum out of the retroperitoneum (Kocher maneuver) can be useful to approximate the injured ends of the bile duct. End-to-end repair is avoided, however, if the ductal injury is near the hepatic duct bifurcation.

For proximal injuries, or if the injured segment of bile duct is >1 cm long, the distal bile duct is oversewn, and the proximal bile duct is debrided of injured tissue and anastomosed end to side to a Roux-en-Y jejunal limb. Use of a Roux-en-Y jejunal limb is preferable to anastomosis to the duodenum.

Elective Repair of Established Strictures

The following are the principles of repair of a biliary stricture:

- Exposure of healthy proximal bile ducts that provide drainage of the entire liver
- Preparation of a segment of intestine that can be brought to the area of the stricture without tension, most frequently a Roux-en-Y jejunal limb
- Construction of a direct biliary–enteric mucosa-to-mucosa anastomosis

In almost all patients, hepaticojejunostomy to a Roux-en-Y limb of jejunum is the preferred procedure.

A transanastomotic stent is helpful in almost all patients. In the early postoperative period, a stent is used to decompress the biliary tree and provide access for cholangiography. If the injury involves the common bile duct or the common hepatic duct at least 2 cm distal to the hepatic duct bifurcation, and adequate proximal bile duct mucosa

can be defined, long-term use of biliary stents is not necessary. In these situations, the preoperatively placed percutaneous transhepatic catheter or surgically placed T tube is used to decompress the biliary–enteric anastomosis for 4 to 6 weeks postoperatively.

When adequate proximal bile duct is not available for a good mucosa-to-mucosa anastomosis, long-term stenting of the biliary–enteric anastomosis with a polymeric silicone transhepatic stent is recommended. For strictures at the hepatic duct bifurcation, both the right and left main hepatic ducts are stented. One surgical technique involves preoperative placement of percutaneous transhepatic catheters, insertion of transhepatic stents, and biliary reconstruction by means of end-to-side hepatojejunostomy (Fig. 43-3). An alternative technique for management of bile duct strictures that involve the bifurcation and one or both of the hepatic ducts is side-to-side anastomosis of the left hepatic duct to the Roux-en-Y limb. This procedure allows anastomosis to normal mucosa, even though there may be fibrosis and stricture at the bifurcation of the ducts and within the distal portion of the hepatic duct. This technique may obviate postoperative stenting.

Results

Complications of repair of bile duct strictures include the usual postoperative complications, such as hemorrhage, cardiopulmonary problems, urinary tract infection, and wound infection. Complications specific to the repair of bile duct strictures include anastomotic leaks at the site of the biliary–enteric anastomosis, cholangitis, and hepatic insufficiency due to biliary cirrhosis. Most anastomotic leaks documented with postoperative cholangiography or bilious drainage from surgical drains can be managed without surgical treatment. Transhepatic stenting diverts biliary secretions to the outside and is one of the advantages of this technique.

The operative mortality for repair of bile duct strictures is <5%. Factors associated with mortality include advanced age, coexistent disease, and a history of severe biliary tract infection. Underlying liver disease, however, is the most important determinant of operative morbidity and mortality. In patients with advanced biliary cirrhosis and portal hypertension, operative mortality can approach 30%, most deaths being caused by liver failure.

Nonsurgical Management

Percutaneous Balloon Dilation

This procedure is performed with local anesthesia and intravenous sedation. The stricture is traversed with a guide wire under fluoroscopic guidance and dilated with angioplasty balloon catheters. After the procedure, a transhepatic stent is left in place across the stricture to allow access to the biliary tree for follow-up cholangiography, repeat dilation, and maintenance of a lumen during healing. Numerous dilations usually are required.

Complications of balloon dilation are:

- Cholangitis
- Hemobilia
- Bleeding, usually from the hepatic parenchyma
- Sepsis due to cholangitis, which can occur despite antibiotic prophylaxis

Endoscopic Dilation

Endoscopic balloon dilation is feasible only in patients with primary bile duct strictures or with strictures at a choledochoduodenal anastomosis. The procedure begins with ERC and endoscopic sphincterotomy. The stricture is traversed retrograde with an atraumatic guide wire, and

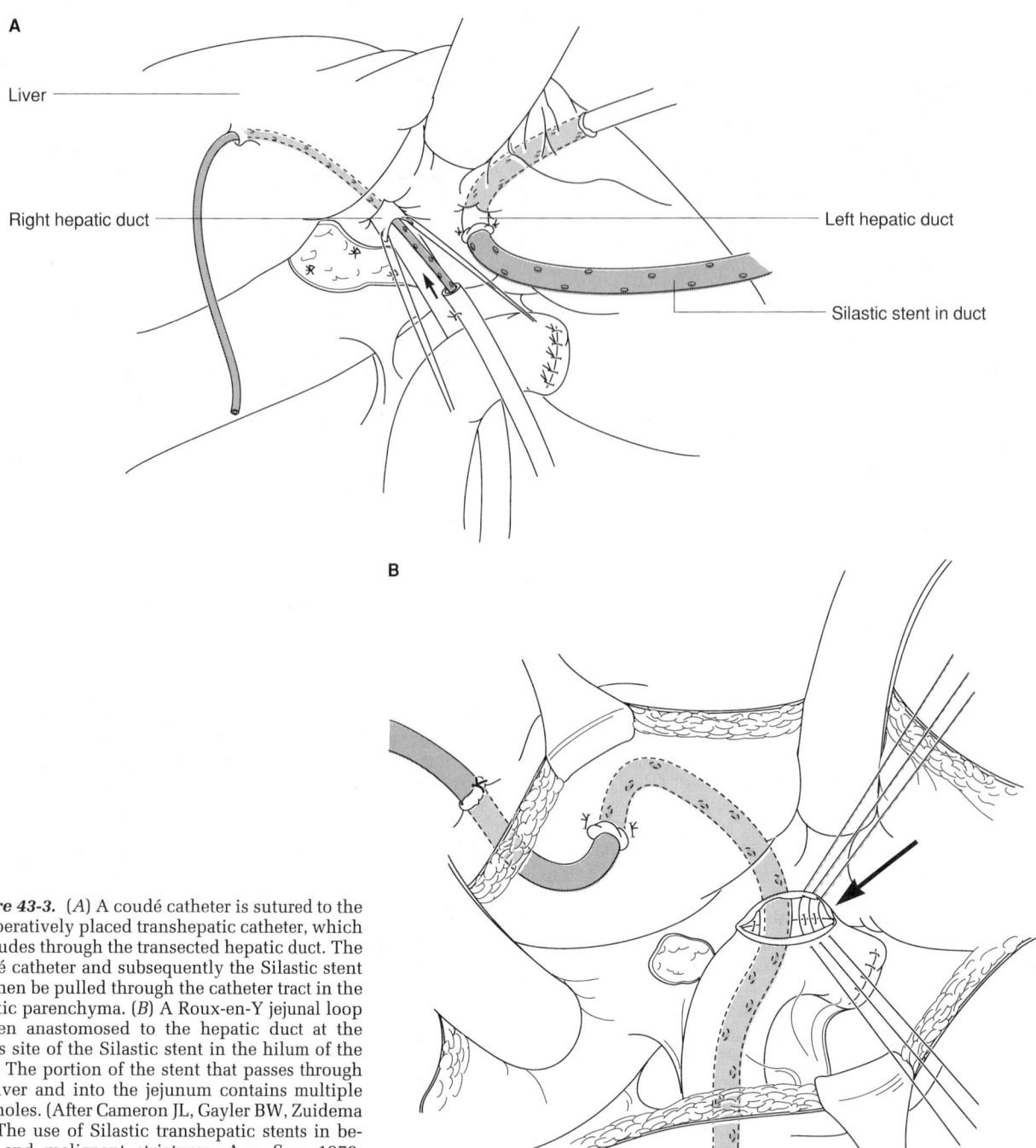

Figure 43-3. (*A*) A coudé catheter is sutured to the preoperatively placed transhepatic catheter, which protrudes through the transected hepatic duct. The coudé catheter and subsequently the Silastic stent can then be pulled through the catheter tract in the hepatic parenchyma. (*B*) A Roux-en-Y jejunal loop is then anastomosed to the hepatic duct at the egress site of the Silastic stent in the hilum of the liver. The portion of the stent that passes through the liver and into the jejunum contains multiple side holes. (After Cameron JL, Gayler BW, Zuidema GD. The use of Silastic transhepatic stents in benign and malignant strictures. Ann Surg 1978; 188:552)

sequential balloon dilation is performed. Follow-up cholangiography is performed every 3 to 6 months. Redilation is performed as necessary. In most patients, an endoprosthesis is left in place after dilation for at least 6 months.

PRIMARY SCLEROSING CHOLANGITIS

Primary sclerosing cholangitis is an idiopathic disease characterized by intrahepatic and extrahepatic inflammatory strictures of the bile ducts. It may be an autoimmune reaction because it is associated with other autoimmune diseases (Table 43-1). The clinical features are:

- Intermittent jaundice, which begins insidiously in the fourth or fifth decade of life
- Right-upper-quadrant pain, pruritus, fever, weight loss, fatigue
- Cyclic remissions and exacerbations
- History of biliary manipulation or operation
- Bilirubin levels that fluctuate with the remissions and exacerbations of the disease and the extent of hepatic injury
- Alkaline phosphatase elevated out of proportion to serum bilirubin
- Diagnosis confirmed with cholangiography

Medical therapy is not effective for primary sclerosing cholangitis. An aggressive surgical approach is advocated. The options are:

Table 43-1. DISEASES ASSOCIATED WITH PRIMARY SCLEROSING CHOLANGITIS

Disease	Frequency (%)
Ulcerative colitis	40–60
Pancreatitis	12–25
Diabetes mellitus	5–10
Retroperitoneal fibrosis	Rare
Riedel thyroiditis	Rare
Crohn's disease	Rare
Histiocytosis X	Rare
Sicca complex	Rare
Rheumatoid arthritis	Rare
Hypertrophic osteoarthropathy	Rare
Sarcoidosis	Rare
Angioimmunoblastic lymphadenopathy	Rare
Acquired immunodeficiency syndrome	Rare

- In patients with a dominant stricture at the hepatic duct bifurcation, resection of the bifurcation and long-term transhepatic stenting with polymeric silicone stents
- Hepatic transplantation

BILE DUCT STRICTURE DUE TO CHRONIC PANCREATITIS

Transient partial obstruction of the distal common bile duct due to inflammation and edema occurs in patients with *acute* pancreatitis. With *chronic* pancreatitis, however, the problem is distal bile duct obstruction due to inflammation and parenchymal fibrosis. These strictures involve the entire intrapancreatic segment of the common bile duct and are associated with dilatation of the entire proximal biliary tree.

The clinical presentation of common bile duct strictures due to chronic pancreatitis is variable, and it can be:

- No symptoms, the diagnosis of bile duct strictures suggested only by abnormal liver function tests
- Elevated serum alkaline phosphatase
- Abdominal pain, with or without jaundice

The definitive diagnostic modality is endoscopic retrograde cholangiopancreatography (ERCP) or PTC. A long (2

to 4 cm), smooth, gradual tapering of the common bile duct is most compatible with a benign stricture due to chronic pancreatitis.

The indications for surgical treatment of common bile duct strictures due to chronic pancreatitis are pain, jaundice, or cholangitis. Biliary bypass is performed by means of choledochoduodenostomy or Roux-en-Y choledochojejunostomy.

MISCELLANEOUS CAUSE OF BILE DUCT STRICTURES

Benign strictures of the bile duct can result from:

- Chronic inflammation associated with gallstones in the gallbladder or common bile duct
- Excessive surgical manipulation at bile duct exploration with forceps, scoops, or catheters
- Stenosis of the sphincter of Oddi, or papillitis
- Cholangiohepatitis due to *Opisthorchis sinensis* or other parasites
- Intrahepatic arterial infusion of 5-fluorouracil used in the treatment of hepatic metastases of colorectal carcinoma
- Acquired immunodeficiency syndrome

SUGGESTED READING

Branum G, Schmitt C, Baille J, et al. Management of major biliary complications after laparoscopic cholecystectomy. Ann Surg 1993;17:53.

David PHP, Tanka AKF, Rauws EAJ, et al. Benign biliary strictures: Surgery or endoscopy? Ann Surg 1993;217:237.

Geenen DJ, Geenen JE, Hogan WJ, et al. Endoscopic therapy for benign bile duct strictures. Gastrointest Endosc 1989;35:367.

Lillemoe KD, Pitt HA, Cameron JL. Primary sclerosing cholangitis. Surg Clin North Am 1990;70:1381.

Marsh JW Jr, Iwatsuki S, Makowka L, et al. Orthotopic liver transplantation for primary sclerosing cholangitis. Ann Surg 1988;207:21.

Mueller PR, van Sonnenberg E, Ferrucci T Jr, et al. Biliary stricture dilatation: multicenter review of clinical management in 73 patients. Radiology 1986;160:17.

Pitt HA, Kaufman SL, Coleman J, et al. Benign postoperative biliary strictures: Operate or dilate? Ann Surg 1989;210:417.

Stahl TJ, O'Connor A, Ansel M, et al. Partial biliary obstruction caused by chronic pancreatitis: an appraisal of indications for surgical biliary drainage. Ann Surg 1988;207:26.

COLON, RECTUM, AND ANUS

ESSENTIALS OF SURGERY: SCIENTIFIC PRINCIPLES AND PRACTICE,
edited by Lazar J. Greenfield, Michael W. Mulholland, Keith T. Oldham, Gerald B. Zelenock,
and Keith D. Lillemoe. Lippincott–Raven Publishers, Philadelphia, © 1997.

CHAPTER 44

COLONIC ANATOMY AND PHYSIOLOGY

THOMAS A. MILLER

The function of the gastrointestinal (GI) tract is to absorb water, nutrients, and substances, such as electrolytes, minerals, and vitamins. The role of the colon is mixing, temporary storage, and slow distal propulsion of luminal contents.

ANATOMY OF THE COLON

General Considerations

The colon consists of appendix, cecum, ascending colon, transverse colon, descending colon, sigmoid colon, rectum, and anal canal (Fig. 44-1). The *right colon* consists of the cecum, the ascending colon, the hepatic flexure, and the proximal transverse colon. The *left colon* comprises the distal transverse colon, the splenic flexure, the descending

colon, the sigmoid colon, and the rectosigmoid. Total colonic length is 4.5 to 6 feet (135 to 180 cm).

The transverse and sigmoid colons are suspended in the peritoneal cavity by mesenteries. The ascending and descending segments are fixed to the retroperitoneum. The diameter of the colon decreases from cecum to sigmoid. The colonic wall contains four layers— mucosa, submucosa, muscularis, and serosa (Fig. 44-2).

Arteries

Two arterial systems supply the colon (Fig. 44-3). The *right colon* is supplied by the *superior mesenteric artery.* The branches of this artery that perfuse the right colon include the *ileocolic artery,* which supplies the ileocecal junction; the *right colic artery,* which supplies the ascending colon; and the *middle colic artery,* which supplies the hepatic flexure and the transverse colon to its midpoint. The *left colon* is supplied by the *inferior mesenteric artery,* which originates from the abdominal aorta. The distal transverse colon and the descending colon obtain their blood supply from the *left colic branch* of the inferior mesenteric artery. The sigmoid colon obtains its blood supply from *sigmoidal arteries.* Throughout the colon, the *marginal artery* forms an anastomosis between the superior mesenteric artery and the inferior mesenteric artery. Complete anastomosis is present only 15% to 20% of the time.

Veins

The veins of the colon accompany the arteries (Fig. 44-4). Veins that drain the right colon enter the *superior mesenteric vein,* and those that drain the left colon form

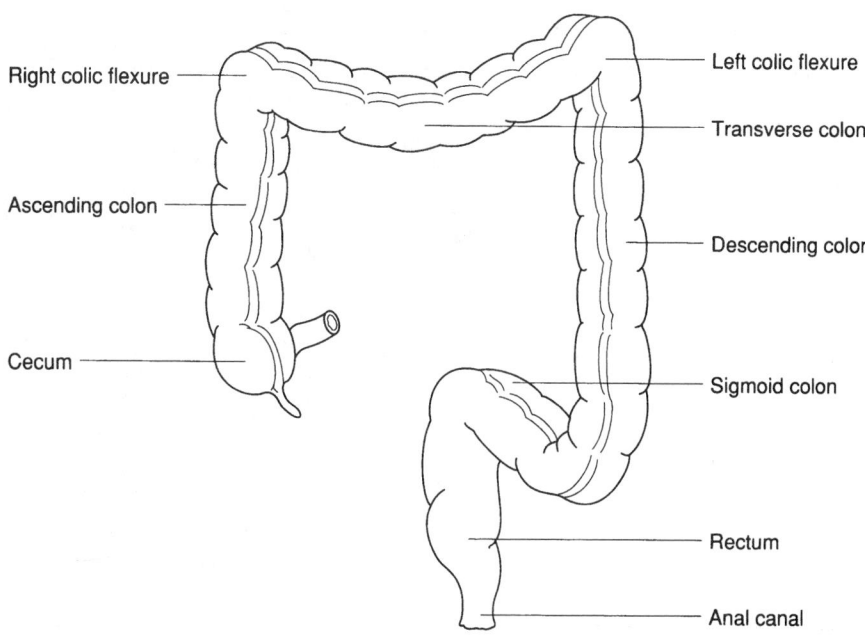

Figure 44-1. Anatomic components of the colon.

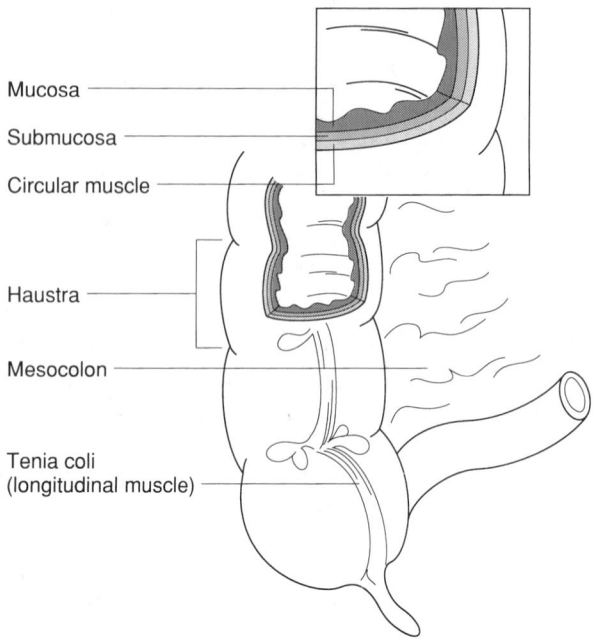

Mucosa

Submucosa

Circular muscle

Haustra

Mesocolon

Tenia coli
(longitudinal muscle)

Figure 44-2. Layers of the colonic wall.

the *inferior mesenteric vein.* Both these veins empty into the *portal vein,* which drains into the liver.

Lymphatic vessels

Lymphatic plexuses in the submucosal and subserosal layers of the intestine drain into lymphatic vessels and lymph nodes that accompany the veins and arteries (Fig. 44-5).

Colonic Epithelium

The mucosal surface of the colon consists of columnar epithelium that is less sophisticated than small-intestinal epithelium. There are no villi in the colon, and the colonic mucosa is flat. Along the mucosal surface, crypts of Lieberkühn open into the colonic lumen. The epithelium of the lower portion of the crypts consists of undifferentiated mucus-secreting goblet cells, scattered endocrine cells, and columnar cells. The upper part of the crypts is composed of differentiated columnar cells, goblet cells, and a few endocrine cells. The mucosa between the crypts is columnar.

Muscular Structure of the Colonic Wall

The colon contains smooth muscle in three layers. The innermost layer, below the epithelium, is *muscularis mucosae.* The muscularis mucosae has an inner circular and an outer longitudinal layer, and the two are fixed so that the muscle bundles are tightly interwoven. Surrounding the muscularis mucosae is a thick layer of *circular smooth*

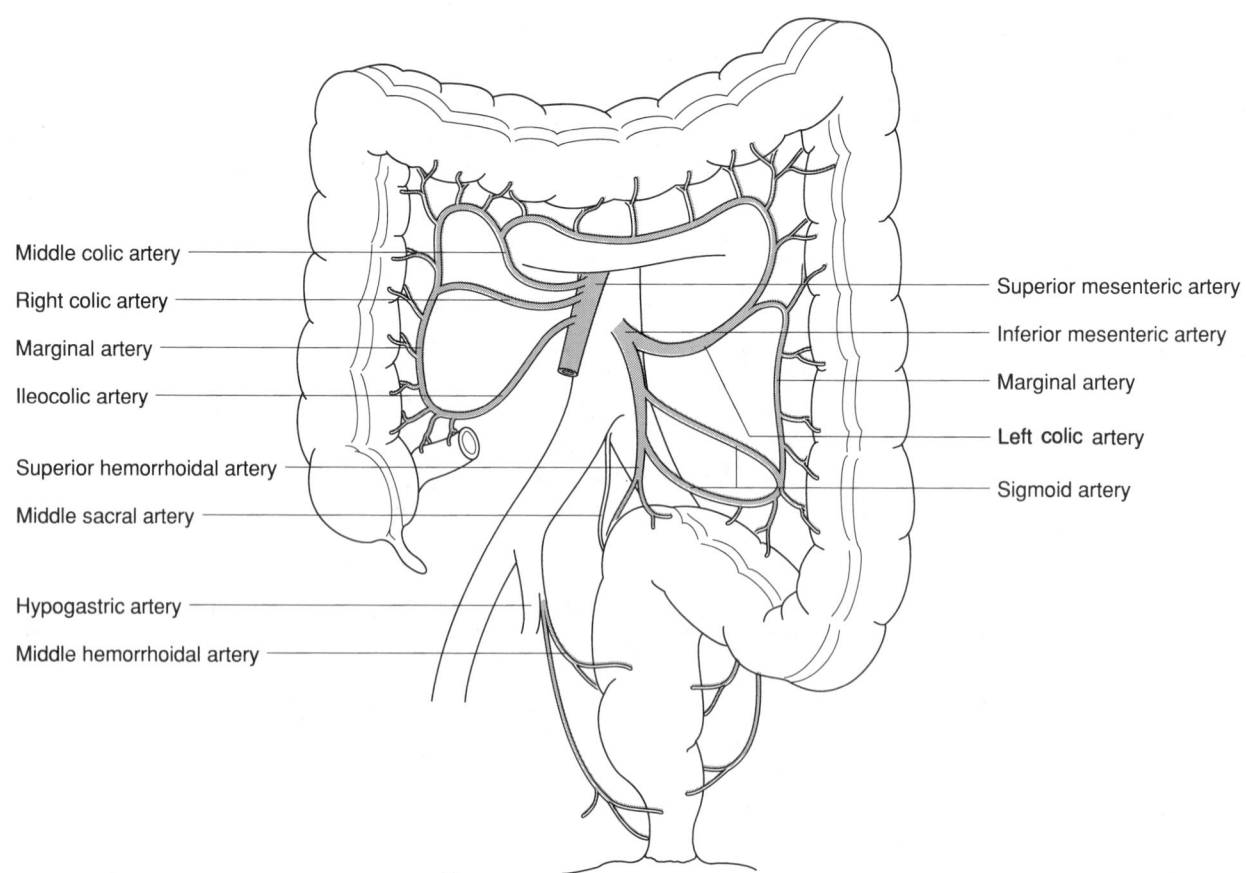

Middle colic artery

Right colic artery

Marginal artery

Ileocolic artery

Superior hemorrhoidal artery

Middle sacral artery

Hypogastric artery

Middle hemorrhoidal artery

Superior mesenteric artery

Inferior mesenteric artery

Marginal artery

Left colic artery

Sigmoid artery

Figure 44-3. Arterial blood supply of the colon.

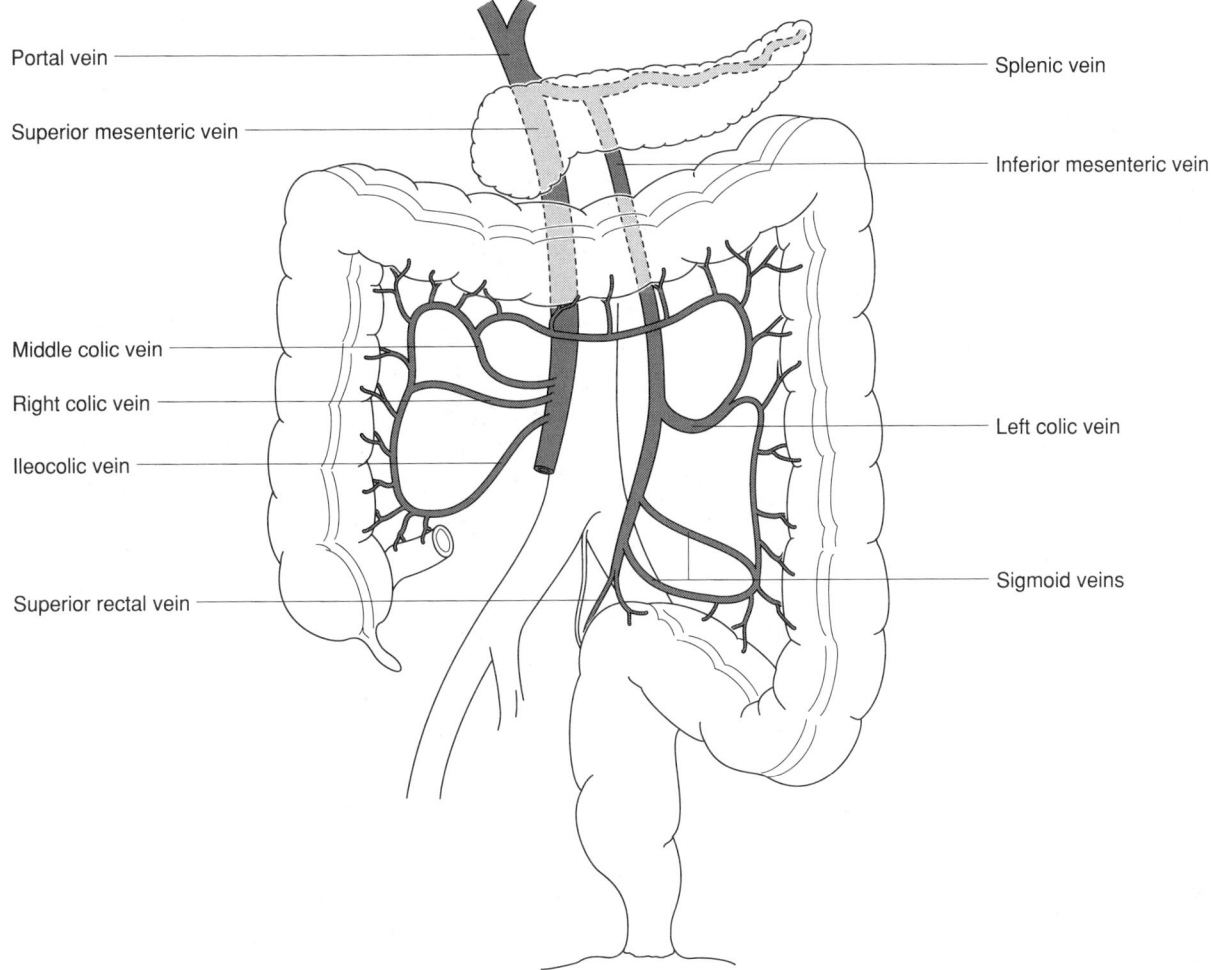

Portal vein

Superior mesenteric vein

Middle colic vein

Right colic vein

Ileocolic vein

Superior rectal vein

Splenic vein

Inferior mesenteric vein

Left colic vein

Sigmoid veins

Figure 44-4. Venous drainage of the colon by the portal vein.

muscle that subtends the entire circumference of the colon. A layer of *longitudinal muscle* surrounds the circular muscle.

The longitudinal muscle layer of the colon is grouped into three thick bands, called *taeniae.* This configuration of the longitudinal muscle gives rise to the sacculated appearance of the colon known as *haustration.* The three taeniae begin in the cecum and continue throughout the large intestine to the point where the sigmoid colon ends and the rectum begins. At this point, the three taeniae become broad based and fuse so that the longitudinal muscle layer is distributed uniformly around the circumference of the rectum.

Neural Components

Two groups of plexuses exist in the wall of the colon. The submucosal plexus (Meissner plexus) is between the muscularis mucosae and the circular muscle layer of the muscularis propria. Between the circular muscle and the outer longitudinal muscle is the myenteric plexus (Auerbach plexus).

PHYSIOLOGY OF COLONIC CONTRACTION

In men, colonic transit time is about 33 hours; in women, it is about 47 hours. This slow transit allows defecation to occur at socially convenient times and under voluntary control.

Each region of the large intestine appears to have motor activity independent of the other regions. Caudal propulsion of fecal contents occurs slowly as the result of the motor activity of the right colon. The left colon is a storage reservoir for the semisolid to solid feces in its lumen, and its contractile patterns are used for distal movement of feces and defecation.

Individual phasic contractions initiate contractile patterns of both short and long duration. Short contractions last <15 seconds; long contractions last 40 to 60 seconds. Although both types of contractions occur in circular muscle, long contractions originate in the longitudinal muscle, and short contractions emanate from circular muscle. The frequency of short contractions is 2 to 13 per minute; that of long contractions is 0.5 to 2 per minute. These contractions mix colonic contents for absorption and slowly propel the semisolid to solid feces distally. Long contractions appear to be especially important in this role. Underlying each phasic contractile pattern is an electrical pattern in smooth muscle cells that enables each cell to control its contractions and couple them with those of adjacent cells.

In addition to short and long contractions, the colon exhibits ultrapropulsive contractions called *giant migrating contractions* (GMCs). GMCs are of long duration and amplitude and propagate over a substantial length of the colon. GMCs cause mass movement of colonic content and emptying of the area of the colon in which they occur. GMCs occur infrequently (once or twice a day). In the distal

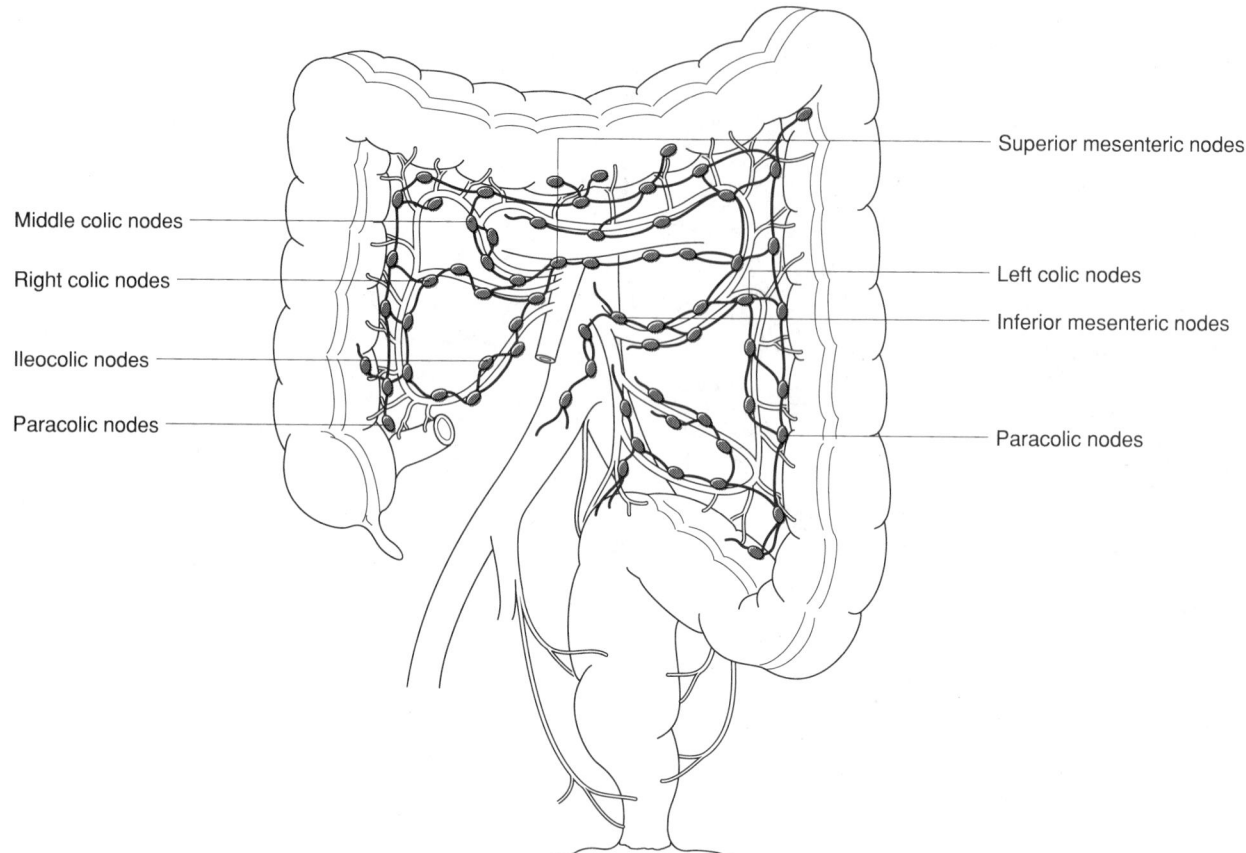

Figure 44-5. Lymphatic drainage of the colon.

colon, GMCs provide the force necessary to propel feces rapidly during defecation.

NEUROHUMORAL CONTROL OF COLONIC MOTILITY

Three levels of neural control influence colonic contractions—the enteric, autonomic, and central nervous systems.

Enteric Nervous System

The enteric nervous system plays a prominent role in the control of colonic motility. The enteric nerves of the colon are organized into the *myenteric plexus* (Auerbach plexus) and the *submucosal plexus* (Meissner plexus). In each plexus, the cell bodies of neurons are grouped into ganglia from which neurons project to the muscle groups they supply. Motor neurons that project to the circular and longitudinal muscle layers are of two types: excitatory and inhibitory. The neurotransmitter of the excitatory neurons is acetylcholine. The neurotransmitters of inhibitory motor neurons, also called nonadrenergic, noncholinergic (NANC) neurons, are not known, but ATP, vasoactive intestinal polypeptide (VIP), and nitric oxide are candidates.

Peptidergic neurons are present in the colonic wall. Most of the transmitters for these neurons are peptides, such as somatostatin, substance P, opioids, calcitonin-gene–related peptide, neuropeptide Y, VIP, and gastrin-releasing peptide. Nonpeptide transmitters, such as γ-aminobutyric acid and serotonin, also may be important. The physiologic

role of these neurons as modulators of colonic motility is not known.

Sensory neurons perceive mechanical and chemical stimuli from luminal content. The axons project to motor neurons and to prevertebral ganglia and higher neural centers. Mediators of such sensory input appear to be substance P and calcitonin-gene–related peptide. The role of these neurons in transmitting sensory information is not known, but because they synapse on the excitatory and inhibitory motor neurons, they probably are important in modulating spontaneous contractions.

Autonomic Nervous System

The vagus and the pelvic nerves are parasympathetic neural inputs, and the lumbar colonic, splanchnic, and hypogastric nerves are sympathetic components. Fibers from these nerves may affect a number of enteric ganglia and provide important pathways for input from the CNS to the colon and for reflex actions and modulation between different portions of the colon and the colon and other organs. Norepinephrine is the primary neurotransmitter of sympathetic nerves in the colon. Through neural transmission, it regulates the release of acetylcholine at presynaptic terminals in the enteric ganglia. Parasympathetic neural transmission is mediated through acetylcholine.

Central Nervous System

The CNS modulates colonic motor function under conditions of stress or during voluntary defecation. Such modulation is transmitted through the autonomic nerves (the vagus, pelvic, hypogastric, lumbar colonic, and splanchnic nerves) to the enteric ganglia. Through such autonomic neural control, the brain stimulates or inhibits colonic contraction by way of motor excitatory and inhibitory neurons.

Peptides may modulate colonic motor activity. Substances such as cholecystokinin (CCK), gastrin, secretin, neurotensin, and pancreatic polypeptide increase after meals. Whether postprandial concentrations of these peptides affect colonic motor activity is not clear. Prostaglandins and motilin are powerful stimulants of intestinal smooth muscle and may have a physiologic role. Bile acids, especially deoxycholic acid, appear to be direct stimulants of colonic motor activity. Drugs such as erythromycin, cisapride, opioids, and serotonin antagonists alter colonic motor activity through a direct increase or decrease in the rate of transit. How these effects are mediated is not known. Some of these drugs may alter neural inputs to colonic motor cells; others may have direct effects on the cells themselves.

PHYSIOLOGIC ALTERATIONS IN COLONIC MOTILITY

Movement of the colon occurs soon after a meal. In some people, ingestion of certain foods almost guarantees an immediate bowel movement. In others, the colonic response to eating is unpredictable, and the extent and magnitude of the response are variable. The colonic response, when it occurs, affects the frequency of colonic contraction and the amplitude of pressure generated. The response is most marked in the sigmoid colon, but the entire colon responds to eating in varying degrees.

The colonic response to eating once was believed to start when food entered the stomach, and thus was called the *gastrocolic reflex.* However, the following observations show that the stomach has a limited role in mediating this response:

- Gastric distention does not elicit the colonic response, which begins slowly and persists after the stomach has emptied its contents
- The colonic response occurs in patients who have undergone complete gastrectomy
- The colonic response is elicited when food is placed directly into the duodenum

Whether the stomach triggers the response and the duodenum and other portions of the proximal intestine sustain it is not known. Different kinds of foods modulate the intensity of the colonic response. Ingestion of fat tends to increase colonic motility, and amino acids inhibit it. Mucosal chemoreceptors appear to be responsible for mediation of the response.

The mechanism by which chemoreceptive sensors effect changes in colonic motility is not known. It appears that neural and humoral pathways have a role. Although an intact cholinergic innervation is necessary to mediate the colonic response, an adrenergic mechanism also may be involved. Whether the response is generated by direct neurogenic muscular contraction or a transient suspension of neurogenic inhibition is not clear.

Also unknown is the role of hormones in mediating the colonic response. For example, gastrin increases colonic motor activity and initiates spike potentials in the sigmoid and rectum. CCK appears to have similar stimulatory effects on colonic motor function. If hormones are involved in the colonic response to eating, release and subsequent colonic motor effects of the hormones are modulated by various components of food as they pass through the GI tract. Gastrin release by food in the stomach may trigger the effect, and CCK release in the proximal intestine may sustain the effect.

COLONIC EPITHELIAL TRANSPORT

The epithelium of the colon is relatively impermeable and requires a long time to absorb the salt, water, and carbohydrate presented to it. Between 500 and 1500 g of a semiliquid material that may contain as much as 100 g of carbohydrate enters the colon each day. Most of this substance is absorbed, yielding a stool output that weighs about 200 g. The reason for this efficient absorptive capacity, despite the relative impermeability of the colonic epithelium, is the close relation between epithelial transport and colonic motor activity.

Transit through the large intestine takes 2 to 3 days. This slow passage provides opportunity for the luminal contents to come into contact with the absorptive epithelium. Sodium and water, which are extracted against high electrochemical and osmotic gradients, are absorbed. The relatively static conditions of the colon allow proliferation of anaerobic bacteria, which break down carbohydrate to volatile fatty acids, which are rapidly absorbed. The more rapid the colonic transit, the less efficient are these absorptive processes.

Ring-like contractions, which move luminal contents antegrade or retrograde or keep the contents stationary, enhance surface contact between luminal slurry and enterocytes, optimizing absorption. These contractions, which produce haustration, ensure that adequate mixing occurs and that the absorptive epithelium comes into direct contact with luminal material, even that in the center of the lumen. Although the viscous nature of the colonic contents makes it difficult for substances in the center of the lumen to gain access to the absorptive epithelium, haustral contraction enhances absorption by bringing the epithelial surface to the material in the colonic bulk.

These patterns appear to mix the *unstirred layer,* a zone of water and mucus adjacent to the epithelium that retards absorption. By generating convection currents, the mixing patterns of the colon disrupt the unstirred layer to enable surface contact between the luminal contents and the epithelial surface so that absorption proceeds without difficulty. The products of carbohydrate fermentation also appear to stimulate salt and water absorption by influencing motor activity through enteric neural reflexes.

Sustained contractions (GMCs) propel the colonic contents into the rectum and toward the anus. Factors that appear to initiate GMCs are fatty acids, bile acids, various indigestible particles, luminal distention, laxatives, and cholinergic stimulation. A balance seems to exist between mass movement that enables regular evacuation of waste and the slower mixing type of contractions that promote absorption of salt and water and bacterial proliferation for carbohydrate salvage. When this balance is disturbed (due to laxative abuse, derangements in bile acid production, excessive delivery of undigested particles to the colon, or disruption of the normal bacterial flora of the colon with inappropriate use of broad-spectrum antibiotics) excessive numbers of long contractions may supervene, causing diarrhea.

DEFECATION

Initiation of defecation appears to be elicited by mechanoreceptors in the anorectal region. These mechanoreceptors probably originate in the mucosa or seromuscular layer. The receptors seem to be more numerous, or at least more sensitive, in the distal than the in proximal part of the rectum. Only an intact distal anorectal region appears to be necessary for defecation to occur. The rectum usually is filled with fecal material in the absence of the urge to defecate. How changes in stool volume and wall pressure excite the anorectal mechanoreceptors to initiate defecation is not known.

The nervous system has a role in defecation. The anal sphincter relaxes; the distal colon contracts to move the fecal contents distally; and ancillary processes (closure of the glottis, descent of the diaphragm, and contraction of the abdominal musculature) raise intraabdominal pressure. Injuries to the cerebral cortex and the spinal cord above the lumbosacral region may disturb defecation, but the disturbance is often transient, and normal function usually is restored.

DISTURBANCES IN COLONIC MOTILITY

Constipation

Constipation is fewer than three bowel movements per week or excessive straining during defecation more than 20% to 25% of the time. It is usually a symptom of an underlying disease (Table 44-1). Because stool volume and frequency are influenced by several factors (age, diet, sex, personality), the causes of constipation are elusive. Most people with constipation respond to simple dietary measures, such as an increase in dietary fiber intake or enhanced physical activity. Patients in whom no underlying cause is identified and who do not respond to these simple management strategies are considered to have *chronic idiopathic constipation,* which is classified as follows.

Colonic Inertia

Colonic inertia, or slow-transit constipation, occurs mainly in young women. Fiber supplementation, large doses of laxatives, and enemas do not relieve the condition. The cause is not known. Explanations include aberration in the neurochemical control of the colon; abnormalities in the neural elements of the myenteric plexus; disturbances in neuromodulation of colonic motility; and disturbances in colonic neurotransmission via humoral agents such as VIP. Diagnosis is by means of assessment

of colonic transit with various radiopaque markers. Total transit time >72 hours is abnormal. Treatment of colonic inertia is difficult; many patients require subtotal colectomy.

Dysfunction of the Pelvic Floor

Pelvic floor function is evaluated with a rectal balloon expulsion examination. If the findings are abnormal, anorectal manometry, electromyography, and a scintigraphic evacuation examination are performed. Depending on the information obtained, treatment is pharmacologic or surgical intervention.

Normal-Transit Constipation

If colonic transit and pelvic floor function are normal in patients with constipation and no cause is identified, the diagnosis is normal-transit constipation. This entity is a variant of irritable colon syndrome. Surgical intervention is not appropriate.

Diarrhea

The mechanisms responsible for diarrhea are poorly defined. Although disordered motility seems to be important, motility patterns depend on whether the diarrhea has an osmotic, secretory, inflammatory, or idiopathic cause. Diarrhea probably occurs because of a hypermotile state (hypomotility causes constipation).

Although colonic transit time decreases during diarrhea, overall motor activity of the colon decreases rather than increases. Loss of phasic activity with a consequent increase in colonic transit, enhancement in the number of large amplitude migrating contractions, or both of these phenomena is the common motility disturbance in most instances of diarrhea.

Emotional stress appears to be linked with alterations in colonic motor function in some patients with diarrhea, but how such aberrations are mediated is not known.

Diverticulosis of the Colon

Diverticulosis of the colon results from high intraluminal pressures that give rise to mucosal herniations through the colonic wall (Figs. 44-6 and 44-7). The pressure in the colonic lumen appears to be a consequence of disordered colonic motility due to thickening of the circular muscle adjacent to the diverticulum with concomitant narrowing of the luminal diameter. Why muscle thickening occurs is unknown.

Patients with diverticulosis have an increased density of nerve tissue in the intramural ganglia. Whether this increase is the cause or consequence of the disease is uncertain. Despite the muscle thickening encountered in patients with diverticulosis, myoelectric activity is the same as in healthy people.

The development of diverticulosis is linked with the low-residue diet consumed in industrialized countries. How such a diet initiates the muscular aberration is not known. One possibility is that the low fecal volume resulting from this diet requires a greater propulsive force to initiate caudal movement and defecation. The muscular thickening may be an attempt to generate propulsive action. Patients with diverticular disease often manage the condition effectively by increasing fiber content in their diet.

Irritable Colon Syndrome

Irritable colon syndrome is a symptom complex of abdominal pain, distention, and abnormal bowel function that ranges from constipation to diarrhea. Often no organic

---

Table 44-1. CAUSES OF CONSTIPATION

FUNCTIONAL
Slow transit
Pelvic floor dysfunction
Dietary
Immobilization
Depression
Irritable bowel syndrome

NEUROLOGIC
Central nervous system (stroke, Parkinson disease, Alzheimer disease)
Spinal (multiple sclerosis, tumor, herniated disc, trauma, myelocele)
Nervi erigentes damage
Aganglionosis (Hirschsprung disease, Chagas disease)

ENDOCRINE
Hypothyroidism
Hypercalcemia
Pheochromocytoma
Diabetes

MEDICATIONS
Narcotics
Anticholinergics
Antacids
Antihypertensives
Antidepressants
Iron
Barium

OBSTRUCTIVE
Tumor
Diverticulitis
Inflammatory bowel disease
Ischemic
Volvulus
Endometriosis

SYSTEMIC
Scleroderma
Uremia
Amyloidosis
Hypokalemia

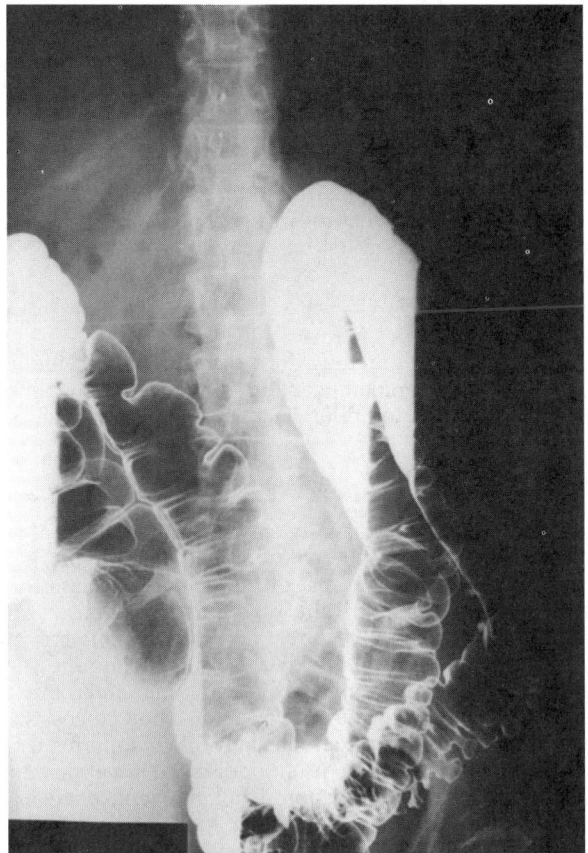

Figure 44-6. Air-contrast barium enema demonstrates extensive sigmoid diverticulosis without colonic narrowing. (Corman ML. Diverticular disease. In: Colon and rectal surgery. Philadelphia, JB Lippincott, 1989:670)

cause is identified. Although it is presumed that this disorder is psychogenic, a large number of patients have no clear psychological abnormality or identifiable stress, depression, or anxiety. Clear-cut motor abnormalities do not occur. Explanations for the altered motility are abnormal colonic myoelectric activity and abnormal GI hormone secretion or sensitivity. Visceral afferent innervation of the intestine appears to be altered in patients with the irritable colon syndrome, causing the pain, fullness, or distention. There is no standard management of irritable colon syndrome.

Postoperative Colonic Motor Dysfunction

Both neural and humoral agents contribute to the intestinal aperistalsis that occurs after an operation. Factors that influence the duration of ileus include:

- Preoperative medications
- Anesthetic and analgesic agents
- The extent to which the intestine is manipulated and handled
- Amount of dissection
- Preoperative and postoperative metabolic status
- Abnormalities in potassium and calcium metabolism
- Protein status of the patient
- Use of meperidine or codeine

Pseudo-obstruction of the Colon

Pseudo-obstruction of the colon is defined as failure of peristalsis without an identifiable mechanical obstructing lesion.

Acute

Acute pseudo-obstruction, or *Ogilvie syndrome* (Fig. 44-8), is the result of a failure of propulsive forces to overcome normal resistances to flow. Acute pseudo-obstruction usually involves the proximal colon but may extend through the transverse colon and, rarely, the descending colon. The cause is unknown. The condition almost always occurs in the critically ill. The most important characteristic of acute pseudo-obstruction is severe abdominal distention without marked pain or tenderness. Later in the disease, symptoms are similar to those of true mechanical obstruction. Radiographs of the abdomen show marked gaseous distention of the colon localized to the right colon.

The most serious problem with pseudo-obstruction of the colon is the risk of cecal perforation. Decompression is performed when the cecum reaches 10 to 12 cm in diameter. Fiberoptic colonoscopy is a successful treatment in almost all patients. If colonoscopy does not work or cannot be performed, cecostomy is performed.

Chronic

Chronic pseudo-obstruction is rare. Causes include visceral myopathy, visceral neuropathy (eg, Hirschsprung disease), connective tissue disorders, generalized nerve diseases, endocrine or metabolic disturbances, and drug use.

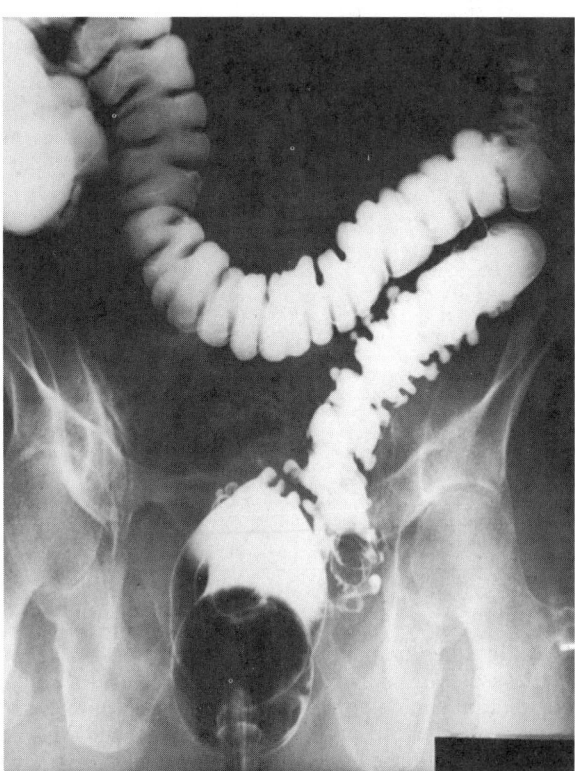

Figure 44-7. Extensive sigmoid diverticular disease with slight spasm but no stigmata of acute inflammation. (Corman ML. Diverticular disease. In: Colon and rectal surgery. Philadelphia, JB Lippincott, 1989:670)

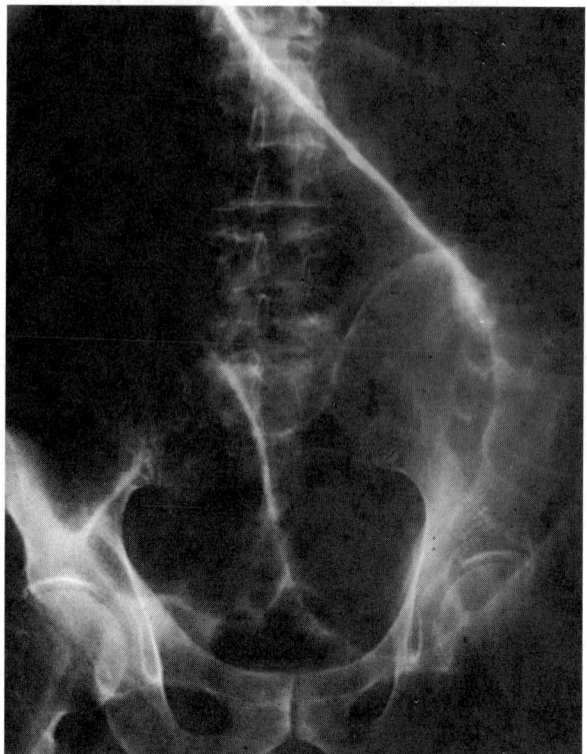

Figure 44-8. Psuedoobstruction of the colon (Ogilvie syndrome). (Corman ML. Miscellaneous colon and rectal conditions. In: Colon and rectal surgery. Philadelphia, JB Lippincott, 1989:977)

SUGGESTED READING

Becker JM. Normal peristalsis and abnormalities in intestinal motility. In: Miller TA, ed. Physiologic basis of modern surgical care. St. Louis, CV Mosby, 1988:347–359.

McIntyre, PB, Pemberton JH. Pathophysiology of colonic motility disorders. Surg Clin North Am 1993;73:1225.

Sarna, SK. Colonic motor activity. Surg Clin North Am 1993; 73:1201.

ESSENTIALS OF SURGERY: SCIENTIFIC PRINCIPLES AND PRACTICE,
edited by Lazar J. Greenfield, Michael W. Mulholland, Keith T. Oldham, Gerald B. Zelenock,
and Keith D. Lillemoe. Lippincott–Raven Publishers, Philadelphia, © 1997.

CHAPTER 45

ULCERATIVE COLITIS

JAMES M. BECKER

Chronic ulcerative colitis (CUC) is a diffuse inflammatory disease of unknown causation that affects the mucosa of the rectum and colon. It features remissions and exacerbations characterized by rectal bleeding and diarrhea and has serious long-term local and systemic effects. Ulcerative colitis and Crohn's disease of the intestine overlap in pathologic features and anatomic distribution. Differentiation is important, because the surgical approaches to the two diseases are quite different.

EPIDEMIOLOGY

The onset of ulcerative colitis occurs at 15 to 40 years of age, but the range extends from infancy to very old age. Males and females are affected about equally. Ten percent to 25% of patients with ulcerative colitis have first-degree relatives with the disease. Geographic and racial differences influence the occurrence of the disease. There is no conclusive evidence regarding the genetic versus the environmental determination of familial patterns.

ETIOLOGY

Theories about the cause of ulcerative colitis include infectious, immunologic, genetic, dietary, environmental, vascular, neuromotor, allergic, and psychogenic factors.

PATHOLOGY

Ulcerative colitis is usually confined to the mucosal and submucosal layers of the colonic wall. The rectum is always involved, and the rest of the colon is diseased to a greater or lesser extent. With severe pancolitis, the terminal ileum may show secondary mild inflammation and dilatation (backwash ileitis). At gross inspection, the colonic mucosa demonstrates healed granular superficial ulcers superimposed on a friable and thickened mucosa with increased vascularity. Patients may have superficial fissures and small, regular pseudopolyps. This appearance is different from the transmural inflammatory changes of Crohn's disease of the colon, in which all layers of the colonic wall may be involved in granulomatous inflammation (Table 45-1).

In the early stages of the disease, the lesions of ulcerative colitis consist of infiltration of round cells and polymorphonuclear leukocytes into the crypts of Lieberkühn at the base of the mucosa, forming crypt abscesses. Light microscopy reveals poor staining and vacuolization of overlying epithelial cells. Swelling of mitochondria, widening of intercellular spaces, and broadening of the endoplasmic reticulum are seen at transmission electron microscopy. As the lesions progress, crypt abscesses coalescence and desquamation of overlying cells form an ulcer. This cryptitis is associated with undermining of adjacent, relatively normal mucosa, which becomes edematous and assumes a polypoid configuration as it becomes isolated between adjacent ulcers.

Collagen and a luxurious growth of granulation tissue occupy the areas of ulceration, which extend down to, but rarely through, the muscularis. Although ulcerative colitis usually is confined to the mucosa and submucosa, in the most severe forms of the disease, especially toxic megacolon, the disease may extend to the deeper muscular layers of the colon and even to the serosa. Rarely, crypt abscesses penetrate the muscularis propria, often extending along a

Table 45-1. PATHOLOGIC FEATURES OF CROHN'S DISEASE AND ULCERATIVE COLITIS

	Crohn's Disease	Ulcerative Colitis
Transmural inflammation	Yes	Uncommon
Granulomas	50–75%	No
Fissures	Common	Rare
Submucosal thickening, fibrosis	Common	No
Submucosal inflammation	Common	Uncommon

Table 45-2. DISTINGUISHING CHARACTERISTICS OF CROHN'S COLITIS AND ULCERATIVE COLITIS

Characteristics	Crohn's Colitis	Ulcerative Colitis
Location	Small bowel involvement	Colon only (rare backwash ileitis)
Anatomic distribution	Asymmetric distribution (skip lesions)	Contiguous involvement beginning distally
Rectal involvement	Rectal sparing common	Involved 90%
Gross bleeding	Absent 25–30%	Universal
Perianal disease	≤75%	Rare, may be severe
Fistulization	Yes	No
Granulomas	50–75%	No

blood vessel. In this situation, the colon may perforate, causing confusion about the diagnosis.

CLINICAL MANIFESTATIONS

Presenting Features

Ulcerative colitis usually presents with bloody diarrhea, abdominal pain, and fever. Most patients seek treatment of a relatively mild attack that occurs as segmental colitis involving the distal colon or as a pancolitis. Some patients with disease limited to the rectosigmoid area show progression that involves most, if not all, of the length of the colon. Some patients present with a moderate attack in which bloody diarrhea is the predominant symptom. In some patients, ulcerative colitis has an acute and catastrophic fulminating course. Such patients experience a sudden onset of frequent bloody bowel movements, high fever, weight loss, and diffuse abdominal tenderness.

Physical findings are directly related to the duration and presentation of the disease. Weight loss and pallor are usually present. In the active phase, the abdomen in the region of the colon is tender to palpation. During acute attacks, or in the fulminating form of the disease, there may be signs of an acute surgical abdomen accompanied by fever and decreased bowel sounds. Patients with toxic megacolon may have abdominal distention. Examination of the skin, tongue, joints, and eyes is important, because the presence of disease in these areas may suggest inflammatory bowel disease (IBD) as a likely cause of the diarrheal illness.

Extraintestinal manifestations of ulcerative colitis are:

- Ocular lesions
  Iritis or uveitis
  Conjunctivitis

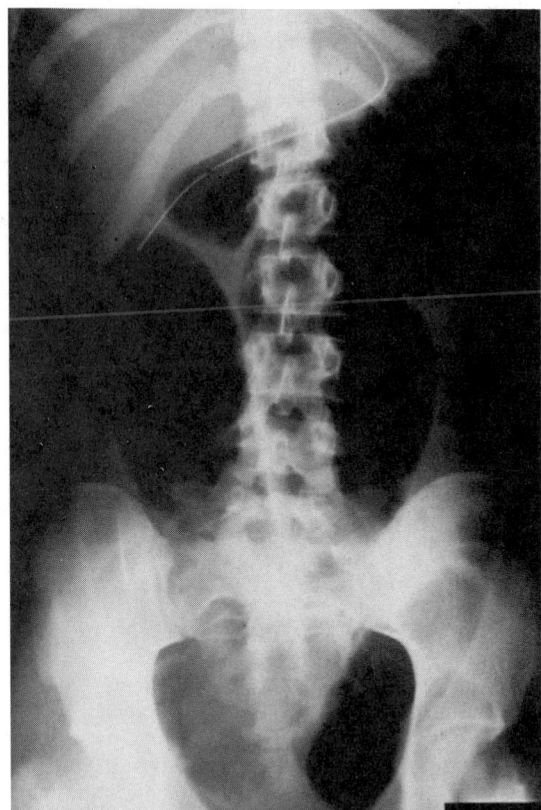

Figure 45-1. Colonic dilation, particularly of the transverse colon, in a patient with toxic megacolon.

    Episcleritis
    Keratitis
    Retinitis
    Retrobulbar neuritis
- Articular disorders
  Peripheral joint disease
  Arthralgia
  Swelling, pain, and redness with migratory involvement
  Ankylosing spondylitis
  Sacroiliitis
- Pyoderma gangrenosum
- Liver and biliary tract disorders
  Pericholangitis
  Fatty infiltration of the liver
  Chronic active hepatitis
  Biliary cirrhosis
  Sclerosing cholangitis
- Thromboembolic disease and vasculitis
- Renal disease, clubbing, bronchial and pulmonary abnormalities, amyloidosis (rare)

DIAGNOSIS

Ulcerative colitis has no pathognomonic laboratory, radiographic, or histologic features. In all patients who present with diarrhea or bloody diarrhea, infection must be excluded. Stool samples and biopsy specimens are evaluated for *Campylobacter* sp., *Salmonella* sp., pathogenic *E. coli, Aeromonas, Plesiomonas* sp., amebas, and *C. difficile.* It is important but difficult to differentiate pseudomembra-

Table 45-3. ENDOSCOPIC FEATURES OF CROHN'S DISEASE AND ULCERATIVE COLITIS

Endoscopic Features	Crohn's Disease	Ulcerative Colitis
Mucosal involvement	Discontinuous	Contiguous
Discrete ulcers (aphthous ulcers)	Common	Rare
Surrounding mucosa	Relatively normal	Abnormal
Longitudinal ulcer	Common	Rare
Cobblestoning	In severe cases	No
Rectal involvement	Sparing common	Involved in 90%
Mucosal friability	Uncommon	Common
Vascular pattern	Normal	Distorted

A

B

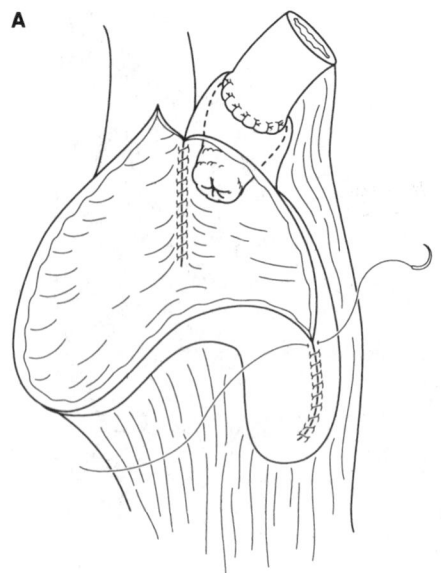

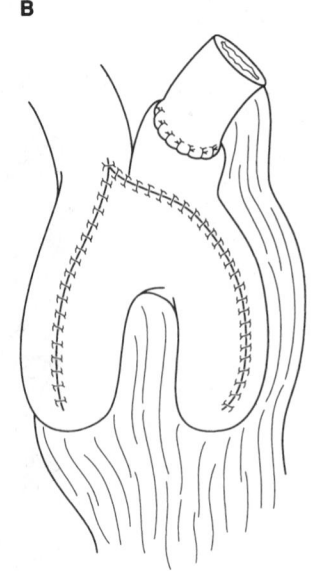

Figure 45-2. The continent ileostomy (Kock pouch) consists of an ileal reservoir and nipple valve constructed by intussuscepting the efferent limb and fixing it in place with sutures or staples. This provides a continent internal intestinal reservoir that the patient can drain by intubating the pouch through the flush cutaneous stoma several times throughout the day.

nous colitis, proctocolitis in homosexual men, traveler's diarrhea, granulomatous colitis, and Crohn's colitis (Table 45-2) from ulcerative colitis.

Flexible sigmoidoscopy is the first step in diagnosis, because ulcerative colitis involves the distal colon and rectum in almost all patients. In advanced disease, areas of ulceration may surround areas of heaped-up granulation tissue and edematous mucosa, so-called pseudopolyps. Colonoscopy may be useful in determining the extent and activity of disease, particularly in patients in whom the diagnosis is unclear or cancer is suspected. Endoscopy is useful in differentiation between ulcerative colitis and Crohn's colitis (Table 45-3).

Barium enema radiographic examination of the colon is useful in most patients, but it is dangerous in patients with toxic megacolon. When ulcerative colitis develops, mucosal granularity and microhemorrhages produce a dif-

fusely reticulated pattern, on which are superimposed countless punctate collections of contrast material lodged in microulcerations. A mild case of acute ulcerative colitis may be manifested by a diffusely granular appearance, which is best seen with air-contrast barium enema examination. In advanced cases, irregular margins develop in the colon with spiculated and undermining collar-button ulcers that are demonstrated at full-column barium enema

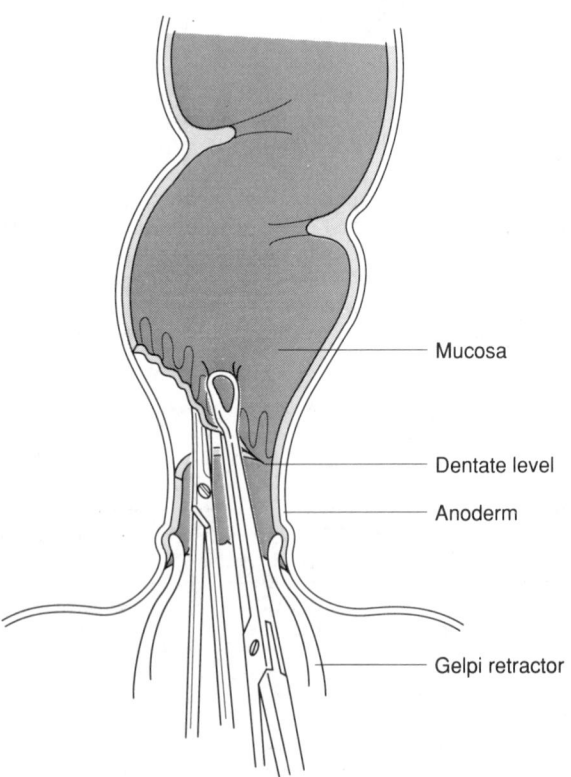

— Mucosa

— Dentate level

— Anoderm

— Gelpi retractor

Figure 45-4. Transanal mucosal proctectomy. A circumferential incision is made at the dentate line, and the rectal mucosa is carefully dissected away from the anal sphincter and the rectal muscularis.

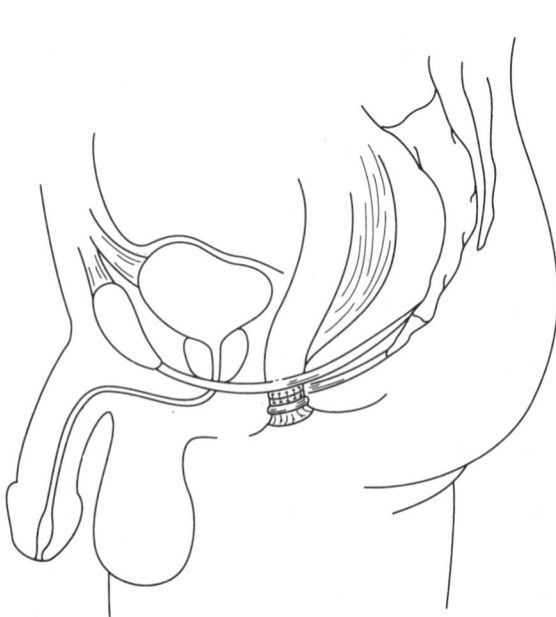

Figure 45-3. End-to-end ileoanal anastomosis after colectomy, mucosal proctectomy, and endorectal ileoanal pull-through.

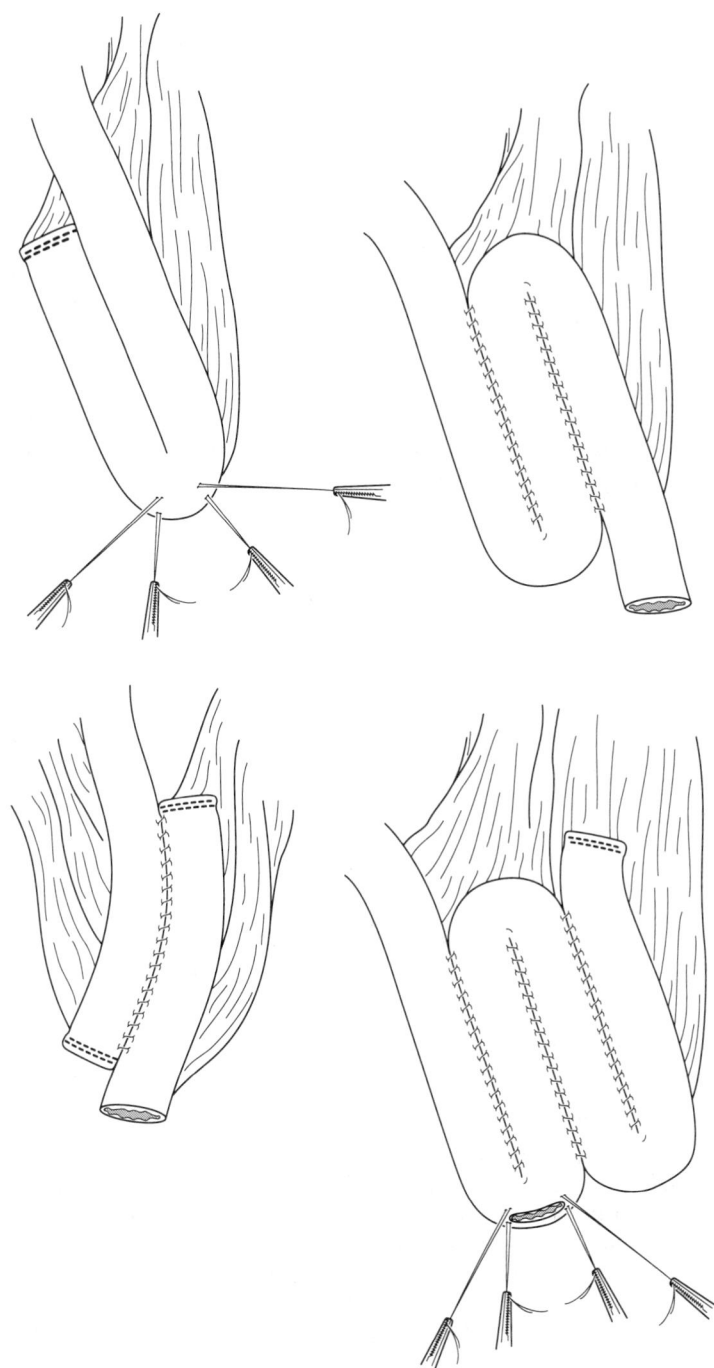

Figure 45-5. Ileal pouch configurations in patients undergoing ileal pouch–anal anastomosis.

examination. End-stage, or burned-out, ulcerative colitis is characterized by shortening of the colon, loss of normal redundancy in the sigmoid region and at the splenic and hepatic flexures, disappearance of the haustral pattern, a featureless mucosa, absence of discrete ulcerations, and narrowed caliber of the intestine. Chronic inflammation may lead to diffuse mucosal atrophy, leaving behind hypertrophic islands of inflamed mucosa and granulation tissue (pseudopolyps). These pseudopolyps may carpet the colon, simulating the polyposis syndrome, or they may be discrete, as in filiform pseudopolyposis.

Plain abdominal radiography may demonstrate colonic dilatation (toxic megacolon) in patients with severe ulcerative colitis (Fig. 45-1). This dilatation is observed in the transverse colon. There may be free air within the peritoneal cavity due to perforation of the diseased colon.

MEDICAL MANAGEMENT OF ULCERATIVE COLITIS

Drug treatment of ulcerative colitis includes:

- Antidiarrheal and antispasmodic agents
- Sulfasalazine and its analogs
- Corticosteroids and corticotropin (ACTH)
- Immunosuppressive antimetabolites

Once the diagnosis of ulcerative colitis is established, the decision regarding treatment depends on the severity

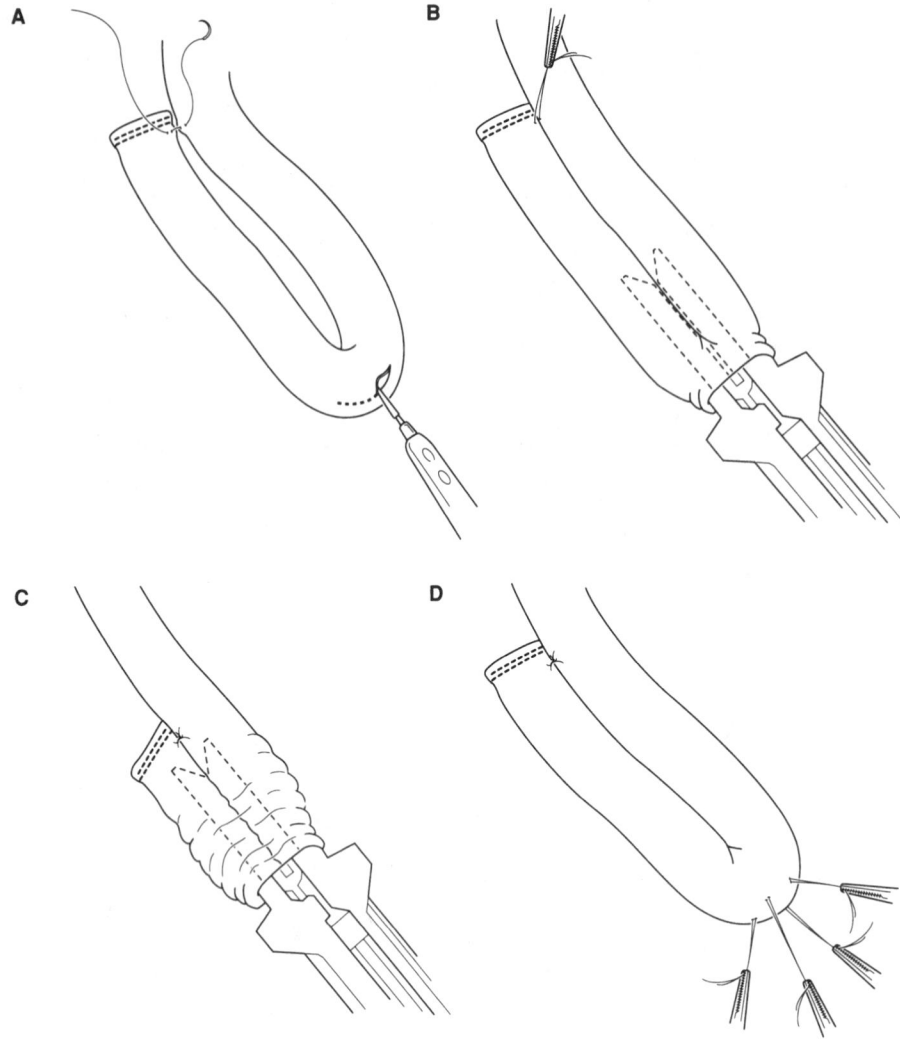

Figure 45-6. Ileal J-pouch construction. (*A*) Using electrocautery, an enterotomy is created at the apex of the 15-cm loop of terminal ileum. (*B*) The forks of an intestinal anastomosing stapler are pressed into the intestinal limbs, and the instrument is fired. (*C*) This is repeated once or twice while the limbs are telescoped onto the stapler, until a 15-cm side-to-side anastomosis is completed. (*D*) The apical enterotomy is closed with a simple pursestring stitch.

of symptoms and the severity and extent of disease, as indicated by radiographic and endoscopic studies.

Some patients with ulcerative colitis have a severe clinical course and require hospitalization. These patients need nutritional support, usually with IV hyperalimentation and correction of anemia. Patients with active disease or toxicity require parenteral hydrocortisone. Total parenteral nutrition (TPN) does not ameliorate the inflammatory response in ulcerative colitis but allows nutritional maintenance and repletion during treatment. During an acute episode of severe colitis, narcotic pain medication and antidiarrheal agents are avoided to prevent toxic megacolon. After responding to therapy, patients begin oral food intake and taking oral steroids while parenteral steroids are tapered. Cyclosporin is used to treat severe, refractory acute ulcerative colitis.

SURGICAL CONSIDERATIONS

Nearly half of patients with CUC undergo surgical treatment within the first 10 years of their illness, mainly because of the chronic nature of the disease and the tendency for relapse. Fulminant complications occur with ulcerative colitis, and there is high risk for malignant degeneration. Indications for surgical intervention are:

- Massive unrelenting hemorrhage
- Toxic megacolon with impending or frank perforation
- Fulminating acute ulcerative colitis unresponsive to steroids
- Obstruction due to stricture
- Suspected or proved cancer of the colon
- Systemic complications
- Intractability
- In children, failure to mature

In most patients with ulcerative colitis, colectomy is performed when the disease enters an intractable, chronic phase and becomes a physical and social burden to the patient. Because a sphincter-sparing operation can be performed in patients with ulcerative colitis, it is critical to avoid conventional proctectomy and to differentiate ulcerative colitis from Crohn's disease.

Indications for Surgical Treatment

Intractable Disease

Intractability is characterized as the severe and persistent impairment of a patient's quality of life, caused by the disease or the treatment of the disease. Elective operations for medically intractable ulcerative colitis are:

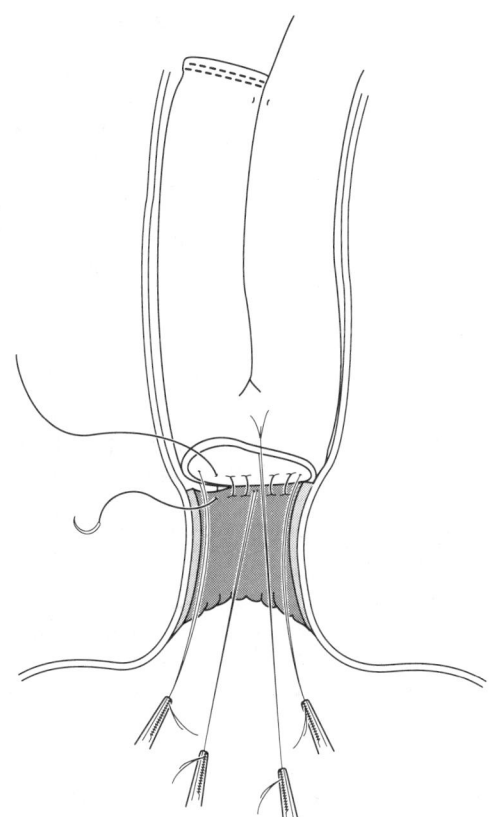

Figure 45-7. Creating the ileal pouch–anal anastomosis. The pouch is secured to the sphincter in each quadrant with a suture. The pursestring stitch closing the enterotomy is cut to allow the apex of the pouch to open. An anastomosis is then created between the apex of the pouch and the anoderm using interrupted absorbable sutures.

- Total proctocolectomy with Brooke ileostomy or continent ileostomy (Kock pouch)
- Subtotal colectomy with ileostomy or ileorectal anastomosis
- Colectomy with mucosal proctectomy and ileoanal anastomosis

Extracolonic Disease

The most common extraintestinal indication for surgical treatment of ulcerative colitis is retardation of growth and development in children and adolescents. Colectomy is of dramatic benefit in these patients. Other extracolonic complications of ulcerative colitis rarely are indications for an operation.

Cancer Prophylaxis

In a patient with long-standing colitis, unequivocal high-grade dysplasia in the absence of acute inflammation is an indication for colectomy. Even low-grade dysplasia, if it is unequivocal and unassociated with inflammation, is an indication for colectomy. The presence of carcinoma is not a contraindication to mucosal proctectomy with ileoanal anastomosis, unless the tumor is of an advanced stage or is located within the rectum. If there is uncertainty about the stage of the tumor at the time of the initial operation, subtotal colectomy with ileostomy and Hartmann closure of the rectum is performed. The stoma can be converted to an ileoanal anastomosis if the patient stays disease free.

Surgical Emergencies

Complications that require urgent operation are:

- Massive, unrelenting hemorrhage
- Toxic megacolon with impending or frank perforation
- Fulminating acute ulcerative colitis unresponsive to steroid therapy
- Acute colonic obstruction from stricture
- Suspicion or demonstration of colonic cancer

Surgical Approaches

Proctocolectomy and Ileostomy

Proctocolectomy is performed in relatively few patients with ulcerative colitis. This surgical treatment is curative; there is no anastomosis to heal; and only one stage is required. It provides the patient with a predictable functional result and eliminates the fear of anal incontinence.

The disadvantage of total proctocolectomy is that it results in permanent fecal incontinence. Patients require an external ileostomy device, which may have to be emptied four to eight times a day. The risks are hemorrhage, contamination and sepsis, and neural injury. Some patients require stoma revision; some have perineal wound problems after a conventional abdominal perineal proctectomy; and some have intestinal obstruction in the postoperative period. Of concern is bladder and sexual dysfunction associated with parasympathetic nerve injury.

Subtotal Colectomy

Although subtotal abdominal colectomy with ileorectal anastomosis usually leaves the patient with full continence, it is not curative. Inflammation persists in the retained rectum in almost all patients, and there is an ongoing risk for malignant growth. Some patients require proctectomy for uncontrollable proctitis, and some because of poor functional results. Even in patients who do well, stool frequency is high in the early postoperative period, eventually averaging four or five stools per 24 hours. The surgical complications include small-intestinal

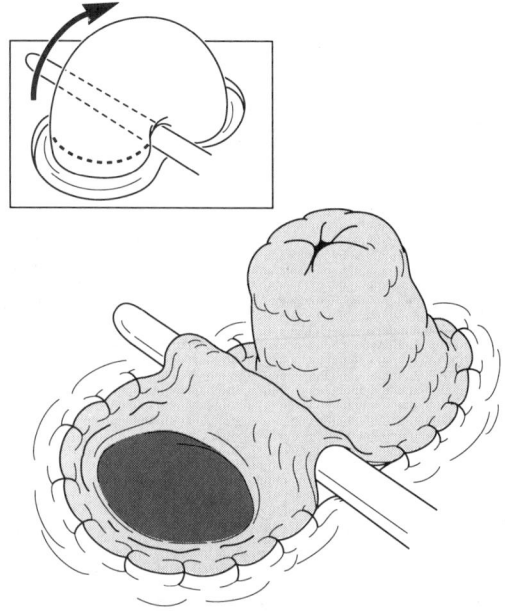

Figure 45-8. A loop ileostomy is constructed 40 cm proximal to the ileal pouch and is matured over a rod.

obstruction and leakage of the anastomosis between the ileum and the disease-bearing rectum. Subtotal colectomy is *contraindicated* in patients with anal sphincter dysfunction, severe rectal disease, rectal dysplasia, or frank cancer. There is little need to perform this operation for ulcerative colitis.

Continent Ileostomy

A continent ileostomy is constructed entirely of terminal ileum. It consists of an intestinal pouch that serves as a reservoir for stool and has an ileal conduit that connects the pouch to a cutaneous stoma (Fig. 45-2). An intestinal nipple valve is constructed between the pouch and the stoma. Patients empty the pouch by passing a soft plastic tube through the valve via the stoma. This operation is curative because it is associated with total proctocolectomy. The patient does not have to use an external appliance.

Continent ileostomy carries a high complication rate. Most of the complications are related to displacement of the nipple valve, producing fecal incontinence, and to difficulty intubating and emptying the pouch. Valve failure and intestinal obstruction occur. The operation carries a risk for bladder dysfunction, impotence, and perineal wound problems. Syndromes of ileostomy dysfunction related to the Kock pouch (stagnant loop syndrome, enteritis, nonspecific ileitis, pouchitis) include malabsorption of fat and vitamin B_{12}, proliferation of anaerobic bacteria, inflammation of the pouch, and incontinence. Fistulas may develop between the pouch and the skin or intestine. Crohn's disease is a *contraindication* to this operation. Despite the complications, patient satisfaction with a continent ileostomy is high.

Ileoanal Anastomosis

In an ileoanal anastomosis, the rectal mucosa is dissected out and removed to the dentate line of the anus. This preserves an intact rectal muscular cuff and anal sphincter apparatus. Continuity of the intestinal tract is reestablished

(Fig. 45-3). The operation eliminates all diseased tissue and is as definitive as total proctocolectomy. Because the pelvic dissection is confined to the endorectal plane, parasympathetic innervation to the bladder and genitalia is preserved. Because abdominal perineal proctectomy is eliminated, long-term drainage of the perineal wound is unnecessary. A permanent abdominal stoma is unnecessary because of the ileoanal anastomosis. Continence is preserved.

In most patients, the surgical procedure is performed in two stages. The first stage consists of abdominal colectomy, mucosal proctectomy (Fig. 45-4), endorectal ileal pouch–anal anastomosis (Fig. 45-5 through 45-7), and diverting loop ileostomy (Fig. 45-8). During the second stage, performed at least 8 weeks after the initial operation, the loop ileostomy is closed (Fig. 45-9). In patients who require emergency colectomy, the procedure has three stages. The first stage consists of abdominal colectomy, ileostomy, and Hartmann closure of the rectum. In the second stage, the rectal mucosa is dissected free, and the ileoanal anastomosis is performed with loop ileostomy. In the third stage, the loop ileostomy is closed.

Poor stool consistency, increased stool frequency, and nocturnal leakage of stool are the most common postoperative problems after ileoanal anastomosis. In an effort to control stool output, patients take loperamide hydrochloride and psyllium hydrophilic mucilloid and eat a high-fiber diet.

An alternative to conventional endoanal rectal mucosal resection eliminates the distal mucosal proctectomy. The rationale for this approach is that when the mucosa of the anal transition zone is preserved, the anatomic integrity of the anal canal is preserved and fecal incontinence improves. Mucosectomy is recommended to patients with rectal dysplasia, proximal rectal cancer, diffuse colonic dysplasia, and familial polyposis.

A proximal diverting ileostomy may not be required at the time of ileal pouch–anal anastomosis for ulcerative colitis. Avoidance of a diverting loop ileostomy eliminates

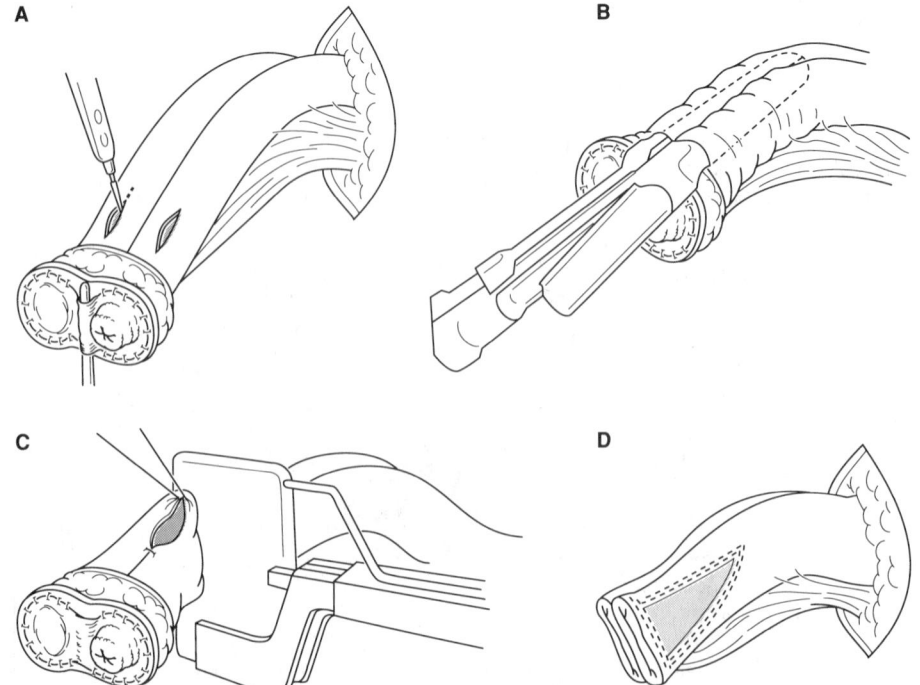

Figure 45-9. Closure of loop ileostomy. (*A*) A transverse elliptical incision is made around the stoma, and the limbs are dissected free. (*B*) The antimesenteric surfaces of the limb are tacked together, and the jaws of an anastomosing stapler are passed through enterotomies and down into the lumen of each of the intestinal limbs. The stapler is then fired to create a side-to-side anastomosis between the afferent and efferent ileal limbs. (*C*) A linear stapler is placed and fired below the former stoma and below the edges of the enterotomy. The stoma and distal limbs are amputated, and the stapler is released. (*D*) The anastomosis is dropped back into the peritoneal cavity, and the peritoneum, fascia, and skin are closed.

the additional surgical intervention needed to close the ileostomy, eliminates the complications of ileostomy and ileostomy closure, and may reduce the rate of diversion enteritis. A diverting ileostomy, however, reduces the risk of leakage from the ileal pouch or ileoanal anastomosis.

Ileoanal anastomosis has a low morbidity and mortality. The most frequent late complication is ileal pouch dysfunction or pouchitis. Pouchitis is an incompletely defined and poorly understood clinical syndrome consisting of increased stool frequency, watery stools, cramping, urgency, nocturnal leakage of stool, arthralgia, malaise, and fever. The cause is not known; speculation includes early Crohn's disease, bacterial overgrowth or bacterial dysbiosis, primary or secondary malabsorption, stasis, ischemia, and nutritional or immune deficiency. Treatment with a short course of metronidazole is successful in most patients.

SUGGESTED READING

Ambroze WL, Pemberton JH, Dozois R, Carpenter HA, O'Rourke JS, Ilstrup DM: The historical pattern and pathological involvement of the anal transition zone in patients with ulcerative colitis. Gastroenterology 1993;104:514.

Kirsner JB, Shorter RG, eds. Inflammatory bowel disease. Philadelphia, Lea & Febiger, 1988.

Luukkonen P, Jarvinen H: Stapled vs hand-sutured ileoanal anastomosis in restorative proctocolectomy. Arch Surg 1993; 128:437.

MacDermott RP, Stenson W, eds. Inflammatory bowel disease. New York, Elsevier, 1991.

Sandborn WJ. A critical review of cyclosporine therapy in IBD. Inflam Bowel Dis 1995;1:48.

Tagran SR, ed. Inflammatory bowel disease: from bench to bedside. Baltimore, Williams & Wilkins, 1994.

Trickson W, Tavery I, Fazio V, Oakley J, Church J, Nilson J. Manometric and functional comparison of ileal pouch anastomosis with and without anal manipulation. Am J Surg 1991;161:90.

ESSENTIALS OF SURGERY: SCIENTIFIC PRINCIPLES AND PRACTICE, edited by Lazar J. Greenfield, Michael W. Mulholland, Keith T. Oldham, Gerald B. Zelenock, and Keith D. Lillemoe. Lippincott–Raven Publishers, Philadelphia, © 1997.

CHAPTER 46

COLONIC POLYPS AND POLYPOSIS SYNDROMES

C. RICHARD BOLAND AND ROBERT S. BRESALIER

A *polyp* is a protrusion of colonic mucosa into the intestinal lumen. It may result from abnormal growth of the mucosa itself or from a submucosal lesion that pushes the mucosa into the lumen. Table 46-1 is a classification of colorectal polyps.

NEOPLASTIC MUCOSAL POLYPS

Carcinoma of the colon and rectum does not originate *de novo*. The mucosal epithelium progresses through a series of molecular and cellular events that alter proliferation and cellular accumulation and produce glandular disarray. The changes become evident in the form of an adenomatous polyp. Genetic alterations produce additional cellular atypia and glandular disorganization (dysplasia),

Table 46-1. CLASSIFICATION OF COLORECTAL POLYPS

MUCOSAL POLYPS

Neoplastic

BENIGN

Adenomatous polyps (dysplastic mucosa)
  Tubular
  Tubulovillous
  Villous

MALIGNANT

Carcinoma in situ
Invasive carcinoma
Polypoid carcinoma

Nonneoplastic

Hyperplastic polyps
Juvenile polyps
Peutz-Jeghers polyps
Inflammatory polyps
Normal epithelium

SUBMUCOSAL POLYPS

Lipomas
Leiomyomas
Colitis cystica profunda
Pneumatosis cystoides intestinalis
Lymphoid aggregates
Lymphoma (primary or secondary)
Carcinoids
Metastatic neoplasms

which may evolve to carcinoma. This is known as the *adenoma-to-carcinoma sequence.*

The epidemiologic features of adenoma of the colon parallel those of carcinoma:

1. Adenoma is rare in geographic regions with a low prevalence of cancer of the colon.
2. The distribution of adenoma in the colon is the same as that of carcinoma.
3. Adenomas in the colon often occur close to carcinomas.
4. Cancer risk is proportional to the number of adenomas present at the same time or at different times in one person.
5. Cancer often is present in polyps removed endoscopically or surgically.
6. The risk for cancer is proportional to the degree of dysplasia or atypia in a polyp.
7. Removal of adenomatous polyps at surveillance proctosigmoidoscopy decreases the risk for death of colorectal cancer.

Pathogenesis

Molecular Biology

Genetic changes that lead to the development of adenomas (and carcinomas) are alterations in protooncogenes, loss of tumor-suppressor gene activity, or abnormalities of genes involved in DNA repair (Fig. 46-1).

Abnormal Proliferation

In a normal colon, DNA synthesis and cellular proliferation occur only in the lower and middle regions of the crypt. Cells that have migrated to the upper crypt become terminally differentiated and can no longer divide. Disordered proliferation and aberrant crypt development are

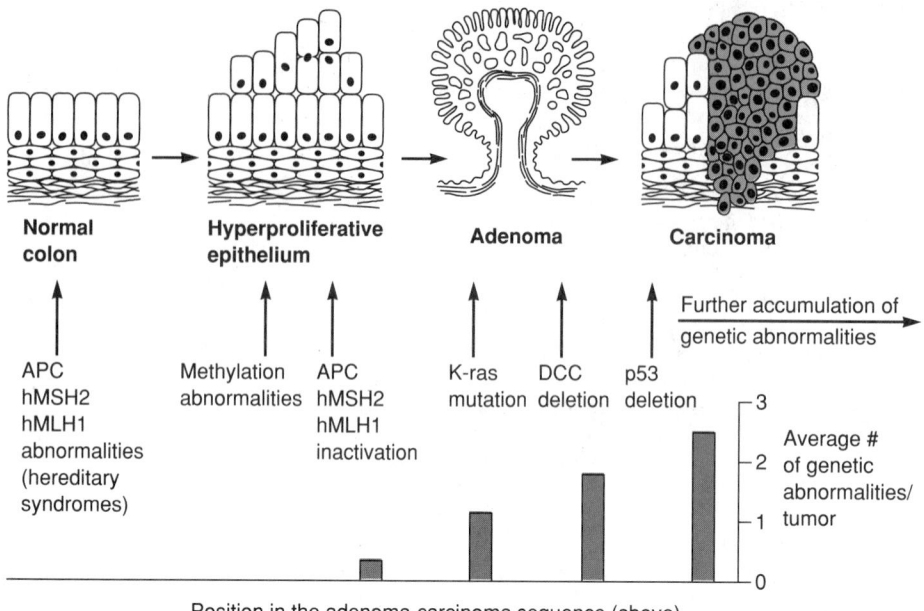

Figure 46-1. Molecular genetic events during the adenoma-to-carcinoma sequence. The progression to adenoma and carcinoma is associated with an accumulation of alterations in oncogenes (k-*ras*), tumor suppressor genes (APC, DCC, p53), and genes involved in maintaining the fidelity of DNA synthesis (DNA repair genes hMSH2, hMLH1). Alterations in APC, k-*ras,* and the DNA repair genes occur as early events in the development of adenomas, while deletion of DCC and p53 occur during the evolution from adenoma to carcinoma. The exact sequence of events is approximate. (Modified from Bresalier RS, Toribara NW. In: Eastwood GL, ed. Premalignant conditions of the gastrointestinal tract. New York, Elsevier 1991)

characteristic of adenoma. The initiating event for adenoma formation appears to be inactivation of the adenomatous polyposis coli (APC) tumor suppressor gene.

Histopathology and Malignant Potential

Adenomatous polyps are characterized by physical characteristics, size, glandular structure, and degree of dysplasia. Polyps may be *sessile,* with a broad-based attachment to the colonic wall, or *pedunculated,* attached to the colonic wall with a fibrovascular stalk. Whether a polyp is sessile or pedunculated determines if it can be removed with endoscopic snare polypectomy. Polyps ≤5 mm in diameter probably do not contain high-grade dysplasia or invasive carcinoma. Malignant potential increases with polyp size.

Adenomas are classified according to their glandular structure. Aberrant (dysplastic) crypts and microadenomas may be the earliest lesions detected in the flat mucosa. These lesions enlarge to become adenomatous polyps. *Tubular adenomas* are characterized by a complex network of branching adenomatous glands. *Villous adenomas* contain glands that extend straight from the surface to the base of the polyp. Both histologic types can coexist in a mixed tubulovillous adenoma. The malignant potential of an adenomatous polyp correlates with the degree of villous architecture.

All adenomas consist of dysplastic mucosa. *Dysplasia* is a term that describes abnormalities in crypt architecture and cytologic detail. Dysplasia may be mild, moderate, or severe, depending on the extent of these characteristics. Severe or high-grade dysplasia represents carcinoma in situ when the basement membrane is intact. Extension into the lamina propria denotes intramucosal carcinoma. Invasion into the muscularis mucosae defines invasive carcinoma and a malignant polyp. The degree of dysplasia often correlates with polyp size and extent of villous architecture.

Although all adenocarcinomas of the colon and rectum originate in adenomatous polyps, not all polyps evolve into carcinoma. The malignant potential of adenomatous polyps is related to polyp size and histologic characteristics. Large polyps and those with a high proportion of villous architecture are more likely to contain carcinoma.

Epidemiology

Prevalence

The prevalence of adenoma among people older than 50 years who do not have symptoms is 20% to 40% and increases with age. Adenoma precedes carcinoma by 5 to 10 years. Advancing age correlates with multiplicity of polyps, polyp size, and higher degrees of dysplasia. Thirty to 50% of people with one adenoma have another elsewhere in the colon.

Anatomic Distribution

Adenomas are uniformly distributed throughout the colon. Large, clinically significant adenomas, however, have a distribution closer to that of carcinoma, ie, left-sided predominance.

Familiality

First-degree relatives of people with colonic adenoma or carcinoma have a two- to threefold higher risk for colon cancer than the general population. Although inheritance appears to determine susceptibility to neoplasia, environmental factors seem to determine in which susceptible people adenoma and carcinoma of the colon develop.

Hereditary nonpolyposis colorectal cancer (HNPCC, Lynch syndrome) is a disease of autosomal dominant inheritance in which cancers originate in discrete adenomas but polyposis (hundreds of polyps) does not occur. The criteria for HNPCC in a family are:

1. At least three relatives have colorectal cancer, one of whom is a first-degree relative of the other two
2. Colorectal cancer involves at least two generations
3. At least one tumor occurs before the person is 50 years of age

Clinical Characteristics

Most colonic adenomas are asymptomatic. If bleeding occurs, it is usually minimal and occult. Very large colonic polyps sometimes cause obstructive symptoms, such as lower abdominal cramping or alteration in bowel habit.

Diagnosis

About 30% of people 50 years or older who undergo colonoscopy because of a positive fecal occult blood test have a polyp detected. Detection and removal of the polyps helps reduce the mortality of colorectal cancer. Beginning at 50 years of age, everyone should undergo *screening sigmoidoscopy* every 3 to 5 years and a *fecal occult blood test* once a year.

Treatment

The Index Polyp

Adenomas are removed with endoscopic snare polypectomy. Polypectomy is safe and easily performed when adenomas are small or pedunculated, but is difficult when polyps are large or sessile. Complications include bleeding and perforation at the polypectomy site. Because 30 to 50% of people with one adenoma have an adenoma elsewhere in the colon, the entire colon is examined at colonoscopy. Polyps <5 mm in diameter carry little malignant potential. If they are too small for snare polypectomy, small polyps can be ablated with a hot biopsy forceps. Sessile villous adenomas >2 cm in diameter have a high potential for malignant degeneration. If such lesions cannot be removed with snare polypectomy, segmental surgical resection may be necessary.

Follow-up After Index Polypectomy

Additional adenomas are likely to develop in patients who undergo removal of an adenoma. Colonoscopic polypectomy and postpolypectomy surveillance reduce the rate of colorectal cancer.

Management of Malignant Polyps

Endoscopic polypectomy is adequate for an adenomatous polyp that contains cancer if the cancer is confined to the head of the polyp (Fig. 46-2). Simple polypectomy may not be adequate when malignant cells invade the stalk. Polypectomy is adequate if a margin >2 mm is present, the cancer is not poorly differentiated, and there is no vascular or lymphatic invasion. These criteria are difficult to assess for sessile polyps. If an adequate margin cannot be demonstrated, surgical intervention is recommended to manage possible regional lymph node metastases.

NONNEOPLASTIC MUCOSAL POLYPS

Hyperplastic Polyps

Hyperplastic polyps are small, usually sessile lesions, most frequently encountered in the distal colon and rectum. Although grossly indistinguishable from small adenomas, hyperplastic polyps carry no potential for malignant degeneration. Hyperplastic polyps are common age-related lesions; they occur in about one-third of people older than 50 years. Because these polyps are asymptomatic and carry no malignant potential, no specific treatment is required. If a hyperplastic polyp is the only lesion detected at index flexible sigmoidoscopy or colonoscopy, no further evaluation is indicated.

Juvenile Polyps

Juvenile polyps, also known as retention polyps, may occur sporadically or as part of a familial polyposis syndrome. These mucosal polyps consist of dilated, cystic, mucus-filled glands, abundant lamina propria, and inflammatory infiltrates. Most occur in children younger than 10 years. These polyps are usually single, pedunculated, and cherry red with a smooth surface and contour. They often cause hematochezia. Rectal prolapse and autoamputation may occur with distal lesions. Intussusception may be precipitated by proximal juvenile polyps in familial syndromes. *Individual* juvenile polyps have no malignant potential, but symptomatic polyps are removed to prevent complications. Juvenile *polyposis* is associated with increased risk for early development of cancer.

Inflammatory Polyps

Inflammatory mucosal polyps are common in idiopathic inflammatory bowel disease (IBD). Marked inflammation and ulceration coexist with granulation tissue in a distorted mucosal architecture that appears polypoid. Healing produces residual islands of mucosa interspersed with de-

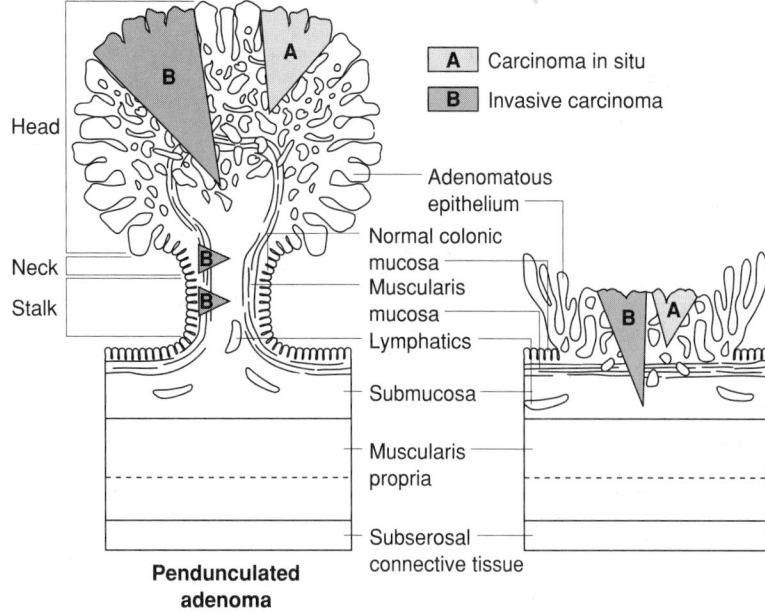

Figure 46-2. Diagrammatic representation of cancer-containing polyps. Pedunculated adenoma is described on the left and a sessile adenoma on the right. In carcinoma in situ, malignant cells are confined to the mucosa. These lesions are adequately treated by endoscopic polypectomy. Polypectomy is adequate treatment for invasive carcinoma only if there is a sufficient margin (perhaps 2 mm), if the carcinoma is not poorly differentiated, and if there is no evidence of venous or lymphatic invasion. (After Haggitt RC, Glotzbach RE, Soffen EE, et al. Prognostic factors in colorectal carcinomas arising in adenomas: implications for lesions removed by endoscopic polypectomy. Gastroenterology 1985;89:328)

nuded epithelium, so-called *pseudopolyps.* Severe chronic inflammation of any kind, including infectious diseases such as tuberculosis, may cause inflammatory polyps that resemble those that occur in the active stages of idiopathic IBD.

SUBMUCOSAL POLYPS

Submucosal masses may expand to push the colonic mucosa into the intestinal lumen. Many submucosal lesions, such as lipomas and leiomyomas, are asymptomatic; their importance is that they be differentiated from neoplastic lesions. Other lesions are malignant, such as lymphomas and metastatic tumors. Many submucosal lesions are not detected with endoscopic mucosal biopsy because a conventional biopsy forceps does not reach beyond the mucosa. If the presence of a submucosal lesion is suspected, multiple biopsies of the same site may sometimes provide tissue for diagnosis. The following are examples of submucosal polyps:

- Lipomas—benign fatty tumors that occur throughout the GI tract, but occur most commonly in the cecum near the ileocecal valve
- Pneumatosis cystoides intestinalis—multiple air-filled cysts in the submucosa
- Colitis cystica profunda—a rare condition in which the intestinal wall is thickened by submucosal mucus-filled cysts of variable size and an accumulation of fibroblasts in the lamina propria
- Carcinoids
- Other lesions—metastatic tumors, such as malignant melanoma; benign lesions such as leiomyoma, fibroma, lymphangioma, hemangioma; endometriosis.

GASTROINTESTINAL POLYPOSIS SYNDROMES

Familial Adenomatous Polyposis

Familial adenomatous polyposis (FAP) is an inherited disease characterized by the development of multiple adenomatous polyps throughout the colon and rectum. The polyps first appear in adolescence. The number of polyps in each patient is variable, and the polyps increase in number and size with advancing age. Cancer develops when patients are in their mid-30s. The genetic basis of FAP is a germ-line mutation in the APC gene located on chromosome 5q. Age at onset, number of polyps, and age at which cancer develops are determined by the location of the mutation in the APC gene (Fig. 46-3).

The extraintestinal manifestations of FAP include:

- Congenital hypertrophy of the retinal pigmented epithelium (CHRPE)
- Osteomas of the mandible, skull, and long bones
- Benign soft-tissue tumors, such as fibromas and lipomas
- Malignant tumors of the colon
- Brain tumors, thyroid tumors, adrenal tumors, benign or malignant tumors of the hepatobiliary tree
- Desmoid tumors

Diagnosis

When FAP is known in a family, relatives at risk undergo surveillance sigmoidoscopy once a year beginning in their mid-teens. When the first adenoma appears, diffuse adenoma development occurs over the next few years. Biopsies must be performed to confirm that the lesions are adenomas. No other disease produces multiple adenomatous polyps in young patients.

The diagnosis of FAP often is made without prior suspicion in an adult. In some patients, the disease occurred in previous generations of relatives, but the correct diagnosis was not made. About 25% of patients may have a germ-line lesion in the APC gene that is not present in either parent.

Treatment

When FAP is recognized, colectomy is performed before cancer develops. The diagnosis of FAP often is made in adolescence, but there is a delay of 20 years or more from the appearance of the first adenomas to the development of cancer. It is usually prudent to wait until a patient reaches full physical maturity before undertaking surgical treatment. The safest surgical approach is a total proctocolectomy with an ileoanal anastomosis. Any residual rectal mucosa is at risk for neoplasia. Even with careful endoscopic surveillance of the rectal segment, invasive carcinoma may develop.

Treatment of Extracolonic Manifestations of FAP

Osteomas, fibromas, and lipomas sometimes degenerate into sarcomas, but so rarely that prophylactic surveillance and surgical treatment are not indicated. CHRPE lesions do not require therapy. Endoscopic surveillance of the stomach is not necessary where gastric carcinoma is uncommon, such as North America.

Two concerns after removal of the colon and rectum are periampullary neoplasia and desmoid tumors. Almost all patients with FAP have one or more adenomas in the duodenum, usually close to the ampulla of Vater. These lesions are subjected to biopsy and destroyed with electrocauterization or laser ablation. The duodenum is examined every 2 years.

Desmoid tumors are aggressive, benign tumors of fibroblasts that can cause life-threatening complications. These tumors grow slowly, and may surround or compress vascular structures, nerves, or the abdominal viscera. Some lesions of the abdominal wall can be treated with simple local excision; there is no uniformly successful management.

Peutz–Jeghers Syndrome

Peutz–Jeghers syndrome is an autosomal dominant familial syndrome characterized by multiple GI polyps and skin lesions. The gene responsible for this disease has not been identified. Carriers of the disorder are predisposed to a number of early-onset cancers.

GI Features

The GI polyps in Peutz–Jeghers syndrome are nonneoplastic hamartomas consisting of a supportive framework of smooth-muscle covered by somewhat hyperplastic epithelium. Peutz–Jeghers polyps can usually be identified as such by the pathologist, and the characteristic cutaneous pigmentation makes this syndrome easily detected.

Skin Lesions

The cutaneous manifestations of Peutz–Jeghers syndrome are dark macular lesions on the mouth (the skin and the buccal mucosa), nose, lips, hands, feet, genitalia, and anus. These lesions usually become less obvious by puberty. Unlike freckles, the cutaneous lesions of Peutz–Jeghers syndrome are present from birth.

Clinical Complications

The principal complication of Peutz–Jeghers syndrome is intestinal obstruction, which may occur in infancy or childhood. GI bleeding also may occur. Cancer in the small

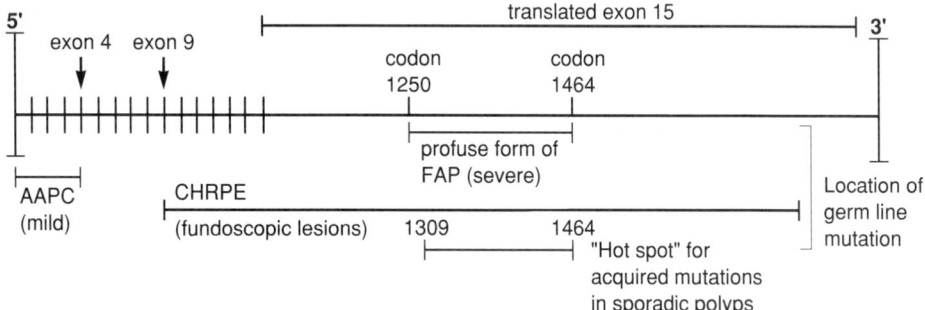

Figure 46-3. This scheme of the APC gene illustrates the genotype-phenotype correlations. Most of the mutations of the APC gene result in premature stop codons; therefore, the site of the mutation usually indicates the relative length of the mutant protein product. Mutations at the 5′ end of the gene produce AAPC, a milder form of the disease. The retinal lesions—CHRPE—occur when the mutations occur between exons 9 and 15. The portion of the APC gene that binds to other cytoskeletal elements in the cell (β-catenins) is represented in the 15th exon. Mutations in a hot spot immediately downstream from the β-catenin–binding site result in a more virulent, profuse form of familial adenomatous polyposis. This site is also the location of most of the acquired mutations in sporadic colorectal neoplasms.

intestine or colon can occur but is uncommon. Prophylactic surgical treatment is not recommended. Patients with Peutz–Jeghers syndrome are at increased risk for cancers outside the GI tract. Organs at risk include the gonads, breasts, pancreas, and the biliary tree. No internal organ is at sufficiently high risk for cancer that a specific screening regimen or prophylactic surgical treatment is indicated.

Treatment

Treatment of Peutz–Jeghers syndrome is removal of the polyps, with endoscopic techniques when possible. Surgical intervention may be required for intussusception caused by small intestinal polyps. Neoplasia is a risk, but prophylactic removal of any section of the GI tract is not indicated. Gonadal neoplasms and breast cancer may necessitate surgical intervention.

Juvenile Polyposis

Multiple juvenile polyps in one person suggests a familial juvenile polyposis syndrome. Three different syndromic presentations occur: familial juvenile polyposis limited to the colon; familial juvenile polyposis throughout the GI tract; and familial juvenile polyposis limited to the stomach.

The manifestations of juvenile polyposis are largely limited to bleeding, intussusception, obstruction, or the passage of autoamputated lesions. Patients with familial juvenile polyposis are at increased risk for the development of colorectal cancer. The presence of mixed juvenile-adenomatous polyps indicates which lesions are premalignant. The pathologist examines the lesions carefully for the presence of adenomatous tissue in the polyps. When mixed lesions are present, patients undergo colonoscopic surveillance, perhaps as often as every 2 years.

Other Familial Polyposis Syndromes

Rare syndromes that may give rise to multiple GI polyps are:

- Cowden syndrome—multiple GI hamartomas, complicated by multiple lesions of the face that originate from follicular epithelium (trichilemmomas)

- Neurofibromatosis (von Recklinghausen syndrome)
- Basal cell nevus syndrome

Nonfamilial Gastrointestinal Polyposis Syndromes

Multiple GI polyps occur in some nonfamilial syndromes and must be differentiated as such. The syndromes include:

- Cronkhite–Canada syndrome
- Inflammatory pseudopolyps with IBD
- Lymphoma
- Pneumatosis cystoides intestinalis
- Multiple lipomas or hyperplastic polyps

SUGGESTED READING

Atkin WS, Morson BC, Cuzick J. Long-term risk of colorectal cancer after excision of rectosigmoid adenomas. N Engl J Med 1992;326:658.

Burt RW. Hereditary polyposis syndromes and inheritance of adenomatous polyps. Semin Gastrointest Dis 1992;3:13.

Cooper HS, Deppisch LM, Gourley WK, et al. Endoscopically removed malignant polyps: clinicopathologic correlations. Gastroenterology 1995;108:1657.

Giardiello FM, Hamilton SR, Krush AJ, et al. Treatment of colonic and rectal adenomas with sulindac in familial adenomatous polyposis. N Engl J Med 1993;328:1313.

Giavannucci E, Rimm EB, Stampfer MJ, et al. Aspirin use and the risk for colorectal cancer and adenoma in male health professionals. Ann Intern Med 1994;121:241.

Marra G, Armelao F, Vecchio FM, Percesepe A, Anti M. Cowden's disease with extensive gastrointestinal polyposis. J Clin Gastroenterol 1994;18:42.

Nagase H, Miyoshi Y, Horii A, et al. Correlation between the location of germ-line mutations in the APC gene and the number of colorectal polyps in familial adenomatous polyposis patients. Cancer Res 1992;52:4055.

Neugat AO, Jacobson JS, Ahsan H, et al. Incidence and recurrence rates of colorectal adenomas: a prospective study. Gastroenterology 1995;108:402.

Powell SM, Petersen GM, Krush AJ, et al. Molecular diagnosis of familial adenomatous polyposis. N Engl J Med 1993;329:1982.

Winawer SJ, Zauber AG, Ho MN, et al. Prevention of colorectal cancer by colonoscopic polypectomy. N Engl J Med 1993; 329:1977.

ESSENTIALS OF SURGERY: SCIENTIFIC PRINCIPLES AND PRACTICE, edited by Lazar J. Greenfield, Michael W. Mulholland, Keith T. Oldham, Gerald B. Zelenock, and Keith D. Lillemoe. Lippincott–Raven Publishers, Philadelphia, © 1997.

CHAPTER 47

COLORECTAL CANCER

ALFRED E. CHANG

Colorectal carcinoma is the second leading cause of cancer-related death. When diagnosed in its early stages, this disease is curable with surgical treatment.

EPIDEMIOLOGY

The incidence of colorectal cancer has broad geographic variation. The difference does not involve genetic factors alone. In populations that migrate from a region of low to a region of high incidence, the rate of colorectal cancer increases. Environmental factors appear to be involved in the pathogenesis of colorectal cancer—industrialized countries appear to have the highest incidence of the disease. Because colorectal cancer may have a dietary connection, it may be responsive to nutritional manipulation and, thus, may be preventable. In the United States, the incidence of colorectal cancer rises steadily from the second to ninth decades of life, and affects men and women at the same rate.

ETIOLOGY

Dietary Factors

Cancer of the colon is associated with intake of animal fat and meat. The proposed mechanism is the interaction between dietary fat and bile acids.

Fiber intake is associated with a low risk for colon cancer. The role of fiber originally was seen simply as providing bulk to dilute potential carcinogens and speed their transit through the colon, but the relation is more complex. Fiber binds mutagens, reducing contact with colonic epithelium, favorably changing the fecal pH and participating in other complex interactions.

Mutagenesis

The first step in carcinogenesis in the colon and rectum involves *initiating factors* that interact with cellular DNA to induce mutations in the genome. The second step is driven by *promotional factors,* which are not mutagenic by themselves but enhance cellular proliferation of mutated cells.

The human diet contains a wide range of mutagens or substances that can be metabolized into mutagens. Such substances are generated from interactions among food, microbial flora, and colonic mucosal enzymes. Fat appears to be a promotional factor in colon cancer. Increased fat intake increases total fecal bile acid load. Bile acids stimulate generation of reactive oxygen metabolites that enhance the conversion of unsaturated fatty acids to compounds that promote cellular proliferation, facilitating emergence of a mutated clone of neoplastic cells. Because of the presence of mutagens in the GI tract, many strategies to reduce colon cancer attempt to interfere with the interaction between mutagens and the target colonic cells.

Molecular Genetics

The development of colorectal cancer is a multistep process in which malignant carcinomas originate from benign adenomas. At least four defined genetic alterations are associated with this process—*ras* gene mutations, and allelic deletions of chromosomes 5q (adenomatous polyposis coli; APC), 17p (p53), and 18q (deleted in colorectal carcinoma; DCC).

One mechanism by which colorectal tumors originate involves germ-line mutations in patients with hereditary nonpolyposis colorectal cancers (HNPCC). A highly conserved family of genes is involved in DNA repair. When this function is altered, DNA repair is disrupted. This leads to somatic mutations and genome instability, which give rise to cancer formation. These genes belong to a family of genes known as *mismatch repair genes.* Five to 10% of all colorectal carcinomas originate in kindreds with HNPCC.

CLINICAL RISK FACTORS
Familial

Familial syndromes (Table 47-1) characterized by numerous adenomatous polyps are associated with a high risk for cancer of the large intestine. The most important is familial polyposis coli, or familial adenomatous polyposis (FAP). Multiple adenomatous colonic polyps develop at a median age of 16 years, and increasing numbers of polyps are detected with increasing age. The disease is inherited as an autosomal dominant trait with essentially 100% penetrance. Unless proctocolectomy is performed in early adulthood, almost all patients with FAP have cancer by 55 years of age. It is extremely important to identify families with FAP so that family members may undergo frequent examinations.

Two types of HNPCC are the Lynch syndromes. *Lynch syndrome I* is inherited as an autosomal dominant trait

---

Table 47-1. CLINICAL RISK FACTORS FOR COLORECTAL CANCER

GENETIC

Polyposis syndromes
  Familial polyposis coli
  Gardner syndrome
  Turcot syndrome (CNS tumors)
  Oldfield syndrome (sebaceous cysts)
  Peutz-Jeghers syndrome (hamartomas)
Nonpolyposis syndromes
  Lynch syndrome I
  Lynch syndrome II (associated extracolonic cancers)
Preexisting disease
  Ulcerative colitis
  Crohn's disease
  Prior colorectal cancer
  Neoplastic polyps
  Pelvic irradiation
  Breast or genital tract cancer

GENERAL

Age >40 y
Family history of colorectal cancer

Table 47-2. NEOPLASTIC COLORECTAL POLYPS

Type	Histologic Features	Incidence (%)	Invasive Malignancy (%)
Adenomatous (tubular adenoma)	Branching tubules embedded in lamina propria	75	5
Villous (villous adenoma)	Finger-like projections of epithelium over lamina propria	10	40
Intermediate (tubulovillous adenoma)	Mixture of adenomatous and villous patterns	15	22

that produces multiple colon cancers 20 to 30 years earlier than colon cancers would be expected. The tumors have a predilection for the proximal colon. *Lynch syndrome II,* also called cancer family syndrome, has the features of Lynch syndrome I, but is characterized by the early onset of carcinoma at other sites, such as the endometrium, ovaries, and stomach. The Lynch syndromes are the most common forms of familial colon cancer.

Relatives of patients with sporadic colon cancer have a risk for cancer of the large intestine two to three times that of the general population. This association does not appear to be a genetic disorder. Familial factors may mediate susceptibility to environmental or dietary risks.

Inflammatory Bowel Disease

Patients with ulcerative colitis or Crohn's disease are at high risk for cancer of the colon. The latter are also at high risk for cancer of the small intestine.

Polyps

Nonneoplastic colorectal polyps, which are hyperplastic, inflammatory, juvenile, or hamartomatous, are not precursors to colorectal cancer.

Neoplastic polyps are adenomas and can develop into malignant tumors. Adenomas occur in one of the following three types:

- Tubular—75% to 100% tubular component
- Tubulovillous—25% to 75% villous component
- Villous—75% to 100% villous component

The most common type is tubular adenoma (adenomatous polyp) (Table 47-2). All adenomas contain some degree of dysplasia or cellular atypia. This dysplasia is graded mild to severe. Carcinoma in situ and severe dysplasia are classified as high-grade dysplasia. In carcinoma in situ, there is no invasion into the muscularis mucosae, as there is in invasive carcinoma (Fig. 47-1). Although villous lesions are much less common than the others, they are more likely to harbor a malignant tumor.

Other Risk Factors

Other risk factors are:

- Age >40 years
- Irradiation for gynecologic cancer
- Previous resection of colorectal cancer
- Cancer of the breast or genital tract

DIAGNOSIS

Symptoms

The symptoms of colorectal cancer are nonspecific. Bleeding may present as melena, usually associated with right colon cancers, or as gross red blood, associated with left colon and rectal cancers. Small amounts of blood can be detected with a fecal occult blood test. Patients with chronic blood loss may have iron-deficiency anemia associated with fatigue.

Malignant obstruction can cause abdominal pain with nausea and vomiting. In the presence of obstruction, there may be a perforation at the site of the tumor or through the proximal uninvolved intestine. With rectal tumors, compromise of the rectal reservoir can cause constipation or decreased stool caliber. With locally advanced rectal cancer, tenesmus, urgency, and perineal pain may occur.

Diagnostic Tests

Digital Examination

Allows localization of distal rectal and anal neoplasms. Stool can be obtained for evaluation of bleeding.

Sigmoidoscopy

Flexible fiberoptic sigmoidoscopy is preferred.

Barium Enema Radiographic Examination

A double-contrast examination with air insufflation is preferred. The apple-core sign is present with cancers of the colon. An advantage of barium enema examination over colonoscopy is visualization of the right colon, which is not possible in 5% to 10% of colonoscopic examinations.

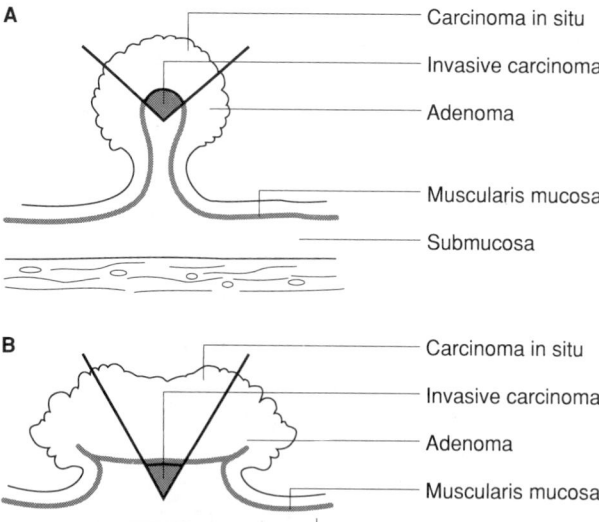

Figure 47-1. Anatomic distinction between carcinoma in situ and invasive malignancy in a pedunculated (*A*) or sessile (*B*) adenomatous polyp. In carcinoma in situ, there is no invasion into the muscularis mucosa.

Proctosigmoidoscopy

Performed to exclude rectal lesions; visualization of the rectum is inadequate with barium enema radiography.

Colonoscopy

Performed for collection of mucosal biopsy specimens and for polypectomy.

Fecal Occult Blood Tests

Several factors affect the utility of these tests:

- Not all colonic cancers or polyps are associated with bleeding, and even when they are, bleeding is often intermittent.
- Patients must be instructed to avoid foods high in peroxidase (rare beef) before testing to avoid false-positive results.
- Use of medications such as iron, cimetidine, antacids, and ascorbic acid may lead to false-negative results.

Screening

First-degree relatives of patients with known hereditary colon cancer syndromes undergo colonoscopy by 20 years of age and regularly thereafter. Patients who have removal of adenomatous polyps undergo colonoscopy once a year until no polyps are found, and then every 3 to 5 years. Patients with ulcerative colitis undergo surveillance colonoscopy after 8 to 10 years of disease activity. For the general population, yearly fecal occult blood tests and flexible sigmoidoscopy every 3 to 5 years beginning at 50 years of age are recommended.

PATHOLOGY

Almost all cancers of the large intestine are adenocarcinomas; the other histologic types are squamous cell carcinomas, adenosquamous carcinomas, lymphomas, sarcomas, and carcinoid tumors. Most adenocarcinomas of the colon are moderately or well differentiated. About 20% of adenocarcinomas are poorly differentiated or undifferentiated, and are associated with a poor prognosis. Ten to 20% of adenocarcinomas are described as mucinous or colloid carcinomas because of abundant production of mucin. These tumors are associated with a poorer 5-year survival rate than nonmucinous tumors. Other histologic features associated with poor prognosis are blood vessel invasion, lymphatic vessel invasion, and absence of a lymphocytic response to the tumor.

STAGING

The most important prognostic factor in colorectal cancer is the depth of invasion of the primary tumor. The staging systems (Fig. 47-2) are:

- Duke's classification
- Modified Astler–Coller staging system
- TNM classification

Equivalent Dukes and modified Astler–Coller stages, according to TNM classification, are defined in Table 47-3.

Prognostic Factors

Pathologic stage is the most important determinant of prognosis, but many factors correlate with survival (Table 47-4).

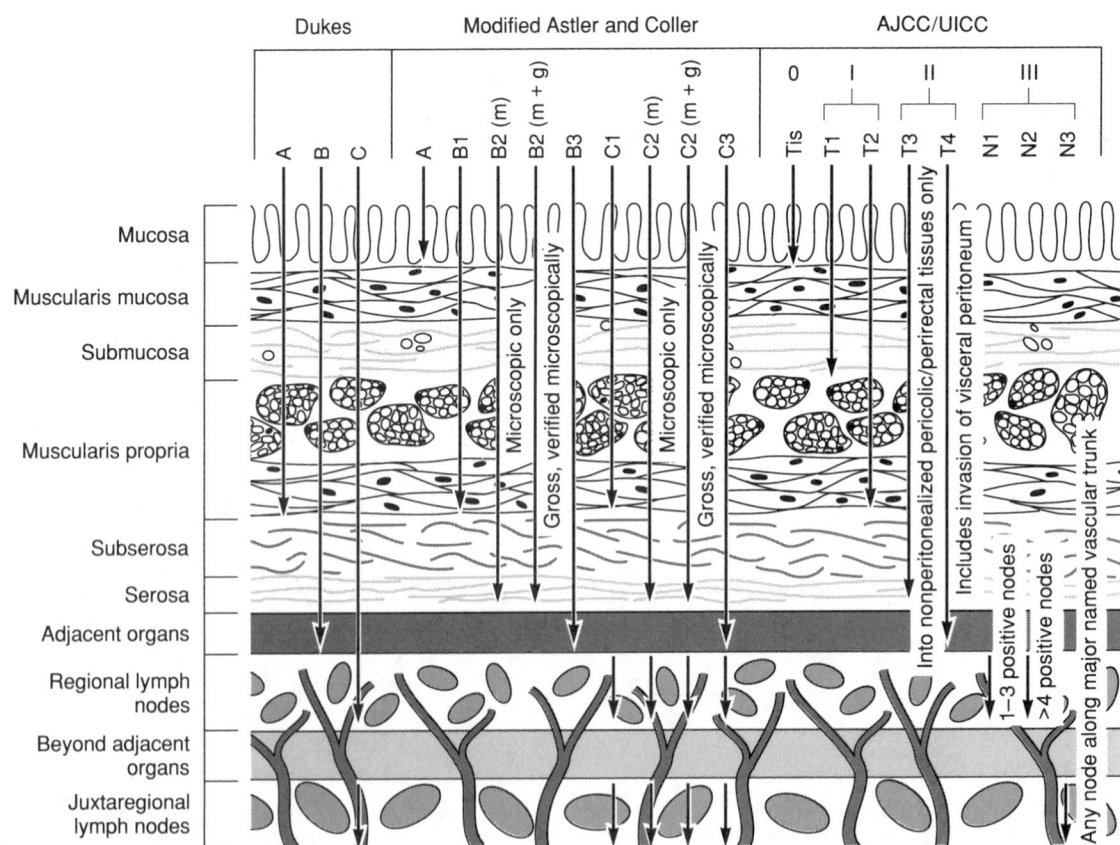

Figure 47-2. Schematic description of the staging systems with respect to depth of invasion.

Table 47-3. STAGING CLASSIFICATION OF COLORECTAL CANCER*

Stage	Description
TNM SYSTEM	
Primary Tumor	
Tx	Primary tumor cannot be assessed
T0	No evidence of tumor in resected specimen (prior polypectomy or fulguration)
Tis	Carcinoma in situ
T1	Invades into submucosa
T2	Invades into muscularis propria
T3/T4	Depends on whether serosa is present
SEROSA PRESENT	
T3	Invades through muscularis propria into subserosa Invades serosa (but not through) Invades pericolic fat within the leaves of the mesentery
T4	Invades through serosa into free peritoneal cavity, or through serosa into a contiguous organ
NO SEROSA (distal two thirds of rectum, posterior left or right colon)	
T3	Invades through muscularis propria
T4	Invades other organs (vagina, prostate, ureter, kidney)
Regional Lymph Node Involvement	
NX	Nodes cannot be assessed (eg, local excision only)
N0	No regional node metastases
N1	1–3 positive nodes
N2	4 or more positive nodes
N3	Central nodes positive
Distant Metastasis	
MX	Presence of distant metastases cannot be assessed
M0	No distant metastases
M1	Distant metastases present
DUKES STAGING SYSTEM CORRELATED WITH TNM	
Dukes A	T1, N0, M0 (stage I)
	T2, N0, M0 (stage I)
Dukes B	T3, N0, M0 (stage II)
	T4, N0, M0 (stage II)
Dukes C	T (any), N1, M0; T (any), N2, M0 (stage III)
Dukes D	T (any), N (any), M1 (stage IV)
MODIFIED ASTLER-COLLER (MAC) SYSTEM CORRELATED WITH TNM	
MAC A	T1, N0, M0 (stage I)
MAC B1	T2, N0, M0 (stage I)
MAC B2	T3, N0, M0 (stage II)
MAC B3	T4, N0, M0 (stage II)
MAC C1	T2, N1, M0; T2, N2, M0 (stage III)
MAC C2	T3, N1, M0; T3, N2, M0 (stage III)
	T4, N1, M0; T4, N2, M0 (stage III)
MAC C3	T4, N1, M0; T4, N2, M0 (stage III)

* In all pathologic staging systems, particularly those applied to rectal cancer, the abbreviations *m* and *g* may be used; *m* denotes microscopic transmural penetration; *g* or *m* + *g* denotes transmural penetration visible on gross inspection and confirmed microscopically.

Natural History

Figure 47-3 is a summary of the natural history of colorectal cancer. The natural progression of adenocarcinoma is:

- Local invasion. Intramural expansion of the tumor into the intestinal lumen is followed by lateral invasion into the intestinal wall. Progression is transverse rather than longitudinal, leading to circumferential involvement of colon.

- Lymphatic spread. The incidence of lymphatic metastasis increases with the extent of local invasion through the intestinal wall.
- Hematogenous spread. The liver is the most common site of hematogenous spread of colorectal cancer, followed by the lung. Tumor involvement of other sites in the absence of liver and lung metastases is unusual.

A possible mode of spread is intra- or extraluminal exfoliation of tumor cells with subsequent implantation. Tumor implantation may occur during surgical resection with spillage of tumor cells, leading to recurrences in intestinal anastomoses, abdominal incisions, or other abdominal sites. When a tumor penetrates the intestinal wall, intraperitoneal implantation of shed tumor cells results in peritoneal carcinomatosis.

TREATMENT OF PRIMARY COLORECTAL TUMORS

Neoplastic Polyps

Endoscopic polypectomy is used to treat neoplastic polyps unless there are medical contraindications. Pedunculated polyps are removed with a snare under endoscopic guidance. Sessile lesions are removed piecemeal, sometimes in several sessions.

If a resected lesion contains a malignant focus, a decision must be made about the need for colectomy. If the lesion *does not penetrate* the muscularis mucosae, it is an in situ malignant tumor that does not have the propensity to metastasize and does not require further surgical treatment. If the lesion *penetrates* the muscularis mucosae (Fig. 47-2), it is an invasive cancer, and colectomy with resection of paracolonic lymph nodes is indicated.

In selected patients with pedunculated polyps, conservative management without colectomy may be undertaken if the lesion does not contain poorly differentiated tumor cells or evidence of vascular invasion and if a negative resection margin is obtained at the level of the stalk. Lesions that are poorly differentiated or show evidence of

Table 47-4. PROGNOSTIC FACTORS FOR PRIMARY COLORECTAL CANCER

Factor	Association
Age	Patients <40 yr old often present with more advanced stage disease
Symptoms	Symptomatic patients tend to have more advanced stage disease
Obstruction and perforation	Poorer prognosis when present
Location of primary	Rectosigmoid and rectal cancers have lower cure rates compared with cancers elsewhere in the colon
Tumor configuration	Exophytic tumors are associated with less advanced stage cancer compared with ulcerative tumors
Blood vessel invasion	Poorer prognosis when present
Lymphatic vessel invasion	Poorer prognosis when present
Perineural invasion	Poorer prognosis when present
Lymphocytic infiltration	Improved prognosis when present
Carcinoembryonic antigen study	Poorer prognosis when elevated before primary tumor resection
Aneuploidy	Poorer prognosis when present

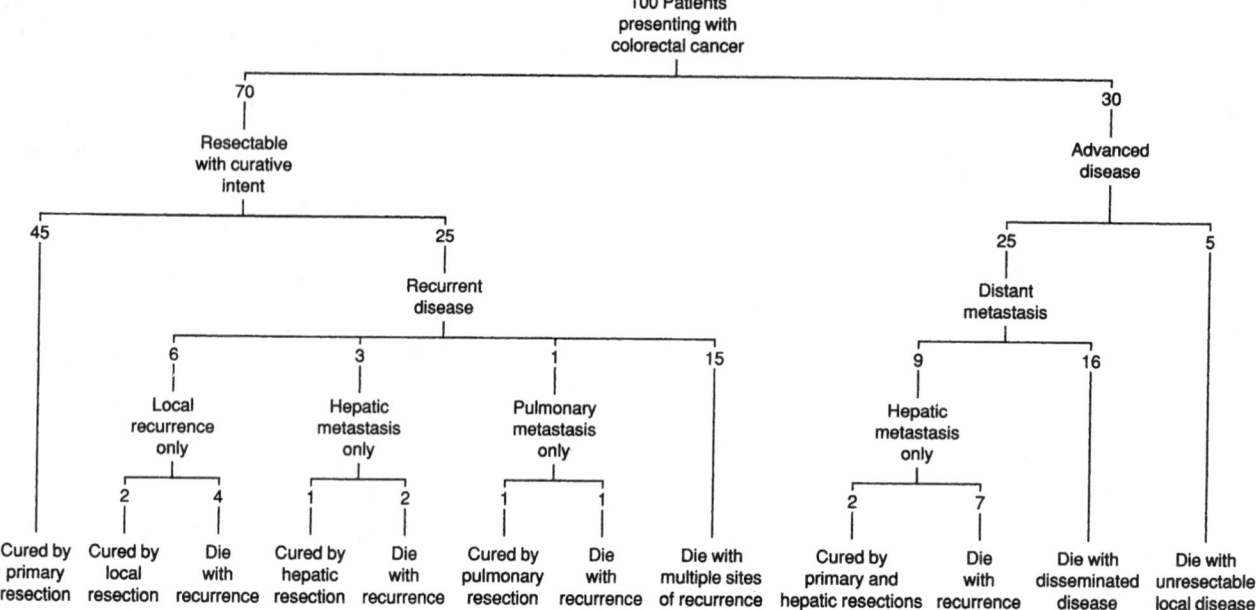

Figure 47-3. Algorithm depicting the natural history of patients with colorectal cancer.

vascular invasion, regardless of a negative surgical margin, are treated with colectomy.

Excision of large villous tumors of the rectum is required for assessment of the presence of invasive cancer. Transanal excision with sphincteric muscle and mucosal approximation is preferred. A procedure such as low anterior resection, coloanal anastomosis, or abdominoperineal resection, however, may have to be performed for total excision of extensive benign rectal lesions.

Invasive Colorectal Cancer

Surgical Treatment

A physical examination finds signs of metastases—hepatomegaly, ascites, or adenopathy. For rectal tumors, distance from the anal verge and tumor mobility are assessed to determine resectability and the type of operation required.

Rectal ultrasonography is used to assess extent of local invasion and the presence of enlarged lymph nodes in the mesorectum.

Laboratory studies include complete blood count, liver function studies, and carcinoembryonic antigen (CEA) determination.

Abnormal liver function studies lead to abdominal computed tomography (CT) to detect liver metastases. The presence of metastatic disease may alter the planned surgical procedure. A low rectal cancer with hepatic metastases may be better palliated with fulguration than with abdominoperineal resection.

Colonoscopy or air-contrast barium enema examination is performed to rule out other primary colorectal polyps or cancers.

The goals in resection of primary colorectal cancer are to:

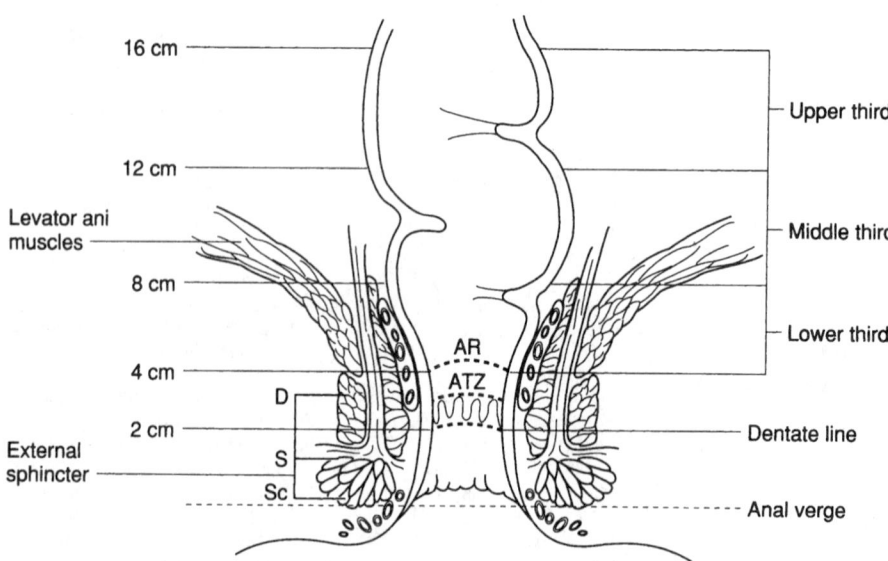

Figure 47-4. Anorectal anatomy with important landmarks. Approximate measurements are relative to the anal verge. D, deep; S, superficial; Sc, subcutaneous; AR, anorectal ring; ATZ, anal transition zone.

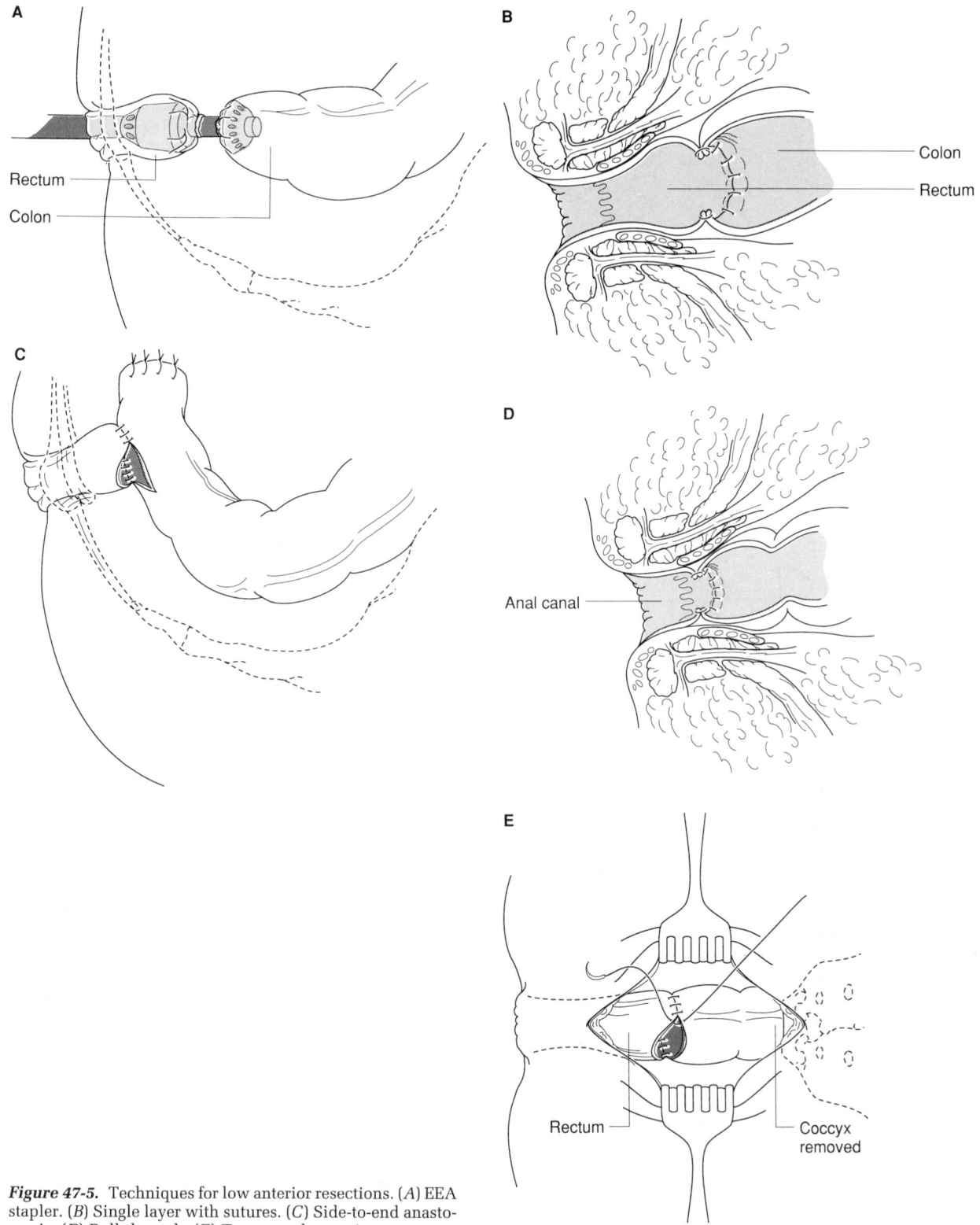

Figure 47-5. Techniques for low anterior resections. (*A*) EEA stapler. (*B*) Single layer with sutures. (*C*) Side-to-end anastomosis. (*D*) Pull-through. (*E*) Transsacral resection.

- Achieve an en bloc resection that encompasses an adequate amount of normal colon proximal and distal to the tumor
- Obtain adequate lateral margins if the tumor is adherent to contiguous structures
- Remove regional lymph nodes

During the operation, the abdominal viscera, particularly the liver and peritoneal surfaces, are examined. If evidence of disseminated disease is apparent, less extensive resection of the primary lesion may be indicated for palliation to avoid obstructive or bleeding complications.

Intraperitoneal Colon and Upper-Third of the Rectum
Resection and Anastomosis. Tumors of the cecum and ascending colon are resected with right hemicolectomy. The ileocolic, right colic, and right branches of the middle

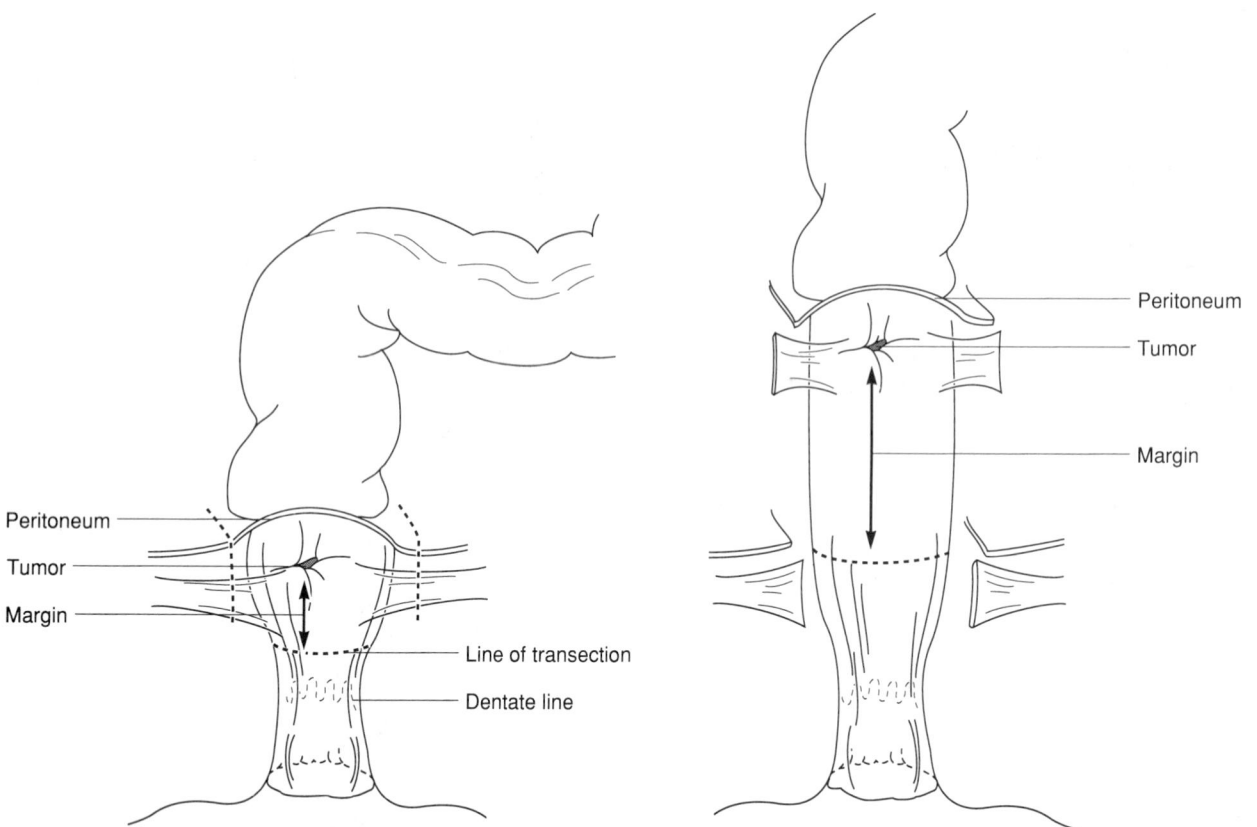

Figure 47-6. Dissection of rectum from pelvic attachments lengthens the distance of distal tumor-free margins and may permit a sphincter-saving procedure.

colic artery are ligated. For tumors at the hepatic flexure, the right hemicolectomy is extended by means of ligation of the middle colic artery near its origin. While mobilizing the ascending colon and hepatic flexure, the surgeon must protect the right ureter, testicular or ovarian vessels, inferior vena cava, superior mesenteric vein, and duodenum.

For lesions of the transverse colon, transverse colectomy is performed with proximal ligation of the middle colic artery. Lesions at the splenic flexure are removed with segmental resection of the flexure in which the mid-transverse colon is anastomosed to the middle descending colon. The left colic artery is divided, and the middle colic artery preserved. The surgeon must protect the spleen while mobilizing the splenic flexure.

Tumors of the descending colon are treated with left hemicolectomy. Intestine is removed from mid-transverse to distal sigmoid colon. High ligation of the inferior mesenteric artery is necessary. For sigmoid cancers, segmental resection is performed with ligation of the sigmoid artery near its origin. Rectosigmoid cancers and tumors confined to the upper-third of the rectum (Fig. 47-4) are removed with anterior resection. The pelvic peritoneum is incised circumferentially around the rectum, and the intestine is mobilized from the presacral fascia. The middle hemorrhoidal vessels are ligated, and the rectum is mobilized from the seminal vesicles and prostate or vagina. The mesenteric vessels are divided at the origin of the sigmoid artery (the origin the inferior mesenteric artery if additional mobilization of the splenic flexure is required to obtain a tension-free anastomosis).

Middle-Third of the Rectum

- Low anterior resection
- Abdominosacral resection

- Coloanal anastomosis
- Abdominoperineal resection
- Local excision or fulguration
- Primary radiation therapy

For cancer 8 to 12 cm from the anal verge (Fig. 47-4), an effort is made to maintain intestinal continuity. Low anterior resection involves resection of the mid-rectum with primary anastomosis. After tumor removal, anastomosis is end-to-end or end-to-side with sutures or staples (Fig. 47-5). A temporary transverse colostomy is performed if there is concern about the integrity of the anastomosis.

Abdominosacral resection allows direct visualization of low hand-sewn anastomoses. The rectum is mobilized through an abdominal approach, and a second incision is made above the anus. The coccyx is resected to allow visualization of the pelvis. A hand-sewn anastomosis is completed through the transsacral incision (Fig. 47-5). This procedure is being supplanted with stapling. Coloanal anastomosis restores intestinal continuity by bringing the colon to the level of the anus and dentate line (Fig. 47-5D).

A controversy surrounding sphincter-saving procedures for rectal tumors is the length of adequate distal mucosal margin. Ideally, a surgical margin of 3 cm, measured on the fresh specimen, is to be achieved. If an EEA stapler is used, a margin of 2 cm plus the additional doughnut specimen obtained with the stapler is adequate. If this margin cannot be obtained, abdominoperineal resection is performed. The segment of rectum between the tumor and pelvic floor can be lengthened as much as 4 cm once the rectum is mobilized from its pelvic attachments (Fig. 47-6).

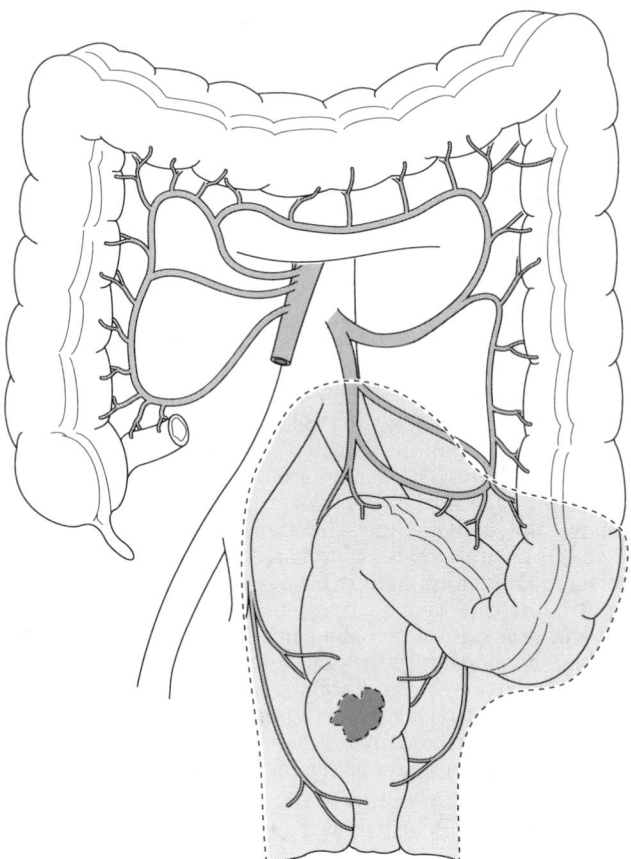

Figure 47-7. Extent of surgery in abdominoperineal resection.

Some small (<3 cm), well-differentiated tumors limited to the intestinal wall can be treated local measures. Full-thickness local excision of the intestinal wall is performed by the transanal route with primary closure of the defect. If negative surgical margins are achieved, adjuvant chemotherapy and radiation are used to optimize locoregional tumor control. If the surgical margins are positive, low anterior resection or abdominoperineal resection is performed.

Ablation with transanal electrofulguration of the tumor in multiple stages is used to treat tumors in patients who cannot undergo surgical therapy. This procedure cannot be performed for circumferential tumors.

Endocavitary irradiation can be used as primary curative therapy for early cancers in some patients. For locally advanced colorectal tumors, Nd:YAG laser therapy is used for palliation of obstructive or bleeding lesions.

Lower-Third of the Rectum

- Abdominoperineal resection
- Local excision or fulguration
- Primary radiation therapy

Cancers between the anorectal ring and 7 to 8 cm from the anal verge (Fig. 47-4) are treated with abdominoperineal resection. The procedure involves wide excision of the rectum to include the lateral attachments and pelvic mesocolon and establishment of a colostomy (Fig. 47-7). When the abdomen is opened, intraabdominal spread is ascertained. If extensive disseminated disease is found, local excision or fulguration to preserve anal function may be appropriate for palliation. If an abdominoperineal resection is performed, the superior hemorrhoidal vessels are ligated at their origin from the left colic artery. The rectum is mobilized and the dissection is carried to the pelvic floor muscles, which are excised en bloc with the anus. An end-sigmoid colostomy is brought out through the rectus sheath. Effort is made to exclude small intestine from a future radiation field by use of uterus, omentum, peritoneum, or absorbable mesh.

Adjuvant Radiation Therapy

The use of radiation therapy is confined to rectal tumors that extend through the intestinal wall or have lymph node involvement. Despite local tumor control, distant metastases occur, but the modality is used to avoid complications associated with tumor recurrence in the pelvis. The effectiveness of radiation therapy is proportional to the total dose. Therapy can be preoperative, postoperative, or combined. Adjuvant radiation therapy for colon cancer can be toxic because of the large amount of small intestine that may lie in the treatment field.

Adjuvant Chemotherapy

Despite adequate local tumor control, patients who die of colorectal cancer do so from disseminated disease. Postoperative adjuvant systemic chemotherapy appears to benefit some patients. The National Institutes of Health (NIH) recommends that patients with stage III *colon cancer* undergo adjuvant chemotherapy to improve survival. The NIH recommends that patients with stage II or III *rectal cancer* undergo postoperative chemotherapy and irradiation.

TREATMENT OF RECURRENT COLORECTAL CANCER

Because some cases of recurrent colorectal cancer can be cured, a comprehensive follow-up program is necessary for patients who have undergone resection of a primary tumor. Fifty percent of cancers that recur do so within 18 months of resection, and almost all recurrences are evident within 3 years. A follow-up program also identifies the 5% of patients in whom another primary tumor of the large intestine develops. Table 47-5 presents guidelines for follow-up care after colorectal resections for cancer.

Hepatic Metastases

The liver is the most frequent site of blood-borne metastases from primary colorectal cancers. Patients who can undergo hepatic resection of metastatic disease have:

Table 47-5. GUIDELINES FOR FOLLOW-UP OF PATIENTS AFTER POTENTIALLY CURATIVE SURGERY

Procedure or Test	Frequency
History and physical examination	Every 6 mo for 3 y, then yearly
Carcinoembryonic antigen study	Every 6 mo for 3 y, then yearly
Fecal occult blood	Every 6 mo for 3 y, then yearly
Liver chemistries	Yearly*
Abdominal CT	Yearly*
Total colonoscopy	Yearly*
Chest radiograph	Yearly*

*After 5 years, if there is no evidence of recurrence, the procedure or test should be performed every 2 to 3 years for the remainder of the patient's life.

- No evidence of extrahepatic tumor
- No medical contraindications to surgical therapy
- Fewer than four lesions amenable to resection with negative surgical margins

Patients with unresectable hepatic metastases that appear to be confined to the liver are treated with regional chemotherapy via the hepatic artery (5-FU, FUDR).

Pulmonary Metastases

Pulmonary metastases develop in about 10% of patients with colorectal cancer, usually in association with widespread metastatic disease. Rectal cancers can spread via the portal or systemic venous systems and give rise to isolated pulmonary metastases. In selected patients, resection of pulmonary recurrences can result in a 20% 5-years survival rate.

Local Recurrence

About 20% of patients experience local recurrence of colon cancer. If the recurrent tumor is isolated to the suture line, resection can be curative. Pelvic recurrences of rectal cancer after low anterior or abdominoperineal resection often are diffuse and associated with disseminated disease. Localized pelvic recurrences are resected—with en bloc partial sacrectomy or pelvic exenteration—if negative surgical margins can be achieved.

Disseminated Disease

Colorectal cancer usually recurs in multiple sites and may not be amenable to surgical resection. Systemic therapy does not appear to improve survival rates but is used for palliation.

SUGGESTED READING

Cannon-Albright LA, Skolnick MH, Bishop T, et al. Common inheritance of susceptibility to colonic adenomatous polyps and associated colorectal cancers. N Engl J Med 1988;319:533.

Kokal WA, Gardine RL, Sheibani K, et al. Tumor DNA content in resectable, primary colorectal carcinoma. Ann Surg 1989; 209:188.

Krook JE, Moertel CG, Gunderson LL, et al. Effective surgical adjuvant therapy for high-risk rectal carcinoma. N Engl J Med 1991;324:709.

Mandel JS, Bond JH, Church TR, et al. Reducing mortality from colorectal cancer by screening for fecal occult blood. N Engl J Med 1993;328:1365.

Steele GD Jr, Augenlicht LH, Begg CB, et al. National Institutes of Health Consensus Development Conference statement: adjuvant therapy for patients with colon and rectal cancer. JAMA 1990;264:1444.

Yeatman TJ, Bland KI. Sphincter-saving procedures for distal carcinoma of the rectum. Ann Surg 1989;209:1.

ESSENTIALS OF SURGERY: SCIENTIFIC PRINCIPLES AND PRACTICE,
edited by Lazar J. Greenfield, Michael W. Mulholland, Keith T. Oldham, Gerald B. Zelenock,
and Keith D. Lillemoe. Lippincott–Raven Publishers, Philadelphia, © 1997.

CHAPTER 48

ANAL CANCER

SANTHAT NIVATVONGS

The anal canal, which extends from the anorectal ring to the anal verge, is lined with several different kinds of epithelium, each of which is susceptible to neoplastic transformation. Below the dentate, or pectinate, line is squamous epithelium, and above the dentate line is columnar epithelium. The change from squamous to columnar epithelium is not abrupt. For a distance of about 1 cm above the dentate line (the transitional or cloacogenic zone) is an area where columnar, cuboidal, transitional, or even squamous epithelium may exist. The anal canal above and below the dentate line has different routes of lymphatic drainage. When the same histologic type of neoplasm develops in these areas, biologic behavior is different. For these reasons, carcinomas of the anal region are classified in two categories in relation to the dentate line: the area above the dentate line is the anal canal; the area below the dentate line is the anal margin.

CARCINOMA OF THE ANAL MARGIN
Squamous Cell Carcinoma

Squamous cell carcinomas of the anal margin, in gross appearance, resemble those of the skin elsewhere on the body. They grow slowly and have rolled, everted edges with central ulceration. Any chronic unhealed or indurated ulceration in the anal area is considered squamous cell carcinoma until biopsy proves otherwise. Squamous carcinomas are usually well differentiated histologically, with well-developed patterns of keratinization (Fig. 48-1). Lymphatic spread from squamous carcinomas of the anal margin is mainly to inguinal lymph nodes.

Despite the superficial location, most lesions are usually diagnosed late, often >24 months after the onset of symptoms. Examination of the inguinal region at regular intervals after excision of the primary lesion is indicated because subsequent metastasis to the lymph nodes of the groin is common.

Treatment

Because squamous cell carcinomas of the anal margin are late to metastasize, wide local excision is used as definitive surgical therapy. If at histologic examination, the carcinoma has invaded the underlying sphincter muscles, metastasis may occur proximally along the superior rectal nodes and laterally along the middle rectal nodes. Abdominoperineal resection is indicated. In some patients, radium implantation therapy is helpful. Radical groin nodal dissection is performed only if metastasis to the inguinal lymph nodes is suspected.

Basal Cell Carcinoma

Basal cell carcinoma of the anal margin is rare. It is more frequent in men than women. The lesions are characterized by central ulceration and irregular, raised edges. Basal cell carcinomas are usually superficial, are not fixed to deeper structures, and rarely metastasize. Although metastases are

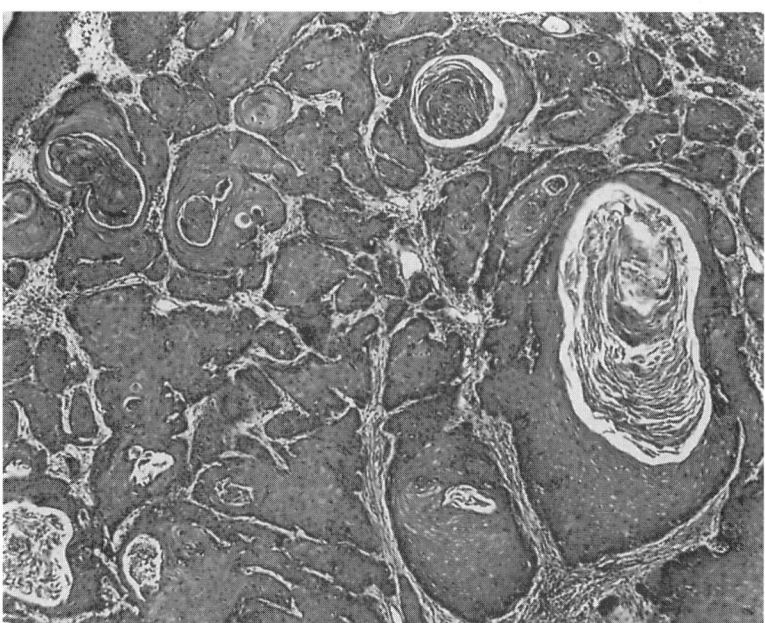

Figure 48-1. Photomicrograph of squamous cell carcinoma of the anal margin.

not common, inguinal lymphadenopathy can develop from reactive inflammation. Almost one-third of basal cell carcinomas of the anal margin are misdiagnosed as hemorrhoids, anal fistulas, or perianal eczema, causing delay in treatment. The patient most frequently presents with mild discomfort, itching, or bleeding.

Treatment

Treatment is local excision with a margin of normal tissue. Local recurrence after excision is common, and re-excision is indicated. Abdominoperineal resection is reserved for large lesions and for uncontrollable local recurrence.

Bowen Disease

Bowen disease of the perianal skin is a rare, slow-growing intraepidermal squamous cell carcinoma. The lesions appear as discrete, scaly, or crusted plaques, sometimes exhibiting a moist surface. The patient may report itching, burning, or spotty bleeding. Although symptoms and gross appearance are suggestive, only a biopsy can confirm the diagnosis. Most patients with Bowen disease already have, or eventually develop, one or more primary internal malignant tumors or primary cancer of the skin with metastasis. An essential part of the diagnostic evaluation is to exclude other primary malignant tumors.

Treatment

Treatment is wide local excision. Microscopic examination is indicated to confirm a clear margin of resection. Bowen disease may extend into the anal canal, necessitating wide excision of anoderm. In this situation, it may be necessary to use flaps to prevent postoperative anal stricture.

Perianal Paget Disease

Paget disease of the perianal area is a rare malignant neoplasm of the intraepidermal portion of the apocrine glands, with or without associated dermal involvement. Paget disease has a long preinvasive phase, but if the disease is not treated, an invasive adenocarcinoma of the apo-

crine gland type develops. The disease is more common in women than men, with the highest incidence in the seventh decade of life.

Most patients with Paget disease have, or subsequently develop, a second primary carcinoma, such as carcinoma of breast or rectum. Intractable anal itching is usually present for many months. The lesion appears as an erythematous scaly or eczematoid plaque, similar to other benign perianal lesions. The correct diagnosis is made with biopsy, which shows characteristic Paget cells—large, pale, vacuolated cells with hyperchromatic eccentric nuclei (Fig. 48-2). The cells invariably contain acid mucosubstances, an important feature in differentiating this lesion from melanoma and Bowen disease.

Treatment

Treatment is wide local excision in the absence of invasive carcinoma. Because of the high incidence of local recurrence and residual tumor, it is vital to obtain an adequate margin of resection. At gross examination, the extent of involvement is ill defined, and multiple punch biopsies may be needed to determine the extent of involvement. For more advanced lesions with underlying carcinoma, abdominoperineal resection is indicated. Inguinal lymph node dissection is performed only if groin lymph nodes are clinically positive for metastasis.

Because diagnosis usually is delayed (average: 4 years), about 25% of patients with perianal Paget disease have metastases when they seek treatment. The sites of metastases, in order of frequency, are inguinal and pelvic lymph nodes, liver, bone, lung, brain, bladder, prostate, and adrenal gland. The prognosis is poor once metastasis has occurred.

CARCINOMA OF THE ANAL CANAL
Adenocarcinoma

The ducts of the anal glands are lined by squamous epithelium close to their opening in the crypts, by transitional epithelium in the middle portion, and, in the depth of the gland, by mucin-secreting columnar epithelium. The histologic features of these lesions may be those of adeno-

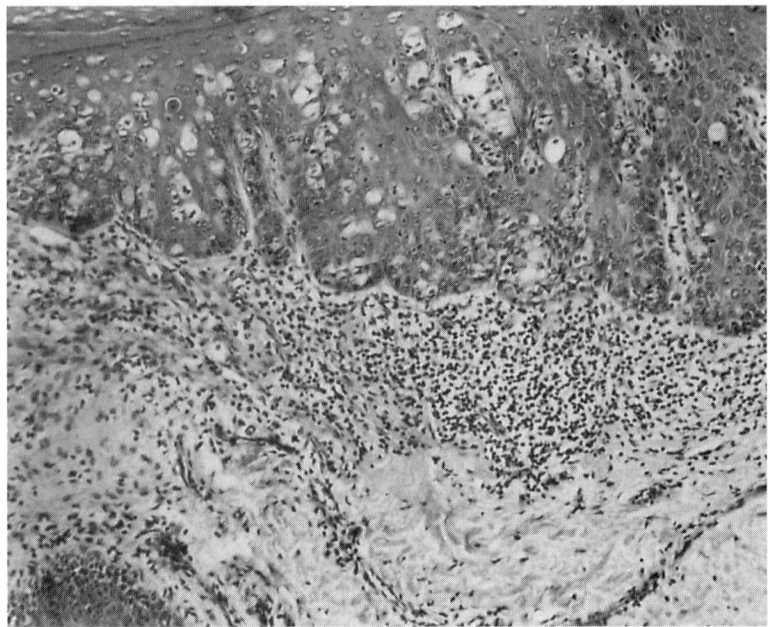

Figure 48-2. Perianal Paget disease. Paget cells are above the basal layer.

carcinoma, mucoepidermoid carcinoma, or basaloid or transitional cell carcinoma. The differentiating feature of ductal carcinoma of the anus is its extramucosal origin. If a break occurs in the surface epithelium, greater perianal involvement or deeper infiltration may be the only clue to the anal-duct origin of these lesions.

Patients with ductal carcinoma of the anus usually report pain, bleeding, and a perianal mass. Symptoms related to a mass in the anal canal are uncommon. Penetration beyond the anal canal may masquerade as perianal or ischioanal abscess or anal fistula. The diagnosis of ductal adenocarcinoma is usually made when the lesion is at an advanced stage, and the disease has frequently spread too far to make cure likely.

Adenocarcinoma sometimes occurs in long-standing anal fistulas. These carcinomas appear to be due to chronic irritation of the epithelium around the internal or external openings of fistulas, or the fistulas may be ductal in origin.

Treatment

Local excision is reserved for carcinomas that are small (≤3 cm in diameter), limited to the submucosa, and have well-differentiated histologic features. For most patients, treatment is abdominoperineal resection. The role of preoperative and postoperative radiation is not defined.

Epidermoid Carcinoma

Types of Tumors

Squamous Cell Carcinoma. Squamous cell carcinoma originates from the cloacogenic area of epithelium. Squamous cancers are typically flat, ulcerating neoplasms. They occur more frequently in women than men. The histologic features resemble those of squamous cell carcinoma of the anal margin, except there is little or no keratin. Minor perianal problems, such as bleeding, occur in about half of patients. Other symptoms include rectal pain and an anal mass. Almost one-third of patients have an initial incorrect diagnosis of benign or inflammatory disease.

Squamous cell carcinomas of the anal canal metastasize to superior rectal lymph nodes in about 40% of patients, and to the inguinal nodes in about 33% of patients.

Basaloid (Cloacogenic) Carcinoma. Basaloid carcinoma is a variant of squamous cell carcinoma and, to some degree, resembles basal cell carcinomas of the skin. *Basaloid* refers to the histologic appearance of palisade nuclei seen in the periphery of clumps of cells that characterize this lesion (Fig. 48-3). The tumor is more frequent in women than men. The mean age at diagnosis is 60 years.

Basaloid carcinoma, also called *transitional cloacogenic carcinoma,* originates from the transitional zone above the dentate line. The clinical features are similar to those of squamous cell carcinomas of the anal canal. As in squamous cell carcinomas of the anal canal, about half of patients already have regional lymph node involvement at operation.

Mucoepidermoid Carcinoma. Mucoepidermoid carcinoma is a variant of squamous cell carcinoma with the same histologic pattern, except for the presence of mucin. Mucin staining varies in amount from lesion to lesion and within different areas of the same lesion. The incidence is slightly higher among women than men. The mean age at diagnosis is 55 years. The behavior and prognosis of these lesions are similar to those of squamous cell or basaloid carcinomas.

Treatment

Local excision is reserved for early or well-differentiated lesions that involve only the submucosa. It also may be considered for patients who are at poor risk for an extensive operation. The recurrence rate is high after local excision.

Abdominoperineal resection is performed with wide excision of perineal tissue. In women, the posterior vaginal wall is excised because the incidence of invasion to the area is high. A high recurrence rate after abdominoperineal resection probably reflects the behavior of the carcinoma and the multiple pathways of the lymphatic network in the anorectum and pelvis. To improve long-term survival and prevent use of a colostomy, combined modality therapy is replacing abdominoperineal resection as the primary treatment of epidermoid carcinoma.

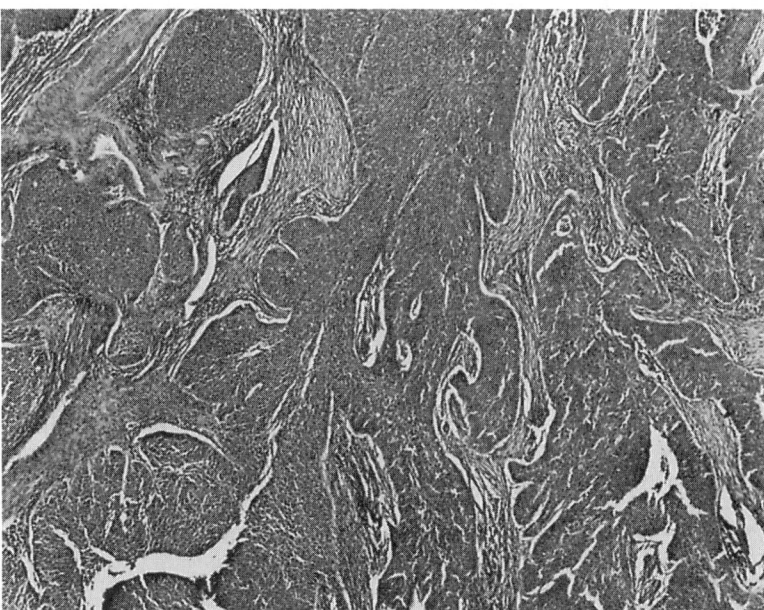

Figure 48-3. Basaloid (cloacogenic) carcinoma of the anal canal.

The following *combined therapy* protocol is designed to contain disease without a radical operation:

- External irradiation, 3000 rad (30 Gy), to the primary tumor, pelvic, and inguinal nodes from day 1 to day 21 (200 rad/d, 5 d/wk)
- Systemic chemotherapy, 5-fluorouracil (5-FU) 1000 mg/m² every 24 hours, as a continuous infusion for 4 days, starting on day 1 of radiation therapy, and repeated on days 28 through 31 of the protocol
- Mitomycin C, 15 mg/m² IV bolus on day 1

If gross examination shows that the lesion has disappeared, and its absence is confirmed with biopsy, no further treatment is necessary. If residual cancer is present, and if there is no evidence of disseminated disease, abdominoperineal resection is performed 4 to 6 weeks after completion of radiation therapy.

Because of the high morbidity of *inguinal lymph node dissection,* the risk of the added procedure outweighs the benefit. Elective radiation of clinically normal inguinal nodes reduces the risk of late node failure and carries little morbidity.

MALIGNANT MELANOMA

Melanoma is a rare malignant tumor of the anal canal. The anal canal, nevertheless, represents the third most common site of melanomas, exceeded only by skin and eyes. Almost all anal melanomas originate from the epidermoid lining of the anal canal. Most melanomas occur adjacent to the dentate line, although a few tumors originate in the rectum.

Rectal bleeding is the most common symptom. Melanoma is suspected when a deeply pigmented lesion is detected. Most tumors, however, are pigmented lightly or are nonpigmented, and they are often misdiagnosed as polyps or epidermoid carcinomas. In amelanotic malignant melanomas, biopsy findings can be misinterpreted as an undifferentiated epidermoid carcinoma.

Anal canal melanomas have a marked tendency to spread submucosally into the rectum, but they rarely invade adjacent organs, probably because most patients die before such spread occurs. Lymphatic spread to the mesenteric nodes has occurred in about one-third of patients by the time of diagnosis; spread to the inguinal nodes is less common. Hematogenous spread to the liver and lung is early and rapid, accounting for most deaths.

Treatment

Melanomas of the anal canal are radioresistant and do not respond to chemotherapy or immunotherapy. The surgical approach to this malignant neoplasm is controversial. Abdominoperineal resection usually is more effective than wide local excision in preventing local recurrence. For patients at low risk, abdominoperineal resection is reasonable treatment for removal of undetected mesenteric lymph node metastases.

SUGGESTED READING

Abel ME, Chiu YSY, Russell TR, Volpe PA. Adenocarcinoma of the anal glands: results of a survey. Dis Colon Rectum 1993; 36:383.

Antoniuk PM, Tjandra JJ, Webb BW, Petras RE, Milsom JW, Fazio VW. Anorectal malignant melanoma has poor prognosis. Int J Colorect Dis 1993;8:81.

Armitage NC, Jass JR, Richman PI, Thomson JPS, Philips RKS. Paget's disease of the anus: a clinicopathological study. Br J Surg 1989;76:60.

Brady M, Kavolius J, Quan SHQ. Anorectal melanoma. Dis Colon Rectum 1994;37:P13.

Deans GT, McAleer JJA, Spence RAJ. Malignant anal tumors. Br J Surg 1994;81:500.

Flaur MS, John MJ, Mowry PA. Definitive combined modality therapy of carcinoma of the anus: a report of 30 cases including results of salvage therapy in patients with residual disease. Dis Colon Rectum 1987;30:495.

Goldman S, Glimelius B, Pahlman L. Anorectal malignant melanoma in Sweden: report of 49 patients. Dis Colon Rectum 1990;33:874.

Jensen SL, Hagen K, Harling H, Shokouh-Amiri MH, Nielsen OV. Long-term prognosis after radical treatment for squamous cell carcinoma of the anal canal and anal margin. Dis Colon Rectum 1988;31:273.

Nigro ND. Multidisciplinary management of cancer of the anus. World J Surg 1987;11:446.

Papillon J, Montbarbon JF. Epidermoid carcinoma of the anal canal: a series of 276 cases. Dis Colon Rectum 1987;30:324.

ESSENTIALS OF SURGERY: SCIENTIFIC PRINCIPLES AND PRACTICE,
edited by Lazar J. Greenfield, Michael W. Mulholland, Keith T. Oldham, Gerald B. Zelenock,
and Keith D. Lillemoe. Lippincott–Raven Publishers, Philadelphia, © 1997.

CHAPTER 49

DIVERTICULAR DISEASE

GORDON L. TELFORD AND MARY F. OTTERSON

Colonic *diverticula* are small pouches in the wall of the large intestine. Most emanate from points of weakness of the wall where mesenteric blood vessels penetrate the circular muscle layer (Fig. 49-1). *Diverticulosis* is an abnormal state in which noninflamed diverticula are present with or without symptoms. *Diverticulitis* is inflammation of one or more diverticula. The inflammation may lead to perforation of the diverticulum with pericolic infection (peridiverticulitis) or abscess formation, free perforation with peritonitis, fistula formation, or obstruction.

PATHOLOGIC ANATOMY

True diverticula involve all layers of the intestinal wall: mucosa, submucosa, and muscularis externa. False diverticula are composed of only mucosa and submucosa that have herniated through the muscularis externa. Most diverticula of the colon are false.

PATHOPHYSIOLOGY

A decrease in fiber in the diet is associated with the high incidence of diverticulosis in Western populations. A perplexing problem is exactly how a diet low in fiber results in the formation of diverticula. One hypothesis is that when circular muscular contractions occur in patients with small amounts of stool in the colon, the colonic lumen becomes occluded. When two such contractions occur close to one another, the lumen of the intervening segment of colon is isolated from the rest of the colon and high pressure is generated in that segment. Increased pressure results in the formation of diverticula by placing increased tension on the colonic wall. In some people, there also appears to be a decrease in tensile strength of the colon wall.

CLINICAL PRESENTATION AND DIFFERENTIAL DIAGNOSES

Diverticulosis

Most colonic diverticula detected at barium enema radiographic examination are asymptomatic or only mildly symptomatic. In patients with abdominal pain and evidence of noninflamed diverticula at barium enema examination, the diverticula are not usually the cause of the pain. One explanation for the pain is the pressure exerted by segmentation of the colon.

In patients with mild to moderate lower abdominal pain, the differential diagnosis of diverticulosis is considered along with that of chronic constipation, diverticulitis, irritable bowel syndrome, and adenocarcinoma of the colon. If pain is severe and constant, a diagnosis of diverticulitis is considered. Irritable bowel syndrome is a prediverticular condition and is a diagnosis made by exclusion. In patients in whom barium enema does not demonstrate diverticula, a diagnosis of irritable bowel or chronic constipation is not made until the diagnosis of carcinoma is eliminated with a colonoscopic examination.

Diverticulitis

The symptoms of diverticulitis are fever, lower abdominal pain, and lower abdominal tenderness. A lower abdominal mass, tachycardia, and an elevated white blood cell (WBC) count with a left shift may also occur.

Diverticulitis with free perforation and generalized peritonitis is difficult to differentiate from perforation of other viscera. Localization of pain to the left lower quadrant and a palpable, tender mass suggest diverticulitis. When free perforation does not occur with diverticulitis, differential diagnoses are perforated colon cancer, acute appendicitis, perforated peptic ulcer, acute ulcerative colitis, acute Crohn's colitis, and ischemic colitis.

Hemorrhage

Hemorrhage may occur with diverticulosis or diverticulitis, but it is more likely with diverticulosis (Fig. 49-2). The differential diagnosis is colonic angiodysplasia.

Obstruction

Diverticulitis and its complications can cause obstruction of the large intestine. Problems in evaluating obstruction of the sigmoid colon are the high incidence of carci-

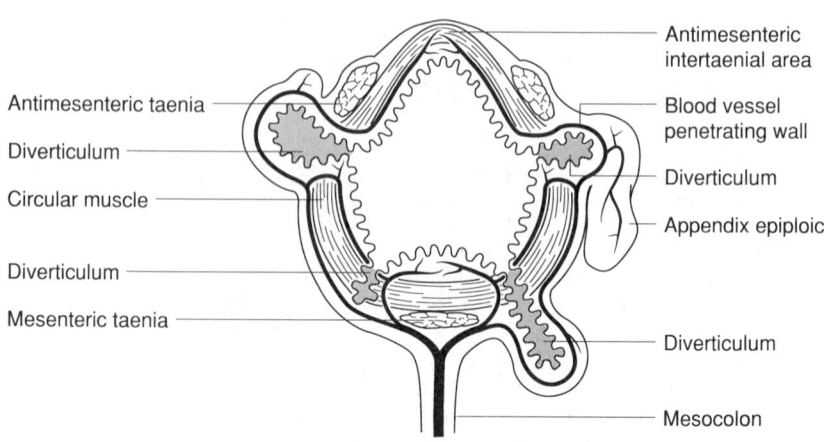

Figure 49-1. Cross section of the colon illustrating the relation of diverticula to the blood vessels penetrating the circular muscle layer, the taeniae, and the appendices epiploicae.

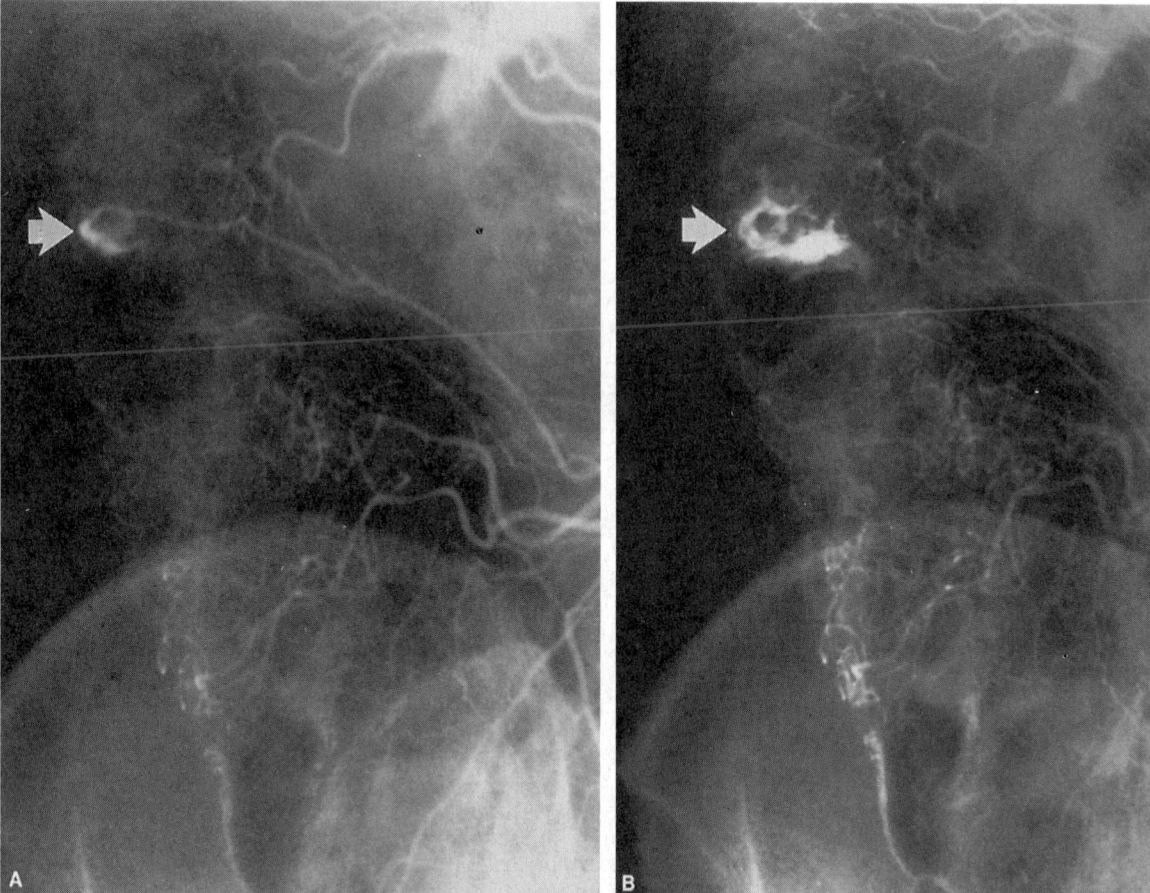

Figure 49-2. Superior mesenteric arteriogram from a patient with bleeding from a right colon diverticulum. (*A*) Early roentgenogram with contrast material outlining the diverticulum (*arrow*). (*B*) Late roentgenogram demonstrating overflow of contrast material into the colonic lumen.

noma in patients with symptomatic sigmoid diverticular disease and difficulty making the diagnosis of carcinoma of the colon when a large, phlegmonous mass is present. Colonoscopy may be helpful, but only if (1) the endoscope can pass the area of obstruction and (2) a biopsy can be performed. Normal colonoscopic findings in a patient with obstruction, inflammation, and edema do not eliminate carcinoma as a diagnosis.

DIAGNOSIS AND THERAPY

Diverticulosis

Patients with a combination of chronic, intermittent, lower abdominal pain and diverticula on barium enema examination are given symptomatic treatment. The diverticula are not considered to be the cause of the pain, and surgical therapy is not indicated. Colectomy is reserved for treatment of complications.

Population studies demonstrate that diverticula can be prevented with a diet high in fiber. It has not been proved, however, that such a diet prevents the complications of diverticulosis. Common-sense recommendations for increasing intake of dietary fiber probably are worthwhile.

In most patients (75%) with diverticular hemorrhage, bleeding stops spontaneously, and does not recur. The 25% in whom bleeding does recur undergo segmental colectomy because they are at risk for subsequent hemorrhage.

Diverticulitis

Diverticulitis is a complication of diverticulosis. There are two theories about how it occurs:

1. Feces become impacted in a diverticulum, obstructing the neck of the diverticulum or abrading the thin-walled diverticulum, thus causing invasive infection.
2. Microperforation occurs as a result of increased intraluminal pressure, leading to spillage of colonic contents.

Either event results in infection of the surrounding pericolic tissues or free perforation. Infection can be asymptomatic or it can become clinically significant and necessitate hospitalization and surgical intervention. If the infection is progressive, the following complications occur.

Peridiverticulitis

Most patients with an episode of acute diverticulitis severe enough to require hospitalization are treated with IV fluids, bowel rest, broad-spectrum antibiotics, and analgesics. Signs and symptoms of severe diverticulitis are fever, tachycardia, leukocytosis with left shift of the differential count, abdominal pain (usually in the left lower quadrant), abdominal tenderness, and a lower abdominal mass.

If nausea, vomiting, or abdominal distention develops, nasogastric suction is instituted. The patient undergoes frequent examinations for signs of progression of disease. If the patient's condition does not improve within 48 hours, complications of diverticulitis probably exist, and further therapy is necessary.

Barium enema radiographic examination performed with water-soluble contrast material aids in the diagnosis of diverticulitis. CT is more useful in delineating the complications of diverticulitis, including perforation and abscess formation (Fig. 49-3). At CT, percutaneous drainage catheters can be placed if an abscess is identified. After CT drainage of an abscess, most patients undergo one-stage segmental colectomy and primary anastomosis. If percutaneous drainage is not feasible, or an abscess is not identified, surgical exploration is performed.

At exploratory laparotomy, if the disease is found to be localized, segmental colectomy is performed. Distal resection extends to the proximal rectum to decrease the risk for recurrence. Proximal resection includes the segment of colon affected by acute disease and any colon with signs of chronic disease or large numbers of diverticula.

The only absolute contraindications to primary anastomosis are free perforation with generalized peritonitis; obstruction with unprepared intestine; and intraoperative conditions that do not warrant primary anastomosis, such as septic shock, ureteral injury, or other conditions that make a prolonged operation inadvisable. If resection is unsafe because of the presence of a massive phlegmon or if the patient's condition is unstable, a diverting end colostomy with mucous fistula and drainage may be performed. Colonic resection is deferred until inflammation subsides.

Obstruction

Fibrotic colonic stricture and obstruction of the large intestine can occur in patients who have had one or more episodes of diverticulitis. When obstruction is diagnosed, it is important to differentiate diverticulitis, colonic carcinoma, and colonic volvulus. All patients undergo sigmoidoscopy or colonoscopy so that biopsies can be performed. Patients also undergo radiography of the colon with water-soluble contrast material to define completeness of obstruction.

The extent of evaluation depends on the patient's condition and the completeness of the obstruction. Patients with incomplete obstruction undergo a thorough but rapid evaluation to secure a preoperative diagnosis. Patients with a complete obstruction require an urgent operation.

If obstruction is *partial*, the patient undergoes complete intestinal preparation, including oral antibiotics, before the operation. These patients do not tolerate rapid intestinal preparation with laxatives or polyethylene glycol and are allowed extra time for complete intestinal cleaning. Once intestinal preparation is complete, the patient undergoes one-stage resection and primary anastomosis. Unless colonic carcinoma is eliminated as a diagnosis, a cancer operation is performed.

Patients with a *complete* obstruction cannot undergo preoperative intestinal preparation, and a one-stage operation is not feasible. The patient undergoes urgent diverting colostomy to relieve the obstruction. Resection of the diseased, obstructed segment of intestine may be performed during this operation or may be deferred until diagnostic evaluation is complete. The evaluation to differentiate carcinoma and diverticulitis is performed after the patient has recovered from the initial operation.

When the patient has recovered from the first operation, which takes at least 1 month, the next operation is performed. The second operation usually is resection of the colostomy and the diseased segment of colon and reestablishment of intestinal continuity with a colocolostomy. When the diseased segment is removed during the first operation, the second procedure is colostomy closure.

Fistula Formation

Diverticular disease may be complicated by the development of fistulas between the diseased colon and other viscera or skin.

Colovesical Fistulas

Most patients with colovesical fistulas have urinary tract symptoms—urgency, dysuria, pneumaturia, and fecaluria. The diagnosis of colovesical fistula is difficult to establish. Recurrent urinary tract infections in an elderly man suggest a fistula. Barium enema examination demonstrates diverticula, or, in some patients, sigmoid narrowing. Only rarely is the fistulous tract filled. After rectal administration of barium, the urine sediment is assessed for barium by means of radiography of a spun urine sample. The presence of barium in the urine is diagnostic of a colovesical fistula. Cystoscopic examination reveals hyperemia and inflammation consistent with chronic cystitis. Although the findings may be localized, indicating the presence of a fistulous communication, the fistula opening is seldom seen. CT with intraluminal contrast material is the most sensitive test for the presence of a colovesical fistula. In almost all patients, air is present in the urinary bladder, and an indurated segment of sigmoid colon is adjacent to a locally thickened bladder wall.

Most patients with colovesical fistulas are treated with

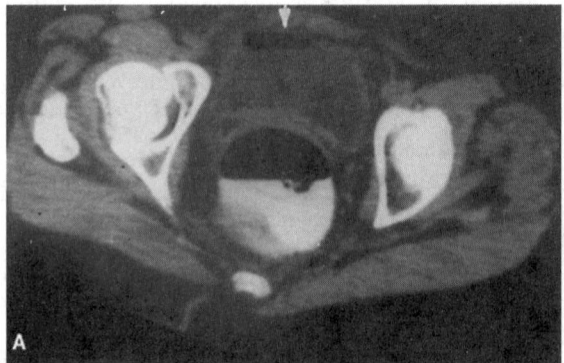 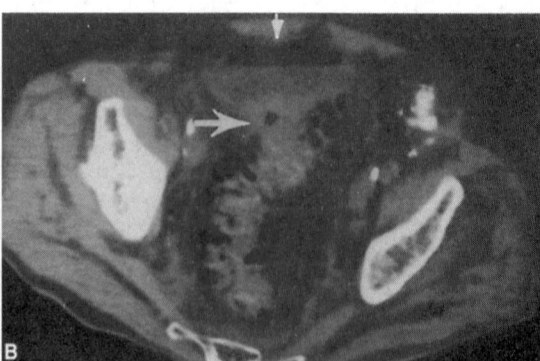

Figure 49-3. (*A*) CT scan demonstrating air in the urinary bladder (*arrow*) in the presence of a colovesical fistula secondary to diverticulitis. (*B*) Air in the urinary bladder (*small arrow*) in association with a paravesical inflammatory mass (*large arrow*). (Sarr MG, Fishman EK, Goldman SM. Enterovesical fistula. Surg Gynecol Obstet 1987;164:2)

one-stage segmental colectomy and closure of the fistula opening in the bladder. The proximal margin of resection includes the entire segment of thickened, contracted colon and any additional colon involved in the acute inflammation. Although it is not necessary to resect all colon involved with diverticulosis, the resection must include enough colon to allow an anastomosis free of diverticula. The distal resection margin is the proximal rectum.

If the fistula opening is not demonstrable, ie, it is very small, the bladder fistula does not have to be identified. Urinary catheter drainage followed by cystographic verification of fistula closure is sufficient therapy.

If the complications of diverticulitis—obstruction, inflammation, abscess, sepsis, or other fistulas—are severe, a two-stage procedure may be necessary. The first stage is segmental colectomy and colostomy formation; the second is closure of the colostomy.

Colovaginal Fistulas

Almost all patients with colovaginal fistulas have undergone a hysterectomy. The only consistent symptom is a feculent vaginal discharge. Some patients have intermittent abdominal pain and distention. A mass may be felt at pelvic examination. At vaginal examination with a speculum, the fistula opening is visible in most patients. The diagnosis may be confirmed with a barium enema radiographic examination.

Unless other complications of diverticulitis are present, a one-stage procedure is performed. The involved colon is resected, and a primary anastomosis is performed. The vaginal defect can be closed, but such defects usually close spontaneously if left open.

Coloenteric Fistulas

Symptoms of diverticular coloenteric fistulas are diarrhea and abdominal pain. The usual signs are abdominal tenderness, abdominal distention, and pelvic mass. Barium enema is diagnostic in most patients.

The preferred surgical management of uncomplicated coloenteric fistula is en bloc resection of the involved segment of small intestine, the fistula, and the diseased segment of colon. Primary anastomoses of both the small intestine and colon are performed. If there are complications, such as other fistulas, intraabdominal abscess, or inadequate intestinal preparation because of obstruction, primary anastomosis of the small intestine, combined with colostomy formation, is performed as the first stage of a two-stage procedure.

DIVERTICULITIS OF THE CECUM AND ASCENDING COLON

When diverticulitis develops in patients with right-sided diverticula, the symptom complex is similar to that of acute appendicitis, and misdiagnosis is frequent. Patients with right-sided diverticulitis are younger (40 to 50 years of age) than patients with left-sided disease and older than most patients with appendicitis. Patients with right-sided diverticulitis have a longer duration of illness than patients with appendicitis, infrequently vomit, and feel pain first in the right lower quadrant rather than the middle abdomen.

CT findings are thickening of the colonic wall, extraluminal mass involving the cecum or ascending colon, and signs of pericolic inflammation. CT is performed in patients with atypical appendicitis who are older than the usual patient with appendicitis and in whom right-sided diverticulitis is being considered as a diagnosis.

At operation, it may be difficult to establish a diagnosis of diverticulitis of the cecum or ascending colon. The presence of an intact, normal appendix eliminates appendicitis as the diagnosis. A large inflammatory mass usually is present that involves the cecum and ascending colon. It often is difficult to differentiate the mass from perforated carcinoma. Right hemicolectomy is performed. If the resection can be performed without contamination of the peritoneal cavity, and mechanical intestinal preparation is complete, a primary anastomosis is performed. If abscess contents have spilled or intestinal preparation was not feasible, an end ileostomy with mucous fistula may be performed.

If the only abnormality identified at laparotomy is an inflamed diverticulum, the diverticulum can be left in situ and treated with broad-spectrum antibiotics. An appendectomy is performed to avoid confusion if right lower quadrant symptoms recur. Most patients treated in this manner do not have recurrent diverticulitis.

If the diagnosis of right-sided diverticulitis is made before an operation, the patient is treated as having sigmoid diverticulitis. If improvement occurs with administration of IV fluids, broad-spectrum antibiotics, bowel rest, and analgesics, therapy is continued and additional testing is performed when the patient has recovered. If the patient's condition does not improve or deteriorates, laparotomy is performed.

SUGGESTED READING

Graham SM, Ballantyne GH. Cecal diverticulitis: a review of the American experience. Dis Colon Rectum 1987;30:821.

Labs JD, Sarr MG, Fishman EK, et al. Complications of acute diverticulitis of the colon: improved early diagnosis with computerized tomography. Am J Surg 1988;155:331.

Mendeloff AI. Thoughts on the epidemiology of diverticular disease. Clin Gastroenterol 1986;15:855.

Stabile BE, Puccio E, van Sonnenberg E, Neff CC. Preoperative percutaneous drainage of diverticular abscesses. Am J Surg 1990;159:99.

Welch CE, Athanasoulis CA, Galdabini JJ. Hemorrhage from the large bowel with special reference to angiodysplasia and diverticular disease. World J Surg 1978;2:73.

Woods RJ, Lavery IC, Fazio VW, et al. Internal fistulas in diverticular disease. Dis Colon Rectum 1988;31:591.

ESSENTIALS OF SURGERY: SCIENTIFIC PRINCIPLES AND PRACTICE, edited by Lazar J. Greenfield, Michael W. Mulholland, Keith T. Oldham, Gerald B. Zelenock, and Keith D. Lillemoe. Lippincott–Raven Publishers, Philadelphia, © 1997.

CHAPTER 50

ACUTE GASTROINTESTINAL HEMORRHAGE

RICHARD H. TURNAGE

The initial management of acute hemorrhage in the gastrointestinal (GI) tract is the same regardless of the cause of hemorrhage. Localization of the site of hemorrhage in relation to the ligament of Treitz (upper or lower GI tract) directs evaluation and therapy. Hemorrhage from the esophagus, stomach, and duodenum accounts for most GI hemorrhage, nearly all of the remainder coming from the colon. The causes of upper and lower GI hemorrhage are listed in Tables 50-1 and 50-2.

CLINICAL PRESENTATION

Hematemesis, the vomiting of blood, indicates hemorrhage proximal to the ligament of Treitz. Aspiration of blood or "coffee grounds" from a nasogastric (NG) tube also suggests an upper GI source. *Melena,* the passage of black tarry stools, is usually associated with an upper GI source of hemorrhage, but lower GI sources also may be associated with melena, particularly small-intestinal and right-colonic lesions. Melena is produced by the breakdown of blood by enteric bacteria. *Hematochezia,* the passage of bright red blood through the rectum, is associated with colonic lesions. Upper GI sources may produce hematochezia in the presence of massive hemorrhage. The *history* may suggest the cause of hemorrhage. Hemorrhage after several days of worsening epigastric or upper abdominal pain suggests peptic ulcer disease. Hematemesis or melena after vomiting or retching suggests Mallory-Weiss tear. Massive, painless upper GI hemorrhage in a patient with cirrhosis suggests variceal hemorrhage. Massive, painless lower GI hemorrhage in an elderly patient suggests bleeding from colonic diverticula.

The presence of cardiac, pulmonary, and renal disease influences outcome. Medication use is reviewed, especially use of nonsteroidal anti-inflammatory agents (NSAIDs), aspirin, corticosteroids, and anticoagulants.

A systematic *physical examination* documents the magnitude of hemorrhage and the patient's ability to compensate. Massive hemorrhage causes shock (cool, clammy, mottled skin, tachycardia, tachypnea, flat jugular veins, oliguria, and perhaps hypotension). Physical examination documents evidence of cirrhosis and portal hypertension (ascites, spider angiomas, hepatosplenomegaly, palmar erythema, and large hemorrhoidal veins). A rectal examination can reveal the presence of bright red blood or melena.

INITIAL EVALUATION AND RESUSCITATION

As soon as a patient presents with GI hemorrhage:

1. Two large-bore intravenous (IV) lines are placed in peripheral veins, and intravascular volume resuscitation is begun with isotonic saline or lactated Ringer solution. Most patients stop bleeding spontaneously,

Table 50-1. DIFFERENTIAL DIAGNOSIS OF ACUTE UPPER GASTROINTESTINAL HEMORRHAGE

Peptic ulcer disease
   Duodenal ulcer
   Gastric ulcer
Acute gastritis
   Stress gastritis
   Alcoholic gastritis
   Drug-induced gastritis
Gastroesophageal varices
Mallory-Weiss tear
Dieulafoy disease
Esophageal, gastric, or duodenal tumors
Aortoduodenal fistula
Esophagitis
Angiodysplasia
Hemobilia
Pancreatitis-induced pseudoaneurysm

Table 50-2. DIFFERENTIAL DIAGNOSIS OF ACUTE LOWER GASTROINTESTINAL HEMORRHAGE

Colonic diverticular disease
Colonic vascular ectasias
Small intestinal diverticular disease
   Meckel's diverticulum
   Pseudodiverticula
Inflammatory bowel disease
   Chronic ulcerative colitis
   Crohn's disease
Colonic neoplasms
Small intestinal neoplasms
Angiodysplasia
Aortoenteric fistula
Colitis
   Infectious
   Ischemic
   Radiation-induced
Internal hemorrhoidal disease

and crystalloid volume resuscitation is all that is required. Massive bleeding necessitates administration of packed red blood cells (RBCs) to restore intravascular volume and oxygen-carrying capacity. The decision to transfuse blood or blood products depends on the needs of the patient and the disease encountered. For example, esophageal varices are likely to continue to hemorrhage, so transfusion is used early in treatment.

2. Blood is drawn for type and crossmatch, complete blood and platelet count, electrolyte levels, liver function tests, and coagulation profiles. At presentation, hematocrit and hemoglobin level do not reflect the magnitude of acute blood loss.

3. An NG tube is placed and the presence of gastric blood determined. Absence of blood in bilious gastric fluid suggests a lower intestinal source. If no bilious fluid is obtained, esophagogastroduodenoscopy is necessary to exclude a duodenal source of hemorrhage. If hemorrhage has been profuse, gastric lavage is used to clear the stomach of clot to facilitate endoscopy. Many patients stop bleeding before or during resuscitation and cleansing of retained blood from the stomach.

4. Hemodynamic monitoring is initiated. Patients who are actively bleeding or who have had recent profuse hemorrhage are admitted to an intensive care unit (ICU) for monitoring of hemodynamic values and signs of continued or recurring hemorrhage. The presence of cardiac, renal, hepatic, or pulmonary insufficiency necessitates invasive cardiac monitoring. A urinary catheter is inserted. Heart rate, blood pressure, gastric aspirate, and mentation are monitored.

DIAGNOSTIC PROCEDURES

Algorithms for the evaluation of acute upper and lower GI hemorrhage are presented in Figures 50-1 and 50-2.

Endoscopy

Esophagogastroscopy

The timing of endoscopy is crucial. Few lesions examined >24 hr after hemorrhage show endoscopic signs of active or recent bleeding. Endoscopy is performed on a hemodynamically stable patient after volume resuscita-

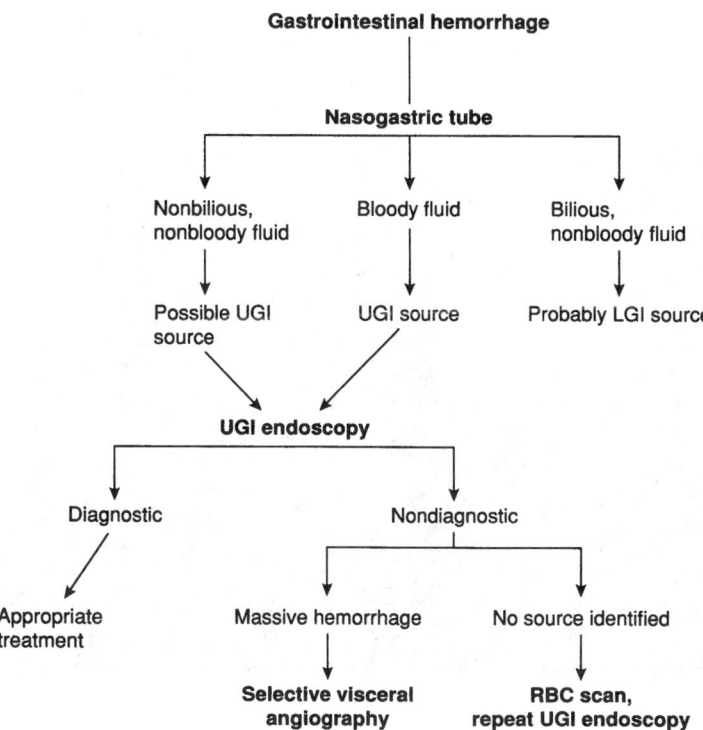

Figure 50-1. Diagnostic steps in the evaluation of acute upper gastrointestinal hemorrhage.

tion. Factors that limit the diagnostic efficacy of endoscopy in actively bleeding patients are impaired visibility, abnormal anatomy, and lesions that simulate ulcers. Complications of emergency or urgent esophagogastroduodenoscopy in an actively or recently bleeding patient include aspiration, recurrent or increased hemorrhage, respiratory depression from sedatives, and perforation of the esophagus, stomach, or duodenum.

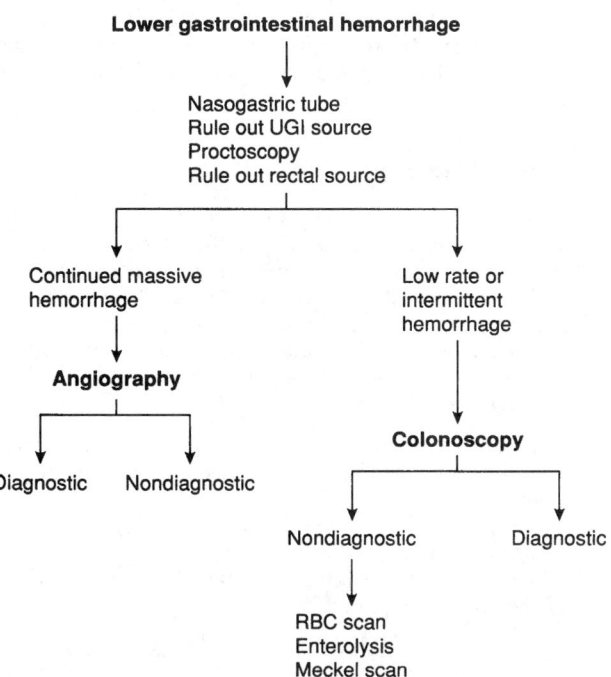

Figure 50-2. Diagnostic steps in the evaluation of acute lower gastrointestinal hemorrhage.

Colonoscopy

Colonoscopy and selective visceral angiography are the most useful diagnostic studies for determining the cause of lower GI hemorrhage. Colonoscopy is performed immediately after the patient is resuscitated and stabilized. It is best if the patient is minimally bleeding at the time of the procedure. Colonic lavage with polyethylene glycol solution clears the lumen of clot and stool, allowing visualization of the mucosa.

Intraoperative Enteroscopy

Intraoperative endoscopy is performed in the rare situation in which there is no clear definition of the site of bleeding before laparotomy. The procedure may allow localization of the site of hemorrhage, limiting extent of resection. Transillumination of the intestine during intraoperative enteroscopy may show angiodysplastic lesions, and insufflation of the intestine may aid in demonstration of small-intestinal diverticula.

Selective Visceral Angiography

In massively bleeding patients, endoscopic visualization is often limited, and selective mesenteric arteriography is often useful for depicting the site of bleeding (Fig. 50-3). Angiographic identification of the source of hemorrhage depends on the presence of active arterial bleeding at the time of the examination. Extravasation of contrast material occurs if the patient is bleeding at rates >0.5 mL/min. Patients are likely to be bleeding at this rate if they need continuous volume infusion to maintain hemodynamic stability.

Radionuclide Scans

Abdominal scintigraphy after injection of radiolabeled erythrocytes is used to localize intermittent bleeding or lesions with slow rates of hemorrhage. This modality can

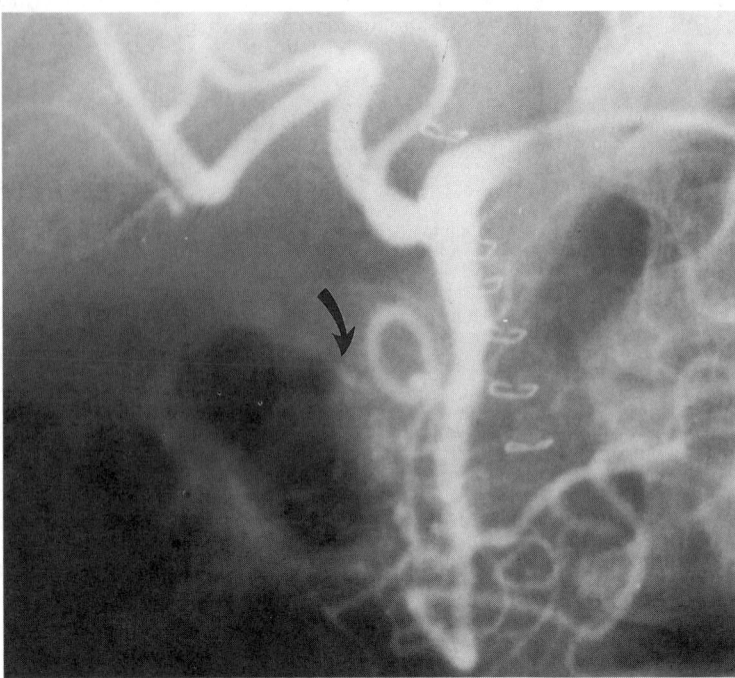

Figure 50-3. Selective celiac arteriography with injection into the common hepatic artery in a patient bleeding from a duodenal diverticulum. Extravasation of contrast from a branch of the gastroduodenal artery can be seen (*arrow*).

be particularly valuable in the evaluation of intermittent lower GI hemorrhage in patients in whom endoscopic findings are inconclusive.

PEPTIC ULCER DISEASE

Peptic ulcer disease is the most common cause of acute upper GI hemorrhage. Hemorrhage is the principal cause of death of peptic ulcer disease and is the most frequent indication for surgical treatment. Complications of peptic ulcer disease are common among older patients, who often have other medical problems.

Duodenal ulcers occur slightly more frequently than gastric ulcers. Penetration of the ulcer through the posterior wall of the duodenal bulb is associated with erosion into the gastroduodenal artery or one of its branches, resulting in brisk hemorrhage. Patients may present with hematemesis of bright red blood and clots or with melena alone. Most patients stop bleeding spontaneously during the initial stages of treatment with volume resuscitation and gastric lavage.

Patients with *gastric ulcers* generally are older than patients with duodenal ulcers and have medical problems that increase morbidity and mortality. Bleeding may occur from any site in the stomach, although ulcers at the incisura are most common. At this site, involvement of the branches of the left gastric artery may result in brisk, if not torrential, hemorrhage.

The clinical presentation of bleeding from gastric ulcers is hematemesis, melena, and hematochezia. Hemorrhage complicating a gastric ulcer is (1) not likely to subside spontaneously, (2) likely to rebleed after endoscopic hemostasis, and (3) likely to necessitate surgical intervention.

An important risk factor for the development of GI hemorrhage and gastroduodenal ulcer formation is the use of NSAIDs. The stomach appears to be more susceptible to injury than the duodenum. NSAID use is associated with a continuum of mucosal injury that ranges from small acute mucosal hemorrhages to large chronic ulcers.

Initial Management

Attentive monitoring and aggressive resuscitation are the first steps in the management of bleeding from peptic ulcer disease. When bleeding stops spontaneously, therapy is initiated, usually with cimetidine or ranitidine.

Endoscopic Therapy

Patients who continue to bleed or who have endoscopic findings that suggest recurrent or continued hemorrhage undergo endoscopic therapy to arrest hemorrhage from bleeding ulcers. Endoscopic techniques stop hemorrhage by inducing coagulation necrosis of the bleeding vessel and surrounding tissue by use of thermal or laser energy or induction of thrombosis or sclerosis of the bleeding vessels.

Surgical Therapy

Open surgical procedures are performed when endoscopy is unsuccessful in arresting hemorrhage. Patients older than 60 years and those with concurrent medical problems undergo surgical intervention early in the course of hemorrhage. These patients do not tolerate continued hemorrhage, recurrent hypotension, or repeated transfusions. Indications for surgical management of bleeding peptic ulcers are:

- Massive hemorrhage unresponsive to resuscitation
- Continued bleeding unresponsive to nonsurgical measures
- Recurrent hemorrhage after pharmacologic or endoscopic control
- Two or more hospitalizations for ulcer hemorrhage
- Coexisting indication for operation

The type of operation depends on the pathologic condition encountered. For bleeding *gastric* ulcers, gastric resection that includes the ulcer is performed, with or without vagotomy, depending on ulcer type. For bleeding *duode-*

nal ulcers, truncal vagotomy, pyloroplasty, and oversewing of the bleeding vessel is the most common operation (Fig. 50-4).

STRESS GASTRITIS

Acute erosion of the gastric mucosa is a common phenomenon among critically ill patients. Stress gastritis is characterized by the appearance of multiple superficial gastric ulcerations within 12 to 14 hours of an acute injury. These lesions, initially localized to the fundus and body of the stomach, later involve the entire gastric surface. Patients at risk include those with sepsis, severe burns, severe trauma, or respiratory, hepatic, or renal insufficiency. Stress gastritis represents the gastric component of multiple-system organ failure. Overt bleeding is often heralded by the appearance of flecks of blood in the gastric aspirate. Hemorrhage is the only symptom of stress gastritis. The superficial nature of the lesions makes perforation unlikely.

Prophylaxis

Prophylaxis of stress gastritis involves prevention of hemorrhage by neutralizing gastric acid, augmenting mucosal defenses, and removing or preventing physiologic stress. Alkalinization of the gastric contents is associated with colonization of the stomach by oral and fecal flora and may increase risk for respiratory complications.

Management

Critically ill patients with overt hemorrhage need blood replacement, intravascular volume restoration, and correction of coagulation defects. Underlying sepsis must be

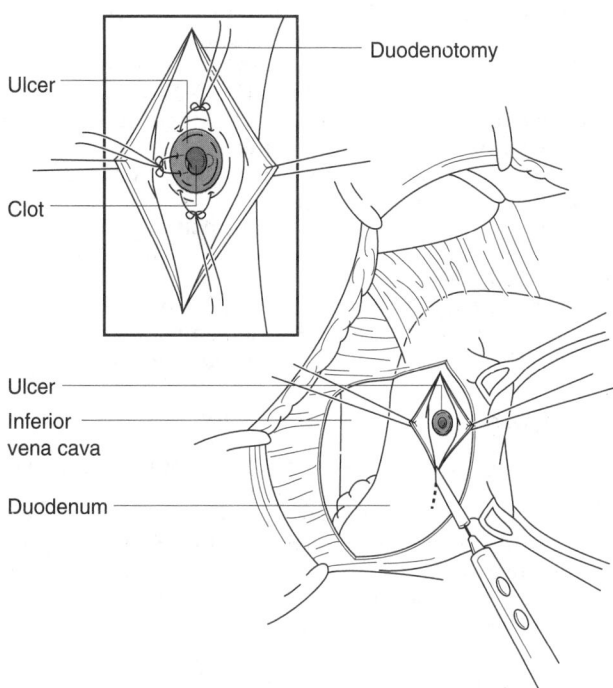

Figure 50-4. Diagram demonstrating the site of hemorrhage and method of ligation used for ulcers penetrating the posterior wall of the duodenal bulb. At this location, ulcers commonly erode into the gastroduodenal artery at the takeoff of the transverse pancreatic artery. Three-point ligation of these vessels (U-stitching) is important to prevent recurrent hemorrhage from the transverse pancreatic artery.

sought and treated. Basic principles of resuscitation and gastric lavage with saline solution usually stop hemorrhage. As soon as resuscitation is complete, endoscopy is performed to determine the cause of the hemorrhage. Antacids or H₂-receptor antagonists can be used for first-line management of hemorrhage due to stress gastritis.

Selective catheterization of the left gastric artery with continuous infusion of vasopressin can be used to arrest hemorrhage in patients not responding to more-conservative methods. Transcatheter arterial embolization may be of greatest benefit to patients at high surgical risk when other treatments have failed and a single bleeding site can be identified.

Surgical Therapy

Only a small number of patients bleeding from erosive gastritis need surgical intervention to arrest hemorrhage. Surgical options include vagotomy and pyloroplasty with oversewing of bleeding sites, vagotomy and hemigastrectomy, total gastrectomy, and gastric devascularization.

GASTROESOPHAGEAL VARICES

Cirrhosis is a leading cause of death, and variceal hemorrhage is the common mode. Patients with bleeding gastroesophageal varices have high rebleeding rates, transfusion requirements, lengths of hospitalization, and risk for death.

Initial Management

Although the basic tenets of resuscitation for massive variceal hemorrhage are similar to those for any source of massive hemorrhage, IV volume resuscitation must be performed with fluids that have minimal sodium. Accurate blood replacement is imperative because overtransfusion increases central venous pressure and worsens portal hypertension, exacerbating hemorrhage. Invasive cardiac monitoring with Swan-Ganz catheterization may be used to guide volume replacement. Coagulation deficits are corrected with administration of fresh frozen plasma. Thrombocytopenia due to hypersplenism or dilution is managed with pooled platelet transfusions. Sedatives are avoided or used sparingly because cirrhosis impairs the ability of the liver to metabolize these drugs. Prophylaxis of delirium tremens is administered.

Endoscopy

Early endoscopy is imperative for bleeding from esophageal varices (Fig. 50-5). Identification of varices alone is not adequate to incriminate them as the source of the hemorrhage. Half of patients with cirrhosis bleed from a source other than varices. Endoscopy may help identify factors associated with heightened risk for variceal hemorrhage. These include the size and number of varices and the presence of red, blue, or other colored spots on the varix. The presence of gastric and duodenal varices and portal hypertensive changes in the gastric mucosa (portal gastropathy) can influence therapy and prognosis.

Vasopressin

Vasopressin is used early in the management of variceal hemorrhage. Infusion is continued for 48 to 72 hours or until bleeding stops, at which time the agent is tapered. If bleeding continues, other treatments are used (sclerotherapy or balloon tamponade).

The risks of vasopressin use are related to cardiovascular

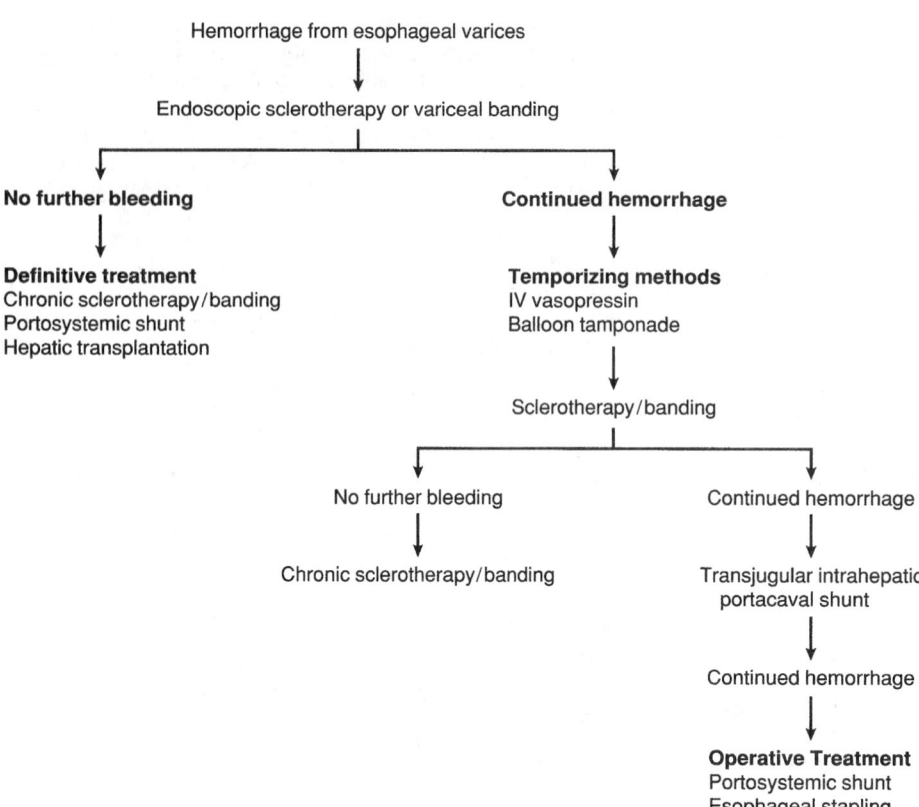

Figure 50-5. Therapeutic maneuvers in the management of acute hemorrhage from esophageal varices.

effects, especially systemic vasoconstriction. Simultaneous administration of nitroglycerin ameliorates many of the adverse hemodynamic effects of vasopressin and may enhance the effectiveness of vasopressin in controlling variceal bleeding. Vasopressin therapy alone is inadequate to manage bleeding esophageal varices, but this treatment may provide initial control of hemorrhage, reduce transfusion requirements, and provide time for resuscitation before definitive treatment.

Balloon Tamponade

Another temporizing method used for massive bleeding is balloon tamponade, utilizing a gastric tube with esophageal and gastric balloons. Pressure from inflation of the balloons tamponades bleeding varices. When the balloons are deflated, however, hemorrhage recurs. The greatest value of the tubes is arresting massive hemorrhage that does not respond to other measures, allowing time for resuscitation before definitive treatment.

The most frequent complication of balloon tamponade is aspiration pneumonitis. Measures to prevent pulmonary complications include endotracheal intubation before tube insertion and placement of an esophageal tube to remove swallowed salivary secretions. Other complications include esophageal rupture or necrosis and airway occlusion due to pharyngeal migration of the balloon.

Sclerotherapy or Banding of Varices

A patient bleeding from esophageal varices undergoes urgent sclerotherapy or banding of varices at the first emergency endoscopy. Sclerotherapy arrests acute variceal hemorrhage in almost all patients. Patients who have stopped bleeding undergo immediate sclerotherapy be-

cause of risk for recurrent hemorrhage. Continued or recurrent hemorrhage after sclerotherapy necessitates temporary control with balloon tamponade and vasopressin followed by urgent surgical intervention.

After control of the initial hemorrhage, sclerotherapy is repeated in 5 to 10 days and then at 1 to 3 weeks intervals until the varices are obliterated. This takes three to five sclerotherapy sessions. During this period, before complete variceal obliteration, risk for recurrent bleeding is highest.

Complications of sclerotherapy include perforation, stricture formation, and ulceration. Systemic complications include fever and sepsis.

Another method of endoscopic control of variceal hemorrhage involves mechanical ligation and strangulation of variceal channels with small, elastic O rings.

Shunting

Nonsurgical decompression of the portal venous system can be accomplished with transjugular intrahepatic portosystemic shunting (TIPS). The procedure involves establishment of a percutaneous channel between a hepatic vein and the portal vein. Expandable metallic stents are used to maintain shunt patency. Complications are shunt occlusion and stenosis.

MALLORY–WEISS TEARS

Mallory–Weiss syndrome is acute upper GI hemorrhage after retching or vomiting. The mechanism of injury is laceration of the gastric cardia. Vomiting raises intragastric pressure to levels capable of mucosal damage. At first the vomitus is gastric content without blood, then hematemesis and melena develop.

Management

Initial management of Mallory–Weiss syndrome entails volume resuscitation, gastric lavage, and gastric decompression. Most patients with Mallory–Weiss tears stop bleeding spontaneously before treatment or after these early measures. Once bleeding has stopped, rebleeding is rare.

Patients who continue to bleed despite the initial maneuvers undergo nonsurgical or surgical therapy. Nonsurgical management consists of endoscopic electrocoagulation or injection therapy. Surgical therapy entails oversewing the laceration through a longitudinal gastrotomy in the middle-third of the stomach.

LOWER GASTROINTESTINAL HEMORRHAGE

Passage of maroon or bright red blood through the rectum suggests a source of hemorrhage distal to the ligament of Treitz. Although numerous potential causes of lower GI hemorrhage are possible (Table 50-2), colonic diverticulosis and vascular ectasia of the colon are the most common. Small-intestinal sources and other colonic abnormalities are unusual causes of acute GI hemorrhage.

Diagnosis

The first step in the diagnosis of lower GI hemorrhage is *gastric aspiration* or *esophagogastroduodenoscopy* to rule out an upper GI source. Anoscopy and flexible or rigid sigmoidoscopy exclude sources of hemorrhage below the peritoneal reflection of the rectum, such as bleeding internal hemorrhoids.

The frequent presence of asymptomatic colonic diverticulosis and vascular ectasia in the elderly make precise determination of the site of hemorrhage imperative. Colonoscopy and selective visceral angiography are used to determine the site of lower GI hemorrhage. The examinations are performed immediately after resuscitation and stabilization. *Colonoscopy* is of greatest value if the patient has stopped bleeding or is bleeding at a slow rate. *Selective visceral angiography* is most valuable if the patient is actively bleeding at a rate that requires IV fluid and blood infusion to maintain hemodynamic stability. *Abdominal scintigraphy* after infusion of ^{99m}Tc-labeled RBCs may delineate the site of hemorrhage in patients with intermittent bleeding or bleeding at rates less than those detectable with angiography.

Preoperative localization of the site of hemorrhage is imperative; only rarely should laparotomy be performed without knowledge of the site of hemorrhage. For some patients, *intraoperative enteroscopy* may be of value in defining the site of hemorrhage.

Colonic Diverticulosis

The prevalence of colonic diverticula increases with age. About half of people in their eighties are affected. Hemorrhage from diverticular disease is massive and is associated with hematochezia and hemorrhagic shock. Patients present with sudden, mild lower abdominal discomfort, rectal urgency, and subsequent passage of a large maroon or melenic stool. Because the colon can contain large volumes of blood, neither the volume nor the frequency of bloody stools is a reliable guide to the rate of hemorrhage. Despite the massive nature of hemorrhage, most patients with diverticular disease stop bleeding spontaneously.

Bleeding associated with diverticular disease comes from a perforated vasa recta at the neck or apex of a diver-

ticulum. The vasa recta penetrates the colonic wall from the serosa to the submucosa through obliquely oriented connective tissue septa. Protrusion of colonic mucosa through this connective tissue plane results in apposition of the diverticulum and the vasa recta. Rupture of the arterial wall produces hemorrhage into the lumen of the intestine.

Diagnosis

The massive hemorrhage associated with diverticular disease limits the usefulness of colonoscopy. Rarely is there a bleeding vessel in a diverticulum, so the presence of blood or clot within diverticula is of no diagnostic benefit. *Selective mesenteric arteriography* may show luminal extravasation of contrast material. Inability to visualize a bleeding point is usually due to cessation of active bleeding.

Management

If bleeding from colonic diverticula stops, the patient is treated expectantly because there is low risk for recurrence. Patients who continue to bleed need surgical treatment. The elderly nature of patients with diverticular hemorrhage necessitates prompt volume replacement.

Nonsurgical methods of arresting lower GI hemorrhage include embolization and endoscopic electrocoagulation. The end artery location of the vasa recta with limited collateral flow limits the usefulness of angiographic embolization. The rapid nature of the hemorrhage and difficulty defining the site of hemorrhage through an endoscope prevent endoscopic treatments from being beneficial for bleeding diverticula.

Surgical Therapy

Patients who continue to bleed from diverticula undergo resection of the colonic segment that contains the site of hemorrhage. If the bleeding diverticulum is in the right colon, right colectomy with ileotransverse colostomy is performed. If the patient continues to bleed massively from the colon and all attempts at preoperative and intraoperative localization are unsuccessful, subtotal colectomy with ileoproctostomy may be required.

Colonic Vascular Ectasia

Vascular ectasias appear to be caused by age-related degeneration of previously normal intestinal submucosal veins and overlying mucosal capillaries. The lesions usually occur in the cecum and ascending colon, but they may be present in the transverse and left colon or rectum. Most patients have multiple lesions.

Vascular ectasias present with hematochezia, melena, occult blood loss, or iron deficiency anemia, depending on the stage of the vascular malformation. Early lesions, characterized by ectatic capillaries and venules, present with low-grade recurrent bleeding and episodic hematochezia or melena. Most early lesions stop bleeding spontaneously and are rarely associated with life-threatening hemorrhage. Advanced lesions, characterized as arteriovenous communications, present with massive hemorrhage and hematochezia that may progress to hemorrhagic shock and death.

Diagnosis

Vascular ectasias may be diagnosed by means of colonoscopy or selective mesenteric angiography. *Colonoscopy* demonstrates most vascular ectasias. The lesions appear as flat or slightly raised red lesions 2 to 10 mm wide. They may be round, stellate, or have sharply circumscribed fern-like margins. A prominent feeding vessel and a surrounding halo may be evident. Colonoscopic diagnosis in actively bleeding patients may be confounded by the presence incidental lesions, including traumatic and suction artifacts produced during the examination. *Selective mesenteric angiography* may depict vascular ectasias and complement colonoscopy, particularly for patients with massive bleeding or for whom colonoscopy is unrevealing or incomplete. Angiographic findings include:

- A densely opacified, slowly emptying, dilated, tortuous vein
- A vascular tuft—cluster of vessels that empties slowly with opacification persisting into the venous phase
- An early-filling vein, usually a segmental vein in the cecum or right colon

Management

Patients bleeding from colonic vascular ectasias can be treated with endoscopic procedures, such as monopolar electrocoagulation, endoscopic injection sclerotherapy, and use of contact probes and lasers. When endoscopic hemostatic methods are unsuccessful the patient can be treated with resection of the colon *after preoperative localization of the bleeding site.*

UNUSUAL CAUSES OF ACUTE GASTROINTESTINAL HEMORRHAGE

The following rare conditions may be the cause of acute GI hemorrhage when the usual causes are excluded:

- Dieulafoy vascular malformation
- Angiodysplasia of the stomach and intestine
- Aortoenteric fistula
- Meckel diverticulum
- Small-intestinal diverticulum
- Inflammatory bowel disease

SUGGESTED READING

Cook DJ, Fuller HD, Guyatt GH, et al. Risk factors for GI bleeding in critically ill patients. N Engl J Med 1994;330:377.

Foutch PG. Angiodysplasia of the GI tract. Am J Gastroenterol 1993;88:807.

LaBerge JM, Ring EJ, Gordon RL, et al. Creation of transjugular intrahepatic portosystemic shunts with the wallstent endoprosthesis: results in 100 patients. Radiology 1993;187:413.

Laine L, El-Newihi HM, Migikovsky B, Sloane R, Carcia F. Endoscopic ligation compared with sclerotherapy for the treatment of bleeding esophageal varices. Ann Intern Med 1993:119:1.

Nagy SW, Marshall JB. Aortoenteric fistulas. Postgrad Med 1993;93:211.

Sacks HS, Chalmers TC, Blum AL, Berrier J, Pagano D. Endoscopic hemostasis: an effective therapy for bleeding peptic ulcers. JAMA 1990;264:494.

Stiegmann GV, Goff JS, Michaletz-Onody PA, et al. Endoscopic sclerotherapy as compared with endoscopic ligation for bleeding esophageal varices. N Engl J Med 1992;326:1527.

Sugawa C, Steffes CP, Nakamura R, et al. Upper GI bleeding in an urban hospital: etiology, recurrence and prognosis. Ann Surg 1990;212:521.

ESSENTIALS OF SURGERY: SCIENTIFIC PRINCIPLES AND PRACTICE, edited by Lazar J. Greenfield, Michael W. Mulholland, Keith T. Oldham, Gerald B. Zelenock, and Keith D. Lillemoe. Lippincott–Raven Publishers, Philadelphia, © 1997.

CHAPTER 51
ANTIBIOTIC-ASSOCIATED COLITIS

F. ROBERT FEKETY

Mild diarrhea is a common side effect of antibiotic therapy. It usually is more a nuisance than a serious problem. Most cases of diarrhea are of unknown causation but are thought to be related to alterations in the ecology of the fecal flora. Diarrhea usually resolves soon after antibiotics are stopped. About 10% to 20% of instances of antibiotic-associated diarrhea, however, are complicated by bacterial toxin-induced colitis. The inflamed colonic mucosa is covered with an adherent nodular exudate (pseudomembrane), which consists of dead leukocytes, mucosal epithelial cells, mucus, and fibrin. Pseudomembranous colitis (PMC) should be suspected in any patient in whom diarrhea develops within 6 weeks after antibiotic therapy, especially if treatment was administered in a hospital. The disease is serious but treatable.

Toxin-producing strains of *Clostridium difficile,* a component of the normal fecal flora, are the cause of almost all cases of antibiotic-associated colitis, but rare cases are attributed to toxigenic *Staphylococcus aureus, Salmonella* sp, *Clostridium perfringens* type C, *Plesiomonas shigelloides, Yersinia enterocolitica, Shigella* sp, *Campylobacter* sp, and *Aeromonas* sp, cytomegalovirus, *Entamoeba histolytica,* and *Listeria monocytogenes.* Pseudomembranes are only rarely detected in association with these organisms. The human immunodeficiency virus (HIV) causes intestinal inflammation that may be confused with *C difficile* colitis when it occurs in patients with AIDS who take antimicrobial agents.

When *C difficile* colitis develops in people with chronic inflammatory bowel diseases, such as Crohn's colitis or chronic idiopathic ulcerative colitis, it may be mistaken for an acute exacerbation of the chronic disease.

PATHOLOGY

The key feature of antibiotic-associated colitis is acute polymorphonuclear inflammation of the colonic mucosa and submucosa. Pseudomembranes may be absent in some patients with colitis, and pseudomembranous plaques may be dislodged during processing of biopsy specimens. The inflammation usually affects only the epithelium and lamina propria, but necrosis and involvement of deeper tissues may occur, and secondary infection may develop. Extensive transmural necrosis may cause toxic dilatation of the colon, perforation, or peritonitis.

The lesions of antibiotic-associated colitis are found throughout the colon, but they are most prominent in the rectosigmoid. In some patients, lesions may be restricted to the cecum or transverse colon. These patients may have little or no diarrhea but have abdominal pain, fever, and leukocytosis. The ileum is rarely involved in *C difficile* colitis, but it is often involved in staphylococcal enterocolitis. *C difficile* diarrhea occurs at all ages but is most common in elderly adults. It also is common in debilitated patients.

PATHOGENESIS AND PREVENTION

C difficile is a spore-forming, gram-positive, obligate anaerobic bacillus present in the normal intestinal flora of 3% to 5% of healthy adults. The organism is ubiquitous in soil and water. Use of antibiotics promotes acquisition and carriage by humans. Transmission usually occurs in hospitals and nursing homes.

C difficile does not produce colitis by invasion of tissues. Colitis results from toxin production in the intestinal lumen and binding of these toxins to the mucosa. The toxins, enterotoxin A and cytotoxin B, attack mucosal cell membranes and microfilaments, causing depolymerization of actin, cytoplasmic contraction, hemorrhage, necrosis of epithelial cells, inflammation, chemoattraction of neutrophils, increased capillary permeability, and loss of protein and fluid into the intestinal lumen. Toxin B interferes with mucosal integrity and protein synthesis. Isolates that produce one toxin produce the other toxin but not to the same degree, which may account for variation in the severity of illness.

The following people are at high risk for PMC after antibiotic therapy:

- Elderly patients
- Patients with cancer, leukemia, uremia, burns, or colonic stasis
- Patients undergoing abdominal operations or cesarean section
- Patients in intensive care units

Antibiotics given for even short periods, as for prophylaxis or treatment of minor infections, may precipitate PMC. The disease may follow oral, intramuscular, IV, or topical administration of antibiotics. The most frequent inciting antimicrobial agents are penicillins and cephalosporins, but almost any antimicrobial agent used to treat infection can cause the disease. The consequence of administration of antimicrobial agents is alteration of an unknown nature in the normal colonic flora that allows *C difficile* to proliferate and produce large amounts of toxin in the intestinal lumen. PMC may not begin until after antibiotics are discontinued, especially if the *C difficile* isolate is susceptible to the antimicrobial agent administered or if the organism is acquired after antibiotics are discontinued.

PMC occurs with unusually high frequency in many hospitals. The organism is transmitted on the hands of personnel after contact with patients who carry the organism or by means of contact with contaminated surfaces. Hospital roommates of carriers are at high risk for colonization with the organism. Perioperative use of prophylactic antibiotics has decreased the frequency of postoperative wound infections, but it has increased the likelihood of antibiotic-associated colitis. Table 51-1 lists measures helpful in the prevention of *C difficile* colitis.

CLINICAL MANIFESTATIONS

Patients with antibiotic-associated colitis usually have watery, mucoid, green, foul-smelling stools; severe, cramping abdominal pain and tenderness; unexplained fever; and leukocytosis. High fever, a high peripheral leukocyte count, dehydration, electrolyte imbalance, and hypoalbuminemia are common with PMC, and indicate colitis rather than benign or simple diarrhea. The symptoms usually begin 3 to 9 days after the patient starts taking antibiotics, but the pattern varies. Some cases of PMC are recognized 1 to 2 days after the start of antibiotic therapy. In some patients, diarrhea does not begin until as long as 6 weeks after antibiotics are discontinued. The stools often

Table 51-1. PREVENTION OF *CLOSTRIDIUM DIFFICILE* COLITIS

GENERAL

Prudent use of antibiotics (narrow spectrum, short courses)
Handwashing between patients
Enteric isolation: single rooms, stool precautions, use of gloves
Immunization with *C difficile* toxoids (future)
Toxin adsorbents: cholestryramine, colestipol sucralfate (still experimental)

OUTBREAK SETTING

Education about the disease
Handwashing before and after each patient
Use of gloves for handling positive patients
Cohorting of affected patients
Treatment of fecal carriers with oral metronidazole, bacitracin, or vancomycin to reduce fecal shedding of *C difficile*
Disinfection of unit and fomites to kill spores and vegetative forms with 2% alkaline glutaraldehyde or hypochlorite solutions (1600 ppm)
Closure of unit (as a last resort)

contain small amounts of blood but are rarely grossly bloody unless the patient has a coagulopathy.

Hypovolemic shock, hypoproteinemia, edema, cecal perforation, toxic dilatation of the colon, secondary sepsis, and hemorrhage are the most serious complications of severe PMC. Toxic dilatation and perforation are surgical emergencies.

Some patients with antibiotic-associated colitis present with localized abdominal pain, signs of peritonitis, and little or no diarrhea. These patients may have disease restricted to the cecum and proximal colon, and the clinical features may be confused with those of pseudo-obstruction of the colon. This atypical, nondiarrheal form of antibiotic-associated colitis is difficult to diagnose without colonoscopy or unless strongly suggested by an abnormal indium-33–labeled leukocyte scan or abnormal computed tomographic (CT) scan of the abdomen (Fig. 51-1). Stool studies for the presence of *C difficile* take too long to be of use to a patient with an acute abdomen.

CLINICAL DIAGNOSIS

The measures most useful in confirming the diagnosis of *C difficile* diarrhea are summarized in Table 51-2.

The differential diagnosis of nonspecific colitis associated with antibiotic use outside a hospital includes Crohn's disease, idiopathic ulcerative colitis, ischemic colitis, gold-induced colitis, chemical colitis, and infection with other intestinal pathogens. When diarrhea develops after a patient is admitted to a hospital and antibiotics are given, stool cultures for other pathogens are not indicated unless tests for *C difficile* are negative.

The diagnosis of PMC is confirmed with flexible sigmoidoscopy or colonoscopy, which are used to detect inflammation and pseudomembranes. The four types of pseudomembranous lesions are:

- Large, adherent pseudomembranes
- Small nodular or plaque-like elevated lesions
- Small, faint, flat circular or ring-like whitish yellow lesions on an erythematous background
- Pseudomembranes visualized with a microscope in biopsy specimens of inflamed mucosa

At microscopic examination, the lesions often appear to erupt from the mucosal surface and are called *volcano* or *summit* lesions. The presence of characteristic nodules and

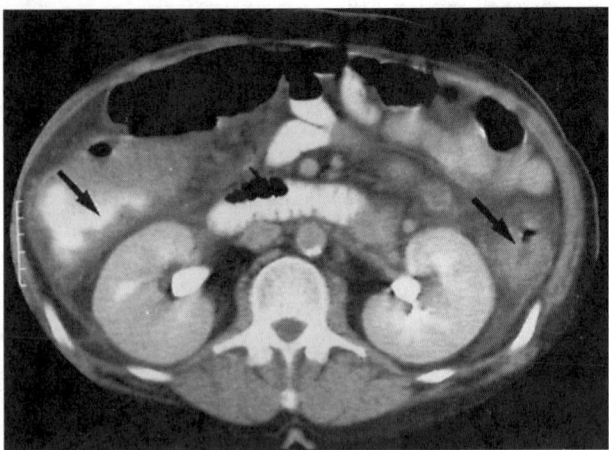

Figure 51-1. CT scan of abdomen in an elderly neurosurgical patient with fever and diarrhea postoperatively. Stools were positive for *Clostridium difficile* cytotoxin. The arrow at left indicates irregularly thickened cecal mucosa; the arrow at right indicates luminal narrowing, mucosal thickening, and edema of the descending colon.

plaques confirms the diagnosis. The lesions usually are most numerous in the distal colon, sigmoid, and rectum. Some patients with PMC have lesions restricted to the cecum or proximal colon. Correct diagnosis may not be possible in these patients unless colonoscopy or CT is performed. Right-sided disease is suspected in a patient with antibiotic diarrhea and toxin-positive stools when no lesions is visualized during sigmoidoscopy. Staphylococcal infection is suspected when the right side of the colon and

the cecum are primarily involved and tests for *C difficile* are negative.

Plain abdominal radiographs suggest ileus, edema, ascites, perforation, or toxic dilatation of the colon. Air-contrast barium enema examination shows thumbprinting, the accordion sign, and other signs of PMC. These findings are not specific and often are not present early in the course of disease. Barium examinations may precipitate toxic megacolon, perforation, and other complications. They are best avoided.

LABORATORY DIAGNOSIS

The tests most useful in the diagnosis of *C difficile* colitis are stool cultures for the organism and stool tests for the presence of *C difficile* toxins. The fecal leukocyte test is a simple, rapid screening measure that sometimes supports the diagnosis of *C difficile* colitis, but it is not specific for *C difficile* (Fig. 51-2). A positive test indicates mucosal inflammation and excludes the benign form of antibiotic diarrhea. No more than one-third of patients with *C difficile* colitis have positive fecal leukocyte tests.

Most adults with antibiotic-associated diarrhea and positive cultures for *C difficile* have colitis. The isolation of *C difficile* from stools of a patient with diarrhea does not prove a patient has colitis caused by *C difficile*. About 25% of isolates of *C difficile* are nontoxigenic and nonpathogenic. At least 3% of healthy adults carry toxigenic isolates of *C difficile* without experiencing symptoms. In hospitals where PMC is frequent, a large percentage adult patients treated with antibiotics carry the organism without experiencing symptoms.

Demonstration of the presence of toxin A (the enterotoxin) or toxin B (the cytotoxin) in stools of adults with

Table 51-2. DIAGNOSING *CLOSTRIDIUM DIFFICILE* COLITIS

Test	Comments
LABORATORY TESTS ON FECES	
Test for fecal leukocytes	A simple screening test but sensitivity only 30–50%. A positive test rules out benign or simple antibiotic diarrhea
Stool culture for *C difficile*	Results delayed. Not diagnostic, since 10–25% of patients in hospitals may carry the organism, and only 75% of isolates produce toxins
Tests for the presence of fecal toxins	
Cytopathic effect of toxin B in tissue cultures	Gold standard laboratory test, but some cell lines are not as sensitive as others, so false-negative results may occur. Time-consuming, expensive, and not widely available. Requires antitoxin neutralization for specificity
ELISA tests for toxins A or B	Rapid, widely available, relatively inexpensive. Sensitivity varies and may be only fair (75–85%). If cut point is chosen to minimize false-negative results, false-positive results become a problem.
Latex agglutination for *C difficile*	Rapid and inexpensive. Detects glutamate dehydrogenase (neither a toxin nor specific for *C difficile*). Many false-positive and false-negative results
RADIOLOGIC STUDIES	
Plain film of the abdomen	Nonspecific and useful only when colitis is far-advanced or complications such as toxic megacolon or perforation are present.
Barium enema	Nonspecific findings. May precipitate perforation or megacolon
Computed tomography	Safe, but expensive, and not highly specific. Can be useful, especially when patients present with an acute abdomen without diarrhea. May demonstrate unsuspected pseudomembranous colitis
Radionuclide scan (indium-labeled white blood cells)	May detect inflammation, but does not diagnose cause
PROCEDURES	
Flexible sigmoidoscopy	Most rapid way to make the diagnosis. Expensive. Misses about 10% of cases (those with only minor or proximal colonic lesions). Biopsy of minor or nonspecific lesions increases yield.
Colonoscopy	Rapid and most sensitive way to make the diagnosis. Expensive and may be hazardous in impending perforation

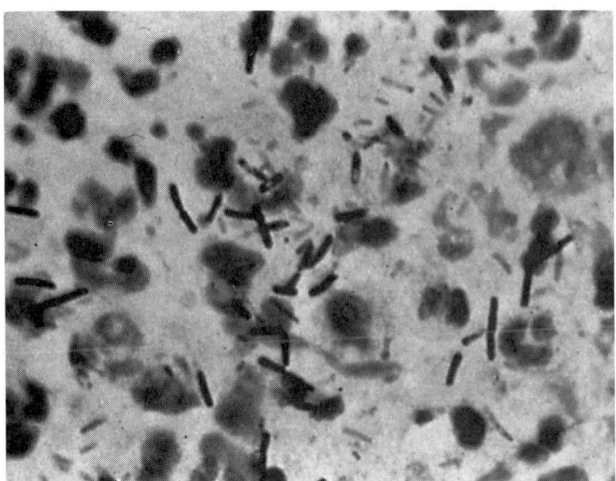

Figure 51-2. Giemsa-stained smear of feces from patient with *Clostridium difficile* colitis. The important finding is that many leukocytes are present. Although organisms resembling clostridia are also numerous, this is often not the case.

diarrhea is helpful, but does not prove a patient has colitis. Some adults (and many colonized infants) may have the toxin in stools and yet be free of symptoms. Cell culture evidence of cytotoxicity with cytotoxin B is the most reliable laboratory aid in the diagnosis of PMC. Almost all adults with antibiotic-associated diarrhea and toxin B-positive stools have colitis. When proctosigmoidoscopy is performed in patients with strongly positive toxin B titers and is normal, it is likely these patients have colitis at a proximal site, such as the cecum, or have mild, nonspecific colitis without pseudomembranes.

An enzyme-linked immunosorbent assay (ELISA) of stools to detect toxin A is used in many hospital laboratories. When one toxin is present, so is the other, with rare exception. Because the results of an ELISA for toxin A can be obtained in a few hours, ELISA is preferred to the cytotoxin B test. However, the end point for reading ELISA tests is arbitrary. One must be aware of the possibility of false-negative or false-positive results when basing management decisions on ELISA tests for the toxins. When an ELISA for toxin A is negative, it may be helpful to repeat it or to perform another test for *C difficile* diarrhea, such as culture, toxin B test in cell cultures, the latex agglutination test, or endoscopy. Use of the polymerase chain reaction (PCR) is under investigation.

MEDICAL TREATMENT

Antibiotics

Oral antimicrobial therapy is more reliable than parenteral therapy for antibiotic-associated colitis. Susceptibility tests rarely are performed, so empiric treatment is based on data from studies with large numbers of isolates of *C difficile*. *C difficile* is susceptible to vancomycin, metronidazole, and bacitracin. Oral vancomycin is the treatment of choice for PMC. If a patient is elderly, debilitated, or likely to have a severe form of the disease, therapy is begun while one awaits results of tests designed to implicate *C difficile*. Empiric therapy is designed to correct fluid and electrolyte imbalances and to prevent hypoproteinemia, edema, toxic colonic dilatation, colonic perforation, and other complications. Vancomycin or metronidazole is used for specific therapy.

Not all patients with antibiotic-associated colitis need

an antimicrobial drug. When a patient has only mild or moderate illness, it may be sufficient to discontinue the precipitating antibiotic and provide supportive therapy with fluid and electrolyte replacement. If the patient's condition improves within a few days, supportive therapy is continued, and diarrhea usually subsides completely in 7 to 10 days. If it does not, an antibiotic is administered, usually for another 7 to 10 days. If the inducing antibiotic must be continued, specific oral antimicrobial treatment with vancomycin or metronidazole is started promptly, even if the symptoms of colitis are mild.

Discontinuation of the inducing antibiotic after recognition of colitis is not essential if specific therapy for PMC is given. The antibacterial effects of vancomycin on *C difficile* in vitro are not antagonized by other antimicrobial agents; vancomycin or metronidazole suppresses the disease despite continuation of antimicrobial agents. Nonetheless, it is a good idea to change to another appropriate antimicrobial regimen to treat the original infection when possible.

Antidiarrheal Agents

Antiperistaltic agents such as loperamide or diphenoxylate with atropine (Lomotil) are best avoided in patients with antibiotic-associated colitis. Although these agents provide symptomatic relief, they do so by causing pooling of fluid in the intestinal lumen. These drugs may improve diarrhea but promote more damage to the colon because toxin-containing fluid pools in the intestinal lumen, possibly causing toxic dilatation of the colon.

The antiperistaltic effects of morphine and related opiates given for relief of postoperative pain may decrease the signs of diarrhea that would alert one to the possibility of PMC and may thus predispose to severe colitis and toxic megacolon.

Treatment of Patients Unable to Take Oral Therapy

Reliance on IV antibiotics for treatment of colitis, to the exclusion of oral or intraluminal therapy, is not recommended. Patients with colitis treated with IV vancomycin or metronidazole may not have therapeutic concentrations of the drug in the intestinal lumen, where it is most needed. When parenteral therapy for PMC is unavoidable (as in patients with paralytic ileus and severe colitis), both IV metronidazole and IV vancomycin are administered and supplemented with vancomycin by means of a nasogastric tube with intermittent clamping, ileostomy or colostomy, enema, or a catheter passed to the cecum at colonoscopy. Nasogastric passage of a long intestinal tube to the distal ileum or through the ileocecal valve into the cecum under fluoroscopic control may be possible in some patients. This procedure allows perfusion of the colon from above under low pressure with vancomycin-containing solutions. Oral metronidazole is not used in this setting, because the drug is absorbed from the small intestine, and little or none reaches the colonic lumen.

SURGICAL TREATMENT

The condition of a patient with PMC may deteriorate rapidly, and life-threatening fulminant colitis, toxic megacolon, or perforation may develop. Urgent subtotal colectomy is necessary to deal with these life-threatening emergencies. Sometimes a colostomy or ileostomy is used to facilitate instillation of vancomycin or metronidazole into the colonic lumen of patients with ileus or obstruction. *C difficile* diarrhea occurs in the small intestine after colostomy, and PMC causes early colostomy dysfunction that may not be suspected until mucosal plaques became apparent on the everted intestine at the colostomy opening.

RECURRENCE OF COLITIS

Most patients with *C difficile* colitis do not experience multiple recurrences. However, 10% to 20% of patients treated with vancomycin, metronidazole, or bacitracin experience another episode of colitis as long as 8 weeks after apparent resolution of the disease. Recurrences usually respond promptly to repeat therapy with vancomycin, metronidazole, or bacitracin. Recurrences may be caused by germination of spores that persist in the colon (relapse) or by acquisition of organisms from environmental or human contacts (reinfection). Relapse is more common than reinfection, but management is the same. The *C difficile* carrier state is not reliably eradicated with antimicrobial agents.

Although most patients with PMC have one recurrence at most, some people experience multiple episodes. Patients may have five to ten intermittent episodes of diarrhea and colitis over 6 to 24 months. Although no entirely satisfactory way to prevent these episodes is known, anecdotal observations and experience support management with short (7 to 10 days) or long (4 to 6 weeks) courses of therapy with oral vancomycin, metronidazole, or bacitracin. Sometimes drug therapy is followed by gradual tapering of the dose for weeks after antibiotic therapy is completed. Oral vancomycin plus rifampin can be used as empiric treatment and prevention of multiple relapses. None of these regimens is better than the others.

The best way to prevent relapses is restoration of the normal fecal flora. Patients with multiple relapses are treated by oral or rectal administration of a nontoxigenic isolate of *C difficile* or a mixture of pure cultures of organisms isolated from stools to suppress *C difficile* and its toxins. Direct attempts at recolonization of the colon include oral administration of yogurt or other Lactobacillus preparations or oral administration of a nonpathogenic yeast, Saccharomyces boulardii.

SUGGESTED READING

Brazier JS. Role of the laboratory in investigations of *C difficile* diarrhea. Clin Infect Dis 1993;16(Suppl 4):S228.

Kuhl SJ, Tang YJ, Navarro L, et al. Diagnosis and monitoring of *Clostridium difficile* infections with the polymerase chain reaction. Clin Infect Dis 1993;16(Suppl 4):S234.

Leung DY, Kelly CP, Boguniewicz M, et al. Treatment with intravenously administered gamma globullin of chronic relapsing colitis induced by *Clostridium difficile* toxin. J Pediatr 1991;118:633.

McFarland LV, Surawicz CM, Greenberg RN, et al. A randomized placebo-controlled trial of Saccharomyces boulardii in combination with standard antibiotic for *Clostridium difficile* disease. JAMA 1994;271:1913.

Mitty RD, LaMont JT. *Clostridium difficile* diarrhea: pathogenesis, epidemiology and treatment. Gastroenterology 1994;2:61.

Stein HD, Sirota RA, Yudis M, et al. Pseudomembranous colitis as a cause of early colostomy dysfunction. J Clin Gastroenterol 1994;18:165.

Teasley PG, Gerding DN, Olson MM, et al. Prospective randomized trial of metronidazole versus vancomycin for *Clostridium difficile*–associated diarrhea and colitis. Lancet 1993;2:1043.

Yankes JR, Baker ME, Cooper C, Gorbatt J. CT appearance of focal pseudomembranous colitis. J Comput Assist Tomogr 1988;12:394.

ESSENTIALS OF SURGERY: SCIENTIFIC PRINCIPLES AND PRACTICE, edited by Lazar J. Greenfield, Michael W. Mulholland, Keith T. Oldham, Gerald B. Zelenock, and Keith D. Lillemoe. Lippincott–Raven Publishers, Philadelphia, © 1997.

CHAPTER 52

ANORECTAL DISORDERS
SANTHAT NIVATVONGS

ANATOMY OF THE RECTUM AND ANAL CANAL
The Rectum

The rectum extends from the level of the promontory of the sacrum to the level of the levator ani muscle. It is 12 to 15 cm long. The outer layer of the rectum is covered circumferentially with longitudinal muscle rather than taeniae. The rectum has two or three lateral curves that form submucosal folds in the lumen (valves of Houston).

The posterior part of the rectum is devoid of peritoneum and is covered with endopelvic fascia (lateral rectal stalks) (Fig. 52-1), which must be cut for full mobilization of the rectum.

Peritoneum covers the upper-two-thirds of the rectum anteriorly and the upper-third of the rectum laterally. The lower-third of the rectum is devoid of peritoneum.

Anal Canal

The anal canal is the terminal portion of the large intestine. About 4 cm in length, it passes through the levator ani muscle and opens to the anal verge. The muscular wall of the anal canal, a thick continuation of the circular muscular layer of the rectum, forms the *internal sphincter*. The anal canal is wrapped by the *external sphincter* muscle and the *puborectalis*, which are arranged in three U-shaped loops (Fig. 52-2):

- The top loop is formed by the puborectalis muscle, which originates from the pubis
- The intermediate loop is the superficial external sphincter muscle; the origin of this loop, at the tip of the coccyx, is the anococcygeal ligament
- The basal loop is composed of the subcutaneous portion of the external sphincter muscle

The upper portion of the anal canal, where the internal sphincter muscle thickens and the puborectalis wraps around it is the *anorectal ring*. From the level of the anorectal ring distally and between the internal and external sphincter muscles, the longitudinal muscle coat of the rectum is joined by fibers of the levator ani and puborectalis muscles to form the conjoined longitudinal muscle (Fig. 52-3).

At about the midpoint of the anal canal, 2 cm from the anal verge, is an undulating demarcation, the *dentate* (or pectinate) *line*. The columns of Morgagni are longitudinal folds of the mucosa above the dentate line. For about 1 cm above the dentate line, the epithelial lining may be columnar, transitional, or stratified squamous epithelium; this area is the *transitional* (or cloacogenic) *zone*. The area above the transitional zone is lined with columnar epithelium; the area below the dentate line is lined with squamous epithelium (Fig. 52-3). The internal hemorrhoidal plexus is in this area.

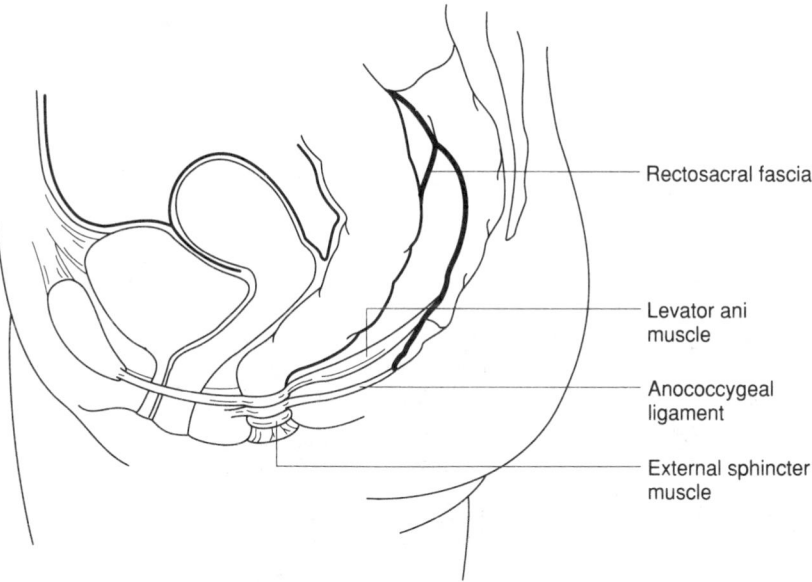

Figure 52-1. Fascial attachments of the rectum.

Pelvic Floor Muscles

The *levator ani* muscle is a broad, thin muscle that forms the floor of the pelvic cavity. The levator ani consists of the *iliococcygeus* and *pubococcygeus* muscles (Fig. 52-4). During defecation, the puborectalis muscle, which is part of the external sphincter, relaxes, and the levator ani contracts.

Perianal and Perirectal Spaces

Surrounding the anorectum are several spaces that are normally filled with areolar tissue or fat. These spaces are important because they are sites of abscess formation. The supralevator spaces communicate posteriorly and may allow spread of infection cephalad into the retroperitoneum.

Arterial Supply of the Rectum and Anal Canal

The *superior rectal* (hemorrhoidal) artery is the continuation of the inferior mesenteric artery. It descends posterior to the rectum, where it bifurcates to supply the rectum and upper portion of the anal canal (Fig. 52-5). The *middle rectal* arteries originate from the internal iliac arteries on each side and enter the lower portion of the rectum anterolaterally at the level of the levator ani muscle. The middle rectal arteries anastomose with the branches of the supe-

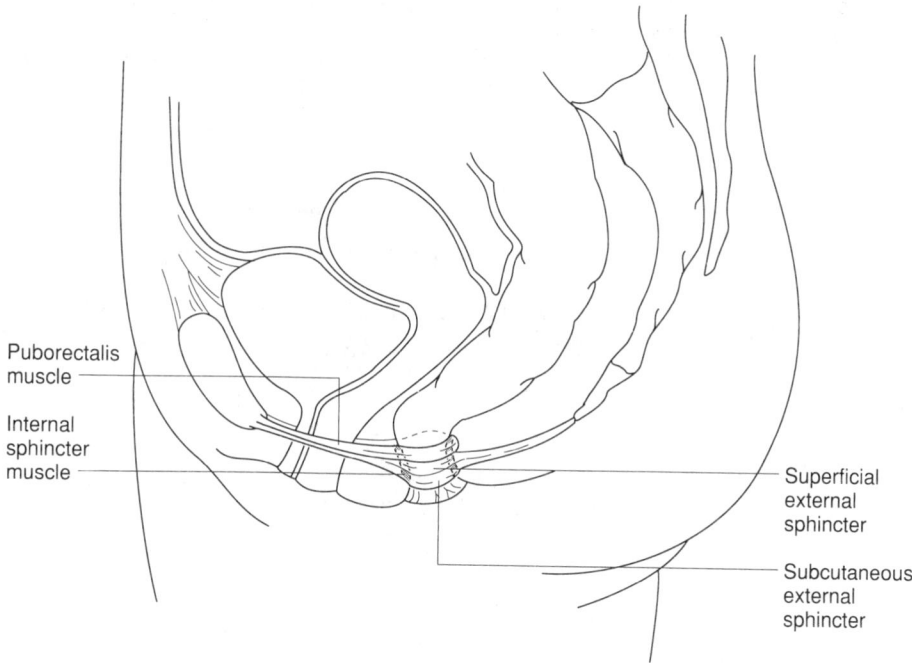

Figure 52-2. Arrangement of the external sphincter muscles.

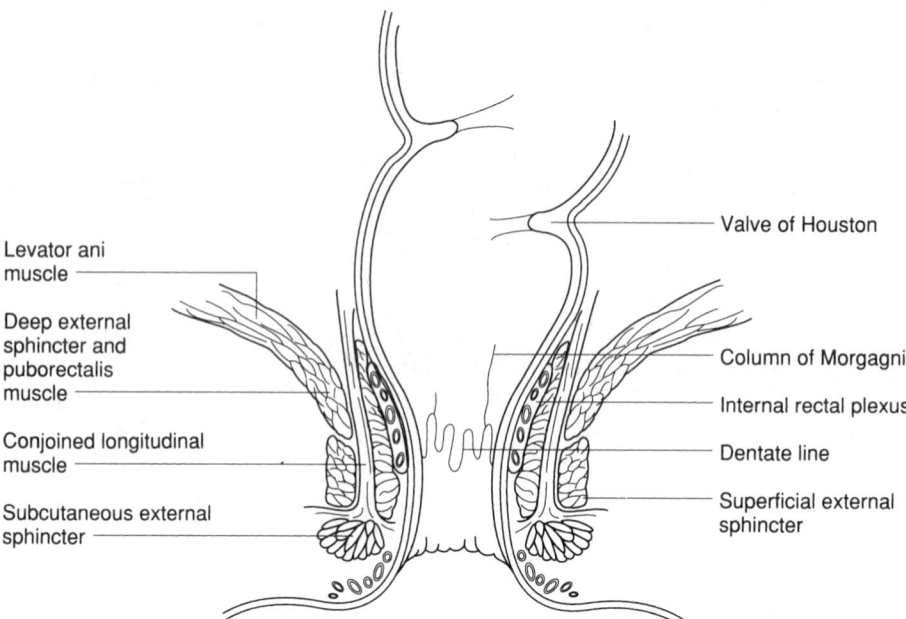

Levator ani muscle

Deep external sphincter and puborectalis muscle

Conjoined longitudinal muscle

Subcutaneous external sphincter

Valve of Houston

Column of Morgagni

Internal rectal plexus

Dentate line

Superficial external sphincter

Figure 52-3. Anatomy of the anal canal.

rior rectal artery. The *inferior rectal* arteries originate from the internal pudendal artery, a branch of the internal iliac artery, and traverse the ischioanal fossa on each side to supply the anal sphincter muscles. The *middle sacral* artery provides a small amount of blood to the rectum. It originates posteriorly above the bifurcation of the aorta and descends over the lumbar vertebrae, sacrum, and coccyx.

Venous Drainage of the Rectum and Anal Canal

Return of the blood from the rectum and the anal canal is portal and systemic (Fig. 52-6). The *superior rectal* vein drains the rectum and upper part of the anal canal into the portal system through the inferior mesenteric vein. The *middle rectal* veins drain the lower part of the rectum and the upper part of the anal canal; they accompany the middle rectal arteries and terminate in the internal iliac veins. The *inferior rectal* veins, following the corresponding arteries, drain the lower part of the anal canal via the internal pudendal veins, which empty into the internal iliac veins.

Lymphatic Drainage of the Rectum and Anal Canal

The lymphatic drainage is depicted in Figures 52-7 and 52-8.

Nerve Supply of the Rectum and Urogenital Organs

Sympathetic and parasympathetic nerves of the autonomic nervous system supply the anorectum and send branches to the adjacent urogenital organs (Fig. 52-9). In women, the sympathetic nerve fibers from the hypogastric plexus are directed toward the uterosacral ligament close to the rectum. In men, the nerve fibers from the hypogastric plexus pass immediately adjacent to the anterolateral wall of the rectum in the retroperitoneal tissue. Nerve trunks are close to the rectum and are prone to injury during mobilization of the rectum, so precautions must be taken to protect the nerves during surgical procedures.

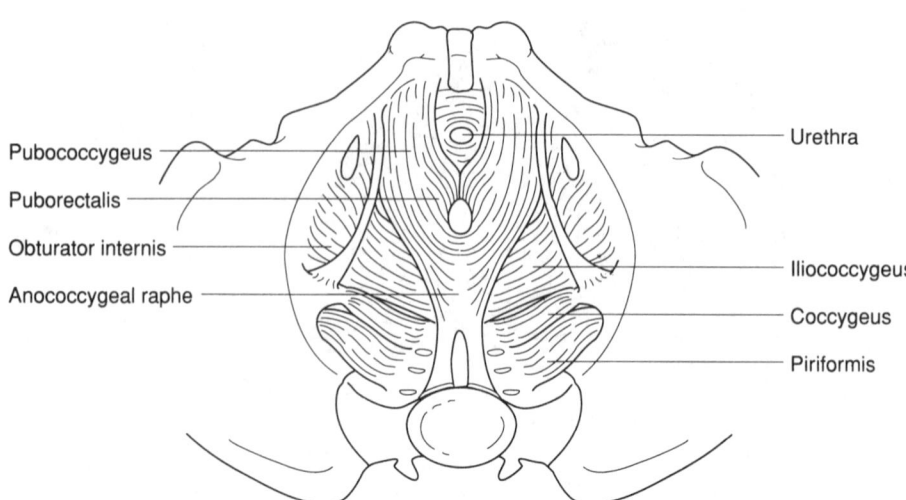

Pubococcygeus

Puborectalis

Obturator internis

Anococcygeal raphe

Urethra

Iliococcygeus

Coccygeus

Piriformis

Figure 52-4. Muscles of the pelvic floor.

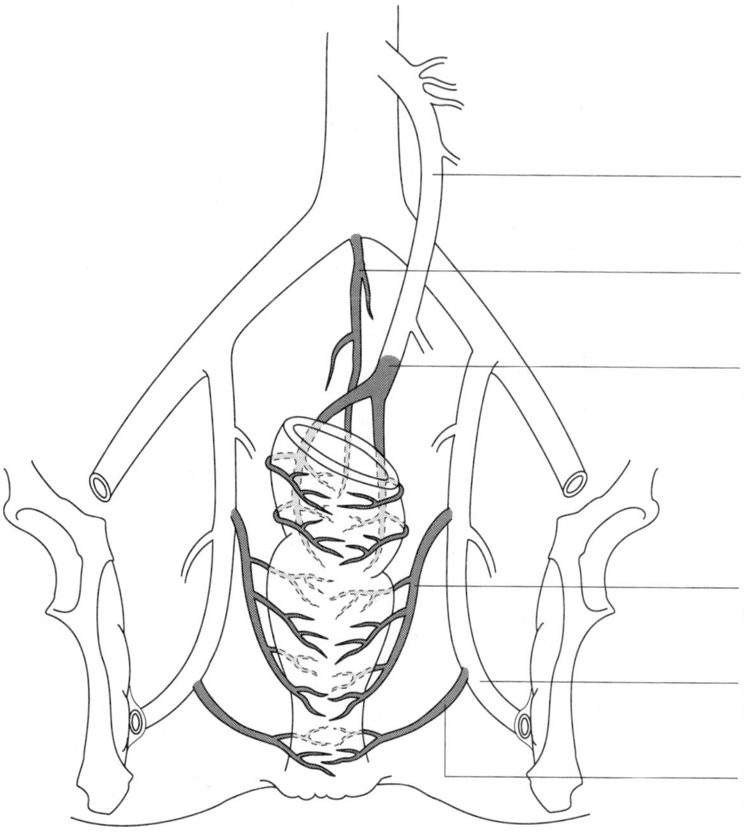
Inferior mesenteric artery
Middle sacral artery
Superior rectal artery
Middle rectal artery
Internal pudendal artery
Inferior rectal artery

Figure 52-5. Arterial supply of the rectum and anal canal.

Nerve Supply of the Anal Canal

The motor innervation of the *internal anal sphincter* is with both sympathetic and parasympathetic nerves. The *external sphincter* is supplied by the inferior rectal branch of the internal pudendal and the perineal branch of the fourth sacral nerve. The *levator ani* is supplied by the pudendal nerve and branches of the third, fourth, and fifth sacral nerves. The sensory nerve supply of the anal canal is the inferior rectal nerve, a branch of the pudendal nerve. The epithelium of the anal canal is profusely innervated with sensory nerve endings, especially near the dentate line.

PHYSIOLOGY OF THE ANORECTUM

Sensation of the Anorectum

Complete anal continence is not possible unless a person senses material in the rectum and discriminates the quality of the substance (feces or gas). The receptors responsible for the appreciation of rectal fullness and impending evacuation are outside the anorectal wall, probably within the levator ani muscle. The nerve-rich epithelium of the anal canal is important in discriminating flatus and feces but it is not critical in anal continence.

Anal Continence

Stool accumulates in the rectum for a variable period of time before the urge to defecate occurs. Continence is maintained by the influence of the pelvic muscles on the shape of the rectum.

The internal anal sphincter is not subject to voluntary control. It is in a continuously tonic state and maintains closure of the resting anal canal. The external anal sphincter contributes to anal pressure only when a bolus of stool is present in the anal canal. The increase in pressure during voluntary contraction is due to the activity of the external sphincter. The high resting pressure in the anal canal is a barrier to prevent leakage of mucus and gas.

When the rectum is distended, the *internal sphincter relaxes* (rectoanal reflex), allowing rectal content to move down to the anal canal. As this happens, the *external sphincter contracts,* preventing rectal content from leaking through the anus. Marked distention of the rectum inhibits external sphincter contraction, and the voluntary act of straining inhibits the external sphincter and the pelvic floor muscles. Although contraction of the external sphincter can be sustained for only short periods, it is the most important mechanism of voluntary continence.

Defecation

Defecation involves both a reflex response and voluntary performance. When a fecal bolus enters the rectum, stretch receptors in the muscles of the pelvic floor register a sensation and an urge to defecate. Distention of the rectum causes reflex relaxation of the internal sphincter and contraction of the external sphincter and puborectalis muscle, allowing the rectal content to make contact with the anal canal. This contact allows the epithelium of the anal canal to sense and discriminate the nature of the material. If rectal distention is maintained, the rectal muscles adapt to decrease rectal pressure. Defecation proceeds when the person squats or sits to straighten the angle between the rectum and the anal canal. The feces is expelled with contraction of the rectum and increased intraabdominal pressure due to the Valsalva maneuver. After defecation, voluntary sphincters contract, and normal postural tone is restored.

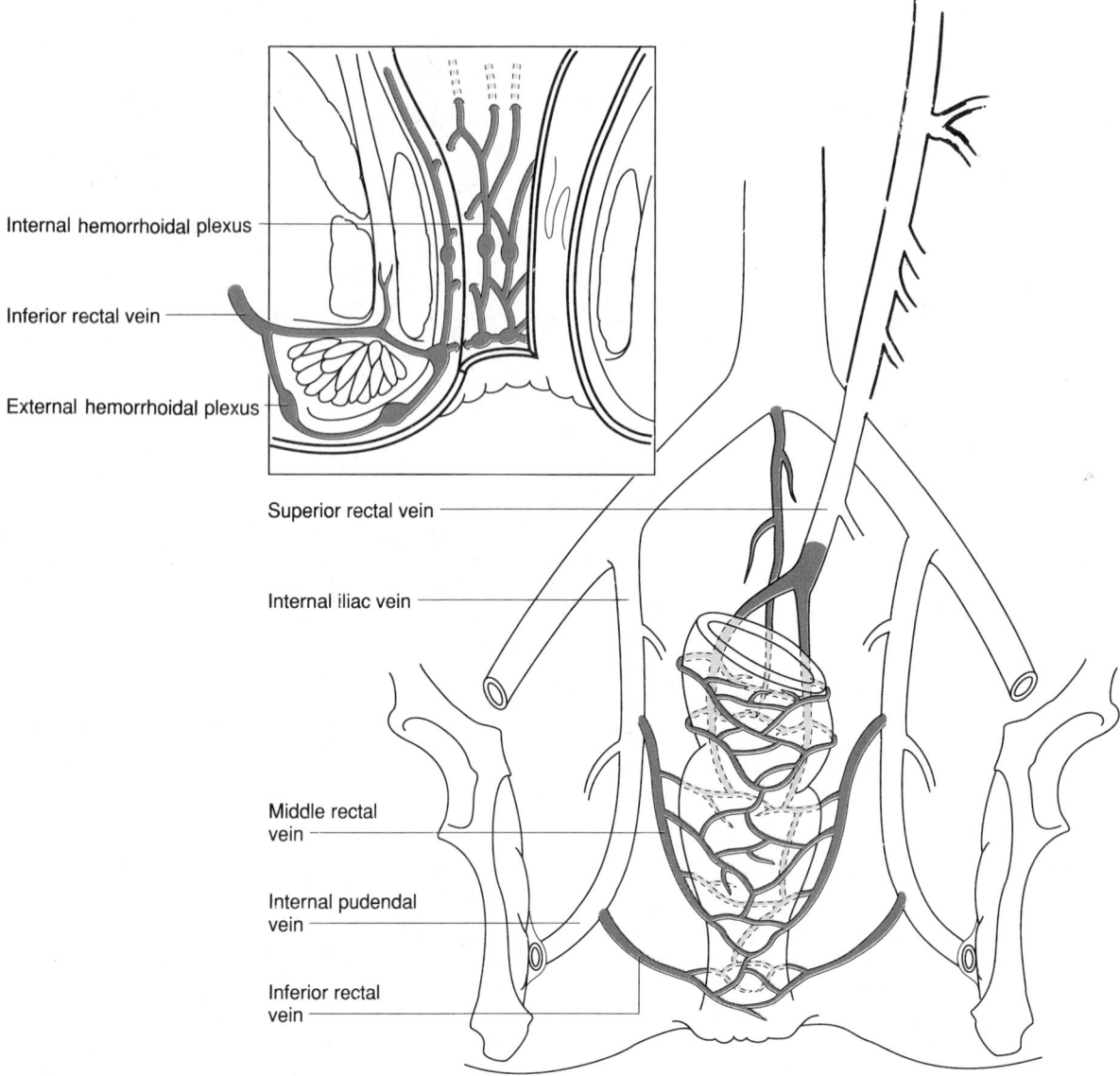

Internal hemorrhoidal plexus

Inferior rectal vein

External hemorrhoidal plexus

Superior rectal vein

Internal iliac vein

Middle rectal vein

Internal pudendal vein

Inferior rectal vein

Figure 52-6. Venous drainage of the rectum and anal canal.

HEMORRHOIDS

In the upper anal canal, cushions of submucosal connective tissue contain venules and smooth muscle fibers. These cushions—left lateral, right anterior, and right posterior—aid in anal continence. During defecation, this tissue becomes engorged with blood, cushions the anal canal, and supports the lining of the canal. The anal cushions are supported by muscles that originate partly from the internal sphincter and partly from the conjoined longitudinal muscles. A *hemorrhoid* is downward displacement of the anal cushion that causes dilatation of the venules inside. Hemorrhoids develop when the supporting muscles deteriorate.

Classification

External hemorrhoids are dilated venules of the inferior hemorrhoidal plexus below the dentate line. *Internal hemorrhoids* are prolapsed anal cushions above the dentate line. Internal hemorrhoids are graded according to the degree of prolapse:

- First degree—the anal cushions slide down beyond the dentate line on straining
- Second degree—the anal cushions prolapse through the anus on straining but reduce spontaneously
- Third degree—the anal cushions prolapse through the anus on straining or exertion and require manual replacement into the anal canal
- Fourth degree—the prolapse is not manually reducible

Clinical Manifestations

The most common manifestation of hemorrhoids is painless, bright red rectal bleeding that occurs with bowel movement. (Burning, itching, swelling, and pain usually are not from hemorrhoids but from conditions such as pruritus ani and anal abrasion.) A feeling of incomplete evacuation is common. In chronic prolapse, exposed rectal mucosa causes perianal irritation and mucous staining on the underwear. Congestion of external hemorrhoids or skin tags can cause discomfort or pain. Symptoms are aggravated by constipation or diarrhea.

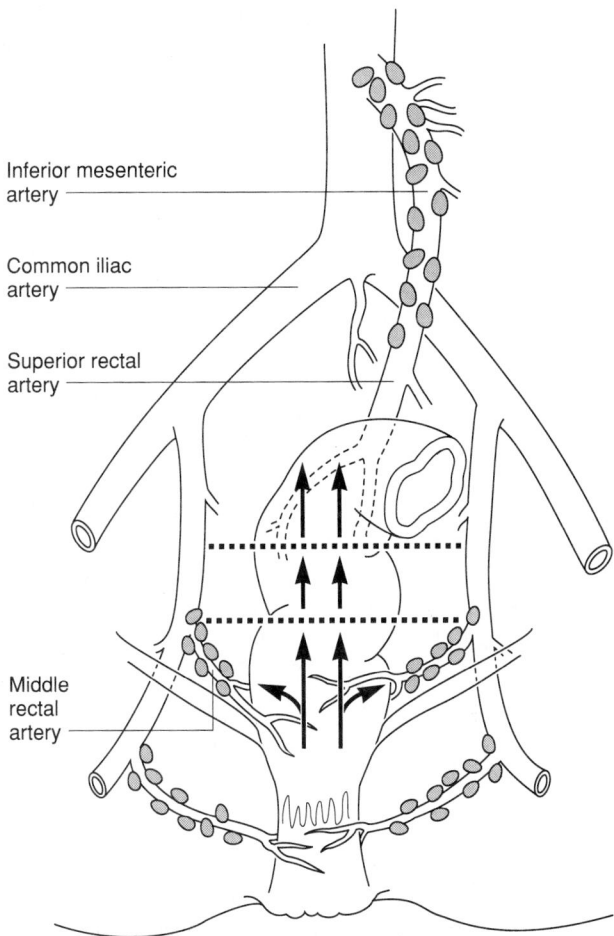

Figure 52-7. Lymphatic drainage of the rectum.

Examination

Definitive diagnosis of hemorrhoids is made at examination. The best and most accurate way to diagnose hemorrhoids is to watch for prolapse while the patient strains as if defecating. Internal hemorrhoids cannot be palpated. Digital examination may help detect anal stenosis and anal scarring. Anal sphincter tone and sphincter squeeze are evaluated subjectively.

Anoscopy is the best way to examine the anal canal. During anoscopy, one must exclude a coexisting anal fissure or fistula. Proctoscopy is performed to rule out coexisting rectal abnormalities, particularly carcinoma and inflammatory bowel disease (IBD). Patients >50 years of age, particularly those with a family history of cancer, undergo a complete colonic examination.

Treatment

A high-fiber diet is prescribed to eliminate straining at defecation. When the high-fiber diet does not work, hemorrhoids are treated with:

* Rubber-band ligation
* Infrared photocoagulation
* Hemorrhoidectomy

Special situations with hemorrhoids are:

* Thrombosed external hemorrhoids—a painful condition in which the skin over the hematoma becomes

necrotic. Treatment is relief of severe pain, prevention of recurrent clot, and prevention of residual skin tag.
* Strangulated hemorrhoids—a prolapsed third-degree hemorrhoid becomes irreducible. Treatment is urgent or emergency hemorrhoidectomy.
* Postpartum hemorrhoids—thrombosed external and internal or strangulated hemorrhoids that occur as the result of prolonged labor. Treatment is the same as for other hemorrhoids.
* Acute hemorrhoidal bleeding due to portal hypertension—suture of the bleeding site must incorporate the mucosa, submucosa, and internal sphincter. Coexisting coagulopathy must be corrected.

RECTAL PROLAPSE

Prolapse of the rectum (procidentia) is an uncommon condition in which the full thickness of the rectal wall turns inside out and passes into or through the anal canal. The extruded rectum is seen as concentric rings of mucosa.

Pathophysiology

Rectal prolapse is an intussusception that usually starts in the anterior part of the lower rectum 6 to 7 cm from the anal verge or at the rectosigmoid junction. Many patients with rectal prolapse have a history of straining associated with intractable constipation, and some have chronic diarrhea. Patients experience impaired resting and voluntary

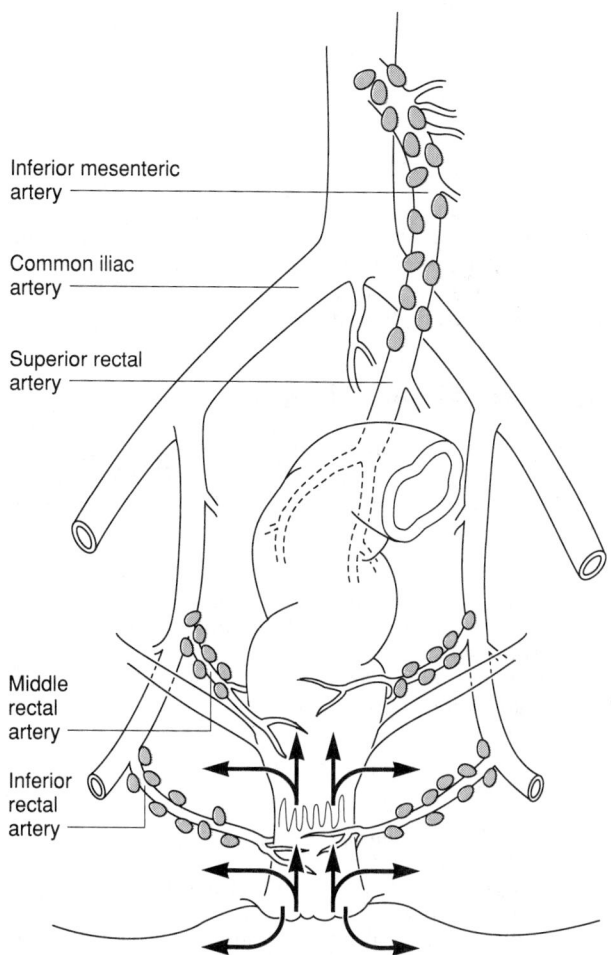

Figure 52-8. Lymphatic drainage of the anal canal.

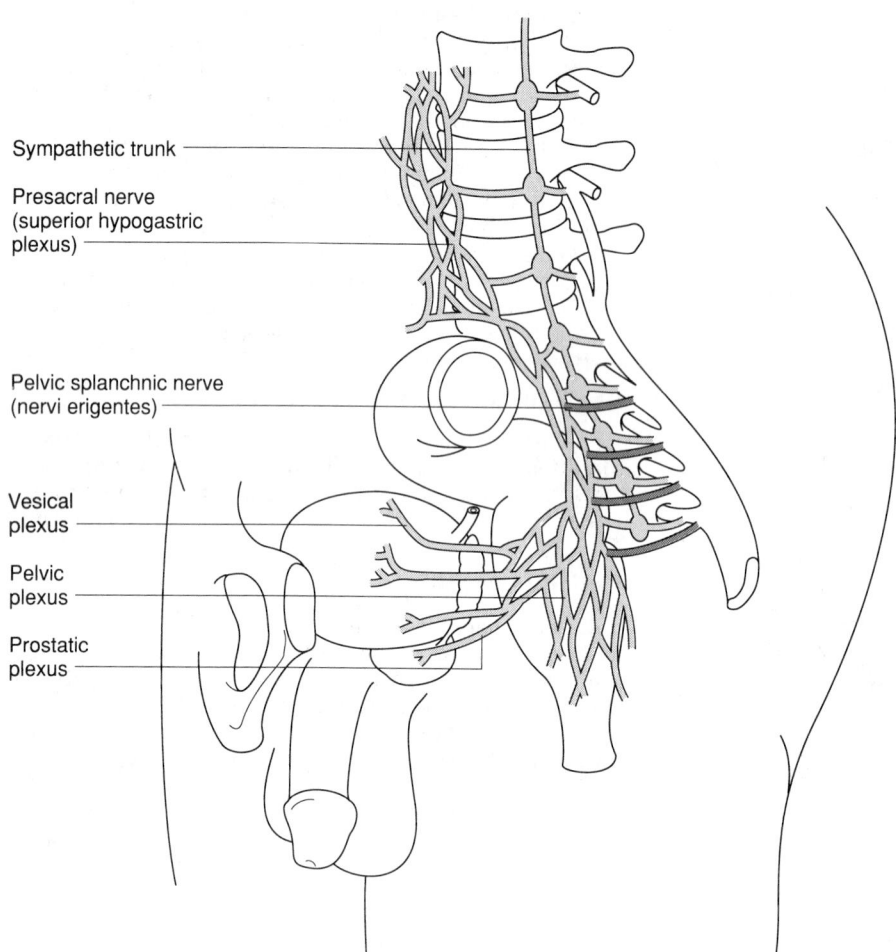

Sympathetic trunk

Presacral nerve
(superior hypogastric
plexus)

Pelvic splanchnic nerve
(nervi erigentes)

Vesical
plexus

Pelvic
plexus

Prostatic
plexus

Figure 52-9. Sympathetic and parasympathetic nerve supply of the rectum.

sphincter activity, decreased rectal capacity, or impaired continence. Some patients experience failure of normal relaxation of the external sphincter and pelvic floor musculature during attempts at defecation.

Anatomic Abnormalities

Prolapse of the rectum occurs more frequently in women than men. Several anatomic defects or abnormalities are consistently demonstrated in patients with chronic rectal prolapse:

- Abnormally deep rectovaginal or rectovesical pouch
- Lax and atonic musculature of the pelvic floor
- Lack of normal fixation of the rectum and an elongated mesorectum
- Redundant rectosigmoid and sigmoid colon
- Lax and atonic sphincters

Classification

Rectal prolapse is classified in the following manner:

- Incomplete (partial) rectal prolapse—prolapse of rectal mucosa only
- Complete rectal prolapse—prolapse involving all layers
  - First degree—occult prolapse

- Second degree—prolapse to, but not through, the anus
- Third degree—protrusion through the anus

Clinical Manifestations

The early symptoms of rectal prolapse are:

- Anorectal discomfort during defecation
- Difficulty in initiating bowel movements
- A feeling of incomplete evacuation

Some patients require digital evacuation of the stool in the rectum; in many patients, the prolapse causes obstruction that leads to chronic constipation. In overt prolapse, the protrusion initially occurs only during or after defecation. As the problem becomes more pronounced, the protrusion may be precipitated by coughing, exertion, or walking. Fecal and urinary incontinence are symptoms of prolapse of long duration.

Diagnosis

Diagnosis of rectal prolapse is easy if the prolapse has come through the anus. The protrusion usually has circumferential mucosal folds. When the prolapse remains in the rectum or anal canal (occult prolapse), diagnosis is difficult. Redness of the rectal mucosa, especially the anterior portion 6 to 7 cm from the anal verge is a sign. Second-degree rectal prolapse is often confused with prolapsed hemorrhoids.

Evaluation

Although not useful for diagnosis of rectal prolapse, a barium enema radiographic examination is indicated to rule out an associated lesion, particularly in patients with a recent episode of constipation. Colonoscopy is an acceptable alternative to barium enema. Anal manometry is helpful for evaluation of incontinence and for follow-up testing of anal sphincteric function after repair. Defecating proctography is useful to confirm the diagnosis.

Treatment

Treatment of rectal prolapse is transabdominal rectosigmoid resection and rectopexy. Perineal rectosigmoidectomy is performed when a prolapse extrudes >3 cm, particularly in elderly patients.

ANAL FISSURE
Definition

Anal fissure is an ulcer in the lower part of the anal canal. Fissures are acute or chronic and primary or secondary. A *primary* fissure occurs without other local or systemic disease. A *secondary* fissure develops in association with diseases such as Crohn's disease, leukemia, aplastic anemia, and agranulocytosis.

Pathophysiology

Most tears of the anal canal are traced to passage of a large, hard stool or explosive diarrhea; trauma to the anus; or tearing during vaginal delivery. Because reflex stimulation of the internal anal sphincter appears to be important in the pathogenesis of anal fissure, surgical approaches are directed at the internal rather than the external anal sphincter.

Clinical Manifestations

Burning, throbbing, or dull aching anal pain, particularly during and after a bowel movement, is the prominent symptom of anal fissure. The pain is severe and incapacitating and may last for several hours. If there is fever, fissure may mimic an intersphincteric abscess. Bleeding is common. Constipation commonly occurs, because the pain makes patients reluctant to have a bowel movement.

Diagnosis

Although pain and bleeding are common characteristics of anal fissure, the diagnosis is confirmed at examination. Inspection of the anus while the patient's buttocks are spread usually reveals the fissure. Digital examination reveals a small, fibrotic defect and tightness of the anal canal. Chronic anal fissure is usually deep, exposing the internal sphincter. Sometimes a chronic anal fissure involves a triad of fissure, sentinel skin tag, and hypertrophied anal papilla. The sentinel tag is the fibrotic or edematous skin adjacent to the fissure.

A small anoscope is useful to visualize the fissure. Proctoscopy or flexible sigmoidoscopy is performed to exclude associated abnormalities of the anal canal and rectum, especially IBD. The examination sometimes must be performed with general anesthesia because of severe pain.

Management

Initial treatment of *acute* anal fissure includes pain relief, anal cleaning, warm sitz baths to relax the anal canal, and use of bulk-forming agents, such as bran or psyllium seed, to relieve constipation. Application of a topical anesthetic jelly directly to the fissure before a bowel movement is helpful. Surgical treatment is not indicated unless the fissure is an exacerbation of a chronic anal fissure.

Chronic anal fissure is unlikely to heal with conservative management. If the pain persists, the fissure is treated with lateral internal sphincterotomy. This outpatient procedure is performed with local, regional, or general anesthesia. The procedure can be closed or open. Fissurectomy with anoplasty and a skin flap to cover the wound is performed when there are markedly redundant skin tags around the fissure.

Secondary Anal Fissure

Fissures or ulcers in Crohn's disease are larger and deeper than primary anal fissures. The skin around the ulcer is edematous, macerated, and erythematous. The pain is not as severe as that of primary fissure; severe pain may be a sign of abscess formation. Treatment is anal cleaning, local care of the lesion, and control of constipation or diarrhea. Surgical intervention is avoided.

Anal fissure or ulcer frequently occurs in patients with leukemia, aplastic anemia, and agranulocytosis. The fissure usually follows a bout of diarrhea or constipation when the patient is neutropenic. The ulcer is extremely painful, usually superficial, and frequently is necrotic at its base. Fever or septicemia is common and is treated with broad-spectrum antibiotics. Treatment is directed at relief of pain with a nonconstipating analgesic drug and perineal cleaning. The ulcer usually heals when the white blood cell count rises above 1000/mL. Surgical intervention is avoided.

ANORECTAL ABSCESSES
Pathogenesis

In the wall of the anal canal, four to ten anal glands lined with stratified columnar epithelium have direct openings into the anal crypts at the dentate line. Infection of these glands is the most common cause of perianal abscesses. Because the glands lie between the internal and external sphincter muscles, an intersphincteric abscess forms, and infection may spread to the spaces (Fig. 52-10). Abscesses, in order of frequency, are perianal, ischioanal, intersphincteric, and supralevator.

Clinical Manifestations

The initial symptom of most anorectal abscesses is severe pain in the anal region. The pain is throbbing or dull aching in character, and is aggravated by walking, straining, coughing, and sneezing. Depending on the location of the abscess, a swollen mass may be felt. Fever or septicemia may occur. Some patients experience urinary retention.

Management

Like an abscess in other parts of the body, an anorectal abscess must be drained as soon as possible. Antibiotics are not necessary after the abscess is adequately drained. However, patients with immune deficiency and those with

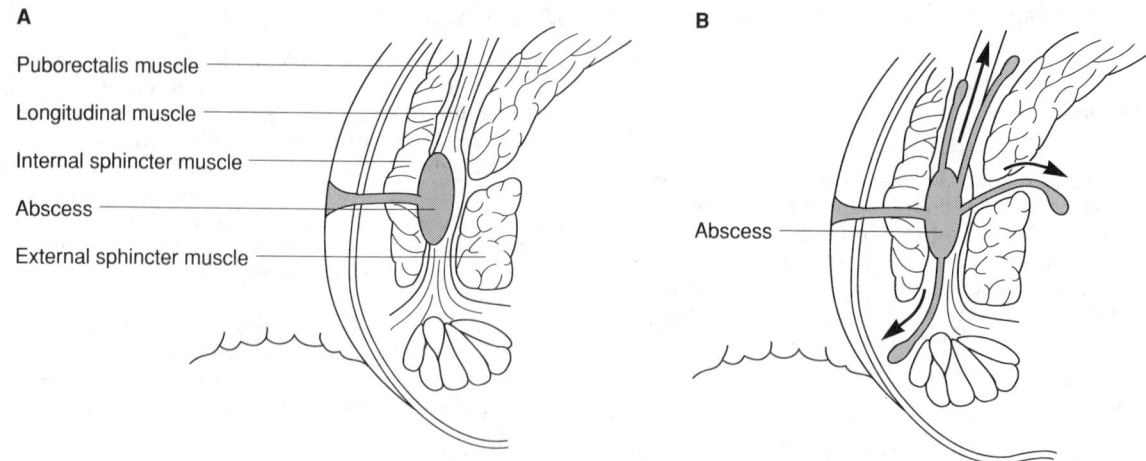

Figure 52-10. Pathways of infection start in the intersphincteric space (*A*) and then spread to perianal spaces, forming perianal abscesses (*B*).

prostheses or cardiac valvular abnormalities do receive antibiotics.

Perianal abscesses are the most superficial and the easiest to treat. The abscess is usually small and can be drained with the patient under local anesthesia. Redundant skin edges are excised to prevent premature closure of the abscess.

An *ischioanal* abscess causes diffuse swelling of the ischioanal fossa. Drainage is the same as with a perianal abscess. Bilateral ischioanal (horseshoe) abscess originates in the deep postanal space, with spread to both sides of the ischioanal space. A horseshoe abscess is drained through the deep postanal space.

Intersphincteric abscesses have no apparent signs of swelling or induration in the perianal area. The diagnosis is suspected when anorectal pain is so severe that rectal examination is impossible. An indurated or bulging mass is felt in the anal wall above the dentate line. Intersphincteric abscesses are drained by means of incision of the anal canal lining and through the internal sphincter muscle. Curettage and irrigation with saline solution continue until the abscess cavity is clean.

A *supralevator* abscess sometimes mimics an acute intraabdominal disorder. Digital examination reveals an indurated or bulging tender mass on either side of the lower rectum or posteriorly above the level of the anorectal ring. It is essential to determine the origin of a supralevator abscess before treatment:

1. Abscess due to upward extension of an intersphincteric abscess are drained into the rectum.
2. Abscess originating from upward extension of an ischiorectal abscess is drained through the ischioanal fossa.
3. Abscess due to intraabdominal disease is drained into the rectum, through the ischioanal fossa, or through the abdominal wall after the primary disease is treated.

FISTULA-IN-ANO

Fistula-in-ano is a chronic form of perianal abscess that is spontaneously or surgically drained, but in which the abscess cavity does not heal completely. The cavity becomes an inflammatory track with a primary opening (internal opening) in the anal crypt at the dentate line and a secondary opening (external opening) in the perianal skin.

The four main forms of fistula-in-ano are based on the relation of the fistula to the sphincter muscles (Fig. 52-11).

Clinical Manifestations

Most patients have a history of anorectal abscess with intermittent drainage. The external opening is usually visible as a red elevation of granulation tissue with purulent or serosanguineous drainage on compression. In superficial fistulas, the track is palpated as an indurated cord. Deep fistulas usually are not palpable.

Anoscopy is performed to identify the internal opening. Proctoscopy or flexible sigmoidoscopy is performed to rule out other lesions and IBD. A fistula probe is introduced into the fistula track to determine the direction of the fistula.

Management

The principles of fistula operations are:

- Unroofing the fistula
- Eliminating the primary opening (infective source)
- Establishing adequate drainage

Anal Fistula Associated With Crohn's Disease

Fistulas associated with Crohn's disease frequently are asymptomatic. Treatment is aggressive medical therapy, including medication for active Crohn's disease. Surgical treatment is indicated only for fistulas associated with an abscess.

PILONIDAL SINUS

Pilonidal sinuses are caused by infection of a hair follicle in the sacrococcygeal area. The average patient with pilonidal disease is a hirsute, moderately obese man 16–25 years of age. Pilonidal disease may present as an acute abscess at the sacrococcygeal area that ruptures spontaneously, leaving unhealed sinuses with chronic drainage. When sinuses develop, pain is usually minimal.

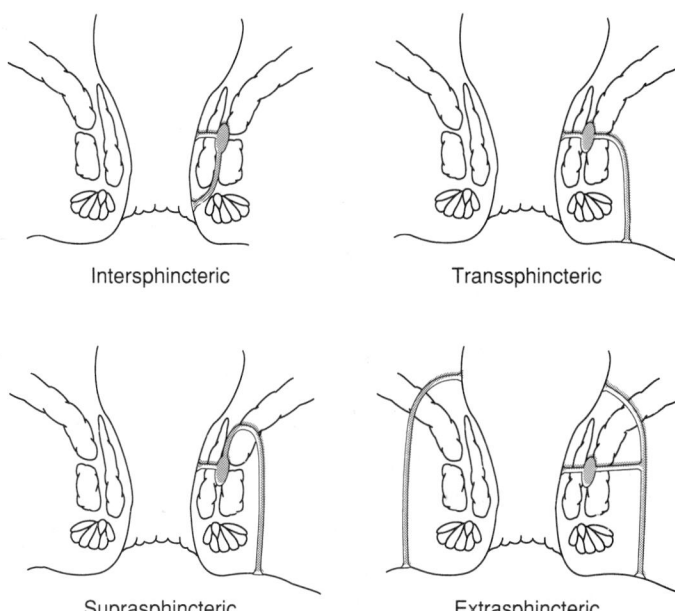

Figure 52-11. The four main anatomic types of fistula.

Diagnosis

A painful and fluctuant mass is the most common presentation of acute pilonidal sinus. In the early stage, only cellulitis may be present. In the chronic stage, the diagnosis is confirmed by the presence of a sinus opening in the intergluteal fold, about 5 cm above the anus. Almost all sinus tracks run cephalad; those that run caudad may be confused with fistula-in-ano or hidradenitis suppurativa. Examination reveals a pit or pits in the midline that represent infected hair follicles.

Treatment

Pilonidal abscesses are incised and drained. All hair in the abscess cavity must be removed. Antibiotics are not indicated. Conservative management of chronic sinuses is minimal excision of midline pits or sinuses and removal of all hair and debris. The cavity is packed and allowed to heal by secondary intention.

The postoperative care of a patient with a pilonidal is as important as the operation. The wound is washed in the bathtub or shower at least once a day. Large cavities are packed with fine gauze. Small cavities are swabbed at least once a day to remove all debris, especially hair.

RECTOVAGINAL FISTULA

Causes of rectovaginal fistula include the following:

- Congenital maldevelopment
- Trauma
  - Obstetric
  - Surgical
  - Blunt and penetrating injury
  - Foreign body
- Infection of anal canal or vaginal septum
- Pelvic irradiation
- Neoplasm

Rectovaginal fistulas are considered *low* if a repair can be performed with a perineal approach and *high* if a trans-

abdominal repair is required (Fig. 52-12). Rectovaginal fistulas may be classified as simple or complex:

Simple
Low to mid-vaginal septum
≤2.5 cm in diameter
Traumatic or infectious cause
Complex
High vaginal septum
≥2.5 cm in diameter
IBD, irradiation, or neoplastic cause

The most common symptom is passage of gas through the vagina. When the fistula is large, vaginal discharge with fecal odor and vaginitis occur. Some patients have fecal incontinence.

Definitive diagnosis of rectovaginal fistula is made at examination. Digital examination of the anal canal reveals scarring and a defect in the anterior wall if the fistula is low. Anoscopy helps locate the opening in the anal canal. Proctoscopy is required to find middle and high fistulas. If the fistula cannot be seen, a tampon is placed in the vagina and methylene blue is instilled into the anorectum. Blue staining of the tampon is evidence of the fistula.

Nonsurgical healing of a rectovaginal fistula depends on the cause and, to a lesser extent, on the size. Half of small rectovaginal fistulas due to obstetric trauma heal spontaneously. Fistulas caused by a foreign body or infection often heal after the object is removed or the infection is treated. Fistulas resulting from Crohn's disease or irradiation rarely heal spontaneously.

For low, simple, and some mid-rectovaginal fistulas, surgical treatment is endorectal advancement of an anorectal flap. If the fistula is associated with incontinence due to injury to the external sphincter, sphincteroplasty is performed.

High and some mid-rectovaginal fistulas necessitate a transabdominal approach. Simple fistulas with healthy surrounding tissues are repaired by means of mobilization of the rectovaginal septum, division of the fistula, and layered closure of the rectal defect without intestinal resection. Complex rectovaginal fistulas are managed with a preliminary colostomy. For elderly or unfit patients, for

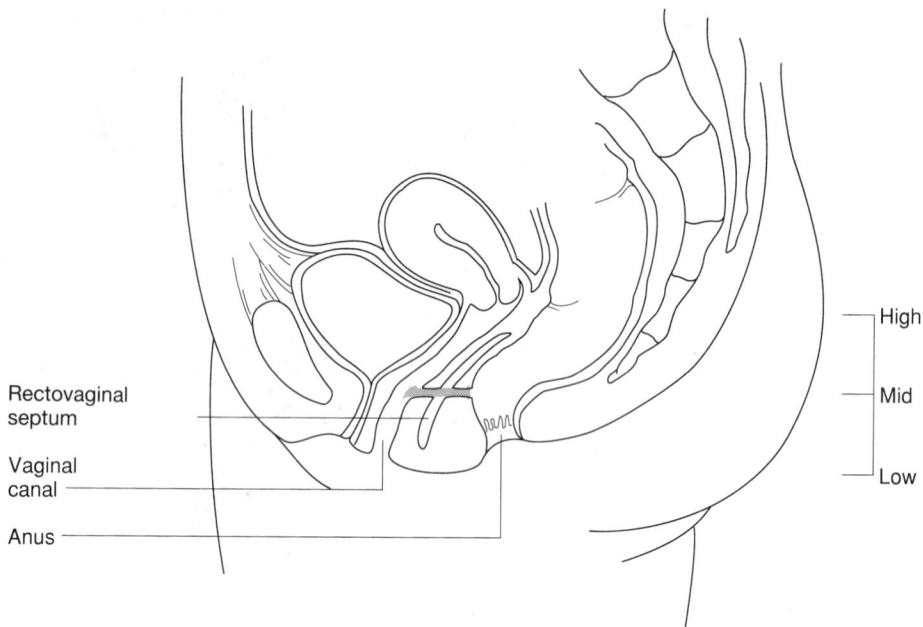

Rectovaginal
septum

Vaginal
canal

Anus

High

Mid

Low

Figure 52-12. Rectovaginal fistula classified by location. Fistulas are low when at or just cephalad to the dentate line, high when near the cervix, and mid when located in between.

most irradiation-induced fistulas, and for Crohn's disease-associated rectovaginal fistulas, a permanent colostomy may be performed.

ANAL INCONTINENCE

Anal incontinence ranges from simple involuntary passage of flatus to loss of sphincter tone with involuntary passage of formed stool. Causes are disturbance of normal anorectal anatomy or physiology, nerve damage that disturbs anorectal sensation, or direct mechanical injury, such as obstetric tear, fistulotomy, hemorrhoidectomy, internal sphincterotomy, anal stretching, and perineal trauma.

Diagnosis

Examination starts with detection of fecal material in the undergarments and evaluation of the degree of perianal skin excoriation. Gaping or laxity of the anus may be apparent and is a sign of neurogenic dysfunction of the sphincter muscles. Abnormal perineal descent, in which downward movement of the anus on straining is >2 cm below the plane of the ischial tuberosities, may indicate damage to the levator ani muscle. A scar or defect in the anal region may indicate surgical injury to the sphincter muscle. Digital examination provides an estimate of the tone of the internal sphincter muscle, and voluntary squeezing of the anal canal provides an estimate of the function of the external sphincter muscles.

Flexible sigmoidoscopy is always performed. Barium enema examination or total colonoscopy is usually indicated. Anal manometry is useful to evaluate the status of the sphincters.

Management

Regulation of bowel habit by decreasing bowel movement to once a day or once every other day, usually improves anal incontinence. A high-fiber diet makes the stool easier to evacuate. Biofeedback is used to retrain the ano-rectum to be aware of the sensation of rectal fullness and to retrain contraction of the sphincteric muscles.

Surgical treatment is provided when conservative management does not work. Sphincteroplasty is most suitable for incontinence due to obstetric injury or injury due to an anorectal operation. For patients who are incapacitated by complete fecal incontinence, a permanent end-sigmoid colostomy is performed.

ANORECTAL DISEASES IN PATIENTS WITH AIDS AND HIV-POSITIVITY
Kaposi Sarcoma

Most Kaposi sarcomas of the colon and rectum are asymptomatic, but bleeding, diarrhea, and obstruction may occur. The lesion has a characteristic red, round, submucosal nodule with central umbilication. A deep biopsy is required. There is no effective medical treatment. Surgical treatment is indicated only to control massive bleeding, perforation, or obstruction.

Cytomegalovirus

CMV enteroproctocolitis occurs in 5% to 10% of patients with AIDS but is responsible for 70% of all deaths among AIDS patients who undergo emergency abdominal operations. Symptoms of CMV enterocolitis are diarrhea, fever, right–lower-quadrant abdominal pain, and weight loss. Opportunistic infection is common. CMV enteroproctocolitis presents with sharply demarcated areas of shallow ulcers, frequently covered with fibrin. Biopsy allows correct diagnosis. The pathognomonic histopathologic feature is large, basophilic intranuclear CMV inclusions. Problems that most commonly necessitate emergency or urgent surgical intervention are bleeding and perforation of CMV ulcers. Medical treatment is with DHPG, ganciclovir, or phosphonoformate.

Lymphoma

Identification of anorectal lymphoma is difficult because the disease usually is extraluminal. The preoperative diagnosis usually is perianal abscess. Correct diagnosis relies on microscopic identification of B-cell immunoblastic configuration of extranodular lymphoma. It is worthwhile to excise the lesion if possible. Radiation and chemotherapy may hasten death by causing additional immunosuppression.

Anal Carcinoma

Squamous cell carcinoma of anus and cervix is caused by oncogenic human papilloma virus (HPV) infection. Patients at high risk for anal carcinoma undergo proctosigmoidoscopic and anoscopic examination. Application of 3% acetic acid helps identify areas of abnormal epithelium for biopsies. High-grade intraepithelial dysplasia is treated with local excision or electrocoagulation. Low-grade dysplasia is examined periodically. Invasive carcinoma is treated with chemoradiation therapy.

Anorectal Ulcers

Most ulcers occur in the posterior midline of the anus, somewhat closer to the dentate line than the usual anal fissure. Ulcers in HIV-positive patients are extremely erosive, dissecting along the submucosal and intersphincteric planes, often skeletonizing the internal sphincter muscle. These erosions produce pockets in which stool and pus collect, causing severe pain, especially on defecation. General anesthesia usually is required for examination of the anorectum. Biopsies are performed and the specimens sent for viral culture and dark field examination. If lymphoma is suspected, the tissue is sent for typing. Pocketing of the ulcers is corrected with débridement and division of a portion of the internal sphincter muscle. In patients with intolerable pain, sigmoid colostomy gives symptomatic relief.

SUGGESTED READING

Gamble B, Midwife RD. Suture rectopexy with colon resection for rectal prolapse. Semin Colon Rectal Surg 1991;2:193.
George BD, Williams NS. Electrically stimulated gracilis neoanal sphincter. Semin Colon Rectal Surg 1992;3:104.
Leff EI. Hemorrhoidectomy: Laser vs. nonlaser—outpatient surgical experience. Dis Colon Rectum 1992;35:743.
Loder PB, Kamm MA, Nicholls RJ, Phillips RKS. Hemorrhoids: pathology, pathophysiology and etiology. Br J Surg 1994; 81:946.
Lowry AC, Jensen LL. Biofeedback for fecal incontinence. Perspect Colon Rectal Surg 1992;5:210.
Palefsky JM. Rising incidence of anal cancer in HIV-positive patients: implications for the colorectal surgeons. Perspect Colon Rectal Surg 1994;7:115.
Schouten WR, Briel JW, Auwerda JJA. Relationship between anal pressure and anodermal blood flow. Dis Colon Rectum 1994;37:664.
Walsh PC, Schlegel PN. Radical pelvic surgery with preservation of sexual function. Ann Surg 1988;208:391.
Williams JG, Rothenberger DA, Midwife RD, Goldberg SM. Treatment of rectal prolapse in the elderly by perineal rectosigmoidectomy. Dis Colon Rectum 1992;35:830.
Wolff BG, Dietzen C. Abdominal resectional procedures for rectal prolapse. Semin Colon Rectal Surg 1991;2:184.

HERNIA, MESENTERY, AND RETROPERITONEUM

ESSENTIALS OF SURGERY: SCIENTIFIC PRINCIPLES AND PRACTICE,
edited by Lazar J. Greenfield, Michael W. Mulholland, Keith T. Oldham, Gerald B. Zelenock, and Keith D. Lillemoe. Lippincott–Raven Publishers, Philadelphia, © 1997.

CHAPTER 53

INGUINAL ANATOMY AND ABDOMINAL WALL HERNIAS

JAMES A. KNOL AND FREDERIC E. ECKHAUSER

ABDOMINAL WALL

The abdominal wall is a lattice of muscles that support, confine, and protect the viscera. It allows variation in intraabdominal pressure for defecation, micturition, vomiting, and coughing. It assists in respiration and erect posture and allows lateral and forward bending. The directions of the muscles, areas of overlap and lack of overlap, and functions of the aponeuroses and tendons are important in understanding incisions, formation and repair of hernias, and reconstruction of the abdominal wall after trauma or tumor excision.

Three sets of muscles—the *external* and *internal obliques* and the *transversus abdominis*—originate from the ribs, spine, and pelvic skeleton, each oriented at an angle to the next. The muscles insert into broad central aponeuroses, which insert into the linea alba (Figs. 53-1, 53-2). The combined force vector of these muscles is in a lateral direction. The aponeuroses of the lateral muscles ensheathe the vertically oriented *rectus abdominis,* which originates on the ribs superiorly and the pubis inferiorly and inserts into transversely oriented tendinous bands along its length. The posterolateral abdominal wall is composed of three layers, comprising a total of eight muscles (Fig. 53-3; Table 53-1).

The blood supply, venous and lymphatic drainage, and innervation of the abdominal wall run at a downward angle from posterior to anterior. The superior epigastric and inferior epigastric arteries and veins form a vascular supply and drainage that course vertically within the rectus abdominis muscle.

Nonmidline incisions that do not run parallel to the nerves sever them. The result is loss of skin sensation and motor innervation that may cause atrophy of the abdominal muscles.

THE INGUINAL AND PELVIC REGIONS

The structure of the inguinal and pelvic regions is illustrated in Figures 53-4 through 53-11. Within the skin and subcutaneous tissues in the region superior to the inguinal crease lie the superficial circumflex iliac, superficial epigastric, and external pudendal arteries and the accompanying veins. The arteries originate from the proximal femoral artery and course superiorly. The external spermatic artery originates from the inferior epigastric artery just inferior to the internal inguinal ring and runs along the spermatic cord.

HERNIA

A hernia is a protrusion of a structure, usually intestine, through tissue that normally contains it. Hernias are caused by:

- Physiologic alterations, such as lack of response of the internal inguinal ring to increases in intraabdominal pressure
- Biochemical and metabolic alterations, such as defects in collagen metabolism
- Chronic overstretching of musculoaponeurotic structures, such as those that occur in sports or pregnancy
- Congenital anatomic variations

Hernias of the Abdominal Wall (Table 53-2)

Inguinal and Femoral Hernias (Fig. 53-12)

Indirect inguinal hernias occur through the internal inguinal ring in a protrusion of peritoneum along the spermatic cord in the internal spermatic fascia. Large, indirect inguinal hernias descend into the scrotum along the spermatic cord. *Direct inguinal hernias* occur through the floor of the inguinal canal separate from the spermatic cord. Direct inguinal hernias occur because of a breakdown of the transversus abdominis aponeurosis and transversalis fascia. *Femoral hernias* occur into the femoral canal.

Hernias of the Anterior Abdominal Wall

Umbilical hernia. Results from an abdominal wall defect at the umbilicus that weakens the fascia. Considered congenital in children, acquired in adults (paraumbilical hernia).

Epigastric hernia. Occurs in the linea alba above the umbilicus.

Spigelian hernia. Rare hernia through the linea semilunaris (Fig. 53-13).

Interparietal hernia. Rare abdominal wall defect in which the hernial sac lies between layers of the abdominal wall. An example is preperitoneal hernia, in which the sac lies between the peritoneum and the transversalis fascia.

Supravesical hernia. Protrudes anterior to the bladder through the transversus abdominis muscle and transversalis fascia and forms a direct inguinal or femoral hernia (Fig. 53-14).

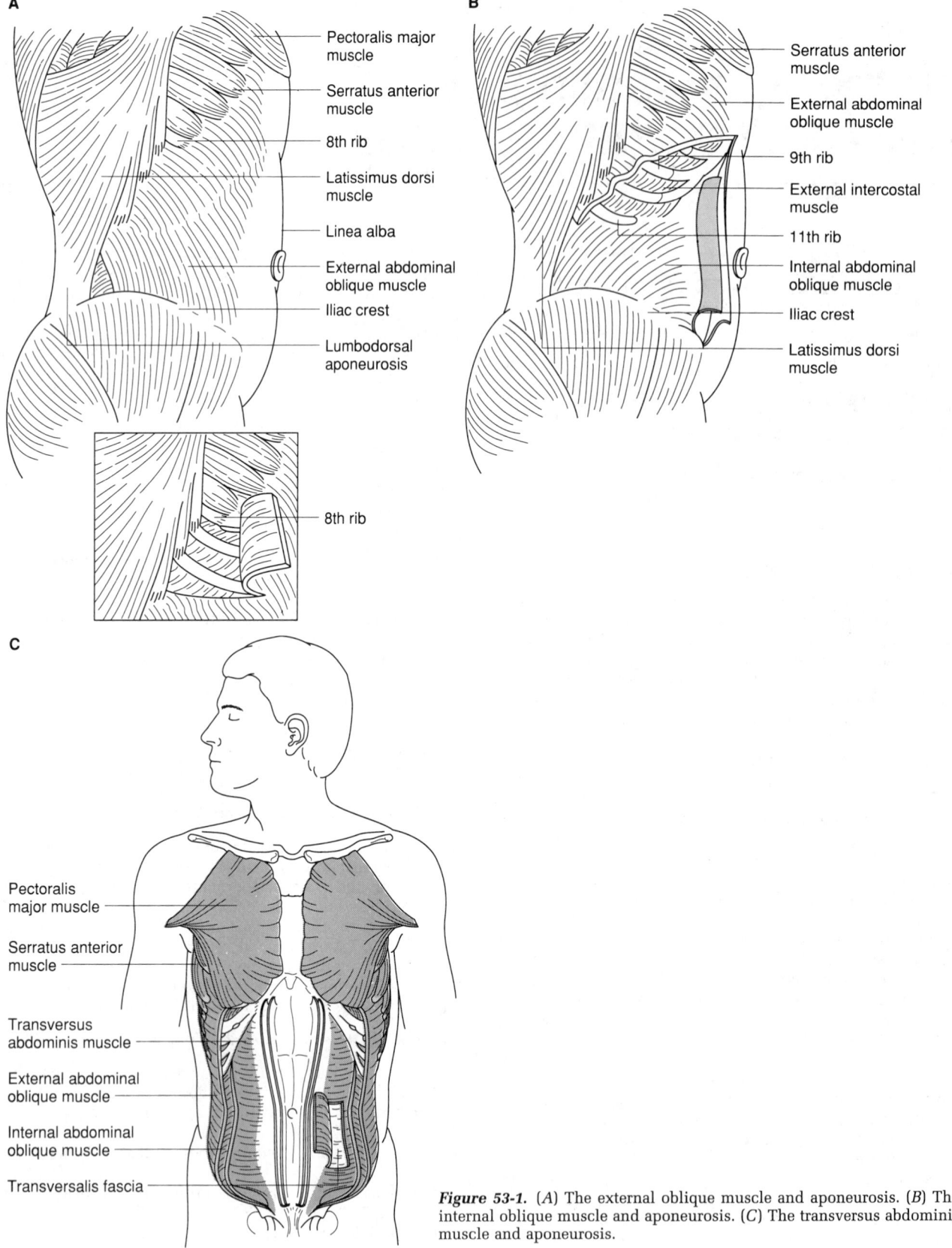

A

Pectoralis major muscle

Serratus anterior muscle

8th rib

Latissimus dorsi muscle

Linea alba

External abdominal oblique muscle

Iliac crest

Lumbodorsal aponeurosis

8th rib

B

Serratus anterior muscle

External abdominal oblique muscle

9th rib

External intercostal muscle

11th rib

Internal abdominal oblique muscle

Iliac crest

Latissimus dorsi muscle

C

Pectoralis major muscle

Serratus anterior muscle

Transversus abdominis muscle

External abdominal oblique muscle

Internal abdominal oblique muscle

Transversalis fascia

Figure 53-1. (*A*) The external oblique muscle and aponeurosis. (*B*) The internal oblique muscle and aponeurosis. (*C*) The transversus abdominis muscle and aponeurosis.

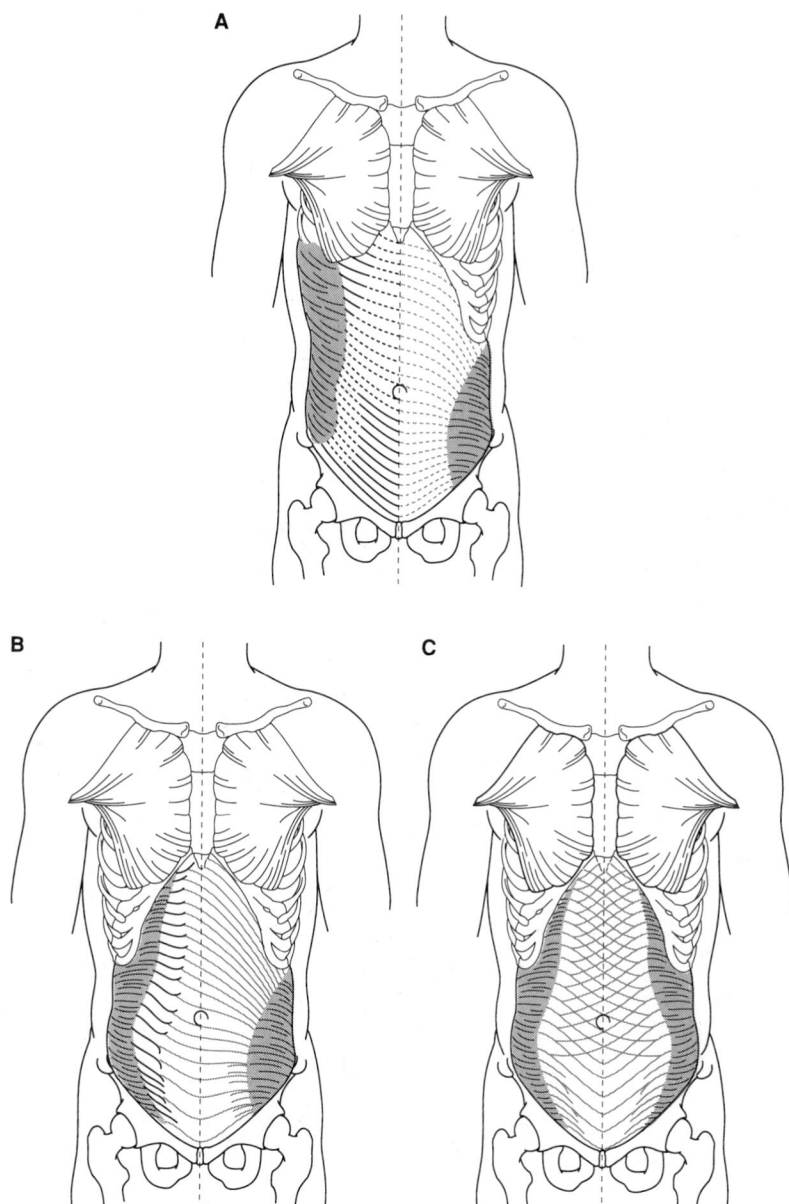

Figure 53-2. Pattern of the crossing of the aponeurotic fascicles of the abdominal wall musculature. (*A*) Fascicles from right external oblique and anterior lamina of left internal oblique. (*B*) Fascicles from right transversus abdominis and posterior lamina of left internal oblique. (*C*) Fascicles between right and left transversus abdominis.

Lumbar and Pelvic Hernias

Lumbar hernia. Occurs between the 12th rib and the iliac crest.

Obturator hernia. Anterior pelvic hernia through the obturator canal. Caused by progressive laxity of the pelvic floor associated with multiparity and increasing age.

Sciatic hernia. Protrusion of a peritoneal sac and contents through the major or minor sciatic foramen (Figs. 53-15, 53-16).

Perineal hernia. Protrusion of tissues through the muscles and fasciae of the pelvic diaphragm. Primary perineal hernias have no discernible cause; secondary perineal hernias occur after trauma to, or operations on, the pelvic floor (Fig. 53-17).

Internal Hernias

Defects in the peritoneum through which intestine and sometimes other viscera pass. No musculoaponeurotic defects are involved.

Paraduodenal hernia. Developmental hernia due to incomplete rotation of the midgut or invagination of the descending mesocolon by jejunum and ileum. Also called *mesocolic* or *mesentericoparietal* hernia.

Mesenteric hernia. Protrusion of peritoneal contents through a defect in the mesentery, omentum, or broad ligament.

Foramen of Winslow hernia. The cecum herniates through the foramen of Winslow.

Incisional Hernias

Incisional hernias often are related to a postoperative wound infection; associated fasciitis or muscle necrosis causes loss of tissue.

Diagnosis

History

The patient is asked about:

- A bulge
- Pain or discomfort

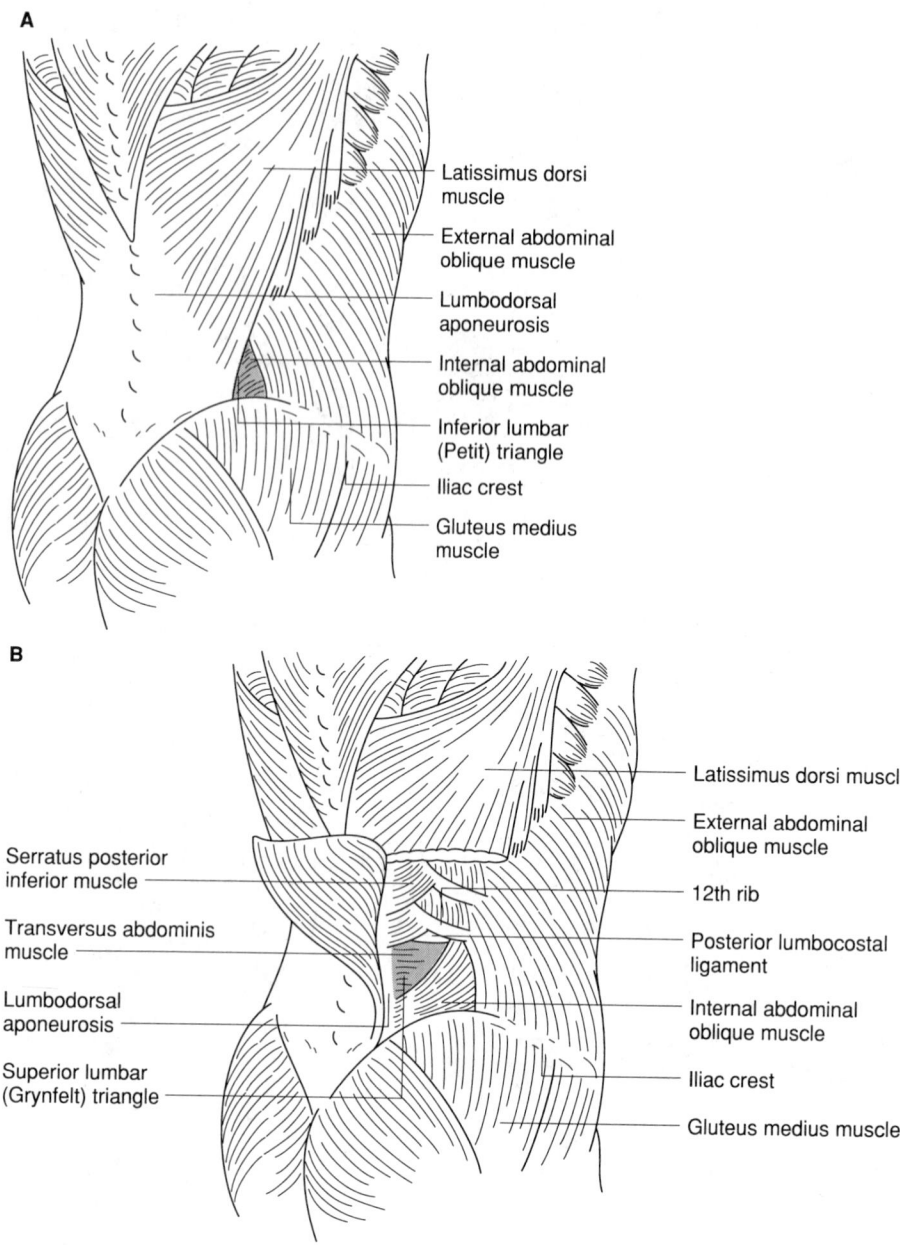

Figure 53-3. The lumbar abdominal wall with the inferior lumbar triangle (*A*) and the superior lumbar triangle (*B*).

Table 53-1. MUSCLES OF THE POSTEROLATERAL ABDOMINAL WALL

DEEP
Quadratus lumborum
Psoas major
Transversus abdominis

MIDLEVEL
Sacrospinalis
Internal oblique
Serratus posterior inferior

SUPERFICIAL
External oblique
Latissimus dorsi

- Symptoms of intermittent intestinal obstruction (distention, bloating, vomiting, and intermittent diarrhea and constipation)
- Previous hernias and repairs
- Use of medication that might retard healing, such as steroids or antineoplastic drugs
- Family history of hernia or connective tissue defects

Physical Examination

The physical examination includes the abdomen and the rectal area. Stool is tested for occult blood. The examination begins with the patient standing so that the abdominal contents exert maximal gravity-induced pressure at possible sites of a hernia. Additional intraabdominal pressure is obtained with a Valsalva maneuver. Palpation is directed toward a bulge that enlarges or appears with the Valsalva maneuver. An attempt is made to reduce the bulge.

If it is not clear whether a mass is reducible or is a hernia, an attempt is made to reduce the hernia with the patient

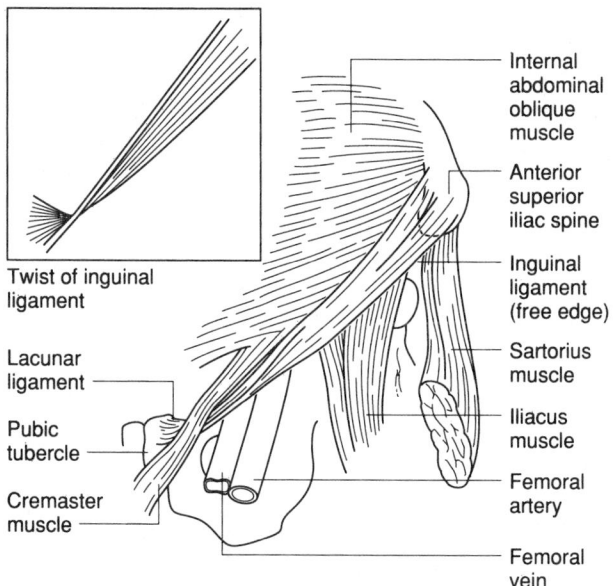

Figure 53-4. The anatomy of the inguinal ligament. The 180-degree twist of the external oblique aponeurosis forms a shelving edge in the lower portion of the ligament.

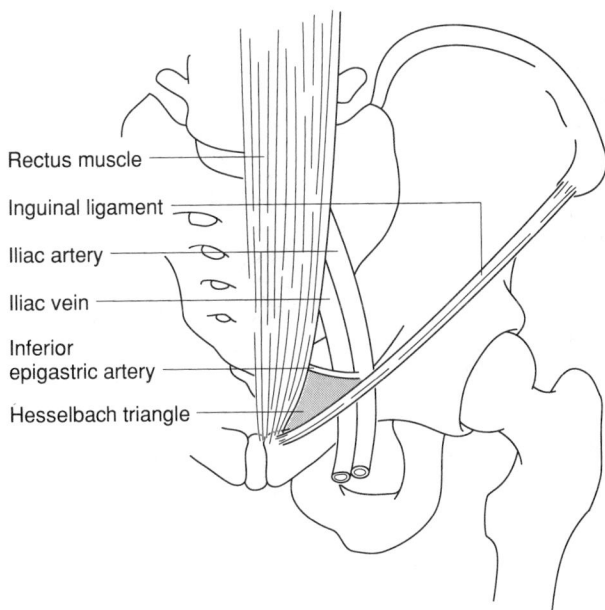

Figure 53-6. Hesselbach triangle.

lying down. Reappearance of the bulge when the patient stands confirms the presence of a hernia. The reducibility of a hernia, the size of the defect, and the proportion of abdominal contents outside the confines of the abdominal cavity are important factors. Previous scars and changes in the overlying skin are meaningful.

Diagnostic Imaging

Plain radiographs of the abdomen may depict gas-containing intestine outside the confines of the abdominal wall. Barium contrast radiographs of the gastrointestinal (GI) tract may show intestine emerging from a defect in

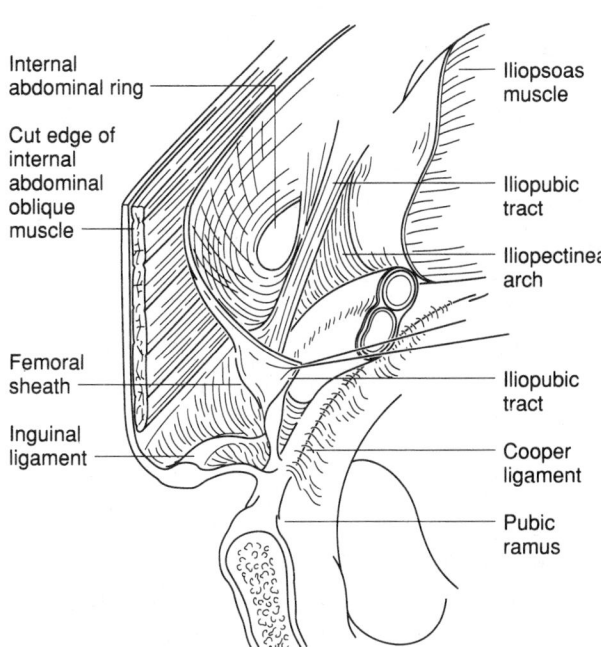

Figure 53-5. The deep aponeurotic layer at the groin.

the abdominal wall, but the abdominal and pelvic walls cannot be visualized.

Ultrasonography (US) may show hernias, abdominal wall structures, and gas or fluid. *Computed tomography* (CT) shows abdominal and pelvic wall structures (usually), abdominal wall defects (sometimes), gas, fluid collections, and contrast material in intestine outside the confines of the abdominal or pelvic walls, particularly if the patient performs a Valsalva maneuver. *Herniography* shows the presence and site of origin of inguinal and pelvic hernias.

Clinical Manifestations
Uncomplicated Hernias

The symptoms of uncomplicated hernias are a dull ache and a bulge. The ache is sometimes described as burning or pain. Patients describe the bulge as being prominent during activity or with any maneuver that increases intraabdominal pressure and as decreasing or nonexistent when the patient is lying down. Some hernias are asymptomatic and discovered in the course of a routine physical examination.

Complicated Hernias

The severe complications of hernias are incarceration, intestinal obstruction, and intestinal strangulation. A complication is more likely to occur when the hernial sac is large relative to the diameter of the hernial defect and in hernias in which the intestine has access to the hernial sac.

Treatment
Nonsurgical Management

Nonsurgical therapy is appropriate for umbilical hernias <3 cm in diameter and for small epigastric hernias in children younger than 4 years, if the hernia is not enlarging or incarcerated. Use of a corset or binder is appropriate for patients who are at greater risk because of concomitant disease or because surgical repair may be dangerous for them than because of complications of the hernia. *Use of*

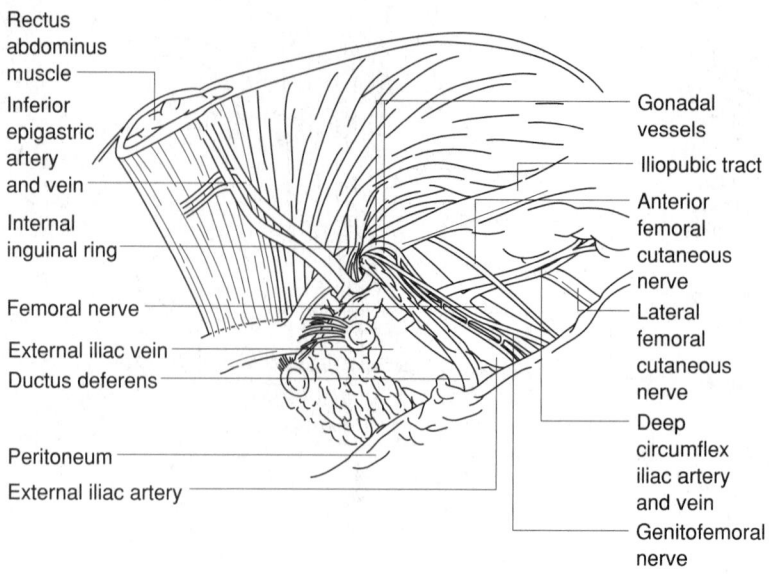

Rectus abdominus muscle
Inferior epigastric artery and vein
Internal inguinal ring
Femoral nerve
External iliac vein
Ductus deferens
Peritoneum
External iliac artery

Gonadal vessels
Iliopubic tract
Anterior femoral cutaneous nerve
Lateral femoral cutaneous nerve
Deep circumflex iliac artery and vein
Genitofemoral nerve

Figure 53-7. Anatomy of the inguinal region from the internal aspect, as seen with the laparoscopic approach.

these devices is contraindicated if the hernia is incarcerated or has a narrow neck relative to the sac.

Surgical Management

Most primary repairs of groin hernias are performed on an outpatient basis with local anesthesia. Complications necessitate an emergency operation.

Surgical repair of a hernia is directed first at the sac and its contents and then at the structural defect, usually in the abdominal wall. To prevent entrapment of visceral contents, a peritoneal sac with a narrow neck is closed at the neck after evacuation of the visceral contents, and excess sac is excised. A sac with a broad entrance is not excised or closed. Repairs of inguinal hernias are shown in Figures 53-18 through 53-21.

Repair of the abdominal wall defect is the most important aspect of hernia repair. The principles of wound closure apply (direct apposition of strong musculoaponeurotic structures without tension). Closure under no tension whatsoever is rarely achieved, so the goal must be to minimize tension at the closure. A relaxing incision is used for this purpose. Grafts of prosthetic material, such as polypropylene mesh, expanded polytetrafluoroethylene sheeting, or tantalum wire mesh, often are used to repair large hernial defects. Musculoaponeurotic or aponeurotic flaps also can be used.

Complications of hernia repair include injury to motor or sensory nerves and nearby organs, including urinary bladder, femoral vein, and intestine; ischemia or necrosis of viscera, if the blood vessels supplying them are injured; and hernia recurrence.

MESENTERY
Anatomy

The mesentery consists of the small-intestinal mesentery, the transverse mesocolon, and the sigmoid mesocolon.

At the base of the small-intestinal mesentery are the ileo-

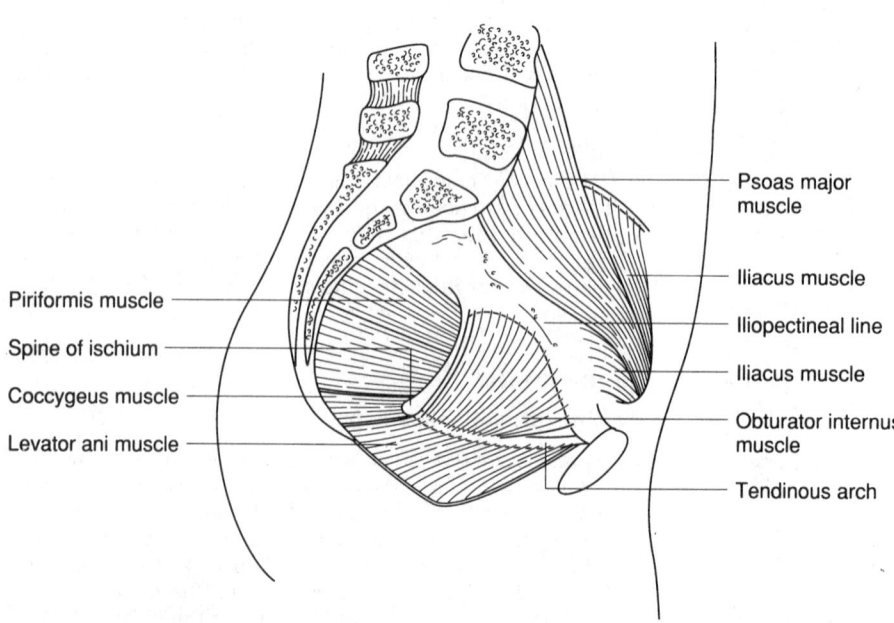

Piriformis muscle
Spine of ischium
Coccygeus muscle
Levator ani muscle

Psoas major muscle
Iliacus muscle
Iliopectineal line
Iliacus muscle
Obturator internus muscle
Tendinous arch

Figure 53-8. Musculature of the pelvis.

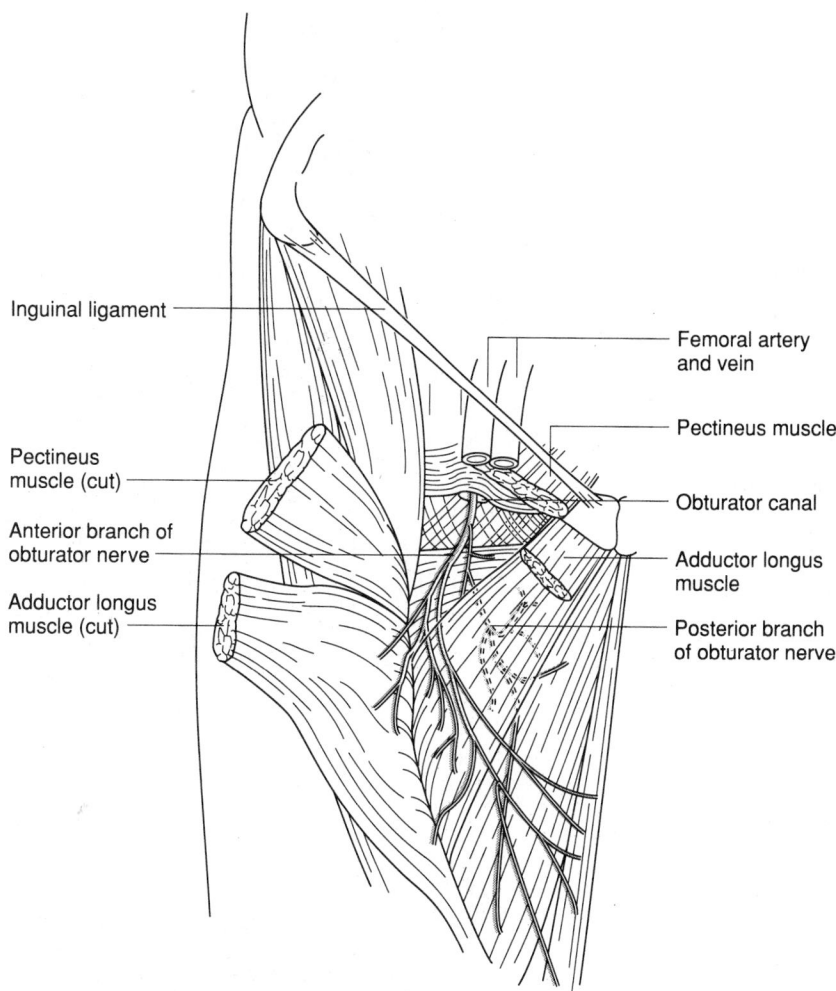

Inguinal ligament

Femoral artery and vein

Pectineus muscle (cut)

Pectineus muscle

Anterior branch of obturator nerve

Obturator canal

Adductor longus muscle (cut)

Adductor longus muscle

Posterior branch of obturator nerve

Figure 53-9. External relations of the obturator canal.

colic artery and vein, which are branches of the superior mesenteric artery (SMA) and vein, which supply blood to the right colon and terminal ileum. The proximal part of the small intestine receives blood through trunks that divide into arcades and anastomose with corresponding arcades from the next most proximal and distal trunk. From these arcades, vasa rectae course directly to the mesenteric margin of the intestine.

The important blood vessels in the *transverse mesocolon* are the middle colic artery, usually the second or third branch of the SMA, and the corresponding vein, which joins with the right gastroepiploic vein to form the gastrocolic trunk, a high tributary into the superior mesenteric vein. Sometimes a supplementary transverse colic artery courses to the left of the middle colic vessels with direct origin from the SMA.

The *sigmoid mesocolon* contains sigmoid arteries, branches of the inferior mesenteric artery, and the sigmoid veins, tributaries of the inferior mesenteric vein.

Lymphatic drainage channels in the mesenteries follow the course of the arteries and drain into the cisterna chyli. Sympathetic and parasympathetic nerves also course along arteries.

Inflammatory Diseases of the Mesentery

Acute Mesenteric Lymphadenitis

Acute mesenteric lymphadenitis is a syndrome of acute, right-lower-quadrant abdominal pain associated with mesenteric lymphatic enlargement and a normal appendix.

The diagnosis of a normal appendix and mesenteric lymphadenitis usually is made at operation for suspected appendicitis. Nodal histologic specimens and cultures are obtained, the terminal ileum is examined, and stool cultures and serologic titers are obtained for tests for microbial agents. Treatment of acute mesenteric lymphadenitis depends on the cause. The course of disease due to some infections is self-limited and resolves before definitive diagnosis is obtained.

Mesenteric Panniculitis

Mesenteric panniculitis is inflammation of the adipose tissue of the mesentery. The small-intestinal mesentery is the most frequent site. Many patients have undergone an abdominal operation. The condition is characterized by a thickened, hard, rubbery or nodular mesentery or by multiple mesenteric masses of similar consistency. Irregular areas of discoloration from gray to reddish brown to pale yellow are scattered throughout the mesentery. The mesentery may be foreshortened and scarred and the intestine distorted.

Symptoms are abdominal pain, vomiting, abdominal mass or swelling, anorexia, weight loss, constipation, diarrhea, and rectal bleeding. Physical examination usually reveals an abdominal mass. Laboratory studies may show an elevated erythrocyte sedimentation rate. Except for leukocytosis in some patients, biochemical or hematologic alterations are unusual.

Barium contrast examination of the small and large

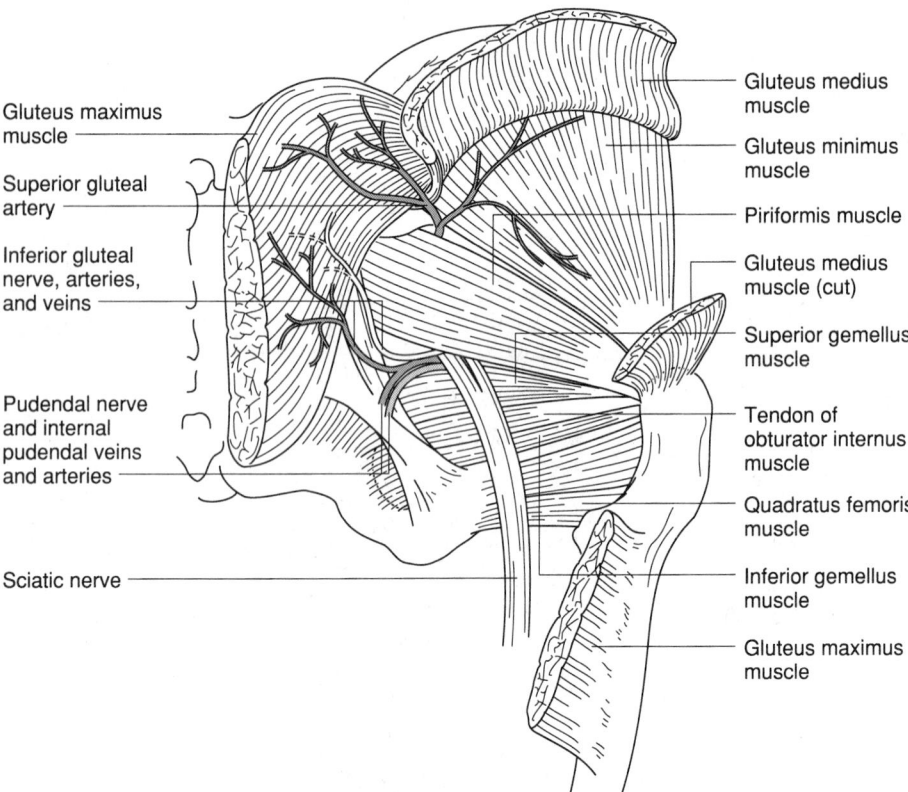

Gluteus maximus muscle

Superior gluteal artery

Inferior gluteal nerve, arteries, and veins

Pudendal nerve and internal pudendal veins and arteries

Sciatic nerve

Gluteus medius muscle

Gluteus minimus muscle

Piriformis muscle

Gluteus medius muscle (cut)

Superior gemellus muscle

Tendon of obturator internus muscle

Quadratus femoris muscle

Inferior gemellus muscle

Gluteus maximus muscle

Figure 53-10. External relations of the sciatic foramens.

intestines often reveals extrinsic displacement of intestinal loops, dilated loops of small intestine, and a spiculated or serrated mucosal surface. Laparotomy for surgical evaluation and biopsy of the mass is necessary for definitive diagnosis. Mesenteric panniculitis rarely requires treatment.

Neoplasms of the Mesentery

Primary tumors of the mesentery are rare. Symptoms of both cystic and solid primary neoplasms of the mesentery occur when the tumor is so large that partial intestinal

obstruction occurs. The most common symptom is abdominal pain, usually cramping and intermittent. Other symptoms are nausea, vomiting, distention, constipation, and diarrhea.

A palpable abdominal mass is the most frequent physical finding and relates to the size of the tumor. Characteristic of mesenteric masses is mobility on palpation in the transverse but not in the craniocaudal axis of the body. A less common abdominal finding is ascites. Complications of mesenteric neoplasms include intestinal obstruction, volvulus of intestine around the tumor with intestinal infarction and peritonitis, torsion of the tumor, hemorrhage

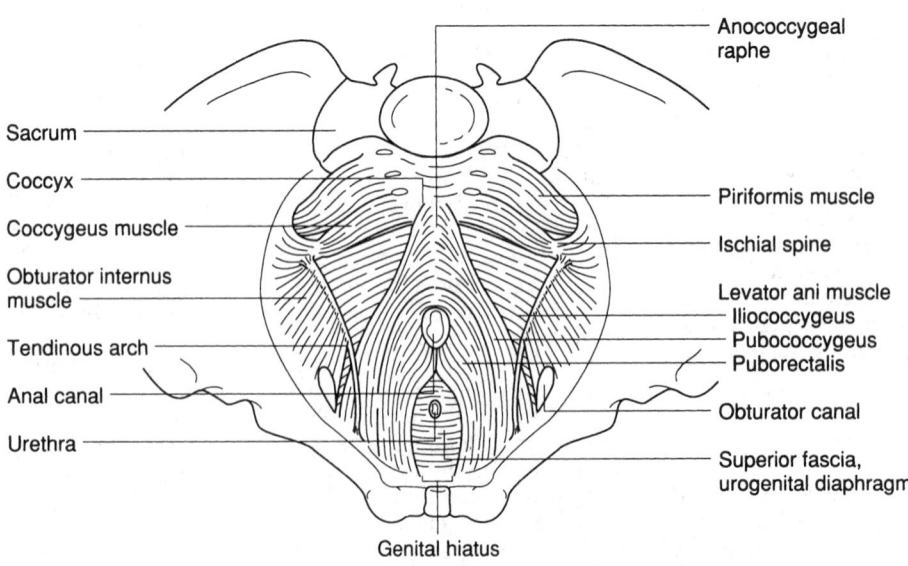

Sacrum

Coccyx

Coccygeus muscle

Obturator internus muscle

Tendinous arch

Anal canal

Urethra

Anococcygeal raphe

Piriformis muscle

Ischial spine

Levator ani muscle
Iliococcygeus
Pubococcygeus
Puborectalis

Obturator canal

Superior fascia, urogenital diaphragm

Genital hiatus

Figure 53-11. Pelvic diaphragm.

Table 53-2. TYPES OF HERNIAS

INGUINAL
Indirect
Direct
Femoral

HERNIAS OF THE ANTERIOR ABDOMINAL WALL
Umbilical
Paraumbilical
Epigastric
Spigelian
Interparietal
Supravesical

LUMBAR AND PELVIC HERNIAS
Lumbar
Obturator
Sciatic
Perineal

INTERNAL HERNIAS
Paraduodenal
Mesenteric
Hernia of the foramen of Winslow

INCISIONAL HERNIAS

into the tumor with rapid enlargement and sometimes anemia, and rupture of cystic tumors.

Laboratory studies are likely to be normal. Plain abdominal radiographs may depict displacement of intestinal gas and sometimes the presence of calcium (in a teratoma). GI contrast studies in the absence of intestinal complications of the neoplasm reveal only displacement of intestinal loops or extrinsic compression of intestine. US shows the internal structure of cystic structures better than CT, and magnetic resonance imaging (MRI) helps locate the tumor. No modality allows differentiation between solid primary and secondary or metastatic tumor or inflammatory lesions. Malignant cystic lesions cannot be differentiated from benign lesions.

Treatment of mesenteric neoplastic lesions is complete excision. Suspected malignant lesions are resected with a wide margin. Small intestine frequently must be resected with the malignant tumor because of encroachment on the vascular supply or involvement of the intestine. Even benign tumors may necessitate intestinal resection for complete excision. Neoplasms of the mesentery recur if excision is less than complete.

Mesenteric Cysts

The common nonneoplastic mesenteric cysts are called *mesothelial cysts.* Most are situated in the small-intestinal mesentery. These cysts may contain chyle when located in the mesentery of the proximal intestine and clear fluid when located in the distal small-intestinal or colonic mesentery.

Symptoms and complications of mesothelial cysts parallel those of cystic neoplasms and correlate with size of the cyst. Diagnostic imaging is with US, CT, or MRI.

Treatment is enucleation of the cyst, which is easy because the mesenteric blood vessels and intestine rarely adhere closely to the wall of the cyst. Internal drainage of the cyst into the peritoneal cavity after excision of a large portion of the cyst wall is an acceptable alternative. The cyst wall is examined for rough, friable, papillary projections that suggest malignancy.

OMENTUM
Anatomy

The omenta are broad, thin structures that extend from the stomach to other organs. They are covered on both surfaces with peritoneum. The *gastrocolic ligament* is the portion of greater omentum that extends from the greater curvature of the stomach to the transverse colon. The *greater omentum* contains mainly adipose and vascular tissue.

The *lesser omentum* extends from the lesser curvature of the stomach to the inferior and medial aspect of the liver at the level of the hilum and extends superiorly anterior to left margin of the caudate lobe. The lesser omentum contains the anterior and posterior vagus nerves to the stomach, the vagus nerves to the liver and gallbladder, the right

(text continues on page 394)

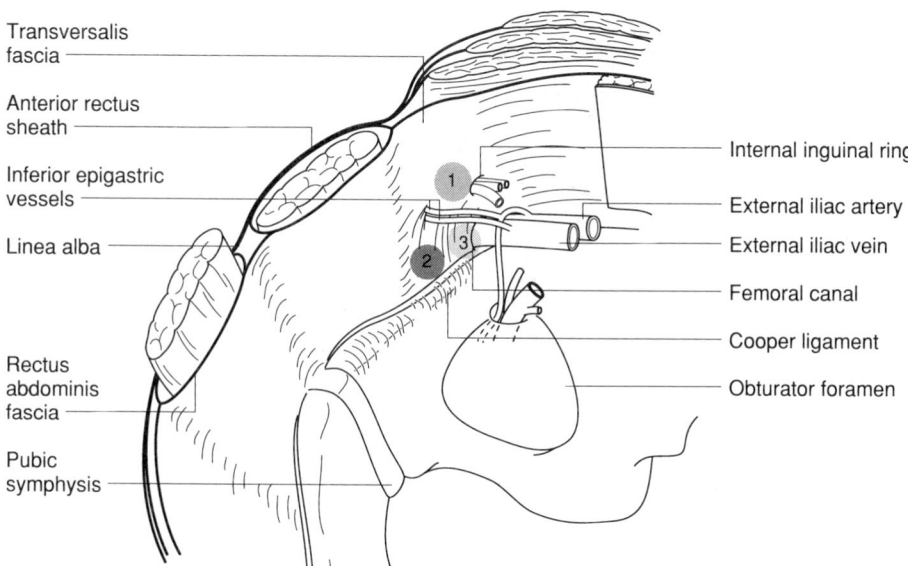

Transversalis fascia
Anterior rectus sheath
Inferior epigastric vessels
Linea alba
Rectus abdominis fascia
Pubic symphysis

Internal inguinal ring
External iliac artery
External iliac vein
Femoral canal
Cooper ligament
Obturator foramen

Figure 53-12. Posterior view of the inguinal region. (1) Site of indirect inguinal hernia, along the spermatic cord. (2) Site of direct inguinal hernia, through the inguinal floor. (3) Site of femoral hernia, the internal orifice of the femoral canal.

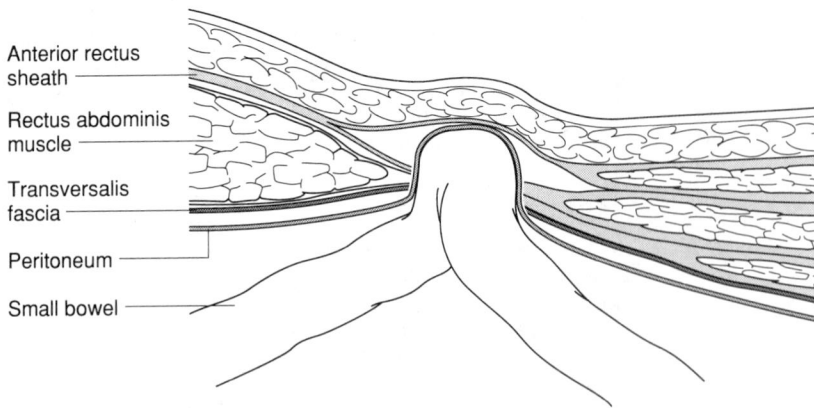

Anterior rectus sheath
Rectus abdominis muscle
Transversalis fascia
Peritoneum
Small bowel

Figure 53-13. Schematic cross section of a spigelian hernia.

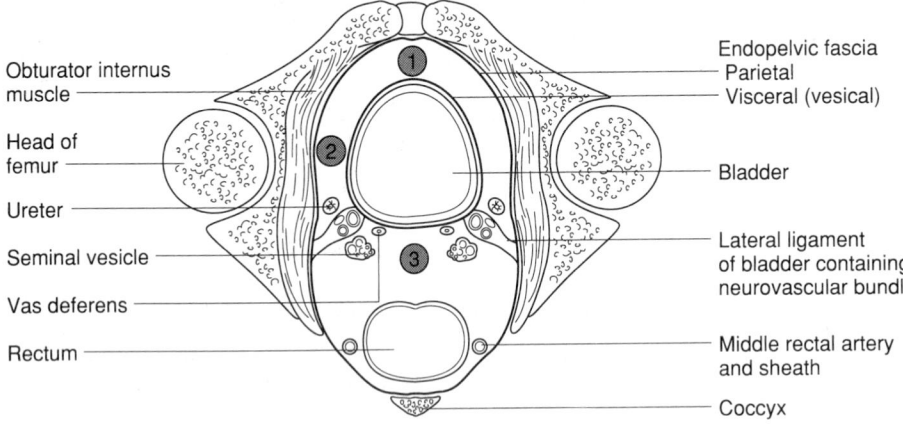

Obturator internus muscle
Head of femur
Ureter
Seminal vesicle
Vas deferens
Rectum

Endopelvic fascia
Parietal
Visceral (vesical)
Bladder
Lateral ligament of bladder containing neurovascular bundle
Middle rectal artery and sheath
Coccyx

Figure 53-14. Anatomic relations in supravesical hernia. (1) Site of anterior internal supravesical hernia. (2) Site of lateral internal supravesical hernia. (3) Site of posterior internal supravesical hernia.

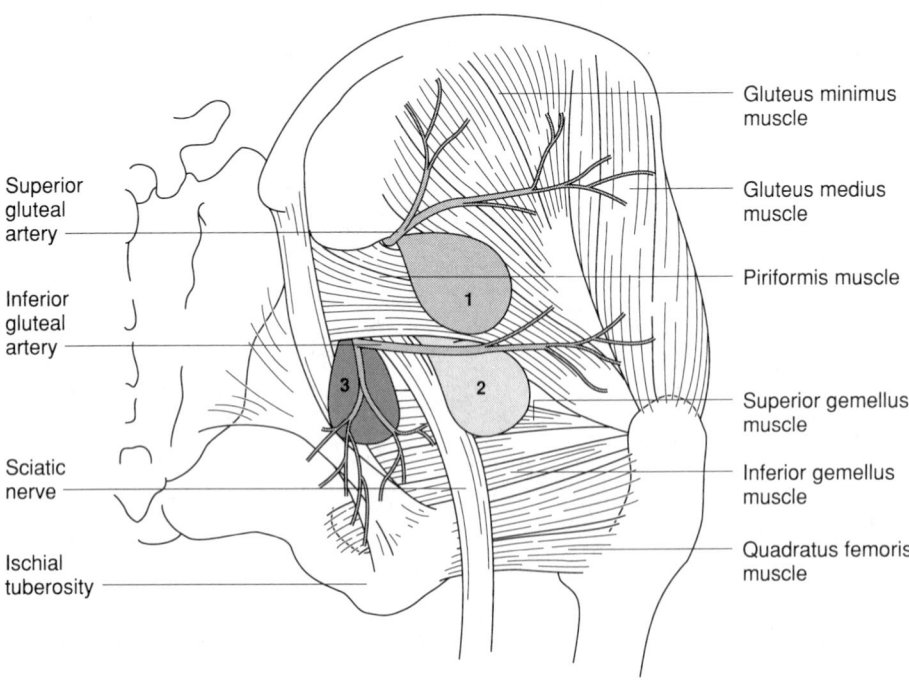

Superior gluteal artery
Inferior gluteal artery
Sciatic nerve
Ischial tuberosity

Gluteus minimus muscle
Gluteus medius muscle
Piriformis muscle
Superior gemellus muscle
Inferior gemellus muscle
Quadratus femoris muscle

Figure 53-15. Anatomic classification of sciatic hernia. (1) Suprapiriform hernia. (2) Infrapiriform hernia. (3) Subspinous hernia.

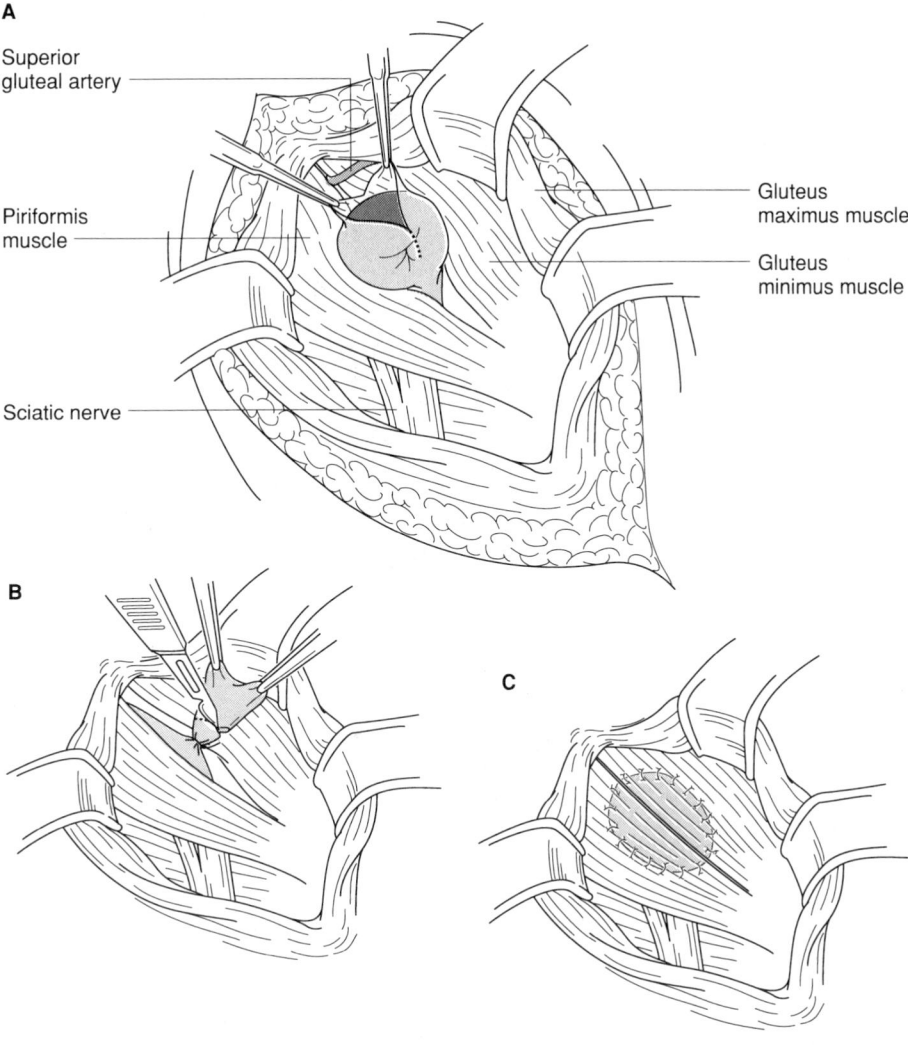

Figure 53-16. Transgluteal repair of sciatic hernia. (*A*) Gluteus maximus separated; sac opened; and ring around neck of sac incised to reduce contents. (*B*) Neck of sac ligated; excess sac excised. (*C*) Mesh prosthesis used to close defect.

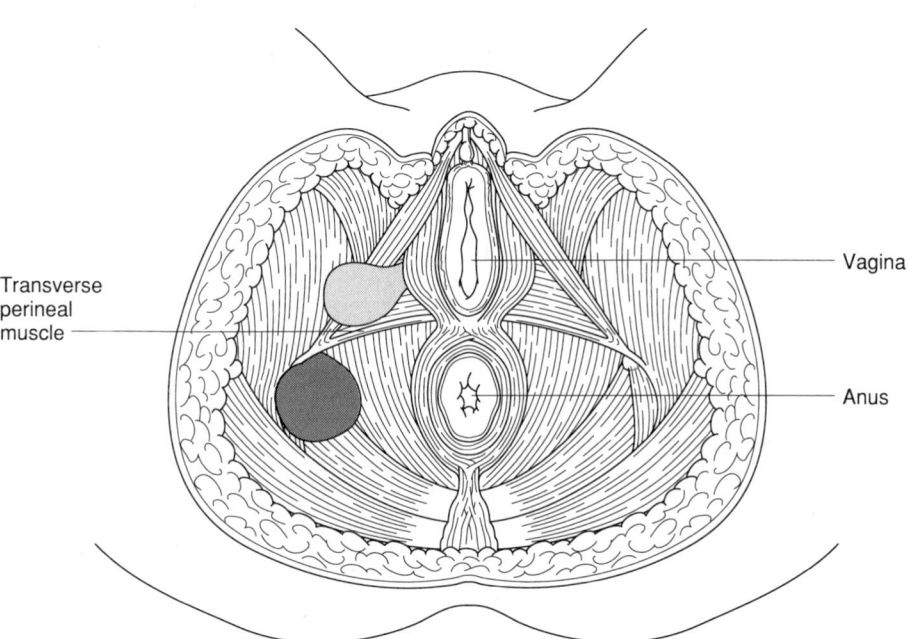

Figure 53-17. Perineal hernia. Transverse perineal muscles distinguish anterior from posterior perineal hernias.

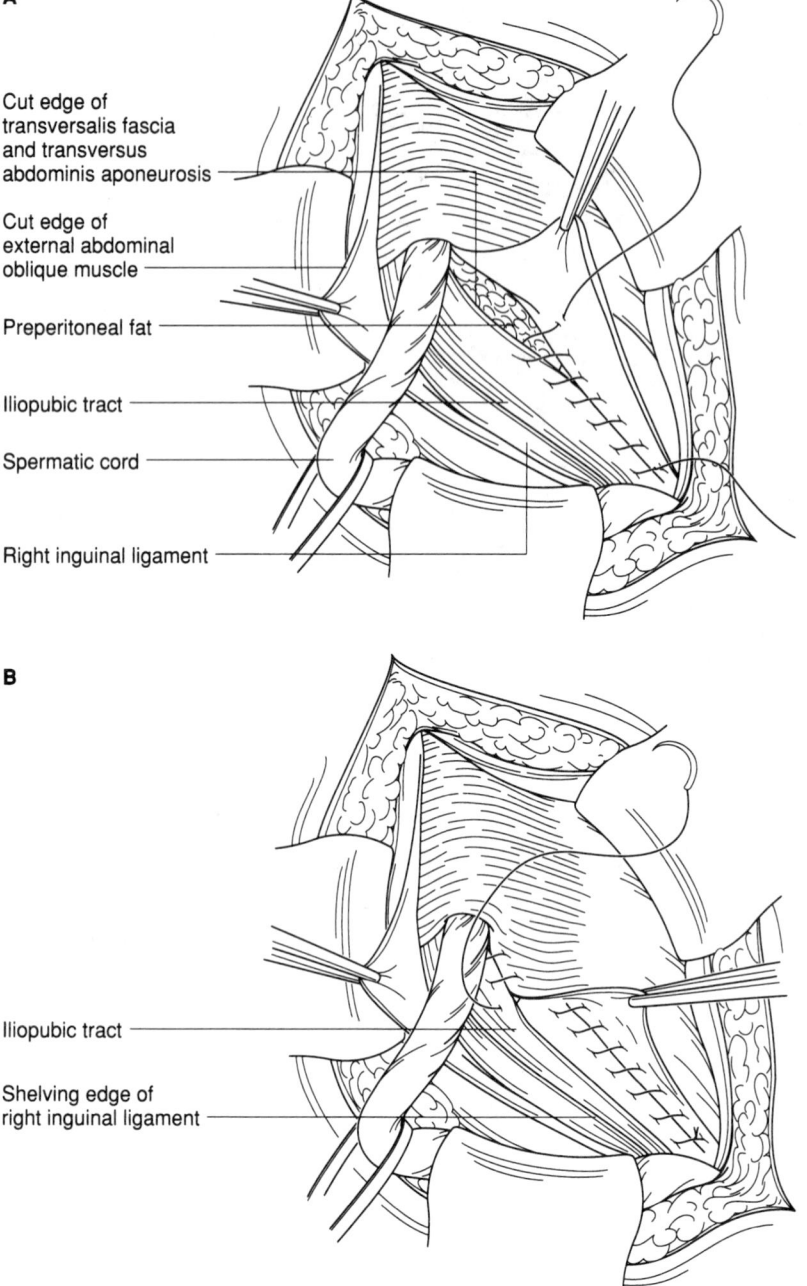

A

Cut edge of
transversalis fascia
and transversus
abdominis aponeurosis

Cut edge of
external abdominal
oblique muscle

Preperitoneal fat

Iliopubic tract

Spermatic cord

Right inguinal ligament

B

Iliopubic tract

Shelving edge of
right inguinal ligament

Figure 53-18. Shouldice inguinal hernia repair.
(*A*) The first of the suture lines approximates
the lateral cut edge of transversus abdominis
aponeurosis and transversalis fascia to the undersurface of these same structures near the
edge of the rectus abdominis muscle. (*B*) The
second suture line joins the medial cut edge
of the inguinal floor to the iliopubic tract and
shelving edge of the inguinal ligament. Two
additional suture lines, approximating progressively more superficial medial to lateral
musculoaponeurotic structures, are frequently
omitted.

gastric artery, the ramifications of the left gastric artery,
and sometimes the left hepatic artery.

Omental Disease

Omental Torsion

Twisting of the omentum causes ischemia and pain.
Torsion may lead to ischemic necrosis of the involved
portion of omentum. Omental torsion is *primary*, no
identifiable cause, or *secondary*, caused by adhesions of
the free end of omentum. Torsion also may be *unipolar*,
the free end of omentum undergoes torsion, or *bipolar*,
the omentum is twisted between its base and an adhesion
at the free end. For example, secondary bipolar omental
torsion occurs when the neck of a hernia is an attachment

point and the intraabdominal portion of omentum becomes twisted.

The symptom of omental torsion is acute, unremitting, mild to severe abdominal pain that usually localizes to the right-lower quadrant. Other symptoms are
nausea and vomiting and low-grade fever. Physical
findings are abdominal tenderness, guarding, mild rebound tenderness usually in the right-lower quadrant,
and sometimes a palpable abdominal mass. *Leukocytosis* is frequent.

Preoperative diagnosis of omental torsion is uncommon.
At *laparotomy*, there may be free serosanguineous fluid in
the abdominal cavity. Omental torsion is suspected when
the appendix is normal and the symptoms and findings of
torsion are present. Treatment is excision of the involved
portion of omentum.

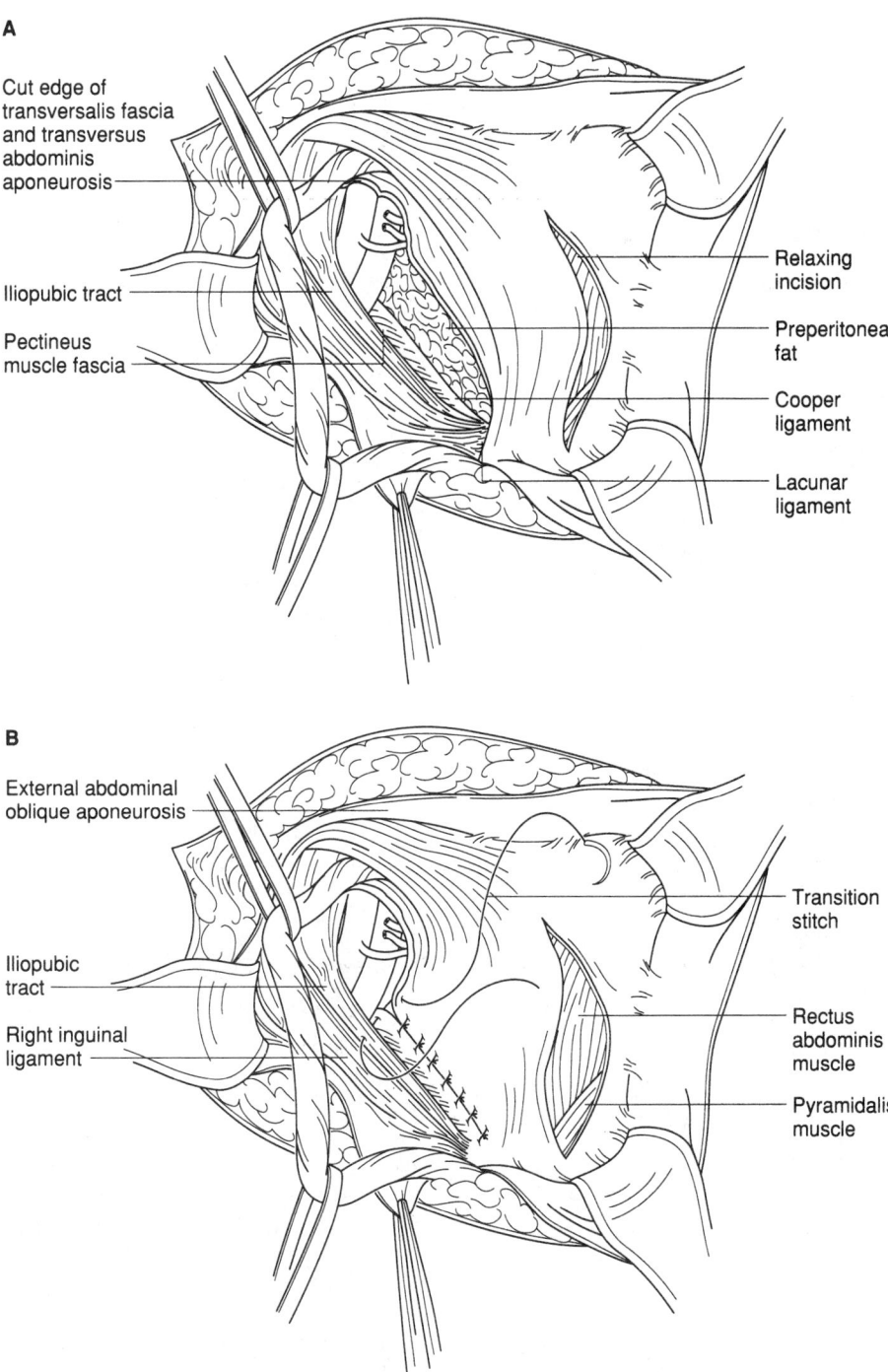

Figure 53-19. Cooper ligament repair. (*A*) Anatomy with the attenuated inguinal floor excised and the relaxing incision made. (*B*) Approximation of the conjoined structures medially to the Cooper ligament laterally, with placement of the transition stitch through conjoined structures, Cooper ligament, pectineus muscle fascia, and iliopubic tract. The internal ring is closed by approximation of transversalis fascia and transversis abdominis muscle medially to iliopubic tract laterally.

Omental Cysts

Omental cysts are similar to mesenteric cysts. Treatment is excision or enucleation. After cyst removal, but before the abdomen is closed, the cyst interior must be examined for papillary projections, which suggest malignant growth.

Omental Neoplasms

Almost all omental neoplasms are metastases. Primary omental tumors are usually benign cystic neoplasms, usually cystic lymphangioma.

The symptoms of omental tumors are abdominal pain, abdominal distention, a sense of weight in the abdomen, and, less frequently, weakness and weight loss, diarrhea, and nausea and vomiting. A *palpable mass* is usually present and is often mobile. The site from which the mass originates may not be apparent, especially with larger masses. The solid or cystic nature of the mass may be determined with abdominal US and CT, but its origin in the omentum usually cannot be found with preoperative studies. Abdominal radiographs and GI contrast studies reveal only displacement of intestine.

When a solid mass is found in the omentum during an operation, the surgeon searches for the primary tumor

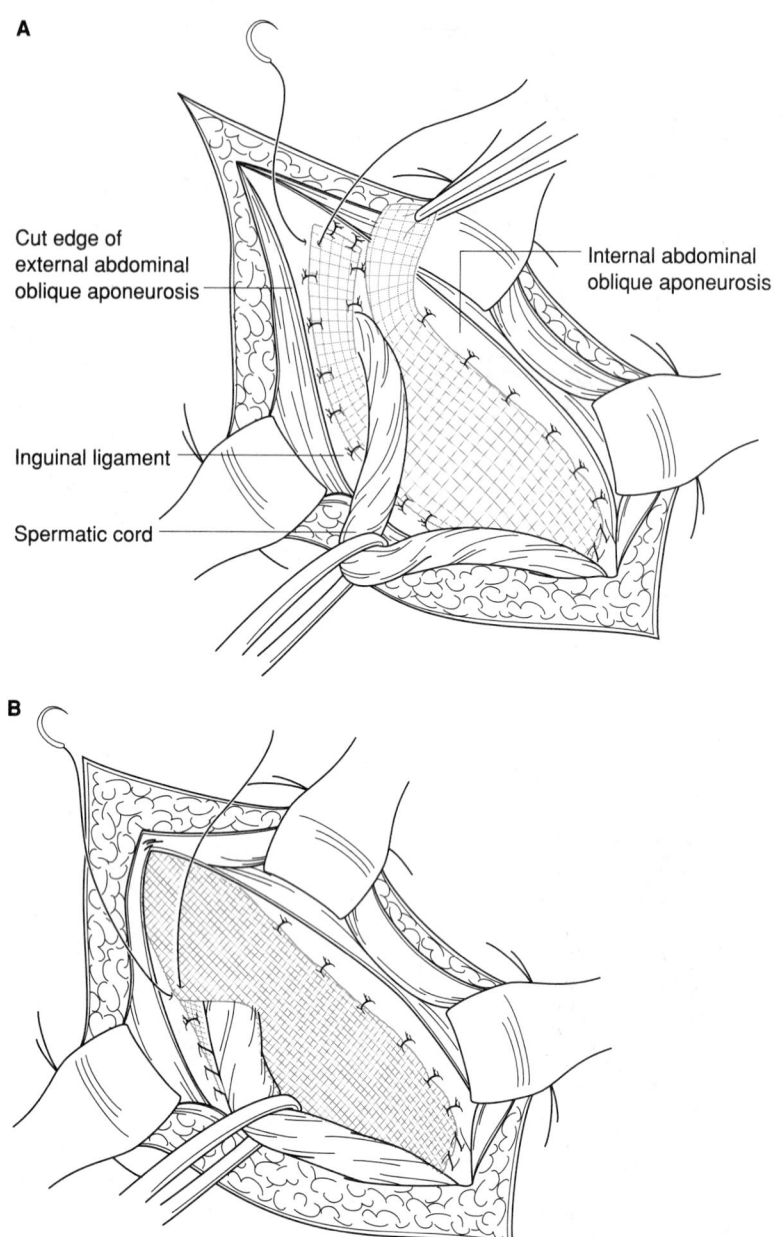

A

Cut edge of
external abdominal
oblique aponeurosis

Internal abdominal
oblique aponeurosis

Inguinal ligament

Spermatic cord

B

Figure 53-20. Placement of mesh in repair of inguinal hernia.

from which it may have metastasized. If the mass is a primary tumor, it is excised with margins. Peritoneal and liver metastases are frequent. Benign tumors are almost always easily excised, but malignant tumors may defy resection.

RETROPERITONEUM

Anatomy

The retroperitoneum is the portion of the torso posterior to the peritoneal cavity. It is contiguous with the mesentery and with soft tissues that lie between the peritoneum and the muscles of the abdominal wall.

Organs in the retroperitoneum are the adrenal glands, kidneys, ureters, bladder, pancreas, second through fourth portions of the duodenum, ascending and descending colon, upper two-thirds of the rectum, upper vagina, ovaries, seminal vesicles, a portion of the vas deferens, the abdominal aorta and iliac arteries, and the abdominal inferior vena

cava and iliac veins and accompanying lymphatic vessels, including the cisterna chyli. The esophagus, upper stomach, liver, and spleen abut the retroperitoneum.

Most of the blood supply, venous drainage (except the liver), and lymphatic drainage below the diaphragm and thoracic dermatomes courses through the retroperitoneum. The retroperitoneum is divided into the lumbar fossa and the iliac fossa.

Retroperitoneal Diseases

Retroperitoneal Abscess

Inflammation spreads widely in the retroperitoneum. The origin of a retroperitoneal abscess may be difficult to pinpoint, even during an operation. CT is used for evaluation of the retroperitoneum, but identification of the origin of inflammation may be impossible. At operation, the retroperitoneum must be widely exposed if the origin of the abscess is to be located.

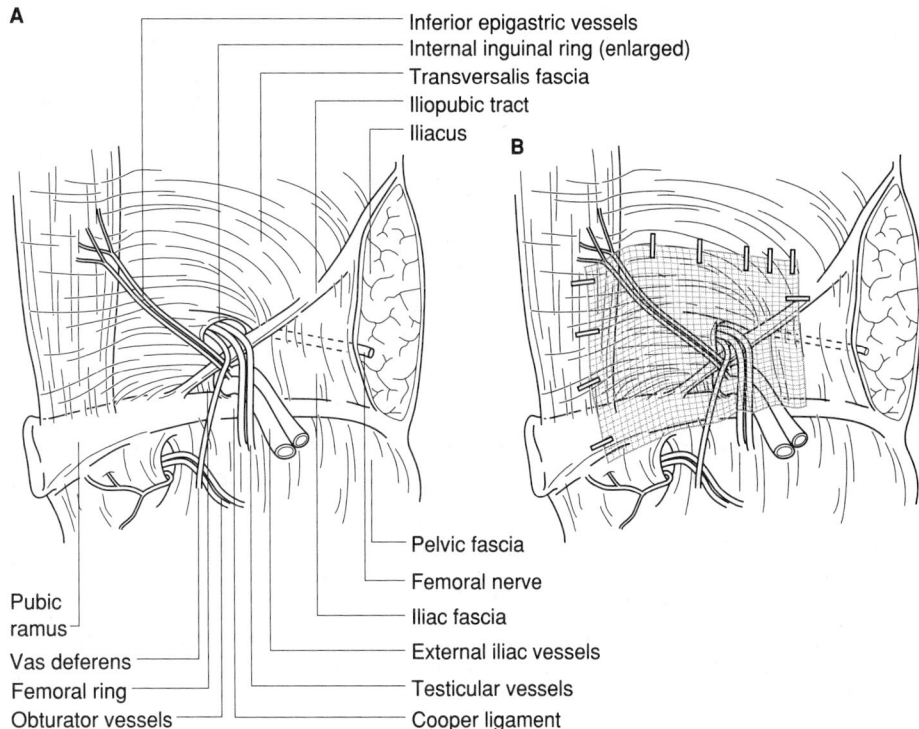

A

Inferior epigastric vessels
Internal inguinal ring (enlarged)
Transversalis fascia
Iliopubic tract
Iliacus

B

Pubic ramus
Vas deferens
Femoral ring
Obturator vessels

Pelvic fascia
Femoral nerve
Iliac fascia
External iliac vessels
Testicular vessels
Cooper ligament

Figure 53-21. Placement of mesh internally in the inguinal region in laparoscopic repair of right groin hernia.

Treatment with surgical or US- or CT-directed percutaneous drainage may be satisfactory when the abscess is localized. A retroperitoneal surgical approach to a retroperitoneal abscess is suitable for localized purulence, but the transabdominal approach is used for extensive abscesses.

Chylous Ascites

Chylous ascites is accumulation in the peritoneal cavity of chyle, a lymphatic fluid with high lipid content. Chylous ascites may result from injury to a lymphatic duct or the cisterna chyli. Spontaneous chylous ascites usually occurs only with extensive occlusion of retroperitoneal lymphatic vessels.

The symptoms of chylous ascites are abdominal distention (almost always); abdominal pain, anorexia, weight loss, and edema (about half the time); and weakness, nausea, dyspnea, weight gain, lymphadenopathy, early satiety, fever, or night sweats (sometimes). Physical examination yields findings of ascites. About half of patients have pleural effusion or peripheral edema.

Diagnostic studies are used to document the lymphatic origin of the abdominal fluid and delineate the cause of the ascites. Paracentesis and analysis of chylous fluid reveal elevated triglyceride, protein, and leukocyte levels with a predominance of lymphocytes. *Lymphangiography* or *lymphoscintigraphy* may help define the site of lymphatic leakage from the cisterna chyli or retroperitoneal lymphatics but not from mesenteric or hepatic lymphatics. CT is useful in nontraumatic chylous ascites. Laparotomy with nodal biopsy often is required for histologic examination and typing of lesions believed to be cancer.

Treatment of chylous ascites is directed at decreasing lymph and triglyceride 1accumulation. A fat-restricted diet is prescribed with added medium-chain triglycerides. Patients with nonneoplastic causes of chylous ascites cease all oral intake and receive total parenteral nutrition.

Retroperitoneal Fibrosis

Retroperitoneal fibrosis is a grayish-white, rubbery, dense thickening in the retroperitoneum. It is several centimeters thick and encompasses all retroperitoneal structures. The usual location is along the lower abdominal aorta, often including the bifurcation. Retroperitoneal fibrosis causes hydronephrosis and kidney damage. It also may obstruct the extrahepatic bile duct, inferior vena cava, or iliac vein and may be associated with malignant retroperitoneal tumors.

The symptoms of retroperitoneal fibrosis are dull, noncolicky pain in the back, flank, or abdomen, weight loss, nonspecific GI symptoms, and lower extremity edema, malaise, and dysuria. Physical signs are a palpable abdominal mass, hypertension, fever, and oliguria or anuria. Most patients have an elevated blood urea nitrogen (BUN) level.

An *intravenous pyelogram* (IVP) shows medial deviation of the ureter, hydroureteronephrosis, and extrinsic ureteral compression. MRI depicts the lesion better than does CT. Exploratory laparotomy with multiple deep biopsies of the retroperitoneal process is essential.

Management of retroperitoneal fibrosis is identification and management of the cause, relief of ureteral obstruction, and reversal of the inflammation and fibrosis. Renal obstruction is relieved with retrograde ureteral stents or percutaneous nephrostomy tubes. Dialysis may be required. A 2- to 3-week trial of corticosteroids may be attempted. Failure of the course of steroids is an indication for surgical treatment.

Retroperitoneal Neoplasms

Tumors of the retroperitoneum are those of its structures, such as the pancreas, kidneys, ureters,and adrenal glands. Metastatic tumors are common because the retroperitoneum contains lymphatic channels. Tumors in the retroperitoneum are asymptomatic until they are large, unless they secrete substances that are active in the body and cause early symptoms. Surgical resection of retroperitoneal tumors often is compromised by the proximity or involvement of multiple important structures.

SUGGESTED READING

Brick WG, Colborn GL, Gadacz TR, Skandalakis JE. Crucial anatomic lessons for laparoscopic herniorrhaphy. Am Surg 1995;61:172.

Clark CP, Vanderpool D, Preskitt JT. The response of retroperitoneal fibrosis to tamoxifen. Surgery 1991;109:502.

Hutchinson R, Sokhi GS. Multicystic peritoneal mesothelioma: not a benign condition. Eur J Surg 1992;158:451.

McDougal WS, MacDonell RC Jr. Treatment of idiopathic retroperitoneal fibrosis by immunosuppression. J Urol 1991;145:112.

Easter DW, Halasz NA. Recent trends in the management of desmoid tumors: summary of 19 cases and review of the literature. Ann Surg 1989;210:765.

McEntee GP, O'Carroll A, Mooney B, Egan TJ, Delaney PV. Timing of strangulation in adult hernias. Br J Surg 1989;76:725.

Monahan DW, Poston WK, Brown GJ. Mesenteric panniculitis. South Med J 1989;82:782.

Nyhus LM, Condon RE, eds. Hernia, ed. 4. Philadelphia, JB Lippincott, 1995.

Shiu MH, Weinstein L, Hajdu SI, Brennan MF. Malignant soft-tissue tumors of the anterior abdominal wall. Am J Surg 1989;158:446.

Zainea GG, Jordan F. Rectus sheath hematomas: their pathogenesis, diagnosis, and management. Am Surg 1988;54:630.

ESSENTIALS OF SURGERY: SCIENTIFIC PRINCIPLES AND PRACTICE, edited by Lazar J. Greenfield, Michael W. Mulholland, Keith T. Oldham, Gerald B. Zelenock, and Keith D. Lillemoe. Lippincott–Raven Publishers, Philadelphia, © 1997.

CHAPTER 54

ACUTE ABDOMEN AND APPENDIX

CARSON D. LIU AND DAVID W. MCFADDEN

ACUTE ABDOMEN

Acute abdomen is a pathophysiologic process of sudden onset that is corrected with surgical manipulation.

In the gastrointestinal (GI) tract, alterations in secretion, absorption, motility, synthesis, digestion, and transport can produce symptoms such as abdominal pain, dysphagia or odynophagia, anorexia, weight loss, nausea and vomiting, bloating or distention, constipation, flatulence, and diarrhea. Signs of disease are demonstrations of a pathologic process. They include tenderness, rigidity, masses, altered bowel sounds, bleeding, malnutrition, jaundice, and stigmata of hepatic dysfunction.

Combining the symptoms elicited from a complete history and the signs from a comprehensive physical examination allows one to establish a differential diagnosis.

Pain

Most diseases of the abdominal viscera cause pain (Fig. 54-1). Abdominal pain is visceral, somatic, or referred.

Visceral Pain

The four classes of visceral stimulation that result in abdominal pain are:

1. Stretching and contraction
2. Traction, compression, and torsion
3. Stretch alone
4. Contact with certain chemicals

The receptors for these responses are located in the walls of hollow organs, on serosal structures (eg, the visceral peritoneum and the capsule of solid organs), within the mesentery (especially associated with large mesenteric vessels and ligaments), and within the mucosa. These receptors are responsive to both mechanical and chemical stimuli.

Somatic Pain

Somatic pain is caused by irritation of the parietal peritoneum. Mediated mainly by spinal nerve fibers that supply the abdominal wall, somatic pain is localized and perceived as originating from one of the four quadrants of the abdominal wall. Somatic pain can be a response to acute changes in pH or temperature, as in bacterial or chemical inflammation. It is perceived as sharp and pricking and is usually constant.

Referred Pain

Referred pain is felt in an area of the body other than the site of origin. It is a characteristic of abdominal pain. Referred pain usually arises from a deep structure, is superficial at its distant presenting location, and often is sharp, localized, and persistent at the distant site.

Two features associated with referred pain are skin hyperalgesia and increased muscle tone of the abdominal wall. A classic example is rupture of the spleen that irritates the left hemidiaphragm, which is innervated by the same cervical nerves as the spleen. In this setting, pain is perceived as originating in the left shoulder (Kehr sign), which is supplied by the same nerves. A knowledge of referred pain and its patterns may help when other evidence of disease is lacking (Table 54-1).

Acute Abdominal Pain

Acute abdominal pain is loosely defined as pain present for <8 hours. The key to treatment is early diagnosis.

History

The history is the most important aspect of diagnosis. It is best if the patient gives the entire history before the physician asks specific questions. The history includes a medical history and information about associated illnesses. A history of previous similar symptoms is sought, as is the presence of any prodromal symptoms.

The character of pain is important. Colicky pain usually indicates an obstructive process, such as intestinal obstruction, ureteral calculus, or acute biliary colic. Between attacks, the pain lessens or disappears. During attacks, the pain is persistent and unrelenting. The pain that occurs with inflammatory conditions, such as appendicitis or diverticulitis, is sustained and worsens over time.

Clues to the cause of pain are provided by the mode of onset. Pancreatitis is usually gradual in onset and commonly follows an episode of alcohol abuse. A perforated hollow viscus, however, produces pain of sudden onset that the patient may be able to time precisely.

The location of pain is helpful in establishing the diagnosis. This is especially true with somatic pain that results from irritation of the parietal peritoneum (Fig. 54-1).

Other factors in the history of abdominal pain include:

History of intraabdominal disease
Previous abdominal operation(s)
Current use of medication(s)
Familial or concomitant disease among family members
Precise menstrual history

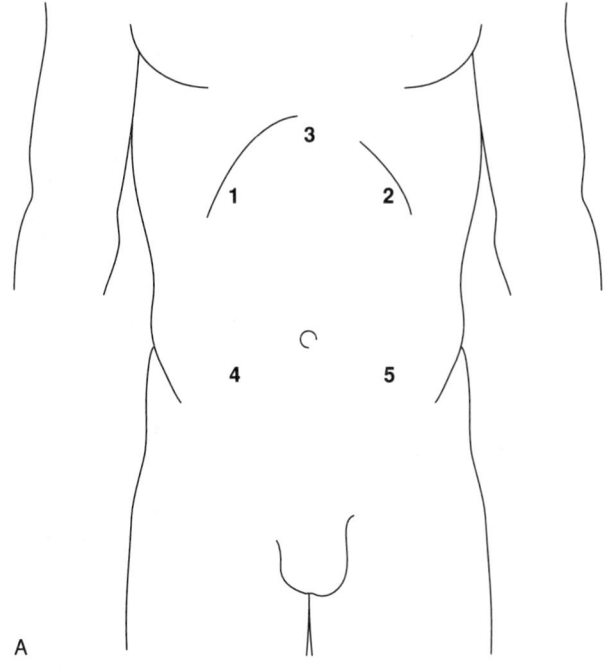

A

Figure 54-1. Abdominal pain map.

B

RIGHT UPPER QUADRANT PAIN (1)

Cholecystitis
Choledocholithiasis
Retrocecal appendicitis
Pancreatitis
Subdiaphragmatic abscess
Hepatic abscess
Hepatitis (A, B, C)
Peptic ulcer
Hepatic metastasis
Choledochocyst
Hepatic vein obstruction
   (Budd-Chiari syndrome)
Herpes zoster
Pneumonia
Hepatomegaly from congestive
   heart failure
Myocardial ischemia
Pericarditis
Pleuritis
Empyema
Pulmonary infarction

LEFT UPPER QUADRANT PAIN (2)

Splenomegaly
Splenic infarction
Splenic artery aneurysm
Splenic rupture (from blunt
   trauma)
Fractured ribs
Gastritis
Peptic ulcer disease
Pancreatitis
Herpes zoster
Pneumonia
Myocardial ischemia
Pericarditis
Pleuritis
Empyema
Pulmonary infarction

EPIGASTRIC PAIN (3)

Pancreatitis
Gastritis
Peptic ulcer disease
Cholecystitis
Reflux esophagitis
Myocardial ischemia
Pericarditis

RIGHT LOWER QUADRANT PAIN (4)

Appendicitis
Ruptured peptic ulcer (Valentino
   syndrome)
Cholecystitis
Intestinal obstruction
Diverticulitis
Crohn's disease
Leaking abdominal aortic
   aneurysm
Ectopic pregnancy
Ovarian cyst
Salpingitis
Ovarian torsion
Endometriosis
Mittelschmerz
Renal calculi
Psoas abscess
Seminal vesiculitis
Abdominal wall hematoma

LEFT LOWER QUADRANT PAIN (5)

Diverticulitis
Appendicitis
Colon cancer
Intestinal obstruction
Splenomegaly
Gastritis
Inflammatory bowel disease
Leaking abdominal aortic
   aneurysm
Ectopic pregnancy
Ovarian cyst
Salpingitis
Ovarian torsion
Endometriosis
Mittelschmerz
Renal calculi
Psoas abscess
Seminal vesiculitis
Abdominal wall hematoma

DIFFUSE PAIN

Early appendicitis
Peritonitis
Gastroenteritis
Pancreatitis
Mesenteric thrombosis
Abdominal aortic aneurysm
Intussusception
Colitis
Intestinal obstruction
Inflammatory bowel disease
Leukemia
Sickle cell crisis
Mesenteric adenitis
Metabolic, toxic and bacterial
   causes

Physical Examination

The first and most important step in the physical examination of a patient with an acute abdomen is observation of the patient's body habitus and facial expression. Unwillingness to change body position suggests peritonitis. Hip flexion with the knees drawn up to maintain comfort suggests abdominal wall and possibly peritoneal irritation. Restriction of diaphragmatic excursion with respiration, evidenced by shallow breathing and use of accessory respiratory muscles, is consistent with peritoneal irritation.

Colicky pain is often manifested by intense movement in an effort to alleviate pain, followed by restful intervals between colicky periods. The abdomen is inspected for hernial bulges, masses, distention, or areas of inflammation. Auscultation of the abdominal cavity for presence or absence and quality of bowel sounds is performed. The presence and location of bruits are recorded. Auscultation of the chest, particularly in the diaphragmatic area, is undertaken to document diaphragmatic movement and to search for basilar pneumonia, which may simulate an acute abdominal condition.

Palpation of all quadrants of the abdomen is performed last. Palpation is gentle and superficial at first, proceeding from the least painful to the most painful area. Peritoneal

Table 54-1. POSSIBLE ORIGINS FOR REFERRED PAIN

RIGHT SHOULDER

Diaphragm
Gallbladder
Liver capsule
Right-sided pneumoperitoneum

RIGHT SCAPULA

Ballbladder
Biliary tree

GROIN OR GENITALIA

Kidney
Ureter
Aorta or iliac artery

BACK—MIDLINE

Pancreas
Duodenum
Aorta

LEFT SHOULDER

Diaphragm
Spleen
Tail of pancreas
Stomach
Splenic flexure (colon)
Left-sided pneumoperitoneum

LEFT SCAPULA

Spleen
Tail of pancreas

signs or masses suggested by the superficial examination may be confirmed with deeper but still gentle palpation.

A percussion test is kinder and more specific than a test for rebound tenderness. Having the patient cough, laugh, or maximally distend the abdomen may localize the disease. A stethoscope test consists of using a stethoscope to depress and release the abdomen. Shaking the pelvis from side to side may elicit true rebound tenderness.

Laboratory Tests

A complete blood count, urinalysis, serum amylase, and, for women with lower abdominal pain, a β-human chorionic gonadotropin (hCG) pregnancy test are requested. Serum electrolytes, blood urea nitrogen (BUN), creatinine, and glucose can be used to determine hydration status, renal function, and basic metabolic state. Liver chemistries are helpful for patients with upper-abdominal pain or stigmata of liver disease. Laboratory tests are not performed unless the results alter the need for additional tests or therapy. At venipuncture, an intravenous cannula often can be inserted and used for hydration or administration of medication.

Diagnostic Imaging

Upright and supine radiographs of the abdomen and upright and lateral radiographs of the chest are obtained. Only a small number of patients with an acute abdomen have abnormalities on screening radiographs, but radiographs are suggested unless a clear-cut diagnosis is established. Pneumoperitoneum, gas-fluid levels, fecaliths, gallstones, ascites, and obliteration of the psoas shadows are all helpful diagnostic findings. Contrast-enhanced GI radiography, ultrasonography (US), computed tomography (CT), and arteriography may be needed.

Gynecologic Causes of the Acute Abdomen

Gynecologic causes of acute abdominal pain include pelvic inflammatory disease (PID), ectopic pregnancy, tuboovarian cysts, torsion, hemorrhage or abscess, and mittelschmerz.

PID must be considered in every woman of reproductive age with lower-abdominal pain. It includes tuboovarian abscess, with or without rupture. PID is usually appreciated bilaterally; an abscess is unilateral. PID becomes apparent as acute pain, fever and chills, or fever and leukocytosis. Pelvic examination usually reveals extreme pelvic tenderness and increased pain with cervical motion. Peritoneal signs in the upper abdomen suggest leakage or rupture of a pelvic abscess, usually necessitating surgical intervention. Differentiation of PID from acute appendicitis is difficult, especially among women of childbearing age (Table 54-2).

Risk factors for ectopic pregnancy include salpingitis, tubal ligation, tubal repair, use of an intrauterine device, or ectopic pregnancy. Pain and abnormal uterine bleeding occur. Human chorionic gonadotropin (hCG) testing and culdocentesis are essential for diagnosis.

Hemorrhage from functional ovarian cysts can simulate an acute surgical abdomen. Symptoms begin at or around ovulation. Pain is severe, abrupt in onset, and often bilateral. A serum hCG pregnancy test differentiates ovarian cyst from ectopic pregnancy. Operation is rarely required to treat hemorrhage associated with rupture of a follicular ovarian cyst.

Adnexal torsion presents with lower-abdominal, sometimes colicky, lateralized pain. US and laparoscopy are used for diagnosis and management.

Urologic Causes of the Acute Abdomen

Acute ureteral or renal pelvic obstruction is the most common condition confused with nonurologic causes of acute abdomen. Urinalysis, plain abdominal radiographs, and an intravenous pyelogram (IVP) usually are confirmatory. Renal and perirenal abscesses may mimic appendicitis, diverticulitis, or cholecystitis. IVP is abnormal, as is urinalysis. Acute testicular torsion and other intrascrotal events present with prominent abdominal pain. Examination of the scrotum usually reveals an elevated testicle on the affected side and profound tenderness.

Acute Abdomen in Specific Conditions

Nonsurgical Problems

Nonsurgical conditions that simulate acute abdomen include pulmonary, cardiac, neurologic, metabolic, toxic, infectious, and hematologic problems (Table 54-3).

Table 54-2. APPENDICITIS DIFFERENTIATED FROM PELVIC INFLAMMATORY DISEASE (PID)

Finding	Appendicitis	PID
Nausea and vomiting	+++	+
Menstrual cycle	No preference	60% in first 14 d
History of venereal disease	+	+++
Mean duration of symptoms	32 h	65 h
Cervical motion or adnexal tenderness	+	+++
Guarding or tenderness	Right lower quadrant	Bilateral

Table 54-3. NONSURGICAL CAUSES OF THE ACUTE ABDOMEN

METABOLIC
Diabetic ketoacidosis
Porphyria
Adrenal insufficiency
Uremia
Hypercalcemia

TOXIC
Insect bites
Venoms (scorpion, snake)
Lead poisoning
Drugs

MISCELLANEOUS
Hemolytic crises
Rectus sheath hematoma

NEUROGENIC
Herpes zoster
Abdominal epilepsy
Spinal cord tumor, infection
Nerve root compression

CARDIOPULMONARY
Pneumonia
Myocardial infarction
Myocarditis
Empyema
Costochondritis

Pediatrics

The differential diagnosis of acute abdominal pain among children is outlined in Table 54-4. In the first few years of life, congenital abnormalities are the most common source of abdominal symptoms.

Histories are almost impossible to obtain from infants and toddlers, and physical examination can be extremely misleading in that no discernible tenderness may be present. Plain abdominal radiographs are used liberally in the treatment of young children. For older children, the history and physical findings are more easily elicited in most cases.

Children with appendicitis or other intraabdominal inflammatory conditions often do not have anorexia. The sigmoid colon is often redundant in children. If the colon is adjacent to an inflamed appendix, diarrhea may predominate, leading to a false diagnosis of gastroenteritis. Microscopic hematuria and pyuria often occur with appendicitis; leukocytosis is less common.

Cardiac Operations

GI bleeding, acute cholecystitis, mesenteric ischemia, pancreatitis, and acute colitis may occur after cardiac operations.

Immunocompromise

Patients receiving allografts, undergoing chemotherapy, taking immunosuppressive drugs for autoimmune disorders, or living with acquired immunodeficiency syndrome (AIDS) may have abdominal complications (Table 54-5).

Nonspecific Pain

Acute, nonspecific abdominal pain is a common final diagnosis.

Abdominal Wall Pain

Causes of abdominal wall pain include iatrogenic peripheral nerve injuries, hernia, myofascial pain syndromes, rib tip syndrome, abdominal pain of spinal origin, and spontaneous rectus sheath hematomas.

Spinal Cord Injury

Acute abdominal conditions are common among, but difficult to diagnose for, patients with spinal cord injuries. The most common conditions are acute cholecystitis, perforated peptic ulcer, and renal disease. Physical examination often is not helpful. Leukocytosis may be present. Plain radiography, CT, oral cholecystography, US, and barium studies aid in diagnosis.

Oral Anticoagulation

Acute abdominal pain in patients taking oral anticoagulants is a difficult clinical situation. The most common diagnosis is intramural hematoma of the intestine. Other diagnoses are intestinal infarction and volvulus. The challenge is to differentiate patients with intramural hematoma from patients who need surgical treatment. Laparotomy or laparoscopy is recommended for patients who do not improve over 24 to 36 hours.

APPENDIX

Acute appendicitis is a sequence of appendiceal inflammation, perforation, abscess formation, and peritonitis. By far the most common cause of appendicitis is luminal obstruction of the appendix itself. Other disorders of the appendix include carcinoid tumors, neuromas, and mucoceles caused by epithelial tumors with appendiceal distention.

The role of the appendix is controversial. Lymphoid aggregations and location distinguish it from colon and cecum. Normally, a pressure gradient exists along the long axis that prohibits entrance of food material into the lumen of the appendix.

Anatomy

The three taeniae of the ascending colon consolidate at the base of the appendix, the anterior taenia serving as a landmark along the anterior cecum. The appendix is connected to the lower aspect of the ileal mesentery by the mesoappendix. Most people have a retrocecal appendix; in the others, the appendix lies over the pelvic brim. Adult appendiceal length averages 9 cm (range: 2 to 20 cm).

Table 54-4. DIFFERENTIAL DIAGNOSIS OF THE ACUTE ABDOMEN IN THE PEDIATRIC POPULATION

Infants	Children	Adolescents
Viral enteritis	Meckel's diverticulitis	Pelvic inflammatory disease
Intussusception	Cystitis	
Pyelonephritis	Viral enteritis	Viral enteritis
Gastroesophageal reflux	Appendicitis	Mittelschmerz
Bacterial enterocolitis	Crohn's disease	Crohn's disease
Pneumonitis	Bacterial enterocolitis	Pancreatitis
Appendicitis		Pneumonia
Pyloric stenosis	Trauma (child abuse)	Hematocolpos
Testicular torsion	Pneumonitis	Bacterial enterocolitis
Mesenteric cysts	Pancreatitis	Psychosomatic illness
Ruptured tumors	Ruptured tumors	Peptic ulcer
Pancreatitis	Poisoning	Poisoning
Meckel's diverticulitis	Pyelonephritis	Trauma
Hirschsprung disease		Ectopic pregnancy
Strangulated hernia		Pregnancy
Poisoning		Cholelithiasis
Trauma (child abuse)		

Table 54-5. ACUTE ABDOMINAL PAIN ASSOCIATIONS IN THE IMMUNOCOMPROMISED PATIENT

CYTOMEGALOVIRUS INFECTION

Interstitial pneumonitis
Mononucleosis
Pancreatitis
Hepatitis
Cholecystitis
Gastrointestinal ulceration

PANCREATITIS

Steroids
Azathioprine
Cytomegalovirus
Pentamidine

HEPATITIS

Hepatitis A, B, and C
Cytomegalovirus
Epstein-Barr virus

CHOLECYSTITIS

Cytomegalovirus
Acalculous cholecystitis
Campylobacter

HEPATOSPLENIC ABSCESS

Fungal
Mycobacterial
Protozoal
Splenic rupture

BOWEL PERFORATION

Lymphoma, leukemia (especially after chemotherapy)
Cytomegalovirus
Colon ulcers
Kaposi sarcoma
Pseudomembranous colitis
Mycobacteria
Iatrogenic

ACUTE GRAFT-VERSUS-HOST DISEASE

PSEUDOACUTE ABDOMEN

FECAL IMPACTION

STANDARD ABDOMINAL PROCESSES

Appendicitis
Cholecystitis
Diverticulitis
Bowel obstruction
Ulcer disease
Pelvic inflammatory disease
Perirectal abscess
Urinary tract infection
Lymphadenitis

NEUTROPENIC ENTEROCOLITIS

The main appendicular artery is a branch of the ileocolic artery that courses behind the ileum, through the mesoappendix, and along the appendiceal wall until it reaches the tip of the organ. The appendicular artery courses along the free border of the mesoappendix until it reaches the distal appendix, where it lies along the wall of the appendix (Fig. 54-2). During acute inflammation, the appendicular artery becomes susceptible to thrombosis as the appendix becomes enlarged.

Lymphatics that drain the appendix include vessels from the body and tip of the appendix that drain posteriorly into the upper and lower ileocolic nodes. Lymph vessels from the base of the appendix drain to the anterior ileocolic nodes. The lymph nodes of the ileocolic chain may be hyperplastic during appendicitis.

The appendix is innervated by the autonomic nervous system without any direct innervation from pain fibers. The absence of pain fibers explains the lack of localized symptoms until an inflamed appendix irritates the peritoneum.

The orifice of the appendix opens to the cecum with a semilunar mucosal fold that forms a valve. The base of the appendix is at about the level of the S-1 vertebral body, the McBurney point (the junction of the middle and lateral thirds of a line drawn from the umbilicus to the right anterior superior iliac spine).

Serosa covers the entire appendix. Longitudinal muscle fibers form an almost complete layer immediately beneath the serosa. At the base, the longitudinal muscles form rudimentary taeniae continuous with the taeniae coli. A layer of circular muscle forms a thicker inner layer. The submucosa contains lymphoid tissue that may hypertrophy and obstruct the lumen during acute appendicitis. The appendix is lined throughout by a mucosal luminal surface. The mucosa has features similar to those of the colon, but lymphoid tissue is concentrated more densely.

Pathophysiology

The most common cause of appendicitis is obstruction of the appendiceal lumen. In children and young adults, the most common cause of luminal obstruction is lymphoid hyperplasia. In older adults, it is a fecalith.

Increased production of mucus stimulated by luminal obstruction and entrapment of bacteria dilate the appendix. Wall tension increases and blood flow becomes compromised, leading to vessel thrombosis and necrosis of the appendiceal wall (Fig. 54-3). When full-thickness necrosis occurs, the appendix perforates, and its fecal and suppurative contents are released into the abdominal cavity. Peritoneal irritation occurs.

Once luminal obstruction occurs and inflammation begins, the stages of acute appendicitis follow (Table 54-6). The increase in intraluminal pressure causes stasis of blood flow, gangrene of the appendix, and rupture.

Diagnosis of Appendicitis

The most useful tools are the history and physical examination. Laboratory and radiologic studies are reserved for questionable presentations of abdominal pain.

History

Periumbilical pain followed by anorexia and minimal nausea is typical before emesis or crescendo somatic pain localized to the right-lower quadrant (RLQ) of the abdomen occurs. The poor innervation of the viscera allows only dull pain until local inflammation irritates the peritoneum in the RLQ.

All patients with appendicitis have abdominal pain and anorexia. Lack of these two symptoms means the diagnosis probably is something other than appendicitis.

Almost all patients with appendicitis have nausea at some point. Alteration in bowel movements is not a reliable historical feature. Almost half of patients have atypical pain. This may include patients with localized RLQ pain from the outset and those with diffuse periumbilical pain. These patients tend to be elderly or taking antibiotics that mask the symptoms.

Physical Examination

Physical findings differentiate appendicitis from other abdominal disorders. The signs of appendicitis are:

• RLQ pain on palpation
• Guarding with peritoneal irritation on percussion

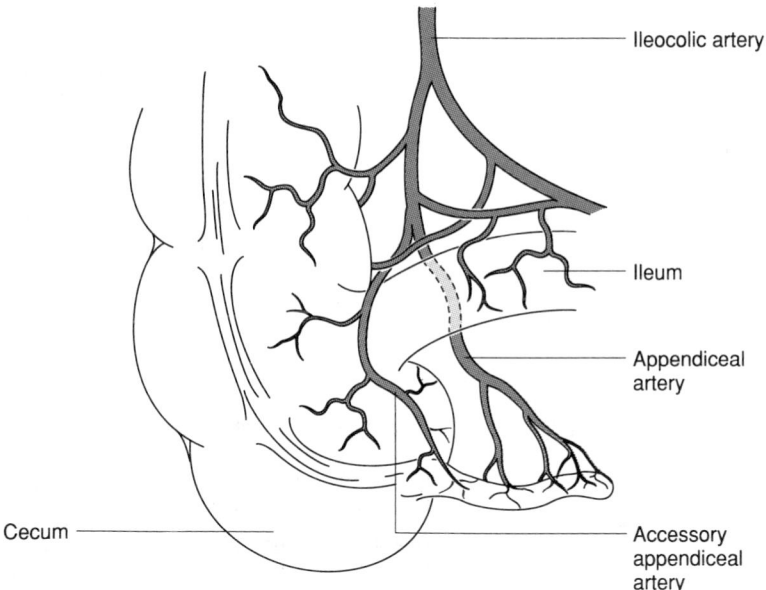

Figure 54-2. Anatomy of and blood supply to the appendix.

- Pain in the RLQ during palpation of the left-lower quadrant (Rovsing sign)
- Increased pain with coughing (Dunphy sign)
- Pain on internal rotation of the hip (obturator sign)
- Pain during extension of the right hip (iliopsoas sign)

The iliopsoas sign is typical of a retrocecal appendix; the obturator sign suggests a pelvic appendix. During a rectal or pelvic examination, focal tenderness is elicited more on the right side in appendicitis; palpation of a tender mass indicates a pelvic abscess.

Laboratory Diagnosis

When the history and physical examination are definitive, no other investigation is required. A white blood cell (WBC) count with a peripheral smear is helpful. About two-thirds of patients have an elevated WBC count but no fever. Almost all patients with acute appendicitis have a predominance of polymorphonuclear leukocytes and lymphopenia. Urinalysis is performed because patients with acute appendicitis often have hematuria, pyuria, or proteinuria.

Radiographs

Abdominal radiographs are rarely useful in the treatment of children. For adults, fecaliths may be visualized with a paucity of gas in the RLQ. Loss of the right psoas shadow usually represents late appendicitis with retroperitoneal inflammation.

Ultrasound

US is valuable after physical examination in the treatment of young women and patients with atypical symptoms. The appendix has a typical target appearance (Fig. 54-4). Findings associated with appendicitis include wall thickening beyond the normal 8 to 10 mm, luminal distention, and lack of compressibility. The visualized appendix usually coincides with the site of localized pain and tenderness.

Advanced appendicitis is depicted on US scans as asymmetric wall thickening, abscess formation, presence of free intraperitoneal fluid, surrounding tissue edema, and decreased local tenderness to compression. Marked wall thickening without distention is present in Crohn's disease of the appendix, often in association with ileal or cecal disease. Rare findings, such as appendiceal neoplasms and mucocele, may be visualized.

Computed Tomography

CT is used to identify obscure inflammatory processes of the abdomen when the diagnosis of appendicitis is not foremost. CT is performed only if US is unavailable or is unrevealing for technical reasons, such as gaseous abdominal distention.

A normal appendix may be difficult to locate on CT scans. CT findings of appendicitis become more prominent with advanced disease. They include a distended, thick-walled, edematous appendix seen as a target structure, inflammatory streaking of surrounding fat, and the presence of an appendicolith. CT findings that suggest appendicitis include a pericecal phlegmon or abscess and small amounts of RLQ intraabdominal free air that signal perforation (Fig. 54-5).

Barium Contrast Studies

A barium study allows assessment of luminal patency of the appendix, examination of the colonic wall for mass effects or secondary effects of appendicitis, and diagnosis of right colonic or terminal ileal mucosal disease that may simulate appendicitis.

When barium fills the appendix, appendicitis is unlikely but not impossible. Barium enema examination complements US and CT in defining mucosal lesions of the cecum and appendix. It is considered when a patient has chronic or recurrent abdominal pain.

Treatment

Laparoscopy

If the diagnosis is not clear, laparoscopy can be used to rule out appendicitis and examine for gynecologic abnormalities. Diagnostic laparoscopy may be performed on all women with symptoms of acute appendicitis to avoid performance of an unnecessary appendectomy. If acute appendicitis is diagnosed at laparoscopy, laparoscopic appendectomy can be performed.

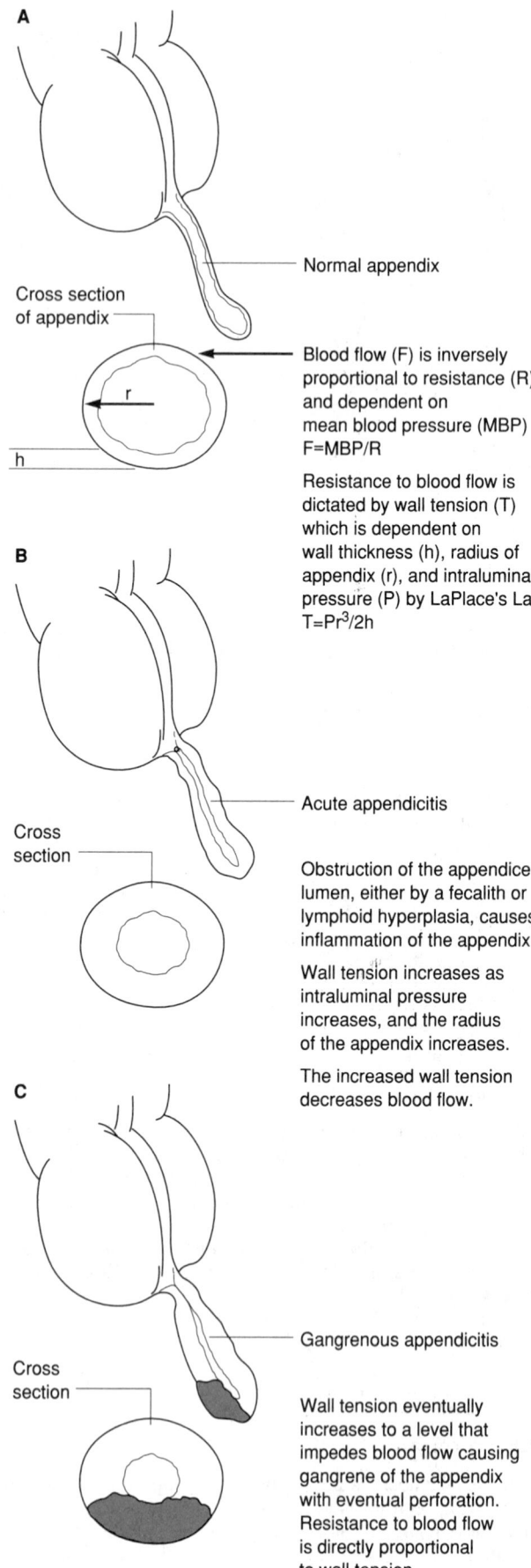

A

Normal appendix

Cross section of appendix

Blood flow (F) is inversely proportional to resistance (R) and dependent on mean blood pressure (MBP)
$$F=MBP/R$$

Resistance to blood flow is dictated by wall tension (T) which is dependent on wall thickness (h), radius of appendix (r), and intraluminal pressure (P) by LaPlace's Law.
$$T=Pr^3/2h$$

B

Acute appendicitis

Cross section

Obstruction of the appendiceal lumen, either by a fecalith or lymphoid hyperplasia, causes inflammation of the appendix.

Wall tension increases as intraluminal pressure increases, and the radius of the appendix increases.

The increased wall tension decreases blood flow.

C

Gangrenous appendicitis

Cross section

Wall tension eventually increases to a level that impedes blood flow causing gangrene of the appendix with eventual perforation. Resistance to blood flow is directly proportional to wall tension.

Figure 54-3. Pathophysiologic stages of appendicitis.

Table 54-6. CHARACTERIZATION OF DIFFERENT STAGES OF APPENDICITIS

Stage	Characteristics
Acute nonperforated appendicitis	Acute inflammation
Acute focal appendicitis	Focal inflammation with localized abscess of mixed flora within the appendix
Gangrenous appendicitis	Worsening edema with arterial occlusion with persistent infection causing necrosis of the appendiceal wall
Acute perforated appendicitis	Elevated intraluminal pressure leading to perforation through the gangrenous portion of the appendix

Laparotomy

The standard for management of appendicitis is open appendectomy by way of a limited RLQ incision. Before induction of anesthesia, the surgeon notes the point of maximal tenderness. While the patient is under anesthesia, a mass is palpated, if possible. The McBurney point does not universally mark the tip of the appendix, and palpation without guarding may help place the incision. An inferior incision below the maximal tender area helps in rotating the cecum into the wound. All incisions are performed with a muscle-splitting technique.

The base of the appendix lies at the confluence of the three taeniae. The cecum and appendix are mobilized into the wound as adhesions are bluntly dissected. The meso-appendix is ligated from the distal tip to the base of the appendix. The appendiceal stump is cauterized to prevent mucocele formation. Copious irrigation with saline solu-

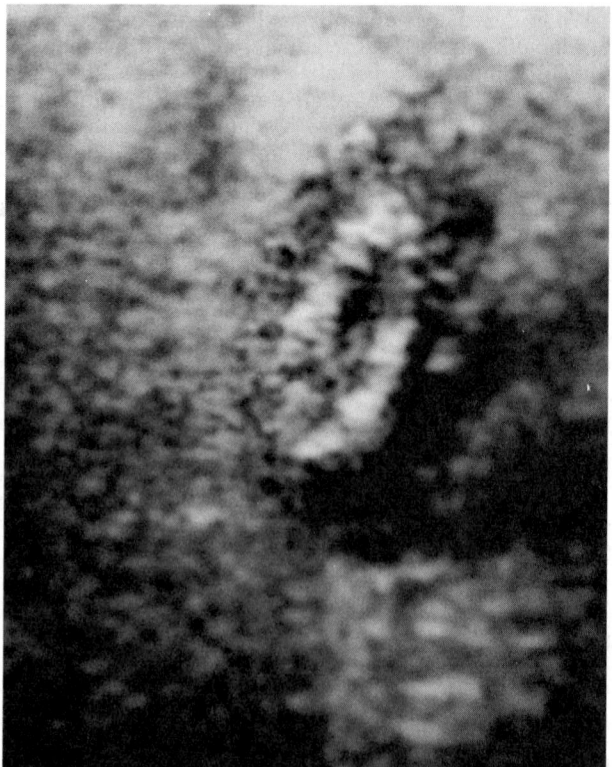

Figure 54-4. Target appearance of an acutely inflamed appendix as seen on ultrasound scan.

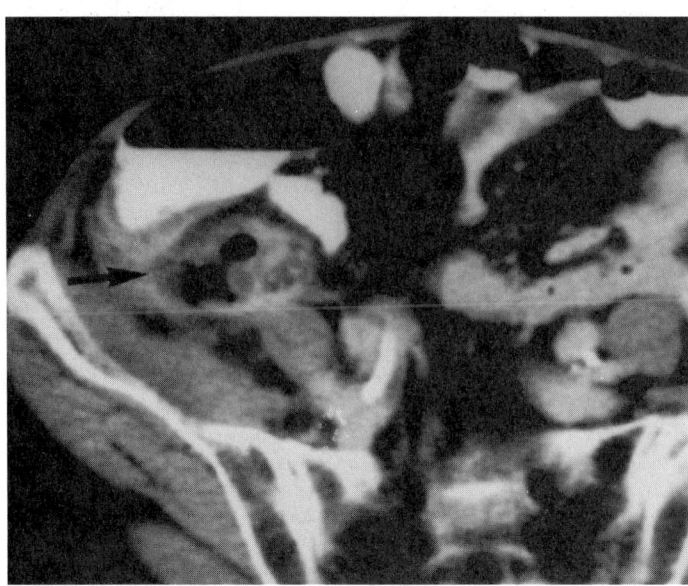

Figure 54-5. CT appearance of appendicitis with perforation and abscess formation.

tion is performed if the appendix has perforated in order to prevent formation of a pelvic or subhepatic abscess. The peritoneum and muscular fasciae are closed. The skin can be closed if the appendix has not perforated. Delayed primary closure is used for ruptured appendicitis.

If a normal appendix is found during appendectomy, the terminal ileum and pelvic structures (ovaries, fallopian tubes, uterus) are visualized to rule out other surgically treatable problems. A Meckel diverticulum or Crohn's disease of the terminal ileum may be discovered. If a normal appendix is found but Crohn's disease affects the terminal ileum, appendectomy is warranted.

Nonsurgical Treatment

If a distinct mass is palpated in the right iliac fossa and the patient has no systemic manifestations, such as fever or peritonitis, nonsurgical management can be undertaken. This method can be used to treat nontoxic patients with a clear diagnosis of appendiceal abscess. The patient fasts while intravenous fluids are administered. Broadspectrum antibiotics are given to cover enteric organisms while pulse is closely monitored. Increasing pain, progressive tachycardia, and lack of response after 24 to 48 hours are factors that necessitate surgical intervention.

Patients with well-formed periappendiceal abscesses can undergo CT-guided placement of drainage catheters to help resolve the abscess rapidly. If the abscess is palpable, percutaneous drainage may be possible. If symptoms of pain and abscess persist after catheter drainage, surgical drainage with appendectomy may be warranted. This approach is followed by interval appendectomy.

Interval Appendectomy

Most surgeons wait 6 weeks to 3 months after nonsurgical management of a perforated appendix to perform interval appendectomy. The benefit is that the operation is conducted in the absence of frank purulence. Interval appendectomy after appendiceal rupture is standard practice.

Antibiotic Treatment

A patient with appendicitis needs hydration and antibiotics. Usual therapy is short-course (<24 hours) antimicrobial prophylaxis. For a presumably ruptured appendix, a second-generation, broad-spectrum cephalosporin, such as cefotetan, is used before definitive surgical treatment.

Special Considerations

Children

Children cannot give an accurate history of symptoms, and abdominal pain from other causes is common. Nausea, vomiting, and abdominal tenderness are frequent signs of extraabdominal disease. The differential diagnosis includes:

- Meningitis
- Otitis media
- Pneumonia
- Viral gastroenteritis
- Mesenteric lymphadenitis
- Intussusception
- Primary peritonitis
- Typhlitis (acute cecal inflammation)

For neutropenic patients with RLQ tenderness, the mainstay of treatment is systemic administration of antibiotics until the neutropenia is resolved. Surgical exploration is associated with an extremely high mortality.

Children may be brought to the emergency department several times and not have acute appendicitis diagnosed until gangrene or perforation occurs. These children may have nonsurgical treatment of the appendiceal mass. Congenital abnormalities include agenesis or hypoplasia of the appendix, appendix multiplex, and horseshoe anomalies.

Elderly Patients

Elderly patients with appendicitis have a high rate of perforation. These patients may not report pain, or the pain may be described as dull RLQ pain. Localization to the RLQ is delayed. WBC count may not be elevated. A large number of elderly patients are found at operation to have a ruptured appendix. Elderly patients tend to have multiple medical problems that delay appendectomy. When a patient >60 years of age undergoes appendectomy, the right colon is inspected for carcinoma.

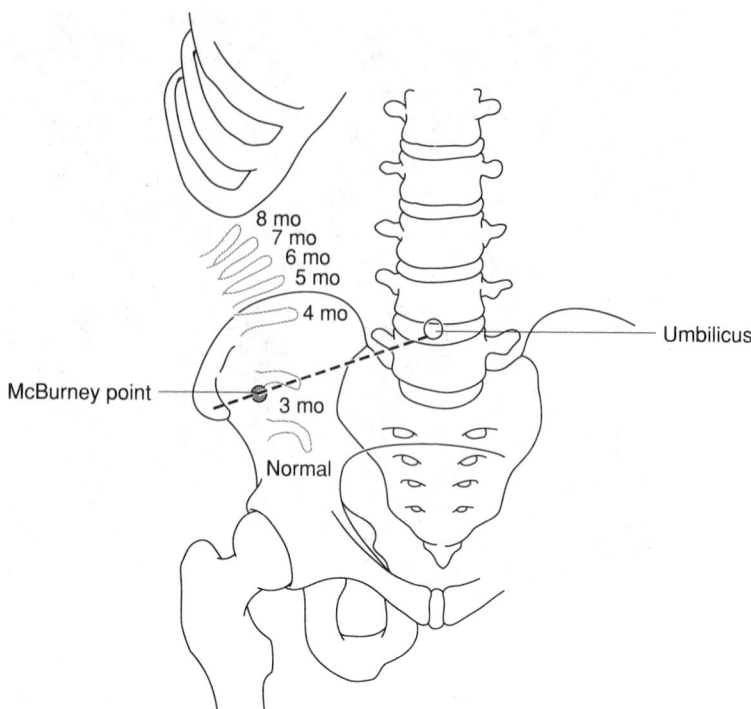

Figure 54-6. Location and orientation of the appendix in pregnancy.

Pregnancy

Anatomic and physiologic changes alter the presentation of appendicitis during the second and third trimesters of pregnancy (Fig. 54-6). Nausea and vomiting may be difficult to differentiate from symptoms of pregnancy. Localizing RLQ tenderness, however, is a reliable sign. Fever is not common, and leukocytosis is difficult to interpret because it is a normal feature of pregnancy.

US may be helpful in differentiating obstetric problems from appendicitis. Peritoneal signs in late pregnancy usually signify perforation and may have grave consequences. Urgent exploration is undertaken once the diagnosis of appendicitis is made.

AIDS

Although patients with AIDS are susceptible to cytomegalovirus-related intestinal perforation, there is no evidence that they have a higher rate of acute suppurative appendicitis. Diagnosis is difficult because opportunistic infection causing enterocolitis may mimic acute appendicitis. Some patients with AIDS have primary Kaposi sarcoma of the appendix, which elicits symptoms similar to those of acute appendicitis. When pathology reports after apparently routine appendectomy show rare opportunistic infections, evaluation for AIDS may be needed.

Incidental Appendectomy

Incidental appendectomy is prophylactic removal of a normal appendix during laparotomy for another condition. Incidental appendectomy is controversial for a child or young adult, but is *not indicated* for the elderly. The argument in favor of incidental appendectomy is that it reduces

the morbidity of an additional operation and eliminates the possibility of perforation later.

Neoplasms of the Appendix

Neoplasms of the appendix are rare. Carcinoid tumors are the most common, followed in frequency by benign and malignant mucoceles.

SUGGESTED READING

Connor TJ, Garcha IS, Ramshaw BJ, et al. Diagnostic laparoscopy for suspected appendicitis. Am Surg 1995;61:187.

Cox MR, McCall JL, Padbury RT, Wilson TG, Wattchow DA, Toouli J. Laparoscopic surgery in women with a clinical diagnosis of acute appendicitis. Med J Aust 1995;162:130.

Dhillon AP, Williams RA, Rode J. Age, site and distribution of subepithelial neurosecretory cells in the appendix. Pathology 1992;24:56.

Hopkins JA, Wilson SE, Bobey DG. Adjunctive antimicrobial therapy for complicated appendicitis: bacterial overkill by combination therapy. World J Surg 1994;18:933.

McFadden DW, Zinner MJ. Manifestations of gastrointestinal disease. New York, McGraw-Hill, 1994.

Ortega AE, Hunter JG, Peters JH, Swanstrom LL, Schirmer B. A prospective, randomized comparison of laparoscopic appendectomy with open appendectomy: Laparoscopic Appendectomy Study Group. Am J Surg 1995;169:208.

Poole GV. Anatomic basis for delayed diagnosis of appendicitis. South Med J 1990;83:771.

Sebastiano PD, Fink T, Weihe E, Friess H, Beger HG, Buchler M. Changes of protein gene product 9.5 (PGP 9.5) immunoreactive nerves in inflamed appendix. Dig Dis Sci 1995;40:366.

Tsuji M, Puri P, Reen DJ. Characterization of the local inflammatory response in appendicitis. J Pediatr Gastroenterol Nutr 1993;16:43.

Wade DS, Nava HR. Neutropenic colitis. Cancer 1992;69:17.

ESSENTIALS OF SURGERY: SCIENTIFIC PRINCIPLES AND PRACTICE,
edited by Lazar J. Greenfield, Michael W. Mulholland, Keith T. Oldham, Gerald B. Zelenock,
and Keith D. Lillemoe. Lippincott–Raven Publishers, Philadelphia, © 1997.

CHAPTER 55

SPLEEN

ANTHONY A. MEYER

SPLENIC ANATOMY

The spleen lies in the left-upper quadrant, posterior to the stomach (Fig. 55-1). It is an elliptic, lobulated solid organ with a convex surface that abuts the diaphragm and a concave surface that faces the stomach and the tail of the pancreas. A normal adult spleen weighs 125 to 175 g. It measures about 15 cm along its cranial–caudal axis and 8 cm along its elliptic axis. The spleen is 2 to 3 cm thick.

The spleen has lobulations on the anterior or ventral edge, closest to the hilum. Splenic parenchymal tissue is enveloped by an outer capsule, which is fibrous but quite thin. This capsule can be stripped easily from the splenic substance, which may result in continuous oozing of blood from the exposed surface.

Blood Supply

Blood flow to the spleen accounts for as much as 5% of cardiac output. Because of this large blood flow, the spleen may function as a reservoir, providing intravascular volume expansion, if needed. The spleen is perfused by the *splenic artery,* a primary branch of the celiac axis. The splenic artery is a tortuous vessel that passes posterior and superior to the pancreas. After it enters the splenic hilum, the splenic artery separates into two or three branches that penetrate the splenic parenchyma.

The spleen has no consistent segmental arterial anatomy, and arterial collaterals exist, which prevents partial splenectomy based on blood supply. One to three arterial branches from the left gastroepiploic artery form the *vasa brevia* (short gastric vessels). These enter the spleen superior to the splenic artery but are within the same hilar area invested by the peritoneum. These short gastric arteries are sufficient for splenic survival if the splenic artery must be sacrificed.

The short gastric arteries are accompanied by *veins* that may penetrate the splenic substance itself or join with other vascular branches at the splenic hilum. These veins provide collateral systemic–portal venous drainage.

The *splenic vein* originates from the confluence of secondary and tertiary veins that drain the splenic hilum, originating within 1 to 2 cm of the splenic substance. The individual branches are arrayed linearly from cephalad to caudad. The splenic vein passes posterior and inferior to the pancreas, joining the inferior mesenteric vein and the superior mesenteric vein to form the portal vein (Fig. 55-2).

Histology

The spleen is composed of red pulp, an area predominantly populated with erythrocytes, and white pulp, an area characterized by a predominance of lymphocytes and macrophages. The volume of the spleen is about 75% to 85% red pulp and 20% white pulp. Unlike any other solid organ, the spleen has no discrete compartments, lobes, or segments.

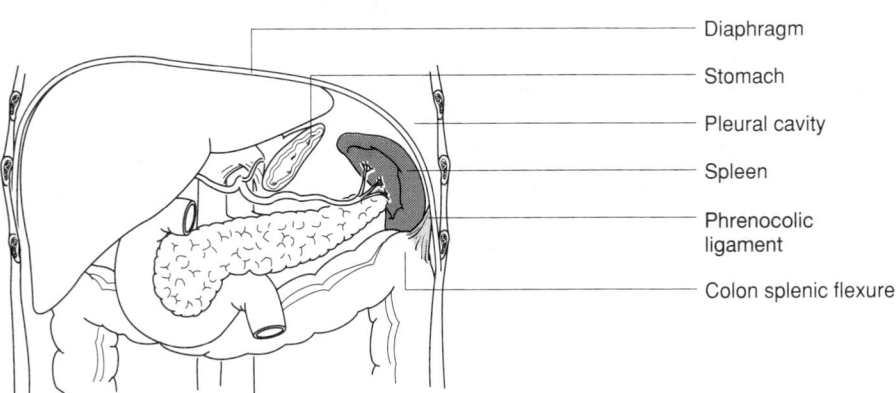

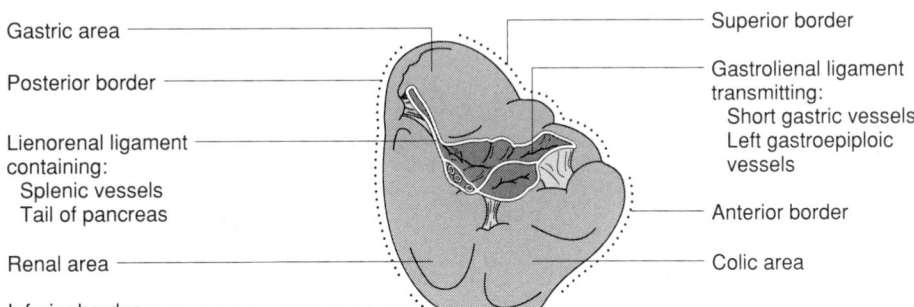

Visceral surface of spleen

Figure 55-1. Anatomic relation of the spleen to the liver, diaphragm, pancreas, colon, and kidney. The stomach is sectioned to illustrate the anatomic relation in situ.

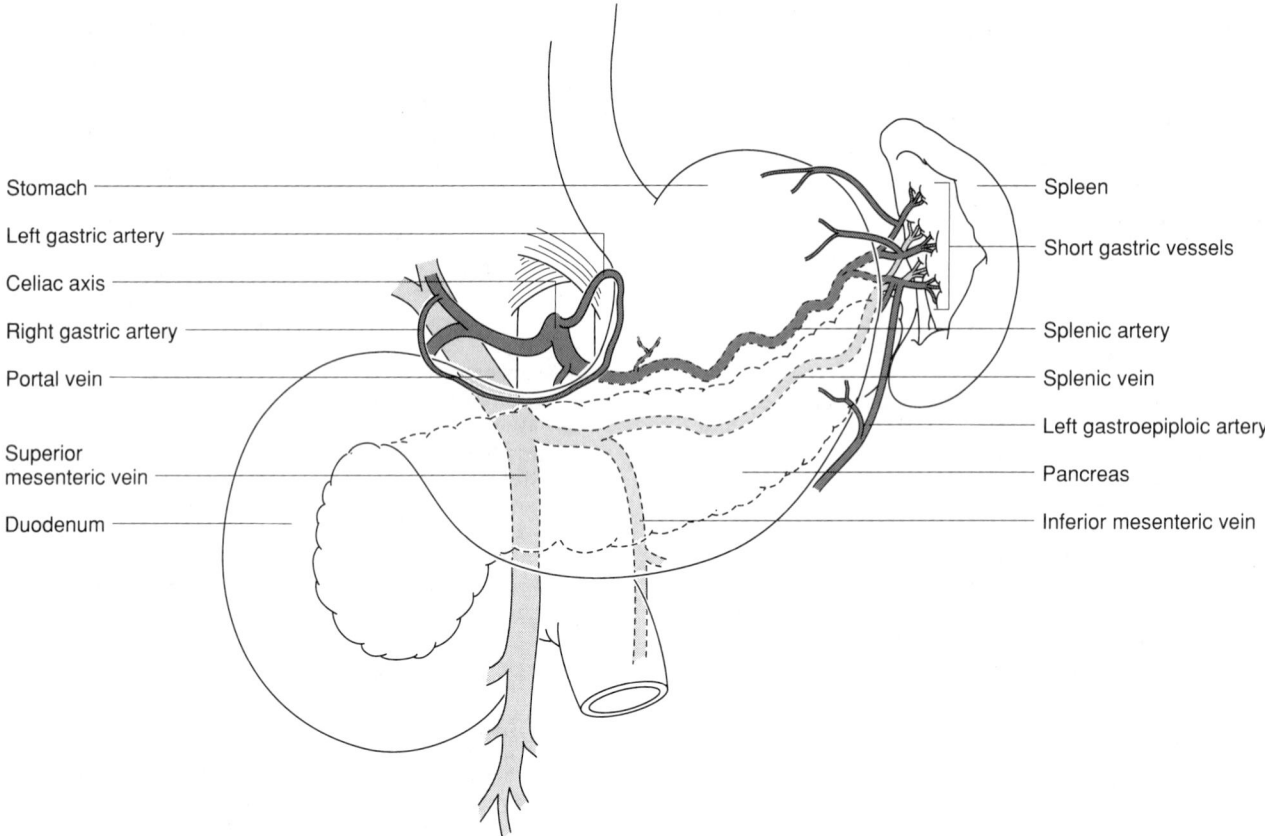

Stomach
Left gastric artery
Celiac axis
Right gastric artery
Portal vein
Superior mesenteric vein
Duodenum

Spleen
Short gastric vessels
Splenic artery
Splenic vein
Left gastroepiploic artery
Pancreas
Inferior mesenteric vein

Figure 55-2. The arterial blood flow to the spleen is derived from the splenic artery, the left gastroepiploic artery, and the short gastric arteries (vasa brevia). The venous drainage into the portal vein is also shown.

The fibrous splenic skeleton consists of collagen trabeculae that have a random, incomplete framework extending from the hilum to the capsule. Blood vessels penetrate the substance of the spleen within these trabeculae. Trabecular arteries and arterioles give rise to capillaries surrounded by macrophages. This high density of macrophages in contact with the capillaries and the cellular blood elements facilitates antigen processing by the spleen.

Blood elements pass through splenic capillaries to follow one of the two routes. The *closed circulation* is characterized by blood cells passing through the capillaries directly into venous sinusoids. The *open circulation* is characterized by blood cells passing through splenic capillaries into the splenic red pulp. The blood then passes through lakes of RBCs with loosely organized cords of white cells. The RBCs move slowly into the sinusoids, which empty into the trabecular veins. Almost all splenic blood flow is through the open system.

SPLENIC PHYSIOLOGY
Erythrocyte Maintenance

The spleen repairs RBCs damaged during circulation. Erythrocytes that cannot be repaired are destroyed in the red pulp. Exaggerated erythrocyte destruction can lead to problems in the spleen. For example, congestion of the spleen with hemoglobin S (sickle) erythrocytes can lead to segmental infarcts.

Immune Function

Immune function in the spleen has two components—nonspecific and specific. *Nonspecific* immune function is characterized by removal of particulate matter by the mac-

rophages. The spleen contains 25% of the fixed tissue macrophage population in the body. The spleen also serves as a principal source of nonspecific opsonins. These include tuftsin, properdin, and fibronectin. *Specific* immune function is related to antigen processing. The lymphocyte population of the spleen is exchanged nearly 50 times each day, although not all cells circulate. The lymphoid cells are located largely in the white pulp. The spleen is the largest producer of IgM.

Vascular Capacity

The spleen serves as an intravascular reservoir. Incorporation of splenic blood into the circulating blood volume occurs by means of vasoconstriction of the splenic artery and diminution of the splenic blood pool by increased venous outflow.

CLINICAL SYNDROMES
Anemia

Erythrocytes are removed from the circulation in the senescent spleen. Anemia associated with increased RBC destruction rather than inadequate erythrocyte production necessitates evaluation of the spleen. Anemias can be congenital or acquired.

Evaluation for anemia includes: (1) assessment of RBC morphology by means of inspection of a peripheral blood smear, (2) hemoglobin electrophoresis to examine the structure of the hemoglobin itself, (3) tests of erythrocyte survival with ^{51}Cr-labeled RBCs, and (4) serum haptoglobin levels to assess hemolysis.

Immune (Idiopathic) Thrombocytopenic Purpura

ITP is a disorder diagnosed on the basis of its symptoms, which include petechiae, gingival bleeding, and soft tissue ecchymoses. An initial blood test identifies a low circulating platelet count. Bone marrow aspirate or core biopsy demonstrates normal or increased levels of megakaryocytes. If antiplatelet antibody is present and no other cause of thrombocytopenia is identified, the diagnosis of ITP is made.

The many causes of ITP include congenital and acquired disorders with immune and nonimmune causes. ITP occurs most commonly among young women, but it is not limited to them. People with human immunodeficiency virus (HIV) infection and acquired immunodeficiency syndrome (AIDS) are at high risk for ITP.

At physical examination, patients with ITP may have persistent evidence of bleeding but do not have abdominal findings. The spleen is not enlarged. A palpable spleen in a patient with apparent ITP leads to a search for another cause of splenomegaly and thrombocytopenia.

The initial treatment of ITP consists of systemic glucocorticoids, usually prednisone. The dosage is reduced over several weeks, and platelet count is monitored. Patients with thrombocytopenia from causes other than ITP continue to have normal or near-normal platelet counts. Patients whose platelet counts begin to drop after cessation of steroids are considered to have chronic ITP and become candidates for splenectomy.

ITP in children requires a different management strategy. In most children < 10 years of age, ITP resolves spontaneously and requires no specific therapy. Splenectomy in children is reserved for those who have consequences of abnormal bleeding, such as intracranial hemorrhage.

Splenectomy is the principal therapy for ITP. Because the spleen is the site of most platelet sequestration in ITP, splenectomy eliminates this source of platelet consumption. Splenectomy also removes a large source of antiplatelet IgG production.

If thrombocytopenia does not respond to splenectomy, another form of therapy may be needed. If corticosteroid therapy is continued, the dosage required is usually lower than before splenectomy. Other medical regimens include immunosuppressive drugs, such as vincristine, danazol, azathioprine, and cyclophosphamide.

Thrombotic Thrombocytopenic Purpura

Thrombotic thrombocytopenic purpura (TTP) is a relatively rare syndrome with no definitive diagnostic test or clinical characteristic. The principal features of TTP are thrombocytopenic purpura, fever, microangiopathic hemolytic anemia, mental status changes with possible peripheral neuropathy, and renal dysfunction.

TTP appears to result from loss of an inhibitory mechanism for platelet aggregation. This results in multiple focal areas of thrombosis and tissue infarction, often involving the brain. A circulating substance that binds platelets may be responsible. TTP is associated with medication reactions, infection, and inflammatory or autoimmune diseases.

The management of TTP is focused on removal of the plasma constituents that lead to platelet aggregation. Plasmapheresis is the principal treatment. Splenectomy may be considered if plasmapheresis is ineffective.

Hemolytic uremic syndrome is a disease of children associated with systemic vasculitis. Like patients with TTP, children with hemolytic uremic syndrome have clinical problems that include thrombocytopenia, renal failure, microangiopathic hemolytic anemia, and changes in mental status. The pathogenic mechanisms are unclear. Treatment is nonspecific supportive care and the disease is often self-limited, although it can be lethal. Splenectomy is rarely indicated for these patients.

Postsplenectomy Sepsis

Patients who have undergone splenectomy are at increased risk for systemic infection. This includes routine bacterial infections and overwhelming systemic sepsis, predominantly associated with gram-positive encapsulated bacteria, such as streptococcal organisms. Risk for overwhelming infection from poorly opsonized bacteria is due to a decrease in specific immune response to bacterial antigens and to reduced capacity to clear bacteria from the blood.

The highest prevalence of postsplenectomy sepsis (PSS) occurs among patients who have undergone splenectomy for malignant lesions and those who have undergone incidental splenectomy during other surgical procedures. Children most at risk for PSS are those who undergo splenectomy for congenital or acquired anemia. Any patient who has undergone splenectomy or who has hyposplenism is at risk for PSS.

The clinical course of PSS has no identifiable initiating event. Patients have symptoms of sepsis, including hypotension, coagulopathy, and multiple organ failure. Blood cultures are usually positive. Because of risk for PSS, the spleen is preserved after trauma or incidental injury, if possible. Splenectomy is reserved for instances in which splenic repair or nonsurgical management is unsuccessful.

Management of PSS is nonspecific. It includes supportive care and administration of broad-spectrum systemic antibiotics. Prevention is the goal. Efforts are focused on partial splenectomy when possible and vaccination with prophylactic antibiotics when total splenectomy is necessary.

Hypersplenism

Hypersplenism is not a specific disease but is a physiologic state characterized by splenomegaly, a decrease in circulating levels of some blood cells or platelets, bone marrow hypertrophy in response to a decrease in circulating blood elements, and improvement with splenectomy.

Primary hypersplenism usually develops in women. A diagnosis of primary hypersplenism can be made only after a thorough search for other physiologic abnormalities. The presence of splenic enlargement alone is insufficient evidence for the diagnosis of hypersplenism. Splenectomy is indicated for true primary hypersplenism. Patients rarely respond to glucocorticoid therapy, and prolonged courses of steroids are not indicated.

Diseases associated with *secondary hypersplenism* include:

Increased venous pressure
Portal hypertension
Splenic venous thrombosis
Severe congestive heart failure
Malignant disease
Leukemias (especially chronic)
Lymphoma
Chronic inflammatory diseases
Felty syndrome
Systemic lupus erythematosus
Sarcoidosis

Metabolic abnormalities
Amyloidosis
Gaucher disease
Niemann–Pick disease
Infection
Mononucleosis
Bacterial endocarditis
Parasites
Fungus
Other
Myelofibrosis with myeloid metaplasia
Polycythemia vera

Hyposplenism

Hyposplenism is the condition in which the peripheral blood has elements that suggest an asplenic state despite the anatomic presence of a spleen. This occurs in patients with sickle cell disease, inflammatory bowel disease, collagen vascular diseases, and other autoimmune processes. The spleen in a patient with hyposplenism may be any size—small, normal, or enlarged.

The classic peripheral blood smear findings of hyposplenism include Howell–Jolly bodies and spur cells (acanthocytes). These findings in the presence of a spleen are diagnostic of hyposplenism. Hyposplenism is associated with increased risk for systemic infection, including PSS. Failure of the erythrocyte maintenance mechanisms of the spleen appears to be associated with abnormalities of the specific and nonspecific immune functions of the spleen.

Neoplastic Disease

As the largest single lymphoid organ in the body, the spleen becomes involved with many lymphoid malignant neoplasms. It is also secondarily affected by malignant neoplasms in other parts of the body. Another possibility is metastatic deposition of solid tumors from nonlymphoid sources into the spleen.

Despite the high blood flow through the spleen and a microanatomy designed to trap circulating cells, the spleen is a relatively rare site of solid-tumor metastatic disease compared with the liver. This may be the result of effective local defenses that destroy abnormal cells. Another mechanism of splenic involvement with malignant disease is the rare primary nonlymphoid tumor that originates in the spleen.

Primary Tumors of the Spleen

Hemangiomas are the most common primary nonlymphoid tumors of the spleen. They usually present as a single lesion and may be large by the time of diagnosis. Multiple lesions also occur. Hemangiomas of the spleen often are associated with hemangiomas of other organs, especially the liver. The primary risks of splenic hemangiomas are rupture and platelet sequestration. Coagulopathies are associated with large hemangiomas of the spleen.

Although hemangiomas are benign tumors, a tissue diagnosis cannot be made until the spleen is removed. It is unclear whether partial splenectomy has a role in the management of these lesions because of risk for recurrence in the remaining splenic tissue. The entire spleen is removed.

Hamartomas of the spleen originate from the white pulp. These lesions usually are incidental findings. Hamartomas can be cystic or solid. Hamartomas have no specific clinical consequences, except those related to size and mass effect. Differentiation of a splenic hamartoma from other lesions may be difficult or impossible with imaging evalua-

tion alone. Splenectomy is usually performed as a diagnostic maneuver.

Lymphangiomas of the spleen are cystic lesions that do not cause primary symptoms but may lead to secondary splenic abnormalities, such as hypersplenism. Splenic lymphangiomas are usually associated with liver lymphangiomas and involve multiple areas of the body. Lung, skin, and bone involvement occurs. As with other splenic lesions, the disease is identified at splenectomy.

Angiosarcoma is an extremely rare malignant disorder of the spleen. It is uncommon without similar tumors in other organs, usually the liver. Splenectomy is performed for diagnosis, and is the only therapy required. At operation, other areas of angiosarcoma involvement can be identified. Additional therapy is dictated by the extent of disease at other sites of involvement.

Hodgkin Disease

Hodgkin disease is the result of a malignant lymphoid neoplasm. Its relatively unusual characteristics are localized origin and limited regional spread. Systemic dissemination of this disease is a relatively late occurrence. Hodgkin disease is pathologically defined by the presence of giant, multinucleated Sternberg–Reed cells in the abnormal lymphoid tissue. The exact cell of origin of this disease varies among individuals. It is unclear whether the cell type is consistent from patient to patient. Macrophages and T cells are likely. Hodgkin disease can develop in any lymphoid tissue. In some patients, the spleen is the primary site. The role of staging splenectomy in Hodgkin disease is controversial.

Non-Hodgkin Lymphoma

Unlike Hodgkin disease, other lymphomas are systemic diseases at the time of diagnosis. Primary disease limited to the spleen is rare. Splenectomy has a limited role in the management of lymphoma. Lymphomas are classified by aggressiveness and the morphologic appearance of the tumor cells:

Low-grade aggressiveness
Small lymphocytic
Follicular small cleaved cell
Follicular mixed cell
Intermediate-grade aggressiveness
Follicular large cell
Diffuse small cell
Diffuse mixed cell
Diffuse large cell
High-grade aggressiveness
Lymphoblastic
Small noncleaved cell
Immunoblastic

Hairy Cell Leukemia

Hairy cell leukemia is a lymphocytic leukemia characterized by abnormal B cells in almost all patients and abnormal T cells in the rest. It is initially diagnosed morphologically on the basis of the ruffled leukocyte cell membranes seen at light and electron microscopic examination. The diagnosis is enhanced with selective staining for tartrate-resistant acid phosphatase, which is present in almost all patients with hairy cell leukemia. The hairy cells are seen predominantly in the red pulp. The spleens of these patients are enlarged and have white surface deposits that resemble a sugar coating.

Patients with hairy cell leukemia have splenomegaly and pancytopenia. Hairy cell leukemia is more common among men and most often occurs after age 50. The pancytopenia is the result of sequestration of all blood elements in the spleen, marrow replacement by leukemic cells, and diminished production of blood cellular components. Hairy cell leukemia is seen with coexistent malignant neoplasms in some patients; there is also a high rate of coexisting infections.

The role of splenectomy in hairy cell leukemia is controversial. Splenectomy for symptomatic hypersplenism is beneficial in most patients. It improves all cell counts and lessens risk for hemorrhage.

Chronic Myelogenous Leukemia

Chronic myelogenous leukemia (CML) occurs most often in the third and fourth decades of life and is slightly more common among men than women. CML is associated with the Philadelphia chromosome. Most CML progresses to acute myelogenous leukemia 1 to 4 years after the diagnosis of CML is established. Splenectomy is performed for symptoms of splenomegaly or exaggerated splenic sequestration of cellular elements and does not affect the survival of patients with CML.

Chronic Lymphocytic Leukemia

Chronic lymphocytic leukemia is a B-cell leukemia that is predominantly a disease of the elderly. It is more common among men than women. It presents as adenopathy and splenomegaly with exaggerated peripheral lymphocyte counts. Some patients have a second malignant tumor, and some have acute hemolytic anemia.

Treatment involves different forms of chemotherapy and sometimes corticosteroids. Splenectomy decreases peripheral lymphocyte count in most patients. Transfusion requirements are decreased after splenectomy because of prolonged RBC survival and better primary cellular production.

Treatment of Malignant Hematologic Disease

Patients who undergo bone marrow transplantation for leukemia or lymphoma may need splenectomy before transplantation. Splenectomy is performed several weeks before bone marrow transplantation to allow the patient time to recover.

Splenic Cysts

True splenic cysts are uncommon. They can be either congenital or acquired. Acquired cysts usually occur after traumatic injury. Pseudocysts of the spleen may result from pancreatitis. These cysts often resolve spontaneously, and can be treated with simple aspiration. Splenectomy can be performed if the cyst persists or becomes symptomatic.

Some splenic cysts are caused by parasitic or nonparasitic infection, particularly from hydatid disease. Primary management is directed at killing all the parasites. The residual cyst can be surgically removed if it presents a problem after nonsurgical treatment of the infection. Nonparasitic cysts of the spleen are rare and usually present with pain. The presence of a parenchymal defect on CT usually results in splenectomy to rule out other causes.

Splenomegaly

The causes of splenomegaly are:

Increased RBC destruction
Inflammatory processes
Autoimmune hemolytic anemia
Infectious problems
Metabolic disorders
Congestion
Elevated venous pressure
Malignant disease
Leukemia
Myelofibrosis
Extramedullary hematopoiesis
Myelofibrosis with myeloid metaplasia

Splenomegaly is not itself an indication for splenectomy. It usually is transient and has no deleterious effects. The finding of splenomegaly leads to an evaluation that includes complete blood and platelet counts with examination of the peripheral blood smear. The spleen is imaged, most effectively with CT, to assess its size, parenchymal abnormalities, and relations to other intraabdominal structures. Liver—spleen scans are used to assess the ability of the spleen to take up particulate matter, but these scans are relatively insensitive.

SURGICAL MANAGEMENT OF SPLENIC DISEASE

Possible indications for surgery include:

Thrombocytopenia
ITP
TTP
Malignant disease
Hairy cell leukemia
Hodgkin disease
Non-Hodgkin lymphoma
Other primary splenic tumors
Metastatic or locally invasive tumor
Anemia
Autoimmune hemolytic anemia
Hereditary hemolytic anemia
Medullary fibrosis with myeloid metaplasia
Hypersplenism
Primary hypersplenism
Other causes of hypersplenism
Miscellaneous
Leukopenias
Metabolic disorders
Gaucher disease
Granulomatous disease
Cysts
Abscesses
Idiopathic splenomegaly
Trauma

Partial splenectomy is performed for some diseases in which splenic involvement is limited. In such circumstances, preservation of a small segment of the spleen must not allow recurrence of the original problem.

Splenic salvage techniques are used routinely in the management of splenic trauma. This is standard procedure if the spleen is minimally injured or when partial resection is possible. Isolated splenic trauma detected on an abdominal CT scan after injury is managed nonsurgically. Total splenectomy is almost always performed for nontraumatic disorders of the spleen.

Technique

The technique of splenectomy is shown in Figures 55-3 and 55-4. The spleen is approached through an upper midline or left subcostal incision. After entry into the peritoneum, abdominal exploration is routine. The spleen is inspected visually and then palpated to estimate size and degree of attachment to the diaphragm and surrounding structures. The lesser sac can be opened for examination and ligation of the splenic vessels.

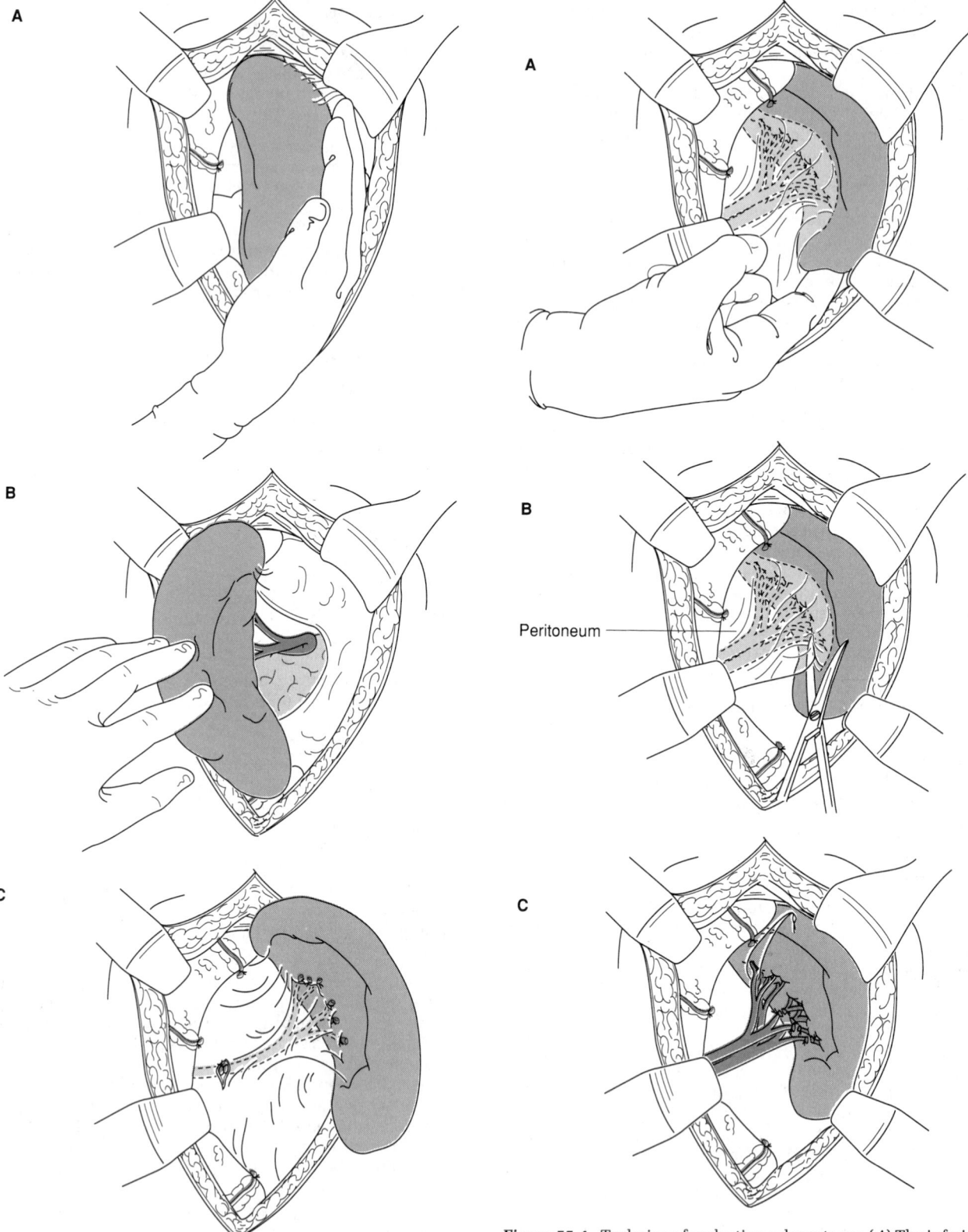

A

B

C

A

B

Peritoneum

C

Figure 55-3. (*A* and *B*) Rapid mobilization of a bleeding spleen can be accomplished in most patients by blunt dissection of the lateral attachments. (*C*) The splenic hilum can then be quickly controlled.

Figure 55-4. Technique for elective splenectomy. (*A*) The inferior pole is reflected laterally by the assistant's fingers, exposing the lower edge of the hilar peritoneal envelope. (*B*) The hilar peritoneum is opened, here shown progressing from inferior to superior. (*C*) Individual vessels are identified and suture ligated.

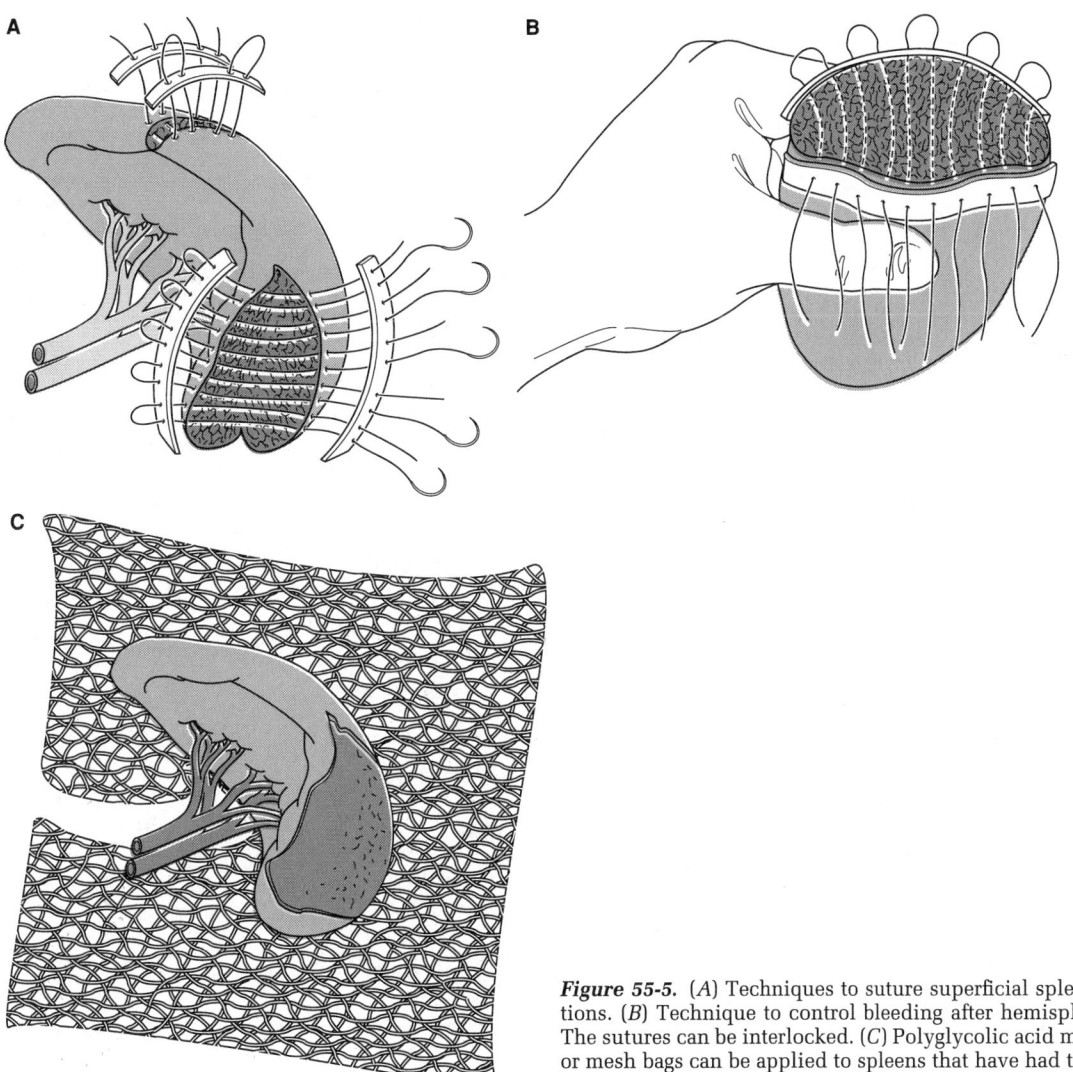

A

B

C

Figure 55-5. (*A*) Techniques to suture superficial splenic lacerations. (*B*) Technique to control bleeding after hemisplenectomy. The sutures can be interlocked. (*C*) Polyglycolic acid mesh sheets or mesh bags can be applied to spleens that have had the capsule stripped away.

Accessory spleens are sought along the cephalad and caudal edges of the pancreas behind the stomach and around gastrohepatic ligament. The greater omentum and splenic hilum also are examined for accessory spleens. It is unclear how much these accessory spleens function, but total splenectomy includes a search for, and excision of, any accessory spleens.

Once the splenic attachments are divided, the spleen is brought into the abdominal wound. If the spleen is ruptured or otherwise abnormal, rapid mobilization can be accomplished by delivering the spleen into the wound by hand.

Massive bleeding during splenectomy is encountered when the splenic vessels are perforated during dissection of the hilum. This sometimes occurs because of traction on the splenic or hilar vessels during dissection. It is best not to blindly place a clamp on the hilum of the spleen. The tail of the pancreas is usually in the immediate area, and pancreatic injury may result in pseudocyst or fistula formation. If bleeding occurs, it is better to occlude the vessels between thumb and finger while the vessels are dissected.

Massive bleeding also can occur from lateral attachments or accessory vessels if portal hypertension is present. This is anticipated before the procedure is begun, and all attachments are divided and tied.

Bleeding from the short gastric vessels can occur late postoperatively from dislodgment of a tie or transection without ligature. It is important to inspect the short gastric vessels on the greater curvature of the stomach and the splenic hilum after the spleen is removed.

Partial splenectomy and *splenorrhaphy* are accomplished with similar principles to total splenectomy (Fig. 55-5). Mobilization of the spleen into the wound for careful inspection and repair of injuries is essential. Mesh bags are used to apply pressure to a fragmented spleen and control hemorrhage. Laparoscopic splenectomy is an alternative for some patients.

Complications

Thrombocytosis is common postoperatively. It is unclear whether risk for thrombosis or embolism increases with platelet count. Patients with myelofibrosis and myeloid metaplasia appear to be vulnerable to thrombotic complications after splenectomy.

Preoperative pneumococcal immunization is provided, when possible, to limit the risk for *PSS*. Immunizations are most effective when given preoperatively, but they can be given at the time of the operation. Regardless of immunization status, prophylactic penicillin is considered for all children and all patients with sickle cell disease and hematologic diseases. Acceleration of *atherosclerosis* can occur after splenectomy. This appears to be due to the increased number of circulating platelets or other immune mechanisms in atherosclerosis.

The most common complication after splenectomy is *bleeding*, mostly in patients with very large spleens.

SUGGESTED READING

Becker CD, Spring P, Glattli A, Schweizer W. Blunt splenic trauma in adults: Can CT findings be used to determine the need for surgery? AJR Am J Roentgenol 1994;162:343.

Carroll BJ, Phillips EH, Semel CJ, et al. Laparoscopic splenectomy. Surg Endosc 1992;6:183.

Duke BJ, Modin GW, Schecter WP, Horn JK. Transfusion signifi-cantly increases the risk for infection after splenic injury. Arch Surg 1993;128:1125.

Kohn JS, Clark DE, Isler RJ, Pope CF. Is computed tomographic grading of splenic injury useful in the nonsurgical management of blunt trauma? J Trauma 1994;37:870.

Lankisch PG. The spleen in inflammatory pancreatic disease. Gastroenterology 1990;98:509.

Lucas CE. Splenic trauma: choice of management. Ann Surg 1991;213:98.

Pisters PW, Pachter HL. Autologous splenic transplantation for splenic trauma. Ann Surg 1994;219:225.

Skandalakis PN, Colborn GL, Skandalakis LJ, Richardson DD, Mitchell WE Jr, Skandalakis JE. The surgical anatomy of the spleen. Surg Clin North Am 1993;73:747.

Taddeo F, Sessa R, Sessa E, Minelli S. Video laparoscopic treatment of spleen injuries: report of two cases. Surg Endosc 1994;8:910.

Uranus S, Kronberger L, Kraft-Kine J. Partial splenic resection using the TA-stapler. Am J Surg 1994;168:49.

SURGICAL ENDOCRINOLOGY

ESSENTIALS OF SURGERY: SCIENTIFIC PRINCIPLES AND PRACTICE,
edited by Lazar J. Greenfield, Michael W. Mulholland, Keith T. Oldham, Gerald B. Zelenock,
and Keith D. Lillemoe. Lippincott–Raven Publishers, Philadelphia, © 1997.

CHAPTER 56

THYROID GLAND

NORMAN W. THOMPSON

ANATOMY

The lobes of the thyroid are adjacent to the thyroid cartilage and anterolateral to the larynx and trachea. They are united by an isthmus just below the cricoid cartilage. The anterior portion of the thyroid is covered by the infrahyoid muscles and their fasciae. Posterolaterally, the lobes are bounded by the carotid sheath.

The thyroid is supplied by two paired main arteries: the superior thyroid arteries and the inferior thyroid arteries. The venous drainage is from three veins—superior, middle, and inferior—these freely anastomose on the surface of the gland.

The thyroid is richly endowed with lymphatics, and the flow drains in many directions from the gland. The regional nodes include the paraglandular or capsular nodes; the pretracheal lymph nodes superior to the isthmus; the paratracheal nodes; the recurrent laryngeal nerve chain; the anterosuperior mediastinal nodes; the upper, middle, and lower jugular nodes; and the retropharyngeal and esophageal nodes.

The critical anatomic relations during thyroidectomy are between the thyroid and the recurrent laryngeal nerve (RLN; Fig. 56-1), superior laryngeal nerve, and parathyroid glands. Injury to the laryngeal nerves paralyzes the vocal cords on the ipsilateral side, the most serious consequences of which are loss of voice and airway obstruction. Injury to the blood supply of, or removal of, the parathyroid glands results in hypocalcemia.

FUNCTIONAL DISORDERS
Hyperthyroidism

Hyperthyroidism has many causes. The most common are Graves disease, toxic nodular goiter, and a single toxic nodule.

Graves Disease

Graves disease (toxic diffuse goiter) is an autoimmune disease with clinical manifestations due to the presence of thyroid-stimulating immunoglobulins and other tissue-specific antibodies. These antibodies bind to the thyroid-stimulating hormone (TSH) receptors on the follicular cell and stimulate thyroid function. Hereditary factors, female sex, and emotional trauma are implicated in the pathogenesis of Graves disease. Graves disease is more common among women than men.

The *clinical manifestations* of Graves disease include thyrotoxicosis, diffuse goiter, exophthalmos, and, infrequently, pretibial myxedema. The systemic manifestations of hyperthyroidism are heat intolerance, thirst, increased appetite, weight loss, sweating, palpitations, and tremors. These symptoms develop most commonly in young patients, but the disease can occur at any age. The ocular findings of Graves disease include exophthalmos with proptosis, spasm of the upper lid, lid retraction, and supraorbital and infraorbital swelling. A large number of patients have extrinsic ocular muscle weakness that is particularly apparent with upward gaze. Severe eye disease is characterized by venous congestion and edema. The initial manifestation of Graves disease in older patients may be atrial fibrillation or myocardial dysfunction (eg, angina pectoris and congestive heart failure). These patients may not have obvious goiters, and if ocular signs are absent, the diagnosis may be overlooked. The thyroid may be diffusely enlarged, symmetric, and smooth, which is characteristic, but it may also be irregular.

In a small number of patients, the thyroid is of normal size. In addition to elevated thyroxine (T_4) or triiodotyrosine (T_3) levels, or both, uptake of radioiodine by the thyroid is markedly elevated. Diffuse, increased uptake of ^{131}I within a symmetrically enlarged gland is diagnostic and differentiates Graves disease from other causes of thyrotoxicosis.

Therapy for Graves disease includes thionamide drugs, radioactive iodine, and thyroidectomy. These modalities are complementary.

Toxic Multinodular Goiter

Hyperthyroidism with multinodular goiter usually affects women >50 years, but it can occur in younger patients. Most patients have had a nontoxic nodular goiter for many years. Enough nodules eventually become autonomous so that hyperthyroidism develops insidiously. In some patients, hyperthyroidism is so mild that it is not suspected until the patient starts thyroid-suppression therapy for the enlarging goiter. Even low doses of thyroid medication may cause overt hyperthyroidism. Toxic goiter also can be precipitated or exacerbated by iodides in contrast media. Older patients may have cardiac findings such as atrial fibrillation, tachycardia, congestive heart failure, or unexplained or accelerated angina. Unexplained weight loss, anxiety, and insomnia also may occur.

Management of most toxic multinodular goiters is thyroidectomy after preparation renders the patient euthyroid. ^{131}I may be an alternative for patients at poor risk with goiters not causing airway compression. ^{131}I does not reduce goiter size and may cause acute enlargement. The operation performed is bilateral subtotal thyroidectomy. Remnant size is not as important as excision of all autonomous nodules. Alternative procedures are total lobectomy, isthmectomy and contralateral subtotal lobectomy, or total thyroidectomy.

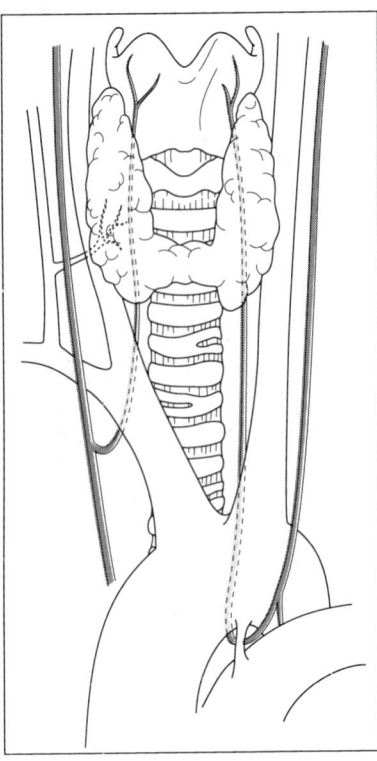

Figure 56-1. Normal course of recurrent laryngeal nerve.

Solitary Toxic Nodule

Patients with autonomous functioning nodules causing thyrotoxicosis are usually younger than those with toxic multinodular goiters. Most patients are women. The nodules are invariably at least 3 cm in diameter. Smaller solitary hot (functioning) nodules are not usually associated with hyperthyroidism. These nodules enlarge, develop central necrosis, and become cold (nonfunctioning). Only about 20% of all autonomous hot nodules eventually enlarge to the point at which clinical hyperthyroidism develops.

Thyroiditis

Hashimoto Disease (Chronic Lymphocytic Thyroiditis)

Hashimoto disease is an autoimmune disease most common among middle-aged women. Most patients have high levels of circulating antimicrosomal and antithyroglobulin antibodies. Both humoral and cell-mediated immunity are involved in the inflammatory response. The tendency of Hashimoto disease and Graves disease to occur in members of the same family suggests genetic predisposition. Environmental factors also appear to have an etiologic role. Hashimoto thyroiditis is common among patients who received irradiation in infancy or childhood.

Hashimoto thyroiditis causes defective hormone synthesis characterized by a lack of organification of trapped iodine. The reduced functional capacity of the thyroid increases TSH secretion, and a goiter develops. Palpation of the gland may suggest a nodular goiter or a neoplasm. Although a goiter is characteristic, some patients may have a smaller than normal but firm and rubbery thyroid.

Hashimoto disease is the most common cause of spontaneous *hypothyroidism* among adults, but many patients may have the disease for years with normal thyroid function. The disease may cause mild thyrotoxicosis, especially during the acute phase when there may be excessive release of thyroid hormone. This phase can be managed antithyroid drugs or propranolol.

Clinical and laboratory findings, particularly an elevated antimicrosomal antibody titer, establish the diagnosis of Hashimoto thyroiditis. *Treatment* with thyroid hormone (0.15 mg levothyroxine daily) should result in regression of the goiter. Despite TSH suppression, the goiter may continue to enlarge and cause compression or cosmetic deformity in some patients. Partial thyroidectomy may be indicated. Hashimoto thyroiditis may coexist with an adenomatous goiter or solitary nodule within a diffusely enlarged or normal-sized gland. Thyroidectomy may be indicated for a solitary nodule, particularly if it is cold (nonfunctioning), definitely malignant, or solid, and if fine-needle aspiration (FNA) biopsy findings are indeterminate.

Well-differentiated carcinoma does occur in glands involved with thyroiditis. Even if the diagnosis of Hashimoto disease is made, a suspicious nodule is evaluated as if the underlying thyroiditis did not exist.

Subacute Thyroiditis

Subacute thyroiditis usually occurs among young women within weeks of an upper respiratory or other viral infection. There may be systemic manifestations such as weakness, depression, easy fatigability, neck pain in the region of the thyroid, or referred pain to the ear or angle of the jaw. The thyroid is usually tender to palpation, and the diagnosis often can be made without laboratory studies or biopsy. The disease is usually self-limited for a few weeks, during which symptomatic relief can be achieved with salicylates or possibly corticosteroids. In some patients, the disease may persist for several months or longer. Recovery is associated with restoration of normal thyroid function. In some patients, the disease may be confined to one lobe and produce a firm, slightly tender mass, suggesting carcinoma. Lobectomy may be indicated to rule out malignancy. Total thyroidectomy may be performed for persistent painful thyroiditis if months of steroid therapy do not alleviate the disease.

Riedel Struma

Goiter with a woody or fibrous component involving the adjacent strap muscles and carotid sheaths is known as *Riedel struma*. The cause is unknown, but the syndrome is associated with other fibrotic processes, such as retroperitoneal fibrosis, sclerosing cholangitis, and fibrosing mediastinitis. The process involves both lobes of the thyroid and the isthmus. It resembles infiltrative undifferentiated thyroid carcinoma or lymphoma, and cannot be differentiated without biopsy. Airway compression is managed by means of open biopsy and excision of the isthmus and as much of the fibrotic process as possible without endangering the recurrent laryngeal nerve (RLN). Tracheostomy may be needed. For patients who do not need urgent decompression of the airway, treatment with steroids may be beneficial.

SOLITARY THYROID NODULE

Diagnosis

History review and *physical examination* are the most important aspects of the diagnosis of thyroid nodules. Half of asymptomatic nodules are discovered during routine physical examination. The patients often are unaware of thyroid enlargement or symptoms, even after the nodule is identified. The other asymptomatic nodules are usually discovered by patients.

Irradiation during infancy or childhood is associated with thyroid carcinoma, and many patients with this exposure seek thyroid evaluation. This relation must be discussed in the history review. Growth of a nodule in a patient taking thyroid hormone for suppression suggests that the nodule is autonomous and may be malignant.

Examination of the neck can often determine whether a nodule is likely to be thyroid carcinoma. Large, firm lymph nodes in the lower third of the neck, particularly in children and young adults, suggest papillary carcinoma. Lymphadenopathy in association with an ipsilateral thyroid nodule is considered due to malignant neoplasia until proved otherwise. Fixation of a nodule to surrounding structures suggests malignancy.

The palpable consistency of a solitary nodule is not always helpful. A firm nodule with an irregular outline usually suggests malignancy. Hoarseness without RLN palsy may occur with benign or malignant nodules. Paralysis of the RLN on the side of a thyroid nodule always suggests carcinoma.

Evaluation of the entire thyroid is important. A search is made for evidence of Hashimoto disease, diffuse enlargement, and other nodules. Presence of other nodules, absence of adenopathy, normal vocal cord function, and no history of irradiation, reduce the probability of malignancy.

Thyroid scintiscans are used to supplement the findings of physical examination. Only rarely is a warm or hot nodule a well-differentiated thyroid carcinoma.

Needle biopsy is performed on any palpable thyroid nodule. Fine-needle aspirate (FNA) cytologic biopsy enables differentiation between nonneoplastic and neoplastic nodules and identification of the type of malignant tumor. In addition to cytologic evaluation, FNA is used in the diagnosis of cystic lesions of the thyroid. When a nodule is found to be a cyst, the fluid is aspirated and physical examination repeated. If a nodule is still present, a specific FNA cytologic test is performed on the solid component. When nothing is palpable after aspiration, an operation can be avoided if the cyst does not recur.

TSH suppression by means of administration of thyroid hormone causes half of benign thyroid nodules to shrink or disappear. Thyroid suppression is used as a diagnostic maneuver and as therapy for thyroid nodules. Most nodules that disappear with thyroid hormone therapy are actually lobulations of the gland or diffuse enlargement of a lobe associated with Hashimoto disease or a goiter. Well-differentiated thyroid cancer, however, may shrink after TSH suppression. Unless the lesion resolves completely, carcinoma cannot be ruled out.

Surgical Treatment

Total extracapsular thyroid lobectomy with isthmectomy is the procedure of choice for surgical removal of a thyroid nodule. The entire lobe with the isthmus is subjected to frozen-section pathologic examination if FNA has not produced a definitive diagnosis of carcinoma. A nodule in the isthmus may be excised with a margin of normal thyroid tissue on both sides for the biopsy. During total lobectomy, both ipsilateral parathyroid glands must be preserved with their blood supply.

THYROID CARCINOMA

Thyroid carcinomas are classified as papillary, follicular, Hürthle cell, medullary, and anaplastic. Lymphomas also can occur as primary neoplasms originating from the thyroid. Only papillary and follicular carcinoma are well differentiated.

Papillary Carcinoma

Papillary carcinomas are divided into three groups, based on size and local extent of the primary tumor: minimal, intrathyroidal, and extrathyroidal (invasion through the true thyroid capsule). *Minimal thyroid carcinoma* is papillary carcinoma <1 cm in diameter and not associated with any clinically apparent lymph node metastases. Most of these microscopic carcinomas are a few millimeters in diameter, but they may be associated with microscopic cervical lymph node metastases. They are found during pathologic examination after operations for benign disease, and usually no additional surgical treatment is necessary. However, if the original operation was subtotal lobectomy, the rest of the lobe may have to be removed at a second operation. The decision depends on age, tumor margins, history of irradiation, and whether there are multiple tumor sites. Therapy for tumors 0.5 to 1 cm in diameter is total lobectomy with isthmectomy.

Most clinically significant papillary carcinomas are 1 to 4 cm in diameter and are *intrathyroidal* (contained within the thyroid capsule). Multicentricity is common. Metastases in the central compartment, anterior mediastinum, or lateral cervical lymph nodes are present in about one-third of patients with papillary carcinoma. The presence of lymph node metastases does not correlate as closely to the size of the tumor as it does to the age of the patient. The younger the patient, the greater the likelihood of metastatic lymph node involvement.

Extension of a primary papillary carcinoma through the thyroid capsule *(extrathyroidal),* even when there are no lymphatic metastases indicating biologic aggressiveness of the tumor. Tumors as small as 1 cm in diameter may invade the capsule into the RLN or other surrounding structures.

Surgical resection of papillary carcinoma is the cornerstone of treatment. The minimal operation for such tumors is total lobectomy and isthmectomy. If previous head or neck irradiation is confirmed, total or near-total thyroidectomy is performed. Children with bilateral thyroid lobe involvement and anterior mediastinal lymph node involvement undergo regional or modified neck dissection and routine excision of the anterior mediastinal lymph nodes through the cervical incision.

Occult pulmonary metastases can be detected and treated with a ^{131}I scan within 6 weeks of operation. Regardless of the extent of resection, all patients with papillary carcinoma are given thyroid replacement therapy sufficient to suppress TSH. When follow-up scintiscans show no residual uptake after total thyroidectomy, it is possible to assure patients that recurrence is unlikely. This cannot be done until all remaining normal thyroid tissue is ablated with large doses of ^{131}I or total thyroidectomy.

Follicular Carcinoma

Follicular carcinomas are classified as those with macroinvasion and those with microinvasion of the capsule or tumor vessels. The diagnosis usually is made after study of permanent sections.

Microinvasive encapsulated follicular carcinomas are rarely associated with metastatic lymph nodes, and distant metastases involving bone are rare.

Macroinvasive follicular carcinomas are usually large and often show invasion of perithyroidal and lateral neck veins at the time of diagnosis. They may already have metastasized to distant sites, most often to bone. These tumors are readily diagnosed at operation because the perithyroidal veins are white and enlarged. Tumor thrombus within the vein can be detected with gentle palpation. The primary tumor may extend into the contralateral lobe or through the thyroid capsule into surrounding structures, such as the trachea or RLN.

Follicular carcinomas of the thyroid are treated by means of total thyroidectomy. Lymphatic dissection usually is not needed. Therapy for bone or pulmonary metastases is radioactive iodine. If a low-grade encapsulated neoplasm is found at permanent section evaluation after total lobectomy, completion thyroidectomy is usually not performed. The patient undergoes close follow-up observation after performance of a [99mTc] bone scan to rule out occult bone metastases. Patients with follicular carcinoma treated by total thyroidectomy undergo a ^{131}I scan 6 weeks after the operation.

Medullary Carcinoma

Medullary carcinoma of the thyroid (MCT) accounts for only a small percentage of malignant tumors of the thyroid. MCT is a more aggressive tumor than papillary or follicular carcinoma, particularly among young patients. MCT metastasizes at an early age to perithyroidal lymph nodes and eventually may involve multiple distant sites, including the liver, lung, and bones.

MCT appears in three clinical settings: sporadic tumor; multiple endocrine neoplasia (MEN IIa) syndrome, with or without adrenal medullary disease (pheochromocytomas) or hyperparathyroidism (C-cell hyperplasia); and MEN IIb syndrome, with or without bilateral adrenal medullary disease and always with the facies and autonomic nervous system dysplasia expressed as a ganglioneuromatosis from the lips to the anus.

The diagnosis of MCT is made most often with preoperative FNA cytology. Calcitonin is a biologic marker of MCT. A serum assay and pentagastrin-stimulated plasma level are obtained. Plasma catecholamine levels also are determined.

Minimal management of MCT is total thyroidectomy. In patients with sporadic tumors, this allows excision of any intraglandular lymphatic spread and immunohistopathologic examination (for C-cell hyperplasia) of the contralateral lobe. If no changes are found, the need for evaluation of other family members is obviated. Sporadic MCT usually presents as a solitary nodule in the upper half of the lateral lobe on either side. Metastatic lymph nodes may be detected, although the primary tumor is occult.

Most patients with sporadic disease have lymph node metastases at diagnosis, and central compartment dissection sparing the parathyroid glands is indicated. If lateral lymph nodes are involved, modified neck dissection is performed. Capsular invasion of the lymph nodes with involvement of contiguous structures may necessitate formal radical dissection.

Patients with the MEN II syndromes must be examined for possible pheochromocytomas before treatment of MCT. Operations for pheochromocytoma take precedence over neck procedures. Total thyroidectomy is essential in patients with MEN IIa disease.

Patients with the MEN IIb disease need total thyroidectomy as soon as the syndrome is recognized, preferably by age 2. In familial cases, the characteristic findings are sufficient to justify operation even without calcitonin testing. If the diagnosis is not made until adolescence or later, central compartment involvement and lateral node involvement necessitate neck dissection. Older patients may have liver or bone involvement, which prevents surgical attempts at cure.

Hürthle Cell Carcinoma

Hürthle cell neoplasms are uncommon. These tumors do not take up iodine or synthesize thyroid hormones—characteristics that differentiate them from follicular carcinoma. Hürthle cell carcinoma infiltrates lymphatic vessels early and metastasizes to the lymph nodes in many patients. It also metastasizes hematogenously, most often to the bone and lung. With the use of FNA cytology, more Hürthle cell neoplasms are encountered at an early stage. The presence of any nodule composed entirely of Hürthle cells is an indication for lobectomy and more definitive evaluation of the neoplasm and its capsule.

A definitive diagnosis of Hürthle cell adenoma is not always possible because some lesions are associated with lymph node or distant metastases. Total thyroidectomy is unnecessary when a diagnosis of adenoma can be made. Hürthle cell carcinomas, verified according to standard histopathologic criteria, are managed by means of total thyroidectomy.

There is no satisfactory adjunctive therapy for this neoplasm. If the tumor recurs with lymphatic involvement, central compartment dissection on the ipsilateral side is indicated. If lateral nodes are involved, modified radical neck dissection to clear all nodes is essential.

Anaplastic Carcinoma

Most anaplastic carcinomas of the spindle or giant cell type originate in differentiated thyroid cancers present for a long time. Although most are follicular carcinomas, the tumor can occur in patients with papillary carcinoma, Hürthle cell carcinoma, and, rarely, MCT. Anaplastic carcinoma usually occurs among older patients with longstanding goiters. Anaplastic carcinoma is rapidly lethal; most tumors are too far advanced for surgical management when first diagnosed. The diagnosis can usually be made on the basis of physical findings and FNA cytology. If an early anaplastic thyroid cancer is confined within the thyroid, total thyroidectomy offers the only possibility of cure.

RADIOACTIVE IODINE

Radioactive iodine is used only to manage follicular and papillary thyroid carcinomas. It is of no value in the treatment or follow-up care of patients with Hürthle cell or medullary carcinomas. An ^{131}I scintiscan is obtained 6 weeks after total thyroidectomy. Thyroid hormone is withheld for the 6 weeks between operation and scan. TSH levels are measured and are usually markedly elevated during the latter part of the 6-week period. A therapeutic dose of ^{131}I is administered. Localized uptake of radioactive iodine indicates metastatic disease. When the ^{131}I scan is positive for lymph node disease, it must be determined whether these metastases can be surgically excised or adequately treated with ^{131}I. Surgical excision is recommended if the lymph nodes are palpable.

Therapeutic administration of ^{131}I necessitates 2 to 3 days of hospitalization, after which replacement doses of levothyroxine are administered. For patients who do not need ^{131}I, levothyroxine therapy is started immediately and continues for life. After a therapeutic dose of radioactive iodine, a follow-up scan is obtained within 1 year; if the scan is normal, no further ^{131}I is administered. If there is evidence of residual disease, a second dose of ^{131}I is administered. A follow-up scan is obtained during the next year.

In some patients, particularly those with pulmonary metastases apparent on chest radiographs or CT scans, cure may not be possible with radioactive iodine. When the disease can be detected only with ^{131}I after total thyroidectomy, eradication of all pulmonary metastases is often possible. Pulmonary metastases are eradicated with timely treatment. The most common site of distant metastatic follicular carcinoma is bone. Although these metastases are resistant to ^{131}I therapy, palliation can be achieved for long periods.

SUGGESTED READING

Bergman DA. Thyroid physiology and immunology. Otolaryngol Clin North Am 1990;23:231.

Decker RA, Peacock ML, Borst MJ, et al. Progress in genetic screening of multiple endocrine neoplasia type IIa: Is calcitonin testing obsolete? Surgery 1995;118:256.

Lennquist S, Smeds S. The hypermetabolic syndrome: hyperthyroidism. In: Friesen SR, Thompson NW, eds. Surgical endocrinology: clinical syndromes, ed. 2. Philadelphia, JB Lippincott, 1990;127.

Lloyd RV. The thyroid. In: Lloyd R, ed. Endocrine pathology. New York, Springer-Verlag, 1990;37.

Spiliotis JD, Chalmoukis A, Androulakis JA, et al. Thyroxine suppressive therapy of benign solitary thyroid nodules: some problems. World J Surg 1991;15:304.

Thompson NW. Surgery for medullary thyroid carcinoma. In: Fee WE Jr, Goepfert H, Johns ME, Strong EW, Ward PH, eds. Head and neck cancer. Philadelphia, BC Decker, 1990;2.

Wells SA, Chi DD, Toshima K, et al. Predictive DNA testing and prophylactic thyroidectomy in patients at risk for multiple endocrine neoplasia type IIa. Ann Surg 1994;220:237.

ESSENTIALS OF SURGERY: SCIENTIFIC PRINCIPLES AND PRACTICE, edited by Lazar J. Greenfield, Michael W. Mulholland, Keith T. Oldham, Gerald B. Zelenock, and Keith D. Lillemoe. Lippincott–Raven Publishers, Philadelphia, © 1997.

CHAPTER 57

PARATHYROID GLANDS

GERARD M. DOHERTY AND SAMUEL A. WELLS, JR.

ANATOMY

There are four parathyroid glands—two superior and two inferior (Fig. 57-1). Normal parathyroid glands are flat, ovoid, and reddish brown to yellow. They measure 5 to 7 mm × 3 to 4 mm × 0.5 to 2 mm, and weigh 30 to 50 mg each. The lower glands are usually larger than the upper glands. The upper glands are most often embedded in the fat on the posterior surface of the upper lobe of the thyroid near the site where the recurrent laryngeal nerve enters the larynx. The lower glands are more ventral and lie close to, or within, the portion of the thymus gland that extends from the inferior pole of the thyroid into the chest. Supernumerary parathyroid glands may exist, most often in the thymus.

The *arterial supply* to both the superior and inferior parathyroid glands is usually from the inferior thyroid artery, although it may originate from the superior thyroid or thyroidea ima arteries or from the rich anastomoses of vessels that supply the larynx, trachea, and esophagus. The inferior, middle, and superior thyroid *veins,* which drain the parathyroid glands, empty into the internal jugular vein or the innominate vein.

In adults a normal parathyroid is about half parenchyma and half stroma, including fat cells. In children, the gland is almost entirely composed of parenchymal chief cells.

PHYSIOLOGY
Mineral Metabolism

The parathyroid glands regulate calcium and phosphate metabolism. Average daily exchanges of these ions from the gastrointestinal (GI) tract, bone, and kidney are shown in Figure 57-2. Maintenance of calcium and phosphate homeostasis depends on contributions from the GI tract, the skeleton, and the kidneys, with minor contributions from the skin and liver. The primary hormonal regulators of this metabolism are parathyroid hormone (PTH), vitamin D, and calcitonin (Table 57-1).

Under normal conditions, serum calcium and phosphate levels vary minimally over the course of the day. Regulation occurs through PTH and a series of feedback loops involving vitamin D and calcitonin (Fig. 57-3). A decrease in serum-ionized calcium level increases PTH secretion and stimulates production of calcitriol. Increases in serum calcium level inhibit PTH secretion and the formation of active calciferol.

HYPERCALCEMIA

The symptoms of hypercalcemia are listed in Table 57-2.

Differential Diagnosis

Although most patients with hypercalcemia have primary hyperparathyroidism, all causes of hypercalcemia must be considered and excluded. They include:

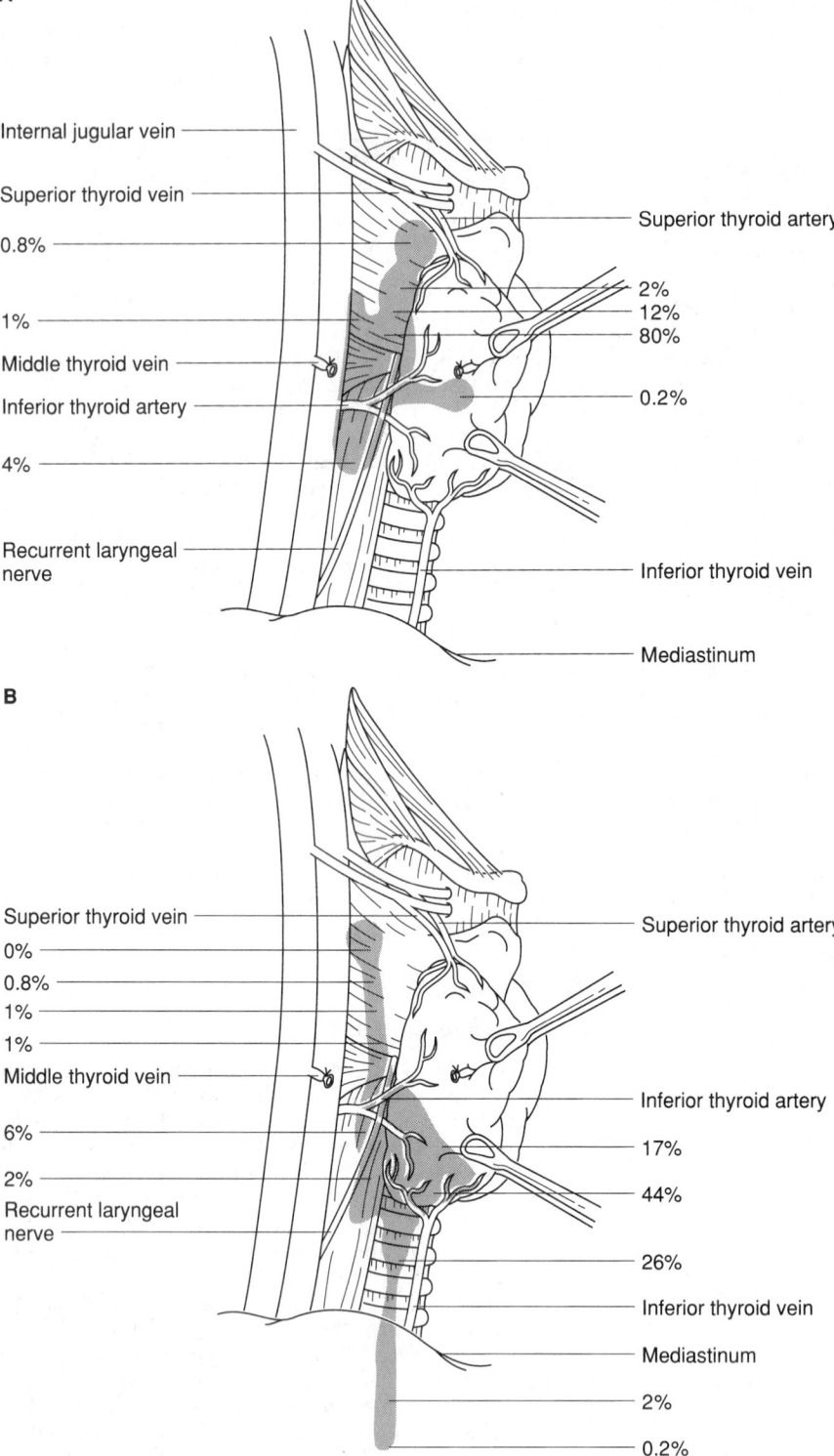

A

Internal jugular vein

Superior thyroid vein

0.8%

1%

Middle thyroid vein

Inferior thyroid artery

4%

Recurrent laryngeal nerve

Superior thyroid artery

2%
12%
80%

0.2%

Inferior thyroid vein

Mediastinum

B

Superior thyroid vein

0%

0.8%

1%

1%

Middle thyroid vein

6%

2%

Recurrent laryngeal nerve

Superior thyroid artery

Inferior thyroid artery

17%

44%

26%

Inferior thyroid vein

Mediastinum

2%

0.2%

Figure 57-1. Location of the superior (*A*) and inferior (*B*) parathyroid glands from 503 autopsy studies. The more common locations are indicated by the shaded areas. The numbers represent the percentage of glands found at each location. Typically, the glands were found posterolateral to the thyroid and above or below the junction of the inferior thyroid artery with the recurrent laryngeal nerve. (After Akerstrom G, Malmaers J, Bergstrom R. Surgical anatomy of human parathyroid glands. Surgery 1984;95:14)

- Hyperparathyroidism
- Malignant disease
- Vitamin A or D intoxication
- Thiazide diuretic therapy
- Hyperthyroidism
- Milk–alkali syndrome
- Sarcoidosis and other granulomatous diseases
- Familial hypocalciuric hypercalcemia
- Immobilization

- Paget disease
- Lithium therapy
- Addisonian crisis
- Idiopathic hypercalcemia of infancy

Medical Treatment

Therapy is tailored to the cause of hypercalcemia, but several general measures may be effective. For mild hypercalcemia, a decrease in dietary calcium is indicated. A

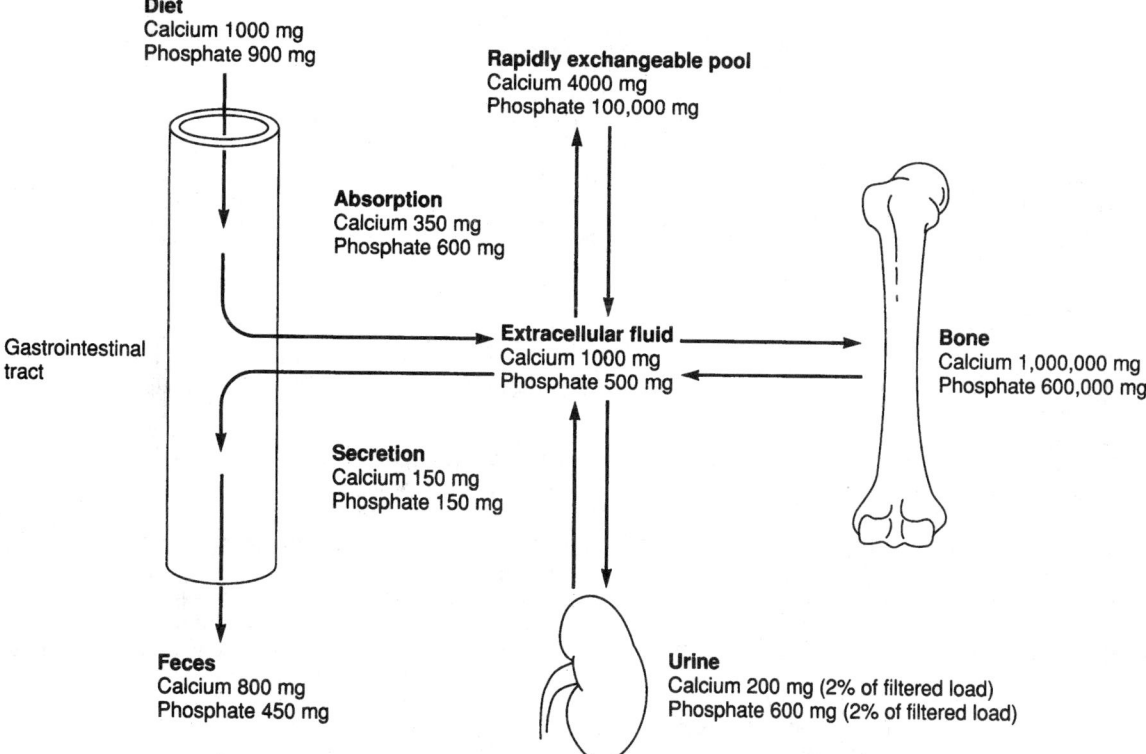

Figure 57-2. Average daily calcium and phosphate turnover in humans. (After Aurbach GD, Marx SJ, Spiegel AM, et al: Parathyroid hormone, calcitonin, and the calciferols. In: Textbook of endocrinology, ed 7. Philadelphia, WB Saunders, 1985:1144)

reduction in intake of milk and other dairy products is suggested, along with discontinuation of thiazide diuretics and vitamin D preparations. Mobilization prevents bone demineralization.

Patients with marked hypercalcemia or severe symptoms are admitted to the hospital for observation. Patients with severe hyperparathyroidism undergo neck exploration when calcium level is close to normal. The principal therapy is IV hydration, preferably with enough normal saline solution to maintain urine output. Saline diuresis usually is effective when hypercalcemia results from hyperparathyroidism or a benign lesion. The hypercalcemia of malignant disease may produce severe symptoms associated with extremely high serum calcium levels. In this setting, other measures may be considered (Table 57-3).

HYPOCALCEMIA

Hypocalcemia is a consequence of a variety of acquired and hereditary diseases. These disorders produce a deficiency of, or a defect in, the action of PTH or vitamin D.

Hypocalcemia is most often a problem after operations for thyroid disease. Vitamin D deficiency is associated with compensatory PTH excess. The result is rickets in children and osteomalacia in adults.

Clinical Features

The signs and symptoms of hypocalcemia (Table 57-4) are a direct consequence of a reduction in plasma-ionized calcium, which produces increased neuromuscular excitability. The earliest clinical manifestations are numbness and tingling around the mouth and in the fingers and toes. Patients become anxious, depressed, or confused. Tetany may develop.

Differential Diagnosis

The causes of hypocalcemia are:

* Hypoparathyroidism
* Vitamin D deficiency

Table 57-1. HORMONAL REGULATION OF CALCIUM AND PHOSPHATE METABOLISM

	Parathyroid Hormone	Vitamin D	Calcitonin
Gastrointestinal tract	No direct effect	Stimulates calcium and phosphate absorption	No direct effect
Skeleton	Stimulates calcium and phosphate resorption	Stimulates calcium and phosphate transport	Inhibits calcium and phosphate resorption
Kidneys	Stimulates calcium resorption Inhibits phosphate resorption	No direct effect	Inhibits calcium and phosphate resorption

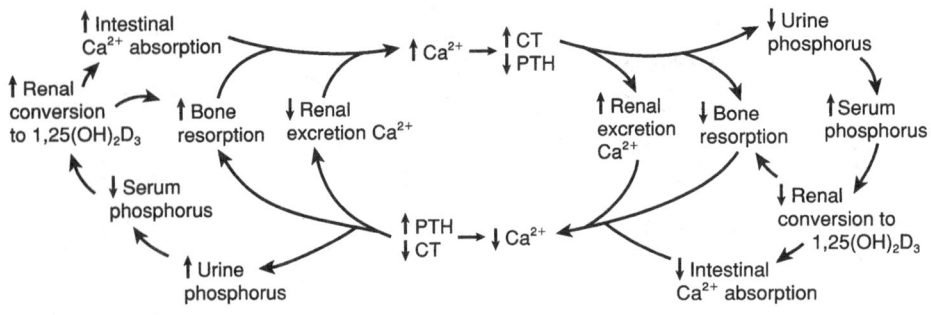

Figure 57-3. Feedback loops involved in the regulation of serum calcium and phosphorus. PTH, parathyroid hormone; CT, calcitonin.

- Pseudohypoparathyroidism
- Hypomagnesemia
- Malabsorption
- Pancreatitis
- Hypoalbuminemia
- Chelation of calcium
- Osteoblastic metastases
- Toxic shock syndrome
- Hyperphosphatemia

Medical Treatment

Treatment of hypocalcemia is as follows:

- Administration of calcium gluconate or chloride
- Diphenylhydantoin for symptomatic tetany
- Correction of hypomagnesemia with magnesium chloride
- Vitamin D supplementation
- Long-term therapy
- Calcium carbonate
- Low phosphate, oxalate diet
- Parathyroid grafting (immunosuppressed)

HYPERPARATHYROIDISM

Definitions

Primary hyperparathyroidism is disturbance in control of serum calcium that causes increased autonomous production of PTH. The condition involves both benign single- and multiple-gland enlargement and parathyroid carcinoma.

Secondary hyperparathyroidism is an increase in parathyroid function in compensation for a defect in mineral homeostasis. It occurs most commonly in response to renal disease but may develop as a consequence of hypocalcemia associated with disease of the GI tract, bone, or other endocrine organs.

Tertiary hyperparathyroidism is a condition in which hyperfunctioning parathyroid glands are no longer physiologically responsive to increased ionized calcium levels. This state develops most commonly after renal transplantation.

Etiology

The cause of primary hyperparathyroidism is unknown. Most patients have disease of a single parathyroid gland rather than multiple glands. Hyperparathyroidism is most common in postmenopausal women—the population group with the most marked alterations in calcium and phosphate metabolism. Loss of renal function with aging is associated with elevations in PTH and decreases in phosphate clearance. Hyperparathyroidism can occur in several familial forms. It is a component of the multiple endocrine neoplasia (MEN) syndromes types I and IIa.

Pathology

Single-Versus Multiple-Gland Disease

The cell most commonly involved in primary hyperparathyroidism is the chief cell. Diseased glands have an increased number of stromal cells and a decreased amount of stromal fat. Patients with multiple-gland disease may have one gland that appears to have an adenoma and another that appears diffusely involved or even histologically normal with gross enlargement.

Carcinoma

Parathyroid carcinoma is rare, and histologic diagnosis is difficult. The surgeon may suspect the diagnosis when he or she encounters dense invasion and scarring. Pathologic criteria are marked mitotic activity, dense fibrous stroma, and evidence of local invasion into the capsule or surrounding vessels. The only reliable criteria for malignancy are metastases and true local invasion.

Systemic Effects

Hyperparathyroidism occurs in three ways (Table 57-5):

1. Renal disease, slow onset of symptoms, low serum calcium

Table 57-2. CLINICAL FEATURES OF HYPERCALCEMIA

NEUROLOGIC	CARDIOVASCULAR
Lethargy	ECG changes (short QT, widened T)
Confusion	Bradycardia
Coma	Heart block
Headache	Hypertension
Depression	
Paranoia	**RENAL**
Muscle weakness	Polyuria
Hyporeflexia	Uremia
Incontinence	Renal colic
Memory loss	Nephrocalcinosis
Hearing loss	
Ataxia	**OTHER**
	Band keratopathy
GASTROINTESTINAL	Conjunctivitis
Constipation	Change in vision
Anorexia	Pruritus
Nausea and vomiting	Thrombosis
Polydipsia	Myalgia
Weight loss	
Pancreatitis	
Peptic ulcer	
Abdominal pain	

Table 57-3. **TREATMENT OF HYPERCALCEMIA**

THERAPY OF PRIMARY DISEASE

Tumor resection (hypercalcemia of malignancy)
Parathyroidectomy (primary hyperparathyroidism)

EXPANSION OF EXTRACELLULAR VOLUME

Saline infusion

ENHANCEMENT OF URINARY CALCIUM EXCRETION

Extracellular volume expansion
Loop diuretics (furosemide and ethacrynic acid)

INHIBITION OF BONE RESORPTION

Calcitonin
Glucocorticoids
Plicamycin (Mithramycin)
Bisphosphonates
Gallium nitrate

REDUCTION OF INTESTINAL CALCIUM ABSORPTION

Low-calcium diet
Glucocorticoids

OTHER

Dialysis
Mobilization
Oral phosphate
Estrogens or progestogens (postmenopausal women with primary hyperparathyroidism)
Chloroquine (sarcoidosis)

(Modified from Attie MF. Treatment of hypercalcemia. Endocrinol Metab Clin North Am 1989; 18:802)

2. Bone disease, rapid onset of symptoms, high serum calcium
3. No symptoms, minimally active disease

No histologic or physiologic characteristics of the parathyroids allow for differentiation between renal disease and bone disease. The early symptoms of hyperparathyroidism are often the vague symptoms of hypercalcemia—

Table 57-4. **CLINICAL FEATURES OF HYPOCALCEMIA**

NEUROLOGIC

Circumoral parethesia
Light-headedness
Depression
Anxiety
Confusion
Chvostek sign
Trousseau sign
Irritability
Laryngeal spasm
Seizures

MUSCULOSKELETAL

Tetany
Cramps
Involuntary twitching
Osteomalacia

CARDIOVASCULAR

ECG changes (prolonged QT interval, T-wave peaking)
Arrhythmia
Tachycardia, hypotension

OTHER

Lenticular cataracts

Table 57-5. **AGE- AND GENDER-SPECIFIC INCIDENCE OF PRIMARY HYPERPARATHYROIDISM**

Age (y)	New Cases per 100,000	
	Men	Women
<39	5	8
40–50	26	104
>60	92	189
Total	18	56

(After Heath H III, Hodgson SF, Kennedy MA. Primary hyperthyroidism: incidence, morbidity, and potential economic impact in a community. N Engl J Med 1980; 302:189)

muscle weakness, anorexia, nausea, constipation, polyuria, and polydipsia. Some patients have evidence of chronic disease that involves the kidney or skeleton.

Renal Manifestations

Renal complications develop because hypercalcemia increases urinary calcium excretion and because PTH increases the excretion of phosphate and produces urinary alkalosis. Both of these events lead to *stone formation.* Urinary stones may be treated with a surgical procedure or lithotripsy. Treating hyperparathyroidism reduces the likelihood of stone recurrence. *Nephrocalcinosis* causes more severe renal damage than nephrolithiasis. The more severe the renal damage, the less likely it is that nephrocalcinosis will improve after parathyroidectomy. *Hypertension* may be the most important cause of morbidity in hyperparathyroidism. The degree of hypertension correlates with the degree of renal impairment. Hypertension sometimes improves after parathyroidectomy.

Skeletal Manifestations

The most severe parathyroid bone disease, osteitis fibrosa cystica, seldom occurs. More common are bone pain and pathologic fractures. Findings in the skull and long bones are bone cysts, localized proliferations of osteoclasts (brown tumors), and diffuse demineralization or granularity.

GI Manifestations

Hypercalcemia is associated with nonspecific GI symptoms, such as nausea, vomiting, constipation, and anorexia. Hypercalcemia is a stimulus for increased gastric acid secretion and is associated with pancreatitis. The incidence of cholelithiasis increases slightly in patients with hyperparathyroidism, presumably because of the higher concentrations of calcium in bile.

Neuromuscular Manifestations

Fatigability and proximal muscle weakness are among the most debilitating neuromuscular symptoms of hypercalcemia. Sensory symptoms include dysesthesia, reduced vibratory sense, and stocking-glove sensory deficits.

Psychologic Manifestations

Emotional disturbances range from depression or anxiety to psychosis. Coma can result without therapy.

Other Manifestations

Other manifestations of hyperparathyroidism include nonspecific arthralgia, particularly of the proximal interphalangeal joints of the hands; chondrocalcinosis; pruritus; vascular and cardiac calcification; and band keratopathy of the cornea.

Diagnosis

Only the skeletal changes of hyperparathyroidism are pathognomonic. Evaluation usually focuses on the differential diagnosis of an elevated serum calcium concentration.

Physical Findings

Except for patients with the classic deformities of advanced bone disease, a physical examination is seldom helpful. Diseased parathyroid glands rarely are palpable, except in patients with parathyroid carcinoma. A mass in the anterior part of the neck in a patient with primary hyperparathyroidism is usually a thyroid nodule.

Laboratory Findings

Calcium. Hypercalcemia is the single most important diagnostic finding in hyperparathyroidism. However, serial analysis may show fluctuations in and out of the normal range.

Parathyroid Hormone. Demonstration of an elevated plasma PTH concentration alone does not establish the diagnosis of hyperparathyroidism. Coincident with an elevated serum calcium level, however, this finding is virtually diagnostic.

Phosphate. PTH increases renal phosphate excretion and sometimes produces hypophosphatemia. In the presence of renal disease, serum phosphate levels may be normal or elevated.

Bicarbonate. PTH increases bicarbonate excretion such that patients may experience hyperchloremic metabolic acidosis. A serum chloride to phosphate ratio >30 is considered highly suggestive of hyperparathyroidism.

Magnesium. When both hypocalcemia and hypomagnesemia occur after parathyroidectomy, it may be difficult to correct the calcium level until the serum magnesium level is corrected.

Other Tests. Additional tests include 24-hour urinary calcium excretion, measurement of tubular reabsorption of phosphate, and measurement of urinary cyclic adenosine monophosphate (cAMP).

Localization

Preoperative localization of the parathyroid glands in patients who have not undergone a neck operation is rarely indicated.

Treatment

Estrogen therapy may be useful in postmenopausal women with mild hyperparathyroidism. Otherwise, the only practical therapeutic option is surgery. Nephrolithiasis, bone disease, and neuromuscular symptoms all respond well to surgical therapy. Parathyroidectomy for renal failure, hypertension, and psychiatric symptoms is not as successful in reversing these symptoms, although it benefits some patients and is usually indicated for all patients, except those at highest risk.

Asymptomatic Hyperparathyroidism

Many patients with hyperparathyroidism have no symptoms. Indications for the surgical treatment of these patients are listed in Table 57-6. Patients not treated surgically are examined every 6 months.

Surgical Exploration

Important landmarks include the tracheoesophageal groove, the recurrent laryngeal nerve, the inferior and superior thyroid arteries, and the middle thyroid vein (Fig. 57-4). Variations in the path of the recurrent laryngeal nerve make it susceptible to injury.

All four glands must be identified because of the possibility of multiple-gland disease. Supernumerary glands are sought. If, after meticulous exploration, three or four parathyroid glands are definitively identified, none of which is enlarged, the operation is terminated. Although frozen section is not helpful in differentiating diseased from normal glands, it is essential for confirmation of the presence or absence of parathyroid tissue.

Extent of Resection

Single-gland disease is treated with simple excision. Any combination of two- or three-gland enlargement is treated with resection of the diseased tissue, and the normal glands are left in place. Four-gland hyperplasia is treated with subtotal parathyroidectomy (removal of three and one-half glands) or total parathyroidectomy with autotransplantation of some parathyroid tissue into the nondominant forearm. In both operations, parathyroid tissue is cryopreserved to allow later autografting if the patient has persistent postoperative hypoparathyroidism.

Special Situations

Persistent or Recurrent Hyperparathyroidism

Persistent hyperparathyroidism usually occurs when a single diseased gland remains in the neck or mediastinum. *Recurrent* disease develops after an interval of normocalcemia and may be the result of regrowth of diseased tissue, implantation from tumor spill at the initial procedure, or recurrent parathyroid carcinoma.

Review of the original operative notes and pathology reports may provide clues to the position of missed glands. Localization studies are performed. Angiographic ablation of mediastinal parathyroid tissue can be undertaken for

---

Table 57-6. CLINICAL CHARACTERISTICS OF PATIENTS WITH PRIMARY HYPERPARATHYROIDISM

Characteristics*	Percentage of Population
Urolithiasis	4
Hypercalciuria (>250 mg/d)	22
Emotional disorder	20
Osteoporosis	12
Diminished renal function	14
Hyperparathyroid bone disease	8
Peptic ulcer disease	8
No problems related to hyperparathyroidism	51

* Listed are problems generally accepted as potentially caused or aggravated by hypercalcemia or hyperparathyroidism
(After Heath H III, Hodgson SF, Kennedy MA. Primary hyperthyroidism: incidence, morbidity, and potential economic impact in a community. N Engl J Med 1980;302:189)

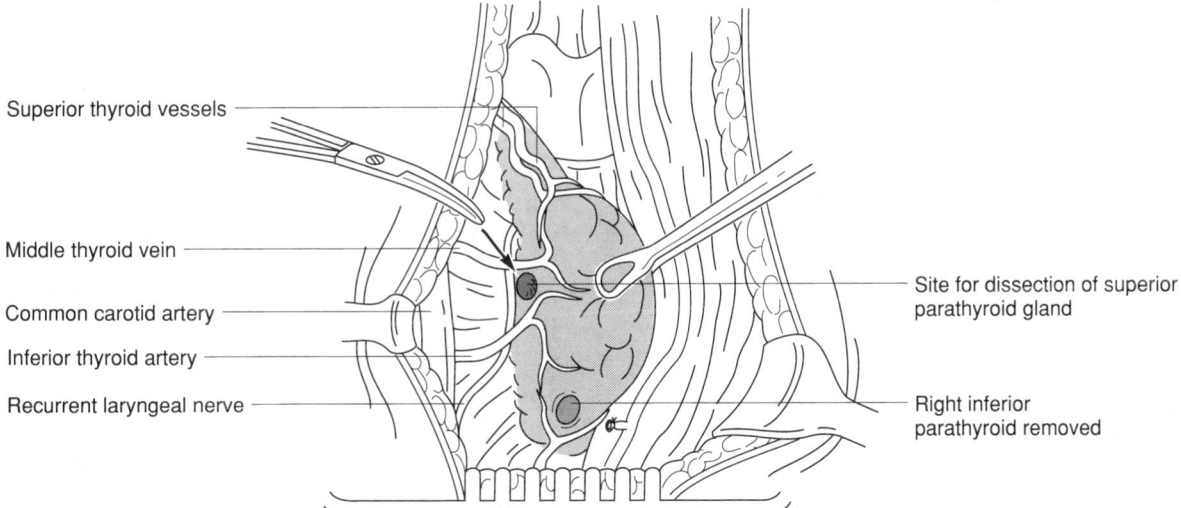

Figure 57-4. Lateral view of the right side of the neck after rotation of the thyroid lobe, emphasizing the important anatomic landmarks.

mediastinal parathyroid adenoma if the patient is at high surgical risk and has other functional parathyroid tissue.

Surgical reexploration is difficult. If a gland is not identified in the neck, the mediastinum is examined. If mediastinal exploration is negative, the area posterior and lateral to the trachea is explored. Superior parathyroid glands may be as far posterior as the esophagus and as far superior as the pharynx. Excised tissue is cryopreserved to allow autotransplantation if hypoparathyroidism develops.

Hypercalcemic Crisis

Some patients with hyperparathyroidism may experience severe, acute hypercalcemia. Patients may experience rapidly developing muscle weakness, nausea and vomiting, lethargy, fatigue, and even coma. If the diagnosis of hyperparathyroidism is in question, ultrasonography (US) or computed tomography (CT) may help identify the enlarged gland. Definitive treatment is resection of the diseased parathyroid tissue.

Hyperparathyroidism in Pregnancy

Hyperparathyroidism in pregnancy is a rare disorder in which the mother experiences hypercalcemia. It is associated with high fetal morbidity and mortality. Newborns are at risk for neonatal tetany. The mother undergoes an operation in the second trimester.

Neonatal Hyperparathyroidism

Neonatal hyperparathyroidism occurs in infants who are homozygous for a mutation of the calcium-sensing receptor. It is characterized by hypotonia, poor feeding, constipation, and respiratory distress. Each parent is affected by familial hypocalciuric hypercalcemia. Total parathyroidectomy with autotransplantation is the treatment.

Secondary Hyperparathyroidism

Secondary hyperparathyroidism develops as a consequence of chronic renal failure. Therapy is control of hyperphosphatemia by means of dietary restriction and phosphate-binding gels, calcium supplementation by mouth and in the dialysate bath, correction of acidosis, administration of vitamin D sterol, and reduction in aluminum intake in both the dialysate and the diet. Indications for surgical therapy (subtotal or total parathyroidectomy with heterotopic autotransplantation) are persistent, symptomatic hypercalcemia that cannot be controlled medically, particularly in prospective renal transplant patients; bone pain and fractures; ectopic calcification; and intractable pruritus.

Parathyroid Carcinoma

Parathyroid carcinoma is rare. The diagnosis is made only on the basis of local invasion or distant metastases. Serum calcium, PTH, and alkaline phosphatase levels are elevated, and patients often have an elevated human chorionic gonadotrophin (hCG) level. Patients may have both renal disease and bone disease. The affected gland is palpable in almost half of patients. Initial treatment is radical resection of the involved gland, the ipsilateral thyroid lobe, and the regional lymph nodes. Neither chemotherapy nor radiation therapy is of benefit. If the disease recurs, an attempt is made to resect the tumor, because untreated patients usually die of uncontrolled hypercalcemia.

MULTIPLE ENDOCRINE NEOPLASIA

Multiple endocrine neoplasia is a familial disorder inherited in an autosomal dominant manner. The tumors tend to be multicentric, may be benign or malignant, metachronous or synchronous. MEN I is characterized by parathyroid hyperplasia, pancreatic islet cell tumors, and pituitary adenomas. MEN IIa consists of medullary thyroid carcinoma (MTC), pheochromocytoma, and parathyroid hyperplasia. MEN IIb includes MTC, pheochromocytoma, mucosal neuromas, and a marfanoid habitus.

MEN I

MEN I develops in the third and fourth decades of life; there is no gender predilection. Almost all patients have hyperparathyroidism, but islet cell neoplasms and pituitary tumors also occur.

Parathyroid Disease

Hypercalcemia secondary to hyperparathyroidism is usually the first biochemical abnormality detected in MEN I and is the best screening tool for members of an affected kindred. Many of these patients have no symptoms and have relatively mild hypercalcemia. When symptoms do develop, they involve the urinary tract rather than the skeleton. Patients usually have four-gland disease, which may be particularly difficult to manage. Treatment is total parathyroidectomy with heterotopic autotransplantation.

Pancreatic Tumors

Patients with pancreatic tumors have multicentric and diffuse hyperplasia of the pancreatic islets, which may occur in areas distant from any grossly evident tumor. In the absence of symptomatic disease, screening for these tumors in an affected kindred does not appear to be of benefit. In patients with hyperparathyroidism, measurement of serum gastrin is helpful because gastrinomas are the most common islet cell lesion. Measurement of serum concentrations of pancreatic polypeptide may provide a screening measure for a variety of islet cell tumors.

Pituitary Adenomas

Prolactin-secreting tumors are most common, although some patients have Cushing's disease or acromegaly. Symptoms may result from compression of the optic chiasm, which produces bitemporal hemianopsia, or from prolactin excess, which produces amenorrhea and galactorrhea in women and hypogonadism in men.

Other Tumors

MEN I sometimes is associated with adrenocortical tumors and benign thyroid adenomas. Lipomas and carcinoid tumors may occur.

MEN IIa and IIb

Medullary Carcinoma of the Thyroid

Bilateral MTC occurs in every patient with MEN IIa or IIb. It is usually the first tumor that develops and appears in the second or third decade of life. Tumors develop in multiple areas of the middle and upper portions of the thyroid. Signs and symptoms include a neck mass, hoarseness, dysphagia, and palpable cervical adenopathy. MTC may produce calcitonin, corticotropin, prostaglandin, or serotonin. With genetic screening, MTC can be identified early.

Residual MTC after thyroidectomy is detected with provocative testing. Reoperation includes mediastinal dissection, which appears to normalize elevated plasma calcitonin levels in some patients. Patients with unresectable metastases have few therapeutic options.

In MEN IIa, MTC is often indolent, and patients have long survival, even in the presence of metastatic disease. The tumors of MEN IIb occur at an early age and are aggressive.

Pheochromocytoma

Pheochromocytoma is usually diagnosed during the initial screening or follow-up examinations of patients with MTC. The tumors appear in the second or third decade of life, and most are bilateral. They usually are benign but multicentric and almost always originate in the adrenal medulla. Pheochromocytomas may be asymptomatic, but most patients have symptoms that may include pounding frontal headaches, episodic diaphoresis, palpitations, anxiety, and hypertension.

Parathyroid Disease

Hyperparathyroidism develops in about one-third of patients with MEN IIa, but it is usually asymptomatic. Some patients have nephrolithiasis. Bone disease is unusual. Enlarged parathyroid glands often are found at operation for

MTC, although the patient is still normocalcemic. Multiglandular chief cell hyperplasia is the predominant histologic finding in MEN IIa. Parathyroid disease rarely develops in MEN IIb. Hypercalcemic MEN IIa is managed with total parathyroidectomy and heterotopic autotransplantation. Normocalcemic MEN IIa is managed with total parathyroidectomy and heterotopic autotransplantation at the time of thyroidectomy for MTC.

Nonendocrine Manifestations of MEN IIb

In addition to MTC and pheochromocytoma, patients with MEN IIb have marked abnormalities of the nervous and musculoskeletal systems. The phenotype is thick lips and a thin, marfanoid habitus. Skeletal abnormalities include kyphosis, pectus excavatum, pes planus or cavus, and congenital dislocation of the hip. Neurologic abnormalities include diffuse autonomic nervous hypertrophy; mucosal neuromas on the tongue, eyelids, lips, and pharynx; hypertrophied corneal nerves; and ganglioneuromatosis in the submucosal and myenteric plexuses of the GI tract. Constipation is common; radiographic findings may suggest megacolon or Hirschprung disease.

SUGGESTED READING

Arnold A. Molecular mechanisms of parathyroid neoplasia. Endocrinol Metabol Clin North Am 1994;23:93.
Doherty GM, Doppman JL, Miller DL, et al. Results of a multidisciplinary strategy for management of mediastinal parathyroid adenoma as a cause of persistent primary hyperparathyroidism. Ann Surg 1992;215:101.
Larsson C, Friedman E. Localization and identification of the multiple endocrine neoplasia type 1 disease gene. Endocrinol Metabol Clin North Am 1994;23:67.
Nussbaum SR. Pathophysiology and management of severe hypercalcemia. Endocrinol Metabol Clin North Am 1993;22:343.
Roth SI. Recent advances in parathyroid gland pathology. Am J Med 1994;50:612.
Skogseid B, Rastad J, Oberg K. Multiple endocrine neoplasia type 1: Clinical features and screening. Endocrinol Metabol Clin North Am 1994;23:1.
Wells SA, Leight GS, Hensley M, Dilley WG. Hyperparathyroidism associated with the enlargement of two or three parathyroid glands. Ann Surg 1994;202:533.

ESSENTIALS OF SURGERY: SCIENTIFIC PRINCIPLES AND PRACTICE, edited by Lazar J. Greenfield, Michael W. Mulholland, Keith T. Oldham, Gerald B. Zelenock, and Keith D. Lillemoe. Lippincott–Raven Publishers, Philadelphia, © 1997.

CHAPTER 58

ADRENAL GLANDS

H.H. NEWSOME, JR.

ANATOMY

The adrenal glands are paired structures on each side of the body above the kidneys. They are flat and triangular and weigh about 5 g. Each gland has two distinct regions: the outer, bright-yellow, lipid-laden *cortex;* and the thin, dark gray *medulla* (Fig. 58-1).

There are three sets of adrenal *arteries:* the superior adrenal artery is a branch of the inferior phrenic artery; the middle adrenal artery originates from the aorta; and the inferior adrenal artery originates from the renal artery. Most of the *venous* drainage is through a single, well-

A

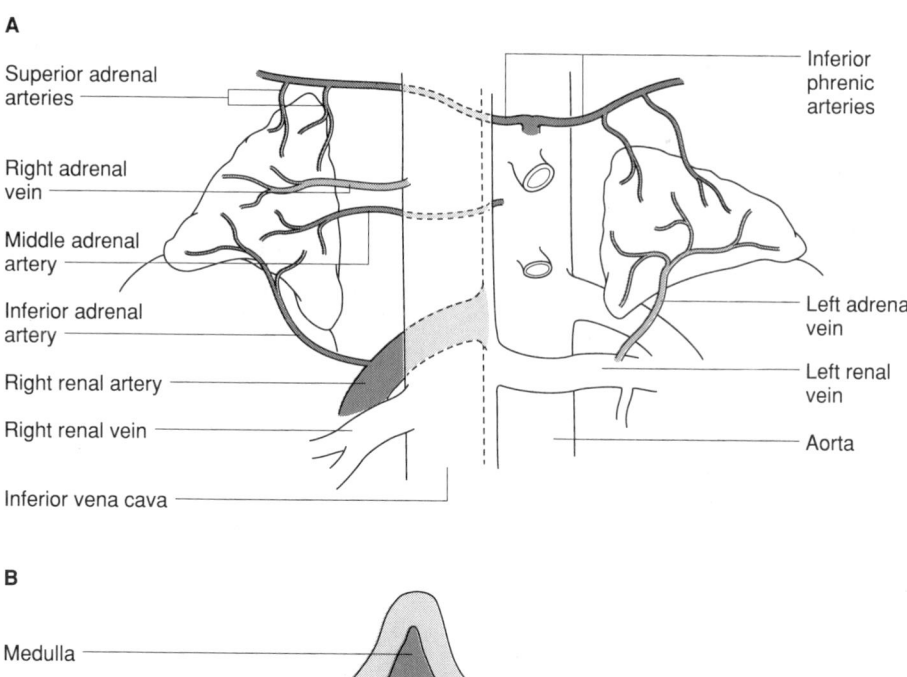

Superior adrenal
arteries

Right adrenal
vein

Middle adrenal
artery

Inferior adrenal
artery

Right renal artery

Right renal vein

Inferior vena cava

Inferior
phrenic
arteries

Left adrenal
vein

Left renal
vein

Aorta

B

Medulla

Cortex

Figure 58-1. (*A*) The arterial and venous anatomy of the right and left adrenal glands. (*B*) Division of the gland into the outer cortex and inner medulla.

defined central vein, which empties into the renal vein on the left and into the vena cava on the right. Blood flow within the gland is predominantly from the cortex through the medulla into the central medullary venous system, forming the large adrenal vein.

PHYSIOLOGY

Adrenocortical Secretion

The steroidogenic pathway is common to all steroids. Cholesterol is converted to δ5-pregnenolone, progesterone, and 17-OH progesterone, then to the adrenal androgens or cortisol.

Control of Cortisol Secretion

Cortisol production is stimulated by adrenocorticotropic hormone (ACTH), also called corticotropin. ACTH originates from the anterior pituitary gland and is regulated by corticotropin-releasing hormone (CRH). Stimulation of CRH is under neural control: The increased cortisol production during fear or other emotional stress indicates central nervous system regulation. The increase in cortisol secretion during pain and physical trauma shows that peripheral sensory pathways also stimulate cortisol production. Release of CRH is under negative-feedback inhibition by cortisol. The secretion of adrenal androgens, which are converted to estrogens, is controlled by the same mechanisms as cortisol secretion. The estrogens and androgens secreted by the gonads are regulated by different pituitary peptides.

Control of Aldosterone Secretion

Control of aldosterone secretion is by angiotensin II (Fig. 58-2). The rate of renin secretion and therefore angiotensin II and aldosterone secretion is stimulated by a decrease in afferent arteriolar pressure in the renal cortex, a decrease

in sodium content in the renal tubule, an increase in serum potassium concentration, and by ACTH secretion.

Adrenomedullary Secretion

Catecholamines are produced in the adrenal medulla. In the systemic circulation, the catecholamines undergo neuronal uptake and degradation, enzymatic degradation by other sites, or excretion in the urine. The catecholamines taken up by neurons are metabolized predominately by monamine oxidase, and they eventually yield vanillylmandelic acid (VMA).

Factors that stimulate adrenal medullary secretion are those that increase sympathetic activity throughout the body. These are assumption of an upright position, pain, emotional stress, hypotension, cold, hypoglycemia, and many others. Mechanisms that diminish the stimulatory effects are feedback inhibition by norepinephrine on the presynaptic, preganglionic α_2 receptors and suppression of tyrosine hydroxylase activity by high concentrations of norepinephrine.

PATHOPHYSIOLOGY

Pathologic conditions that affect the adrenal glands include tumor formation and the steroidogenic enzymatic defects of congenital adrenal hyperplasia. Overproduction of hormones is a key underlying problem. The pathologic condition is caused by the effects of steroids and catecholamines on peripheral tissues.

Steroids

After secretion into the blood, most steroid molecules are bound to specific plasma proteins and are present only to a limited degree in unbound, or free, form. Except in unusual situations in which steroid-binding proteins are

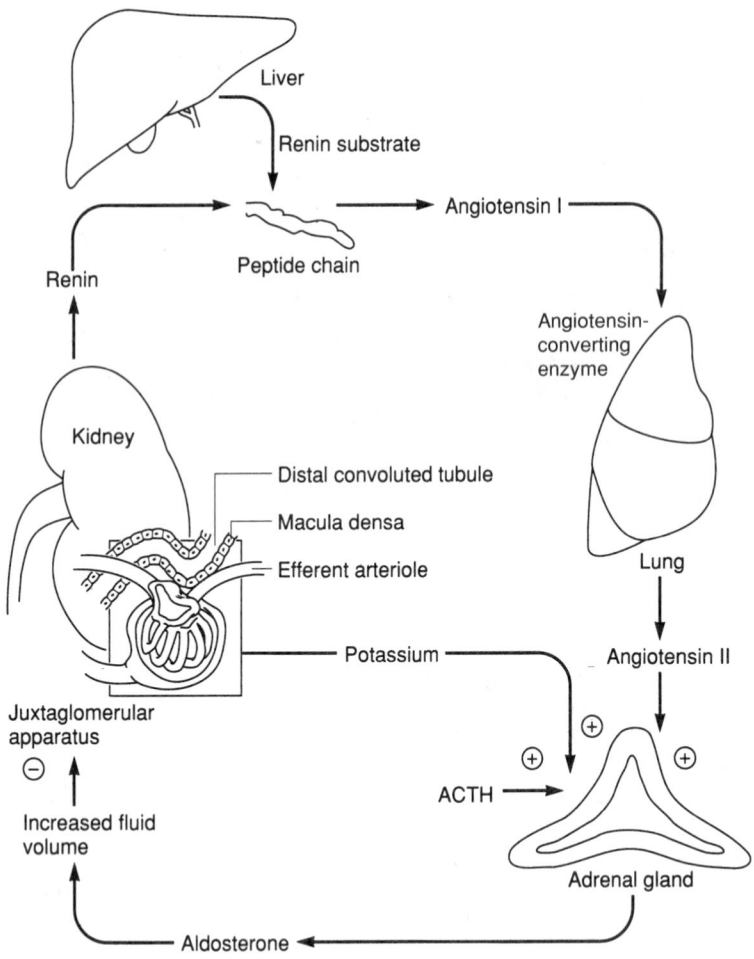

Figure 58-2. The relations of renin, angiotensin I, angiotensin II, and their anatomic sites of production and enzymatic conversion.

in excess, an increased level of total circulating hormone accurately reflects increased secretion. This is usually seen with stress, functioning tumors, and congenital adrenal hyperplasia.

Circulating unbound steroid molecules pass freely through the cellular membrane of a target cell, where binding with a specific cytosolic receptor occurs. It is the distribution of receptors specific for each of the steroids among various cell populations that determines the effects of steroids on tissues. *Cortisol* has receptors in almost all tissues of the body. *Androgen* and *estrogen* receptors are restricted in distribution; key cell populations are in the breast, prostate, and external genitalia. The distribution of *mineralocorticoid* (eg, aldosterone and deoxycorticosterone) receptors is limited to target tissues such as the renal tubule, salivary glands, and colonic mucosa.

Cortisol

Table 58-1 lists the effects of normal and excess cortisol secretion. Cortisol excess produces *Cushing's syndrome.* The causes are:

Exogenous administration of steroids
Cushing's disease (pituitary ACTH excess)
Ectopic production of ACTH
Adrenal adenoma or carcinoma
Micronodular pigmented hyperplasia
Macronodular hyperplasia
Steroid-dependent adrenal hyperplasia

Androgens and Estrogens

The important adrenal androgens are dehydroepiandrosterone, androstenedione, and testosterone. Androstenedione is the principal androgen converted in peripheral tissues to estrogens, and testosterone is the most potent masculinizing steroid. Table 58-2 lists the effects of normal and excess androgen secretion. Excess androgen

Table 58-1. SYSTEMIC EFFECTS OF CORTISOL

Function	Normal Amounts	Excessive Amounts
Metabolic		
Protein	Proteolysis	Muscle wasting
Glucose	Gluconeogenesis	Hyperglycemia
Fat	Low-use peripheral lipolysis	Limb thinness
	Central lipogenesis	Truncal obesity
Gastrointestinal	Mucosal cells	Ulceration
	Prostaglandin	Pancreatitis(?)
Cardiovascular	Chronotropic, inotropic	Hypertension
	Vascular resistance	
Renal	Sodium resorption	Hypertension
Bone	Osteoblastic development	Osteoporosis
Inflammatory and immune	Circulating cells	Infection
	Soluble mediators	
	Antigen processing	
Wound healing	Fibroblasts	Striae
	Epithelial cells	Dehiscence

Table 58-2. EFFECTS OF ANDROGEN SECRETION

Normal Secretion	Excess Secretion
Deepening of voice	Boys and Men
Male hair distribution	Precocious puberty
Coarsening of skin	Girls and Women
Toughening and darkening of facial hair	Masculine features
Protein deposition in muscles	Clitoral hypertrophy
Development of male sex organs	Menstrual cessation

or estrogen production by the adrenal gland almost always arises from carcinoma. In the rare adrenal carcinoma that produces estrogen, menstrual irregularities may be the only symptoms experienced by women. Men may experience loss of libido, enlargement of breast tissue, and female distribution of hair.

Enzymatic defects in the steroidogenic pathway produce *congenital adrenal hyperplasia.* This syndrome appears in the neonatal period as sexual ambiguity. The enzymatic defects lower cortisol secretion, increasing ACTH production and stimulation. The specific enzyme defects determine the clinical form of the syndrome. The most common form is 21-hydroxylase deficiency. This defect and 11β-hydroxylase deficiency cause excess androgen production in utero and masculinization with ambiguous genitalia of newborn girls. Masculinizing effects in boys may not be detected until precocious puberty becomes obvious. Salt wasting or sodium loss in the urine are common and may allow early detection, because they lead to symptomatic hypovolemia.

Aldosterone

Aldosterone is the primary mineralocorticoid. The principal site of action is the distal renal tubule. Table 58-3 lists the effects of normal and excessive aldosterone secretion. *Primary aldosteronism* occurs with conditions in which secretion is excessive and autonomous: adrenal adenoma, primary hyperplasia of the zona glomerulosa, and adrenal carcinoma that produces aldosterone. *Secondary aldosteronism* is related to increased renin secretion due to renal artery stenosis, congestive heart failure, and renal salt wasting.

Catecholamines

The two important catecholamines, norepinephrine and epinephrine, mediate their effects through cellular membrane receptors. α-Receptors mediate contraction of smooth muscle, and β-receptors regulate relaxation (Table 58-4).

Pheochromocytomas are tumors of the adrenal medulla. *Nonfunctioning* pheochromocytomas do not secrete active

substances of any kind. *Functioning* pheochromocytomas produce catecholamines, always autonomously and usually in great excess. Although some tumors produce only epinephrine or norepinephrine, most produce the two catecholamines in combination. The clinical effects are hypertension, tachycardia, nervousness, and sweating.

The secretory effects of functioning pheochromocytomas have one of three patterns:

1. Sustained hypertension without episodic increases in blood pressure or any other signs of excessive secretion
2. Normal blood pressure with episodes of increased secretion manifested by tachycardia, hypertension, or flushing
3. A combination of the other two patterns, with sustained baseline hypertension and superimposed attacks of episodic hypertension

Pheochromocytomas may be asymptomatic because the active products are metabolized on site; few, if any, active products reach the systemic circulation. Diagnostic sensitivity improves when metabolites and catecholamines in the urine are measured.

DIAGNOSIS

A patient with a functioning adrenal lesion usually seeks treatment because of:

- A condition such as hypertension or hypokalemia
- Changes in appearance, such as abdominal striae or redistribution of fat
- Symptoms such as palpitations or muscular weakness
- The incidental finding of a lesion during radionuclide, magnetic resonance, computed tomographic, or ultrasonic imaging

Functional Assessment

1. Screen the urine or plasma for secretory products
2. Identify the pathologic condition with functional tests that manipulate the feedback mechanisms
3. Perform scans and obtain images to differentiate the lesions

Hypercortisolism (Cushing's Syndrome)

Table 58-5 lists the steps in the diagnosis of hypercortisolism.

Sex Steroid Excess

Evidence of androgen excess is clinically apparent only in women. Although an ovarian source of androgen production must be sought, the predominant adrenal lesion is

Table 58-3. EFFECTS OF ALDOSTERONE SECRETION

Tubular Action	Normal Amounts	Excessive Amounts
Increased resorption of sodium	Protects against low-volume states	Hypertension Positive sodium balance Hyporeninemia
Decreased resorption of potassium	Protects against hyperkalemia	Hypokalemia Metabolic alkalosis Hyperglycemia Nocturia, polyuria Muscle weakness

Table 58-4. CATECHOLAMINE EFFECTS

Receptor Class	Normal Amounts	Excessive Amounts
β_1	Chronotropic, inotropic	Tachycardia
	Sweat glands	Sweating
	Decreased glucose use	Hyperglycemia
β_2	Smooth muscle relaxation	Hypotension
α_1	Smooth muscle contraction	Hypertension
	Gluconeogenesis	
	Glycogenolysis	Hyperglycemia
	Suppressed insulin effects	
α_2	Smooth muscle contraction	Pallor
	Platelet aggregation	

Table 58-5. STEPS IN THE DIAGNOSIS OF CUSHING SYNDROME

SCREENING TESTS

Plasma cortisol—random and diurnal
Urinary 17-OH corticosteroids
Urinary free cortisol
Overnight low-dose dexamethasone

DETERMINING THE CAUSE

Standard dexamethasone suppression
  Positive—pituitary cause
  Negative—adrenal or ectopic cause
Corticotropin-releasing hormone stimulation
  Accentuated—pituitary cause
  No response—adrenal or ectopic cause
Petrosal sinus sampling
  Lateralizing—pituitary cause
  Nonlateralizing—adrenal or ectopic cause

Table 58-7. STEPS IN THE DIAGNOSIS OF ALDOSTERONISM

SCREENING TESTS

Serum potassium concentration—low
Urinary potassium excretion—high
Urinary aldosterone excretion—high
Plasma renin—low
Oral sodium loading

CONFIRMING TESTS

Plasma and urinary aldosterone
  Saline infusion
  Captopril
  Integrated plasma values
Plasma renin
  Negative sodium balance

TUMOR VERSUS HYPERPLASIA

Upright posture—plasma aldosterone and renin levels
  Tumor—remain suppressed
  Hyperplasia—slight rise
18-OH-corticosterone—high with tumor

a cortical carcinoma. Men whose features become feminine probably have *adrenocortical carcinoma*. Precocious puberty in boys or virilization in girls suggests carcinoma. The differential diagnosis in children includes 21-OH deficiency, 11β-OH deficiency, and primary ovarian tumors. Table 58-6 presents the steps in the diagnosis of an adrenal source of excessive sex steroids. The dexamethasone suppression test is used to determine if one is dealing with autonomous secretion of 17-ketosteroids by a tumor or an enzymatic defect in the steroidogenic pathway.

Congenital adrenal hyperplasia comes to the attention of physicians because of ambiguous genitalia of a girl at birth or salt wasting in a boy or girl. It is important to make the diagnosis early. For girls, there is the critical need for gender assignment. For boys and girls, prompt treatment of the salt wasting may be life-saving.

Hyperaldosteronism

The steps in the diagnosis of aldosteronism are presented in Table 58-7.

Catecholamines

The urinary and plasma tests for determining the presence of a pheochromocytoma are listed in Table 58-8.

The following events, substances, and emotional states influence plasma and urinary catecholamine levels:

Endogenous release
- Pain
- Hypotension
- Hypoglycemia
- Psychic distress
- Drug withdrawal
- Surgical intervention

Interfering drugs
- Catecholamines: calcium-channel blockers, captopril, α-agonists, β-blockers, α-blockers, methenamine mandelate
- VMA or metanephrine: clofibrate, nalidixic acid, methylglucamine
- Catecholamines and metabolites: labetalol, levodopa, tricyclic antidepressants, phenothiazines, methyldopa, monoamine oxidase inhibitors

Localization Studies

CT is used because it is noninvasive, easy to perform, and sensitive. MRI provides information about the nature of nonfunctioning tumors. NP-59 (^{131}I-labeled cholesterol) scintigraphy is useful in the diagnosis of Cushing's syndrome and hyperaldosteronism. MIBG (a norepinephrine analog) scintigraphy may be required to detect multiple, extraadrenal, recurrent, or metastatic pheochromocytomas. Vena caval sampling of catecholamines may be helpful. Adrenal venous sampling is used for questionable cases of primary aldosteronism (Table 58-9).

TREATMENT

Adrenal Hypercortisolism

Nonoperative Treatment

Functioning benign lesions of the adrenal cortex that are not ACTH dependent, such as adenomas or macronodular hyperplasia, are treated with metyrapone and aminoglutethimide, which inhibit enzymes in the adrenal steroido-

Table 58-6. STEPS IN THE DIAGNOSIS OF AN EXCESS OF SEX STEROIDS

SCREENING

Measurement of urinary 17-ketosteroids
Measurement of urinary estrogens (feminine boys)

DETERMINING THE CAUSE

Dexamethasone suppression test
Measurement of 17-OH progesterone
Measurement of 11-deoxycortisol

Table 58-8. DIAGNOSIS OF PHEOCHROMOCYTOMA

Urinary excretion
  Catecholamines
  Metanephrine, normetanephrine
  VMA
Plasma epinephrine, norepinephrine
Clonidine suppression test
DHPG/norepinephrine ratio

Table 58-9. USE OF LOCALIZATION PROCEDURES

Procedure	Characteristics
RADIOGRAPHIC SCANS	
CT	Good first test; sensitive but not very specific
MR	Can identify some types of pathology and defines anatomy well; competes with scintigraphy in nonfunctioning tumors; lower sensitivity than CT; expensive
SCINTIGRAPHIC SCANS	
NP-59	Adrenocortical imaging can distinguish unilateral from bilateral disease in most instances; dexamethasone can add specificity, potential for identifying carcinomas in nonfunctioning tumors
MIBG	Adrenal medulla imaging can supplement CT scan when extraadrenal, recurrent, or metastatic pheochromocytomas are suspected
INVASIVE STUDIES	
Adrenal venous sampling	Greatest use in distinguishing adenoma from hyperplasia in primary aldosteronism; technically demanding; adrenal venography can cause hemorrhage
Vena cava sampling	Largely replaced by MIBG in search for extraadrenal pheochromocytomas
Arteriography	Can be dangerous with pheochromocytomas; largely replaced by noninvasive scanning

genic pathway. These agents are not satisfactory for long-term use because of the high incidence of drug reactions, lack of patient compliance, and continued growth of lesions. The drugs may be useful when surgical intervention must be delayed.

Functioning malignant tumors are treated by means of surgical debulking, but chemotherapeutic agents, such as mitotane, can be used for adjunctive therapy.

Nonoperative treatment is definitive for *congenital adrenal hyperplasia*, although surgical genitoplasty often is required. Cortisone acetate is the agent used. For salt-losing hyperplasia, IV steroids sometimes are required for short-term therapy until the salt-losing tendency is under control with cortisone treatment.

Operative Treatment

Indications. An operation is clearly indicated for a *unilateral functioning* adrenal tumor. For a *unilateral nonfunctioning* adrenal tumor, the need for surgical treatment is related to the size of the tumor and its rate of growth. In adults, a tumor >6 cm in diameter is removed. Some surgeons recommend that the acceptable size limit be 3 cm, especially when MRI suggests carcinoma or when functional studies suggest activity. When nonoperative therapy is chosen, the patient undergoes regular adrenal scans to assess growth of the lesion. If the tumor grows, surgical removal is indicated.

For *bilateral functioning* adrenocortical lesions, the pituitary–adrenal axis is assessed with the dexamethasone suppression test and CRH stimulation. If the pituitary gland is not the source of the hypercortisolism, bilateral adrenalectomy is indicated. For *bilateral nonfunctioning* adrenal lesions, the probability of metastasis to the adrenal gland is high, and image-guided needle biopsy is performed.

Preparation. Preoperative preparation for adrenalectomy includes administration of enzyme inhibitors and steroid replacement.

Approach. The surgical approach is determined by the position and size of the lesion. For small unilateral lesions like adenomas, a posterior approach through the bed of the 12th or 11th rib is used. An alternative approach is through the flank, with the patient in the lateral decubitus position. The bilateral posterior approach is reserved for small, hyperplastic glands, as in micronodular hyperplasia or hyperplasia of Cushing's disease in which pituitary treatment has failed.

Complications. The most serious intraoperative complications are avulsion of the right adrenal gland from the inferior vena cava or direct tear of the vena cava. The posterior approach is particularly hazardous because it is difficult to extricate a large tumor through the small posterior aperture. Large tumors may be carcinomas, and the transabdominal approach allows wide resection of lymph node-bearing areas and perhaps partial removal of attached surrounding structures. Other complications related to the incision are pneumothorax for the posterior approach, pancreatitis for the left abdominal approach.

Postoperative Care. The postoperative course involves tapering the exogenous steroid doses to maintenance levels after bilateral adrenalectomy or to cessation after unilateral adrenalectomy. One simple regimen is administration of 100 mg hydrocortisone IV every 6 hours for 48 hours, and then to halve the dose every 48 to 72 hours, if tolerated. The pituitary–adrenal axis remains suppressed for 6 to 12 months after the operation. Even patients with normal contralateral adrenal glands cannot stop steroid replacement until after that time. Complications in the postoperative period include wound infection, pancreatitis, and thromboembolism.

Hyperaldosteronism

Nonoperative Treatment

The only drug used for hyperaldosteronism is spironolactone. This drug inhibits sodium–potassium exchange in the distal renal tubule, normalizes serum potassium level, and, if tolerated, for a period of time, lowers blood pressure. Oral potassium chloride helps correct hypokalemia. Because of gynecomastia and other side effects, long-term use of spironolactone is troublesome to some patients.

Operative Treatment

Indications. Primary aldosteronism due to an adrenal adenoma is best managed with surgical removal of the adenoma. When the syndrome arises from adrenal hyperplasia, surgical removal of the adrenal gland is seldom curative. Every effort is made to differentiate the two causes. Surgical treatment is indicated only for adenomas and for forms of hyperplasia that behave as adenomas at dynamic testing.

Preparation. Preoperative preparation is potassium replenishment. Correction of hypokalemia may be aided with short-term use of spironolactone. Because the tumors usually are small and rarely malignant and hyperplasia is minimal, a unilateral or bilateral posterior approach is used. If bilateral adrenalectomy is anticipated, hydrocortisone is administered.

Approach. Because these adenomas may be very small, it sometimes is necessary to mobilize the adrenal gland and examine it with bidigital palpation. Pneumothorax and vena caval bleeding may occur, but the tissues are not as friable as in chronic hypercortisolism.

Postoperative Care. Because of hyporeninemia, the remaining zona glomerulosa is usually temporarily suppressed, and relative hypoaldosteronism may follow removal of an adenoma. The symptoms are low blood pressure and hyperkalemia, which usually respond to administration of a mineralocorticoid, such as fludrocortisone. Bilateral adrenalectomy necessitates exogenous cortisol administration, which usually can be tapered to maintenance levels during the recovery period.

Pheochromocytoma

Nonoperative Treatment

Nonoperative treatment of pheochromocytoma is generally unsatisfactory. It entails pharmacologic blockade of the effects of catecholamines.

Operative Treatment

Preparation. Patients with pheochromocytoma are prone to wide swings in blood pressure and other effects of chronic catecholamine secretion; therefore, surgical resection is routinely advised. α-Adrenergic blockade is instituted 2 to 3 weeks before the operation. This helps control blood pressure and allows restoration of blood volume. For patients who require β-adrenergic blockade, it is essential to first establish good α-adrenergic blockade. These patients are especially prone to cardiac failure induced by β-adrenergic blockade due to cardiomyopathy. β-Adrenergic blockade in a patient with cardiomyopathy, if the afterload is not first reduced with α-adrenergic blockade, can precipitate cardiac failure.

In the operating room, pulmonary artery monitoring is optional, but intraarterial blood pressure must be monitored. With catecholamine excess, the peripheral pulse may disappear, and auditory monitoring of blood pressure is unreliable. The following drugs must be immediately available:

Agents that lower blood pressure, such as phentolamine (Regitine) or nitroprusside
β-Adrenergic blockers, such as esmolol
Antiarrhythmic agents, such as lidocaine
Blood pressure support agents, such as norepinephrine, to counteract possible postoperative hypotension

Approach. Pheochromocytomas are approached by the transabdominal route, usually through a bilateral, subcostal rooftop incision. The technical principles are to minimize manipulation of the tumor and to isolate and ligate the adrenal vein as soon as possible in the dissection.

Once the tumor is removed, blood pressure may fall precipitously. This can be counteracted immediately with administration of an α-adrenergic agonist, such as norepinephrine. A preexisting low blood volume may contribute to hypotension, and transfusion of one or two units of blood may be required.

If blood pressure does not decrease at least to normal when the tumor is removed, a second pheochromocytoma or metastases may be present. A thorough intraabdominal search along the vertebral bodies, aorta, contralateral adrenal gland, and urinary bladder is conducted before closure.

Postoperative Care. Once hypotension is corrected, the patient usually has an uneventful recovery.

Nonfunctioning Adrenal Tumors

Indications for surgical treatment of nonfunctioning adrenal tumors are diameter >6 cm, growth of small tumors during a period of observation, and questionable functional status. Because carcinomas <6 cm in diameter do occur, some clinicians remove any tumors >3 cm in diameter. The surgical approach is much the same as for functioning tumors. Tumors >5 to 6 cm in diameter are probably best approached through the flank or by way of the transabdominal route. Small tumors with a low likelihood of malignancy can be removed with a posterior approach.

SUGGESTED READING

Bravo EL, Gifford RW. Pheochromocytoma. Endocrinol Metab Clin North Am 1993;22:329.
Gordon, RD. Primary aldosteronism: a new understanding. Med J Aust 1993;158:729.
Lamki LM, Haynie TP. Role of adrenal imaging in surgical management. J Surg Oncol 1990;43:139.
Merrell RC. Aldosterone-producing tumors (Conn's syndrome). Semin Surg Oncol 1990;6:66.
Perry RR, Nieman LK, Cutler GB, et al. Primary adrenal causes of Cushing's syndrome: diagnosis and surgical management. Ann Surg 1989;210:59.
Suzuki K, Kageyama S, Ueda D. Laparoscopic adrenalectomy: clinical experience with 12 cases. J Urol 1993;150:1099.
Wooten MD, King DK. Adrenal cortical carcinoma. Cancer 1993;72:3145.

ESSENTIALS OF SURGERY: SCIENTIFIC PRINCIPLES AND PRACTICE, edited by Lazar J. Greenfield, Michael W. Mulholland, Keith T. Oldham, Gerald B. Zelenock, and Keith D. Lillemoe. Lippincott–Raven Publishers, Philadelphia, © 1997.

CHAPTER 59
PITUITARY GLAND
WILLIAM F. CHANDLER AND RICARDO V. LLOYD

The hypothalamus of the brain is the principal organ for regulation of the internal environment of the body. The pituitary gland links the hypothalamus to organs outside the nervous system.

ANATOMY AND PHYSIOLOGY

In adults, the pituitary gland is 6×9×12 mm, and weighs about 0.6 g. The adenohypophysis (anterior pituitary gland) constitutes 80% of the gland. The neurohypophysis (posterior pituitary gland) is considered an extension of the hypothalamus.

The neurohypophysis and adenohypophysis are connected to the base of the brain by a common stalk. The stalk transports hormone-enriched portal blood to the adenohypophysis and nerve fibers to the neurohypophysis. The optic chiasm lies directly above the pituitary gland, just anterior to the stalk; thus, it is vulnerable to compression by a pituitary tumor.

The median eminence is where blood destined for the adenohypophysis picks up its hormonal contribution (Fig. 59-1). Blood enters this region from the superior hypophyseal artery and enters small capillary plexes, which pick up hormones in the median eminence. This blood is transported in a portal system to influence secretory cells in the adenohypophysis. These cells secrete hormones into the circulation to stimulate end organs. The following hormones are transported:

- Thyrotropin-releasing hormone (TRH) to stimulate secretion of thyroid-stimulating hormone (TSH)

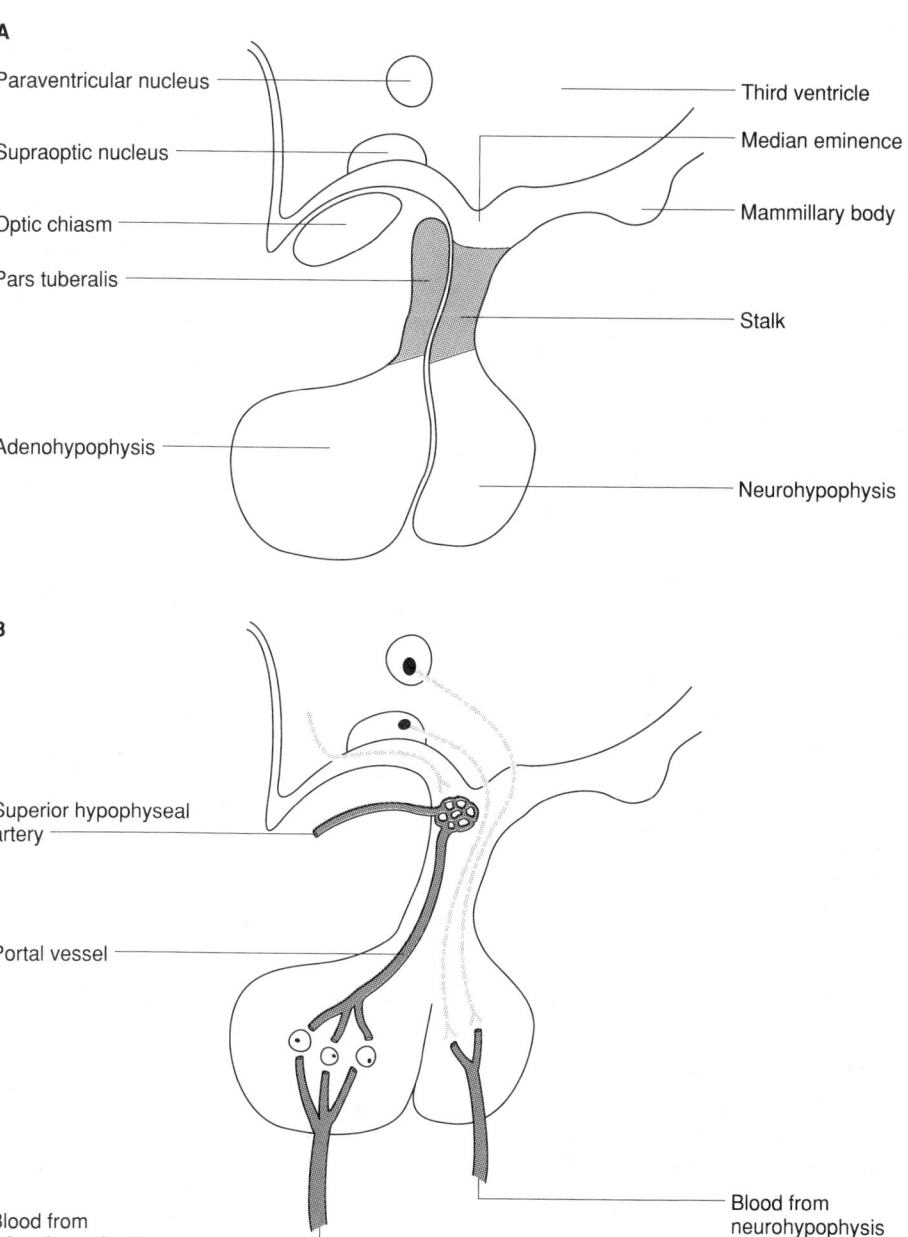

A

Paraventricular nucleus

Supraoptic nucleus

Optic chiasm

Pars tuberalis

Adenohypophysis

Third ventricle

Median eminence

Mammillary body

Stalk

Neurohypophysis

B

Superior hypophyseal artery

Portal vessel

Blood from adenohypophysis

Blood from neurohypophysis

Figure 59-1. (*A*) Schematic diagram of pituitary and floor of the third ventricle as seen in midline sagittal view. Anterior is to the left. (*B*) Diagram on same schematic drawing of physiology of hormone release. The adenohypophysis receives releasing hormones through a portal venous system, and the neurohypophysis receives hormones directly from hypothalamic nuclei by means of neurons.

- Corticotropin-releasing hormone to stimulate secretion of adrenocorticotropic hormone (ACTH)
- Growth hormone-releasing hormone to stimulate secretion of growth hormone (GH)
- Gonadotropin-releasing hormone to stimulate secretion of luteinizing hormone (LH) and follicle-stimulating hormone (FSH)
- Prolactin-inhibitory factor (dopamine) to inhibit secretion of prolactin

The neurohypophysis differs from the adenohypophysis in that its hormonal control is not in the portal system but is direct transport of hormones through nerve fibers. These fibers carry both antidiuretic hormone (ADH; vasopressin) and oxytocin. ADH in the bloodstream causes the kidneys to absorb free water. ADH excess causes water retention and hyponatremia; ADH shortage (diabetes insipidus) causes water loss and hypernatremia. Surgical loss of the neurohypophysis does not usually result in diabetes insip-

idus, because the stalk still secretes ADH into the circulation. Oxytocin functions only during pregnancy.

The pituitary gland sits within the bony confines of the sella turcica. It is bordered laterally by the cavernous sinuses (venous), inferiorly and anteriorly by the sphenoid sinus (air), posteriorly by the dorsum sella, and superiorly by the membranous diaphragma sella. The cavernous sinuses contain the siphon region of the internal carotid artery and portions of cranial nerves III, IV, V, and VI, all within a venous plexus. The optic chiasm lies immediately above the diaphragma sella. Directly below the anterior and inferior portions of the sella is the sphenoid sinus.

METHODS OF CELL ANALYSIS

Pituitary adenomas are classified as acidophilic, basophilic, and chromophobic. However, because adenomas show a variable staining pattern with hematoxylin and eosin dyes, it is difficult to classify adenomas on the basis of these stains (Table 59-1). Immunohistochemical staining of pituitary adenomas with antibodies is used to classify adenomas according to the hormones produced. Ultrastructural immunohistochemistry defines the site of storage of hormones in secretory granules and the subcellular sites of production and processing in the rough endoplasmic reticulum and Golgi bodies. mRNA localization of protein hormones is used in the study and classification of pituitary adenomas.

IMAGING OF THE PITUITARY GLAND AND PARASELLAR REGION

Magnetic resonance imaging (MRI) is often the only examination needed. With IV infusion of a paramagnetic substance such as gadolinium, MRI depicts intrasellar masses as small as 5 mm and shows the growth pattern of large tumors. MRI reveals the extent of suprasellar and sphenoid sinus extension and lateral extension into the cavernous sinuses. Cysts and hemorrhage can be differentiated, as can blood flow within an aneurysm.

Computed tomography (CT) depicts calcification better than does MRI and thus is often helpful in imaging craniopharyngioma. CT, even with IV administration of contrast material, cannot be used to identify an aneurysm. MRI or angiography must be performed.

Skull radiography is not needed if the diagnosis is made with CT or MRI, but radiographs are important for incidental detection. The finding of enlargement of the sella turcica on a plain lateral skull radiograph obtained for reasons such as trauma is an indication for MRI or CT.

Angiography is performed only if an aneurysm is suspected or if a lesion is so large that occlusion or compression of the internal carotid artery is a possibility.

CLINICAL AND ENDOCRINE EVALUATION

Clinical Manifestations

Patients with pituitary lesions may present with symptoms and signs related to a mass effect on the pituitary gland and its surrounding structures, hypersecretion of hormones by the lesion, or a combination of both.

Tumors or other mass lesions usually are >1 cm in diameter before they produce symptoms of compression. Compression may cause loss of function of the pituitary gland, usually manifested by a decrease in secretion of hormones from the adenohypophysis:

- A decrease in TSH causes hypothyroidism
- A decrease in ACTH causes Addison's disease
- A decrease in LH and FSH causes amenorrhea
- A decrease in GH impedes normal growth in children

Pituitary compression may *increase* prolactin level, because release of prolactin inhibitory factor (dopamine) from the hypothalamus may be compromised.

When mass lesions in the region of the pituitary gland enlarge, they compress or invade nearby structures, causing a number of symptoms unrelated to endocrine function. *Lateral* tumor growth compresses cranial nerves III, IV, or VI, causing diplopia, or cranial nerve V, causing ipsilateral facial numbness. Invasion or constriction of the carotid artery may cause carotid occlusion. *Upward* tumor growth compresses the optic chiasm, causing bitemporal hemianopsia. Extensive upward intracranial growth compresses the third ventricle, causing hydrocephalus. Rarely, intracranial extension results in cortical irritation and seizures. *Downward* tumor growth into the sphenoid sinus is common but causes no clinical symptoms or signs.

The syndromes associated with hypersecretion of pituitary hormones include Cushing's disease (ACTH), acromegaly (GH), hyperprolactinemia (prolactin), and Nelson's syndrome (ACTH after adrenalectomy). TSH-secreting adenomas are rare. Although secretion of these hormones may not cause clinical symptoms or signs, they may serve as a marker for the presence of the tumor before and after treatment.

General Endocrine Evaluation

The extent of endocrine evaluation of a pituitary lesion depends on the urgency of the situation (eg, the situation is urgent if vision is impaired) and whether a hypersecretory state is suspected. If time allows, endocrine status is evaluated, including testing of pituitary reserve. Pituitary endocrine evaluation includes baseline values for prolactin, GH, LH, FSH, testosterone or estrogen, cortisol, ACTH, electrolytes, glucose, and thyroid function tests, including TSH.

Because baseline values may not reflect the ability of the pituitary gland to respond to stress, it is important to test

---

Table 59-1. FUNCTIONAL PITUITARY ADENOMAS: PATHOLOGIC FINDINGS

Adenoma Type	Incidence (%)	Staining*	Immunoreactivity	Ultrastructure
PRL-secreting				
Sparsely granulated	28	C	PRL	Few SG 150–500 nm misplaced exocytosis
Densely granulated	1	A	PRL	SG 400–1200 nm
GH-secreting				
Sparsely granulated	5	C–A	GH	SG 300–600 nm, fibrous bodies
Densely granulated	5	A	GH	SG 100–250 nm
Mixed GH cell–PRL cell	5	A–C	GH, PRL	Variable pattern
Mixed GH cell–PRL cell	1	A	GH, PRL	SG 150–450 nm and 350–1000 nm
ACTH-secreting	10	B	ACTH	SG 250–700 nm Prominent type I microfilaments
Gonadotroph cell adenoma	7–10	C–B	FSH, LH	SG 50–150 nm Distinct female pattern of honeycomb Golgi region
Thyrotroph cell adenoma	1	C–B	TSH	SG 50–250 nm

ACTH, adrenocorticotropic hormone; FSH, follicle-stimulating hormone; GH, growth hormone; LH, luteinizing hormone; PRL, prolactin; SG, secretory granules; TSH, thyroid-stimulating hormone.
* Conventional hematoxylin–eosin staining: A, acidophil; B, basophil; C, chromophobe.

the reserve capacity of the gland. If urgent surgical decompression is indicated, baseline values are obtained, and the patient is prepared for an operation with sufficient hydrocortisone to cover inadequate cortisol reserve.

Postoperative evaluation is conducted to determine if long-term replacement therapy is needed. If the patient receives postoperative radiation therapy, the status of the pituitary gland is checked periodically over the following years, because pituitary function may decline after radiation exposure.

If diabetes insipidus is suspected, urine specific gravity, serum sodium, and fluid intake and output are measured.

Cushing's Disease

The findings in hypercortisolism (Cushing's syndrome) are central obesity, hypertension, hirsutism, fatigue, bruisability, striae, moon-like facies, dorsal fat pad, and sometimes depression or other mental changes. Less common abnormalities are headache, osteoporosis, diabetes mellitus, galactorrhea, peripheral edema, and amenorrhea. Some patients do not have the classic cushingoid appearance and report only severe fatigue or depression.

The cause of hypercortisolism in 80% of patients is an ACTH-secreting pituitary adenoma (Cushing's disease). The other 20% have an adrenocortical tumor or an ectopic neoplasm that secretes ACTH or corticotropin-releasing factor. Pituitary-dependent hypercortisolism is more common in women, and ectopic neoplasms are more common in men.

Imaging is not helpful in the diagnosis of pituitary hypercortisolism. Endocrine testing is required (Fig. 59-2).

The most specific diagnostic study is transfemoral catheterization with simultaneous measurement of ACTH levels in both inferior petrosal sinuses and determination of pe-

ripheral ACTH level. This study produces information about the existence of an ACTH-secreting pituitary tumor and the laterality of the tumor.

CT of the adrenal glands and thorax is performed to detect adrenal or lung tumors.

Acromegaly

The diagnosis of acromegaly is apparent when patients present in advanced stages of the disease. In the early stages, enlargement of facial features and acral enlargement may be subtle and the presenting symptoms may be nonspecific headaches, fatigue, arthralgia, decreased libido, or amenorrhea. Patients often have hypertension, diabetes mellitus, and early-onset atherosclerotic cardiovascular disease. The cause of acromegaly almost always is a GH-secreting pituitary adenoma. The tumors may be small or large and invasive. Patients with large tumors may experience loss of vision.

Endocrine diagnosis rests on serum GH levels. Most patients have levels >10 ng/mL. Normal GH level in a resting, nonstressed person is <5 ng/mL. Somatomedin C, or insulin-like growth factor I, which mediates the effect of GH on peripheral tissues, is measured whenever GH excess is suspected. When acromegaly is apparent, but consistently elevated GH levels are not obtained, the glucose suppression test is the most useful diagnostic procedure (Fig. 59-3).

Hyperprolactinemia

Hyperprolactinemia in women usually causes amenorrhea and often galactorrhea. These signs compel women to seek treatment early, and the tumors are detected as microadenomas. Men do not have an early warning sign,

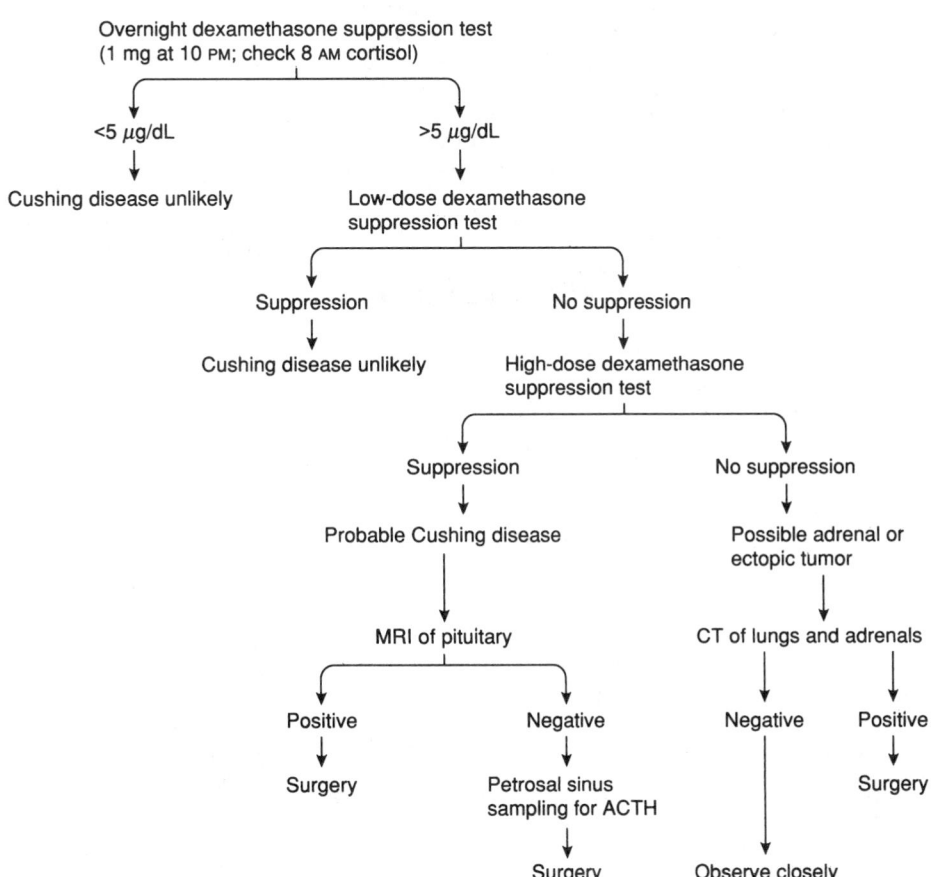

Figure 59-2. Workup and treatment of Cushing disease.

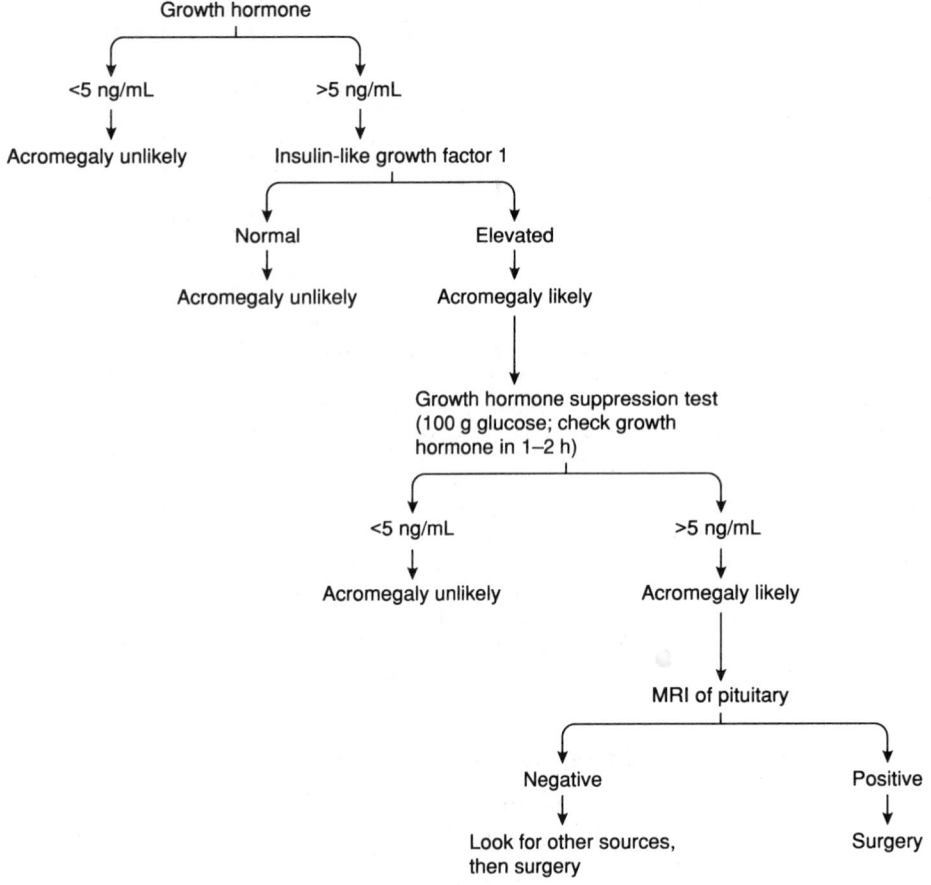

Figure 59-3. Workup and treatment of acromegaly.

and they present with macroadenoma, usually associated with loss of libido, infertility, or loss of vision. Table 59-2 lists other of hyperprolactinemia. Compression of the pituitary stalk by any type of mass lesion results in increased secretion of prolactin.

If serum prolactin level is >150 ng/mL, a pituitary tumor is almost always the cause. The size of the tumor correlates with the degree of prolactin elevation. No reliable, provocative test differentiates prolactinoma from other causes of hyperprolactinemia, so the diagnosis is based on exclusion of other causes and imaging of the adenoma (Fig. 59-4).

Nelson's Syndrome

Nelson's syndrome is progressive hyperpigmentation, visual field loss, and amenorrhea associated with elevated ACTH levels related to functional pituitary adenoma in a patient who has undergone bilateral adrenalectomy for hypercortisolism.

DIFFERENTIAL DIAGNOSIS

Table 59-3 lists the possible lesions that may occur within the sella or in the parasellar region. Pituitary adenomas are the most common lesion in this region and constitute 8 to 10% of all brain tumors. Occasionally, they are cystic and confused with other lesions.

TREATMENT

The treatment of primary pituitary adenoma is surgical, although some exceptions exist. Even with modern imaging techniques, the unequivocal diagnosis of adenoma is not reached until tissue is obtained. In addition to surgical removal or decompression of a pituitary adenoma, radiation therapy or medical therapy is often indicated. Pre- and posttreatment pituitary function is assessed to determine if hormone replacement is needed.

Almost all pituitary adenomas are approached by the transsphenoidal route, usually through a sublabial incision

---

Table 59-2. CAUSES OF HYPERPROLACTINEMIA

Pituitary disease
  Prolactinoma
  Growth hormone-secreting adenoma
  Pituitary stalk section
  Empty sella syndrome
Hypothalamic disease
  Tumors
  Sarcoidosis
  Radiation
Hypothyroidism
Chronic renal failure
Hepatic disease
Drugs
Phenothiazines
  Tricyclic antidepressants
  Estrogen
  Opiates
  Reserpine
  Verapamil
  Others
Pregnancy
Stress

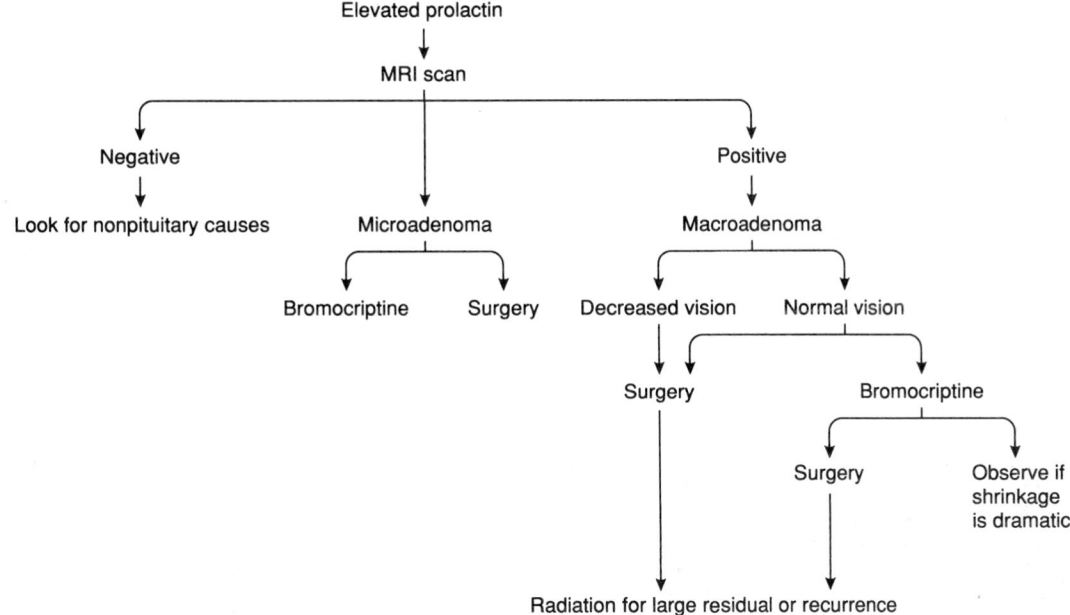

Figure 59-4. Diagnostic tests and treatment of hyperprolactinemia.

and a transseptal approach to the sphenoid sinus. Once the sinus is entered, the anterior wall of the sella is drilled away and the dura surrounding the pituitary gland is identified. The dura is opened. If it is a macroadenoma, the tumor is usually seen immediately beneath the dura. If the tumor is a microadenoma, one must dissect around and often through the pituitary gland to identify the lesion.

Contraindications to a transsphenoidal approach, and therefore indications for a craniotomy, are:

- Massive suprasellar extension
- Extensive lateral intracranial extension
- A dumbbell-shaped tumor with the constriction at the level of the diaphragma sella

If craniotomy is necessary, a right subfrontal approach to the optic nerve and chiasm is required, and the tumor is removed piecemeal with the aid of an operating microscope and microinstruments.

Table 59-3. DIFFERENTIAL DIAGNOSES OF INTRASELLAR AND PARASELLAR LESIONS

Tumors	Cysts
Pituitary adenoma	Rathke cleft cyst
Craniopharyngioma	Pituitary cyst
Meningioma	Inflammatory and granulomatous
Lymphoma	lesions
Germinoma	Bacterial abscess
Chordoma	Sarcoidosis
Granular cell tumor	Eosinophilic granuloma
(choristoma)	(histiocytosis X)
Neuroma (arising from	Tuberculosis
cranial nerve V)	Mycoses
Metastatic	Granulomatous hypophysitis
Optic nerve glioma	Aneurysm
Epidermoid	Hamartoma
Dermoid	Empty sella syndrome
Infundibuloma	Pituitary apoplexy
Hypothalamic glioma	

Nonfunctioning Adenomas

Because patients with nonfunctioning adenomas usually present with the effects of a mass lesion, these tumors are rarely microadenomas. Although they may be exclusively intrasellar or may have extensive intracranial involvement, almost all these tumors are approached by the transsphenoidal route.

The following are the goals of surgical treatment of nonfunctioning macroadenomas:

- Establishment of the diagnosis
- Decompression of surrounding structures
- Removal of all tumor tissue if possible

There is no medical therapy for nonfunctioning adenomas.

Cushing's Disease

Treatment of Cushing's disease is transsphenoidal exploration of the pituitary gland. Because less than half of patients have abnormal imaging findings, many patients require systematic exploration of the sellar contents. Microadenomas that secrete ACTH may be very small and are often located deep within the gland. If a tumor is not evident when the dura is opened and all surfaces of the pituitary gland are examined, incisions are made into the gland, and internal exploration is conducted. These microadenomas are usually in one side of the pituitary gland; the decision as to which side to explore is guided by the results of preoperative petrosal sinus sampling for ACTH levels.

If no tumor is identified, all or a portion of the pituitary gland is resected. If endocrine studies strongly suggest the tumor is pituitary, and the patient does not want to bear children, total hypophysectomy is performed. If petrosal sinus sampling shows laterality of ACTH secretion, hemiresection of the pituitary gland is performed. Macroadenomas are treated with maximum tumor resection, but endocrine remission is difficult.

Adrenal or ectopic tumors are resected. In about 75% of

patients, a microadenoma is the source of ACTH secretion. Treatment of microadenoma is selective microsurgical tumor resection.

Ten to 20% of patients who undergo exploration have macroadenomas, and the postoperative remission rate is high. Most patients require postoperative radiation therapy, which leads to remission in some patients in whom surgical therapy has failed. When remission does not occur, adrenalectomy or medical suppression of adrenal function is necessary. In some patients who undergo adrenalectomy, pituitary tumors continue to grow and secrete ACTH, producing Nelson's syndrome.

Acromegaly

Acromegaly threatens the life of the patient. For this reason, it must be treated aggressively, even at the expense of normal pituitary function. No one treatment lowers GH levels, and often a combination of treatments is necessary. The goals are to lower circulating GH or somatomedin C level to normal range and to reduce the size of the mass causing compression-related symptoms.

Only 20% to 34% of GH-secreting tumors are microadenomas, making microsurgical tumor resection ineffective. When a microadenoma is removed transsphenoidally, endocrine remission occurs in 80% to 88% of patients.

When a macroadenoma is resected, immediate postoperative remission is reported in 30% to 68% of patients. The rate of remission is inversely related to preoperative GH levels and invasiveness of the tumor. Preoperative treatment of macroadenomas with a somatostatin analog may improve postoperative remission rates. Radiation therapy is moderately effective as a primary mode of treatment and in conjunction with partial surgical resection.

Administration of bromocriptine, a dopamine receptor agonist, does not appear to be effective as primary treatment of acromegaly. It may help control GH and somatomedin C levels as adjuvant therapy.

Octreotide, a somatostatin analog, reduces GH and somatomedin C levels in most patients and normalizes values in 50% of patients. This treatment provides only minimal tumor shrinkage, and GH levels rise immediately after cessation of the drug. Octreotide may prove useful for preoperative treatment or for therapy when surgical treatment fails. If remission is to be achieved, treatment is tumor resection and radiation therapy. Somatostatin analog may be used for 2 to 3 months of preoperative treatment. It also is used to reduce GH levels in patients who have undergone unsuccessful surgical treatment and are awaiting the effects of radiation therapy.

Prolactinoma

The treatment options for prolactin-secreting adenomas are medical therapy, usually with bromocriptine, transsphenoidal surgical resection, radiation therapy, and no treatment.

Macroadenomas

The goal in treating large, prolactin-secreting adenomas is to decompress the optic pathways, to reduce prolactin level, and to control growth of the tumor.

Treatment of macroadenomas with bromocriptine al-

most always brings about marked reduction in prolactin level. In most patients, the size of the tumor decreases. The tumor returns to its original size when bromocriptine is stopped.

The role of surgical treatment of prolactin-secreting macroadenomas is limited to situations in which the tumor does not respond to bromocriptine or the patient cannot tolerate medical therapy. Other indications for surgical debulking of the tumor are:

* Rapid decline in vision unresponsive to bromocriptine
* Marked intratumor hemorrhage
* CSF leak due to skull-base erosion
* In a patient with macroprolatinoma who wants to become pregnant, avoidance of vision loss due to tumor growth during pregnancy

If the residual tumor is not controlled with bromocriptine, focused radiation therapy is administered. Follow-up evaluation with CT or MRI is required for the lifetime of the patient.

Microadenomas

The surgical treatment of prolactin-secreting microadenomas results in postoperative remission in a high percentage of patients. Bromocriptine appears to induce fibrosis within the tumor, and the lower remission rate is related to this fibrosis. Primary medical treatment is safe and effective but may lessen the likelihood of long-term surgical cure by causing fibrosis. Long-term therapy is indicated, because prolactin levels rise rapidly with cessation of dopamine agonists. Pregnancy is not a great risk to a patient with a microadenoma because tumor expansion and vision loss are rare. Radiation therapy is not used to treat microadenomas unless tumor recurrence is aggressive.

The role of surgical exploration in patients with suspected microadenoma is unclear. Most patients with hyperprolactinemia and normal imaging studies do not undergo surgical exploration. Once other causes of hyperprolactinemia are ruled out, dopamine agonists are administered to lower prolactin levels. These patients need lifetime follow-up evaluation with imaging studies and measurements of prolactin level.

SUGGESTED READING

Barkan AL, Lloyd RV, Chandler WF, et al. Preoperative treatment of acromegaly with long-acting somatostatin: shrinkage of invasive pituitary macroadenomas and improved surgical remission rate. J Clin Endocrinol Metab 1988;67:1040.

Black PM, Zervas NT, Ridgeway EC, Martin JB, eds. Secretory tumors of the pituitary gland. New York, Raven, 1984.

Chandler WF, Schteingart DE, Lloyd RV, McKeever PE. Surgical treatment of Cushing's disease. J Neurosurg 1987;66:204.

Ebersold MJ, Quast LM, Laws ER, Scheithauer B, Randall RV. Long-term results in transsphenoidal removal of nonfunctioning pituitary adenomas. J Neurosurg 1986;64:713.

Lloyd RV, Cano M, Chandler WF, Barkan AL, Horvath E, Kovacs K. Human growth hormone and prolactin secreting pituitary adenomas analyzed by in situ hybridization. Am J Pathol 1989;134:605.

Oldfield EL, Chrousos GP, Schulte HM, et al. Preoperative lateralization of ACTH-secreting pituitary adenomas by bilateral and simultaneous inferior petrosal venous sinus sampling. N Engl J Med 1985;312:100.

ESSENTIALS OF SURGERY: SCIENTIFIC PRINCIPLES AND PRACTICE,
edited by Lazar J. Greenfield, Michael W. Mulholland, Keith T. Oldham, Gerald B. Zelenock,
and Keith D. Lillemoe. Lippincott–Raven Publishers, Philadelphia, © 1997.

CHAPTER 60

BREAST

DAVID A. AUGUST AND VERNON K. SONDAK

ANATOMY

Functional Architecture

The fascia enveloping the breast abuts the fascia of the pectoralis major and serratus anterior muscles. Projections of the fascia (suspensory ligaments of Cooper) course through the breast to the skin, forming a supporting framework for the breast parenchyma. The breast is divided into lobular and ductal elements (Fig. 60-1).

The areola is a somewhat flat area of pigmented skin that is usually well demarcated from the surrounding breast skin. The surface of the areola contains Montgomery tubercles, numerous small protuberances that lubricate the nipple during lactation. Beneath the skin of the areola is a compact layer of circular smooth muscle, and there are similar fibers in the nipple. These are responsible for nipple erection. The entire breast, especially the nipple, is richly supplied with sensory nerves.

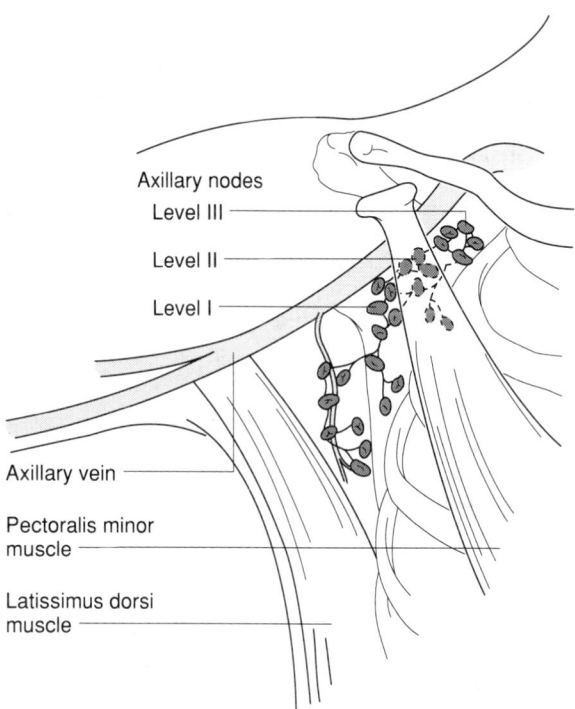

Figure 60-2. Anatomic classification of axillary lymph nodes into three levels based on their relation to the pectoralis minor muscle. Level I nodes are lateral to the edge of the muscle, level II nodes lie beneath the muscle, and level III nodes are medial to the muscle. Rotter nodes (*not shown*) are found between the pectoralis major and minor muscles, anterior to the axillary space.

Blood Vessels

The arterial supply to the medial and central breast comes from perforating branches off the internal mammary artery. The lateral thoracic artery, branches of the thoracodorsal and subscapular arteries, and perforating branches of the intercostal arteries nourish the lateral breast. The breast contains a plexus of veins that begins in the subareolar region and drains into the intercostal, internal mammary, and axillary veins.

Lymphatic Drainage

Almost all lymphatic flow from the breast is into the axilla; the rest courses to the internal mammary nodes. In the axilla, lymphatic vessels terminate in lymph nodes embedded within the axillary fat pad (Fig. 60-2). Isolated lymph nodes are present between the pectoralis major and minor muscles (Rotter nodes) and within or alongside the lateral edge of the breast (intramammary nodes). The axillary lymph nodes are situated in an area bordered laterally by the latissimus dorsi muscle, superiorly by the axillary vein, and medially by the chest wall.

PHYSIOLOGY

Cell Regulation

Breast growth, development, and function are orchestrated by a variety of hormones and growth factors, including estrogens, progestins, prolactin, oxytocin, corticosteroids, thyroid hormone, and growth hormone. Binding of these substances to specific cellular receptors triggers the effects.

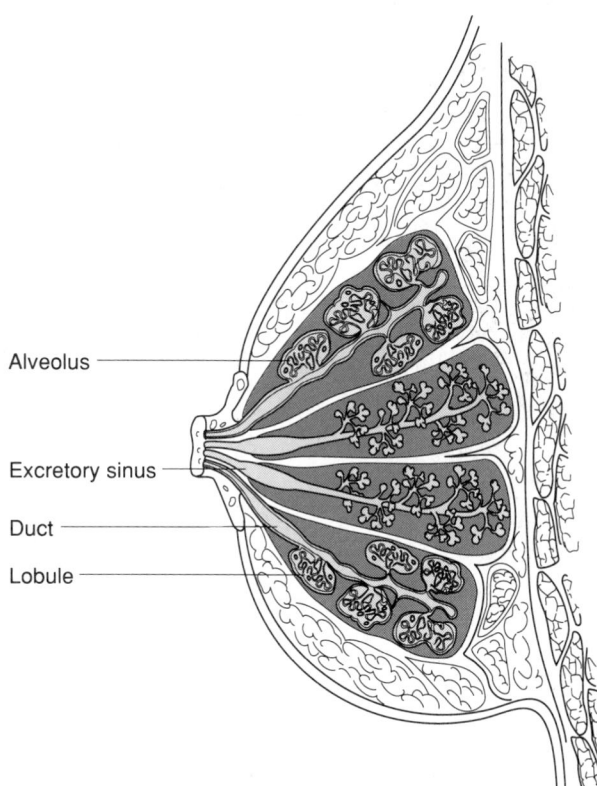

Figure 60-1. The basic functional unit of the breast is the lobule. Each lobule contains 10 to 100 elongated terminal ducts called *alveoli*. Ducts draining 20 to 40 lobules coalesce to form larger ducts, and ultimately an excretory duct. Each excretory duct dilates just beneath the nipple to form an excretory sinus. Ten to 20 excretory ducts drain the entire breast.

Estrogens are important in breast development, growth, and differentiation. Because they are lipid-soluble, estrogens gain entry to breast cells by diffusing through the cell membrane. Once inside a cell, estrogens bind to the estrogen receptor (ER). Both normal and malignant breast cells contain ER. The estrogen–ER complex binds with nuclear chromatin and influences transcription of messenger RNA (mRNA). This mRNA is translated into proteins, such as progesterone receptor (PR), and perhaps growth factors that alter and regulate breast cell growth and metabolism. Tamoxifen works, at least in part, by preventing the binding of hormones and growth factors to the target receptors.

Menstruation

Cyclic changes associated with the menstrual cycle influence breast structure and function (Fig. 60-3). Breast engorgement and tenderness are at a minimum 5 to 7 days after menstruation. At this point in the cycle, breast palpation is most sensitive for detection of masses and most comfortable for the patient. Ductal, secretory, and vascular events and interlobular edema cause the breast swelling, engorgement, and tenderness of the premenstrual phase. At the onset of menstruation, a rapid decline in circulating sex hormone levels leads to breast involution, and the cycle begins anew.

Pregnancy

During pregnancy, ductal, lobular, and alveolar growth occurs under the influence of estrogen, progesterone, placental lactogen, prolactin, and human chorionic gonadotropin (hCG). These changes prepare the breasts for milk production at parturition. Early in the first trimester, ducts sprout and lobules form. Later in the first trimester, noticeable breast enlargement occurs, the superficial veins dilate, and the pigmentation of the nipple–areolar complex deepens. During the second trimester, colostrum collects within the lobular alveoli. By parturition, vascular engorgement, epithelial proliferation, and colostrum accumulation may triple the size of the breast.

Lactation

The withdrawal of placental lactogen and sex hormones at delivery leaves the breasts under the influence of prolactin. The alveolar cells produce and secrete colostrum, which is followed in 4 to 5 days by milk rich in lipid, protein, carbohydrate, and immunoglobulin. Milk production is maintained during lactation by ongoing secretion of prolactin by the anterior pituitary gland. An infant's stimulation of the nipple–areolar complex prompts this pituitary activity. Oxytocin elaboration by the posterior pituitary gland also results from nipple–areolar stimulation. Oxytocin increases intramammary ductal pressure, helping to eject milk from the lobules into the ducts.

Throughout lactation, the breasts remain engorged and nodular, making examination and assessment difficult. The presence of milk throughout lactation makes the ductal lumina a fertile environment for bacterial overgrowth. Obstructive mastopathy due to areolar inflammation accounts for suppurative mastitis that occurs during lactation.

Postlactational Involution

Postlactational involution of the breast occurs during the 3 months after cessation of nursing. Regression of the extralobular stroma is the primary feature of this period, but there is also glandular and ductal atrophy. The breast gradually returns to its nulliparous state, but this process is not complete because some glandular hypertrophy persists indefinitely.

Menopause

Mammary involution with menopause involves loss of glandular tissue. Although some lobules remain, the postmenopausal breast consists largely of fat, connective tis-

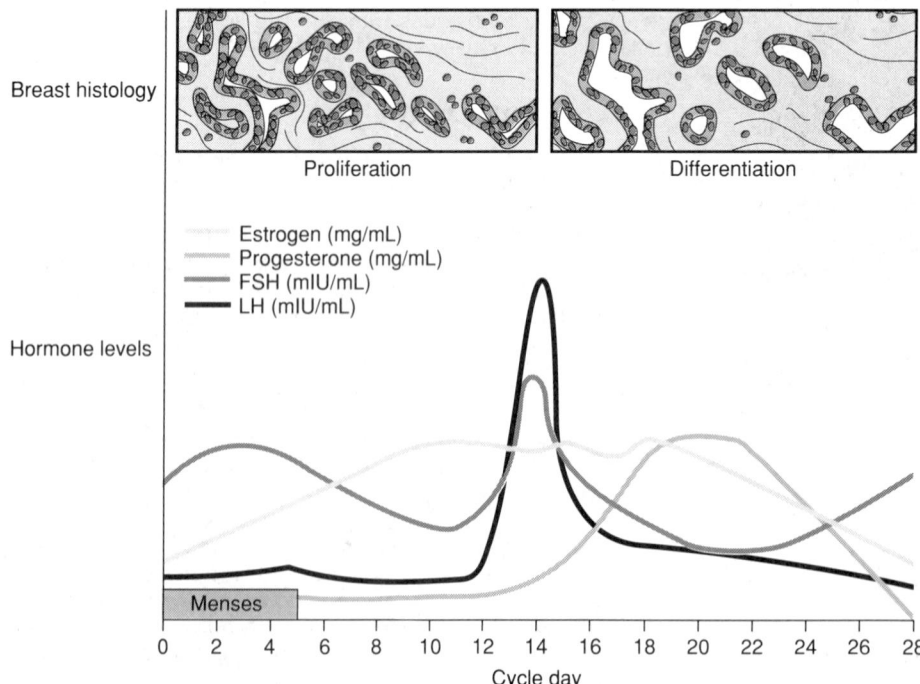

Figure 60-3. The effect of cyclic hormonal changes on the breast. FSH, follicle-stimulating hormone; LH, luteinizing hormone.

sue, and mammary ducts. Fat replacement of lobular elements helps maintain the breast contour. The breasts may become ptotic if lobular volume is not replaced with adipose tissue.

BREAST EXAMINATION
History

Most patients seek medical attention because of breast tenderness or a lump. Others have had a mammogram showing a nonpalpable lesion. It is important to elicit symptoms such as pain, tenderness, and nipple discharge. Pain, tenderness, or nodularity that vary with the menstrual cycle suggest a benign cause. Cancer is often asymptomatic. Patients are asked about findings at BSE.

The timing and nature of previous breast problems and operations are clarified. Histologic findings from prior biopsies are reviewed; pathology reports, slides, or cell blocks are obtained. A history of breast cancer confers risk for new breast cancer. Previous breast cysts or abscesses may have recurred.

A family history that reveals combinations of multiple first-degree relatives, multiple generations, or multiple occurrences of bilateral or premenopausal breast cancer strongly suggest a genetic predisposition to breast cancer. Women in families in which the autosomal dominant gene BRCA-1 (breast cancer gene 1) is present have a 50% chance of inheriting this gene from their mother or father.

Other factors addressed are menstrual history, reproductive history, and radiation exposure. Estrogens may alter the texture of the breast at examination and influence development or regression of benign breast disease. Use of hormones is recorded.

Physical Examination

Physical examination of the breast is easiest during the week after menses, when tenderness and engorgement are at a minimum. Palpation of the supraclavicular and anterior and posterior cervical lymph node chains initiates the examination. Skin changes, dimpling, or nipple abnormalities are important. Palpation of the axillae, including lymph nodes and the mammary tissue in the axillary tail, is performed while the patient is sitting. The number, size, consistency, and mobility of any palpable lymph nodes are recorded.

Palpation of the breast also is performed with the patient supine, with her ipsilateral hand behind her head. Palpation proceeds in a systematic way to ensure that the whole breast is examined. Subtly thickened areas may be compared with the contralateral breast. Discrete or dominant nodules and thickenings are described according to location (clock face position and distance from nipple), consistency, borders, and size. Tender areas are documented. Breast palpation is completed with gentle squeezing of the nipple–areolar complex to detect subareolar masses and latent nipple discharge. If a discharge is evident, the duct of origin is examined. Milky, serous, or green–brown discharges are almost always benign. Bloody discharge may indicate cancer.

The breast examination ends with a discussion of BSE. BSE is best performed immediately after menstruation (monthly for nonmenstruating women). Emphasis is on detection of changes rather than interpretation of findings.

Imaging

Imaging is a complement to, not a substitute for, the history and physical examination. Mammography, ductography, ultrasonography (US), computed tomography (CT),

and positron emission tomography (PET) are the modalities used for breast imaging.

The American Cancer Society recommends that mammographic screening begin at age 40. Mammography may help establish the diagnosis of a palpable mass or other clinical abnormality. Mammography is performed before biopsy for all women >30 years of age to detect synchronous, nonpalpable disease.

Only about one-fourth of nonpalpable lesions detected on mammograms are found to be malignant at biopsy. A spicular density with ill-defined margins on a mammogram is almost certainly malignant (Fig. 60-4). The following features suggest but are not diagnostic of cancer:

- Clustered microcalcifications
- Asymmetric density
- Ductal asymmetry
- Distortion of normal breast architecture
- Skin or nipple distortion

EVALUATION OF BREAST MASSES

Figure 60-5 outlines the evaluation of a palpable breast mass.

BENIGN BREAST DISORDERS
Fibrocystic Disease

Nodular (lumpy) or tender breasts without symptoms or with minimal symptoms have *fibrocystic changes*. The only treatment is reassurance. A condition that causes

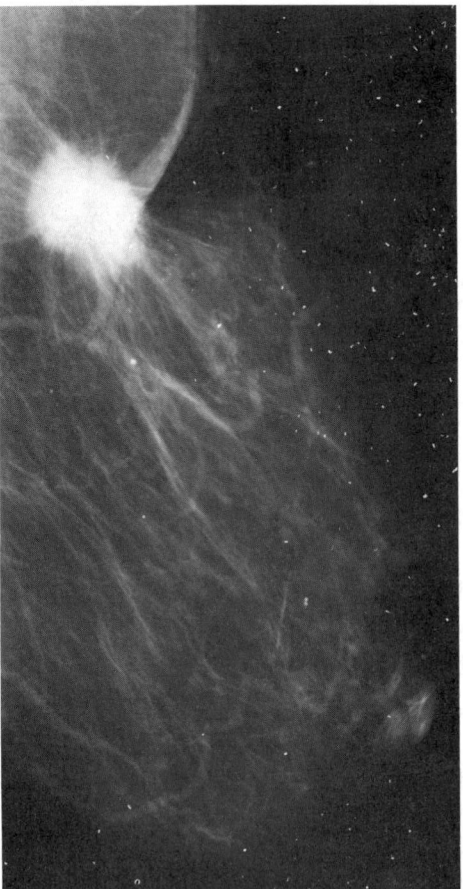

Figure 60-4. Left mediolateral mammogram revealing a 3.5-cm spiculated mass in the upper outer quadrant with associated skin thickening and retraction. Excisional biopsy demonstrated infiltrating ductal carcinoma. (Courtesy of Debra Ikeda, MD; from the Division of Breast Imaging, University of Michigan Medical School, Ann Arbor)

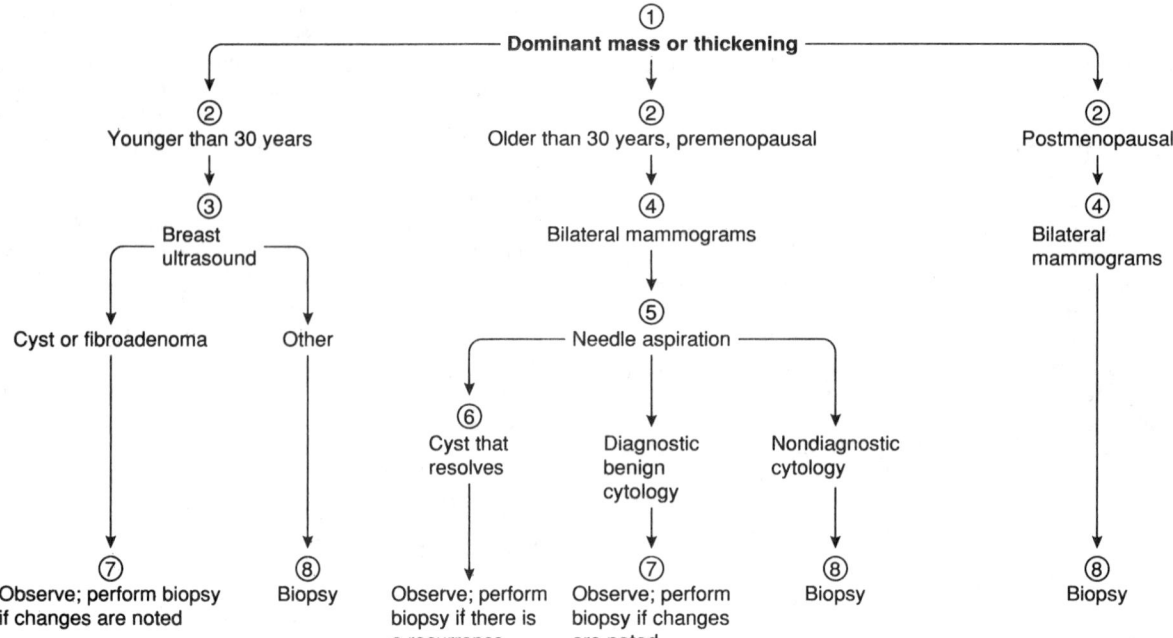

Figure 60-5. Algorithm for evaluation of a discrete breast mass.

(1) A *dominant mass* is a discrete area of breast parenchyma that is distinct in density or consistency from surrounding tissue in three dimensions. A *thickening* is a region of breast tissue that is not discrete but that is clearly distinguishable from the patient's other breast tissue. Recognition of a dominant mass or thickening may be aided by examining the corresponding location in the opposite breast; if the findings are symmetric, further evaluation may not be required.

(2) Age and menopausal status determine the workup of a dominant mass or thickening. Only 2% of breast cancers occur before the age of 30 years, whereas 70% are diagnosed after 50 years of age. In a young woman, if other factors corroborate an impression of a benign mass, observation may be warranted. All lesions in women older than 30 years (whether premenopausal or postmenopausal) must be assumed to be cancer until proved otherwise. In the presence of known major risk factors for breast cancer, evaluation in any woman should follow the algorithm for postmenopausal women, regardless of age.

(3) In women younger than 30 years, an ultrasound scan that corroborates a clinical impression of a simple cyst or fibroadenoma supports observation. Breast ultrasound is indicated after 30 years of age only when confirmation of a mammographic impression of a simple cyst is needed. The accuracy of breast ultrasound is not sufficient to allow its use to avoid the need for biopsy in women older than 30 years.

(4) The sensitivity and specificity of mammography for detecting malignant lesions improve with increasing age. Additionally, although the radiation exposure risk is low at any age, the risk decreases with age. Mammograms are rarely helpful before 30 years of age.

(5) Fine-needle aspiration is useful in premenopausal women older than 30 years. Aspiration may resolve a simple cyst or establish an unequivocally benign tissue diagnosis, obviating the need for further evaluation. If a lesion that is not a simple cyst is to be observed, the cytology must be both diagnostic and benign. Equivocal cytologic readings (eg, acellular, blood only, normal fat and mammary cells) require further workup (generally formal biopsy).

(6) Simple cysts that resolve completely after aspiration of nonbloody fluid may be observed. If they do not recur after aspiration, they may be assumed to be benign. A recurrent or enlarging cyst should undergo biopsy.

(7) Observation must be active, not passive. Reevaluation should occur in 2 to 3 months if it is elected to follow a discrete mass, and it should be repeated at least once thereafter. In women younger than 30 years, a decision to observe can be made if a clinical impression of benignity is substantiated by ultrasound or aspirate findings. In premenopausal women older than 30 years, a decision to observe should be made only with more stringent corroborative evidence—namely, a normal or benign-appearing mammogram *and* an aspirate that reveals either a simple cyst or unequivocally benign cytology. In postmenopausal women, tissue diagnosis of a discrete mass or thickening is mandatory. If observation is to be sensitive and useful, the baseline findings (location, size, consistency, tenderness) must be completely and accurately recorded and available for review by the same examiner at subsequent visits.

(8) *Biopsy* refers to a definitive tissue diagnosis made from unequivocally diagnostic fine-needle cytology or definitive histology from a sample obtained with a core-needle, incisional, or excisional biopsy.

moderate or severe symptoms is *fibrocystic disease.* Fibrocystic disease is classified as mastodynia (breast pain), a breast mass, or a nipple discharge. Treatment involves confirming that the process is fibrocystic rather than a benign or malignant entity, providing symptomatic relief, and giving reassurance.

Abnormalities such as adenosis, cysts, and fibrosis are present in the breast tissue of women without symptoms. These nonspecific histologic findings are *fibrocystic features.* If the same patient were to undergo biopsy at another point in the menstrual cycle, some of these changes might no longer be present. Other histologic findings, such as ductal and lobular hyperplasia, are clear pathologic entities.

The finding of fibrocystic features in a breast biopsy specimen does not increase risk for breast cancer. The presence of fibrocystic changes, however, may impair palpation or mammography. Because of changes during the menstrual cycle, repeated BSE is necessary to discern changes. Any new palpable mass is evaluated even if mammography is normal.

Epidemiology and Risk Factors

Almost every woman of reproductive age has cyclic breast discomfort. Most benign breast problems occur in menstruating women. Mastodynia usually occurs among young women (late teens and 20s) and among women about to undergo menopause. Users of estrogen replacement therapy (ERT) may experience symptoms. Oral contraceptive use, especially high-progesterone formulas, by premenopausal women decreases risk for benign breast disease.

Clinical Evaluation

Mastodynia

One of the most common presenting symptoms of benign breast disease is mastodynia (mastalgia), which may be cyclic (waxing or waning with the menstrual cycle) or continuous. Breast pain, especially cyclic mastodynia, is rarely associated with malignant neoplasms of the breast. Cyclic mastodynia is most severe just before, and least severe or absent immediately after, menstruation. The pain may be referred to the axilla, the undersurface of the upper arm, or the scapula. Continuous pain may be caused by acute or subacute infection or a single, large cyst. Once physical and mammographic findings rule out a mass lesion, reassurance is the only treatment needed. Mastodynia that begins as cyclic but becomes constant and severe suggests disease that necessitates specific therapy. Costochondritis of the upper ribs may be perceived by the patient as breast pain.

Breast examination reveals tender, nodular breasts, suggesting fibrocystic disease. The examiner must determine whether a dominant mass, distinct from the surrounding breast tissue, is present. Such a mass can represent a cyst or confluent area of fibrocystic changes or a malignant tumor that is not the cause of the pain but is an incidental finding.

After the presence of malignancy is ruled out, treatment of mastodynia is to reassure the patient that she does not have breast cancer. For most patients, nonprescription analgesics are the only drug therapy. Symptoms severe enough to require stronger drugs mandate more extensive evaluation and therapy.

Patients with mastodynia are advised to eliminate caffeinated beverages as much as possible for 2 to 3 months. At the end of that time, the patient can judge whether the pain has improved. Patients also are urged to stop smoking because nicotine is purported to worsen mastodynia.

Breast Mass

A palpable breast mass may be a cyst. Cysts can be aspirated with a fine needle or observed to see if they resolve. Persistent or enlarging cysts are aspirated. If cyst fluid is obtained and the lesion disappears, the only management is observation for recurrence. If aspiration yields no fluid, the mass must be presumed to be a solid lesion, and cytologic examination of the aspirate is performed. Bloody cyst fluid or a palpable mass that persists after aspiration of fluid suggests the possibility of cancer within a cyst. Excisional biopsy is mandated to exclude malignancy. Any palpable cyst that recurs after complete aspiration is excised.

Fibrocystic changes may present as a palpable mass in the absence of a macroscopic cyst. Physical examination reveals a palpable area of asymmetry rather than a true dominant mass. Reexamination at a different point in the menstrual cycle may reveal regression of the area, indicating that the patient may undergo observation. Fibrocystic changes are rare among postmenopausal women unless the patient is taking exogenous estrogen.

Nipple Discharge

The most common physiologic basis for nipple discharge is *lactation.* Milk may be secreted intermittently for as long as 2 years after breastfeeding. Evaluation is indicated if the discharge is spontaneous or blood tinged.

If a discharge is caused by subareolar *infection,* the fluid is purulent and the nipple erythematous and tender. Therapy is antibiotics and drainage.

A milky-white discharge, usually bilateral, not related to lactation or breast stimulation is *galactorrhea.* The presence of bilateral galactorrhea prompts evaluation for an endocrinopathy causing increased prolactin secretion by the pituitary gland.

Nipple discharges associated with *fibrocystic changes* are green, yellow, or brown. The brownish discharge of fibrocystic disease can be confused with old blood. A guaiac test or dabbing the discharge with a gauze pad and examining the stain can differentiate the two.

A bloody or blood-tinged discharge must be evaluated promptly to exclude *carcinoma.* A contrast ductogram may be obtained.

Specific Entities

Fibroadenoma is a palpable breast mass that must be differentiated from cancer. Women <30 years old with physical and US findings of fibroadenoma may undergo observation; the lesion is removed only if it enlarges or changes in character. After 30 years of age, cytologic diagnosis of fibroadenoma is obtained with FNAB.

Other benign breast masses are:

Sclerosing adenosis
Radial scar
Fat necrosis
Periductal mastitis (mammary duct ectasia)
Lactational mastitis
Galactocele
Mondor disease (thrombophlebitis of a superficial vein of the breast)
Intraductal papilloma

Diseases of the nipple are unusual. They are important because they must be differentiated from malignant processes that may involve the nipple. Nipple retraction is a common sign of breast carcinoma, and malignancy must be excluded whenever nipple retraction occurs in an adult.

BREAST CANCER

The factors associated with risk for breast cancer are summarized in Table 60-1. Most patients with breast cancer have no identifiable risk factor. Any woman older than 25 years with a palpable mass or abnormal mammogram is at risk.

Inherited Breast Cancer Syndromes

Women with a family history of breast cancer are at high risk. Four syndromes appear to be important:

1. Li-Fraumeni syndrome, attributed to mutations in the p53 tumor-suppressor gene
2. A mutation on the short arm of chromosome 2 in a gene associated with DNA repair
3. Inheritance of the BRCA-1 gene, located on the long arm of chromosome 17
4. Inheritance of the BRCA-2 gene, located on a small region of chromosome 13q12-13

The only accepted method of prevention of breast cancer is bilateral mastectomy. This may not even be of value because even small remnants of breast tissue left behind may pose substantial risk. When women at risk experience their first breast cancer, bilateral mastectomy is considered. In BRCA-1 families, bilateral oophorectomy also is considered.

Pathology

If malignant growth is found at breast biopsy, the following features are determined:

* Tumor size
* ER and PR status
* Status of excision margins
* Histologic type
* Status of pathologic prognostic features (nuclear grade, angiolymphatic invasion, host lymphocytic response)

Table 60-1. BREAST CANCER RISK FACTORS

DEMOGRAPHIC FACTORS

Age more than 30 yr
Female gender (130:1 female/male ratio)

GREATLY INCREASED RISK

Known carrier of breast cancer susceptibility gene
Strong family history—two or more first-degree relatives with bilateral or premenopausal breast cancer
Atypical ductal or lobular hyperplasia or lobular carcinoma in situ
Ductal carcinoma in situ, risk limited to ipsilateral breast

MODERATELY INCREASED RISK

Family history—one or more relatives with breast cancer, not bilateral or premenopausal
Menstrual history—menarche before age 12 yr, menopause after age 55 yr
Parity—nulliparity or first live birth after age 30 yr
Radiation—exposure to low-dose ionizing radiation in childhood or adolescence
Previous breast cancer—low-grade, node-negative, or receptor-positive; lobular histology
Other cancers—colon or endometrial cancer
Diet—high-fat or high-calorie diet

Invasive Carcinoma

Once the diagnosis of malignant disease is made, the most important prognostic feature is the presence or absence of invasion through the basement membrane. Invasive carcinoma is capable of regional and distant metastasis. Even tiny invasive cancers are fatal.

Invasive Ductal Carcinoma. Although the breast is composed of both lobular and ductal elements, most breast cancer originates in the ductal elements. Invasive ductal carcinoma (infiltrating ductal carcinoma) accounts for most cases of breast cancer. Invasion of nerves, blood vessels, and lymphatic channels in the breast parenchyma at the edges of a lesion may be present. These findings carry a poorer prognosis.

A number of uncommon types of breast cancer originate from the ductal epithelium. Histologic criteria for classifying these lesions must be met throughout the entire tumor. These variants include medullary carcinoma, tubular carcinoma, mucinous carcinoma (colloid carcinoma), and secretory carcinoma.

Invasive Lobular Carcinoma. The clinical features, epidemiology, and risk factors for lobular carcinoma are similar to those for ductal carcinoma. Lobular carcinoma, however, does not form microcalcifications and is extensively infiltrative, so mammographic detection is difficult. There is a high incidence of bilateral cancer among patients with invasive lobular cancer. The contralateral breast may be involved synchronously or metachronously.

Other Histologic Types of Breast Cancer

Metaplastic carcinoma, squamous and pseudosarcomatous
Carcinosarcoma
Squamous carcinoma
Apocrine carcinoma (cancer originating from the sweat gland elements of the breast)
Adenoid cystic carcinoma

Staging

Breast cancer staging is summarized in Table 60-2.

Treatment Planning

Biopsy—procedures to obtain tissue for diagnostic and prognostic purposes (FNAB, core-needle biopsy, incisional or excisional surgical biopsy)
Breast conservation—treatment undertaken to gain regional control of breast cancers in a manner that preserves an aesthetically acceptable breast (usually surgical excision of the tumor with radiation therapy to the rest of the breast)
Lumpectomy—en bloc tumor resection with sufficient margins to ensure removal of all tumor without contamination of surrounding, normal tissue
Reexcision lumpectomy—lumpectomy undertaken after a previous procedure (biopsy or lumpectomy) during which the cancer was not completely removed
Total mastectomy—removal of all breast tissue, including the nipple–areolar complex
Subcutaneous mastectomy—removal of the bulk of the breast tissue with preservation of the nipple–areolar complex
Axillary lymph node dissection (ALND)—removal of level I and II axillary lymph nodes en bloc with the axillary fat pad
Radical mastectomy—en bloc excision of the breast, overlying skin, pectoralis major and minor muscles,

Table 60-2. TNM CLASSIFICATION FOR STAGING OF CANCER OF THE BREAST

TNM DEFINITIONS

Primary Tumor

TX	Primary tumor cannot be assessed
T0	No evidence of primary tumor
Tis	Carcinoma in situ
T1	Tumor 2 cm or less in greatest dimension
T2	Tumor more than 2 cm but not more than 5 cm in greatest dimension
T3	Tumor more than 5 cm in greatest dimension
T4	Tumor of any size with direct extension into chest wall (not including pectoral muscles) or skin edema or skin ulceration or satellite skin nodules confined to the same breast or inflammatory carcinoma

Regional Lymph Node Involvement

NX	Regional lymph nodes cannot be assessed
N0	No regional lymph node involvement
N1	Metastasis to movable ipsilateral axillary lymph node(s)
N2	Metastasis to ipsilateral axillary lymph node(s) fixed to one another or to other structures
N3	Metastasis to ipsilateral internal mammary lymph nodes

Distant Metastasis

MX	Presence of distant metastasis cannot be assessed
M0	No distant metastasis
M1	Distant metastasis present (including ipsilateral supraclavicular lymph nodes)

STAGE GROUPING

Stage 0	Tis, N0, M0
Stage I	T1, N0, M0
Stage IIA	T0–1, N1, M0
	T2, N0, M0
Stage IIB	T2, N1, M0
	T3, N0, M0
Stage IIIA	T0–2, N2, M0
	T3, N1–2, M0
Stage IIIB	T4, N1–2, M0
	Any T, N3, M0
Stage IV	Any T, any N, M1

Beahrs OH, Henson DE, Huller RVP, Kennedy RJ. Manual for staging of cancer, ed 4. Philadelphia, JB Lippincott, 1992:149

level I, II, and III axillary nodes, and sacrifice of the long thoracic and thoracodorsal nerves
Modified radical mastectomy (MRM)—total mastectomy combined with ALND. Conserves the pectoralis major muscle and its innervation from the medial pectoral nerve
Breast reconstruction—procedures to alleviate breast and chest wall deformities after breast cancer operations

The formulation of a treatment plan for a woman with newly diagnosed primary operable (stage I or II) breast cancer is simplified by separate consideration of local control, regional control, adjuvant therapy for occult metastatic disease, and function and cosmesis (Table 60-3).

Surgical Management of Primary Operable Breast Cancer

Surgical therapy for primary operable breast cancer establishes local tumor control and allows staging. Surgical excision is the most important method of establishment of local control. When mastectomy is performed, failure to remove all tumor is likely to lead to local recurrence, even

Table 60-3. TREATMENT OPTIONS FOR PRIMARY OPERABLE BREAST CANCER

Objective	Options
Local control	Lumpectomy
	Lumpectomy with breast irradiation
	Mastectomy
Regional control	Axillary lymph node dissection
	Regional irradiation
Control of occult micrometastatic disease	Chemotherapy
	Hormone therapy
Improved function and cosmesis	Breast-conserving therapy
	Reconstruction (immediate or delayed)

if adjuvants are used. Breast conservation is more likely to be successful if all known tumor is surgically removed before initiation of radiation therapy.

Breast-conserving Procedures

A breast-conserving procedure is suitable for all women with primary operable breast cancer, unless a contraindication exists (Table 60-4). A breast-conserving operation is almost always followed by radiation therapy to the entire breast to reduce risk for local recurrence. ALND is performed through a separate incision from the tumor excision with fresh instruments, so that tumor cells are not spread to the axilla.

Table 60-4. MASTECTOMY VERSUS BREAST-CONSERVING THERAPY FOR PRIMARY OPERABLE BREAST CANCER

FACTORS FAVORING BREAST-CONSERVING THERAPY
Patient preference for breast conservation
Tumor size and location in breast favorable for good aesthetic result
Unifocal tumor
Small or absent intraductal component of tumor
Postlumpectomy breast anticipated easy to follow by physical examination and mammography
Patient inability to tolerate general anesthesia

FACTORS FAVORING MASTECTOMY
Patient preference for mastectomy
Tumor size and location in relation to breast not favorable for good aesthetic result with breast conservation
Multifocal tumor
Extensive intraductal component of tumor
Inability to closely observe patient postoperatively
Inability to achieve negative margins on lumpectomy
Contraindication to radiotherapy (eg, prior chest irradiation, pregnancy, severe pulmonary disease, patient inability to keep appointments)

FACTORS IRRELEVANT TO CHOICE
Size of tumor (if it can be totally excised with acceptable aesthetic result)
Breast size (if tumor can be totally excised with acceptable aesthetic result)
Node status
Tumor histology
Anticipated need for adjuvant chemotherapy
Patient age

Mastectomy

Total mastectomy is used to establish local control of stage 0, I, or II breast cancer. It is indicated when the patient prefers mastectomy over other options or when breast-conserving therapy is contraindicated (Table 60-4). Mastectomy can be used for local control of stage III and stage IV breast cancer only when used in conjunction with radiation and chemohormonal therapy.

MRM is performed when total mastectomy is needed for local control and when ALND is indicated for staging. MRM includes division of the pectoralis minor muscle at the coracoid process to expose the axillary space and allow thorough removal of the highest lymph nodes.

Early complications of MRM include wound infection, necrosis of the skin flaps, and seromas under the skin flaps or in the axilla. These are prevented by limiting rehabilitation exercises until after the drains are removed and leaving the drains in until output has decreased to <40 mL/d (as long as 4 weeks). Seromas can be treated with aspiration. Reinsertion of a closed-suction drain under sterile conditions is needed if the seroma recurs after two or three aspirations.

The most common late complication after ALND is *lymphedema* of the arm. This is managed with nighttime elevation and activity restriction. Severe lymphedema may necessitate use of a fitted support glove and arm stocking or intermittent compression device. Lymphedema can predispose a patient to cellulitis.

Axillary Lymph Node Dissection

The indications for ALND are staging and removal of clinically involved axillary nodes. Lumpectomy and ALND are not performed through the same incision.

Breast Reconstruction

Breast reconstruction is performed at the time of mastectomy (immediate) or later (delayed). Most patients undergo immediate reconstruction. Postponement is warranted when the need for radiation therapy is uncertain, risk for complications that may delay adjuvant chemotherapy is high, or the patient is uncertain about reconstruction.

Breast reconstruction techniques involve use of autogenous tissue or synthetic prostheses to produce a new breast mound. Autogenous tissue is ideal for use in previously irradiated fields or to manage skin and muscle defects caused by prior therapy. The most common procedure involves use of a transverse rectus abdominis musculocutaneous (TRAM) flap.

Prosthetic reconstruction involves subpectoral placement of a saline- or silicon gel-filled implant. Maintenance of a subpectoral pocket for an implant requires preservation of the pectoralis fascia and the medial pectoral nerve during mastectomy. A subpectoral tissue expander can be placed during mastectomy to provide enough skin for reconstruction.

Whatever the method for restoring the breast mound, breast reconstruction often involves a second, delayed procedure, such as reconstruction of a nipple–areolar complex or modification of the reconstructed or contralateral breast to establish symmetry. Tissue sources for nipple–areolar reconstruction include local skin, a portion of the contralateral nipple–areolar complex, or pigmented skin from the upper inner thigh or labia minora.

Radiation Therapy for Primary Operable Breast Cancer

Radiation Therapy After Lumpectomy

Contraindications to breast irradiation that may preclude breast-conserving therapy are:

The presence of tumor in two or more widely separated locations within the breast

Prior lung, chest wall, or breast irradiation
Pregnancy
Inability to achieve negative lumpectomy margins

Any technique used for postlumpectomy irradiation of the breast must cover the volume at risk, deliver a homogeneous dose throughout the target tissues, avoid overlapping or inadequate apposition of fields, and minimize the dose reaching the heart and lungs.

Acute complications of radiation therapy include fatigue, breast edema, and skin erythema. These are almost always self-limiting and resolve over weeks (fatigue) to months (erythema) or years (edema). The most common long-term problems are rib fractures and arm edema.

Radiation Therapy After Mastectomy

Postmastectomy irradiation is used to prevent regional treatment failure in patients at high risk for recurrent regional disease (those with multiple involved axillary nodes, extracapsular extension of nodal tumor, or locally advanced primary tumors). Because risk for arm edema is high among women who undergo ALND and axillary irradiation, this combination is avoided.

Adjuvant Systemic Therapy

Adjuvant Hormonal Therapy

Advanced breast cancer often responds to hormonal manipulation, which is usually well tolerated. Although hormonal therapy alters the growth rate of breast cancer cells, it may not entirely eradicate them. Hormonal intervention may be ablative or additive. *Ablative* measures include oophorectomy or ovarian irradiation, adrenalectomy or hypophysectomy, and antiestrogenic drugs such as tamoxifen (Table 60-5). *Additive* measures involve pharmacologic doses of estrogen or progestin, although corticosteroids and testosterone derivatives can be used.

Adjuvant Cytotoxic Chemotherapy

Breast cancer is sensitive to chemotherapy. The cyclophosphamide, methotrexate, and 5-fluorouracil (CMF) regimen leads to objective responses in more than half of premenopausal women with metastatic breast cancer. Other active regimens for these patients include CMF plus vincristine and prednisone (CMFVP) and doxorubicin-containing regimens, such as Adriamycin plus cyclophosphamide (AC) and cyclophosphamide, Adriamycin, and 5-fluorouracil (CAF). These regimens have activity in postmenopausal women but to a slightly lesser degree than in premenopausal women (Table 60-5).

Neoadjuvant chemotherapy is preoperative use of cytotoxic drugs. It is used to shrink large tumors to allow resection. But even for resectable tumors, it might be advantageous to begin systemic chemotherapy as soon as the diagnosis of cancer is made.

Breast-conserving procedures that involve postoperative radiation therapy necessitate consideration of the problem of coordinating chemotherapy and radiation. With longer-duration chemotherapy regimens, radiation is usually integrated into the chemotherapy schedule. One or two initial cycles of chemotherapy are given, and concurrent radiation is delivered with the next two cycles. At the conclusion of radiation therapy, chemotherapy resumes until completion of the prescribed dose. Doxorubicin is avoided during radiation therapy.

Management of Locally Advanced Breast Cancer

Neoadjuvant therapy for locally advanced breast cancer is initiated with combined chemohormonal therapy and continues until maximal clinical response is achieved. The

Table 60-5. **CURRENT RECOMMENDATIONS FOR ADJUVANT THERAPY IN STAGE I AND II BREAST CANCER**

Tumor	Premenopausal Patient		Postmenopausal Patient	
	ER-Positive	ER-Negative	ER-Positive	ER-Negative
<1 cm, negative nodes	NT	NT	NT	NT
≥1 cm, negative nodes	Tam ± chemo	Chemo	Tam	Chemo
Positive nodes	Chemo	Chemo	Tam	Chemo

ER, estrogen receptor; PR, progesterone receptor; NT, no treatment indicated outside of a clinical study; Tam, treatment with tamoxifen for at least 5 years indicated; chemo, chemotherapy may be indicated for some patients in addition to or instead of tamoxifen; Chemo, chemotherapy is indicated.

tumors are restaged clinically, radiographically, and pathologically, including repeat breast biopsy. Patients with no tumor in the rebiopsy specimen undergo breast irradiation to consolidate local control. If residual tumor is found, the patient undergoes MRM and postoperative radiation therapy.

Management of Recurrent Disease

Almost all women who have a recurrence of breast cancer die of the disease. Breast cancer recurrences can be divided into three broad categories—local, involving the breast or chest wall; regional, involving the first draining lymph nodes (axillary or internal mammary); and distant, involving secondary node groups and distant sites.

For local recurrence after mastectomy radiation therapy is attempted. Women with in-breast recurrences after breast-conserving therapy have a better prognosis than women with recurrence after mastectomy. Treatment is total mastectomy. Regional node recurrence is rare. Management is more radical dissection, if possible, radiation therapy to the entire involved node basin, or systemic therapy.

Management of Metastatic Disease

For most patients with metastatic breast cancer, treatment is palliative. The treatment options are systemic chemotherapy, hormonal manipulation, and localized radiation therapy (Table 60-6). The choice is based on site, hormonal sensitivity, and aggressiveness of the metastatic disease and on age, overall state of health, and menstrual status.

Noninvasive Breast Carcinoma

Noninvasive (in situ) cancer is a neoplastic entity confined within its epithelium of origin and without invasion through the basement membrane. Noninvasive cancer has no access to lymphatic or vascular elements and cannot metastasize. Mammography enables detection of microscopic, noninvasive cancers. Like invasive breast cancer, noninvasive cancer originates from ductal or lobular elements. The clinical presentation and behavior of ductal carcinoma in situ (DCIS) and lobular carcinoma in situ (LCIS) differ markedly (Table 60-7).

Management of Ductal Carcinoma In Situ

Although total mastectomy is the standard for management of DCIS, breast conservation can be performed with the understanding that recurrence can be in the form of invasive cancer, which has a worse prognosis than noninvasive cancer. When breast conservation is chosen for management of DCIS, lumpectomy is combined with radiation therapy. Breast conservation may be performed if the entire tumor can be surgically removed with negative his-

Table 60-6. **OPTIONS FOR THE TREATMENT OF METASTATIC BREAST CANCER**

CHEMOTHERAPY
Doxorubicin
Cyclophosphamide
Methotrexate
5-Fluorouracil
Vincristine
Vinblastine
Cisplatin
Paclitaxel

RADIOTHERAPY
Localized radiotherapy to discrete, symptomatic sites of disease or weight-bearing bone metastases
Whole-brain radiotherapy for intracranial metastases

HORMONE THERAPY
Surgical ablation
  Oophorectomy
  Adrenalectomy
  Hypophysectomy
Diethylstilbestrol (estrogen)
Tamoxifen
Megestrol acetate
Fluoxymesterone
Prednisone

Table 60-7. **CLINICAL FEATURES OF DUCTAL CARCINOMA IN SITU VERSUS LOBULAR CARCINOMA IN SITU**

	Ductal	Lobular
Age distribution	<50% Premenopausal (same as invasive ductal cancer)	75% Premenopausal
Palpable mass	Rare	Never
Radiographic findings	Microcalcifications	Usually none
Node involvement	<1%	None
Subsequent cancer risk	Invasive ductal cancer	Invasive ductal or lobular cancer
	Same breast	Either breast
	Same quadrant	Any quadrant

(Modified from Harris JR, Hellman S, Henderson IC, Kinne DW, eds. Breast diseases. Philadelphia, JB Lippincott, 1987:365)

tologic margins and the remaining breast tissue can be reliably assessed. The presence of extensive microcalcifications throughout the breast is a contraindication to breast conservation. These calcifications may represent DCIS, and even if they do not, their presence can impair mammographic detection of recurrence.

Management of Lobular Carcinoma In Situ

Both breasts are at equal risk, so both breasts are treated the same way. Resection of all areas of LCIS with breast conservation is not possible because of the multifocality of the disease. The treatment options are observation of both breasts to detect cancer development or bilateral total mastectomy. A well-informed patient makes the decision.

Bilateral, total mastectomy, usually with immediate reconstruction obviates long-term follow-up observation. This is the choice for patients who cannot or prefer not to undergo an observation follow-up regimen that includes annual mammography, twice-yearly physical examinations, and monthly self-examination. Bilateral mastectomy may be preferable for patients with LCIS with family histories of breast cancer, who are at high risk for invasive cancer. Most informed, motivated patients choose follow-up observation rather than bilateral mastectomy.

Prophylactic Mastectomy

The only treatment that can reliably prevent breast cancer is total mastectomy. However, risk for cancer is rarely so great as to justify prophylactic removal of a normal breast. In the few situations in which it does merit consideration, prophylactic mastectomy may be life-saving and life-affirming. The indications for prophylactic mastectomy are summarized in Table 60-8. The only established alternative to bilateral mastectomy for women at high risk is close observation with frequent physical examinations and screening mammography.

Cystosarcoma Phyllodes and Sarcomas of the Breast

Mesenchymal tumors originating in the breast are rare. Recognition is important because therapy for breast sarcomas differs markedly from that for breast carcinomas. Mesenchymal breast tumors are stratified into two groups—phyllodes tumors, which are unique to the breast, and soft tissue sarcomas of the breast that can occur elsewhere in the body.

Paget Disease of the Nipple

Paget disease is characterized by a weeping, eczematoid lesion of the nipple. There is often accompanying edema and inflammation. Biopsy of the nipple reveals malignant cells within the milk ducts. The lesion is invariably associated with invasive or in situ ductal carcinoma. The cancer sometimes can be detected at mammography. The prognosis of Paget disease is that of the underlying cancer. Treatment is mastectomy; ALND is performed only if invasive carcinoma is present.

Breast Cancer During Pregnancy and Lactation

Diagnosis of breast cancer in pregnant or lactating women is frequently delayed because of breast engorgement, tenderness, and nodularity. Therapy for breast cancer during lactation involves cessation of breastfeeding and treatment as for nonlactating patients. Pregnancy makes the treatment choices more problematic. Termination of pregnancy and suppression of lactation in and of themselves are not therapeutic, although they may simplify therapy. *Radiation therapy is contraindicated with a fetus in utero.* If breast conservation is performed, the pregnancy must be terminated or radiation therapy delayed until after delivery. Mastectomy is safe during pregnancy and lactation. Adjuvant chemotherapy or hormonal therapy is rarely administered to pregnant or lactating women because of risk of fetal exposure. Adjuvant therapy may be delayed, or if the risk for recurrence is low, omitted completely. There are no known direct effects of breast cancer on the fetus. Subsequent pregnancy poses no risk, although delay of pregnancy for 3 to 5 years is suggested.

Occult Breast Cancer Presenting as Axillary Metastases

Breast cancer may present with enlarged axillary lymph nodes as the first sign of disease. Sometimes physical examination and mammography do not detect a primary tumor in the breast even after lymph node biopsy reveals metastatic adenocarcinoma. Evaluation focuses on pathologic examination of the nodal tissue and a brief search for other primary tumors. If these endeavors are unrevealing, an occult breast primary tumor may be assumed. Breast examination and mammography are performed. A complete physical examination includes skin and thyroid assessment and testing for fecal occult blood. Laboratory and radiographic investigation in the absence of suggestive physical findings are complete blood count, liver function tests, carcinoembryonic antigen determination, and chest radiograph.

Women with adenocarcinoma in the axillary lymph nodes and no known primary tumor undergo mastectomy. A complete axillary dissection is performed. Therapy is mastectomy or breast conservation. Adjuvant therapy is recommended.

BREAST DISEASES OF EXTRAMAMMARY ORIGIN

Derangements of hormonal regulation elsewhere in the body can affect the breast as an endocrine target organ. These include:

Diseases of the skin over the breast
Benign and malignant soft tissue tumors
Fibromatosis (desmoid tumors)
Fat necrosis
Foreign-body reactions
Sarcoidosis
Lymphoma
Infections

Table 60-8. CRITERIA FOR CONSIDERATION OF PROPHYLACTIC MASTECTOMY

ONE OF THE FOLLOWING

Strong family history of breast cancer
Lobular carcinoma in situ
Atypical hyperplasia and a family history of breast cancer

PLUS ANY ONE OF THE FOLLOWING

High anxiety about cancer development
Limited access to follow-up
Difficult to follow clinically or radiographically
Patient preference for prophylactic surgery

Because the breast is responsive to hormonal influences, endocrine abnormalities may produce mammary sequelae; most common is *galactorrhea* resulting from abnormal elaboration of prolactin due to pituitary adenoma, thyroid disorder, or medication. New-onset fibrocystic changes in postmenopausal women suggest a hormone-producing ovarian neoplasm.

MALE BREAST DISEASES

Gynecomastia

Gynecomastia is palpable enlargement of the male breast. Nonspecific breast enlargement from fat deposition in obese patients must be differentiated from true gynecomastia, in which a distinct disk of breast tissue is palpable immediately under the nipple–areolar complex. Gynecomastia may be caused by changes in the normal male hormonal milieu. At the onset of puberty, the estrogen-to-testosterone ratio may be high in some boys, and this condition can persist for several years. Asymptomatic gynecomastia is a common finding among adolescents, probably because of this relative imbalance. Among elderly men, declining serum levels of testosterone in the presence of physiologic estrogen levels may be associated with gynecomastia.

Gynecomastia can be drug-induced (androgens, cimetidine, among others) or caused by syndromes such as Klinefelter syndrome, testicular feminization, secondary testicular failure, ectopic estrogen secretion, or hepatic failure. Drug-related gynecomastia can be unilateral or unequal between the two breasts. Discontinuing the drug does not always resolve the condition.

Clinical evaluation of the gynecomastia patient begins with a history and systems review aimed at uncovering hormonal, pharmacologic, or pathologic causes. Physical examination may reveal signs of an underlying disorder, such as liver dysfunction, Klinefelter syndrome, or a testicular tumor.

Palpation of the breast tissue is critical to verify the presence of gynecomastia and to exclude the possibility of cancer. Benign gynecomastia feels disk-shaped or spheric, firm, and rubbery. The breast tissue is symmetric and centered directly below the nipple. Irregular masses or those not immediately below the nipple–areolar complex are likely to be malignant. Mammography is performed. Testicular US is performed only if the testes are not normal to palpation. Liver function tests and a chest radiograph can help exclude some causes of gynecomastia.

Management of gynecomastia involves correction or elimination of the cause combined with reassuring the patient about the benignity of the condition. For most patients, particularly older men with bilateral disease, exclusion of malignant neoplasia is all that is required. Surgical management of gynecomastia is subcutaneous mastectomy under local anesthesia.

Male Breast Cancer

Men with breast cancer present at a more advanced stage than women. This is attributable to delay in presentation and to the smaller amount of breast tissue, which allows early invasion into the chest wall. Men have few clear risk factors for breast cancer. The presence of gynecomastia is not associated with development of cancer, yet protracted hyperestrogenemic states, which are associated with gynecomastia, are linked to breast cancer development.

Radiation to the chest wall, particularly in childhood or adolescence, is associated with risk for breast cancer. Female relatives of men with breast cancer do not appear to have a higher breast cancer risk than the general population.

Because a normal male breast does not have lobular elements, male breast cancer is almost always ductal in origin. All other histologic types of breast cancer occur in men, as do inflammatory breast cancer and Paget disease. Most male breast cancers are ER-positive.

The most common presentation of male breast cancer is a hard, painless breast lump. Bloody nipple discharge and skin ulceration are more common than in female patients. Unlike gynecomastia, male breast cancer is usually hard, asymmetric, and fixed to the skin or chest wall. Is is associated with axillary adenopathy. Mammography and biopsy are performed if clinical findings indicate. Male patients who have had cancer in one breast undergo mammography of the other breast to detect a second primary tumor.

Most tumors can be managed with modified radical mastectomy; en bloc excision of pectoralis major without complete removal of the muscle may be necessary. Postoperative radiation therapy improves local control. Metastases to the axillary nodes are frequent with male breast cancer. Adjuvant systemic chemotherapy is advocated.

When metastatic disease develops in a man with breast cancer, endocrine manipulations are the first therapy. Most patients respond to hormone therapy. ER-positive tumors are far more likely to regress with hormonal therapy than ER-negative tumors. Treatment includes orchiectomy, pharmacologic doses of estrogen (diethylstilbestrol), tamoxifen, progestational agents, antiandrogens, and adrenalectomy. Patients who are ER-negative, do not respond to first-line therapy, or have serious visceral disease (usually liver involvement) undergo combination chemotherapy.

SUGGESTED READING

Ayash LJ. High dose chemotherapy with autologous stem cell support for the treatment of metastatic breast cancer. Cancer 1994;74:532.

Biesecker BB, Boehnke M, Calzone K, et al. Genetic counseling for families with inherited susceptibility to breast and ovarian cancer. JAMA 1993;269:1970.

Bland KI, Copeland EM, eds. The breast: comprehensive management of benign and malignant diseases. Philadelphia, WB Saunders, 1991.

Fisher B, Constantino J, Redmond C, et al. Lumpectomy compared with lumpectomy and radiation therapy for the treatment of intraductal breast cancer. N Engl J Med 1993;328:1581.

Futreal PA, Liu Q, Shattuck-Eidens D, et al. BRCA1 mutations in primary breast and ovarian carcinomas. Science 1994;266:120.

Gasparini G, Weidner N, Bevilacqua P, et al. Tumor microvessel density, p53 expression, tumor size, and peritumoral lymphatic vessel invasion are relevant prognostic markers in node-negative breast carcinoma. J Clin Oncol 1994;12:454.

Kerlikowske K, Grady D, Rubin SM, et al. Efficacy of screening mammography: a meta-analysis. JAMA 1995;273:149.

Schnitt SJ, Abner A, Gelman R, et al. The relationship between microscopic margins of resection and the risk of local recurrence in patients with breast cancer treated with breast-conserving surgery and radiation therapy. Cancer 1994;74:1746.

Vasconez LO, Lejour M, Gamboa-Bobadilla M. Breast reconstruction. Philadelphia, JB Lippincott, 1991.

Wooster R, Neuhausen SL, Mangion J, et al. Localization of a breast cancer susceptibility gene, BRCA2, to chromosome 13q12. Science 1994;265:2088.

SECTION K

THORAX

ESSENTIALS OF SURGERY: SCIENTIFIC PRINCIPLES AND PRACTICE,
edited by Lazar J. Greenfield, Michael W. Mulholland, Keith T. Oldham, Gerald B. Zelenock,
and Keith D. Lillemoe. Lippincott–Raven Publishers, Philadelphia, © 1997.

CHAPTER 61

LUNG NEOPLASMS

VALERIE W. RUSCH

LUNG CANCER

Lung cancer is the second most common malignant disease and the most common cause of cancer-related death among both men and women. Causes include cigarette smoking, genetic predisposition (people with lung cancer may have genetic abnormalities that limit their ability to detoxify the carcinogens in tobacco smoke), abnormalities of the cytochrome P450 enzyme system, exposure to environmental carcinogens such as radon and asbestos (which also may interact synergistically with cigarette smoke), occupational exposure to carcinogens, such as arsenic, chromium, nickel, copper, beryllium, vinyl chloride, benzene, and uranium.

Pathologic Classification

Eighty percent of lung cancers are non–small-cell cancers, and 20% are small cell cancers. The two types differ in histologic features and clinical behavior, but frequent admixtures of small cell and non–small-cell carcinoma in tumors suggest a common origin of all lung cancers. The criteria for the histologic classification of lung tumors are shown in Table 61-1.

Non–Small-Cell Lung Cancers

Non–small-cell lung cancers are subdivided into squamous cell cancers, adenocarcinomas, and large cell cancers (Table 61-2).

Most squamous cell tumors originate centrally, in the main-stem, lobar, or segmental bronchi, but a third type occurs in the small bronchi of lung tissue. Adenocarcinoma originates peripherally in the pulmonary parenchyma. Large cell cancers are the least common form of non–small-cell lung cancer.

Bronchioloalveolar carcinoma, a subtype of adenocarcinoma, is characterized by growth of malignant cells along the walls of alveoli without destruction of the normal pulmonary architecture. Despite this uniform histologic appearance, bronchioloalveolar carcinomas have varying biologic behaviors. They can present as indolent, well-circumscribed, small, peripheral pulmonary nodules or as aggressive tumors with diffuse pneumonic involvement. Bronchioloalveolar carcinoma is more likely to be multifocal than are the other types of non–small-cell lung cancer.

Early-stage squamous cell cancers, adenocarcinomas,

Table 61-1. HISTOLOGIC CLASSIFICATION OF LUNG TUMORS

WHO*	WPL-LCSG†
	01 Carcinoma in situ
1. Squamous cell carcinoma (epidermoid carcinoma) Variant:	10 Squamous cell carcinoma
	11 Well-differentiated
	12 Moderately differentiated
a. Spindle cell (squamous carcinoma)	13 Poorly differentiated
2. Small cell carcinoma	20 Small cell
a. Oat cell carcinoma	21 Lymphocyte-like or oat cell
b. Intermediate cell type	22 Intermediate
c. Combined oat cell carcinoma	
3. Adenocarcinoma	30 Adenocarcinoma
a. Acinar adenocarcinoma	31 Well-differentiated
b. Papillary adenocarcinoma	32 Moderately differentiated
c. Bronchioloalveolar carcinoma	33 Poorly differentiated
d. Solid carcinoma with mucus formation	34 Bronchiolar or alveolar
4. Large cell carcinoma Variants:	40 Large cell undifferentiated
a. Giant cell carcinoma	41 Giant cell
b. Clear cell carcinoma	
5. Adenosquamous carcinoma	50 Poorly differentiated carcinoma
6. Carcinoid	60 Bimulticomponent or multidifferentiated
7. Bronchial gland carcinoma	70 Carcinoid
a. Adenoid cystic	
b. Mucoepidermoid carcinoma	
c. Others	
8. Others	80 Bronchial gland tumors
	81 Adenoid cystic
	82 Mucoepidermoid
	83 Mixed tumors

* World Health Organization. Adapted from: Histological typing of lung tumours. Tumori 1981;67:253.
† Working Party for the Study of Lung Cancer. Modified by Lung Cancer Study Group, National Cancer Institute.

and large cell cancers differ in clinical behavior, but almost half of non–small-cell lung tumors show more than one of the three cell types, again suggesting a common origin for all lung cancers.

Small-Cell Lung Cancer

Small-cell lung cancers are part of the larger family of neuroendocrine tumors that originate in many different areas of the body. In the lung and bronchial tree, neuroendocrine tumors include a spectrum of lesions ranging from well-differentiated, indolent, typical carcinoid tumor, to aggressive, atypical carcinoid tumor, to large-cell neuroendocrine carcinomas, to small-cell cancer.

Table 61-2. **FREQUENCY OF HISTOLOGIC CELL TYPES FROM TWO LARGE SCREENING PROJECTS***

Cell Type	Memorial Sloan-Kettering (%)	Mayo Clinic (%)	
		Prevalence	Incidence
Adenocarcinoma	45	27	24
Squamous cell carcinoma	33	43	30
Undifferentiated carcinoma			
Small cell	16	13	26
Large cell	6	17	19

* Based on results from 20,000 screened patients.
(Petts SB Jr, Wernly JA, Akl BF. Lung Cancer: current concepts and controversies. West J Med 1986;J145:52).

Light microscopic examination allows differentiation between two subtypes of small-cell lung cancer: oat-cell carcinoma, a tumor composed of small round uniform cells, and intermediate small-cell cancer, a tumor composed of less regular, polygonal cells. These two categories are characterized in small-cell lung cancer cell lines as classic and variant subtypes. *Classic* cell lines express a panel of four biomarkers, including L-dopa decarboxylase, neuron-specific enolase, creatine kinase, and bombesin-like immunoreactivity. *Variant* cell lines express creatine kinase and low amounts of neuron-specific enolase but not the other two markers. Variant cell lines also reveal amplification and expression of the oncogene c-*myc*, whereas classic cell lines do not. The variant cell line or intermediate form of small-cell cancer is associated with malignancy.

Biology

Tumors develop as a result of multiple events, including activation of oncogenes and inactivation of tumor suppressor genes. At least three abnormalities that occur in overt tumors also exist in dysplastic bronchial epithelium. These are probably early steps in lung tumorigenesis. The precise sequence of these and other events leading to transformation of normal bronchial epithelial cells to metaplasia, dysplasia, carcinoma in situ, or invasive and metastatic cancer is not known.

Primary tumors, even when histologically similar, manifest disparate cellular abnormalities, which affect cell function at the cell surface (EGFR and its ligands), within the cytoplasm (K-*ras*), and ultimately within the nucleus (Rb and p53). Some genetic changes affect only tumor initiation or growth; others affect tumor progression (metastasis) or act at several stages in lung tumorigenesis. Primary tumors with p53 mutations or overexpression rarely show K-*ras* point mutations or inactivation of Rb. Different cellular pathways may lead to clinically similar outcomes. For example, EGFR activation leads to activation of the *ras* pathway or may induce transcription by activation of a group of proteins (the Stat proteins) through tyrosine phosphorylation. p53 May promote cell proliferation by activating the EGFR promoter in the nucleus.

NON–SMALL-CELL LUNG CANCER

Table 61-3 shows the staging of non–small-cell lung cancer.

Clinical Presentation and Diagnosis

Early-stage non–small-cell lung cancers cause hemoptysis, atelectasis, or postobstructive pneumonia, if they are located centrally. Peripheral tumors that extend into the chest wall, spine, or brachial plexus cause pain. Most patients are referred to a surgeon because of an asymptomatic nodule or mass on a chest radiograph. Old chest radiographs are helpful. If the lesion has not grown in 2 years, it is likely to be benign. Radiographic characteristics, such as a smooth contour, dense homogeneous calcification, or "popcorn" calcification, suggest diseases other than lung cancer.

Tissue diagnosis can be established at bronchoscopy for centrally located lesions or percutaneous needle aspiration for peripheral masses. Exploratory thoracotomy without a preoperative diagnosis is acceptable if the history and radiographic findings strongly suggest lung cancer or if attempts to obtain a tissue diagnosis have failed and there is no evidence of distant disease. An algorithm for the management of solitary pulmonary nodules is shown in Figure 61-1.

Selection of Treatment

Therapy for non–small-cell lung cancer is based on stage of disease at diagnosis and overall medical condition (Table 61-4). The aims of the initial evaluation for non–small-cell lung cancer are to determine whether distant metastatic disease is present and to assess the extent of intrathoracic disease. Common metastatic sites include the brain, supraclavicular nodes, contralateral lung, bone, liver, and adrenal glands.

History and physical examination, plain chest radiography, and baseline laboratory data (complete blood count and serum sodium, calcium, alkaline phosphatase, and lactate dehydrogenase levels) may suggest the presence of metastatic disease. Abnormal findings are investigated with radionuclide imaging, computed tomography (CT), or magnetic resonance imaging (MRI) and needle aspiration or open biopsy to prove extent of disease.

If there is no clinical evidence of extrathoracic disease, it is important to determine whether mediastinal nodal metastases (N2 or N3 disease) are present. This is accomplished with CT and mediastinoscopy. Mediastinal nodes ≤1 cm in diameter on a CT scan are almost always benign. Mediastinal nodes >1.5 cm in diameter often are malignant but sometimes are enlarged because of underlying pulmonary disease or postobstructive pneumonia. Peripheral tumors without associated mediastinal adenopathy on CT scans are unlikely to be nodal metastases and do not require mediastinoscopy. More centrally located tumors or tumors with mediastinal adenopathy on CT scans warrant mediastinoscopy. Mediastinoscopy is crucial to avoiding thoracotomy for patients with unresectable disease.

Patients with early-stage non–small-cell lung cancer must be examined to determine whether pulmonary function and medical condition allow pulmonary resection. The patient's cardiac status is assessed if history, physical examination, or baseline electrocardiogram suggests cardiac dysfunction. Patients who smoke must stop for at least 2 weeks before the operation. Patients undergo intensive bronchodilator therapy and are treated with appropriate antibiotics if they have chronic bronchitis. These measures reduce risk for postoperative atelectasis or pneumonia.

Surgical Resection of Stage I and II Disease

The goals of pulmonary resection are complete removal of the primary tumor and staging (Figs. 61-2, 61-3). The extent of pulmonary resection is dictated by the location and size of the primary tumor and whether there is involvement of the adjacent bronchopulmonary nodes. Pneumo-

Table 61-3. TNM CLASSIFICATION FOR STAGING SYSTEM OF NON–SMALL CELL LUNG CANCER

TNM DEFINITIONS

Primary Tumor

TX	Tumor proved by the presence of malignant cells in bronchopulmonary secretions but not visualized roentgenographically or bronchoscopically, or any tumor that cannot be assessed as in a retreatment staging
T0	No evidence of primary tumor
Tis	Carcinoma in situ
T1*	A tumor that is 3 cm or less in greatest dimension, surrounded by lung or visceral pleura, and without evidence of invasion proximal to a lobar bronchus at bronchoscopy
T2	A tumor more than 3 cm in greatest dimension, or a tumor of any size that either invades the visceral pleura or has associated atelectasis or obstructive pneumonitis extending to the hilar region. At bronchoscopy, the proximal extent of demonstrable tumor must be within a lobar bronchus or at least 2 cm distal to the carina. Any associated atelectasis or obstructive pneumonitis must involve less than an entire lung
T3	A tumor of any size with direct extension into the chest wall (including superior sulcus tumors), diaphragm, or the mediastinal pleura or pericarium without involving the heart, great vessels, trachea, esophagus, or vertebral body, or a tumor in the main bronchus within 2 cm of the carina without involving the carina
T4†	A tumor of any size with invasion of the mediastinum or involving the heart, great vessels, trachea, esophagus, vertebral body, or carina or presence of malignant pleural effusion

Regional Lymph Node Involvement

N0	No demonstrable metastasis to regional lymph nodes
N1	Metastasis to lymph nodes in the peribronchial or the ipsilateral hilar region, or both, including direct extension
N2	Metastasis to ipsilateral mediastinal lymph nodes and subcarinal lymph nodes
N3	Metastasis to contralateral mediastinal lymph nodes, contralateral hilar lymph nodes, ipsilateral or contralateral scalene lymph nodes, or supraclavicular lymph nodes

Distant Metastasis

M0	No (known) distant metastasis
M1	Distant metastasis present—specify sites

STAGE GROUPING

Occult carcinoma	TX, N0, M0
Stage 0	Tis, carcinoma in situ
Stage I	T1, N0, M0
	T2, N0, M0
Stage II	T1, N1, M0
	T2, N1, M0
Stage IIIa	T3, N0, M0
	T3, N1, M0
	T1–3, N2, M0
Stage IIIb	Any T, N3, M0
	T4, any N, M0
Stage IV	Any T, any N, M1

* The uncommon superficial tumor of any size with its invasive component limited to the bronchial wall that may extend proximal to the main bronchus is classified as T1.

† Most pleural effusions associated with lung cancer are due to tumor. There are, however, some few patients in whom cytopathologic examination of pleural fluid (on more than one specimen) is negative for tumor and in whom the fluid is nonbloody and is not an exudate. In cases in which these elements and clinical judgment dictate that the effusion is not related to the tumor, the patient should be staged T1, T2, or T3, excluding effusion as a staging element.

nectomy, lobectomy, or bilobectomy provides microscopically negative vascular and bronchial margins. Limited resection, wedge resection, or segmentectomy may be adequate for some early-stage (T1, N0) tumors.

Tumors with direct extension into the chest wall, diaphragm, or pericardium are resected with the involved structure en bloc with the pulmonary resection, and reconstruction is performed. Tumors that have extensive endobronchial disease without involvement of the surrounding vascular or lymphatic structures can sometimes be completely removed by means of lobectomy with segmental resection of the bronchus (sleeve resection), preserving lung function.

Patterns of Recurrence

The predominant mode of relapse for all stages of non–small-cell lung cancer after surgical resection is distant metastasis. Local recurrence is more common with squamous cell carcinoma than with nonsquamous tumors. The brain is the single most common site of relapse. Most recurrences develop within 2 years of surgical intervention. Follow-up care includes history, physical examination, serial chest radiographs, and screening blood tests, including complete blood count and chemistry profile.

Adjuvant Therapy

Immunotherapy with intrapleural bacillus Calmette-Guérin (BCG) might improve survival after resection of stage I lung cancer. Adjuvant management of stage II tumors is postoperative radiation therapy.

Therapy for Stage IIIa Disease

Role of Surgical Resection

Stage IIIa non–small-cell lung cancer includes a heterogenous group of tumors with widely varying survival rates after surgical resection. T3, N0 tumors involving the chest

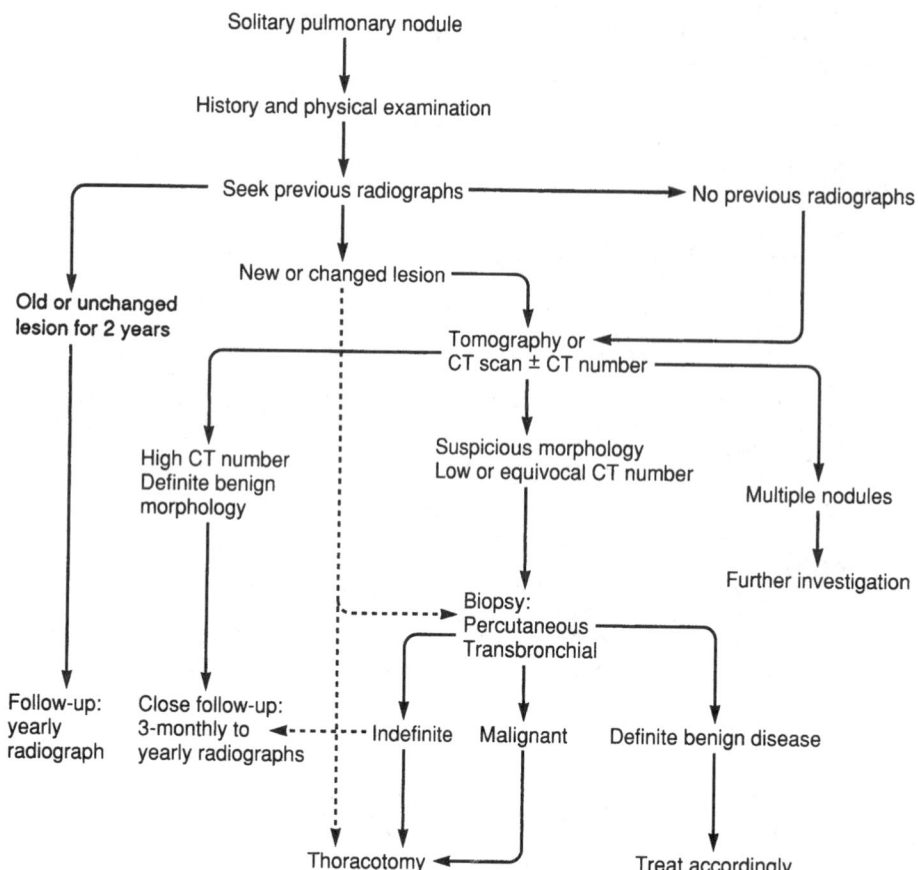

Figure 61-1. Algorithm for decision making for patients who present with solitary pulmonary nodules.

wall, pericardium, diaphragm, or main-stem bronchi are the most favorable stage IIIa tumors. Exclusion of the presence of N2 mediastinal nodal disease at mediastinoscopy is mandatory before thoracotomy.

The most controversial and complex part of therapy for stage IIIa non–small-cell lung cancer is management of N2 disease. This variation reflects extent of mediastinal nodal involvement, T status of the primary tumor, and ability to perform complete resection. With respect to mediastinal nodal involvement, adverse prognostic factors include presence of extracapsular nodal disease, multiple levels of involved lymph nodes, and presence of superior mediastinal nodal metastases. Usually only T1 or T2 primary and single-level, intranodal N2 disease are resected.

Rationale for Neoadjuvant Therapy

Neoadjuvant regimens are grouped into two categories: (1) chemoradiation therapy without surgical resection and (2) chemotherapy or chemoradiation therapy followed by surgical resection. For patients with stage III non–small-cell lung cancer who cannot undergo surgical resection, chemoradiation therapy is standard care. Although a few patients with minimal N2 disease benefit from surgical resection as the primary form of therapy, most patients have more extensive nodal involvement and cannot undergo surgical treatment. High-dose, continuous irradiation yields the best chance of local control.

NEUROENDOCRINE TUMORS

Neuroendocrine tumors of the lung have a common histogenesis but varying clinical behaviors, from indolent (typical carcinoid) to rapidly growing and aggressive (small-cell lung cancer).

Carcinoid Tumors

Carcinoid tumors originate from the neuroendocrine stem cells of the bronchial epithelium. *Typical* carcinoids consist of uniform round cells with small nuclei and fine granular chromatin. Mitoses and lymph node metastases are infrequent. *Atypical* carcinoids are pleomorphic and may have areas of increased cellularity with disorganization of the architecture and tumor necrosis. Mitoses are present within the context of a recognizable carcinoid pattern. Lymph node metastases occur in about half of patients.

Diagnosis

Some carcinoids are located centrally and may be diagnosed at bronchoscopy. The bronchoscopic appearance is typically a pink or purple friable endobronchial mass cov-

Table 61-4. MANAGEMENT OF NON-SMALL CELL LUNG CANCER

Stage	Treatment
I, II	Surgical resection
IIIA	Combination of chemotherapy, surgical resection, radiation therapy
	Sometimes surgical resection alone
IIIb	Radiation therapy or combined chemoradiation therapy
IV	Chemotherapy

About half of patients have symptoms, which include hemoptysis, postobstructive pneumonitis, and dyspnea. Carcinoid syndrome is rarely associated with bronchial carcinoids and occurs primarily in the few patients with metastatic disease, particularly liver metastases. Other endocrinopathies occur rarely, including Cushing syndrome, inappropriate antidiuretic hormone secretion, and hypoglycemia.

Management

Therapy for bronchial carcinoids is complete surgical resection with mediastinal lymph node sampling or dissection. Some patients need lobectomy. Segmentectomy or sleeve resection is adequate for some patients. Endoscopic resection is used only as for palliation in patients whose medical condition precludes thoracotomy and pulmonary resection.

Large Cell Neuroendocrine Carcinomas

Large cell neuroendocrine carcinoma is characterized by a neuroendocrine appearance at light microscopic examination but with large cells, low nuclear-to-cytoplasmic ratio, high mitotic rate, and necrosis. These tumors do not appear to be responsive to chemotherapy or radiation therapy. Management of large cell neuroendocrine carcinoma is identical to that of non–small-cell lung cancer.

Small-Cell Lung Cancer

Small-cell lung cancers grow rapidly and disseminate widely by the time of diagnosis. They are rarely managed surgically. They are responsive to chemotherapy, but the response is not durable. Chemoradiation may be possible for early-stage (limited) disease.

Percutaneous needle aspiration for the diagnosis of coin lesions often reveals early-stage small-cell lung cancer. Surgical resection is considered after distant disease is excluded with a metastatic evaluation that includes a bone scan and CT of the chest, abdomen, and brain. Mediastinal nodal disease must be excluded by means of mediastinoscopy. Adjuvant postoperative chemotherapy is provided. If surgical resection is complete, radiation is not administered.

BRONCHIAL ADENOMAS

Bronchial adenomas constitute only a small number of lung neoplasms. The term *adenoma* is misleading because these tumors constitute a group of tumors that can be of low- or high-grade malignancy. This group includes cystic carcinoma, mucoepidermoid carcinoma, and mucous gland adenoma (the only truly benign tumor).

The presenting signs and symptoms of these tumors depend on location. Peripheral tumors are asymptomatic, presenting as a nodule on a routine chest radiograph. Proximal tumors present with hemoptysis or signs of airway obstruction, including cough, recurrent infection, wheezing, or stridor. Because of the slow growth of these tumors, signs and symptoms may develop over a period of years. Incompletely obstructing tumors frequently masquerade as asthma for prolonged periods of time.

Diagnosis

Peripheral tumors are diagnosed by means of percutaneous needle aspiration biopsy or at thoracotomy. Tumors in major airways are diagnosed at bronchoscopy. Other studies, such as CT scans, are rarely required to make the diagnosis but may be of value in planning therapy.

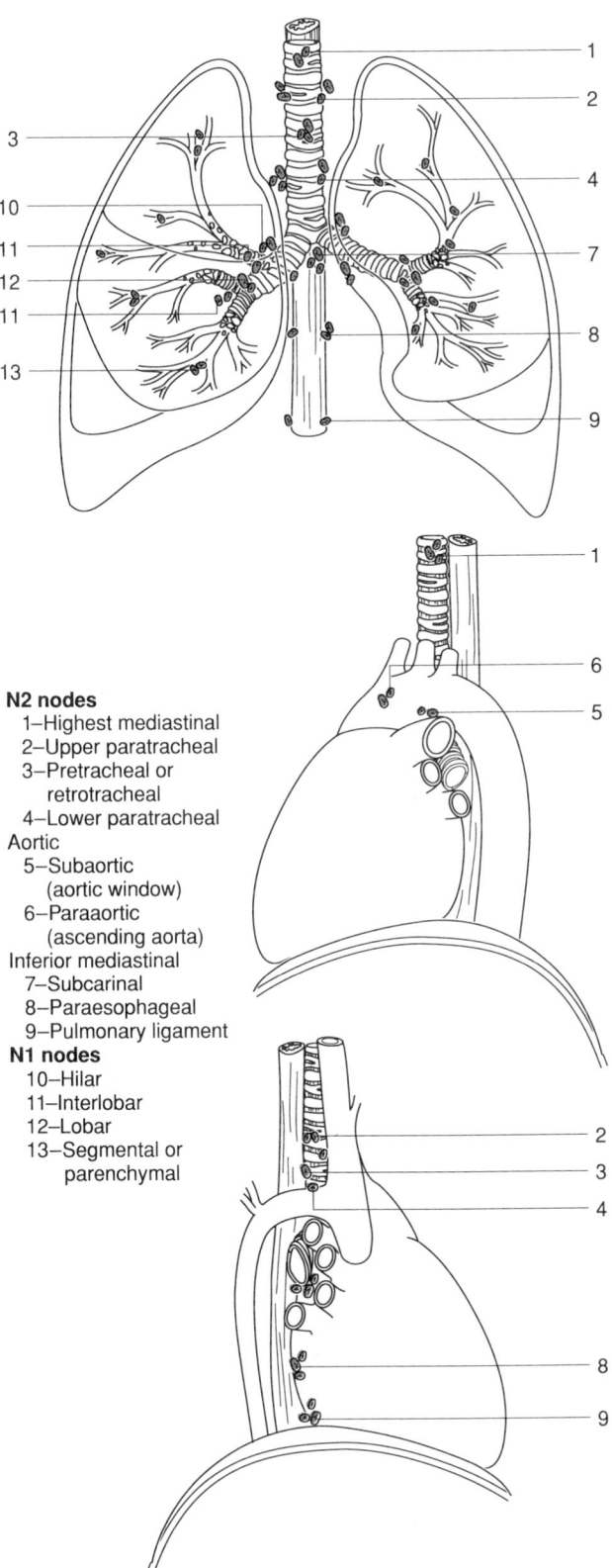

N2 nodes
1–Highest mediastinal
2–Upper paratracheal
3–Pretracheal or retrotracheal
4–Lower paratracheal
Aortic
5–Subaortic (aortic window)
6–Paraaortic (ascending aorta)
Inferior mediastinal
7–Subcarinal
8–Paraesophageal
9–Pulmonary ligament
N1 nodes
10–Hilar
11–Interlobar
12–Lobar
13–Segmental or parenchymal

Figure 61-2. Naruke lymph node map. (After Manual for staging of cancer, ed 3. Philadelphia, JB Lippincott, 1988:115)

ered by intact epithelium. Other carcinoids appear as well-circumscribed nodules on chest radiographs. Typical carcinoids occur more frequently in the central or lobar airways than do atypical carcinoids.

A

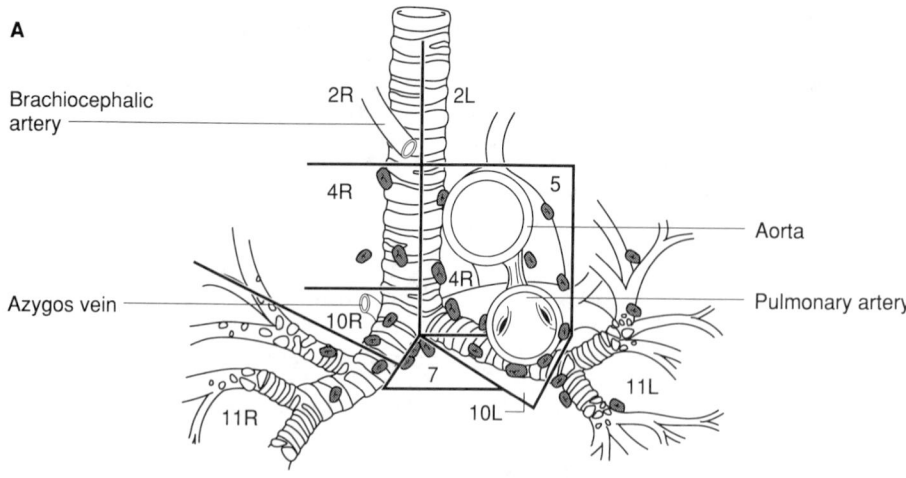

N2 nodes
Superior mediastinal nodes
2 [2R–*Right upper paratracheal:* Between intersection of caudal margin of innominate
        artery with trachea and the apex of the lung (suprainnominate nodes)
    2L–*Left upper paratracheal:* Between top of aortic arch and apex of
       the lung (supraaortic nodes)
4 [4R–*Right lower paratracheal:* Between intersection of caudal margin
       of innominate artery with trachea and cephalic border of azygos vein
    4L–*Left lower paratracheal:*Between top of aortic arch and carina
10 [10R–*Right tracheobronchial:* From cephalic border of azygos vein to origin of RUL bronchus
    10L–*Left tracheobronchial:* Between carina and LUL bronchus
       (medial to ligamentum arteriosum)
Aortic nodes
    [5–*Aortopulmonary:* Subaortic and paraaortic nodes; lateral to the ligamentum arteriosum
        (proximal to first branch of left PA)
    [6–*Anterior mediastinal:* Anterior to ascending aorta or innominate artery
Inferior mediastinal nodes
    [7–*Subcarinal:* Caudal to carina of the trachea
    [8–*Paraesophageal:* Dorsal to posterior wall of the trachea and to right
       or left of the midline of the esophagus
    [9–*Pulmonary ligament:* Within the pulmonary ligament
N1 nodes
    [11–*Interlobar*
    [12–*Lobar*
    [13–*Segmental*
    [14–*Subsegmental*

B

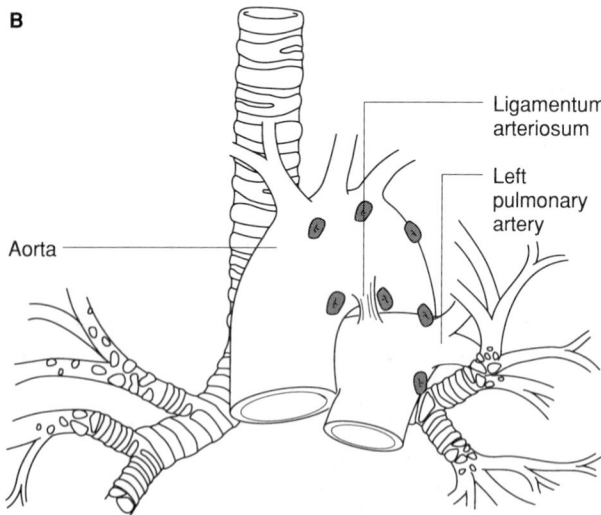

Figure 61-3. American Thoracic Society lymph node map. Compared with the Naruke map in Figure 61-2, this newer map has more strictly defined anatomic boundaries for each lymph node region. This allows easy correlation between findings at operation and findings on the chest CT scan. (After Am Rev Resp Dis 1983; 127:659)

Management

Because most of these tumors do not metastasize, complete excision preserving as much pulmonary tissue as possible is the goal. Whenever possible, sleeve resection of main bronchi is performed to preserve pulmonary tissue.

Adenoid Cystic Carcinoma

Adenoid cystic carcinomas are slowly growing malignant tumors that originate from the submucosal glands of the trachea and main bronchi. These tumors spread in the submucosal plane along the perineural lymphatics, well beyond the apparent endoluminal component of the tumor.

Management

Whenever possible, therapy is total excision by means of tracheal resection or tracheobronchial resection. This is not always possible because of the extensive submucosal spread of the tumor. Postoperative radiation therapy is indicated. When surgical resection is not feasible because of the extent of the lesion, palliative treatment is endoscopic laser removal followed by radiation therapy.

Mucoepidermoid Carcinoma

Mucoepidermoid carcinomas are rare bronchial tumors. They occur in people of all ages. Mucoepidermoid carcinomas may be of low- or high-grade malignancy. Low-grade tumors have a large proportion of mucous cells; high-grade tumors have a large proportion of squamous cells.

Management

Therapy for mucoepidermoid tumors is similar to that for carcinoid tumors. Highly malignant tumors, however, are managed as bronchogenic carcinoma. Complete surgical resection is the mainstay of treatment.

Mucous Gland Adenoma

Mucous gland adenomas are rare submucosal tumors that originate from mucous glands. They are also known as bronchial cysts and papillary cystadenoma. Because of their totally benign behavior, these lesions can usually be treated by means of endoscopic excision. Thoracotomy and surgical resection are indicated only if the distal lung is destroyed by chronic infection or if endoscopic removal is contraindicated or incomplete.

BENIGN TUMORS OF THE LUNG

The lung is composed of epithelial, mesodermal, and endodermal cells. Benign tumors may originate from any of these cells. They present as endobronchial lesions or peripheral nodules. Endobronchial tumors present with signs and symptoms of airway obstruction or bleeding. Tumors originating in peripheral airways or in association with pulmonary parenchyma present as undiagnosed asymptomatic solitary pulmonary nodules. The many types of benign lung tumors are listed in Table 61-5.

Hamartoma

The most frequently occurring benign tumors are hamartomas. A hamartoma consists of an unusual arrangement of normally occurring cells. In the lung, the most frequent component is cartilage. A hamartoma usually presents as a solitary pulmonary nodule with an extremely slow growth pattern.

Diagnosis

The radiographic appearance of hamartoma is a well-circumscribed nodule that may contain popcorn calcification. Previous chest radiographs show that the tumor has been present for many years. The growth pattern is variable but slow. If calcification is demonstrated, the diagnosis of hamartoma can be made with CT. Needle aspiration is frequently diagnostic of a cartilaginous benign lesion.

Table 61-5. TYPES OF BENIGN LUNG TUMORS CLASSIFIED ACCORDING TO THEIR CELLULAR ORIGIN

EPITHELIAL
Polyps
Papilloma

MESENCHYMAL
Nerve
Granular cell myoblastoma
Neurilemoma
Neurofibroma
Chemodectoma
Muscle
Leiomyoma
Others
Lipoma
Chondroma
Plasma cell granuloma
Teratoma

ENDOTHELIAL
Sclerosing hemangioma
Glomus tumor
Arteriovenous malformation

Management

Whether hamartomas should be excised for pathologic diagnosis is controversial. Excision is not necessary unless the lesion is proximal and causes symptoms of endobronchial obstruction or unless carcinoma cannot be ruled out. If transthoracic needle aspiration biopsy confirms the nature of these hamartomas, the patient may be followed with annual chest radiographs rather than surgical excision. Growth during the observation period may necessitate excision.

Arteriovenous Malformations

Arteriovenous (AV) malformations are the result of direct connection between branches of the pulmonary artery and pulmonary vein. They are congenital and often present as symptomatic pulmonary nodules. Most occur in the lower lobes, and they sometimes are identified because of an enlarged draining pulmonary vein running from the lesion to the mediastinum. Multiple AV malformations are associated with Osler-Weber-Rendu disease. The lesions are usually not recognized until at least the second decade of life. Often they enlarge progressively in response to increasing flow.

Diagnosis

Symptoms include dyspnea due to AV shunting and hypoxemia, parenchymal hemorrhage, hemoptysis, and neurologic sequelae related to emboli.

Management

Therapy for AV malformations is embolic via percutaneous catheters, using embolization coils or balloons.

Other Benign Tumors

Other benign tumors may present as endobronchial lesions (fibromas, lipomas, chondromas, and granular cell myoblastomas). These tumors may be removed endoscopically but may necessitate surgical excision when the diagnosis is in doubt or when endoscopic excision is incomplete. Peripheral tumors often are removed for diagnosis.

OTHER MALIGNANT TUMORS OF THE LUNG

Malignant tumors originating from epithelial, mesodermal, or endodermal cell lines can occur in the lung. Sarcomas originating from soft tissue or large vessels and carcinosarcomas are managed in a manner similar to that for sarcomas elsewhere. Primary pulmonary lymphomas usually are excised for confirmatory diagnosis. Other rare tumors include primary melanomas of the bronchus, malignant teratomas, and pulmonary blastomas. Therapy is complete surgical resection.

PULMONARY METASTASES

Clinical Presentation and Diagnosis

Pulmonary metastases are asymptomatic most of the time and are usually detected on routine chest radiographs. Patients who have undergone resection of a primary tumor known to be prone to pulmonary metastases undergo chest radiography as part of their routine follow-up care. On a chest radiograph, metastases usually are well-circumscribed, spherical solid masses with well-defined borders (Fig. 61-4). Cavitation may occur in large lesions that have central necrosis.

Metastases to the lung usually originate in the pulmonary parenchyma. Endobronchial disease represents extension of contiguous parenchymal disease. The extent of endobronchial tumor can affect the approach to surgical resection. Endobronchial metastases are uncommon and occur most often with renal cell, colon, and breast cancers.

Hilar or mediastinal nodal involvement sometimes accompanies pulmonary metastases. Lymphangitic spread can occur with or without concomitant pulmonary nodules. This occurs most often with breast cancer, and produces a characteristic radiographic appearance of diffusely increased interstitial markings and a clinical presentation of severe dyspnea out of proportion to the radiographic findings. When a chest radiograph suggests pulmonary metastases, CT is performed to determine number, location, size, and resectability.

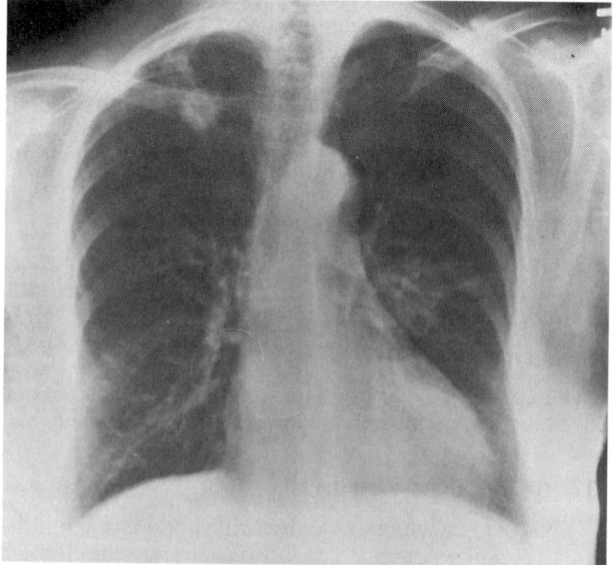

Figure 61-4. Chest radiograph of a patient with bilateral pulmonary metastases from endometrial cancer. The right upper lobe mass is well circumscribed and has the radiographic appearance typical of a metastasis.

Multiple pulmonary nodules in the setting of previously treated malignant disease rarely pose a diagnostic problem. Solitary pulmonary nodules are troublesome. A solitary lesion is likely to be a metastasis if the primary tumor was a sarcoma or a melanoma. If the primary tumor originated in the head, neck, or breast, the solitary lesion is likely to be new primary lung cancer. It is equally likely to be metastatic or a new primary if the initial tumor was of gastrointestinal or genitourinary origin.

Percutaneous fine-needle aspiration biopsy usually yields a tissue diagnosis. The question of need for biopsy of a solitary lesion is difficult. If the patient fits the selection criteria for resection, biopsy may be an excisional biopsy. Because the findings at needle biopsy do not alter recommendations for excision of a solitary lesion, this procedure is performed only if the patient cannot undergo surgical treatment, if an alternative method of treatment is indicated, or if the patient wants to know the diagnosis before consenting to surgical therapy.

Criteria for Surgical Resection

Therapy for pulmonary metastases from many solid tumors that cannot be managed with chemotherapy is surgical resection. These include colon cancer, renal cell cancer, melanoma, some head and neck tumors, and endometrial cancer. Surgical removal of pulmonary metastases is widely accepted, but effective chemotherapy is available for some cancers.

Resection is undertaken only if complete resection is considered technically feasible. Several guidelines must be met before a patient is considered for resection of pulmonary metastases: control of the primary tumor is achieved, absence of extrathoracic metastases, general medical condition that allows thoracotomy, pulmonary function that allows complete resection of all metastases, and lack of more effective systemic treatment.

If the metastatic lesion is found at the same time as a recurrence of the primary tumor, the recurrent primary tumor is managed before the metastatic disease to prevent further seeding of the metastatic site. When the primary tumor and the metastasis are diagnosed simultaneously, lung resection may precede the operation for the primary disease if doubt exists about whether the pulmonary disease can be completely resected. Immediate subsequent resection of the primary tumor is planned.

When a patient meets the criteria for resection of one or more pulmonary metastases, consideration must be given to the natural history of the tumor and whether effective systemic therapy is available. For example, because effective systemic therapy is available for breast cancer, surgical resection of pulmonary metastases is rarely indicated.

Chemotherapy is the primary form of management of germ cell cancer. Surgical resection is reserved for patients who have gross residual disease after the initial chemotherapy and whose serum tumor markers (β-human chorionic gonadotropin and α-fetoprotein) have fallen to normal levels. Persistent elevation of tumor markers signifies residual active tumor and is an indication for continuing chemotherapy. Negative tumor markers in the presence of gross disease on chest radiograph or CT scan suggest residual benign teratoma. Removal of teratoma is performed to prevent degeneration to a malignant germ cell tumor and to avoid the complications of local tumor growth. Surgical resection is strictly adjunctive therapy for malignant germ cell tumors.

The timing of an operation in relation to chemotherapy depends on the number, size, and location of pulmonary metastases at diagnosis and whether the patient has undergone previous chemotherapy. Often surgical resection is performed between several cycles of chemotherapy, with the aim of controlling both gross and micrometastatic disease. This approach allows assessment of the sensitivity of the patient's tumor to chemotherapy and determines the advisability of continuing the regimen postoperatively.

Preoperative Evaluation

Pulmonary function is assessed with pulmonary function tests, arterial blood gases, and, if necessary, ventilation–perfusion lung scan to ensure that the patient has sufficient reserve to tolerate complete resection of the metastases. Patients who received chemotherapy may have substantial reduction in their pulmonary function. Patients must stop smoking. Patients who smoke up to the time of operation are at risk for postoperative atelectasis and pneumonia.

Medical condition and cardiovascular status are assessed. Older patients may have coronary artery disease that requires preoperative treatment and additional perioperative monitoring. Patients who previously received chemotherapy may have impaired cardiac function. A preoperative radionuclide scan or echocardiogram is obtained to determine left ventricular ejection fraction and whether intraoperative hemodynamic monitoring is necessary. Some drugs can impair renal or neurologic function and may influence perioperative management.

For patients who have recently undergone chemotherapy, therapy is timed so that the operation is not performed when the patient is neutropenic or thrombocytopenic. Resumption of chemotherapy is timed so that it does not compromise wound healing.

Surgical Technique

The surgical approach to resection of pulmonary metastatic lesions follows two guidelines—complete resection of the disease and maximal sparing of functioning lung tissue. Wedge resection is performed when possible. This can be done with staples, electrocautery, or laser. Lobectomy or pneumonectomy is performed only when wedge resection will not provide complete resection.

Unilateral disease is approached via an anterolateral or a posterolateral thoracotomy incision. Patients with bilateral pulmonary metastases undergo simultaneous resection of the bilateral lesions, if technically feasible. This can be accomplished by means of median sternotomy or a clamshell incision (bilateral anterior thoracotomy with transverse sternotomy). Bilateral pulmonary nodules may necessitate sequential posterolateral thoracotomy if the lesions are centrally located.

SUGGESTED READING

Bonney GE. Interactions of genes, environment, and life-style in lung cancer development. J Natl Cancer Inst 1990;82:1236.

Fowler WC, Langer CJ, Curran WJ Jr, Keller SM. Postoperative complications after combined neoadjuvant treatment of lung cancer. Ann Thorac Surg 1993;55:986.

Martini N, Yellin A, Ginsberg RJ, et al. Management of non–small-cell lung cancer with direct mediastinal involvement. Ann Thorac Surg 1994;58:1447.

Martini N, Zaman MB, Bains MS, et al. Treatment and prognosis in bronchial carcinoids involving regional lymph nodes. J Thorac Cardiovasc Surg 1994;107:1.

McCormack PM, Ginsberg KB, Bains MS, et al. Accuracy of lung imaging in metastases with implications for the role of thoracoscopy. Ann Thorac Surg 1993;56:863.

Mehran RJ, Deslauriers J, Piraus M, Beaulieu M. Survival related to nodal status after sleeve resection for lung cancer. J Thorac Cardiovasc Surg 1994;107:576.

Rodenhuis S, Slebos RJC. Clinical significance of *ras* oncogene activation in human lung cancer. Cancer Res 1992;52:2665s.

Rosell R, Gómez-Codina J, Camps C, et al. A randomized trial comparing preoperative chemotherapy plus surgery with surgery alone in patients with non–small-cell lung cancer. N Engl J Med 1994;330:153.

Shah SS, Thompson J, Goldstraw P. Results of operation without adjuvant therapy in treatment of small-cell lung cancer. Ann Thorac Surg 1992;54:498.

Yashar J, Weitberg AB, Glicksman AS, Posner MR, Feng W, Wanebo HJ. Preoperative chemotherapy and radiation therapy for stage IIIa carcinoma of the lung. Ann Thorac Surg 1992;53:445.

ESSENTIALS OF SURGERY: SCIENTIFIC PRINCIPLES AND PRACTICE, edited by Lazar J. Greenfield, Michael W. Mulholland, Keith T. Oldham, Gerald B. Zelenock, and Keith D. Lillemoe. Lippincott–Raven Publishers, Philadelphia, © 1997.

CHAPTER 62

CHEST WALL, PLEURA, MEDIASTINUM, AND NONNEOPLASTIC LUNG DISEASE

MARK D. IANNETTONI AND MARK B. ORRINGER

ANATOMY

Respiration

The primary muscles of inspiration are the diaphragm, which contributes 75% to 80% of ventilation during quiet respiration, and the intercostal muscles, which are responsible for 20% to 25% of respiratory movement. At the end of quiet inspiration, when contraction of the inspiratory muscles has expanded the rib cage maximally against atmospheric pressure, elastic recoil of the lungs and rib cage results in a rise of intrapulmonic pressure that forces air out of the lungs until intrapulmonic pressure equals atmospheric pressure. Expiration that occurs is facilitated by contraction of the abdominal wall musculature that forces abdominal viscera against the diaphragm.

Skeletal Support

The chest wall is made up of the sternum, 10 pairs of ribs and their costal cartilages, two pairs of ribs without cartilages, and 12 thoracic vertebrae and their intervertebral disks. These bony elements surround the thoracic cavity, which extends from the thoracic inlet above to the outlet below.

The boundaries of the *thoracic inlet* are the manubrium of the sternum anteriorly, the first ribs laterally, and the first thoracic vertebra posteriorly. The anterior border of the thoracic inlet is 2 to 3 cm below its posterior border. The endothoracic fascia makes up the roof of the thoracic inlet and extends into the base of the neck with the parietal pleura, which is just beneath it. The *thoracic outlet* is bounded by the xiphoid process anteriorly, the fused 7th through 10th costal cartilages anterolaterally, and portions of the 11th and 12th ribs and the 12th thoracic vertebra posteriorly. It is separated from the abdomen by the diaphragm.

The adult sternum is 15 to 20 cm long and consists of

three sections—the manubrium, the body, and the xiphoid process. Wider in its upper half than in its lower half, the *manubrium* articulates along its upper border with the clavicles and laterally with the cartilages of the first and upper halves of the second ribs. The *body* of the sternum, somewhat more than twice the length of the manubrium, articulates with the lower half of the second costal cartilages and the cartilages of the third through seventh ribs. The lower end of the body of the sternum articulates with the xiphoid process and is at the lateral level of the 10th or 11th thoracic vertebrae. The *xiphoid* cartilage ends in the rectus sheath.

Each *intercostal space* is made up of three layers of muscle and their respective deep fascia.

Blood Supply, Venous Drainage, and Lymphatics

Each intercostal space receives blood from anterior and posterior intercostal *arteries*. Except for the first two interspaces, in which the posterior intercostal arteries originate as branches of the subclavian arteries, the posterior intercostal arteries originate from the thoracic aorta and constitute the bulk of the blood supply to all but the very anterior end of the interspace. The anterior intercostal arteries, two in each space, are branches of the internal thoracic (internal mammary) arteries; one branch passes toward the rib above and the other toward the rib below. Both branches anastomose with terminal branches of the posterior intercostal arteries.

The intercostal *veins* follow the course of the posterior intercostal arteries and are tributaries of the azygos or hemiazygos systems.

The *lymphatic vessels* of the intercostal spaces communicate freely with those of the mediastinum. The upper four or five intercostal spaces drain to lymph nodes along the internal thoracic chain, which communicate with bronchomediastinal channels. Posteriorly, lymphatics drain to nodes at the vertebral ends of the interspaces and communicate with pleural lymphatics and with the thoracic duct above and the cisterna chyli below.

Chest wall *innervation* is derived from 12 pairs of thoracic spinal nerves, each of which is formed from a dorsal and a ventral root from the spinal cord that fuse before exiting the normal foramen.

Muscles

The thoracic muscles are depicted in Figure 62-1.

CHEST WALL TUMORS
Diagnosis

Posteroanterior and lateral chest radiographs assist in localizing the mass, determining the presence of rib destruction, identifying associated pulmonary disease such as lung metastases, and defining the presence of a pleural effusion that merits thoracentesis and cytologic evaluation.

Computed tomography (CT) is used to demonstrate the relation between the mass and contiguous structures, define the dimensions and consistency of the tumor, identify the presence of synchronous metastases to the lungs, assess the mediastinum for adenopathy, and demonstrate associated pleural tumor or fluid. CT includes chest and abdominal views so that the kidneys and liver can be assessed.

For chest wall tumors near the axilla, *angiography* may be used to define involvement of the axillary artery. When a muscle flap from a previously irradiated field may be needed, angiography is used to define the integrity of the vascular pedicle.

A *bone scan* is performed on all patients with tumors of the chest wall, ribs, or sternum to rule out other sites of metastatic disease that might preclude resection.

Baseline *pulmonary function testing* and determination of arterial blood gases are used to assess the surgical risk when removal of a major portion of the lung is anticipated.

Physical examination of patient with a chest wall tumor identifies possible sites of primary tumors. The thyroid gland is palpated, breast and abdominal masses are excluded, and urine and stool are examined for occult blood.

Biopsy of a chest wall mass is performed through an incision that can be excised when skin flaps are raised at a later date. Multiple core-needle biopsies are performed. The tissue obtained at biopsy is subjected to permanent histopathologic assessment, immunohistochemical studies, and electron microscopic study.

Primary Tumors of the Ribs and Sternum

Therapy for most of the following tumors of the ribs and sternum is wide excision or resection:

Benign rib tumors
Osteochondroma
Chondroma
Fibrous dysplasia
Histiocytosis X
Malignant rib tumors
Chondrosarcoma
Ewing sarcoma
Osteogenic sarcoma
Plasmacytoma

Tumors of the Sternum and Clavicles

Almost all tumors of the sternum are malignant. They include chondrosarcoma, plasmacytoma, malignant lymphoma, and osteogenic sarcoma. Carcinomas of the breast, thyroid, and kidney metastasize to the sternum. Clavicular tumors are extremely rare, and almost all are malignant. Management of sternal and clavicular tumors is wide resection of the entire involved bone with a 4-cm margin.

Soft Tissue Sarcomas

The most common histologic types of soft tissue sarcoma are fibrosarcoma, leiomyosarcoma, liposarcoma, synovial sarcoma, neurofibrosarcoma, and malignant fibrous histiocytoma. Sarcomas are surrounded by a pseudocapsule of compressed normal tissue that is inevitably invaded by the tumor. Sarcomas metastasize, particularly to the lungs, within 2 years of diagnosis. Therapy is wide resection, followed by irradiation and multidrug chemotherapy for some types of tumors.

Chest Wall Resection and Reconstruction

Full-thickness skeletal defects of the chest wall <5 cm in diameter require no reconstruction. Posterior thoracic defects <10 cm in diameter, particularly those involving the upper ribs, are covered by the overlying scapula and do not require reconstruction. Replacement of the bony thorax is used in the reconstruction of anterior and anterolateral chest wall defects. Prosthetic material often is needed for stabilization of the chest. For relatively small chest wall defects that do not require skeletal reconstruc-

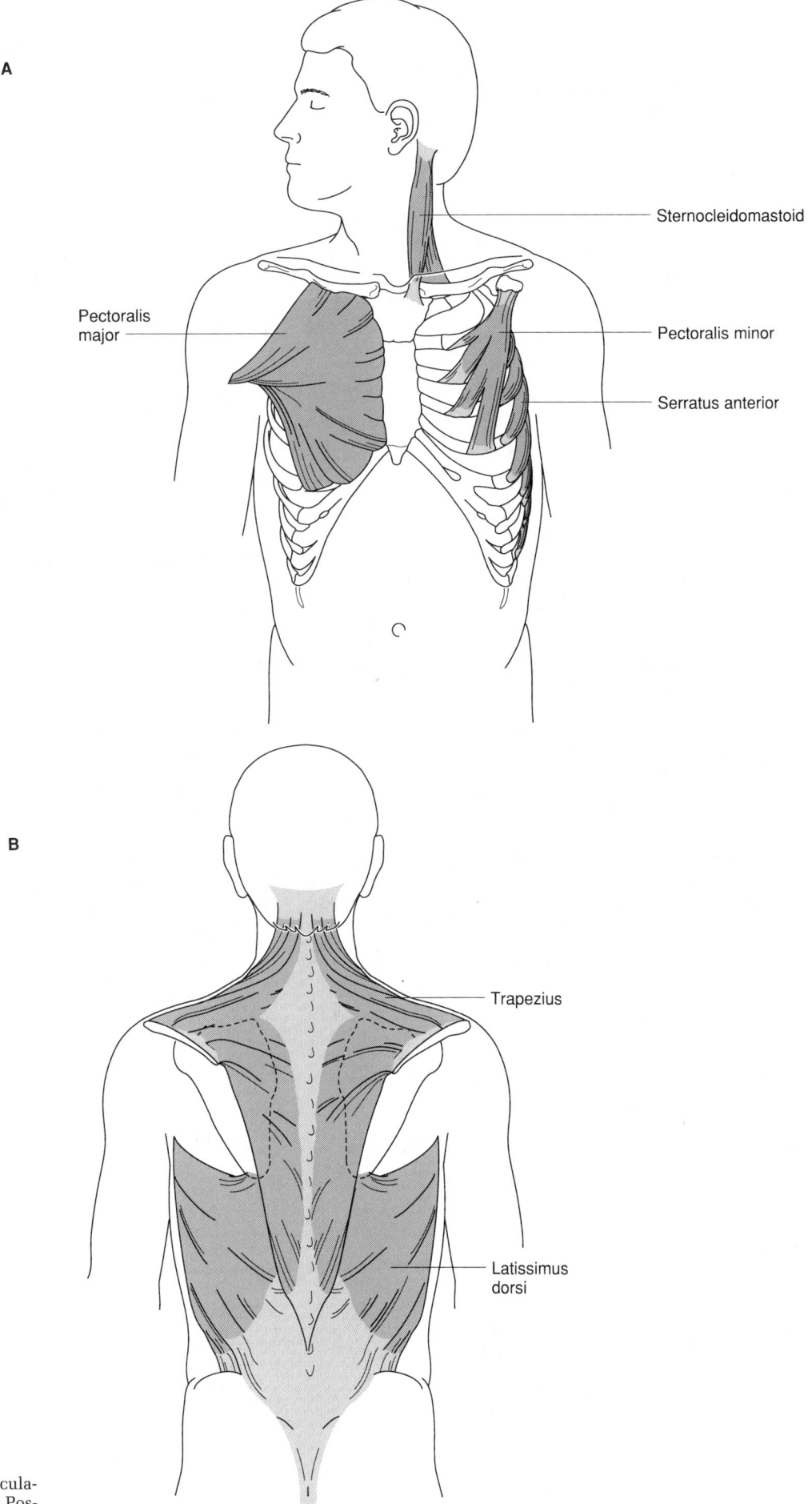

A

Sternocleidomastoid

Pectoralis major

Pectoralis minor

Serratus anterior

B

Trapezius

Latissimus dorsi

Figure 62-1. Thoracic musculature. (*A*) Anterior view. (*B*) Posterior view.

tion, and for situations in which it is desirable not to use prosthetic material, full-thickness chest wall defects can be managed by transposition of a variety of muscle and musculocutaneous flaps.

PLEURA
Anatomy

The pleural space is a closed serous sac. The pleura consists of two parts: the parietal pleura, which is applied to the thoracic wall, and the visceral pleura, which covers the surface of the lung and is intimately applied to it. Each of these pleural surfaces is lined by a mesothelial layer that secretes a small amount of lubricating fluid.

The parietal pleura has four subdivisions:

1. Costal, against the ribs and intercostal muscles
2. Diaphragmatic, covering the thoracic surface of the diaphragm
3. Mediastinal, investing the mediastinum
4. Cervical, at the apex of the pleural space

The *parietal pleura* receives its arterial supply from the intercostal, internal thoracic (internal mammary), superior phrenic, and anterior mediastinal arteries. The venous drainage corresponds to these arteries. The *visceral pleura*, is supplied by tributaries of the bronchial and pulmonary arteries. Venous drainage is into the pulmonary veins.

The central portion of the diaphragmatic pleura and the mediastinal pleura are innervated by the *phrenic nerves.* The *intercostal nerves* innervate the costal and peripheral diaphragmatic pleurae. The parietal pleura is much more sensitive to contact than the visceral pleura.

An extensive network of *lymphatic vessels* in the connective tissue beneath the pleural mesothelial cells drains the pleura. The lymphatics of the visceral pleura coalesce with the superficial efferent lymphatics of the lung and form a subpleural lymphatic plexus that drains to mediastinal, intercostal, substernal, phrenic, and anterior and posterior mediastinal lymph nodes. There is also communication at the apex of the chest between cervical and costal pleural lymphatics and axillary lymph nodes. The parietal and visceral pleural lymphatics drain into the right lymphatic duct; those on the left drain into the left thoracic duct.

Pleural Effusions

A pleural effusion is a sign of systemic or pleural disease. The symptoms are chest pain and dyspnea. Tumors involving the parietal pleura produce constant dull pain. Large pleural effusions interfere with expansion of the lung and produce dyspnea, shortness of breath, and atelectasis.

Pleural fluid normally flows from the parietal pleura into the pleural space and to the visceral pleura, where it is absorbed. Lymphatic drainage also removes fluid from the pleural space. Pleural fluid may accumulate in the chest if there is:

Increased hydrostatic pressure (eg, congestive heart failure)
Increased capillary permeability (eg, pneumonia)
Decreased plasma colloid oncotic pressure (eg, hypoalbuminemia)
Increased negative intrapleural pressure (eg, atelectasis)
Impaired drainage of the pleural space by lymphatics obstructed by tumor

Pleural effusions are transudates or exudates (Table 62-1). *Transudates* are the result of abnormal formation or absorption of pleural fluid and do not indicate primary pulmonary disease. *Exudates* result from diseased pleura or pleural lymphatics.

Diagnosis

Lateral decubitus radiographs that allow fluid to shift to the dependent portion of the thoracic cavity help differentiate fluid in the costophrenic angle from pleural thick-

---

Table 62-1. DIFFERENTIAL DIAGNOSIS OF PLEURAL EFFUSIONS

TRANSUDATIVE PLEURAL EFFUSIONS
Congestive heart failure
Pericardial disease
Cirrhosis
Nephrotic syndrome
Peritoneal dialysis
Superior vena cava obstruction
Myxedema
Pulmonary emboli
Sarcoidosis
Urinothorax

EXUDATIVE PLEURAL EFFUSIONS
Neoplastic diseases
  Metastatic disease
  Mesothelioma
Infectious diseases
  Bacterial infections
  Tuberculosis
  Fungal infections
  Viral infections
  Parasitic infections
Pulmonary embolization
Gastrointestinal disease
  Esophageal perforation
  Pancreatic disease
  Intraabdominal abscess
  Diaphragmatic hernia
  Postabdominal surgery
  Endoscopic variceal sclerotherapy
Collagen vascular diseases
  Rheumatoid pleuritis
  Systemic lupus erythematosus
  Drug-induced lupus erythematosus
  Immunoblastic lymphadenopathy
  Sjögren syndrome
  Wegener granulomatosis
  Churg-Strauss syndrome
Postcardiac injury syndrome
Asbestos exposure
Sarcoidosis
Uremia
Meigs syndrome
Yellow nail syndrome
Drug-induced pleural disease
  Nitrofurantoin
  Dantrolene
  Methysergide
  Bromocriptine
  Procarbazine
  Amiodarone
Trapped lung
Radiotherapy
Electrical burns
Urinary tract obstruction
Iatrogenic injury
Ovarian hyperstimulation syndrome
Chylothorax
Hemothorax

(Data from Light RW. The physiology of pleural fluid production and benign pleural effusion. In: Shields TW, ed. General thoracic surgery, ed 4. Malvern, PA, Williams & Wilkins, 1994:676)

ening and fibrosis, which do not change configuration with a shift in patient position. Accumulation of pleural fluid between the lung and the diaphragm is called *subpulmonic effusion* and gives the false impression of an elevated hemidiaphragm. When pleural fluid is trapped within a fissure of the lung, its spheric contour may result in a masslike pseudotumor. CT indicates the presence of a pleural effusion.

The cause of most large pleural effusions that fill one hemothorax is a malignant tumor of the pleura. Massive effusions also may be caused by tuberculosis, empyema, or transudates from congestive heart failure or cirrhosis.

Management of Malignant Pleural Effusions

For patients with large malignant effusions adversely affecting cardiorespiratory dynamics, thoracentesis may provide palliation. When thoracentesis is needed, the effusion is tapped dry. Subsequent chest radiographs are used to determine if the lung expands fully or if it has become trapped down by tumor, fibrosis, or a proteinaceous layer. Resolution requires apposition of visceral and parietal pleural surfaces.

If after evacuation of a large amount of fluid from the pleural cavity, a follow-up chest radiograph shows that the lung has not reexpanded, fluid is likely to reaccumulate in the pleural dead space. If a chest tube is used to evacuate the fluid, and chest radiographs obtained during the next 1 to 2 days show the lung has not expanded, the chest tube is removed before the pleural space becomes infected. Alternative forms of therapy are initiated or thoracentesis is repeated.

If the lung expands after thoracentesis, but the effusion recurs, management is chemical pleurodesis, which produces inflammatory pleuritis with obliteration of the pleural space. If further intervention is needed, pleurectomy is performed. This operation necessitates thoracotomy and involves removal of as much of the diseased visceral and parietal pleura as is possible so that expansion of the lung and symphysis between the two pleural surfaces can occur.

Thoracic Empyema

Accumulation of pus in the pleural space is thoracic empyema. Empyema can be acute or chronic, localized or diffuse, unilateral or bilateral. Pus is the fluid product of inflammation and contains leukocytes and the debris of dead cells and tissues. Tube drainage is needed if the fluid is too thick or viscous to be aspirated with a thoracentesis needle. At least half of empyemas are due to pneumonia (Table 62-2).

Table 62-2. CAUSES OF EMPYEMA

Cause	Frequency (%)
Pyogenic pneumonia	50
Postsurgical	25
Subphrenic abscess extension	10
Posttraumatic	3–5
Lung abscess rupture	1–3
Generalized sepsis	1–3
Pulmonary tuberculosis	1
Pulmonary mycotic infection	1
Spontaneous pneumothorax	<1
Parasitic infection	<1
Retained tracheobronchial foreign body	<1

(Modified from Miller JI Jr. Infections of the pleura. In: Shields TW, ed. General thoracic surgery, ed 3. Philadelphia, Lea & Febiger, 1989:634)

Patients with empyema have chest pain and a feeling of heaviness or discomfort on the affected side. Fever, cough with purulent sputum production, and shortness of breath are common. Physical examination reveals decreased breath sounds and dullness to percussion on the affected side. Complications include the following:

- Empyema necessitatis, in which the intrathoracic infection works its way through the chest wall to the skin surface as a draining sinus
- Costochondritis and osteomyelitis of the ribs
- Bronchopleural fistula
- Mediastinal or pericardial infection
- Disseminated infection, such as a brain or renal abscess

Diagnosis

Conventional posteroanterior and lateral chest radiographs are obtained. The finding of pneumonia with a large pleural effusion or complete opacification of one hemothorax is common. Air–fluid levels or multiple loculations also may be seen. With large effusions, the trachea and mediastinum may be shifted to the contralateral side. Most parapneumonic empyemas are posterior and lateral and extend to the diaphragm. The aerated lung can be seen anteriorly.

Differentiation between lung abscess and empyema may necessitate additional diagnostic studies, such as bronchoscopy, bronchography, or CT. CT is used to demonstrate the extent of the empyema and areas of loculation. Thoracentesis in which pus is recovered from the pleural cavity confirms the diagnosis. The fluid is subjected to Gram-stain, culture and sensitivity testing, and analysis of pH, white-cell count with differential, sugar, protein, and LDH. Thin, watery parapneumonic effusions that are infected may be treated with repeated thoracentesis and specific antibiotic therapy.

Management

An algorithm for the management of parapneumonic or nonsurgical empyema is shown in Figure 62-2.

Spontaneous Pneumothorax

The cause of spontaneous pneumothorax is unknown in many patients. The presenting symptoms are chest pain and shortness of breath. Spontaneous pneumothorax in young, otherwise-healthy patients can be well tolerated, even when the lung is almost collapsed, as long as tension does not develop. Patients who do not have symptoms of pneumothorax are treated with an apical chest tube. Indications for surgical intervention for pneumothorax are:

History of a previous pneumothorax,
Continued air leak or lack of reexpansion of the lung after a chest tube has been in place for 3 to 5 days,
Massive air leak with inability to reexpand the lung within 24 hours; bilateral pneumothoraces simultaneously or at different times,
Occupation for which recurrent pneumothorax constitutes a threat to life (eg, airline pilot, diver),
Residence in a remote area,
Demonstrable large pulmonary bullae.

Operations to manage pneumothorax can be performed with any of the following approaches: anterior thoracotomy, lateral thoracotomy, median sternotomy, transaxillary minithoracotomy, or thoracoscopy.

Tension pneumothorax results from a tangential tear in the visceral pleura that allows air to enter the pleural space during inspiration but closes during exhalation. The re-

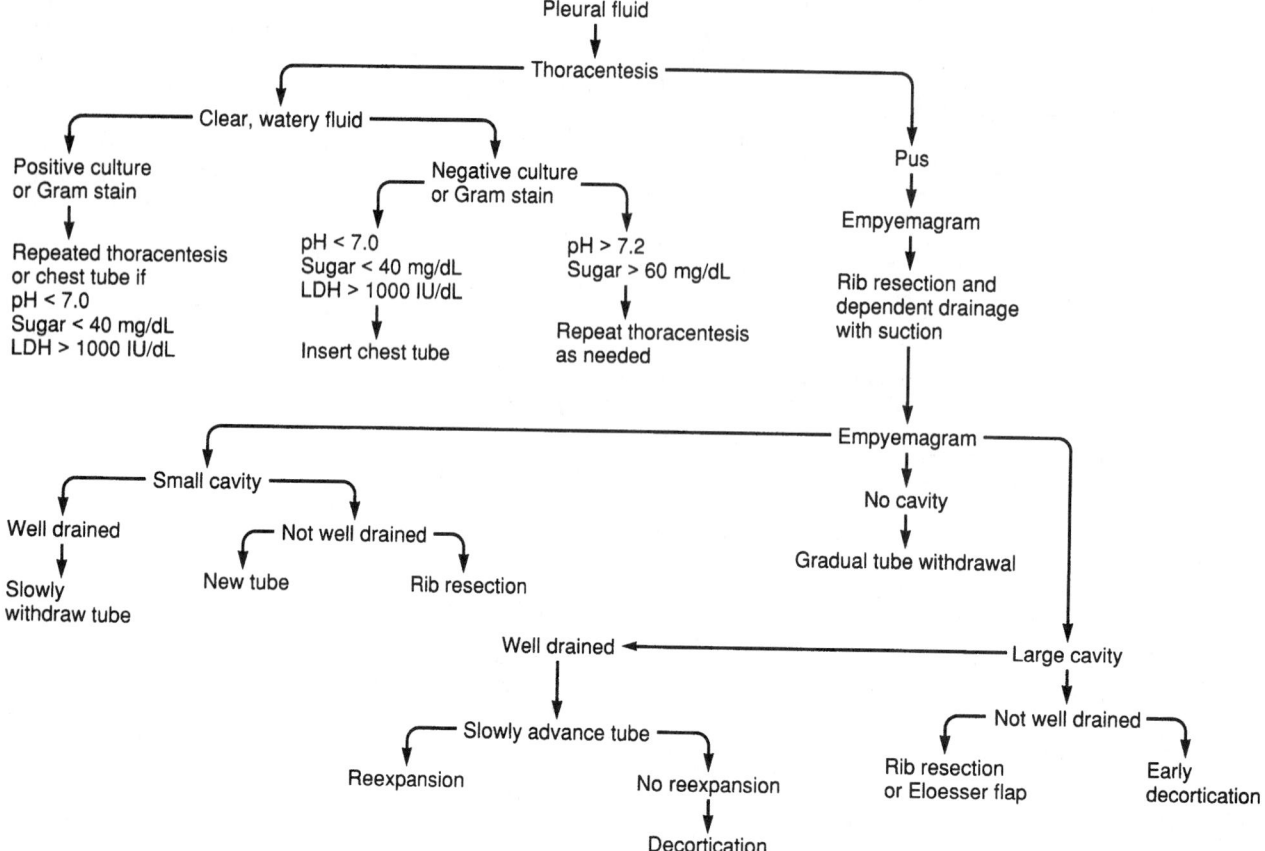

Figure 62-2. Management of empyema. (After Miller JI Jr. Infections of the pleura. In: Shields TW, ed. General thoracic surgery, ed 3. Philadelphia, Lea & Febiger, 1989:637)

sulting increased pressure within the pleural cavity causes shift of the mediastinum to the contralateral side with compression of the uninvolved lung, diminished venous return to the heart, and eventually decreased cardiac output. This condition is incompatible with life. The signs are those of marked respiratory distress; decreased breath sounds over one hemothorax, which is hyperresonant to percussion; and shift of the trachea toward the contralateral side.

When tension pneumothorax is suspected, immediate action must be taken. A large-bore needle is inserted into the second interspace anteriorly. A hiss of air under pressure is heard as pressure within the pleural cavity is relieved. The patient's condition improves dramatically.

Chylothorax

Injury to the thoracic duct (Fig. 62-3) and leak of chyle into the pleural space (chylothorax) can occur with penetrating or blunt trauma, hyperextension injuries to the spine, forceful vomiting, violent coughing, and posterior mediastinal tumors. Iatrogenic thoracic duct injury can occur during operations in the left thorax involving the aortic arch or esophagus or operations involving cervical or abdominal lymph nodes or the lungs.

When the thoracic duct is injured, chyle accumulates in the posterior mediastinum until the mediastinal pleura ruptures into the chest. Accumulation of chyle in the pleural space compresses the lung and mediastinum and may produce chest discomfort and dyspnea. The diagnosis of chylothorax is apparent when opalescent, milky pleural fluid is obtained during thoracentesis. In the first few post-

operative days, however, the pleural fluid may appear clear or serosanguineous.

The diagnosis of a chylothorax in a patient who can eat may be made by staining the pleural fluid with Sudan red, which stains the fat globules normally present in chyle. The diagnosis of chylothorax is confirmed when milky fluid is identified. High concentrations of lymphocytes are expected as well. Injuries to the thoracic duct below T-5 to T-6 result in a right-sided chylothorax. Injuries above this level cause left-sided chylous effusions.

Chylothorax has a variety of causes (Table 62-3). Chylothorax unassociated with trauma to the thoracic duct may respond to nonsurgical therapy, such as intravenous hyperalimentation, chemical pleurodesis, and mediastinal irradiation. With postoperative chylothorax, loss of large amounts of chyle from a chest tube can cause substantial fluid shifts, electrolyte imbalance, loss of serum protein and albumin, and decrease in peripheral lymphocytes with an altered immune response. After an extensive surgical procedure, if prolonged or excessive serosanguineous chest tube drainage suggests thoracic duct injury, administration of cream by mouth or feeding tube changes the character of the drainage to the milky fluid of chyle.

Surgical management involves a transthoracic approach to the injured thoracic duct, usually on the same side as the pleural drainage. A double-lumen endotracheal tube allows one-lung anesthesia and ventilation of the contralateral side during visualization of the site of injury to the thoracic duct, which is ligated and suture ligated above and below this point. Because of the abun-

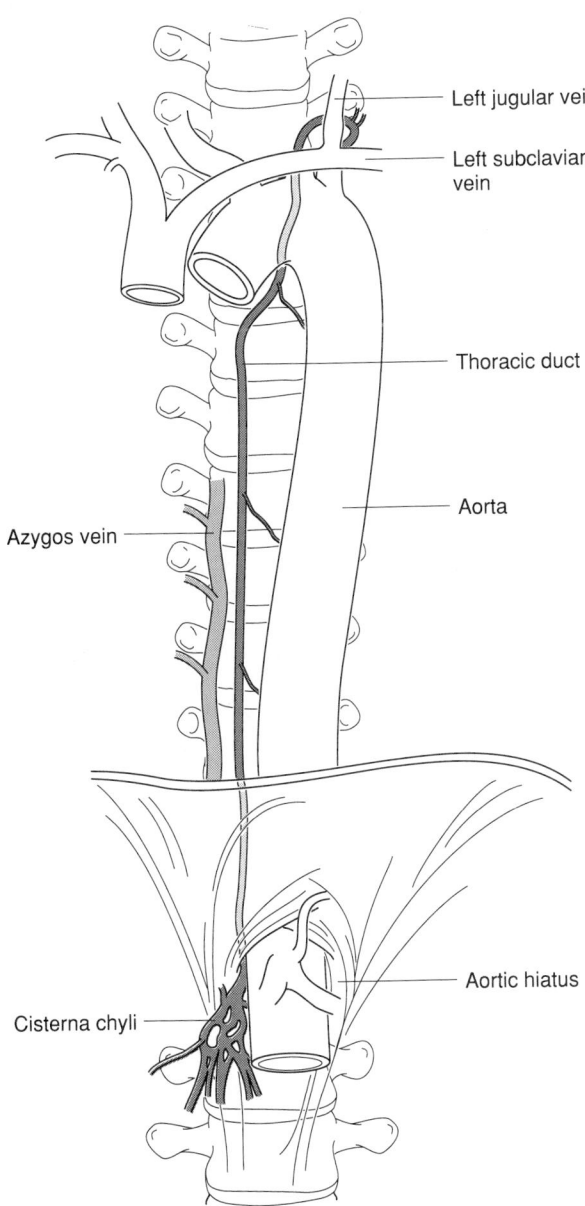

Figure 62-3. Course of the thoracic duct.

dance of alternative collateral pathways for lymphatic drainage in the chest, thoracic duct ligation has no adverse consequences.

Tumors of the Pleura

Benign tumors of the pleura are exceedingly rare. They include lipomas, endotheliomas, and angiomas. They originate from the subpleural tissues of the chest wall, and are resected when they present as an asymptomatic mass on chest radiograph. Cysts of the pleura occur predominantly at the pleuropericardial reflection. They originate from the parietal pleura. The chest radiographic appearance is a rounded mass adjacent to the right-sided heart border. CT is used to determine the cystic nature of these lesions, and CT-guided transthoracic aspiration is performed for cytologic assessment of the fluid. Follow-up chest radiographs are obtained.

Mesothelioma is the most common primary tumor of the pleura. There is a relation between asbestos exposure and development of mesothelioma. Mesotheliomas can be dif-

fuse or localized. Diffuse mesothelioma almost always is malignant. The TNM staging of mesothelioma is shown in Table 62-4.

Localized mesotheliomas, benign and malignant, are removed by means of application of a surgical stapler across the lung parenchyma 1 cm from the stalk of the tumor. Management of diffuse mesothelioma is combined chemotherapy and radiation therapy followed by radical pleuropneumonectomy.

The pleura may be involved with metastatic disease. Among men, lung cancer and lymphoma account for most malignant effusions. Among women, cancers of the breast, genital tract, and lung are responsible.

MEDIASTINUM

The mediastinum is the central portion of the chest. It extends from thoracic inlet to diaphragm. It is bounded anteriorly by the sternum, laterally by the mediastinal pleura, and posteriorly by the vertebral bodies. The contents of the mediastinum are:

Superior mediastinum
Thymus gland
Aortic arch and great vessels
Upper trachea
Upper esophagus
Anterior mediastinum
Thymus gland
Lymph nodes
Middle mediastinum
Pericardium
Heart
Tracheal bifurcation
Main-stem bronchi

Table 62-3. CAUSES OF CHYLOTHORAX

CONGENITAL
Thoracic duct atresia
Thoracic duct fistula
Birth trauma

TRAUMA
Blunt
Penetrating
Surgical
   Cervical (lymph node biopsy or radical neck dissection)
   Thoracic
      Aortic operations (patent ductus arteriosus, coarctation repair, operations for vascular ring, resection of aneurysm)
      Pulmonary resection
      Esophagectomy
      Mediastinal tumor excision
      Sympathectomy
   Abdominal
      Lymph node dissection
      Sympathectomy
Diagnostic procedures (translumbar aortogram, subclavian vein catheterization)

TUMORS

INFECTIONS
Granulomatous lymphadenitis or mediastinitis
Filariasis

OTHER
Vena cava or subclavian vein thrombosis
Pulmonary lymphangiomyomatosis

(Modified from DeMeester TR, Lafontaine E. The pleura. In: Sabiston DC Jr, Spencer FC, eds. Surgery of the chest, ed 5. Philadelphia, WB Saunders, 1990:456)

Table 62-4. TNM CLASSIFICATION FOR STAGING OF MESOTHELIOMA

TNM DEFINITIONS
Primary Tumor

Tx Primary tumor cannot be assessed
T0 No evidence of primary tumor
T1 Primary tumor limited to ipsilateral parietal, or visceral pleura, or both
T2 Tumor invades any of the following: ipsilateral lung, endothoracic fascia, diaphragm, pericardium
T3 Tumor invades any of the following: ipsilateral chest wall muscle, ribs, mediastinal organs or tissues
T4 Tumor extends to any of the following: contralateral pleura or lung by direct extension, peritoneum or intraabdominal organs by direct extension, cervical tissues

Regional Lymph Node Involvement

Nx Regional lymph nodes cannot be assessed
N0 No regional lymph node metastases
N1 Metastases in ipsilateral bronchopulmonary or hilar lymph nodes
N2 Metastases in ipsilateral mediastinal lymph nodes
N3 Metastases in contralateral mediastinal, internal mammary, supraclavicular, or scalene lymph nodes

Distant Metastasis

Mx Presence of distant metastasis cannot be assessed
M0 No known distant metastasis
M1 Distant metastasis present

STAGING GROUPING*

Stage I	T1, N0, M0
	T2, N0, M0
Stage II	T1, N1, M0
	T2, N1, M0
Stage III	T3, N0, M0
	T3, N1, M0
	T1, N2, M0
	T2, N2, M0
	T3, N2, M0
Stage IV	Any T, N3, M0
	T4, any N, M0
	Any T, any N, M1

* Staging solely on clinical measures is designated cTNM. Staging that can be done in clinical pathologic information is designated as pTNM. Clinical and pathologic groups are identical.
(Adapted from Rusch VW, Ginsberg RJ. New concepts in the staging of mesotheliomas. In: Deslaurier J, Lacquet LK, eds. Thoracic surgery. St Louis, CV Mosby, 1990:340)

Subcarinal and peribronchial lymph nodes
Ascending aorta
Posterior mediastinum
Esophagus
Descending aorta
Nerves (sympathetic, parasympathetic, and intercostal)

Infection

Infection after median sternotomy for a cardiac operation is a serious complication, especially if the patient has prosthetic aortic graft material at the base of the wound. Mediastinitis in this setting is heralded by sternal instability, drainage from the wound, and fever. Surgical management is sternal and mediastinal débridement and one-stage reconstruction with a rotated muscle flap or omentum.

Descending necrotizing mediastinitis is a lethal form of acute mediastinitis in which infection originating in the oropharynx spreads to the mediastinum. Symptoms are fever, pleuritic chest pain, dysphagia, and airway obstruc-

tion. Patients may experience exsanguination from erosion of the great vessels of the neck and mediastinum, aspiration, cranial nerve paralysis, brain abscesses, and necrotizing fasciitis. Tracheostomy is needed. Management is transcervical and subxiphoid or transthoracic drainage and broad-spectrum aerobic and anaerobic antibiotic coverage followed by culture-specific antibiotics.

Granulomatous infections of the chest involve paratracheal and subcarinal mediastinal lymph nodes. Histoplasmosis is the most common cause. Management is resection of large, acutely inflamed mediastinal lymph nodes. A complication of mediastinal granulomatous disease is necrosis of the esophageal and tracheobronchial walls with bronchoesophageal fistula. Management is identification and division of the fistulous opening, closure of the tracheal and esophageal openings, and interposition of a flap of pleura or mediastinal fat.

Mediastinal Tumors and Cysts

Although mediastinal tumors can originate primarily, secondary metastases to mediastinal lymph nodes and direct invasion of the mediastinum by tracheobronchial, esophageal, or other malignant tumors are common. The differential diagnosis of a mediastinal mass includes neoplasms and congenital cysts, which are not neoplastic. Most mediastinal masses are neurogenic tumors, followed in frequency by thymomas, cysts, and lymphomas. The locations of tumors in the various mediastinal compartments are as follows:

Anterior mediastinum
Thymoma
Teratoma
Carcinoma
Lymphangioma
Hemangioma
Lipoma
Superior mediastinum
Thymoma
Lymphoma
Thyroid adenoma
Parathyroid adenoma
Posterior mediastinum
Neurogenic tumor
Enteric cyst
Middle mediastinum
Pericardial cyst
Bronchogenic cyst
Lymphoma

Mediastinal masses cause symptoms (chest pain, cough, or dyspnea) in most patients. Nearly half of symptomatic mediastinal tumors are malignant. Almost all asymptomatic mediastinal masses discovered on routine chest radiographs are benign. Malignant mediastinal tumors are more common among children than adults. Patients with mediastinal masses and evidence of involvement of adjacent structures are likely to have malignant disease. For example, hoarseness is indicative of recurrent laryngeal nerve invasion, and back pain may be indicative of chest wall invasion with intercostal nerve involvement.

Contrast-enhanced CT provides information about the location of the mediastinal mass, its vascularity, relation to adjacent mediastinal structures, and consistency (cystic, solid, or fat). Aortography may be needed to differentiate a mediastinal tumor from an aneurysm. Fine-needle aspiration or core-needle biopsy of mediastinal masses under CT or fluoroscopic guidance may provide enough tissue for cytologic or pathologic diagnosis. With a flexible fiberoptic bronchoscope and fluoroscopic guidance, transbronchial needle aspiration of subcarinal or paratracheal lymphadenopathy may establish a diagnosis while avoiding a major operation. Mediastinoscopy provides access to paratracheal and subcarinal lymph nodes for the purpose of biopsy. One-lung anesthesia and thoracoscopic biopsy are used if a diagnosis is needed before complete excision. For most newly diagnosed mediastinal masses, unless there is strong evidence to suggest unresectability, diagnosis is made with excisional biopsy.

Mediastinal Emphysema (Pneumomediastinum)

Air may enter the mediastinum, tracheobronchial tree, neck, or abdomen. Mediastinal emphysema is caused by penetrating wounds of the mediastinum and blunt chest trauma. Compression injuries of the thorax may cause a marked rise in intrathoracic pressure, rupture of peripheral alveoli, and the initiation of dissection of air in the interstitial planes of the lung toward the hilum and into the mediastinum. A forceful sneeze or bout of asthma can produce mediastinal emphysema in the same way (spontaneous mediastinal emphysema).

Mediastinal emphysema may have a dramatic clinical presentation but is usually not life-threatening. Patients often describe retrosternal discomfort and have subcutaneous crepitus at the base of the neck. As air continues to dissect upward from the mediastinum into the subcutaneous tissue planes, cervical, fascial, thoracic, truncal, scrotal, and extremity swelling and crepitus can develop. Air within the periorbital tissues may cause sufficient swelling to prevent the patient from opening the eyelids. A precordial crunch is heard during systole (Hamman sign). This is characteristic of air in the mediastinal tissue planes, along the pericardium, and in the soft tissues of the neck, chest, and upper abdomen. Tension pneumomediastinum may interfere with venous return to the heart and cause cardiovascular collapse.

Spontaneous mediastinal emphysema usually is self-limiting and requires little treatment other than sedation and supplemental oxygen. If pneumothorax is identified, tube thoracostomy is performed. If the patient is distressed about the inability to open their eyes, decompressing incisions can be made in the skin folds of the eyelids or neck to allow air to escape, permitting the patient to open their eyes.

Superior Vena Cava Syndrome

Superior vena cava (SVC) syndrome is caused by obstruction of the SVC. It presents clinically as facial and upper extremity edema, distention of the veins of the head, neck, arms, and upper thorax, and a dusky rubor of these areas suggesting cyanosis. Symptoms are periorbital swelling, a full feeling in the head, and a roaring in the ears aggravated by lying supine or bending. Most adult patients with SVC syndrome have malignant disease within the mediastinum that compresses the SVC, most often bronchogenic carcinoma involving the right-upper lobe. SVC obstruction also is caused by lymphoma and metastatic carcinoma within the mediastinum. One-fourth of patients with SVC syndrome have a benign cause, such as mediastinal granulomatous disease, idiopathic mediastinal fibrosis, goiter, or bronchogenic cysts.

Clinical presentation leaves little doubt about the diagnosis. SVC obstruction is evaluated with magnetic resonance imaging (MRI) or magnetic resonance angiography (MRA). Most instances of SVC syndrome due to malignant disease cannot be cured because of the extent of mediasti-

nal invasion by the tumor. Tissue diagnosis is important, however, because it may alter therapy. Radiation therapy and chemotherapy can be provide rapid relief of SVC obstruction due to malignant disease. Surgical therapy is seldom indicated. Chest wall and mediastinal venous collaterals gradually develop in most patients with SVC obstruction from benign disease, so the symptoms improve with time.

TRACHEA

The trachea is 11 cm long from the inferior border of the cricoid cartilage to the carina. The vocal cords are 1.5 to 2 cm above the inferior border of the cricoid cartilage.

Primary Tumors

Primary tumors of the trachea (excluding the larynx and main bronchi) are uncommon; the most frequent types are squamous cell carcinoma, adenoid cystic carcinoma (cylindroma), and carcinoid adenoma. Tracheal tumors produce stridor, cough, dyspnea, hemoptysis, and recurrent pneumonia.

Squamous carcinoma of the trachea can occur in an exophytic or ulcerative form, and mediastinal or pulmonary metastases are present in one-third of patients at the time of diagnosis.

Adenoid cystic carcinoma spreads within the tracheal wall for a distance greater than that evidenced on gross inspection. Frozen-section confirmation of adequate margins is important at the time of operation. The goal of resection is to remove gross tumor only. Regional lymph

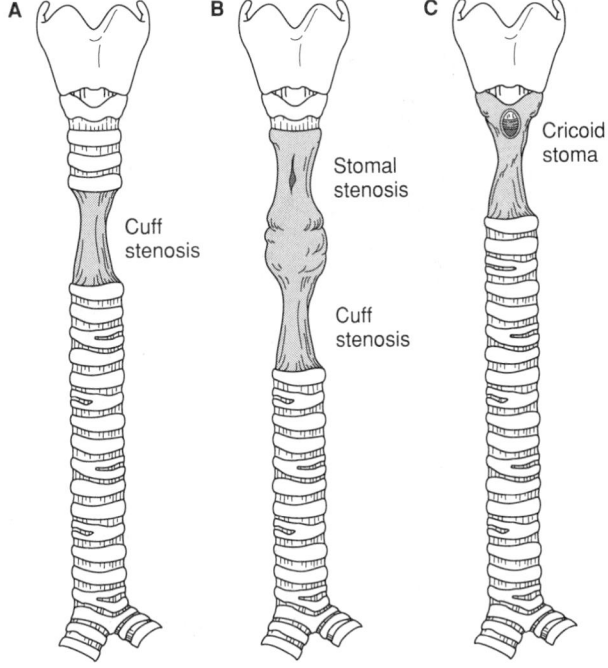

Figure 62-4. Postintubation tracheal injuries. (*A*) Stenosis at site of endotracheal tube cuff. Pressure necrosis by the cuff typically results in a circumferential injury and stenosis. (*B*) Injuries due to tracheostomy tubes include stenosis at the level of the stoma and cuff stenosis (generally lower than with an endotracheal tube). The segment between the two injuries may be malacic. (*C*) Subglottic stenosis resulting from either too high a tracheostomy or erosion of the tracheostomy tube through the cricoid cartilage.

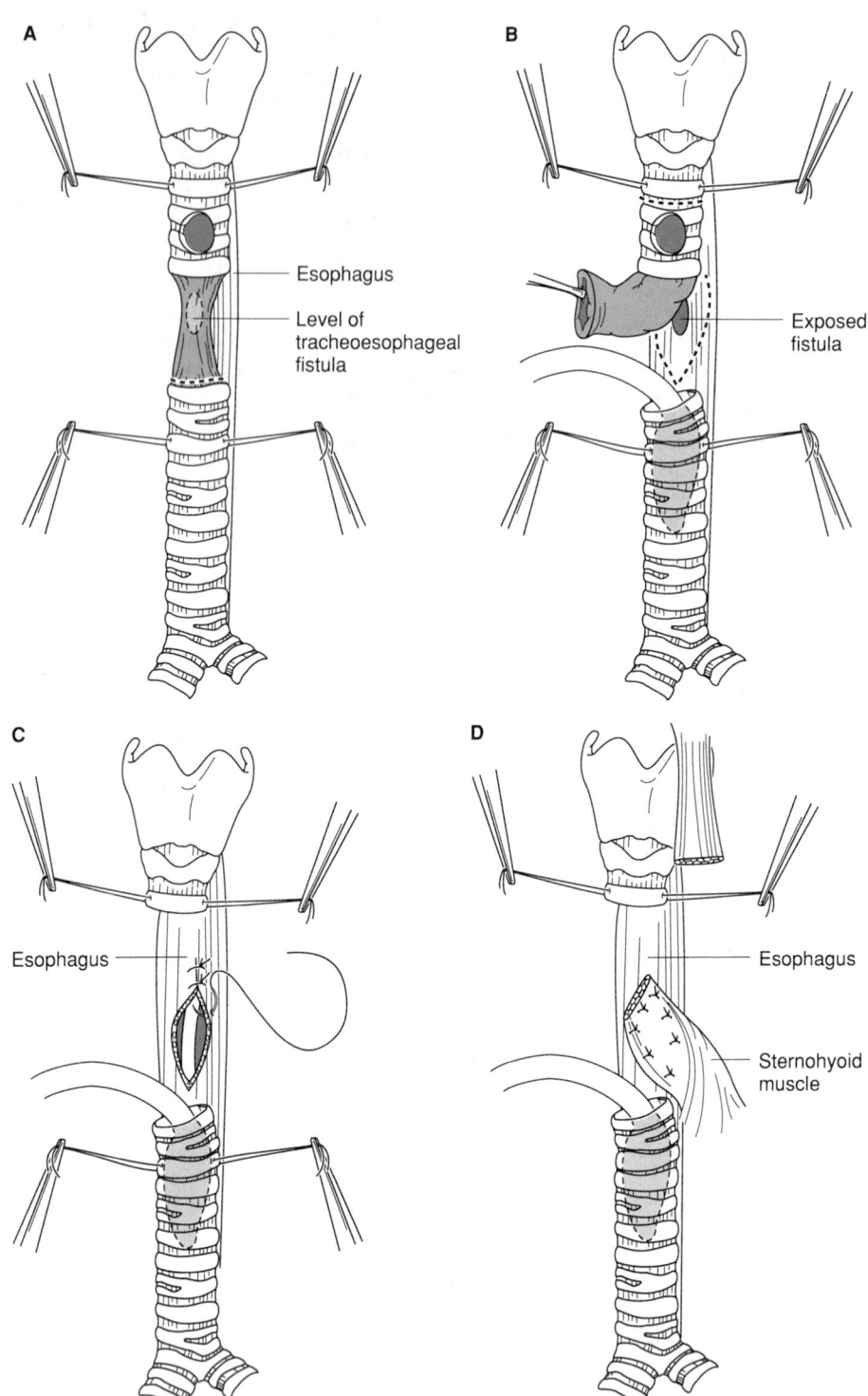

A

Esophagus

Level of tracheoesophageal fistula

B

Exposed fistula

C

Esophagus

D

Esophagus

Sternohyoid muscle

Figure 62-5. Management of postintubation tracheoesophageal fistula. (*A*) Only the length of damaged trachea to be resected (usually including the tracheostomy stoma) is circumferentially mobilized above and below the fistula to avoid devascularizing the remaining trachea. Stay sutures secure the trachea above and below this segment. (*B*) The trachea is transected, the distal trachea intubated across the field, and the fistula identified by elevating the damaged tracheal segment. (*C*) The stenotic tracheal segment is resected and closure of the esophageal fistula begun, being certain to invert the mucosa. A two-layered closure is completed. (*D*) After interposing the mobilized sternohyoid muscle and suturing it over the esophageal closure, an end-to-end tracheal anastomosis is performed.

node involvement is common. Management of adenoid cystic carcinoma is postoperative radiation therapy.

Secondary Tumors

Carcinomas of the esophagus, lung, thyroid, and larynx may involve the trachea. Contiguity of the posterior membranous trachea with the cervical and upper thoracic esophagus accounts for involvement by esophageal carcinoma. All patients with cancers involving the upper and midesophagus to the level of the carina undergo preopera-

tive bronchoscopy to rule out tracheobronchial invasion. Bronchogenic carcinoma may extend up the major bronchi and involve the trachea. Involvement of the trachea by esophageal or lung cancers represents surgically incurable disease. Thyroid carcinoma may invade the trachea and sometimes is amenable to radical resection.

Extrinsic Compression

Large goiters that descend retrosternally and cause chronic compression of the trachea in the thoracic inlet and superior mediastinum may be associated with chon-

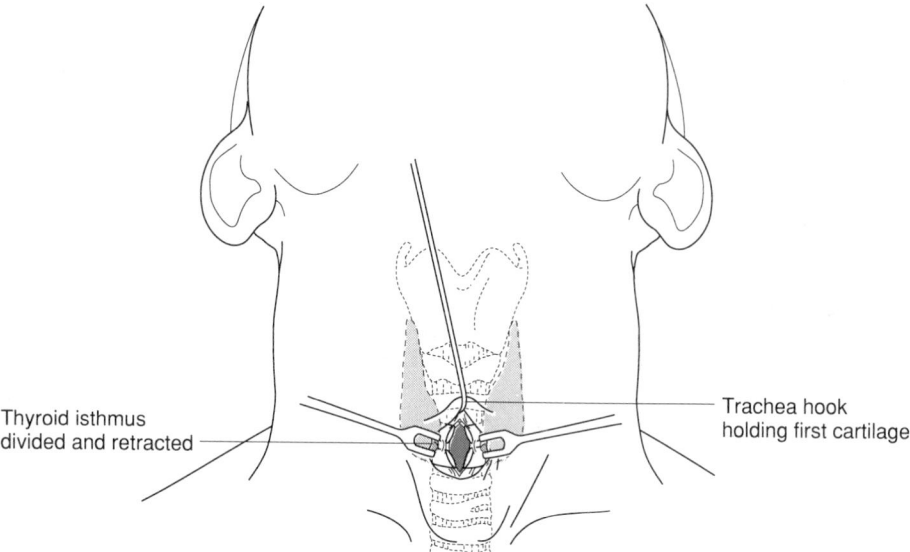

Thyroid isthmus
divided and retracted

Trachea hook
holding first cartilage

Figure 62-6. Standard tracheostomy using a vertical incision
through the second and third tracheal rings.

dromalacia and respiratory distress after removal, which
may necessitate temporary tracheostomy. Congenital vascular rings, aneurysms of the innominate (brachiocephalic)
artery, or an anomalous subclavian artery passing behind
the trachea and esophagus also may produce tracheal
compression.

Inflammatory Stenosis

Tracheal strictures may follow healing of endotracheal
tuberculosis, severe diphtheria, and sclerosing mediastinitis. Management of tracheal lacerations or disruptions
from blunt trauma is control of the airway, bronchoscopic
evaluation of the extent of the injury, and primary repair.
Stenosis at the injury site may necessitate later tracheal
resection and reconstruction.

The possibility of postintubation tracheal trauma (Fig.
62-4) exists for any patient with signs of upper-airway
compromise within the first few months after extubation.
Severe postintubation tracheal stenosis may be asymptomatic. The airway problem does not manifest itself until the
patient becomes active after discharge from the hospital.

Diagnosis of Tracheal Disorders

The following procedures are used:

- Conventional chest radiographs
- Lateral radiographs of the neck
- Tracheal laminograms
- Spiral or helical CT

Instrumentation of a critical tracheal stenosis during
bronchoscopy may precipitate local edema and complete
airway obstruction. Granulation tissue at the site of a tracheostomy stoma or the tip of a tracheostomy tube may be
excised with biopsy forceps through a rigid bronchoscope.
Respiratory distress due to obstructing tracheal tumor may
be relieved by coring out the tumor through a rigid
bronchoscope.

Tracheoinnominate Artery Fistula

A tracheostomy tube may erode into the innominate
(brachiocephalic) artery, producing life-threatening hemorrhage. A sign of impending tracheoinnominate artery

erosion is return of bright-red blood during suctioning of
an indwelling tracheal tube. The diagnosis is confirmed
when temporary deflation of the tracheal cuff causes profuse hemorrhage. Immediate management is overinflation
of the tracheal cuff against the innominate artery or finger
compression on the artery against the sternum through the
tracheostomy stoma. Pressure is maintained as the patient
is transported to the operating room.

Surgical treatment is resection of the involved segment
of innominate artery. Both ends are oversewn, and the
suture lines are covered with adjacent mediastinal or thymic fat or muscle. If a low tracheostomy stoma is identified,
muscle flap closure of the stoma is performed and a higher
new stoma developed. Tracheal resection is unnecessary.

Acquired Tracheoesophageal Fistula

A patient who needs prolonged mechanical ventilation
may have a tracheoesophageal fistula caused by erosion at
the site of the cuffed tracheal tube. This is more common
when there is an indwelling esophageal feeding tube and
the common wall between the esophagus and trachea becomes compressed between the two tubes. Circumferential
tracheal injury is caused by pressure from the cuff. A
marked increase in tracheal secretions, difficulty ventilating the patient, and abdominal distention may be observed.
Gastroesophageal reflux may cause aspiration pneumonia.
The diagnosis is established with bedside bronchoscopy
and inspection of the posterior tracheal wall in the region
of the tracheal cuff as the tube is gradually withdrawn.

Acute tracheoesophageal fistulas are not repaired until
mechanical ventilatory assistance is discontinued. During
mechanical ventilation, the esophageal tube is removed
and the tracheal tube replaced with a large-volume, low-
pressure cuffed tube, below the fistula, if possible. A gastrostomy is performed to decompress the stomach and to
prevent gastroesophageal reflux. Feeding jejunostomy is
performed for alimentation.

Tracheal resection is performed at the time of fistula
repair (Fig. 62-5). A sternohyoid muscle flap is interposed
between the two suture lines. No tracheostomy tube is used
postoperatively.

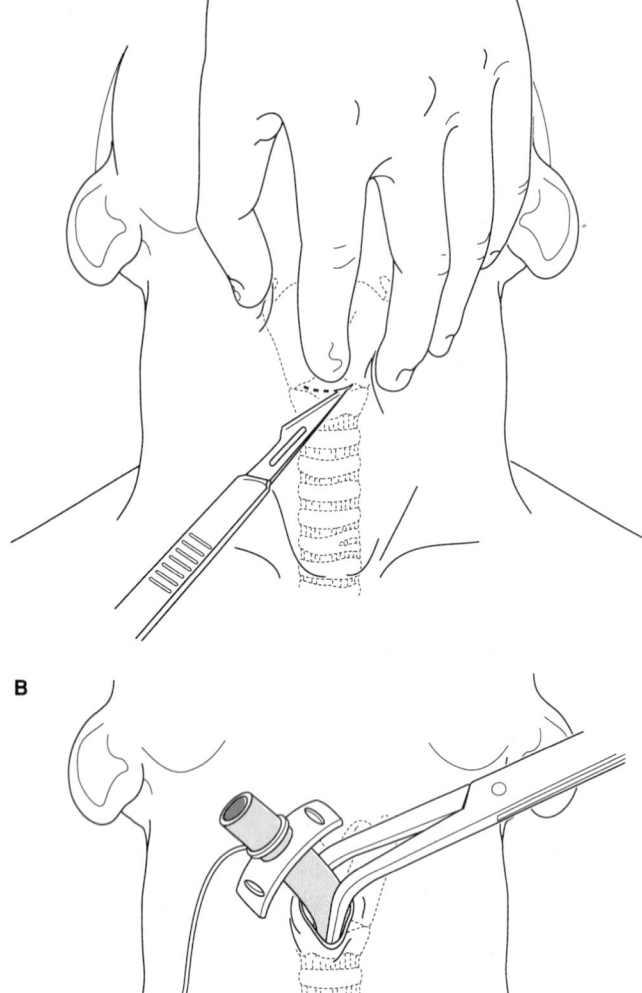

A

B

Figure 62-7. Cricothyroidotomy. (*A*) Identification of the cricothyroid membrane by palpation and incising the membrane transversely. (*B*) Insertion of a tracheostomy tube through the cricothyroid membrane, which is spread with a tracheal dilator.

Tracheostomy

Tracheostomy is not performed as an emergency. The airway is restored with an endotracheal tube or rigid ventilating bronchoscope. An endotracheal tube must be in place before tracheostomy is begun. The steps of tracheostomy are:

1. Skin incision over the second or third tracheal ring
2. Division of subcutaneous tissue and platysma muscle
3. Separation of the strap muscles
4. Retraction of the thyroid isthmus (division, if necessary)
5. Retraction of the trachea
6. Incision of the trachea (Fig. 62-6)
7. Insertion of tracheostomy tube and withdrawal of endotracheal tube

At the end of the procedure, the tube balloon is tested, the trachea is suctioned through the tube. Ventilation of both sides of the chest is assessed. The flange of the tracheostomy tube is sutured to the skin and tied in place with tracheal ties around the neck to ensure that the tube does not dislodge before the tracheostomy is sufficiently matured.

In *percutaneous tracheostomy,* a transtracheal guide wire is placed in the airway under bronchoscopic guidance. The tracheal opening is progressively dilated and a tracheostomy tube inserted without an open procedure.

Cricothyroidotomy

Cricothyroidotomy is an alternative to tracheostomy. The advantage is that the thyroid isthmus and blood vessels in the lower neck are avoided. The disadvantage is risk for vocal cord injury. The procedure is performed after placement of an endotracheal tube. The steps are as follows:

1. Transverse skin incision over the thyroid cartilage (Fig. 62-7)
2. Blunt dissection and puncture of cricothyroid membrane
3. Enlargement of opening in the cricothyroid membrane as endotracheal tube is withdrawn
4. Insertion and anchoring of cuffed tracheostomy tube

LUNG
Abscess

Pulmonary infection rarely progresses to abscess formation now. Surgical management is used for complications, such as pleural spread with empyema and a residual parenchymal cavity. Opportunistic pulmonary infections due to immunosuppression cause a large number of pulmonary abscesses associated with fungal or multiple organisms.

Pathogenesis

The common causes of most lung abscesses is aspiration of infected material and a compromised neurologic state. Pulmonary abscesses are associated with anaerobic infections in patients who have poor oral hygiene, decayed teeth, or gingival disease. The aspirated material becomes lodged in the bronchial tree, an area of local necrosis develops, and suppurative cavity infection rapidly follows. These areas of infarction often are found in the posterior segment of the upper lobe or in the superior segment of the lower lobe. Liquefaction necrosis from anaerobic organisms rarely allows identification of the causative agent because of poor culture technique or initiation of antibiotic therapy before culture.

Presentation

Patients have upper respiratory tract infection, fever, and sepsis with expectoration of purulent material and possibly hemoptysis. If the cavity cannot drain and remains internalized, rupture, pyopneumothorax, and septic shock follow. Patients may have a chronic indolent course with episodes of productive sputum during the drainage phase and a relatively nonproductive cough between episodes.

With bronchial drainage of the cavity, an air–fluid level and thick cavitary wall are identified on radiographs. Isolates are anaerobic in most instances.

Treatment

Initial management of any pulmonary abscess is antibiotic therapy and drainage. Penicillins or clindamycin are most effective. Drainage is achieved with pulmonary physiotherapy and postural drainage. Bronchoscopy is performed to determine whether an endobronchial lesion, foreign body, or extrinsic disorder is the cause of inadequate drainage. When inadequate drainage is found, endobronchial drainage is established with rigid bronchoscopy. Contralateral airway protection must be provided to prevent surgical drainage into the opposite lung.

Surgical treatment rarely is needed. Indications are overwhelming sepsis, abscess >6 cm in diameter, bronchopleural fistula, life-threatening hemoptysis, and empyema. For a chronic abscess, surgical treatment is indicated if there is no resolution or if a cavity persists for >5 weeks. In these situations therapy is pulmonary resection. External drainage with rib resection may be needed for uncontrolled disease. CT-guided percutaneous drainage with irrigation of the cavity through the catheter is an alternative. Expandable metal stents also can be used.

Bronchiectasis

Bronchiectasis results from chronic or recurrent infection of the distal bronchi, most commonly in the basilar segments, with dilatation and destruction of the bronchial walls. This results in fibrosis, poor drainage, and destruction of the lung and airways. Bronchiectasis can be congenital or acquired. Common causes of congenital bronchiectasis are cystic fibrosis, congenital cystic bronchiectasis, and α_1-antitrypsin deficiency. Acquired bronchiectasis can result from any cause of chronic airway obstruction. This leads to distal infection with retained purulent bronchial secretions, mucous plugs, and further injury to the distal conducting airways. This cycle leads to dilatation of the distal small airways, mucous and fluid collection, and further tissue destruction with airway collapse.

Pathogenesis

Bronchiectasis is classified as follows:

- Cylindric—dilated bronchi of regular configuration
- Varicose—dilatation and irregularity
- Saccular or cystic—aneurysmal-type dilatation in the periphery; the bronchi may be filled with fluid collections

Diagnosis

Patients have a chronic productive cough with recurrent pulmonary infections. Foul-smelling sputum, fever, and hemoptysis are common. Hemoptysis results from increased bronchial collateral circulation, intimately associated with tissue destruction in the bronchial tree and occurs in about half the patients who have acquired chronic bronchiectasis. A chest radiograph may show increased bronchial markings with areas of overinflation. High-resolution and dynamic CT are used to evaluate the lung parenchyma. Exhalation CT provides information about air trapping. Bronchoscopy is used to determine whether the disease is due to intrinsic abnormality of the airways or other endobronchial abnormalities, such as a foreign body, neoplasia, or extrinsic compression. Bronchoscopy also facilitates culture acquisition and drainage of diseased segments.

Management

Management of bronchiectasis is supportive. It consists of antibiotics to control infection and aggressive pulmonary physiotherapy to promote drainage of the diseased segments. Surgical therapy is reserved for failures of medical treatment and consists of resection of segmental or lobar areas with advanced disease and little physiological function.

SUGGESTED READING

Antman KH, Pass HI, Delaney T, et al. Benign and malignant mesothelioma. In: DeVita V, Hellman S, Rosenberg SA, eds. Principles and practices of oncology, ed. 2. Philadelphia, JB Lippincott, 1993.

Barker AF. Bronchiectasis. Semin Thorac Cardiovasc Surg 1995: 7:112.

Blumberg D, Port JL, Weksler B, et al. Thymoma: a multivariate analysis of factors predicting survival. Ann Thorac Surg 1995;60:908.

Cole FH, Cole FH, Khandekar A, Maxwell JM, Pate JW, Walker WA. Video-assisted thoracic surgery: primary therapy for spontaneous pneumothorax? Ann Thorac Surg 1995;60:931.

Dulmet EM, Macchiarini P, Suc B, Verley JM. Germ cell tumors of the mediastinum: a 30-year experience. Cancer 1993;72:1894.

Light RW, ed. Pleural diseases, ed. 2. Philadelphia, Lea & Febiger, 1990.

Sabiston DC Jr, Spencer FC, eds. Surgery of the chest, ed. 6. Philadelphia, WB Saunders, 1995.

Shields TW, ed. Mediastinal surgery. Philadelphia, Lea & Febiger, 1991:254.

Waller DA, Morritt GN, Forty J. Video-assisted thoracoscopic pleurectomy in the management of malignant pleural effusion. Chest 1995;107:454.

Wiedemann HP, Rice TW. Lung abscess and empyema. Semin Thorac Cardiovasc Surg 1995;7:119.

ESSENTIALS OF SURGERY: SCIENTIFIC PRINCIPLES AND PRACTICE,
edited by Lazar J. Greenfield, Michael W. Mulholland, Keith T. Oldham, Gerald B. Zelenock,
and Keith D. Lillemoe. Lippincott-Raven Publishers, Philadelphia, © 1997.

CHAPTER 63

CONGENITAL HEART DISEASE AND CARDIAC TUMORS

RALPH S. MOSCA, FLAVIAN M. LUPINETTI,
AND EDWARD L. BOVE

ATRIAL SEPTAL DEFECT

Atrial septal defect (ASD) is a hole in the atrial septum (Fig. 63-1). ASDs usually occur in the central aspect of the septum. The defect may range from a simple patent foramen ovale to complete absence of the septum primum.

ASDs cause increased pulmonary blood flow due to left-to-right shunting through the defect. Blood flow is directed from the left atrium to the right atrium because of the greater diastolic compliance and lower diastolic pressures in the right ventricle. Symptoms occur when pulmonary flow is twice that of the systemic circulation (Qp/Qs ratio >2). The most common symptoms are fatigue, shortness of breath, and recurrent respiratory infection. Atrial dysrhythmias are common in adults.

Diagnosis

Physical findings with large ASDs are:

- Normal first heart sound
- Wide, fixed splitting of second heart sound
- Soft ejection flow murmur across the pulmonary valve
- Diastolic flow murmur audible across the tricuspid valve
- Prominent right ventricular lift and increased intensity of pulmonary component of the second sound with pulmonary hypertension.

Chest radiographs depict enlargement of the right atrium, right ventricle, and pulmonary artery. Pulmonary vascular markings are increased. An *electrocardiogram (ECG)* shows right axis deviation and an incomplete right bundle branch block pattern. When right bundle branch block is associated with a leftward or superior axis, atrioventricular septal defect (AVSD) is likely. Two-dimensional (2D) *echocardiography* is used to visualize the ASD and anomalies of pulmonary venous return. Right ventricular volume overload with a flat or reversed septal motion suggests a large volume of left-to-right shunting.

Treatment

Any ASD with a large left-to-right shunt that produces volume overload is closed surgically. This occurs with a Qp/Qs ratio ≥ 1.5. Elective repair is advised before school age for patients with moderate to large ASDs. ASD also may be repaired by means of transcatheter closure with an umbrella device.

VENTRICULAR SEPTAL DEFECT

Most ventricular septal defects (VSDs) are single and occur high in the ventricular septum just beneath the aortic valve, but they can occur anywhere in the septum (Fig. 63-2). Associated lesions are common with VSD, and the defect itself is often a part of a more complex lesion. Prolapse of the aortic valve with aortic insufficiency may be caused by VSD. VSD may be associated with left heart obstructive lesions, such as aortic stenosis, mitral stenosis, and coarctation.

Isolated VSDs cause left-to-right shunting with increased pulmonary blood flow. Hemodynamics and symptoms depend on the size of the defect and the magnitude of the shunt. As the normally elevated PVR of a neonate falls during the first few weeks of life, the degree of left-to-right shunting increases, causing congestive heart failure (CHF) (Table 63-1).

Diagnosis

Large VSDs usually become apparent at 6 weeks to 2 months of age, when the normally elevated PVR falls, allowing an increase in left-to-right shunting. Symptoms of CHF are tachypnea, tachycardia, diaphoresis with poor feeding, and inadequate weight gain. The diagnosis of VSD may be made with 2D *echocardiography*. Color flow imaging provides information about the location, size, and number of VSDs. Associated lesions, such as aortic stenosis, coarctation, and mitral stenosis, may be evaluated. Complete evaluation of a large VSD includes *cardiac catheterization* to assess pulmonary blood flow and pressure and PVR.

Treatment

All VSDs are first managed medically with digoxin and diuretics to control CHF. The most common indication for operative closure of a large VSD is CHF that causes failure to thrive. By 6 months of age, the likelihood of spontaneous closure of large defects diminishes, and PVR may be elevated. In favorable situations, PVR decreases and Qp/Qs ratio increases, and an operation is advisable. If Qp/Qs ratio remains >1.5 with a R_p/R_s ratio >0.6 to 0.7, an operation is contraindicated.

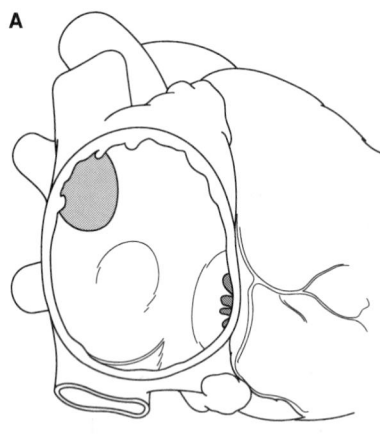

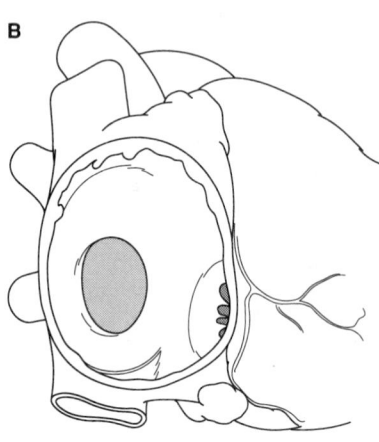

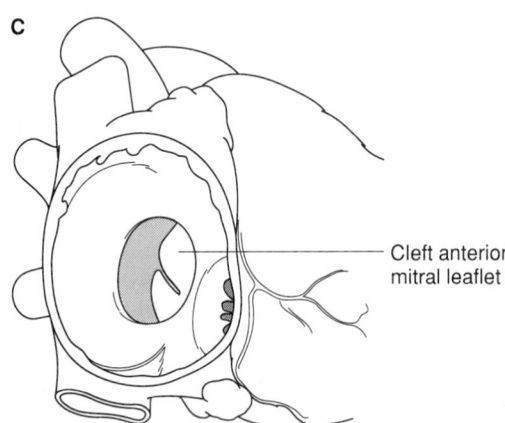

Cleft anterior
mitral leaflet

Figure 63-1. The anatomy of atrial septal defects. In the sinus venosus type (*A*), the right upper and middle pulmonary veins frequently drain to the superior vena cava or right atrium. (*B*) Secundum defects generally occur as isolated lesions. (*C*) Primum defects are part of a more complex lesion and are best considered as incomplete atrioventricular septal defects.

AORTIC STENOSIS

Obstruction to left ventricular outflow may occur at multiple levels (Fig. 63-3).

Valvar Aortic Stenosis

Valvar aortic stenosis is caused by abnormalities of aortic valve development, most commonly a bicuspid aortic valve with fusion of the commissures. The most common lesions associated with aortic stenosis are coarctation of the aorta, VSD, and mitral stenosis.

Diagnosis

Most cases of valvar aortic stenosis are diagnosed during childhood with the finding of an asymptomatic murmur. The classic symptoms of aortic stenosis are CHF, angina, and syncope. The physical findings include low pulse volume, precordial thrill, and an ejection systolic murmur at the cardiac base that radiates into the neck. A systolic ejection click means the stenosis is valvar. Severe stenosis may be accompanied by a fourth heart sound and paradoxic splitting of the second sound. An ECG usually shows left ventricular hypertrophy but may be normal. Two-dimensional echocardiography is extremely useful in determining the site and severity of the lesion. The left ventricular outflow tract gradient may be estimated with Doppler ultrasound.

Treatment

A neonate with aortic stenosis and CHF needs urgent operative intervention. Many patients have severe low cardiac output and metabolic acidosis. Their condition may be improved with endotracheal intubation and inotropic support. An infusion of prostaglandins opens the ductus arteriosus and allows increased systemic blood flow. Symptoms are rare after infancy, but if CHF, angina, or syncope occurs with a left ventricular outflow tract gradient ≤50 mmHg, an operation is indicated. Even without symptoms, a gradient >75 mmHg is considered severe. Patients with an aortic valve gradient between 50 and 75 mmHg and no symptoms may undergo observation. If an ECG demonstrates left ventricular strain or ischemia at rest or with exercise, an operation is indicated.

Subvalvar Aortic Stenosis

Subvalvar aortic stenosis occurs beneath the aortic valve. In the *discrete* type, a fibrous membrane is present immediately beneath the aortic valve leaflets. In the *diffuse* form, a long, tunnel-like obstruction exists beneath the valve and may extend for a considerable distance toward the apex of the left ventricle.

Supravalvar Aortic Stenosis

Supravalvar aortic stenosis is an obstruction that begins distal to the aortic valve. The discrete form is localized to the supravalvar area just above the aortic valve commissures. This produces an hourglass deformity of the ascending aorta. The discrete form is more common than the diffuse form. Diffuse vascular abnormalities involve thickening of the aortic wall that extends distally into the aortic arch and its branches.

Diagnosis

The signs and symptoms of supravalvar aortic stenosis are similar to those of other forms of left ventricular outflow tract narrowing. The diagnosis is established with cardiac catheterization and angiography. These studies are necessary to define the extent of obstruction and associated anomalies. The most common associated condition is peripheral pulmonary artery stenosis, which may be diffuse and severe.

Treatment

Operation is indicated for supravalvar aortic stenosis with outflow tract gradients >50 mmHg.

TETRALOGY OF FALLOT

The four components of tetralogy of Fallot (Fig. 63-4) are:

1. Hypoplasia of the right ventricular outflow tract and pulmonary valve annulus due to anterior displacement of the infundibular septum

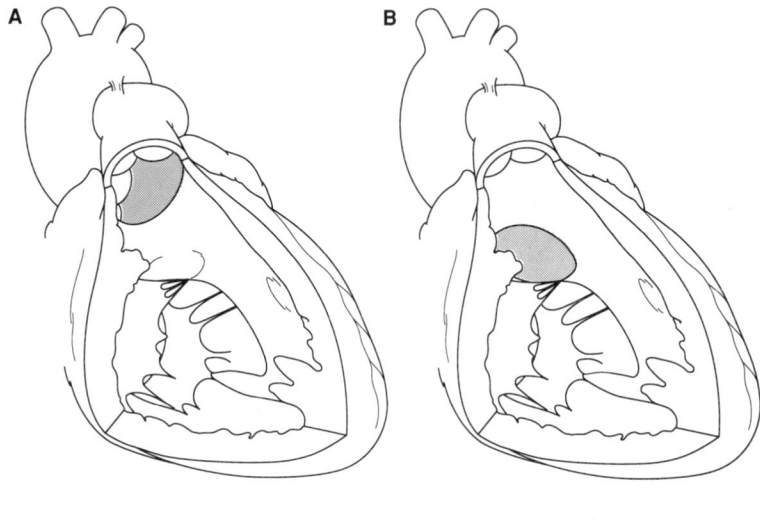

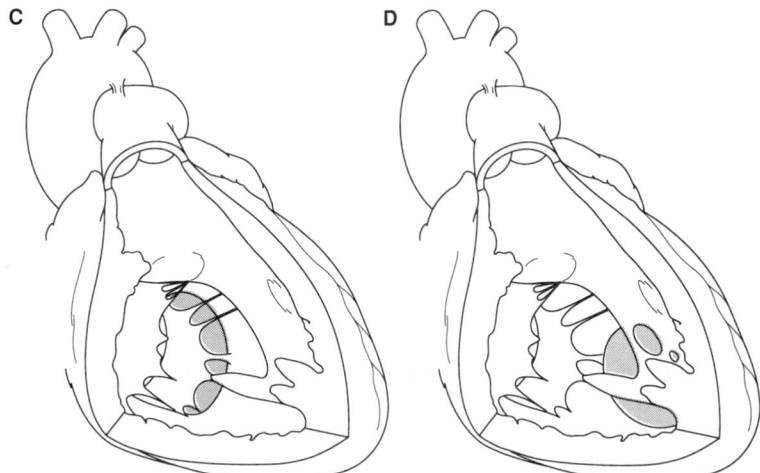

Figure 63-2. The anatomy of ventricular septal defects (VSDs) as seen through the right ventricle. (*A*) Subarterial VSDs, or high type, are generally bordered superiorly by the pulmonary valve annulus. (*B*) Perimembranous VSDs are the most common, extending from the membranous septum into the infundibular septum. (*C*) Inlet defects are located predominantly beneath the septal leaflet of the tricuspid valve. (*D*) Muscular VSDs are situated away from the valves, toward the cardiac apex.

2. Large malalignment VSD
3. Overriding of aorta
4. Right ventricular hypertrophy due to outflow tract obstruction

Diagnosis

Physical examination reveals cyanosis. Older patients may have clubbed fingers and toes. The precordium is quiet, without thrill, and the second sound may appear to

Table 63-1. SIZE OF VENTRICULAR SEPTAL DEFECT AND DEGREE OF LEFT-TO-RIGHT SHUNTING

Size of Defect	Pressure Relation	Qp/Qs Ratio
Large (size of defect approximates size of aortic annulus)	Systemic or near systemic right ventricular pressure	>2.5–3
Moderate	Right ventricular pressure about half systemic pressure or less	1.5–2.5
Small	Normal right ventricular pressure	<1.5

be single because of the soft pulmonic component. A mid-intensity systolic ejection murmur occurs, which may decrease in intensity with increasing degrees of outflow tract obstruction. Continuous murmurs may be audible over the back because of collaterals. CHF is rare.

Chest radiography may demonstrate a classic boot-shaped heart sign with a concave pulmonary outflow tract and an upward-tipped apex. Heart size is normal, and pulmonary vascular markings are decreased. There may be a right aortic arch.

Two-dimensional echocardiography shows the position and nature of VSD and outflow tract obstruction and can be used to visualize the branch pulmonary arteries and proximal coronary arteries. Echocardiography often is the only preoperative procedure needed.

Cardiac catheterization sometimes is necessary to outline the anatomy of the pulmonary arteries and the presence of important coronary abnormalities.

Treatment

The most common indications for operative intervention are increasing cyanosis and the occurrence of cyanotic spells. Spells may be managed with propranolol, but more definitive surgical intervention is indicated. Palliation is accomplished with a conventional or modified Blalock-Taussig shunt. Complete repair involves VSD closure

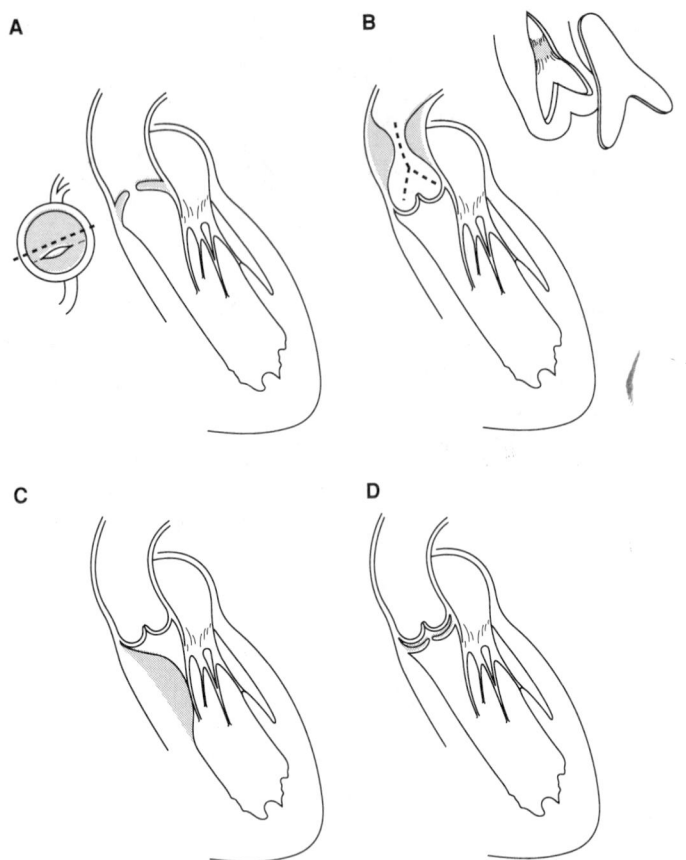

Figure 63-3. The anatomy of the types of congenital aortic stenosis. (*A*) Valvar aortic stenosis. (*B*) Supravalvular aortic stenosis and its repair (*inset*). (*C*) Tunnel-type subvalvar aortic stenosis. (*D*) Membranous subvalvar aortic stenosis.

and relief of right ventricular outflow tract obstruction. The VSD is closed transatrially, often avoiding a ventriculotomy.

TRANSPOSITION OF THE GREAT ARTERIES

In transposition of the great arteries (TGA), the aorta originates from the right ventricle and the pulmonary artery originates from the left ventricle (Fig. 63-5). Oxygen-

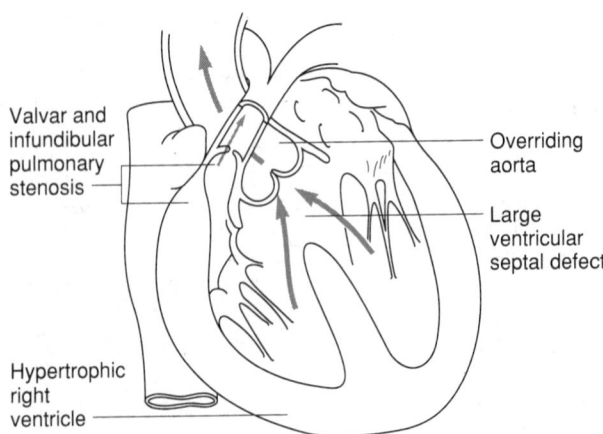

Valvar and infundibular pulmonary stenosis

Overriding aorta

Large ventricular septal defect

Hypertrophic right ventricle

Figure 63-4. The four anatomic features of the tetralogy of Fallot. The primary morphologic abnormality, anterior and superior displacement of the infundibular septum, results in the malalignment ventricular septal defect, overriding of the aortic valve, and obstruction of right ventricular outflow. The right ventricular hypertrophy is a secondary occurrence.

ated pulmonary venous blood is returned to the lungs and desaturated systemic blood to the body. Mixing may occur at several levels, but it occurs most commonly at the atrial level through an ASD or patent foramen ovale. A fixed shunt does not occur in one direction without an equal amount of blood passing in the other direction, or one circulation would empty into the other. The amount of desaturated blood that reaches the lungs (effective pulmonary blood flow) equals the amount of saturated blood that reaches the aorta (effective systemic blood flow).

Diagnosis

A newborn with TGA has cyanosis within hours of birth. There may be no other abnormal physical findings. The ECG is normal at birth, demonstrating the typical pattern of right ventricular dominance. The classic chest radiographic appearance of an egg on its side may be seen, but this finding is often obscured by an enlarged thymic shadow. Echocardiography shows that the posterior great vessel originating from the left ventricle is a pulmonary artery that bifurcates soon after its origin. The anterior great vessel is the aorta and originates from the right ventricle. Cardiac catheterization may be helpful to define anatomy, discern associated lesions, and improve cardiac mixing with balloon atrial septostomy.

Treatment

An infant with TGA and severe cyanosis needs prompt treatment to improve mixing and increase arterial oxygen saturation. This is best accomplished with early surgical repair or balloon atrial septostomy. Patients with large VSDs have clinically significant CHF and pulmonary hypertension early in life. Banding of the main pulmonary

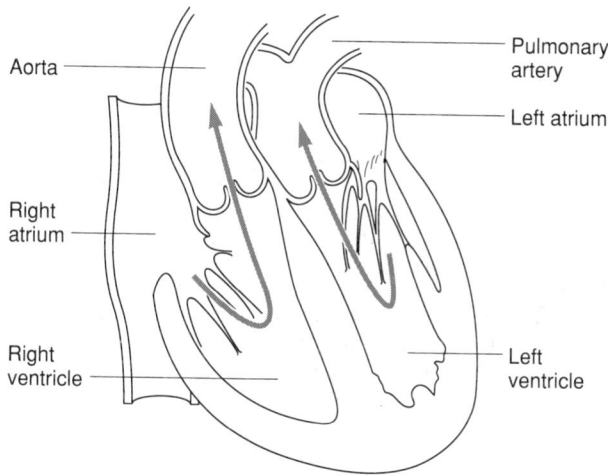

Figure 63-5. The anatomy of the most common type of transposition of the great arteries. The ascending aorta is usually located anterior and to the right of the pulmonary artery.

artery may be performed to reduce distal pulmonary artery pressure and prevent pulmonary vascular occlusive disease. About 25% of patients with hemodynamically large VSDs may have changes of pulmonary vascular disease by 3 months of age; early reduction of pulmonary artery pressure is essential. The arterial-switch procedure is used to manage TGA.

DOUBLE-OUTLET RIGHT VENTRICLE

Double-outlet ventricle includes a variety of malformations in which both great arteries originate from one ventricle. Double-outlet right ventricle (DORV) is far more common than double-outlet left ventricle. A VSD usually is present with DORV. Other defects include discordant ventriculoarterial connections, valvar or subvalvar stenosis of the pulmonary artery, and aortic outflow and single ventricle.

The physiologic consequences of DORV vary with the associated defects. The three most critical factors determining the net effects on the circulation are the size of the VSD, the presence or absence of pulmonary stenosis, and the presence and degree of left-sided obstruction. DORV clinically may resemble isolated VSD, tetralogy of Fallot, or TGA.

TRUNCUS ARTERIOSUS

Truncus arteriosus is rare. A single arterial vessel originates from the heart, overriding the ventricular septum and giving rise to the systemic, coronary, and pulmonary circulations. Most cases of truncus arteriosus are associated with a VSD similar to that of tetralogy of Fallot, except the superior margin of the defect is formed by the truncal valve. Other associated lesions include patent foramen ovale, atrial septal defect, persistent left superior vena cava, mitral valve anomalies, interrupted aortic arch, and coronary artery abnormalities. Lethal noncardiac abnormalities also occur.

The anatomy of truncus arteriosus allows mixing of the systemic and pulmonary venous blood at the level of the VSD and truncal valve. Systemic arterial saturation depends on the volume of pulmonary blood flow, determined by PVR. As PVR begins to fall, pulmonary overcirculation occurs, causing pulmonary congestion.

Diagnosis

Newborn infants with truncus arteriosus have signs of CHF and collapsing peripheral pulses. Chest radiography shows marked cardiomegaly, pulmonary plethora, often with minimal thymus shadow, and a right aortic arch. An ECG shows biventricular hypertrophy. Echocardiography demonstrates the truncal vessel, the structure and function of the truncal valve, associated lesions such as interrupted aortic arch, and often the pulmonary artery anatomy. Cardiac catheterization is reserved for situations in which the anatomy is unclear, more 1information is needed about the status of the truncal valve, or the status of the pulmonary vessels is unclear.

Treatment

Truncus arteriosus is treated with surgical therapy. Medical therapy is directed at control of CHF with fluid restriction, diuretics, digitalis, and afterload reduction. The onset of tachypnea can be used a marker to identify declining PVR and the optimal timing of repair.

CORONARY ARTERY ANOMALIES

Anomalies of coronary artery anatomy are divided into three categories on the basis of functional importance:

1. Abnormalities of no functional importance detected incidentally at cardiac catheterization (eg, origin of the circumflex coronary artery from the right coronary sinus or as a branch of the right coronary artery)
2. Anomalies with no intrinsic physiologic effects that because of their association with other cardiac defects alter surgical management (eg, abnormal course of the left anterior descending coronary artery associated with tetralogy of Fallot)
3. Anomalies that by their very existence produce adverse effects on the myocardium (eg, coronary arteriovenous fistula)

Coronary Arteriovenous Fistula

Cardiac catheterization or echocardiography and Doppler ultrasound are used for diagnosis. Because of the possible increase in size and possible predilection for subacute bacterial endocarditis or rupture, most surgeons recommend obliteration of the fistula unless the shunt is not clinically significant.

Origin of a Coronary Artery From the Pulmonary Artery

Symptoms first occur at about 6 weeks to 3 months of life. *Angiography* is needed to establish the diagnosis. *Echocardiography* can be used to define the origin and course of the coronary arteries.

Surgical correction is performed promptly when origin of a coronary artery from the pulmonary artery is identified. When collaterals are extensive, simple ligation of the anomalous vessel at its origin eliminates the steal into the pulmonary circulation. The optimal surgical approach is direct connection between the aorta and the anomalous coronary artery by means of direct implantation or construction of a tunnel within the pulmonary artery.

Origin of Coronary Artery From Coronary Sinus

A dangerous abnormality exists when the *left main coronary artery originates from the right coronary sinus* and passes between the pulmonary artery and the aorta. Fatal complications may occur when the *right coronary artery originates from the left coronary sinus* and passes between the great arteries, particularly when the right coronary artery is dominant. This condition often causes sudden death during vigorous physical exertion by young, otherwise-healthy people. This abnormality necessitates surgical intervention. Coronary artery bypass with the internal mammary artery can be performed easily with low operative risk.

PATENT DUCTUS ARTERIOSUS

In some newborn infants, the ductus arteriosus does not close because of cardiac or pulmonary conditions associated with abnormally low arterial oxygen. Patent ductus arteriosus (PDA) also may occur as an isolated lesion, most frequently in premature infants. PDA becomes apparent in older children as an asymptomatic murmur.

Indomethacin administration can cause the ductus to close, but pharmacologic closure of a PDA is rarely successful after the neonatal period, and surgical closure is needed. An operation is indicated for isolated PDA in almost all instances to prevent pulmonary vascular changes and CHF. Even a hemodynamically insignificant small ductus is closed to prevent the complications of endocarditis. PDA is closed by means of thoracoscopic ligation or transcatheter closure.

ATRIOVENTRICULAR SEPTAL DEFECT

Defects in embryologic development of the endocardial cushions may cause a variety of morphologic abnormalities in the AV valves and the atrial and ventricular septa. These anomalies encompass primum ASD, complete AVSD (or AV canal defect), and a range of intermediate forms. PDA and tetralogy of Fallot sometimes occur with these defects. A high percentage of patients with abnormalities of the AV structures have Down syndrome.

Diagnosis

Physical examination demonstrates increased precordial activity and fixed splitting of the second heart sound. A chest radiograph shows increased pulmonary vascularity and cardiomegaly. An ECG shows right ventricular or biventricular hypertrophy. Echocardiography is used to assess anatomy, define the presence or absence of valvar insufficiency, and provide information about the relative sizes of the ventricles. If pulmonary arterial resistance is high, it is important that it be remeasured while the child is breathing 100% oxygen. If pulmonary resistance falls, much of the elevated resistance is dynamic and can be managed in the perioperative period with vigorous ventilation and supplemental oxygen. Markedly elevated pulmonary resistance that does not respond to oxygen administration may constitute a contraindication to repair.

Treatment

Operative treatment is almost always necessary as soon as symptoms occur to prevent more clinical deterioration. Even if there are no symptoms, an operation is best performed before 6 months of age. The immediate operative results are good, especially if the patient is treated before pulmonary vascular disease develops. Patients with severe preoperative valvar regurgitation, those with clinically significant associated defects, and those with pulmonary vascular disease fare less well.

COARCTATION OF THE AORTA

Coarctation of the aorta (COA) is narrowing that most commonly occurs in the upper descending aorta just distal to the left subclavian artery. COA varies in the degree of luminal stenosis and the length of aorta affected. There usually is a shelf-like projection of aortic media and intima at the area of tightest obstruction. COA may be associated with tubular hypoplasia of the more proximal aortic arch or with Turner syndrome. The most common cardiac anomalies associated with COA are bicuspid aortic valve, VSD, and severe aortic stenosis.

Diagnosis

A prominent feature of COA is extensive development of collateral arteries. Extensive flow through the collaterals causes the physical findings of pulsation under the ribs and near the scapula, as well as diffuse bruits over the chest wall. Echocardiography demonstrates the anatomy and allows estimation of the pressure gradient. *Aortography* with pressure measurement may be used when the diagnosis is not clear. It allows definition of other possible cardiac anomalies and is useful to demonstrate the presence or absence of collaterals.

Newborns

COA may become apparent as profound CHF. The onset of symptoms may coincide with closure of the ductus arteriosus. Physical findings are a hyperdynamic precordium, a harsh murmur audible over the left chest and back, and diminished or undetectable femoral pulses. Radiographs do not show rib notching, but they do show cardiomegaly.

Older Children

There almost always are no symptoms. COA is usually diagnosed because of upper extremity hypertension with diminished or absent lower extremity pulses. Radiographs show rib notching and the typical *3* shadow in the aortic knob.

Adults

Symptoms are severe hypertension and CHF.

Treatment

Neonates with COA and CHF undergo operative repair as a life-saving measure. Older children undergo repair of COA to prevent the long-term sequelae of hypertension, CHF, endocarditis, aortic rupture, and intracranial vascular lesions.

Treatment after repair of COA involves control of hypertension. Abdominal discomfort in the postoperative period may be a symptom of mesenteric arteritis. This complication, which can be fatal, is preventable with control of blood pressure. It is advisable to forbid oral intake until bowel sounds are active.

UNIVENTRICULAR HEART

Univentricular heart (UVH) is a congenital anomaly characterized by the presence of only one ventricular chamber connected to the atria. In the most common form, both the mitral and tricuspid valves connect to a morphologic left ventricle, which ejects blood through a hypoplastic outlet chamber and then to the aorta. UVH is frequently

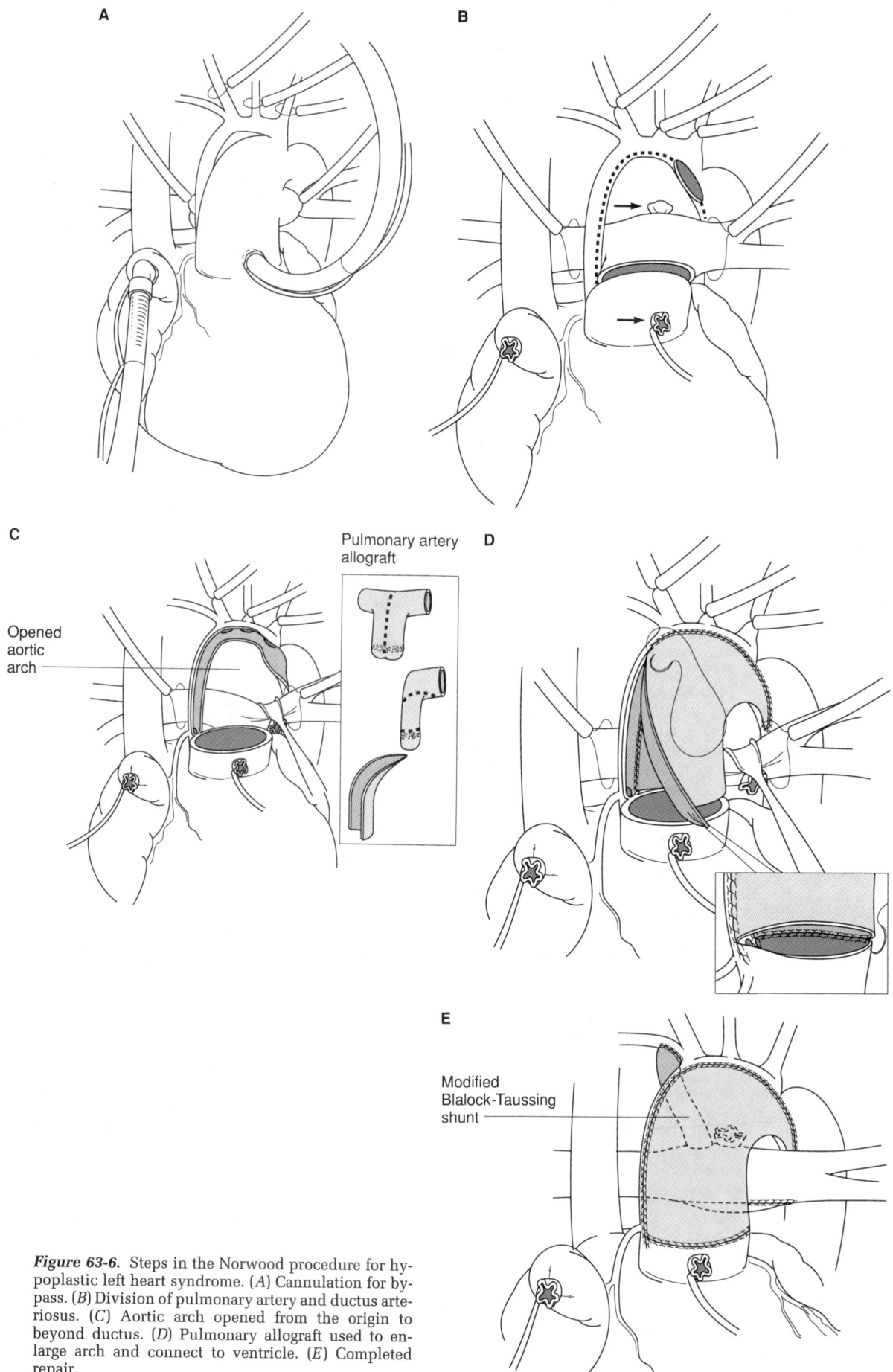

Figure 63-6. Steps in the Norwood procedure for hypoplastic left heart syndrome. (*A*) Cannulation for bypass. (*B*) Division of pulmonary artery and ductus arteriosus. (*C*) Aortic arch opened from the origin to beyond ductus. (*D*) Pulmonary allograft used to enlarge arch and connect to ventricle. (*E*) Completed repair.

associated with TGA and varying degrees of obstruction to pulmonary blood flow.

The signs and symptoms of UVH vary. When pulmonary flow is excessive, cyanosis may be mild. Here, the dominant feature is CHF. Pulmonary stenosis decreases pulmonary blood flow, and the degree of cyanosis increases. Associated lesions, such as COA, subaortic stenosis, or restrictive ASD, complicate the situation. Most patients undergo surgical intervention with a ventricular septation procedure early in life to reduce pulmonary blood flow if excessive (and prevent pulmonary vascular obstructive disease) or increase flow in the presence of severe pulmonary stenosis.

HYPOPLASTIC LEFT HEART SYNDROME

Hypoplastic left heart syndrome is a group of defects that may include aortic valve stenosis or atresia, mitral valve stenosis or atresia, and severe underdevelopment of the left ventricle. Initial management includes prostaglandin infusion to maintain ductal patency and correction of metabolic acidosis. The limited supply of donor hearts for transplantation necessitates surgical reconstruction (Fig. 63-6).

PRIMARY NEOPLASMS OF THE HEART AND PERICARDIUM

Diagnosis

The signs and symptoms of cardiac tumors include CHF, angina, syncope, pulmonary hypertension, pulmonary or systemic emboli, arrhythmias, and hemolysis. Initial diagnostic studies for patients with cardiac neoplasms are rarely specific. Some tumors calcify, facilitating radiographic diagnosis. An ECG may show nonspecific chamber enlargement or rhythm disturbances. Two-dimensional echocardiography assists in diagnosis, although differentiating tumor from thrombus may be difficult.

Benign Cardiac Tumors

Myxomas occur in either sex, at any age, in any cardiac chamber, and with a familial predilection. Most myxomas originate in the left atrium; a small percentage are multiple. The lesions rarely extend deeper than the endocardium. Malignant degeneration does not seem to occur. Because they commonly originate in the left atrium, myxomas may occur with symptoms of mitral valve disease murmurs, atrial arrhythmias, systemic emboli, and CHF. One striking symptom is dyspnea that varies dramatically with posture, especially dyspnea aggravated by assumption of an upright position.

Rhabdomyomas become apparent before the age of 1 year. Most occur in the left or right ventricle, and often protrude into the ventricular lumen, where they obstruct blood flow.

Other benign tumors of the heart are papillary fibroelastomas, fibromas, lipomas, hemangiomas, and teratomas.

Malignant Cardiac Tumors

The most common primary malignant neoplasm of the heart is *angiosarcoma*. Most originate from the right atrium or pericardium and cause CHF. Surgical excision is rarely possible. Radiation and chemotherapy may provide palliation, but few patients survive more than 1 year after diagnosis. Other malignant cardiac tumors, such as rhab-

domyosarcomas, mesotheliomas, fibrosarcomas, and osteosarcomas, also carry a poor prognosis.

SUGGESTED READING

Alvarez-Tostado RA, Millan MA, Tovar LA, et al. Thoracoscopic clipping and ligation of a patent ductus arteriosus. Ann Thorac Surg 1994;57:755.

Hanley FL, Heinemann MK, Jonas RA, et al. Repair of truncus arteriosus in the neonate. J Thorac Cardiovasc Surg 1993; 105:1047.

Hawkins JA, Thorne JK, Boucek MM, et al. Early and late results in pulmonary atresia and intact ventricular septum. J Thorac Cardiovasc Surg 1990;100:492.

Iannettoni MD, Bove EL, Mosca RS, et al. Improving results with the first stage reconstruction of hypoplastic left heart syndrome. J Thorac Cardiovasc Surg 1994;107:934.

Rome JJ, Keane JF, Perry SB, et al. Double umbrella closure of atrial septal defects: initial clinical applications. Circulation 1990:82:751.

Sealy WC. Paradoxical hypertension after repair of coarctation of the aorta: a review of its causes. Ann Thorac Surg 1990;50:323.

Weintraub RG, Brawn WJ, Venables AW, Mee RBB. Two-patch repair of complete atrioventricular septal defect in the first year of life: results and sequential assessment of atrioventricular valve function. J Thorac Cardiovasc Surg 1990;99:320.

ESSENTIALS OF SURGERY: SCIENTIFIC PRINCIPLES AND PRACTICE, edited by Lazar J. Greenfield, Michael W. Mulholland, Keith T. Oldham, Gerald B. Zelenock, and Keith D. Lillemoe. Lippincott–Raven Publishers, Philadelphia, © 1997.

CHAPTER 64

VALVULAR HEART DISEASE

O. WAYNE ISOM AND TODD K. ROSENGART

ANATOMY

The *atrioventricular* (AV) valves—the mitral and tricuspid—bridge the systolic pressure gradients between the atria and ventricles. The *semilunar* valves—the aortic and pulmonary—bridge the diastolic gradients between the ventricles and the peripheral circulation (Fig. 64-1).

The tricuspid and mitral valves are fibrous structures lined by endocardium. The *tricuspid valve* guards the right AV orifice. It consists of a large anterior leaflet attached to the anterior wall of the heart, a posterior leaflet at the right margin of the heart, and a septal leaflet attached to the interventricular septum. The *mitral (bicuspid) valve* guards the left AV orifice. It consists of a large anterior (aortic) leaflet in continuity with the posterior wall of the aorta and a smaller posterior (mural) leaflet in continuity with the the posterior wall of the heart at the AV groove.

The *semilunar valves, aortic and pulmonary,* guard the outlets of the two ventricles. The aortic valve bears important anatomic relations to the mitral valve, interventricular septum, and conduction system (Fig. 64-2).

PATHOLOGY

Aortic valvular stenosis is the most common type of valvular lesion, followed by mitral stenosis (Tables 64-1 through 64-5).

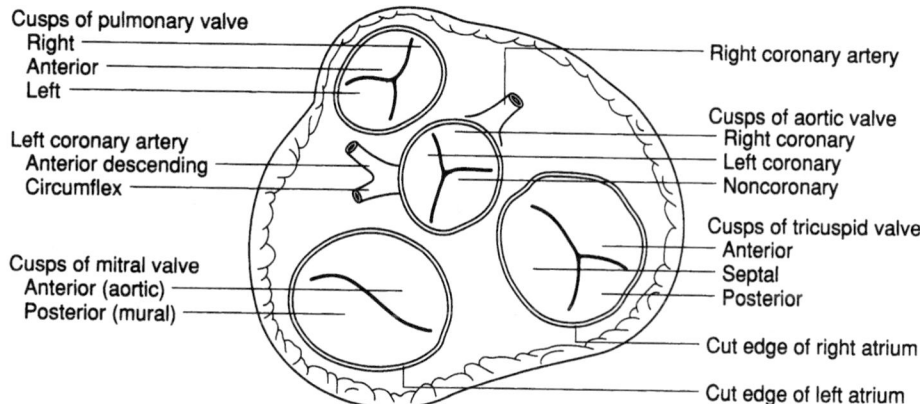

Figure 64-1. Cross-sectional representation of the normal anatomic relations of the semilunar (aortic and pulmonary) and atrioventricular (mitral and tricuspid) valves.

PATHOPHYSIOLOGY

Valvular dysfunction stresses the heart in two ways: volume overload and pressure overload. Both represent increased cardiac afterload, ie, increased systolic wall stress. Huge cardiac reserves exist in patients with valvular heart disease. Valvular disease may be asymptomatic until severe valvular and ventricular dysfunction develops. Patients with acute valvular dysfunction without gradual adaptation may die rapidly of severe heart failure. The following mechanisms allow the heart to adapt to gradual valvular dysfunction:

Chamber enlargement
Shifts in ventricular contractility as a function of left ventricular end-diastolic volume (LVEDV)
Myocardial hypertrophy
Increased adrenergic stimulation

Increased diastolic filling of the ventricle increases myocardial sarcomere length (preload). This improves ventricular ejection as a function of ventricular filling, shown as a shift in length-active tension relation, or the Frank-Starling curve (Fig. 64-3). According to Laplace's law, wall stress increases with increasing ventricular radius (preload) but is inversely related to wall thickness. Ventricular hypertrophy, another compensatory mechanism, decreases wall stress.

CONGESTIVE HEART FAILURE

Heart failure is the end point in the natural history of valvular dysfunction. Heart failure is the inability of the heart to pump blood at a level adequate for the metabolic demands of the body. In patients with valvular dysfunction, heart failure may initially be caused by abnormal hemodynamic loads in the presence of normal myocardial function. *Systolic heart failure* is pump failure. *Diastolic heart failure* is impaired ability of the ventricle to fill properly because of chamber stiffness and abnormal relaxation. Venous congestion, pulmonary or systemic, occurs in the circulation upstream from the failing ventricle.

In congestive heart failure (CHF), pulmonary congestion is caused by damming of blood behind the ineffectively contracting left ventricle. High pulmonary hydrostatic

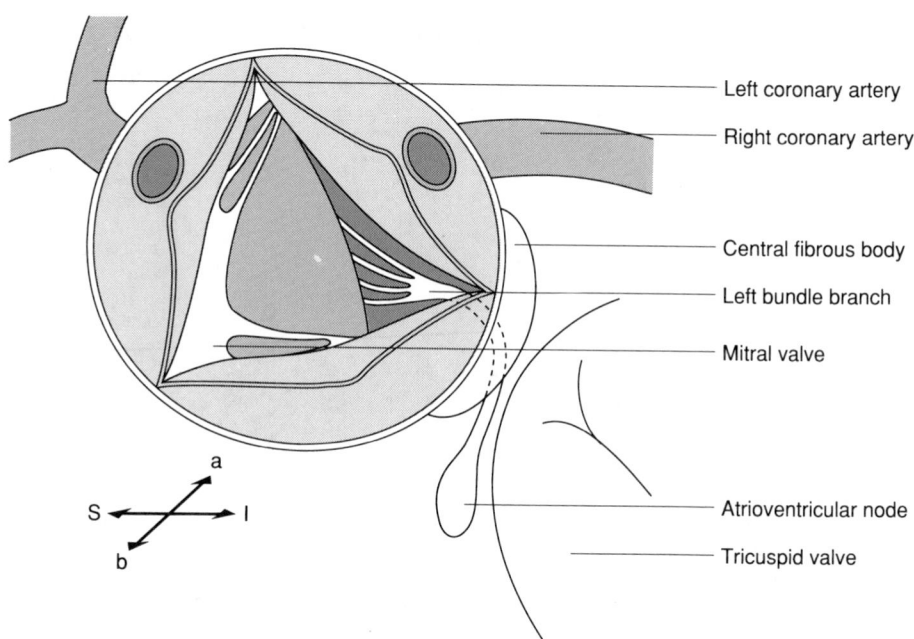

Figure 64-2. Schematic diagram of the anatomic relations of the aortic valve showing the mitral valve posterolaterally and the septum medially. (After Wilcox BR, Anderson RN. Surgical anatomy of the heart. New York, Raven Press, 1985)

Table 64-1. CAUSES OF MITRAL STENOSIS

VALVULAR

Rheumatic disease
Nonrheumatic disease
  Infective endocarditis
  Congenital mitral stenosis
  Single papillary muscle (parachute valve)
  Mitral annular calcification

SUPRAVALVULAR

Myxoma
Left atrial thrombus
Other

pressure overwhelms the counterbalancing osmotic pressure gradient. Edema fluid escapes into the interstitial space from the pulmonary capillaries, causing pulmonary congestion and reduced vital capacity. Air in the lungs is replaced by interstitial and intraalveolar fluid and engorged vessels. The lungs stiffen as intraparenchymal fluid decreases compliance. The work of breathing increases; intrapleural pressures must increase to expand collapsed airways and stiff lungs. Tidal volume decreases and respiratory frequency increases. Patients become aware of these changes when they experience dyspnea. Skeletal muscle fatigue from increased work of breathing may heighten the sensation.

DIAGNOSIS

Physical Examination

Cardiac examination includes careful palpation, auscultation, and provocative maneuvers. Peripheral arterial pulses and jugular venous pattern are evaluated, and a thorough search is conducted for systemic findings, such as edema, ascites, or jaundice. The signs are as follows:

Table 64-2. CAUSES OF LEFT VENTRICULAR OUTFLOW TRACT OBSTRUCTION

VALVULAR (AORTIC STENOSIS)

Acquired
  Rheumatic disease
  Degenerative (fibrocalcific) disease
    Tricuspid valve
    Congenital bicuspid valve
  Infective endocarditis
  Other
Congenital
  Tricuspid valve with commissural fusion
  Unicuspid unicommissural valve
  Hypoplastic annulus

SUPRAVALVULAR

Membranous
Hourglass
Hypoplastic

SUBVALVULAR

Hypertrophic cardiomyopathy
Discrete (membranous) subaortic stenosis
Tunnel subaortic stenosis

Table 64-3. ETIOLOGY OF AORTIC INSUFFICIENCY

	Pathology		
Cause	Leaflet	Aortic Root	Loss of Commissural Support
COMMON			
Rheumatic disease	+	−	−
Congenital disease	+	−	±
Endocarditis	+	−	±
LESS COMMON			
Syphilis	±	+	−
Connective tissue disease (eg, Marfan syndrome)	+	+	+
Aortic dissection	−	+	+
UNCOMMON			
Trauma	+	+	+
Hypertension	±	±	±
Inflammatory disease (ankylosing spondylitis, Reiter syndrome)	+	+	−

(Modified from Greenberg BH. Acquired aortic valve disease. In: Greenberg BH, Murphy E, eds. Valvular heart disease. Littleton, MA, PSG Publishing, 1987:157)

Aortic Stenosis

Pulsus parvus et tardus—a late-peaking, low-pulse pressure impulse
Midsystolic murmur—best heard at the base of the heart, usually radiates to both carotid arteries

Table 64-4. CAUSES OF MITRAL REGURGITATION

DISORDERS OF THE MITRAL VALVE LEAFLETS

Loss of contracture of valvular tissue
  Rheumatic fever
  Endocarditis
  Systemic lupus erythematosus
Congenital
  Cleft leaflet (isolated)
  Endocardial cushion defect
Connective tissue disorders
Other

DISORDERS OF THE MITRAL ANNULUS

Calcification
Dilatation
Destruction

DISORDERS OF THE CHORADAE TENDINEAE

Rupture of the chordae tendineae
  Endocarditis
  Myocardial infarction
  Connective tissue disorder
  Other
Thickening or fusion of the chordae tendinae
Elongation of the chordae tendineae

DISORDERS OF THE PAPILLARY MUSCLES

Dysfunction of rupture of papillary muscle
  Ischemia or infarction
  Endocarditis
  Inflammatory disorder
Malalignment
  Left ventricular dilatation
  Hypertrophic cardiomyopathy
  Infiltrative cardiomyopathy
Other

(Modified from Silverman ME, Hurst JW. The mitral complex: clues to its afflictions. Cardiovasc Clin North Am 1973;5:35)

Table 64-5. CAUSES OF RIGHT-SIDED VALVULAR DYSFUNCTION

TRICUSPID VALVE	PULMONIC VALVE
Regurgitation	Regurgitation
RV or annular dilatation	Annular dilatation
RV infarct	Pulmonary hypertension
RV hypertension	Marfan syndrome
RV failure	Other
Marfan syndrome	Congenital defects
Congenital	Endocarditis
Ebstein anomaly	Carcinoid heart disease
AV canal	Iatrogenic or other
Rheumatic heart disease	Stenosis
Tricuspid valve prolapse	Congenital pulmonic stenosis
Papillary muscle	Rheumatic heart disease
dysfunction	Carcinoid heart disease
Infective endocarditis	Cardiac tumors
Carcinoid heart disease	Other
Right atrial myxoma	
Endomyocardial fibrosis	
Other	
Stenosis	
Rheumatic disease	
Congenital tricuspid atresia	
Right atrial tumors	
Carcinoid heart disease	
Constrictive pericarditis	
Other	

AV, atrioventricular; RV, right ventricular.

Gallavardin phenomenon—radiation of a high-pitched component to the cardiac apex with an intervening quiet area
Palpable, sustained, forceful, nondisplaced apical impulse (PMI)
Thrills—palpable vibrations in the aortic auscultation area
Carotid shudder

Aortic Insufficiency

High systemic arterial pulse pressure with low diastolic pressure
Corrigan water-hammer pulse
Musset sign—head bobbing in time with heart beat
Quincke sign—capillary pulsation in fingertips, detected with light compression
PMI displaced laterally and bounding
Cardiac auscultory findings
* High-pitched, decrescendo diastolic murmur heard best at the left sternal border with the patient leaning forward and exhaling
* Austin Flint murmur—apical, mid to late diastolic rumble
* Short diastolic murmur (acute aortic insufficiency)

Mitral Regurgitation

Brisk, laterally displaced PMI
* Unremarkable peripheral findings
* Cardiac auscultory findings
* Widely split S_2 due to early aortic valve closure
* Holosystolic murmur constant and blowing, heard best at apex and usually radiating to the axilla
* Little beat-to-beat variation of murmur
* No increase in murmur with inspiration
* Variable mid to late systolic click murmur heard with provocative maneuvers, such as a Valsalva maneuver or standing

Mitral Stenosis

PMI nondisplaced and possibly of low intensity
* Opening snap and accentuated S_1
* Diastolic rumble at apex
* Presystolic accentuation of diastolic murmur at auscultation
* Rales
* Late signs of pulmonary hypertension

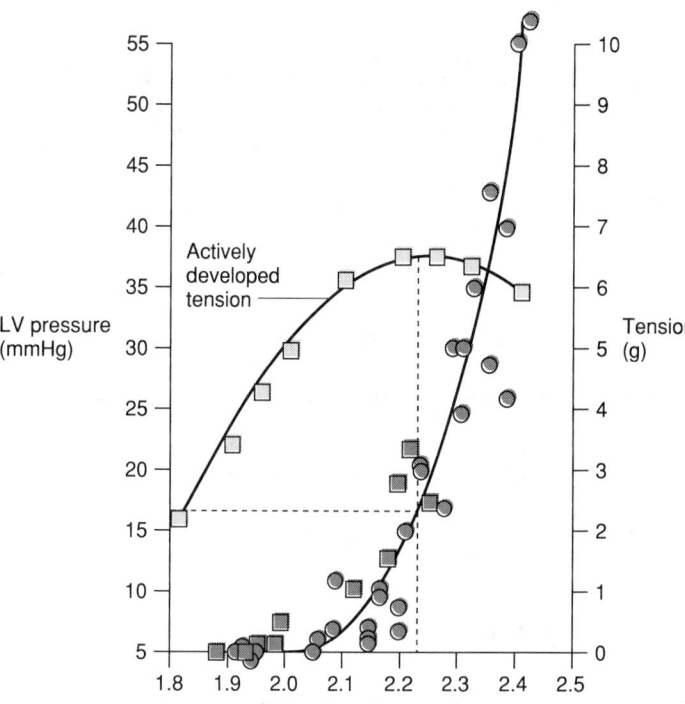

Figure 64-3. Frank-Starling relation describing ventricular contractility as a function of left ventricular (LV) end-diastolic volume. Data are derived from animal studies. The upper curve represents myocardial tension development as a function of sarcomere length; the lower curve represents resting ventricular pressure as a function of sarcomere length. (After Spotnitz JH, Sonnenblick EH, Spiro D. Relationship of ultrastructure to function in the intact heart: sarcomere structure relative to pressure-volume curves of the intact left ventricles of dog and cat. Circ Res 1966;18:57)

Tricuspid Regurgitation

Pulsatile liver

- Ascites, edema
- Right ventricular heave
- Jugular venous distention with bounding v waves (c-v waves)
- Pansystolic murmur localized to left lower sternal border that increases with inspiration (Carvello sign)

Tricuspid Stenosis

Cardiac findings masked by associated mitral stenosis

- Diastolic murmur at left lower sternal border, increases with inspiration
- Marked jugular venous distention with prominent a wave, ascites, or anasarca in the presence of clear lung fields

Electrocardiogram

A 12-lead ECG is used to assess rhythm disturbances and the specific chamber enlargement associated with valvular disease.

Radiography

Chest Radiography

Posteroanterior and lateral chest radiographs provide information about cardiac chamber enlargement and pulmonary congestion that may help in assessment of the physiologic effects of valvular heart disease. Kerley B lines, dense, short, horizontal lines at the costophrenic angles, usually correlate with high pulmonary wedge pressures and are a sign of valvular disease.

Radionuclide Angiography

Radionuclide cineangiography provides visual and numeric data about cardiac function and valvular disease.

Echocardiography

Mitral stenosis is quantified with 2D imaging. Direct measurement of orifice size correlates with catheterization data. Decreased range of mitral valve excursion on the M-mode study (E-F slope), thickened leaflets, and decreased diastolic leaflet separation also yield useful information. The structural causes of *mitral regurgitation,* such as a ruptured chordae or flail leaflet, may be visualized, but quantification of mitral regurgitation depends on Doppler analysis.

Echocardiographic assessment of the *aortic valve* yields data about orifice size and abnormality such as a bicuspid valve. Leaflet thickening and orifice narrowing are characteristic of aortic *stenosis.* Aortic *insufficiency* may be suggested by diastolic fluttering of the mitral or aortic leaflet. Prognostic data about LV diameter can be collected.

In Doppler echocardiography, the velocity of red blood cells is measured in a targeted area. Continuous-wave Doppler ultrasound is used to measure high-speed blood flow, as in aortic stenosis. Pulsed Doppler ultrasound is used to assess flow at a specific point.

Cardiac Catheterization

Intracardiac pressures and hemodynamic measurements are obtained by means of selective catheter positioning with fluoroscopy (Table 64-6; Fig. 64-4).

Table 64-6. NORMAL CARDIAC HEMODYNAMIC PRESSURES AND VALUES

	Systolic	End-Diastolic	Mean
PRESSURE (mmHg)			
Right atrium			0–8
Right ventricle	15–30	0–8	
Pulmonary artery	15–30	3–12	9–16
Pulmonary artery wedge/ left atrium			1–10
Left ventricle	100–140	3–12	
Aorta	100–140	60–90	70–105
CARDIAC OUTPUT INDEX (L/min/m²)		2.6–4.2	
RESISTANCE (dynes·sec/cm⁵)			
Pulmonary		20–130	
Systemic		700–1600	

(Modified from Grossman W, Barry WH. Cardiac catheterization. In: Braunwald E, ed. Heart disease: a textbook of cardiovascular medicine. Philadelphia, WB Saunders, 1988:287)

MEDICAL MANAGEMENT

Medical therapy for valvular heart disease is based on correction of the physiologic abnormalities and therapy for CHF. The three determinants of ventricular function must be optimized: preload, afterload, and myocardial contractility (Table 64-7).

Specific Considerations

Aortic Stenosis

The ventricle of a patient with aortic stenosis tends to be noncompliant, causing large changes in LVEDP with small volume changes. Incremental adjustment of volume status may be needed. Negative inotropic agents must be avoided. Reduced output associated with atrial fibrillation may necessitate pharmacologic or electrical cardioversion.

Aortic Insufficiency

Peripheral vasodilators are used to manage aortic insufficiency. They produce a pressure gradient that favors blood flow to the periphery. Use of vasoconstricting drugs or an intraaortic balloon pump is contraindicated. Valve replacement is often the only effective therapy.

Mitral Stenosis

Symptoms of dyspnea and pulmonary fluid overload may improve with sodium restriction and diuresis, but dehydration must be avoided. Ventricular rate must be controlled by management of atrial fibrillation with digitalis or calcium channel or β-blockers. Antiarrhythmic therapy may be indicated for frequent premature atrial contractions. Cardioversion may be indicated for atrial fibrillation, especially if hemodynamic compromise develops.

Mitral Regurgitation

Ventricular preload reduction with diuretics or nitrates improves pulmonary congestion. Preload and afterload reduction with vasodilators helps reduce the degree of mitral regurgitation. Positive inotropes may be used to shrink the regurgitant orifice. For acute, severe mitral regurgitation, aggressive afterload reduction with nitroprusside or balloon counterpulsation may be used to stabilize the patient's condition before surgical correction.

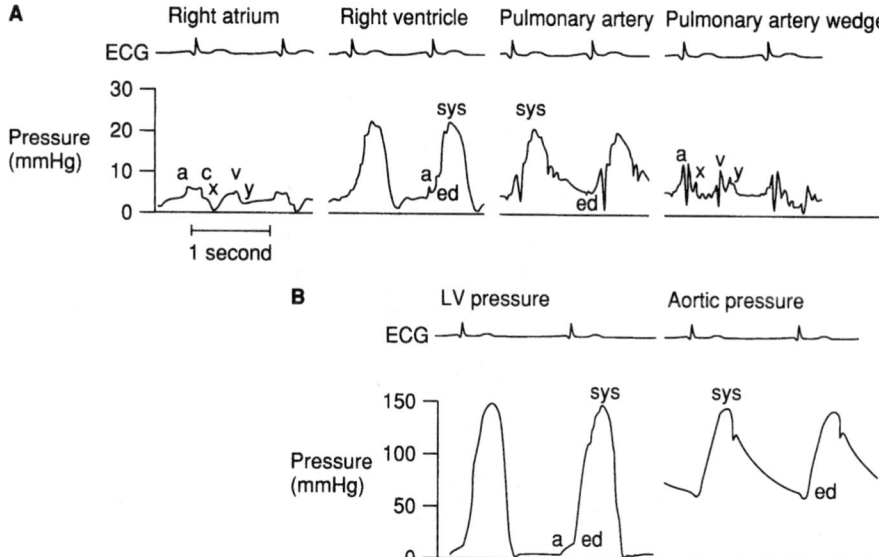

Figure 64-4. Normal pressure tracings from the right (*A*) and left (*B*) sides of the heart. (After Grossman W, Barry WH. Cardiac catheterization. In: Braunwald E, ed. Heart disease: a textbook of cardiovascular medicine, ed 3. Philadelphia, WB Saunders, 1988:250)

Tricuspid Disease

Stenosis and regurgitation are treated with aggressive diuresis. Tricuspid valve excision may be tolerated if right ventricular systolic pressure is normal.

SURGICAL MANAGEMENT

Surgical treatment of valvular heart disease is indicated for deterioration in ventricular function or functional class. An open heart operation with aortic valve replacement is the option for most patients with *aortic stenosis.* Balloon aortic valvuloplasty may be used as a bridging technique if the patient is critically ill. Mitral commissurotomy can be used to treat patients with *mitral stenosis* but may be limited by extensive calcification, leaflet stiffness, chordal fusion, or mitral regurgitation. Tricuspid valve annuloplasty is used to manage secondary *tricuspid regurgitation.*

Preoperative Care

Screening for occult infection is performed to prevent prosthetic valve endocarditis and contamination of valvular prostheses. Dental abscesses are treated, if cardiac status allows. Bleeding history and risk for coagulopathy are assessed because of the need for intraoperative and postoperative anticoagulation. GI bleeding is evaluated. Aspirin and other agents that may alter coagulation are discontinued 1 week before the operation. Patients with respiratory compromise receive pulmonary therapy. Cigarette

Table 64-7. THERAPY OF HEART FAILURE

Abnormality	Treatment
Preload	Diuretics
	Venous dilators
Afterload	Arterial vasodilators
	Angiotensin-converting enzyme inhibitors
Contractility	Positive inotropic agents

(Schlant RC, Sonnenblick EH. Pathophysiology of heart failure. In: Hurst JW, ed. The heart, ed 6. New York, McGraw-Hill, 1986:319)

smoking is discontinued preoperatively. Nutritional therapy is provided.

Surgical Technique

Technique at the outset of the procedure is similar for valve repair and valve replacement. A median sternotomy allows the best access to the heart. After the pericardium is opened, the tricuspid valve is palpated and tricuspid regurgitation assessed through an incision in the right atrial appendage. The aorta is assessed for calcification before cannulation for cardiopulmonary bypass. Aortic calcification may dictate an alternative site for bypass return. Heparin is administered, and the ascending aorta is cannulated to allow total bypass (Fig. 64-5). The heart is arrested by means of cross-clamping the ascending aorta and injection of cardioplegic solution into the aortic root.

Mitral Valve Repair

After the heart is cooled and arrested, a longitudinal left atrial incision is made, and retraction is applied. In mitral commissurotomy, the fused commissures are divided to a point a few millimeters from the valve annulus; attachments to the chordae tendineae are left intact to prevent mitral insufficiency (Fig. 64-6). Mitral reconstruction for insufficiency may involve mitral annuloplasty or mitral reconstruction (Fig. 64-7).

Valve Replacement

Mitral valve replacement (Fig. 64-8) begins with excision of the diseased valve 3 to 4 mm from the annulus. The posterior leaflet or at least some chordae to the posterior annulus are preserved. After valve removal and débridement of calcium to allow passage of sutures into compliant tissue, the valve orifice is sized. Valves at least 29 mm in diameter allow reasonable flow. The prosthesis is sewn to the annulus. The valve is lowered into place and the sutures are tied down. The valve annulus must be seated properly to avoid paravalvular leaks.

Aortic valve replacement is illustrated in Figure 64-9. After a transverse aortotomy, the aortic valve is excised and stray pieces of calcium are removed. The valve orifice is sized and the valve sewn into place.

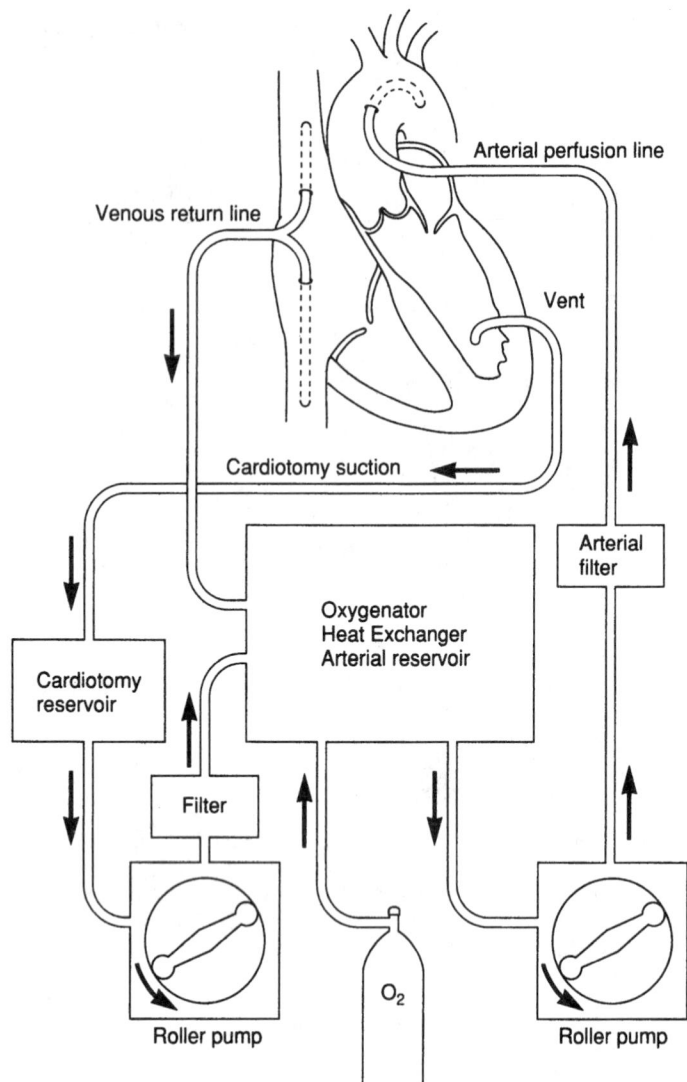

Figure 64-5. Schematic depiction of the main components of the pump oxygenator (heart-lung machine). (After Callaghan JC, Wartak J. Open heart surgery: theory and practice. New York, Praeger Press, 1986)

Closure

The patient's temperature is restored with rewarmed blood, and the aortotomy or atriotomy incision is oversewn. Air is evacuated from the left side of the heart, usually during electrical fibrillation. If this step is not taken, arterial air embolism may occur. After the aortotomy or atriotomy incision is closed, protamine is given to neutralize the heparin dose, and atrial and ventricular epicardial pacing wires are placed.

Prosthetic Valves

Design

Most bioprosthetic valves are porcine heterografts fixed in glutaraldehyde. Mechanical valve designs are as follows:

Ball in cage (Starr–Edwards)
• Tilting disk (Björk–Shiley)
• Tilting disk with pivoting bileaflet mechanism that eliminates the need for retaining struts (St. Jude)

Mechanical valves are recommended for most patients. Tissue valves are used for tricuspid valve replacement.

Complications

The main disadvantage of *tissue valves* is early calcific degeneration, which leads to stenosis or insufficiency. Emergency replacement may be needed. *Mechanical valve* dysfunction usually is caused by valvular thrombosis. Thrombotic occlusion of the tilting-disk leaflet leaves it in a half-open, half-closed position, causing severe stenosis and insufficiency.

Auscultation is an effective way to screen for prosthetic valve dysfunction, although dysfunction may occur without changes in auscultatory findings. Diminution of prosthetic heart valve sounds may represent tissue ingrowth or thrombus formation. New or changed murmurs suggest valvular dysfunction. Evaluation also may involve fluoroscopic examination of mechanical valve leaflet motion, echocardiographic and Doppler echocardiographic studies, or cardiac catheterization.

Therapy for prosthetic valvular dysfunction may be urgent or emergency surgical valve replacement. Open thrombectomy sometimes is possible. Intraaortic balloon counterpulsation may stabilize the condition of patients with prosthetic mitral insufficiency. Fibrinolytic therapy may be used to manage acute thrombotic occlusion of prosthetic valves, especially the tricuspid valve.

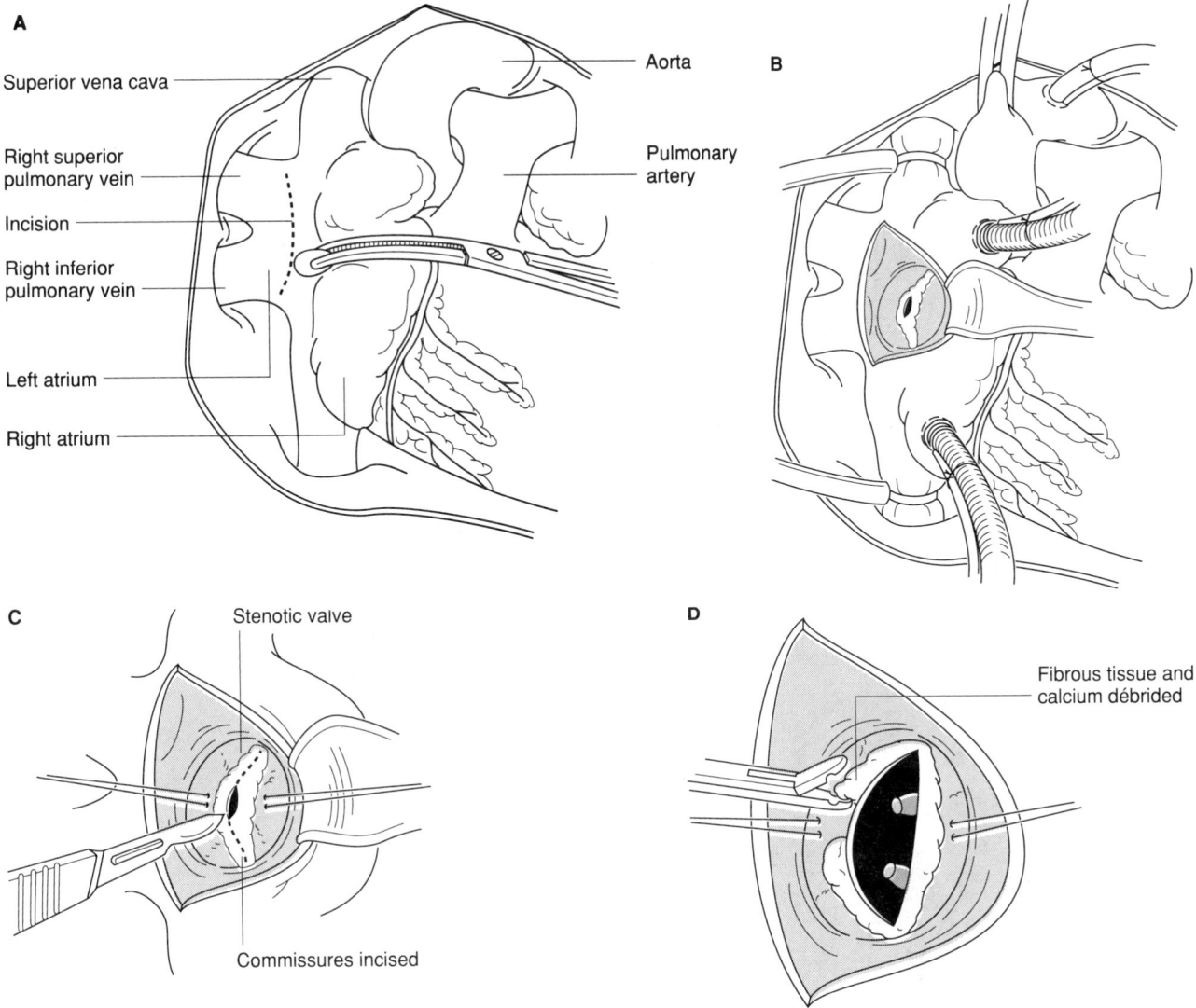

Figure 64-6. Mitral valve repair for stenotic disease. (*A* and *B*) Left atrial incision. (*C*) Mitral commissurotomy showing incision of fused commissures. (*D*) Débridement of excessive calcium.

Hemolysis is a complication of the use of mechanical valves. It may be severe enough to produce jaundice and necessitate transfusion, but it usually resolves with time. Other complications of valve replacement are endocarditis, atrial and ventricular arrhythmias, coronary ostial obstruction (aortic valve), LV rupture, AV groove tear (mitral valve), postpericardiotomy syndrome, and ventricular outflow tract obstruction.

Postoperative Care

The goal after a valve operation is cardiac output sufficient for nominal systemic perfusion. Qualitative assessment of cardiac function is made by means of observation of mental status and of the color and temperature of the extremities. Urine output is often high immediately after bypass but later is a good indicator of organ perfusion. Systemic blood pressure is a poor indicator of hemodynamic function. A pulmonary arterial thermodilution catheter allows direct quantification of cardiac index, which should be >2 L/min/m². Mixed venous gas pressure or saturation is a physiologic index of adequate perfusion;

PVO_2 should be >30 mmHg. Treatment of low cardiac output may involve volume resuscitation to increase preload, administration of positive inotropic agents, or the use of vasodilators to decrease afterload (Fig. 64-10).

Complications

Pulmonary dysfunction—common after bypass. Therapy is diuresis, pulmonary toilet, and ventilatory support.
- Renal dysfunction—reduced with early implementation of hemodialysis or peritoneal dialysis. Furosemide and mannitol are used to promote diuresis.
- Transient deterioration in intellectual ability and neurologic function—clears in hours to days. Treatment is supportive.
- Metabolic acidosis
- Hypothermia—resolves within 6 hours of the operation
- Sodium and water retention—physiologic diuresis is usually assisted by administration of exogenous di-

(text continues on page 491)

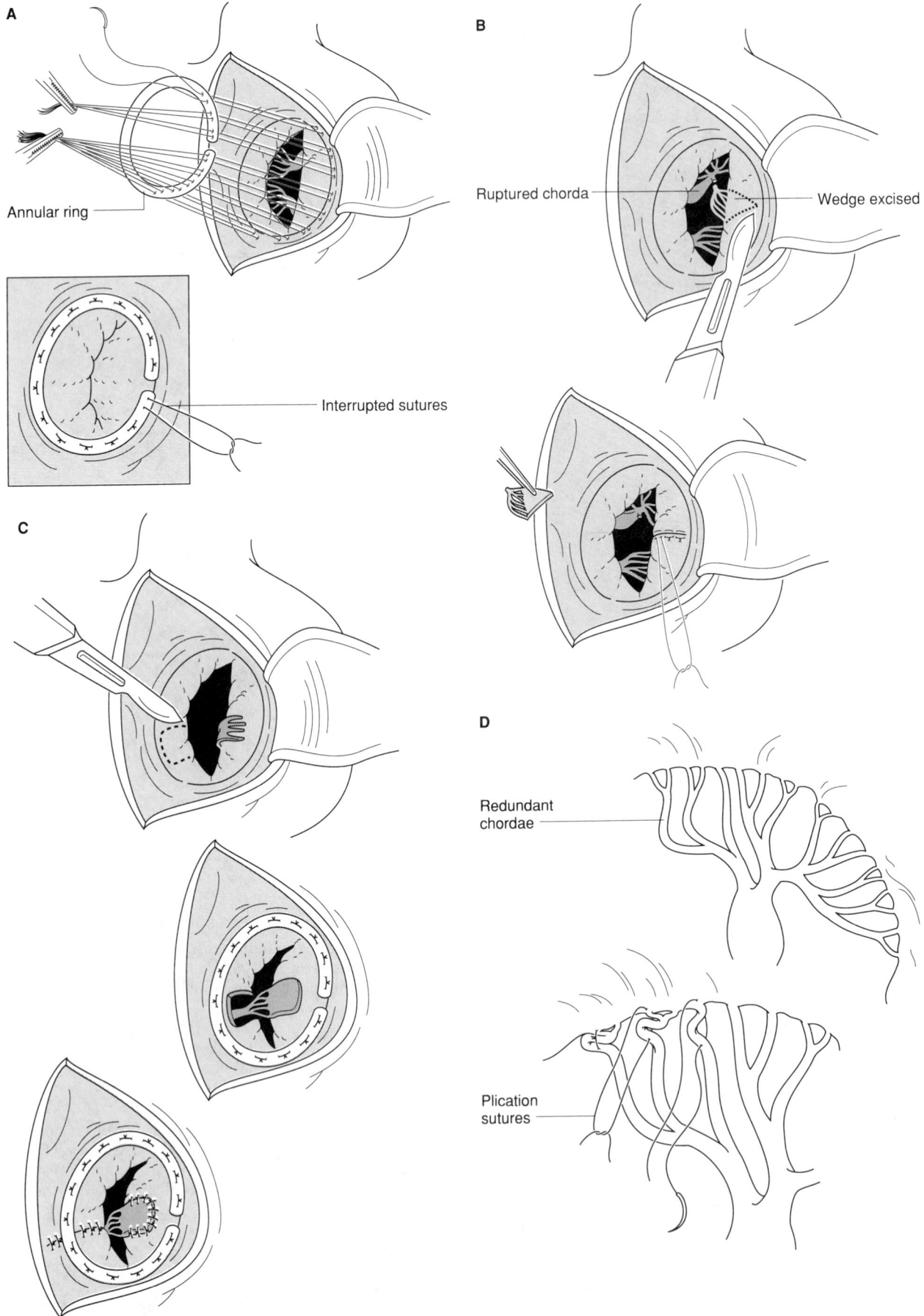

A

Annular ring

Interrupted sutures

B

Ruptured chorda

Wedge excised

C

D

Redundant chordae

Plication sutures

Figure 64-7. Mitral valve repair for regurgitant disease. (*A*) Annuloplasty. (*B*) Leaflet resection. (*C*) Chordal transposition. (*D*) Chordal plication. (After Galloway AC, Colvin SB, Baumann FG, et al. Current concepts of mitral valve reconstruction for mitral insufficiency. Circulation 1988;78:1087)

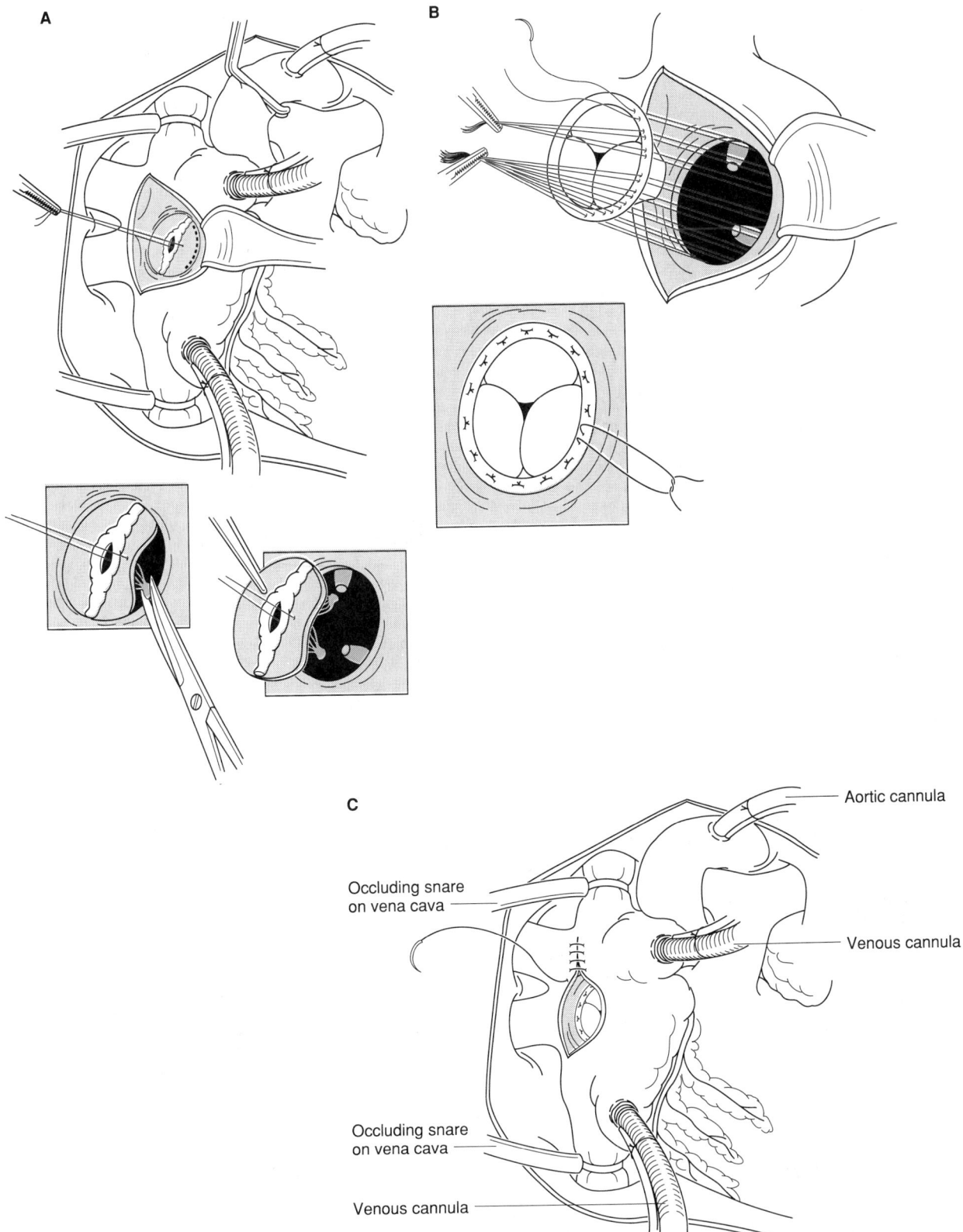

Figure 64-8. Mitral valve replacement. (*A*) Excision of diseased valve. (*B*) Suturing appropriately sized prosthesis. (*C*) Atriotomy closure.

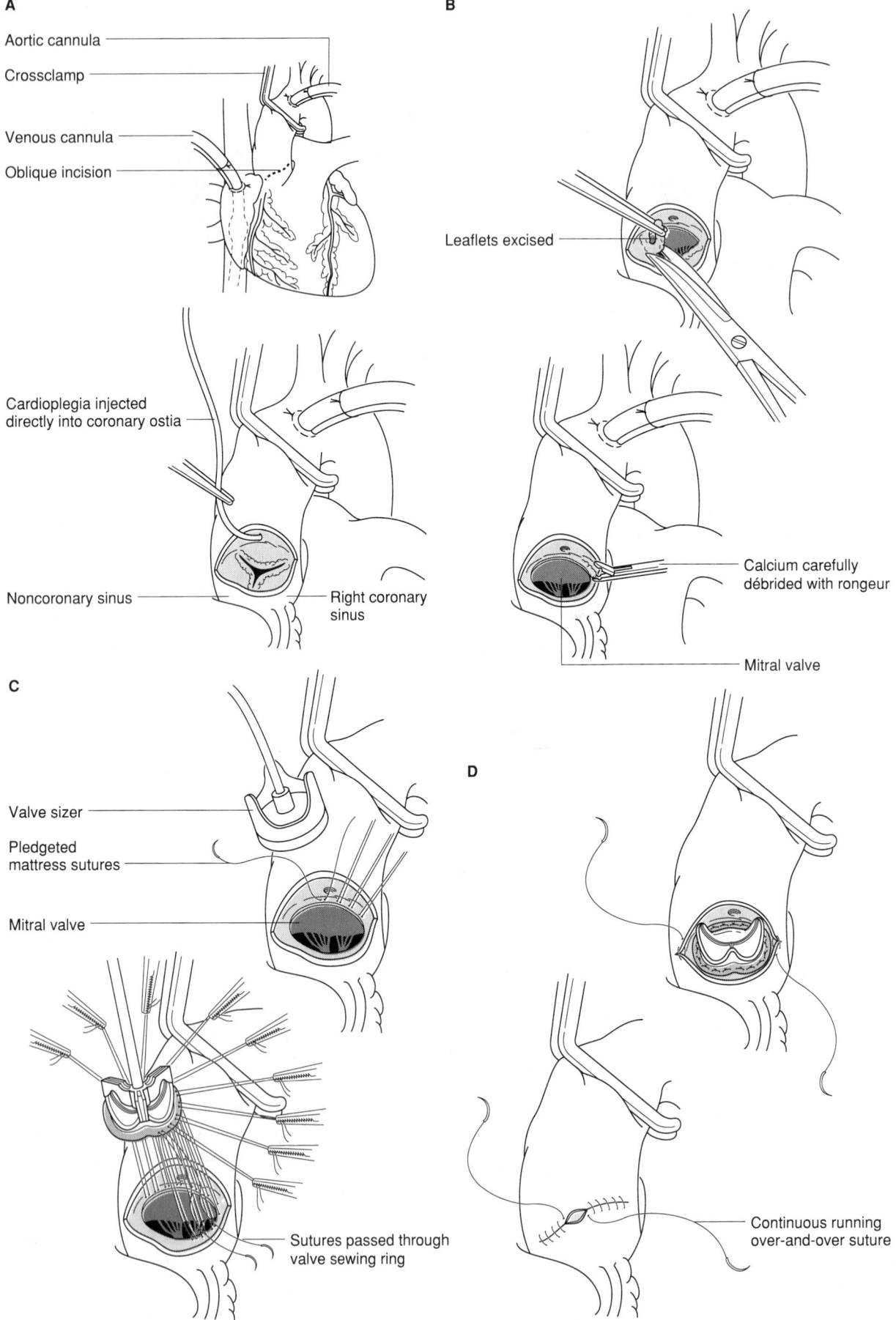

A

Aortic cannula

Crossclamp

Venous cannula

Oblique incision

Cardioplegia injected
directly into coronary ostia

Noncoronary sinus

Right coronary
sinus

B

Leaflets excised

Calcium carefully
débrided with rongeur

Mitral valve

C

Valve sizer

Pledgeted
mattress sutures

Mitral valve

Sutures passed through
valve sewing ring

D

Continuous running
over-and-over suture

Figure 64-9. Aortic valve replacement. (*A*) Aortotomy below crossclamp and aortic cannula. (*B*) Excision of heavily calcified valve. (*C*) Suturing of valve prosthesis. (*D*) Closure of aortotomy.

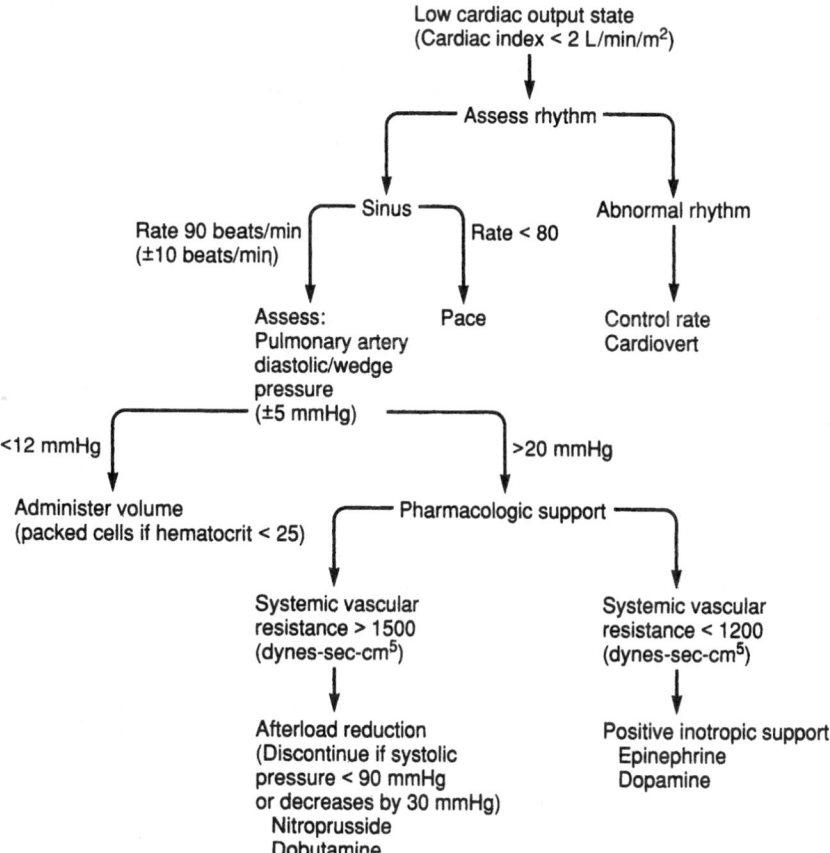

Figure 64-10. Algorithm for treatment of postoperative low cardiac output syndrome. Indicated pressures vary depending on ventricular compliance and other factors.

uretic agents. Hyperthermia and leukocytosis are exacerbated after cardiopulmonary bypass, and are not useful as guides to infection. Anemia, thrombocytopenia, and depletion of clotting factors present risk for bleeding and cardiac tamponade.

- Mediastinitis
- Acute abdominal complications—jaundice, acalculous cholecystitis, pancreatitis, GI bleeding, peptic ulcer disease, intestinal ischemia, probably related to poor organ perfusion during bypass

ANTICOAGULATION

Anticoagulation is indicated when the risk for thromboembolism exceeds the morbidity of hemorrhagic complications caused by anticoagulant therapy (Table 64-8). Anticoagulant therapy is recommended for patients with atrial fibrillation and systemic emboli, atrial fibrillation and mitral valve disease, and atrial fibrillation with cardiomyopathy.

Anticoagulant therapy is contraindicated for patients who:

Have a predisposition to bleeding complications, as from systemic disease (eg, active ulcer disease) or coagulopathy
- Are likely to incur trauma through occupation or pasttime
- Are unlikely to comply with treatment
- Want to become pregnant

ENDOCARDITIS

Prosthetic heart valves and diseased native valves are at high risk for endocarditis, and infection of normal valves is occurring with increasing frequency. Hypertrophic car-

diomyopathy, mitral valve prolapse associated with a murmur, and mitral annular calcification are predisposing factors.

Diagnosis

Endocarditis becomes apparent as fever, chills, or sweats, and septic emboli may occur. Although most patients with endocarditis have a murmur at some point, almost one-third have no murmur when the infection presents itself. Blood cultures are the mainstay of diagnosis of endocarditis. Two-dimensional echocardiography is a useful adjunct, but small lesions may not be detected.

Management

Bacterial endocarditis is prevented with antibiotic prophylaxis. Medical therapy is IV administration of antibiotics at bacteriocidal levels for 4 to 6 weeks. However, continued medical therapy for valvular endocarditis and cardiac deterioration carries an extremely high mortality rate. The chief cause of death is CHF due to aortic insufficiency.

Surgical intervention may be necessary if a new aortic insufficiency murmur develops, especially if it is accompanied by CHF. Other indications for surgical treatment are failure of antimicrobial therapy, valvular insufficiency, perivalvular abscess, and pericarditis. Surgical intervention usually is required for aortic valve endocarditis. Excision of the diseased valve, débridement of perivalvular abscesses, and valve replacement are the usual treatment. Surgical treatment of tricuspid disease may be performed

Table 64-8. ANTICOAGULANT RECOMMENDATIONS

Indication	Recommended Prothrombin Time Elevation With Warfarin Administration
PROSTHETIC HEART VALVES	
Mechanical	1.5–2
Bioprosthetic	1.3–1.5 (3 mo postoperatively)
NATIVE VALVE DISEASE	
Rheumatic mitral valve	
Previous embolism	1.5–2 (1.3–1.5 after 1 yr)
Atrial fibrillation	1.3–1.5
Dilated left atrium	
(>55 mm in diameter)	1.3–1.5
Aortic valve disease	No treatment*
Mitral valve prolapse	No treatment*
Mitral annular calcification	No treatment*
Infective endocarditis	No treatment*
ATRIAL FIBRILLATION	
Previous embolism	1.5–2 (1.3–1.5 after 1 yr)
Mitral valve disease	1.3–1.5
Cardiomyopathy	
Dilated	1.3–1.5
Hypertrophic	1.3–1.5
Thyrotoxicosis	1.3–1.5†
Lone atrial fibrillation	No treatment*
Cardioversion	1.3–1.5†

* Unless other indications exist.

† Maintain therapy for 2 to 4 weeks after conversion to sinus rhythm.

without valve replacement, although valve replacement is preferable.

SUGGESTED READING

Akins CW, Hilgenberg AD, Buckley MJ, et al. Mitral valve reconstruction versus reoperation for degenerative or ischemic mitral regurgitation. Ann Thorac Surg 1994 (suppl)S8668.

Cohn LH, Couper GS, Arlaki SF, et al. Long term results of mitral valve reconstruction for regurgitation of the myxomatous mitral valve. J Thorac Cardiovasc Surg 1994;107:143.

Cohn LH, Couper ES, Kinchla NM, et al. Decreased operative risk of surgical treatment of mitral regurgitation with or without coronary artery disease. J Am Coll Cardiol 1990;16:1575.

David TE, Bos J, Christakis GT, Brofman PR, Wong D, Feindel CM. Heart valve operations in patients with active infective endocarditis. Ann Thorac Surg 1990;49:701.

Smedira NG, Ports TA, Merrick SH, Rankin JS. Balloon aortic valvuloplasty as a bridge to aortic valve replacement in critically ill patients. Ann Thorac Surg 1993;55:914.

Turi ZG, Reyes VP, Raju BS, et al. Percutaneous balloon valvuloplasty versus surgical closed commissurotomy for mitral stenosis: a prospective, randomized trial. Circulation 1991;83:1179.

Tuzcu EM, Block PC, Palacios IF. Comparison of early versus late experience with percutaneous mitral balloon valvuloplasty. J Am Coll Cardiol 1991;17:1121.

ESSENTIALS OF SURGERY: SCIENTIFIC PRINCIPLES AND PRACTICE, edited by Lazar J. Greenfield, Michael W. Mulholland, Keith T. Oldham, Gerald B. Zelenock, and Keith D. Lillemoe. Lippincott–Raven Publishers, Philadelphia, © 1997.

CHAPTER 65

ISCHEMIC HEART DISEASE

GLENN J.R. WHITMAN AND VERDI J. DISESA

CORONARY ARTERY DISEASE

Coronary Circulation

Coronary Arteries

The right and left coronary arteries originate from the aorta just above the aortic valve cusps (Fig. 65-1). The right and left coronary cusps are in the sinuses of Valsalva. The third cusp is the noncoronary cusp.

The *left main coronary artery* courses posterolaterally to the left behind the pulmonary artery and divides (usually within 10 mm) into two main branches, the *left anterior descending (LAD) coronary artery* and the *left circumflex coronary artery.*

The LAD emerges from behind the pulmonary artery to course anteriorly within the interventricular groove down to the cardiac apex, sometimes wrapping around it onto the posterior interventricular groove. The initial tributaries of the LAD are usually the *first diagonal,* which emerges at an acute angle and runs over the anterolateral surface of the left ventricle, and the *first septal perforator,* which emerges at a right angle from the LAD and penetrates the interventricular septum. The continuation of the LAD may have several more diagonal and septal branches. This pattern means that the LAD nourishes the anterior, anterolateral, septal, and apical walls of the left ventricle.

The *circumflex coronary artery* descends posteriorly from the left main coronary artery and runs within the posterior atrioventricular (AV) groove. It usually ends in branches to the posterolateral wall of the left ventricle. Sometimes the circumflex artery extends to the crux of the heart and gives off the *posterior descending coronary artery* (PDA), which follows the posterior interventricular groove. The branches of the circumflex artery are the *obtuse marginals.* They cover myocardium where the lateral and posterior walls of the heart form an angle >90°.

The *right coronary artery* descends in the right AV groove to the crux, where it usually gives off the PDA but occasionally continues and ends in posterior left ventricular branches. The right ventricular free wall is fed by *acute marginal branches* from the right coronary artery.

The artery (right coronary or left circumflex) that supplies the PDA determines whether the coronary circulation is called *right dominant* or *left dominant.* The PDA gives off the *AV nodal artery.* Occlusion of the PDA can cause heart block.

Coronary Veins

Three venous systems drain the coronary circulation:

1. The coronary sinus, located in the posterior AV groove, receives blood from the great, middle, and small cardiac veins and the posterior veins of the left ventricle. It empties into the right atrium. The *great cardiac vein* ascends along the LAD in the interventricular groove and then turns posteriorly to follow the circumflex coronary artery to empty into the coronary sinus. The *middle cardiac vein* returns from the

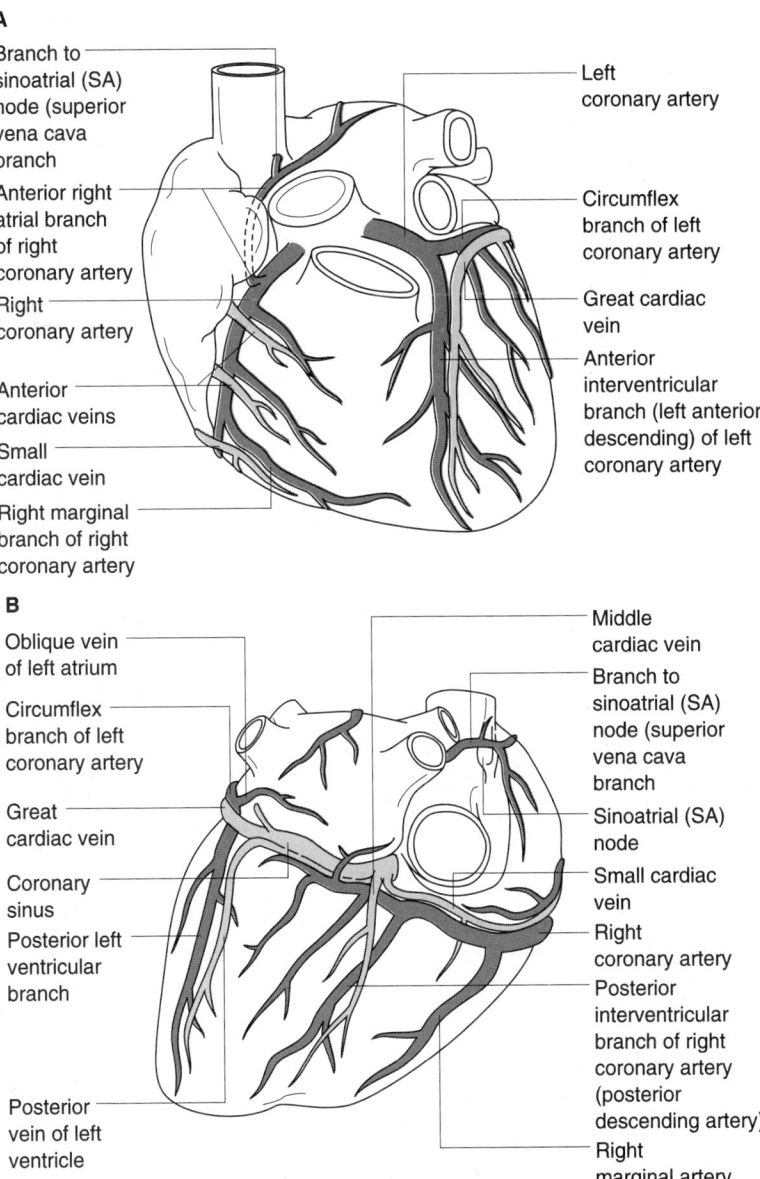

A

Branch to sinoatrial (SA) node (superior vena cava branch

Anterior right atrial branch of right coronary artery

Right coronary artery

Anterior cardiac veins

Small cardiac vein

Right marginal branch of right coronary artery

Left coronary artery

Circumflex branch of left coronary artery

Great cardiac vein

Anterior interventricular branch (left anterior descending) of left coronary artery

B

Oblique vein of left atrium

Circumflex branch of left coronary artery

Great cardiac vein

Coronary sinus

Posterior left ventricular branch

Posterior vein of left ventricle

Middle cardiac vein

Branch to sinoatrial (SA) node (superior vena cava branch

Sinoatrial (SA) node

Small cardiac vein

Right coronary artery

Posterior interventricular branch of right coronary artery (posterior descending artery)

Right marginal artery

Figure 65-1. Cardiac anatomy depicting the coronary arteries and cardiac veins. The origin of the left main coronary artery is left lateral and somewhat posterior with respect to the aorta, coursing behind the pulmonary artery and then dividing into the left anterior descending and circumflex coronary arteries. The right coronary artery comes off almost directly anterior, running in the atrioventricular groove. The great, middle, and small cardiac veins all come together at the level of the coronary sinus, which lies in the left inferior atrioventricular groove and empties into the right atrium.

apex along the posterior interventricular groove. The *small cardiac vein* follows the right coronary artery. Both veins empty at the level of the crux into the *coronary sinus.*

2. The *thebesian veins* are small venous orifices that drain the myocardium by emptying into any of the chambers of the heart.

3. The *anterior cardiac veins* drain the right ventricular coronary system. They traverse the free wall of the right ventricle and cross the AV groove to empty directly into the right atrium or a correlating vein at its base.

Regulation of Coronary Blood Flow

Physical Factors.   Perfusion pressure determines blood flow. Most myocardial blood flow occurs in diastole; as aortic diastolic pressure increases, so does myocardial perfusion. At low diastolic pressure, dilatation of the coronary arteries decreases vascular resistance and increases blood flow. During systole, increased cavitary pressure compresses intramyocardial vessels, eliminating forward flow.

Coronary flow may decrease as a result of coronary spasm, intramural clot, or coronary atherosclerosis.

Metabolic Factors.   The coronary circulation increases blood supply in proportion to increases in myocardial O_2 requirements. The most important metabolic regulator of this phenomenon is *adenosine,* a breakdown product of adenosine triphosphate (ATP). Increased myocardial O_2 demands increase ATP utilization and increase adenosine concentration. The result is coronary vasodilatation and increased O_2 delivery.

Prostaglandins decrease coronary vascular resistance, but only *thromboxane A_2* is considered an important coronary vasoconstrictor. Thromboxane A_2 is released by platelets, particularly in angina and myocardial infarction (MI).

Stimulation of cardiac sympathetic nerves constricts coronary arteries. This effect is usually overwhelmed by the autoregulatory vasodilatory response to increased myocardial O_2 demand caused by sympathetic stimulation.

Although *acetylcholine* causes coronary vasodilation, it lowers heart rate and decreases contractility, decreasing O_2 requirements and causing vasoconstriction.

Coronary Atherosclerosis
Pathology

Atherosclerosis causes proliferation of smooth muscle; formation of a tissue matrix of collagen, elastin, and proteoglycans; and accumulation of intra- and extracellular lipids. The lesions occur within the intima (innermost wall of the artery) and progress from a benign fatty streak to a complicated plaque (Fig. 65-2).

Advanced atherosclerotic lesions are caused by aging fibrous plaques. The necrotic core of the plaque may enlarge and become calcified. Hemorrhage into the plaque may disrupt the smooth fibrous surface, causing thrombogenic ulcerations. Organization of clot on the plaque surface increases protrusion into the arterial lumen, further decreasing blood flow.

Risk Factors

Risk factors for atherosclerosis include advanced age, genetic predisposition, male sex, hypertension, diabetes mellitus, hyperlipidemia, and cigarette smoking.

Diagnosis
Symptoms

Angina pectoris is the classic presentation of coronary artery disease. Patients describe angina as pressure or heaviness in the middle of the chest, sometimes radiating to the left shoulder and down the left arm. Patients often clench their fists in the middle of the chest as they describe this discomfort. Other symptoms include abdominal pain, nausea, belching, back pain, pain in one or both shoulders, jaw pain, and hand heaviness or numbness.

Stable angina pectoris is brought on by reproducible increases in myocardial demand for oxygen. Patients report that certain levels of activity or emotional stress or excitement trigger angina, which is relieved with rest or relaxation.

In unstable angina pectoris symptoms may occur during rest or sleep. Patients have myocardial ischemia without demonstrable changes in myocardial oxygen demand. Unstable angina also describes new-onset angina pectoris or

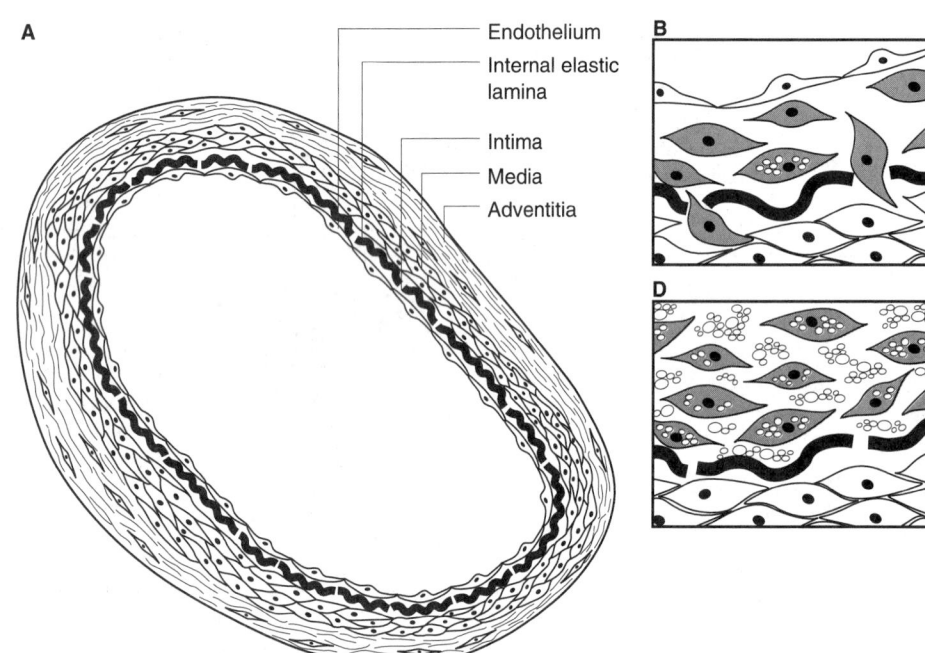

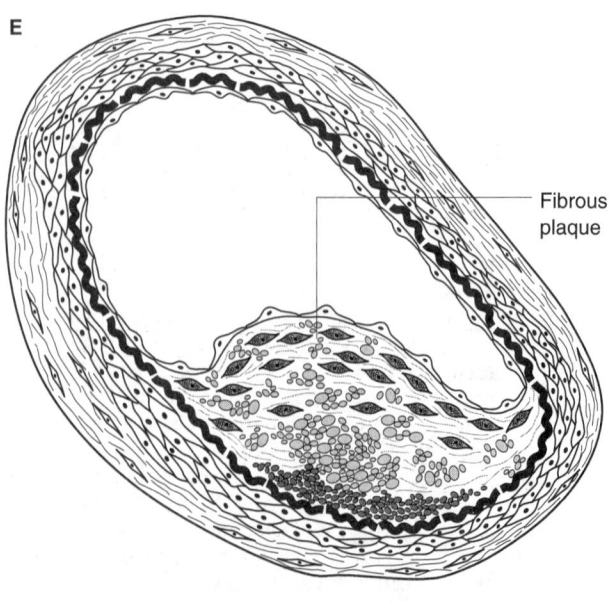

Figure 65-2. Developmental stages of the lesions of atherosclerosis. (A) The normal muscular artery consists of an internal intima with endothelium and internal elastic lamina. The smooth muscle of the vessel wall is in the media and the thin adventitial layer contains connective tissue and vasa vasorum. With age, the thin and sparsely muscled intima increases in thickness and smooth muscle cell content. (B) In the first phase of an atherosclerotic lesion, there is focal thickening of the intima with smooth muscle cells and extracellular matrix. There is also initial accumulation of intercellular lipid deposits. (C) Extracellular lipid may also develop. (D) When both intercellular and extracellular lipid is present in the earliest phase, it is referred to as a *fatty streak*. (E) A fibrous plaque results from continued accumulation of fibroblasts covering proliferating smooth muscle cells laden with lipids and cell debris. The lesion becomes more complex as continuing cell degeneration leads to ingress of blood constituents and calcification. (After Glomset JA, Ross R. Atherosclerosis and the arterial smooth muscle cells. Science 1973;180:1332)

an increase in the frequency or severity of angina after a stable period.

Angina often is graded according to the New York Heart Association description of the severity of heart failure:

Class I—no symptoms of heart failure
Class II—symptoms at exertion
Class III—symptoms at mild exertion, such as normal daily activities
Class IV—symptoms at rest

The differential diagnosis of angina includes esophagitis due to gastrointestinal reflux, peptic ulcer disease, biliary colic, visceral artery ischemia, pericarditis, pleurisy, thoracic aortic dissection, and many musculoskeletal disorders.

Physical Examination

Physical examination usually shows no detectable signs of coronary artery disease, but evidence of associated conditions such as peripheral vascular disease may exist. Patients may have loss of pulses or bruits in the carotid arteries, abdomen, or femoral arteries. Other signs include ocular xanthomas and hypertensive retinal changes.

Diagnostic Studies

Laboratory Studies. Tests are conducted for cardiac risk factors, such as diabetes mellitus, hyperlipidemia, and hyperthyroidism. Anemia in the presence of coronary obstruction may precipitate angina because of myocardial ischemia.

Electrocardiogram. The diagnosis of myocardial ischemia requires documentation of ECG changes of ischemia during chest pain or exercise testing (Fig. 65-3). An ECG often is normal but may reveal evidence of an old MI. These changes include Q waves or loss of R-wave progression in the precordial leads. Chronic ST-segment and T-wave changes may suggest underlying coronary disease, but these signs are not specific.

Stress Testing. A stress test may be used to detect the presence of coronary disease or assess the functional importance of coronary lesions. The test is positive if the patient has signs or symptoms of angina pectoris with typical ischemic ECG changes. ECG changes used to confirm the diagnosis are downward sloping depressions in the ST segment. The specificity of a stress test may improve with thallium injection during exercise. If a patient has coronary ischemia, the involved area of myocardium does not take up thallium initially, and a defect appears on a myocardial scan. As the patient recovers from exercise and the ischemia is relieved, the defect fills. A defect that does not

fill throughout thallium scanning is a sign of irreversibly scarred, nonviable myocardium.

Coronary Arteriography. Coronary arteriography is the only way to make the definitive diagnosis of coronary disease. It is indicated for patients with atypical presentations and borderline or normal stress tests and when a patient is a candidate for surgical treatment of valvular or coronary artery disease.

Medical Management

Controllable risk factors are identified and reduced by means of weight reduction, smoking cessation, blood pressure control, and limitation of dietary fats. Hyperthyroidism or anemia, which may exacerbate angina, is corrected.

The goal of therapy for angina pectoris is to decrease the imbalance between myocardial oxygen supply and demand. Most medications used to manage angina pectoris have a greater effect on reducing myocardial oxygen demand than on increasing supply. These drugs include nitroglycerin, nitrate compounds, β-adrenergic blocking agents, and calcium-channel blocking agents such as nifedipine and diltiazem.

ACUTE MYOCARDIAL INFARCTION

Acute MI is caused by interruption of the blood supply to the myocardium. It is the result of *loss of oxygen supply* not of increased myocardial oxygen demand. MI usually is caused by coronary artery thrombosis at a site of stenosis over a complicated plaque. Thrombosis may be caused by plaque rupture, hemorrhage, or coronary spasm.

One determinant of prognosis after acute MI is the amount of ventricular myocardium that undergoes necrosis. Loss of 25% of ventricular myocardium leads to symptomatic cardiac dysfunction. Acute loss of >40% frequently is associated with cardiogenic shock and death. Treatment during MI focuses on immediate improvement in blood flow to the area at risk to decrease myocardial loss. Collaterals may supply enough flow to limit the amount of myocardium lost.

Diagnosis

Symptoms

Pain is the most common symptom of MI. It is deep and visceral, and frequently described as heavy or crushing. However, some patients feel no pain. The combination of substernal chest pain that lasts >20 to 30 minutes and

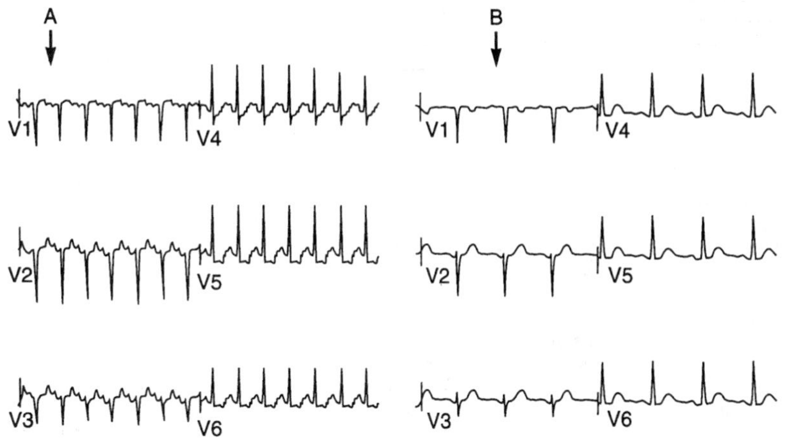

Figure 65-3. ECG from a 60-year-old man during an exercise test showing the standard precordial leads, V_1 through V_6. During exercise (*A*) ST segment depression and ischemia are seen in leads V_4 through V_6, which resolved after the exercise was stopped (*B*). (After Wagner GS. Ischemia due to increased myocardial demand. In: Marriott's practical electrocardiography, ed 9. Baltimore, Williams & Wilkins, 1994)

diaphoresis strongly suggests MI. Anterior MIs (involving the LAD) produce sympathetic hyperactivity with tachycardia and hypertension. Inferior infarctions (involving the RCA) frequently cause parasympathetic activity with bradycardia and hypotension.

ECG Findings

The classic ECG signs of acute MI are the development of Q waves and elevated ST segments in leads that reflect the affected area (Fig. 65-4). Clinicians often characterize MIs by ECG changes. For example, transmural infarctions produce Q waves. Subendocardial or nontransmural infarctions produce transient ST-segment changes with evolving T-wave inversion but without the development of Q waves.

Laboratory Studies

Serum levels of creatine kinase, a cardiac enzyme involved in high-energy phosphate metabolism, increase after myocardial cell death and rise within 8 to 24 hours, returning to normal within 1 to 2 days. Because creatine kinase has several tissue-specific isoenzymes, it is crucial to measure the specific isoenzyme in cardiac tissue (CK-MB) when ruling out MI.

Management

Immediate Care

In the 4 to 6 hours after the onset of continuing chest pain, it may be unclear whether the patient has unstable preinfarction angina or a process leading to irreversible myocardial injury. The ECG may be unrevealing, and cardiac isoenzyme studies may not be feasible. In this situa-

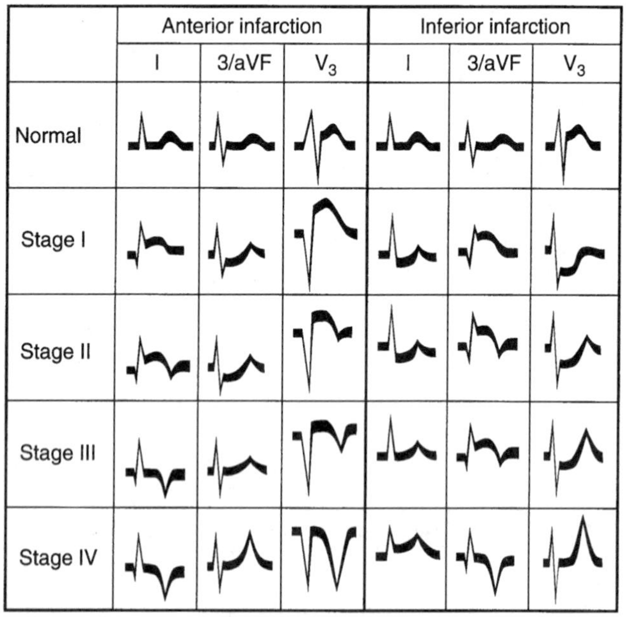

Figure 65-4. The pattern of evolution of the ECG in acute myocardial infarction. In the first stage, acute ST elevations are present in leads reflecting the affected area of myocardium. There are reciprocal ST depressions in leads away from the site of the infarct. Stage 2 T-wave inversion begins, which deepens in stage 3. ST segment elevations are no longer present. A Q wave may develop early, but by stage 4, Q waves are present and persistent T-wave inversions, which may be deep, are seen. (After Marriott HJL. Myocardial infarction. In: Practical electrocardiography, ed 7. Baltimore, Williams & Wilkins, 1983:379).

Table 65-1. INDICATIONS FOR CORONARY BYPASS SURGERY

ANATOMY
Left main coronary artery disease
Triple-vessel disease involving the proximal left anterior descending coronary artery with normal or diminished ejection fraction
Double-vessel disease involving the proximal left anterior descending coronary artery with normal or diminished ejection fraction

SYMPTOMS
Unstable (crescendo) angina
Post-myocardial infarction angina
Acute coronary occlusion after percutaneous transluminal coronary angioplasty
Symptoms unsuccessfully controlled with medical therapy
Controlled symptoms, but with unacceptable life style

tion, oxygen is administered, heart rhythm is monitored, and lidocaine is given to prevent ventricular fibrillation. At this point, ischemic myocardium can be salvaged before irreversible necrosis occurs.

Initial treatment is control of pain, most often with IV *morphine.* Decreasing anxiety and pain may have a therapeutic effect, decreasing myocardial oxygen demand and limiting infarct size. IV *nitroglycerin* begun at a low dose to prevent the side effects of hypotension and headache may diminish infarct size, decrease the likelihood of sudden death, and lower the incidence of congestive heart failure. *β Blockers* limit infarct size and decrease the likelihood of early mortality.

Thrombolysis

Thrombolytic agents are used to dissolve coronary thrombi, reversing the process that leads to MI. The earlier the treatment, the greater is the effect; the greatest benefit is achieved within 1 to 2 hours of the onset of symptoms. Complications of thrombolytic therapy include allergic reactions, hemorrhage, and stroke.

Surgical Treatment After Acute Myocardial Infarction

Indications

Postinfarction angina
Cardiogenic shock
Ventricular septal defect
Acute mitral regurgitation
Free wall rupture

Percutaneous Transluminal Coronary Angioplasty

PTCA is a cardiac catheterization technique used to reduce the degree of coronary stenosis and improve regional blood flow.

Indications. The ideal lesion for PTCA is symmetric focal stenosis in an epicardial vessel. PTCA is *contraindicated* if there is substantial disease in the left main coronary artery, if the target coronary artery is <2 mm in luminal diameter, if multiple obstructive lesions are present in the same artery, or if there are complex lesions, such as those involving or straddling arterial bifurcations.

Technique. Under fluoroscopic guidance, a catheter is directed into the coronary artery to be treated. A guide wire is then placed across the obstructing lesion. A balloon catheter is passed over the guide wire and the balloon positioned in the mid-portion of the lesion. The balloon is inflated, sometimes several times, to widen the lumen of the aorta. After the catheter is withdrawn, coronary angiography is performed to assess the degree of dilation and to identify dilation-related complications.

Complications. The primary risk of angioplasty is dissection of the coronary artery. MI may occur but these patients can be treated with immediate surgical revascularization. Other risks include cerebral vascular accident and local arterial trauma.

Coronary Artery Bypass Operation

Indications The indications for coronary artery bypass grafting (CABG) are listed in Table 65-1. Emergency CABG is indicated as soon as it is apparent that an acute coronary occlusion has occurred, an event heralded by the onset of chest pain, ECG changes, or hemodynamic instability. The presence and nature of an acute coronary occlusion can be verified with immediate coronary angiography.

Preoperative Care. During evolving MI, ischemic injury can be attenuated and hemodynamic stability achieved if intraaortic balloon counterpulsation is established promptly in the catheterization laboratory before transport to the operating room. If the patient has severe hemodynamic instability despite balloon pump support, portable cardiopulmonary bypass perfusion may allow sufficient stabilization for transport to the operating room.

Cardiopulmonary bypass is initiated as quickly as possible to begin cardioplegic arrest and myocardial cooling and to prevent extension of the infarction (Fig. 65-5).

Surgical Technique. In CABG, a diseased coronary artery is bypassed with an alternative conduit for delivery of blood beyond the stenosis. Most patients require multivessel grafting, and typically have a combination of vein grafts and a mammary artery graft (Fig. 65-6). *[handwritten: Saphenous internal Thoracic artery]*

If diffuse atherosclerotic changes are found during CABG, or if the site chosen for a distal anastomosis is heavily diseased, the surgeon may perform an endarterectomy to improve flow and facilitate the anastomosis. Endarterectomy is reserved for patients with distal disease so severe that flow otherwise is impossible.

Postoperative Care. Hemodynamic monitoring is provided in an intensive care unit. Arterial blood pressure, central venous pressure, pulmonary capillary wedge pressure, cardiac output, and urine output are monitored. Arterial blood gases, complete blood counts, electrolyte levels, and ECG are performed at intervals.

A chest radiograph is obtained when the patient arrives at the ICU to check for the position of the endotracheal tube, nasogastric tube, chest tubes, and Swan–Ganz catheter. Pleural effusion, pneumothorax, and mediastinal widening are ruled out, and a follow-up chest radiograph is

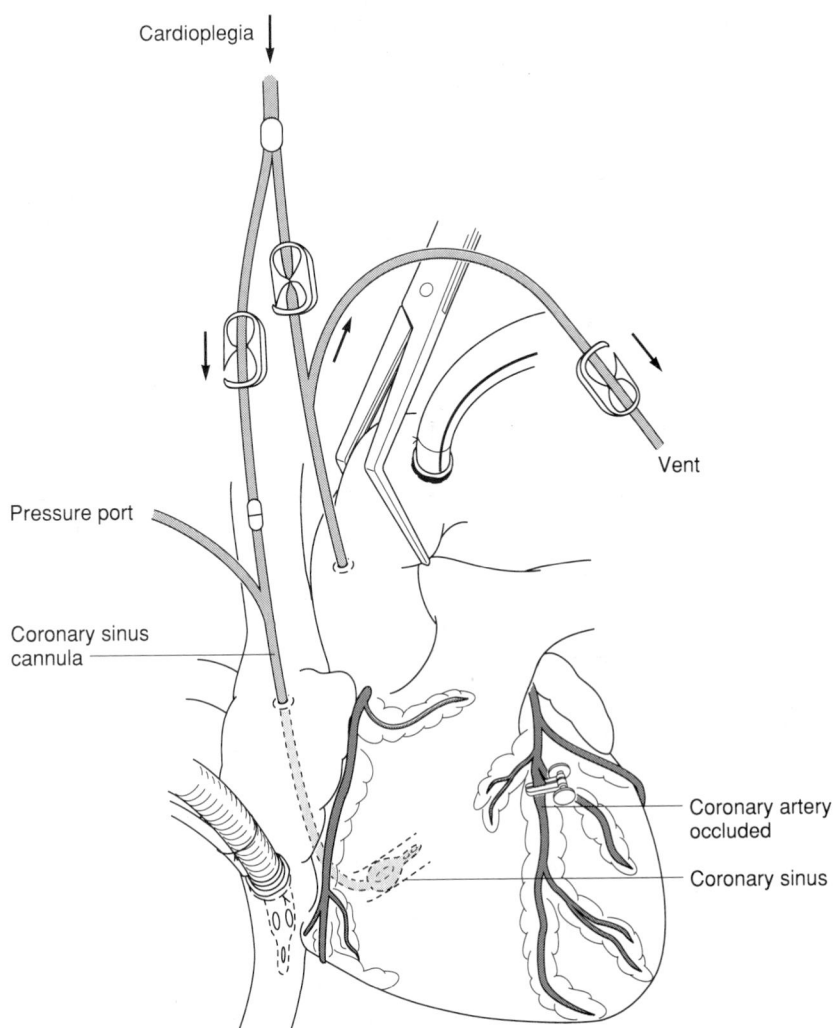

Cardioplegia

Pressure port

Coronary sinus cannula

Vent

Coronary artery occluded

Coronary sinus

Figure 65-5. Cardiac instrumentation for retrograde cardioplegic administration through the coronary sinus. A catheter with an occlusive balloon tip has been placed within the coronary sinus through the right atrium. The cardioplegic solution can be administered by means of the coronary sinus or the aortic root (antegrade). There is a pressure-measuring side port on the coronary sinus catheter that can be used to prevent overdistention of the coronary venous system. (After Partington MT, et al. Studies of retrograde cardioplegia I. J Thorac Cardiovasc Surg 1989;97:613)

obtained 8 to 12 hours later. Mediastinal and chest tube drainage is recorded hourly.

The patient is weighed for fluid management. All patients have a capillary leak syndrome after cardiopulmonary bypass. Fluid accumulation with a marked increase in total body sodium and weight gain of 5 to 10 kg is typical.

After extubation, which occurs 4 to 12 hours postoperatively, pulmonary toilet is vigorous. Most patients who undergo CABG can be transferred to a stepdown unit the day after the operation. There they undergo monitoring for arrhythmias and gradual diuresis to return to preoperative weight. They also begin eating a regular diet and start walking.

Complications. *Low cardiac output.* Patients are vigorously rewarmed, given adequate crystalloid or colloid solution, and are often treated with a vasodilator. Arrhythmias and bradycardia are managed with atrial or AV pacing.

Bleeding. Platelet function and blood clotting factors may not return to normal for up to 36 hours. Average postoperative blood loss is 400 to 800 mL, and much of this shed blood can be reinfused. Bleeding at a rate >200 mL/hr for ≥4 hours postoperatively is considered excessive, and abnormalities in coagulation are corrected aggressively. Reexploration is needed if bleeding continues after correction of coagulopathy.

Sudden cessation of excessive bleeding is a sign of *cardiac tamponade.* Transesophageal echocardiography is used to establish this diagnosis and assess ventricular function and preload.

The serious *wound complications* are sternal infection, dehiscence, and mediastinitis. Staphylococcus usually is the pathogen, and often is methicillin resistant. Risk factors are preoperative hospital stay >2 days, chronic ob-

structive pulmonary disease with prolonged ventilator support, use of bilateral internal mammary artery grafts, and low cardiac output.

Stroke is due to atherosclerotic emboli that probably originate from the aorta and are loosened by cannulation, cross clamping, or construction of the proximal anastomoses.

Postpericardiotomy syndrome is a delayed pericardial inflammatory reaction characterized by fever, anterior chest pain, and pericardial friction rub. Treatment with nonsteroidal anti-inflammatory drugs usually eliminates the symptoms.

Risk factors for operative mortality are listed in Table 65-2.

Table 65-2. PREDICTION OF THE RISK FOR OPERATIVE MORTALITY*			
	Low	Medium	High
Age	60 yr	75 yr	75 yr
Gender	Male	Female	Female
Diabetes	No	Yes	Yes
Unstable angina	Yes	No	Yes
Ejection fraction	65%	35%	25%
Three-vessel disease	Yes	Yes	Yes
Operative incidence	First	First	Redo
Predicted mortality rate	0.8%	3.4%	12%

* Based on The Society of Thoracic Surgery National Cardiac Database Risk Stratification Algorithm.

SUGGESTED READING

Akins CW. Controversies in myocardial revascularization: coronary artery surgery for single-vessel disease. Semin Thorac Cardiovasc Surg 1994;6:109.

Green MA, Gray LA Jr, Slater AD, Ganzel BL, Mavroudis C. Emergency aortocoronary bypass after failed angioplasty. Ann Thorac Surg 1991;51:194.

Grover FL, Johnson RR, Marshall G, et al. Factors predictive of operative mortality among coronary artery bypass subsets. Ann Thorac Surg 1993;56:1296.

Lawrie, GM, Morris GC Jr, Earle N. Long-term results of coronary bypass surgery: analysis of 1698 patients followed 15 to 20 years. Ann Surg 1991;213:355.

Lytle BW, Loop FD, Taylor PC, et al. The effect of coronary reoperation on the survival of patients with stenoses in saphenous vein bypass grafts to coronary arteries. J Thorac Cardiovasc Surg 1993;105:605.

Myers WO, Schaff HV, Gersh BJ, et al. Improved survival of surgically treated patients with triple vessel coronary disease and severe angina pectoris. J Thorac Cardiovasc Surg 1989;98:487.

Nwasokwa ON, Koss JR, Friedman GH, Grunwald AM, Bodenheimer MM. Bypass surgery for chronic stable angina: predictors of survival benefit and strategy for patient selection. Ann Intern Med 1991;114:1035.

Rosengart TK, Krieger K, Lang SJ, et al. Reoperative coronary artery bypass surgery: improved preservation of myocardial function with retrograde cardioplegia. Circulation 1993;88:II330.

Smith JM, Rath R, Feldman DJ, Schreiber JT. Coronary artery bypass grafting in the elderly: changing trends and results. J Cardiovasc Surg 1992;33:468.

White HD, Rivers JT, Maslowski AH, et al. Effect of intravenous streptokinase as compared with that of tissue plasminogen activator on left ventricular function after first myocardial infarction. N Engl J Med 1989;320:817.

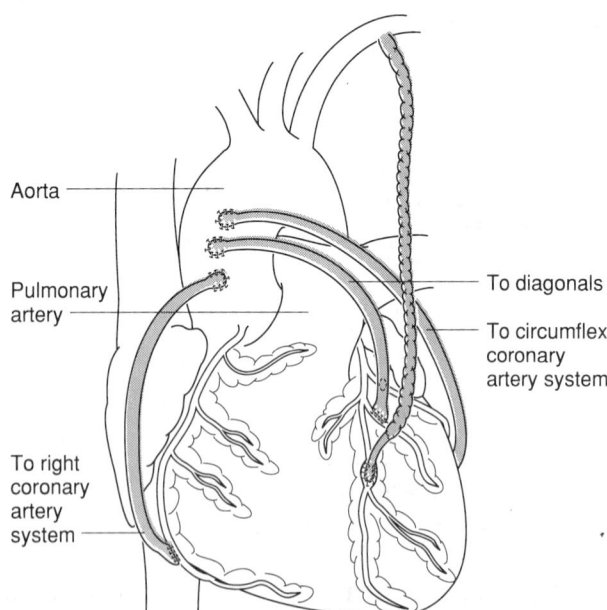

Figure 65-6. Most patients require multivessel grafting and typically have a combination of vein grafts and a mammary artery graft. The most common site for use of the left internal mammary artery is the left anterior descending artery.

ESSENTIALS OF SURGERY: SCIENTIFIC PRINCIPLES AND PRACTICE,
edited by Lazar J. Greenfield, Michael W. Mulholland, Keith T. Oldham, Gerald B. Zelenock,
and Keith D. Lillemoe. Lippincott–Raven Publishers, Philadelphia, © 1997.

CHAPTER 66

MECHANICAL CIRCULATORY SUPPORT

JOHN S. SAPIRSTEIN AND WILLIAM S. PIERCE

Mechanical circulatory support is needed when the heart can no longer safely meet the perfusion requirements of the body. Severe cardiac dysfunction may be the result of an acute event such as myocardial infarction (MI) or of a chronic process, such as idiopathic cardiomyopathy. A variety of devices, ranging from the intraaortic balloon pump (IABP) to the permanent total artificial heart (TAH), are used to treat patients with failing hearts.

INTRAAORTIC BALLOON PUMP

Myocardial oxygen consumption is a function of ventricular wall tension. The time during which wall tension develops is a determinant of oxygen consumption. The *tension–time index* (TTI), the area under the arterial pressure tracing, reflects consumption of oxygen by the heart muscle. Decreasing TTI supports a failing heart.

An IABP withdraws blood from the arterial tree just before ventricular systole and returns it to the circulation during diastole. A catheter-mounted balloon is passed into the aorta and inflated during ventricular diastole, augmenting diastolic blood flow. Deflation just before ejection decreases the afterload of the heart and work during systole. Percutaneous insertion allows timely insertion of an IABP without a surgical procedure.

The benefits of use of an IABP rely on modification of the oxygen supply and demand equilibrium of the heart. Deflation of the intraaortic balloon just before ventricular ejection increases aortic compliance, resulting in a lower ventricular afterload (Fig. 66-1). The reduction decreases myocardial oxygen demand, manifested by a lower TTI or

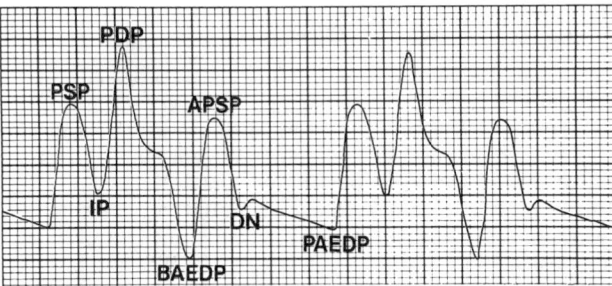

Figure 66-1. Aortic pressure tracing during intraaortic balloon pump support. Balloon counterpulsation is occurring after every other heartbeat (1:2 counterpulsation). With correct timing, balloon inflation (IP) begins immediately after aortic valve closure, signaled by the dicrotic notch (DN). Compared with unassisted ejection, the pump augments diastolic blood flow by increasing peak aortic pressure during diastole (PDP). Balloon deflation before systole decreases ventricular afterload, with lower aortic end-diastolic pressure (BAEDP versus PAEDP) and lower peak systolic pressure (APSP versus PSP). (Courtesy of St Jude Medical, Inc., Cardiac Assist Division, Minneapolis)

a smaller pressure–volume area. Inflation of the balloon during diastole increases aortic root pressure. The increased pressure gradient between the intraventricular cavity and the coronary orifices (diastolic pressure–time index) augments coronary perfusion and oxygen supply. Benefits of the IABP as an adjunct to coronary vessel reperfusion derive from the mechanics of increased intraluminal flow and pressure.

Indications

Myocardial Infarction

An IABP is used to manage cardiogenic shock due to acute MI. The combination of hypotension (systolic blood pressure <90 mmHg) and hypoperfusion (altered mental status, decreased urine output, cool, clammy skin) is the hallmark of cardiogenic shock, a syndrome that complicates about 8% of MIs. Myocardial injury extends beyond the acutely infarcted muscle. The volume of myocardial injury decreases when an IABP is used after coronary vessel occlusion. Infarction size does not decrease, however. Emergency coronary artery bypass grafting in the setting of cardiogenic shock after MI dramatically improves survival, and better outcomes are achieved when IABP support is instituted before revascularization.

The role of an IABP during thrombolysis or percutaneous transluminal coronary angioplasty (PTCA) is to provide hemodynamic stabilization. Ameliorating the oxygen supply-to-demand balance with an IABP immediately after reperfusion seems to salvage more of the "stunned" myocardium. Use of an IABP also reduces the likelihood of reocclusion of coronary vessels after thrombolytic therapy for acute MI and after emergency PTCA.

Cardiac Operations

Low-output syndrome results from ventricular dysfunction after a technically adequate cardiac surgical procedure. This syndrome manifests itself when a patient's condition does not allow discontinuation of cardiopulmonary bypass (CPB). Contributing factors include inadequate myocardial preservation during the procedure, long bypass periods (>2 hours), and poor ventricular function before the operation. For patients for whom pharmacologic therapy is insufficient, mechanical support with an IABP is effective.

Ventricular septal rupture and *acute mitral regurgitation* are surgical emergencies that can occur after acute MI. Ischemia involving the posteromedial papillary muscle is the most common cause of acute mitral regurgitation; nonischemic causes include rupture of chordae tendineae and endocarditis. Pulmonary edema is a frequent finding. Ventricular septal rupture usually develops within 1 week of the MI. It is characterized by a large left-to-right shunt. An IABP can provide stabilization in both situations before definitive surgical repair. Modulation of oxygen supply and demand theoretically prevents rapid deterioration of ischemic myocardium associated with the mitral valve apparatus. Lowering ventricular afterload with an IABP can decrease the fraction of left heart output shunted into the low-pressure right heart.

Cardiogenic shock can be caused by nonischemic insults such as viral myocarditis. An IABP can assist the injured heart until ventricular function improves. If adequate recovery does not return, the patient can undergo heart transplantation. The IABP is a first-step, short-term bridging device when a donor heart is not immediately available.

Noncardiac Operations

Noncardiac operations place elderly patients at high risk for MI. Prophylactic placement of an IABP can be attempted for carefully selected patients. The physician must weigh any added margin of safety against the morbidity associated with use of an IABP.

Septic Shock

The pathophysiologic aspects of septic shock are markedly more complex than those of cardiogenic shock. There may be hemodynamic benefit to counterpulsation for patients with septic shock, but this is not standard therapy.

Insertion and Operation of Intraaortic Balloon Pumps

The common femoral artery is entered by means of a skin puncture about 3 cm below the inguinal ligament. This anatomic site allows hemostasis by means of direct compression during catheter removal. It also limits distal limb ischemia associated with cannulation of the smaller superficial femoral artery.

After passage of a flexible guide wire, the soft tissue track and vessel are dilated until an appropriately sized sheath can be inserted. A catheter is passed proximally until the tip rests in the thoracic aorta just distal to the left subclavian artery, at about the level of the left second intercostal space. Fluoroscopic guidance can aid the procedure. A chest radiograph is used to confirm positioning.

Direct surgical placement sometimes is necessary (eg, for obese patients). The catheter is inserted through a pursestring suture in the vessel or an anastomosed prosthetic graft. Alternative access sites, such as the axillary artery, sometimes are used. The balloon catheter also can be placed directly into the aorta during a thoracic surgical procedure.

Counterpulsation can be timed with an electrocardiogram (ECG) or arterial pressure tracing. The goal is to achieve balloon inflation immediately after aortic valve closure and deflation just before ventricular ejection. Anticoagulation protocols vary; heparin or low–molecular-weight dextran usually is used. Meticulous wound management is needed to prevent local and systemic infection, and patients must stay at bed rest.

Discontinuation of IABP support involves a gradual increase in heartbeat-to-counterpulsation ratio. Back-bleeding during catheter removal decreases the likelihood of distal ischemic events. Removal may necessitate a surgical procedure, particularly if the catheter was placed surgically; embolectomy usually is performed in this situation.

Complications

Complications of IABP use are:

Ischemia distal to the catheter insertion site (the most common)
Infection and localized hematoma
Vessel perforation with extensive hemorrhage
Aortic dissection from catheter passage below the intima
Pseudoaneurysm formation at the vessel puncture site
Peripheral nerve damage
Lymphatic disruption with fistula formation

The balloon can occlude branches of the aorta and, depending on the extent of preexisting vascular disease, cause ischemia of the tissues supplied by these vessels. Examples of this are intestinal "angina" from occlusion of the mesenteric vessels and upper extremity symptoms when the balloon impinges on the left subclavian artery. Cardiac function worsens if the catheter tip traverses the aortic valve.

The relatively small volumes of gas in the balloon yield minimal sequelae in the rare event of intraluminal balloon rupture. The high solubility of carbon dioxide in blood makes it preferable to helium in an IABP.

EXTRACORPOREAL MEMBRANE OXYGENATION AND VENTRICULAR ASSIST DEVICES

If the left ventricle cannot produce a baseline systemic pressure—because of profound cardiogenic shock, physical injury to the heart, or severe dysrhythmias—IABP support is ineffective. In such situations, more elaborate measures to support the circulation are needed. Circulatory support beyond use of an IABP most often involves use of a ventricular assist device (VAD). Some devices are appropriate for short-term applications in an acutely failing heart; others are used for long-term bridging to cardiac transplantation.

Extracorporeal Membrane Oxygenation

Because CPB is limited to a maximum of 6 hours, the CPB circuit includes membrane oxygenation. Designed to manage pulmonary dysfunction, extracorporeal membrane oxygenation (ECMO) entails use of a venovenous or venoarterial bypass circuit. The circuit involves cannulation of the common carotid or common femoral artery and the internal jugular vein, femoral vein, or both.

Effective balloon counterpulsation is difficult in children because their aortas are highly elastic and because IABPs sized for very small patients are not widely available. ECMO is an effective intervention for children, and it may be possible to use ECMO to treat adults with cardiogenic shock unresponsive to use of an IABP. There appears to be a synergism when ECMO and IABP are combined in the immediate management of MI.

The *disadvantages* are that ECMO may cause hematologic changes and that a whole-body inflammatory response occurs in response to circulatory bypass. Although any mechanical circulatory support device with interfaces between blood and artificial surface can promote these reactions, the likelihood appears higher with ECMO, because of the interactions between the blood and the oxygenator surface. The complexity of ECMO mandates continuous intensive care, often with the patient pharmacologically paralyzed, and the circuit requires high levels of anticoagulation.

Ventricular Assist Devices

Many types of VAD exist. Some can be applied only to the left ventricle, and others can be used for either or both ventricles. Delivered flow is pulsatile or nonpulsatile. Although some devices are better suited than others for particular situations, all systems are indicated only for treatment of patients with severe, refractory cardiac dysfunction. The predominant indications for use of a VAD are postcardiotomy cardiogenic shock (PCCS) and bridging to cardiac transplantation.

General inclusion criteria for VAD implantation are listed in Table 66-1. Left ventricular assistance is the most common type of support used. Isolated right heart failure in adults is rare. Right ventricular failure, when present, usually becomes evident after mechanical support of the failing left ventricle is initiated. If right ventricular failure does develop, pharmacologic support with inotropic agents and pulmonary vasodilators (isoproterenol, prostaglandin E_1, and nitric oxide) can be tried. Persistent dysfunction may necessitate use of a right VAD.

Table 66-1. CHARACTERIZATION OF VENTRICULAR FAILURE

LEFT VENTRICULAR FAILURE
Cardiac index <1.8 L/min/m^2
Left atrial pressure >20 mmHg
Peak systolic aortic pressure <90 mmHg
Scant urine output
Poor tissue perfusion

RIGHT VENTRICULAR FAILURE
Cardiac index <1.8 L/min/m^2
Right atrial pressure >20 mmHg
Left atrial pressure <15 mmHg

Implantation of a VAD usually necessitates CPB. Complications of use of the devices include perioperative bleeding, infection, thromboembolism, and hemolysis. Hemolysis results from physical trauma to erythrocytes caused by the mechanical pumps. Risk for bleeding depends, in part, on the anticoagulation requirements of the specific device. Excessive bleeding may necessitate transfusion of blood products, predisposing the patient to infection with blood-borne pathogens.

Of particular concern for patients awaiting transplantation is transmission of cytomegalovirus, infection with which can severely complicate posttransplantation management. Exposure to foreign antigens also makes location of an antigenically acceptable organ difficult. Infection in a transplant recipient about to undergo induction immunosuppression is dangerous.

Patients who need mechanical circulatory support are at high risk for infection for several reasons. At the time of device placement, these patients are in hemodynamically unstable condition, which compromises their immune response. The implanted components of the systems are a large potential nidus for infection.

Nonpulsatile Devices

There are three types of nonpulsatile VAD: roller-head pumps, centrifugal pumps, and axial flow pumps. These devices are not actuated in a phasic manner; their pumps operate in a continuous, unidirectional manner.

The pumps are mechanically simple. The continuous, high-speed nature of these systems, however, tends to produce substantial blood trauma. An empiric law of fluid mechanics, the "no-slip" condition, requires that blood immediately adjacent to a pump surface be stationary. The change in the velocity of blood flow away from the stationary surface is the *shear rate*. Stress on the blood and all the elements suspended within it is directly proportional to the shear rate. Shear rates and the resulting shear stresses are produced by all types of pumps, but the shearing caused by nonpulsatile pumps is particularly high. The stress imposed on erythrocytes can lead to membrane instability and hemolysis with release of free hemoglobin into the bloodstream.

Shear stresses have profound effects on platelets and the clotting cascade. Shearing can elicit changes in the expression and functionality of platelet membrane glycoproteins, inducing the binding of von Willebrand factor and fibrinogen. These events are critical to activation and aggregation of platelets and the formation of platelet thrombi. Shearing also causes platelet fragmentation, exposing more cellular surface on which catalytic amplification of the clotting cascade can occur.

Nonpulsatile pumps can cause thrombus formation and subsequent risk for embolic events, in part, because of the high shear stresses. Thrombus formation and relatively high levels of hemolysis and operational constraints have limited nonpulsatile ventricular support to short-term use (several days to a week). Nonpulsatile pumps are not optimal for bridging to transplantation. They are, however, well suited to temporary support of patients with PCCS.

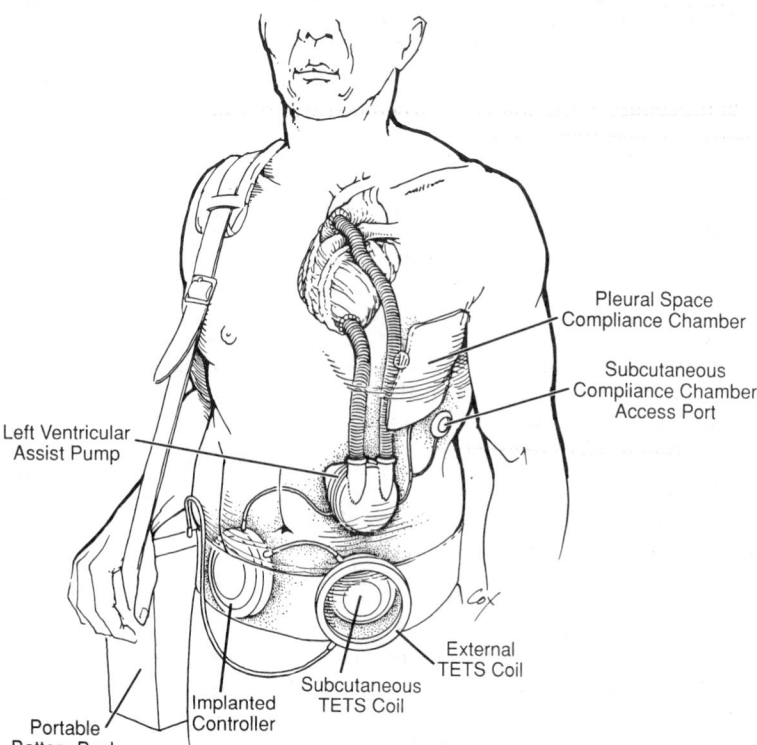

Figure 66-2. Penn State electric left ventricular assist device. This diagram shows the anticipated placement in a human recipient. All implanted components except the cannulas and compliance chamber are positioned subcutaneously. There are no percutaneous wires or external vents for this system. Battery packs are designed to power the system using the transcutaneous energy transmission system (TETS) for 8 hours before recharging.

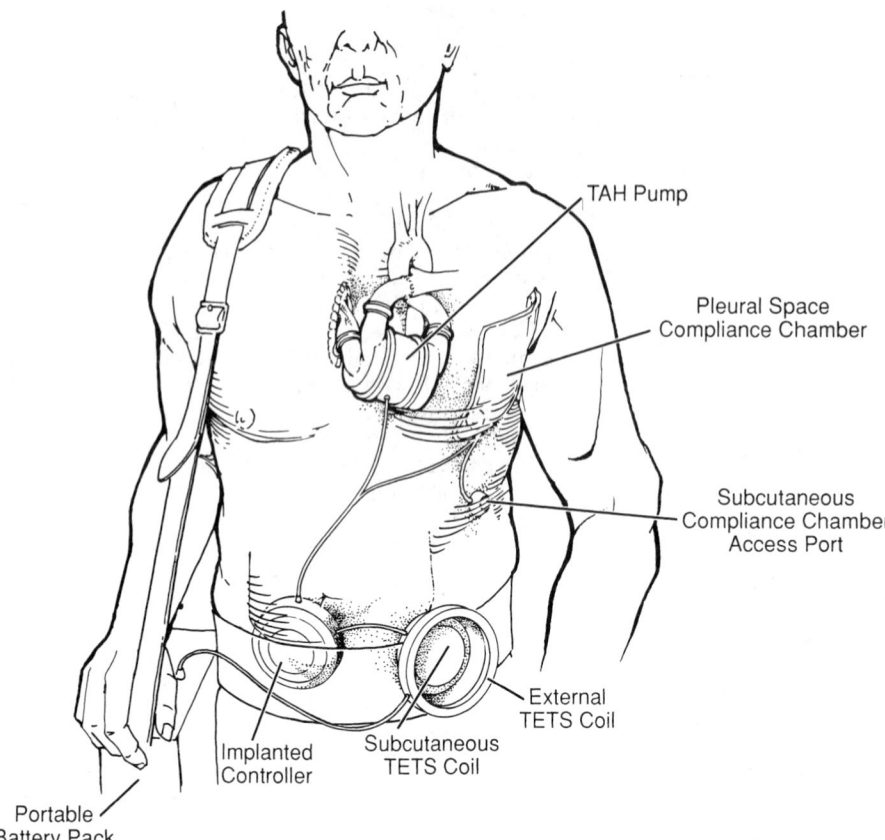

TAH Pump

Pleural Space
Compliance Chamber

Subcutaneous
Compliance Chamber
Access Port

External
TETS Coil

Subcutaneous
TETS Coil

Implanted
Controller

Portable
Battery Pack

Figure 66-3. PSU/Sarns electric total artificial heart (TAH). This diagram shows the anticipated placement in a human recipient. As with the permanent electric left ventricular assist device, this completely implantable system contains no percutaneous lines or vents. Similar designs are employed for the Abiomed/THI and CCF/Nimbus hearts. TETS, transcutaneous energy transmission system.

Pulsatile Devices

Pulsatile VADs contain blood-pumping chambers that are completely isolated from their actuating mechanisms. The need for biocompatible seals and bearings is greatly reduced, and the systems are suited to long-term pumping. For this reason, pulsatile VADs are particularly advantageous for bridging to heart transplantation. The issue of nonphysiologic blood flow is also less important than with nonpulsatile pumps.

TOTAL ARTIFICIAL HEARTS

A total artificial heart (TAH) consists of orthotopically positioned blood pumps that physically and functionally replace the left and right ventricles. The main indication for placement of a TAH is biventricular failure in a transplantation candidate that cannot be corrected with use of a left VAD and pharmacologic support of the right ventricle. This situation might also be managed by means of implantation of bilateral VADs. When the heart is extremely dilated and lacking much contractility, there may be an advantage to excising the thrombogenic ventricles.

A TAH can be used to treat a small number of patients with left-sided heart failure whose myocardium is so compromised that placement of a VAD would be unsafe or ineffective. This includes transplantation candidates with ischemic cardiomyopathy who experience ventricular rupture or who have an irreparable ventricular septal defect with a large shunt.

The decision to use a TAH as opposed to a VAD is not trivial; implantation of the more complicated TAH puts the patient at high risk for perioperative morbidity. The procedure, which involves cardiectomy, carries a high risk for bleeding. If the device fails, there is no residual native

heart function to even minimally sustain the circulation while corrective measures are taken.

Control of a TAH is intrinsically more difficult than control of a VAD. A VAD maximizes its output in direct proportion to the preload of the pump, a function of intravascular volume status. The blood volumes pumped out of the native left and right ventricles are not in equilibrium. The discrepancy is due in part to left-to-left shunt of bronchial blood and to differing characteristics of the great vessels. Passive pulmonic perfusion, or right-to-left pass-through flow, can occur in the TAH. The TAH control algorithm must respond to differing left and right volume requirements if adequate perfusion is to be maintained. Two TAHs, both pneumatically driven, are under clinical investigation.

PERMANENT CIRCULATORY SUPPORT SYSTEMS

Limited donor heart availability means that 10% to 40% of patients die awaiting transplantation. A permanently implanted device—one that provides its recipient with good quality of life at an acceptable cost—may ameliorate the supply-demand disparity in transplantation.

A permanent VAD offers several advantages over a permanent TAH. Many candidates for a support device may not need replacement of both right and left ventricles. Residual heart function can provide a safety net if a mechanical device fails. If univentricular support suffices, implantation of a TAH is inappropriate. Although nonpulsatile blood pumps for longer-term use are being developed, the systems specifically targeted as permanent substitutes for transplantation deliver pulsatile blood flow. Figure 66-2 shows an example of an implanted left VAD.

The goal in developing a long-term, implantable TAH is to produce a tether-free device that offers recipients a reasonably normal life style. The device must have no percutaneous lines, and the system must respond to the varying circulatory demands of everyday activity. The TAH must supply an output of 8 L/min from each ventricle, given physiologic preloads and afterloads. Because the system must work for at least 5 years, biocompatibility is essential.

Each TAH system has orthotopically positioned blood pumps that alternately eject blood into the pulmonary and systemic vasculature. All four systems in development use brushless direct-current motors that are powered by a transcutaneous energy transmission system (TETS). Implanted nickel-cadmium batteries drive the system if the external coils detach. A TAH converts the movements of a motor into the pulsatile pumping of blood. The control schemes of TAH systems demonstrate so-called Starling behavior to the extent that increased venous return elicits a commensurate increase in left pump output until maximum output is reached. Figure 66-3 illustrates placement of a TAH system in an average-sized patient.

SUGGESTED READING

Barnett MG, Swartz MT, Peterson GJ, et al. Vascular complications from intraaortic balloons: risk analysis. J Vasc Surg 1994; 19:81.

Dembitsky WP, Moore CH, Holman WL, et al. Successful mechanical circulatory support for noncoronary shock. J Heart Lung Transplant 1992;11:129.

Gurbel PA, Anderson RD, MacCord CS, et al. Arterial diastolic pressure augmentation by intraaortic balloon counterpulsation enhances the onset of coronary artery reperfusion by thrombolytic therapy. Circulation 1994;89:361.

Ishihara M, Sato H, Tateishi H, et al. Intraaortic balloon pumping as the postangioplasty strategy in acute myocardial infarction. Am Heart J 1991;122:385.

Lazar HL, Treanor P, Yang XM, et al. Enhanced recovery of ischemic myocardium by combining percutaneous bypass with intraaortic balloon pump support. Ann Thorac Surg 1994; 57:663.

Magovern GJ Jr, Magovern JA, Benckart DH, et al. Extracorporeal membrane oxygenation: preliminary results in patients with postcardiotomy cardiogenic shock. Ann Thorac Surg 1994; 57:1462.

Mueller HS. Role of intraaortic counterpulsation in cardiogenic shock and acute myocardial infarction. Cardiology 1994; 84:168.

Phillips ST. Resuscitation for cardiogenic shock with extracorporeal membrane oxygenation systems. Semin Thorac Cardiovasc Surg 1994;6:131.

Pifarre R, Sullivan H, Montoya A, et al. Comparison of results after heart transplantation: mechanically supported versus nonsupported patients. J Heart Lung Transplant 1992;11:235.

ESSENTIALS OF SURGERY: SCIENTIFIC PRINCIPLES AND PRACTICE, edited by Lazar J. Greenfield, Michael W. Mulholland, Keith T. Oldham, Gerald B. Zelenock, and Keith D. Lillemoe. Lippincott–Raven Publishers, Philadelphia, © 1997.

CHAPTER 67

CARDIAC ARRHYTHMIAS AND PERICARDIUM

STEVEN F. BOLLING AND JAMES R. STEWART

CARDIAC ARRHYTHMIAS

Physiology of Arrhythmias

All arrhythmias are caused by automaticity, re-entry, or a combination of these mechanisms.

Automaticity

Myocardial tissue that depolarizes, reaches threshold, and fires an action potential (Fig. 67-1) is *automatic,* and stimulation of the surrounding myocytes generates an automatic rhythm. Automatic rhythms are normal in the sinoatrial (SA) and atrioventricular (AV) nodes. Abnormal automaticity occurs because a pathologic condition moves the resting membrane potential toward threshold, allowing lesser stimuli to achieve threshold and making cardiac muscle hyperexcitable or irritable.

Reentry

Cardiac tissue has a long refractory period; few myocytes remain excitable at the end of a beat. Myocardial ischemia, fibrosis, and necrosis slow electrical conduction and produce nonconductive areas that interrupt conduction waves. These areas of differential myocardial conduction

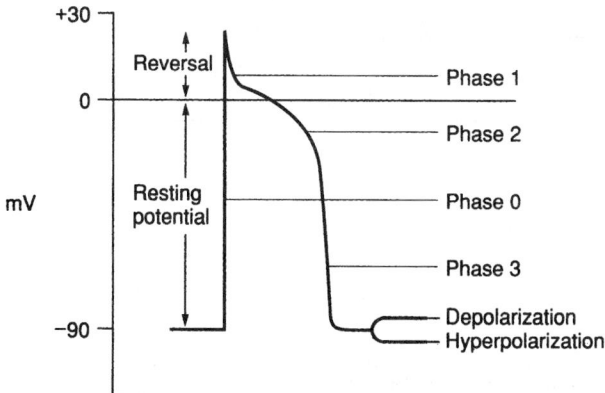

Figure 67-1. A cardiac action potential with a resting potential of −90 mV with respect to the outside. At the peak of the action potential, the inside of the cell becomes about 30 mV positive with respect to the outside. The upstroke of the action potential is called phase 0. The initial rapid repolarization is phase 1, the plateau or period of persisting depolarization is phase 2, and the period of more rapid repolarization is phase 3. A change in membrane potential away from the resting potential toward zero represents depolarization; a change in the membrane potential that makes the inside of the cell more negative is hyperpolarization. (After Cranefield, Erinson. Cardiac arrhythmias: the role of triggered activity in other mechanisms. Mt Kisko, NY, Futura, 1988)

(Fig. 67-2) can form a *reentry* circuit if the conduction time through this abnormal area exceeds the normal impulse. When a slowed electrical impulse finally leaves the area of abnormal conduction, the surrounding tissue may be stimulated again, setting up an abnormal circuit. Slow conduction of the SA and AV nodes, a shortened refractory period, and anatomic heterogeneity after infarction all favor reentry arrhythmias.

Electrophysiologic Testing

Electrophysiologic studies are used to document that an arrhythmia is automatic or reentry, or of ventricular or supraventricular origin. Electrophysiologic testing is performed in a specialized cardiac catheterization laboratory with multiple invasive catheters on both the venous and arterial sides. The tests are performed in the fasting state, and all antiarrhythmic medications are discontinued at least 24 hours before the procedure.

For supraventricular arrhythmias, electrophysiologic studies can establish the presence of a Kent bundle causing Wolff–Parkinson–White (WPW) syndrome. Other arrhythmias of atrial origin, including atrial fibrillation and AV nodal reentry tachycardia, can be diagnosed.

Electrophysiologic testing for ventricular arrhythmias involves introduction of one to three ventricular stimuli. The goal is to induce sustained ventricular arrhythmia or multiple episodes of nonsustained ventricular tachycardia.

Drug Therapy

Antiarrhythmic drug therapy is the fundamental management of arrhythmias and precedes surgical therapy. Antiarrhythmic drugs are classified according to their action

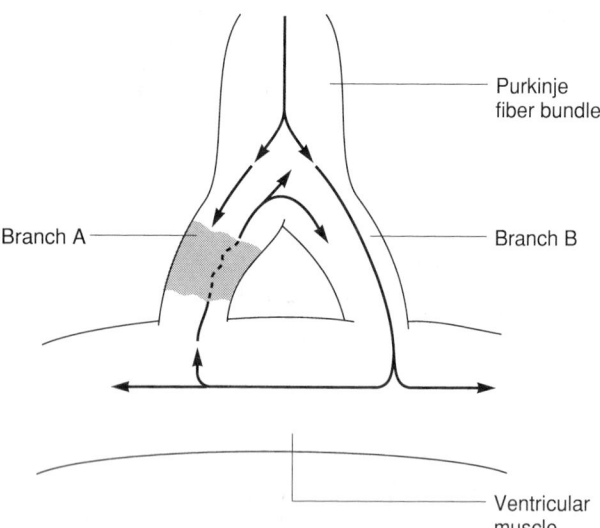

Figure 67-2. Diagram of reentry and circus movement consisting of a fiber bundle that divides into two branches (A and B). Branch A is an area of ischemic injury through which an impulse will not conduct in an antegrade direction but will conduct slowly in a retrograde direction. When an antegrade impulse arrives, it will block in A but will conduct normally through B to activate the ventricular muscle and will enter A in a retrograde fashion. Because retrograde conduction through the area of injury is slowed, the previously depolarized tissue has time to repolarize and become reexcitable. Therefore, when the impulse finally gets through the area of injury, it produces another beat, a ventricular extrasystole (premature ventricular beat). If the impulse continues to go around this reentrant circuit, it will produce a ventricular tachycardia reentrant rhythm. (After Schmitt, Erlanger. J Physiol 1929;87:326)

(Table 67-1). Serial drug testing can be performed during electrophysiologic testing to assess the effects of pharmacologic intervention on arrhythmias.

Supraventricular Arrhythmias

Supraventricular arrhythmias are caused by automatic or reentry factors in normally present, although diseased, myocardial tissue or by abnormal anatomy. The diagnosis is made with electrophysiologic testing. Catheters placed in the heart generate a His bundle electrogram, which allows identification of the presence and type of accessory pathway.

Postoperative supraventricular arrhythmias (atrial flutter, paroxysmal atrial tachycardia, or atrial fibrillation) are the most common arrhythmias encountered in surgical practice. A long rhythm strip or an atrial lead tracing differentiates these arrhythmias from sinus tachycardia. Each of these arrhythmias can cause hypotension and myocardial ischemia.

Patients with compromised vital signs, hypotension, heart rate >150 beats/min, or electrocardiographic (ECG) or clinical evidence of myocardial ischemia need emergency treatment. Patients with stable vital signs can be treated in a less urgent manner. The goals are ventricular rate control and conversion to normal sinus rhythm. Once rhythm is identified, atrial overdrive is attempted for paroxysmal atrial tachycardia or atrial flutter. For recovering cardiac surgical patients, this can be accomplished with temporary wires in place. This may result in conversion to normal sinus rhythm.

Administration of verapamil is the most effective method of rate control, and often causes cardioversion. Digoxin is given to adult patients once their potassium level is normal. Diltiazem is used for ventricular rate control. Rarely are patients so severely compromised by rapid supraventricular tachyrhythmia that emergency cardioversion is required. Cardioversion of patients receiving digoxin is undertaken carefully because these patients are prone to ventricular fibrillation.

Rate control of supraventricular arrhythmias is achieved when ventricular response rate is 80 to 110. At this point, most patients convert to normal sinus rhythm without other drugs. If the supraventricular arrhythmia continues after 48 hours, a class 1A drug is added for cardioversion. For patients with supraventricular arrhythmias, a ventricular-demand pacemaker should be available in case of bradycardia.

Wolff–Parkinson–White Syndrome

The pathophysiologic source of WPW syndrome is the Kent bundle. Kent bundles conduct up to 400 beats/min and can degenerate to ventricular tachycardia or ventricular fibrillation with lethal consequences.

The clinical features of WPW syndrome include an a wave with short PR interval (<0.12 seconds) on ECG. Most patients present with supraventricular tachycardia (SVT), including paroxysmal atrial tachycardia, atrial fibrillation, and atrial flutter. Some present with ventricular tachycardia or ventricular fibrillation.

Medical therapy for WPW syndrome includes procaine, quinidine, propranolol, verapamil, and amiodarone, but it is not particularly successful. The mainstay of treatment is catheter-delivered radiofrequency ablation or surgical interruption of the Kent bundle. The indication for ablation is recurrent SVT in patients at acceptable risk.

Table 67-1. CLASSIFICATION OF ANTIARRHYTHMIC DRUGS

Class	Example	Action
1	Membrane-stabilizing local anesthetics	Sodium channel blockade, which inhibits rapid influx of sodium ions Reduction in velocity in phase 0 of the action potential or rate of membrane depolarization, which slows impulse conduction throughout the myocardium (increased QRS interval) Prolongation of refractory period Reduction of membrane excitability Decrease in phase 4 spontaneous depolarization, which reduces automaticity
1A	Quinidine, disopyramide, procainamide	Moderate slowing and mild prolongation of QRS interval Prolongation of action potential and QT interval
1B	Lidocaine, mexiletine, phenytoin, moricizine, tocainide	No effect on membrane depolarization No change in QRS interval Prolongation of repolarization
1C	Flecainide, encainide, lorcainide, propafenone	Marked reduction in velocity and impulse conduction Prolongation of QRS
2	β Blockers	Antiarrhythmic Adrenergic blockade, which inhibits β-receptor stimulation through the sympathetic nervous system and circulating catecholamines
3	Bretylium, amiodarone, N-acetylprocainamide	Effect on membrane properties Inhibition of potassium influx into cells Prolongation of action potential duration (phase 2 and 3) and membrane repolarization Slow, channel-dependent pacemaker effect (SA and AV nodes)
4	Calcium-channel blockers Verapamil, nifedipine, diltiazem	Generation of slowed action potential mediated by calcium ion influxes into the myocardium (Digitalis, although not a slow-calcium calcium blocking drug, also exerts its effects in pacemaker tissue)

AV Nodal Reentry Tachycardia

Catheter ablation of the His bundle is the most rapid and reliable method of producing permanent AV block.

Atrial Fibrillation

A series of atrial incisions *(maze procedure)* can be made to prevent atrial reentry and allow sinus node impulses to activate the entire atrial myocardium. The maze procedure for atrial fibrillation restores atrial ventricular synchrony and preserves atrial transport function.

Ventricular Arrhythmias

Ventricular arrhythmias during acute MI are common, easily managed, and do not alter prognosis. Late ventricular arrhythmias (after 48 hours) are less common, are difficult to manage, and have a poor prognosis. Refractory ventricular tachycardia after MI is the most common rhythm found at electrophysiologic testing, regardless of the rhythm, causing sudden cardiac death.

The most commonly encountered ventricular arrhythmias are those caused by both reversible and nonreversible ischemic damage. Ventricular arrhythmia caused by reversible ischemia is a diagnosis of exclusion. Patients have coronary artery disease but no MI or irreversible damage, no ventricular wall motion abnormality, and essentially normal left ventricular function. In these patients, ventricular arrhythmias are not induced by electrophysiologic study but can be associated with angina or induced by treadmill testing.

Far more common are ventricular arrhythmias caused by ischemic damage from previous infarctions. The mechanism for ventricular tachycardia in these patients is usually microreentry in the nonhomogeneous ischemic border zones of previous infarctions, where normal myocardial fibers are interspersed with scarring. This morphologic substrate for arrhythmias may be worsened by stress caused by an aneurysm and subendocardial scarring, which extends beyond the aneurysm.

Other causes of ventricular arrhythmias include:

Idiopathic ventricular tachycardia with no other evidence of cardiac disease
Nonischemic cardiomyopathy caused by coxsackievirus or sarcoid
Arrhythmogenic right ventricular dysplasia
Uhl syndrome
Long QT-interval syndrome

Catheter Technique

Catheter ablation for ventricular tachycardia is disappointing.

Surgical Resection

Monomorphic ventricular tachycardia is the arrhythmia most amenable to surgical resection. Some patients who also have inducible ventricular fibrillation can undergo surgical treatment, if the arrhythmia is converted to a monomorphic tachycardia with antiarrhythmic drug therapy.

Indications for surgical therapy are that the patient's condition be refractory to medical treatment; arrhythmia be inducible at electrophysiologic testing; acceptable risk; and an apparent scar or aneurysm. *Contraindications* are inability to induce arrhythmia at electrophysiologic testing; ventricular failure; poor surgical risk; and recent MI.

Preoperative and intraoperative electrophysiologic mapping is used to identify the specific site of origin of the arrhythmia. Coronary angiography and ventriculography are used to determine risk and to determine whether other procedures are needed (CABG, valve operation). During the operation, ventricular tachycardia is induced by means of programmed stimulation after initiation of cardiopulmonary bypass.

The operations used to manage ventricular arrhythmia include encircling endocardial ventriculotomy or extended endocardial resection. Favorable intraoperative factors include generalized resection, which is more effective than localized resection; map-guided resection; and mapping of the warm, beating heart.

Implantable Devices

Implantable devices allow treatment of patients with ventricular tachycardia or fibrillation who have unfavorable anatomy or unsuitable arrhythmias for direct surgical therapy. An automatic internal cardioverter-defibrillator (AICD) is effective for patients with both sustained ventricular tachycardia and fibrillation.

An AICD includes an arrhythmia detection circuit, a power source, and capacitors to store and release electrical current. Electrodes are used for cardioversion and defibrillation, rate sensing, and ventricular pacing. The leads are implanted by a sternotomy, thoracotomy, or subxiphoid approach, and are tunneled to the generator in a subcutaneous abdominal pouch. Arrhythmia detection by an AICD is based on rate criteria or ECG morphologic analysis.

AICD implantation is indicated for drug-refractory ventricular tachycardia and globally depressed left ventricular function without aneurysm, arrhythmia noninducible at electrophysiologic study, and frequent ventricular tachycardia in a patient who cannot undergo direct resection.

Complications of AICDs include programming errors, component failures, and technical problems, including infection, generator migration, and skin erosion. Inappropriate shock also may occur.

PERICARDIUM
Anatomy

The pericardium is the membrane that covers the heart and great vessels. The apex ends in continuity with the adventitia of the great vessels, and the base is attached to the central tendon of the diaphragm. The pericardium is attached to the posterior surface of the sternum by the superior and inferior sternopericardial ligaments, which secure the heart in the thorax, but is separated from the sternum by the lungs and thymus, except for a small area corresponding to the fourth and fifth interspaces anteriorly.

The *serous pericardium* lines the outer fibrous pericardium and consists of a single layer of mesothelial cells. The *visceral pericardium* (epicardium) covers the heart and great vessels. The pericardium folds on itself to form the oblique sinus, a cul-de-sac of serous pericardium behind the left atrium. The space between the aorta and main pulmonary artery anteriorly and the right and left atria posteriorly forms the transverse sinus. The arterial supply to the pericardium is from the internal thoracic arteries and the descending thoracic aorta. Venous drainage is via the azygos system. The pericardium is innervated by the vagus and phrenic nerves and both sympathetic trunks.

Physiology

The function of the pericardium is not known. The pericardium may protect the heart, prevent acute distention, distribute force, or enforce diastolic coupling of the ventricles. The pericardium also serves as an absorptive surface.

Absorption of fluid from the pericardial space occurs predominantly through the thoracic duct, but some fluid passes to the pleural space and is absorbed by the right lymphatic duct.

Pericardial Diagnostic Studies

Two-dimensional *echocardiography*, surface or transesophageal, provides information about the location, size, distribution, and physiologic effects of effusions. Cardiac tamponade is suggested by a lack of inspiratory collapse of the inferior vena cava, early diastolic collapse of the right ventricle, and late diastolic collapse of the right atrium. The heart can be visualized swinging within the excess pericardial fluid.

Doppler estimation of superior vena cava (SVC), hepatic venous, and transvalvular flow may show characteristic abnormalities of tamponade. Echo Doppler flow patterns may also be useful in screening for constrictive or restrictive physiologic disorders.

Echocardiography also may help differentiate pericardial constriction and restrictive cardiomyopathy.

Computed tomography (CT), including spiral, ultrafast, and gated studies, provides information regarding pericardial thickness and is used to quantitate and localize pericardial effusions. Because tissue attenuation coefficients vary, CT may elucidate the composition of effusions (eg, chyle, blood, and exudate). CT also may identify other thoracic lesions that involve the pericardium.

Magnetic resonance imaging (MRI) can be used in pericardial disease. Although effusions are detected with a high degree of sensitivity, MRI may not be helpful in determining pericardial thickness. Radionuclide ventriculography is helpful in evaluating constriction and tamponade.

Congenital Abnormalities

Congenital absence or defects of the pericardium may be associated with anomalies of the pleura, heart, lung, peritoneum, or kidney. They usually involve asymptomatic partial absence of the pericardium, particularly on the left side. With right-sided pericardial defects, herniation of the right atrium, right ventricle, and lung may be associated with ECG changes and a murmur. Congenital absence of the pericardium is usually asymptomatic and an incidental finding at autopsy or operation for another condition. Management is completion pericardiectomy or replacement of the absent portion with a substitute.

When the embryonic pericardial lacunae do not fuse, a *pericardial cyst* occurs. Most cysts occur at the right cardiophrenic angle and are detected on routine chest radiographs. A communication to the pericardium becomes a diverticulum. Pericardial cysts are usually asymptomatic, but they can cause life-threatening respiratory or hemodynamic compromise in neonates. The diagnosis can be made with CT. Other conditions in the differential diagnosis include foramen of Morgagni hernia, bronchogenic cyst, lipoma, and other homogeneous benign or malignant lesions of the mediastinum. Surgical exploration and removal are undertaken if the diagnosis is in doubt, if the lesion appears to be enlarging, or if it becomes symptomatic.

Neoplasms

Primary malignant neoplasms of the pericardium are rare. They include sarcomas, teratomas, pheochromocytomas, and mesotheliomas, which usually present with constriction. Benign tumors include lipomas, hemangiomas, lymphangiomas, leiomyomas, neurofibromas, and thymomas. The pericardium may be involved by direct extension of lung, esophageal, or primary mediastinal malignant tumors and present as constriction or tamponade. Diagnosis is made with CT or MRI.

Metastatic involvement of the pericardium is the most common form of neoplasm. It is seen most frequently with lymphoma and lung, breast, and ovarian carcinoma. Treatment is with radiation therapy, but antineoplastic agents can be instilled into the pericardium. Tetracycline is used for chemical pericardiodesis. Management is to relieve effusion and tamponade and confirm the diagnosis of malignant pericardial disease. Malignant pericardial disease that presents as cardiac tamponade is an indication for surgical intervention but carries a low survival rate. For patients expected to have prolonged survival, surgical treatment may minimize risk for recurrence or cardiac encasement by metastatic tumor.

Pericarditis

The diagnosis of pericarditis can be difficult, but it is of utmost importance that pericarditis be differentiated from myocardial ischemia. The chest pain of acute pericarditis differs from ischemic pain in that it can last for days, is pleuritic, and is aggravated by breathing, lying flat, or turning; it is relieved by sitting or leaning forward. A diphasic (systolic and diastolic) pericardial friction rub often is heard over the entire precordium and sounds like walking on snow.

Causes

The causes and types of pericarditis are as follows:

Metastatic neoplasm
Idiopathic or nonspecific factors, probably viral illness
Uremic pericarditis
Acute infectious pericarditis
Parasitic pericarditis
Tuberculous pericarditis
Complications of AIDS
Association with MI (Dressler syndrome)
Complication of pericardiotomy for a cardiac operation
Iatrogenic pericarditis related to drugs or procedures
Connective tissue disease

Management

Acute tamponade is uncommon with pericarditis, but large pericardial effusions may develop. Early diagnosis and treatment are important to avoid later fibrous constriction. Acute infectious pericarditis is managed with a combination of drainage and specific antimicrobial therapy. Drainage can be accomplished with pericardiocentesis, but more complete drainage is ensured with surgical placement of a subxiphoid tube. In some infections (pneumococcal pneumonia), pericardial involvement is incidental and resolves as the patient responds to treatment of the primary infection. In others, there may be cardiac tamponade or persistent infection in the pericardium.

Specific types of pericarditis are treated for the underlying cause. Chest pain may be relieved with aspirin, indomethacin, or ibuprofen. For severe pain, narcotics may be required. When the pain does not respond to these agents, prednisone nearly always relieves symptoms. Pericardiectomy is performed for relapsing or refractory pericarditis.

Cardiac Tamponade

Cardiac tamponade occurs when adequate filling of the heart is prevented by compression from fluid or blood in the pericardial space, restricting ventricular filling during diastole, reducing stroke volume and cardiac output, and increasing systemic and pulmonary venous pressure.

Causes and Diagnosis

Cardiac tamponade is caused by metastatic malignant tumors, idiopathic pericarditis, renal failure, infection, connective tissue disease, anticoagulants, and complications of procedures. The diagnosis of cardiac tamponade is suggested when a patient with a pericardial effusion has elevated systemic venous pressure, dyspnea, and tachycardia. Three clinical signs (Beck triad) occur in acute tamponade:

1. The heart is small and quiet
2. Venous pressure is elevated
3. Systemic blood pressure is depressed

With acute tamponade, shock is evident with a rapid and paradoxic pulse. Cyanosis, especially in the face, may be a manifestation of venous stasis. Systemic blood pressure may be normal, low, or elevated in previously hypertensive patients. The neck veins are visibly distended and Kussmaul sign (lack of variation of venous filling with respiration) is present. Heart sounds are sometimes faint but may be normal. The cardiac apical impulse is usually not palpable, and cardiac murmurs

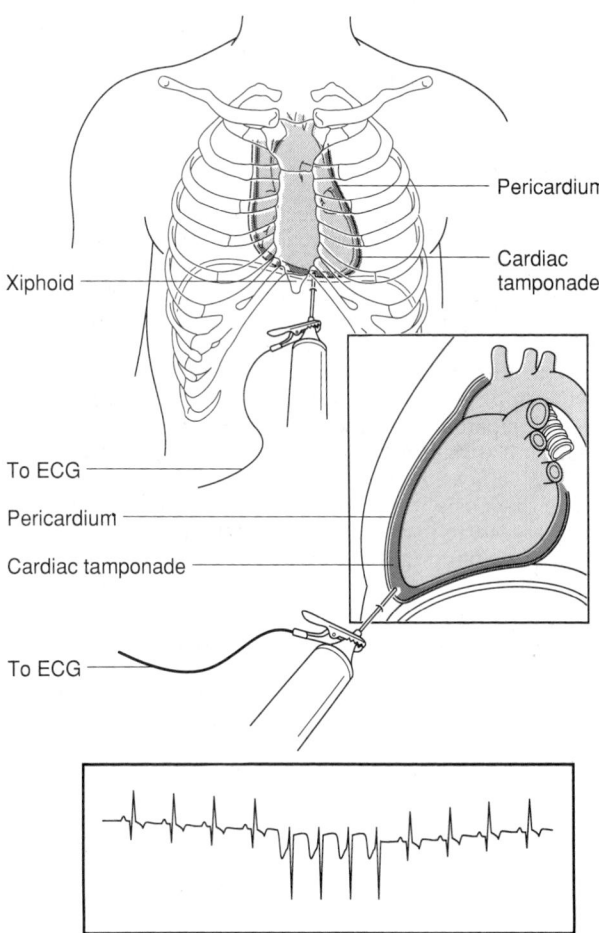

Figure 67-3. Pericardiocentesis. The needle is inserted to the left of the xiphoid and directed toward the left shoulder or midscapular area, posteriorly at a 45-degree angle. The ECG lead is attached to the needle, and the negative deflection of the QRS complex represents contact with the epicardium. (After Ebert PA, Najafi H. In: Sabiston DC Jr, Spencer FC, eds. Gibbon's surgery of the chest, ed 5. Philadelphia, WB Saunders, 1990:1234)

and gallop rhythm are absent. The diagnosis of cardiac tamponade is proved when removal of pericardial fluid relieves the symptoms.

Although the diagnosis of tamponade is made clinically, echocardiographic findings may be helpful. Moderate to large effusions may be present both anterior and posterior to the heart. Two-dimensional echocardiography is useful in needle pericardiocentesis.

Tamponade Related to Surgical Intervention

Although rising filling pressures and falling systemic pressure, urine, and cardiac output may be a manifestation of postoperative myocardial dysfunction, cardiac tamponade can occur early or late after open heart operations and is included in the differential diagnosis of low cardiac output. Diagnostic signs favoring tamponade include high elevation of the central venous pressure in relation to pulmonary capillary wedge pressure, poor response to vasopressors and diuretics, enlarging cardiac silhouette, and abrupt increase or cessation of mediastinal drainage. Late postsurgical tamponade is common among patients taking anticoagulants.

Treatment of cardiac tamponade depends on the cause and the clinical manifestations. When blood pressure is decreasing, emergency pericardiocentesis must be performed. Needle pericardiocentesis under hemodynamic and echocardiographic monitoring may be done when the diagnosis is known. When the diagnosis is unclear, surgical drainage is a better choice. The patient is observed for recurrence of cardiac tamponade. Recurrent tamponade is usually an indication for a pericardial window or pericardial resection.

Constriction

Constrictive pericarditis occurs when the heart is compressed by fibrosis of the pericardium, obliterating the pericardial space. The pericardium may contain fluid between the fibrotic, thickened visceral and parietal pericardium. The condition usually progresses slowly, producing elevated venous pressure over months to years. Patients present with effort dyspnea, fatigue, abdominal swelling or discomfort, orthopnea, cough, elevated venous pressure, edema, hepatomegaly, ascites, pleural effusion, Kussmaul sign, pericardial knock, pulsus paradoxus, and refractory congestive heart failure despite diuretics.

The diagnosis of constriction is made only when coronary disease, hypertension, and valvular disease are ruled out. Constriction is likely if heart size is normal and the

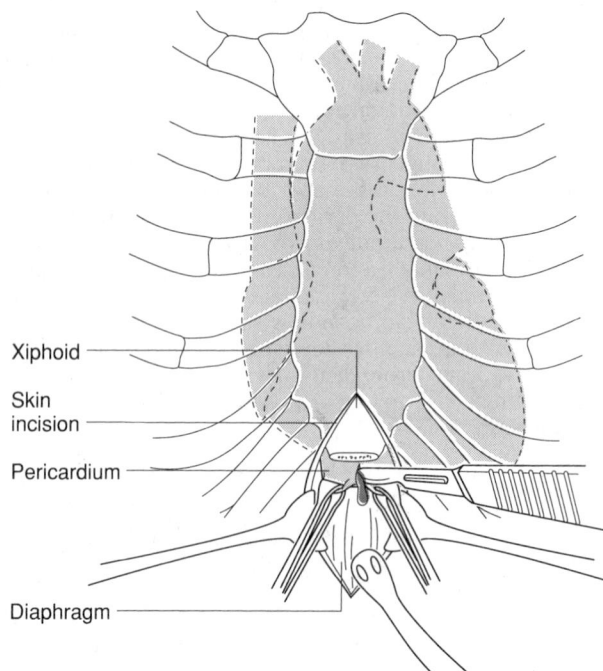

Figure 67-4. The xiphoid is exposed through a midline incision and either retracted or removed. Limited exposure to the pericardium is achieved, and biopsy or drainage is performed. (After Hood RM. Techniques in general thoracic surgery. Philadelphia, WB Saunders, 1985:58)

lung fields are clear on a chest radiograph. The diagnosis is almost certain if there is pericardial calcification, but calcification is present in less than half of patients with constriction.

Although any type of acute pericarditis can cause constriction, a common cause is radiation. Other causes are amyloidosis, scleroderma, hemochromatosis, infiltrative neoplasms, sarcoidosis, myocarditis, endomyocardial fibrosis, and pseudoxanthoma elasticum. Pericardial con-

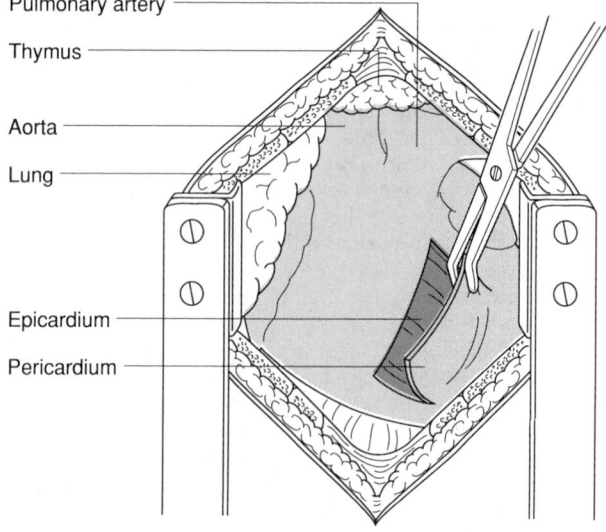

Figure 67-5. The pericardium is exposed through a median sternotomy. The pericardium is incised, and the dissection plane established between the pericardium and epicardium. (After Ebert EA, Najafi H. In: Sabiston DC Jr, Spencer FC, eds. Gibbon's surgery of the chest, ed 5. Philadelphia, WB Saunders, 1990:1242)

Table 67-2. FINDINGS OF PERCARDIOCENTESIS

Disorder	Finding in Pericardial Aspirate
Tuberculous pericarditis	Acid-fast bacilli
Uremic pericarditis	Blood
Cholesterol pericarditis	Cholesterol crystals
Rheumatic pericarditis	High in protein and leukocytes and low in glucose
	Complement levels depressed; immune complexes possibly present
Pericarditis complicating systemic lupus erythematosus	Normal or slightly reduced glucose content
	Low complement level
	Possibly lupus cells
Other connective tissue diseases	Fluid straw colored
	No antibodies, immune complexes, or complement

striction with effusion is common in suppurative, malignant, and uremic pericardial disease.

Diagnosis

Ventriculography shows accelerated left ventricular filling in early diastole. During the first third of diastole, left ventricular filling averages 80% in patients with constrictive pericarditis. ECG shows low-voltage and nonspecific T-wave changes. Some patients have atrial fibrillation or flutter. Sometimes there is a pattern of right ventricular hypertrophy due to fibrotic obstruction of the right ventricular outflow tract or narrowing of the mitral orifice.

Echocardiographic changes are not specific. The ventricles are small with preserved systolic function. There is

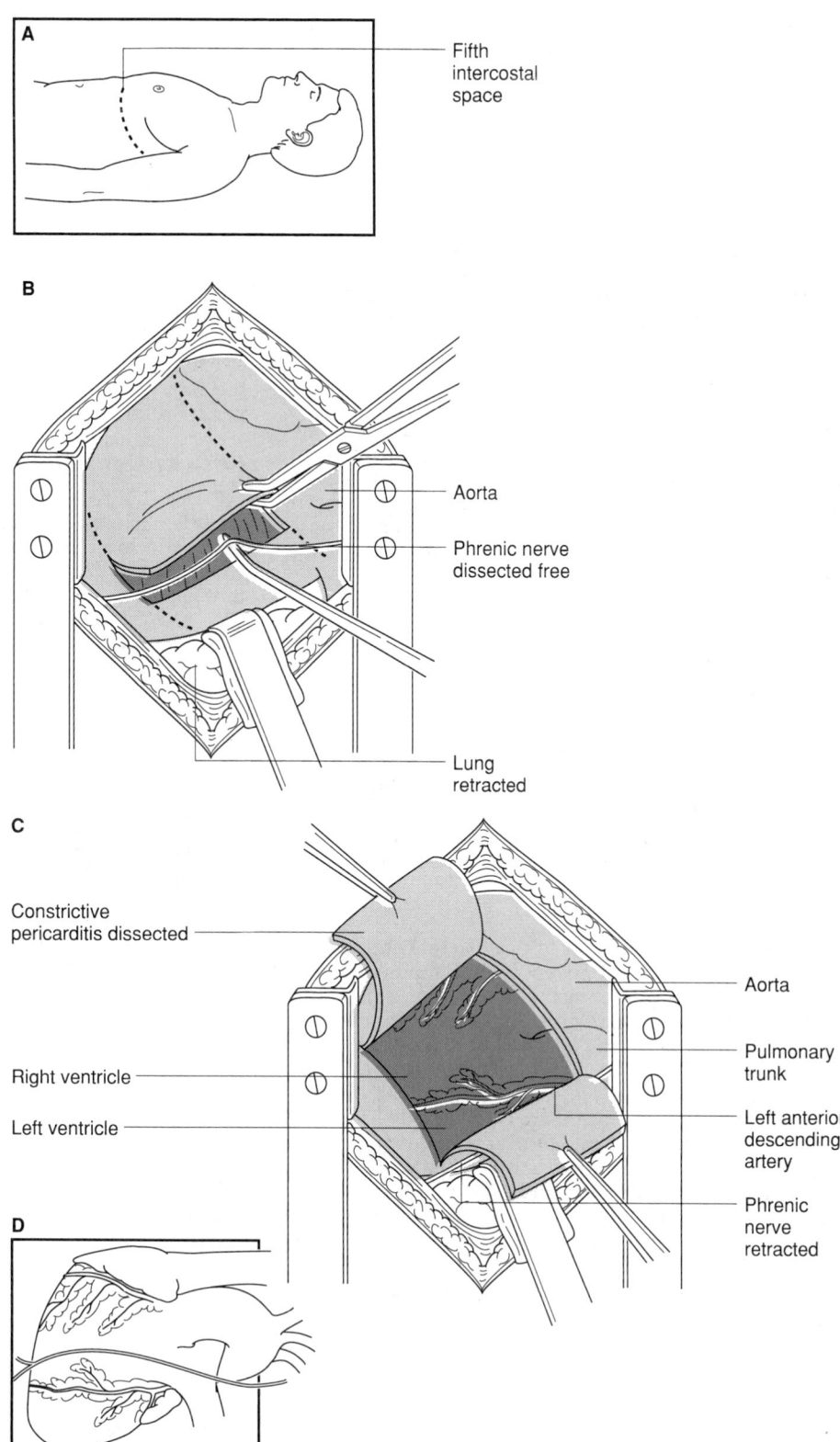

Figure 67-6. Pericardiectomy through an anterolateral left thoracotomy. The heart is exposed through the fifth interspace. The appropriate dissection plane is established and the phrenic nerve mobilized to allow removal of the posterolateral pericardium. (After Kirklin JW, Barratt-Boyes BG. Cardiac surgery. New York, John Wiley & Sons, 1986:1438)

abrupt halting of ventricular expansion during early diastole, with diastolic flattening of the left ventricular posterior wall. The inferior vena cava is dilated. Findings at Doppler echocardiography are an abnormal inspiratory increase in tricuspid flow and abnormal inspiratory decrease in mitral valve flow.

In patients with effusive-constrictive pericarditis, pericardial fluid collects between the fibrotic visceral and parietal pericardium. The heart is larger on chest radiographs than it is with constrictive pericarditis. In effusive-constrictive pericarditis, atrial and ventricular pressure curves resemble those of cardiac tamponade. If the pericardial fluid is removed with a needle, the pressure tracings resemble those of constrictive pericarditis.

The diagnosis of constrictive pericarditis is made from the hemodynamic findings in the presence of pericardial thickening confirmed with CT or MRI. Right atrial and pulmonary wedge pressures may be equal, and there may be an early diastolic dip in the pressure tracings of both left and right ventricles. Sometimes pericardial biopsy may be necessary to confirm the diagnosis because long-standing constriction with ascites and peripheral edema may be confused with primary liver disease.

Management

Although diuretics may offer improvement, pericardiectomy is definitive therapy for constrictive pericarditis. Operation may be deferred in patients in New York Heart Association (NYHA) functional class I who have a satisfactory quality of life. Patients with constrictive pericarditis caused by radiation or connective tissue disease may respond poorly because of associated restrictive cardiomyopathy.

Pericardiocentesis

Indications

Acute cardiac tamponade and rapidly falling blood pressure

Purulent pericarditis suggested by fever or high white cell count

Diagnostic purposes when a patient has continued fever or unresolved or progressive pericardial effusion

Technique

A subxiphoid (Fig. 67-3) or left parasternal approach is used. The needle is slowly advanced until fluid is encountered or an ECG shows contact with the heart (injury current). Air bubble (echocardiography) or radiopaque (fluoroscopy) contrast agent can be injected to see if the tip of the needle is in the right ventricle or the pericardial space. The aspirated fluid is saved for bacteriologic, cytologic, and chemical analysis. A drainage catheter may be passed through the aspirating needle or over a guide wire.

Complications of pericardiocentesis include myocardial or coronary arterial laceration, induction of ventricular arrhythmias, perforation of the lung with pneumothorax, and penetration of abdominal viscera. The use of 2D echocardiography to localize the pericardial effusion before attempted aspiration reduces the risk of the procedure.

Results

Pericardiocentesis is both therapeutic and diagnostic. Infections may be cultured. Viral or nonspecific pericarditis is usually diagnosed by excluding other specific causes. Fluid findings are summarized in Table 67-2.

Pericardial Biopsy and Drainage

When pericardiocentesis does not establish a diagnosis or the patient does not have a large effusion, open biopsy may be performed from either the subxiphoid or the anterior thoracotomy approach (Fig. 67-4). The sternum is elevated and a segment of pericardium is excised for pathologic examination. Fluid is aspirated and saved for bacteriologic or cytologic evaluation. In effusion, a tube is placed into the pericardium through the defect. If the biopsy is through a left anterior thoracotomy, the defect is drained into the pleural space, which is evacuated with a tube thoracostomy.

Open drainage of the pericardium is often required in malignant effusion and acute pyogenic pericarditis, in which drainage through a catheter may be incomplete. The subxiphoid approach provides drainage and avoids contamination of the pleura. For malignant disease or chronic effusion, drainage into the pleura may be desirable, and the anterior approach is used. A large segment of anterior pericardium is excised for intrapleural communication.

Pericardiectomy

Pericardial resection is performed for constrictive pericarditis, constrictive effusion, and malignant effusion. Pericardiectomy can be used for pericarditis resistant to conventional therapy. The operation may be performed through an anterior thoracotomy or median sternotomy (Fig. 67-5). Cardiopulmonary bypass is used to facilitate removal of the thickened pericardium when dissection is difficult and extensive manipulation of the heart is required. A left anterolateral thoracotomy through the fifth intercostal space, with or without transection of the sternum, is an alternative approach (Fig. 67-6).

SUGGESTED READING

Bolling SF, Deeb GM, Morady F, et al. AICD: new bridge to transplantation. J Heart Lung Transplant 1991;10:562.

Cox JL, Boineau JP, Schuessler RB, Kater KM, Lappas DG. Five-year experience with the maze procedure for atrial fibrillation. Ann Thorac Surg 1993;56:814.

Fowler NO. Recurrent pericarditis. Cardiac Clin 1990;8:621.

Hancock EW. Neoplastic pericardial disease. Cardiac Clin 1990;8:673.

Hazelrigg SR, Mack MJ, Landreneau RJ, Acuff TE, Seifert PE, Auer JE. Thoracoscopic pericardiectomy for effusive pericardial disease. Ann Thorac Surg 1993;56:792.

McCarthy PM, Castle LW, Maloney JD, et al. Initial experience with the maze procedure for atrial fibrillation. J Thorac Cardiovasc Surg 1993;105:1077.

Moran JM. Surgery for ventricular arrhythmias. Ann Thorac Surg 1990;49:837.

Spodick DH. Pericarditis in systemic diseases. Cardiac Clin 1990;8:709.

Tuna IC, Danielson GK. Surgical management of pericardial diseases. Cardiol Clin 1990;8:683.

Zipes DP, ed. Cardiac electrophysiology: from cell to bedside. Philadelphia, WB Saunders, 1990.

SECTION M

ARTERIAL SYSTEM

BASIC CONSIDERATIONS
IN VASCULAR DISEASE

ESSENTIALS OF SURGERY: SCIENTIFIC PRINCIPLES AND PRACTICE,
edited by Lazar J. Greenfield, Michael W. Mulholland, Keith T. Oldham, Gerald B. Zelenock,
and Keith D. Lillemoe. Lippincott–Raven Publishers, Philadelphia, © 1997.

CHAPTER 68

ATHEROSCLEROSIS AND THE PATHOGENESIS OF OCCLUSIVE DISEASE

ALEXANDER W. CLOWES

Atherosclerosis is a disease of the intima of large arteries that causes luminal narrowing, thrombosis, and occlusion with ischemia of the end organ. Throughout much of its course, the disease is not readily detectable. Thrombosis, including vascular occlusion and embolization, produces myocardial infarction, stroke, and ischemic gangrene of the extremities. The high prevalence of asymptomatic arterial lesions, the chronicity of the process, the suddenness of the terminal vascular events, and the lack of a single etiologic factor make it impossible to give a simple explanation for atherogenesis and atherosclerosis.

NORMAL STRUCTURE OF BLOOD VESSELS

An artery is not just an inert conduit for blood. It is an organ, the structure and function of which are carefully modulated by interactions among vascular wall cells and between vascular wall cells and the blood. Normal arteries and veins, both large and small, are formed from endothelium, smooth muscle, and extracellular matrix (ECM) synthesized by the cells of the vascular wall. The vascular wall is organized into layers (Fig. 68-1). The *intima,* the part of the wall between the blood and the internal elastic lamina, is composed of a monolayer of endothelium at the luminal surface and can overlie one or more layers of smooth muscle. The *media,* beneath the intima, constitutes the bulk of the vessel and contains smooth muscle cells arranged in layers and dispersed in a matrix of elastin, collagen, and proteoglycan. The *adventitia* lies outside the external elastic lamina and forms the outer coat. It is composed of loose connective tissue, fibroblasts, capillaries, neural fibers, and a few leukocytes.

In large arteries with more than 28 elastic layers, a microvasculature *(vasa vasorum)* penetrates the media from the adventitial side and provides the bulk of the nutrient supply to the the vessel (there is some supply due to luminal surface). In thickened, atherosclerotic vessels, the vasa vasorum are extensive and penetrate into the diseased intima.

REGULATION OF LUMINAL AREA

The foregoing description of the usual arterial wall anatomy gives no clue how a vessel adjusts its mass and dimensions in response to external stimuli (hypertension, increased blood flow, vascular injury) or how it maintains a nonthrombogenic state at the luminal surface. For this, the array of possible physiologic processes of the wall and its cellular components must be considered under normal and abnormal conditions.

Blood vessels, both large and small, enlarge during growth and development and as a compensatory mechanism to increased blood flow (velocity) (Fig. 68-2). A vessel undergoing stenosis experiences an increase in blood velocity at the point of luminal narrowing. When the stenosis is due to intimal thickening or atherosclerotic plaque, the vessel dilates at the site of the lesion. For example, a diseased coronary vessel dilates and can maintain the correct luminal dimensions despite changes in wall structure, as long as the intimal lesion does not occupy >40% of the area inside the internal elastic lamina (Fig. 68-3). At this point, pathologic narrowing begins to take place. The cells in the wall, particularly the endothelium, may sense changes in blood velocity and can translate this biomechanical information into biochemical signals that regulate the contractile state of the artery.

Endothelial cell secretory products are critical in smooth muscle cell function. They secrete vasodilating substances (prostaglandin I_2 and E_2, adenosine, endothelium-dependent relaxing factor [EDRF]) and vasoconstricting substances (endothelin). When endothelium is damaged or absent, adherent platelets release the vasoconstrictor thromboxane A_2. EDRF appears to be a particularly important regulator in normal and diseased vessels. A number of factors stimulate endothelial cells to secrete EDRF, including thrombin, acetylcholine, bradykinin, serotonin, and products of platelet release.

When endothelium is present and functional, neighboring thrombotic events are likely to cause vasodilation. When the endothelium is absent or dysfunctional, these same factors cause vasoconstriction. When the endothelium is missing, the vessel does not respond normally to changes in blood flow in the short or long term, and changes in blood flow affect wall mass.

Various factors that affect smooth muscle contraction or relaxation also modulate growth (nitric oxide, endothelin, thrombin, prostaglandins). Transient signals that affect the diameter of vessels may have permanent effects on wall structure. Pathologic conditions in which endothelium is

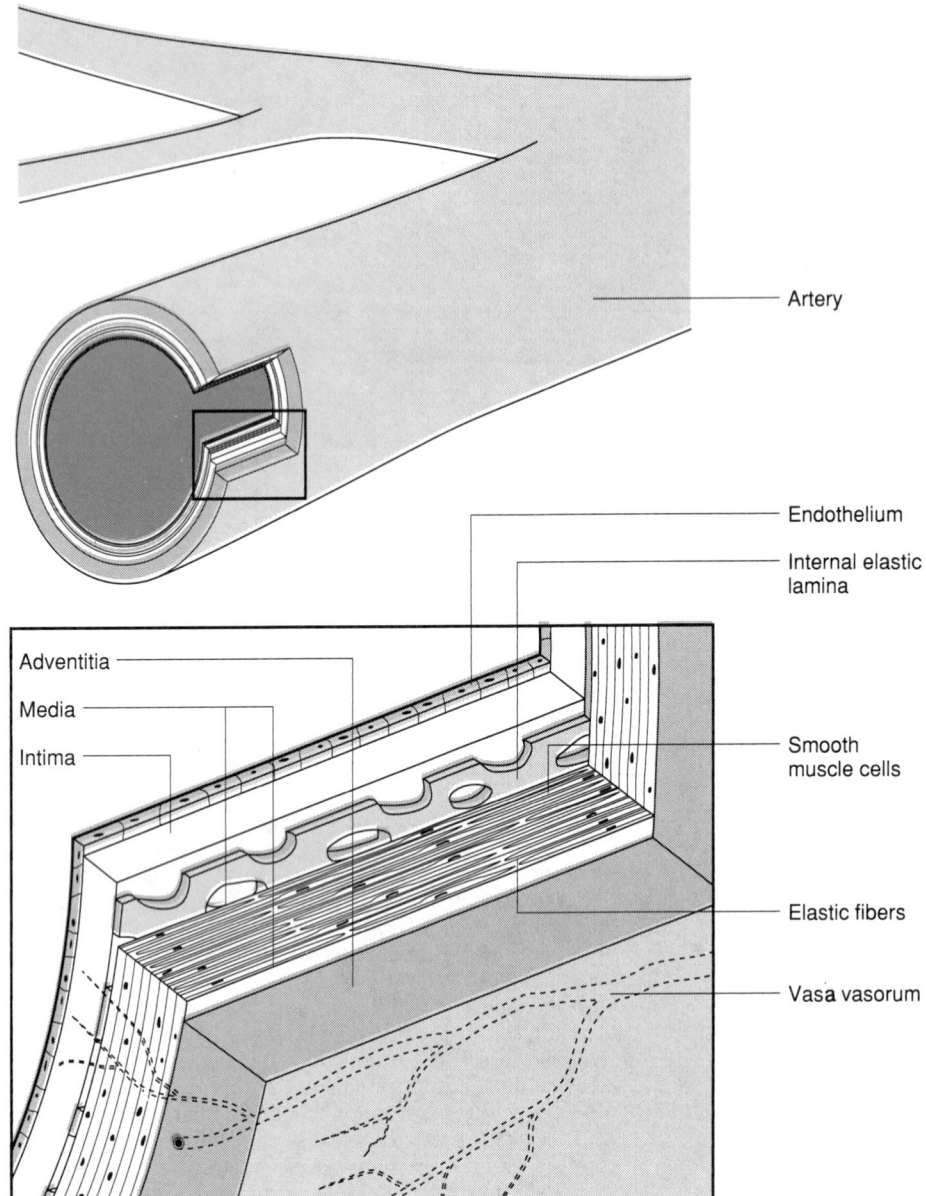

Artery

Endothelium

Internal elastic
lamina

Adventitia

Media

Intima

Smooth
muscle cells

Elastic fibers

Vasa vasorum

Figure 68-1. The artery wall is made of multiple layers (intima, media, and adventitia) that vary in composition depending on the artery.

missing or abnormal are associated with acute and chronic vasospasm. The acute problems of atypical angina (coronary vasospasm) and cerebrovasospasm after cerebral hemorrhage may be manifestations of abnormal endothelial function and decreased EDRF.

REGULATION OF MEDIAL AND INTIMAL THICKENING

In hypertension, arteries exhibit medial thickening, but after endothelial denudation or in the presence of hypercholesterolemia, a thick intima develops. How these responses are regulated is unclear, although it is certain that proliferation of smooth muscle cells and accumulation of ECM are important components. In patients with hypercholesterolemia, accumulation of lipid and lipid-filled macrophages contributes to the intimal lesion.

Vessel wall mass is largely determined by accumulation of smooth muscle cells and matrix synthesized by smooth muscle cells. Under normal circumstances, smooth muscle cells proliferate in the vessels and enter a quiescent state at maturity.

Although hypertension has its greatest impact on the small resistance vessels, large arteries also are affected. In response to increased pressure, the wall thickens. This increase is largely a medial process and involves all components of the vessel wall, including the mass of smooth muscle cells and matrix. In some forms of hypertension, the number of smooth muscle cells increases; in others, there is an increase in DNA content per cell.

How a change in pressure might induce smooth muscle cells to proliferate, change their ploidy, or synthesize matrix is not known. In some circumstances (severe hypertension, vein grafting), a small amount of endothelium is lost, but this is not typical of moderate or chronic forms of hypertension. Increased tension and stretch have a direct effect on matrix protein synthesis but not on cell proliferation. Increased wall tension affects the endothelium, and the endothelium might secrete factors that regulate smooth muscle mass.

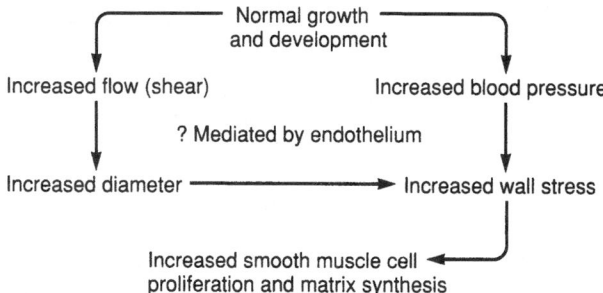

Figure 68-2. Changes in blood flow and pressure can have profound effects on arterial wall structure. In part, the response to hemodynamic changes may be mediated by the endothelium. (After Clowes AW. Theories of atherosclerosis. In: White RA, ed. Atherosclerosis and arteriosclerosis: human pathology and experimental animal methods and models. Boca Raton FL, CRC Press, 1989:3)

There may be a link between smooth muscle proliferation and platelet granule release. Among the proteins released are several growth factors, including platelet-derived growth factor (PDGF), transforming growth factor β (TGFβ), and an epidermal growth factor (EGF)-like protein. Where these granule proteins go after being released from the platelets is not known. They may accumulate in the arterial wall and stimulate smooth muscle growth. Platelet products participate in the movement of smooth muscle cells from one vascular compartment to the next (media to intima) but do not affect the initiation of proliferation.

Little is known about what starts or stops intimal thickening. Endothelium may suppress smooth muscle growth and migration from the media to the intima. It is known that smooth muscle growth inhibitors can be extracted from the vessel wall, endothelium can synthesize a heparin-like molecule that inhibits smooth muscle cell growth in vitro, and heparin can suppress proliferation and migration of smooth muscle cells. Endothelium appears to inhibit smooth muscle proliferation. The quiescent state of smooth muscle cells in normal arteries might be actively maintained rather than attributable to the lack of growth factors.

REGULATION OF SMOOTH MUSCLE GROWTH

Platelets are the main source of mitogen for proliferating smooth muscle. Smooth muscle cells, however, can proliferate in injured and hypertensive arteries when platelets are absent. If platelet factors are not essential, one of the following may be the stimulus for smooth muscle growth: (1) growth factors from vascular wall cells or resident leukocytes; (2) exogenous, neuroendocrine factors; or (3) loss of local inhibitors of smooth muscle proliferation.

REGULATION OF THE ANTICOAGULATED STATE

Blood does not clot in normal arteries even when flow is stopped for prolonged periods. Endothelial injury or loss, however, provokes a dramatic thrombotic response. This observation defines the importance of the endothelial layer in maintenance of the anticoagulated state. Endothelial cells also have several procoagulant functions. The balance between procoagulant and anticoagulant functions is regulated by signals from the blood and from neighboring cells.

On the *anticoagulant* side of the balance, the endothelium synthesizes membrane-associated heparan sulfate, which like heparin increases the affinity of antithrombin III for

thrombin. Endothelial-derived heparan sulfate can impede two aspects of the injury response: activation of the clotting cascade and stimulation of smooth muscle proliferation. Endothelial cells also can inhibit clotting along the protein C pathway. Endothelial cells can inhibit platelet adhesion and aggregation through the synthesis of prostaglandin I_2 and can degrade formed fibrin by activating plasminogen to plasmin.

On the *procoagulant* side, endothelial cells synthesize and secrete tissue factor, platelet-activating factor, a plasminogen-activator inhibitor, and von Willebrand factor. They also express a number of receptors for factors of the clotting cascade.

When exposed to a variety of inflammatory mediators derived from the blood or from resident macrophages (endotoxin, IL-1, tumor necrosis factor [TNF]), endothelial cells respond by changing the balance of anticoagulant-procoagulant activities to favor coagulation. The cells synthesize and express IL-1, which can affect the underlying smooth muscle cells. Lymphocytes also are present in atherosclerotic plaque. The ability of the vascular wall cells to maintain the anticoagulant state at the luminal surface has direct bearing on the thrombotic complications associated with end-stage atherosclerosis.

THEORIES OF ATHEROSCLEROSIS
Theories About the Lesions

Lipid Streaks

Atherosclerosis is a disease of the intima, characterized by accumulation of smooth muscle cells and lipids. The earliest lesion appears to be local accumulation of lipid in the vessel wall in the ECM or inside foam cells. Fatty or lipid streaks occur even in young children. Lipid streaks are equally com-

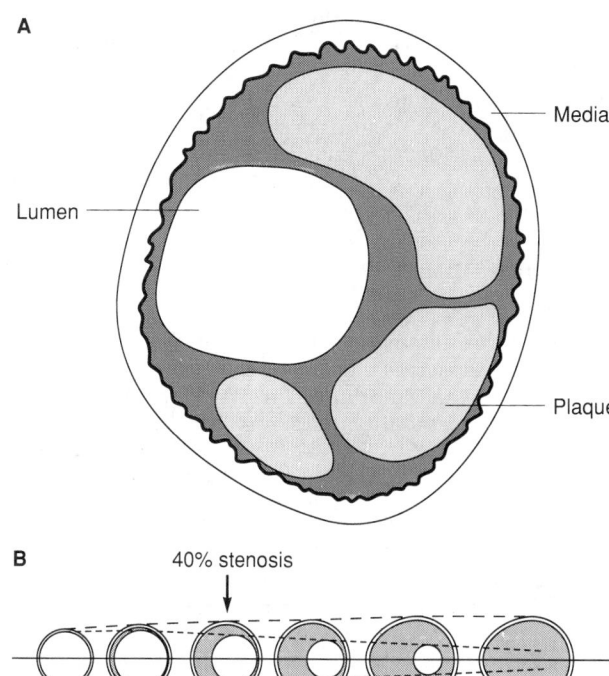

Figure 68-3. (A) Coronary arteries dilate as atherosclerotic plaques form and maintain normal luminal dimensions. Luminal narrowing begins only after the plaque occupies more than 40% of the cross-sectional area within the internal elastic lamina and bulges outward at sites of medial atrophy. (B) The course of lesion formation and luminal narrowing. (After Glagov S, Weisenberg E, Zarins CK, Stankunavicius R, Kolettis GJ. Compensatory enlargement of human atherosclerotic coronary arteries. N Engl J Med 1987;316:1371)

mon among women and men, although atherosclerosis is more prevalent among men. Even though the lipid streaks are distributed throughout the aorta, end-stage disease usually is confined to the abdominal segment. If fatty streaks are precursors of advanced lesions, there must be a selection process, or else the whole concept is wrong.

Intimal Cell Mass

An alternative precursor of atherosclerotic plaques is the *intimal cell mass*. These focal accumulations of smooth muscle cells are present in the vessels of children in locations where fibrous plaques later develop. Although the concept of an intimal cell mass as the initial lesion is attractive, there are several problems with it. First, this initial lesion is present in people throughout the world regardless of eventual risk for atherosclerosis. Second, gradual thickening of the intima throughout the arterial tree is part of aging; this has little to do with atherosclerosis.

Plaques

Whatever the initial lesion in atherosclerosis, the lesions characteristic of late atherosclerosis are fibrous and complicated plaques.

Fibrous plaques are characterized by a thick, fibrous luminal cap that contains smooth muscle cells and leukocytes over a central core of necrotic debris and lipid (atheroma). There might be denudation or nondenuding injury of the endothelium at the surface. Macrophages, by becoming "foamy," participate in the metabolism of lipid, and activated macrophages secrete a range of factors that modulate the metabolic and growth states of the vascular wall cells. Macrophages also proliferate locally in the lesions. Other leukocytes, particularly T lymphocytes, also are present.

Complicated plaques are fibrous plaques with the addition of ulceration, luminal thrombosis, calcification, and wall hemorrhage. They are the source of the thromboembolism associated with symptomatic disease. Inflammatory cells and the release of mediators of inflammation participate in the development of complicated lesions. Growth factors for smooth muscle are liberated from platelets and are synthesized and secreted by macrophages and the vascular wall cells. Cytokines, such as IL-1, TNF, and γ-interferon alter the growth state and metabolism of the vascular wall cells.

Theories About the Evolution of Atherosclerosis

Each of the following hypotheses attempts to explain one or more aspects of atherogenesis. Each might be applicable at a different time during the development of a lesion (Fig. 68-4). Susceptibility to atherosclerosis might be determined by both intrinsic factors (numbers of intimal masses) and extrinsic factors (hypercholesterolemia, hypertension, diabetes, cigarette smoking).

Lipid Insudation Hypothesis

The lipid in an atherosclerotic lesion is derived from lipoproteins in the blood. This hypothesis links the risk factor hypercholesterolemia directly to the development of plaque foam cells (the atheroma) and, eventually, the complicated lesion. The lipid in the plaques probably comes from the blood. Although this hypothesis provides a concept for how lipid accumulates, it does not explain other features of the lesion, including smooth muscle proliferation and thrombosis.

Encrustation Hypothesis

Plaque initiation and progression are the consequence of repeated cycles of thrombosis and remodeling. However, thrombosis is not the initial event in atherogenesis; it ap-

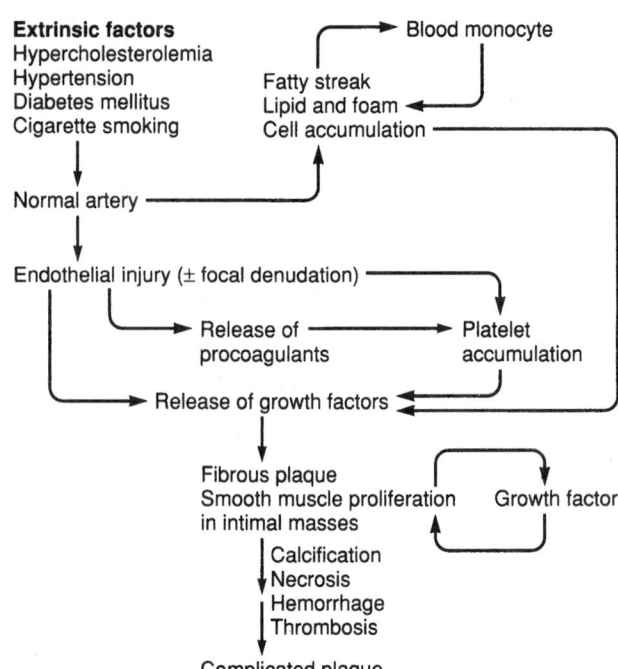

Figure 68-4. Atherogenesis and progression of atherosclerosis are probably the consequences of multiple factors acting on the arterial wall. (After Clowes AW. Theories of atherosclerosis. In: White RA, ed. Atherosclerosis and arteriosclerosis: human pathology and experimental animal methods and models. Boca Raton, FL, CRC Press, 1989:3)

pears to be a feature of advanced disease. This hypothesis is applicable only to the problem of plaque progression. It also does not explain how lipid and smooth muscle cells accumulate in the lesion.

Reaction-to-Injury Hypothesis

The initial event in atherosclerosis is injury to the endothelium. In regions denuded of endothelium, platelets adhere and release growth factors; these growth factors accumulate in the wall and stimulate medial smooth muscle proliferation and migration into the intima. A modified version of this theory is that injuries to the endothelium that do not produce denudation might also cause smooth muscle growth by stimulating damaged endothelium to synthesize and release growth factors. This hypothesis suggests a possible mechanism for the accumulation of connective tissue cells and matrix; it does not explain lipid accumulation or the monoclonal nature of advanced atherosclerotic plaques.

Monoclonal Hypothesis

The cells of a plaque are likely to arise as a clone from a single progenitor smooth muscle cell. At a certain moment in time, single cells might be stimulated to enter the growth cycle and undergo several rounds of division, leading to formation of a monoclonal lesion. Carcinogens or viruses may be etiologic agents, which might explain the link between cigarette smoking and atherosclerosis. An alternative to carcinogenesis as an explanation for monoclonality is the possibility of activation of a susceptible population of stem cells.

Intimal Cell Mass Hypothesis

Accumulations of intimal smooth muscle cells are one of the possible initial lesions in atherosclerosis. How the cells get to the site of the lesion is unclear, nor is it evident what makes the masses susceptible to atherogenic stimuli. These cells may be primordial rests and really a form of stem cell capable of responding to external mitogenic stimuli. Because the intimal cell masses are found in the vessels of children throughout the world regardless of the prevalence of atherosclerosis, atherosclerotic change probably is largely determined by extrinsic risk factors such as hypercholesterolemia.

SUGGESTED READING

Davies PF, Tripathi SC. Mechanical stress mechanisms and the cell: an endothelial paradigm. Circ Res 1993;72:239.

Ferns GAA, Raines EW, Sprugel KH, Motani AS, Reidy MA, Ross R. Inhibition of neointimal smooth muscle accumulation after angioplasty by an antibody to PDGF. Science 1991;253:1129.

Gibbons GH, Dzau VJ. The emerging concept of vascular remodeling. N Engl J Med 1994;330:1431.

Lindner V, Reidy MA. Proliferation of smooth muscle cells after vascular injury is inhibited by an antibody against basic fibroblast growth factor. Proc Natl Acad Sci USA 1991;88:3739.

Majesky MW, Lindner V, Twardzik DR, Schwartz SM, Reidy MA. Production of transforming growth factor β_1 during repair of arterial injury. J Clin Invest 1991;88:904.

Resnick N, Collins T, Atkinson W, Bonthron DT, Dewey CF Jr, Gimbrone MA Jr. Platelet-derived growth factor B chain promoter contains a cis-acting fluid shear-stress-responsive element. Proc Natl Acad Sci USA 1993;90:4591.

Lupu F, Bergonzelli GE, Heim DA, et al. Localization and production of plasminogen activator inhibitor in human healthy and atherosclerotic arteries. Arterioscler Thromb 1993;13:1090.

O'Brien ER, Alpers CE, Stewart DK, et al. Proliferation in primary and restenotic coronary atherectomy tissue: implications for antiproliferative therapy. Circ Res 1993;73:223.

Schneiderman J, Sawdey MS, Keeton MR, et al. Increased type 1 plasminogen activator inhibitor gene expression in atherosclerotic human arteries. Proc Natl Acad Sci USA 1992; 89:6998.

Wolf YG, Rasmussen LM, Ruoslahti E. Antibodies against transforming growth factor-β_1 suppress intimal hyperplasia in a rat model. J Clin Invest 1994;93:1172.

ESSENTIALS OF SURGERY: SCIENTIFIC PRINCIPLES AND PRACTICE, edited by Lazar J. Greenfield, Michael W. Mulholland, Keith T. Oldham, Gerald B. Zelenock, and Keith D. Lillemoe. Lippincott–Raven Publishers, Philadelphia, © 1997.

CHAPTER 69

NONATHEROSCLEROTIC VASCULAR DISEASE

LLOYD M. TAYLOR, JR., RAYMOND W. LEE, E. JOHN HARRIS, JR., AND JOHN M. PORTER

FIBROMUSCULAR DYSPLASIA

Fibromuscular dysplasia (FMD) is characterized by multiple areas of eccentric arterial stenosis alternating with segments of arterial dilatation. It probably is a developmental abnormality. Multiple stenoses are present in sequence (string of beads angiographic sign; FMD rarely causes a single focal stenosis. FMD usually involves the renal arteries, most commonly, the right renal artery. The carotid and iliac arteries are next most frequently affected. Almost all patients are women.

The cause of FMD is unknown. Theories include hormonal imbalance, primarily estrogenic; embryologic maldevelopment; immunologic phenomena; injury from arterial stretching; and abnormal distribution of the vasa vasorum with mural ischemia. Four variants of FMD are based on differences in histologic appearance—intimal fibroplasia, medial fibroplasia, medial hyperplasia, and perimedial dysplasia.

The *clinical findings* in FMD are related to the vascular bed involved. Many patients have no symptoms. Hypertension caused by renal arterial stenosis and transient cerebral ischemic attacks caused by internal carotid artery stenosis are frequent with FMD.

Surgical *therapy* is indicated for FMD because of symptomatic arterial stenoses. Surgical management may be indicated for true, false, or dissecting aneurysms in areas of FMD. Procedures include arterial dilation, arterial patch angioplasty, and interposition arterial bypass grafting with autogenous or prosthetic materials. Percutaneous transluminal balloon angioplasty can be used for FMD lesions of the main renal artery.

BUERGER'S DISEASE

Buerger's disease (thromboangiitis obliterans) is characterized by extensive segmental thrombotic occlusion of small and medium arteries in the lower and upper extremities, accompanied by prominent inflammatory cell infiltration of the arterial wall. Most patients with Buerger's disease are young male smokers who seek treatment because of distal limb ischemia, often accompanied by gangrene of the toes or fingers. About half of patients with Buerger's disease have a history of superficial migratory thrombophlebitis; others may exhibit Raynaud syndrome. Buerger's disease usually is limited to vessels distal to the elbow and knee, although cerebral, coronary, and visceral arterial involvement can occur.

The acute pathologic lesion of Buerger's disease is nonnecrotizing panarteritis associated with intraluminal thrombus. The internal elastic lamina is intact. The chronic phase of Buerger's disease includes a decline in hypercellularity, production of perivascular fibrosis, and frequent recanalization of the luminal thrombus. Adjacent veins and nerves are frequently involved in the perivascular inflammation.

Diagnostic criteria for Buerger's disease are:

Onset of distal extremity ischemic symptoms before 45 years of age
Absence of an underlying proximal embolic source
Absence of trauma
Absence of autoimmune disease (all serologic tests normal)
Absence of diabetes
Absence of hyperlipidemia
Absence of hypercoagulable state
Normal arteries proximal to popliteal and brachial arteries
Arteriographic, plethysmographic, or pathologic evidence of distal arterial occlusion and absence of disease in proximal arteries

Vascular laboratory testing for Buerger's disease consists of plethysmography of the fingers and toes, combined with segmental proximal limb pressures and Doppler analog waveform recording. Plethysmographic evidence of digital arterial obstruction in all four extremities, combined with normal proximal vessels, is sufficient evidence of intrinsic small artery obstructive disease, and arteriography is not required.

Patients with unilateral digital plethysmographic abnormalities undergo *arteriography* to rule out proximal arterial lesions as an embolic source of the distal digital ischemia. Arteriography also is advised for patients with vascular laboratory findings that localize the disease to the distal feet and toes in the presence of normal hand and finger plethysmography to rule out a proximal arterial em-

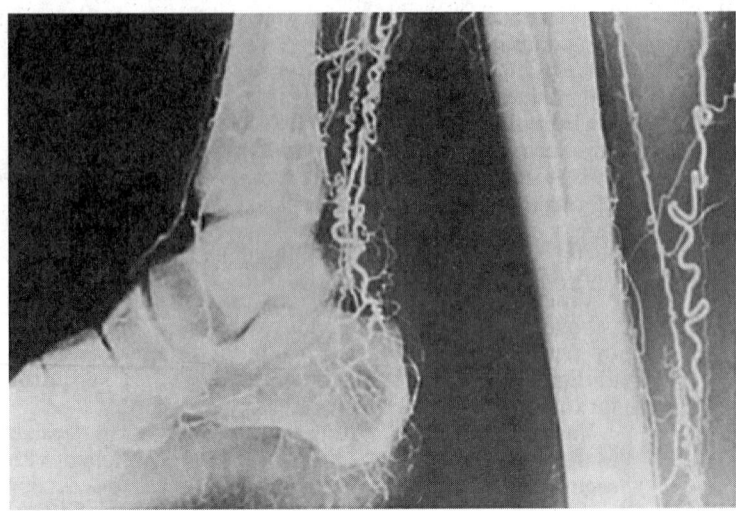

Figure 69-1. Typical arteriogram of patient with Buerger's disease showing abrupt occlusion of proximal normal tibial vessel and characteristic corkscrew collaterals. (Mills JL, Taylor LM Jr, Porter JM. Buerger's disease in the modern era. Am J Surg 1987;154:123)

bolic source of the ischemia. Although not pathognomonic, characteristic arteriographic findings of Buerger's disease are as follows. The arterial tree appears normal proximal to the popliteal and distal brachial levels. Distally, there is an abrupt transition to occlusion, which is most often segmental rather than diffuse. Extensive digital, palmar, and plantar arterial occlusions are common. The collaterals have a characteristic appearance *(corkscrew collaterals)* (Fig. 69-1).

Management of Buerger's disease centers on abstinence from tobacco. Buerger's disease undergoes remissions and relapses correlated with cessation and resumption of tobacco use.

Management of *upper-extremity* Buerger's disease consists of minor local débridement of ischemic segments, including partial excision of exposed phalangeal bone and soap and water scrubs of ischemic ulcers and antibiotic use as indicated by culture results. Extensive tissue loss is rare in upper-extremity Buerger's disease, and is virtually unknown if patients stop smoking. *Lower-extremity* involvement with Buerger's disease often leads to limb loss and amputation. Some patients have arteriographically patent distal arterial segments in the calf and foot, suggesting arterial bypass grafting may be possible.

DISEASES OF THE ARTERIAL MEDIA

Several conditions affect the amount, strength, and stability of collagen and elastin, which provide strength and resilience to the arteries.

Cystic Medial Necrosis

Cystic medial necrosis is characterized by uniform hyaline degeneration of the arterial media with replacement by a mucoid-appearing basophilic substance associated with aortic dissection. The most common manifestation of cystic medial necrosis is aortic dissection; spontaneous arterial rupture and diffuse aneurysm formation occur less frequently. Metabolic aberrations occur in many patients with cystic medial necrosis.

Most patients with cystic medial necrosis have a syndrome characterized by a heritable disorder of collagen metabolism. The most frequent are Marfan syndrome and Ehlers–Danlos syndrome.

Marfan Syndrome

Marfan syndrome is a heterogeneous disorder characterized by ocular abnormalities (myopia and lens dislocation), skeletal disproportion (tall stature, chest wall defor-

mities, arachnodactyly, scoliosis), and cardiovascular abnormalities (mitral valve prolapse, aortic dissection with aortic aneurysm formation). Inheritance of Marfan syndrome is autosomal dominant. It appears to be caused by a mutation in the genes that control production and use of type I collagen. Recent evidence points to a specific abnormality of fibrillin, the main component of extracellular microfibrils. The defective gene is located on the long arm of chromosome 15.

Almost all patients with Marfan syndrome have dilatation of the aortic root that leads to development of an ascending aortic aneurysm (Fig. 69-2), which can progress to aortic valvular incompetence. Some patients have mitral valve prolapse and mitral insufficiency. The life expectancy of untreated patients with Marfan syndrome is about 40 years; almost all deaths are related to cardiovascular complications.

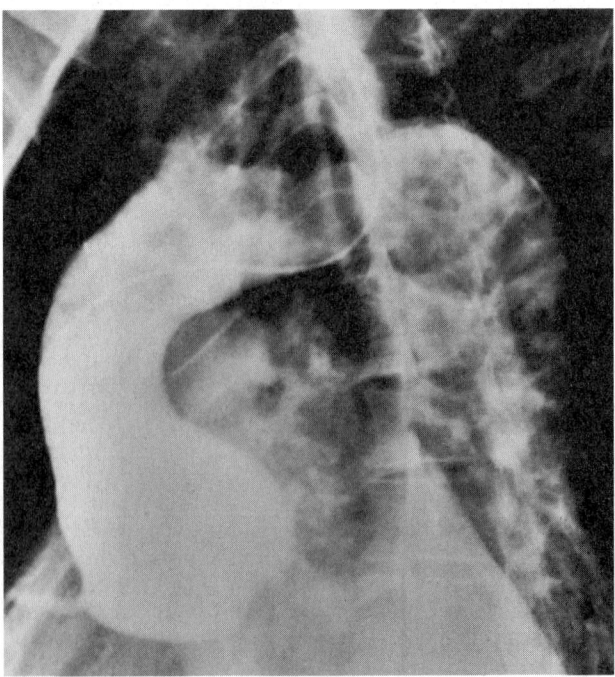

Figure 69-2. Aortogram of a patient with Marfan syndrome showing marked dilation of aortic root and aortic valvular insufficiency. (Porter JM, Taylor LM Jr, Harris EJ Jr. Nonatherosclerotic vascular disease. In: Moore WS, ed. Vascular surgery: a comprehensive review. Philadelphia, WB Saunders, 1994:136)

Medical and surgical *management* can be used for prophylaxis against aortic dissection and aortic insufficiency. The medical regimens center on use of β-adrenergic blockers in a regimen designed to decrease the force of cardiac contraction and reduce blood pressure to protect the weakened ascending aorta. Surgical treatment is replacement of the ascending aorta and aortic valve with a composite graft. Elective repair is performed before severe aortic insufficiency compromises left ventricular function or the diameter of the ascending aorta reaches 55 to 60 mm, at which point risk for dissection and rupture increases.

Ehlers–Danlos Syndrome

Ehlers–Danlos syndrome is a group of generalized connective tissue disorders characterized by hyperextensible skin, hypermobile joints, fragile tissues, and bleeding diathesis related to fragile vessels. There are more than ten types of Ehlers–Danlos syndrome. It is important to identify the various types because the natural histories differ.

Three types of Ehlers–Danlos syndrome—types I, III, and IV—frequently have arterial complications. Patients with Ehlers–Danlos syndrome type IV produce little or no type III collagen, which is of structural importance to blood vessels, viscera, and skin.

Clinical features of Ehlers–Danlos syndrome are thin, translucent skin, easy bruisability, and varicose veins. The main vascular complication is arterial rupture; aneurysm formation and acute aortic dissection also occur. Spontaneous arterial rupture can lead to stroke, intraabdominal or intrathoracic bleeding, and compartment syndromes in the extremities. The most common site of spontaneous arterial rupture is the abdominal cavity; visceral arteries are more commonly involved than the aorta. Repair of the ruptured vessels is difficult because of their extreme friability. Arteriography is not performed because of risk for vessel laceration and hemorrhage.

Whenever possible, *management* of spontaneous arterial rupture in Ehlers–Danlos syndrome type IV is nonsurgical, consisting of compression and transfusion. If nonsurgical intervention is unsuccessful, the treatment objective is ligation to control hemorrhage. If tissue loss is expected, arterial reconstruction can be attempted.

Pseudoxanthoma Elasticum

Pseudoxanthoma elasticum is a group of genetic disorders that involve the elastic fibers. The disorder is characterized by yellow xanthoma-like cutaneous papules and loose, baggy skin in areas such as the axilla, antecubital fossa, and groin. The disorder involves the skin, eyes, and arteries. The basic pathologic change in the arterial wall is that normal medial elastic fibers are replaced with calcium deposits.

The *clinical features* of pseudoxanthoma elasticum are stenoses or occlusion, or a combination of the two, of the peripheral, cerebral, or coronary arteries. Diminished arterial elasticity and resistance to distention are expressed as weak or absent pulses, which have characteristic plethysmographic tracings. Arterial occlusive disease occurs at an early age, usually before 40 years. Plain radiographs often depict vascular calcification. Hypertension is common. Diffuse arterial elastin degeneration can involve the visceral arteries, and gastrointestinal (GI) hemorrhage is common. *Management* is with autogenous venous bypass, endarterectomy, or coronary artery bypass.

Arteria Magna Syndrome

Arteria magna syndrome is a peculiar condition of the aorta and iliofemoral arteries that presents as diffuse arterial elongation, dilatation, and/or tortuosity. Findings range from generalized ectasia to contiguous aneurysms from the thoracic aorta to the popliteal trifurcation. The arterial media is devoid of the usual elastic tissues.

The relation between arteria magna and typical atherosclerosis is not clear. Aneurysms associated with arteria magna are pathologically similar to typical degenerative aneurysms. The histologic appearance is fragmentation of the internal elastic membrane and a profound decrease in the elastic tissue content of the media. There is no inflammatory component in the arterial wall. Although intimal atheromatous changes often are present, they are minimal in comparison with the extensive nature of the medial changes.

Arteriographic findings include arterial widening and tortuosity, markedly diminished arterial flow velocity with delayed distal arterial filling, and multiple aneurysms. Aneurysms are detected by means of physical examination and ultrasound screening of abdominal, femoral, and popliteal sites.

Management of arteria magna syndrome is arterial replacement. Localized aneurysms 2 to 2.5 times the diameter of the artery are replaced. Embolisms of intraaneurysmal thrombus and thrombotic arterial occlusions are common complications of this diffuse aneurysmal disease and are indications for arterial replacement. Coronary artery disease is common among patients with arteria magna syndrome, even though there is no typical arterial occlusive disease elsewhere in the body.

ADVENTITIAL CYSTIC DISEASE

Adventitial cystic disease is a rare condition characterized by single or multiple synovial-like cysts in the subadventitial layer of the arterial wall with arterial stenosis. The mucin-filled cysts are similar to ganglion cysts. The disease is most often bilateral and usually affects men about 40 years of age. The popliteal artery and its branches are most frequently affected, but adventitial cystic disease also occurs in the femoral, radial, and ulnar arteries. The disease appears to be caused by the development of true ganglia in the adventitia that originate from an adjacent joint capsule or tendon sheath.

The most frequent *symptom* is intermittent claudication. Physical examination rarely reveals a palpable cyst, and signs of generalized arterial insufficiency are not present. Palpable pulses change with knee flexion and extension, presumably because of luminal compression that varies with position. Diagnosis is possible with computed tomography (CT), magnetic resonance imaging (MRI), and ultrasonography. Arteriograms demonstrate a scimitar sign of luminal encroachment by the cyst.

When the vessel is not occluded, *management* is simple cyst excision, enucleation, or aspiration. When the vessel is occluded, the occluded segment can be resected with the cystic mass, and primary end-to-end anastomosis can be performed. Interposition grafting usually is required, however, and is best done with autogenous saphenous vein. CT-guided aspiration of popliteal artery cysts also can be attempted.

RADIATION-INDUCED ARTERIAL INJURY

Arterial injury can be caused by tumoricidal external-beam irradiation of regional malignant tumors. There are three pathologic forms:

1. Early posttreatment period, intense arterial inflammatory reaction with endothelial sloughing and luminal thrombosis
2. One to 10 years after radiation therapy, the healing

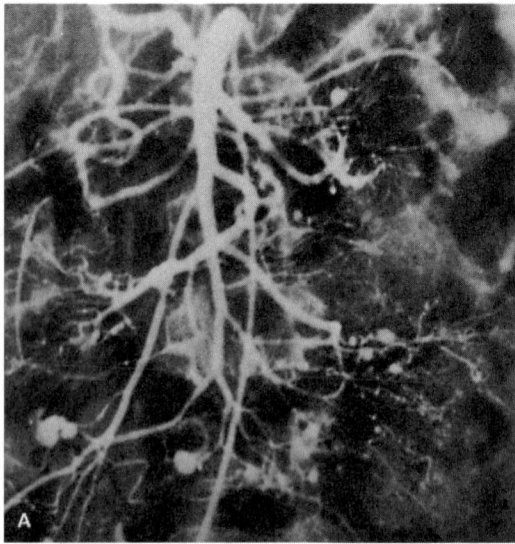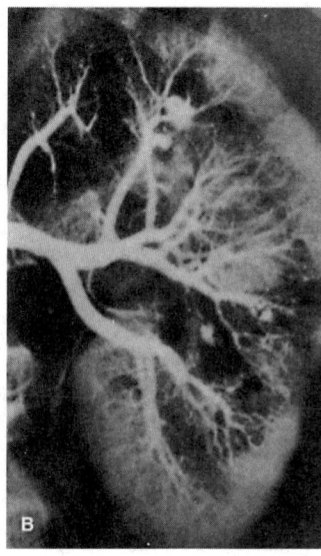

Figure 69-3. Arteriogram showing typical aneurysm formation in medium-sized visceral (*A*) and renal (*B*) arteries in a patient with polyarteritis nodosa. (Porter JM, Taylor LM Jr, Harris EJ Jr. Nonatherosclerotic vascular disease. In: Moore WS, ed. Vascular surgery: a comprehensive review. Philadelphia, WB Saunders, 1994:111)

phase of the arterial inflammatory response to radiation injury; intense fibrosis and scar formation within the arterial wall resulting in areas of arterial stenosis
3. Two to 30 years after radiation therapy, accelerated atherosclerosis

Vascular operations on these irradiated arteries are performed with standard techniques. Prosthetic and autogenous bypass grafts and endarterectomy can be used.

IMMUNE ARTERITIS

The terms *arteritis* and *vasculitis* apply only to necrotizing transmural inflammation of the arterial wall. Most immune vasculitis is associated with deposition of antigen-antibody immune complexes on the endothelium, followed by damage to the arterial wall. Leukocyte lysosomal enzymes, including elastase and collagenase, released within the arterial wall appear to be the primary cause of the arterial wall necrosis. Thrombosis, aneurysm formation, hemorrhage, and arterial occlusion follow or accompany the transmural arterial enzymatic injury. Immune arteritis is classified as follows:

Polyarteritis nodosa group (medium muscular arteries)
Classic polyarteritis nodosa (PAN)
Kawasaki disease
Cogan syndrome
Behçet syndrome
Hypersensitivity angiitis group (small arteries)
Hypersensitivity angiitis
Arteritis of collagen diseases
Mixed cryoglobulinemia
Arteritis associated with malignant tumors
Giant cell arteritis (large arteries)
Temporal arteritis
Takayasu arteritis

Polyarteritis Nodosa Group

Polyarteritis Nodosa

PAN is a systemic disease characterized by focal necrotizing arterial inflammatory lesions of small- and medium-sized muscular arteries. Most patients are men in the fifth decade of life. Aneurysm formation is associated with inflammatory destruction of the media. Although renal arterial involvement is most common with PAN, the heart,

lung, liver, GI tract, and skin arterials also can be involved (Fig. 69-3). Extensive lower extremity arterial involvement occurs. Aneurysms associated with PAN usually regress with steroid therapy. Vascular complications include aneurysm rupture and arterial stenosis or thrombosis with ischemia. Spontaneous rupture of a visceral arterial aneurysm affected by PAN is a surgical emergency because of intra- or retroperitoneal hemorrhage. Interventional radiologic techniques can be used to occlude bleeding vessels. GI complications in ischemic segments include hemorrhage, perforation, and segmental gangrene.

Kawasaki Disease

Kawasaki disease (mucocutaneous lymph node syndrome) is a form of arteritis that occurs among infants and children; it is similar to PAN. Although arterial involvement is widespread, the most striking feature is diffuse fusiform and saccular aneurysm formation in the coronary and, sometimes, the brachiocephalic arteries (Fig. 69-4).

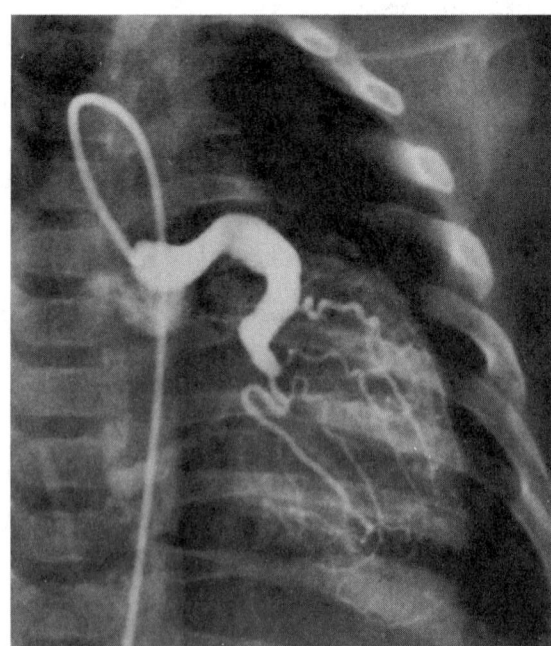

Figure 69-4. Selective coronary arteriogram showing typical aneurysm in a child with Kawasaki disease.

The coronary artery abnormality consists of areas of active arteritis, thrombosis, calcification, and stenosis. Although coronary artery rupture can occur, patients usually die of acute cardiac arrhythmia or myocardial infarction.

Cogan Syndrome

Cogan syndrome is a rare condition consisting of non-syphilitic interstitial keratitis associated with vestibuloauditory symptoms. It affects people in their 20s. The vasculitis, present in less than half of patients, is aortitis. Aortic insufficiency sometimes occurs.

Daily administration of high-dose corticosteroids can be used to reverse the visual and auditory symptoms of Cogan syndrome. Corticosteroids are indicated when aortitis is present. Aortic valve replacement is performed if hemodynamic function is compromised.

Behçet Syndrome

The features of Beçet syndrome are iritis and oral and genital mucocutaneous ulcerations. The predominant pathologic lesion is nonspecific panarteritis. This systemic disease largely affects the populations of the Mediterranean area and Japan, suggesting an environmental or genetic factor. There appear to be both bacterial and viral infectious causes. Autoimmune dysfunction is likely.

The lesions of Behçet can cause aneurysmal or occlusive disease, although occlusion is rare. The aorta is the most frequent site of aneurysm formation, although the carotid, subclavian, iliac, femoral, and popliteal arteries also are affected. Arterial puncture can lead to the development of pseudoaneurysms in Behçet disease, rendering diagnostic arteriography hazardous.

Immunosuppressive agents, including azathioprine, can be used for nonarterial symptoms, as can corticosteroids. Although corticosteroids can suppress symptoms, especially arthritic and ophthalmic symptoms, they do not alter the course of the underlying disease. No satisfactory therapy exists for Behçet disease, but early diagnosis and aggressive reconstruction of arterial aneurysms provides long-term limb salvage, despite arterial graft complications. The arterial aneurysms are likely to recur after repair, necessitating numerous operations.

Hypersensitivity Angiitis Group

Hypersensitivity angiitis is a large and heterogeneous group of syndromes characterized by involvement of small arteries. The syndromes include hypersensitivity angiitis, arteritis of collagen vascular disease, mixed cryoglobulinemia arteritis, and arteritis associated with malignant tumors. Involved arteries have a thickened basement membrane, swelling of the collagenous and elastic connective tissues, and fragmentation of the elastic fibers. The result is vascular occlusion, which can lead to regional ischemia. This process appears to be caused by deposition of immune complexes within the small arteries. Sometimes the inciting antigen can be identified, such as a drug or chemical, a virus, or a tumor antigen.

Clinical features include rash, fever, and symptoms of organ dysfunction. Plethysmography and arteriography help identify widespread palmar and digital arterial occlusions, which are frequently associated with digital ischemia. Although some patients have autoimmune disorders, a large number have no serologic evidence of autoimmune disease, no clinical evidence of any systemic disease, and present only with the acute onset of hand arterial occlusion and finger ischemia.

Treatment is local wound care and limited débridement. Vasodilator therapy, principally with calcium-channel blockers, may be tried. Healing of digital ischemic ulcers appears to improve with use of pentoxifylline.

Giant Cell Arteritis Group

Two disease patterns occur within the giant cell arteritis group—temporal arteritis and Takayasu arteritis. These two conditions may be different expressions of the same disease. Both consist of localized periarteritis with inflammatory mononuclear infiltrates and giant cells, along with disruption and fragmentation of the elastic fibers of the arterial wall.

Temporal Arteritis

Most patients with temporal arteritis (systemic giant cell arteritis) are white women older than 55 years. It is a systemic disease characterized by chronic inflammation of the aorta and the carotid artery. The disease also can cause aneurysms or stenoses of the aorta and its main branches. Thoracic aortic aneurysms and aortic dissection occur, and they can be managed by means of surgical replacement.

The most frequent presenting *symptom* is headache—severe pain along the course of the temporal artery, frequently bilateral. At onset, the patient has febrile myalgia, usually involving the back, shoulder, and pelvis. The headache is accompanied by tenderness and nodularity of the temporal artery with overlying skin erythema. More than half of patients have severe visual disturbances caused by ischemic optic or retrobulbar neuritis or occlusion of the central retinal artery. A large number of patients experience permanent partial or complete loss of vision, which can be prevented with early administration of steroids.

The *angiographic features* of giant cell arteritis are long segments of smooth stenosis interspersed with normal segments, smoothly tapered occlusions, absence of irregular plaques and ulcerations, and distribution of abnormalities among the subclavian, axillary, and brachial arteries (Fig. 69-5).

Early high-dose corticosteroid *therapy* may minimize the likelihood of aortic lesions but also may increase risk for aneurysmal rupture. Surgical procedures often fail unless accompanied by high-dose steroid administration.

Takayasu Arteritis

Takayasu arteritis is a rare, primary arteritis of unknown cause that affects the aorta, its principal branches, and the pulmonary artery. Most patients are girls and women, 3 to 35 years of age. Takayasu arteritis can produce stenosis, occlusion, dilatation, or aneurysm formation of the involved artery. Elastic fibers in the arterial wall are involved in intense periarteritis, characterized by granulomatous inflammation with mononuclear cell infiltration and formation of multinucleated giant cells.

Patients have *symptoms* of cerebral, visceral, or extremity ischemia. The course of Takayasu arteritis has two stages. The first stage is characterized by nonspecific symptoms of fever, myalgia, and anorexia. The second stage can follow closely and consists of a pulseless phase with multiple arterial occlusions and cardiovascular symptoms related to disease location. Hypertension is common and might be due to aortic coarctation or renal arterial stenosis. Neurologic symptoms can result from hypertension or central nervous system ischemia associated with arterial stenosis or occlusion. Coronary artery involvement is rare. The most frequent cardiac pathologic condition is heart failure due to systemic and pulmonary hypertension.

Takayasu disease is characterized by a pattern of cardiovascular involvement:

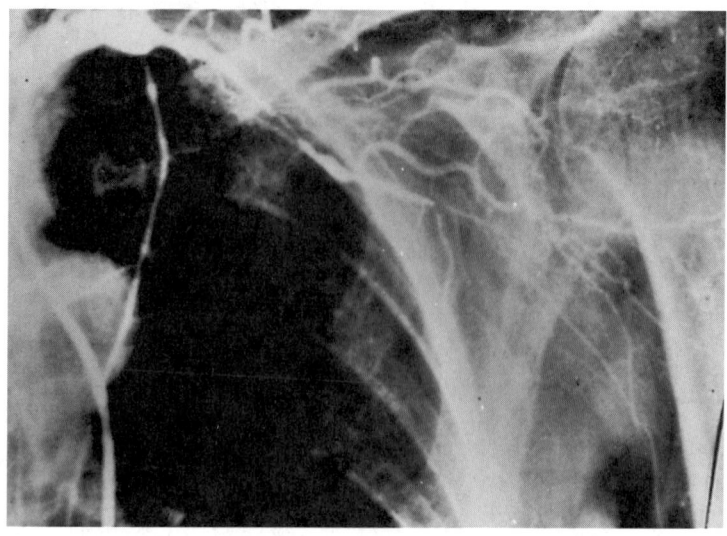

Figure 69-5. Typical tapered stenosis of left axillary artery in giant cell arteritis.

Type I—involvement of the aortic arch and arch vessels

Type II—involvement of the descending thoracic and abdominal aorta

Type III—the most common; involvement of the arch vessels and the abdominal aorta and its branches

Type IV—pulmonary artery involvement with or without the other types

Angiographic findings are stenosis in the aorta and its branches and occlusion in the pulmonary artery.

Corticosteroids are the key to *management* of Takayasu arteritis. Surgical reconstruction has a selective role. End-arterectomy is not recommended. Surgical treatment is implantation of a bypass graft into disease-free arterial segments and continuation of corticosteroid therapy.

HOMOCYSTINURIA

Homocystinuria is an inborn error of metabolism in which homocysteine accumulates abnormally in plasma and tissues and is excreted in large quantities in the urine. Patients have multiple abnormalities, including ectopia lentis, mental retardation, rapidly progressive arteriosclerotic vascular disease, and thromboembolic disorders. All forms of homocysteine accumulation are associated with premature atherosclerosis, frequently complicated by thrombosis. The arteriosclerotic plaques are typical fibrous plaques. Homocystinuria is associated with premature atherosclerosis and thrombosis, but the exact mechanism is not known.

HYPERVISCOSITY SYNDROMES

Hyperviscosity syndromes are characterized by an increase in blood viscosity that causes arterial or venous thromboembolism. These syndromes can be divided into two categories:

1. Pathophysiologic conditions, in which a primary blood abnormality causes an increase in the formed elements of the blood, such as the myeloproliferative disorders

2. Pathologic conditions that elevate serum proteins, such as myeloma, benign monoclonal gammopathy, macroglobulinemia, cryoglobulinemia, and neoplasia

Hyperviscosity syndromes cause thrombosis most frequently in the venous system, next most often in the small peripheral arteries (hands and fingers), and least often in the large arteries.

Management of hyperviscosity syndromes is directed at correction of the underlying disorder with appropriate anticoagulation therapy as needed. Vascular operations rarely are needed.

SUGGESTED READING

Bartlett ST, McCarthy WJ, Palmer AS, et al. Multiple aneurysms in Behçet's disease. Arch Surg 1988;123:1004.

Francfort JW, Gallagher JF, Penman E, et al. Surgery for radiation induced symptomatic atherosclerosis. Ann Vasc Surg 1989; 3:14.

Gott VL, Pyeritz RF, Magovern GJ, et al. Surgical treatment of aneurysms of the ascending aorta in the Marfan syndrome: results of composite graft repair in 50 patients. N Engl J Med 1986;314:1070.

Hall S, Barr W, Lie TE, et al. Takayasu arteritis: a study of 32 North American patients. Medicine 1985;64:89.

Harris EJ Jr, Taylor LM Jr, Malinow MR, et al. The association between elevated plasma homocysteine and symptomatic peripheral arterial disease. Surg Forum 1989;40:307.

Joyce JW. The giant cell arteritides: diagnosis and the role of surgery. J Vasc Surg 1986;3:827.

MacFarlane R, Livesey SA, Pollard S, Dunn DC. Cystic adventitial arterial disease. Br J Surg 1987;74:89.

Mills JM, Porter JM. Buerger's disease. In: Cameron JL, ed. Current surgical therapy III. Philadelphia, BC Decker, 1989;575.

Olszewski AJ, Szostak WB, Bialkowska M, et al. Reduction of plasma lipid and homocysteine levels by pyridoxine, folate, cobalamin, choline, riboflavin, and troxerutin in atherosclerosis. Atherosclerosis 1989;75:1.

Takagi A, Kajiura N, Tada Y, Ueno A. Surgical treatment of nonspecific inflammatory arterial aneurysms. J Cardiovasc Surg 1986;27:117.

ESSENTIALS OF SURGERY: SCIENTIFIC PRINCIPLES AND PRACTICE,
edited by Lazar J. Greenfield, Michael W. Mulholland, Keith T. Oldham, Gerald B. Zelenock,
and Keith D. Lillemoe. Lippincott–Raven Publishers, Philadelphia, © 1997.

CHAPTER 70

OCCLUSIVE DISEASE: THROMBOSIS

G. PATRICK CLAGETT, JR.

Hemostatic mechanisms prevent hemorrhage at breaks in the vascular system. By localizing the clotting of blood at the site of injury, hemostatic mechanisms also maintain blood fluidity and circulation through the vessel. Imbalances between hemostatic reactions and protective mechanisms lead to formation of thrombi, which may obstruct the circulation.

LOCATION OF THROMBI

Thrombi form in the arteries, veins, heart, and microcirculation. *Arterial thrombi* cause tissue ischemia with organ dysfunction or infarction due to local obstruction of the vessel or distal embolism. Irregularity in the vessel wall due arterial disease, usually atherosclerosis, forms a nidus for arterial thrombus formation. One of the most common manifestations is ischemic heart disease. Rupture of coronary atherosclerotic plaque with thrombosis is felt to be the underlying mechanism in most patients with unstable angina, myocardial infarction, and sudden death from ischemic heart disease.

Most *venous thrombi* occur in the lower extremities. They originate from tiny clots in venous valve sinuses, an area where blood pools during periods of immobility, such as after an operation. Many venous thrombi are clinically silent, but some cause pain and swelling due to inflammation of the vessel wall or obstruction, or they embolize to the pulmonary circulation.

Intracardiac thrombi form on damaged heart valves, infarcted endocardium, or prosthetic valves. Flow disturbances contribute to intracardiac thrombus growth in areas of relative stasis and blood pooling behind obstructed valve orifices, in areas of ventricular dysfunction or aneurysm formation, or during dysrhythmia. Cardiac thrombi are usually asymptomatic until they embolize and produce symptoms according to site of lodgment. Most patients with cardiac embolism experience stroke, blindness, or transient ischemic attacks (TIAs).

In the *microcirculation,* widespread thrombosis is usually a manifestation of disseminated intravascular coagulation (DIC). This may lead to ischemic necrosis and generalized organ failure or consumption of hemostatic elements and secondary diffuse microvascular bleeding.

HISTOLOGIC COMPOSITION OF THROMBI

Histologic composition differs in arterial and venous thrombosis. Thrombi are composed of fibrin and red blood cells (RBCs), leukocytes, and platelets.

Arterial thrombi form under conditions of high flow, and are frequently composed of platelet aggregates bound loosely by fibrin strands. Because of flow conditions and the relatively small amounts of fibrin that bind them, arterial thrombi break off easily and tend to continually embo-

lize small fragments, producing symptoms such as unstable angina or cerebral TIAs.

Venous thrombi form in areas of sluggish blood flow. They are composed of RBCs, large amounts of fibrin, and few platelets. Venous thrombi grow large and fragment, resulting in pulmonary embolism.

Thrombi undergo constant structural change as they age. Leukocytes are attracted by chemotactic factors released from platelets and incorporate into the thrombus. Aggregated platelets fuse and undergo autolysis, and are replaced by fibrin lysed by plasma-borne fibrinolytic enzymes and leukocyte proteases. Infiltration of the thrombus by fibroblasts and smooth muscle cells leads to remodeling and incorporation into the architecture of the vessel wall. This may contribute to growth of atherosclerotic plaque in the arterial circulation.

Central portions of atherosclerotic plaques have cross-linked fibrin and platelet antigens, suggesting that arterial thrombus is present early in the growth of the plaque. Organization of venous thrombus may lead to recanalization of the lumen and scarring of the venous wall and valves, rendering them incompetent and leading to chronic venous insufficiency.

MECHANISMS THAT PROTECT AGAINST THROMBOSIS

Protective mechanisms that limit hemostatic reactions and prevent thrombus formation include: antithrombotic properties of vascular endothelium, inhibitory substances in blood that counteract coagulation reactions or lyse clots, and maintenance of normal laminar blood flow, which washes away activated coagulation enzymes and platelets and prevents excessive buildup of clot.

Impairment of the protective mechanisms affects coagulation and platelet reactions. Therapy is designed to prevent thrombosis or restore vascular patency after thrombus has formed. Rarely does the loss of a single protective factor lead to thrombosis. For example, one factor that causes postoperative deep venous thrombosis (DVT) is sluggish venous blood flow with pooling of blood in the lower extremities, but perioperative decreases in antithrombin III, defective fibrinolysis, and venous endothelial damage can be equally important factors.

Derangements in combinations of protective mechanisms also stimulate arterial thrombosis. A hemodynamically significant atherosclerotic plaque that causes disturbed, nonlaminar blood flow is not particularly thrombogenic as long as its surface is covered with healthy endothelium. When endothelial defenses are impaired or endothelium is lost, as occurs with plaque rupture, thrombogenesis occurs. The combination of major rheologic disturbance, loss of endothelium, and exposure of blood to thrombogenic plaque components can cause thrombotic occlusion, distal embolization, or both.

Endothelium and Vessel Wall Reactions

Endothelial Physiology

Endothelial cells are important in the regulation of coagulation, fibrinolysis, vascular tone, cellular growth and differentiation, and immune and inflammatory responses. Normal, intact endothelium is nonthrombogenic and reacts with neither platelets nor blood coagulation factors. Antithrombotic properties of endothelium are shown in Figure 70-1.

Endothelial cells synthesize prostaglandin I_2 (prostacyclin), which inhibits platelet aggregation and causes

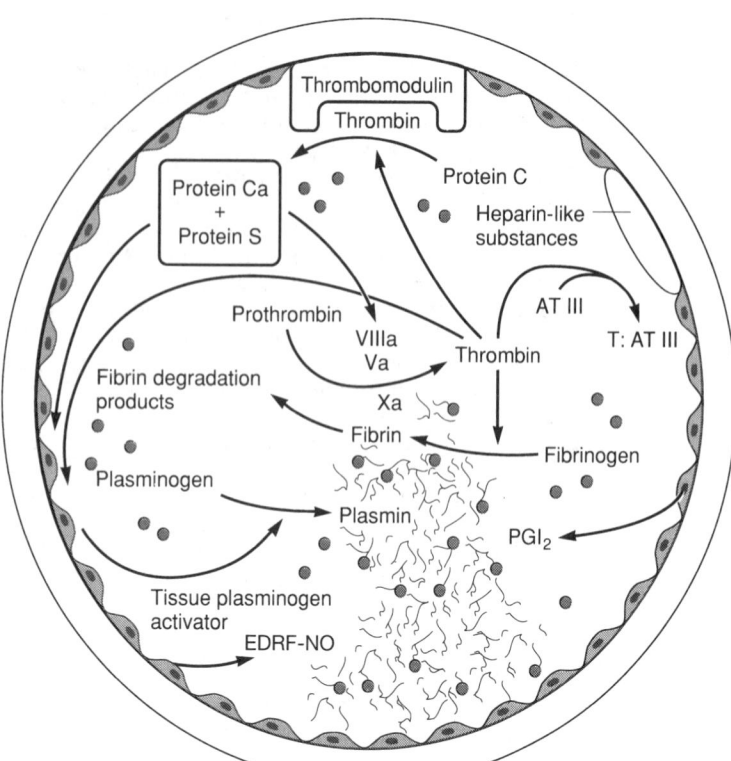

Figure 70-1. Major antithrombotic properties of vascular endothelium.

smooth muscle relaxation and vasodilatation. Vasodilatation caused by prostacyclin may lead to local increases in blood flow that help wash away newly formed platelet aggregates. Prostaglandin metabolism produces enzymes that inhibit smooth muscle cell contraction, inhibit platelet aggregation, stimulate disaggregation, inhibit platelet and monocyte adhesion to endothelial surfaces, and inhibit smooth muscle cell proliferation.

Endothelium counteracts coagulation enzymatic reactions. Endothelial cells synthesize heparin-like glycosoaminoglycans that possess anticoagulant activity. Endothelial heparan sulfate activates circulating antithrombin III, which neutralizes activated factors XII, XI, X, IX, and II (thrombin). The principal action of this system is to limit thrombin production by binding to thrombomodulin. Thrombin bound to thrombomodulin loses its ability to activate coagulation factors.

Thrombin complexed with thrombomodulin can activate protein C, which destroys factors Va and VIIIa and stimulates release of plasminogen activator. Binding of thrombin to thrombomodulin causes loss of the coagulant effects and enhancement of the ability to activate protein C and inhibit thrombogenesis. Thrombin stimulates endothelial production of prostacyclin and expression of fibrinolytic activity.

Endothelium synthesizes and secretes plasminogen activator and is the principal source of tissue plasminogen activator (tPA). tPA Converts plasminogen to plasmin, which lyses fibrin. Endothelial cells release tPA and possess surface receptors that bind plasminogen and enhance the efficiency of local fibrinolytic mechanisms. Endothelial cells are the source of plasminogen activator inhibitor (PAI-1), a protein that neutralizes tPA. Endothelium can stimulate or down-regulate local fibrinolytic activity, depending on the stimulus.

Vessel Wall Damage

Damage to the vessel wall can lead to loss of endothelium and thrombus formation. *Direct* endothelial trauma includes blunt and penetrating vascular trauma, surgical intervention (injury from application of vascular clamps, endarterectomy, vascular suturing, manipulation of blood vessels), interventional endovascular therapy (balloon angioplasty, atherectomy), and extreme thermal conditions (burn injury, frostbite). *Indirect* endothelial injury may be caused by immune complexes, viruses or bacteria, hemodynamic stress from localized jetlike flows, tobacco products, high blood cholesterol, elevated blood homocystine, and enzymes released from platelets and leukocytes in inflammatory states.

Loss of endothelium exposes underlying thrombogenic tissues to platelet and coagulation factors. Endothelial dysfunction causes loss of antithrombotic properties, and activation of endothelial mechanisms that can promote thrombosis (Fig. 70-2).

Platelet Reactions

Platelet reactions critical to thrombogenesis (Fig. 70-3) are:

- Platelet adhesion—platelets adhere to nonendothelialized surfaces
- Platelet secretion—platelets undergo shape change and release their granular contents
- Platelet aggregation—platelets aggregate to form clumps
- Platelet coagulant activity—a property of activated platelets that accelerates coagulation reactions

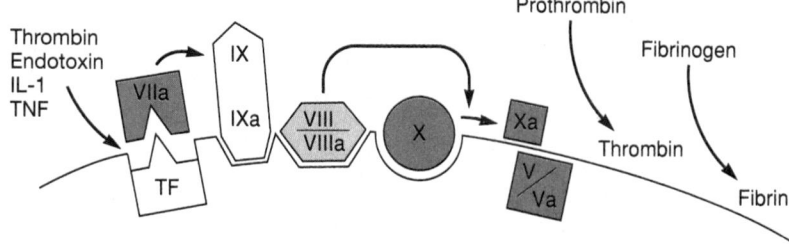

Figure 70-2. Procoagulant properties of vascular endothelium. Endothelial procoagulant activity is induced by bacterial endotoxin, thrombin, and interleukin-1. Perturbed endothelial cells not only express tissue factor (TF), but also possess specific binding sites for factors VII, IX, VIII, and X. In addition, endothelial cells can synthesize factor V. Binding and activation of these factors results in local thrombin generation.

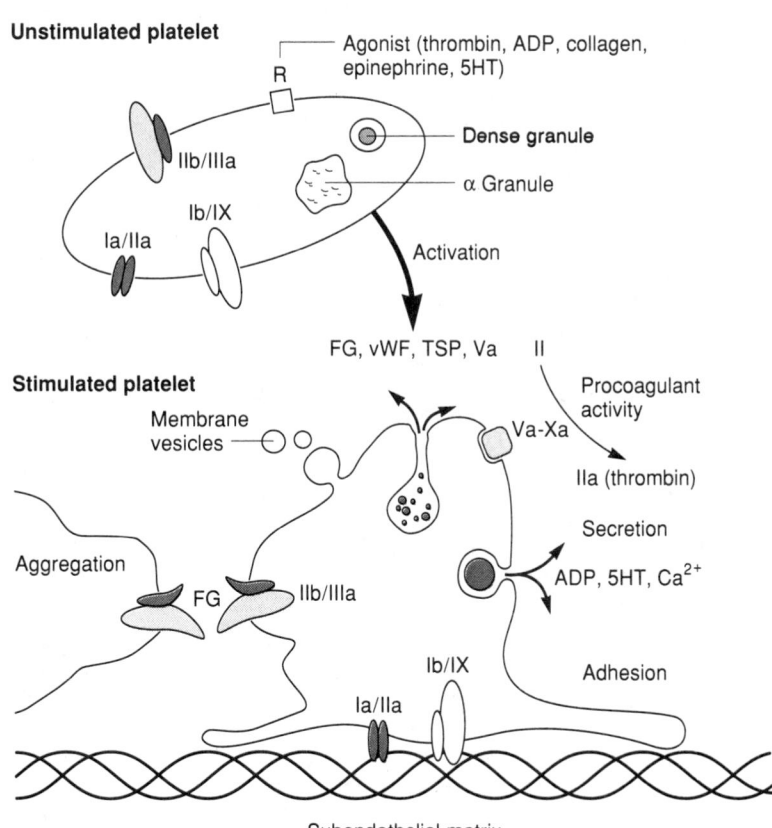

Figure 70-3. The receptor-mediated events of platelet activation, adhesion, secretion, and aggregation. R, receptor; ADP, adenosine diphosphate; 5HT, serotonin; FG, fibrinogen; vWF, von Willebrand factor; TSP, thrombospondin.

Coagulation Reactions

Blood coagulation caused by activation of the intrinsic and extrinsic pathways occurs during thrombogenesis. Activation of the intrinsic pathway is initiated by conversion of factor XII to enzymatic factor XIIa when blood comes into contact with a nonendothelialized vascular surface after vessel wall damage. Factor XII also is activated when blood contacts a prosthetic device or other biomaterial. The extrinsic pathway is initiated when factor VII, activated by tissue thromboplastin, is expressed by damaged endothelial cells or is released into the bloodstream during extensive tissue damage, as may occur during an operation or generalized trauma.

Circulating Inhibitory Proteins and the Fibrinolytic System

Serine Protease Inhibitors

Activated coagulation factors are serine proteases neutralized by circulating protease inhibitors, the most important of which is *antithrombin III*. This inhibitor scavenges activated blood-clotting enzymes that are free in the microenvironment of a growing clot, limiting its size.

Antithrombin III neutralizes thrombin, factor Xa, and factor IXa and is a relatively weak inhibitor of factors XIIa and XIa. Reduction of antithrombin III to <50% of normal values predisposes to venous thrombosis. The rate of inhibition of these activated coagulation factors by antithrombin III is dramatically accelerated by heparin and, to a lesser extent, heparan sulfate on the surface of endothelial cells.

Protein C is a vitamin K-dependent protein activated by thrombin. This process is facilitated when thrombin is bound to the endothelial cell surface receptor, thrombomodulin. Activated protein C acts as an anticoagulant by destroying coagulation factors Va and VIIIa, especially when these factors are bound to platelet and endothelial membranes. Activated protein C also limits clot formation by facilitating fibrinolysis. Enhancement of fibrinolysis by activated protein C may be due in part to its ability to bind to plasminogen activator inhibitor (PAI-1).

Protein S is a vitamin K-dependent plasma protein necessary for expression of the anticoagulant activity of activated protein C.

Fibrinolytic System

Fibrinolytic activity occurs in circulating blood when plasminogen is converted to plasmin by a number of plasminogen activators synthesized by endothelial cells and other tissues or during systemic thrombolytic therapy.

Interactions between components of the fibrinolytic system take place primarily within a blood clot. During fibrin formation, both plasminogen and tPA, derived from adjacent endothelium, bind to fibrin. tPA Converts the clot-bound plasminogen to plasmin. When fibrinolysis occurs, plasmin is released into the blood, where it is rapidly neutralized by α_2-antiplasmin. Excess plasmin is inactivated by α_2-macroglobulin. If both inhibitors are overwhelmed, as may happen during thrombolytic therapy, degradation of plasma coagulation factors and fibrinogen occurs.

Endothelium is important in modulating physiologic fibrinolysis. Endothelial cells produce tPA and specifically bind this protein. Endothelial cells also oppose fibrinolysis by synthesizing PAI-1.

Hypercoagulable Syndromes

Prothrombotic or hypercoagulable states can be hereditary or acquired. They occur under the following circumstances:

- Deficiencies of serine proteases or natural anticoagulants
- Imbalances in the fibrinolytic system
- The presence of substances that accelerate coagulation or platelet reactions
- Diffuse endothelial dysfunction exists

Congenital Hypercoagulable States

The hereditary or congenital coagulation abnormalities are often referred to as *inherited thrombotic disorders.* The biochemical abnormalities are fixed and persistent, but the thrombotic events are episodic. The congenital hypercoagulable states are:

- Antithrombin III deficiency
- Protein C deficiency
- Resistance to activated protein C
- Protein S deficiency
- Congenital fibrinolytic disorders
- Dysfibrinogenemia
- Homocystinuria (cystathionine synthase deficiency)
- Presence of lipoprotein(a)

Inherited thrombophilic disorders are frequently characterized by venous thrombosis, especially in unusual sites. The following suggest an underlying congenital hypercoagulable disorder:

- Unexplained venous thrombosis in a person younger than 45 years
- Recurrent venous thromboembolism
- Thrombosis of mesenteric, hepatic, portal, renal, or cerebral veins or the inferior vena cava
- Diffuse cutaneous microvascular thrombosis
- Family history of thrombosis

Acquired Hypercoagulable States

Acquired hypercoagulable states often accompany another illness. Acquired hypercoagulable states are far more common than congenital thrombophilias. They may present with venous or arterial thrombosis. The acquired hypercoagulable states are as follows:

- Lupus anticoagulant and related antiphospholipid antibodies
- Heparin-induced thrombocytopenia and thrombosis
- Myeloproliferative disorders (polycythemia vera, chronic myelogenous leukemia, myeloid metaplasia, and essential thrombocythemia)
- Malignant disease (acute promyelocytic leukemia, myeloproliferative disorders, primary tumors of the brain, mucin-secreting adenocarcinomas of the pancreas, gastrointestinal tract, lung, and ovary)
- Postoperative and inflammatory states, such as inflammatory bowel disease, rheumatoid arthritis, and chronic infections, pregnancy, use of oral contraceptives, increased levels of fibrinogen and factor VII, and nephrotic syndrome

Blood Flow and Thrombosis

Normal, nondisturbed, laminar blood flow discourages thrombogenesis. *Laminar flow* is the type of motion in which the fluid moves as a series of individual layers, each stratum moving at a different velocity from its neighboring layers (Fig. 70-4A). Because blood is viscous, its flow near solid boundaries is shear flow. *Shear* refers to the sliding motion between contiguous planes. Because of frictional resistance at the blood-vessel wall interface, flow velocity is greater in midstream than at the luminal surface.

Movement of cells and molecules in blood occurs by means of two principal transport processes—convection

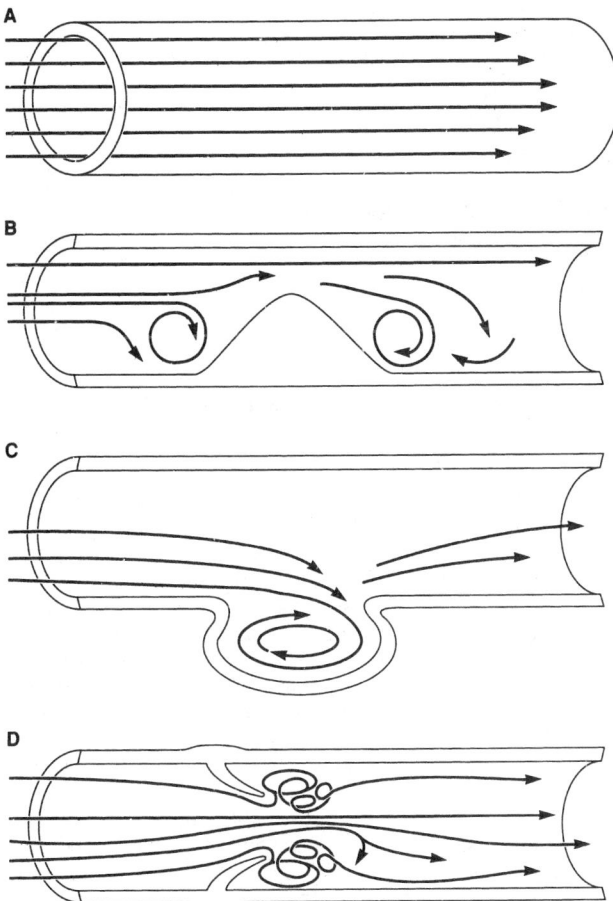

Figure 70-4. (*A*) Nondisturbed laminar blood flow. (*B*) Blood flow at a site of irregularity or stenosis. There are vortices (zones of recirculation) on both sides of the stenosis. In addition, the shear rate is highest at the maximum point of stenosis. (*C*) Vortices occurring in an area of lumen expansion. Arterial pathology causing such areas would include an aneurysm and the crater of an ulcerated atherosclerotic plaque. (*D*) Zone of recirculation formed within a venous valve sinus.

- Activated platelets and coagulation factors have prolonged residence times at one site
- Platelets collide with each other and other cells and undergo secretion and aggregation
- There is a lack of dilution and clearing of these elements by normal blood-containing inhibitors

Platelets and platelet aggregates are transported toward the vessel wall by means of convective diffusion, especially under conditions of high shear. Diffusion of platelets toward the wall is enhanced at high shear rates by the paddling effect of RBCs that transport platelets radially. In the presence of localized endothelial dysfunction, absence of endothelium, or presence of a reactive surface, disturbed flow in areas of high shear favors platelet thrombogenesis.

Extreme levels of shear stress exist close to each other at the most prominent portion of an atherosclerotic plaque that produces hemodynamically significant narrowing of the lumen. In vessels with intimal injury, platelet deposition increases with increasing stenosis, indicating shear rate-induced cell activation. Platelet deposition is greatest at the apex of the stenosis and not the flow recirculation zone distal to the apex.

In veins, blood flow is slow and shear rates are low. At low shear rates, blood becomes viscous because of attraction between RBCs in the presence of fibrinogen. Blood, in essence, thickens as flow rates decrease.

Sluggish blood flow in veins favors thrombosis primarily because of the prolonged residence time of activated coagulation factors, which allow reactions to proceed to fibrin formation. These reactions are accelerated if there are deficiencies in serine protease inhibitors, defective fibrinolytic activity, or excess activation of coagulation factors. Disturbed, nonlaminar flow may promote these effects at specific sites. The fluid in the center stream is accelerated, whereas vortices and areas of flow separation form in the pockets (Fig. 70-4D). This area becomes isolated from the already sluggish venous circulation and is the site of nascent venous thrombi.

THERAPEUTIC IMPLICATIONS

Venous Thrombosis

Because it depends on coagulation reactions that result in fibrin formation, venous thrombosis is treated with the anticoagulants heparin and warfarin sodium. These drugs in small doses prevent the onset of venous thrombosis and can be used as prophylaxis against postoperative DVT. Agents that are pure inhibitors of platelet function, such as aspirin, are much less successful in prophylaxis against postoperative venous thrombosis.

Methods that prevent venous pooling and stasis of blood in the lower extremities help prevent DVT. Augmentation of venous emptying by application of intermittent pneumatic compression boots is as effective as use of anticoagulants.

Dextran, an effective agent in reducing venous thromboembolism, increases blood volume (increasing venous flow) by interfering with fibrin polymerization so clots are more susceptible to lysis and by weakly inhibiting platelet function.

Besides preventing the onset of venous thrombosis, anticoagulants inhibit the growth, propagation, and embolization of established thrombi. These agents are the mainstay of treatment of patients with active venous thrombosis who are at risk for pulmonary embolism. Aspirin and other antiplatelet agents are not effective in the management of active venous thrombosis.

and diffusion. *Convection* occurs because cells and molecules move with the fluid surrounding them. *Diffusion* occurs when molecules or particles move relative to the motion of the surrounding medium. When convection and diffusion operate simultaneously, transport is said to occur by *convective diffusion.*

In blood, all cells, particles, and molecules are transported by means of convective diffusion. Convective diffusion in vessels relies on a combination of convection (to effect transport over relatively long distances) and diffusion (to effect transport over relatively short, radial distances).

When blood flow does not follow unidirectional, predictable, or stable linear paths, it becomes nonlaminar and is said to be *disturbed*. In arteries, disturbed blood flow occurs at vessel orifices, branches, bifurcations, stenoses, irregularities in the vessel wall, and sudden expansions in the radius of the lumen, as with an aneurysm (Figs. 70-4B,C). Thrombus formation occurs at these sites in part because of complex flow patterns. These patterns include areas of flow separation (a portion of the fluid volume moves separately from the main flow), vortices, and zones of recirculation. Thrombogenesis is favored under these conditions of flow because:

Intracardiac Thromboemboli

Intracardiac thromboemboli are responsive to anticoagulant treatment. Immediate treatment with heparin and long-term therapy with warfarin sodium reduce risk for symptomatic emboli from intracardiac thrombi.

Arterial Circulation

Antiplatelet agents prevent thrombogenesis in areas of abnormal shear and disturbed flow in the arterial circulation. This most commonly involves the surface irregularity or stenoses caused by atherosclerotic plaque. *Aspirin* is the most widely used antiplatelet agent and prevents myocardial infarction among patients with unstable angina and stable coronary disease; stroke and TIAs among patients with cerebrovascular arteriosclerosis or after carotid endarterectomy; venous graft thrombosis after coronary artery bypass; and prosthetic bypass thrombosis among patients with femoropopliteal reconstruction. Aspirin retards platelet thrombogenesis on the surface of atherosclerotic plaque, but it does not appear to prevent plaque formation.

Ticlopidine is an antiplatelet agent used to prevent platelet-dependent arterial thromboembolism. For cerebrovascular disease, ticlopidine is more effective than aspirin.

Fibrinolytic agents include streptokinase, recombinant tPA, and urokinase, all of which accelerate conversion of plasminogen to plasmin. These substances are most effective in the treatment of patients with acute myocardial infarction. Because fibrinolytic agents dissolve hemostatic clots along with pathologic clots (thrombi), they cause more bleeding complications than anticoagulants.

SUGGESTED READING

Allaart CF, Poort SR, Rosendaal FR, et al. Increased risk of venous thrombosis in carriers of hereditary protein C deficiency defect. Lancet 1993;341:134.

Dahlback B. The protein C anticoagulant system: inherited defects as basis for venous thrombosis. Thromb Res 1995;77:1.

DeLoughery TG, Goodnight SH. The hypercoagulable states: diagnosis and management. Semin Vasc Surg 1993;6:66.

Kassis J, Hirsh J, Podor TJ. Evidence that postoperative fibrinolytic shutdown is mediated by plasma factors that stimulate endothelial cell type I plasminogen activator inhibitor biosynthesis. Blood 1992;80:1758.

Kirchhofer D, Sakariassen KS, Clozel M, et al. Relationship between tissue factor expression and deposition of fibrin, platelets, and leukocytes on cultured endothelial cells under venous blood flow conditions. Blood 1993;81:2050.

Rubin BG, Santoro SA, Sicard GA. Platelet interactions with the vessel wall and prosthetic grafts. Ann Vasc Surg 1993;7:200.

Svensson PJ, Dahlback B. Resistance to activated protein C as a basis for venous thrombosis. N Engl J Med 1994;330:517.

Ware JA, Heistad DD. Platelet-endothelium interactions. N Engl J Med 1993;328:628.

ESSENTIALS OF SURGERY: SCIENTIFIC PRINCIPLES AND PRACTICE, edited by Lazar J. Greenfield, Michael W. Mulholland, Keith T. Oldham, Gerald B. Zelenock, and Keith D. Lillemoe. Lippincott–Raven Publishers, Philadelphia, © 1997.

CHAPTER 71

PERIPHERAL ARTERIAL EMBOLISM

LOUIS M. MESSINA

ACUTE ARTERIAL EMBOLISM

Source and Etiology

The potential sources of acute arterial emboli are illustrated in Figure 71-1; however in 5% to 10% of patients, the site of origin is never identified.

Thrombus forms on the endocardial surface of the heart and is most commonly associated with atrial fibrillation. Ischemic and rheumatic heart disease are the common underlying *heart diseases* that cause intracardiac thrombus formation. Ventricular aneurysm formation, a complication of acute MI, can be a source of arterial emboli. Cardiomyopathy and CHF are other, less common causes of mural thrombus formation as a source of peripheral arterial emboli.

Arterial aneurysms are a noncardiac source of peripheral arterial embolism. Thrombus forms along the dilated portion of the artery, and layers of thrombus increase as the aneurysm enlarges. Fragments of this laminated thrombus break loose and obstruct the downstream arterial circulation. The most common arterial aneurysms associated with peripheral arterial embolism are infrarenal abdominal aortic, and femoral and popliteal arterial aneurysms.

In patients with *bacterial endocarditis,* valvular vegetations fragment and embolize into the arterial circulation, obstructing small arteries, such as the palmar or plantar arches or the digital arteries.

Prosthetic heart valves can be an important source of arterial emboli. The mitral valve is a more common source of emboli than the aortic valves. Most emboli lodge in the cerebral circulation; some are fatal.

Cardiac tumor fragments from an atrial myxoma or angiosarcoma can embolize. Because bacterial endocarditis and atrial myxoma often present as an acute arterial embolism, specimens of acute emboli must be subjected to microscopic analysis and culture after they are removed during surgical embolectomy. Emboli can originate from the surface of *atherosclerotic plaques.*

Trauma may be a cause of peripheral arterial embolism. A bullet that enters the heart or great vessels can cause embolism downstream from the point of entry. After a bullet embolus is identified, the site at which the bullet entered the vascular tree must be identified. The injury at the site of entry usually is more life-threatening than the ischemia that develops downstream from the bullet obstruction.

Trauma due to surgical manipulation or diagnostic or therapeutic vascular catheterization can cause arterial embolism. These emboli originate from thrombus that forms on the surface of catheters, particularly those that have been in place for a long time. The catheters themselves also can fracture and embolize.

Portions of *malignant tumors* can fragment and embolize into the arterial circulation. Most are primary or metastatic tumors of the lung. Embolism of lung tumor fragments

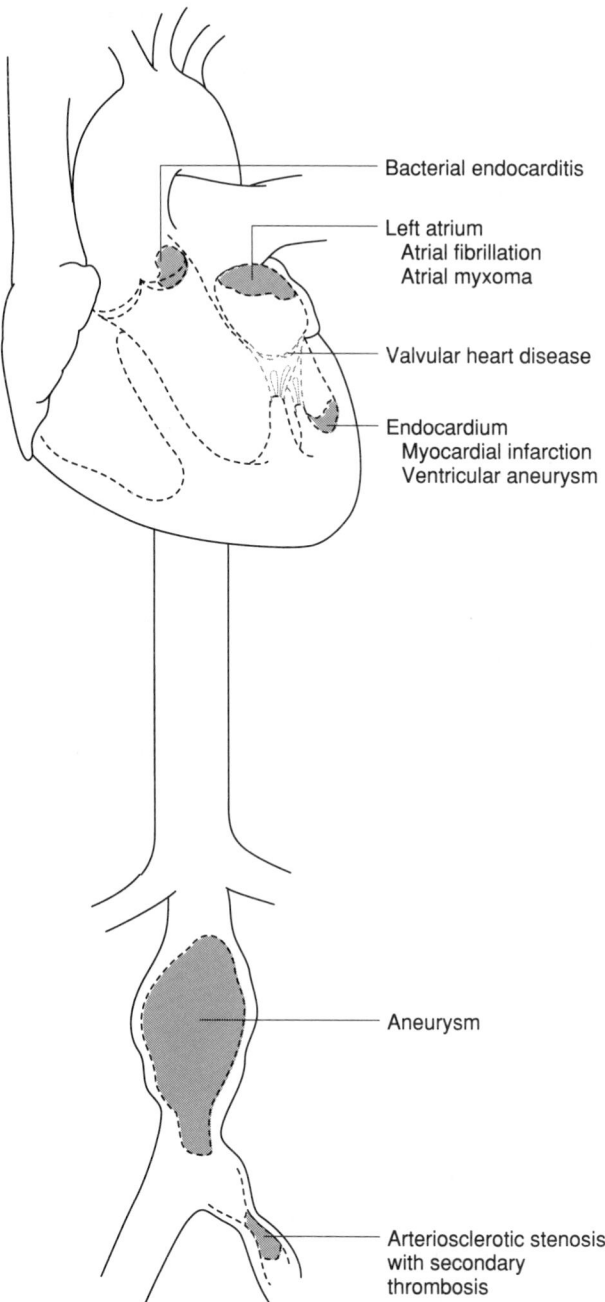

Figure 71-1. Common sources of arterial emboli.

Distribution

Arterial emboli do not distribute in the arterial circulation proportionate to the flow rate of a particular artery. Factors that influence the distribution in the arterial tree include: the size and density of the embolus, arterial diameter, arterial branch angle, and the shape of arterial bifurcations.

About half of arterial emboli go to the cerebral circulation. The frequency of cerebral embolism differs with the type of heart disease. Patients who have rheumatic heart disease complicated by mitral valve disease and atrial fibrillation are at high risk for cerebral embolism and strokes.

Most arterial emboli lodge at arterial bifurcations, where there is a sudden change in arterial diameter (Fig. 71-2).

Pathophysiology

The pathophysiologic process of acute limb ischemia due to arterial embolism reflects changes in skeletal muscle after ischemia and after embolectomy during reperfusion. Skeletal muscle is more tolerant of ischemia than other organs. The extent of skeletal muscle necrosis is a function of the duration and severity of ischemia, the metabolic rate of the muscle, and the type and duration of reperfusion. Under resting conditions and normothermia, skeletal muscle can tolerate 1 to 3 hours of ischemia.

The manifestations of skeletal muscle reperfusion injury are a direct reflection of cellular and metabolic changes. Reperfusion syndrome is characterized by metabolic acidosis, hyperkalemia, myoglobinuria, acute renal tubular necrosis, and muscle edema. Other manifestations of reperfusion syndrome are acute tubular necrosis and compartment syndrome.

occurs during surgical manipulation of the tumor or in the immediately postoperative period.

Arterial embolism can originate from a site of *venous thrombosis* (paradoxic embolus). The embolus passes through a patent foramen ovale, an atrial septal defect, a patent ductus arteriosus, or a pulmonary arteriovenous fistula. After pulmonary embolism, pulmonary and right ventricular hypertension can occur, and right atrial pressure exceeds left atrial pressure. This interarterial pressure gradient facilitates passage of venous emboli into the arterial circulation. Paradoxic emboli usually occur in patients who already have symptomatic acute pulmonary embolism or chronic pulmonary hypertension. A patient who has acute arterial embolism in the absence of a condition that predisposes to arterial embolism should be evaluated for possible paradoxic embolism.

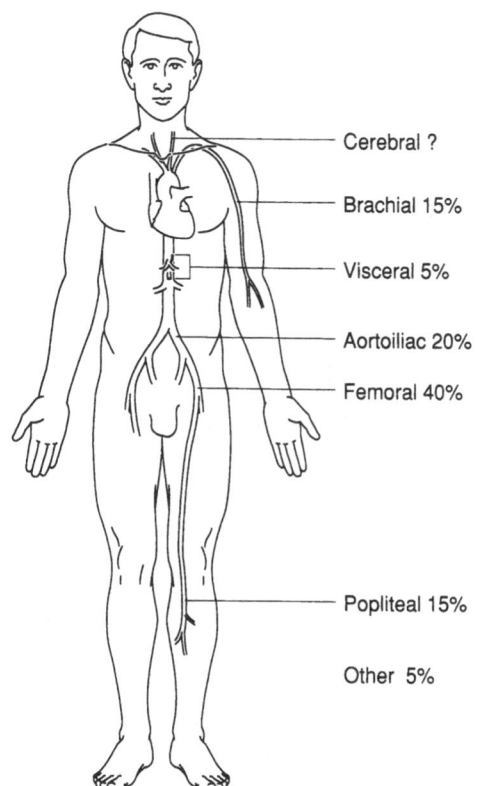

Figure 71-2. Approximate distribution of arterial emboli based on pooled data.

Clinical Manifestations

Sudden occlusion of a peripheral artery by an acute embolus causes the five Ps of acute limb ischemia: pain, pallor, pulselessness, paresthesia, and paralysis. These signs and symptoms occur in a characteristic distribution, often allowing localization of the arterial embolus on the basis of physical examination alone (Fig. 71-3). The signs and symptoms of acute ischemia progress as the duration of ischemia increases.

The *pain* caused by acute arterial occlusion is so sudden and severe that the patient can recall the precise time of onset. The pain is described as severe and deep, well localized and unremitting. The pain does not dissipate until arterial circulation is restored or irreversible ischemic injury to the sensory nerves occurs.

Paresthesia appears soon after the arterial occlusion. Because small nerve fibers are sensitive to ischemia, the first loss of sensation is light touch.

Pallor of the limb appears immediately after the onset of ischemia. It is caused by diminished skin blood flow due to arterial obstruction and reflex vasoconstriction as a secondary response to tissue ischemia.

Although some weakness of the involved extremity can be present soon after the onset of ischemia, *paralysis* of any muscle group is a late feature. The limb is cool, the temperature changes becoming greater in areas distal to the arterial occlusion.

Localization of an embolus is based on the level of *absent pulses* and the level of change in skin temperature and color. The change in skin temperature is the most sensitive sign of ischemia and is present one skeletal segment below the level of arterial obstruction. Changes in skin color occur one to two skeletal segments below the level of arterial obstruction.

For example, acute occlusion of the distal infrarenal aorta, a so-called saddle embolus, is manifest by the absence of femoral pulses bilaterally. The decrease in skin temperature starts on the upper thigh, and changes in skin color beginning at the knee. Occlusion of the common femoral artery is manifest by a decrease in skin temperature on the lower thigh and a change in skin color starting at midcalf.

Other factors that influence the manifestations and diagnosis of acute arterial embolism are the general condition of the patient, the presence of synchronous arterial embolism, and the metabolic consequences of the tissue ischemia. Many patients with acute arterial embolism have severe medical illnesses, such as acute CHF complicated by peripheral edema, acute MI, chronic obstructive pulmonary disease, and pneumonia. General debility and the presence of concurrent systemic illness can obscure the signs and symptoms of acute limb ischemia.

Some patients seek treatment weeks or months after the embolic event. Most of these patients have evidence of subacute limb ischemia inconsistent with acute embolic occlusion or chronic occlusive disease. Some have a his-

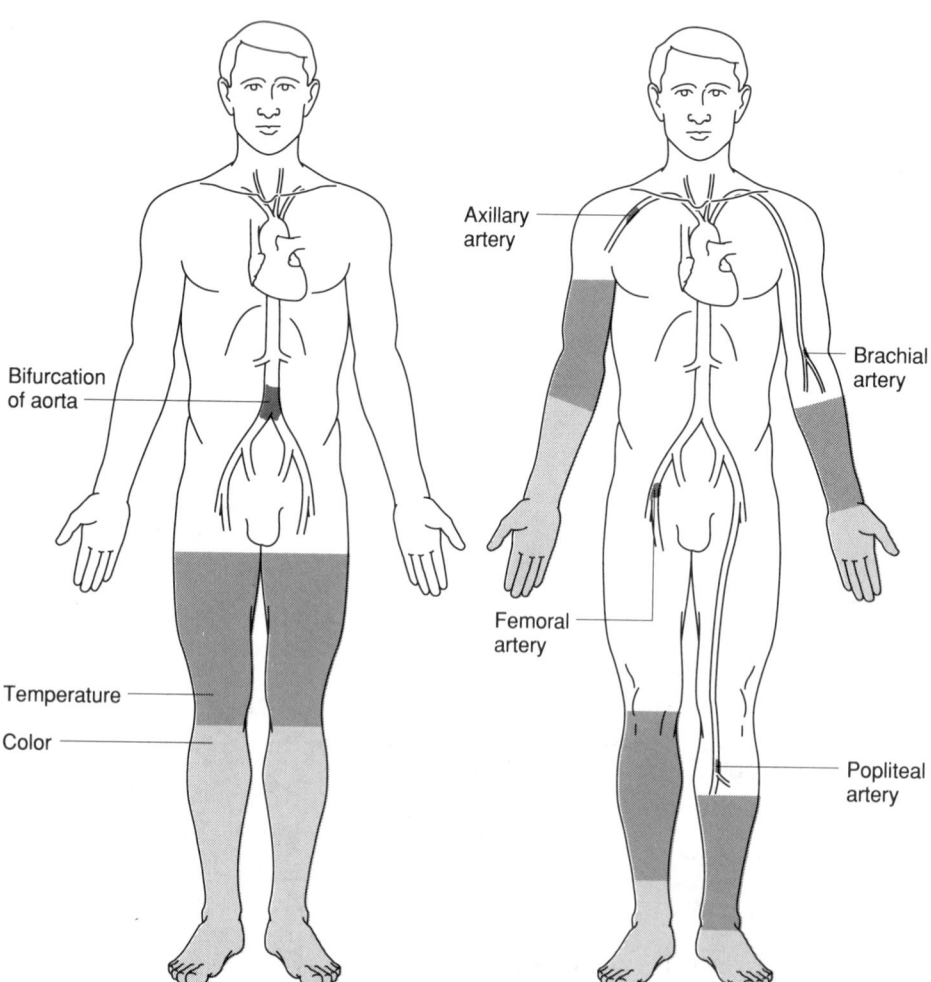

Figure 71-3. The location of an acute arterial embolus can usually be determined precisely based on physical examination of the patient.

tory of a sudden onset of calf claudication or ischemic limb pain. Some patients are referred for evaluation for presumptive diagnosis of acute deep venous thrombosis. The diagnosis of acute arterial embolism is usually made after arteriography discloses findings consistent with embolic occlusion. Even if a long time has elapsed since the onset of symptoms, most patients can undergo embolectomy.

Differential Diagnosis

The differential diagnosis of acute limb ischemia includes acute arterial embolism, acute arterial thrombosis, acute aortic dissection, acute venous thrombosis, and arterial spasm. The most important differential diagnosis is between acute arterial embolism and acute arterial thrombosis (Table 71-1).

The diagnosis of acute arterial embolism can be established with the history and physical examination. Patients with the classic signs of acute limb ischemia and a readily identifiable cardiac abnormality, such as atrial fibrillation or acute MI, need no further evaluation. When the diagnosis is in doubt, angiography is performed.

Management

Most patients cannot tolerate 4 to 6 hours of acute limb ischemia before serious nerve and muscle injury occurs. Prompt diagnosis and expeditious evaluation and treatment are necessary to preserve limb function.

The first step in the management of acute limb ischemia is administration of *heparin.* Heparin prevents proximal and distal propagation of thrombus, maintains patency of collateral vessels, and can reduce the extent of ischemic injury.

The next step is *thromboembolectomy* with arterial embolectomy catheters. Because the perioperative morbidity and mortality for this operation are high, patients at poor risk, such as those who have had acute MI and those who have intractable, severe CHF, undergo nonsurgical treatment with heparin. The surgeon must use the smallest catheter that is effective. Important technical points include never passing the catheter against resistance and never withdrawing it under excessive tension. Although complete embolectomy is important, repetitive passage of the catheter increases the frequency of complications.

When ischemia lasts >4 hours, four-compartment fasciotomy can be performed. The consequences of reperfusion of ischemic skeletal muscle are not fully manifested until 12 to 24 hours after the operation. Long fasciotomy incisions through relatively small skin incisions can prevent development of compartment syndrome.

Before leaving the operating room, the patient must have adequate arterial circulation to maintain limb viability and

Table 71-2. MANAGEMENT OF SKELETAL MUSCLE REPERFUSION SYNDROME

Clinical Manifestation	Treatment
Lactic acidosis	Sodium bicarbonate
Hyperkalemia	Insulin and glucose
Myoglobinuria or acute tubular necrosis	Alkalinization of urine to prevent precipitation of myoglobin in renal tubules
Muscle edema or compartment syndrome	Fasciotomy

function. This usually can be ascertained by means of continuous-wave Doppler probe evaluation of the pedal pulses. When the viability of the extremity is threatened or when there are no Doppler signals in the distal extremity, intraoperative arteriography or angioscopy is performed.

Postoperative care involves close monitoring. Patients usually have severe medical illnesses and are at risk for complications associated with reperfusion of an ischemic limb (Table 71-2). These complications can be minimized by the use of fasciotomy, hydration, administration of mannitol to maintain renal diuresis, and intravenous sodium bicarbonate sufficient to alkalinize the urine. Heparin is reinstituted 6 to 12 hours after the operation because of a high rate of recurrent embolism.

Complications after arterial embolectomy are myocardial, pulmonary, renal, and recurrent arterial emboli. Anticoagulation with heparin or warfarin reduces the rate of recurrent embolism and associated limb loss and mortality. Complications due to the use of balloon catheters include intimal injury, arterial perforation, vessel wall disruption, arteriovenous fistulas, pseudoaneurysms, and arterial stenosis.

ATHEROEMBOLISM

Atheroembolism is caused by the release of cholesterol-rich atheromatous debris from ulcerated atherosclerotic plaques. Most atheroemboli are composed of cholesterol crystals that obstruct the arterioles. Some occlude large vessels. The most familiar syndrome of atheroembolism is *blue toe syndrome,* obstruction of the digital arteries of the toes.

The *signs and symptoms* of atheroembolism are summarized in Figure 71-4 and Table 71-3. Atheroembolism can produce organ-specific symptoms or signs and symptoms of multisystem organ failure. Atheroembolism can occur by at least three mechanisms: spontaneously, sometimes as a consequence of coughing, tenesmus, or lifting; precipitated by surgical manipulation of the aorta or its branches; and induced by catheter manipulation during angiography.

Pathophysiology

Atheroembolism is caused by sudden rupture of an atherosclerotic plaque, resulting in showers of cholesterol-rich atheromatous debris into the distal arterial circulation. Depending on the size and concentration of particles, these emboli can pass through the microcirculation or obstruct a vessel. Most episodes of atheroembolism do not have detectable clinical sequelae. When an embolus is large, tissue infarction occurs. The emboli gradually become incorporated into the vessel wall, and obliterative endarteritis, including intimal and medial thickening and fibrosis, occurs. Cholesterol crystals that have penetrated

Table 71-1. CLINICAL DISTINCTIONS BETWEEN ACUTE ARTERIAL EMBOLISM AND ACUTE ARTERIAL THROMBOSIS

Embolism	Thrombosis
Arrhythmia	No arrhythmia
Sudden onset	Sudden onset
No prior claudication or rest pain	History of claudication or rest pain
Normal contralateral pulses	Contralateral pulses absent
No physical findings of chronic limb ischemia	Physical findings of chronic limb ischemia

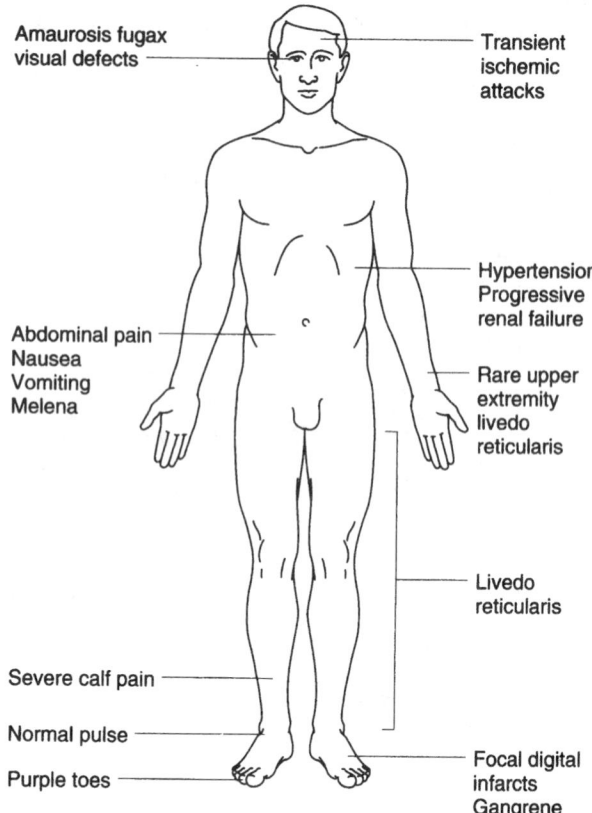

Figure 71-4. Clinical manifestations of multiple cholesterol emboli. (After Kalter X, et al. Livedo reticularis due to multiple cholesterol emboli. J Am Acad Dermatol 1985;13:235)

through microvascular walls incite perivascular granulomatous inflammation.

Clinical Syndromes

Arterial Catheter-related Atheroembolism

Atheroembolism is a serious complication of angiography caused by manipulation of angiographic catheters. Distal embolism also can be caused by dilation of a balloon during angioplasty. The complication often does not occur for a long time after the procedure. Signs of atheroembolism include those of livedo reticularis and digital infarction in the feet. When diffuse atheroembolism occurs, signs and symptoms are those of episodic or sustained hypertension, fever, and eosinophilia. Acute renal failure due to renal atheroembolism is often not detectable until 1 to 4 weeks after angiography.

Lower-extremity Atheroembolism

Lower-extremity atheroembolism is manifest by sharply demarcated areas of focal ischemia of the lower leg or foot, usually the toes (Fig. 71-4). Livedo reticularis sometimes extends from the umbilicus to the feet. Thigh and calf myalgia are common and are caused by atheroembolism in muscle. The areas of focal ischemia are characterized by purplish discoloration of the skin and surrounding petechial hemorrhages. These lesions represent blue toe syndrome and are intensely painful. Pedal pulses may be present.

Atheroembolism of the lower extremities can cause large-vessel obstruction that has features indistinguishable from those of emboli of cardiac origin. Usually the diagnosis is not made until inspection of the embolus. A large percentage of patients with atheroembolism of an extremity have tissue loss. Amputation often is necessary.

Patients with lower-extremity atheroembolism undergo prompt arteriography to delineate possible sources of emboli. The most common source of embolism is stenotic or ulcerated lesions of the distal superficial femoral artery. Management of arterial lesions is removal of the lesion by means of endarterectomy or excision of the diseased portion of the vessel. When these techniques cannot be used, bypass and exclusion of the lesion are an alternative.

Gastrointestinal Microembolism

The stomach, small intestine, pancreas, and gallbladder are affected by atheroembolism to the GI tract. Atheroembolism causes occlusion of multiple submucosal arterioles, which leads to variable degrees of mucosal ischemia. Transmural necrosis of the intestinal wall can develop, or there can be a pattern of diffuse ulceration. These ulcers undergo cycles of healing and breakdown.

The manifestations of atheroembolism to the GI tract are diffuse abdominal pain, paralytic ileus, bleeding, and, rarely, small-intestinal obstruction. Atheroembolism may cause perforation of the intestine or gallbladder. There is an association between cholesterol embolism and angiodysplasia. Biopsy shows cholesterol emboli, granuloma formation, subepithelial ectasia of vessels, and epithelial atrophy. The only therapy is resection of the involved portion of the GI tract.

Coronary Atheroembolism

Atheroembolism of the coronary arteries can cause acute MI. It occurs during cardiopulmonary resuscitation, after strenuous exercise, and as a cause of perioperative MI during coronary artery bypass grafting. Atheroembolism is caused by plaque rupture and release of cholesterol crystals and other debris into the circulation. Inflammation of the vessel walls is characterized in its later stages by eosinophilic infiltration. The vasculitis is attributed to a hypersensitivity reaction to noncholesterol constituents of atheroma.

Renal Atheroembolism

The kidney is the organ most often affected by atheroembolism. There is extensive occlusion of the arcuate and interlobar arteries, and there can be hyalinization of glomeruli. Variable degrees of inflammation occur in vessel walls and around cholesterol outside the vessel walls. Renal atheroembolism can be a complication of angiography, can be caused by manipulation of the aorta or its branches during an operation, or can occur as a spontaneous event.

Table 71-3. LABORATORY ABNORMALITIES ASSOCIATED WITH MULTIPLE CHOLESTEROL EMBOLI

Elevated erythrocyte sedimentation rate
Eosinophilia
Leukocytosis
Abnormal urinalysis—proteinuria, hematuria, albuminuria, granular or hyaline casts
Elevated amylase
Elevated creatinine phosphokinase, aldolase
Azotemia
Findings of disseminated intravascular coagulopathy (rare)
Biopsy of skin, muscle, or kidney—cholesterol clefts in small arteries

(Kalter X, et al. Livedo reticularis due to multiple cholesterol emboli. J Am Acad Dermatol 1985;13:235)

The clinical situation is acute, subacute, or chronic renal failure. Patients have a recent onset of episodic hypertension or exacerbation of preexisting hypertension. Erythrocyte sedimentation rate is elevated and peripheral eosinophilia occurs. The urine contains protein, white blood cells, and red blood cells. The diagnosis is suggested by predisposing factors among patients with subacute renal failure. Renal biopsy can be performed to confirm the diagnosis.

If the patient recovers from the renal failure, angiography is performed to determine if the offending lesion can be removed. For other patients, treatment involves dialysis and management of hypertension.

Diffuse Atheroembolism

Diffuse atheroembolism results from showers of cholesterol emboli sufficient to obstruct the microcirculation of multiple organs. Diffuse atheroembolism can mimic many other illnesses, especially polyarteritis nodosa. Diffuse atheroembolism often is misdiagnosed as systemic necrotizing vasculitis. Diffuse atheroembolism is not a rare finding at autopsy of patients with severe atherosclerotic disease of the aorta.

Common signs and symptoms are abdominal pain, lower-extremity pain, livedo reticularis, blue toes, neurologic dysfunction, melena, and azotemia. Acute or chronic renal failure may occur. The differential diagnosis includes infection, especially bacterial endocarditis, disseminated neoplasm, and vasculitis.

Laboratory studies show elevated erythrocyte sedimentation rate, hematuria, thrombocytopenia, and depletion of complement. Diagnosis is based on suspicion of the syndrome and biopsy of the skin, muscle, or kidney. Angiography can induce further complications. Aortic atherosclerosis usually extends over the thoracic and abdominal aorta. Thoracoabdominal aortic resection often is required.

SUGGESTED READING

Baxter-Smith D, Ashton F, Slaney G. Peripheral arterial embolism: a 20 year review. J Cardiovasc Surg 1988;29:453.

Bowles CR, Olcott CW, Pakter RL, et al. Diffuse arterial narrowing as a result of intimal proliferation: a delayed complication with the Fogarty catheter. J Vasc Surg 1988;7:487.

Dobrin PB. Mechanisms and prevention of arterial injuries caused by balloon embolectomy. Surgery 1989;106:457.

Kaufman JL, Stark K, Brolin RB. Disseminated atheroembolism from extensive degenerative atherosclerosis of the aorta. Surgery 1987;102:63.

Messina LM. In vivo assessment of microvascular injury after reperfusion of ischemic anterior tibialis of the hamster. Surg Res 1990;48:615.

Messina LM, Faulkner JA. The skeletal muscle. In: Zelenock GB, D'Alecy LG, Fantone JC, et al., eds. Clinical ischemic syndromes. St. Louis, CV Mosby, 1990:457.

Petersen P. Thromboembolic complications in atrial fibrillation. Stroke 1990;21:4.

Schwarcz TH, Dobrin PB, Mrkvicka R, et al. Balloon embolectomy catheter-induced arterial injury: a comparison of four catheters. J Vasc Surg 1990;11:382.

Takolander R, Lannerstad O, Bergqvist D. Peripheral arterial embolectomy, risks and results. Acta Chir Scand 1988;154:567.

Wingo JP, Nix ML, Greenfield LJ, et al. The blue toe syndrome: hemodynamics and therapeutic correlates outcome. J Vasc Surg 1986;3:475.

Wright JG, Kerr JC, Valeri R, et al. Heparin decreases ischemia-reperfusion injury in isolated canine gracilis muscle. Arch Surg 1988;123:470.

ESSENTIALS OF SURGERY: SCIENTIFIC PRINCIPLES AND PRACTICE, edited by Lazar J. Greenfield, Michael W. Mulholland, Keith T. Oldham, Gerald B. Zelenock, and Keith D. Lillemoe. Lippincott–Raven Publishers, Philadelphia, © 1997.

CHAPTER 72

ARTERIAL COMPRESSION SYNDROMES

LLOYD A. JACOBS

Compression of vascular structures can produce ischemic injury and cellular death, leading to organ loss or extremity dysfunction.

THORACIC OUTLET SYNDROMES

Thoracic outlet syndrome (TOS) occurs when bones or ligaments impinge on upper-extremity neurovascular structures in the thoracic outlet or costoclavicular space (Fig. 72-1). The common causes of TOS are:

- Skeletal abnormalities, such as a cervical rib or an elongated C-7 transverse process
- Muscular abnormalities (Fig. 72-2)
- Acquired lesions, such as excessive callus formation or deformity from a clavicular fracture
- Cervical trauma, such as a whiplash deceleration injury

Many patients with TOS have multiple anomalies, such as compression of the axillary artery by the humeral head during the subluxation that occurs in some athletic activities.

Diagnosis

Symptoms

Patients with TOS have a long, prodromic history of intermittent and vague but progressive neurologic symptoms including: pain; paresthesia; weakness in the neck, shoulder, or hand, which may be exacerbated by certain activities, postures, or unusual exercise. Irritation of the brachial plexus is the most common presentation of TOS. It produces symptoms related to the nerves and nerve roots involved. Compression of the lower portion of the brachial plexus produces symptoms in the ulnar nerve distribution; compression of the upper portion of the brachial plexus produces symptoms in the radial nerve distribution. Both areas can be involved, and there may be neck, back, anterior chest, or posterior paraspinous symptoms.

Venous compression can produce a chronic syndrome characterized by intermittent venous obstruction with an increase in upper-extremity volume and cyanosis exacerbated by certain movements. Acute compression can contribute to axillary or subclavian venous thrombosis related to strenuous physical activity. Acute venous thrombosis can cause pain, cyanosis, or edema, and can lead to chronic upper-extremity venous insufficiency or pulmonary embolism. The acute symptoms lessen as compensatory circulation is established.

Arterial complications of thoracic outlet obstruction are rare but serious. They are almost always caused by long-standing compression, usually by a bony or fibrous abnormality and in the costoscalene or costoclavicular passage.

A

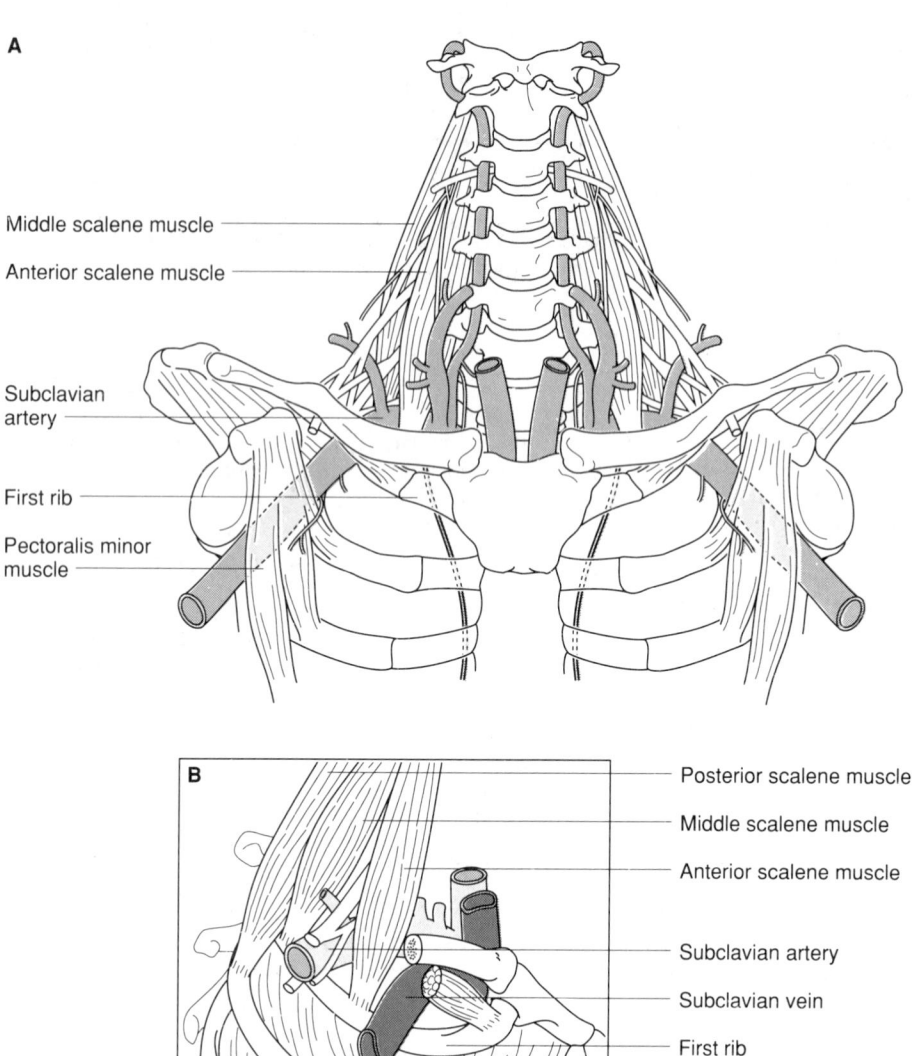

Middle scalene muscle

Anterior scalene muscle

Subclavian artery

First rib

Pectoralis minor muscle

B

Posterior scalene muscle

Middle scalene muscle

Anterior scalene muscle

Subclavian artery

Subclavian vein

First rib

Figure 72-1. The normal anatomy of the thoracic outlet in anteroposterior (*A*) and oblique (*B*) views. The brachial plexus and subclavian artery traverse the narrow triangle formed by the anterior and middle scalene muscles and the first rib. The subclavian vein lies anteriorly. (After Zelenock GB. Nonpenetrating subclavian artery injuries. Arch Surg 1985;120:685)

Physical Findings

Most patients with thoracic outlet syndrome have a normal neurologic examination or weakness and/or atrophy of the triceps or hand muscles. Direct palpation in the supraclavicular fossa or axilla and/or provocative positioning may reproduce the symptoms. Acute venous obstruction causes a swollen, tender, congested, and plethoric arm and, possibly, a pattern of collateral veins across the anterior chest. In the rare patient with acute arterial thrombosis, diminished pulses and a pale or mottled, cool extremity that fatigues rapidly with exercise are readily apparent.

Diagnostic Imaging

Radiographs of the chest, clavicle, shoulder, and cervical and upper-thoracic spine are obtained. Plain radiographs in anteroposterior and lateral projections show a cervical rib, abnormal first thoracic rib, or nonunion or hypertrophic callus formation from a clavicular fracture.

Myelograms, electromyograms, nerve conduction studies, computed tomography (CT), magnetic resonance imaging (MRI), and somatosensory evoked potentials are used to exclude causes of the symptoms other than TOS.

Arterial lesions resulting from TOS are diagnosed with *arteriography*. Selective injection of the appropriate subclavian artery is performed, but adequate visualization

may require multiple views, subtraction techniques, or positional maneuvers. Diagnosis is easy when large impingements are associated with an abnormal first thoracic rib or cervical rib. In such situations, poststenotic dilatation may be obvious and may have progressed to aneurysmal proportions. The presence of mural thrombus in an aneurysm or associated with an intimal lesion dictates early surgical intervention.

Treatment

Treatment of patients with *arterial* complications of TOS is always surgical. An emergency operation sometimes is required because of the presence of upper-extremity ischemia, continued embolism, or free-floating thrombus in the area. The operation manages the underlying arterial compression and the complications of aneurysm formation or thromboembolism. Intraarterial thrombolytic therapy followed by definitive surgical repair is used for distal small-vessel thromboses and emboli that are difficult to manage with conventional surgical approaches.

Decompression of the thoracic outlet is achieved with transection or resection of the anterior scalene muscle and excision of cervical ribs, abnormal fibrous bands and the first thoracic rib. Arterial aneurysms are resected, as are

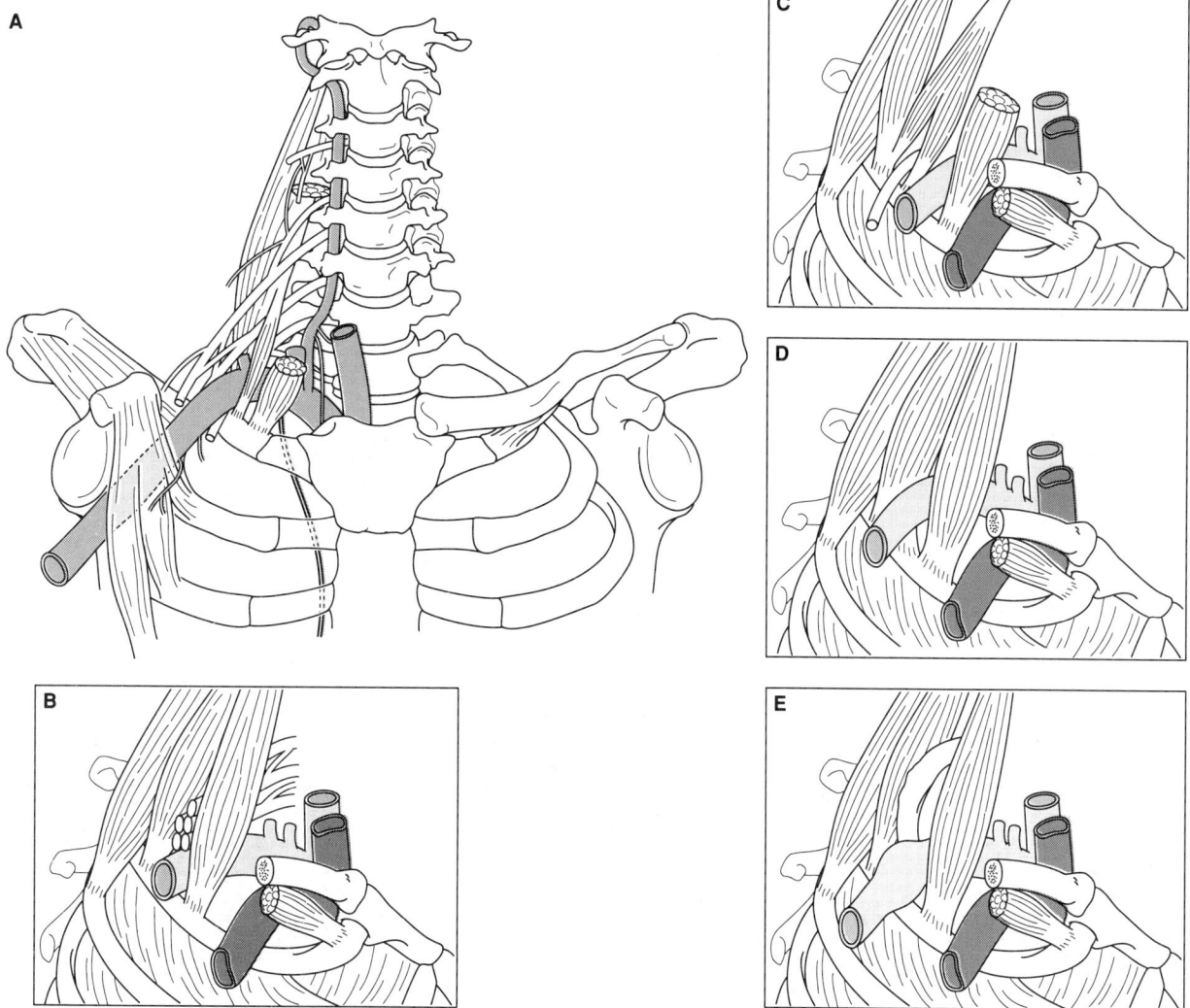

Figure 72-2. (*A*) The anomalous scalene minimus muscle can irritate lower brachial plexus trunks. (*B*) Hypertrophied, fibrosed, and foreshortened scalene muscles elevate the first rib and compress the brachial plexus. (*C*) Unnamed anomalous muscle slips from either the anterior or middle scalene muscle can cause a variable pattern of nerve root compression. (*D*) A broad insertion of the tendon of the middle scalene muscle along the superior aspect of the first rib. (*E*) An anomalous cervical rib or fibrous band is the most common cause of arterial compression. Note the poststenotic subclavian artery aneurysm (see Fig. 72-3). (After Wylie EJ. Manual of vascular surgery, vol 2. New York, Springer-Verlag, 1986)

areas of artery having arteriographic evidence of mural thrombosis or intimal ulceration. Arterial reconstruction with saphenous vein or prosthetic conduits is performed. Balloon catheter embolectomy may be needed during these procedures. When microembolism is present, upper-extremity sympathectomy can be performed. Intraoperative infusion of urokinase is successful in clearing multiple small-vessel occlusions.

Therapy for upper-extremity *venous* thrombosis is varied. It usually involves heparin-coumadin anticoagulation and may involve clot lysis with urokinase injection into the clot or throracic decompression.

VERTEBRAL ARTERY COMPRESSION

Abnormally low entry of the vertebral artery into the vertebral canal at the level of C-7 is associated with compression of the artery by tendinous structures in the low neck. Osteophytic spurring and subluxation of the cervical vertebrae cause chronic compression (Fig. 72-3). Repeated trauma to the vessel causes intimal lesions or permanent and nonexpandable cicatricial narrowing. In extreme situations, the vertebral artery is completely occluded.

Diagnosis

Vertebral artery compression can cause vertebrobasilar insufficiency, although isolated symptomatic vertebral artery compression is rare. A combination of arteriosclerotic lesions and compression often occurs in patients whose symptoms are produced by positional changes of the head and neck. One vertebral artery can be occluded by atherosclerotic disease, and the other compressed when the person rotates his or her head.

The symptoms of vertebrobasilar insufficiency are vague. Dizziness, vertigo, and paresthesia are common but

A

B

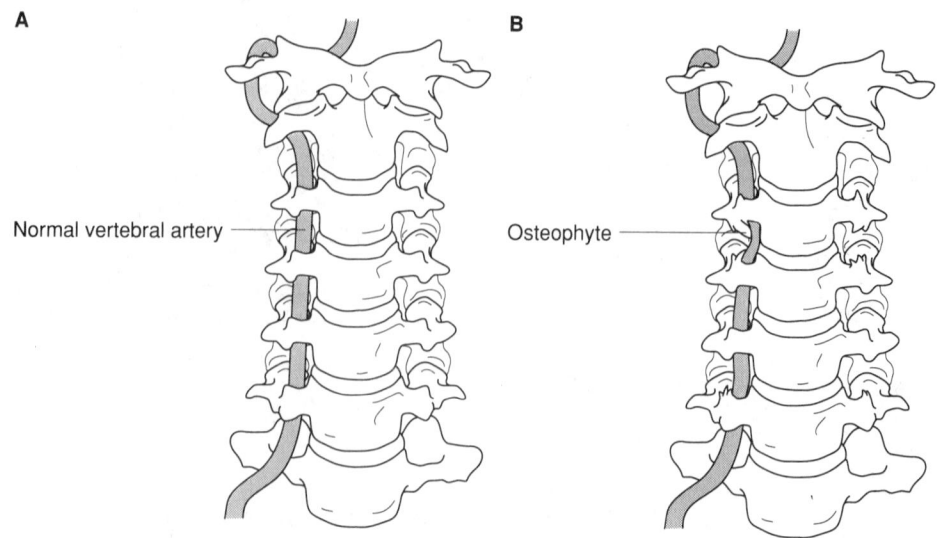

Normal vertebral artery

Osteophyte

Figure 72-3. (*A*) A normal vertebral artery lying within the vertebral canal. (*B*) A large osteophyte compresses the vertebral artery at the level of C-3. Rotation or flexion-extension can exacerbate the compression.

are easily confused with those of other syndromes; therefore, evaluation of the symptoms is systematic and methodical. One must rule out orthostatic and drug-induced hypotension, middle-ear labyrinthine disease, and cardiac problems.

Arteriography to study vertebrobasilar insufficiency involves examination of the entire cerebral vasculature, but is indicated only after careful exclusion of other causes of the symptoms. The carotid and intracranial arteries and the vertebral blood vessels must be completely visualized. Arteriographic findings are atherosclerotic lesions of the vertebral arteries or other sites in the vertebral system or diffuse extracranial cerebrovascular disease. Evidence of extrinsic compression of the vertebral artery may necessitate use of special views and orientations, subtraction techniques, and maneuvers to reproduce the symptoms.

Treatment

Treatment of patients with symptomatic extrinsic compression of the vertebral artery is surgical when indicated because of symptoms or when there is evidence of emboli in the posterior circulation. Relief of the extrinsic compression may necessitate resection of osteophytes, unroofing of the transverse process foramina, or transection of musculotendinous bands associated with the cervical muscles. Damage to the vertebral artery necessitates vascular reconstruction.

POPLITEAL ARTERY ENTRAPMENT SYNDROME

Popliteal artery entrapment syndrome is an uncommon problem. It usually appears as unilateral calf claudication in a young person and tends to occur in heavily muscled men.

Diagnosis

Calf claudication is episodic, but patients frequently relate the onset of symptoms to specific and intense exercise such as running. During this phase, the artery is compressed intermittently, producing claudication. An acute phase starts when repeated trauma damages the intima or when scar tissue envelops the artery and arterial thrombosis occurs. Acute ischemia of the lower limb develops, and

the patient has a pulseless, cold, painful, and paralyzed extremity.

Patients with popliteal artery entrapment syndrome usually do not have the risk factors for, or secondary signs of, atherosclerotic occlusive disease. Those with entrapment but without an occluded popliteal artery frequently have normal foot pulses. These pulses may disappear on passive dorsiflexion of the foot or active plantar flexion against resistance. The sensitivity of this portion of the physical examination can be enhanced with detection of a decreased Doppler signal or decreased ankle pressures in the noninvasive vascular laboratory.

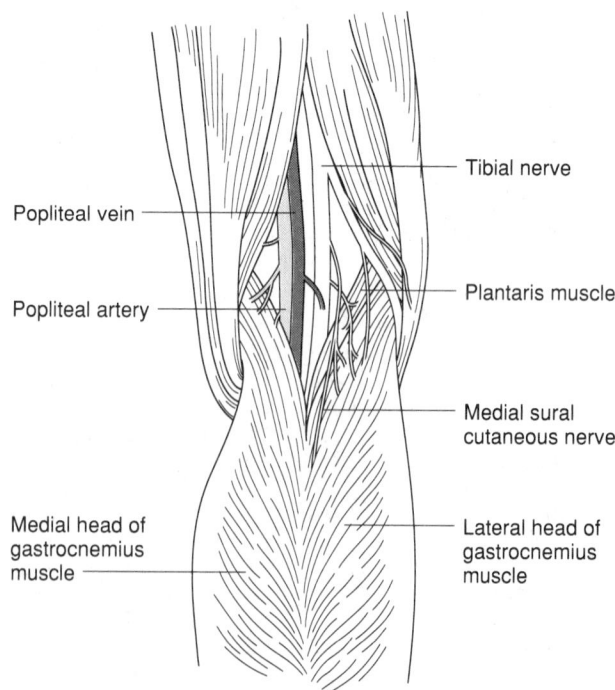

Tibial nerve

Plantaris muscle

Popliteal vein

Popliteal artery

Medial sural cutaneous nerve

Medial head of gastrocnemius muscle

Lateral head of gastrocnemius muscle

Figure 72-4. The normal anatomy of the popliteal fossa. The popliteal artery and vein and the tibial nerve lie between the medial and lateral heads of the gastrocnemius. The peroneal nerve courses lateral to the head of the gastrocnemius and the head of the fibula.

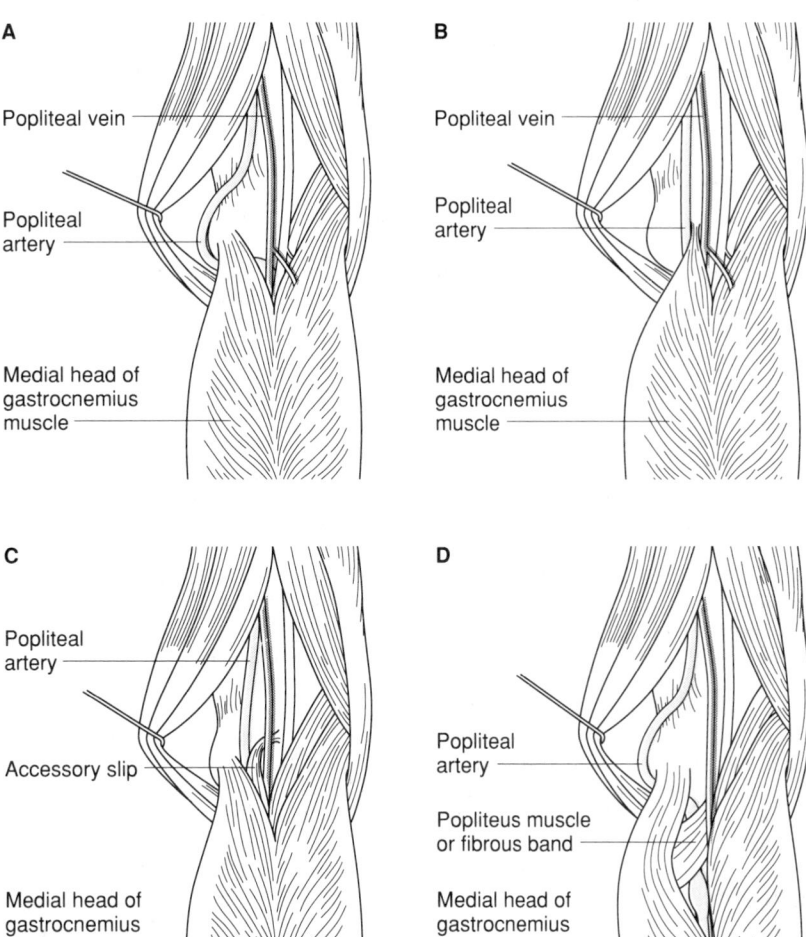

Figure 72-5. (*A*) Posterior view of right popliteal fossa. Normally located medial head of gastrocnemius with deviant medial pathway of popliteal artery (type I). (*B*) In the type II anomaly, an abnormally lateral origin of the medial head of the gastrocnemius muscle places traction on an otherwise normally placed popliteal artery. (*C*) An accessory slip of the gastrocnemius muscle compressing the popliteal artery. (*D*) Medial deviation of the popliteal artery and compression by the popliteus muscle. (After Whelan TJ. Popliteal artery entrapment. In: Rutherford RB, ed. Vascular surgery, ed 3. Philadelphia, WB Saunders, 1989)

Popliteal artery entrapment syndrome usually is associated with a congenital anomaly. A normal popliteal artery passes through the adductor canal and traverses the popliteal space between the medial and lateral heads of the gastrocnemius muscle (Fig. 72-4). Congenital variations of the popliteal artery are classified into four types (Fig. 72-5).

The definitive diagnosis of popliteal artery entrapment syndrome is confirmed with *arteriography*. Arteriography is performed bilaterally, because the anomaly is frequently found in the leg without symptoms. Medial deviation of the popliteal artery, occlusion of the popliteal artery, and stenosis with poststenotic dilatation may confirm the presence of popliteal artery entrapment syndrome.

Treatment

The high rate of limb loss due to acute popliteal artery occlusion warrants surgical release of the entrapped artery, even when symptoms are minimal or absent. Transection of the compressing part of the medial head of the gastrocnemius or fascial band relieves the entrapment and usually is all that is needed. When an intimal lesion, stenosis, or occlusion occurs, arterial reconstruction is performed, usually with autogenous saphenous vein.

ADVENTITIAL CYSTIC DISEASE OF THE POPLITEAL ARTERY

Adventitial cystic disease of the popliteal artery causes intermittent claudication in young, physically active people. It can cause debilitating symptoms and irreversible damage if the vessel becomes occluded (Fig. 72-6).

Diagnosis

Pulses may be normal in the foot, particularly at rest. *CT* helps differentiate popliteal artery entrapment syndrome from a Baker or synovial cyst in the popliteal space. *Arteriography* is performed, particularly if there is a question about distal embolism or thrombosis of the artery. Uncom-

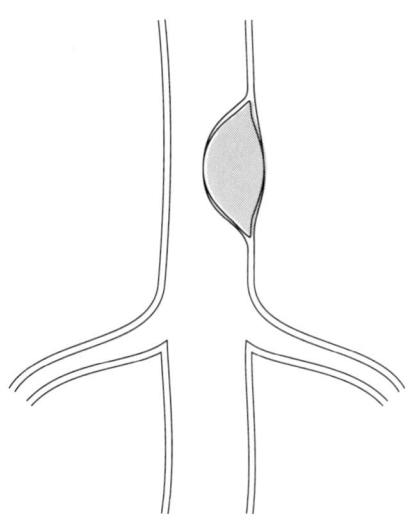

Figure 72-6. Adventitial cystic disease of the popliteal artery causes luminal compromise.

plicated adventitial cysts of the popliteal artery may be difficult to visualize at angiography. A lateral projection typically demonstrates a smooth indentation into the column of contrast material and is noteworthy for the lack of atherosclerotic lesions.

Treatment

Management of symptomatic adventitial cystic disease of the popliteal artery is surgical. The artery and cystic area are exposed. The cyst itself is unilocular or multilocular, and some cysts appear to contain old blood. The cyst is incised and the contents removed. This completes the operation. Cicatricial stenosis of the artery, poststenotic dilatation, or thrombosis may necessitate additional procedures.

COMPARTMENT SYNDROMES

Compartment syndromes are encountered when high tissue pressure in a limited anatomic space compromises circulation. For example, in the leg there are four compartments—a deep posterior compartment, a superficial posterior compartment, a lateral compartment, and an anterior compartment (Fig. 72-7); each is nonexpandable and delineated by thick fascia. The compartment syndrome is caused by an increase in the volume of the contents of a compartment, as with hemorrhage due to trauma, or by a reduction in compartmental capacity, as by a tight plaster cast. The most common compartment syndromes are associated with interruption and restoration of blood flow to an extremity made ischemic by embolism, thrombus, trauma, or prolonged unusual positioning.

Diagnosis

The *symptoms* of compartment syndromes include throbbing and unrelenting pain and loss of neuromuscular function. The forearm and leg are the most frequent sites of compression, and each compartment of the forearm and leg contains at least one important peripheral nerve (Fig. 72-7).

Examination of the hand or foot may disclose neurologic deficits. Subtle sensory changes or paresthesias may occur before clear signs of ischemia. Movement or stretching of the involved muscle by means of passive motion of the wrist or ankle produces pain. The only objective signs are a compartment that is tense, tender, or swollen at direct palpation and subcutaneous edema or hematoma. Distal pulses are assessed, but capillary or venous compression usually precedes cessation of arterial inflow; tissue damage can occur before intracompartmental pressure exceeds arterial perfusion pressure (Fig. 72-7C). Paralysis of the involved muscles suggests the compression is advanced.

All patients with trauma or crush injury or who have undergone embolectomy or prolonged vascular reconstruction undergo *repeated neurovascular examinations* of the involved limb for 48 to 72 hours after the injury or operation. If the patient is unconscious, intermittent or continuous measurement of intracompartmental pressure is conducted. Normal compartmental pressure is about 10 mmHg. Pressures >20 mmHg are considered abnormal; those >40 mmHg are dangerous and necessitate decompression.

Treatment

Fasciotomy is performed on the forearm or leg. Decompression of all four compartments of the *leg* is the goal. The anterior and lateral compartments are decompressed through an anterior lateral incision and the posterior compartments through a posteromedial incision. These longitudinal incisions are left open for delayed primary closure or skin grafting when the edema subsides. Ankle and foot fasciotomy, as an adjunct to leg fasciotomies, is performed when continued foot swelling and tension over the medial

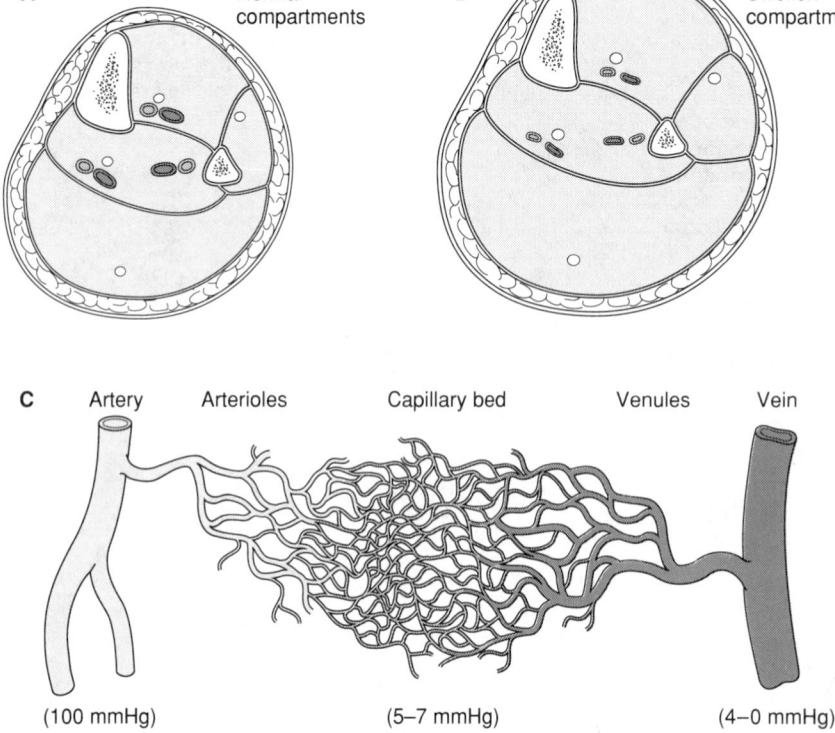

Figure 72-7. (*A*) Compartments of the leg at midcalf. The anterior, lateral, and both the deep and superficial posterior compartments contain major nerves. (*B*) When cellular swelling and interstitial edema develop within the fixed confines of the various compartments, pressure necrosis of the compartment's contents may result. The tissue most sensitive to ischemia is the peripheral nerve. (*C*) As compartment pressures rise to 20 to 40 mmHg, obstruction to flow occurs first at the capillary-venule level. Profound ischemia may then result despite normal distal arterial pulses. (After Mubarak SJ, Hargens AR. Compartment syndromes and Volkmann's contracture. Philadelphia, WB Saunders, 1981)

aspect of the proximal foot are encountered. Ankle and foot fasciotomies may be performed during prolonged reconstructive vascular procedures for arteriosclerotic disease.

Most compartmental syndromes in the *forearm* are decompressed with one long volar incision from the antecubital fossa to the proximal palm. Carpal tunnel release is usually included in this procedure, and sometimes a second incision directly over the dorsal compartment of the forearm is necessary. These incisions, like those in the lower extremity, are left open for delayed primary closure or skin grafting as appropriate.

Some patients with compartment syndrome have a slow, progressive course of skeletal muscle death, with shrinkage and fibrosis of the muscle, despite adequate and timely decompression, resulting in Volkmann contracture. The goal of fasciotomy is a functional extremity. Rehabilitative therapy is critical.

OTHER COMPRESSION SYNDROMES

Processes such as retroperitoneal fibrosis, Baker cysts, and primary or metastatic neoplasms cause compression of nearby vascular structures. An example is involvement of the carotid bifurcation with metastatic head and neck cancer. In the treatment of some patients with extensive laryngeal or oropharyngeal cancer, resection and reconstruction of the carotid artery can be performed with radical excision of the tumor.

SUGGESTED READING

Ascer E, Strauch B, Calligaro KD, Gupta SK, Veith FJ. Ankle and foot fasciotomy: an adjunctive technique to optimize limb salvage after revascularization for acute ischemia. J Vasc Surg 1989;9:594.

Berguer R, Caplan LR. Vertebrobasilar arterial disease. St. Louis, Quality Medical, 1992.

Collins PS, McDonald PT, Lim RC. Popliteal artery entrapment: an evolving syndrome. J Vasc Surg 1989;10:484.

Cormier JM, Amrane M, Ward A, Laurian C, Gigou F. Arterial complications of the thoracic outlet syndrome: fifty-five operative cases. J Vasc Surg 1989;9:778.

Forrest I, Lindsay T, Romaschin A, Walker P. The rate and distribution of muscle blood flow after prolonged ischemia. J Vasc Surg 1989;10:83.

Jay GD, Ross FL, Mason RA, Giron F. Clinical and chemical characterization of an adventitial popliteal cyst. J Vasc Surg 1989;9:448.

Khalil IM. Bilateral compartmental syndrome after prolonged surgery in the lithotomy position. J Vasc Surg 1987;5:879.

Machleder HI, Moll F, Nuwer M, Jordan S. Somatosensory evoked potentials in the assessment of thoracic outlet compression syndrome. J Vasc Surg 1987;6:177.

Williams LR, Flinn WR, McCarthy WJ, Yao JST, Bergan JJ. Popliteal artery entrapment: diagnosis by computed tomography. J Vasc Surg 1986;3:360.

ESSENTIALS OF SURGERY: SCIENTIFIC PRINCIPLES AND PRACTICE, edited by Lazar J. Greenfield, Michael W. Mulholland, Keith T. Oldham, Gerald B. Zelenock, and Keith D. Lillemoe. Lippincott–Raven Publishers, Philadelphia, © 1997.

CHAPTER 73

TISSUE ISCHEMIA

GERALD B. ZELENOCK AND LOUIS G. D'ALECY

Ischemic heart and brain disease (myocardial infarction and stroke) are the first and third leading causes of death, respectively. More than 570,000 vascular operations, 1.2 million cardiac procedures, and hundreds of thousands of other operations are performed annually to alleviate ischemia; of note, the procedures themselves are associated with risk for ischemic injury.

Ischemic injury is a concern in transplantation and donor preservation, resuscitation from shock and trauma, the use of tourniquets and other techniques to obtain a bloodless field, reconstructive surgical procedures with translocation of flaps, and the integrity of anastomoses in gastrointestinal and genitourinary operations. Ischemia occurs in strangulation infarction due to hernia, volvulus, adhesions, and other forms of intestinal obstruction.

The cause of ischemic cell death is probably multifactorial and may be different in various tissues. The following mechanisms characterize ischemic injury (Fig. 73-1):

- Energy failure
- Direct parenchymal cell injury
- Vascular (endothelial) injury
- Activation of soluble and cellular inflammatory systems
- Activation of secondary cascades, such as complement, prostaglandins, and coagulation
- Reperfusion effects

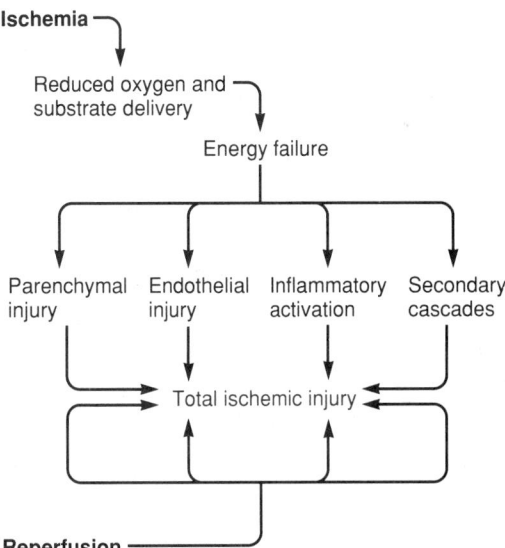

Figure 73-1. Ischemia produces multiple adverse effects. Lack of oxygen and substrate cause failure of energy production for essential cellular processes, resulting in parenchymal and vascular injury, as well as activation of the inflammatory system and secondary cascades. The injury process continues throughout the reperfusion phase.

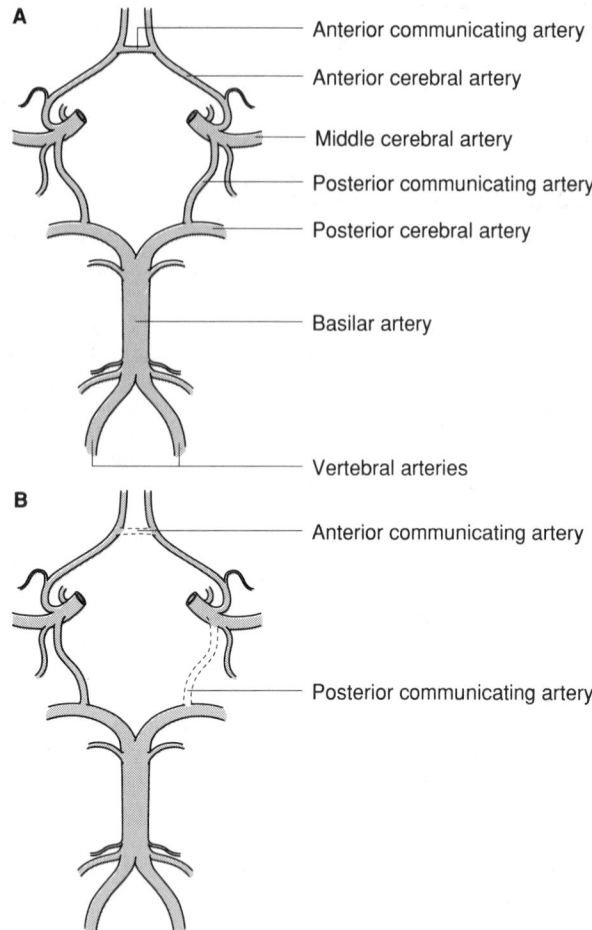

Figure 73-2. (*A*) The normal circle of Willis provides an efficient collateral circulation in the event of internal carotid artery occlusion or clamping. (*B*) An isolated hemisphere with inadequate anterior and posterior communicating arteries places the brain at risk when internal carotid artery occlusion or clamping occurs.

TOLERANCE

Ischemia leads to cellular and tissue injury, organ failure, tissue necrosis, and death. The duration and severity of ischemia influence outcome. The ability of various tissues and organs to tolerate ischemic injury lasts from minutes (brain) to several hours (skeletal muscle). Tolerance is influenced by:

- The duration and severity of ischemic insult
- Resting metabolic rate
- Temperature
- Ability of an organ or tissue to decrease metabolic demand
- The substrate being metabolized during the ischemic episode
- Ability to use alternative substrate (phosphocreatinine, glycogen, ketone)
- Anaerobic glycolysis
- Availability of subtypes of key metabolic enzymes
- Rapidity of development of ischemia
- Efficiency of existing collateral blood vessels (Fig. 73-2)
- Potential for development of collateral circulation
- Availability of antioxidants, scavengers, and other defenses

- The manner in which reperfusion occurs (Figs. 73-3, 73-4)
- Potential for regeneration

Inherent metabolic factors may influence ischemic tolerance. Cells and organs with direct, continuous activity, constant energy demand, and high basal oxygen extraction, such as myocardium, are less prepared to meet the demands of ischemic insult than is skeletal muscle, which can diminish activity, use glycogen stores, and increase oxygen extraction.

The substrate metabolized during ischemia is important. Enhanced or exclusive use of glucose during central nervous system (CNS) ischemia worsens neurologic outcome. Brain ischemia is better tolerated when ketone is used as

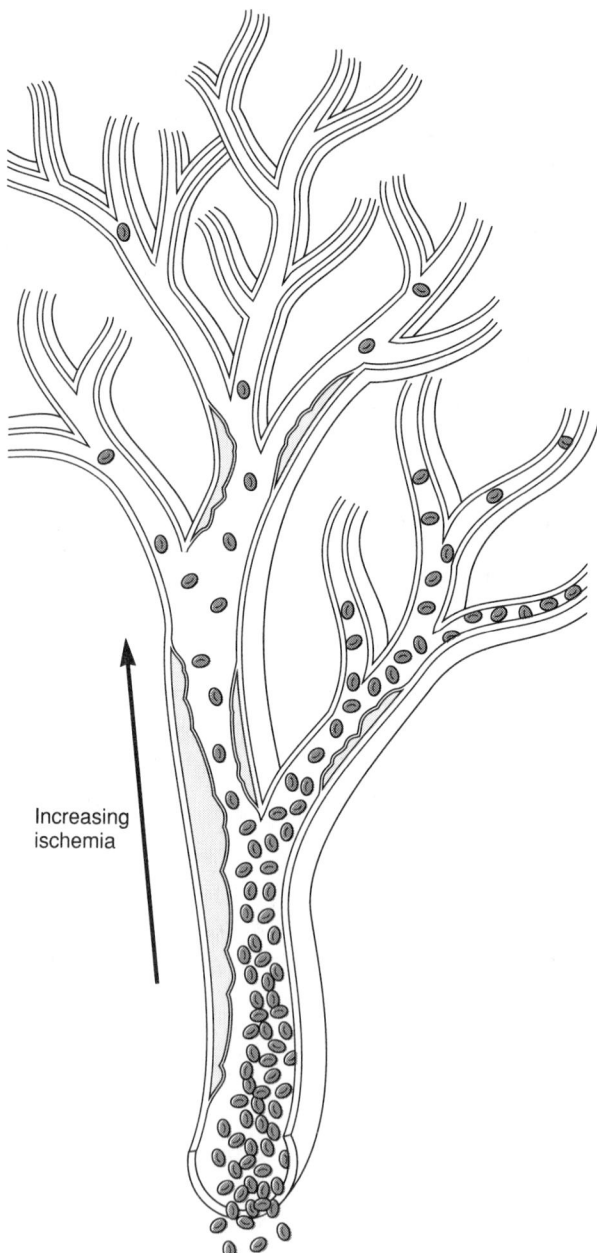

Figure 73-3. Tissues supplied by end arteries may experience watershed infarcts as the most distal tissues become ischemic. The normal decrease in perfusion pressure as one proceeds to the periphery becomes critical as a result of more proximal lesions or periods of systemic hypotension.

(within image) Increasing ischemia

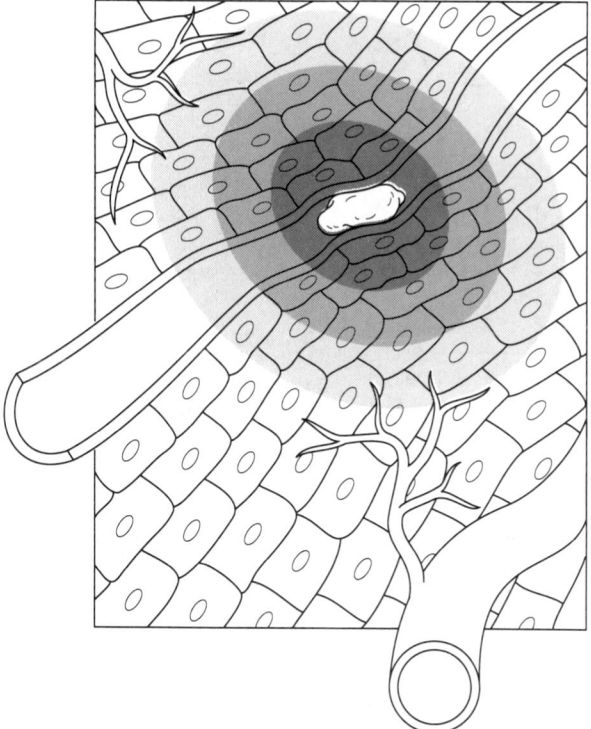

Figure 73-4. The ischemic penumbra concept recognizes zones of ischemic injury around a vascular occlusion. Some tissues are inadequately perfused and die, some are relatively well perfused and survive, and others are marginally perfused, perhaps by collateral flow from adjacent vascular beds. This last zone may potentially be salvaged by timely and appropriate interventions.

the metabolic fuel. Lowering blood glucose level by means of administration of insulin appears to enhance CNS but not renal tolerance to ischemic stress. The tolerance of an organ may be influenced by the presence of specific isoenzymes that continue to function under ischemic conditions and allow continued energy production, despite a decline in pH.

The severity of an ischemic event can be assessed on the basis of:

* Symptoms
    Pain (angina pectoris, claudication)
    Neurologic status (paralysis, amaurosis fugax)
* Physiologic findings
    Pulse–pressure ratios (ankle–brachial index)
    Waveform analysis
    Velocity profiles
* Imaging findings
    Angiography
    Duplex ultrasound scans

Preoperative assessment of large-vessel occlusive disease is possible, but is difficult in cases of small-vessel disease. The severity of ischemia (or blood-flow restriction) may be a result not only of an increase in large-vessel resistance or obstruction, as in atherosclerotic occlusive disease or coarctation, but also of the extent of small-vessel involvement, as in diffuse arteritis. Surgical intervention is restricted to alleviation of large-vessel involvement. The degree of success of such operations depends on the relative contributions of the large and small vessels to the overall ischemic event.

Recognition of an ischemic event occurs at a point when normal physiologic reserves are near exhaustion, even

though the severity of ischemia, in terms of functional loss, is just becoming apparent (Fig. 73-5). In lower-extremity arterial occlusive disease, the occurrence of pain at rest versus exercise-induced claudication indicates exhaustion of vasodilator reserve and severe disease. The range over which tissues tolerate changes in blood flow varies. Skin and kidney are tolerant; heart and brain are not.

The many paradoxes of ischemic injury are summarized in Table 73-1. The most difficult is that a substantial portion of the injury during an ischemic event occurs during reperfusion. This paradox is ascribed to the following mechanisms:

* Formation of oxygen radicals (in the endothelium, white blood cells [WBCs], parenchymal cells)
* Endothelial cell swelling or intramural edema
* Platelet and leukocyte adherence
* Irretrievable loss of diffusible nucleotide bases
* Consumption of energy due to reformation of ATP

Severe, unrelieved ischemia always produces necrosis. *Concern regarding reperfusion injury should not delay revascularization attempts.*

Although ischemia is not equivalent to hypoxia, the dose or severity of ischemia can be characterized by the ratio of oxygen delivery (Do_2) to oxygen consumption (Vo_2). The normal systemic ratio is 5:1, that is, 20% of the delivered oxygen is extracted; oxygen extraction (Vo_2/Do_2) equals 0.2. The systemic supply of oxygen is inadequate when the ratio of delivery to consumption is $\leq$2:1 (Fig. 73-6).

ENERGY FAILURE

Life depends on the ready availability of free energy. Essential cellular processes such as membrane stability, ion gradients, electrical activity, biosynthesis, and mechanical work must be maintained. All energy-dependent processes balance production and utilization, for the most part, through the ATP cycle. Regulation occurs by hormonal mechanisms, genetic regulation of enzyme synthesis, feedback loops of key enzymes, and cellular factors.

Normal oxygen metabolism is relatively efficient (Fig. 73-7, left). About 44% of the available energy in one molecule of glucose is captured by various mechanisms, producing 38 mol of ATP. In anaerobic metabolism (Fig. 73-9, right), rather than 38 mol of ATP, only 2 mol is produced, a 94% reduction in the efficiency of energy production for essential cellular processes.

Glucose is dominant in normal cellular energy metabolism. Ketones and, to a lesser extent, proteins also are metabolized for energy whenever they are available to the cell. When energy failure is a component of ischemia, carbon source and oxygen availability must be considered. Various substrates influence the ability of an organ's ability to tolerate ischemic insult. Continued or enhanced use of glucose may adversely affect the outcome in CNS, spinal cord, and renal ischemia. Provision of an alternative substrate (ketone) may be beneficial.

PARENCHYMAL CELL INJURY

Hypoxic metabolism is more than inefficient; if allowed to continue, it is injurious. Direct parenchymal cell injury occurs as a result of the ischemic insult. Accumulation of lactic acid has many adverse effects, including direct injury to organelles. Lesser degrees of lactic acid accumulation with resultant pH changes alter crucial enzyme activity and the shape and configuration of macromolecules. Lactic acid enhances cytokine production by activated macrophages.

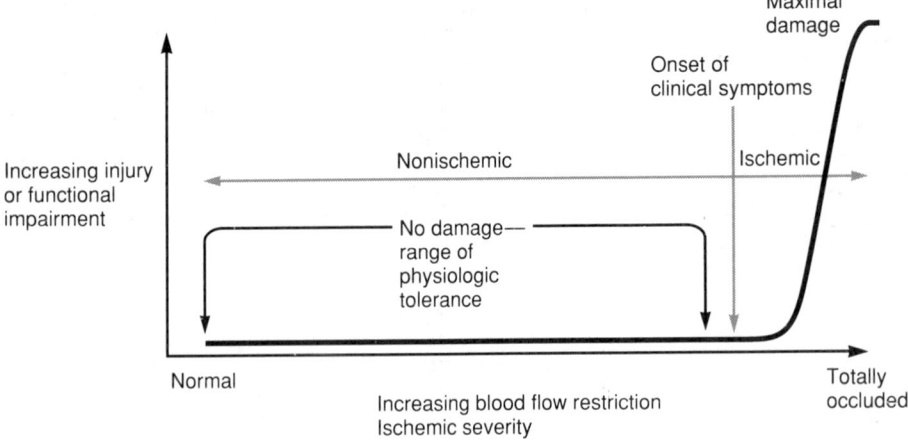

Figure 73-5. Increasing blood flow restriction is usually well tolerated until blood flow restriction becomes severe. Symptoms develop as physiologic reserves are depleted.

Failure of essential energy-requiring cellular functions produces an inability to maintain ionic gradients, resulting in cell swelling, increased diffusion distances, and disruption of cell membranes. Leakage of enzymes and other vital components and the continued drop in pH cause structural and functional changes. Release of proteases, lipases, and other autolytic enzymes causes irreparable damage. Lack of maintenance of ionic gradients leads to local accumulation of calcium. The precise compartmentalization of intracellular Ca^{2+} and the extracellular to intracellular gradient are lost, allowing large increases in free intracellular Ca^{2+} (Fig. 73-8). The essential structure of cellular membranes comes under direct attack. In addition to loss of essential cell structure and release of autolytic enzymes, membrane disruption releases arachidonic acid and activates secondary cascades, such as prostaglandin, thromboxane, and eicosanoids (Fig. 73-9).

Parenchymal cell injury in ischemia depends on tissue temperature. From cold-water drowning to hypothermic cardiac arrest, profound hypothermia has a salutary effect on ischemia. This profound cooling is relevant to organ preservation for transplantation and to total circulatory arrest during repair of complex cardiovascular defects, but it has little applicability to naturally occurring ischemic events or most operations. Even slight reductions in tissue temperature (1 to 2°C) can have profound protective effects on the extent of damage to ischemic tissue. Moderate local cooling can be accomplished without incurring myocardial irritability or compromising hemostasis, offering a nonspecific and safe approach to attenuating intraoperative ischemic injury.

Table 73-1. CLINICAL CAVEATS AND MECHANISTIC PARADOXES IN ISCHEMIA AND REPERFUSION

Hypoxia ≠ ischemia.
Injury continues during reperfusion.
Concern regarding reperfusion injury should not delay prompt relief of ongoing ischemia.
Low flow may be more harmful than no flow.
Oxygen excess is harmful.
Significant reduction in cardiovascular events occurs with control of metabolic factors (ie, cholesterol and homocysteine) despite little change in anatomic severity of stenosis.
Attenuating ischemia and reperfusion injury will probably not be a "silver bullet," but rather a multifaceted approach targeted at basic mechanisms.

The cellular origin of the damaging agents in ischemia and reperfusion is not known. Lipid peroxidation and other direct effects induced by toxic oxygen species, including the superoxide anion and hydroxyl radical, are likely.

ENDOTHELIAL INJURY

In many organs, the tissue most susceptible to ischemic insult is blood vessel, specifically endothelial tissue. Ischemic stress that causes only limited injury to parenchymal cells may severely injure the endothelium and smooth muscle of the associated blood vessels (Fig. 73-10). Activated platelets and WBCs adhere to vascular endothelium, causing release of cytokines, procoagulants, proteases, oxygen radicals, lysosomal enzymes, and arachidonic acid derivatives. The exposure of highly thrombogenic subendothelial material, such as collagen, results in enhanced accumulation of platelets and other formed elements in the blood.

WBCs are important in localized destruction and amplification of injury. Aside from direct injurious effects, adherence of granulocytes in the microcirculation in association with swelling of the endothelial and smooth muscle cells of the vessel wall cause obstruction and luminal narrowing, which may impede postischemic blood flow after ischemic injury. After ischemia, initial hyperemia is replaced by a prolonged period of limited blood flow. This no-reflow phenomenon increases the number of WBCs that adhere to the luminal surface of the blood vessel. The luminal compromise caused by swelling and granulocyte adherence increases ischemic stress on the parenchymal cell.

An additional means by which endothelial vascular injury produces parenchymal cell injury is altered production of substances by normal endothelial cells. Vascular endothelium is an important and active physiologic tissue, not a simple thromboresistant lining for distributing conduits. Many complex interactions between endothelial cells and blood elements occur. Release of biologically active compounds, including tissue plasminogen activator, heparin sulfate, fibronectin, interleukin-1, prostacyclin, endothelium-derived relaxing factor, nitric acid, endothelin-1, and other small molecules occurs in response to physiologic or pathologic stimuli. Several of these molecules may be important in conditions as diverse as hypertension, diabetes, atherosclerosis, endotoxin shock, and subarachnoid hemorrhage, as well as in ischemia and reperfusion.

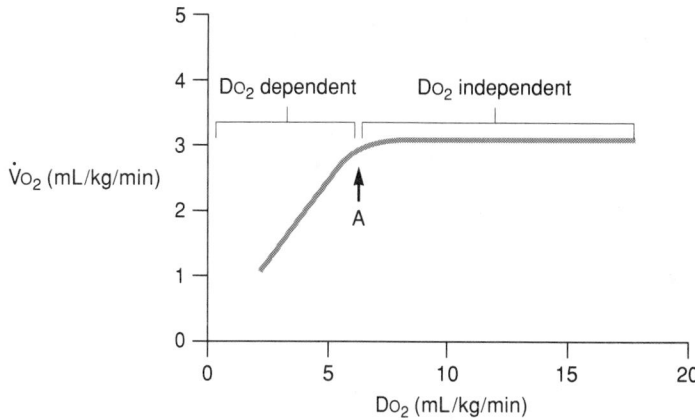

Figure 73-6. The point at which oxygen consumption depends on delivery characterizes ischemia.

Simplified metabolic scheme

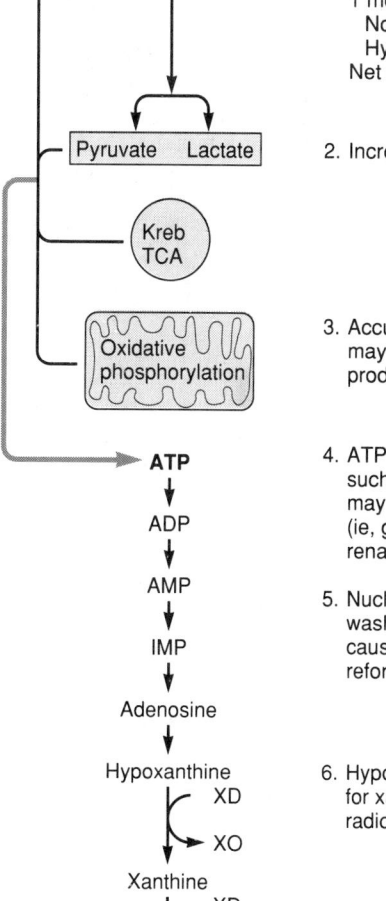

Potential mechanisms of ischemic damage

1. Decreased efficiency of ATP production
   1 mol of glucose:
   Normoxic metabolism → 38 ATP
   Hypoxic metabolism → 2 ATP (net)
   Net reduction of ATP → Loss of intracellular homeostasis, ion pump dysfunction, and intracellular ion translocations

2. Increased lactate accumulation

3. Accumulation of NADH and NADPH may facilitate the initiation reactions, producing toxic oxygen species

4. ATP degradation products such as adenosine are diffusable and may have adverse systemic effects (ie, generalized arterial dilation and renal vasoconstriction)

5. Nucleotide base loss washout of diffusable nucleotide bases causes net loss of substrate pool for reforming ATP

6. Hypoxanthine and xanthine are the substrates for xanthine oxidase–catalyzed oxygen radical formation

7. Reformation of ATP during reperfusion costs energy, which is diverted from essential cellular processes

Figure 73-7. (*Left*) Metabolism under normoxic conditions is reasonably efficient. Almost half of the available energy in a molecule of glucose is captured by glycolysis, Krebs cycle, and oxidative phosphorylation, producing 38 mol of ATP. (*Right*) Ischemic metabolism has multiple potential mechanisms to produce cellular, tissue, and organ injury.

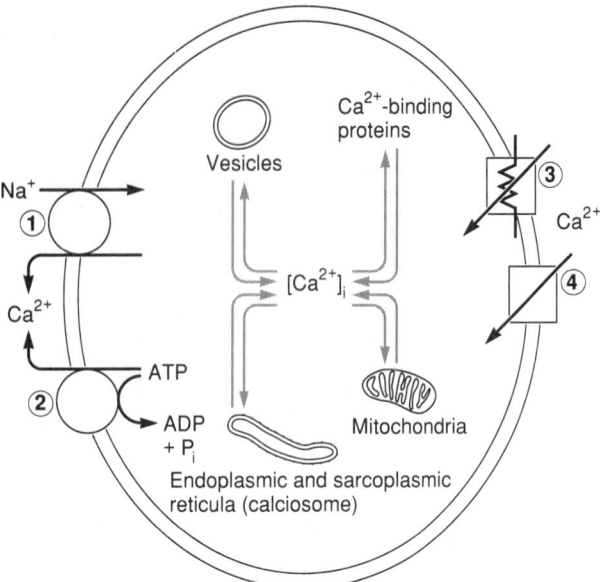

Figure 73-8. The extracellular-to-intracellular Ca^{2+} gradient is approximately 10^4 and is highly regulated (extracellular $[Ca^{2+}]$ is approximately 10^{-3} mol, whereas the intracellular free $[Ca^{2+}]$ is approximately 10^{-7} mol). Calcium can leave cells against this large gradient by Na^+-Ca^{2+} exchange energized by the Na^+ gradient established by the Na^+-K^+-ATPase pump (1). Ca^{2+} can also leave by means of Ca^{2+} ATPases located at the plasma membrane (2). Ca^{2+} can enter cells through voltage-dependent (3) or voltage-independent pathways (4). Within the cell, free Ca^{2+} can exchange with Ca^{2+} in vesicles, endoplasmic and sarcoplasmic reticula, or mitochondria. In addition, dynamic equilibrium exists between free Ca^{2+} and Ca^{2+} associated with Ca^{2+}-binding proteins in the cytosol and intracellular membrane compartments. (After Bonventre JV. Calcium. In: Zelenock GB, ed. Clinical ischemic syndromes mechanisms and consequences of tissue injury. St. Louis, CV Mosby, 1990)

INFLAMMATORY SYSTEMS

After the initial ischemic insult and metabolic failure with injury to the parenchymal cell and vascular endothelium, the soluble and cellular inflammatory systems are activated. Adherence molecules, chemoattractants, and other mediators amplify or attenuate this complex process (Fig. 73-11). The cellular inflammatory system activated by the ischemic process results in WBC accumulation and adherence to vascular endothelium. Migration of the cells through the blood vessels into the parenchymal matrix and release of proteases, reactive oxygen metabolites, interleukin-1, TNF, and other active mediators results in continued destruction. WBCs are involved in many abnormal processes and are a source of toxic oxygen species and cytokines. Removal of injured cells can be escalated to a widespread, uncontrolled effect and contribute to overall parenchymal injury. The role of oxygen radicals is summarized in Table 73-2.

Oxygen radicals are highly reactive and tend to propagate in chain reactions. Although radicals are continuously produced in normal metabolic processes, when present in excess of the capacity of the normal quenching and scavenging systems, they are extremely toxic, affecting virtually all cellular processes. They cross-link membrane proteins, cleave peptide bonds, promote DNA disruption and base modification, cause lipid peroxidation, and alter the function of glycosaminoglycans.

ACTIVATION OF SECONDARY CASCADES

Interactions occur among parenchymal cells, vascular (endothelial) cells, and inflammatory cells (Fig. 73-11). Membrane disruption due to phospholipase A_2 activation causes release of arachidonic acid. Subsequent metabolism can produce prostacyclin, thromboxanes, and eicosanoids (Fig. 73-9).

In the ischemic environment, the normally fine balance between prostacyclin and thromboxane effects is dis-

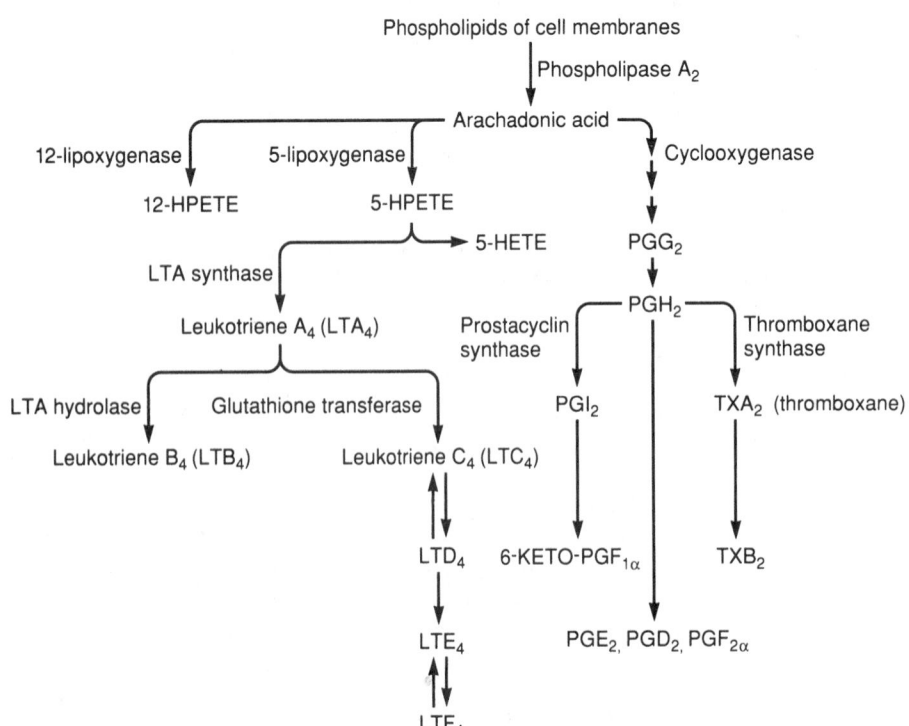

Figure 73-9. Phospholipase activation causes phospholipid degradation and triggers arachidonic acid metabolite cascades.

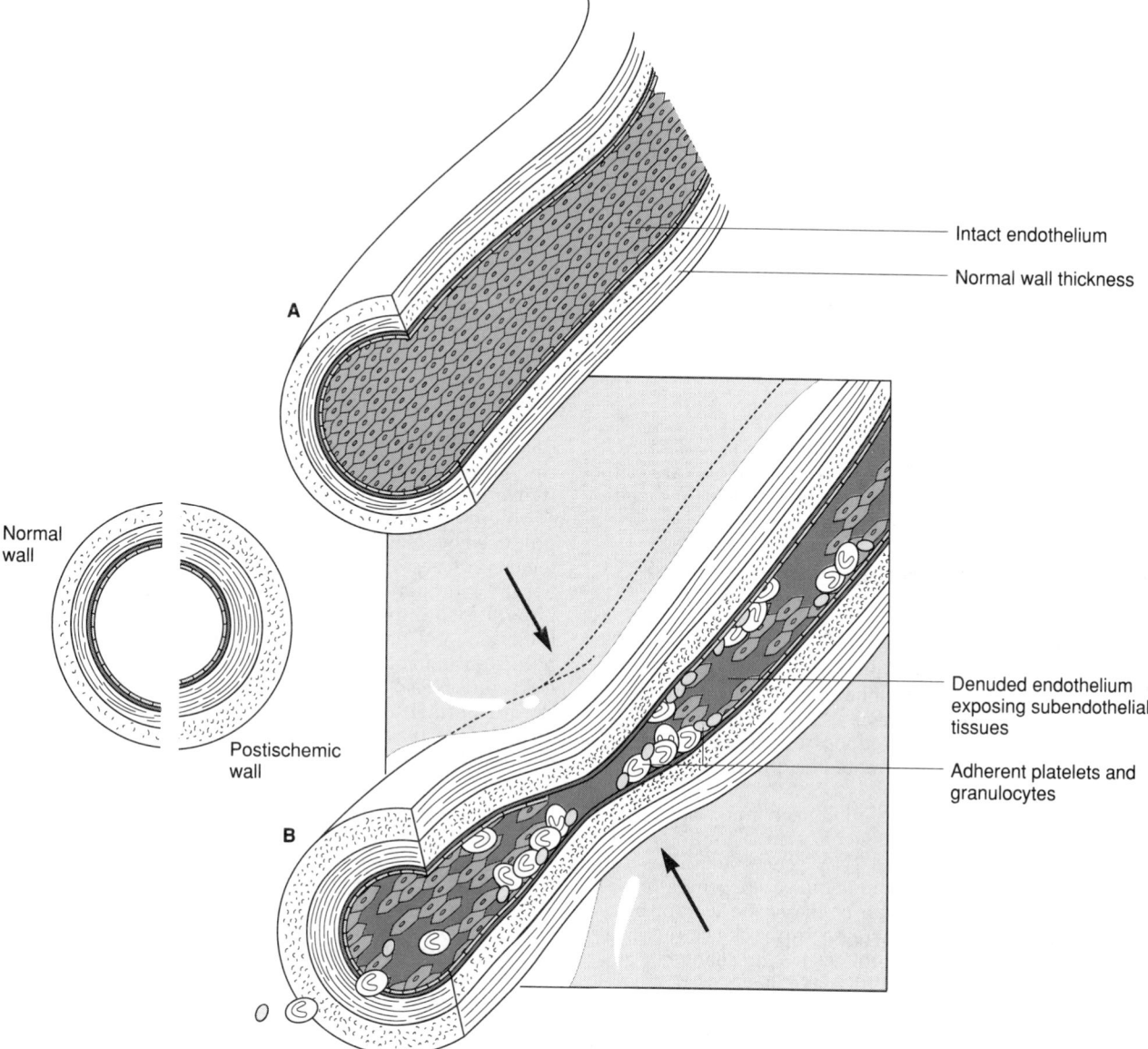

Figure 73-10. (*A*) Normal blood vessel showing normal diameter and wall thickness. The endothelium is intact, produces normal quantities and types of mediators, and resists adherence by granulocytes and platelets. (*B*) Postischemic blood vessel exhibits reduced luminal diameter and increased wall thickness as a result of intramural cell swelling and edema. Sloughing of endothelial cells exposes highly thrombogenic subendothelial tissues, especially collagen. Denuded or injured endothelium results in altered production of mediators with potential adverse effects (ie, loss of PGI_2 and HO and enhanced production of thromboxane A_2 and procoagulants). Granulocyte and platelet adherence result in luminal plugging, reduced flow, and continued injury. Injury to the parenchymal tissues enveloping the blood vessels produces extrinsic compression and reduced flow, exacerbating the original injury.

rupted. Enhanced production of thromboxane causes vasoconstriction and platelet adherence, leading to continued ischemic injury. Thromboxane A_2 (TXA_2) is implicated in the systemic and remote effects of lower torso ischemia, particularly the noncardiogenic pulmonary edema associated with aortic reconstruction. This effect of TXA_2 may be initiated by leukotriene B_4 or other mechanisms. It requires WBCs but not complement. The coagulation cascade is locally activated by exposure of collagen after desquamation of endothelial cells, causing platelet adherence and activation and, by means of release of tissue factor from injured cells, activating the extrinsic pathway.

REPERFUSION EFFECTS

Reperfusion is a widespread phenomenon that involves other mechanisms (Figs. 73-7, 73-10; Table 73-2). Increased generation of oxygen radicals occurs with reoxygenation. The result is the same, whether such an increase occurs from parenchymal cells, endothelial cells lining the microvasculature, or locally attracted leukocytes.

Continued injury during reperfusion may result from swelling of the cells in the vessel wall and from platelet and WBC adherence to the luminal surface. Irretrievable loss of nucleotide bases may limit the supply of substrate

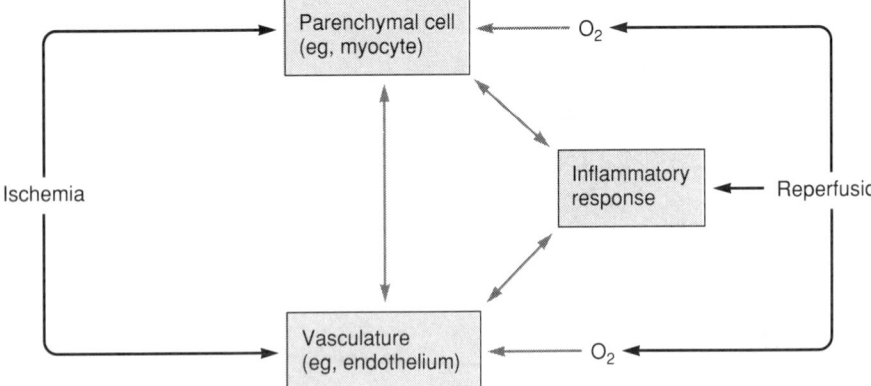

Figure 73-11. Complex cellular interactions occur in ischemia and reperfusion injury involving the parenchymal cells, the vasculature (especially the endothelium), and inflammatory cells. (After Fantone JC. Pathogenesis of ischemia-reperfusion injury: an overview. In: Zelenock GB, ed. Clinical ischemic syndromes: mechanisms and consequences of tissue injury. St Louis, CV Mosby, 1990)

for ATP reformation. ATP re-formation is an energy-consuming process. At a time when energy stores are critically low, re-formation of ATP stores competes for available energy with vital cellular processes.

REMOTE OR SYSTEMIC EFFECTS OF ISCHEMIA

Aortic operations with lower torso ischemia are associated with renal failure and pulmonary dysfunction. Profound skeletal muscle ischemia with rhabdomyolysis as occurs in the crush syndrome or delayed treatment of thrombosis or embolism produces oliguria and uremia. The effect of ischemia on remote organ function involves specific mediators.

TXA_2 and WBC-mediated pulmonary injury are linked with leg and lower torso ischemia. These findings were correlated with an increase in TXA_2 generation (measured as TXB_2, its stable metabolite). Increased generation of TXA_2 begins with application of the aortic clamp; however, a clamp-associated increase in prostacyclin (measured as 6-keto-PGF_{1a}) does not occur. The change in pulmonary status appears to be WBC dependent and mediated by TXA_2 and leukotriene B_4. Complement does not appear to be involved.

Other mechanisms that occur with ischemia may have adverse systemic effects or compromise the performance of distant organs. As ATP degrades, adenosine release may contribute to systemic hypotension, because in most vascular beds it is a potent vasodilator. Adenosine causes renal and pulmonary vascular vasoconstriction. Such effects may contribute to declamping hypotension and to the renal and pulmonary compromise that occurs with aortic clamping and declamping, as in aortic reconstruction.

CELLULAR AND MOLECULAR ASPECTS OF ISCHEMIA

Hypoxia, ischemia-reperfusion sequences, and surgical stress activate the hypothalamic-pituitary-adrenal axis, the sympathetic nervous system, and acute-phase reactants. After activation, the latter three modulate gene expression by formation of transcription factors that interact with certain DNA sequences, affecting the rate of transcription and production of complementary mRNA. Altered transcription results in variable production of protein effectors.

Transcription factors are proteins encoded by genes and are subject to regulatory processes. Some transcription factors are constitutively expressed, some are inducible, and some accelerate and some inhibit transcription. Multiple transcription factors exist, including heat-shock transcrip-

tion factor, which is produced by vascular smooth muscle cells in response to several stresses, including shock and ischemia-reperfusion sequences.

Atherosclerosis causes ischemic events. Nitric oxide produced by intact endothelial cells is integral to the maintenance of vessel wall smooth muscle vasodilator tone. Nitric oxide plays a part in hypertension, appears to be important in intimal hyperplasia and smooth muscle proliferation, and probably is important in postischemic reperfusion injury and other physiologic and pathophysiologic processes. Lowering an elevated cholesterol level toward normal appears to allow endothelium to secrete products, such as nitric oxide, which allows maintenance of normal vasomotor tone, inhibition of platelet activity, maintenance of the balance between thrombosis and fibrinolysis, and regulation of the recruitment of inflammatory cells into the vascular wall. The paradoxic vasoconstriction that occurs with infusion of acetylcholine in "diseased coronary arteries" is eliminated and returned toward the normal vasodilator response after hypercholesterolemia is controlled. Lowering cholesterol may result in a lesser degree of plaque activation.

Elevated plasma homocysteine level correlates with arteriosclerotic vascular disease. Elevated homocysteine levels may account for a large portion of the vascular disease in the United States. The relation seems consistent for cerebrovascular disease, peripheral vascular occlusive disease, and coronary artery disease. Elevated homocysteine impairs the production of endothelium-derived relaxing factor, stimulates proliferation of smooth muscle cells, and has a prothrombotic effect by changing the expression of thrombomodulin and activation of protein C. Elevated homocysteine levels can be reduced to normal with simple provision of folate and vitamins B_{12} and B_6. Patients with high homocysteine levels are at high risk for cardiovascular disease.

THERAPY

Therapeutic strategies for ischemia aimed at the underlying pathophysiologic condition are being devised. Pretreatment to lessen ischemic damage is relevant to surgeons who must clamp blood vessels or interrupt blood flow to a tissue or organ during a reconstructive procedure. Pretreatment protocols also may be used in transplantation and organ preservation.

Treatment during or after an ischemic event is difficult because most spontaneously occurring ischemic events present as emergencies with little or no warning. Ability to attenuate ischemic injury or retard its progression will be of benefit, because even if initial therapy only slows the

Table 73-2. ISCHEMIA AND REPERFUSION, FREE RADICALS, AND TOXIC OXYGEN SPECIES

1. Free radical is any species capable of independent existence that contains one or more unpaired electrons (electrons normally associate in pairs and move in precise relations around the nucleus).
2. Free radical reactions tend to proceed as chain reactions; when reacting with nonradicals (giving up the unpaired electron, removing an electron from the nonradical species, or combining with a nonradical), this still results in an unpaired electron (ie, a radical).
3. Radicals may be involved in biologic processes in addition to ischemia and reperfusion: autoimmune or inflammatory reactions, cancer, heavy metal overload, brain and CNS disorders, vitamin E deficiency, AIDS, eye disorders (retrolental fibroplasia, cataracts, posthemorrhage visual deteriorations), and exposure to various toxins (ozone, asbestos, cigarette smoke).
4. Radicals may have physiologic or beneficial effects.
    $NO^{\bullet}$ relaxes vascular smooth muscle, resulting in vasodilation
    $O_2^{\bullet-}$ participates in the killing and disposal of unwanted material by phagocytes; may serve as a growth regulator; may react with $NO^{\bullet}$ to produce nonradical products and oppose vasodilation
5. Radicals may be formed under physiologic or pathologic circumstances and have a variety of sources.
    Reactive oxygen metabolites

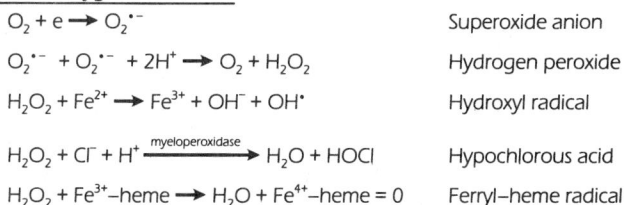

$$O_2 + e \longrightarrow O_2^{\bullet-} \qquad \text{Superoxide anion}$$
$$O_2^{\bullet-} + O_2^{\bullet-} + 2H^+ \longrightarrow O_2 + H_2O_2 \qquad \text{Hydrogen peroxide}$$
$$H_2O_2 + Fe^{2+} \longrightarrow Fe^{3+} + OH^- + OH^{\bullet} \qquad \text{Hydroxyl radical}$$
$$H_2O_2 + Cl^- + H^+ \xrightarrow{\text{myeloperoxidase}} H_2O + HOCl \qquad \text{Hypochlorous acid}$$
$$H_2O_2 + Fe^{3+}\text{-heme} \longrightarrow H_2O + Fe^{4+}\text{-heme} = 0 \qquad \text{Ferryl-heme radical}$$

Sources of reactive oxygen species during reperfusion

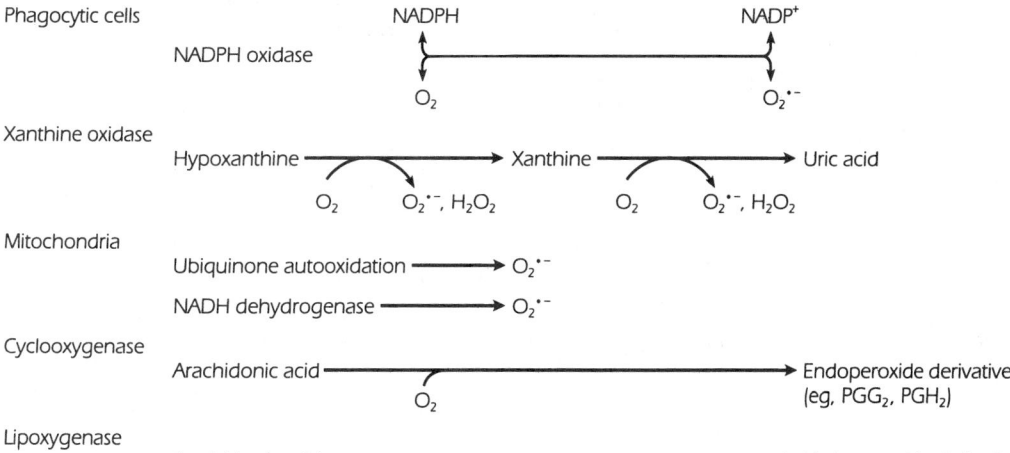

Phagocytic cells — NADPH oxidase
Xanthine oxidase: Hypoxanthine → Xanthine → Uric acid
Mitochondria: Ubiquinone autooxidation → $O_2^{\bullet-}$; NADH dehydrogenase → $O_2^{\bullet-}$
Cyclooxygenase: Arachidonic acid → Endoperoxide derivatives (eg, PGG_2, PGH_2)
Lipoxygenase: Arachidonic acid → Hydroperoxide derivatives (eg, 15-HPETE)

6. Antioxidant defenses:
    Antioxidant enzymes
$$O_2^{\bullet-} + O_2^{\bullet-} + 2H^+ \xrightarrow{\text{superoxide dismutase}} O_2 + H_2O_2$$
$$2H_2O_2 \xrightarrow{\text{catalase}} 2H_2O + O_2$$
$$H_2O_2 + 2GSH \xrightarrow{\text{glutathione peroxidase}} 2H_2O + GSSG$$
$$ROOH + 2GSH \longrightarrow ROH + GSSG + H_2O$$
    Minimization of amount of free metal ions (ie, iron and copper)
        Transferrin
        Ferritin
        Ceruloplasmin
        Desferrioxamine
    Antioxidant and quenching reactions
        α-Tocopherol (lipid soluble)
        β-Carotene
        Phytofluene
        Lycopene
        Ascorbic acid
7. Adverse effects of radicals and toxic oxygen species:
    Alter the function of certain enzymes and structural proteins, depolymerization, cleavage of peptide bonds, intramolecular and intermolecular cross-linking of membrane proteins
    Glycosaminoglycan oxidation
    Promote DNA scission and base modifications
    Promote lipid peroxidation

(Modified from Fantone JC. Pathogenesis of ischemia-reperfusion injury: an overview. In: Zelenock GB, ed. Clinical ischemic syndrome: mechanisms and consequences of tissue injury. St. Louis, CV Mosby, 1990; and Halliwell B. Lipid peroxidation, free radical reactions, and human disease. In: Current concepts. Kalamazoo, Upjohn, 1991)

progression of injury or temporarily stabilizes a precarious episode of critical ischemia, it may allow time for diagnostic studies and preparation for conventional intervention.

A single pharmacologic intervention is unlikely to be effective. Intervention must be aimed at several points in the ischemic cascade and at the various mechanisms of ischemic injury.

SUGGESTED READING

Fong Y, Moldawer LL, Shires GT, Lowry SF. The biologic characteristics of cytokines and their implication in surgical injury. Surg Gynecol Obstet 1990;170:363.

Jensen JC, Buresh C, Norton JA. Lactic acidosis increases tumor necrosis factor secretion and transcription in vitro. J Surg Res 1990;49:350.

Levine GN, Keaney JF, Vita JA. Cholesterol reduction in cardiovascular disease: clinical benefits and possible mechanisms. N Engl J Med 1995;332:512.

Moncada S. Higgs A. Mechanisms of disease: the L-arginine-nitric oxide pathway. N Engl J Med 1993;329:2002.

Selhub J, Jacques PF, Bostom AG, et al. Association between plasma homocysteine concentrations and extracranial carotid-artery stenosis. N Engl J Med 1995;332:286.

Udelsman R, Holbrook NJ. Endocrine and molecular responses to surgical stress. Curr Probl Surg 1994;31:657.

Vane JR, Anggard EE, Botting RM. Regulatory functions of the vascular endothelium. N Engl J Med 1990;323:27.

Walsh TR, Rao PN, Makowka L, Starzl TE. Lipid peroxidation is a nonparenchymal cell event with reperfusion after prolonged liver ischemia. J Surg Res 1990;49:18.

Zelenock GB, D'Alecy LG, Fantone JC III, Shlafer M, Stanley JC, eds. Clinical ischemic syndromes: mechanism and consequences of tissue injury. St. Louis, CV Mosby, 1990.

ESSENTIALS OF SURGERY: SCIENTIFIC PRINCIPLES AND PRACTICE, edited by Lazar J. Greenfield, Michael W. Mulholland, Keith T. Oldham, Gerald B. Zelenock, and Keith D. Lillemoe. Lippincott–Raven Publishers, Philadelphia, © 1997.

CHAPTER 74

ARTERIAL HEMODYNAMICS AND VASCULAR DIAGNOSTICS

JACK L. CRONENWETT, MARK F. FILLINGER, AND DAVID S. SUMNER

ARTERIAL HEMODYNAMICS

Arterial Structure and Function

The arterial wall is composed of endothelial cells, smooth muscle cells, collagen, and elastin. These elements are organized into three layers of the vessel wall—intima, media, and adventitia.

The *intima* is composed of endothelial cells and internal elastic lamina. The *media* is composed of collagen, elastin, and smooth muscle cells arranged in bundles oriented along the lines of greatest tension (circumferentially). It carries most of the tensile load. The *adventitia* is composed of fibrous connective tissue, vasa vasorum for nutrient supply to the outer layers of larger arteries, and nerve fibers that regulate medial smooth muscle cell tone. The adventitia carries little of the tensile load. When it does perform a support function (eg, in the proximal visceral arteries),

the adventitia has a larger number of collagen and elastin fibers.

The *endothelium* is much more than an antithrombotic barrier that interacts with platelets to promote hemostasis at the site of physical injury. The most important hemodynamic function of endothelial cells is interaction with smooth muscle cells to regulate luminal diameter.

The arterial wall is subject to a number of *hemodynamic stresses,* and its structure must accommodate all of them (Fig. 74-1). These stresses are controlled by intraluminal blood pressure, blood flow velocity, arterial diameter, and wall thickness.

Blood Flow Control

Blood flow is controlled by the following mechanisms:

- Local control—blood flow remains constant in most organs despite changes in perfusion pressure. The *myogenic theory* of control is that vascular smooth muscle contracts in response to stretch caused by increases in intravascular pressure, and relaxes in response to decreased stretch when perfusion pressure falls. The *metabolic theory* is that tissue blood flow parallels metabolic activity.
- Nervous system control—the sympathetic nervous system has primary neural control of vascular smooth muscle tone
- Local humoral control—humoral substances affect vascular smooth muscle tone (eg, epinephrine, vasopressin, prostaglandins)
- Flow-related control—blood flow regulates arterial diameter

Arterial Pressure and Energy

Determinants of the Arterial Pressure Curve

Systemic arterial pressure is the result of interaction among cardiac pump, aortic valve, compliance of large central arteries, peripheral vascular resistance, and total vascular volume. The pressure wave transmitted after systolic contraction is a result of the stroke volume of the heart and of the compliance (distensibility) of the aorta and proximal arteries. Expansion of large central arteries reduces systolic pressure, and contraction helps sustain diastolic pressure.

Pressure and Energy

Blood flow is controlled by energy gradients. Arterial pressure makes the largest contribution to these gradients. Total energy in the circulation results from the sum of potential energy (PE) and kinetic energy (KE). PE is the sum of intraarterial pressure and gravitational energy. KE

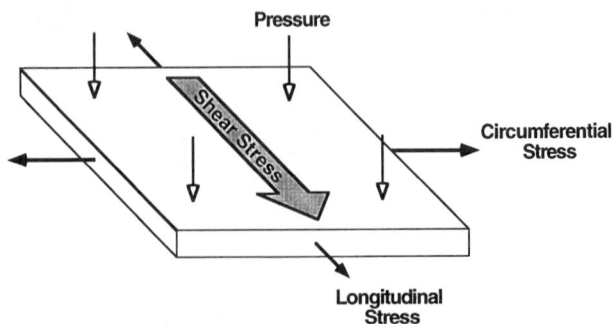

Figure 74-1. Stresses imposed on the arterial wall.

derives from the ability of flowing blood to perform work based on its velocity.

Arterial Flow and Energy Loss

Viscosity and Laminar Blood Flow

Friction develops between the layers of a flowing fluid. *Viscosity* is the lack of slipperiness between adjacent lamina. An ideal fluid with no viscosity (ie, no internal friction between layers) and flowing in a frictionless conduit would have all fluid particles traveling at the same velocity, resulting in a *flat velocity profile* (Fig. 74-2A).

In a real system, cohesive attraction forces develop between the conduit wall and the fluid in contact with the wall, preventing the outermost layer of fluid from moving. Although some molecular exchange occurs between the outermost fluid layer and the inner fluid layers, no actual movement or slippage of the outermost fluid layer occurs along the conduit wall. Because of net fluid movement in the conduit, there must be a velocity gradient across the conduit, so maximal velocity is attained at the greatest distance from the conduit wall, the axial center of the tube. Proceeding from this center toward the conduit wall, there is a progressive decrease in velocity of each layer (lamina) of fluid. Zero velocity is reached at the conduit wall, resulting in a *parabolic profile* for laminar flow of real liquids (Fig. 74-2B).

Real arteries are not smooth, straight tubes, however. Atherosclerotic plaques, branches, vessel curvature, and pulsatile flow cause departures from the parabolic velocity profile of laminar flow. Blood flow disturbances result in disruption of the parallel streamlines characteristic of laminar flow and produce *turbulence* (Fig. 74-2C).

Averaged over time, turbulent flow produces a mean velocity profile similar to that of laminar flow, only *blunted* (Fig. 74-2D). The conditions of physiologic blood flow are too stable for true turbulence. Flow disturbances do occur, but they tend to dampen over short distances.

Stress or force per unit area required to overcome the friction between adjacent fluid layers is defined as *shear stress. Shear rate* is the velocity gradient that develops between fluid layers divided by the distance between adjacent layers. Shear rate is proportional to velocity.

Viscosity is the ratio of shear stress to shear rate. Viscosity is the tangential force required to maintain a constant velocity between two adjacent laminas with area and distance constant. Viscosity is conceptualized as the thickness of a liquid. A Newtonian fluid (eg, water) is one in which viscosity is constant despite changes in velocity (shear rate). Although plasma may be considered newtonian in behavior, blood may not, primarily because of red blood cells (RBCs). At low shear rates, RBCs aggregate and increase viscosity, particularly in the presence of large plasma proteins, such as fibrinogen. At high shear rates, RBCs are drawn into the central high-velocity portion of the flow pattern, which reduces viscosity.

Blood viscosity depends on shear rate (ie, velocity), hematocrit, and plasma protein concentration. Hematocrit, or packed cell volume (PCV), is proportional to the logarithm of viscosity. Hematocrit >45% cause disproportionately large increases in viscosity.

Viscous Energy Loss

As a real fluid flows through a rigid, straight tube, energy is lost in proportion to fluid viscosity as heat generated by friction between layers of the fluid. Because vascular resistance cannot be directly measured, it is calculated from direct measurements of pressure (P) and flow (Q), according to the relation $R = P/Q$. Resistance is expressed in mmHg/cm³/min and is defined as a peripheral resistance unit. The units mmHg/cm³/sec are expressed in standard resistance units (dynes/sec^{-1}/cm⁵).

Inertial Energy Loss

Changes in pressure in straight tubes are proportional to changes in flow. At high flow rates, turbulence disrupts the laminar flow pattern of parallel streamlines when flow rate reaches a critical value. Turbulence in an artery may result in an audible noise, or *bruit,* as a result of vibration of the arterial wall. Severe wall vibration in superficial arteries may be palpated as a *thrill.* Turbulence is more likely with increased velocity and decreased viscosity.

In addition to viscous energy losses, fluids lose inertial (kinetic) energy because of changes in velocity that cause turbulence or flow disturbance. These changes are impossible to measure in vivo, so energy losses cannot be calculated. At low flow velocities, viscous forces predominate, and pressure gradients are more linearly proportional to flow (Poiseuille's law). At high flow velocities, inertial energy losses predominate because of rapidly increasing velocity.

Local Effects of Turbulent Flow

Changes in geometry at an arterial bifurcation result in altered velocity vectors that produce subtle but important local turbulence or disturbed flow. At a bifurcation where there is sudden change in direction of flow, local pressure gradients develop, and the laminar velocity profile becomes skewed with higher velocities toward the central flow divider. This produces a region of zero velocity separate from the arterial wall *(boundary layer separation)* (Fig. 74-3).

Increased particle residence time at sites of boundary layer separation accelerate atherosclerosis because of the prolonged contact between the arterial wall and blood-borne stimulants derived from platelets and other blood elements. Low shear is also a stimulus for endothelial cells to increase production of biologic mediators that induce narrowing of the vessel lumen through vasoconstriction, smooth muscle cell proliferation, and extracellular matrix production.

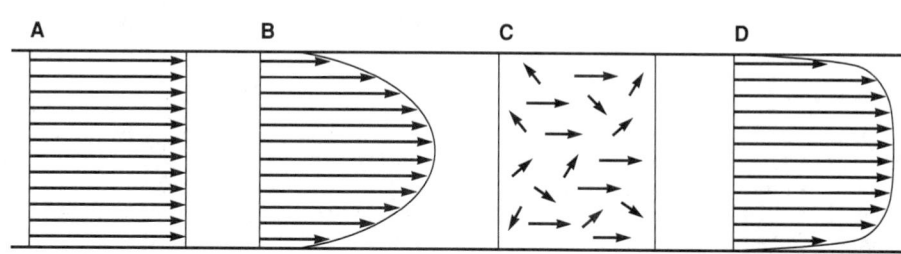

Figure 74-2. (*A*) Flat velocity profile of an ideal fluid (zero viscosity) in a straight, rigid tube. (*B*) Parabolic laminar flow profile of a real, newtonian fluid. (*C*) Turbulent flow of a real fluid at high Reynolds number. Velocity vectors at any moment in time are random. (*D*) Time-averaged velocity profile for turbulent flow has a blunted profile when compared with laminar flow.

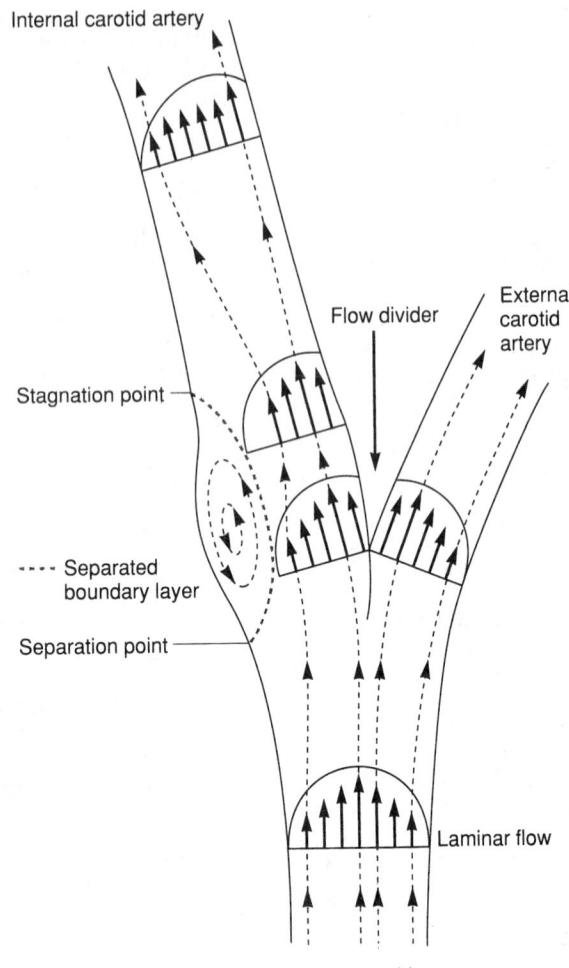

Internal carotid artery

Flow divider

External carotid artery

Stagnation point

Separated boundary layer

Separation point

Laminar flow

Common carotid artery

Figure 74-3. Alteration in flow at the human carotid artery bifurcation resulting in boundary layer separation and stagnant flow along the outer wall of the internal carotid artery. This corresponds to the region of development of atherosclerotic plaque. (After Zarins CK, Giddens DP, Bharaduaj BK, Sottiurai VS, Mabon RF, Glagov S. Carotid bifurcation atheroscleroses: quantitative correlation of platelet localization with flow velocity profiles and wall shear stress. Circ Res 1983;53:502)

Arterial Stenosis

Energy Loss

Atherosclerotic occlusive disease affects the circulation through energy loss at arterial stenoses or occlusions. As blood flow encounters a fixed stenosis in an artery, velocity increases across the stenosis to maintain constant flow. Estimates of inertial and viscous energy lost at an arterial stenosis allow one to predict that 50% reduction in luminal diameter would cause at least a 16-fold energy loss. Inertial effects (turbulence) contribute more to this energy loss than do viscous effects. The energy lost at any fixed stenosis increases exponentially with increasing blood flow or velocity.

Critical Stenosis

An arterial stenosis is *critical* at the point at which it reduces distal pressure or flow. This point depends on the blood flow (velocity) in the artery. A stenosis not critical at lower flow might become critical at high flow *(subcritical)* stenosis. Flow-limiting stenosis occurs at about 50% diameter reduction, and becomes worse beyond that point.

Subcritical Stenosis

A stenosis *subcritical* during resting conditions (low blood flow) may become critical during the increased blood flow associated with exercise. If flow increases across a fixed stenosis (resistance), the pressure gradient across the stenosis increases accordingly. This reduces distal blood pressure, which limits the blood flow increase to meet the increased metabolic demands of exercise. Inadequate blood flow leads to metabolite accumulation and pain (claudication). Only when exercise stops is resting blood flow sufficient to remove accumulated metabolites and relieve pain.

If lower-extremity arterial stenosis is subcritical at rest, systolic cuff pressure measured at the ankle demonstrates no gradient compared with central arterial pressure (*ankle–brachial index,* ABI). The distal blood pressure reduction that results from increased flow across a subcritical stenosis can be used to detect such a stenosis. Immediately after or during exercise, ABI decreases in proportion to reduction in blood flow, returning gradually toward normal after cessation of exercise. This principle is used to detect subcritical stenoses and verify the presence of early arterial occlusive disease in patients with claudication who do not have reduced resting blood pressure.

Multiple Stenoses

Because atherosclerotic occlusive disease is a diffuse process, it is unlikely that an isolated arterial stenosis occurs but is likely that multiple sequential stenoses develop. Multiple factors, such as distance between stenoses, stenosis contour, and stenosis severity, do not allow calculation of the contribution of sequential stenoses in a real arterial system. Multiple sequential stenoses have an additive effect, although each subsequent stenosis contributes less resistance. In practice, the single most critical stenosis determines limitation of blood flow. Multiple subcritical stenoses can produce the effect of a single critical stenosis.

It is clinically expedient to divide the lower extremity into three major subsegments—the aortoiliac, femoropopliteal, and distal (below-the-knee) circulations. Stenoses can occur in more than one of these segments, resulting in complex influences on distal arterial pressure. It is important to determine the hemodynamic significance of stenoses in each of these areas to reconstruct arterial occlusive disease and achieve maximal clinical effects with minimal intervention.

Although arteriography provides an anatomic representation of atherosclerotic disease, it is frequently impossible to measure the severity of stenoses because of irregularities in geometry and three-dimensional asymmetry. Measurement of segmental pressure gradients in the lower extremity by means of placement of blood pressure cuffs at different levels is an important part of clinical evaluation.

Collateral Circulation

Assessment of an arterial stenosis by measuring the pressure gradient is complicated by the presence of collateral arteries that may improve blood flow around a stenosis or occlusion. Blood flow through collateral arteries results when an energy gradient occurs across the stenosis in a major artery, inducing flow through collaterals from the proximal, higher energy level to the distal, lower energy level. Clinical pressure and flow measurements cannot differentiate the contribution of flow across the stenosis and the collateral flow. They determine overall flow reduction and pressure gradient.

Because collateral arteries are much smaller than the primary diseased vessel, a large number of collateral vessels are needed to compensate for the resistance change due to stenosis of a large artery. Resistance is an inverse function of the radius to the fourth power; 50% stenosis in a 0.5-cm artery would require 625 collateral arteries 1 mm in diameter to compensate completely for this stenosis. Inability to achieve this compensation necessitates surgical bypass or endovascular intervention to restore conduit diameter and relieve symptoms.

Arterial Aneurysms

Aneurysm expansion occurs as a result of tangential stress in the wall of an aneurysm. Rupture occurs when tangential stress exceeds wall tensile strength. Increased arterial blood pressure and aneurysm size are linearly proportional to wall tensile stress and to risk for aneurysm expansion and rupture. Aneurysm wall thickness is inversely proportional to wall stress, making thin aneurysms more prone to rupture than thick-walled aneurysms.

The wall thickness (and strength) of aneurysms is not homogeneous and cannot be accurately measured. However, the tensile stress in an aneurysmal wall is inversely related to the size of the native (proximal) aorta if wall thinning occurs during aneurysm expansion. A 6-cm aneurysm arising from a 1-cm aorta would experience three to four times greater wall stress than a 6-cm aneurysm arising from a 3-cm aorta.

VASCULAR DIAGNOSIS
Vascular Laboratory

Ultrasound

Doppler *flow detectors* emit a US beam at a frequency of 2 to 10 MHz. When the beam encounters a moving RBC, its frequency is changed in proportion to the velocity of the moving particle and the cosine of the angle (I) between beam and velocity vector. Because the frequency shift is audible, listening to the Doppler signal provides a quick,

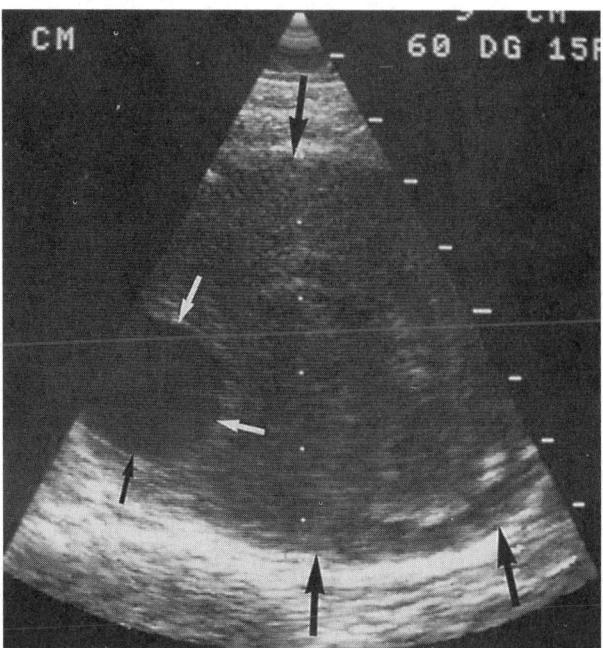

Figure 74-5. Real-time B-mode scan of cross section of a 5.6-cm abdominal aortic aneurysm. Lumen is largely filled with clot; hypoechogenic residual lumen is clearly defined. (Sumner DS. Ultrasonic screening for the detection of abdominal aortic aneurysms. Surg Clin North Am 1989;69:715)

simple method for transcutaneous assessment of blood flow.

Additional information can be obtained by subjecting the Doppler signal to *spectrum analysis*. The spectra are depicted graphically with frequency on the vertical axis, time on the horizontal axis, and amplitude as increasing intensity of a gray scale. The display shows the direction and contour of the flow pulse and flow disturbances (Fig. 74-4).

Real-time B-mode US devices measure the time required for a pulse of US to reach an acoustic interface and return to the transducer. Intensity of the echoes is shown on a gray scale, and time is shown on an axis perpendicular to the probe. As the sound beam is swept over the area of interest, a two-dimensional image appears on a screen. It corresponds to a "slice" of the underlying tissue (Fig. 74-5). The interface between vessel wall and blood is imaged.

Duplex scanning, which combines real-time B-mode imaging and Doppler flow detection, allows accurate placement of Doppler sample volume, and the Doppler signal facilitates identification of the vessel being imaged. *Color-flow imaging* superimposes in real time a flow map on the B-mode image. Color identifies the direction of flow, and color saturation corresponds to velocity. Slow flow has a deep color, and high velocities are pale. Color-flow scanning helps differentiate arteries and veins and allows immediate identification of areas of increased velocity and flow disturbances.

Plethysmography

Plethysmographs measure volume change. Because volume changes in all organs (except the lungs) are a function of blood content, plethysmography can be used to measure fluctuations in venous blood volume and arterial pressure pulsation.

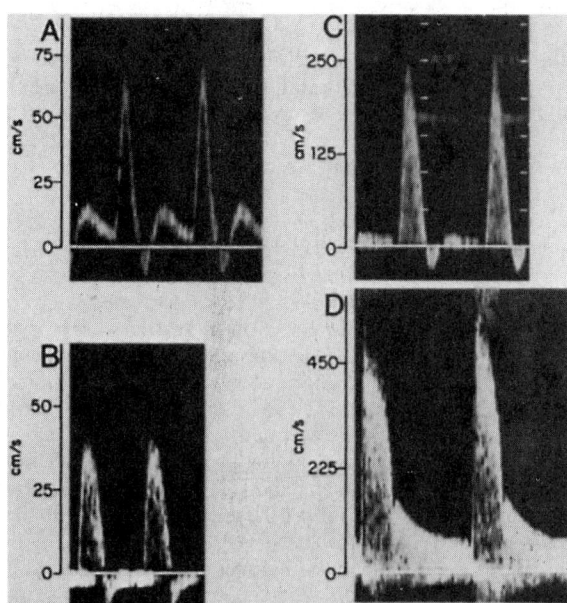

Figure 74-4. Spectral analysis of Doppler flow signals: (*A*) normal, (*B*) 1% to 19% stenosis, (*C*) 20% to 49% stenosis, and (*D*) 50% to 99% stenosis. (Kohler TR, Nance DR, Cramer MM, Vandenburghe N, Strandness DE. Duplex scanning for diagnosis of aortoiliac and femoropopliteal disease: a prospective study. Circulation 1987;76:1075)

Other Vascular Laboratory Methods

Polarographic electrodes applied to the skin are used to measure oxygen tension (T_{CPO_2}) or carbon dioxide tension (T_{CCO_2}) in the underlying cutaneous vascular bed. A *laser Doppler flowmeter,* which amplifies shifts in frequency of monochromatic light caused by motion of RBCs, provides qualitative assessment of cutaneous blood flow.

Imaging

Computed Tomography

Computed tomography (CT) displays the dimensions and anatomic relations of large vessels, especially in the abdomen and chest. It is used to assess the anatomic extent of ischemic lesions in the brain and for demonstrating intracranial hemorrhage, vascular malformations, and tumors. Spiral (helical) CT allows construction of three-dimensional displays of vascular structures. By manipulating the image on a computer screen, one can obtain views in multiple projections. Spiral CT may be helpful in evaluation of anatomic relations between abdominal aortic aneurysms and associated visceral arteries, obviating arteriography. Other applications include assessing disease in renal and visceral arteries.

Magnetic Resonance Imaging

Magnetic resonance imaging (MRI) does not involve use of ionizing radiation and is completely noninvasive. The images are comparable with CT scans and often are superior. Cross-sectional, sagittal, and coronal displays can be obtained. MRI can be used to assess blood flow. MR angiography (MRA) generates an image of the flow stream that closely resembles a conventional arteriogram. Cross-sectional and longitudinal images can be obtained in any plane.

Physiologic Measurements

Indirect Measurement of Blood Pressure

Measurement of peripheral arterial blood pressure is the most informative diagnostic method. A pneumatic cuff is wrapped around the limb, and a Doppler probe is positioned over a peripheral artery (usually the radial artery at the wrist or the dorsalis pedis or posterior tibial artery at the foot). The cuff is inflated to supersystolic pressure, then slowly deflated. The pressure in the cuff when flow resumes equals systolic pressure in the arteries under the cuff.

Ankle Pressure.   Resting ankle pressure normally exceeds brachial blood pressure. Because ankle systolic blood pressure varies with central aortic pressure, values may be normalized by dividing the ankle pressure by the brachial blood pressure. This ratio (ABI) normally averages about 1.1. An ABI <0.92 signifies the presence of hemodynamically significant arterial disease. Absolute ankle pressures <40 mmHg indicate severe arterial compromise, regardless of ABI.

Toe Pressure.   A small pneumatic cuff is wrapped around the proximal part of the toe, and a photoplethysmograph distal to the cuff is used to sense return of blood flow. Toe pressures are valuable for identifying lesions confined to the pedal or digital arteries and are more reliable than ankle pressures in diabetic extremities. A toe pressure <30 mmHg indicates severe ischemia.

Segmental Leg Pressures.   Arterial pressures are estimated in the upper thigh, above the knee, and upper calf by placement of pneumatic cuffs. Comparison of pressures measured at the same level in the two legs or between levels in the same leg may help identify the location of obstruction. A difference of 20 to 30 mmHg is hemodynamically significant.

Upper-Extremity Pressure Measurements.   A pressure difference >15 mmHg between arms at the brachial, forearm, or wrist level signifies proximal arterial obstruction. Finger pressures are measured with cuffs around the proximal part of the finger and a photoplethysmograph attached to the fingertip. The finger-brachial index is calculated by dividing finger pressure by ipsilateral brachial pressure. If there is no arterial obstruction, finger-brachial index averages 0.97. Values <0.8 suggest obstruction of the digital, palmar, or more proximal arteries.

Direct Measurement of Blood Pressure

Arterial pressure is measured with a needle or cannula connected by a length of plastic tubing to a pressure transducer. At the level of the common femoral artery, normal systolic femoral-systemic pressure index is >0.9. Lower values indicate critical proximal arterial stenosis. To increase the sensitivity of the test, 30 mg of papaverine (a vasodilator) may be injected into the common femoral artery, while blood flow velocity is monitored with a Doppler flow detector. A 15% decrease in femoral-systemic pressure index confirms hemodynamically significant stenosis.

Plethysmography

Plethysmographic pulses normally have a rapid upslope, a sharp peak, and a downslope that bows toward baseline. Distal to an obstruction, the pulse is rounded, has a slow upslope, and has a downslope that bows away from the baseline (Fig. 74-6). In severe ischemia, pulses may be imperceptible.

One performs segmental plethysmography by applying air-filled cuffs to the thigh, calf, and ankle. These studies *(pulse volume recordings)* provide information about the location of disease (Fig. 74-7). More useful is *digital plethysmography,* in which mercury strain gauges or photoplethysmographic transducers are applied to the tips of the fingers or toes to act as volume sensors. An abnormal or absent plethysmographic tracing signifies disease in the digital arteries or more proximal vessels. Digital plethysmography is used with digital pressures for assessing disease distal to the wrist or ankle. The amplitude of the digital pulse, which is roughly proportional to blood flow, provides an index of local tissue perfusion.

Flow Studies

Normal peripheral arterial flow pulse is characterized by rapid acceleration in early systole that culminates in a sharp peak velocity. It is followed by a rapid deceleration phase, during which velocity falls to zero, a short period of flow reversal in early diastole, and a low-level forward flow phase extending throughout the remainder of diastole (Fig. 74-8). These fluctuations in velocity produce a characteristic triphasic audible *Doppler signal.* Beyond an obstruction, the flow pulse becomes rounded, the acceleration phase is less rapid, the peak is less clearly defined, the reversed flow component disappears, and velocities remain well above baseline levels throughout diastole (Fig. 74-8). Audible signals have a lower peak frequency, are noisy, and become monophasic. As the Doppler probe is passed over a stenotic area, the frequency of the signal increases with the increase in velocity. Absence of a signal indicates total occlusion of the artery.

Spectral analysis of the Doppler flow signal, usually performed with duplex scanning, is used to assess blood flow patterns (Fig. 74-4). In peripheral arteries and bypass

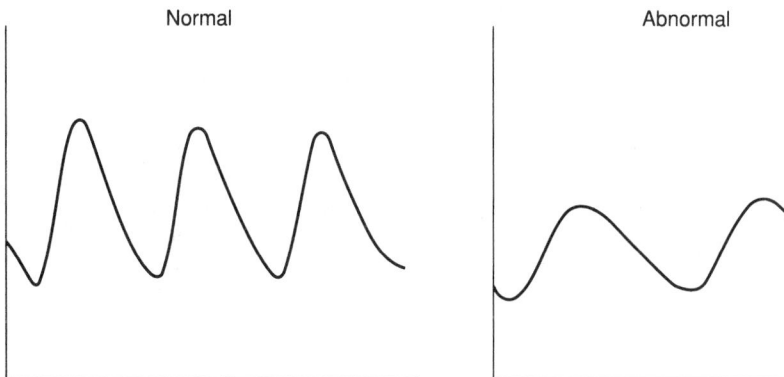

Figure 74-6. Toe plethysmographic pulses, normal and abnormal (distal to an arterial obstruction). Tracings on the right were recorded at a sensitivity twice that of those on the left.

grafts, an increase in velocity ≥100% and loss of the reversed flow component identifies the presence of a stenosis with a diameter reduction >50%. The presence of spectral broadening in the absence of a velocity increase differentiates normal from minimally diseased arteries (1% to 19% stenosis). A velocity increase of 30% to 100% suggests moderate stenosis (20% to 50% diameter reduction). Different criteria are applied to studies of the carotid circulation.

Color-coded flow mapping is used for rapid identification of areas of flow disturbance or increased velocity. Spectral analysis must still be performed for accurate assessment of the degree of arterial stenosis. *Laser Doppler tracings* of arterial obstruction show attenuated pulse waves, decreased mean velocity, and reduced vasomotor waves.

Oxygen Tension

The quantity of oxygen available for diffusion to the skin depends on the quantity delivered by the influx of blood and that extracted to meet metabolic demands. $TcPO_2$ pro-

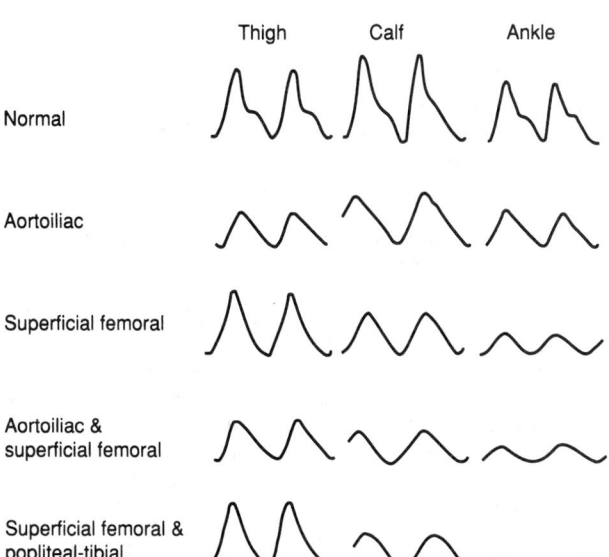

Figure 74-7. Segmental plethysmographic pulses from normal limbs, limbs with obstruction confined to the aortoiliac and superficial femoral segments, and limbs with multilevel obstruction involving the aortoiliac and superficial femoral arteries and superficial femoral and popliteal-tibial arteries. (After Rutherford RB, Lowenstein DH, Klein MF. Combining segmental systolic pressures and plethysmography to diagnose arterial occlusive disease of the legs. Am J Surg 1979;138:216)

vides an index of the adequacy of tissue perfusion. Measurements may be made from any region, usually the dorsum of the foot or the upper calf. Peripheral measurements are compared with $TcPO_2$ from a well-perfused central area, such as infraclavicular skin. In normal limbs, $TcPO_2$ averages 60 mmHg (about 90% of the infraclavicular value).

Exercise Testing

Walking on a treadmill at 2 mph at a 10% grade provides an estimation of the severity of claudication. Healthy people can walk for 5 minutes without experiencing leg pain; patients with arterial obstruction usually stop after 2 to 3 minutes. In normal legs, ankle pressures remain unchanged after exercise. A decrease in ankle pressure immediately after exercise indicates arterial obstruction, the severity of which is roughly proportional to the pressure drop and to the time required for pressure to return to preexercise levels (>20 minutes for severely diseased extremities).

Reactive Hyperemia

Reactive hyperemia is a substitute for treadmill testing. Hyperemia is produced when a pneumatic cuff placed around the limb is inflated to supersystolic pressures for 3 to 5 minutes and quickly deflated. The increase in blood flow is commensurate with the ability of the terminal arterioles to dilate in response to ischemia. Digital plethysmographic pulse reaches peak amplitude in a few seconds, and maximum excursion is more than double that measured during the control period. In limbs with arterial obstruction, pulse reappearance time is delayed, and there is little increase in pulse amplitude.

CLINICAL APPLICATIONS

Not every patient needs every test. Tests are dictated by history and physical findings and are designed to answer questions pertinent to diagnosis, prognosis, or treatment.

Lower-Extremity Peripheral Arterial Obstruction

The approach to intermittent claudication is shown in Figure 74-9, and to rest pain, nonhealing ulcers, or gangrene in Figure 74-10. One must identify the presence of arterial disease, determine its severity, and assess potential for healing.

Locating Sites of Obstruction. Duplex scanning and color-flow imaging are used to identify and evaluate the severity of arterial stenoses. These studies can help differentiate extensive occlusions that require surgical management from short stenoses that can be managed with transluminal angioplasty. Once the decision to intervene is

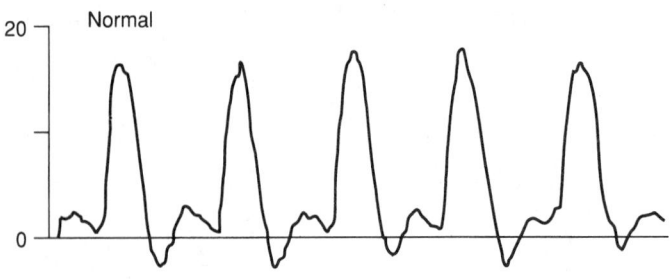

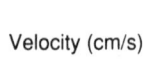

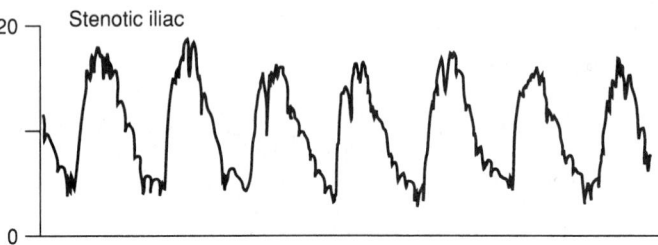

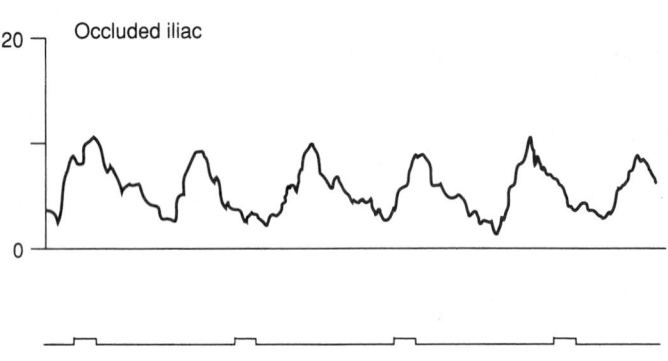

Figure 74-8. Analogue recordings of Doppler signals obtained from the common femoral artery of a normal subject, a patient with an iliac artery stenosis, and a patient with occlusion of the iliac artery. (After Strandness DE Jr, Sumner DS. Hemodynamics for surgeons. New York, Grune & Stratton, 1975:257)

made, arteriography is performed. Arteriography, however, provides no physiologic information.

Acute Arterial Obstruction and Trauma

When occlusion is embolic, a Doppler survey usually identifies the site of obstruction and obviates arteriography. If Doppler signals are present in the terminal arteries of the involved extremity, and if distal pressures (ankle or wrist) are >30 mmHg, it is safe to delay surgical intervention, if the symptoms are not severe. The time gained may be used to administer thrombolytic therapy.

Low pressure and reduced or absent Doppler signals in arteries distal to the site of penetrating or blunt trauma indicate arterial trauma or spasm. Arteriography or surgical exploration must be undertaken. Normal noninvasive studies do not exclude arterial trauma when severe hemorrhage, hematoma formation, fractures, or penetrating wounds exist near a major artery.

Vasospastic Disease

Vasospasm of the digital arteries in response to cold or to emotional stimuli (Raynaud phenomenon) is a common symptom. Digital arterial pressures and digital plethysmographic waveforms are used to identify or rule out arterial obstruction. Careful Doppler surveys of the wrist, palmar, and digital arteries may locate the site of obstruction and suggest a cause.

Cerebrovascular Disease

Noninvasive testing is the initial diagnostic procedure for extracranial carotid arterial disease. Cervical bruits are unreliable. Duplex scanning, with or without color-flow imaging, is used to detect plaques at the carotid bifurcation and provides information about the degree of stenosis. If a duplex scan confirms disease in a patient with symptoms or depicts a highly stenotic plaque in a patient without symptoms, arteriography is performed before the patient undergoes carotid endarterectomy. Sometimes duplex findings alone are sufficient.

B-mode US is used to evaluate the morphology, surface characteristics, and composition of arterial plaques. Duplex scanning shows vertebral arteries and is used to evaluate flow pattern. These studies are facilitated by color-flow mapping.

Transcranial Doppler studies also can be performed.

Visceral Arterial Obstruction

Duplex scanning allows noninvasive study of the visceral and renal arteries. Absence of flow identifies total occlusion, and marked spectral broadening and a ratio of renal artery to aortic peak systolic velocity >3.5 indicate 60% of diameter stenosis. Duplex scanning may not show accessory renal arteries. Duplex scanning is used as the initial screening technique for renal arterial hypertension and for monitoring renal arterial reconstruction.

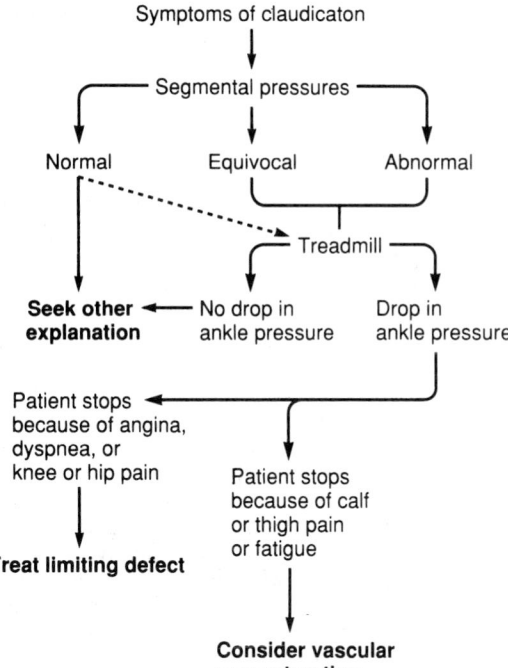

Figure 74-9. Diagnostic approach to patients with intermittent claudication. (After Sumner DS, Lambeth A, Russell JB. Diagnosis of upper extremity obstructive and vasospastic syndromes by Doppler ultrasound, plethysmography, and temperature profiles. In: Puel P, Boccalon H, Enjalbert A, eds. Hemodynamics of the limbs, vol 1. Toulouse, France, GEPESC, 1979:369)

Flow reversal in early diastole is present in the superior mesenteric artery during the fasting state, but is absent in the celiac axis. Severe stenoses are identified by the presence of a high-velocity jet with high systolic and diastolic frequencies. Peak systolic velocities >200 cm/sec in the celiac axis or 275 cm/sec in the superior mesenteric artery correlate with diameter reductions of ≥70%.

Aneurysms

MRI and CT are used to evaluate the dimensions of aneurysms or dissections of the thoracic and abdominal aorta. B-mode US is used to detect and size abdominal and peripheral aneurysms (Fig. 74-5). Coupled with color-flow imaging, B-mode US helps differentiate femoral, popliteal, and upper extremity true and false aneurysms from hematomas, cysts, enlarged lymph nodes, and other masses. If the decision is made not to operate, the aneurysm is monitored noninvasively to detect growth. Arteries peripheral to the aneurysm are evaluated to detect and locate any concomitant atherosclerotic stenoses or emboli. Findings may affect the decision to operate and the design of the operation.

When the relation between an abdominal aortic aneurysm and the renal or visceral arteries requires better definition, or when obstructive disease of these arteries or the iliofemoral vessels is suspected, arteriography is necessary. MRA may provide sufficient detail in patients who cannot undergo arteriography.

Follow-up Studies

Duplex scanning is used to monitor bypass grafts. A localized increase in systolic velocity >100% of that in the graft, above or below the lesion, identifies a diameter reduction >50%. Peak systolic velocities <40 cm/sec throughout the graft are an ominous sign. To preserve graft

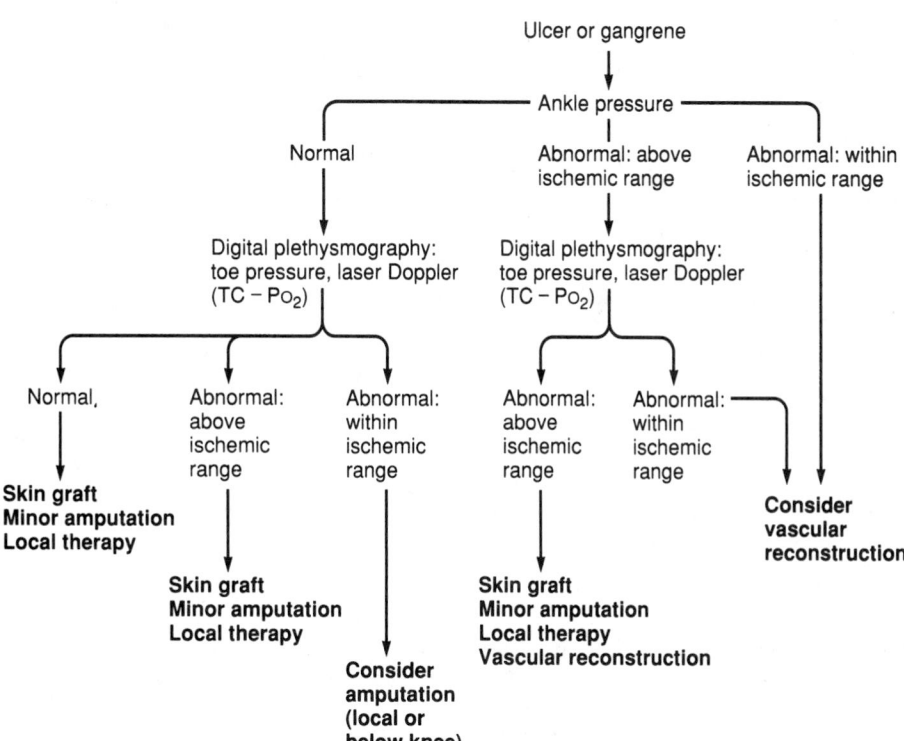

Figure 74-10. Diagnostic approach to patients with foot ulcers or gangrene.

function when either of these findings is present, arteriography is performed and the lesion corrected. Arteriovenous fistulas associated with in situ bypass grafts produce a pattern of localized flow disturbance, increased velocity at the site of the fistula and above, and decreased velocity below. These changes are recognized with duplex scanning or color-flow imaging.

SUGGESTED READING

Bernstein EF, ed. Vascular diagnosis, ed. 4. St. Louis, CV Mosby, 1993.

Carpenter JP, Baum RA, Holland GA, Barker CF. Peripheral vascular surgery with magnetic resonance angiography as the sole preoperative imaging modality. J Vasc Surg 1994;20:861.

Faught WE, Mattos MA, van Bemmelen, et al. Color-flow duplex scanning of carotid arteries: new velocity criteria based on receiver operator characteristic analysis for threshold stenoses used in the symptomatic and asymptomatic carotid trials. J Vasc Surg 1994;19:818.

Giddens DP, Zarins CK, Glagov S. Response of arteries to near-wall fluid dynamic behavior. Appl Mech Rev 1990;43:S96.

Gomes MN, Davros WJ, Zeman RK. Preoperative assessment of abdominal aortic aneurysm: the value of helical and three-dimensional computed tomography. J Vasc Surg 1994;20:367.

Hatsukami TS, Primozich JF, Zierler RE, et al. Color Doppler imaging of infrainguinal arterial occlusive disease. J Vasc Surg 1993;16:527.

Moneta GL, Lee RW, Yeager RA, et al. Mesenteric duplex scanning: a blinded prospective study. J Vasc Surg 1993;17:79.

Prince MR, Narasimham DL, Stanley JC, et al. Gadolinium-enhanced magnetic resonance angiography of abdominal aortic aneurysms. J Vasc Surg 1995;21:656.

Rutherford RB, ed. Vascular surgery, ed. 4. Philadelphia, WB Saunders, 1995.

Tennant WG, Hartnell GG, Baird RN, Horrocks M. Radiologic investigation of abdominal aortic aneurysm disease: comparison of three modalities in staging and the detection of inflammatory change. J Vasc Surg 1993;17:703.

CHAPTER 75

DIAGNOSTIC ANGIOGRAPHY

DAVID M. WILLIAMS AND KYUNG J. CHO

Angiography is the visualization of blood vessels. In conventional angiography, radiographs are made as blood is displaced by contrast medium injected through a catheter placed in an artery or vein. When the lumina of vessels become visible as branching columns of contrast medium, inferences can be made about the vessels, their surroundings, and the organs or tumors they supply. Angiography is used to demonstrate vascular anatomy, to identify abnormalities of the vascular wall and lumen, and to guide interventional vascular radiologic procedures.

Angiographic detail can be enhanced with: photographic

subtraction (Fig. 75-1), digital subtraction angiography (DSA) (Fig. 75-2), helical computed tomographic (CT) angiography (Fig. 75-3), or magnetic resonance angiography (MRA) (Fig. 75-4).

COMPLICATIONS

Puncture site complications include hematoma, dissection, pseudoaneurysm, arteriovenous (AV) fistula, thrombosis, and graft infection. The frequency and severity of these complications depend on the experience of the angiographer, attention to postprocedure hemostasis, size of the catheter or sheath, choice of puncture site, number of catheter exchanges, and duration of the procedure. Patients with uncontrolled hypertension, severe atherosclerosis, precariously compensated renal or cardiac disease, spasm-prone vessels, poor coagulation status, or those who are obese, are at risk for complications.

Catheterization and injection complications include arterial dissection, perforation, and embolism (including stroke). Risk depends on the experience of the angiographer, anatomic variations affecting ease of selective catheterization, vessel catheterized, and intrinsic arterial disease. Embolic stroke is associated with catheter manipulation or contrast injection in the aortic arch or brachiocephalic arteries. The gravity of a complication, such as arterial dissection or thrombosis, depends on the vessel involved and the integrity of collaterals.

Contrast medium complications include renal failure, fluid overload, congestive heart failure, transverse myelitis, and anaphylaxis. Complications can be minimized with hydration, careful catheter placement, and use of a steroid preparation before the procedure or use of nonionic contrast medium.

CONTRAINDICATIONS

There are no absolute contraindications to angiography. Relative contraindications include severe hypertension, poor coagulation status, severe renal or cardiac failure, and a history of severe reaction to contrast material. Reversible medical conditions that affect risk are corrected before the angiographic procedure.

ANATOMIC VARIATIONS THAT SIMULATE DISEASE

Anatomic variations and artifacts of an angiographic procedure can simulate arterial occlusion, arterial encasement, and parenchymal perfusion defects. Lack of filling of the expected arterial pattern of an organ or limb may be due to arterial occlusion or an avascular mass. It also may occur when contrast material does not fill aberrant or accessory arteries. Catheter- and guide wire-induced spasm can mimic neoplastic encasement. Selective catheterization is preceded by proximal arterial injections to demonstrate true arterial narrowing. For example, aortography precedes renal arteriography, and celiac arteriography precedes gastroduodenal arteriography.

Contrast injection sometimes demonstrates *standing waves,* in which the arterial lumen is differentiated by smooth, regular, alternating bands of mild narrowing and expansion (Fig. 75-5). This condition is differentiated from drug-induced (Fig. 75-6) or hypovolemic vasoconstriction and from arterial fibrodysplasia on the basis of the monotonous regularity of the alternating bands.

The high specific gravity of contrast material compared with blood contributes to incomplete mixing of contrast material during injection. When mixing is incomplete,

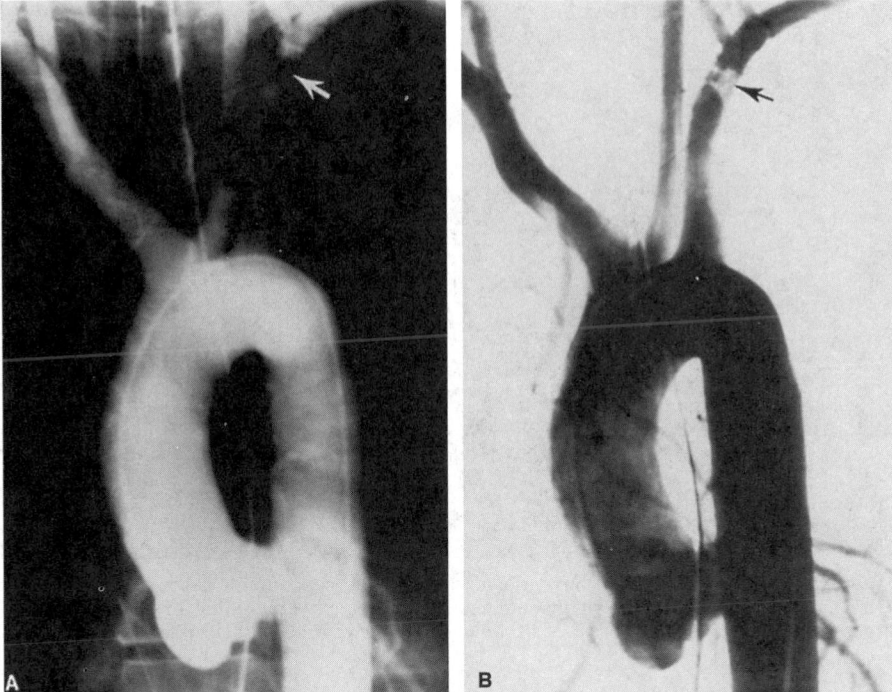

Figure 75-1. Value of photographic subtraction technique in thoracic aortography in a patient with chest trauma. An intimal injury in the left subclavian artery is barely appreciable on the conventional angiogram (*A*), but it is evident after photographic subtraction (*B*).

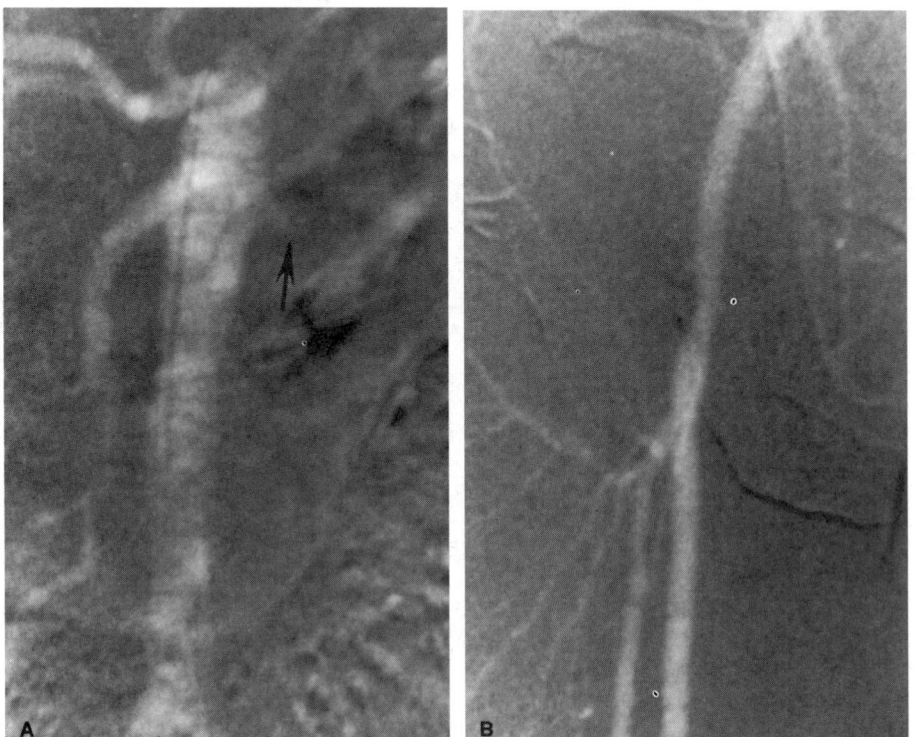

Figure 75-2. Carbon dioxide gas used as a contrast medium. A lumbar aortogram (*A*) and right common femoral arteriogram (*B*) were made during hand injection of carbon dioxide gas using digital subtraction angiography. The renal and lumbar arteries, which course posteriorly, are generally not filled by the buoyant gas with the patient in the supine position. The left renal artery is incompletely opacified (*arrow*).

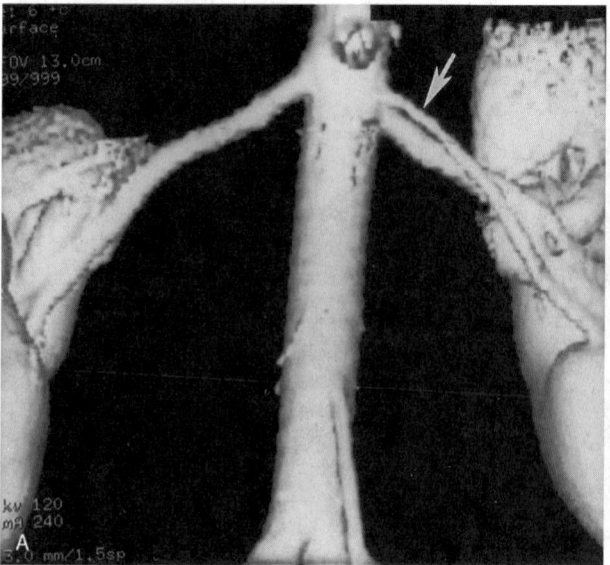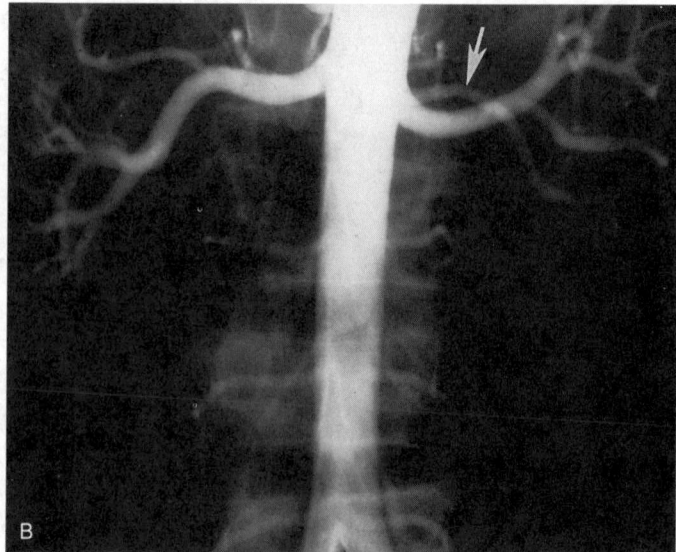

Figure 75-3. Helical CT (*A*) and conventional transcatheter (*B*) abdominal aortograms in a prospective renal donor. Both images demonstrate renal artery anatomy, including an accessory left renal artery (*arrows*). (Courtesy of Joel F. Platt, MD, University of Michigan Hospitals, Ann Arbor)

contrast material tends to pool along the dependent surface of large vessels, such as the aorta or along the mural surface of small arteries. This layering of contrast material is responsible for visualization of lumbar arteries on abdominal aortograms after visceral and renal arteries have cleared (Fig. 75-7).

In small arteries, mural layering of contrast material with nonopacified blood flowing in the center of the lumen can simulate an embolus (Fig. 75-8).

DIAGNOSTIC ANGIOGRAPHY: INDICATIONS AND FINDINGS

Indications for Diagnostic Angiography

Hemorrhage
Ischemia
Demonstration of vascular anatomy before surgical or transcatheter intervention
Venous thromboembolism

The clinical presentation of ischemia depends on the organ involved. It includes stroke, angina, renovascular hypertension, mesenteric ischemia, and limb claudication. The prototypical ischemic diseases are macroembolism and nonaneurysmal atherosclerosis.

Macroembolism

Angiography is indicated in acute ischemia to document the cause of acute occlusion (eg, arterial emboli), show arterial anatomy proximal and distal to large occlusions, and demonstrate associated or incidental pathologic conditions.

If emboli are documented, the angiographer searches for an aortic or arterial source, such as an aneurysm or atherosclerotic plaque or ulcer (Fig 75-9). The search for a cardiac source of emboli requires echocardiography. The appropriateness of intraarterial lytic therapy is considered at diagnostic angiography. If no emboli are found, other causes of acute ischemia are considered, including mesenteric arterial spasm or in situ thrombosis due to a low flow state.

Dissection and trauma may cause acute ischemia but are usually suggested by the clinical history.

Contrast agent around the leading or trailing edge of an arterial clot indicates acute occlusion, either embolic or thrombotic (Fig. 76-10). It may be impossible to differentiate acute embolism from thrombosis unless multiple sites of acute occlusion due to random embolism are demonstrated. The distinction between acute and chronic occlusion is based on the size of the collaterals bridging the occlusion; they are small when the occlusion is acute and large when the occlusion is of long standing.

If history and presentation suggest embolic disease, angiographic evaluation includes thoracic and biplanar abdominal aortography to locate a source of emboli and selective arteriography tailored to the clinical problem (eg, mesenteric, renal, lower extremity).

Nonaneurysmal Atherosclerosis: Renal, Mesenteric and Peripheral

Atherosclerosis is a progressive, systemic disease that mainly affects large and medium-sized arteries. The ischemic syndrome varies with the organ involved and severity of disease. Renal arteriosclerosis may present as hypertension or renal failure; mesenteric ischemia as postprandial epigastric pain, weight loss, or intestinal infarction; and peripheral occlusive disease as claudication, rest pain, or gangrene.

The purposes of angiography are to (1) document hemodynamically significant occlusive disease, (2) show the arterial anatomy of the donor and receptor sites of a prospective revascularization graft, and (3) demonstrate associated or incidental pathologic conditions.

The appropriateness of transcatheter interventional procedures, such as percutaneous angioplasty, is considered at diagnostic angiography.

Atherosclerosis is characterized at angiography by ulcers (pocket-like collections of contrast medium communicating with the arterial lumen), irregular or smooth narrowing and occlusions of large and medium-sized arteries, and the presence of collaterals. Atherosclerotic stenoses

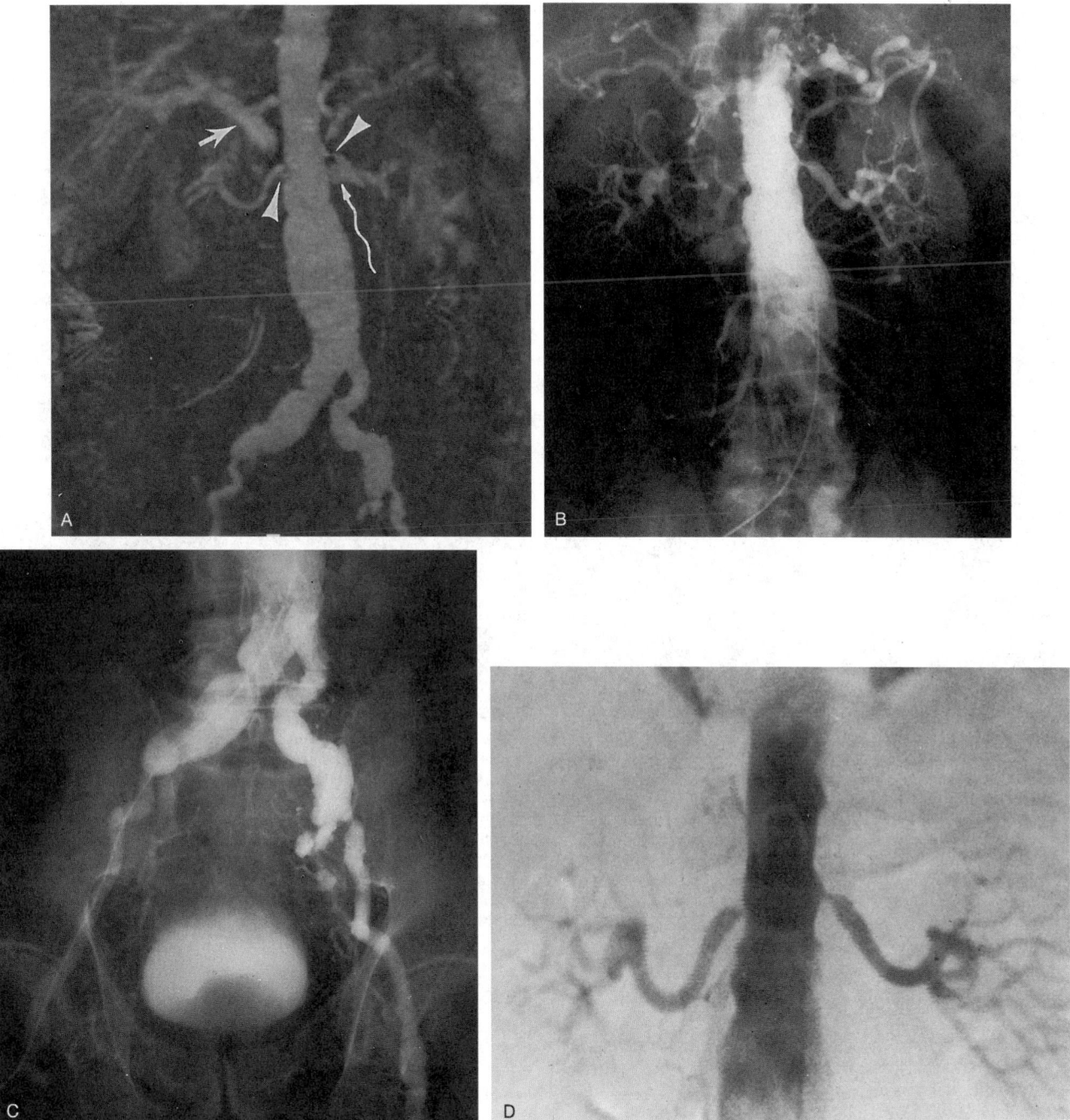

Figure 75-4. (*A*) Gadolinium-enhanced MR abdominal aortogram shows, in a coronal reconstruction, an infrarenal aortic aneurysm with proximal stenoses involving bilateral single renal arteries (*arrowheads*). Iliac artery aneurysms are also present. The celiac and superior mesenteric artery origins were demonstrated on a sagittal reconstruction of the dataset (not shown). Gadolinium has reached the portal (*straight arrow*) and left renal (*wavy arrow*) veins, but in this instance the study is not compromised. (*B* and *C*) Transcatheter aortography (using three injections) confirms the extent of the aneurysm. (*D*) Digital subtraction angiography with rapid image acquisition rate confirms the renal artery anatomy. (*continues*)

may be confused with neoplastic encasement or arterial fibrodysplasia.

Angiographic features of *stenosis* that suggest atherosclerosis are eccentricity, calcification, a tendency to involve the ostium or branch points, evidence of atherosclerosis in other vessels, and normal associated veins. Arterial stenosis is considered hemodynamically significant when associated with bridging collaterals, poststenotic dilata-

tion, a pressure gradient >10 mmHg, or ipsilateral renal vein renin hypersecretion. Stenosis of questionable hemodynamic significance at angiography during baseline blood flow is reassessed after augmentation of flow with pharmacologic or physiologic stimulation, such as vasoactive drugs or postischemic hyperemia.

Vasospasm (diffuse narrowing of an arterial bed) is differentiated from severe diffuse arteriosclerotic narrowing

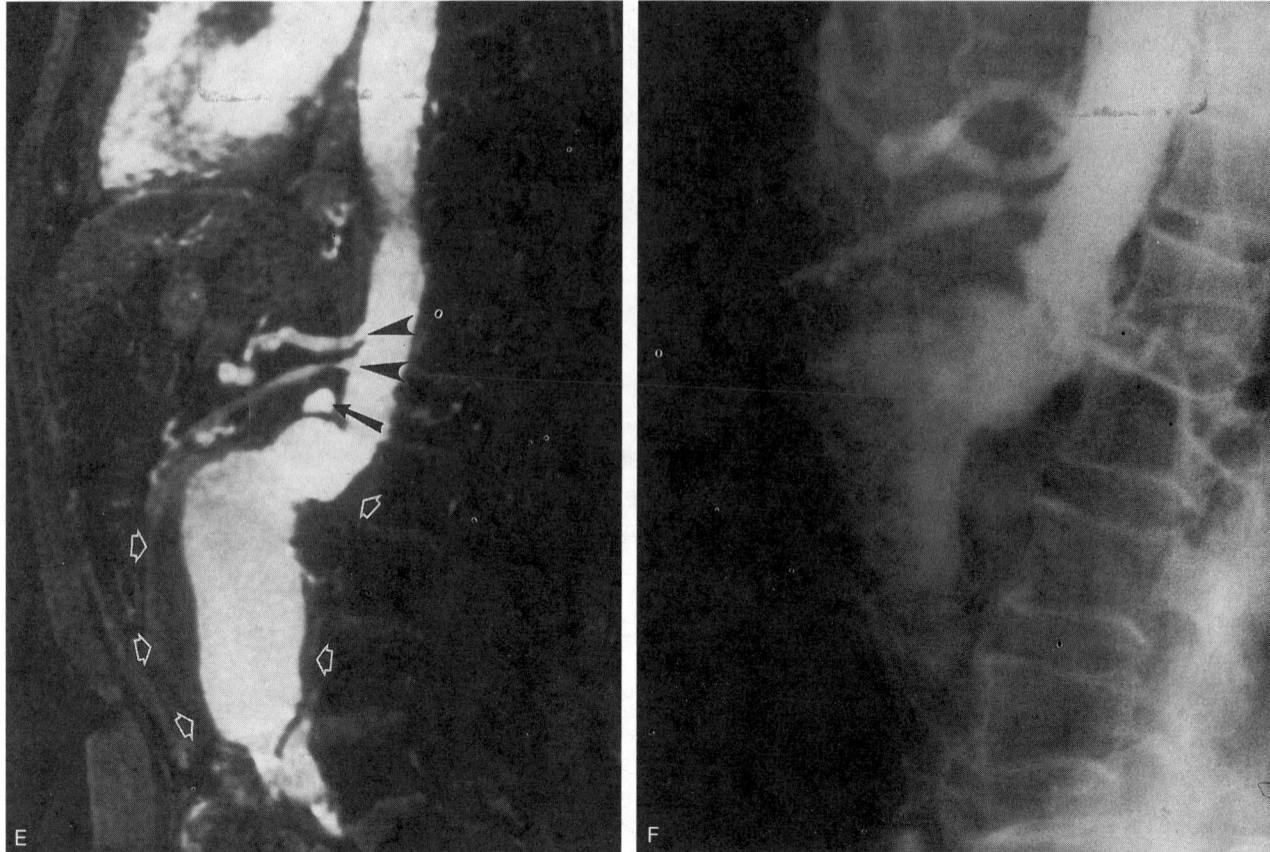

Figure 75-4. *(Continued) (E)* In another patient, gadolinium-enhanced MR abdominal aortogram shows the celiac and superior mesenteric origins *(arrowheads)* in profile. At the level of the left renal vein *(straight arrow),* an infrarenal aortic aneurysm buckles anteriorly; other reconstructions showed that the aneurysm extended to the bifurcation (not shown). Mural thrombus is apparent anteriorly and posteriorly *(open arrows). (F)* Conventional aortogram confirms visceral artery anatomy, but the caudal extent of the aneurysm is poorly opacified, even on later films in this sequence, because of contrast medium layering in the dependent posterior aspect of the aorta. *(A* to *D* from Prince M, Narasimham D, Stanley J, et al. Gadolinium-enhanced magnetic resonance angiography of abdominal aortic aneurysms. J Vasc Surg 1995;21:656; *E* and *F* from Prince M. Gadolinium-enhanced MR aortography. Radiology 1994;191:155. Courtesy of Martin R. Prince, MD, University of Michigan Hospitals, Ann Arbor)

by its involvement of collaterals and branch arteries in the affected distribution, which are relatively spared in arteriosclerosis. Vasospasm is not a prominent finding on angiograms of atherosclerosis and suggests drug toxicity (eg, ergot, digitalis), Raynaud phenomenon, cellulitis or compartment syndrome, heavy smoking, or other conditions with increased vascular tone.

Renovascular occlusive disease resulting in hypertension or renal failure is most commonly due to atherosclerosis (Fig. 75-11). Other causes include arterial fibrodysplasia, abdominal or thoracic aortic coarctation, neurofibromatosis, aortic dissection, and trauma. The indication for angiography is to document a hemodynamically adequate conduit from the aortic root to the renal parenchyma. If aortic coarctation or arterial stenosis is present, angiography is used to document hemodynamic significance and demonstrate vascular anatomy necessary for planning revascularization or angioplasty.

For older adults, an abdominal aortogram that demonstrates all renal artery origins in profile along the aorta or iliac artery is sufficient to rule out surgically correctable stenosis. For children and young adults, hypertension may be due to renal arterial branch stenosis, which can require selective renal artery injections with magnification filming for documentation.

Hypertension also may be due to aortic coarctation. Revascularization in the presence of densely calcified or severely ulcerated aortic and iliac vessels may necessitate use of the splenic, hepatic or gastroduodenal artery. A lateral aortogram must be obtained to rule out celiac artery stenosis.

Mesenteric ischemia may be acute or chronic, occlusive or nonocclusive. Biplane aortography demonstrates the celiac artery and SMA origins. It is useful in documenting proximal stenosis and embolic occlusion and in demonstrating mesenteric collateral flow. Selective injections into the celiac artery, SMA, and inferior mesenteric artery (IMA) may be necessary to demonstrate distal emboli, branch occlusions, or unsuspected neoplasms mimicking ischemic bowel disease. Mesenteric injection rates should be high enough to document patency of the mesenteric and portal veins. Acute embolic occlusion appears as a filling defect in the contrast column, usually at branch points.

Angiography in nonocclusive mesenteric ischemia may show diffuse vasoconstriction of the SMA and branches with slowing of blood flow and decreased accumulation

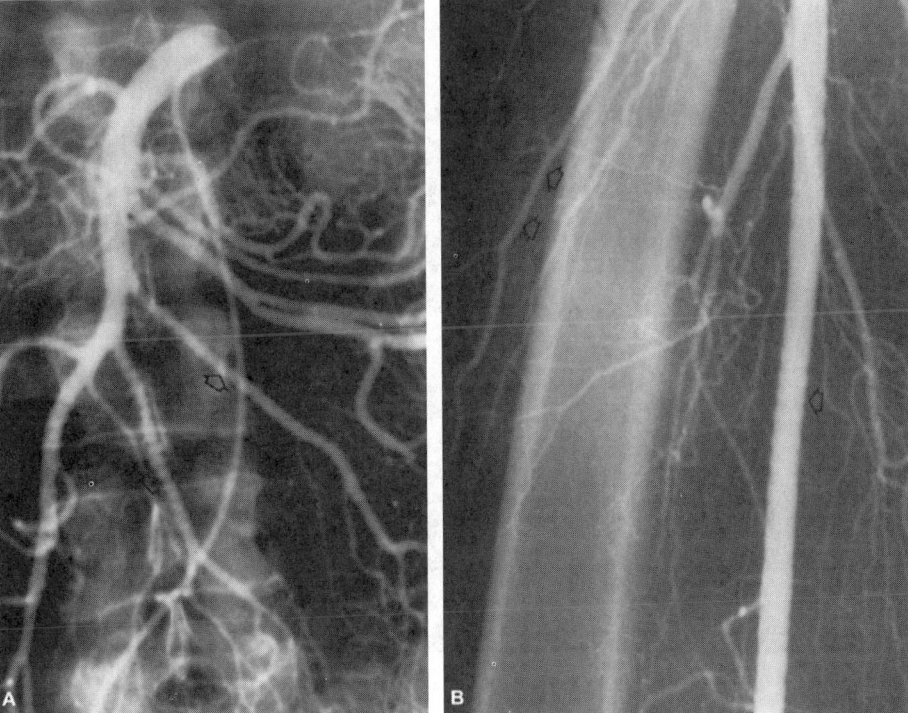

Figure 75-5. Arterial standing waves. Smooth repetitive bands of mild narrowing (*open arrows*) are demonstrated in branches of the superior mesenteric (*A*) and superficial femoral (*B*) arteries during contrast injection.

of contrast agent in the intestinal wall, or it may be normal (Fig. 75-12). Isolated celiac artery or SMA occlusion is common and is usually asymptomatic because of abundant, short peripancreatic collaterals. Angiography shows collateral supply to the intestine.

Lower-extremity ischemia can be documented noninvasively with blood pressure measurements and pulse wave-

forms. Angiography is reserved for planning surgical or percutaneous revascularization. It demonstrates distribution of disease, distribution of relatively healthy arteries (necessary for surgical bypass), and the status of collaterals. A complete study consists of an aortogram to demonstrate renal arterial anatomy and distal aortic disease, one or both oblique pelvic arteriograms to display the iliac and

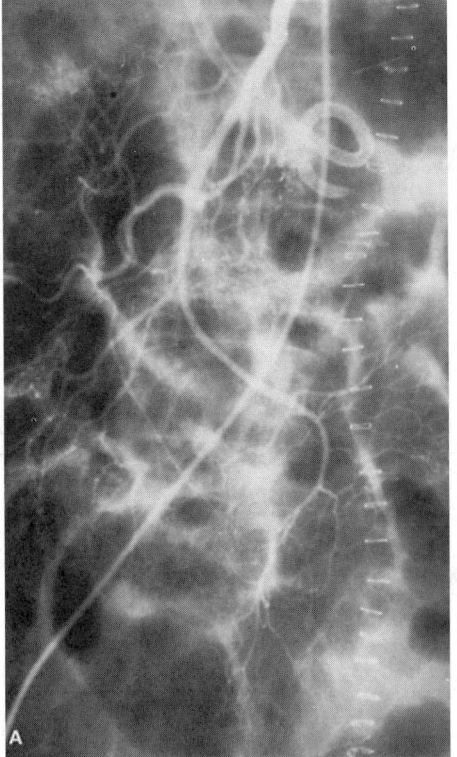
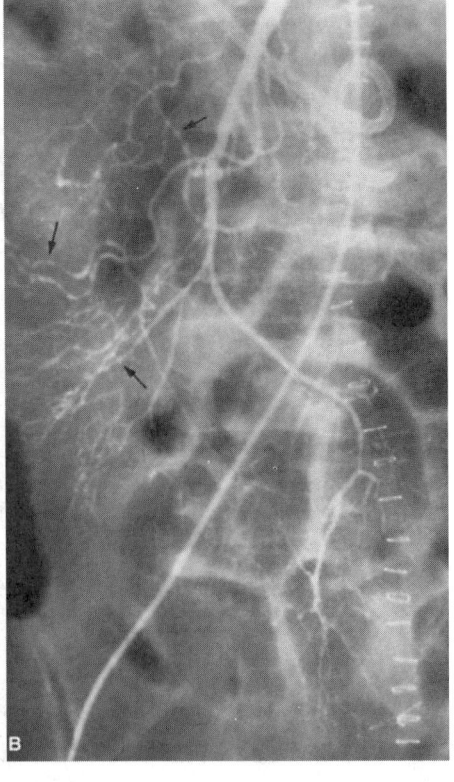

Figure 75-6. Vasopressin-induced arterial spasm in a woman with gastrointestinal bleeding and multiple vascular ectasias in the small bowel. (*A*) Celiac and superior mesenteric arteriograms show no vascular abnormalities. (*B*) A second mesenteric arteriogram after 12 hours of vasopressin infusion into the superior mesenteric artery (0.2 IU/min) shows diffuse arterial vasoconstriction. Multiple focal vasodilated segments (*small arrows*) reflect uneven response to vasopressin.

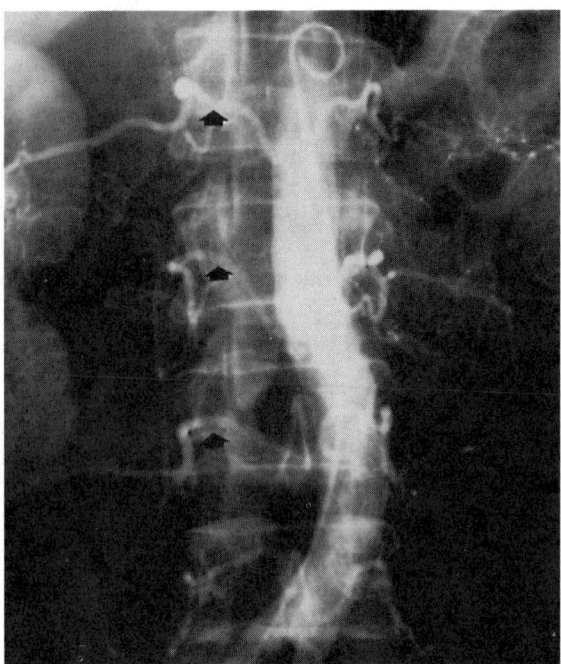

Figure 75-7. Dependent layering of contrast material. Late arterial phase of a lumbar aortogram demonstrates contrast material pooling along the posterior surface of the aorta in a patient in the supine position. Contrast material continues to fill lumbar arteries (*arrows*) after it has cleared from renal and mesenteric branches.

femoral artery bifurcations, and a lower-extremity outflow study to demonstrate thigh and calf vessels.

Aneurysmal Disease

The indication for angiography in aneurysmal disease is to show the origin of the aneurysm and its relation to nearby vessels (Fig. 75-13). Deployment of stent grafts re-

quires accurate depiction of aneurysm dimensions, the location of critical aortic branch origins, and the length of the aneurysm necks between the margins of the aneurysm and branch vessel origins.

Three-dimensional rendering of aneurysms and *periaortic inflammation* is best seen with CT. *Mycotic aneurysms* have no distinctive angiographic appearance other than an unusual location and configuration (Fig. 75-14).

Rupture of an atherosclerotic thoracic or abdominal aortic aneurysm is an indication for emergency surgical intervention. The patient's condition is usually too unstable to allow angiography, which in any case, is less sensitive than CT in demonstrating the periaortic hematoma.

At angiography, aneurysms appear as dilatations in the arterial lumen. With extensive mural thrombus, the caliber of the lumen may be normal, and the presence of the aneurysm may only be inferred from mural calcification or stereotypical thrombosis of arterial branches, such as lumbar arteries.

Large atherosclerotic aneurysms of the thoracic and abdominal aorta may distort the axis of the aorta and quickly dilute the bolus of contrast medium. Additional contrast injections or filming projections may be required to demonstrate branch artery anatomy. In this setting, there is an important clinical compromise to be made between a thorough anatomic study and contrast-medium load.

A thoracic aortogram shows the coronary and brachiocephalic artery origins. An abdominal aortogram shows the visceral and renal artery origins, with focus on multiple renal arteries. Thoracic aortic aneurysms are studied from aortic root to diaphragm, and abdominal aortic aneurysms from diaphragm to inguinal ligaments. If clinical findings suggest infrainguinal arterial disease, an arterial runoff study is performed.

Renal or visceral arterial aneurysms are studied with selective injections of the parent artery, often in multiple projections. Angiography demonstrates the relation of the aneurysms to nearby branch arteries. When relevant, the adequacy of collateral arteries should be demonstrated in

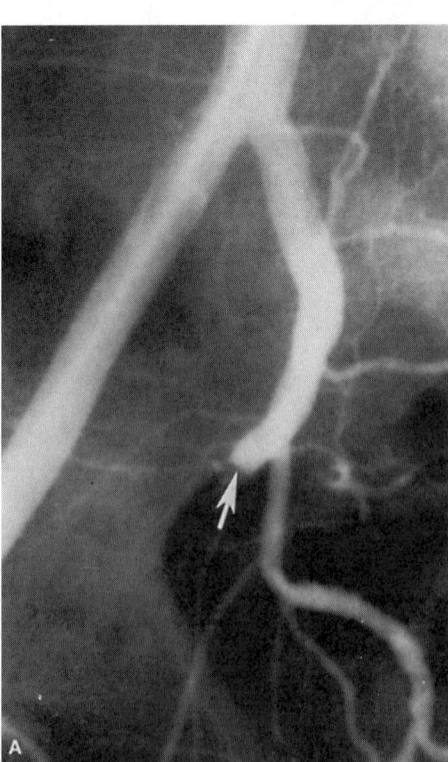
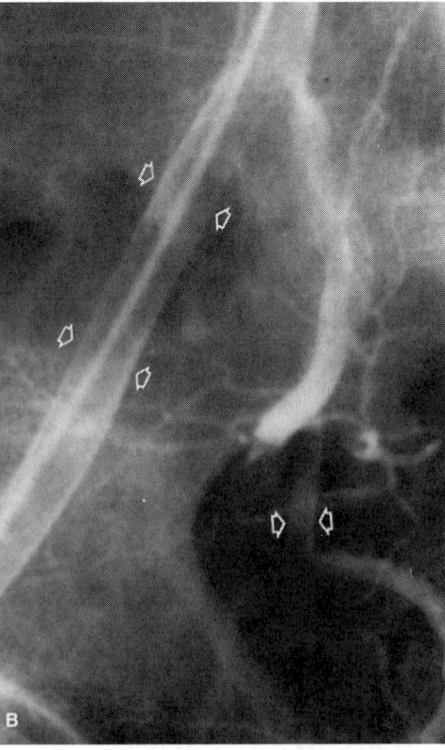

Figure 75-8. Residual contrast material simulating thrombosis in an artery. (*A*) Right common iliac arteriogram demonstrates embolic occlusion of the superior gluteal artery (*arrow*). (*B*) Later in the filming sequence, after unopacified blood has replaced the center of the contrast column, residual contrast outlines the walls of the external iliac artery and anterior division of the internal iliac artery, simulating thrombus (*open arrows*). This artifact can be confusing when the artery in question has been underinjected or receives collateral blood supply from unopacified arteries.

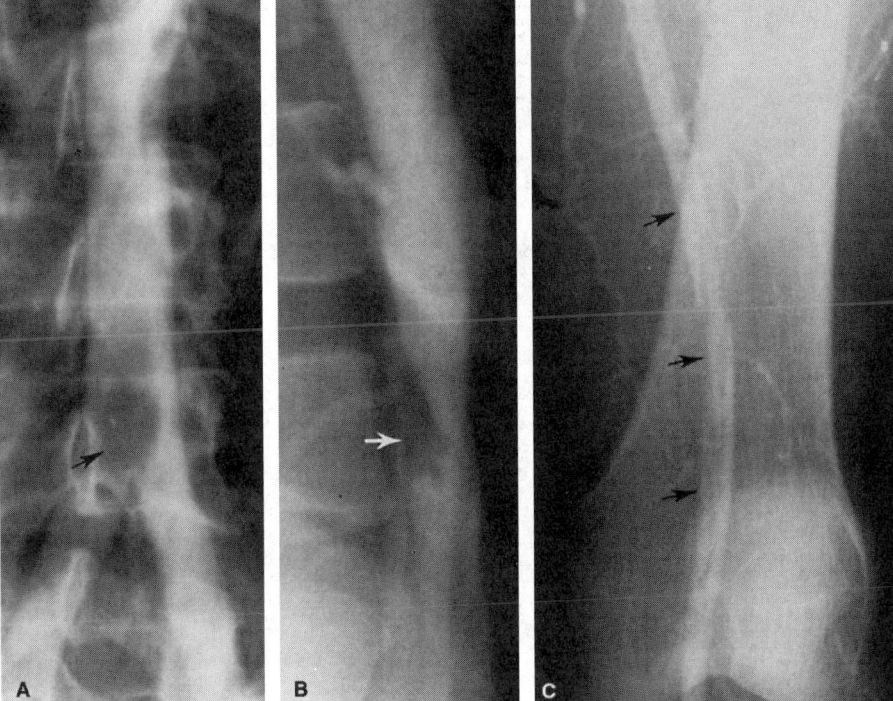

Figure 75-9. Recurrent lower extremity macroemboli from an atherosclerotic plaque in a man with recurrent lower extremity emboli, in whom surgical embolectomy failed to restore peripheral pulses. Biplanar aortogram shows a large irregular posterior plaque (*arrow*) at the aortic bifurcation, subtle on the frontal film (*A*) but evident on the lateral film (*B*). (*C*) A detail from the lower extremity outflow study shows extensive thromboemboli (*arrows*) in the left popliteal artery.

sufficient detail to allow planning of surgical reconstruction, resection, or percutaneous embolization (Fig. 75-15).

Arterial Dissection

The diagnosis of aortic dissection (Fig. 75-16) and its classification with respect to involvement of the ascending aorta are established with transesophageal echocardiogra-

phy, CT, or MRA. The indications for transcatheter aortography are to (1) resolve equivocal findings from cross-sectional imaging, (2) evaluate the hemodynamic significance of branch vessel compromise by the dissection, and (3) plan and perform endovascular management of ischemic and aneurysmal complications of dissection.

The angiographic appearance of *aortic dissection* depends on the site of contrast injection and the characteris-

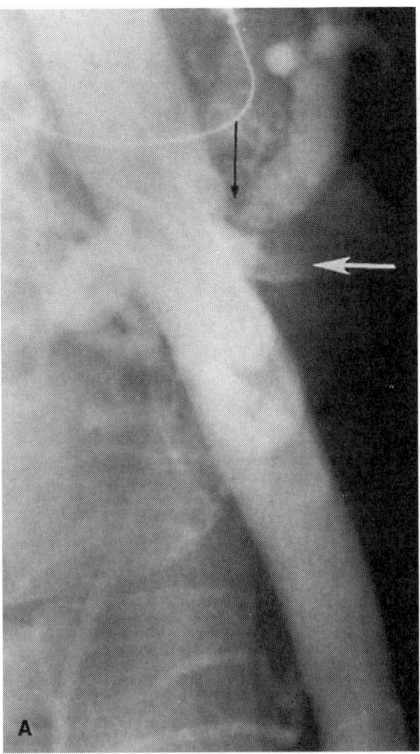
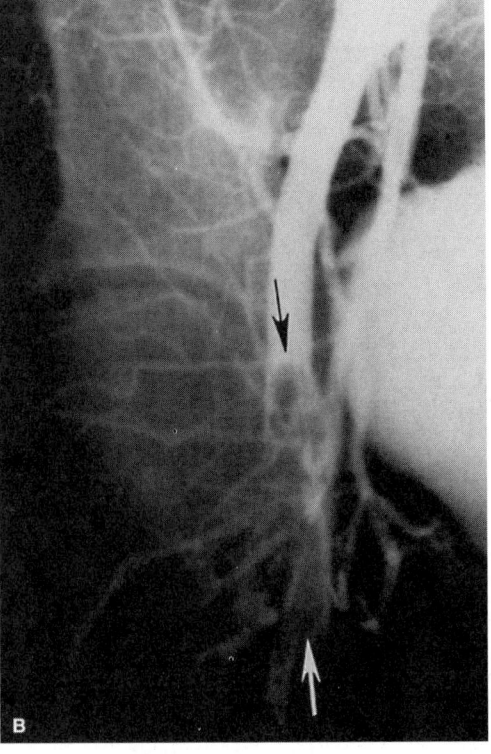

Figure 75-10. Arterial emboli in a woman with right lower extremity ischemia. (*A*) Lateral aortogram shows median arcuate ligament compression on the celiac axis (*black arrow*) and an embolus in the superior mesenteric artery (*white arrow*). (*B*) An embolus is also visible at the bifurcation of the common femoral artery (*arrows*).

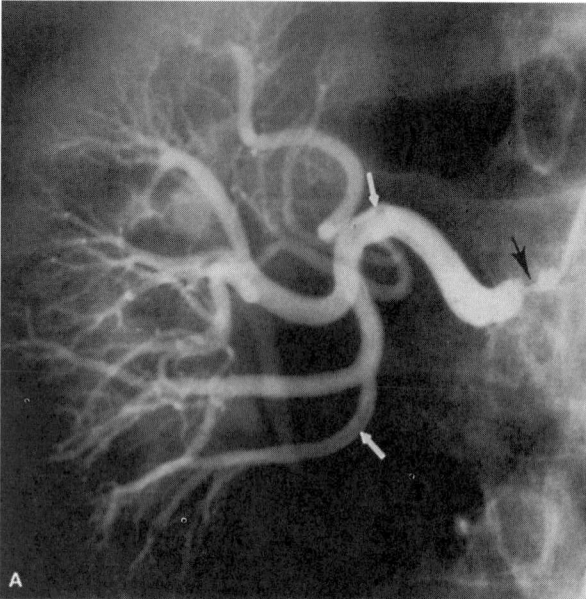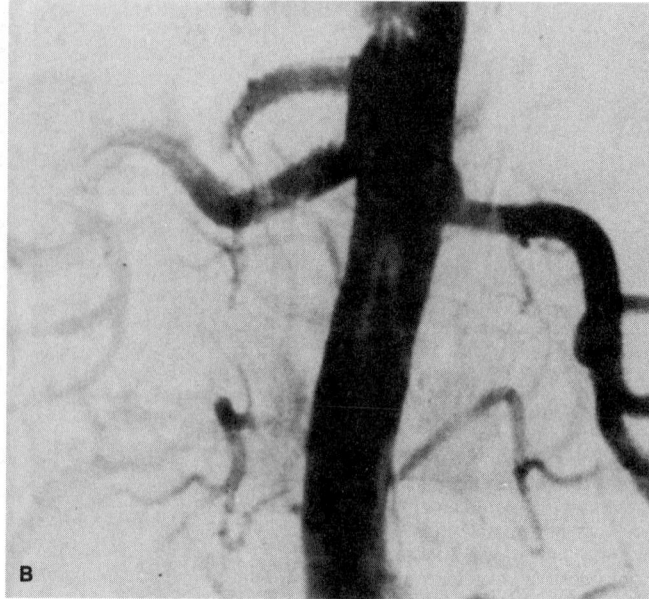

Figure 75-11. Atherosclerotic renal artery stenosis. (*A*) Right renal arteriogram shows a tight concentric proximal stenosis of the renal artery (*black arrow*). The linear filling defects in the main renal artery and its segmental branches (*white arrows*) represent flow defects caused by unopacified blood flowing retrograde from nonparenchymal renal artery branches. The presence of collateral flow to the kidney indicates that the stenosis is hemodynamically significant. (*B*) Lumbar aortogram after percutaneous angioplasty shows significant improvement in the caliber of the arterial lumen.

tics of the dissection. If injection is upstream from the intimal tear or reentry point, it fills the true and false lumina, usually at different rates, and outlines the intervening septum as a linear filling defect in the contrast column. If the injection is remote from a transseptal communication and fills one lumen, the margins of the lumen are variable, smoothly scalloped in profile, and normal or possibly aneurysmal elsewhere.

Involvement of aortic branches may be difficult to demonstrate unless the lumen perfusing the branches in question can be catheterized directly. Manometry, interpreted in the context of peripheral limb pressures, may help determine the hemodynamic significance of a branch arterial stenosis.

In dissection of the *renal* or *visceral arteries,* angiography documents the hemodynamic significance of arterial narrowing, the extent of the dissection, the relation of the

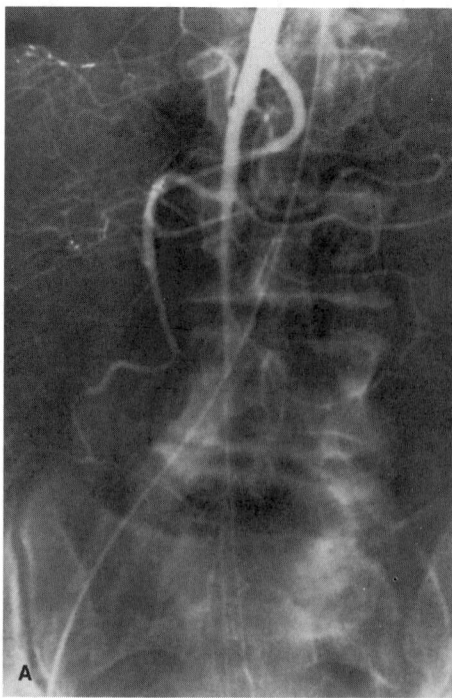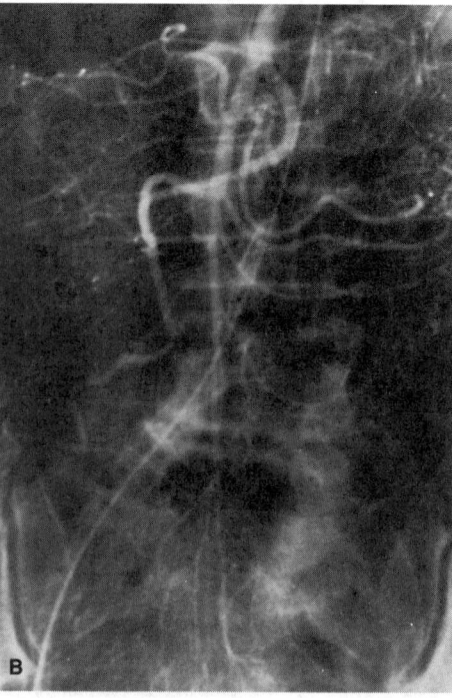

Figure 75-12. Nonocclusive mesenteric ischemia. (*A*) Superior mesenteric angiogram shows diffuse arterial vasoconstriction without occlusion. (*B*) A second arteriogram after injection of 50 mg of tolazoline into the superior mesenteric artery shows decreased vasoconstriction.

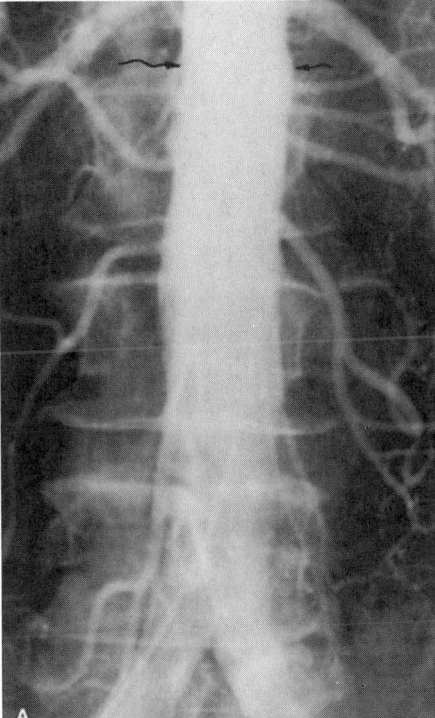

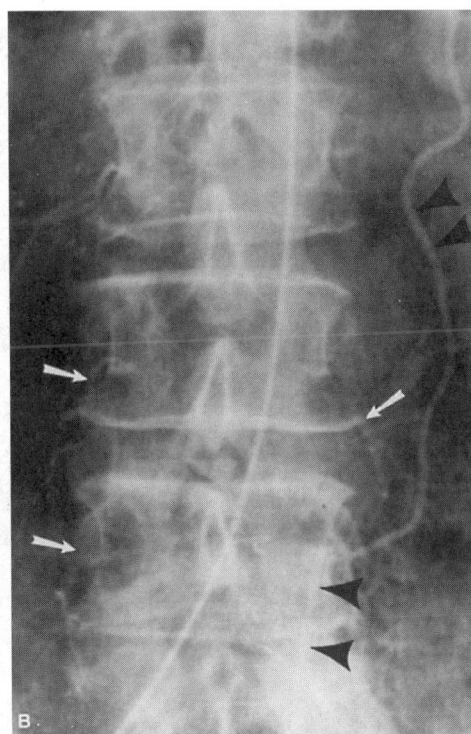

Figure 75-13. Abdominal aortic aneurysm in a 74-year-old man. (A) Lumbar aortogram shows subtle widening of the infrarenal aortic lumen (*wavy arrows*). Renal and superior mesenteric artery branches are normal, but infrarenal aortic branches are apparently missing. (B) A later film shows filling of lumbar (*arrows*) and inferior mesenteric (*arrowheads*) arteries through collaterals, as a result of occlusion of these vessels by mural thrombus in the aneurysm.

dissection to nearby normal branches, and the integrity of the collateral circulation. Dissection in these medium-sized arteries appears as long, smooth narrowings of the artery, with smooth sigmoid contour changes or dead ends that reflect the spiral course of the dissection, which usually terminates at a branch point of the parent artery. A double lumen is not always seen.

Sometimes an atherosclerotic ulcer penetrates the media and bleeds with *intramedial dissection* by the resulting hematoma. This penetrating ulcer may be associated with a pseudoaneurysm or a false lumen and may simulate classic dissection clinically. The dissecting hematoma or pseudoaneurysm of a penetrating aortic ulcer tends to originate in the distal thoracic aorta.

Iatrogenic dissection results from intraarterial manipulation of guide wires or catheters, percutaneous angioplasty, and cannulation of the aorta during bypass (Fig. 75-17). The hemodynamic significance of these dissections depends on the vessel involved, the status of the collateral circulation, and the direction of dissection with respect to blood flow.

Arterial Fibrodysplasia

The indications for angiography for arterial fibrodysplasia are the same as those for atherosclerosis, aneurysms, and dissection. The classic angiographic appearance of arterial fibrodysplasia is the "string of beads" appearance of medial fibroplasia, the most common histologic type (Fig. 75-18). Angiographic findings in renal arteries that suggest fibrodysplasia include; long, smooth narrowing; long, irregular, beaded narrowing, often with poststenotic dilatation or large aneurysms: discrete, weblike stenoses; spontaneous dissections; and involvement of the middle and distal thirds of the main trunk that often extends into segmental arteries.

Arteritis

The indications for angiography in inflammatory arteritis are to determine the extent of disease and demonstrate the status of the proximal and distal circulation for a prospective vascular reconstruction procedure.

Angiography sometimes is helpful in the primary diagnosis of inflammatory arteritis. The angiogram may demonstrate diffuse spasm or microaneurysms in active disease. Arterial stenosis, occlusion, and prominent collaterals may be present in active or quiescent disease.

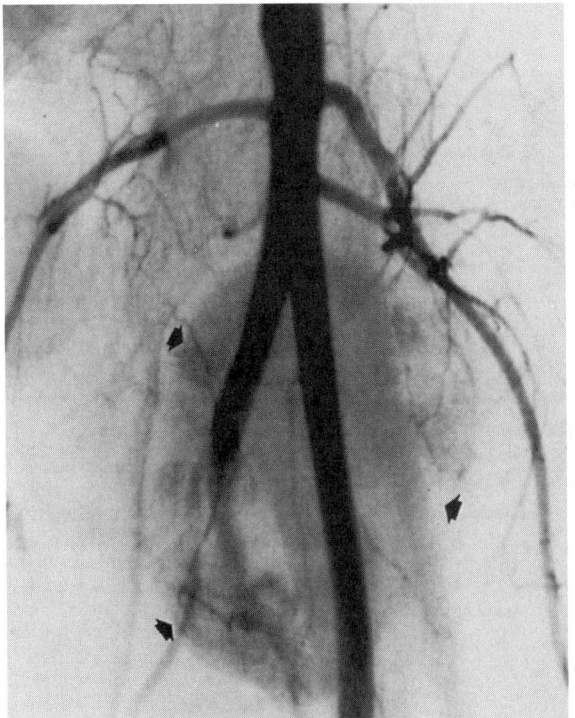

Figure 75-14. Mycotic pseudoaneurysm. Left common femoral arteriogram shows a saccular pseudoaneurysm (*arrows*) originating from the deep femoral artery.

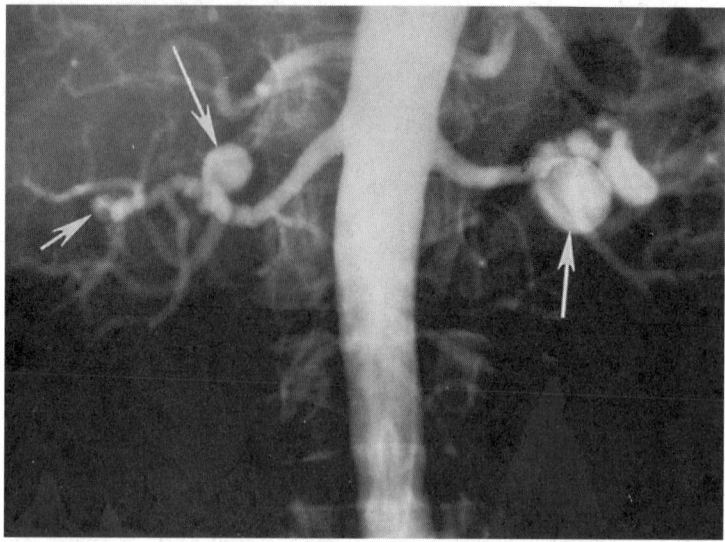

Figure 75-15. Renal artery aneurysms. Lumbar aortogram in a normotensive woman demonstrates multiple bilateral renal artery aneurysms (*arrows*) associated with renal arterial fibrodysplastic disease.

Trauma

Blunt and penetrating trauma can cause acute ischemia or hemorrhage, either immediately or later. Deceleration injuries (motor vehicle accidents, falls) are associated with injury to the thoracic aorta and brachiocephalic vessels. Penetrating wounds are associated with vascular injuries along the track of the foreign body (knife, low-speed bullets).

The role of angiography in trauma is to demonstrate the extent of arterial injury and the status of the proximal and distal normal circulation. Angiographic findings include pseudoaneurysm, arterial or venous occlusion, AV fistula, and extravasation of contrast medium, which indicates active hemorrhage.

Aortic rupture is shown with thoracic aortography in the right posterior oblique projection (Fig. 75-19). The diagnosis of a subtle injury can be difficult in the presence of an unusual ductus diverticulum or atherosclerotic plaque (Fig. 75-20). Multiple views of the aorta may help clarify variants. Thoracic aortography is followed with routine supine radiography of the abdomen to evaluate the kidneys and bladder. If renal injury is suspected, abdominal aortography is performed (Fig. 75-21).

In the angiographic evaluation of traumatic hemorrhage, therapeutic considerations may necessitate extension of the diagnostic examination. For example, if occlusive therapy is being considered (either surgical ligation or transcatheter embolization), the status of the collateral cir-

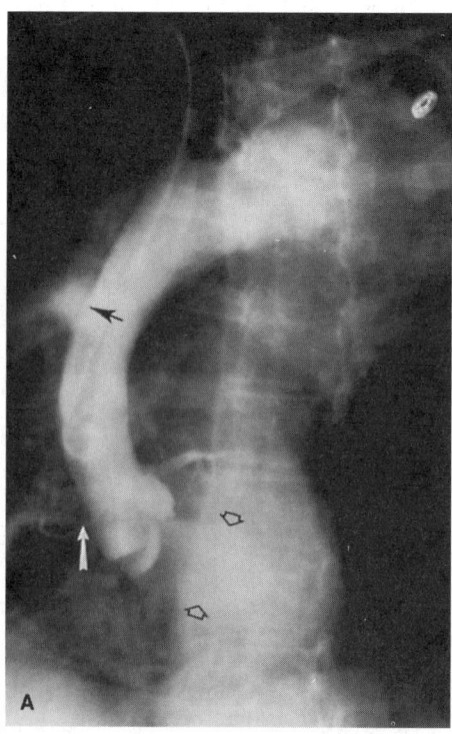

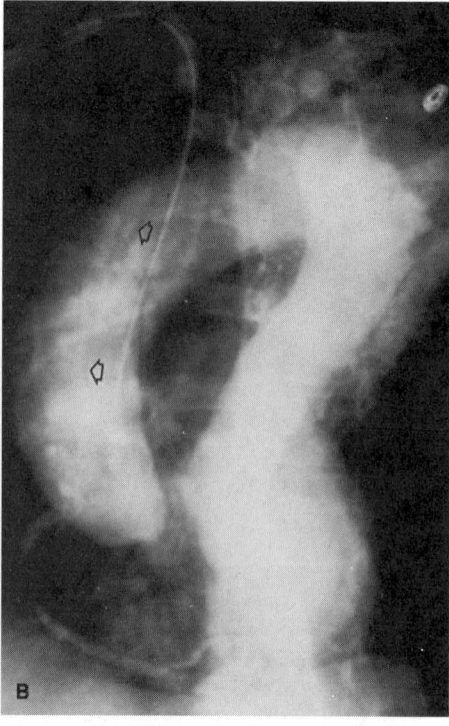

Figure 75-16. Type I aortic dissection in an 86-year-old hypertensive woman with acute onset of back pain. (*A*) Arch aortogram, performed from a right brachial artery approach, shows early opacification of the true lumen. The jet of contrast material is opacifying the intimal tear that initiated the dissection (*black arrow*). The false lumen extends retrograde, compressing the ascending aorta along its right lateral margin, narrowing the origin of the right coronary artery (*white arrow*), and undermining the aortic valve leaflets with loose-secondary aortic insufficiency (*open arrows*). (*B*) A few seconds later, the entire false lumen is opacified, and the dissection septum appears as a radiolucent line (*open arrows*) between the false and true lumens. The dissection extends into the descending aorta with involvement of the innominate artery.

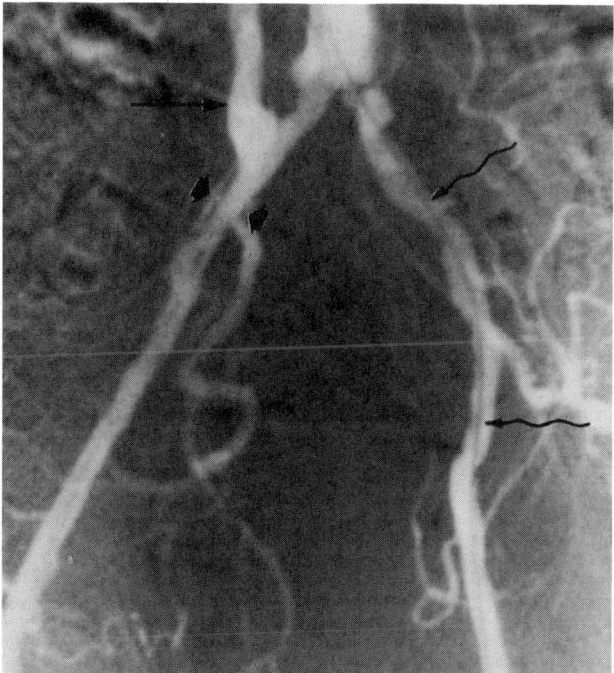

Figure 75-17. Iatrogenic dissection during cardiac catheterization in a 70-year-old woman with cholesterol emboli. Pelvic arteriogram performed with digital subtraction angiography demonstrates a linear collection of contrast medium outside the arterial lumen, representing a dissection. The dissection extends into the common iliac artery (*solid arrows*), stopping short of the origin of the iliorenal bypass graft (*straight arrow*). The linear filling defect in the left iliac artery (*wavy arrows*) is produced by the angiographic catheter.

culation and arterial bed distal to the arterial injury is evaluated.

Hemangiomas and Vascular Malformations

In the presence of possible hemangiomas and vascular malformations, angiography is used to assess the arterial supply to the lesion and nearby structures. In the extremities, venography is often performed to demonstrate the deep veins. CT and MRI are useful to demonstrate the three-dimensional relation between the malformation and the normal structures.

Angiographic findings in an AV malformation consist of tortuous and enlarged feeding arteries, a nidus of innumerable small arteries, and large draining veins (Fig. 75-22). When rapid flow throughout the malformation is demonstrated, venography is not indicated. In a venous malformation, the arterial phase of the angiogram may be normal. Veins are large and tortuous with slow flow; sometimes large venous lakes are present. The venous malformation is studied with closed-system venography or direct injection of contrast material into the malformation (Fig. 75-23).

Neoplasms

Angiography is usually performed after CT or MRI has defined the location of the primary tumor or the presence of metastases. Angiography is used to provide a vascular "road map" before resection of abdominal neoplasms, document vascular invasion by nonresectable tumors, answer questions about resectability, and aid transcatheter chemotherapy.

Neoplasms are characterized at angiography as avascu-

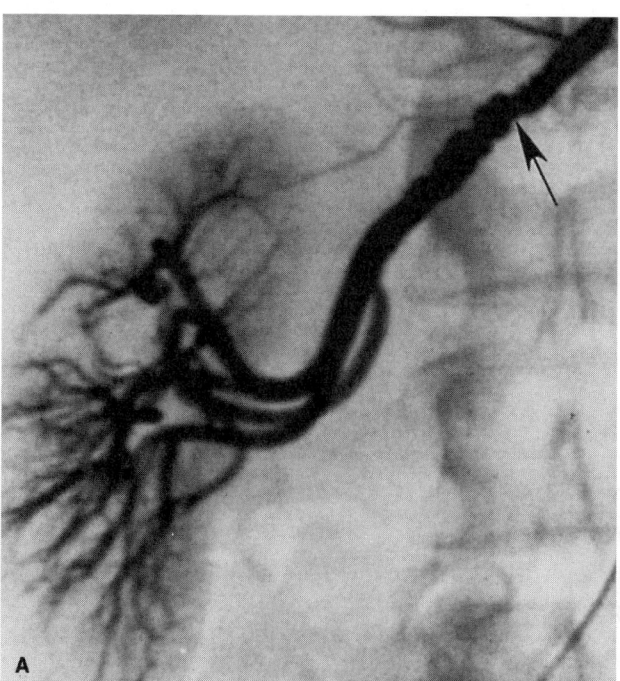 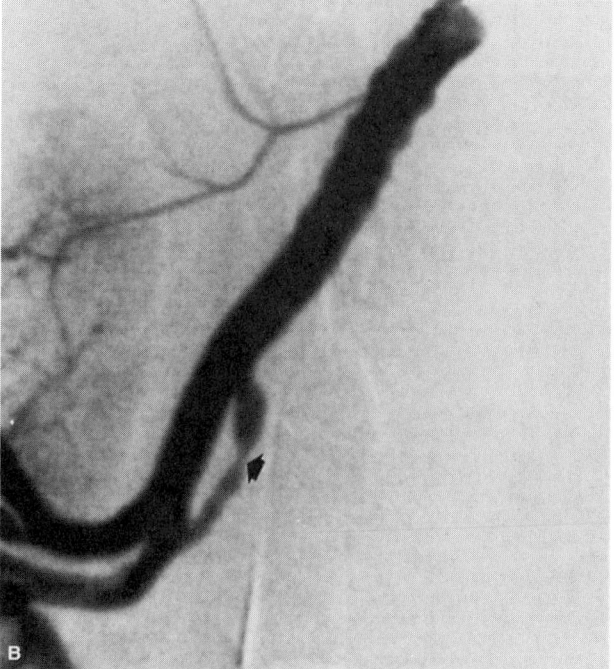

Figure 75-18. Fibrodysplasia of the renal artery in a 51-year-old hypertensive woman. (*A*) Digital subtraction angiogram of the right renal artery shows a ptotic kidney with alternating bands of narrowing and dilation in the middle third of the main renal artery (*arrow*), in the so-called string-of-beads configuration of medial fibroplasia. (*B*) A second arteriogram made after percutaneous transluminal angioplasty shows improvement in the arterial lumen. Irregularity in the small branch of the renal artery (*solid arrow*) represents transient guide wire-induced spasm. (Courtesy of James Shields, MD, St Joseph Mercy Hospital, Ann Arbor)

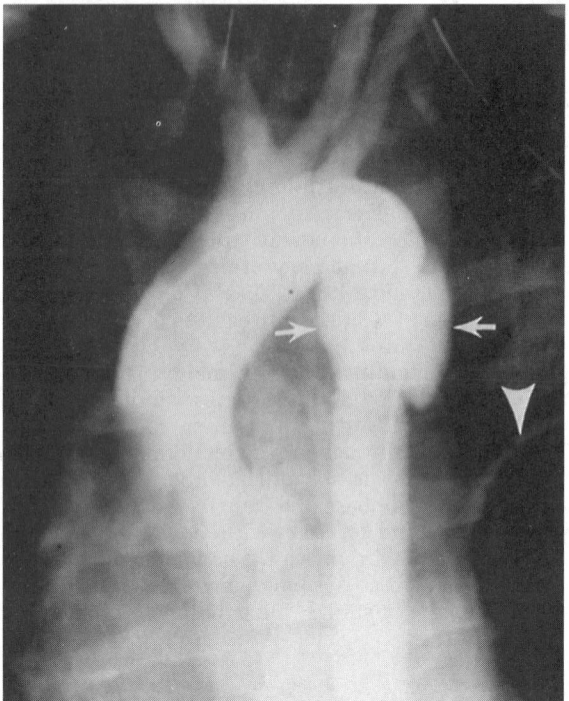

Figure 75-19. Traumatic thoracic aortic rupture in a 30-year-old man involved in a motor vehicle accident. Arch aortogram shows a contained rupture of the proximal descending aorta (*arrows*), just distal to the origin of the left subclavian artery. A ruptured left hemidiaphragm with herniation of the stomach (*arrowhead*) is visible.

lar, hypovascular, or hypervascular. Tumor vessels are disorderly and meandering compared with normal parenchymal vessels, which branch systematically. The contour of tumor vessels may be smooth, somewhat beaded, or highly irregular and serrated. Early or intense venous opacification is common with hypervascular tumors, such as hepatoma, hypernephroma, and leiomyoma (Fig. 75-24).

Postsurgical Follow-up Care

Angiography is performed after surgical procedures to establish a vascular baseline (after revascularization), rule out a surgical complication (after transplantation, revascularization, or a shunt operation), and demonstrate progression of disease.

Vascular complications include stenosis, occlusion, dissection, pseudoaneurysm, and AV fistula. The angiographic evaluation is tailored to the clinical signs, the surgeon's impression of a specific complication, and the known preoperative anatomy. Multiple views may be necessary to show vascular anastomoses in profile to exclude arterial strictures (especially after renal revascularization or transplantation).

Peripheral Venous Disease

Venography is used to diagnose deep venous thrombosis (DVT) and incompetent lower-extremity venous valves. It also is used to demonstrate venous anatomy in vascular malformations or hemangiomas or before dialysis shunt construction or venous reconstructive procedures. When injections are in a peripheral vein, venography can depict deep and superficial veins of an extremity. For the diagnosis of DVT, conventional contrast venography has been replaced by duplex or color-flow ultrasonography for the

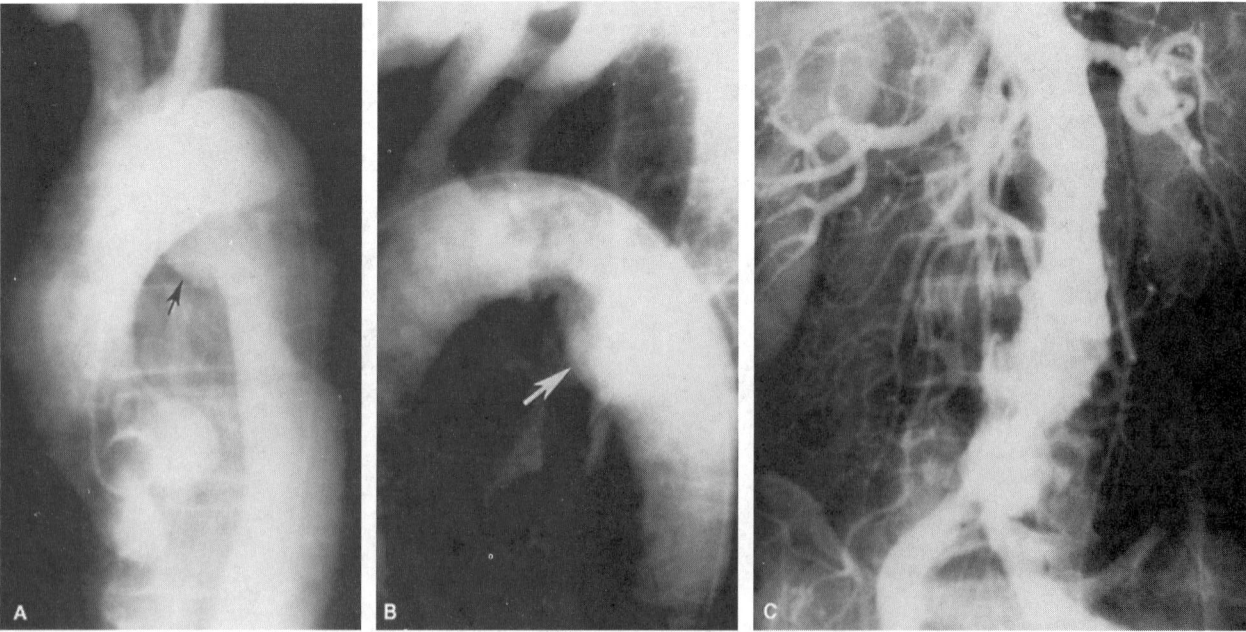

Figure 75-20. Prominent ductus bump simulating a posttraumatic aortic pseudoaneurysm in a man with septic peripheral emboli. (*A* and *B*) Biplanar arch aortograms show focal bulging from the anteromedial surface of the descending aorta at the ligamentum arteriosum (*arrow*). (*C*) Abdominal aortogram shows an irregular infrarenal aneurysm with mural debris. At exploration, the thoracic aorta was normal, and a mycotic abdominal aortic aneurysm was resected. Angiographically, this mycotic aneurysm cannot be distinguished from a bland atherosclerotic aneurysm.

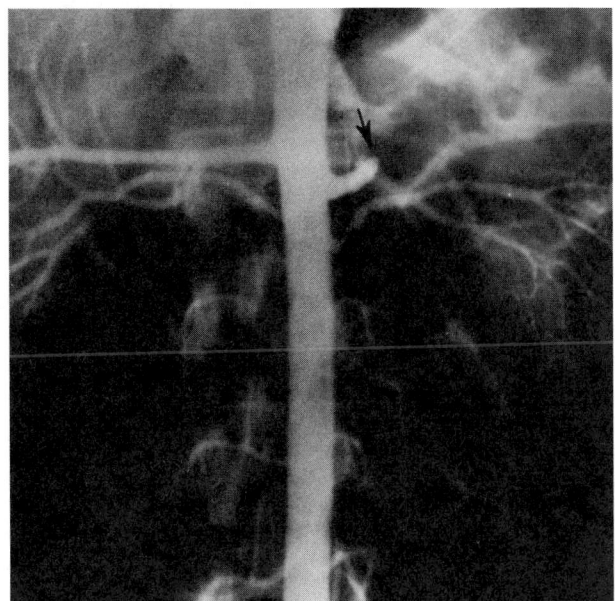

Figure 75-21. Traumatic renal artery occlusion in a 20-year-old male victim of a motor vehicle accident. Abnormal nephrogram was demonstrated on an abdominal film obtained after arch aortography. A subsequent lumbar aortogram confirmed left renal artery occlusion (*arrow*). The lower pole artery, fortuitously originating separately from the aorta, is irregular and deformed secondary to a retroperitoneal hematoma.

extremities and magnetic resonance venography for the iliocaval, portal, and renal systems.

At lower-extremity *ascending* venography, acute DVT appears as a castlike filling defect in the contrast column within the deep veins (Fig. 75-25A). Acute thrombosis may be so extensive that contrast material does not enter the deep system. Absence of deep-vein filling in acute DVT is

differentiated from that in chronic DVT on the basis of the size of the superficial veins and venous collaterals. They are small with acute disease and large with chronic disease. For patients with chronic DVT, venography demonstrates linear or weblike intraluminal filling defects that represent organized thrombus, occluded deep veins with large collaterals, or, rarely, no abnormality (Fig. 75-25B).

Lower-extremity *descending* venography is performed to evaluate the competence of the valves in the saphenous, femoral, and popliteal veins. Reflux in the greater saphenous, deep femoral, and superficial femoral veins is assessed and graded from 0 (no reflux) to 4 (reflux below the knee). A global view of venous anatomy (required if venous bypass or valvuloplasty is planned) necessitates ascending venography.

Closed-system extremity venography may be needed for demonstration of the extent of a venous malformation or hemangioma (Fig 75-23B).

Pulmonary Embolism

The diagnosis of pulmonary embolism often requires confirmation with pulmonary angiography because of the low specificity of ventilation and perfusion scans in some clinical settings. In addition to documenting the presence of pulmonary emboli, angiography can demonstrate other pathologic conditions that explain abnormalities on chest radiographs or ventilation and perfusion scans. Pulmonary arterial injections are preceded by measurement of pulmonary arterial pressure, because the risk of sudden cardiac decompensation increases in the presence of right ventricular or pulmonary arterial hypertension.

The angiographic findings of *acute* pulmonary embolism consist of intraarterial filling defects, arterial cutoffs, and perfusion defects (Fig. 75-26). The angiographic findings of *chronic* pulmonary embolism are intraluminal webs, arterial stenoses and cutoffs, collateral reconstitution of occluded vessels, and perfusion defects.

Figure 75-22. Arteriovenous malformation in a 50-year-old schizophrenic woman. Cardiac output measured 16 L/min. (*A*) The arterial phase of the pelvic angiogram shows gross asymmetry of the common iliac arteries, with a massively dilated left internal iliac artery supplying a large nidus of innumerable small arteries (*arrows*). Other arterial injections documented contributions from the left external, deep femoral, and right internal iliac arteries. (*B*) A large tangle of tortuous veins (*arrows*) empties into dilated left iliac veins.

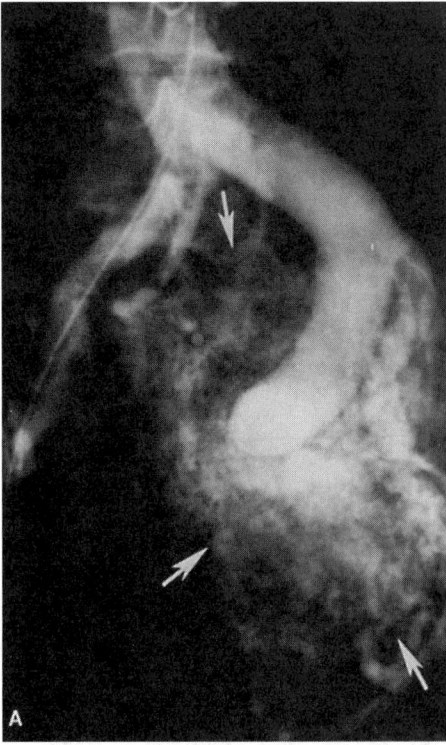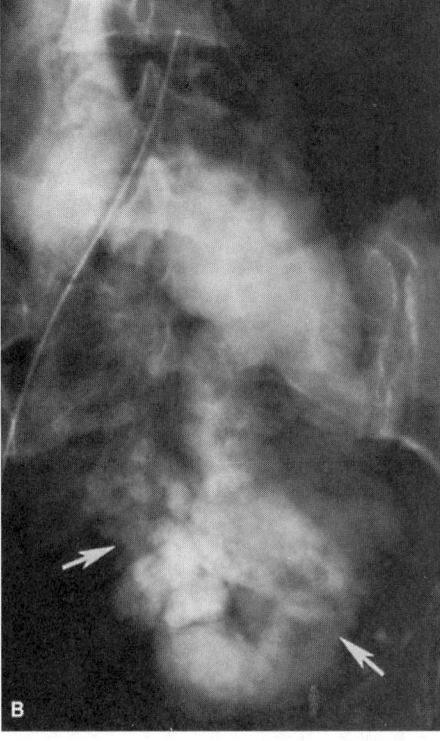

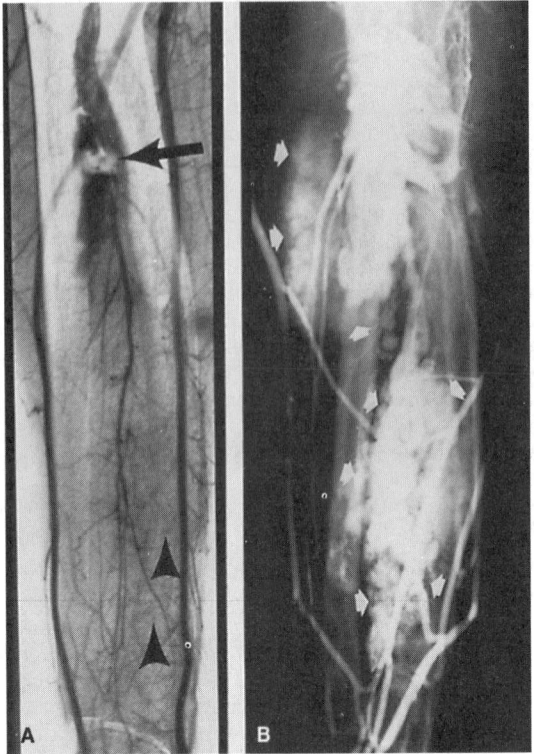

Figure 75-23. Venous angioma in a 19-year-old woman with symptoms of recurrent right forearm venous thrombosis and a mass noticed at age 6 years. (*A*) Photographic subtraction arteriogram of the capillary phase of the forearm shows normal radial, ulnar, interosseous, and muscular arteries; faint scattered punctate areas of contrast pooling (*arrowheads*); and draining vein containing thrombus (*arrow*). (*B*) A closed-system venogram provides much better documentation of the component of the angioma (*solid arrows*).

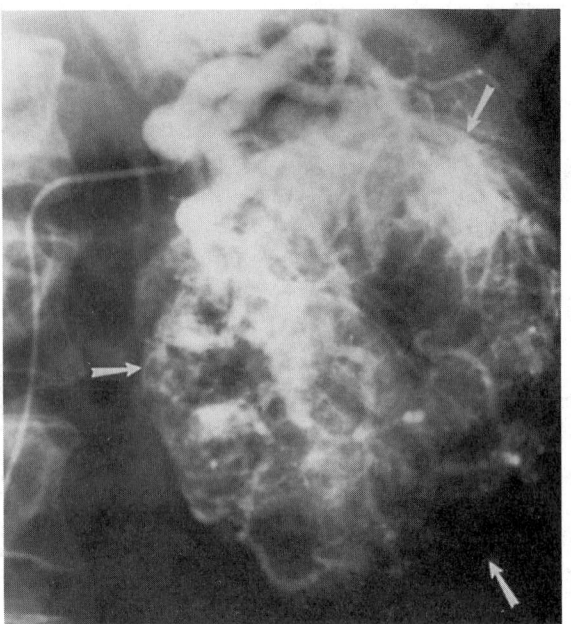

Figure 75-24. Tumor neovascularity in a 52-year-old man with a hypernephroma. Left renal arteriogram demonstrates a large hypervascular tumor in the lower pole of the left kidney (*arrows*) with abundant neovascularity and intense contrast accumulation (tumor stain).

INTERVENTIONAL ANGIOGRAPHY
Angioplasty

Percutaneous transluminal angioplasty (PTA) is used to manage arterial and venous occlusive lesions. PTA entails crossing the stenosis or occlusion with a guide wire. After the intraluminal position of the guide wire is confirmed,

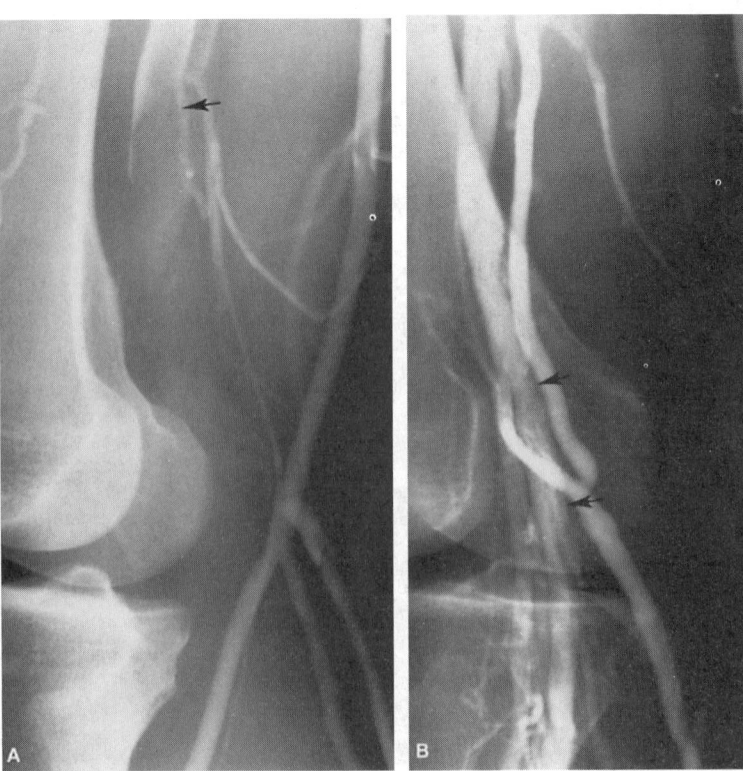

Figure 75-25. Acute and chronic deep venous thrombosis in a 19-year-old man who presented with acute right calf swelling. (*A*) An ascending leg venogram shows acute thrombus in the popliteal vein. The patient was examined 25 months later for right calf pain. (*B*) A second venogram shows recanalization of the popliteal vein with residual linear filling defects (*arrows*), representing organized clot. No valves are seen in this segment of popliteal vein.

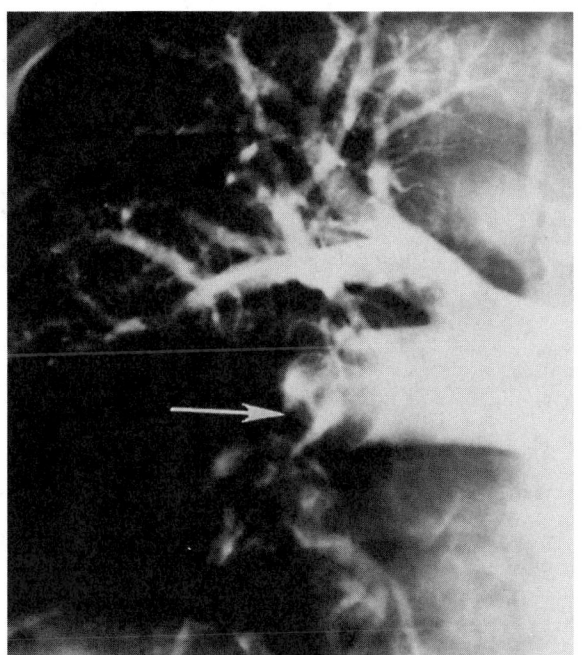

Figure 75-26. Acute pulmonary embolism in a 39-year-old man with a renal transplant. A selective right pulmonary arteriogram shows a large saddle embolus in the right main pulmonary artery with occlusion of the middle lobe arteries and a cast of thrombus (*arrow*) in the lower lobe arteries.

a balloon is advanced over the wire across the stenosis or occlusion and inflated. Inflation is assessed with fluoroscopy. Dilation is assessed with intraarterial manometry, ankle–brachial pressure indices, or improvement in the luminal diameter of the vessel at post-PTA angiography (Fig. 75-27). The ideal PTA lesions are renal fibromuscular dysplastic lesions without associated aneurysms (Fig. 75-18) and concentric, nonostial, noncalcified atherosclerotic lesions. Complications of PTA include thrombosis, perforation, dissection, and distal embolism.

Thrombolytic Therapy

Embolic or thrombotic occlusion of vascular conduits often is managed with thrombolytic therapy. Diagnostic angiography being used to define vascular anatomy is performed before lytic therapy. Angiography being used to identify the cause of arterial occlusion or graft failure follows lytic therapy (Fig. 75-28). Judicious choice of the initial puncture site (based on the patient's symptoms and, if known, arterial and bypass anatomy) may simplify placement of the infusion catheter in the occluded conduit and percutaneous management of the cause of occlusion.

Acute embolic occlusion of a vessel presents additional considerations. Emboli are often multiple, precluding efficient lysis, even when they are accessible by catheter. Emboli may be composed of organized material less susceptible to lytic agents. A symptomatic embolus in the leg may mask a more serious embolus in the intestine or kidney, and a cardiac source of emboli may shower additional emboli during the lytic state.

Close clinical monitoring of the patient, laboratory determination of coagulation status, and frequent angiographic inspection of progress are important to avoid complica-

Figure 75-27. Percutaneous transluminal angioplasty of a superficial femoral artery occlusion in a 60-year-old man with claudication. Superficial femoral arteriograms before (*A*) and after (*B*) recanalization and angioplasty of a distal superficial femoral artery occlusion. The caliber of the popliteal artery (*arrow*) is increased after inflow has been improved.

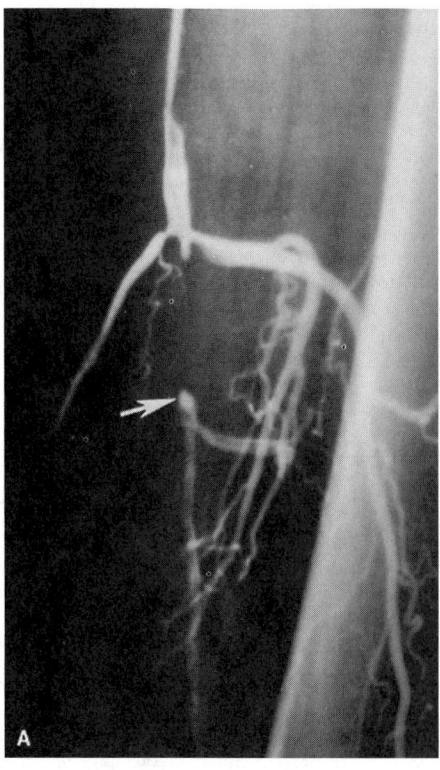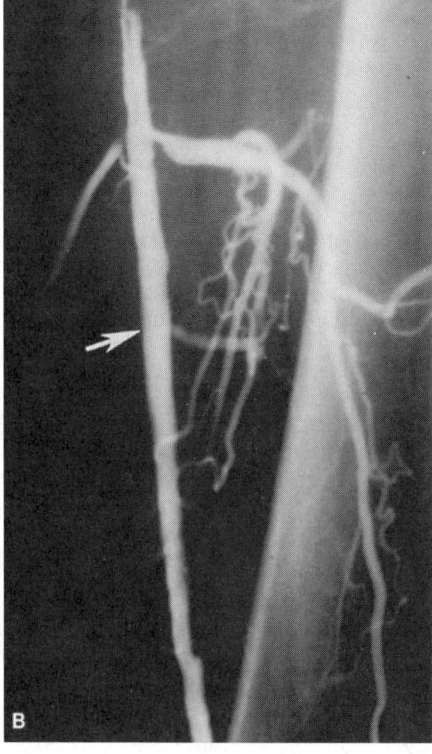

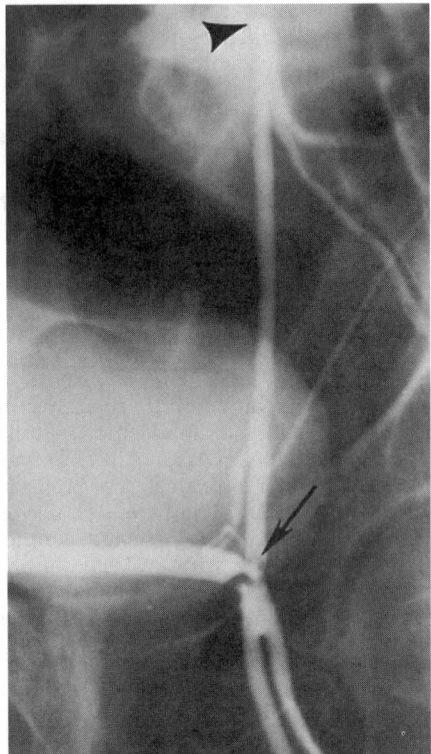

Figure 75-28. Lytic therapy with urokinase. A 50-year-old man presented with occluded right axillofemoral and right-to-left femorofemoral bypass grafts. With use of a right brachial artery approach, flow in the axillofemoral graft was reestablished after 12 hours of urokinase infusion at 2000 IU/min. With use of a right femoral artery approach, flow in the femorofemoral graft was reestablished after 6 hours of urokinase infusion at 2000 IU/min through a catheter with the tip just distal to the graft origin. Angiogram made at the termination of the procedure shows narrowing of the distal graft lumen and a filling defect in the left common femoral artery (*arrow*). Because of the angle of the graft insertion site (nearly 90 degrees) and the filling defect above and below the anastomosis, this lesion is not suitable for angioplasty or atherectomy from the right femoral approach. A mound of intimal hyperplasia was removed during surgical revision of the anastomosis. The left internal iliac artery fills through retrograde flow in the external iliac artery (*arrowhead*).

tions of lytic therapy and maintain surface contact between the catheter tip and the remaining thrombus. Infusion is terminated when complete recanalization of the vessel is achieved, as long as no complication supervenes. If an underlying lesion is found, endovascular or open surgical treatment is undertaken.

Embolotherapy

Transcatheter delivery of embolic agents is used in the management of life-threatening hemorrhage and in some devascularization procedures. With the use of steerable guide wires and coaxial catheter systems, superselective catheterization of vessels as small as 1 mm in diameter is possible. Embolotherapy is preceded by diagnostic angiography to document the vascular anatomy and to predict the hemodynamic effect of embolization with respect to target organ infarction, recanalization of vessels, and recruitment of collaterals.

Indications for embolotherapy include management of gastrointestinal or traumatic hemorrhage (Fig. 75-29), man-

agement of vascular malformation and AV fistula, and tumor therapy (devascularization or vascular redistribution to optimize perfusion therapy).

The complications of embolotherapy (besides those of selective angiography) include abscess formation and infarction of normal tissue due to reflux of embolic material. A postinfarction syndrome of fever, pain, and leukocytosis may follow extensive embolic procedures in solid organs. Antibiotic coverage depends on the immune status of the patient, the level of occlusion, and the amount and type of tissue infarcted.

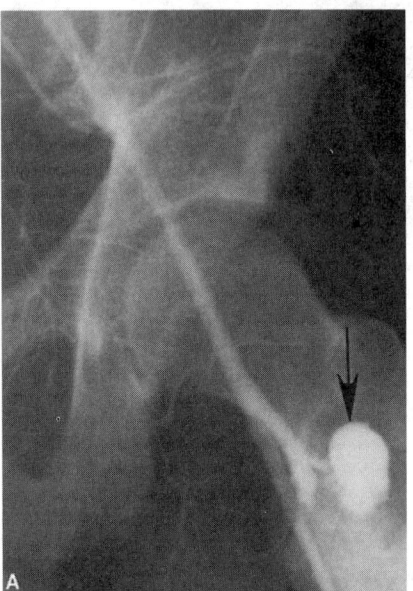

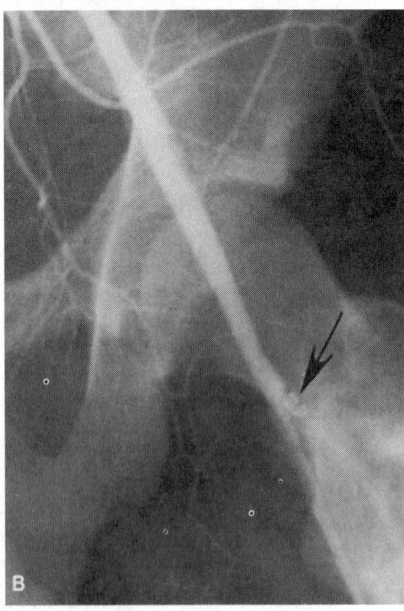

Figure 75-29. Posttraumatic hemorrhage. A 17-year-old male presented with an enlarging left groin hematoma after a gunshot wound. (*A*) Left pelvic arteriogram shows extravasation of contrast medium (*arrow*) from the deep femoral artery. The deep femoral artery was selectively catheterized from the right femoral artery approach and occluded with Gelfoam pledgets and two 3-mm Gianturco steel coils. (*B*) Pelvic arteriogram after embolization shows the coil in the proximal deep femoral artery with arrest of the bleeding. The superficial femoral artery remains patent.

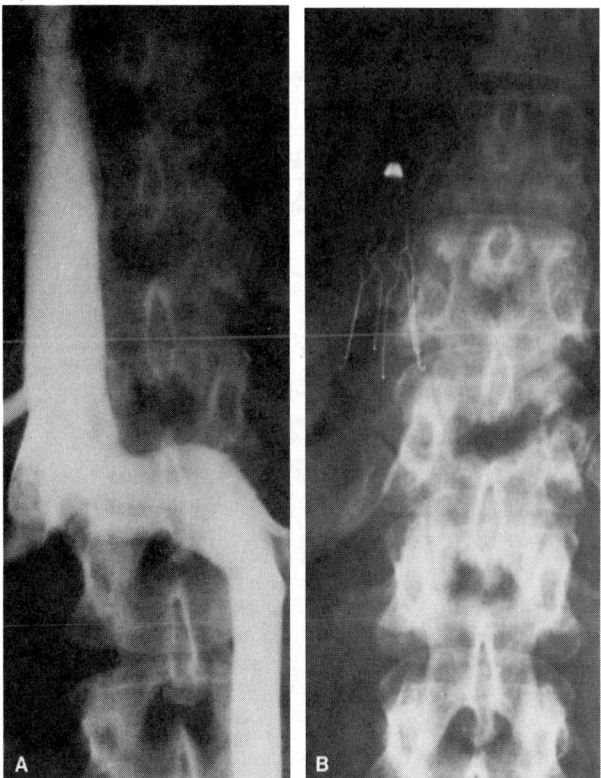

Figure 75-30. Suprarenal Greenfield filter placement through the left inferior vena cava. (*A*) Vena cavogram demonstrates a left-sided inferior vena cava joining the left renal vein and suprarenal cava. A 24F carrier was advanced into the suprarenal cava with use of the percutaneous left transfemoral approach. (*B*) Abdominal film after filter placement shows the filter in satisfactory position.

Caval Interruption

Before an IVC filter is placed, cavography is performed to identify IVC anomalies and variants in the renal veins (Fig. 75-30).

Transjugular Intrahepatic Portosystemic Shunt

In the transjugular intrahepatic portosystemic shunt (TIPS) procedure, a conduit is made between intrahepatic portal and hepatic venous branches (usually the right hepatic and right portal veins) through a percutaneous transjugular approach and buttressed open with intravascular stents. Indications for TIPS include: variceal bleeding unresponsive to medical and endoscopic therapy (sclerotherapy or banding); recurrent variceal bleeding not controlled with endoscopic therapy; and intractable ascites.

Restenosis of a TIPS, usually at the hepatic venous end, occurs in more than half of patients by 6 months. This usually responds to repeat angioplasty and stenting.

Miscellaneous Interventional Procedures

Percutaneous *retrieval of catheter fragments* in the arterial or venous system is straightforward (Fig. 75-31).

Indwelling *central venous access* devices may be placed under fluoroscopic guidance for: localization of the venous entry; optimal catheter placement in the right atrium or superior vena cava-atrium junction; and guidance across chronic thromboses or venous strictures.

Venous access procedures are preceded by diagnostic venography to ensure venous patency.

Percutaneous *management of the ischemic complications* of aortic dissection includes fenestration of the aortic septum, balloon dilation of a compressed true lumen, and

Figure 75-31. Knotted Swan-Ganz catheter. (*A*) Chest film shows an overhand loop (*arrow*) in the shaft of a right transfemoral Swan-Ganz catheter. The catheter tip is in the main pulmonary artery (*open arrow*); the knot is in the right atrium. (*B*) From the right groin, the catheter knot was retracted into the iliac vein confluence, where the knot (*open arrows*) was engaged and teased loose by a left transfemoral catheter (*arrow*).

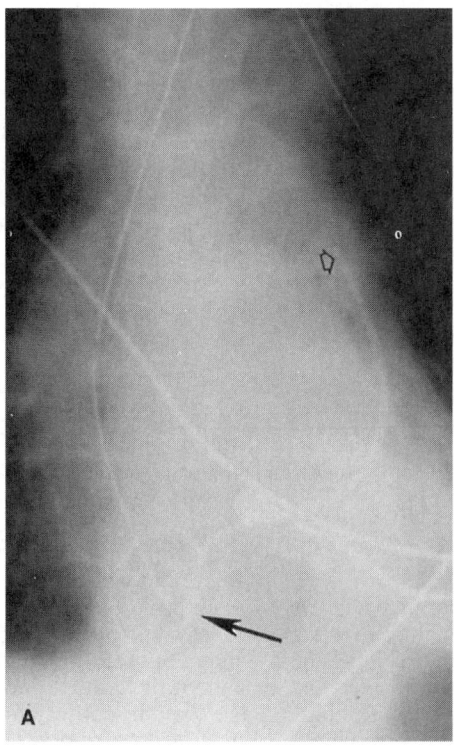

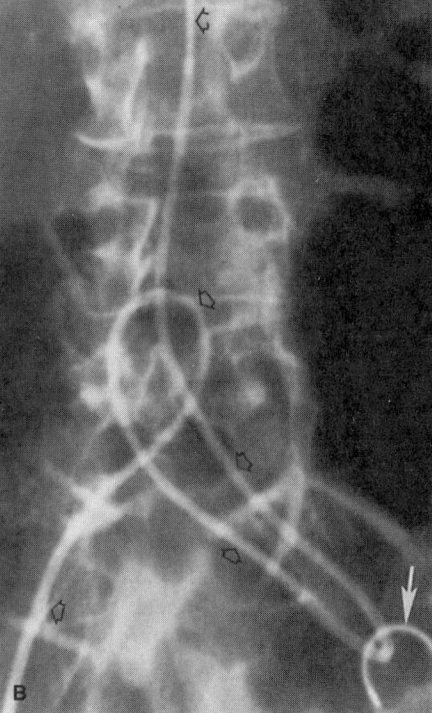

internal stenting of the aortic true lumen or affected branch arteries.

SUGGESTED READING

Andrews J, Walker-Andrews S, Ensminger W. Long-term central venous access with a peripherally placed subcutaneous infusion port: initial results. Radiology 1990;176:45.

Becker G. Intravascular stent. General principles and status of lower-extremity arterial applications. Circulation 1991; 83:I122.

Coldwell D, Ring E, Rees C, et al. Multicenter investigation of the role of transjugular intrahepatic portosystemic shunt in management of portal hypertension. Radiology 1995;196:335.

Katayama H, Yamaguchi K, Kozuka T, Takashima T, Seez P, Matsuura K. Adverse reactions to ionic and nonionic contrast media. Radiology 1990;175:621.

Kerlan R, LaBerge J, Gordon R, Ring E. Transjugular intrahepatic portosystemic shunts: current status. Am J Roentgenol 1995;164:1059.

Martin E. Percutaneous therapy in the management of aortoiliac disease. Semin Vasc Surg 1994;7:17.

Prince M. Gadolinium-enhanced MR aortography. Radiology 1994;191:155.

Prince M, Narasimham D, Stanley J, et al. Gadolinium-enhanced magnetic resonance angiography of abdominal aortic aneurysms. J Vasc Surg 1995;21:656.

Rubin G, Dake M, Semba C. Current status of three-dimensional spiral CT scanning for imaging the vasculature. Radiol Clin North Am 1995;33:51.

Williams D, Brothers T, Messina L. Relief of mesenteric ischemia in type III aortic dissection by percutaneous fenestration of the aortic septum. Radiology 1990;174:450.

ESSENTIALS OF SURGERY: SCIENTIFIC PRINCIPLES AND PRACTICE, edited by Lazar J. Greenfield, Michael W. Mulholland, Keith T. Oldham, Gerald B. Zelenock, and Keith D. Lillemoe. Lippincott–Raven Publishers, Philadelphia, © 1997.

CHAPTER 76

NONOPERATIVE TREATMENT OF ATHEROSCLEROSIS

JOSEPH H. RAPP, LINDA M. REILLY, AND WILLIAM C. KRUPSKI

RISK FACTORS FOR ATHEROSCLEROSIS

Risk factors are behavioral or metabolic. The two main behaviors that increase risk for atherosclerosis are consuming a diet high in animal fat and smoking cigarettes. The metabolic factors are hyperlipidemia, hypertension, diabetes, and homocystinuria.

Hyperlipidemia

Much of the confusion regarding the role of lipids in atherosclerosis results from a lack of appreciation of what constitutes a physiologically normal cholesterol level. In countries where total plasma cholesterol level averages 150 mg/dL (3.88 mmol/L), atherosclerosis is not a public health problem. U.S. citizens of European descent have a mean cholesterol level >210 mg/dL (5.43 mmol/L) at 50 years of age.

Lipoproteins

Although a high level of low-density lipoprotein (LDL) cholesterol is an important risk factor for atherosclerosis, levels of apolipoprotein B, the primary protein constituent of LDL, very low-density lipoprotein (VLDL), and chylomicrons, correlate more accurately with risk for atherosclerosis. VLDL is a triglyceride-rich lipoprotein secreted by the liver and possibly the intestine. High-density lipoproteins (HDLs) oppose deposition of cholesterol by participating in centripetal transport of cholesterol to the liver. Low levels of HDL correlate with reduced centripetal transport of cholesterol and increased risk for atherosclerosis.

Lipid Disorders

Type I Hyperlipidemia. Accumulation of chylomicrons in plasma constitutes type I hyperlipidemia. Chylomicrons are the largest of the lipoproteins. They are formed in the intestine primarily from dietary fat. Taken to the blood via the thoracic duct, chylomicrons release their triglyceride load by interacting with lipoprotein lipase in the endothelium. After removal of the triglyceride, cholesterol ester-enriched chylomicron remnants form. This is a rare genetic disorder and does not appear to increase risk for atherosclerosis.

Type IIa Hypercholesterolemia and Type IIb Hyperlipidemia. Elevations of LDL alone constitute type IIa (familial) hypercholesterolemia. Type IIb (familial combined) hyperlipidemia is characterized by elevations of both LDL and VLDL. Both IIa and IIb are associated with coronary artery disease; some patients also have peripheral vascular lesions.

People with type IIa hypercholesterolemia have defective cellular apolipoprotein B receptors and, therefore, reduced clearance of LDL. People with this rare genetic abnormality have plasma cholesterol levels ≥350 mg/dL (9.05 mmol/L). Type IIb hyperlipidemia is more frequent than type IIa and is probably caused by overproduction of VLDL.

Type III Hyperlipidemia. Accumulations of chylomicrons and VLDL remnants characterize type III hyperlipidemia, an unusual condition that includes both premature peripheral vascular disease and coronary heart disease. A combination of metabolic influences and abnormal apolipoprotein E levels reduces the affinity of the lipoprotein for the apolipoprotein-B E receptor.

Type IV Hyperlipidemia. Type IV hyperlipidemia results from overproduction of VLDL rather than a clearance defect. Type IV is a common condition among persons with diabetes, and may be the most common lipid abnormality in peripheral vascular disease.

Lipid-lowering Therapy

Lipid lowering affects the angiographic structure of lesions in the coronary circulation. Lipid effects on the arterial wall are a key element in atherosclerosis, but lipids also affect platelet aggregation, fibrinogen level, and vascular reactivity. All these factors may be important in the clinical manifestations of atherosclerosis, making the benefits of an aggressive treatment of hyperlipidemia all the more important.

For many people, aggressive dietary change alone is adequate. Substantial dietary change is difficult without high patient motivation and support, however, and many clinics provide both dietetic and behavioral counseling. Restriction of saturated fat and cholesterol intake can lower cholesterol levels ≥20%. Caloric restriction can normalize triglyceride levels.

Drug therapy for hypercholesterolemia includes the *bile acid-binding resins* cholestyramine and colestipol. These drugs interrupt the enterohepatic recycling of bile acids, increase synthesis of bile acids from cholesterol in the liver, and increase the receptor clearance of LDL. These agents may also increase production of VLDL, the precursor of LDL. Therefore, combination therapy with niacin, which reduces VLDL production, is effective.

Niacin can be used as a single agent and in combination therapy. The decreased VLDL level that occurs with niacin therapy is associated with a rise in HDL levels. Niacin also may affect thrombogenicity. Flushing is the most common side effect. Although serious hepatic toxicity is rare, elevated transaminase levels are common. Patients with gout or diabetes mellitus may have to avoid niacin because it can raise uric acid and glucose levels.

The *fibric acid derivatives* reduce plasma VLDL levels, probably by increasing lipoprotein lipase activity. They are used to manage hypertriglyceridemia and type III hyperlipidemia. In some instances, LDL levels may rise and HDL levels minimally increase. Clofibrate and gemfibrozil are the fibric acid derivatives available in the United States.

Lovastatin is a structural analog of HMG CoA reductase that inhibits synthesis of cholesterol. Lovastatin is the most effective lipid-lowering agent and allows single-drug therapy for moderate hypercholesterolemia. Lovastatin, in combination with bile salt-binding resins or niacin, normalizes lipid values in heterozygous familial hypercholesterolemia. Side effects of lovastatin are elevations in liver enzyme levels and hepatitis. Mild elevations in creatine kinase are common, and some patients have painful, tender muscles. Risk for this myopathic syndrome increases with concomitant use of cyclosporine, fibric acid derivatives, erythromycin, or niacin. Although rare, these complications are not trivial; anyone taking lovastatin needs close follow-up care.

There is a relation between a reduction in lipoprotein risk profile and a reduction in cardiac events. A 20% reduction in LDL cholesterol yields a >30% reduction in coronary events. This reduction can be achieved with *cholestyramine*. *Gemfibrozil* works by increasing HDL level.

Smoking

Risk

Cigarettes cause one in six deaths in the United States. Most of the deaths are due to cardiovascular disease. Smokers have 70% more coronary artery disease than nonsmokers. Risk increases with duration of smoking, quantity of cigarettes smoked, and depth of inhalation of smoke.

The cardiovascular risks of smoking multiply other coronary risk factors, such as hypertension, hypercholesterolemia, diabetes, and use of oral contraceptives. A 40-year-old smoker with a serum cholesterol level >260 mg/dL (6.72 mmol/L) and a diastolic blood pressure >95 mmHg has >2.5 times the risk for MI than a smoker without the other risk factors.

Smoking is an especially important risk factor in peripheral vascular occlusive disease. Patients with established peripheral vascular disease who smoke cigarettes are more likely to have disease progression and graft failure than those who do not. The amputation rate among patients with claudication who smoke is 11 times that of patients who do not smoke.

Tobacco smoking also induces formation of abdominal aortic aneurysms. Smokers are two to three times more likely to die of aneurysms than are nonsmokers.

Smokers are at higher risk for stroke than nonsmokers. People who smoke >40 cigarettes per day are almost twice as likely as nonsmokers to have strokes, independent of the presence of hypertension. Use of tobacco and oral contraceptives is a particularly dangerous combination.

Mechanism

The mechanisms by which smoking exerts its deleterious effects on blood vessels are complex. Because tobacco smoke contains more than 2000 substances, identification of a single toxic agent is not likely. Smoking is believed to increase risk for atherosclerosis by means of direct effects on the vascular wall and on circulating lipoproteins. Vasoconstriction, increased heart rate, increased blood pressure, decreased regional myocardial blood flow, and a negative inotropic effect result from cigarette smoking and influence acute and chronic symptoms of vascular disease.

Tobacco smoke affects platelets, red blood cells, leukocytes, and fibrinogen. The net result is a tendency toward thrombosis through increases in these elements and blood viscosity and through increased platelet aggregation accompanied by decreased platelet sensitivity to prostacyclin.

Smoking cessation results in rapid reduction in risk for stroke. This suggests that smoking precipitates the acute event rather than promoting atherosclerosis.

Therapy

Almost all cigarette smokers want to stop smoking, and most have tried unsuccessfully to stop several times. Inability to stop smoking is attributable, in large part, to the addictive properties of nicotine. The six main smoking cessation methods are:

Behavior modification
Educational and commercial programs
Hypnosis
Acupuncture
Multiple risk factor reduction programs
Drug therapy

Regardless of the cessation method chosen, physicians must identify patients who smoke and motivate them to stop. Brief counseling achieves smoking cessation among only a small percentage of otherwise-well patients, but is effective for patients with smoking-related illnesses.

Pharmacologic management of tobacco dependence is based on the symptoms that occur after smoking cessation: craving for cigarettes, irritability, anxiety, difficulty concentrating, coughing, and constipation. Because it blocks withdrawal symptoms, nicotine gum assists smokers in long-term abstinence. When combined with behavioral counseling in smoking cessation clinics, nicotine gum doubles cessation rates. Some patients have difficulty discontinuing use of nicotine gum after the recommended 2 to 6 months therapy period.

Clonidine, an α-noradrenergic agonist first used as an antihypertensive agent, may help smokers stop. The transdermal patch form of the medication decreases side effects. Clonidine reduces the intensity of tobacco craving and the severity of tobacco-withdrawal symptoms, presumably by means of its effect on the adrenergic receptors of the central nervous system.

Hypertension

Even mild elevations in blood pressure convey considerable disease risk, and the risk increases with the degree of hypertension. This morbidity is due to the strong relation

Table 76-1. AGE-ADJUSTED INCIDENCE OF CARDIOVASCULAR EVENTS ACCORDING TO SEX AND DIABETIC STATUS*

Type of Arterial Disease	Men		Women	
	Diabetic	Nondiabetic	Diabetic	Nondiabetic
Cerebrovascular	4.7	1.9	6.2	1.7
Coronary	12.6	3.3	8.4	1.3
Claudication	24.8	14.9	17.8	6.9

* Incidence per 100 patient-years
(Adapted from Kannel WB, McGee DL. Diabetes and cardiovascular disease: the Framingham study. JAMA 1979;241:2035)

between hypertension and stroke, but hypertension also promotes the development of peripheral and coronary atherosclerosis. Although blood pressure reduction is of clear benefit in reducing the incidence of stroke, renal failure, and congestive heart failure, the incidence of MI is not affected if other risk factors, particularly hyperlipidemia, are not controlled. However, β-adrenergic receptor-blocking agents and thiazide diuretics, the most commonly used antihypertensive agents, can have negative effects on a patient's lipid profiles. Blood pressure reduction is important in decreasing cardiovascular events in the long term and in promoting regression of lesions.

Diabetes Mellitus

Atherosclerotic occlusive disease is more prevalent among persons with insulin-dependent (type I) or non–insulin-dependent (type II) diabetes than the general population (Table 76-1). Atherosclerosis is the most common complication and cause of death among persons with diabetes. After MI, persons with diabetes have a higher in-hospital mortality rate than persons without diabetes and have a higher 5-year mortality rate. The long-term survival rate among persons with diabetes with claudication is less than among persons without diabetes. Late survival of persons with diabetes after virtually any type of revascularization procedure is worse than for persons without diabetes (Table 76-2). The situation is less clear with respect to risk for impaired glucose tolerance (chemical or borderline diabetes), although a strong association exists between vascular disease and mild hyperglycemia.

The effect of diabetes on risk for cardiovascular complications diminishes with age at onset, suggesting that duration of exposure may be a factor in the development of atherosclerosis. Severity of diabetes and degree of control

appear to have little relation to the development of vascular disease. The effect of diabetes on cardiovascular risk is greater for women than for men (Table 76-1). Among men, diabetes has the smallest effect of all the risk factors; among women, the impact exceeds that of cigarette smoking. Although diabetes increases risk for atherosclerosis at almost any anatomic site, the most dramatic effect occurs in the arteries of the lower extremities.

In addition to influencing the pattern of atherosclerotic disease, diabetes influences the severity of the disease. Occlusive arterial lesions develop in persons with diabetes about 10 years earlier than in persons without diabetes. Inoperable coronary artery disease is more frequent among persons with diabetes. The prevalence of lower-extremity ulceration or gangrene at presentation is almost twice as great among persons with diabetes as among persons without diabetes. Patients with claudication who have diabetes are more likely to require amputation (Table 76-2). After distal arterial reconstruction, patients with diabetes are less likely to have long-term graft patency or limb salvage.

Control of hyperglycemia appears to correct many of the metabolic abnormalities that occur in diabetes. Improved glycemic control of type I diabetes reduces abnormally elevated plasma triglyceride and cholesterol levels and restores normal LDL internalization and degradation by fibroblasts. HDL cholesterol level rises with control of type II diabetes. Abnormally elevated plasma fibrinogen levels and fibrinogen turnover rates decrease toward normal with treatment. Abnormalities of platelet function in persons with diabetes sometimes are corrected with improved diabetic control.

Despite the foregoing observations, there is little evidence that oral hypoglycemic agents or insulin treatment reduce the prevalence of cardiovascular sequelae among persons with diabetes. Tight glycemic control is feasible for many persons with diabetes because of the availability of home blood-glucose monitoring, infusion pumps, and multiple-dose insulin regimens, but it may not diminish risk for atherosclerosis. More is to be gained with risk factor intervention than with attention to early detection and control of hyperglycemia alone.

Homocysteine

Elevated levels of homocysteine, a thiol-containing amino acid formed from the metabolism of methionine, may play a role in atherosclerosis. Homocystinuria is an inborn error of metabolism in which homocysteine and related compounds accumulate and are excreted in the urine. Patients have severe and usually fatal atherosclerosis in childhood. Moderate increases in plasma homocysteine levels can be treated simply. In general, simple folate

Table 76-2. SURVIVAL AND AMPUTATION RATES ACCORDING TO TREATMENT AND DIABETIC STATUS

Patient Category	Follow-Up (yr)	Survival Rate (%)		Amputation Rate (%)	
		Diabetic	Nondiabetic	Diabetic	Nondiabetic
Claudication	9	54.4	75.7	27.1	3.8
	6	50.0	74.0	12.8	0.5
	6	—	—	46.0	1.0
Revascularization					
Aortic	9	36.0	73.0	—	—
Femoropopliteal	10	8.0	35.0	—	—
Femorotibial	6	66.0	79.0	—	—

normalizes levels whether or not the patient is folate deficient.

NONSURGICAL MANAGEMENT OF CLAUDICATION

Exercise

Exercise is effective in the management of intermittent claudication, although the mechanism of symptomatic improvement is unknown. Trained muscle extracts more oxygen. An increase in aerobic metabolism is manifested by decreased venous lactate levels, increased incorporation of glucose into glycogen and lipids with decreased incorporation into lactate, and increased muscle succinic oxidase activity. Exercise also reduces blood viscosity and red cell aggregation. The only contraindications to the use of exercise in managing claudication are the presence of advanced limb ischemia (rest pain or gangrene) and comorbid conditions. Exercise does require a high degree of patient commitment over a prolonged period.

Pharmacologic Management of Claudication

Pentoxifylline

Pentoxifylline increases the flow of erythrocytes through capillaries by increasing red blood cell ATP content, improving erythrocyte deformability. It also reduces platelet aggregation and hyperactivity. It is presumably because of these changes that pentoxifylline reduces blood viscosity. Perhaps as a result of improved viscosity, limb blood flow increases. Tissue PO_2 in ischemic muscle increases after treatment with pentoxifylline. This agent may be appropriate for patients with severely impaired walking who are not candidates for revascularization or exercise treatment because of anatomic constraints or serious comorbid conditions.

Levocarnitine

Levocarnitine is a metabolic agent believed to enhance pyruvate oxidation, and energy production, by stimulating the activity of pyruvate dehydrogenase. Production of lactate decreases and generation of adenosine triphosphate (ATP) increases. The ability of levocarnitine to improve energy production might improve muscle function in ischemic limbs.

Aspirin

Aspirin, the most frequently used antiplatelet agent, inhibits platelet aggregation by blocking cyclooxygenase. Aspirin also prevents the vasoconstriction caused by thromboxane A_2. PGI_2 and thromboxane A_2 exert opposite effects on platelets, and therapeutic strategies are directed at using these different actions to achieve a balance that favors production of PGI_2 and inhibition of thromboxane A_2 synthesis. Low doses of aspirin achieve this favorable balance. Indications for aspirin treatment are grouped into three broad categories: (1) prevention of complications of atherosclerosis; (2) therapy for established disease; and (3) improvement in results of invasive procedures for atherosclerosis.

Other Agents

Dipyridamole indirectly increases platelet cyclic adenosine monophosphate (cAMP) levels by blocking phosphodiesterase, which converts cAMP to AMP. Resultant increased levels of cAMP inhibit platelet aggregation caused by adenosine diphosphate (ADP). *Calcium channel block-ers* may interfere with the effect of calcium flux on the release of phospholipase from the platelet membrane. *Imidazole* blocks thromboxane synthetase, reducing production of thromboxane A_2. *Ticlopidine* is a platelet antiaggregant that functions primarily as an inhibitor of the ADP pathway of platelet aggregation.

SUGGESTED READING

Blankenhorn DH, Nessim SA, Johnson RL, et al. Beneficial effects of combined colestipol-niacin therapy on coronary atherosclerosis and coronary venous bypass grafts. JAMA 1987;257:3233.

Brevetti G, Chiariello M, Ferulano G, et al. Increases in walking distance in patients with peripheral vascular disease treated with L-carnitine: a double-blind, cross-over study. Circulation 1988;77:767.

Brown G, Albers JJ, Fisher LD, et al. Regression of coronary artery disease as a result of intensive lipid-lowering therapy in men with high levels of apoprotein B. N Engl J Med 1990;323:1289.

Buchwald H, Varco RL, Mattis JP, et al. Effect of partial ileal bypass surgery on mortality and morbidity from coronary heart disease in patients with hypercholesterolemia: report of the program on the surgical control of the hyperlipidemias (POSCH). N Engl J Med 1990;323:946.

Glassman AH, Stetner F, Walsh BT, et al. Heavy smokers, smoking cessation, and clonidine: results of a double-blind, randomized trial. JAMA 1988;259:2863.

Hass WK, Easton JD, Adams HP, et al. A randomized trial comparing ticlopidine hydrochloride with aspirin for the prevention of stroke in high-risk patients. N Engl J Med 1989;321:501.

Kane JP, Malloy MJ, Ports TA, et al. Regression of coronary atherosclerosis during treatment of familial hypercholesterolemia with combined drug regimens. JAMA 1990;264:3007.

Radack K, Wyderski RJ. Conservative management of intermittent claudication. Ann Intern Med 1990;113:135.

Steering Committee of the Physicians' Health Study Research Group. Preliminary report: findings from the aspirin component of the ongoing physicians' health study. N Engl J Med 1988;29:318.

Steinberg D, Parthasarathy S, Carew TW, et al. Beyond cholesterol: modifications of low density lipoprotein that increase its atherogenicity. N Engl J Med 1989;320:915.

ESSENTIALS OF SURGERY: SCIENTIFIC PRINCIPLES AND PRACTICE, edited by Lazar J. Greenfield, Michael W. Mulholland, Keith T. Oldham, Gerald B. Zelenock, and Keith D. Lillemoe. Lippincott–Raven Publishers, Philadelphia, © 1997.

CHAPTER 77

VASCULAR INFECTIONS

DENNIS F. BANDYK

Vascular infection is an uncommon and dreaded clinical condition. Delays in recognition and treatment lead to sepsis, arterial wall erosion into adjacent organs, and hemorrhage after aneurysmal rupture. Infection can occur after arterial reconstruction or cannulation of arteries or veins for drug administration, pressure monitoring, diagnostic studies, or therapeutic endovascular procedures (transluminal angioplasty, atherectomy, placement of a stent or vena caval filter).

CLASSIFICATION

Mycotic Aneurysms
Intravascular
Extravascular

Embolomycotic
Cryptogenic
Vascular Graft Infection
Perigraft (early vs late appearing)
Graft-enteric erosion or fistula
Aortic stump sepsis

Suppurative (Septic) Thrombophlebitis

Mycotic aneurysms encompass pseudoaneurysms caused by arterial infection and true aneurysms that are secondarily infected. Mycotic aneurysms occur by three mechanisms:

1. Direct extension of an adjacent suppurative focus (extravascular)
2. Bacterial colonization of diseased arterial segments (intravascular)
3. Septic embolism as a result of endocarditis (embolomycotic) or septicemia with organisms entering the

vessel wall at sites of damaged endothelium or the vasa vasorum (cryptogenic)

Vascular graft infections are classified according to:

Anatomic signs (perigraft, graft-enteric erosion or fistula)
Mode of onset (early or late)
Pathogen involved

Aortic stump sepsis is a vascular lesion caused by residual arterial wall infection after excision of an infected aortic graft or aneurysm and ligation of the aorta.

Suppurative thrombophlebitis involves the venous system. Infection usually develops at the site of intravenous cannulation, but it can occur in the deep veins of the pelvis, leg, and neck.

ANATOMIC DISTRIBUTION

Most mycotic aneurysms are extravascular or intravascular in origin, the most frequent being the result of direct trauma (drug abuse, endovascular procedures) and con-

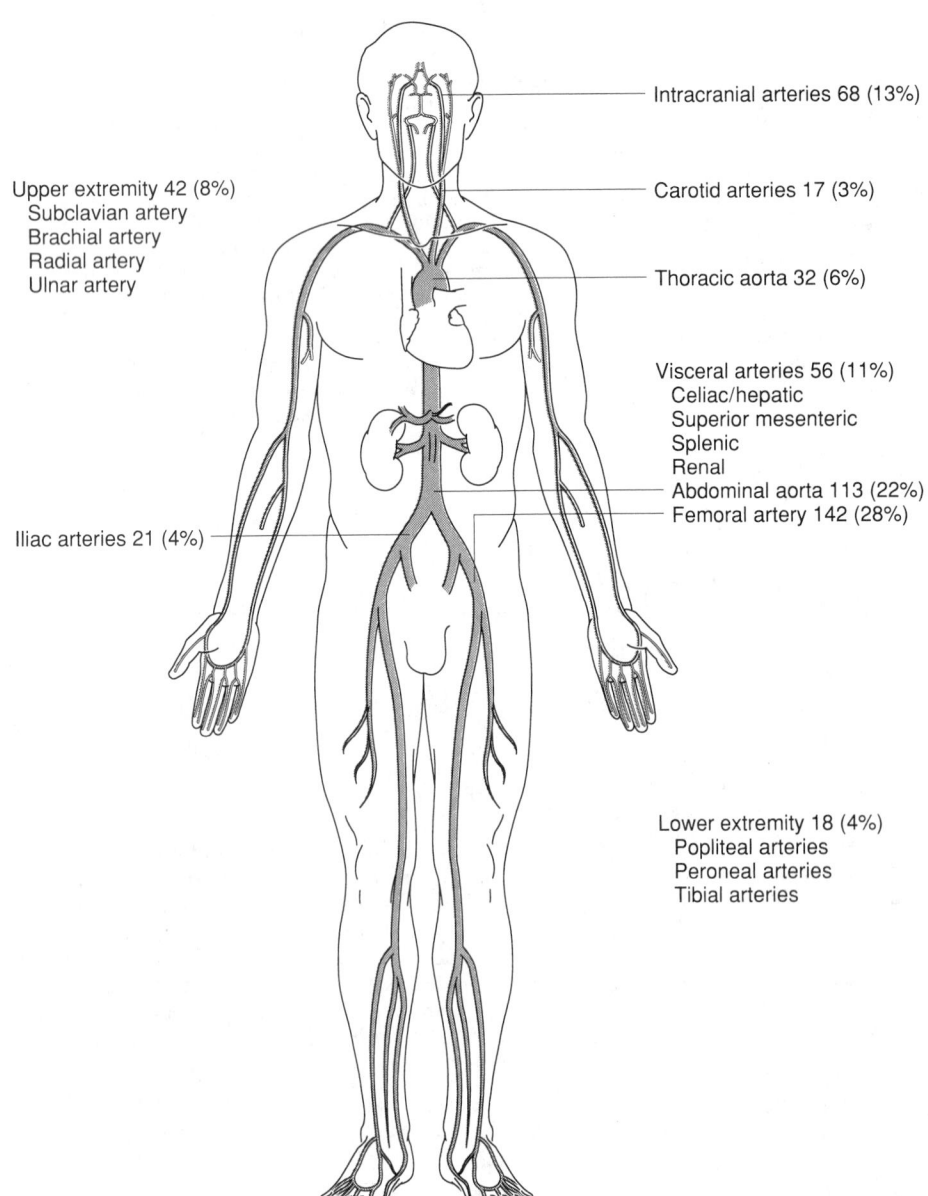

Intracranial arteries 68 (13%)

Carotid arteries 17 (3%)

Thoracic aorta 32 (6%)

Upper extremity 42 (8%)
Subclavian artery
Brachial artery
Radial artery
Ulnar artery

Visceral arteries 56 (11%)
Celiac/hepatic
Superior mesenteric
Splenic
Renal
Abdominal aorta 113 (22%)
Femoral artery 142 (28%)

Iliac arteries 21 (4%)

Lower extremity 18 (4%)
Popliteal arteries
Peroneal arteries
Tibial arteries

Figure 77-1. Anatomic distribution of 510 mycotic aneurysms from collected series.

comitant bacterial contamination. The femoral artery is the main location, followed by the abdominal aorta and visceral vessels (Fig. 77-1). Mycotic aortic aneurysms tend to be saccular and develop in the transverse aortic arch or thoracoabdominal aorta, especially posterior to the origin of the visceral vessels.

Infection can follow any vascular reconstructive procedure but is more common when prosthetic material is used and when the grafting procedure extends into the groin. Most vascular graft infections originate from a wound infection. Infection after placement of an aortic graft confined to the abdomen is rare. Those that occur follow repair of a ruptured abdominal aortic aneurysm or a postoperative abdominal complication (intestinal ischemia or perforation, cholecystitis, appendicitis).

CLINICAL MANIFESTATIONS

Mycotic Aneurysm

- Triad of back or groin pain, pulsatile mass, and fever
- History of bacterial endocarditis, other source of septicemia, or recent penetrating trauma
- In extremities, a palpable mass
- Petechial skin lesions and septic arthritis
- Systolic bruit over the lesion
- Fever of unknown origin (deep infection; aneurysm not palpable)
- Abdominal pain (35% of patients with abdominal aortic aneurysms)
- Myalgia, arthralgia, fever and chills, or progressive weakness that persists for weeks
- Lateralizing hemispheric deficits due to rupture or lethargy and confusion due to abscess formation (intracerebral aneurysms)

Vascular Graft Infection

General Manifestations

- Anastomotic false aneurysm
- Anastomotic or gastrointestinal (GI) hemorrhage (aortoenteric fistula)
- Graft thrombosis
- Signs (local or systemic) of infection

Early Graft Infections (within 4 months of operation)

- Sepsis (fever, leukocytosis, bacteremia)
- Draining or pulsatile mass in the incision
- Graft-artery anastomotic dehiscence
- Graft material visible in wound after drainage of an abscess (indicates diffuse involvement of a vascular prosthesis)

Infection of Grafts Confined to the Abdomen (aortic interposition, aortoiliac)

Unexplained sepsis
- Prolonged postoperative ileus
- Abdominal distention and tenderness

Aortic Graft Infection

- Recognized >1 year after graft implantation
- Inflammation (sinus tract, perigraft exudate) of the groin incision of an aortofemoral graft or anastomotic false aneurysm
- Erosion into the upper or lower GI tract
- Acute bleeding episodes (hematemesis or melena) accompanied by hypotension

Suppurative Thrombophlebitis

- Mimics aseptic venous thrombosis
- Swelling, erythema, induration along involved vein or at sites of cutdown and cannulation
- Purulence at site of cannulation
- Persistent fever and chills

Systemic sepsis with positive blood culture occurs when suppuration involves the thrombosed segment of vein. At this stage, the entire vein is inflamed, extremely painful, and fluctuant.

PATHOPHYSIOLOGY

Infection has a predilection for atherosclerotic lesions, aneurysms, vascular reconstructions in which a prostheses is implanted, and sites of iatrogenic, accidental, or self-induced penetrating arterial trauma. A common infection is of a surgical arteriovenous fistula used for long-term hemodialysis.

Inoculation of the vessel wall can occur at the time of injury or surgical manipulation, from a contiguous septic process via periarterial lymphatics or vasa vasorum, or by means of embolism of septic microemboli to arterial branch points or arterial vasa vasorum. Intercurrent bacteremia from any source can establish infection in any intimal defect, especially vessels with atherosclerotic plaque and mural thrombus. Whether an infection becomes established depends on the quantity and virulence of the pathogens and host resistance. Traumatized tissue and collections of blood can provide nourishment, and foreign bodies (vascular prostheses) adversely affect local host defense mechanisms.

Organisms adhere to the surface of a foreign body and form a bacteria-laden biofilm that protects enclosed organisms against antibiotics, antibodies, and phagocytes. Gram-positive organisms, such as *Staphylococcus* sp., produce extracellular mucin, which promotes adherence and biofilm formation. The addition of suture lines and mural thrombus increases bacterial adherence. Once a prosthetic graft is incorporated with surrounding tissue, and a lumi-

Table 77-1. BACTERIOLOGY OF VASCULAR INFECTIONS

Microorganism	Incidence from Collected Series (%)		
	Mycotic Aneurysm	Graft Infection	Suppurative Thrombophlebitis
Streptococcus sp.	10	10	5
Staphylococcus aureus	28	36	50
Staphylococcus epidermidis	<5	25	10
Salmonella sp.	20	<1	—
Pseudomonas sp.	10	2	1
Escherichia coli	10	12	20
Proteus sp.	4	4	2
Klebsiella sp.	3	6	5–30
Enterobacter sp.	3	4	5
Enterococcus group	2	1	2
Serratia sp.	3	3	2
Candida sp.	2	1	5
Mycobacterium tuberculosis	1	—	—
Other species	5–10	2–5	<5
Culture-negative	15–20	15–25	

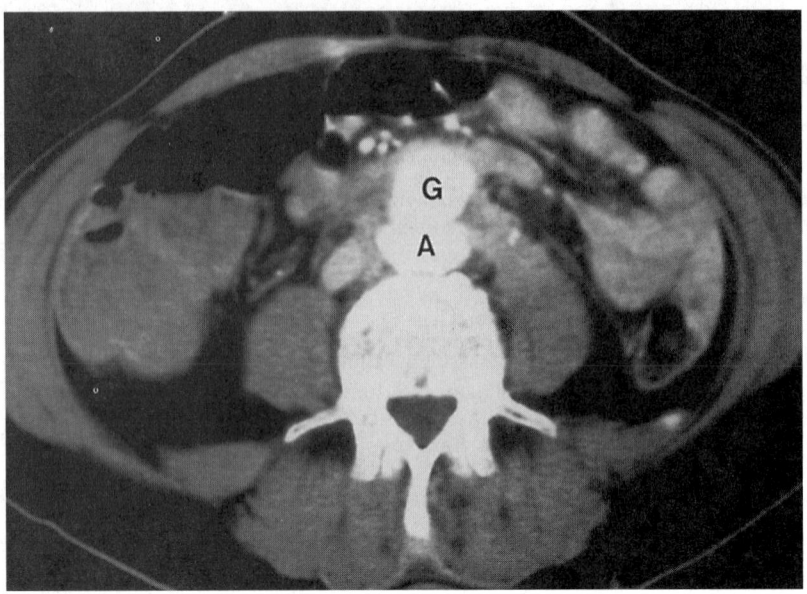

Figure 77-2. CT scan of infected aortic aneurysm with gas (*arrow*) present within the aorta and adjacent soft tissue. Infected, confined aneurysmal rupture was found at operation.

nal pseudointima is established, the graft is less susceptible to colonization by means of bacteremia or adjacent infection.

The ultimate manifestation of arterial or vascular graft infection is disruption and hemorrhage of the vessel wall or anastomosis. Tissue invasion by the microorganism into vessel walls with accompanying inflammation weakens tensile strength. Aneurysm formation or local, contained rupture can cause deposition of mural thrombus, forming a septic nidus for continuous bacteremia.

Predisposing Factors

- **Arterial Trauma**
  Accidents
  Surgical manipulation

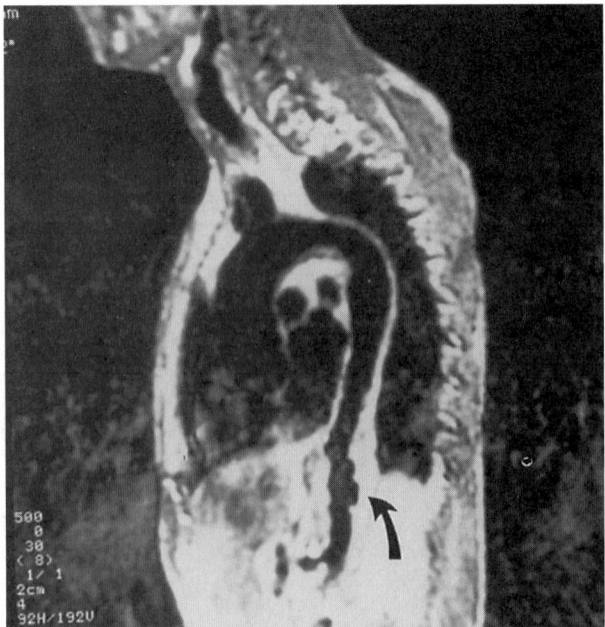

Figure 77-3. MR image of thoracic and suprarenal aorta in a patient with tuberculous aortitis. Saccular dilatation of aorta was demonstrated in the sagittal view (*arrow*).

  Parenteral drug abuse
  Invasive diagnostic procedures
  Endovascular procedures
- **Depressed Immunocompetence**
  Malignant neoplasms
  Lymphoproliferative disorders
  Chronic alcoholism
  Corticosteroid administration
  Chemotherapy
  Chronic renal failure
  Autoimmune disease
  Diabetes mellitus
- **Bacterial Endocarditis**
- **Concurrent Sepsis**
  Salmonella bacteremia
  Tuberculous lymphadenitis
  Syphilitic gumma
- **Wound Healing Complications**
  Hematoma
  Lymphocele
  Dermal necrosis
- **Vascular Prosthesis**
- **Congenital Cardiovascular Defects**
  Patent ductus arteriosus
  Coarctation of the thoracic aorta
- **Emergency Arterial Revascularization**

Bacteriology

Any organism can infect the vascular system, but *Staphylococcus aureus* is the prevalent pathogen. About 80% of early postoperative vascular infections are caused by staphylococcal or streptococcal species (Table 77-1). Aneurysms infected with gram-negative organisms have a higher rupture rate than infections due to gram-positive organisms.

Infections due to *Pseudomonas* sp. are particularly virulent because the organism produces destructive endotoxins (elastase, alkaline protease) that act against elastin and collagen in arterial and venous graft walls to compromise structural integrity.

Salmonella sp. are the infecting pathogen in most intravascular mycotic aneurysms that involve the thoracic or

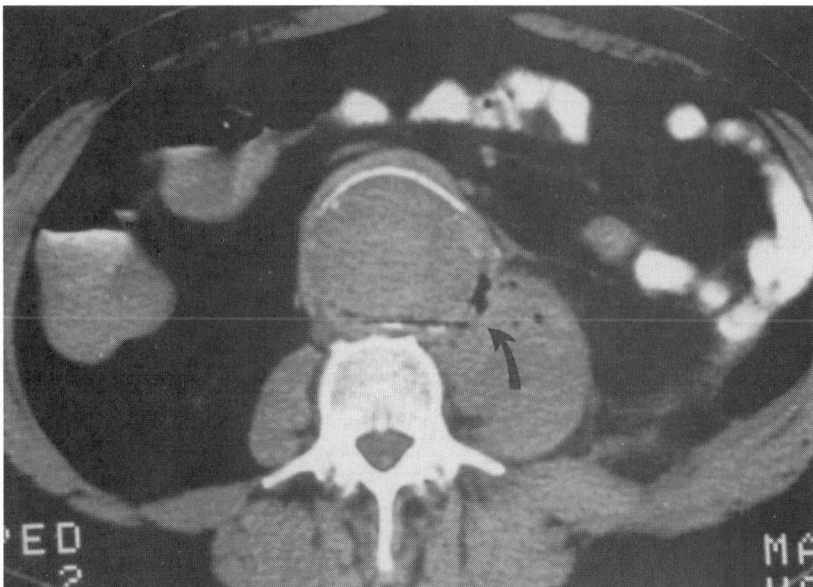

Figure 77-4. Contrast-enhanced CT scan of an aortic interposition graft in a patient with gastrointestinal bleeding. False aneurysm at graft (G) to aorta (A) anastomosis and perigraft inflammation were consistent with diagnosis of graft-enteric erosion. The corresponding aortograms are shown in Figure 78-5.

abdominal aorta; staphylococci and other gram-positive cocci are second. Contaminated water, poultry, and meat products are the most important sources of these gram-negative bacteria, which have a predilection for diseased arterial walls. The portal of entry is the GI tract and the biliary tree.

DIAGNOSIS

Blood cultures usually are positive in mycotic infections, but this is not true of vascular graft infections. Leukocytosis and a high erythrocyte sedimentation rate are common but nonspecific findings in vascular infections. All

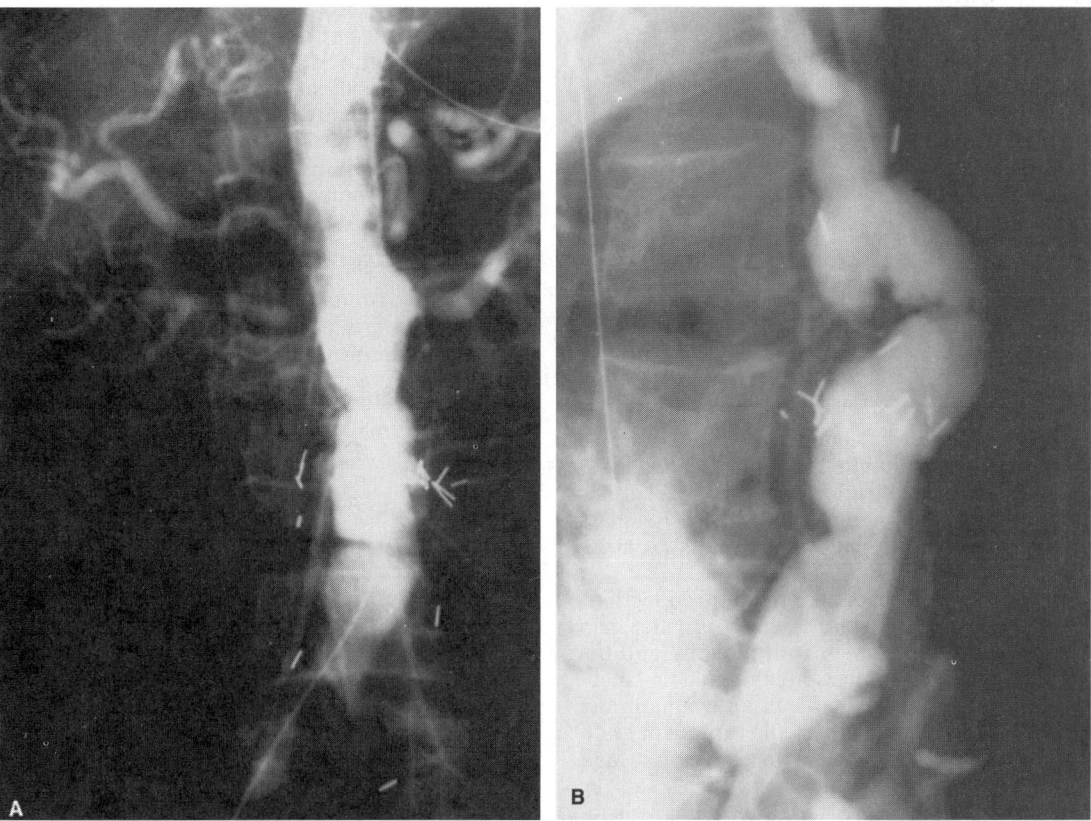

Figure 77-5. Anteroposterior (A) and lateral (B) aortograms of an interposition graft 11 months after aortic endoaneurysmorraphy. False aneurysm is present at the distal anastomosis with kinking of the graft. Graft-enteric erosion was found at operation.

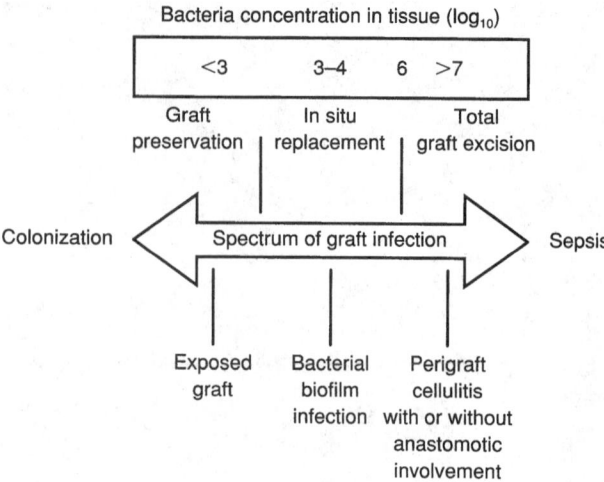

Figure 77-6. The spectrum of vascular graft infection. Clinical manifestation and treatment options depend on the bacteria virulence and concentration in tissue.

laboratory findings may be normal in patients with late-appearing perigraft infections due to *Staphylococcus epidermidis.*

Vascular imaging is vital in evaluating vascular infection. Both anatomic and functional diagnostic imaging techniques may be necessary to help confirm the presence of infection and assess surgical sites for residual or recurrent infection.

Ultrasonography

Ultrasonography is used to locate aneurysms and identify the presence of perigraft fluid. Color Doppler flow imaging is used to evaluate pulsatile masses to differentiate fluid collection or hematoma from a false aneurysm. US is used to verify vessel patency and size and to assess pulsatile masses adjacent to peripheral vessels and grafts, especially in the groin and limbs. US of the venous system helps identify saphenous and femoral veins to be used as autologous grafts.

Computed Tomography

Contrast-enhanced CT is used to evaluate infection of the aorta, visceral arteries, or abdominal vascular grafts. Diagnostic criteria for infection include well-localized vessel dilatation with little calcification; abnormal collections of fluid or air around vessels or grafts; or an encasing mass that contains air, adjacent vertebral osteomyelitis, or juxta-aortic retroperitoneal abscess.

CT-guided needle aspiration of perigraft fluid collections is used to identify the infecting pathogen. CT is better than US in the assessment of aneurysm wall integrity and the detection of inflammation or infection involving the aneurysmal sac (Fig. 77-2). CT is fast enough for evaluation of symptomatic but hemodynamically stable rupture or graft-enteric fistula or erosion. Many hemorrhagic, embolic, and ischemic complications of surgical treatment can be avoided with preliminary CT. Arterial segments not involved in inflammation can be located and are used as initial sites for dissection, vascular control, and placement of occluding clamps.

Magnetic Resonance Imaging

MRI allows anatomic delineation in multiple planes (transverse, sagittal, and coronal) (Fig. 77-3) and provides information about tissue characteristics (eg, presence of fluid, inflammation). MRI provides better resolution between tissue and fluid interfaces than does CT and is better than CT in assessing the presence and extent of infection of aortic grafts. Multiplanar reconstruction of vascular anatomy allows evaluation of complex aortic aneurysms and infectious complications after operations on the aorta. Information includes luminal dimensions, rate of blood flow, quality of the aortic wall, cephalad and caudal extension, and involvement of branch vessels and neighboring structures.

Angiography

Biplanar angiography is performed on all patients with confirmed or suspected arterial infection. Angiograms depict pseudoaneurysms and help one assess patency of involved vessels or grafts to evaluate the status of proximal and distal vessels (Figs. 77-4, 77-5). A saccular or lobulated aneurysm of the aorta with otherwise normal vasculature is pathognomonic of a mycotic aneurysm. The diagnosis of intracranial or visceral mycotic aneurysms can be made reliably only with angiography.

For most patients with arterial or vascular graft infections, angiography is used to aid in planning surgical therapy and to answer questions about results of clinical examination or CT and MRI. Intraarterial digital subtraction arteriography is the preferred angiographic technique.

Functional Imaging Techniques

Radionuclide scans with ^{99m}Tc-labeled leukocytes, ^{111}In-labeled leukocytes, or polyclonal human IgG show accumulation at sites of infection. Functional imaging studies can be used with MRI and CT to delineate the extent of infection. If a patient has no symptoms after aortic graft placement, a positive radioisotope scan but normal CT scan indicates a low-grade infection; parenteral antibiotic administration followed by detailed serial physical examinations is recommended.

Microbiologic Testing

Recovery of microorganisms from sites of suspected vascular infection is necessary to confirm the diagnosis and to select antibiotic therapy. Gram stain of tissue or perigraft fluid showing no organisms is insufficient to exclude the

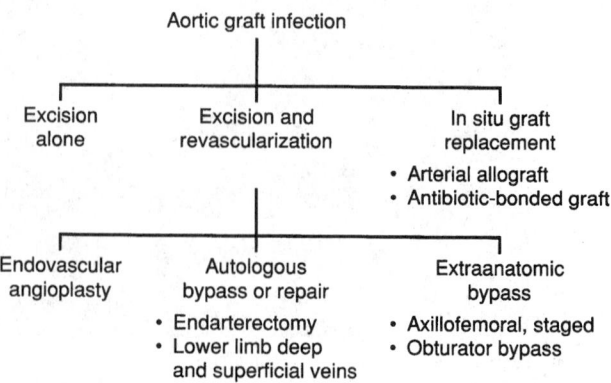

Figure 77-7. Treatment options for vascular graft infections.

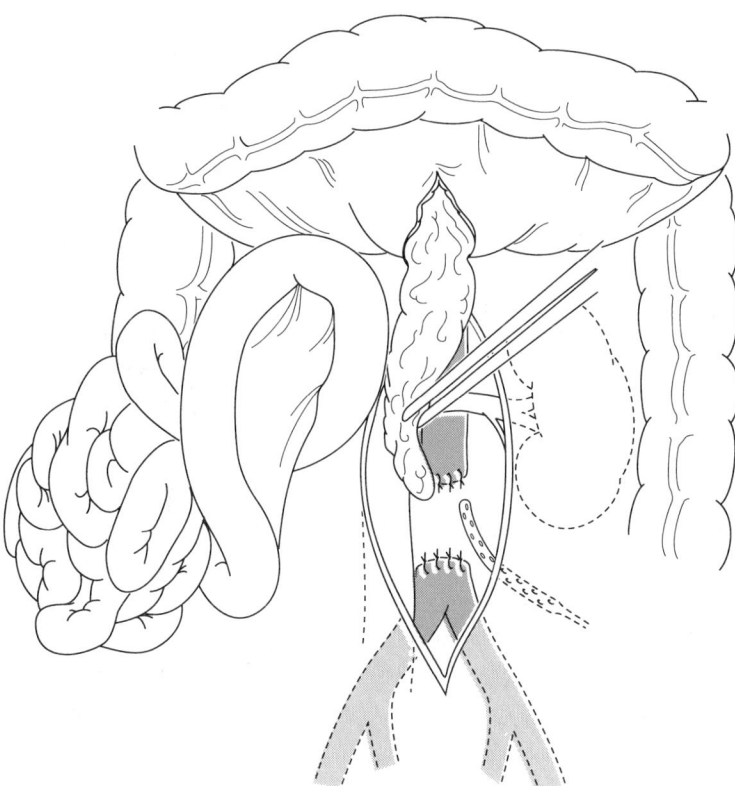

Figure 77-8. Schematic representation of the retroperitoneum after excision of an aortic mycotic aneurysm or infected aortic graft and closure of the aorta. Pedicle of omentum is brought through transverse mesocolon and interposed between the aortic stump and bowel. Closed suction drain is placed in the graft bed and brought out the left flank.

presence of infection. Use of tryptic soy broth media and mechanical (tissue grinding) or ultrasonic disruption of explanted tissue or graft material increases the recovery of microorganisms.

MANAGEMENT

Mycotic aneurysms and most vascular graft infections are fatal if not controlled with aggressive surgical and antibiotic therapy. Therapy is based on clinical presentation and the anatomic and microbiologic characteristics of the infection (Figs. 77-6, 77-7).

Eradication of the infection and maintenance of distal circulation are the principles of management. Systemic antibiotics that kill the bacteria recovered from blood or wound cultures, aspirated perigraft fluid, or expected pathogens are administered. Patients must be physiologically and psychologically prepared for an operation. Surgical control of infection is a priority when sepsis is present, because antibiotic administration alone is insufficient.

Ruptured aneurysms or graft-enteric fistulas require immediate surgical intervention. The infected artery, aneurysm, or vascular graft must be totally excised and arterial reconstruction, if necessary, meticulously performed as a staged or simultaneous procedure. Surgical principles are:

Wide débridement of infected tissue, including the artery adjacent to the infection
- Antibiotic irrigation and placement of drains
- Reconstruction of vital arteries through uninfected tissue planes
- Prolonged postoperative antibiotic administration

Aorta

For infrarenal aortic infections, preliminary axillobifemoral bypass is performed if the patient is in hemodynamically stable condition and if the diagnosis can be estab-

lished. This approach avoids leg ischemia and the necessity for heparinization during excision of the aortic aneurysm or graft and closure of the aortic stump. The aorta is débrided to normal-appearing tissue and closed with monofilament sutures. A pedicle of omentum is positioned around the aortic stump and bed of excised aorta and graft (Fig. 77-8). Closed suction drains are left in the retroperitoneum and brought out of the flank opposite the axillofemoral graft.

In situ prosthetic reconstruction can be performed for both primary and secondary aortic infection, but relapsing infection is common with gram-negative infections, especially with *Salmonella*. In situ graft replacement is used to manage primary and secondary aortoenteric fistulas. Patients with graft-enteric erosion and minimal retroperitoneal infection fare best. When infection involves thoracic or suprarenal aorta and branches, in situ graft replacement is the only practical approach.

Femoropopliteal Arterial Segment

Collateral circulation is usually sufficient to maintain limb viability after excision and ligation of infected femoral artery aneurysms. Autologous reconstruction with saphenous vein or extraanatomic obturator canal bypass can be used to reconstitute arterial flow to the leg when the entire femoral artery bifurcation must be excised (Fig. 77-9).

Most infections of extremity grafts necessitate complete graft removal, autologous patch closure of anastomotic sites, muscle flap coverage of the artery, and if necessary to maintain limb viability, autologous reconstruction or endovascular angioplasty.

Carotid Artery

Ligation without reconstruction is safe management of infected carotid or innominate artery aneurysms, if carotid stump systolic pressure is >70 mmHg. Autologous recon-

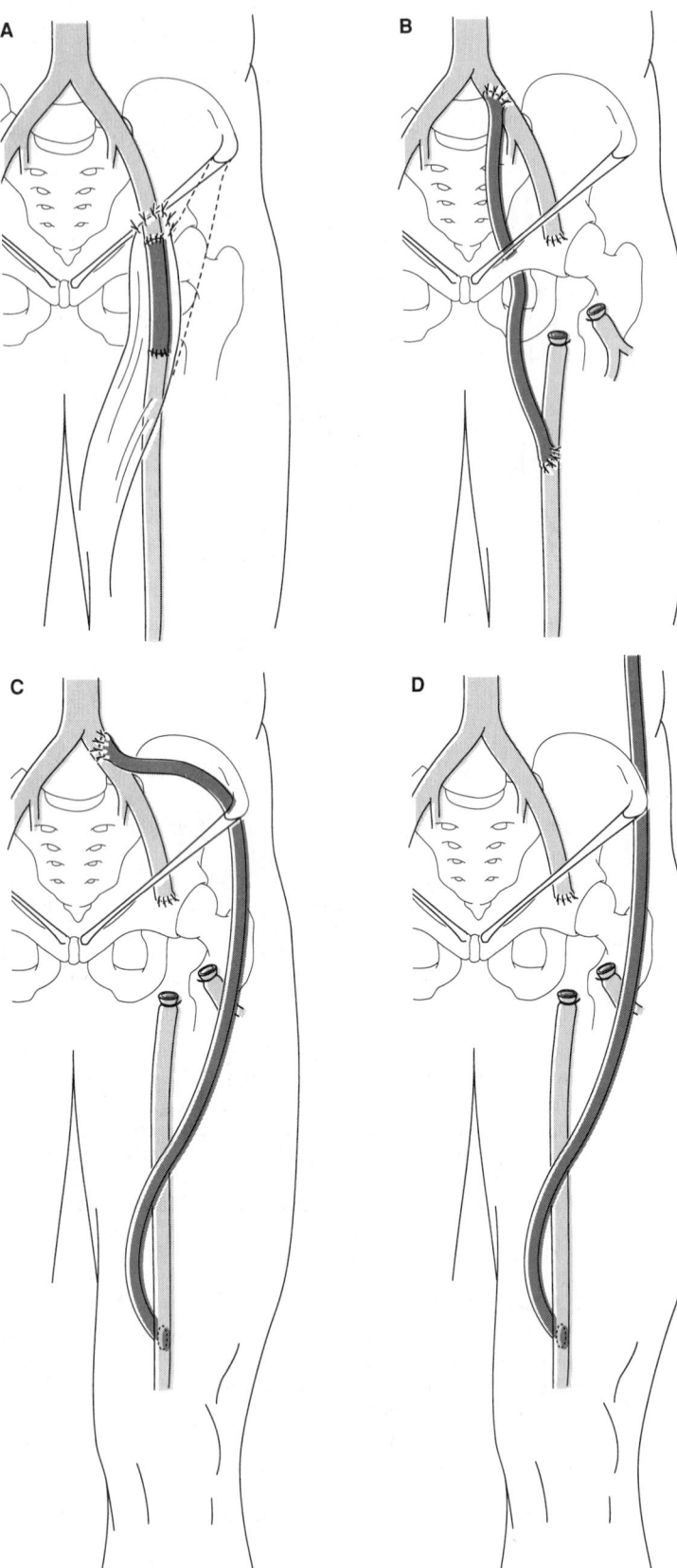

Figure 77-9. Methods of femoral artery reconstruction after excision and ligation of femoral mycotic aneurysm. (*A*) Interposition vein autograft with sartorius muscle flap coverage. (*B*) Obturator bypass. (*C*) Lateral femoral bypass. (*D*) Unilateral axillofemoral bypass. (After Reddy DJ, Smith RF, Elliott JP Jr, et al. Infected femoral artery false aneurysms in drug addicts: evolution of selective vascular reconstruction. J Vasc Surg 1986;3:718)

struction with saphenous vein or extracranial to intracranial bypass may be needed to maintain cerebral circulation in patients with poor hemispheric collaterals, depending on the extent of infection in the neck.

Visceral Artery

Management of mycotic aneurysms involving the visceral or renal arteries is based on angiographic findings. Proximal and distal arterial control is obtained and the aneurysm is excised, if possible. Endoaneurysmorrhaphy with oversewing of the orifices of afferent and efferent vessels is used when excision is not possible and for management of saccular aneurysms without purulence. Aneurysm excision and ligation of superior mesenteric, hepatic, celiac, and splenic arteries is performed. Renal artery reconstruction is needed to maintain organ function.

Suppurative Thrombophlebitis

Wide excision of the infected vein to normal-appearing, patent vein and débridement of all devitalized tissue are needed for local control of infection. Surgical wounds are left open and packed with sterile, saline-soaked gauze. Secondary closure is performed when the infection is resolved and granulation tissue develops. Systemic anticoagulation with heparin is necessary. Antibiotics are administered if suppurative thrombophlebitis involves deep veins of the pelvis or extremities. If pulmonary septic emboli develop, venous ligation distal to the infected deep venous segment may be performed. An alternative is surgical drainage or thrombotomy with insertion of a Greenfield filter.

SUGGESTED READING

Calligaro KD, Veith FJ, Schwartz ML, et al. Differences in early versus late extracavitary arterial graft infections. J Vasc Surg 1995;22:680.

Clagett GP, Bowers L, Lopez-Viego MA, et al. Creation of a neo-aortoiliac system from lower extremity deep and superficial veins. Ann Surg 1993;218:239.

Fiorani P, Speziale F, Rizzo L, et al. Detection of aortic graft infection with leukocytes labelled with technetium 99m hexametazime. J Vasc Surg 1993;17:87.

Kieffer E, Bahnini A, Koskas F, et al. In situ allograft replacement of infected aortic prosthetic grafts: results in forty-three patients. J Vasc Surg 1993;17:349.

Mertens RA, O'Hara PJ, Hertzer NR, et al. Surgical management of infrainguinal arterial prosthetic graft infections: review of a 35-year experience. J Vasc Surg 1995;21:782.

Schmitt DD, Seabrook GR, Bandyk DF, et al. Graft excision and extra-anatomic revascularization: the treatment of choice for the septic aortic prosthesis. J Cardiovasc Surg 1990;327.

Torsello G, Sandmann W, Gehrt A, et al. In situ replacement of infected vascular prostheses with rifampin-soaked vascular grafts: early results. J Vasc Surg 1993;17:768.

Towne JB, Seabrook GR, Bandyk DF, et al. In situ replacement of arterial prostheses infected with bacterial biofilms: long-term followup. J Vasc Surg 1994;19:226.

ESSENTIALS OF SURGERY: SCIENTIFIC PRINCIPLES AND PRACTICE, edited by Lazar J. Greenfield, Michael W. Mulholland, Keith T. Oldham, Gerald B. Zelenock, and Keith D. Lillemoe. Lippincott–Raven Publishers, Philadelphia, © 1997.

CHAPTER 78

ENDOVASCULAR SURGICAL TECHNIQUES

RODNEY A. WHITE

Endovascular surgical therapy involves the use of minimally invasive procedures to revascularize ischemic tissues. This therapy is beneficial to patients with cardiovascular disease because they are at high risk during conventional operations. A controversial advantage of endovascular therapy is its use to manage lesions that produce minimal symptoms, such as claudication, that are not considered indications for a conventional operation.

An endoluminal approach can be used to remove arterial occlusions in the management of atherosclerotic disease. Plaque is removed by means of endarterectomy with metal strippers or intramural or intraplaque introduction of gas to separate the lesion from the vessel wall. Endovascular therapies enlarge the vessel lumen by dilating the vessel, compacting the lesion, or lysing its constituents. In comparison with dilation, endarterectomy yields a more durable repair. Patency rates with endarterectomy are not as good as those with reconstructive operations.

Endovascular surgical procedures can be used to manage selected lesions, but successful recanalization is limited by early recurrence. Guidance techniques, such as angioscopy and intraluminal ultrasonography (US), reduce the likelihood of perforation or inability to cross the lesion, and allow preservation of sufficient vessel wall to prevent aneurysm formation.

DISTRIBUTION OF ATHEROSCLEROTIC LESIONS

Most coronary and peripheral lesions develop in an eccentric position within the vessel so that the residual lumen is usually off center in relation to the walls of the artery (Fig. 78-1). Endarterectomy relies on the eccentric localization of lesions to allow complete removal through an incision in the anterior surface of the artery. The plaque is removed with a smooth transition to the adjacent luminal surface. Eccentric positioning of the atherosclerotic le-

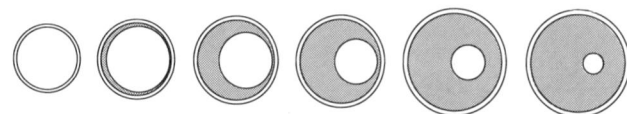

Figure 78-1. Diagrammatic representation of a possible sequence of changes in atherosclerotic arteries leading eventually to lumen narrowing. The artery enlarges initially (left to right in diagram) in association with plaque accumulation to maintain an adequate, if not normal, lumen area. Early stages of lesion development may be associated with overcompensation. At more than 40% stenosis, however, the plaque area continues to increase to involve the entire circumference of the vessel, and the artery no longer enlarges at a rate sufficient to prevent narrowing of the lumen. (After Glagov S, Weisenberg E, Zarins C, et al. Compensatory enlargement of human atherosclerotic coronary arteries. N Engl J Med 1987;316:1374)

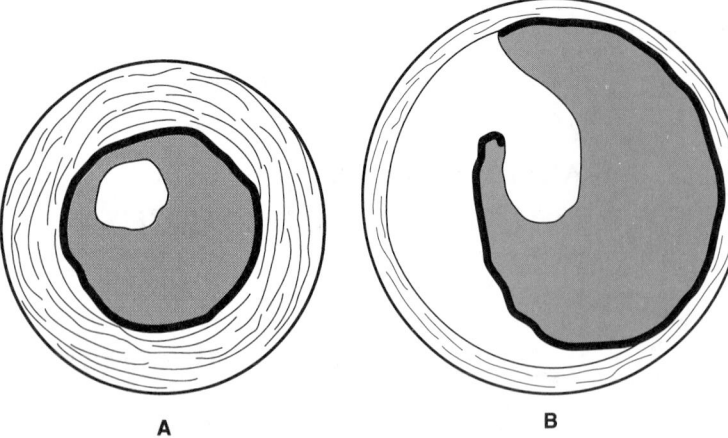

A   B

Figure 78-2. Mechanism of balloon dilation of an arterial stenosis. (*A*) Eccentric atherosclerotic arterial lesion. (*B*) The weakest point of the eccentric lesion is fractured and displaced by expansion of the balloon.

sions within the arterial wall predisposes to controlled fracture of the thinner portion of the plaque during balloon dilation, displacing most of the mass to produce a neolumen (Fig. 78-2).

Another factor that facilitates transluminal recanalization is the localized nature of atherosclerotic lesions in the artery. Clot and soft, organized material fill the lumen proximal and distal to the lesion up to the site of patent branch arteries (Fig. 78-3). With most long occlusions, large portions of the vessel are obstructed by acute and chronic thrombosis. The length of many vascular lesions can be markedly reduced with thrombolytic therapy. The large component of soft material in an arterial occlusion enables guide wires to cross long obstructions. However, failures of therapy are related to imprecise passage and guidance of devices and inadequate debulking of lesions in segments occluded by fibrotic or calcified material (Fig. 78-4).

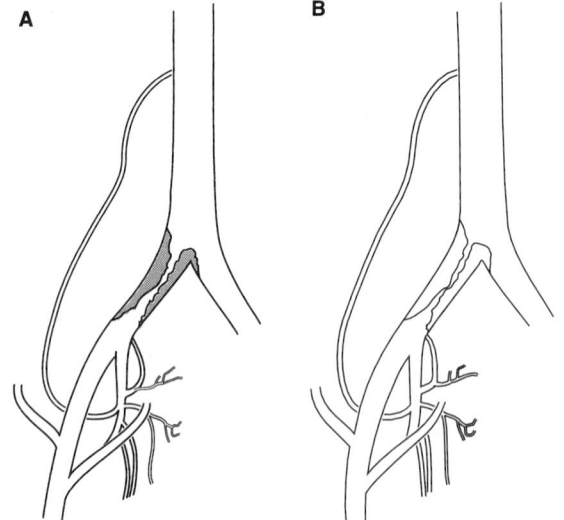

A   B

Figure 78-3. (*A*) Schematic drawing of a localized fibrocalcific atherosclerotic lesion in the right common iliac artery. (*B*) Occlusion of the artery proximal and distal to the lesion with clot and softer organized thrombus (*blue area*) to the site of patent branch arteries. (After White RA, White GH. The atherosclerotic lesion and balloon angioplasty. In: Color atlas of endovascular surgery. London, Chapman & Hall, 1990:13)

INTRALUMINAL ACCESS TECHNIQUES

Access to an artery being treated with an endovascular device is gained by means of percutaneous catheter techniques or surgical exposure and opening of the vessel. For percutaneous vascular access, a small skin incision is made and a needle is introduced through the arterial wall. The needle is slowly withdrawn until return of arterial blood is achieved. A guide wire is introduced through the lumen of the needle and positioned under fluoroscopic control. For many procedures, an introducer sheath is threaded over the guide wire after passage of a vascular dilator. Guide wires establish a channel through the lesion and facilitate introduction and atraumatic passage and exchange of endovascular devices. Angiographic catheters are used to introduce or exchange guide wires or inject contrast material.

Access for many percutaneous procedures is obtained by means of cannulation of the common femoral artery. Lesions of the infrarenal aorta, iliac bifurcation, and iliac arteries are most effectively approached by means of ipsilateral retrograde puncture of the femoral artery. Lesions of the infrainguinal vessels often are approached antegrade by way of the ipsilateral femoral artery. Alternative approaches include the axillary, brachial, superficial femoral, and popliteal arteries or direct puncture of bypass grafts.

ENDOVASCULAR SURGICAL DEVICES AND TECHNIQUES

Table 78-1 summarizes the mechanisms and applicability of various endovascular surgical modalities.

Transluminal Dilation

Balloon angioplasty is effective for localized, short stenotic lesions or short occlusions of the iliac arteries. The procedure is likely to be successful if there are patent arteries in the distal vascular bed.

Dilation of atherosclerotic lesions is achieved with a Fogarty balloon embolectomy catheter. After placement of the balloon at the site of narrowing, the weakest point in the plaque is fractured by means of expansion of the balloon, which enlarges the arterial lumen. Measurement of pressure gradients across a lesion before and after dilation is helpful to determine the success of angioplasty. Pressure gradients across a lesion are measured simultaneously

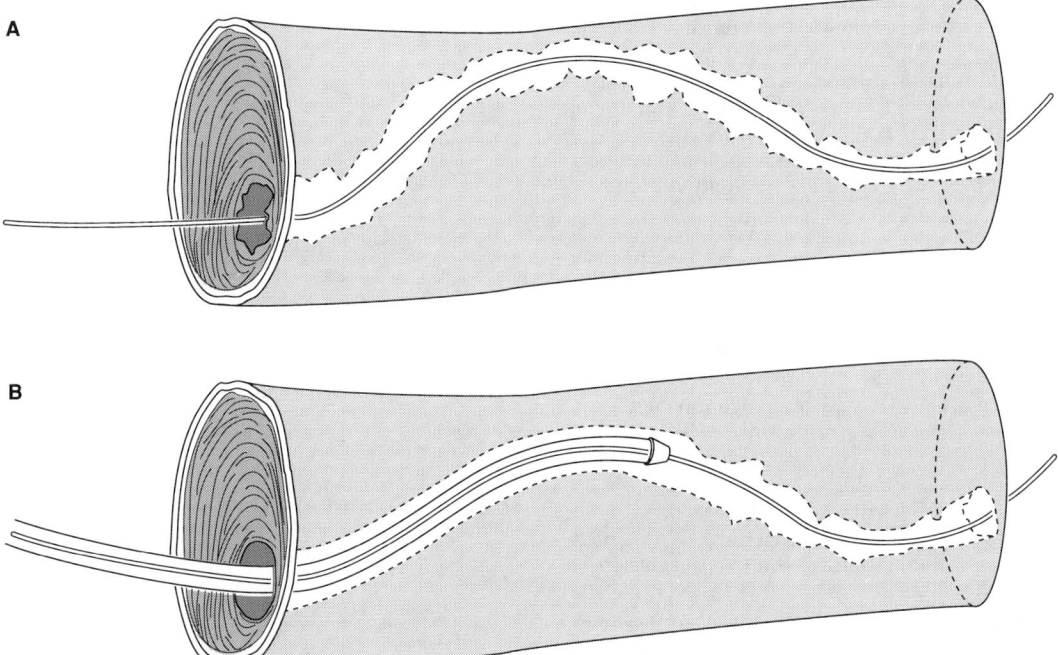

Figure 78-4. Placement of a guide wire through the meandering, eccentric lumen of an atherosclerotic vessel (*A*) limits the ability of a device passed over the guide wire (*B*) to adequately remove the lesion without causing vessel wall perforation as a result of being maintained in the eccentric position by the guide wire.

with dual catheters, or separately by means of measurement of pressure as a catheter is passed through the lesion.

Balloon angioplasty can be used to manage disease in the branches of the abdominal aorta, particularly the renal and mesenteric arteries. Renovascular disease is amenable to dilation if there is short, focal stenosis of the renal artery that does not involve the ostium. Lesions of the orifice of the renal artery formed by an extension of aortic plaque are more difficult to manage, as are totally occlusive lesions of the renal artery.

Atherectomy

Atherectomy is used to remove atherosclerotic plaque from a vessel by means of cutting, drilling, or pulverizing the atheroma. This produces a luminal surface different from that of balloon dilation or open surgical endarterectomy. Some atherectomy devices have mechanisms for extracting the fragments, and others reduce the plaque to microparticles, which are circulated in the bloodstream and removed by the lungs and reticuloendothelial system.

Most atherectomy devices are suitable only for stenotic lesions, and are inserted over a guide wire. If the stenotic arterial lumen is not sufficiently enlarged after atherectomy, balloon dilation can be performed. Similarly, complications of balloon angioplasty, such as dissection or acute occlusion or inadequate vessel recanalization, may improve with passage of an atherectomy catheter.

Other Techniques

Laser angioplasty is an investigational method. Indications include arterial stenoses and short occlusions, iliac lesions, chronically occluded polytetrafluoroethylene (PTFE) grafts, high risk for conventional surgical treatment, or the likelihood that interval patency may improve operability at a later date.

Nonlaser thermal angioplasty systems, such as radiofre-

Table 78-1. ENDOVASCULAR SURGERY MODALITIES

Method	Mechanism	Applications	Advantages
Thrombolysis	Clot lysis	Thromboses of variable lengths	Thrombis removal without a surgical procedure
Balloons	Lesion displacement	Stenoses and short occlusions	Cost-effective
			Percutaneous angioplasty
Lasers	Tissue ablation	Stenoses and occlusions	Tissue removal
			Miniature delivery systems
Atherectomy	Tissue removal	Stenoses and some occlusions	Tissue removal
Stents	Maintain lumen patency by fixed lesion displacement	Stenoses, occlusions, dissections, lesion recoil, etc	Maintains luminal patency and treats some complications of other devices

quency and electric and catalytic thermal systems, may be alternatives to laser thermal devices, if thermal ablation is acceptable.

Ultrasonic ablation of atherosclerotic plaques can be used to remove abnormal tissue, while preserving normal arterial wall. Pulsed and continuous forms of energy are delivered to plaques via wire probes. Another method of plaque dissolution is use of a pulsatile, high-velocity water jet.

THROMBOLYTIC THERAPY

The fibrinolytic system, which is responsible for clot lysis, is activated when plasminogen is converted to plasmin by mediators such as tissue-type plasminogen activator. Fibrinolysis can be initiated by exogenous activators such as urokinase (UK) and streptokinase (SK). Plasmin degrades fibrin and fibrinogen into fragments, some of which have antithrombotic activity.

Thrombolytic agents, particularly UK, are used extensively as adjuncts to endovascular procedures. These drugs are useful for lysis of acute and chronic thrombus in occluded vessels to localize atherosclerotic lesions that may be amenable to balloon dilation, another recanalization procedure, or use of an intravascular stent.

Another possible application of thrombolysis is use of lytic agents as an alternative to conventional surgical management of acute arterial occlusions. Thrombolytic agents may be useful as an adjunct to endoluminal and conventional surgical management of vascular lesions.

Complications of thrombolytic therapy include allergic reactions; localized bleeding and bruising; systemic fibrinolysis causing diffuse hemorrhage, gastrointestinal hemorrhage, or cerebral bleeding; and embolism of dislodged clot to distal arteries.

Endovascular Implants

Vascular stents have three basic designs—stainless steel spring-loaded stents, thermally expanded memory metal stents, and balloon-expandable stents. The latter is the most popular type because it can be inserted during balloon angioplasty.

Stents are most beneficial in large-diameter, high-flow vessels, such as the iliac arteries and veins and superior vena cava. The value of stents is to manage acute reclosure of angioplasties because of residual thrombotic material, flaps, dissections, or recoil of the vessel wall. Use of stents can save patients whose coronary balloon angioplasties close abruptly by restoring patency and preventing myocardial infarction. Balloon angioplasty, with and without stenting, has been proposed as an alternative to carotid endarterectomy, and there is considerable interest in prospective randomized trials.

Vascular lesions can be repaired with intraluminal devices deployed by catheter delivery systems. The prosthesis is fixed in the arterial lumen with an intravascular stent (Fig. 78-5). Transluminal placement of a prosthetic graft-stent can be used to manage lesions such as thoracic aortic aneurysms or dissections. Studies regarding the efficacy of various devices for endovascular aortic abdominal aneurysm repair are ongoing.

INTRALUMINAL IMAGING TECHNIQUES

Imaging is needed to guide devices through high-resistance, occlusive lesions during angioplasty. A high degree of precision is required to enable passage of devices

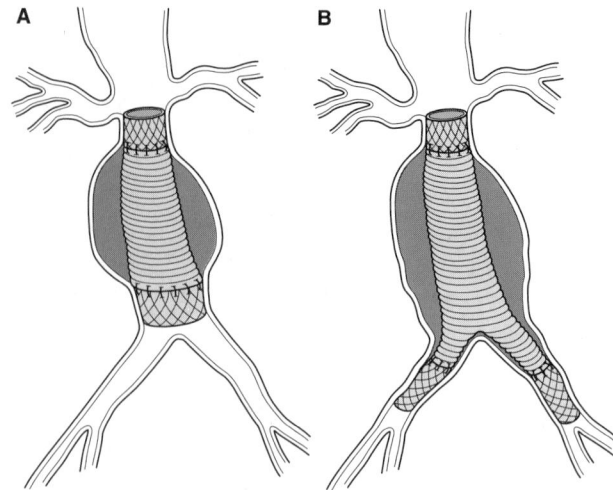

Figure 78-5. Schematic of an intraluminal prosthesis for treatment of abdominal aortic aneurysms in tubular (*A*) and bifurcated (*B*) configurations. Fixation at the ends of the prostheses is by intravascular metal stents.

through a vessel without causing perforation or a false aneurysm.

Cinefluoroscopy

Cinefluoroscopy often is used to perform endovascular procedures. It provides a detailed outline of the location and severity of stenoses and occlusions and is used to guide devices and determine the success of interventional procedures.

Digital subtraction angiography (DSA) increases contrast-material sensitivity and allows detection of low levels of iodinated contrast agent. Many digital units have freeze-frame and road-mapping features that allow superimposition of a subtracted contrast image of a vessel on a live fluoroscopic image.

Cinefluoroscopy is limited as a diagnostic and therapeutic guidance method during endovascular procedures, because atherosclerotic occlusions of arteries develop with eccentric positioning within the vessel lumen in most coronary and peripheral lesions. Because of the asymmetric location of the residual lumen, contrast radiography varies in estimation of percentage of luminal stenosis, because it depicts the vessel in only one dimension. An additional consequence of the eccentric positioning of atherosclerotic lesions is that angiography does not depict the transmural component of a lesion.

Angioscopy

Angioscopy is endoscopic examination of the luminal anatomy of blood vessels. It is used to establish the diagnosis and cause of vascular diseases, to evaluate the technical accuracy of vascular reconstruction, and to visualize intraluminal instrumentation.

Percutaneous angioscopy is used to define the mechanisms and accuracy of angioplasty and to evaluate vessel trauma when angiograms provide equivocal information. Access to the lumen is obtained by means of passage of the scope through an introducer catheter. Control of proximal blood flow in the area being examined can be achieved by means of inflation of a balloon on the tip of the catheter. Rapid flow of irrigating solution through the delivery catheter is required to control blood from collateral vessels.

Angioscopic Thrombectomy

Embolectomy and thrombectomy of peripheral vessels are enhanced with angioscopy. Unless the whole length of a vessel is occluded, the angioscope can be introduced through an arteriotomy to allow inspection of the lumen, definition of the site and extent of thrombosis or embolism, and determination whether there is atherosclerotic disease. Fogarty catheters are passed beside the angioscope, if the arterial lumen is large enough to accommodate both devices. Balloon inflation and detachment and removal of thrombus and debris are visually monitored.

Direct visual observation of the degree of balloon inflation is important because it determines the amount of balloon distention needed to remove the lesion without injury to the vessel wall. Balloon catheters often slide over thrombi that adhere to the wall, leaving large fragments that may or may not be removed with repeated passes and that often are not depicted on completion arteriograms.

When adherent thrombus is found, retrieval is attempted by means of positioning the balloon just distal to the clot and oscillating it back and forth over the site. If this is not successful, one must decide whether further attempts at extraction are warranted with other instruments, such as a flexible grasping forceps, rotary atherectomy device, or vascular brush. An alternative is intraoperative use of fibrinolytic agents.

When thromboembolectomy is considered complete, a final angioscopic inspection is made of the entire artery. Angiographic examination of the smaller runoff vessels is performed with injection of contrast medium through the fluid channel of the angioscope before the scope is withdrawn. An advantage of angioscopy is that complications and technical errors, such as retained thrombus or intimal flaps, can be corrected while the arterial lumen is open and before blood flow is restored.

In prosthetic grafts, extensive buildup of neointimal hyperplasia may be difficult to differentiate from chronic thrombus. Instruments such as forceps, curettes, and brushes to extract intraluminal lesions can be used more safely in prostheses than in native vessel. Inspection of the distal anastomosis is important because this is often the site of hyperplastic stenosis. Twists or kinks of the graft can be identified by means of angioscopic inspection.

During angioscopic thrombectomy, infusion of irrigating fluid simulates blood flow, giving a dynamic representation of potential flaps and loose debris. Sometimes severe dissection or atherosclerotic stenosis or occlusion identified with endoscopy cannot be managed with an endoluminal technique. The best therapy then is to perform immediate vascular bypass rather than persist with unproductive attempts at thrombectomy.

Angioscopy-assisted In Situ Vein Bypass

Being able to see the completeness of a valvulotomy during in situ vein bypass improves the accuracy of the procedure and reduces operative time by ensuring complete incompetence of valve cusps. A valvulotome is inserted through a side branch of the upper segment of the saphenous vein or through the venous lumen at the distal end. It is passed proximally from the distal vein through the most proximal valve, and the angioscope is inserted proximally and passed distally until the valvulotome can be seen at the valve site. The competency of valve cusps is tested under direct vision by means of distention of the vein with saline infusion and compression of the venous lumen with external pressure. As valve cusps are serially disrupted, the valvulotome and angioscope are advanced distally to the next valve.

Intraluminal identification of tributary veins during the procedure can help limit dissection and isolation of the vein and prevent tears in the vein caused by hooking a side branch with the valvulotome. During the procedure, extreme care must be taken to prevent damage to the vein by the intraluminal instruments.

Angioscopic Monitoring of Angioplasty Procedures

Angioscopy is better than arteriography in monitoring angioplasty because it removes the hazards of radiation exposure and contrast-material reactions and allows immediate detection and correction of technical complications. Angioscopic inspection under magnification and video control enables placement of angioplasty devices without deviation into collateral vessels. Angioscopy after angioplasty is helpful in determination of adequacy of recanalization and inspection of the surface for fragments.

Angioscopic inspection of the treated arteries often shows intimal flaps, mural thrombus, balloon dilation cracks, and other intraluminal features not apparent with angiography. An additional benefit of angioscopy during angioplasty is that the examination is conducted before restoration of blood flow and may help prevent embolism of arterial wall or thrombus fragments.

Intravascular Ultrasound

Intravascular US generates images of the transmural anatomy of blood vessels. US images are generated from piezoelectric transducers by means of rotation of an echotransducer or a mirror on the tip of a catheter or by means of scanning an array of stationary elements.

Intraluminal US can be performed in any procedure in which introduction of a 5F-9F catheter is possible. The modality can be used to identify intraluminal thrombus, intimal flaps, and arterial wall dissections. In muscular arteries, distinct layers of the vessel wall may be visible; the lumen and adventitia are more echogenic than the media.

The intravascular US features of plaques are as follows: hypoechoic images denote a deposit of lipid, soft echoes reflect fibromuscular tissue (intimal proliferation) and lesions that consist of fibromuscular tissue and diffusely dispersed lipid, bright echoes denote collagen-rich fibrous tissue, and bright echoes with shadowing behind the lesion represent calcium.

During intravascular US, careful positioning of catheter tips and appropriate ratios of probe size to vessel size are required to optimize visualization. Image quality is best when the catheter is perpendicular to the vessel wall; minor angulations may affect image quality. Eccentric positioning makes the near wall appear more echogenic and thicker than the far wall.

The benefits of intravascular US are that it helps define the distribution of disease within the arterial lumen by allowing visualization of transmural anatomy, and provides cross-sectional information about luminal and wall structure before, during, and after catheter-based interventions.

SUGGESTED READING

Cavaye DM, White RA. Intravascular ultrasound imaging. New York, Raven Press, 1993.

Chuter T, Donayre C, White R, eds. Endoluminal vascular prostheses. Boston, Little, Brown, 1995.

Clagett GP, Genton E, Salzmon E. Antithrombotic therapy in peripheral vascular disease. Chest 1989;95:1285.

Diethrich EB. Endovascular techniques for abdominal aortic occlusions. Int Angiol 1993;12:270.

Glagov S, Weisenberg E, Zarins C, et al. Compensatory enlargement of human atherosclerotic coronary arteries. N Engl J Med 1987;316:1371.

Johnson KW. Balloon angioplasty: predictive factors for long-term success. Semin Vasc Surg 1989;2:113.

Ouriel K, Shortell CK, DeWeese JA, et al. A comparison of thrombolytic therapy with operative revascularization in the initial treatment of acute peripheral arterial ischemia. J Vasc Surg 1994;19:1021.

Palmaz J, Rivera F, Encarnacion C. Intravascular stents. In: Whittemore A, et al, eds. Advances in vascular surgery. St. Louis, Mosby-Year Book, 1993:107.

Zimmerman JH, Fogarty TJ. Adjunctive intraoperative dilatation (angioplasty). In: Wilson SE, Veith F, Hobson R, et al., eds. Vascular surgery: principles and practice. New York, McGraw-Hill, 1986:297.

Occlusive Disease Involving Specific Vascular Territories

ESSENTIALS OF SURGERY: SCIENTIFIC PRINCIPLES AND PRACTICE, edited by Lazar J. Greenfield, Michael W. Mulholland, Keith T. Oldham, Gerald B. Zelenock, and Keith D. Lillemoe. Lippincott–Raven Publishers, Philadelphia, © 1997.

CHAPTER 79

CEREBROVASCULAR OCCLUSIVE DISEASE

LOUIS M. MESSINA AND GERALD B. ZELENOCK

Stroke is the third most common cause of death in the United States, and atherosclerotic occlusive disease of the extracranial arteries is the most common cause of stroke. Of the patients who survive stroke, two-thirds are disabled by and one-third need prolonged hospitalization because of paralysis, blindness, and aphasia. Risk factors for the development of carotid atherosclerosis are the same as those for coronary artery disease—age, hypertension, diabetes mellitus, hyperlipidemia, hypercoaguable states, family history, and tobacco use.

ANATOMY

Because of the high oxygen requirement of neural tissue, the brain has a rich blood supply. Although the brain constitutes only 2% of total body weight, it uses 17% of cardiac output and 20% of the available oxygen supply. The implication of the high oxygen requirement is that necrosis of neural tissue can occur within minutes of loss of arterial circulation.

The ascending aorta originates from the left ventricle and courses anteriorly in the mediastinum. The branches of the aortic arch are the brachiocephalic artery, the left common carotid artery, and the left subclavian artery. These arteries supply the head and neck, both upper extremities, and the torso.

The aortic arch crosses the upper mediastinum obliquely from right anterior to left posterior. The *brachiocephalic artery* is the first and most anterior branch of the aortic arch. Beneath the head of the right clavicle, the brachiocephalic bifurcates to form the *right subclavian artery* and the *right common carotid artery*. The *left common carotid artery* originates within 1 cm of the brachiocephalic artery

and courses posteriorly into the base of the left side of the neck. In some people, the left common carotid artery originates directly from the brachiocephalic artery. The *left subclavian artery* originates from its posterior location at the distal end of the aortic arch.

The brain is supplied by the paired *internal carotid arteries* anteriorly and the *vertebral arteries* posteriorly (Fig. 79-1). The carotid arteries supply 80% to 90% of total cerebral blood flow, and the vertebral arteries supply 10% to 20%.

The *common carotid artery* bifurcates at the angle of the mandible into the internal and external carotid arteries. The branches of *external carotid artery* include the ascending pharyngeal, which supplies the hypopharynx and oropharynx; the superior thyroid; the lingual; the occipital; and the posterior auricular. The terminal branches are the internal maxillary and superficial temporal arteries.

The *internal carotid artery* has four segments: cervical, intrapetrosal, intracavernous, and supraclinoid. The cervical, extracranial portion of the internal carotid artery has no branches. The intracavernous and supraclinoid portions are called the *carotid siphon*. The first branch of internal carotid artery is the ophthalmic artery. The supraclinoid portion of the internal carotid artery gives rise to the branches of internal carotid artery, including the ophthalmic, posterior communicating, and anterior choroidal arteries.

The internal carotid artery bifurcates into its terminal branches: the anterior cerebral and the middle cerebral arteries. The *anterior communicating artery* joins the anterior cerebral arteries from their respective hemispheres. The *posterior communicating arteries* are continuous with the posterior cerebral branches of the *basilar artery*, and connect the internal carotid system with the vertebrobasilar system via the posterior communicating artery, thus forming the circle of Willis (Fig. 79-2). Variations in the anatomy of the circle of Willis occur in a large segment of the population.

The *vertebral arteries* originate from the first portion of the subclavian artery and enter the transverse cervical process at the level of the sixth cervical vertebra and ascend in the transverse foramen, eventually piercing the posterior allantoid-occipital membrane and coursing into the posterior fossa through the foramen magnum. The vertebral arteries course along the lateral border of the medulla and unite to form the *basilar artery*. The extracranial portion of the vertebral artery has segmental spinal and muscular branches. The basilar artery terminates as the right and

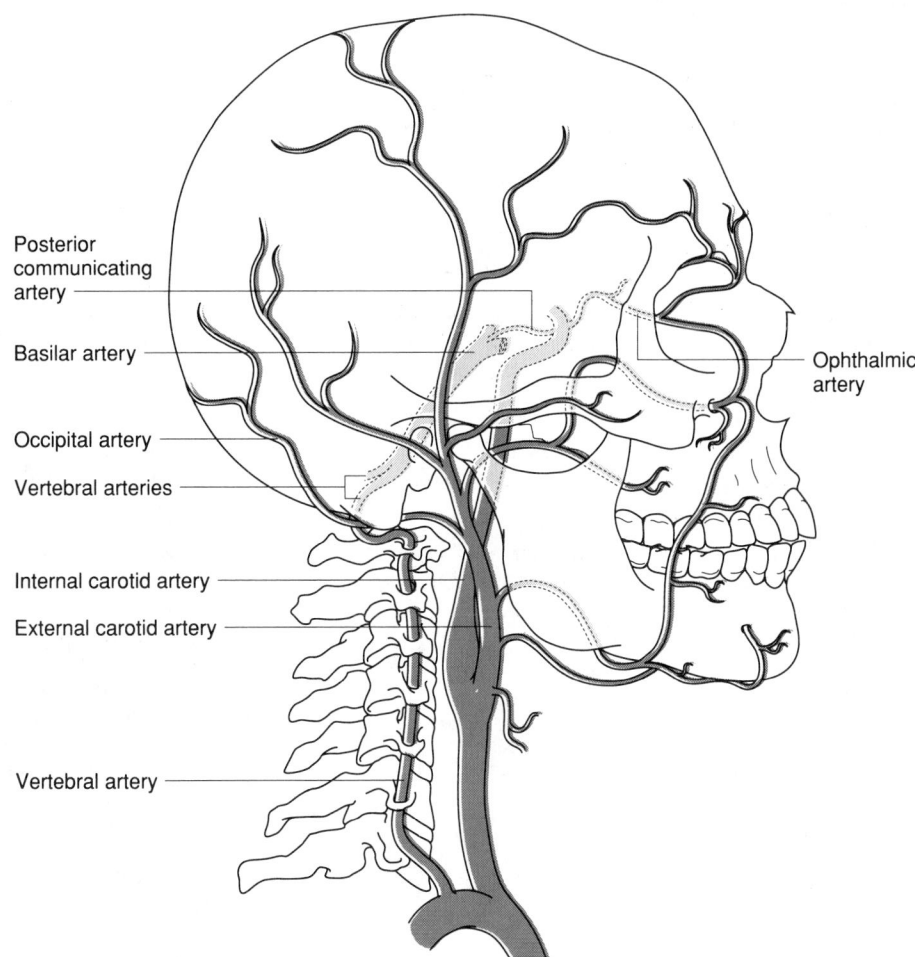

Figure 79-1. The arterial blood supply to the brain is from the paired carotid and vertebral arteries. Extensive extracranial collaterals between the external carotid and vertebral systems allow antegrade perfusion when either vessel has a proximal occlusion. Likewise, periorbital collateral allows retrograde flow through the ophthalmic artery to the internal carotid artery in the presence of a cervical internal carotid artery occlusion. Extensive side-to-side collateral exists between the right and the left external carotids and the right and left vertebral arteries.

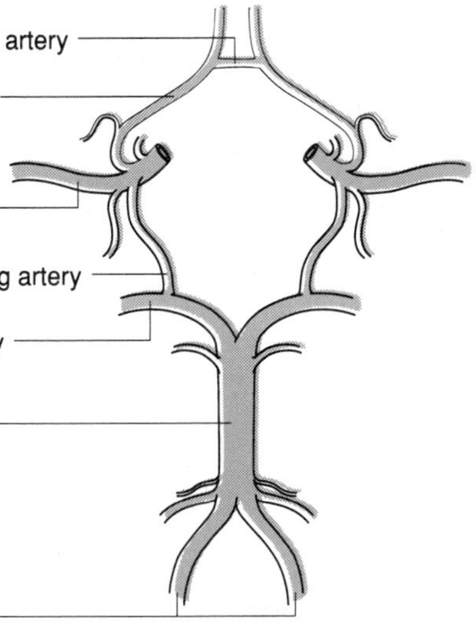

Figure 79-2. The circle of Willis is a highly efficient intracranial collateral network; however, multiple important variations occur, and an incomplete circle producing an isolated hemisphere is not uncommon.

left *posterior cerebral arteries,* from which originate the posterior communicating arteries of the circle of Willis.

A number of *collateral pathways* exist between cerebral arteries. These collaterals are important sources of arterial flow to the brain when arterial occlusive disease develops in one of the four main arteries supplying blood to the brain. Communication between the external carotid artery branches and the ophthalmic artery branch of internal carotid artery is the most important collateral network.

The vertebral artery gives rise to numerous muscular branches in the neck. If the proximal vertebral artery is occluded, collateral arteries from the external carotid may anastomose to the distal vertebral artery via these branches. A person who experiences common carotid artery occlusion may receive blood flow from the vertebral artery through the external carotid artery branches into the internal carotid artery.

PATHOPHYSIOLOGY

The causes of stroke are listed in Table 79-1. Atherosclerosis is the most common cause. Less common processes include aneurysms of the internal carotid artery; anatomic abnormalities such as coils and kinks; fibromuscular dysplasia; Takayasu arteritis; and temporal arteritis.

Atherosclerosis causes most symptoms of cerebrovascular insufficiency (Table 79-2). The cause of atherosclerosis in the cerebral arterial circulation, or any portion of the

Table 79-1. CAUSES OF CEREBRAL ISCHEMIA AND INFARCTION

ISCHEMIC

Atherothromboembolic

High-grade stenoses and occlusions
Emboli
Plaque
Platelet-fibrin debris
Intraplaque hemorrhage

Cardioembolic

Arrhythmias (atrial fibrillation; other arrhythmias)
Myocardial infarction with mural thrombus
Mitral valve prolapse; calcified annulus
Rheumatic heart disease (valvular, nonvalvular)
Prosthetic heart valves
Other (myopathy, atrial myxoma, subacute bacterial endocarditis, paradoxical emboli)

Systemic

Cardiac arrest and resuscitation
Profound shock
Cardiopulmonary bypass

Venous Thromboses

Dural venous sinuses
Bilateral jugular vein occlusions

Miscellaneous Causes

Lacunar infarcts
Lipohyalinosis
Fibrinoid necrosis
Charcot-Bouchard aneurysms
Migraine and vasospasm
Diabetes
Moyamoya
Kawasaki syndrome
Amyloid degeneration
Fibromuscular disease
Giant cell arteritis
Spontaneous dissections
Trauma (extracranial cerebral vessels)
  Blunt
  Penetrating
Hypercoaguable states
Binswanger encephalopathy
Substance abuse

HEMORRHAGIC

Intraparenchymal Hemorrhage

Hypertensive encephalopathy
Amyloid angiography
Arteriovenous malformation
Trauma

Subarachnoid Hemorrhage

Berry aneurysms
Arteriovenous malformation
Trauma

EXTRACRANIAL

Atherosclerosis
  Great vessels
  Carotid artery
Fibromuscular dysplasia
Trauma
Aortic aneurysms
  Dissecting
  Atherosclerotic
  Traumatic
Takayasu panarteritis
Temporal arteritis
Carotid dissections
  Spontaneous
  Trauma associated
Carotid aneurysms

(Modified from Zelenock GB. The brain. In: Clinical ischemic syndromes: mechanisms and consequences of tissue injury. St Louis, CV Mosby, 1990)

systemic arterial circulation, is not understood. Atherosclerosis is a segmental disease, usually developing at areas of local turbulence, such as vessel bifurcations, and causes focal vessel wall injury. The carotid bifurcation is the most common location of atherosclerosis in the cerebral circulation. Turbulent blood flow at the carotid bifurcation produces areas of low shear stress and increased particle residence time.

Atherosclerotic plaque appears as a fatty streak, which is largely an intimal lesion, characterized by fat deposition and some mononuclear and foam cell infiltration. Fatty streaks do not cause hemodynamically significant steno-

ses, and not all fatty streaks develop into complex plaques. As plaques enlarge, they may intermittently ulcerate or cause intraplaque hemorrhage; both processes can cause emboli or thrombosis of the artery.

Mature atherosclerotic plaques are characterized by endothelial cell damage and denudation, intimal hyperplasia due to smooth muscle cell proliferation, and gradual increased deposition of collagen matrix and extensive intracellular and extracellular lipid accumulation. Mature atherosclerotic plaques are usually covered by a fibrous cap. Disruption of the fibrous cap can cause a plaque to become symptomatic. Fibrous caps can be disrupted by progressive growth of the atherosclerotic lesion, increased blood flow velocity and shear stress, hemorrhage into the plaque, or rupture of vasa vasorum.

Loss of a fibrous cap due to intraplaque hemorrhage or surface disruption due to mechanical forces causes a loss of endothelial cell coverage, exposing the underlying necrotic core of the plaque to the circulating blood. These changes promote platelet deposition and thrombus formation on the ulcerated surface. Disrupted mature, complex plaques may cause stroke by means of embolization of atheromatous debris or platelet-fibrin aggregates. Thrombosis of the artery can cause ischemic necrosis when there is insufficient collateral blood flow.

Stroke due to cerebrovascular disease occurs by two distinct mechanisms—ischemia due to low-flow states and embolism. Cerebral *ischemia* due to low-flow states is the result of development of hemodynamically significant stenosis, often involving multiple cerebral arteries, or of stenosis in an artery supplying a vascular territory for which is there is a poor collateral network. Most strokes caused by carotid artery occlusive disease are due to cholesterol or platelet-fibrin *emboli* that dislodge from atherosclerotic plaques within the extracranial carotid artery and occlude distal branches of the internal carotid artery.

CLINICAL PRESENTATION

The common presentations of cerebrovascular occlusive disease are transient ischemic attack (TIA) and hemispheric stroke.

Table 79-2. CLASSIFICATION OF SYMPTOMS

HEMISPHERIC

Contralateral hemiparesis
Contralateral paresthesias or hemisensory changes
Ipsilateral monocular visual changes
Aphasia

NONHEMISPHERIC

Vertigo
Ataxia
Diplopia
Bilateral visual symptoms
Shifting pareses or paresthesias
Drop attacks
Dysarthria
Syncope
Dizziness
Light-headedness
Decreased mentation
Headache
Personality change
Tinnitus
Seizures

Transient Ischemic Attack

A TIA is a focal neurologic deficit of sudden onset that resolves completely within 24 hours. TIAs due to atheroemboli usually last <15 minutes. TIAs can occur as transient hemispheric ischemic attacks or transient mononuclear blindness. *Transient hemispheric attacks* present as contralateral motor and sensory deficits or as a pure motor or pure sensory deficit. *Transient mononuclear blindness* (amaurosis fugax) is transient loss of vision due to mechanical obstruction of a branch of the retinal artery.

A TIA can affect the distal distribution of the posterior circulation of the brain, causing transient vertebrobasilar insufficiency. This can present as binocular visual loss; drop attacks, in which the patient does not lose consciousness but collapses to the floor; dysarthria; vertigo; dysphasia; incoordination; and other signs of cerebellar insufficiency.

The differential diagnosis of TIA includes cerebral tumor, hypoglycemia, hyponatremia, hypercalcemia, and hepatic or renal failure. Vasospasm, particularly associated with migraine headache, can present as transient ischemia.

Stroke

A stroke is an acute neurologic deficit that lasts >24 hours. Like TIAs, most strokes are due to embolic occlusion of a branch of the middle cerebral artery by atheromatous debris or a platelet-fibrin aggregate. The characteristics of strokes according to area affected are summarized in Table 79-3.

Lacunar strokes are usually characterized by pure motor or sensory dysfunction in the contralateral limb in patients with hypertension. *Lacunar* describes the appearance of the infarcted tissue within the brain at gross examination. Lacunar strokes are caused by disease of arterioles. *Vertebrobasilar strokes* cause ipsilateral cranial nerve deficits; contralateral sensorimotor deficits; and signs of cerebellar insufficiency, including ataxia, vertigo, nystagmus, diplopia, and drop attacks.

Table 79-3. **CHARACTERISTICS OF STROKE ACCORDING TO DISTRIBUTION OF AFFECTED ARTERY**

Artery	Characteristics of Stroke
Middle cerebral	Sensorimotor deficits in the contralateral limbs Homonymous hemianopsia
Internal carotid	Contralateral sensorimotor deficit more pronounced in proximal than distal limb Proiminent visual field defect Aphasia Partial inattention
Anterior cerebral	Weakness, paralysis, numbness, or tingling contralateral limbs, sparing of the face Dyspraxia Abnormalities of higher cerebral function due to frontal lobe involvement manifested by the presence of a grasp reflex, behavior disorder, poor concentration, and slowness of response
Anterior choroidal	Contralateral hemiplegia, hypesthesia, and homonymous hemianopsia

DIAGNOSIS

Examination

Diagnosis of symptomatic cerebrovascular occlusive disease centers on *neurologic examination* performed before any diagnostic studies. It is crucial to differentiate focal from nonfocal neurologic deficits, such as dizziness. The history and examination localize the area of cerebral ischemia responsible for the neurologic deficit. After the neurologic examination, a complete *physical examination* is conducted to determine the presence of vascular occlusive disease in the coronary or peripheral arteries and to define other risk factors for stroke, such as acute arrhythmia.

Ultrasound

Color-flow duplex scanning entails real-time B-mode ultrasound (US) and color-enhanced pulsed Doppler flow measurement to determine the extent of the carotid stenosis, localize the disease, and determine the presence or absence of calcification within the plaque. Carotid duplex scanning is most accurate in the estimation of carotid artery stenosis that causes >50% reduction in luminal diameter.

Transcranial Doppler US takes advantage of the thinness of the temporal bone to focus a directional low-frequency Doppler probe on the anterior, middle, and posterior cerebral arteries. This modality is of value to patients experiencing vasospasm after subarachnoid hemorrhage. For patients with cerebrovascular disease, transcranial Doppler US complements duplex scanning by allowing assessment of the presence of intraarterial stenoses and patterns of collateral flow.

Angiography

Angiography is the standard for the diagnosis of cerebrovascular disease because it allows complete and detailed visualization of the intracranial and extracranial arterial circulation. The disadvantages are that angiography is painful and has risks, such as dye allergy, renal toxicity, chronic renal insufficiency, and neurologic complications such as stroke. Digital subtraction angiography (DSA) reduces the need for selective carotid artery catheterization and thus reduces risk for neurologic complications.

Computed Tomography

Computed tomography (CT) of the brain is valuable for patients with TIA or stroke. Contrast-enhanced CT can be used to assess density changes, the presence of edema, the presence of mass effect, and the location and extent of a stroke. CT also helps one differentiate between cerebral hemorrhage and infarction. Hemorrhage is associated with areas of increased density on a CT scan. Infarction is associated with areas of decreased density that do not appear until at least 8 hours after the occurrence of the stroke.

Magnetic Resonance Imaging

Magnetic resonance imaging (MRI) and angiography (MRA) are highly sensitive techniques for the evaluation of symptomatic cerebrovascular disease. MRI is more sensitive than CT in the detection of acute stroke. MRI can depict a stroke immediately after the infarction, whereas CT cannot. CT is more useful in identifying cerebral hemorrhage. MRA allows evaluation of the extra- and intracranial cerebral circulation. MRA is inferior to conventional angiography in determination of extent of stenosis.

MANAGEMENT

Medical Treatment

Carotid artery occlusive disease almost always is caused by atherosclerosis, a systemic disease. It is important to modify risk factors to prevent progression of disease. The most important risk factor for stroke that can be controlled is hypertension. Cessation of smoking, management of lipid disorders, attainment of ideal body weight, and regular exercise are undertaken.

No drug has been found to reduce risk for stroke among patients with asymptomatic carotid artery occlusive disease. There is no definitive evidence that systemic antico-agulant therapy reduces risk for stroke among patients with carotid artery occlusive disease who experience a TIA and stroke. Aspirin, by reducing platelet adhesion and aggregation, reduces morbidity and mortality from symptomatic coronary artery occlusive disease. Thus, when stroke and death are endpoints in studies of cerebrovascular disease, aspirin seems beneficial.

Surgical Treatment

The indications for reconstruction of the cerebrovascular arteries are hemispheric TIA, stroke that leaves minimal residual neurologic deficit, and high-grade asymptomatic

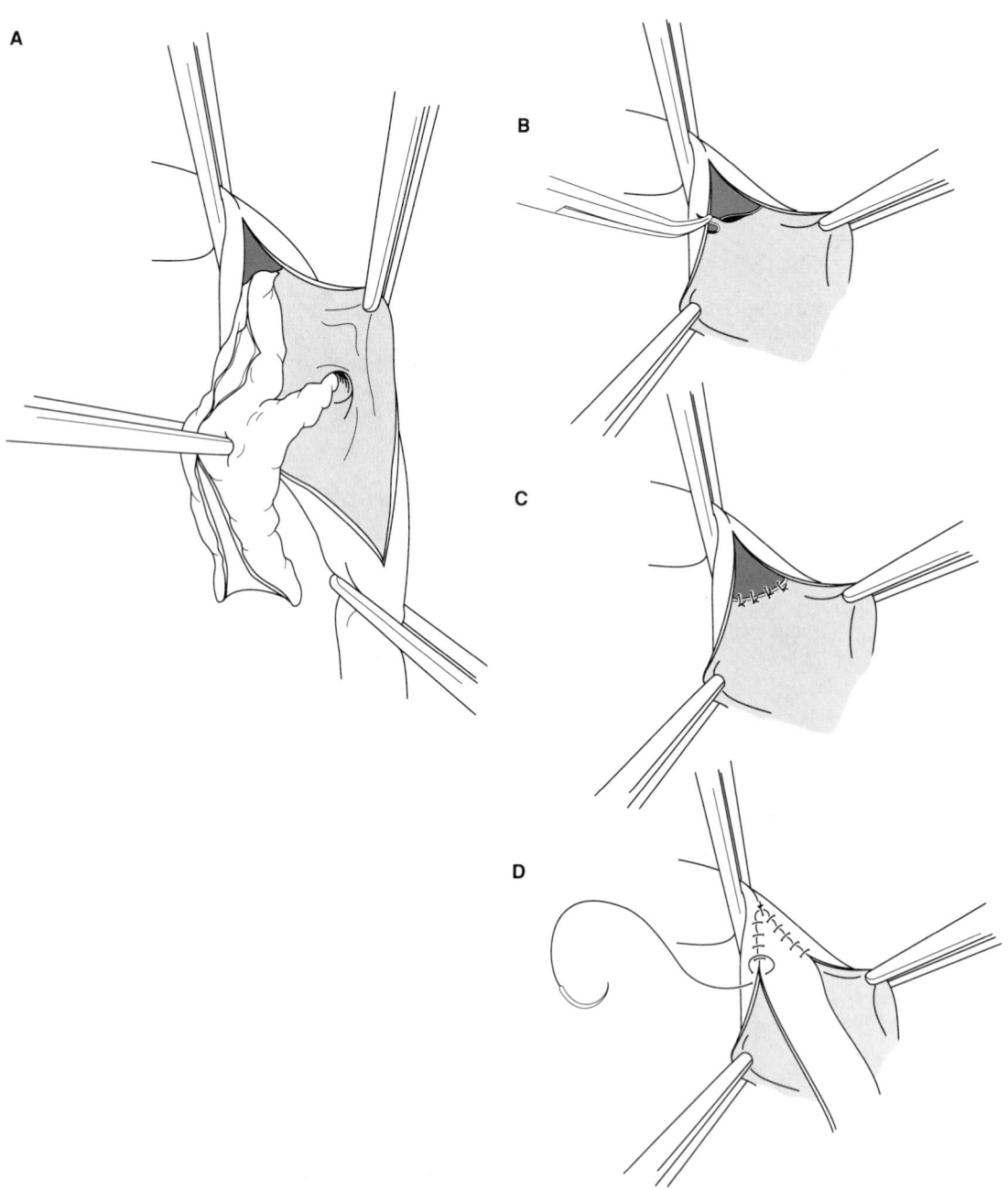

Figure 79-3. Carotid endarterectomy. (*A*) The atheroma is transected proximally and teased out of the external and internal carotid arteries. The distal internal carotid endpoint must be directly visualized to ensure that it feathers into normal intima. (*B*) Any loose pieces of atheroma or strands of media are removed. (*C*) If necessary, the distal normal intima is tacked in place with vertically oriented stitches. (*D*) Although direct closure is often possible, patch angioplasty may be required when the carotid is small or in cases of reoperation.

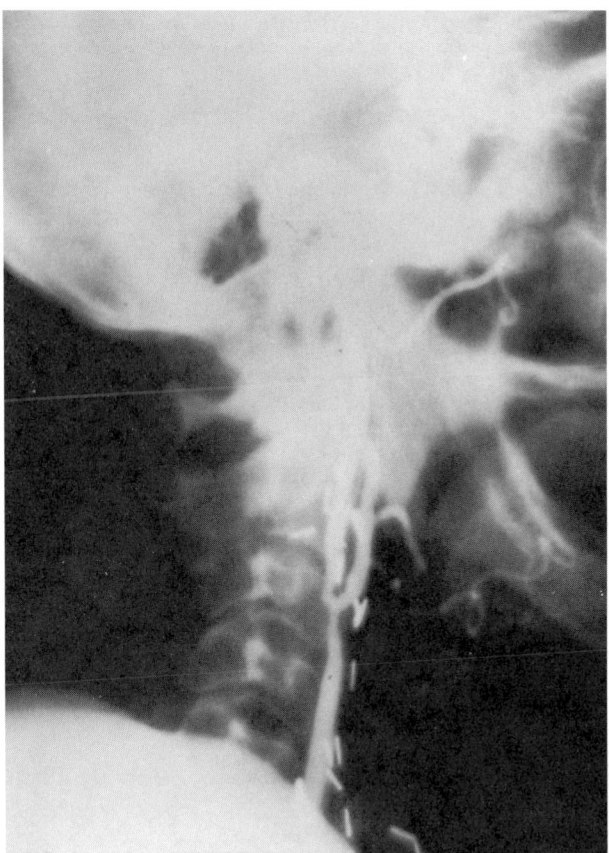

Figure 79-4. Angiogram showing recurrent carotid stenosis.

ing sutures are placed to avoid a raising a flap during restoration of blood flow.

The carotid arteriotomy is closed with a running suture. If the internal carotid artery is small, patch angioplasty can be performed (Fig. 79-3). The patency of the endarterectomy is assessed with continuous-wave Doppler B-mode US or intraoperative arteriography.

Complications of Carotid Endarterectomy

Neurologic Complications. *Stroke* can occur during or after carotid endarterectomy. Mechanisms include inadequate collateral blood flow to the brain during temporary internal carotid artery occlusion, embolization during dissection of the carotid artery, or embolism or thrombosis of the reconstruction during the early postoperative period. *Thrombosis* after carotid endarterectomy is caused by sudden intimal dissection due to a loose flap or inadequate distal endarterectomy endpoint. *Embolization* is caused by formation of platelet aggregates on the surface of the endarterectomized vessel. Stroke also can be caused by *intracerebral hemorrhage,* which seems to be more common among patients with multivessel involvement preoperatively; it tends to occur on the second or third postoperative day.

Postoperative *cranial nerve dysfunction* occurs in a large number of patients undergoing carotid endarterectomy. Common cranial nerve injuries include dysfunction of the recurrent laryngeal nerve (causing hoarseness), dysfunction of the hypoglossal nerve (causing deviation of the tongue toward the side of the injury), and superior laryngeal nerve dysfunction (causing easy fatigability of the voice).

carotid artery stenosis. Carotid endarterectomy is highly beneficial to patients with recent hemispheric or retinal TIAs or nondisabling strokes and ipsilateral high-grade carotid stenosis. When symptomatic high-grade carotid arterial stenosis is identified, evaluation for surgical treatment must begin immediately.

Technique of Carotid Endarterectomy

Anesthesia for carotid endarterectomy can be general endotracheal anesthesia, regional cervical block, or local anesthesia. Surgical exposure of the carotid artery can be achieved through an incision along the medial border of the sternocleidomastoid muscle or an oblique transverse incision through a skin crease. During dissection and mobilization of the common carotid artery and its branches, it is important that dissection be gentle and manipulation of the carotid bulb be minimal to prevent embolization from the atherosclerotic plaque.

After heparin is administered, the carotid artery is occluded, and a lateral arteriotomy is made from just proximal to the plaque in the common carotid artery to just beyond the distal extent of the plaque in the internal carotid artery (Fig. 79-3). The cleavage plane for the endarterectomy is at the thickest part of the plaque, usually in the carotid bulb. This plane is extended proximally and circumferentially, and the proximal plaque is transected. As the endarterectomy extends toward the internal carotid artery, the transition zone of the plaque from within the deep media to the intima must be identified.

The operation is completed with eversion endarterectomy of the part of the plaque that extends into the external carotid artery. Any loose fragments of arterial wall are removed. If there is any residual shelf or loose intima, tack-

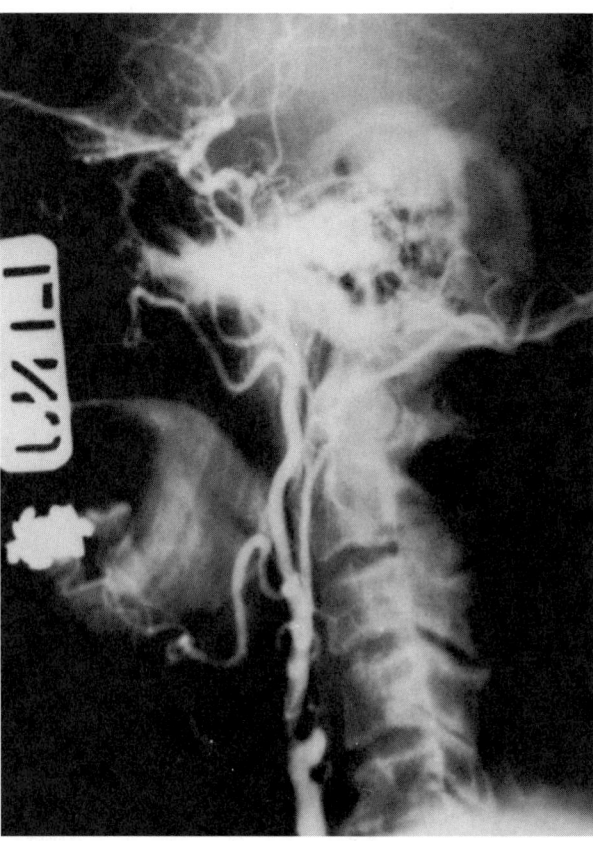

Figure 79-5. A totally occluded internal carotid artery with a residual stump may be a source of emboli. Note the periorbital collateral circulation.

Nonneurologic Complications. *Hemorrhage* can occur after carotid endarterectomy, mainly among patients undergoing perioperative aspirin therapy. *Hypotension* and *bradycardia* occur because of increased baroreceptor reflex activity during dissection of the carotid artery or stimulation of the sinus nerve after removal of a rigid atheromatous plaque. *Hypertension* may be caused by interruption of the carotid sinus nerve due to transection or changes in arterial wall compliance. Severe hypertension or hypotension is associated with increased risk for neurologic deficits. *Myocardial infarction* is the most common source of non−stroke-related morbidity and mortality after carotid endarterectomy.

Recurrent carotid stenosis (Fig. 79-4) is a common complication after carotid endarterectomy, but usually is not serious. Recurrent carotid stenosis that occurs within 6 months of the initial endarterectomy usually is due to intimal hyperplasia. It is characterized by proliferation of vascular smooth muscle and increased matrix deposition. When recurrent stenosis develops ≥2 years after endarterectomy, recurrent atherosclerosis is usually found at reoperation. Risk for recurrent carotid stenosis is higher among women and patients with hypercholesterolemia.

External Carotid Endarterectomy

External carotid endarterectomy is recommended for patients with ipsilateral internal carotid artery occlusion and evidence of retinal or hemispheric TIAs or stroke. Many of these patients have a large cul-de-sac in the proximal internal carotid artery that may serve as a source of emboli (Fig. 79-5).

Direct Aortic Arch Reconstruction

Atherosclerotic lesions at the origin of the great vessels can cause TIA or stroke. Most commonly involved is the brachiocephalic or left common carotid artery. When identified, these lesions can be repaired by means of direct reconstruction through a median sternotomy. For brachiocephalic artery lesions, an option is endarterectomy or aortobrachiocephalic bypass with a synthetic graft. Often it is necessary to undertake revascularization of both the brachiocephalic and left common carotid arteries.

Vertebral Artery Reconstruction

Atherosclerosis at the origin of the vertebral arteries can be symptomatic, causing TIA or stroke in the posterior cerebral circulation. When appropriate indications exist, the vertebral arteries can be reconstructed. Vertebral artery endarterectomy can be undertaken through an arteriotomy in the subclavian artery. The vertebral artery can be ligated at its origin and replanted into normal ipsilateral common carotid artery. Some distal vertebral artery reconstructions are accomplished with a carotid-vertebral bypass with saphenous vein.

Nonanatomic Bypass

Patients with atherosclerotic stenosis at the origin of the aortic arch vessels may have neurologic implications and symptoms related to ischemia of the upper extremities. Patients who cannot undergo direct aortic arch reconstruction can undergo a bypass, such as a subclavian-carotid, carotid-subclavian, axillary-axillary, carotid-carotid, or femoral-axillary. Synthetic grafts seem to have better patency than saphenous vein grafts.

SUGGESTED READING

CASANOVA Study Group. Carotid surgery vs medical therapy in asymptomatic carotid stenosis. N Engl J Med 1993;328:221.
European Carotid Surgery Trialists' Collaborative Group. MRC European Carotid Surgery Trial: interim results for symptomatic patients with severe (70−99%) or with mild (0−29%) carotid stenosis. Lancet 1991;337:1235.
Executive Committee for the Asymptomatic Carotid Atherosclerosis Study. Endarterectomy for asymptomatic carotid artery stenosis. JAMA 1995;273:1421.
Hobson RW II, Weiss DG, Fields WS, et al. Efficacy of carotid endarterectomy for asymptomatic carotid stenosis. N Engl J Med 1993;328:221.
Mayberg MR, Wilson SE, Yatsu F, et al., for the Veterans Affairs Cooperative Studies Program 309 Trialist Group. Carotid endarterectomy and prevention of cerebral ischemia in symptomatic carotid stenosis. JAMA 1991;266:3289.
McCann RL. Surgical management of carotid artery atherosclerotic disease. South Med J 1993;86:2S23.
Moneta GL, Edwards JM, Chitwood RW, et al. Correlation of North American Symptomatic Carotid endarterectomy trial (NASCET) angiographic definition of 70% to 99% internal carotid artery stenosis with duplex scanning. J Vasc Surg 1993;17:152.
Norris JW, Zhu CA. Silent stroke and carotid stenosis. Stroke 1992;23:483.
Ross R. The pathogenesis of atherosclerosis: a perspective for the 1990's. Nature 1993;362:801.
Selhub J, Jaques PF, Bostom AG, et al. Association between plasma homocysteine concentrations and extracranial carotid artery stenosis. N Engl J Med 1995;332:286.

ESSENTIALS OF SURGERY: SCIENTIFIC PRINCIPLES AND PRACTICE, edited by Lazar J. Greenfield, Michael W. Mulholland, Keith T. Oldham, Gerald B. Zelenock, and Keith D. Lillemoe. Lippincott−Raven Publishers, Philadelphia, © 1997.

CHAPTER 80

UPPER EXTREMITY OCCLUSIVE DISEASE

JAMES S.T. YAO

Upper-extremity arterial occlusive disease encompasses a wide spectrum of diseases that cause ischemic symptoms. Diagnosis requires a thorough history, careful physical examination, and liberal use of ancillary diagnostic tests. Surgical treatment depends on the location of the occlusive lesion and the nature of the underlying occlusive process. Proximal arterial lesions of the subclavian, axillary, and brachial arteries are amenable to surgical reconstruction as are some distal lesions.

DIAGNOSIS
History

The history is the most important initial step in the evaluation of upper extremity ischemia. The patient is asked about symptoms; occupational, pharmacologic, and athletic risk; and pertinent medical history (Table 80-1).

Symptoms

The presenting symptoms of upper-extremity occlusive disease include evidence of arterial emboli, Raynaud phenomenon, pain, and exercise-related forearm fatigue. Embolic symptoms include gangrene of the tips of the fingers, petechiae of the skin, splinter hemorrhages of the nail bed, and livedo reticularis.

Raynaud phenomenon is episodic digital color changes

Table 80-1. CONDITIONS AND RISKS FOR UPPER EXTREMITY ISCHEMIA

OCCUPATIONAL INJURY

Vibration syndrome
  Pneumatic tools
  Chain saws
  Grinders
Electrical burns
Hypothenar hammer syndrome
  Mechanical work or auto
    repair
  Lathe operation
  Carpentry
  Electrical work
Occupational acroosteolysis-
    polyvinylchloride
    exposure

ATHLETIC ACTIVITIES

Thoracic outlet compression
  Baseball pitching
  Kayaking
  Weight lifting
  Rowing
  Butterfly swimming
  Golfing
Hand ischemia
  Baseball catching
  Frisbee
  Karate
  Handball

PHARMACOLOGIC HISTORY

Ergot poisoning
β-Blockers
Drug abuse, cocaine use
Cytotoxic drugs
Dopamine overdose

MEDICAL CONDITIONS

Atherosclerosis
Arteritis
  Collagen disease
    Scleroderma
    Rheumatoid arteritis
    Systemic lupus
      erythematosus
    Dermatomyositis
  Allergic necrotizing arteritis
  Takayasu disease
  Giant cell arteritis
Blood dyscrasias
  Cold agglutinins
  Cryoglobulins
  Polycythemia vera
Behçet syndrome
Antiphospholipid syndrome
Thoracic outlet syndrome
Congenital arterial wall defects
  Pseudoxanthoma elasticum
  Ehlers-Danlos syndrome
Fibromuscular dysplasia
Iatrogenic injury
  Arterial blood gas and
    pressure monitoring
  Cardiac catheterization
  Arteriography
Frostbite
Renal transplantation and related
    problems
  Azotemic arteriopathy
  Hemodialysis shunts
Radiation
  Breast carcinoma
  Hodgkin disease
Aneurysms of the upper
    extremity

provoked by stimuli, such as cold or emotion. The digits exhibit pallor followed by cyanosis and reactive hyperemia. The changes in color from white to blue to red are caused by digital ischemia (due to vasospasm) followed by desaturation of hemoglobin (which produces cyanosis) and reactive hyperemia. Raynaud *phenomenon* is a secondary process; Raynaud *disease* is a primary disease without known cause. *Unilateral* Raynaud phenomenon suggests organic arterial occlusive disease. *Bilateral* symptoms are often due to systemic disease that causes vasospasm.

The diagnosis of primary Raynaud disease is made only after exclusion of all the etiologic factors in Table 80-1 and after symptoms persist for at least 2 years in the absence of other causal conditions. *Raynaud syndrome* is episodic vasospastic disease of the hands of any cause. It must be differentiated from acrocyanosis, which is painless, persistent, diffuse cyanosis of the fingers and hands.

Physical Examination

Physical examination includes the thoracic outlet and the entire upper extremity. Palpation of the supraclavicular region may help detect a subclavian aneurysm or cervical rib. Auscultation of the subclavian artery with a stethoscope placed just below the midclavicular region and listening for a bruit with the arm placed in neutral (or

abduction) and external rotation (or hyperabduction) help establish the diagnosis of thoracic outlet compression to the artery.

Pulse palpation begins with the subclavian artery in the supraclavicular fossa and continues with the axillary artery under the armpit, the brachial artery at the upper arm and elbow, and the radial and ulnar arteries at the wrist. A decreased or absent pulse at any site other than the supraclavicular fossa indicates arterial occlusion. A readily palpable pulse in the supraclavicular fossa can represent subclavian artery aneurysm.

The examination must include an *Allen test*. The examiner stands beside or facing the patient. The radial and ulnar arteries of one wrist are compressed by the examiner's fingers. The patient is asked to open and close the hand rapidly for 1 minute to empty blood from the hand and then to extend the fingers quickly. The radial or the ulnar artery is released, and the hand is observed for capillary refilling and return of color. The test is negative if refilling of the hand is complete within a short period (<6 seconds). If any portion of the hand does not blush, the arch lacks continuity. Hyperextension of the fingers must be avoided because it produces a false-positive result.

The palm is palpated for a pulsatile mass or excess scar tissue. Assessment of the patency of digital arteries by means of palpation is difficult and unreliable. Upper-extremity digital capillary refill is nearly instantaneous in healthy people.

Noninvasive Examination

Doppler ultrasound examination consists of audible signal interpretation, waveform recording with spectral analysis, and systolic pressure measurements. Bilateral examinations are performed for comparative purposes. Because many diseases of the hand are symmetric, the hand without symptoms often also has disease. This is especially true among patients with systemic disease that causes hand ischemia.

Because both the axillary and brachial arteries are superficial, they lend themselves to Doppler examination. Any change from normal signals (triphasic) to abnormal signals (monophasic) indicates the presence of an occlusive lesion. Between the elbow and wrist, arterial signals are difficult to obtain. At the wrist, both the radial and ulnar arteries again become superficial. Palpation of the ulnar artery can be difficult, and Doppler examination is helpful in determining the patency of this artery.

In the hand, Doppler examination of the palmar arches is performed best at the midthenar and hypothenar regions. The common digital vessels are examined at the base of the fingers at their division into the proper digital arteries, which lie along the shaft of the proximal phalanx of each finger. Waveform recording is useful in both analysis and record keeping.

For segmental upper-extremity pressures, a pneumatic cuff is placed on the upper arm, as in routine blood pressure recording. Brachial artery blood pressure reflects all proximal arteries and should be within 10 to 20 mmHg of that in the opposite extremity. A greater difference means innominate, subclavian, axillary, or brachial stenosis. If brachial artery occlusion is suspected, a pressure cuff is applied to the forearm and the pressure recorded in a similar manner and the radial artery used for signal detection. A pressure drop of 20 to 30 mmHg means obstruction distal to the brachial artery. For finger pressure measurement, a 2.5-cm cuff is placed at the base of the finger, and the return of Doppler signals after cuff deflation is monitored at the fingertip. Arterial occlusion distal to the palmar arch is defined by a pressure gradient between the fingers >15 mmHg or a wrist-to-digit difference of 30 mmHg.

The Doppler technique is valuable in determining palmar arch patency in a patient who is unconscious or is uncooperative during the Allen test. Before arterial line placement, this test may help avoid hand ischemia. In the modified Allen test, the Doppler probe is placed over the radial artery while the ulnar artery is compressed. If the signal disappears, the arch depends on the ulnar artery for supply. If the signal stays strong, the arch is complete. A similar maneuver is repeated over the ulnar artery while the radial artery is compressed.

Plethysmography is used to record finger pulse contours for analysis and to differentiate normal, obstructive, and vasospastic disease. *Duplex scanning* is helpful in establishing the diagnosis of aneurysms.

Laboratory Examination

In severe bilateral hand ischemia, a systemic cause of the arterial lesions is sought. Laboratory tests include these serologic, immunologic, and hematologic studies:

- Erythrocyte sedimentation rate (ESR)
- Rheumatoid factor

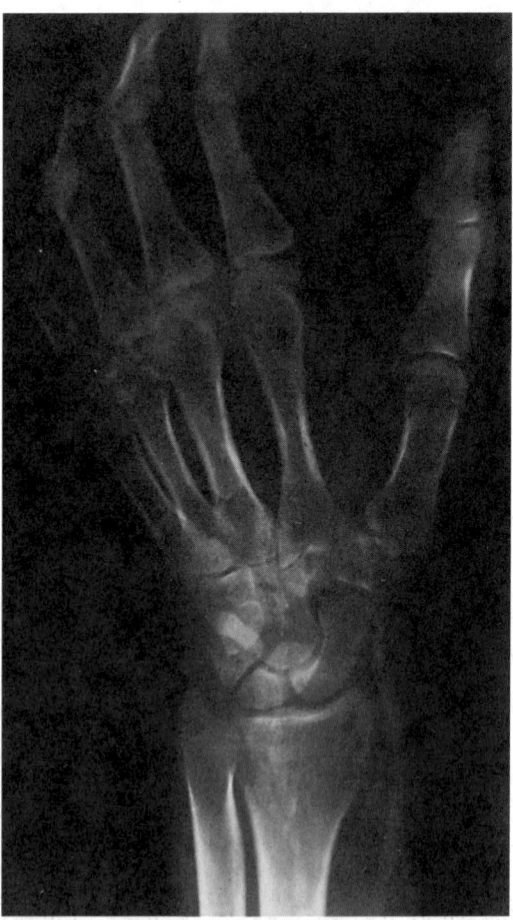

Figure 80-1. Typical appearance of azotemic arteriopathy (calciphylaxis) in a diabetic patient with a renal transplant. All digital arteries are distinctly seen on plain radiography. The radial artery has a pipestem appearance. An arteriogram shows multiple digital artery occlusions. (Yao JST. Arterial surgery of the upper extremity. In: Haimovici H, Callow AD, DePalma RG, et al, eds. Vascular surgery: principles and techniques, ed 3. Norwalk, CT, Appleton & Lange, 1989:863)

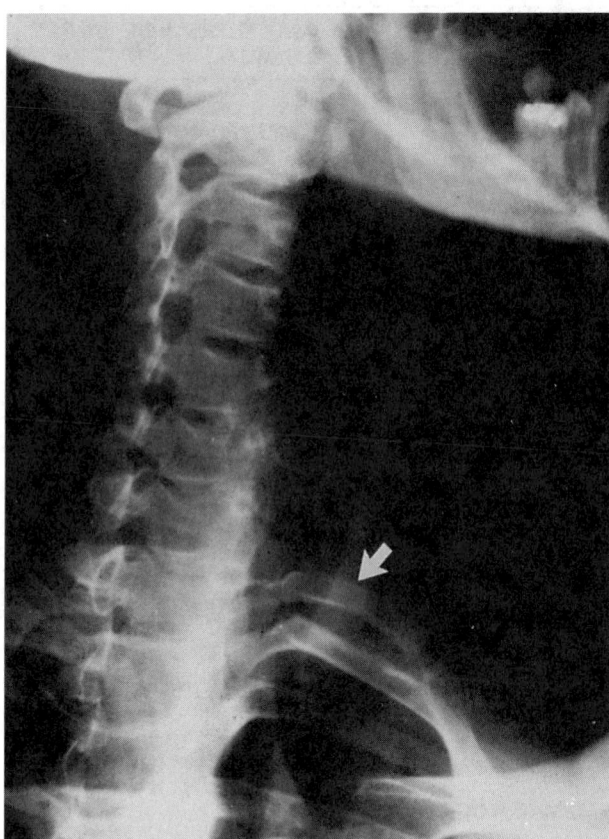

Figure 80-2. Cervical rib (*arrow*) in a patient with subclavian aneurysm caused by thoracic outlet compression.

- Antinuclear antibody
- Immunoglobulin electrophoresis
- Cryoglobulins
- Cold agglutinins
- VDRL test
- Complement (C3, C4)
- Anticardiolipin antibody
- Blood counts

ESR is a screening test to aid in the diagnosis of various forms cf arteritis. A positive *antinuclear antibody* test is helpful in detecting connective tissue disease and other types of arteritis. When the antinuclear antibody titer is abnormal, *immunofluorescent pattern* analysis of antibodies can help establish the diagnosis of various connective tissue disorders. The speckled pattern antibody is more specific for systemic lupus erythematosus. A nucleolar pattern suggests the presence of scleroderma. A positive *anticardiolipin antibody* is diagnostic for antiphospholipid syndrome, which is characterized by thromboembolic events in young adults.

Diagnostic Imaging

A combination of laboratory and radiologic testing may be needed to establish the diagnosis of systemic disease. *Soft-tissue radiography* of the hand may reveal calcinosis, which is diagnostic of the CREST syndrome, or diffuse calcified arteries in diabetic or azotemic arteriopathy (Fig. 80-1). *Chest radiography* is essential to detect bony anomalies of the thoracic outlet, such as cervical ribs (Fig. 80-2), anomalous first ribs, and healed fractures of the first rib or clavicle. Pulmonary fibrosis on a chest radiograph suggests systemic sclerosis.

Arteriography is used to define the vascular anatomy of the hand and to calculate the degree of peripheral ischemia. In investigation of upper-extremity ischemia, arteriography must include all arteries from the aortic arch to the hand. Subtraction techniques, multiple views, and magnification studies provide detail. In addition to the state of the inflow arteries, knowledge of the anatomic features of the palmar arches may aid in determining the degree of hand ischemia. Anatomic variation of upper-extremity arteries, especially the palmar arches (superficial and deep), occurs. Incomplete palmar arches are important in ischemic disease and contribute to digital ischemia.

The deep palmar arch is formed primarily by the terminal part of the radial artery, and the superficial arch by the ulnar artery. Variations of the arches, based on the manner in which the contributing arteries join, are common and may produce complete or incomplete arches. There are

many subtypes and variations of the superficial and deep palmar arches (Fig. 80-3). Because the ulnar artery is usually the dominant artery in the blood supply of the hand, the completeness of the superficial palmar arch is the determining factor in hand ischemia. Unlike the deep arch, there are many variations of the superficial palmar arch.

PROXIMAL ARTERIAL LESIONS
Atherosclerosis

Atherosclerosis is the most common cause of upper-extremity occlusive lesions. The most common site of involvement is the first part of the subclavian artery; the innominate artery is also a common site of disease. Lesions include total occlusion with or without associated steal phenomena, high-grade stenoses, and ulcerating plaques that cause distal embolism.

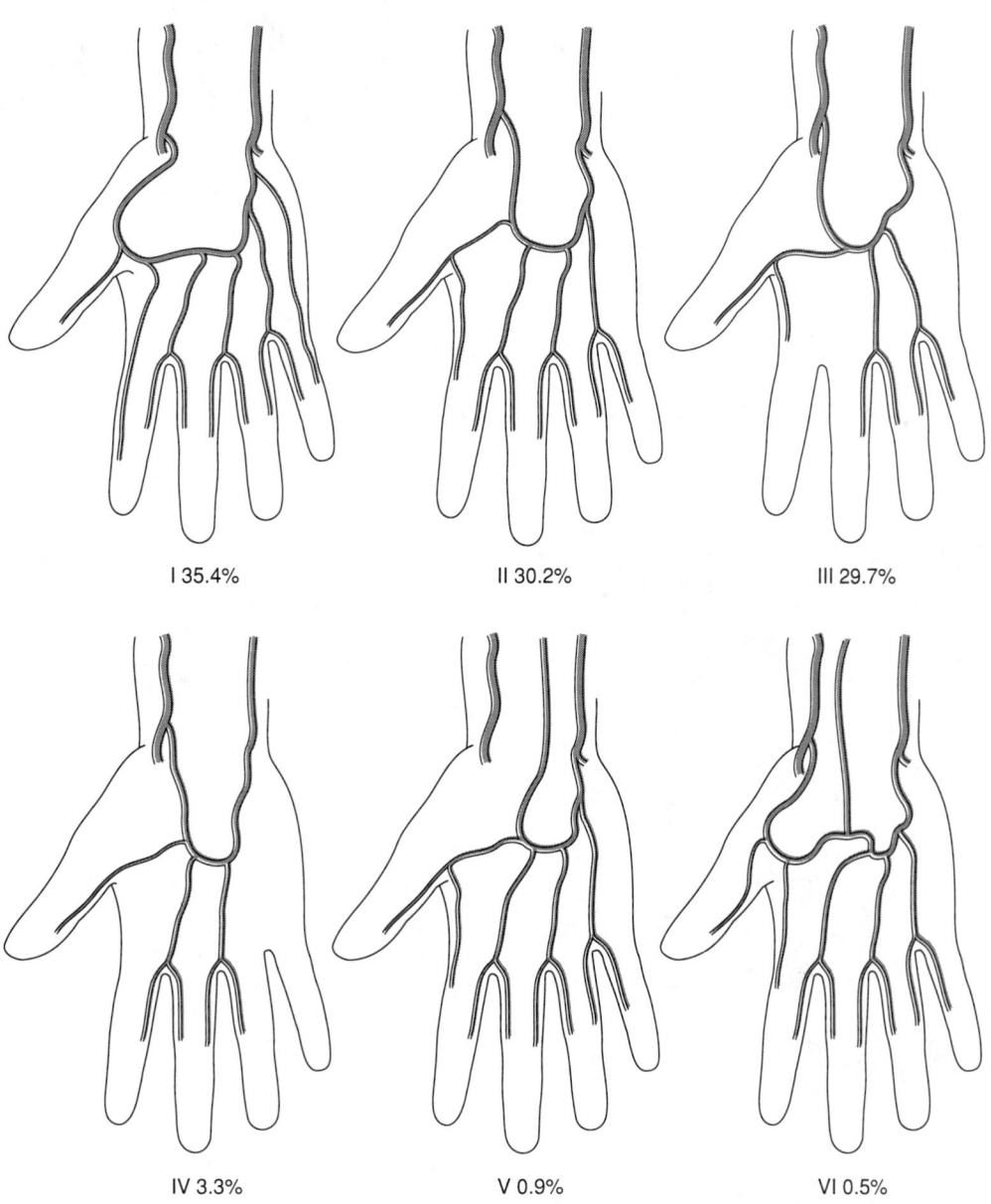

Figure 80-3. Different types of complete superficial palmar arch found on 500 hand arteriograms. (After Janevski BK. Angiography of the upper extremity. The Hague, Amsterdam, Martinus Nijhoff, 1982)

Arteritis

Arteritis that produces upper-extremity ischemic symptoms includes processes such as Takayasu arteritis, giant cell arteritis, temporal arteritis, and polymyalgia rheumatica. *Takayasu arteritis* is nonspecific inflammation of unknown causation that affects the aorta and its main branches. The disease affects carotid, subclavian, axillary, and pulmonary arteries; it occurs most often among women 10 to 30 years of age.

The clinical features of *giant cell arteritis* (cranial, temporal, and granulomatous arteritis) result from involvement of cranial arteries. In *temporal arteritis* and *polymyalgia rheumatica,* the subclavian or axillary arteries are common sites of involvement. In addition to upper-extremity ischemic symptoms, arteritis causes fever, malaise, headache, and joint pain. ESR often is elevated. Some serologic tests are positive, but none is sensitive or specific enough to be diagnostic.

Arteriographic examination of patients with upper-extremity occlusive symptoms often is diagnostic. Multiple artery involvement and a well-developed network of collaterals are characteristic of Takayasu disease; the pulmonary artery is affected in almost half of patients. Characteristic arteriographic findings in giant cell arteritis include long segments of smooth arterial stenosis alternating with areas of normal or increased caliber, smoothly tapered occlusions, and the absence of irregular plaques and ulcerations (Fig. 80-4).

Thoracic Outlet Syndrome

Thoracic outlet syndrome is the most common cause of upper-extremity vascular complications among young adults. Possible compression sites include the costoclavicular space formed by the first thoracic rib and clavicle; the interscalene triangle; the angle between the insertion of the pectoralis minor tendon and the coracoid process in

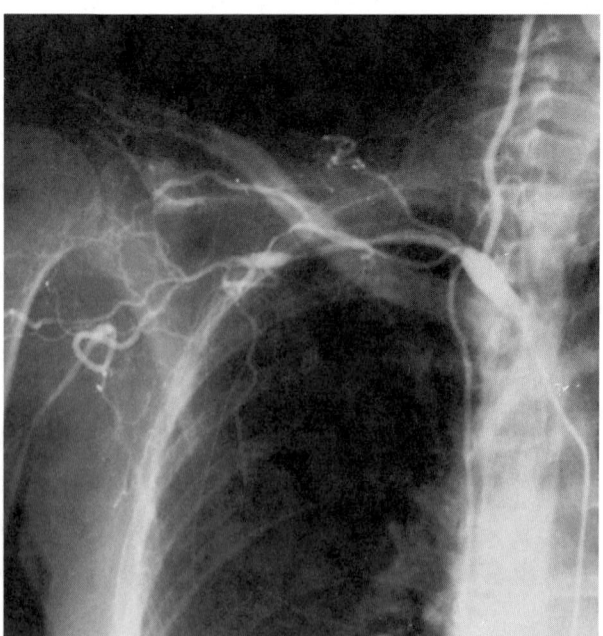

Figure 80-4. Characteristic long segmental narrowing of the subclavian artery in a patient with giant cell arteritis. (Yao JST. Arterial surgery of the upper extremity. In: Haimovici H, Callow AD, DePalma RG, et al, eds. Vascular surgery: principles and techniques, ed 3. Norwalk, CT, Appleton & Lange, 1989:858)

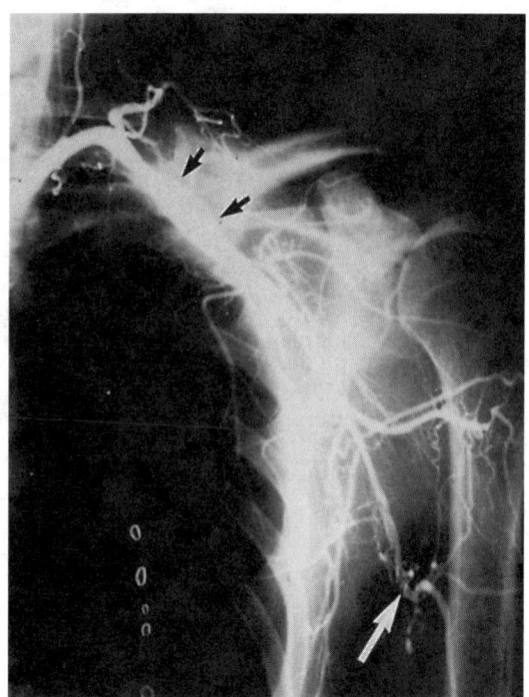

Figure 80-5. Arteriogram of a patient with subclavian aneurysm (*black arrows*) caused by a cervical rib. Multiple distal arterial occlusion has occurred as the result of embolization (*white arrow*).

the axilla; and the humeral head in extreme external rotation.

Thoracic outlet compression may be caused by bony anomalies such as a cervical rib (Fig. 80-5) or an abnormal first thoracic rib, or it may be caused by hypertrophy of the anterior scalene muscle. Arterial complications include aneurysm formation, poststenotic dilatation, thrombosis, and distal embolism. Distal embolism can cause digital gangrene or severe hand ischemia. Aneurysm formation is not confined to the subclavian or axillary arteries; repetitive trauma to branch arteries, such as the posterior circumflex humeral artery, may lead to aneurysm formation in baseball pitchers and volleyball players. In such patients, Raynaud phenomenon is often an initial symptom and is often unilateral. Neurologic symptoms and upper-extremity venous thrombotic complications are more common presentations of thoracic outlet syndrome than are arterial complications, but arterial symptoms are more threatening to limb and function and are always an urgent indication for arteriography.

DISTAL ARTERIAL LESIONS

Several *collagen vascular disorders* produce distal upper-extremity ischemia, including scleroderma, rheumatoid arthritis, systemic lupus erythematosus, polyarteritis nodosa, and dermatomyositis. All have systemic symptoms and present upper-extremity symptoms that range from Raynaud phenomenon to gangrene of the digits. Extensive involvement of the palmar arches or digital arteries is common (Fig. 80-6).

Buerger disease (thromboangiitis obliterans) is digital gangrene without occlusion of larger arteries. It is associated with heavy smoking of a particularly addictive nature. Diagnosis of Buerger disease depends on histologic examination that shows involvement of arteries as well as veins. Venous involvement may manifest itself as migrating phle-

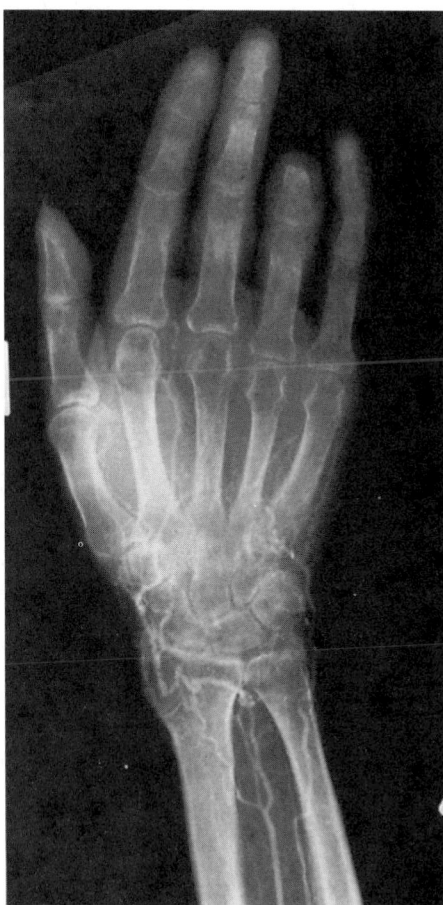

Figure 80-6. Arteriogram of a patient with scleroderma and digital gangrene. The extensive small-artery occlusion involves the palmar arch and digital arteries.

bitis. Characteristic arteriographic findings are occlusion of the small arteries of the digits with abundant collaterals. The typical corkscrew appearance of the collaterals and the lack of large-vessel plaques strongly suggest Buerger disease. In addition to the hand with symptoms, the hand without symptoms may demonstrate digital arterial occlusions.

Cold agglutinins, cryoglobulin, and polycythemia vera are the most common forms of *blood dyscrasia* associated with occlusion of the hand arteries. Small-artery occlusion apparently is caused by local thrombosis or embolism. Immunologic and blood tests help establish the diagnosis.

Catheter injuries with damage to the radial and brachial arteries are common. They are especially troublesome when an incomplete palmar arch is not recognized before a catheter is placed in the radial artery. Gangrene or severe ischemia can occur.

Vibration syndrome (blanching and numbness of the hands after use of pneumatic drills) causes hand ischemia. Repetitive trauma to the digital arteries that initially causes spasm, but ultimately causes thrombosis and permanent occlusion, appears to be the primary factor responsible for ischemic symptoms.

Hypothenar hammer syndrome is a form of occupational trauma common among mechanics and carpenters. The mechanism of injury is repetitive use of the palm of the hand in activities that involve pounding, pushing, or twisting. The location of the ulnar artery at the area of hypothenar eminence places it in a vulnerable position. When this area is repeatedly traumatized, ulnar artery occlusion or

aneurysm formation can occur (Fig. 80-7). Digital arterial occlusion is caused by embolism from the injured artery.

Calciphylactic arteriopathy in patients with diabetes or chronic renal failure can cause heavy calcification of the arteries, which leads to gangrene or severe ischemia of the hand. Calciphylaxis is characterized by calcification of the media of the digital arteries that produces a pipestem pattern on plain radiographs.

TREATMENT

Management of ischemic vascular disorders of the upper extremity is directed at the underlying cause. Patients with *proximal large-vessel stenosis* or lesions likely to lead to embolism usually need surgical therapy. The type of reconstructive procedure depends on the nature and location of the lesion.

Arterial complications due to thoracic outlet obstruction often necessitate a bypass procedure after resection of the subclavian aneurysm and removal of the cervical rib. A bypass graft with autogenous vein (saphenous or cephalic) often relieves occlusion of the brachial artery and its principal branches. Short segmental occlusion of either the radial or ulnar artery is managed by means of thrombectomy or endarterectomy with a vein patch. An aneurysm in the hand can be resected and continuity restored by means of end-to-end anastomosis or an interposed venous graft.

Proximal grafts fare better than distal grafts. Amputation is not often required, even after graft occlusion. Steroid therapy may be needed if there is arteritis with systemic symptoms. Iatrogenic drug-induced ischemia is managed by means of cessation of the drug.

Distal lesions with occlusion at or distal to the palmar arch are unlikely to be amenable to surgical management. Patients undergo conservative treatment with a calcium blocker (eg, nifedipine) to reduce the severity and frequency of attacks.

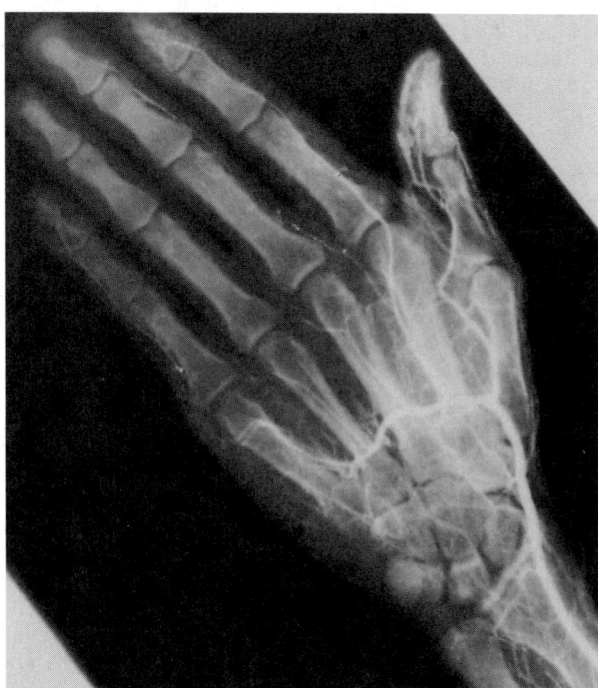

Figure 80-7. Occlusion of the ulnar artery over the hamate bone in a patient with hypothenar hammer syndrome.

All patients with upper-extremity ischemia of any cause must stop smoking. Protective measures such as avoiding exposure to cold and avoiding mechanical trauma can be helpful.

SUGGESTED READING

Durham JR, Yao JST, Pearce WH, Nuber GM, McCarthy WJ. Arterial injuries in the thoracic outlet syndrome. J Vasc Surg 1995;21:57.

Love PE, Santoro SA. Antiphospholipid antibodies: anticardiolipin and the lupus anticoagulant in systemic lupus erythematosus (SLE) and in non-SLE disorders. Ann Intern Med 1990;112:682.

Mesh CL, Yao JST. Upper extremity bypass: five-year follow-up. In: Yao JST, Pearce WH, eds. Long-term results in vascular surgery. Norwalk, CT, Appleton & Lange, 1993:353.

Yao JST, Bergan JJ, Neiman HL. Arteriography for upper extremity and digital ischemia. In: Neiman HL, Yao JST, eds. Angiography of vascular disease. New York, Churchill Livingstone, 1985:353.

Yao JST, Flinn WR, McCarthy WJ, et al. Upper extremity revascularization. In: Bergan JJ, Yao JST, eds. Techniques in arterial surgery. Philadelphia, WB Saunders, 1990:328.

ESSENTIALS OF SURGERY: SCIENTIFIC PRINCIPLES AND PRACTICE, edited by Lazar J. Greenfield, Michael W. Mulholland, Keith T. Oldham, Gerald B. Zelenock, and Keith D. Lillemoe. Lippincott–Raven Publishers, Philadelphia, © 1997.

CHAPTER 81

VISCERAL OCCLUSIVE DISEASE

GERALD B. ZELENOCK

Acute visceral ischemia can be dramatic in presentation. Unattended, the syndromes are life-threatening. Prompt recognition of the clinical syndromes, early and liberal use of diagnostic angiography, urgent or emergency surgical intervention, vigorous resuscitation, and pharmacologic support offer the best chance for survival.

VASCULAR ANATOMY OF THE ABDOMINAL VISCERA

Arteries

The circulation of the abdominal viscera is adapted for absorption and distribution of nutrients.

The *celiac artery* typically gives rise to three branches— the splenic, common hepatic, and left gastric arteries (Fig. 81-1). It also gives rise to the inferior phrenic arteries in about half of people. The *splenic artery* originates from the celiac artery distal to the origin of the *left gastric artery.* The splenic artery is closely associated with the pancreas and provides arterial input to the spleen, pancreas, and stomach by way of the short *gastric* and *left gastroepiploic arteries.* The *common hepatic artery* divides into the gastroduodenal and proper hepatic arteries. Through its *proper hepatic branch,* the hepatic artery gives rise to both the right and left hepatic arteries. In some people, the left hepatic artery is derived from the left gastric artery, and in some, the right hepatic artery has a replaced origin from the superior mesenteric artery (SMA). This replaced state may be complete or partial.

The blood supply to the middle lobe of the liver is from the *right hepatic artery.* The *left hepatic artery* supplies the lateral and medial segments of the left lobe; in almost half of people, it also supplies the middle hepatic lobe. The proper hepatic artery is the origin of the *right gastric artery,* which supplies the distal lesser curvature of the stomach.

The *gastroduodenal artery* is a branch of the common hepatic artery. It has several constant branches—the anterior and posterior superior pancreatoduodenal arteries and the right gastroepiploic artery. The gastroduodenal artery is an important source of large-vessel collateral circulation in the event of occlusion or stenosis of the celiac artery or SMA.

The *superior mesenteric artery* originates from the anterior surface of the aorta within 1 to 2 cm of the celiac trunk (Fig. 81-2). The SMA passes behind the pancreas and above the fourth part of the duodenum. The vessel provides arterial blood to the pancreas through the *inferior pancreatoduodenal artery* to most of the small intestine through *jejunal and ileal branches* and to the ascending and right half of the transverse colon through its *ileocolic, right colic, and middle colic branches.*

There are extensive large-vessel anastomotic arcades among the 10 to 20 jejunal and ileal arteries. Anastomoses between the main branches of the SMA and inferior mesenteric artery (IMA) in the region of the splenic flexure also are important.

The *inferior mesenteric artery* originates 5 to 6 cm distal to the SMA. It supplies the left half of the transverse colon and all of the descending colon through the *left colic artery* (Fig. 81-2). The IMA provides a number of sigmoidal branches and terminates as the paired *superior hemorrhoidal arteries.* Important SMA-to-IMA anastomoses occur between the middle colic and left colic arteries in the region of the splenic flexure and between the superior hemorrhoidal artery and internal iliac branches that supply the pelvis. The marginal artery of Drummond and arch of Riolan are discrete branch vessels that can enlarge. They are important sources of collateral blood supply in the presence of occlusion or stenosis of the proximal visceral vessels.

Veins

The venous anatomy of the gastrointestinal (GI) tract parallels the arterial blood supply and drains into the portal venous system, which perfuses the liver. The *inferior mesenteric vein* drains into the *splenic vein.* The splenic vein anastomosis with the *superior mesenteric vein* forms the origin of the portal vein. The *portal vein* subdivides into right and left portal veins, and by repetitive subdivision, supplies the liver parenchyma. Hepatic venous blood is drained via *right, middle, and left hepatic veins,* which enter the vena cava. Portosystemic anastomoses are common and are important if portal hypertension occurs.

Extensive visceral-visceral and visceral-systemic collaterals and the redundant anatomic patterns in the system afford protection from vascular occlusion (Fig. 81-3). Almost every visceral organ has multiple sources of blood and venous drainage. The extensive collateral circulation is enhanced by the arcade arrangement and frequently encountered collateral patterns. Visceral-systemic collaterals can occur, as between the IMA and the hypogastric artery or between the celiac axis and the systemic vessels via phrenic, esophageal, and intercostal arteries. An extensive intramural plexus and the specialized circulation in the mucosa and tip of the villus allow the intestinal circulation to function and account for the vulnerability of the mucosal tip.

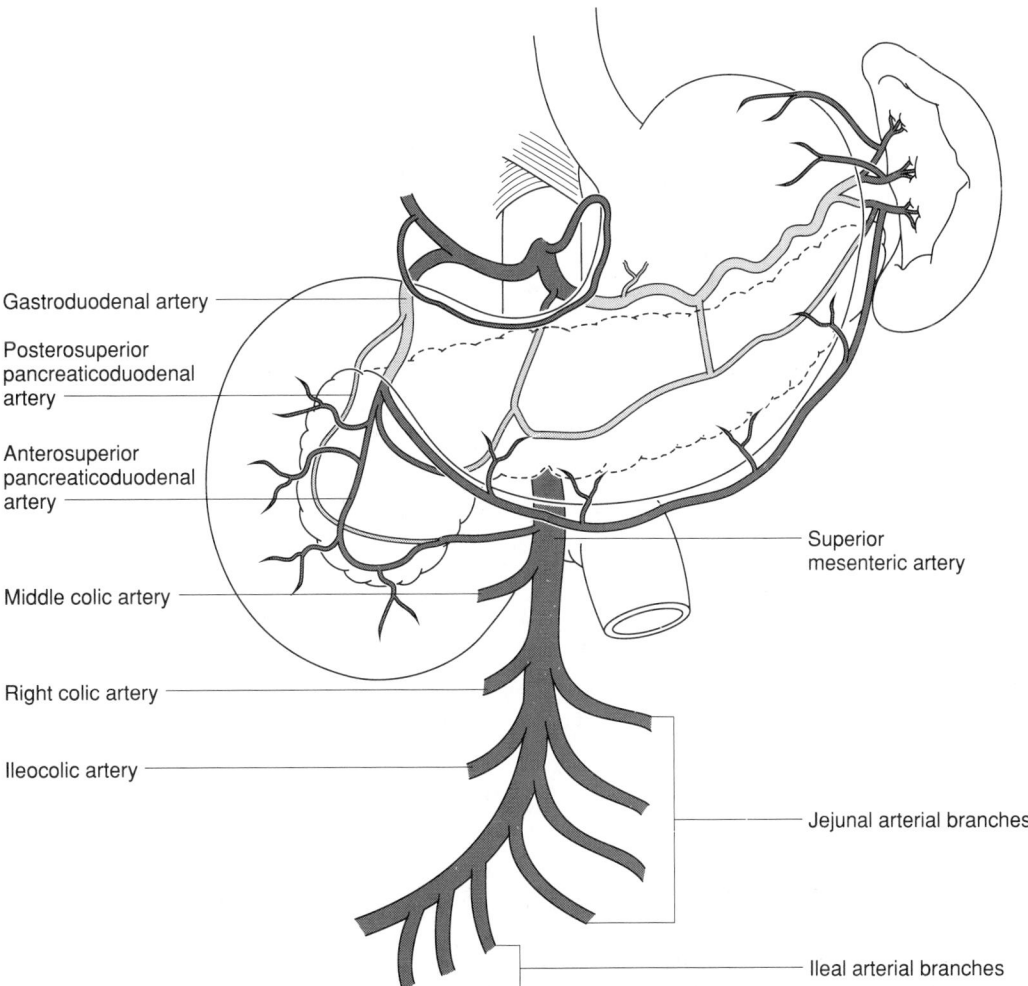

Gastroduodenal artery

Posterosuperior
pancreaticoduodenal
artery

Anterosuperior
pancreaticoduodenal
artery

Middle colic artery

Right colic artery

Ileocolic artery

Superior
mesenteric artery

Jejunal arterial branches

Ileal arterial branches

Figure 81-1. The celiac artery provides blood flow distribution to the stomach, duodenum, pancreas, liver, and spleen and has important collateral branches with the superior mesenteric artery by means of the gastroduodenal artery and the pancreaticoduodenal arcades. The superior mesenteric artery is retropancreatic but crosses anteriorly to the fourth portion of the duodenum. It supplies blood to the duodenum and head of the pancreas, the jejunum, the ileum, and the ascending and right half of the transverse colon (see Fig. 82-3). There are large anastomotic arcades among the jejunal and ileal branches.

Measurement of Blood Flow

Large-vessel intestinal blood flow is 500 to 1200 mL/ min, or about 10% to 20% of cardiac output. Noninvasive vascular diagnostic techniques allow visualization and volume flow determinations within the celiac artery and SMA. Duplex scanning is used to calculate flow volume, knowledge of which is useful in the diagnosis of intestinal vascular disorders. Blood flow values are shown in Table 81-1. Small changes in celiac artery blood flow occur with all meal types; increases in SMA flow occur 20 to 30 minutes after eating and persist for as long as 90 minutes after ingestion.

Within the wall of the intestine, most blood flow is to the mucosa. This tissue, 50% of the mass of the intestine, receives about 75% of resting blood flow. The muscular and serosal layers receive the other 25%. Control of blood flow in the splanchnic circulation is affected by the sympathetic nervous system and by metabolic, myogenic, and extrinsic factors. Stimulation of sympathetic nerves increases vascular tone and decreases splanchnic blood flow. Parasympathetic nerve fibers seem to have little direct effect on blood flow. Numerous intrinsic hormonal regula-

tors (eg, secretin, gastrin, cholecystokinin, glucagon, and vasoactive intestinal peptide) and substances such as histamine, serotonin, bradykinin, and prostaglandins may help regulate blood flow. Circulating hormones and regulatory substances (eg, epinephrine, norepinephrine, and angiotensin) and many drugs affect splanchnic circulation (Table 81-2).

PATHOPHYSIOLOGY OF ISCHEMIC INJURY

In the intestinal tract, in addition to ischemia and reperfusion, which are common to all ischemic events, translocation of bacteria and absorption of toxins and mediators have adverse effects. These effects exacerbate intestinal injury and have indirect systemic effects, such as myocardial depression and increased capillary permeability with edema formation and organ dysfunction. Loss of mucosa, which functions as a barrier to prevent luminal transfer of bacteria, endotoxin, and cytokines, occurs in shock, burns, trauma, and multiorgan failure.

Mucosal barrier function is lost in the visceral ischemic

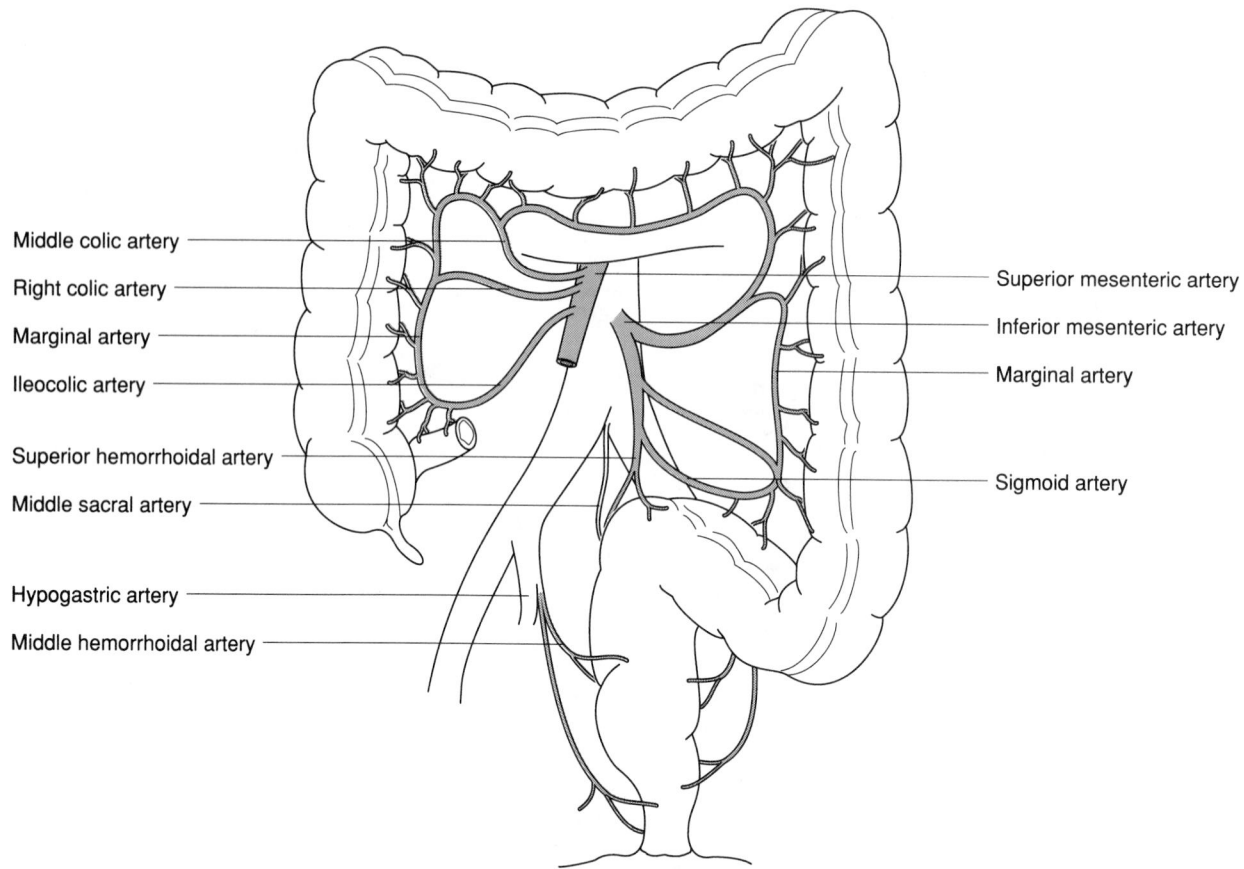

Figure 81-2. The inferior mesenteric artery (IMA) provides blood to the left half of the transverse colon and all of the descending colon, including the sigmoidal and superior hemorrhoidal branches. The left branch of the middle colic artery from the superior mesenteric artery and the ascending portion of the left colic artery from the IMA form a collateral network in the region of the splenic flexure. The IMA serves as an important source of collateral blood supply when the proximal two visceral vessels are occluded.

syndromes. Three factors appear to predispose to loss of intestinal mucosal barrier function: (1) physical disruption of the mucosa, (2) change in normal intestinal microflora (usually from treatment with broad-spectrum antibiotics), and (3) impaired host immune defenses. The first two always are present in patients with visceral ischemia; the third often is present in patients with extreme weight loss and malnutrition. Repair of locally damaged mucosa and enhancement of host defenses appear to be facilitated by early enteral feeding, provision of specific nutrients, such as glutamine, and perhaps by growth factors and GI trophic hormones.

CLINICAL SYNDROMES

Acute Visceral Ischemic Syndromes

Mesenteric Embolism

Mesenteric embolism accounts for about half of instances of acute mesenteric ischemia. Atrial fibrillation or myocardial infarction with mural thrombus formation usually is the source of the embolus, but almost any arrhythmia or anatomic cardiac defect may cause a mesenteric embolus.

Diagnosis. *Symptoms* are sudden, severe epigastric or midabdominal pain, followed promptly by emesis or explosive diarrhea. The patient feels well before the pain

occurs and often can pinpoint the onset of the pain. Many patients have experienced previous embolic events in other vascular territories.

Physical examination may reveal the underlying cardiac disorder. An irregularly irregular rhythm indicating atrial fibrillation, the murmur of mitral stenosis, or an enlarged heart all support the diagnosis of mesenteric embolism. The abdominal examination may reveal an acute abdomen or be normal. Slight to moderate abdominal distention is common. Bowel sounds are highly variable, as are findings at palpation. In acute mesenteric insufficiency, the severity of abdominal symptoms often is out of proportion to the physical findings. Peritoneal signs or blood in the stool are late findings that suggest severe ischemia with infarction.

There are no pathognomonic *laboratory* tests. An electrocardiogram may confirm cardiac abnormalities suggested by the history and physical examination, or a cardiac echocardiogram or ultrasound scan may show mural thrombus. Such tests are helpful but not diagnostic. Hematologic and biochemical evaluations are not useful early in the clinical course. Late evaluation may show hemoconcentration, acidosis, leukocytosis, or serum phosphorus or transaminase elevations.

Diagnosis depends on clinical suspicion followed by *angiography*. Emboli tend to lodge at branch points of the SMA. The origin of the SMA is spared, and the lodging point is close to the origin of the inferior pancreatoduodenal artery or the middle colic artery.

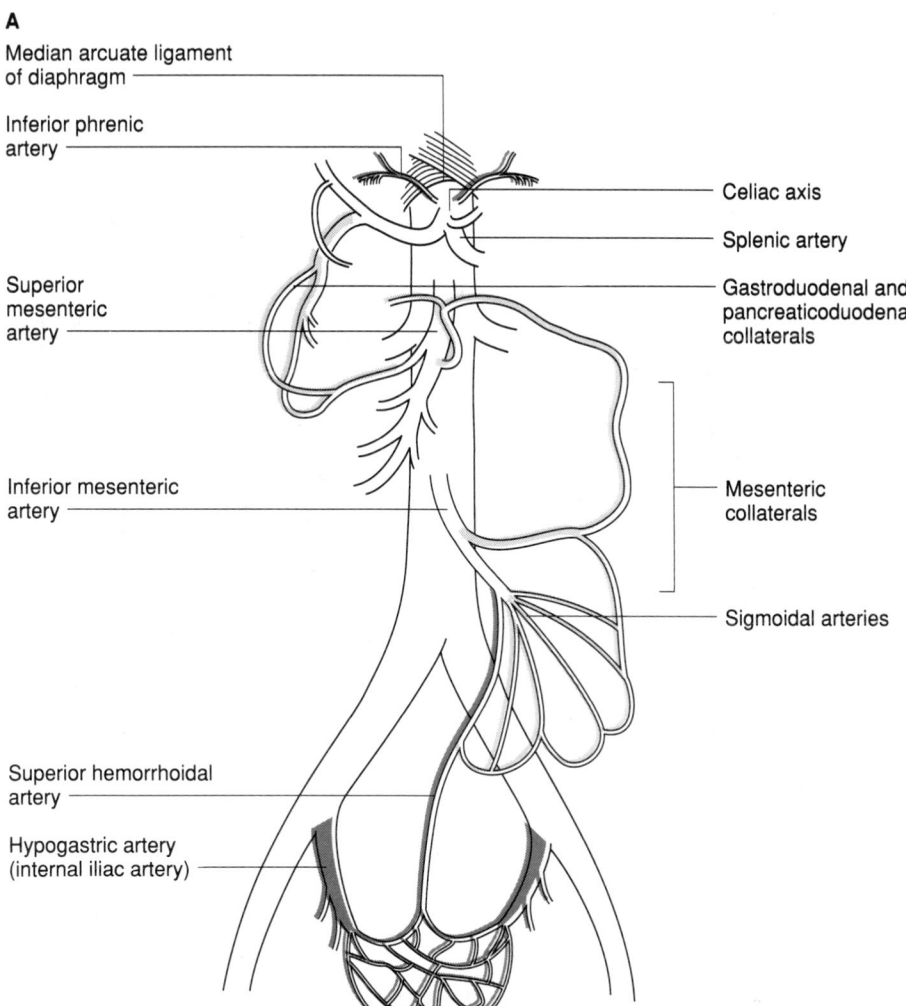

A

Median arcuate ligament
of diaphragm

Inferior phrenic
artery

Superior
mesenteric
artery

Inferior mesenteric
artery

Superior hemorrhoidal
artery

Hypogastric artery
(internal iliac artery)

Celiac axis

Splenic artery

Gastroduodenal and
pancreaticoduodenal
collaterals

Mesenteric
collaterals

Sigmoidal arteries

Figure 81-3. (*A*) The collateral circulation to the intestine occurs at several levels. Well-recognized visceral-visceral and visceral-parietal collateral branches and anastomoses are important. The unnamed intestinal arcades (*B*) and the intramural anastomoses (*C*) are effective short-segment collaterals.

Management. After diagnosis, heparin is administered, volume resuscitation is provided, and emergency surgical treatment is begun. Prophylactic antibiotics and full hemodynamic monitoring are necessary. The SMA is approached beneath the transverse mesocolon. Proximal and distal control is obtained, and Fogarty catheter embolectomy is performed through a transverse or longitudinal arteriotomy. This approach allows prompt return of visceral blood flow. Intestinal viability is assessed. After restoration of blood flow, an important concern is the possibility of multiple emboli in distal branches of the SMA.

Mesenteric Thrombosis

The presentation of mesenteric thrombosis is an acute intestinal catastrophe with progressive development of severe midabdominal pain. Acute symptoms may be superimposed on subacute intestinal angina or may occur without antecedent symptoms. If the patient has a history of postprandial abdominal pain associated with meals, extreme weight loss is common. The weight loss is caused by fear of eating, which precipitates pain. A history of motility disturbances that cause nausea, diarrhea, or constipation is much more common than malabsorption syndromes. Often the patient has undergone an extensive diagnostic evaluation for a malignant GI tumor.

Diagnosis. Urgent visceral *angiography* includes lateral aortography and anteroposterior views. The occlusive process is more widespread than may be apparent at angiography.

Management. The viscera must be reperfused. Reperfusion for temporary maintenance of intestinal viability may be accomplished with infusion of thrombolytic agents or other angioplastic techniques. If blood flow is restored, vigorous hyperalimentation optimizes the patient's condition and allows an elective operation. *This approach is never appropriate when frankly necrotic intestine must be resected.*

Operations for acute mesenteric thrombosis must be individualized. Emergency revascularization procedures involve multiple-vessel revascularization and use of short antegrade conduits (prosthetic or vein), when possible. For acute ischemia, single-vessel revascularization or venous and retrograde conduits can be used. If frankly necrotic intestine necessitates resection, autogenous conduits are used.

Low-flow Nonocclusive Mesenteric Ischemia

Vasoconstriction in mesenteric blood vessels is the underlying mechanism most commonly cited as the cause of low-flow nonocclusive ischemia. This vasoconstriction occurs in response to diminished cardiac output, shock, hypovolemia, dehydration, and the use of drugs known to diminish splanchnic blood flow (Table 81-2). Most patients are critically ill and in intensive care units. Patients often have unstable hemodynamic measurements because of shock, congestive heart failure, cardiac arrhythmia, recent myocardial infarction, or valvular insufficiency. These problems often coexist with renal or hepatic disease.

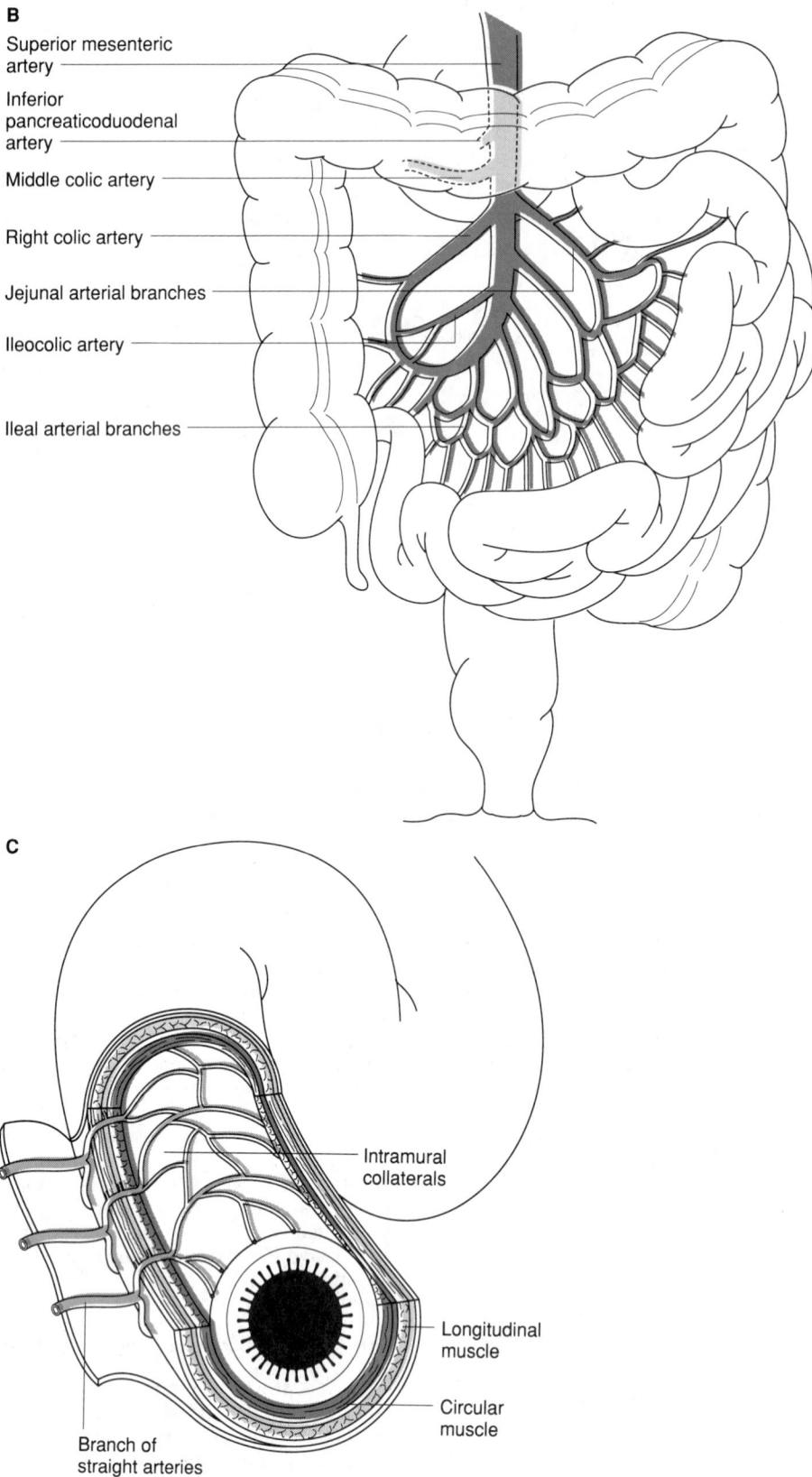

B

Superior mesenteric artery

Inferior pancreaticoduodenal artery

Middle colic artery

Right colic artery

Jejunal arterial branches

Ileocolic artery

Ileal arterial branches

C

Intramural collaterals

Longitudinal muscle

Circular muscle

Branch of straight arteries

Figure 81-3. *(Continued)*

Table 81-1. DUPLEX MEASUREMENT OF INTESTINAL BLOOD FLOW

Vessel	Average Diameter (Range)	Characteristics on Duplex Scan	Calculated Fasting Volume Flow (mL/min)	Calculated Volume Flow Change From Fasting by Type of Meal* (%)					
				Mixed	Cholesterol	Fat	Protein	Mannitol	Water
Celiac artery	0.66 cm (0.4– 0.8 cm)	Continuous forward flow; no reverse flow; end-diastolic velocity about $^1/_3$ peak systolic velocity No significant changes with meals	1083 ± 75	18 ± 4	1 ± 4	10 ± 8	21 ± 6	37 ± 19	14 ± 5
Superior mesenteric artery	0.59 cm (0.44– 0.68 cm)	Early diastolic flow reversal; forward diastolic flow; end-diastolic velocity about 0 After eating, loss of reverse flow and increased peak systolic and end-diastolic velocities are noted	538 ± 37	164 ± 30	118 ± 23	117 ± 25	78 ± 15	48 ± 11	24 ± 8

* Calculated volume flow changes that occurred after meals were not significantly increased in the celiac artery but were significantly increased with all meals except water in the superior mesenteric artery.
(Moneta GL, Taylor DC, Heiton WS, et al. Duplex ultrasound measurement of postprandial intestinal blood flow: effect of meal composition. Gastroenterology 1988;95:1294)

Diagnosis. Blood or guaiac-positive secretions may be seen in nasogastric aspirates. *Angiography* may be needed.

Management. There is no definitive surgical therapy other than resection of necrotic intestine, so the focus of intervention is pharmacologic support of the circulation with relief of splanchnic vasoconstriction. Treatment includes optimization of hemodynamic and volume status, correction of contributing medical conditions, and discontinuation, when possible, of adverse drugs. Under some circumstances, a vasodilator can be infused. Papaverine requires use of selective intraarterial infusion to avoid systemic hypotension. Glucagon, which selectively increases splanchnic blood flow, may be given by means of peripheral venous infusion and has positive inotropic effects; it may be more suitable in some settings.

Iatrogenic Visceral Ischemia

This condition can occur after operations, diagnostic procedures, or with the use of some drugs. Digitalis preparations clearly decrease intestinal blood flow, as do ergotamines and pressor agents. Diagnostic or therapeutic angiography may cause iatrogenic visceral ischemia due to embolization, and selective mesenteric angiography may cause intimal flap formation or dissection.

Aortic aneurysm resection is the surgical procedure most commonly associated with iatrogenic intestinal ischemia. Compromise of the colonic and sometimes the intestinal circulation may occur, with or without ligation of the IMA. Intestinal ischemia is more common with ruptured aneurysms, when occlusive and aneurysmal disease coexist, and when important collateral vessels are compromised by the aortic procedure. After aneurysm repair, colonic ischemia occurs in some patients.

Diagnosis. Patients present with diarrhea, often bloody or guaiac positive. When hemorrhagic diarrhea occurs, immediate *colonoscopy* is indicated.

Management. When ischemia is confined to the mucosa and submucosa and heals, the patient survives, but stricture formation occurs. When the ischemia is more serious and transmural infarction occurs, resection is performed. The incidence of colonic ischemia after aortic operations can be decreased with use of aggressive colonic and pelvic revascularization. Operations such as extensive resection for GI and genitourinary cancer can compromise intestinal blood flow.

Table 81-2. EFFECTS OF VARIOUS SUBSTANCES ON MESENTERIC CIRCULATION AND MOTOR ACTIVITY

Substance	Intestinal Blood Flow	Intestinal O_2 Uptake	Intestinal Motility
Acetylcholine	Increase	Increase	Increase
Adenosine	Increase	Variable	—
Angiotensin II	Decrease	—	Increase
Bradykinin	Variable	—	Increase
Ca^{2+}, high levels	Decrease	—	Increase
Ca^{2+} antagonists	Increase	—	Decrease
Dopamine	Variable	Decrease	—
Epinephrine	Variable	Variable	—
Gastrin	Increase	Increase	Increase
Glucagon	Increase	Increase	Decrease
Histamine	Increase	Increase	Increase
Isoproterenol	Increase	Variable	—
K^+ high levels	Decrease	—	Increase
Mg^{2+}	Increase	—	—
Nitroprusside	Increase	—	—
Norepinephrine	Decrease	Decrease	—
Papaverine	Increase	No change	—
PGE_1	Increase	Increase	—
$PGF_{2\alpha}$	Decrease	Variable	Increase
PGI_2	Increase	—	—
Secretin	Variable	No change	—
Serotonin	Variable	Variable	Variable
Somatostatin	Decrease	—	Decrease
Vasopressin	Decrease	Decrease	Variable
Vasoactive intestinal polypeptide	Increase	Increase	—

(Wakefield TW, Stanley JC. The intestine. In: Zelenock GB, D'Alecy LG, Schlafer M, et al, eds. Clinical ischemic syndromes: mechanisms and consequences of tissue injury. St Louis. CV Mosby, 1990)

Miscellaneous Causes of Acute Visceral Ischemia

Acute visceral ischemia can occur with aortic dissection, traumatic injuries, inflammatory arteriopathy, or vasculitis (Table 81-3). The clinical presentation depends on the underlying cause, with superimposed symptoms of abdominal distention, acute abdomen, or GI bleeding. *Diagnosis* depends on recognition of risk for intestinal ischemia and often is confirmed with angiography. *Treatment* is highly individualized. Branch revascularization in the setting of acute aortic dissection is essential when ischemia is profound. Traumatic injuries necessitate immediate surgical intervention. Inflammatory arteriopathy and vasculitis necessitate therapy for the underlying medical condition; surgical intervention is reserved for resection of clearly nonviable segments of intestine.

Recognition of Intestinal Viability

Any urgent intervention for visceral occlusive disease raises the issues of intraoperative recognition of viability, limits of resection, and need for a second-look procedure.

Recognition of Viable vs. Nonviable Intestine

When critical lengths of intestine are compromised, decisions must be made about how much to resect. Color, spontaneous peristalsis, and the presence or absence of palpable pulses are not sensitive or specific enough to allow confident clinical decisions. Adjunctive techniques to assess intestinal viability range from straightforward but

---

Table 81-3. MISCELLANEOUS CAUSES OF VISCERAL ARTERY OCCLUSION

MECHANICAL CAUSES
Aortic dissection
Blunt and penetrating trauma

COLLAGEN VASCULAR AND INFLAMMATORY VASCULOPATHY
Polyarteritis
Dermatomyositis
Rheumatoid arthritis
Sjögren syndrome
Henoch-Schönlein purpura
Essential mixed cryoglobulinemia
Wegener granulomatosis
Giant cell arteritis
Hepatitis B–associated antigens
Typhoid
Inflammatory bowel disease

LOCALIZED INJURY
Cholesterol embolization
Radiation
Enteric-coated potassium salts

SYSTEMIC VASCULOPATHY
Diabetes mellitus
Polycythemia vera
Köhlmeier-Degos syndrome

REACTIVE VASCULOPATHY
Estrogen–progesterone compounds
Pheochromocytoma
Carcinoid syndrome
Ergotism
Buerger disease
Associated with renal vascular hypertension or accelerated phase of malignant hypertension

---

Table 81-4. TECHNIQUES FOR ASSESSING INTESTINAL VIABILITY

COMMONLY USED
Clinical assessment
Intraoperative Doppler
Fluorescein dye or Wood lamp

INFREQUENTLY USED
Surface oximetry
Laser Doppler
Radiolabeled microspheres
Ultrasonography of intestinal wall
Intraluminal tonometry
Electronic contractility monitor (ECM)

SECOND-LOOK PROCEDURES
Surgery
Laparoscopy or peritoneoscopy

---

insensitive to sensitive but so complex they cannot be used for an acute problem (Table 81-4).

Limits of Resection

Margins of resection usually are determined with Doppler ultrasonography. This modality shows blood flow signals and not necessarily viability. Fluorescein dye or Wood lamp examination also can be used.

Second-look Procedures

If large segments of ischemic small intestine are resected, short-bowel syndrome can occur, in which insufficient intestinal mucosal surface remains for adequate nutrient absorption. All definitely and marginally viable intestine is left in the patient; only unequivocally necrotic tissue is resected. A second-look operation is planned, and the patient is prepared to undergo another operation in 24 to 48 hours for additional evaluation of the status of the intestine. Laparoscopy and peritoneoscopy also may be performed.

Subacute Visceral Ischemic Syndromes

Visceral Angina

Arteriosclerotic occlusive disease of the splanchnic trunks causes midepigastric pain 30 to 45 minutes after eating. The anatomic lesions usually involve the origins of at least two of the three visceral vessels, but the occlusive process also is relatively widespread throughout the mesenteric arcades. Patients have atherosclerosis or a severe cigarette smoking habit. Smoking causes proliferative overflow of aortic intima into the origins of the visceral vessels.

Patients have "food fear." Some avoid solid food altogether. Others consume small amounts each time they eat; they may describe themselves as "eating all the time." Patients with subacute visceral ischemia experience extreme weight loss due to avoidance of food because of pain rather than to malabsorption. GI contrast studies, endoscopies, and scans often are normal. Some patients have undergone exploratory laparotomy with normal findings.

Progression from symptoms to infarction is unpredictable. Many patients with intestinal infarction are found in retrospect to have had symptoms of visceral angina. Although recognition usually is delayed, diagnosis and treatment must proceed quickly because progress from symptomatic visceral angina to visceral thrombosis with transmural infarction is deadly.

Diagnosis. Expeditious screening of patients with postprandial pain and weight loss may enable timely diagnosis. *Aortography,* including anteroposterior and lateral views, confirms clinical suspicion. Multiple proximal vascular trunks are totally occluded or are affected by high-grade, hemodynamically significant stenosis. Although diseased, the IMA often is the main intestinal blood supply.

Management. Elective but urgent intestinal revascularization is performed. The most common procedures involve multiple-vessel revascularization with short, antegrade conduits of autogenous saphenous vein or prosthetic material. A variety of techniques, however, may be used (Fig. 81-4).

Mesenteric Venous Thrombosis

A vague prodrome of crampy abdominal pain, abdominal distention, nausea, and malaise may occur over a few days to several weeks. With widespread venous occlusion, the presentation may be more acute. Mesenteric venous thrombosis may be caused by an underlying condition or occur without recognized cause. Associated conditions include intraabdominal inflammatory processes, peritonitis, portal hypertension, hypercoagulable states, and the use of oral contraceptives.

Diagnosis. Plain *radiographs* reveal edema of the intestinal wall. *Computed tomography* may show thrombus within the portal vein or superior mesenteric vein. The venous phase of selective mesenteric *arteriography* may

reveal the thrombus. The diagnosis usually is made at *surgical exploration,* which reveals:

- Bloody ascites
- Intestine that looks dusky; feels thick and rubbery
- Palpable arterial pulses in the mesentery
- Mesenteric veins that feel cordlike and exude clot when cut

Management. Surgical therapy involves resection of nonviable intestine, sometimes large-vessel venous thrombectomy, and use of anticoagulants. Predisposing causes are corrected, and hypercoagulability states are investigated. Postoperative anticoagulant therapy is continued indefinitely because of risk for recurrent venous thrombosis.

Median Arcuate Ligament Syndrome

Symptoms include postprandial abdominal pain that may be caused by visceral ischemia. Another mechanism may be irritation of neural tissue over the origin of the celiac artery. Patients seek treatment because of abdominal pain, and in the course of the diagnostic evaluation, arteriography shows compression of the celiac axis by the median arcuate ligament of the diaphragm (Fig. 81-5). Other visceral vessels seldom show involvement with an occlusive process. Lysis of the overlying median arcuate ligament and surrounding neural tissue often relieves symptoms, if other causes of the symptoms have been thoroughly evaluated.

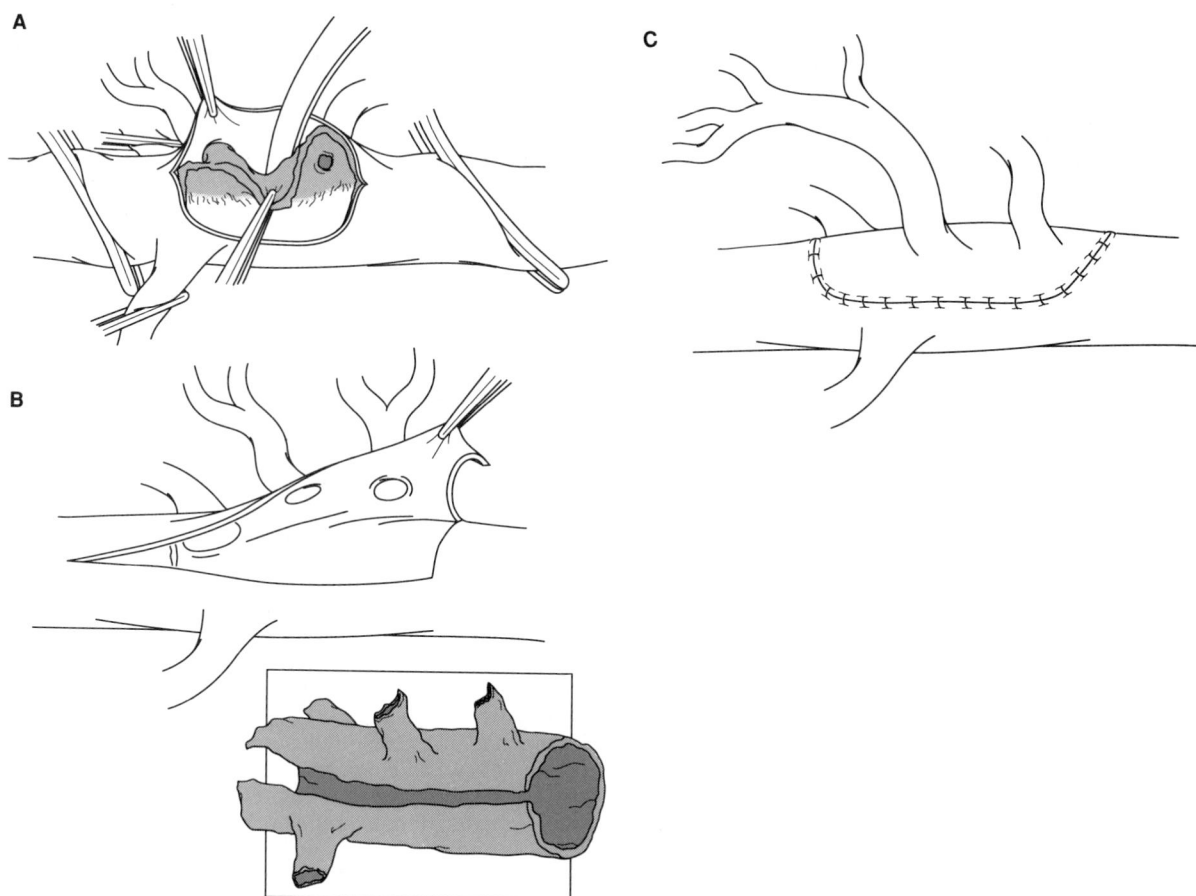

Figure 81-4. Endarterectomy of the celiac and superior mesenteric arteries is performed through a longitudinal trapdoor aortotomy. (After Wylie EJ. Manual of vascular surgery, vol 1. New York, Springer-Verlag, 1980)

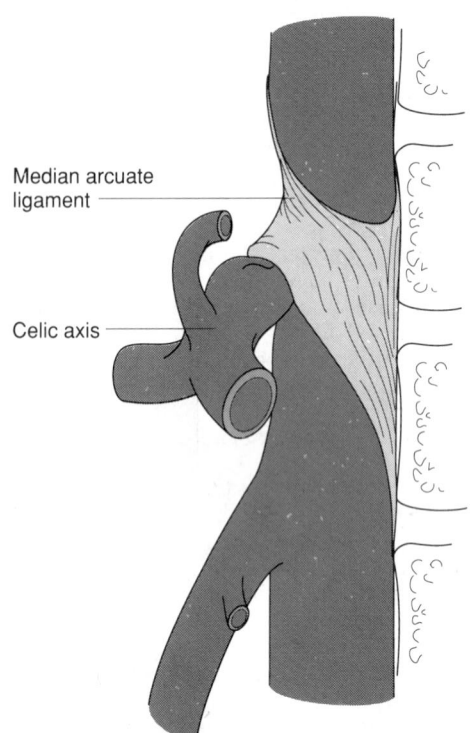

Median arcuate
ligament

Celic axis

Figure 81-5. The median arcuate ligament syndrome is controversial, but the anatomic structure is very real. This firm, fibrous connection between the crura of the diaphragm is extraordinarily strong and may significantly narrow the celiac axis.

SUGGESTED READING

Landreneau RJ, Fry WJ. The right colon as a target organ of nonocclusive mesenteric ischemia. Arch Surg 1990;125:591.

Levy PJ, Krausz MM, Manny J. Acute mesenteric ischemia: improved results—a retrospective analysis of ninety-two patients. Surgery 1990;107:372.

Levy PJ, Krausz MM, Manny J. The role of second-look procedures in improving survival time for patients with mesenteric venous thrombosis. Surg Gynecol Obstet 1990;170:287.

Mesh CL, Gewertz BL. The effect of hemodilution on blood flow regulation in normal and postischemic intestine. J Surg Res 1990;48:183.

Park PO, Haglund U, Bulkley GB, et al. The sequence of development of intestinal tissue injury after strangulation ischemia and reperfusion. Surgery 1990;107:574.

Stoney RJ, Schneider PA. Technical aspects of visceral arterial revascularization. In: Bergan JJ, Yao, JST, eds. Techniques in arterial surgery. Philadelphia, WB Saunders, 1990.

Taylor LM Jr. Mesenteric ischemia. Semin Vasc Surg 1990;3:141.

ESSENTIALS OF SURGERY: SCIENTIFIC PRINCIPLES AND PRACTICE, edited by Lazar J. Greenfield, Michael W. Mulholland, Keith T. Oldham, Gerald B. Zelenock, and Keith D. Lillemoe. Lippincott–Raven Publishers, Philadelphia, © 1997.

CHAPTER 82

RENAL ARTERIAL OCCLUSIVE DISEASE

JAMES C. STANLEY

Renovascular hypertension due to renal arterial occlusive disease is the most common form of surgically correctable hypertension. Systemic blood pressure elevations follow reductions in renal perfusion with activation of the renin-angiotensin system. Although this physiologic response tends to restore renal circulation toward normal, it does so in a pathologic way by producing hypertension in the systemic circulation.

PATHOPHYSIOLOGY OF RENOVASCULAR HYPERTENSION

Increased renin release and its effects on angiotensin and aldosterone cause renovascular hypertension (Fig. 82-1). *Renin* is produced by the juxtaglomerular apparatus of the kidney. It is a proteolytic enzyme active at neutral pH on its only known substrate, *angiotensinogen*. At normal sodium balance, the sum of renin activity in both renal veins is 48% greater than in the infrarenal vena cava or peripheral arterial and venous circulation. Renin levels in the peripheral circulation appear to be in a steady state because of this constant 48% contribution of renin from the kidneys. The liver is the primary site of removal and clearance of renin.

The biochemistry of the *renin–angiotensin system* is diagramed in Figure 82-2. The primary, if not sole, function of renin is hydrolysis of renin substrate (angiotensinogen) to form angiotensin I. *Angiotensinogen* is produced in the liver. *Aldosterone* is secreted from the zona glomerulosa of the adrenal cortex, and represents the volume element of renovascular hypertension. Aldosterone increases renal conservation of sodium and water, which is followed by extracellular fluid volume expansion and an increase in blood pressure.

Angiotensin-converting enzyme (ACE) is responsible for producing angiotensin II from angiotensin I. The highest concentration of ACE is in the endothelium of the pulmonary circulation. Conversion of angiotensin I to angiotensin II occurs in a single passage through the lungs. ACE is present at low levels in the blood and kidney and in other vascular beds. ACE is important in metabolism of the vasodepressor *bradykinin*.

The most common way to determine *plasma renin activity* is measurement of angiotensin I generation with a modified radioimmunoassay. Renin activity is expressed as hourly amount of angiotensin I generated per volume of plasma assayed. The assay involves two phases: incubation of plasma to generate angiotensin I, and radioimmunoassay of generated angiotensin I. Renin secretion is calculated as renal arteriovenous difference in renin activity multiplied by renal plasma flow. It is expressed as nanograms per mL per hour.

The effects of angiotensin on cardiac activity, vascular smooth muscle reactivity, and sodium and water metabolism contribute to increased arterial pressure (Fig. 82-3).

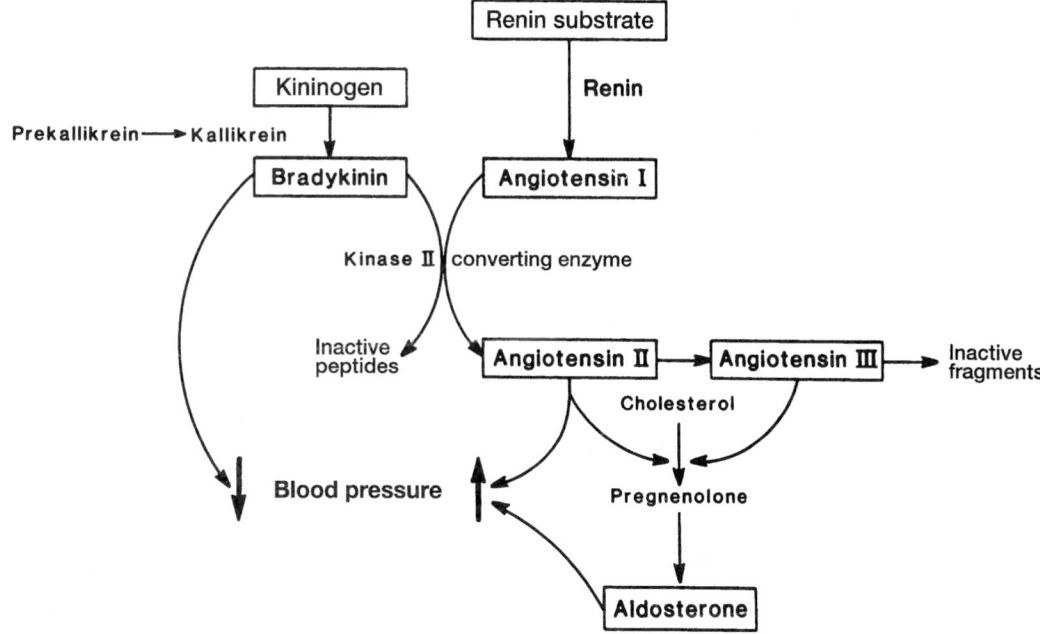

Figure 82-1. Renin-angiotenin system interrelation with aldosterone and bradykinin in regulation of blood pressure. (After Stanley JC, Graham LM, Whitehouse WM Jr. Renovascular hypertension. In: Miller TA, Rowland BJ, eds. Physiologic basis of modern surgical care. St Louis, CV Mosby, 1988:734)

The most important consequence of renal arterial occlusive disease is production of angiotensin II, a potent pressor substance. Angiotensin II acts directly on the arteriolar smooth muscle of nearly all vascular beds; the splanchnic, renal, and cutaneous circulations are most sensitive to its effects.

Hemodynamic responses to an activated renin-angiotensin system depend on the rate of alteration in renal blood flow and on whether one or both kidneys are affected. Acute reductions in renal blood flow cause rapid increases in plasma renin production and blood pressure. In unilateral renovascular disease with a normal opposite kidney, hypertension is characterized by renin hypersecretion from the affected kidney and suppression of renin production in the other kidney. Sodium retention within the affected kidney is counterbalanced by continuous sodium

excretion from the normal kidney, causing relative intravascular volume depletion. This vasoconstrictive form of hypertension is angiotensin II dependent, and responds to ACE inhibitors.

Pathophysiologic alterations in bilateral renovascular disease or unilateral disease of a solitary kidney relate to changes other than vasoconstriction. Angiotensin II causes sodium retention, diminutions in glomerular filtration, stimulation of aldosterone production, and stimulation of norepinephrine release from the adrenergic nervous system. In chronic bilateral or unilateral renovascular hypertension in patients with only one kidney, sodium retention accounts for late reductions in renin secretion. Blood pressure elevations do not seem to depend on the renin-angiotensin system in sodium-replete chronic renovascular hypertension. ACE inhibitors are effective in reducing blood pressure with sodium depletion.

PATHOLOGY OF RENAL ARTERIAL OCCLUSIVE DISEASE

Arteriosclerosis

Arteriosclerotic renal arterial occlusive disease accounts for 95% of cases of renovascular hypertension. The disease most commonly occurs during the sixth decade of life; men are affected twice as often as women. Arteriosclerotic renal arterial stenotic disease affects nearly half of the elderly population, but it is not always associated with high blood pressure.

Arteriosclerotic renal arterial occlusive disease affects the proximal third of the vessel in the form of eccentric or concentric stenoses. These lesions usually are spillover of diffuse aortic atherosclerosis. Arteriosclerotic renal arterial lesions usually are bilateral. When unilateral, the lesions affect the right and left renal arteries with equal frequency, although the left renal artery often is more severely diseased. Intimal and medial accumulations of cholesterol-laden foam cells and fibrous tissue are typical of these

```
Asp – Arg – Val – Tyr – Ile – His – Pro – Phe – His – Leu – R
```

Renin substrate
α_2-Globulin
↓
Angiotensin I
Decapeptide
↓
Angiotensin II
Octapeptide
↓
Angiotensin III
Heptapeptide

Figure 82-2. Biochemical composition of renin substrate and the angiotensins. (After Stanley JC, Graham LM, Whitehouse WM Jr. Renovascular hypertension. In: Miller TA, Rowland BJ, eds. Physiologic basis of modern surgical care. St Louis, CV Mosby, 1988:734)

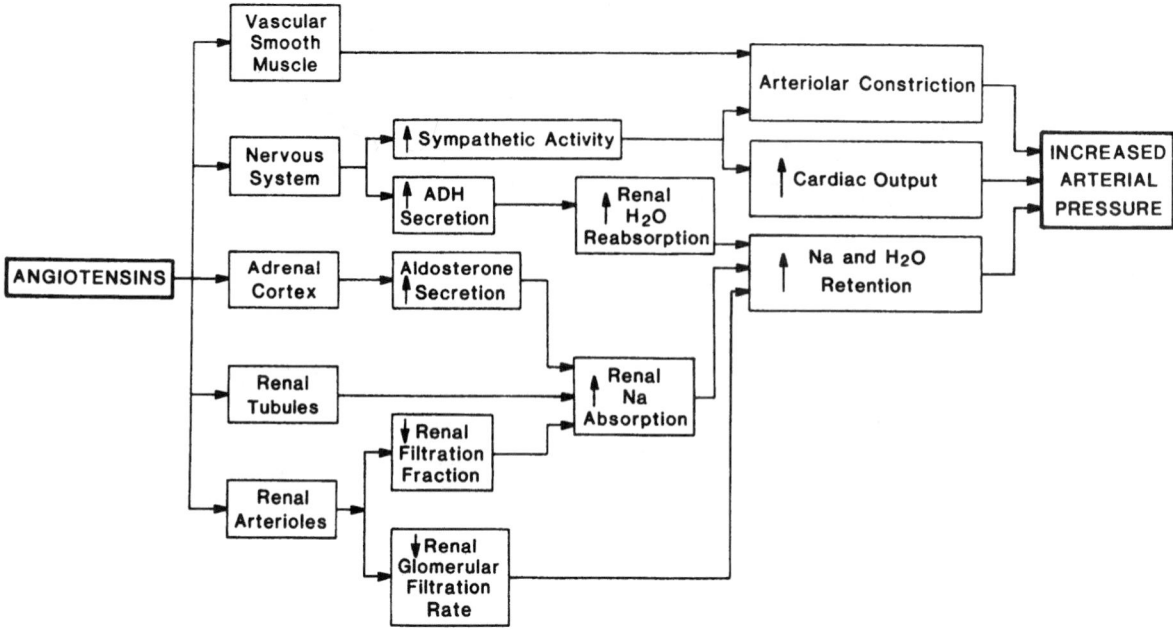

Figure 82-3. Effects of angiotensins contributing to increased arterial pressure. (After Stanley JC, Graham LM, Whitehouse WM Jr. Renovascular hypertension. In: Miller TA, Rowland BJ, eds. Physiologic basis of modern surgical care. St Louis, CV Mosby, 1988:734)

lesions. Necrosis, hemorrhage, calcification, and luminal thrombus are characteristic of complicated atherosclerotic plaques associated with advanced disease.

Arterial Fibrodysplasia

Arterial fibrodysplasia is the second most common type of renal artery disease, but it accounts for only 5% of cases.

Intimal fibroplasia accounts for about 5% of dysplastic renal artery stenoses. It is more common among children and young adults than the elderly; it affects both sexes equally. The cause of *primary* intimal fibroplasia may be related to persistent embryonic myointimal cushions. *Secondary* intimal fibroplasia is attributed to flow disturbances, blunt abdominal trauma during childhood, and the sequelae of arteritis, as occurs with rubella. Progression of intimal fibroplasia may cause turbulent blood flow and an accelerated fibroproliferative response that rapidly compromises the arterial lumen.

Intimal fibroplasia usually presents as a smooth, focal stenosis of the distal main renal artery. Some lesions produce long, tubular stenoses, and some produce webs that affect segmental arteries. Proximal ostial lesions usually represent the secondary form of this disease, which is associated with abdominal aortic hypoplasia and coarctation. Subendothelial accumulations of irregularly arranged mesenchymal cells surrounded by loose fibrous connective tissue are typical of all intimal fibrodysplastic lesions. The internal elastic lamina is usually intact, but partial fragmentation may occur. Medial and adventitial structures are normal in primary intimal fibrodysplasia.

Medial fibroplasia is the most commonly diagnosed dysplastic renal artery disease, accounting for 85% of lesions. Medial fibroplasia affects women 25 to 45 years of age. Medial fibroplasia appears to be a systemic arteriopathy; the internal carotid and external iliac arteries are the extrarenal vessels most often affected. The causes of medial fibroplasia appear to be modification of smooth muscle to myofibroblasts due to estrogenic stimulation during the

reproductive years, unusual traction forces on affected vessels, and mural ischemia from impairment of blood flow in the vasa vasorum. Physical forces contributing to medial fibroplasia appear to be ptotic kidneys with stretching of the renal arteries (Fig. 82-4).

The morphologic appearance of medial dysplasia ranges from solitary stenoses to multiple constrictions with intervening mural dilatations of the middle and distal main

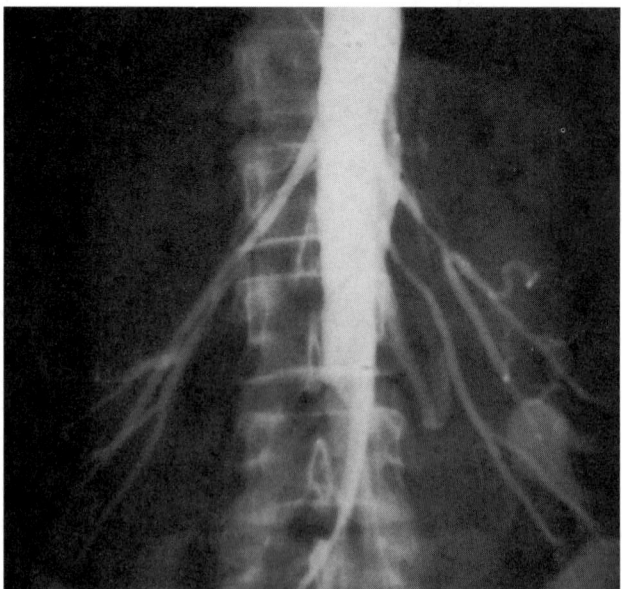

Figure 82-4. Medial fibrodysplasia manifest as irregular narrowings to ptotic kidneys (*arrows*) affecting the mid-portion of the main renal arties, which appear stretched during upright aortography. (Stanley JC, Wakefield TW. Arterial fibrodysplasia. In: Rutherford RB, ed. Vascular surgery, Philadelphia, WB Saunders, 1995:264)

renal artery ("string of beads" sign). Stenotic disease of segmental branches occurs about 25% of the time. Bilateral disease affects more than half of patients, and is usually more severe on the right. Unilateral lesions affect the left renal artery 10% of the time, the right renal artery 30%.

Gradations in medial fibroplasia include diffuse and peripheral forms of the disease in the same vessel. *Diffuse* medial fibroplasia is typified by severe disorganization of medial smooth muscle cells, which appear to be transformed to myofibroblasts, which generate accumulations of ground substance that encroach on the vessel lumen. These stenoses often alternate with areas of medial thinning and mural dilatation. *Peripheral* medial fibroplasia is typified by limitation of fibroproliferation to the outer portion of the media, causing stenoses less severe than those of diffuse disease.

Perimedial dysplasia occurs among women 30 to 50 years of age. Perimedial dysplasia is bilateral in 20% of patients, and appears to be more progressive than medial fibrodysplasia. Perimedial dysplasia is characterized by solitary or multiple constrictions without intervening dilatations. Most stenoses involve the distal main renal artery without segmental branch involvement. Some histologic features are common to perimedial dysplasia and medial fibroplasia, and they may represent different manifestations of the same disease. Unusual accumulations of elastic tissue in inner adventitial regions is the most prominent abnormality in perimedial dysplasia, but increases in medial ground substance may accompany this type of dysplastic disease.

Developmental Renal Arterial Disease

Developmental renal arterial stenoses are a rare cause of renovascular hypertension. These lesions are encountered most often in children and young adults. About 40% of children with renovascular hypertension have developmental renal artery stenoses. Nearly 20% of adults with intimal fibroplastic renal artery disease have stenoses that can be attributed to developmental defects. Both sexes are affected equally. These stenotic lesions represent true hypoplasia of the renal artery, and have an external hourglass appearance.

Developmental lesions usually occur at the aortic origin of the artery. Sparse medial tissue, intimal fibroplasia, fragmentation and duplication of the internal elastic lamina, and disproportionate excesses in adventitial elastic tissue are the most common histologic abnormalities in these vessels.

Developmental renal arterial narrowing may be attributed to embryonic events that take place as the two fetal dorsal aortas fuse and all but one of their lateral branches to the kidney regress. Abnormal transition of mesenchyme to medial smooth muscle at that time, or later impairment of its growth, can cause aortic and renovascular anomalies. A solitary artery to each kidney evolves from these arteries in most people. Flow changes in the region where single central renal arteries originate may afford hemodynamic advantages that ensure their persistence.

DIAGNOSIS
Clinical Features

Findings suggestive of renovascular hypertension are:

Systolic and diastolic upper-abdominal bruits
Diastolic blood pressures >115 mmHg
Sudden worsening of mild to moderate essential hypertension

Development of hypertension during childhood
Rapid onset of high blood pressure after 50 years of age

Hypertension resistant to drug therapy and malignant hypertension probably are associated with renovascular hypertension. Patients who have deterioration in renal function while taking multiple antihypertensive drugs, especially ACE inhibitors, may have underlying renal arterial stenotic disease. Figure 82-5 is a management algorithm for renovascular hypertension.

Diagnostic Imaging

Conventional *arteriography* is central to the evaluation of renovascular hypertension. Oblique aortography and multiple-plane selective renal arteriography improve recognition of the morphologic character and extent of renal arterial stenosis. Collateral vessels circumventing renal artery stenosis are evidence of the hemodynamic importance of a lesion. A pressure gradient of about 10 mmHg is necessary for development of collateral vessels, and the same degree of pressure change occurs with activation of the renin system. The functional importance of benign-appearing stenosis is established when collateral vessels are evident (Fig. 82-6).

Intraarterial *digital substraction angiography* (DSA) helps assess the presence of renal arterial stenotic disease. Intraarterial DSA requires less contrast material than conventional arteriography or intravenous DSA, decreasing risk for contrast agent-induced nephrotoxicity.

Magnetic resonance angiography (MRA), especially with gadolinium enhancement, provides high-resolution images of diseased renal arteries. Noninvasiveness and lack of nephrotoxicity make MRA a helpful diagnostic test.

Deep abdominal renal arterial *ultrasonography* may depict hemodynamically significant renal arterial narrowing. It also can be used to assess flow velocity patterns through these vessels. Existence of stenosis is likely when peak systolic velocities are 180 to 200 cm/sec and the ratio of these velocities to those in the aorta approaches 3.5. Ultrasonography cannot be used to identify renal arterial stenoses with >60% cross-sectional narrowing. Inability to identify a main renal artery in the absence of parenchymal flow signal suggests occlusion of the main renal artery.

Functional Studies
Renal Vein Renin Activity

One calculates *renal vein renin ratio* (RVRR) by dividing the renin activity in venous blood from the affected kidney by that in blood from the other kidney. An RVRR >1.48 indicates functionally important renovascular stenotic disease. Because this test compares one kidney with the other, it may not be useful to patients with bilateral disease, if both kidneys show elevated but equal degrees of abnormally high renin secretion. One calculates *renal-systemic renin index* (RSRI) by subtracting systemic renin activity from individual renal vein renin activity and dividing the remainder by systemic renin activity. It is an expression of individual kidney renin release.

In patients with essential nonrenovascular hypertension, renal vein renin activity from each kidney is usually 24% higher than systemic activity. The total of both kidneys' activity is usually 48% higher than systemic activity. This figure of 48% represents a steady state of renal renin release.

In renovascular hypertension, the RSRI of the affected kidney is >0.24. In mild degrees of renal arterial disease, an increase in ipsilateral renin release is normally balanced by suppression of renin production in the other kid-

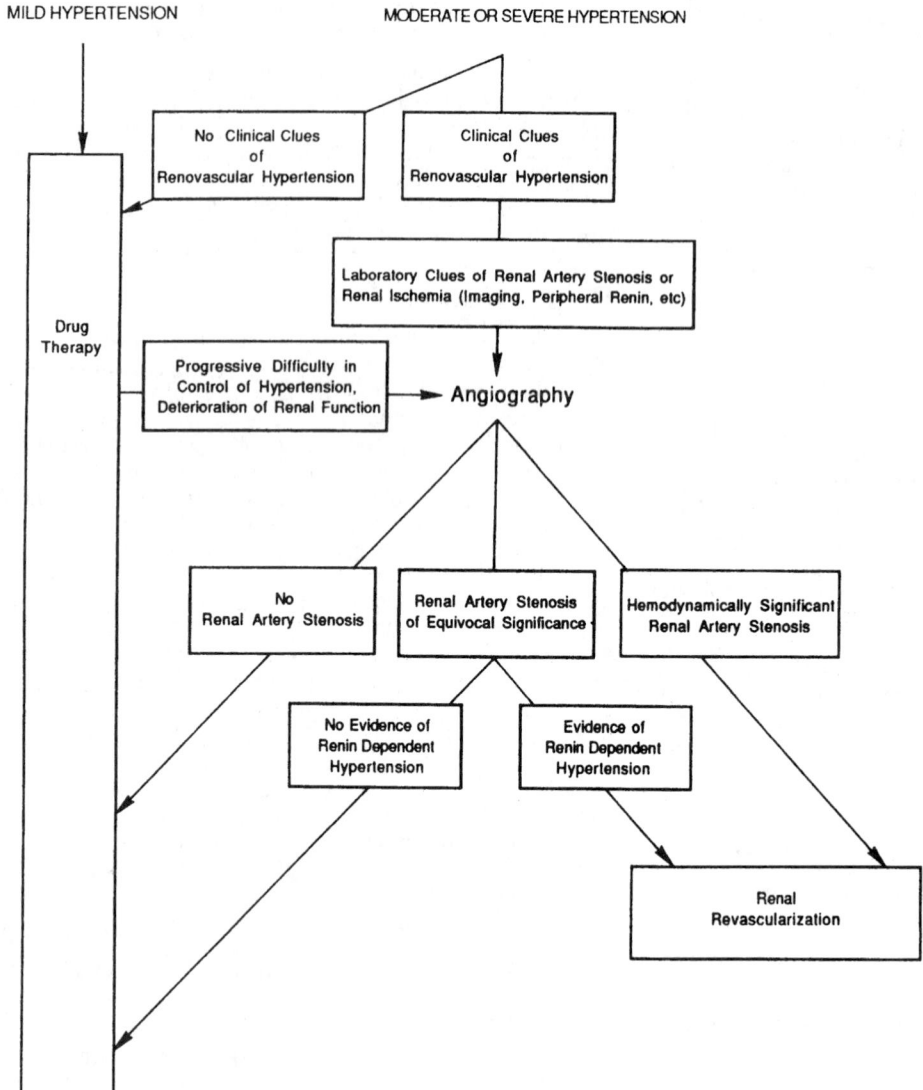

Figure 82-5. Management algorithm for renovascular hypertension. (After Stanley JC. Renal artery stenosis and hypertension. In: Brewster DC, ed. Common problems in vascular surgery. Chicago, Year Book, 1989:187)

ney with a drop in its RSRI to <0.24. Bilateral renal artery disease may cause loss of this mechanism, and the autonomous release of renin from both kidneys may cause the sum of the individual RSRIs to be >0.48. Renin production then exceeds the capacity of normal hepatic degradation, and a hyperreninemic form of hypertension evolves.

Urography

Urography is not a good diagnostic test for renovascular hypertension because of limited sensitivity.

Radionuclide Studies

Isotopic renography allows renal imaging and analysis of the washout curve of a number of radioactive tracers. These studies provide an assessment of renal blood flow and excretory function. Different states of hydration and intrarenal vascular resistance often contribute to flow abnormalities and false-positive results for patients with nonrenovascular hypertension. Administration of ACE inhibitors improves sensitivity and specificity by blocking the compensatory change in glomerular filtration, causing it to fall in the affected kidney.

Split Renal Function Studies

A ureteral catheter is used to sample urine from each kidney. The two common tests are the:

Howard test, which documents reduced urine volume

and increased sodium and creatinine concentration in the affected kidney

Stamey test, which reveals a smaller volume of urine and a greater concentration of paraaminohippurate in the affected kidney

MANAGEMENT

Drug Therapy

Antihypertensive drugs such as the β-blockers propranolol and atenolol are used in the initial management of renovascular hypertension. Refractory hypertension, especially that due to bilateral disease or unilateral lesions with contralateral parenchymal disease, may respond to addition of a thiazide diuretic. If renal function is impaired, use of a loop diuretic such as furosemide is effective.

ACE inhibitors, such as captopril and enalapril, are the most effective drugs in the management of renovascular hypertension. ACE inhibitors may have a deleterious effect on renal function by critically decreasing intrarenal blood pressure and altering intrarenal autoregulation. ACE inhibitors are used cautiously when the entire renal parenchymal mass is at risk, as in patients with bilateral renovascular hypertension or a solitary kidney. Because stenotic disease of the renal artery often progresses with concomitant loss of renal mass and function, a definitive means of

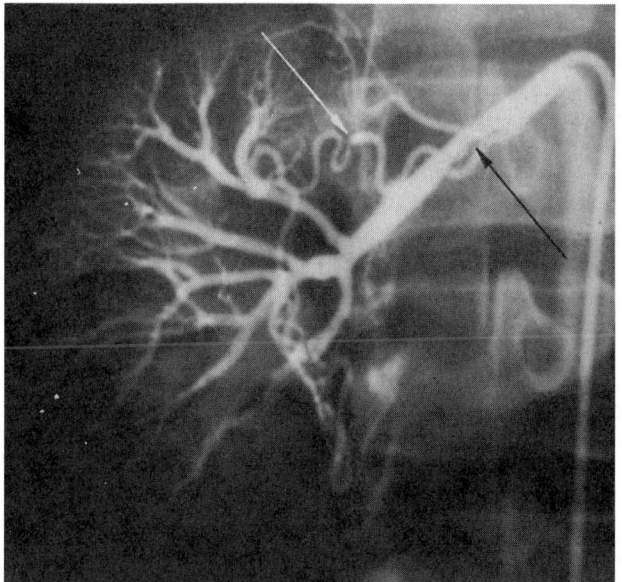

Figure 82-6. Arteriogram of a benign-appearing stenosis (*black arrow*) associated with a large collateral vessel (*white arrow*) circumventing the lesion, defining hemodynamic significance of the stenosis and implicating its functional importance. (Stanley JC, Graham LM, Whitehouse WM Jr. Limitations and errors of diagnostic and prognostic investigations in renovascular hypertension. In: Bernhard VM, Towne JM, eds. Complications in vascular surgery. Orlando, Grune & Stratton, 1984:213)

restoring normal renal blood flow may be more logical therapy than drug treatment once the diagnosis of renovascular hypertension is established.

Percutaneous Transluminal Renal Angioplasty

Renal PCTA is considered alternative therapy for renovascular hypertension. Intimal and medial dysplastic stenoses are most amenable to PCTA. PCTA of atherosclerotic stenoses is limited by the inability to dilate spillover plaque from extensive aortic disease. These aorta-associated lesions are responsible for the high recurrence rate of arteriosclerotic occlusive stenoses after balloon angioplasty. Complications of dilation of arteriosclerotic and fibrodysplastic lesions are uncommon. Extrarenal complications usually relate to hemorrhage at the site of arterial catheterization. This is rarely limb- or life-threatening.

Renal Revascularization

The primary revascularization procedure must be successful. Nephrectomy accompanies nearly half of reoperations performed because of failed initial reconstructions. Careful preoperative assessment of extrarenal occlusive disease in the presence of arteriosclerotic renovascular disease is mandatory to ensure the patient's ability to undergo a complex renal artery operation.

Bypass Procedures

Aortorenal bypass in adults with arteriosclerotic and fibrodysplastic occlusive disease is most often performed with autologous reversed saphenous vein. Dacron or expanded polytetrafluoroethylene (PTFE) conduits also may be used. Because venous grafts in children often become aneurysmal, autologous hypogastric artery grafts and di-

rect aortic reimplantation of the renal artery are favored for children.

Nonanatomic bypass procedures are used to treat many patients with renovascular hypertension. The hepatic or iliac arteries may be used as sites of origin for bypass grafts to the renal artery, especially when originating a graft from the aorta entails unacceptable risk. Use of the splenic artery in situ for left-sided splenorenal bypass is appropriate for adults, but only after one ascertains that this vessel and the celiac trunk are free of stenotic disease. Splenorenal bypasses are not recommended for children.

Renal Artery Reconstruction

Ex vivo renal artery reconstruction is an alternative for some patients with renovascular hypertension, especially those with revascularization of multiple second- or third-order segmental branches. Most renal artery reconstructions can be performed in situ. Disadvantages of ex vivo reconstruction include the necessity to cool the kidney, longer operating time, and disruption of collateral channels.

Arterial Dilation

Surgical arterial dilation, alone or in conjunction with a bypass procedure, is useful in the management of fibrous intraparenchymal stenotic disease. In this setting, sequentially larger metal dilators are advanced through a transverse arteriotomy in the main renal artery after heparin anticoagulation. These dilators must be advanced with care not to overdilate the vessel, lest intimal fracture occur.

Endarterectomy

Endarterectomy is often the preferred means of managing proximal renal arteriosclerotic disease. The techniques most often used are (1) transaortic renal endarterectomy through an axial aortotomy or the transected infrarenal aorta or (2) direct renal arterial endarterectomy. The extent of aortic and renal artery disease and the need to perform aortic reconstruction dictate which procedure is appropriate.

A linear aortotomy begins just to the left of the superior mesenteric artery and extends in the midline to below the renal arteries. The diseased aortic intimal and medial tissues are elevated, and with gentle traction the renal artery atheroma is extracted. This type of endarterectomy is particularly useful in treating patients with bilateral disease or when the disease affects multiple renal arteries. Extensive plaque of the distal part of the renal artery, especially involving bifurcations, may be better managed with direct renal arteriotomy and endarterectomy with a patch graft closure.

SUGGESTED READING

Anderson CA, Hansen KJ, Benjamin ME, et al. Renal artery fibromuscular dysplasia: results of current surgical therapy. J Vasc Surg 1995;22:207.

Cambria RP, Brewster DC, L'Italien G, et al. Simultaneous aortic and renal artery reconstruction: evolution of an eighteen-year experience. J Vasc Surg 1994;21:916.

Dougherty MJ, Hallett JW Jr, Naessens J, et al. Renal endarterectomy vs. bypass for combined aortic and renal reconstruction: Is there a difference in clinical outcome? Ann Vasc Surg 1995;9:87.

Hansen KJ, Thomason RB, Craven TE, et al. Surgical management of dialysis-dependent ischemic nephropathy. J Vasc Surg 1995;21:197.

Hertz SM, Holland GA, Baum RA, et al. Evaluation of renal artery stenosis by magnetic resonance angiography. Am J Surg 1994;168:140.

McNeil JW, String ST, Pfeiffer RB Jr. Concomitant renal endarterectomy and aortic reconstruction. J Vasc Surg 1994;20:331.

Missouris CG, Buckenham T, Cappuccio FP, et al. Renal artery stenosis: a common and important problem in patients with peripheral vascular disease. Am J Med 1994;96:10.

Morris BJ. Molecular biology of renin. I. Gene and protein structure, synthesis and processing. J Hypertens 1992;10:209.

Murray SP, Kent KC, Salvatierra O, Stoney RJ. Complex branch renovascular disease: management options and late results. J Vasc Surg 1994;20:338.

Stanley JC, Zelenock GB, Messina LM, et al. Pediatric renovascular hypertension: a thirty-year experience of operative treatment. J Vasc Surg 1995;21:212.

ESSENTIALS OF SURGERY: SCIENTIFIC PRINCIPLES AND PRACTICE, edited by Lazar J. Greenfield, Michael W. Mulholland, Keith T. Oldham, Gerald B. Zelenock, and Keith D. Lillemoe. Lippincott–Raven Publishers, Philadelphia, © 1997.

CHAPTER 83

AORTOILIAC DISEASE

DAVID C. BREWSTER

Arteriosclerotic occlusive disease that involves the infrarenal abdominal aorta and iliac arteries is a common cause of arterial insufficiency of the lower extremities. Because arteriosclerosis is a generalized process, obliterative disease in the aortoiliac segment often coexists with disease in the infrainguinal vessels. Correction of hemodynamic problems in the inflow system alone often relieves ischemic symptoms in the leg. Evaluation of the adequacy of arterial inflow is important even if the primary difficulty is in the femoropopliteal outflow segment. Despite its generalized nature, chronic arteriosclerosis usually is segmental in distribution and is amenable to surgical treatment.

ANATOMY

The *abdominal aorta* (Fig. 83-1) begins at the aortic hiatus of the diaphragm in front of the lower border of the last thoracic vertebra and descends in front of the vertebral column slightly to the left of midline. As it courses distally, the aorta becomes smaller because many large visceral and parietal branches originate from it. The most important of these branches are the *celiac trunk, superior mesenteric artery* (SMA), right and left *renal arteries, inferior mesenteric artery,* and about four sets of paired *lumbar arteries.* The abdominal aorta terminates at the level of the fourth lumbar vertebra by bifurcating into the common iliac arteries, at about the level of the umbilicus.

Because the aorta is in a deep posterior retroperitoneal location, surgical exposure is difficult, especially of the suprarenal aortic segment from the diaphragm to the renal artery. The aorta is enveloped by the muscular crura of the diaphragm as they insert onto the lumbar vertebrae and is covered anteriorly by the lesser omentum, stomach, pancreas, and left renal vein. The left renal vein crosses the aorta anteriorly but is retroaortic or circumaortic in a small number of people. Mobilization of the suprarenal aorta is further complicated by the origin of the celiac axis and SMA from the anterior wall of the aorta.

Exposure of the infrarenal aorta involves opening the overlying retroperitoneal tissue and displacing the inferior aspect of the duodenum and small-intestinal mesentery. The inferior vena cava often is close to the right side of the infrarenal aorta.

The *common iliac arteries* diverge from the aortic bifurcation and pass downward and laterally. They are usually about 5 cm long before dividing into the internal (hypogastric) and external iliac arteries. The *internal iliac artery* supplies the viscera and parietes of the pelvis; the *external iliac artery* supplies the lower extremity.

The *femoral artery* is the continuation of the external iliac artery. It begins at the level of the inguinal ligament. About 4 to 5 cm below the inguinal ligament, the common femoral artery divides into superficial and deep (profunda femoris) branches. Because patients with aortoiliac disease also are likely to have occlusive disease in the superficial femoral artery, the deep femoral branch is important in revascularization procedures.

Pathways of *collateral circulation* to compensate for aortoiliac disease include visceral and parietal routes, such as internal mammary to inferior epigastric; intercostal and lumbar arteries to circumflex iliac and hypogastric networks; hypogastric and gluteal branches to the common and deep femoral arteries; and superior to inferior mesenteric and superior hemorrhoidal pathways via the marginal artery of Drummond (meandering mesenteric artery) and arch of Riolan (Figs. 83-2, 83-3).

PATHOPHYSIOLOGY

Arteriosclerosis can partially or completely occlude the aorta and iliac arteries. Progressive narrowing of these vessels reduces blood flow to the pelvic viscera and lower extremities, and characteristic symptoms develop. Because arteriosclerosis commonly centers on the aortic bifurcation, disease is usually maximal in the lower infrarenal aorta, aortic bifurcation, and common iliac arteries (Fig. 83-4). The occlusive process often is most pronounced at arterial bifurcations. Plaque is extensive on the posterior arterial wall, causing the distal lumbar arteries and median sacral vessel to be occluded early in the disease.

It is unusual for occlusive disease to involve the suprarenal aorta or aorta immediately distal to the renal arteries.

Because of collateral circulation, blood flow to the lower extremities is rarely critically reduced as long as the occlusive process is restricted to the intraabdominal aortoiliac segment. Claudication and/or sexual impotence are common, but blood flow at rest is adequate, and the viability of the extremity is rarely threatened. Advanced ischemic symptoms nearly always mean additional distal disease.

Symptoms occur when progressive narrowing of the vessel lumen and reduction of distal tissue perfusion outpace the ability of collateral circulation to compensate. Claudication or crampy, aching discomfort with exercise is almost always the earliest manifestation. It occurs because collateral blood flow is sufficient for tissue nutrition at rest but is unable to accommodate the increase in blood flow associated with exercise of a normal leg. Advanced ischemic symptoms, such as pain at rest or tissue necrosis (ulceration or digital gangrene), occur when resting blood flow is insufficient to satisfy the basic metabolic requirements of nonexercising tissue.

With progressive stenosis of a diseased vessel, blood flow may be reduced to the point that total thrombosis of the diseased segment occurs. This often accounts for sudden worsening of symptoms in a patient with previously mild ischemic manifestations. Degeneration or ulceration of plaques can lead to distal embolism of thrombin or platelet aggregates or dislodgment of atherosclerotic debris from the plaque itself *(atheromatous embolism).*

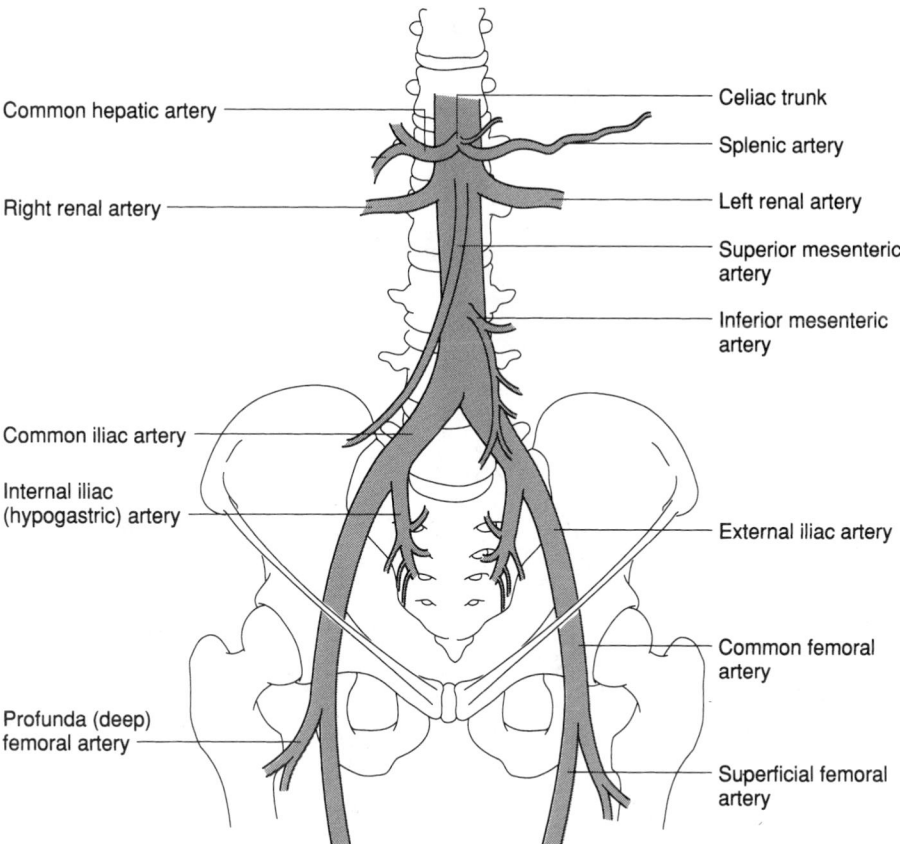

Figure 83-1. Anatomy of the abdominal aorta and iliac arteries.

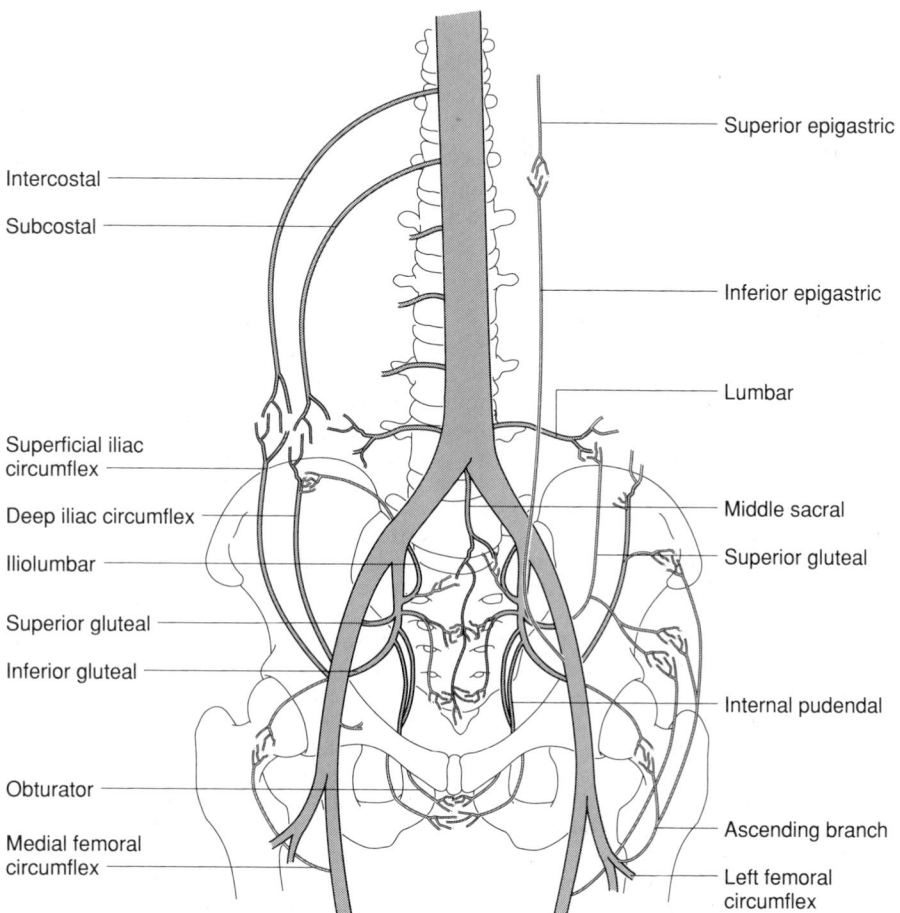

Figure 83-2. Major pathways of parietal collateral circulation in aortoiliac occlusive disease.

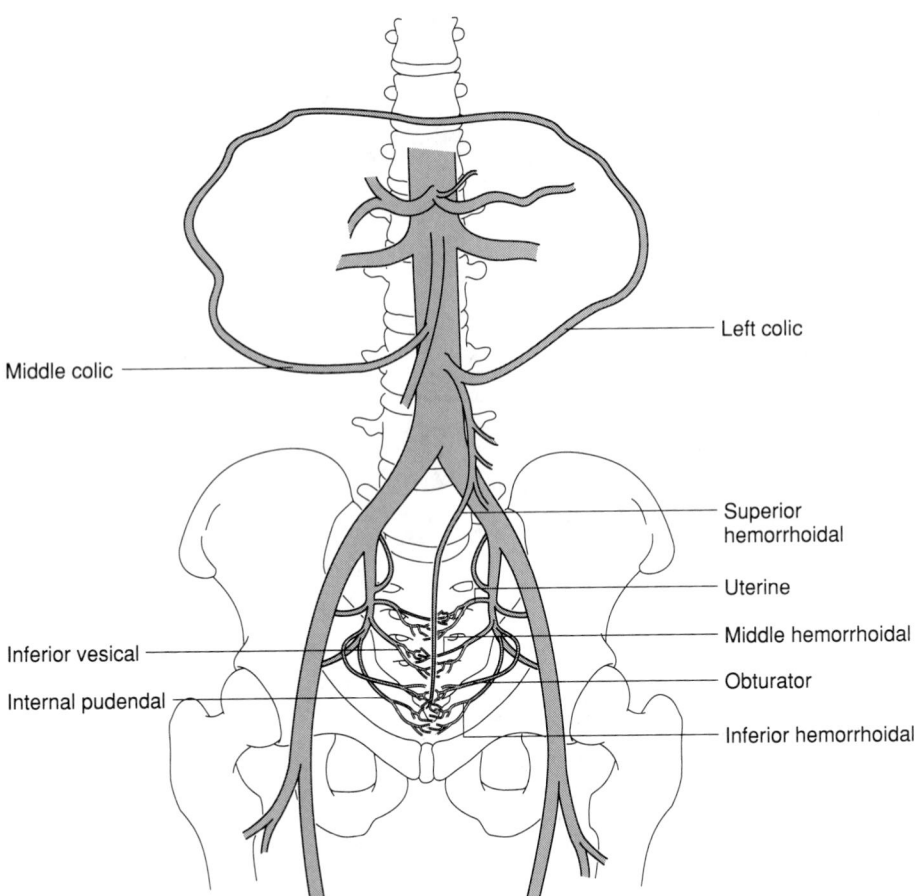

Middle colic

Left colic

Superior hemorrhoidal

Uterine

Middle hemorrhoidal

Inferior vesical

Obturator

Internal pudendal

Inferior hemorrhoidal

Figure 83-3. Major visceral collateral networks available for compensation of aortoiliac disease.

PATTERNS OF DISEASE AND CLINICAL MANIFESTATIONS

The symptoms, natural history, and choice of surgical reconstruction are influenced by the extent and distribution of occlusive disease (Fig. 83-5).

Type I

Most patients seek treatment because of claudication alone, which involves the proximal muscles of the thigh, hip, or buttock. Advanced ischemic symptoms do not occur unless distal atherosclerosis or atheroembolic complications are present. Impotence is an associated symptom. Patients are young with a relatively low prevalence of hypertension or diabetes, but often have abnormal blood lipids. Almost half of patients with localized aortoiliac disease are women, often with small aortic, iliac, and femoral vessels *(hypoplastic aorta syndrome)*. Invasive studies often are not performed.

Disease initially isolated to the bifurcation progresses to occlude one iliac artery or extends to the external iliac or femoral vessels, usually via a posterior tongue of atheroma. Although circulation to both lower extremities may be maintained via hypogastric collateral networks of the stenotic limb, this pattern of disease is unstable. Occlusion of the other common iliac artery can occur with thrombus propagating to the groin, which causes severe ischemia of both lower extremities and precipitates emergency intervention, which rarely is necessary in chronic aortoiliac disease.

Bilateral occlusion of the common iliac arteries leads to propagation of thrombus and total occlusion of the infrare-

nal aorta. Complete aortic occlusion extends to the level of the inferior mesenteric artery. If this vessel has undergone prior obliteration, superimposed thrombus extends proximally to a juxtarenal level, the renal vessels acting as an outflow tract for the proximal aorta. Rarely, further proximal extension of clot compromises the renal arteries or SMA, but this is unusual unless these vessels are stenotic because of associated occlusive disease. About 5% to 10% of patients undergoing aortoiliac operations for occlusive disease have a totally occluded aorta.

Type II

Most patients who are candidates for aortoiliac operations have diffuse disease, in which occlusive disease is confined to the abdominal vessels but also involves the external iliac and, perhaps, common femoral arteries.

Type III

Diffuse occlusive disease involves inflow and infrainguinal outflow arterial segments. Patients with such multilevel disease *(combined segment* or *tandem disease)* are older, typically male and are likely to have diabetes, hypertension, and associated atherosclerotic disease involving the coronary, cerebral, or visceral arteries. Most patients have symptoms of advanced ischemia, such as ischemic pain at rest or varying degrees of actual tissue necrosis. An operation is more often undertaken for limb salvage than simply for relief of claudication. The high incidence of associated atherosclerotic disease and other conditions increases risk of revascularization procedures.

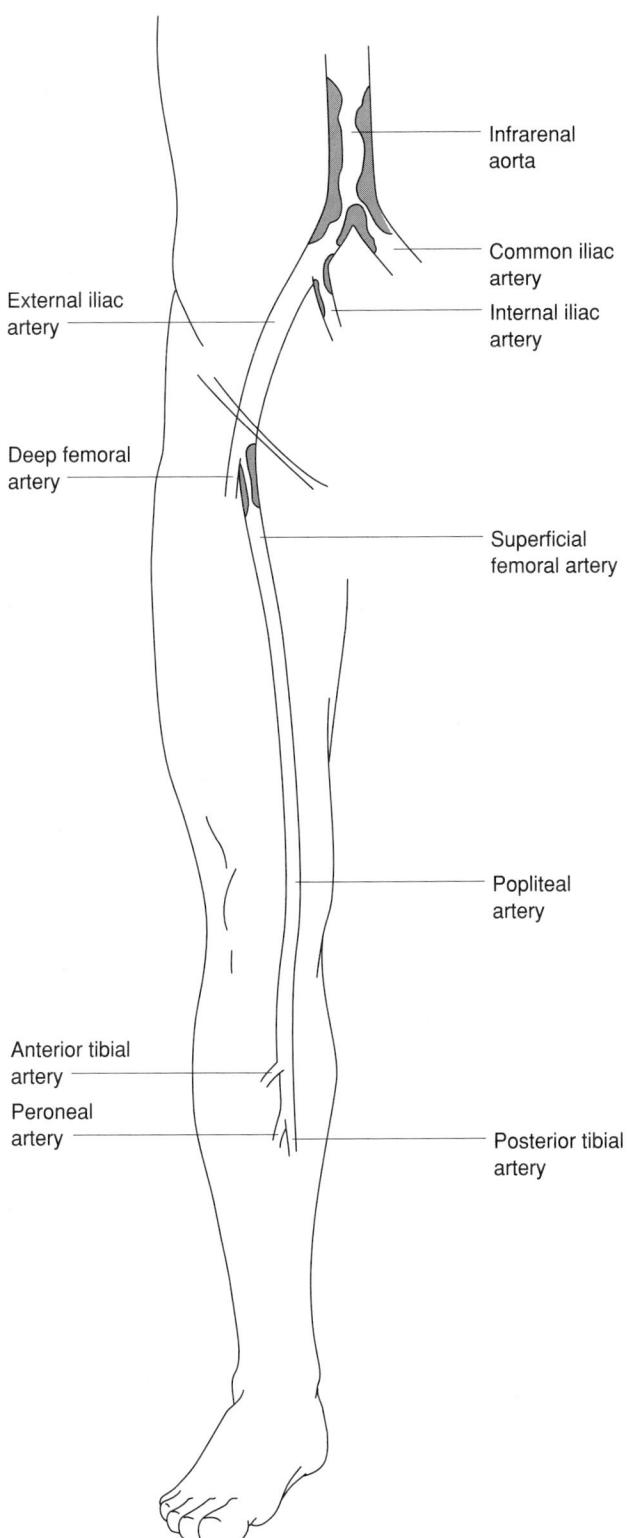

Figure 83-4. Common sites of arteriosclerotic lesions in aortoiliofemoral occlusive disease. Although often a generalized process, partially segmental distribution of major disease, most prominent at arterial bifurcations, usually allows surgical revascularization.

DIAGNOSIS
History and Physical Examination

Findings of the history and physical examination usually establish the diagnosis of aortoiliac disease. A reliable description is claudication in one or both legs, possible

decreased sexual potency among men, and diminished or absent femoral pulses *(Leriche syndrome).*

Although symptoms of claudication in the distribution of thigh, hip, and buttock muscles are usually a reliable indicator of inflow disease, a large number of patients, with aortoiliac disease, particularly multilevel disease, describe only calf claudication. The *physical findings* are as follows:

- Diminished femoral pulses
- Bruits heard over the lower abdomen or femoral vessels, particularly after exercise
- Elevation pallor
- Rubor on dependency
- Shiny, atrophic skin of the distal limbs and feet
- Areas of ulceration, ischemic necrosis, or gangrene, depending on the extent of atherosclerotic impairment

Noninvasive Testing

Use of noninvasive physiologic tests, such as segmental limb Doppler pressure measurements and plethysmography, may be helpful in diagnosis and help quantify the severity of disease. For example, these tests can help one differentiate diabetic neuropathic foot pain from true ischemic rest pain or help one predict the likelihood that a foot lesion may heal without revascularization. Findings of noninvasive studies provide a baseline with which a patient's course can be followed.

Arteriography

If clinical evaluation suggests a patient is a candidate for surgical arterial reconstruction, arteriography provides the anatomic information necessary for selection of the best method of revascularization and for planning an operation. Besides evaluating the anatomic distribution of occlusive disease in the aortoiliac segment and distal vessels, the surgeon examines the arteriograms for anatomic variations or associated occlusive lesions in the renal, visceral, or runoff vessels.

A complete arteriographic survey of the entire intraabdominal aortoiliac segment and infrainguinal runoff vessels is advisable. Runoff views are obtained to at least the level of the mid-calf; these views are also advisable for patients with threatened limbs and advanced disease, distal views, including the ankle and foot.

The most serious risk of contrast angiography is contrast-medium-induced renal dysfunction. This difficulty may be minimized with adequate hydration and limitation of contrast volume. For patients at high risk, such as those with diabetes with chronic renal insufficiency, imaging modalities such as magnetic resonance angiography may be a satisfactory substitute.

Pressure Measurements

Although accurate assessment of occlusive disease is possible by means of clinical evaluation and arteriography, difficulty can exist in the presence of multilevel occlusive disease. Assessment of the hemodynamic significance of occlusive disease at each segmental level is critical in selection of an appropriate reconstructive procedure. For this purpose, femoral arterial pressure is measured. Peak systolic pressure in the femoral artery is compared with distal aortic or brachial systolic pressure. A resting systolic pressure difference >5 mmHg or a fall in femoral artery pressure >15% with reactive hyperemia induced pharmacologically or by means of inflation of an occluding thigh cuff for 3 to 5 minutes

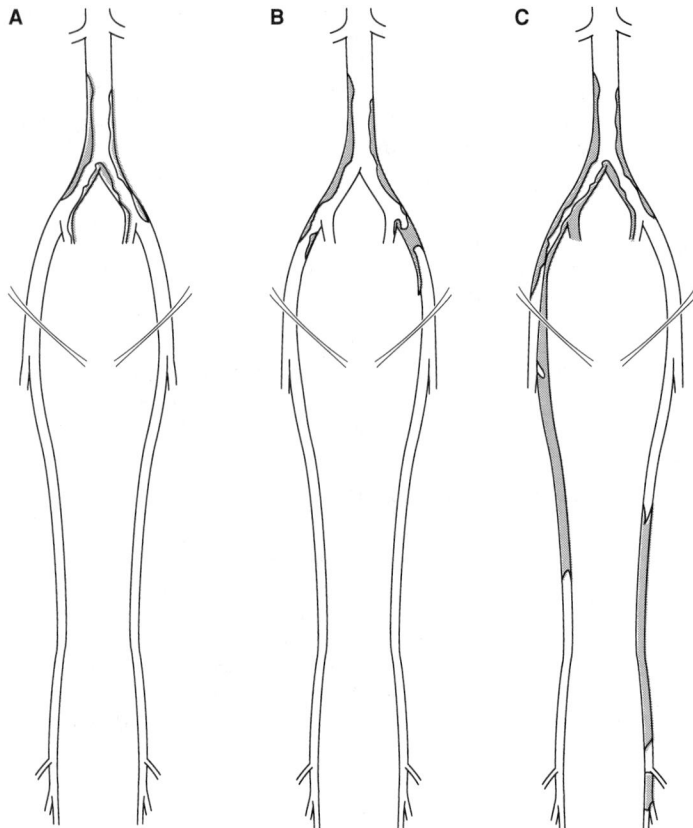

A   B   C

Figure 83-5. Patterns of aortoiliac disease. (*A*) In type I, localized disease is confined to the distal aorta and common iliac arteries. More widespread intraabdominal disease is present in type II (*B*), whereas a type III pattern signifies multilevel disease with associated infrainguinal occlusive lesions (*C*).

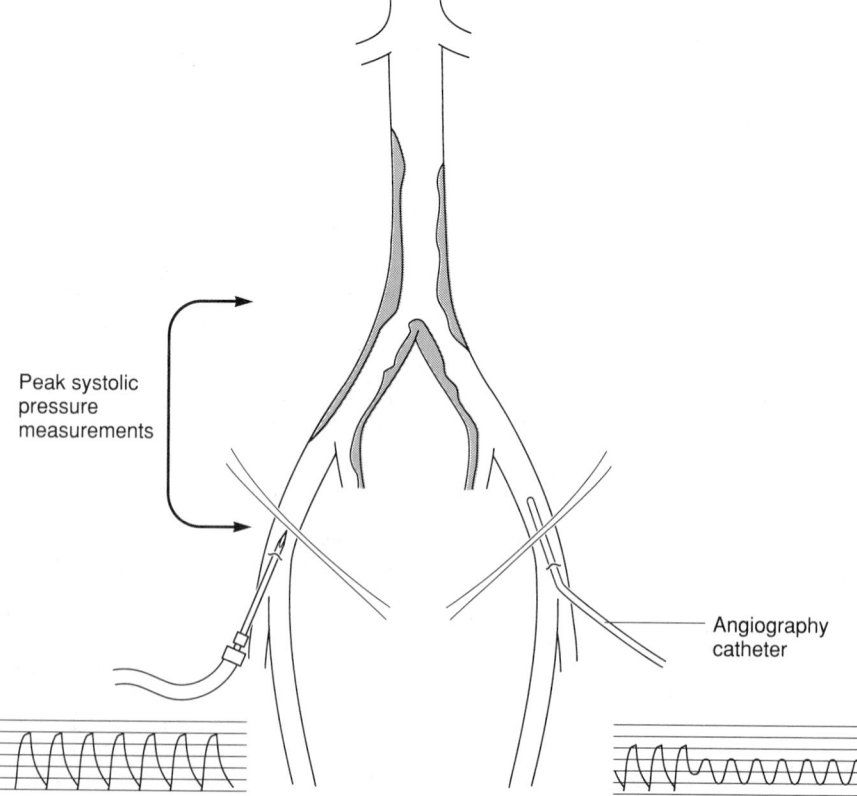

Peak systolic pressure measurements

Angiography catheter

Figure 83-6. Femoral artery pressure measurement to assess hemodynamic significance of aortoiliac disease. A significant decrease in peak systolic pressure is recorded on the left as the catheter is withdrawn across the diseased segment in the left iliac arterial system.

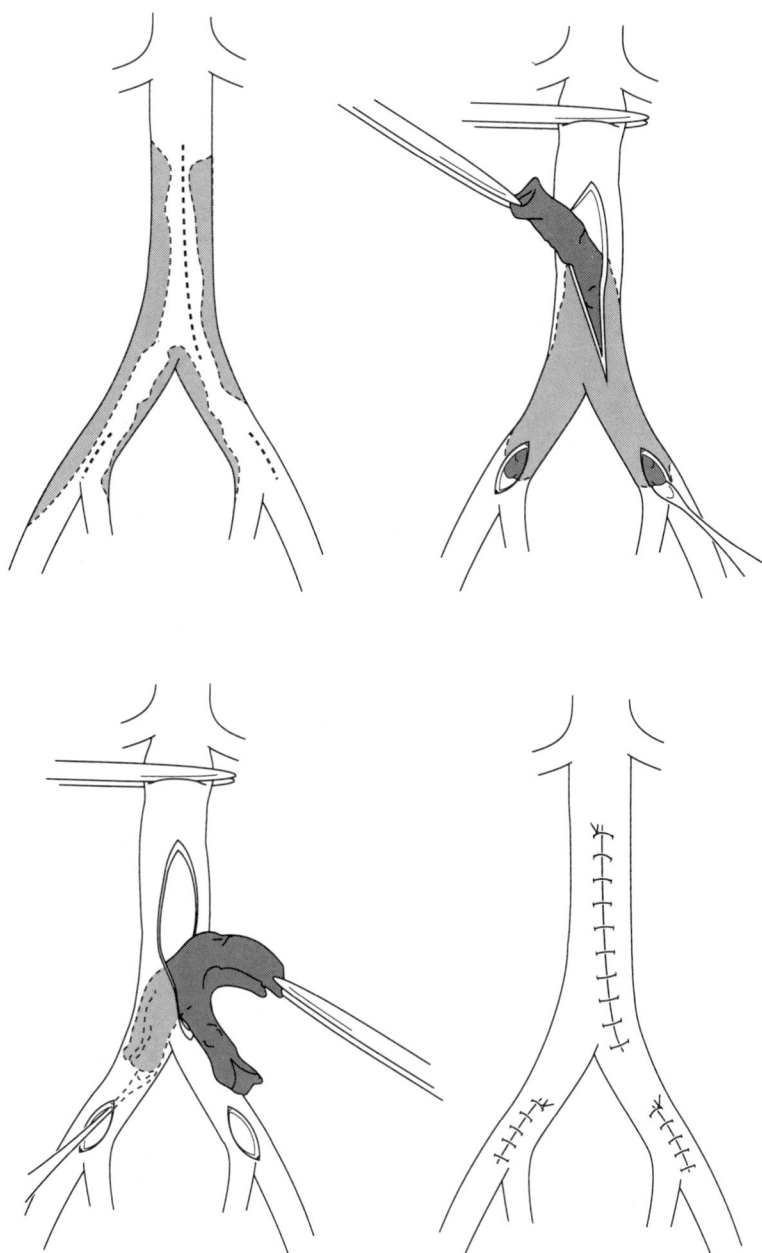

Figure 83-7. Aortoiliac endarterectomy.

implies hemodynamically significant inflow disease (Fig. 83-6). If revascularization is indicated, the inflow lesions are corrected first. If the study is normal, the surgeon can proceed directly with distal revascularization without fear of premature compromise or closure of the distal graft and without having the patient undergo an unnecessary inflow operation.

TREATMENT

Indications for Operation

Ischemic pain at rest or actual tissue necrosis, including ischemic ulcerations or frank digital gangrene, suggests advanced ischemia and threatened limb loss. Although true ischemic rest pain or ulceration sometimes resolves because of collateral development, this is infrequent. An exception is ischemia that occurs after an acute thrombotic

event, such as terminal thrombosis of a previously stenotic artery. Improvement of collateral circulation over a period of days to a few weeks may lessen ischemia and leave only claudication symptoms.

Untreated, most patients with symptoms of limb-threatening ischemia eventually need amputation. These symptoms are clear indications for arterial reconstruction, if anatomically feasible. Age alone is rarely an important consideration.

Decisions concerning operations for claudication symptoms alone must be individualized according to age, associated medical disease, employment requirements, and life-style preferences. Claudication that jeopardizes the livelihood of a patient or impairs the life style of a patient otherwise at low risk may be an indication for surgical correction, if a favorable anatomic situation for operation exists. If this more liberal approach is used, symptoms must be attributed to isolated proximal inflow disease, as

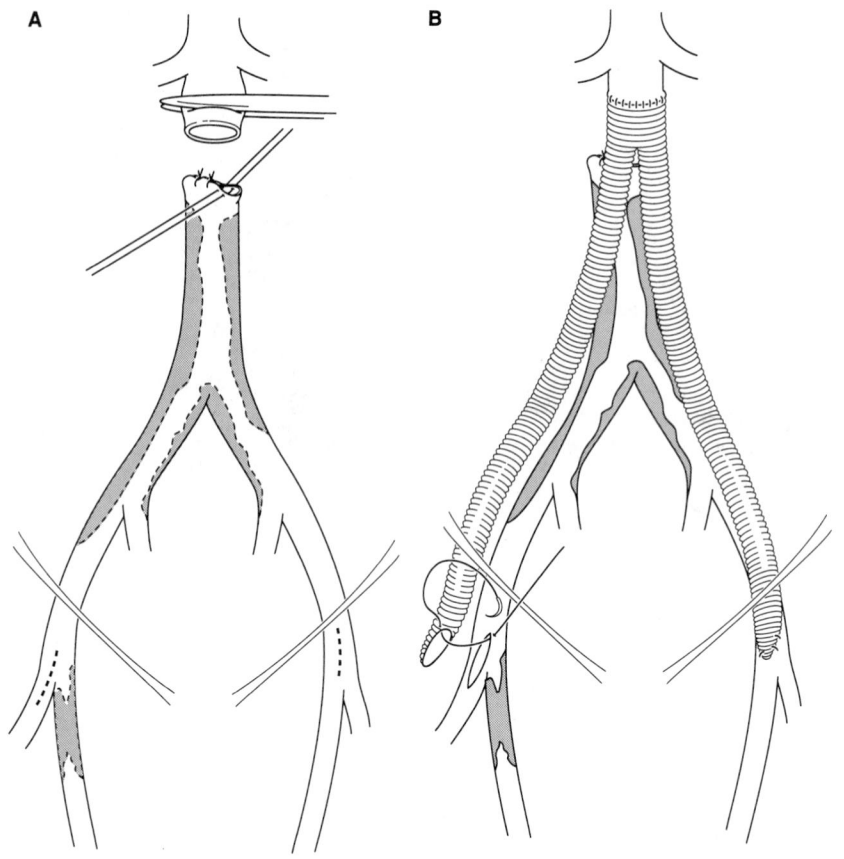

Figure 83-8. Aortobifemoral graft reconstruction. (A) Oversewing distal aorta. (B) Proximal end-to-end anastomosis.

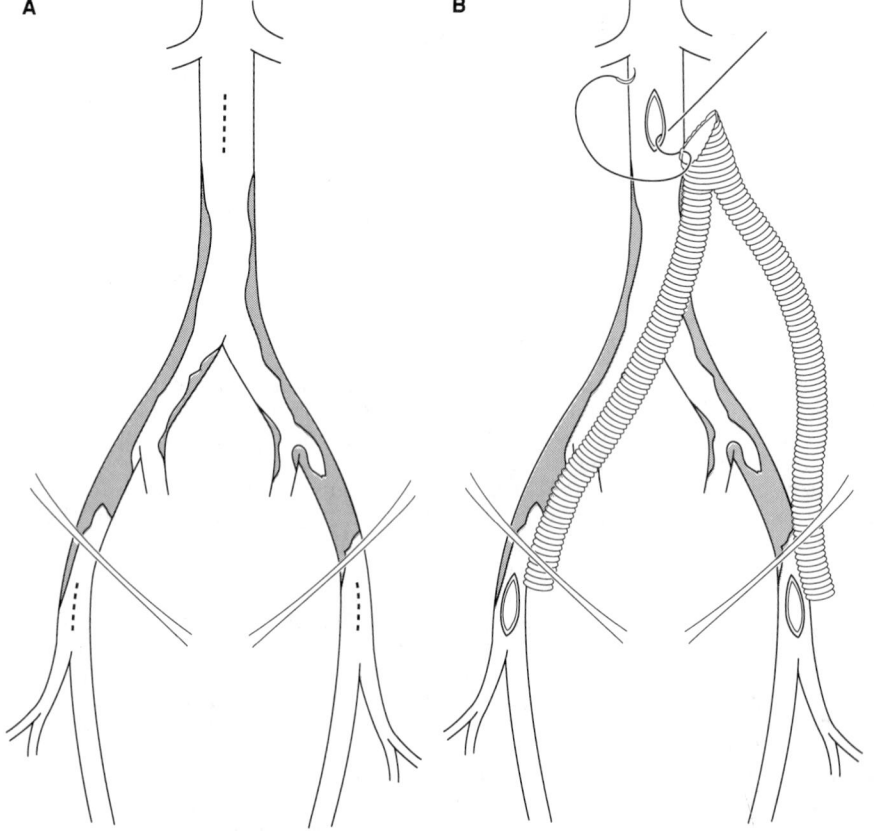

Figure 83-9. (A) Anatomic circumstances favoring end-to-side aortic anastomosis include large accessory renal arteries arising from the lower aorta, an enlarged patent inferior mesenteric artery, or occlusive disease confined largely to external iliac arteries that precludes retrograde pelvic perfusion. (B) Both proximal and distal anastomoses are end to side.

opposed to distal disease in the femoropopliteal arterial segment.

Direct Aortic Reconstruction

Aortoiliac Endarterectomy

Aortoiliac endarterectomy is used to treat a small number of patients with localized disease, particularly patients with a projected life span of 20 to 30 years or patients who might be at high risk for infection with nonautogenous reconstruction (Fig. 83-7).

Aortobifemoral Bypass Grafting

Prosthetic bypass grafting from the infrarenal aorta to femoral arteries (Fig. 83-8) is the most frequently used reconstructive procedure for aortoiliac occlusive disease, and is the most effective and durable method of revascularization.

The proximal aortic anastomosis may be end-to-end or end-to-side. End-to-end anastomosis is indicated in the presence of coexisting aneurysmal disease or complete aortic occlusion up to the renal arteries. End-to-side proximal anastomosis is used to preserve a patent inferior mesenteric artery or sizable accessory renal artery or if the anatomic pattern of disease suggests that end-to-end bypass is likely to devascularize both hypogastric arteries and the pelvic region (Fig. 83-9). Whichever technique is used, the principle is to place the proximal anastomosis as high as possible in the infrarenal aorta. The graft usually is carried to the femoral level, where exposure is optimum, anastomosis is easier, and disease of the deep femoral artery can be assessed and corrected. Establishment of adequate graft outflow through the deep femoral artery is important.

Iliofemoral Grafts

If arteriography confirms largely unilateral iliac disease, limited arterial reconstruction by means of an iliofemoral bypass may be considered. Ipsilateral iliofemoral grafts are useful principally for patients with disease confined to the external iliac artery of the symptomatic extremity with a common iliac artery that can be used for proximal graft anastomosis. A retroperitoneal approach through an oblique lower abdominal incision is used.

Complications

- Bleeding that necessitates reoperation or acute limb ischemia due to graft thrombosis or distal thromboembolism
- Acute renal failure (infrequent with intraoperative provision of adequate fluid volume, optimization of cardiac function, and avoidance of declamping hypotension)
- Spinal cord and intestinal ischemia
- Myocardial infarction
- Pulmonary insufficiency (unusual in the absence of severe preoperative chronic lung disease)
- Anastomotic aneurysm, almost always at the femoral anastomosis
- Graft infection and enteric fistula

Indirect Revascularization Methods

Extraanatomic bypass grafts are routed in remote subcutaneous tissue planes, deliberately avoiding the natural location of the blood supply because of hostile pathologic conditions in the area (infection, prior irradiation, multiple previous operations, abdominal stomas) or because entering the area is likely to increase the risk of an operation (as in the transabdominal direct aortic approach). Long-term patency is less satisfactory than with direct methods of revascularization.

The most frequently used extraanatomic grafts are axillofemoral and femorofemoral bypass or a combination (axillobifemoral bypass). Axillobifemoral grafts are chosen whenever bilateral iliac disease requires an extraanatomic means of inflow restoration. Femorofemoral grafts are used for unilateral iliac disease, if the contralateral iliac artery is free of hemodynamically significant disease and can adequately serve as a donor inflow source. If disease in the contralateral iliac artery is focal, percutaneous transluminal balloon angioplasty on this side may be carried out to establish adequate inflow for a femorofemoral graft. Femorofemoral grafts are used to manage occlusion of one limb of an aortobifemoral graft that cannot be reopened by means of thrombectomy.

SUGGESTED READING

Brewster DC, Cambria RP, Darling RC, et al. Long-term results of combined iliac balloon angioplasty and distal surgical revascularization. Ann Surg 1989;210:324.

Cambria RP, Yucel EK, Brewster DC, et al. The potential for lower extremity revascularization without contrast arteriography: experience with magnetic resonance angiography. J Vasc Surg 1993;17:1050.

Harrington ME, Harrington EB, Haimov N, Schanger H, Jacobson JH. Iliofemoral versus femorofemoral bypass: the case for an individualized approach. J Vasc Surg 1992;16:841.

Piotrowski J, Pearce WH, Jones DN, et al. Aortobifemoral bypass: The operation of choice for unilateral iliac occlusion? J Vasc Surg 1988;8:211.

Rutherford R, Patt A, Pearce WH. Extra-anatomic bypass: a closer view. J Vasc Surg 1987;6:437.

van der Vliet JA, Scharn DM, de Waard J-WD, Roumen RMH, van Roye SFS, Buskens FGM. Unilateral vascular reconstruction for iliac occlusive disease. J Vasc Surg 1994;19:610.

ESSENTIALS OF SURGERY: SCIENTIFIC PRINCIPLES AND PRACTICE, edited by Lazar J. Greenfield, Michael W. Mulholland, Keith T. Oldham, Gerald B. Zelenock, and Keith D. Lillemoe. Lippincott–Raven Publishers, Philadelphia, © 1997.

CHAPTER 84

FEMOROPOPLITEAL AND INFRAPOPLITEAL OCCLUSIVE DISEASE

LLOYD M. TAYLOR, JR., JOHN M. PORTER, AND PHILIPPE A. MASSER

Symptomatic lower-extremity ischemia is frequent among the aging population. Patients with generalized cardiovascular disease, diabetes, and renal failure also are likely to have lower-extremity arterial occlusive disease.

ANATOMY

The *common femoral artery* begins at the inguinal ligament as the direct extension of the external iliac artery. It lies midway between the anterior superior iliac spine and the symphysis pubis (Fig. 84-1). In the proximal thigh, the common femoral artery is superficial, covered by skin and subcutaneous tissue; the femoral nerve is lateral to the artery and the femoral vein is medial. Below the inguinal ligament, the common femoral artery divides into the lateral and posterior *deep femoral artery* and the medial *superficial femoral artery*. The *medial* and *lateral circumflex femoral arteries* and four to six *perforating muscular arteries* to the upper thigh originate from the deep femoral artery, which terminates in the middle thigh.

The superficial femoral artery continues anteromedially beneath the sartorius muscle. In the middle third of the thigh, it enters the adductor (Hunter) canal, which is an aponeurotic tunnel formed by fascial contributions from the vastus medialis, adductor longus, and adductor magnus muscles. The *popliteal artery* emerges from the adductor canal and proceeds posteriorly behind the knee between the lateral and medial heads of the gastrocnemius muscle. The popliteal artery divides into two branches just distal to the knee. The first is the *anterior tibial artery*, which passes laterally, pierces the interosseous membrane between the tibia and fibula, and lies anterior to this membrane in the anterior compartment of the calf, eventually terminating in the foot as the *dorsalis pedis artery*.

The *tibial peroneal trunk* is the direct continuation of the popliteal artery, and quickly divides into the posterior tibial and peroneal arteries. The *posterior tibial artery* continues distally in the calf behind the tibia, entering the foot between the medial malleolus and the Achilles tendon, where it divides into the *medial and lateral plantar arteries*. The *peroneal artery* courses deep in the substance of the calf, descending along the medial aspect of the fibula, and ends in terminal branches above the ankle. All three vessels supply the calf, the anterior tibial and posterior tibial arteries continuing onto the foot to provide its primary blood supply.

COLLATERAL CIRCULATION

Arterial collaterals occur by means of enlargement of preexisting arterial connections rather than by growth of new vessels when obstruction of the large arteries prevents normal lower-extremity blood flow. When the common femoral artery is obstructed, collateral circulation to the upper thigh occurs through the internal pudendal and obturator branches of the internal iliac artery and through the deep circumflex and inferior epigastric branches of the external iliac artery (Fig. 84-2). When the superficial femoral artery is obstructed, the popliteal artery is supplied from the branches of the deep femoral and lateral femoral circumflex arteries and a number of muscular perforating branches. Occlusion of the popliteal artery leads to filling of the tibial vessels by the medial and lateral geniculate arteries. The peroneal artery fills an important collateral bed with reconstitution of the plantar arch when the dorsal pedal and posterior tibial arteries are obstructed at the ankle.

PATHOPHYSIOLOGY
Intermittent Claudication

The collateral arterial circulation of the lower extremity allows a person to tolerate atherosclerotic obstruction of the leg arteries, at least initially. Moderate arterial obstruction does not change resting flow but restricts the ability of arterial flow to increase in response to exercise. The result of this restriction is *intermittent claudication,* defined as lower-extremity muscular pain with exercise that is relieved by short periods (minutes) of rest. The site of the symptoms is always one level distal to the site of arterial obstruction; eg, superficial femoral artery obstruction in the thigh produces calf claudication. Most patients with intermittent claudication have lower-extremity arterial obstruction at one site (Table 84-1).

Ischemic Rest Pain

As atherosclerotic disease intensifies, the lower-extremity arteries become involved at multiple levels in series (eg, superficial femoral artery plus popliteal artery) or in parallel (eg, superficial femoral artery plus deep femoral artery). As the obstruction worsens, resting blood flow may decrease to levels below minimal metabolic requirements, and the foot becomes ischemic at rest. Patients feel pain in the forefoot and toes, which is worse at night when they

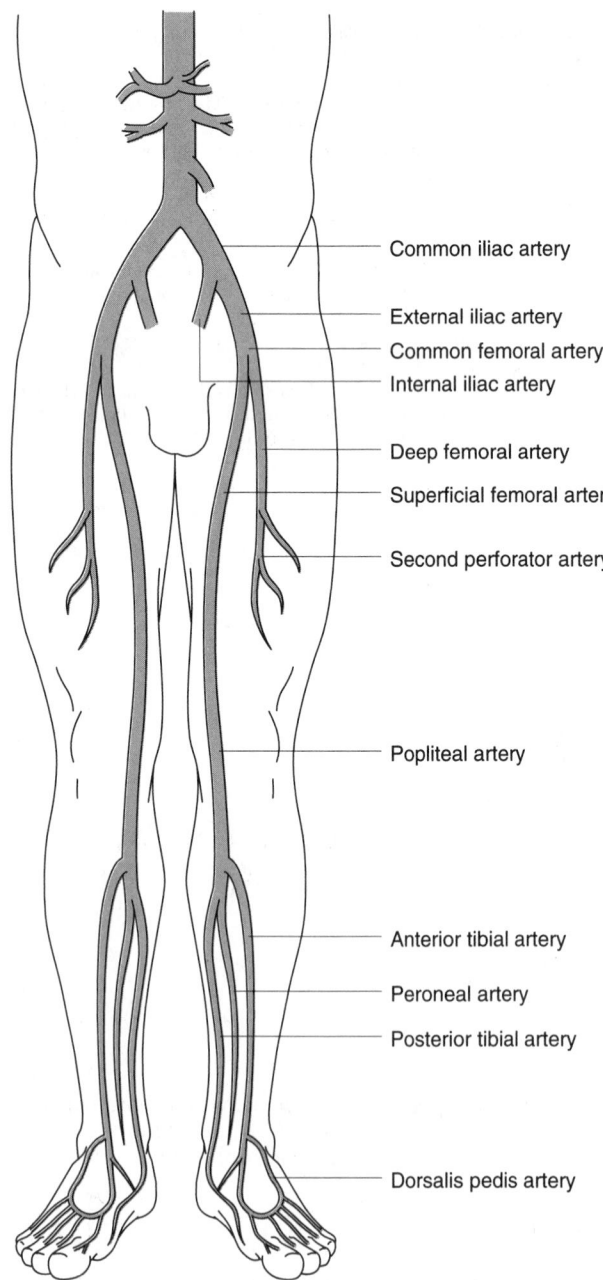

Figure 84-1. Anatomy of the arterial circulation to the lower extremity.

Common iliac artery

External iliac artery
Common femoral artery
Internal iliac artery

Deep femoral artery

Superficial femoral artery

Second perforator artery

Popliteal artery

Anterior tibial artery

Peroneal artery

Posterior tibial artery

Dorsalis pedis artery

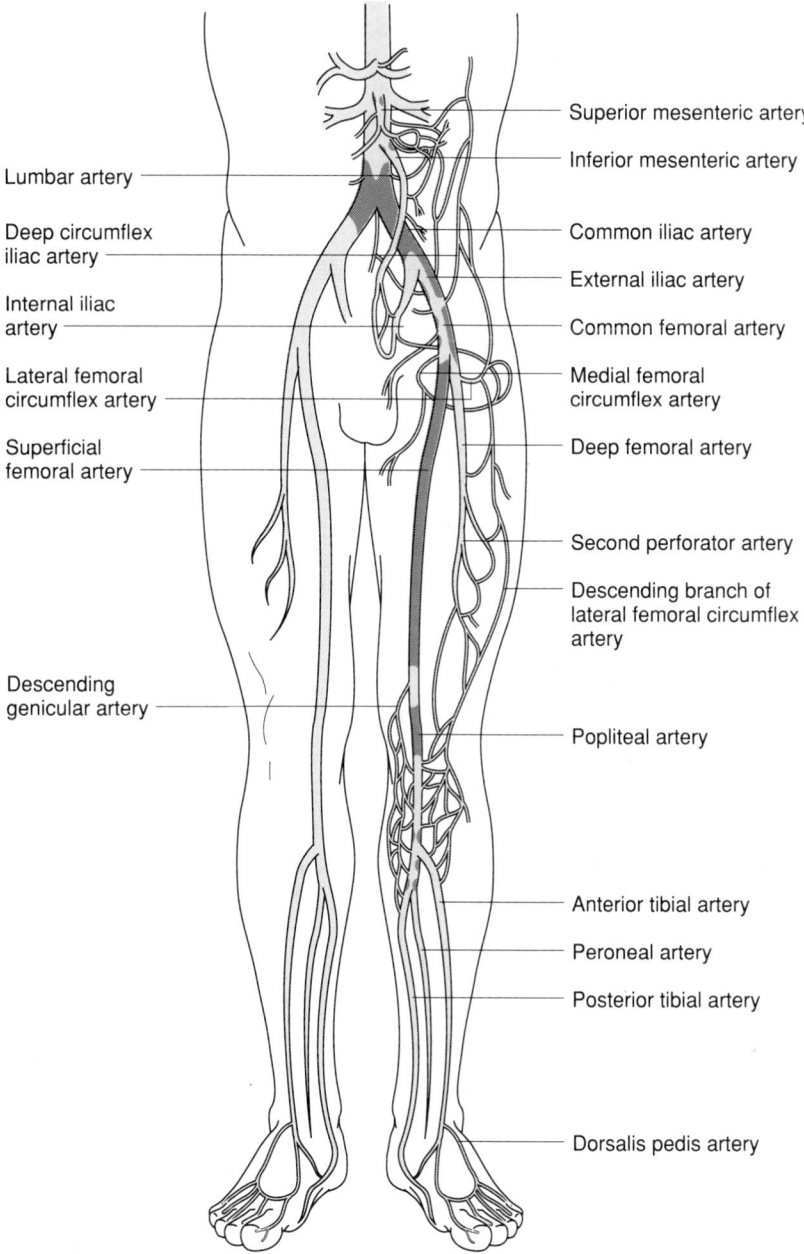

Lumbar artery

Deep circumflex iliac artery

Internal iliac artery

Lateral femoral circumflex artery

Superficial femoral artery

Descending genicular artery

Superior mesenteric artery

Inferior mesenteric artery

Common iliac artery

External iliac artery

Common femoral artery

Medial femoral circumflex artery

Deep femoral artery

Second perforator artery

Descending branch of lateral femoral circumflex artery

Popliteal artery

Anterior tibial artery

Peroneal artery

Posterior tibial artery

Dorsalis pedis artery

Figure 84-2. Major collateral vessels of the lower extremity.

lie down. Patients achieve some relief of ischemic foot pain by placing the foot in a dependent position, as in sitting or walking, presumably because blood flow increases because of increased arterial pressure due to gravity. This syndrome is *ischemic rest pain.*

Ischemic Ulcers

Patients with ischemic rest pain have insufficient blood supply to allow healing of minor traumatic lesions, such as cuts, scrapes, and bruises. These lesions are *ischemic ulcers.*

Table 84-1. SYMPTOMS PRODUCED BY ARTERIAL OBSTRUCTION IN THE LOWER EXTREMITY

Symptom	Site of Arterial Obstruction	Ankle/Brachial Pressure Ratio
Claudication	Single level	>0.5
Ischemic ulcer	Multiple level	0.3–0.5
Gangrene	Multiple level	<0.3

Gangrene

As resting blood flow decreases to its lowest ebb, spontaneous necrosis of the distal toes and forefoot causes *gangrene.*

NATURAL HISTORY OF INFRAINGUINAL ATHEROSCLEROSIS

Patients with claudication and an ankle–brachial arterial pressure index (ABI) <0.5 are more likely to need revascularization than those with higher ABIs. The outcomes for patients with chronic lower-extremity ischemia can be predicted on the basis of severity of disease, as assessed with simple ankle blood pressure measurement. Revascularization is rarely necessary, and amputation is virtually unheard of in patients with ABIs ≥0.55. One of these outcomes is close to inevitable for patients with ABIs <0.3.

Infrainguinal atherosclerosis is an important indicator of systemic atherosclerosis and of the corresponding reduced life expectancy that results from coronary and cerebral atherosclerotic disease. The magnitude of decrease in life expectancy appears to be directly related to the severity of lower-extremity ischemia. The causes of decreased survival rates are summarized in Figure 84-3.

DIAGNOSIS

History

The history of intermittent claudication may include:

- Consistent onset of symptoms when walking
- Reproduction of symptoms during a walk of the same distance
- Reliable relief of symptoms with a few minutes rest
- Symptoms confined to the calf, which suggests occlusive disease limited to the area below the inguinal ligament
- Ischemic rest pain confined to the forefoot and toes, provoked by elevating the foot, and relieved by dependency
- Arterial disease at other sites, especially coronary and cerebral arterial ischemic symptoms
- Angina pectoris, myocardial infarction, coronary bypass, cerebral transient ischemic attacks, stroke, or carotid artery operations

Physical Examination

Physical examination must include palpation of all peripheral pulses. Classic signs of lower-extremity ischemia include pallor, hair loss, dependent rubor, abnormal nail growth, and slow capillary filling. These signs are subjective and may be influenced by environmental conditions. Measurement with a Doppler ultrasound flow detector of blood pressure in both arms and ankles is routine.

Noninvasive Vascular Testing

Noninvasive testing in the vascular laboratory is performed for all patients with suspected infrainguinal occlusive disease. The basic examination consists of *segmental pressure measurements* and *Doppler arterial waveform tracings* from the level of the upper thigh, above the knee,

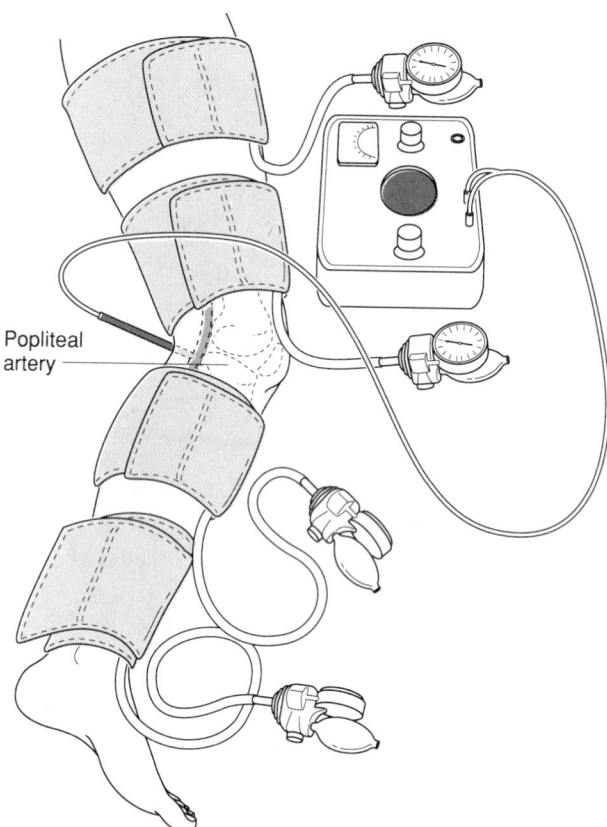

Figure 84-4. Technique of segmental pressure measurements using a Doppler ultrasonic flow detector.

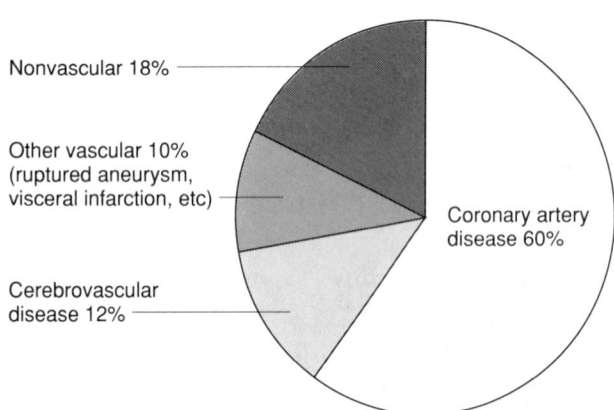

Figure 84-3. Causes of death in patients with chronic lower extremity ischemia. (After Taylor LM Jr. Porter JM. Natural history and nonoperative treatment of chronic lower extremity ischemia. In: Rutherford RB, ed. Vascular surgery, ed 3. Philadelphia, WB Saunders, 1989:653)

below the knee, and at the ankle (Fig. 84-4). Pressures and waveforms from the toes, recorded by means of plethysmography, are useful in the diagnosis of distal arterial disease and extensive calcification of proximal arteries, which makes pressure measurements invalid, a condition frequently present in people with diabetes.

Sometimes *ankle pressure measurements* are repeated immediately after treadmill walking. A decrease in ankle pressure after treadmill walking is abnormal and provides objective confirmation of the diagnosis of claudication. Vascular claudication is always associated with at least a 20% decrease in ABI when symptoms occur (Fig. 84-5). Absence of this finding raises questions about the diagnosis and leads to a search for other causes of leg pain.

Duplex scanning allows evaluation of specific lesions in the lower extremities and determination of location, length, and degree of stenosis.

Because of the frequency of associated coronary and cerebrovascular disease, examination of patients with infrainguinal atherosclerosis includes *assessment of the coronary circulation* and *noninvasive evaluation of the carotid bifurcations.*

NONSURGICAL MANAGEMENT OF LOWER-EXTREMITY ISCHEMIA

Modification of Risk Factors

Exercise

Walking improves symptoms of claudication. The improvement in walking distance resulting from a program of regular exercise averages about 75% after 8 weeks of training. What appears to change is the amount of oxygen

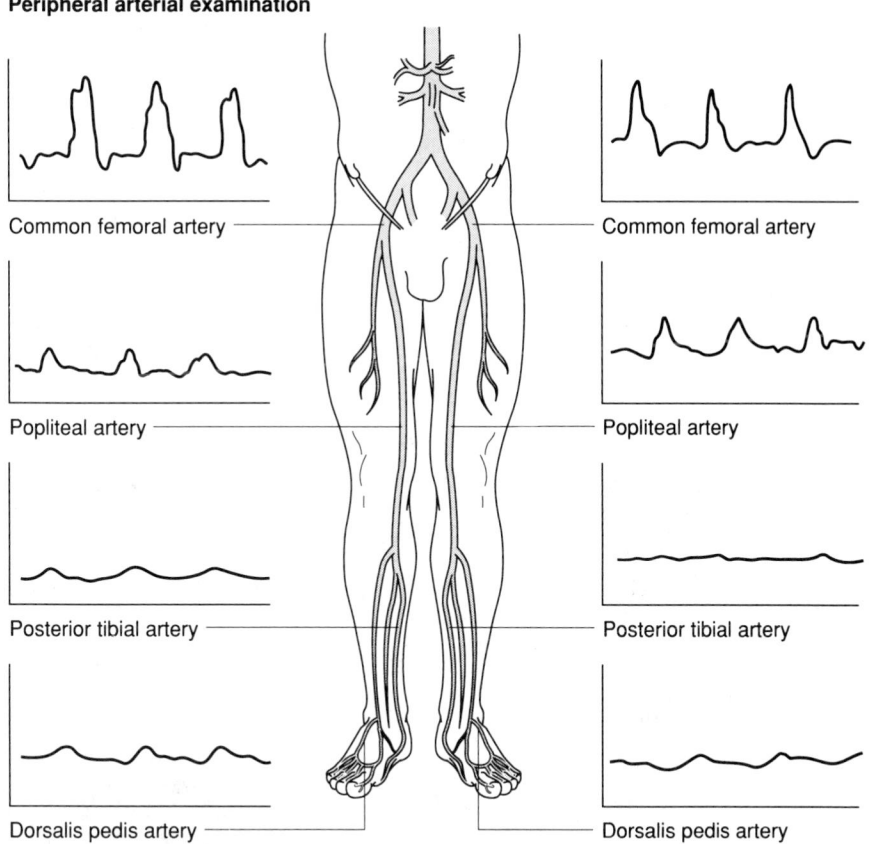

Peripheral arterial examination

Common femoral artery — Common femoral artery

Popliteal artery — Popliteal artery

Posterior tibial artery — Posterior tibial artery

Dorsalis pedis artery — Dorsalis pedis artery

Resting segmental blood pressures

	Right Pressure	Right Leg/arm ratio	Left Pressure	Left Leg/arm ratio
Arm	168		168	
Upper thigh	124	0.74	127	0.76
Above knee	99	0.59	115	0.68
Below knee	88	0.52	100	0.59
Ankle DP	82	0.48	80	0.48
PT	82	0.48	74	0.44
Toe	60	0.36	66	0.39

Treadmill: 1.5 mph at 0% grade
Stopped arbitrarily; no discomfort at 5:00 (202 meters)

Right

Arm	165	150	156	150
Ankle	50	65	70	72

Index (1.2, 1.0, 0.8, 0.6, 0.4, 0.2, 0)
Minutes after exercise (0 2 4 6 8)

Left

Arm				
Ankle	98	90	60	90

Index (1.2, 1.0, 0.8, 0.6, 0.4, 0.2, 0)
Minutes after exercise (0 2 4 6 8)

Figure 84-5. Standard noninvasive vascular laboratory peripheral arterial examination includes results of ankle pressure response to treadmill walking.

extracted from the blood (femoral arterial and venous oxygen difference is increased), which is associated with increased efficiency of muscle function (popliteal venous lactate levels are reduced). Patients are advised to walk at a comfortable pace to the point of claudication, to stop and rest until symptoms are relieved, to walk again, and to repeat this cycle for 1 hour each day.

Cessation of Smoking

Tobacco use is the most important risk factor patients need to modify. The physician must inform patients of the causative relation between smoking and limb ischemia. This information is given to patients in a specific, unqualified, and conclusive manner that leaves no room for rationalization. Patients are simply told: "The cause of your problem is cigarette smoking" at every patient encounter.

Pharmacologic Management of Infrainguinal Ischemia

Hemorrheologic Drugs

Interest in pharmacologic treatment centers on *hemorrheology,* the study of the flow characteristics of blood. In large vessels, the important flow characteristic is viscosity. Reducing blood viscosity by means of hemodilution results in reproducible improvement in walking distance. In the microcirculation, cellular deformability is a critical determinant of blood flow. Erythrocytes must deform considerably to pass through capillaries. Another important determinant of microcirculatory flow is degree of aggregation of erythrocytes, leukocytes, and platelets.

Pentoxifylline appears to affect blood viscosity, cellular deformability, and cellular aggregation, and it appears to act through hemorrheologic mechanisms to improve the symptoms of chronic lower-extremity ischemia, specifically claudication. Pentoxifylline improves treadmill walking distance for many patients with claudication.

Metabolism-enhancing Drugs

Carnitine is a naturally occurring substance that facilitates aerobic metabolism by promoting entry of pyruvate into the citric acid cycle and by enhancing the transport of fatty acids. These effects result in production of large amounts of adenosine triphosphate and in large amounts of energy from the same amount of oxygen. Carnitine helps increase treadmill walking distance and decrease popliteal venous lactate levels.

Antiplatelet Agents

Aspirin affects platelet function by irreversibly acetylating the enzyme cyclooxygenase, blocking the formation of thromboxane A_2, and eliminating an important stimulus of platelet aggregation and release. The use of aspirin by patients with chronic lower-extremity ischemia reduces the mortality rate for vascular disease and the rate of nonfatal stroke and myocardial infarction. Aspirin apparently also enhances the patency of vascular repairs, especially if the drug is begun preoperatively. Many clinicians prescribe aspirin to all patients with symptomatic lower-extremity ischemia unless the drug is contraindicated because of allergy or side effects.

Ticlopidine apparently acts by inhibiting platelet adenosine diphosphate receptors and stimulating adenyl cyclase. It improves treadmill walking distance and ABI.

SURGICAL TREATMENT OF INFRAINGUINAL OCCLUSIVE DISEASE

Nonsurgical measures are sufficient to relieve most instances of symptomatic infrainguinal ischemia. Some patients, however, have symptoms severe enough to necessitate direct restoration of blood flow to ischemic areas—methods include vascular operations and angiographic and interventional techniques, such as transluminal balloon angioplasty, laser-assisted balloon angioplasty, and catheter atherectomy.

Indications

Surgical intervention is indicated for lower-extremity ischemia that is severe enough to threaten limb survival. Clinical symptoms involved are ischemic rest pain, ischemic ulceration, and gangrene. Objective findings that confirm the presence of limb-threatening ischemia usually include an ABI <0.4, nonpulsatile distal extremity plethysmographic waveforms, and a great toe-brachial pressure index <0.25. Surgical treatment of claudication usually is reserved for patients whose symptoms interfere with employment or whose walking distance is less than one block. Such patients nearly always have ABIs <0.55.

Arteriography

Selection of appropriate surgical therapy for lower-extremity arterial disease requires visualization in detail of the obstructive lesions and the proximal and distal vessels. This is achieved by means of arteriography. Selective catheterization of distal vessels, external warming, vasodilator injections, digital subtraction techniques, and femoral occlusion balloon angiography all are used to improve distal arteriographic visualization. It may be necessary to obtain repeat arteriograms to answer questions critical to surgical planning for patients with severe ischemia, once the initial arteriogram has been examined.

Primary Amputation

Some patients have limb ischemia from arterial obstructive disease so advanced that revascularization is impossible. Distal bypass grafts to the ankle and foot arteries are performed. Primary amputation must not be considered until meticulous arteriography shows no distal vessels suitable for bypass (Fig. 84-6). Simple lack of visualization of distal vessels cannot be used as a criterion for inoperability.

Venous Bypass Grafting

Potential sites for saphenous vein bypass grafting extend from the popliteal artery below the knee to the tibial and peroneal arteries of the calf and the arteries of the ankle and foot. Vein bypass is possible if there is arterial inflow to the level of the femoral artery and a patent distal vessel suitable for anastomosis. Two techniques are used to construct lower-extremity vein

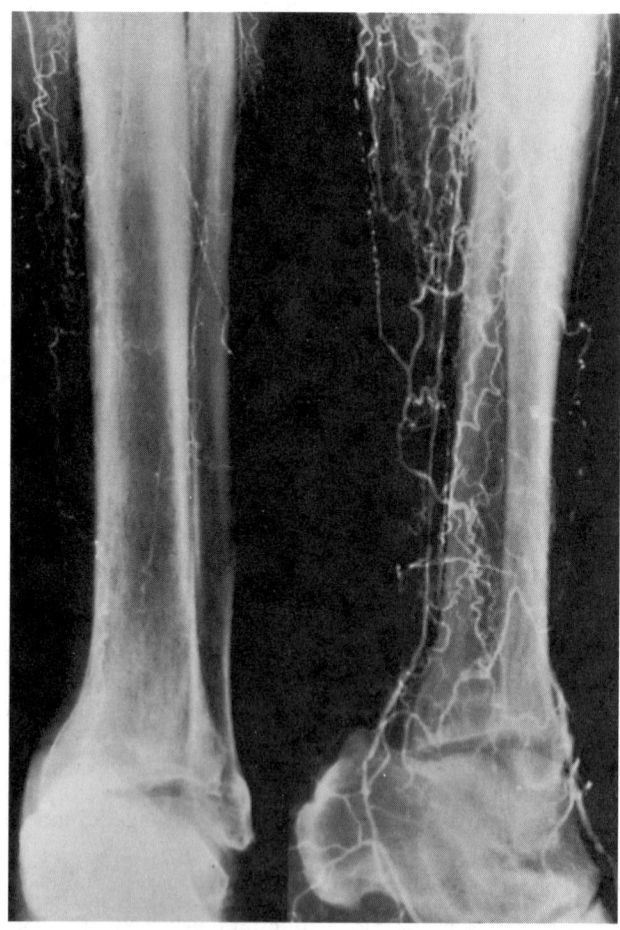

Figure 84-6. (*Left*) Initial arteriogram fails to show graftable distal vessels. The patient was considered to be inoperable. (*Right*) A second arteriogram selective injection, external warming, and intraarterial vasodilator demonstrates graftable distal posterior tibial artery. The patient's foot was salvaged by a successful bypass graft. (Taylor LM Jr, Edwards JM, Phinney ES, Porter JM. Reversed vein bypass to infrapopliteal arteries. Ann Surg 1987;205:90)

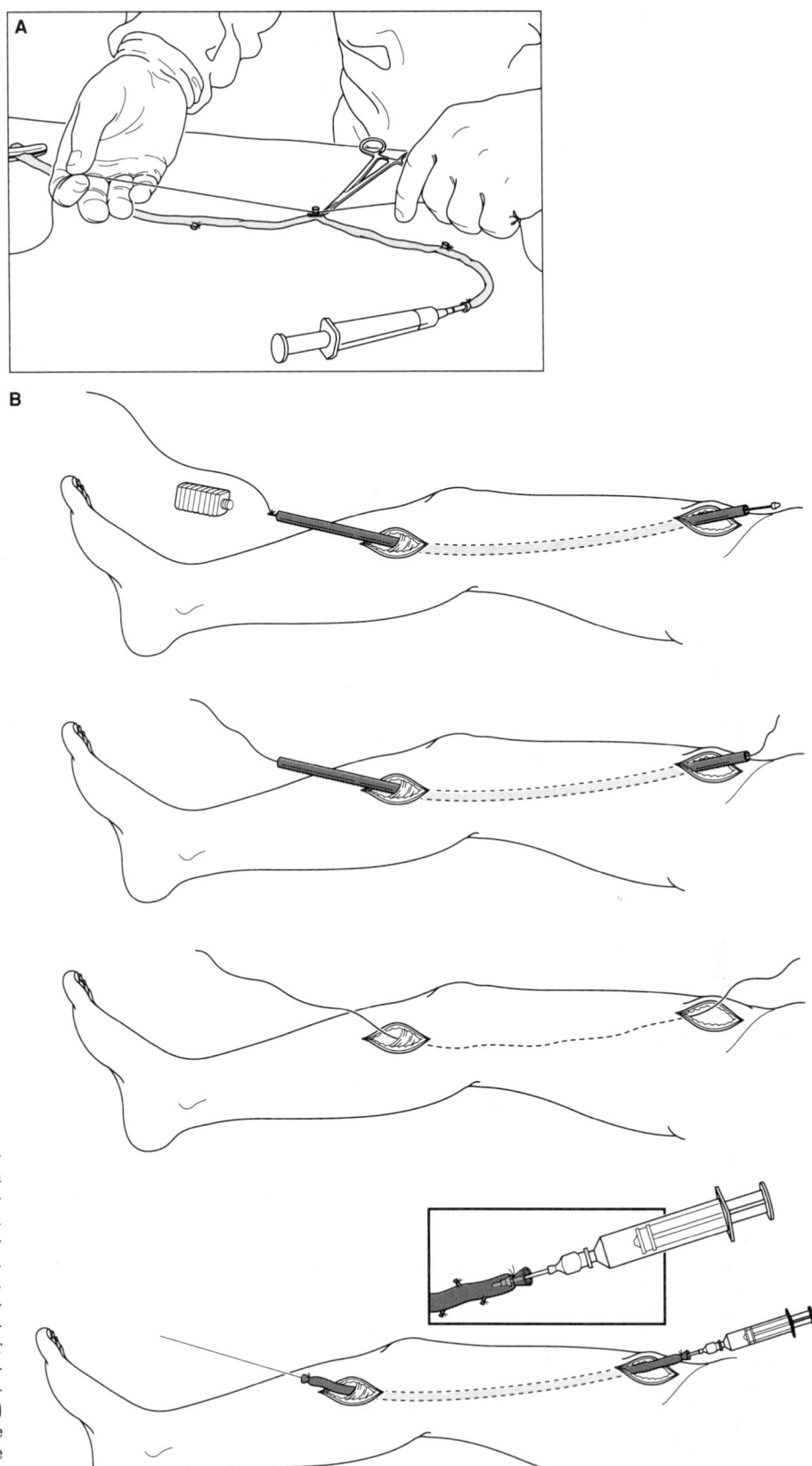

Figure 84-7. (*A*) Technique of side-branch ligation. (*B*) Method of vein graft passage through specially designed tunneling device. The vein graft is passed in a distended condition to avoid twisting or angulation. (*C*) Detail of proximal anastomosis. Use of the adjacent side branch prevents stricture at the site of anastomosis. (*D*) Alternative technique for proximal anastomosis. Vein graft origin serves as a patch for extended profundaplasty after endarterectomy. (*E*) Technique of distal anastomosis. The length of the anastomosis should be 10 to 15 times the diameter of the recipient artery. (*continues*)

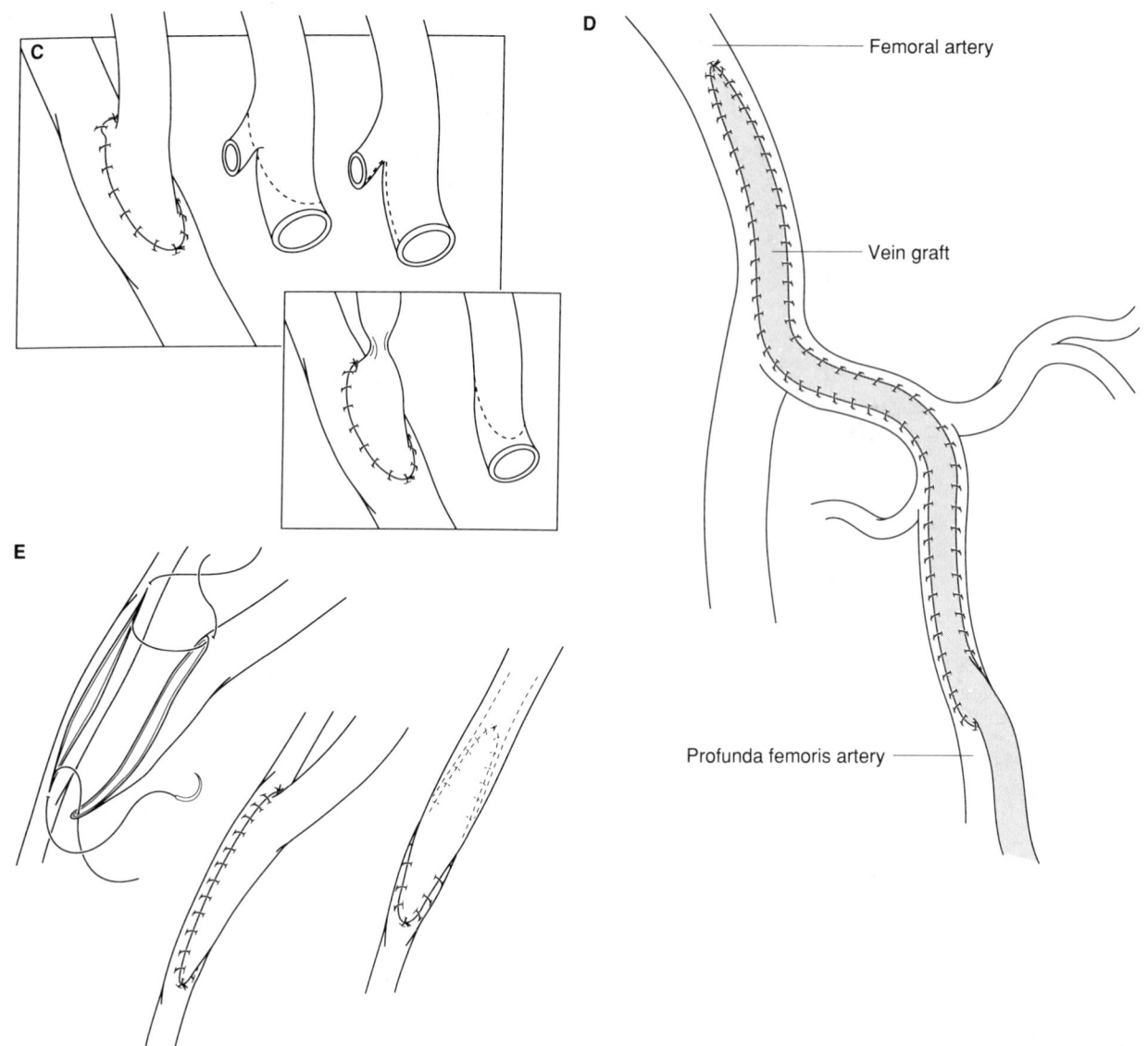

Figure 84-7. (*Continued*)

bypasses—the reversed technique and the in situ technique.

In *reversed vein grafting,* the saphenous vein is removed by means of gentle dissection, reversed in direction to allow blood flow in the direction allowed by the venous valves, distended with physiologic solution, and passed through the leg in a tunnel, after which anastomoses to proximal and distal vessels are performed (Fig. 84-7).

With the *in situ technique,* the upper greater saphenous vein is detached from the common femoral vein and anastomosed to the common femoral artery, after which the vein is allowed to fill with blood under arterial pressure. The valve sites are successively identified and incised until unobstructed arterial flow arrives at the chosen level of distal anastomosis. The saphenous vein branches that become arteriovenous fistulas must be individually occluded (Fig. 84-8).

Whichever technique is used to construct lower-extremity vein grafts, the immediate success of the

procedure is confirmed by use of electromagnetic flow measurements, continuous wave or pulsed Doppler confirmation of normal flow, surgical completion arteriography (Fig. 84-9, or a combination of these procedures.

For patients with absent or unusable greater saphenous veins, grafting by means of the in situ technique is impossible. These patients can undergo reversed vein grafting with alternative vein sources, such as an arm vein, lesser saphenous vein, or superficial femoral vein.

Complications of Lower-Extremity Venous Grafting

Myocardial infarction is the most frequent complication after lower-extremity vein bypass and causes most operative deaths.

Complications related to the extensive incisions needed for vein harvest and preparation and exposure of proximal

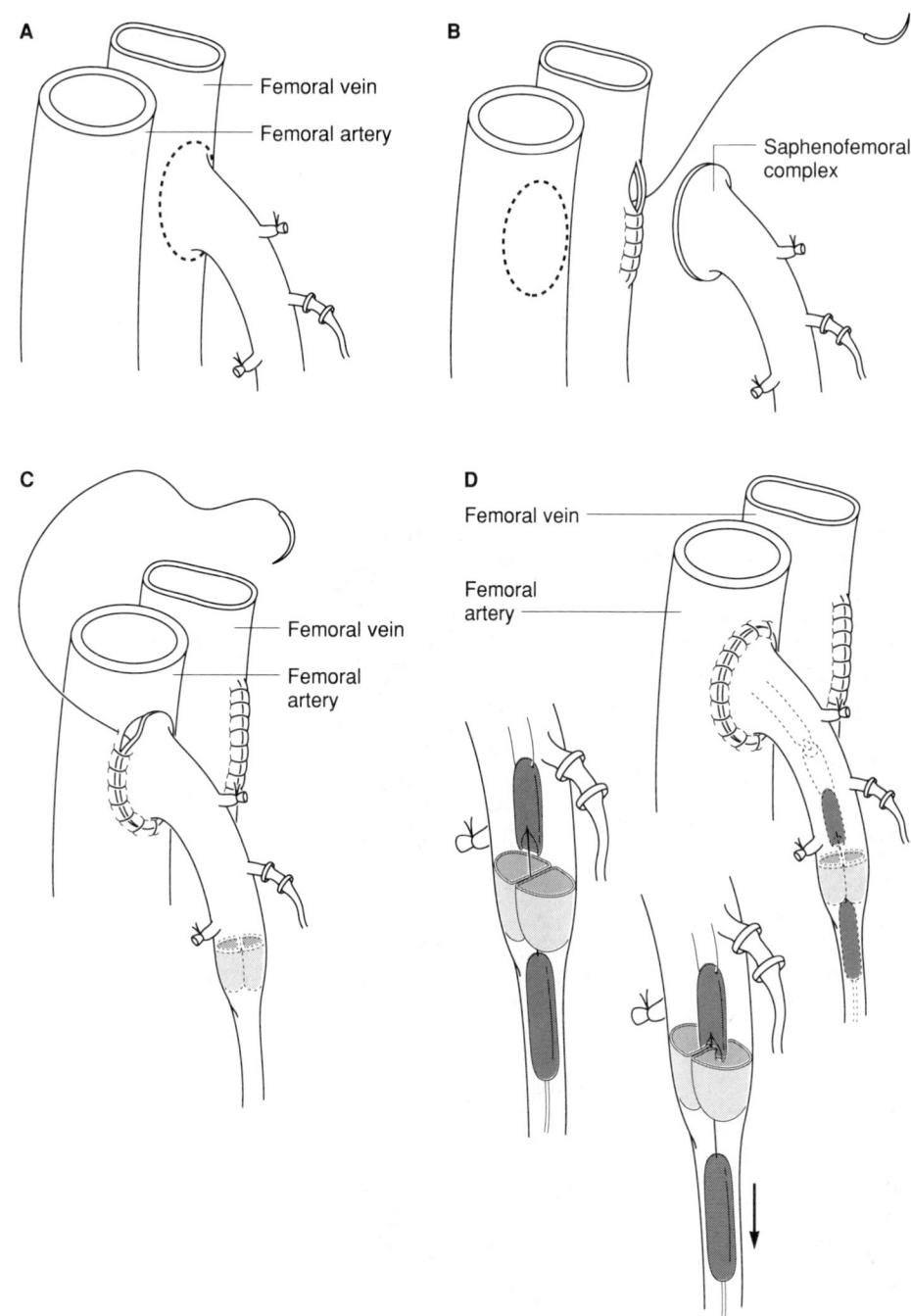

Figure 84-8. (*A*) The sapheno-femoral complex is detached from the femoral vein. (*B*) The femoral vein harvest site is over-sewn. (*C*) The proximal end-to-side anastomosis is completed. The valve is intact. (*D*) The valve cutter is passed retrograde through the valves and pulled distally, engaging and cutting the valves. (After LeMaitre G. In situ grafting made easy. Arch Surg 1988;123:102)

and distal arterial sites include *delayed wound healing* and *skin edge necrosis*. These complications are rarely serious after reversed venous grafting, in which the bypass grafts are tunneled deep within the leg. They may, however, lead to severe complications after in situ grafting, in which the bypass grafts are superficial and may be exposed by wound complications with subsequent graft infection, necrosis, hemorrhage, or occlusion. Preoperative mapping of the saphenous vein in which the course is marked with an indelible pen minimizes undermining of the skin and wound complications.

All patients who undergo lower-extremity bypass grafting have *postoperative leg edema* caused by interruption of leg lymphatics at the groin and knee caused by the multiple incisions.

Many patients have a *neuralgic pain syndrome* con-sisting of painful paresthesia of the medial thigh, knee, and upper calf, which is attributed to injury to the saphenous nerve, medial femoral cutaneous nerve or other sensory cutaneous nerves.

Long-term patency of lower-extremity vein grafts is related to the quality of the vein conduit, the site of the distal anastomosis, the indication for operation, and the experience and skill of the surgical team. There seems to be little difference in patency whether the reversed or in situ technique is used (Table 84-2).

Prosthetic Lower-Extremity Bypass

For some patients, a venous conduit adequate for a bypass may not be present because of:

Previous removal of vein for management of venous disease or use as coronary or peripheral venous grafts

Primary venous disease, such as varicosities or episodes of superficial venous thrombosis

These patients can undergo bypass grafting with prosthetic conduits, usually of polytetrafluoroethylene (PTFE; Teflon). Patency rates with prosthetic conduits at all locations in the lower extremities are lower than those with autogenous vein. Materials besides PTFE include Dacron, nylon, and a variety of biologic materials such as bovine carotid arteries, umbilical veins, and cryopreserved human saphenous veins, which must be treated to increase strength and destroy antigenicity. Long-term warfarin anticoagulation improves the patency of prosthetic lower-extremity grafts, especially with distal anastomoses below the knee. The improvement does not equal the results of autogenous vein grafting and is accompanied by complications of anticoagulation.

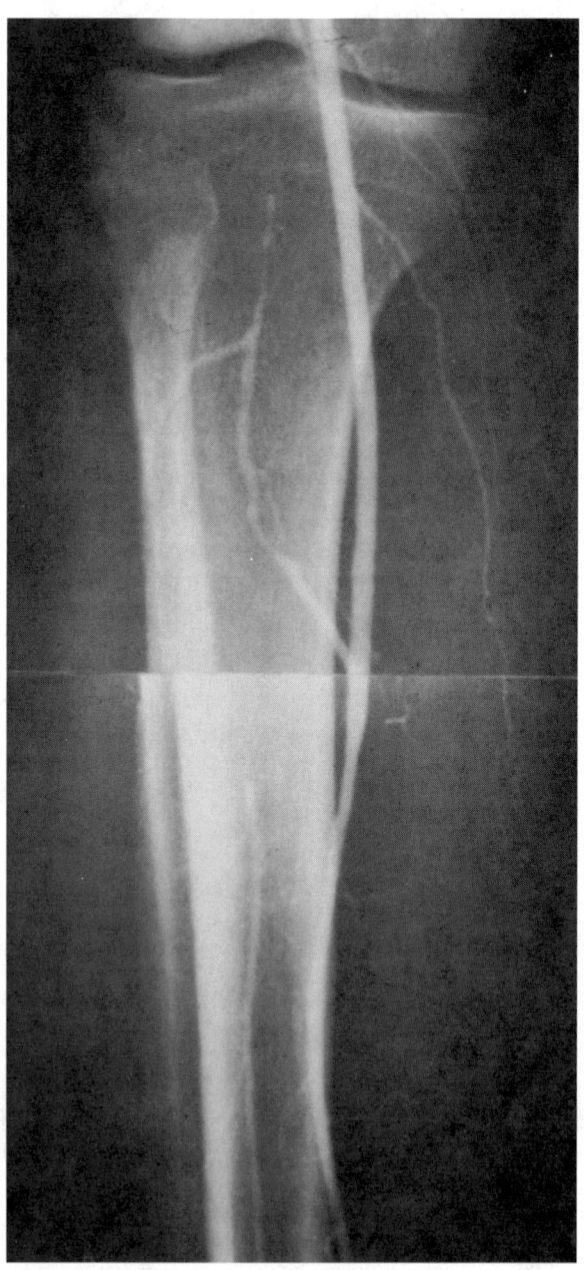

Figure 84-9. Operative completion arteriogram demonstrating a satisfactory reversed saphenous vein graft to the distal posterior tibial artery.

Table 84-2. VEIN GRAFT PATENCY RATES (%)

	1 mo	6 mo	1 yr	2 yr	3 yr	4 yr
ABOVE-KNEE FEMOROPOPLITEAL GRAFTS						
Primary Patency						
RSV	99	91	84	82	73	69
Arm vein	99	—	82	65	60	60
HUV	95	90	82	82	70	70
PTFE	—	89	79	74	66	60
BELOW-KNEE FEMOROPOPLITEAL GRAFTS						
Primary Patency						
RSV	98	90	84	79	78	77
ISVB	95	87	80	76	73	68
Secondary Patency						
ISVB	97	96	96	89	86	81
Arm vein	97	—	83	83	73	70
HUV	88	82	77	70	61	60
PTFE	96	80	68	61	44	40
Limb Salvage						
RSV	100	92	90	88	86	75
ISV	97	96	94	84	83	—
INFRAPOPLITEAL GRAFTS						
Primary Patency						
RSV	92	81	77	70	66	62
ISVB	94	84	82	76	74	68
Secondary Patency						
RSV	93	89	84	80	78	76
ISVB	95	90	89	87	84	81
Arm vein	94	—	73	62	58	—
HUV	80	65	52	46	40	37
PTFE	89	58	46	32	—	21
Limb Salvage						
RSV	95	88	85	83	82	82
ISVB	96		91	88	83	83
RTFE		76	68	60	56	48
AT-KNEE OR BELOW-KNEE GRAFTS						
Primary Patency						
RSV	95	85	81	—	—	—
Secondary Patency						
RSV	96	90	85	81	76	—
ISVB	93	93	92	82	72	—
Foot Salvage	99	94	93	87	84	—

RSV, reverse saphenous vein; HUV, human umbilical vein; PTFE, polytetrafluoroethylene; ISVB, in situ vein bypass.

SUGGESTED READING

Dalman RD, Taylor LM Jr. Basic data related to infrainguinal revascularization procedures. Ann Vasc Surg 1990;4:309.

Dormandy J, Mahir M, Ascady G, et al. Fate of the patient with chronic leg ischemia. J Cardiovasc Surg 1989;30:50.

Flinn WR, Rohrer MJ, Yao JST, et al. Improved long-term patency of infragenicular polytetrafluoroethylene grafts. J Vasc Surg 1988;7:685.

Kim YW, Taylor LM Jr, Porter JM. Circulation enhancing drugs. In: Rutherford RB, ed. Vascular surgery, ed. 4. Philadelphia, WB Saunders, 1995:324.

Taylor LM Jr, Edwards JM, Porter JM. Present status of reversed vein bypass: five year results of a modern series. J Vasc Surg 1990;11:193.

Taylor LM Jr, Porter JM. Natural history and nonoperative treatment of chronic lower extremity ischemia. In: Rutherford RB, ed. Vascular surgery, ed 4. Philadelphia, WB Saunders, 1995:751.

ESSENTIALS OF SURGERY: SCIENTIFIC PRINCIPLES AND PRACTICE,
edited by Lazar J. Greenfield, Michael W. Mulholland, Keith T. Oldham, Gerald B. Zelenock,
and Keith D. Lillemoe. Lippincott–Raven Publishers, Philadelphia, © 1997.

CHAPTER 85

LOWER EXTREMITY AMPUTATION

THOMAS S. HUBER

INDICATIONS

Most lower-extremity amputations are performed for complications of diabetes or arterial insufficiency (Table 85-1). Amputation is indicated for gangrene (dry gangrene), gangrene with infection (wet gangrene), unremitting and unreconstructable rest pain, and nonhealing ulcers. The objectives are to remove all nonviable tissue, relieve the source of ischemic rest pain, ensure primary wound healing, and facilitate rehabilitation. Amputation and revascularization are used to manage dry or wet gangrene. Amputation is performed for rest pain and nonhealing ulceration, if revascularization is precluded or unsuccessful.

Amputation sometimes is primary treatment for lower-extremity trauma. The decision is based on severity of injury, overall status of the patient, and rehabilitation potential. Penetrating and blunt extremity injuries are complicated by nerve, vascular, bone, and soft tissue injuries. The treatment guideline is to perform primary amputation for open tibial fractures with vascular injuries, if the posterior tibial nerve is disrupted in adults or if the injury results from a crush mechanism and the duration of warm ischemia was >6 hours. The Mangled Extremity Severity Score is used to predict the need for amputation, based on the extent of skeletal or soft tissue damage, limb ischemia, shock, and patient age.

PREOPERATIVE MANAGEMENT

Medical Evaluation

Evaluation includes a complete history and physical examination, routine laboratory studies, chest radiography, an electrocardiogram, and additional diagnostic studies and consultations, as indicated. Special attention is directed at the cardiac, respiratory, and renal systems.

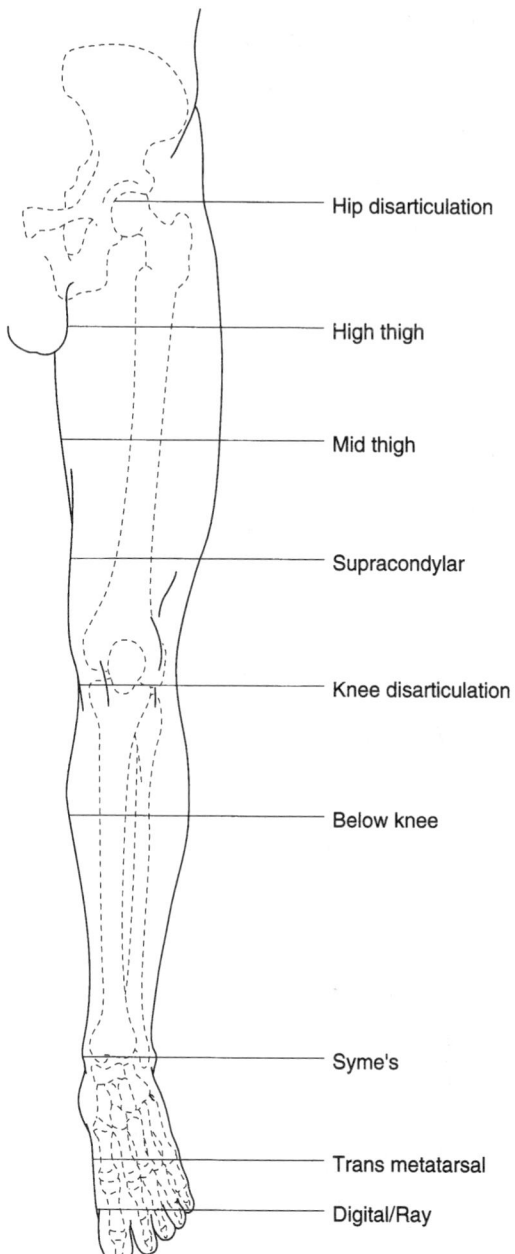

Figure 85-1. Common amputation levels for the lower extremity.

Hip disarticulation
High thigh
Mid thigh
Supracondylar
Knee disarticulation
Below knee
Syme's
Trans metatarsal
Digital/Ray

Table 85-1. INDICATIONS FOR LOWER EXTREMITY AMPUTATION

	Percentage
Complications of diabetes mellitus	60–80
Nondiabetic infection with ischemia	15–25
Ischemia without infection	5–10
Chronic osteomyelitis	3–5
Trauma	2–5
Miscellaneous (neuroma, frostbite, tumor, pain, nonhealing)	5–10

(Malone JM. Lower extremity amputation. In: Moore WS, ed. Vascular surgery: a comprehensive review. Philadelphia, WB Saunders, 1993:810)

Management of Infectious Problems

Foot and lower-extremity infections are common among patients with arterial insufficiency or diabetes. Cellulitis or wet gangrene of the digits, forefoot, or foot is an *emergency*. All wounds are cultured, and empiric administration of broad-spectrum antibiotics effective against gram-negative, gram-positive, and anaerobic organisms is initiated against a presumed polymicrobial infection. The empiric, broad-spectrum antibiotic coverage is narrowed, according to the results of the culture, if the patient's clinical course improves. Plain radiographs of the extremity are obtained to rule out gas in the soft tissue, osteomyelitis, fractures, and foreign bodies.

Management of the extremity depends on the extent of the infection, the presence of systemic signs, and the severity of vascular occlusive disease. *Cellulitis* can be treated

Table 85-2. REHABILITATION ENERGY COST OF AMPUTATION AT VARIOUS LEVELS

Amputation Level	Energy Cost
Digital or ray	Minimal (except first ray)
Transmetatarsal	Minimal during normal walking
Below-knee amputation	30%–60% increase in energy required for ambulation
Above-knee amputation	60%–100% increase in energy required for ambulation
Hip disarticulation	100%–110% increase in energy required for ambulation

Table 85-3. PREOPERATIVE LEVEL SELECTION: TOE AMPUTATION

Selection Criteria	Successful Healing, Primary and Secondary/Total
Empiric	86/115 (75%)
Presence of pedal pulses	357/365 (98%)
Doppler toe pressure >30 mm*	47/60 (78%)
Doppler ankle pressure >35 mm*	44/46 (96%)
Photoplethysmographic digit or TMA pressure >20 min*	20/20 (100%)
^{133}Xe skin blood flow >2.6 mL/100 g tissue/min	5/6 (83%)

* Systolic pressure (mmHg).
TMA, transmetatarsal.
(Durham JR. Lower extremity amputation levels: indications, methods of determining appropriate level, technique, prognosis. In: Rutherford RB, ed. Vascular surgery, ed 3. Philadelphia, WB Saunders, 1989:1693)

successfully with a course of systemic antibiotics, if the extremity is well vascularized. In the presence of peripheral vascular occlusive disease, the blood supply may be inadequate to eradicate the infection, and revascularization is considered. Cellulitis with systemic signs mandates intervention to rule out a plantar space soft tissue abscess as the septic source.

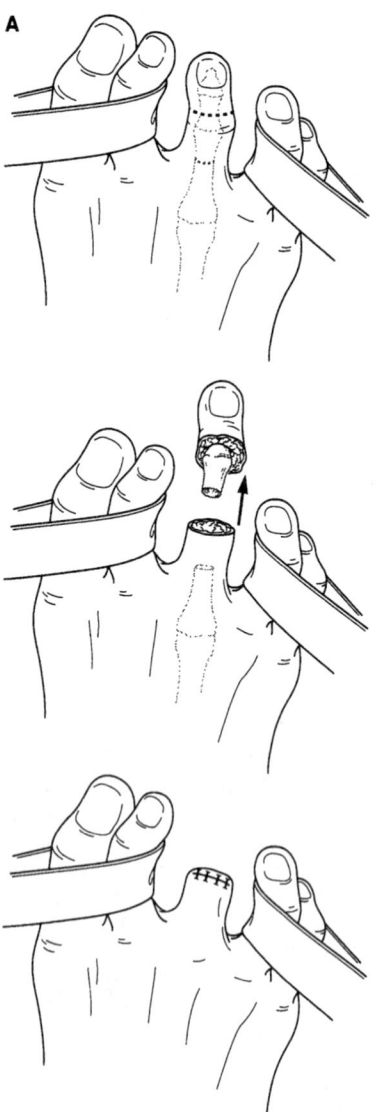

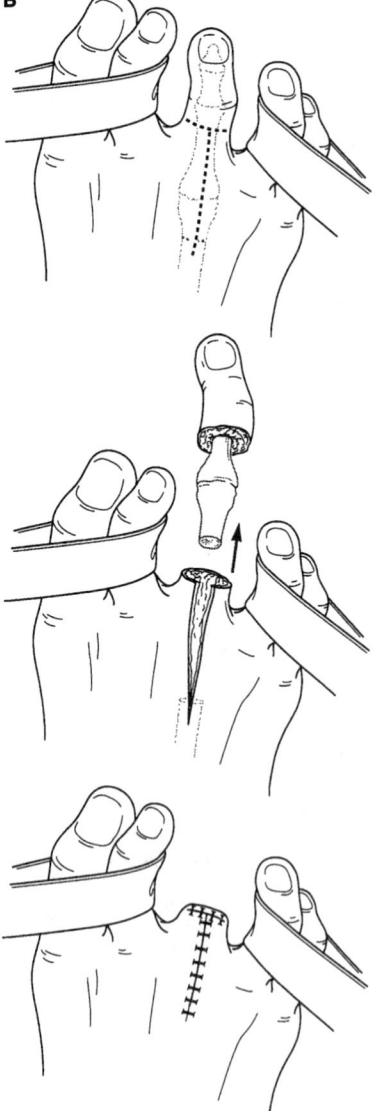

Figure 85-2. (*A*) Digital amputation. A circumferential skin incision is made proximal to the gangrenous process. The proximal phalanyx is transected and the soft tissue approximated. (*B*) Metatarsal head resection (ray amputation). A racquet-shaped skin incision is made with the circular component extending circumferential around the digit and the longitudinal component extending proximal to the metatarsal head. The metatarsal is transected proximal to the head and the soft tissue approximated.

All infected, *gangrenous* tissue of the digits, forefoot, or foot is débrided and cultured. This can be performed at the bedside for limited wounds, especially if the patient has diabetes with peripheral neuropathy and a minimally sensate foot. Extensive involvement necessitates emergency surgical débridement and open drainage. In the presence of extensive wet gangrene of the foot, a guillotine amputation through the distal tibia or fibula may be indicated. Lower-extremity revascularization to salvage ischemic but viable tissue often is necessary for patients with wet gangrene. The presence of gas in the soft tissues of the foot or lower extremity is a life-threatening *emergency* that requires high-dose broad-spectrum antibiotics and aggressive débridement or amputation of all involved tissue.

Patients with diabetes are particularly prone to foot and lower-extremity infections as a result of a compromised immune system, vascular occlusive disease, and peripheral neuropathy. The sensory deficit that occurs with peripheral neuropathy often leads to ulceration of the foot over the metatarsal heads and bony prominences. Although these ulcerations are not necessarily infectious, they may become infected and involve the bone. Management involves stopping the inciting trauma and any weight bearing on the affected surfaces until resolution. Patients are fit with proper shoes before they resume walking. The presence of a peripheral neuropathy complicates selection of amputation level because forefoot amputations in the presence of decreased foot sensation can be ulcerogenic.

Selection of Amputation Level

Amputation level depends on the indication for the procedure, the medical condition of the patient, the rehabilitation potential of the patient, and the potential for wound healing. The goal is to provide the most functional extremity that satisfies the indications for the procedure and does not require additional operations. The common amputation levels are shown in Figure 85-1.

Medical Condition

For patients with arterial insufficiency or diabetes, the goal is to remove all nonviable, painful tissue while ensuring wound healing and maximal rehabilitation. Amputations for extremity trauma are performed proximal to necrotic, nonviable tissue. Most trauma patients do not have underlying vascular disease, so wound healing is likely as long as there is no infection. Selection of amputation level for malignant disease depends on the biologic characteristics of the tumor and the extent of disease.

Rehabilitation

The amputation level selected should provide the greatest likelihood of maintaining walking and independence. If the patient cannot walk, has limited rehabilitation potential, or has overwhelming comorbid medical conditions, amputation level is dictated by wound healing rate. An above-knee amputation is favored in this setting.

The likelihood that a patient will walk on a prosthesis after a lower-extremity amputation varies with amputation level. The energy requirement for walking on a prosthesis increases with proximity of amputation level (Table 85-2). That is, a well-rehabilitated person with bilateral below-knee prostheses has less energy expenditure walking than a person with one above-knee prosthesis.

Wound Healing

The preoperative considerations for wound healing are adequacy of skin and muscle blood flow, surgical technique, nutritional status, and the presence of infection. Failure of a wound to heal necessitates more proximal

amputation. A palpable pulse at the level immediately above the selected amputation site almost always ensures wound healing, but absence of a pulse does not equate with lack of healing. The following tests are helpful: systolic blood pressure measurements; digital pressures; radionuclide imaging; skin blood flow quantification with fluorescein; transcutaneous oxygen and carbon dioxide tension measurement with an electrode; laser Doppler velocimetry; photoplethysmography; skin temperature measurements; and pulse volume recordings.

Timing of Surgical Intervention

Acute Ischemia

Arterial embolism and thrombosis account for most episodes of acute ischemia. The heart is the most common source of peripheral arterial emboli; aortoiliac and peripheral aneurysms account for the rest. The cause of acute ischemia (embolus vs thrombus) can be determined with the history and physical examination. Immediate revascularization is performed by means of embolectomy, distal bypass, or lytic therapy. Revascularization may be precluded by the severity of the patient's medical condition, the extent of ischemia or necrosis, or the presence of systemic signs.

Some patients need emergency amputation but have overwhelming medical problems that preclude surgical intervention. A temporizing medical amputation is indicated

Table 85-4. PREOPERATIVE LEVEL SELECTION: FOOT AND FOREFOOT AMPUTATION

Selection Criteria	Successful Healing, Primary and Secondary/Total
Empiric	11/24 (46%)
	36/50 (72%)
Doppler ankle systolic pressure	
<40 mmHg	5/9 (56%)
>40 mmHg	20/60 (33%)
40–60 mmHg	4/5 (80%)
>50 mmHg	14/21 (66%)
>60 mmHg	68/91 (75%)
>70 mmHg	70/93 (75%)
Doppler toe systolic pressure >30 mmHg	4/5 (80%)
Doppler ankle–brachial pressure index	
>0.45 (nondiabetic)	
>0.50 (diabetic)	58/60 (97%)
Photoplethysmographic toe systolic pressure	
>55 mmHg	14/14 (100%)
>45 and <55 mmHg	2/8 (25%)
<45 mmHg	0/8 (0%)
Fiberoptic fluorometry (dye fluorescence index >44)	18/20 (90%)
Laser Doppler velocimetry	2/6 (33%)
^{125}I iodopyrine skin blood flow >8 mL/100 g tissue/min	18/18 (100%)
^{133}Xe skin blood flow >2.6 mL/100 g tissue/min	23/25 (92%)
Transcutaneous P_{O_2}	
>10 mm (or a >10 mm increase on F_{IO_2} = 1.0)	6/8 (75%)
>28 mmHg	3/3 (100%)
Transcutaneous P_{CO_2} <40 mmHg	3/3 (100%)

(Durham JR. Lower extremity amputation levels: indications, methods of determining appropriate level, technique, prognosis. In: Rutherford RB, ed. Vascular surgery, ed 3. Philadelphia, WB Saunders, 1989:1695)

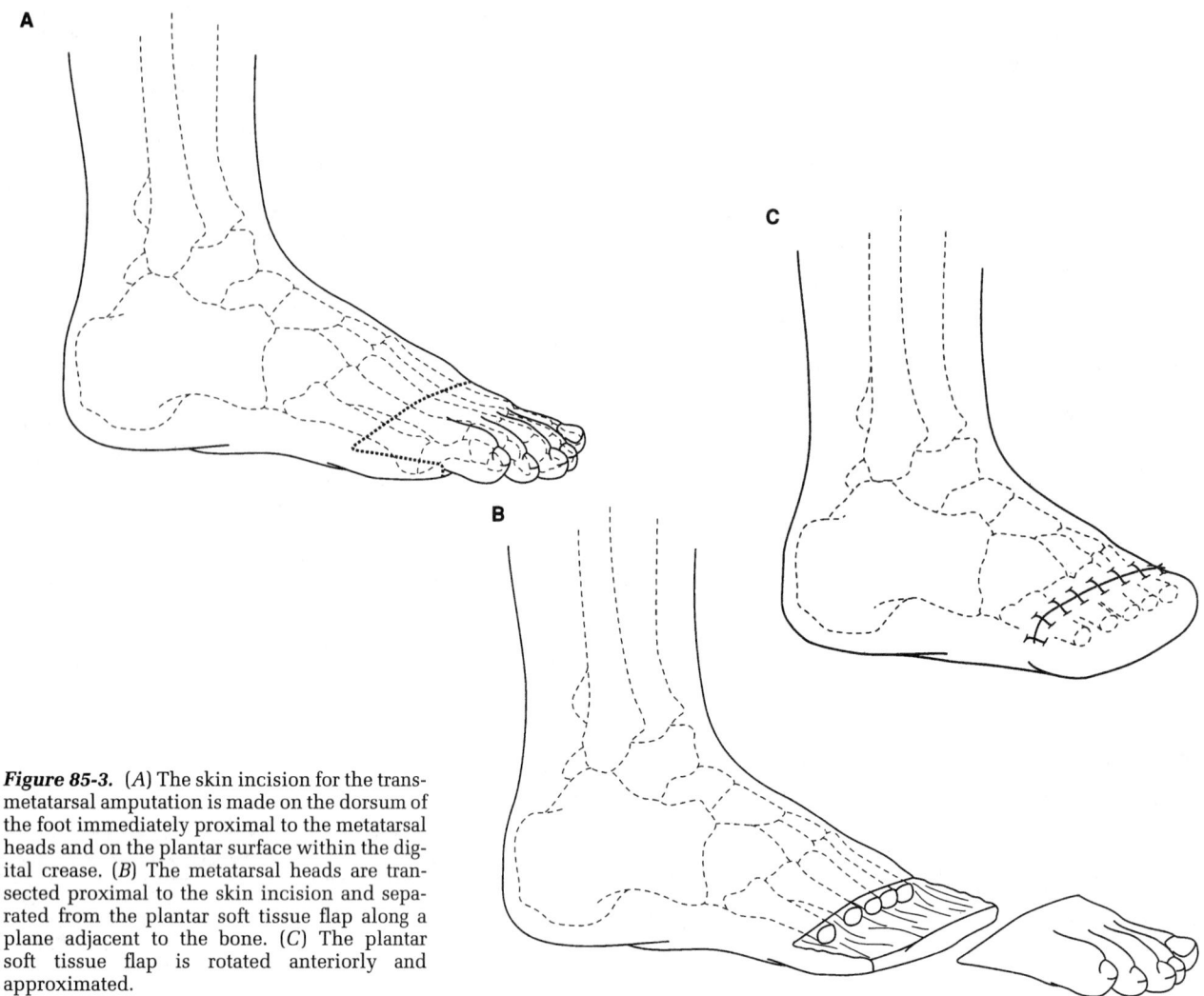

Figure 85-3. (*A*) The skin incision for the transmetatarsal amputation is made on the dorsum of the foot immediately proximal to the metatarsal heads and on the plantar surface within the digital crease. (*B*) The metatarsal heads are transected proximal to the skin incision and separated from the plantar soft tissue flap along a plane adjacent to the bone. (*C*) The plantar soft tissue flap is rotated anteriorly and approximated.

in this setting. A tourniquet is applied proximal to the gangrene or infection, and the extremity is packed in dry ice. This prevents release of systemically active ischemic breakdown products and allows delay of definitive amputation for a few days until the medical condition is stabilized.

Chronic Ischemia

Dry gangrene is noninfectious and does not produce systemic symptoms. All patients with dry gangrene are examined for possible revascularization to salvage additional tissue or allow more distal amputation. Gangrene localized to the digits may be managed surgically, or the digits can be allowed to mummify and autoamputate. Gangrene proximal to the digits is managed surgically.

The infection dictates the timing of amputation for *wet gangrene*. The goal is to manage the infection and salvage the greatest amount of viable tissue. All infected wounds are débrided to remove the necrotic tissue, and parenteral antibiotics are administered. Viable infected tissue is preserved in the hope that the antibiotics are effective. The patient is examined for distal arterial revascularization.

If the infection resolves with débridement and antibiotics, the patient is treated for the resultant dry gangrene, and amputation can be performed after thorough evaluation. The presence of systemic symptoms, extensive infection, or failure of débridement and antibiotic treatment

necessitate emergency amputation. A wide débridement or guillotine amputation is performed as part of a staged procedure to remove additional necrotic or grossly infected tissue. A second-stage definitive amputation is performed after the infection resolves.

SURGICAL MANAGEMENT

General Considerations

The techniques of amputation apply to all levels. All gangrenous tissue is draped outside the surgical field with an adhesive drape or bowel bag. Proximal tourniquets are *not* used for patients with arterial insufficiency or diabetes, but they are helpful for amputations performed for other indications, such as trauma and malignant disease.

Incisions are made perpendicular to the plane of the skin to avoid undermining and destroying the blood supply of flaps. All major blood vessels are identified, dissected free, and suture ligated. The major nerves are placed under tension, transected, suture ligated, and allowed to retract. Ligation prevents bleeding from the vaso nervorum; retraction ensures that the nerve end and the resultant neuroma are not incorporated into the incisional scar or allowed to come in contact with a weight-bearing surface. All tendons are transected sharply under tension and allowed to retract.

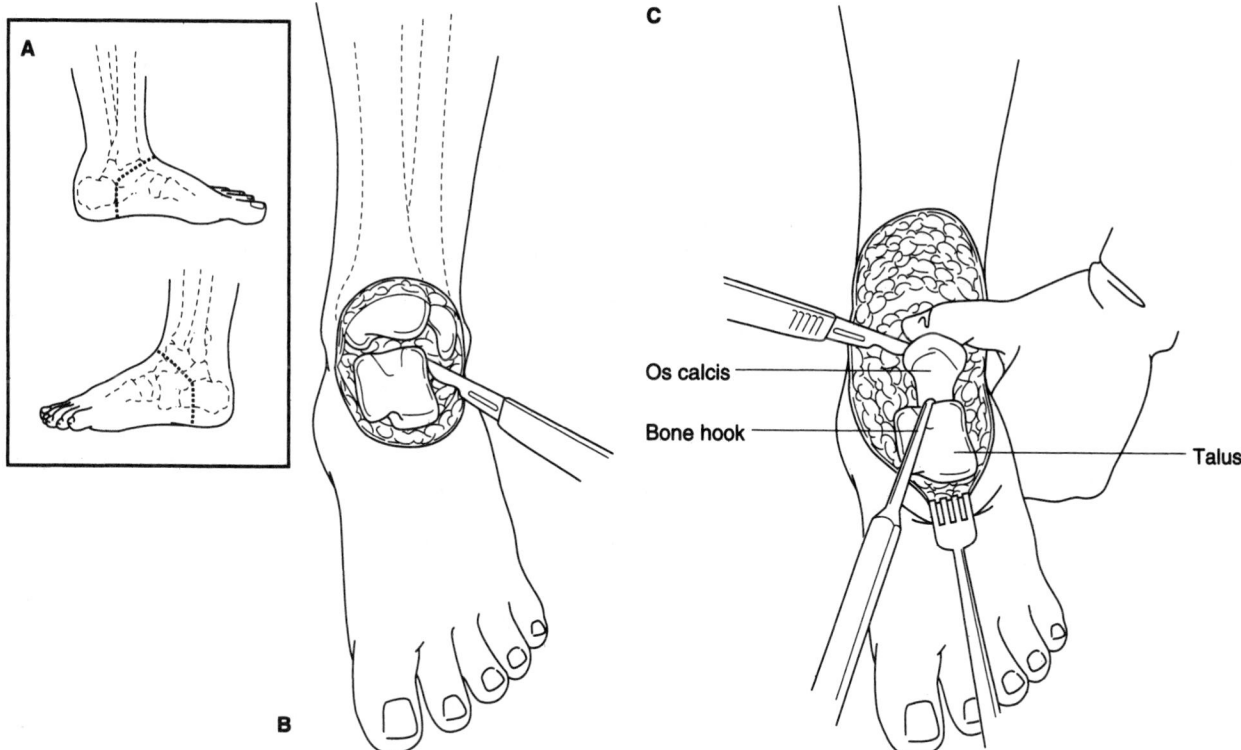

Figure 85-4. (*A*) The skin incision (*black*) for the one-stage Syme amputation connects the medial and lateral malleoli in both the horizontal and vertical planes. The skin incision for the two-stage procedure (*blue*) is located approximately 1.5 cm further distal. (*B*) The incision is extended into the tibial-talar joint space and the foot is placed in forced plantar flexion. (*C*) The calcaneus is sharply dissected from the adherent plantar fascia along a plane adjacent to the bone. (*D*) The heel pad is rotated anteriorly and approximated after the calcaneal dissection in the two-stage procedure and after the additional transection of the medial and lateral malleoli in the one-stage procedure. (*E*) Elliptical incisions are made over the medial and lateral malleoli during a second operation for the staged procedure. The medial and lateral malleoli are transected flush with the ankle joint, and the distal flares of the tibia and fibula are removed. (*F*) The two-stage procedure results in a less bulbous, more cosmetically appealing residual limb. (*continues*)

Amputations through joint articular surfaces are avoided because of poor vascular supply. The periosteum adjacent to the proposed level of bone transection is elevated proximally no more than necessary in an attempt to prevent excessive bone overgrowth. A reciprocating air-driven power saw is used because of the precision of the cut. All bone edges are filed smooth to prevent damage to soft tissue. Prosthetic material from previous bypass procedures is removed.

All wounds are irrigated with saline solution containing antibiotics, and hemostasis is confirmed. Postoperative hematomas can compromise the amputation level and predispose to wound infections. The fascial and skin layers are reapproximated atraumatically without tension. Nonreactive, permanent monofilament sutures or staples can be used for the skin closure. The wound is left open and packed with saline-soaked gauze if there is any concern that the tissues are infected. These open wounds can be allowed to heal by secondary intention, or delayed primary closure is performed.

Digital and Ray Amputations

Digital and ray (metatarsal) amputations are common for gangrene due to diabetes and arterial insufficiency. The selection criteria are shown in Table 85-3.

The choice between digital and ray amputation is deter-

mined by the extent of bone and soft tissue involvement. *Digital* amputation is indicated for gangrene involving the distal or mid-phalanx. *Ray* amputation is indicated for gangrene extending to the digital crease. Ray amputation is contraindicated if multiple digits are involved; in this setting, a transmetatarsal amputation is indicated. The techniques for digital and ray amputation are illustrated in Figure 85-2.

The postoperative course after digital or ray amputation is usually uneventful. A soft incisional dressing is used, and walking may be resumed 2 to 3 weeks after operation.

Transmetatarsal Amputation

Transmetatarsal amputation is indicated when gangrene or infection involves multiple digits or the forefoot. The selection criteria are summarized in Table 85-4. A transmetatarsal amputation is *contraindicated* when the underlying disease extends to the proposed skin incisions or when disease involves the plantar surface of the forefoot. In the latter situation, a guillotine amputation through the metatarsal bones can be performed and allowed to heal by secondary intention or covered with a split-thickness skin graft. The technique of transmetatarsal amputation is shown in Figure 85-3.

The postoperative concerns after transmetatarsal amputation are adherence and healing of the plantar flap. Walk-

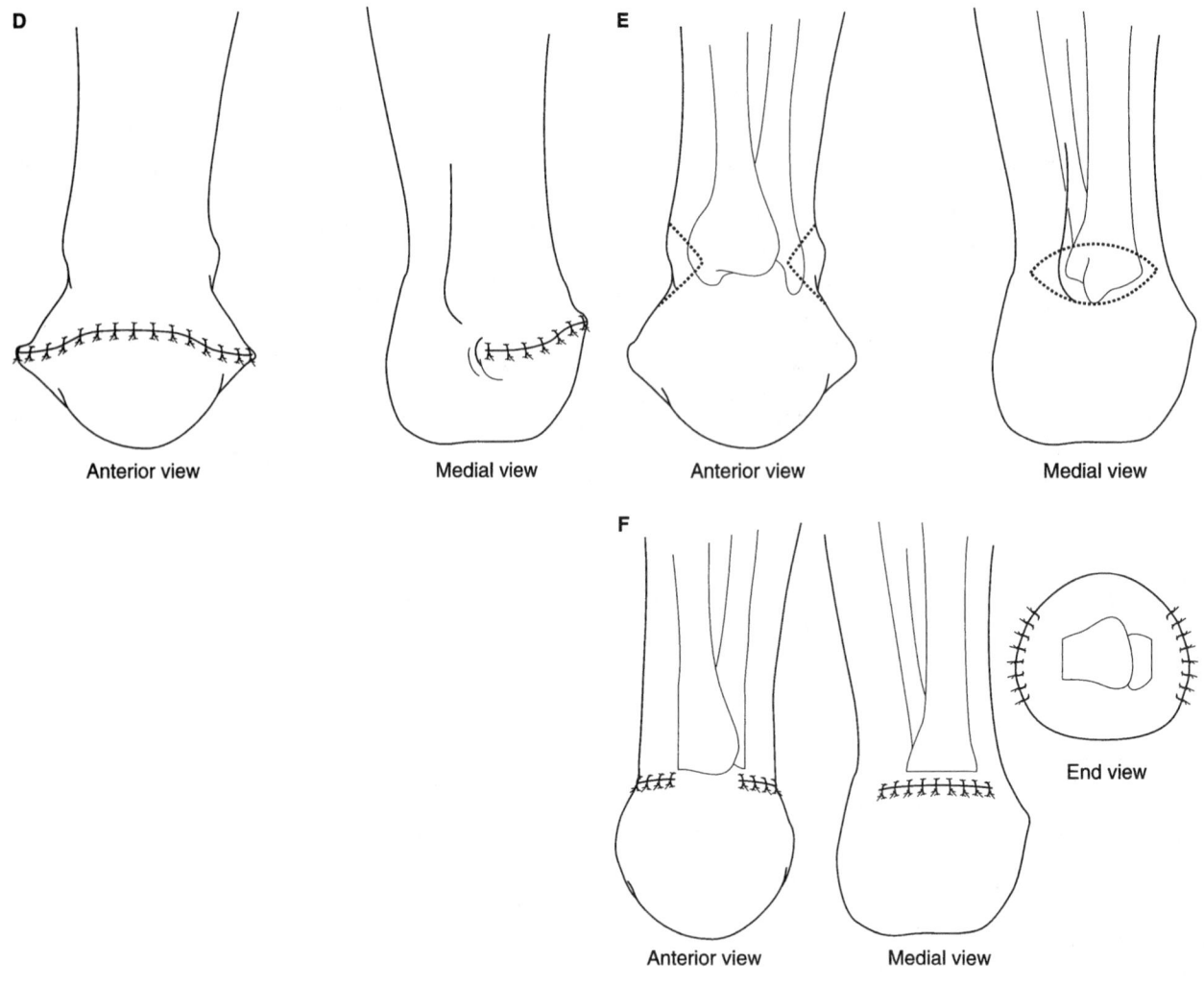

D   Anterior view   Medial view

E   Anterior view   Medial view

F   Anterior view   Medial view   End view

Figure 85-4. (*Continued*)

ing is avoided for 1 month. A soft dressing or a short leg cast is a suitable postoperative dressing.

Syme Amputation

Syme amputation is a foot amputation in which the ends of the tibia and fibula are covered by the preserved heel pad. The selection criteria are the same as for transmetatarsal amputation (Table 85-4). Syme amputation is indicated for extensive foot trauma and for diabetic or dysvascular indications when gangrene or infection precludes transmetatarsal amputation. Syme amputation is useful in the treatment of children because it preserves the epiphyseal growth plates.

The Syme amputation can be performed as a one- or a two-stage procedure (Fig. 85-4). The two-stage procedure results in a square stump that is easier to fit with a prosthesis.

Healing and fixation of the plantar flap are the postoperative concerns. Weight bearing on the heel pad is avoided for at least 1 month to allow fixation. A soft or a rigid short leg cast is used as a postoperative dressing.

Below-knee Amputation

The complications of diabetes and arterial insufficiency are the common indications for below-knee amputations. The inclusion criteria are summarized in Table 85-5. The

technique of below-knee amputation based on a posterior flap is illustrated in Figure 85-5. If disease involves the skin incisions outlined for the posterior flap, a shorter below-knee stump can be made with the same flap design but a more proximal anterior incision.

Although suboptimal, a short below-knee amputation is superior to an above-knee amputation. In the most extreme conditions, a below-knee prosthesis can be fit for a stump in which the tibia is transected at the tuberosity. If the tibia is transected at this level, the fibula is removed to prevent angulation.

A *guillotine below-knee amputation* is performed as part of a staged procedure in the presence of extensive foot infection. A guillotine amputation is essentially a large débridement. A circumferential incision is made in the distal calf and extended through the underlying fascia. The tibia and fibula are dissected free, the periosteum is elevated, and the bones are transected flush with the skin incision. All major neurovascular structures are suture ligated and the remaining soft tissue incised to complete the amputation. The wound is left open, and a second-stage, definitive below-knee amputation is delayed until the infection resolves.

A formal below-knee amputation can be performed in the presence of extensive foot infection and the skin and soft tissue flap left open. The flap can be closed with a delayed primary technique after resolution of the infec-

Table 85-5. PREOPERATIVE LEVEL SELECTION: BELOW-KNEE AMPUTATION

Selection Criteria	Successful Healing, Primary and Secondary/Total
Empiric	794/974 (82%)
Doppler ankle systolic pressure	
>30 mmHg	66/70 (94%)
Doppler calf systolic pressure	
>50 mmHg	36/36 (100%)
>68 mmHg	96/97 (99%)
Doppler thigh systolic pressure	
>100 mmHg	31/31 (100%)
>80 mmHg	104/113 (92%)
Fluorescein dye	24/30 (80%)
Fiberoptic fluorometry (dye fluorescence	
index >44)	12/12 (100%)
Laser Doppler velocimetry	8/8 (100%)
Skin perfusion pressure	
^{99m}Tc pertechnate	24/26 (92%)
^{131}I or ^{125}I antipyrine >30 mm	60/62 (97%)
Photoelectric skin perfusion pressure	
>20 mm	60/71 (85%)
^{133}Xe skin blood flow	
Epicutaneous >0.9 mL/100 g	
tissue/min	14/15 (93%)
Intradermal >2.4 mL/100 g	
tissue/min	83/89 (93%)
Intradermal >1 mL/100 g	
tissue/min	11/12 (92%)
Transcutaneous P_{O_2} = 0	0/3 (0%)
>10 mmHg (or >10 mm increase on	
F_{IO_2} = 1.0)	76/80 (95%)
>10 and <40 mmHg	5/7 (71%)
>20	25/26 (96%)
>35 mmHg	51/51 (100%)
Transcutaneous P_{O_2} index >0.59	17/17 (100%)
Transcutaneous P_{CO_2} <40 mmHg	7/8 (88%)

(Durham JR. Lower extremity amputation levels: indications, methods of determining appropriate level, technique, prognosis. In: Rutherford RB, ed. Vascular surgery, ed 3. Philadelphia, WB Saunders, 1989:1700)

Other Amputation Levels

Amputation of the lower extremity at the level of the *hip* (hip disarticulation) is rare. Indications are malignant disease, trauma, complications of arterial insufficiency, and infected hip prostheses.

Amputation at the level of the *knee* (knee disarticulation) may be indicated when below-knee amputation is not possible. Knee disarticulation allows end weight bearing, proprioception, and prosthetic control. It preserves the epiphyseal growth plates, which makes it advantageous for children.

POSTOPERATIVE CARE

Postoperative care entails management of coexisting medical conditions, care of the extremity, and initiation of rehabilitation. Wound-healing objectives in the postoperative period are to prevent stump edema, allow for stump shrinkage, maintain full range of joint motion, maintain nutrition, and anticipate and manage all complications. The wound is inspected daily, and all hematomas or evidence of cellulitis managed. Edema is prevented with elastic compression wraps or a rigid dressing. Stump shrinkage is expedited by the dressing. Early initiation of joint range of motion exercises is the key to prevention of contractures.

COMPLICATIONS
Stump Complications

Postoperative *wound complications* vary with the indication for the procedure. Risk for wound infection is reduced with staged local débridement or guillotine amputation before the definitive procedure. Postoperative wound infections are managed with a combination of intravenous antibiotics, wound exploration and drainage, and dressing changes.

Wound *hematomas* can become secondarily infected and compromise the amputation level. Hematomas are managed with evacuation, irrigation, and reclosure of the wound. An infected hematoma is managed as an abscess.

tion. The skin and soft tissue flap is left slightly longer than usual in this setting to allow for contraction.

A rigid postoperative dressing is used after below-knee amputation. The knee is positioned in about 10° flexion, and a cast is constructed to high on the thigh with graded compression. The cast is suspended with a strap and waist belt. The wound is examined 10 days after amputation during the first cast change unless the patient has a fever or there are wound concerns. A rigid removable dressing is an alternative to the thigh-high rigid dressing.

Above-knee Amputation

The indications for above-knee amputation are similar to those for below-knee amputation. The selection criteria are shown in Table 85-6. Above-knee amputation can be performed at the distal, middle, or proximal femur, depending on the extent of disease. Above-knee amputation is *contraindicated* if the gangrene or infection extends above the proposed amputation level. Failure of an above-knee amputation to heal can be fatal. The technique for above-knee amputation is illustrated in Figure 85-6.

Postoperative care after above-knee amputation is similar to that after below-knee amputation. Soft dressings with elastic support are applied during the operation.

Table 85-6. PREOPERATIVE LEVEL SELECTION: ABOVE-KNEE AMPUTATION

Selection Criteria	Successful Healing, Primary and Secondary/Total
Empiric	390/430 (91%)
Fiberoptic fluorometry (dye fluorescence	
index >44)	6/7 (86%)
Laser Doppler velocimetry	6/6 (100%)
Photoelectric skin perfusion pressure	
>21 mm	19/19 (100%)
Skin perfusion pressure (^{131}I or	
^{125}I antipyrine)	44/48 (92%)
^{133}Xe skin blood flow intradermal	
>2.6 mL/100 g tissue/min	20/20 (100%)
Transcutaneous P_{O_2}	
>10 mm (or 10 mm increase on	
F_{IO_2} = 1.0)	15/23 (65%)
>20 mm	12/12 (100%)
>23 mm	2/2 (100%)
>35 mm	21/24 (88%)
Transcutaneous P_{CO_2} <38 mm	5/5 (100%)

(Durham JR. Lower extremity amputation levels: indications, methods of determining appropriate level, technique, prognosis. In: Rutherford RB, ed. Vascular surgery, ed 3. Philadelphia, WB Saunders, 1989:1707)

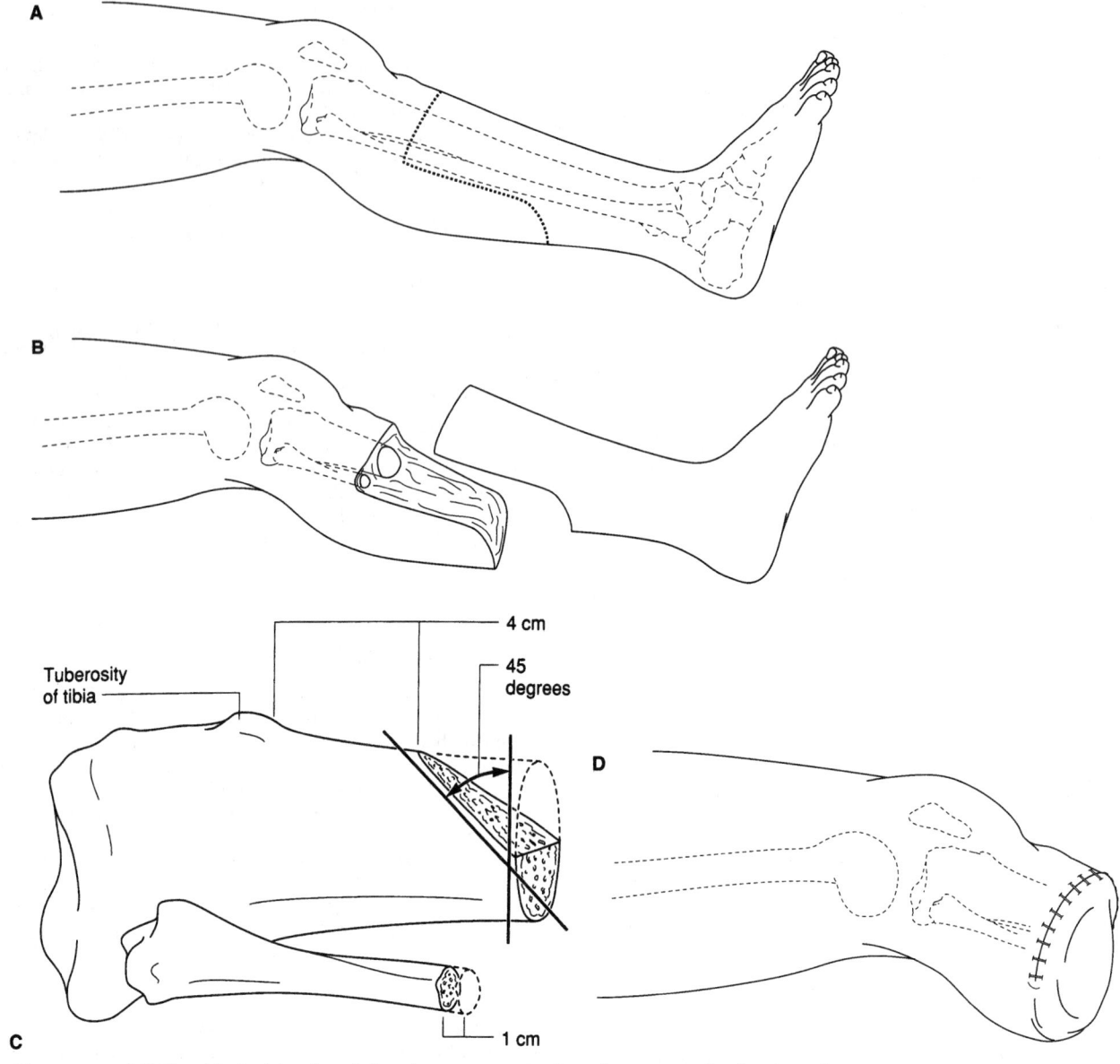

Figure 85-5. (*A*) The skin incision for a below-knee amputation based on a posterior flap is made 11 cm distal to the tibial tuberosity and extended medially and laterally to the mid-point of the calf. The length of the posterior flap is about 2 cm longer than the diameter of the calf at the point of the proximal incision. (*B*) The tibia is transected 1 cm proximal to the skin incision. The fibula is transected an additional 1 cm proximal to the level of the tibial transection, and the posterior calf muscles are incised along the plane of the skin incision. (*C*) The anterior aspect of the tibia is beveled at an angle of about 45 degrees, and the bone edges are filed. (*D*) The posterior flap is rotated anteriorly and approximated.

Strict hemostasis is the key to avoiding postoperative hematomas.

Flexion joint *contractures* can develop rapidly. A flexion contracture of 15° at the knee or 10° at the hip precludes fitting a prosthesis. Prevention is the key to avoiding this complication. Active and passive range of motion is initiated immediately postoperatively and facilitated with pain control. The amputation stump should not be positioned with either the hip or the knee flexed, even though such a position may be more comfortable for the patient.

The skin and soft tissue of the amputation stump are prone to *ulceration* over the bony prominences. These ulcerations result most often from poorly fitting prostheses. They also can occur after above-knee amputation over the

transected femur on the anterior thigh owing to the greater pull of the hip flexors relative to the hip extensors. The ulcerations usually heal with a combination of local wound care, antibiotics, and cessation of walking on the prosthesis. Prosthetic fit is reexamined before the patient begins walking again. Breakdown of the skin and soft tissue with involvement of the underlying bone necessitates revision of the amputation with transection of the exposed bone.

The regenerative mass of nerve tissue *(neuroma)* that results as a physiologic response to transection may cause pain if it becomes trapped within the amputation scar or comes in contact with the prosthesis. This complication may be prevented during the original procedure if the

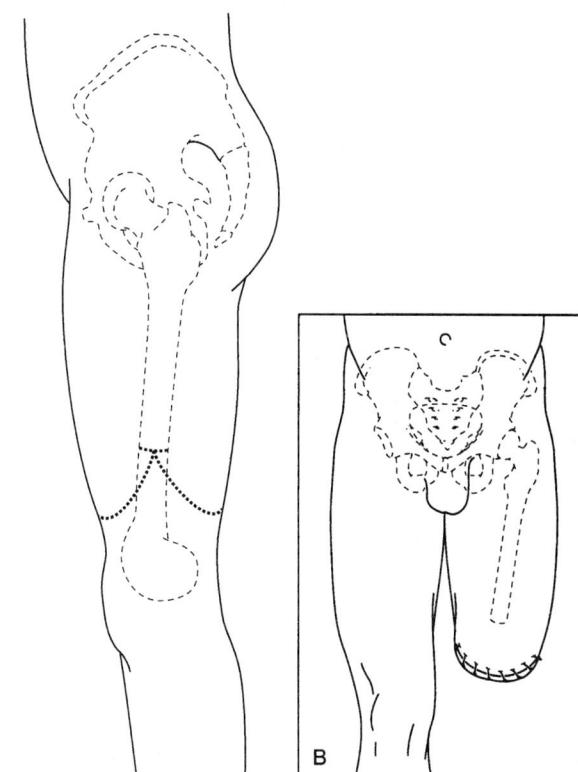

Figure 85-6. (*A*) Equal length anterior and posterior flaps are made for the above-knee amputation, and the femur is transected at the level of the angle formed by the flaps. (*B*) The anterior and posterior thigh soft tissues are incised along the plane of the skin incision, and the flaps are approximated.

nerves are transected under tension and allowed to retract into the wound. Symptomatic neuromas are managed by means of proximal resection of the nerve because excision of the neuroma is rarely adequate.

Phantom extremity pain occurs after almost all lower-extremity amputations. This pain is part of a central pain syndrome and is unrelated to a neuroma or the perception of an intact extremity. There is no effective management of chronic phantom pain. Disabling phantom pain can be reduced with postamputation rehabilitation and immediate fitting of a prosthesis.

Deep Venous Thrombosis and Pulmonary Embolism

Immobility and prior attempts at arterial revascularization with injury to the deep venous system increase risk for thrombosis and pulmonary embolism. Prophylactic measures include subcutaneous administration of heparin, early mobility, and use of pneumatic compression devices.

Additional Limb Loss

Additional limb loss is common among patients with arterial insufficiency or diabetes. This reflects the systemic nature of the underlying disease and emphasizes the importance of foot care, patient education, and close medical surveillance.

SUGGESTED READING

Burnham ST, Wagner WH, Keagy BH, et al. Objective measurement of limb perfusion by dermal fluorometry: a criterion for healing of below knee amputation. Arch Surg 1990;125:513.

Cambria RP, Yucel EK, Brewster DC, et al. The potential for lower extremity revascularization without contrast arteriography: experience with magnetic resonance angiography. Radiology 1993;187:637.

Dwars BJ, Van Den Broek TA, Ravwerda JA, et al. Criteria for reliable selection of the lowest level of amputation in peripheral vascular disease. J Vasc Surg 1992;15:536.

Endean ED, Schwarz TH, Barker DE, et al. Hip disarticulation: factors affecting outcome. J Vasc Surg 1991;14:398.

Frang RD, Taylor LM, Porter JM. Amputations. In: Porter JM, Taylor LM, eds. Basic data underlying clinical decision making in vascular surgery. St. Louis, Quality Medical Publishing, 1994:153.

Johansen K, Daines M, Howey T, et al. Objective criteria accurately predict amputation following lower extremity trauma. J Trauma 1990;30:568.

Leonard JA, Andrews KL. Rigid removable dressings, immediate postoperative prostheses, and rehabilitation of the amputee. In: Ernst CB, Stanley JC, eds. Current therapy in vascular surgery, ed. 2. Philadelphia, BC Decker, 1991:708.

Malone JM. Lower extremity amputation. In: Moore WS, ed. Vascular surgery: a comprehensive review. Philadelphia, WB Saunders, 1993:809.

Mills JL, Porter JM. Acute limb ischemia. In: Porter JM, Taylor LM, eds. Basic data underlying clinical decision making in vascular surgery. St. Louis, Quality Medical Publishing, 1994:134.

Owens RS, Carpenter JP, Baum RA, et al. Magnetic resonance imaging of angiographically occult runoff vessels in peripheral arterial occlusive disease. N Engl J Med 1992;326:1577.

Aneurysmal Disease

ESSENTIALS OF SURGERY: SCIENTIFIC PRINCIPLES AND PRACTICE,
edited by Lazar J. Greenfield, Michael W. Mulholland, Keith T. Oldham, Gerald B. Zelenock,
and Keith D. Lillemoe. Lippincott–Raven Publishers, Philadelphia, © 1997.

CHAPTER 86

PATHOGENESIS OF ANEURYSMS

M. DAVID TILSON, ANIL P. HINGORANI,
AND ANITA K. GREGORY

An aneurysm is a permanent, localized dilatation of a blood vessel, specifically a 50% increase in the diameter of a vessel compared with its expected normal diameter (Fig. 86-1). Aneurysms occur throughout the arterial tree, in central vessels (thoracic and abdominal aorta), peripheral vessels (femoral and popliteal arteries), cerebral vessels, and mesenteric and renal vessels. The most common location for an aneurysm is the infrarenal aorta. Many of the factors in the formation of abdominal aortic aneurysm (AAA) apply to aneurysms of the thoracic aorta and the femoral and popliteal arteries.

Aneurysms have been attributed to atherosclerosis. However, the increasing incidence of AAA combined with the decreasing rate of atherosclerotic disease suggests that aneurysmal disease of the aorta may not have the same cause as stenosing disease. Genetic, biochemical, and immune factors play a role.

About 15,000 deaths each year in the United States are due to AAA disease. White men have a three times higher prevalence of AAA than women and black men. People with first-order relatives who have had an AAA are more likely than other people to have an AAA.

ARTERIAL STRUCTURE

Like the other arteries, the aorta has three layers: intima, media, and adventitia. The *intima* consists of a basal lamina lined with a layer of endothelial cells that form the luminal surface of the vessel. The aortic *media* is arranged in a highly organized system of fibromuscular layers that contain connective tissue matrix and smooth muscle cells. The *adventitia* is the outermost layer of the vessel wall and consists of fibrous tissue and vasa vasorum.

The effects of atherosclerosis, aneurysm, and dissection on aortic structure are shown in Fig. 86-2. Inflammatory infiltrates that occur in AAA include plasma cell infiltrate within the media, a chronic inflammatory component within the adventitia, and more immunoglobulin in aortic aneurysmal tissue than is normal. Inflammation mediates connective tissue proteolysis.

There is substantial loss of medial and adventitial elastin in aneurysms. The decrease in elastin content does not correlate with the size of the aneurysm. Diffuse adventitial elastolysis may be the primary event in arterial dilatation, preceding a clinically apparent aneurysm.

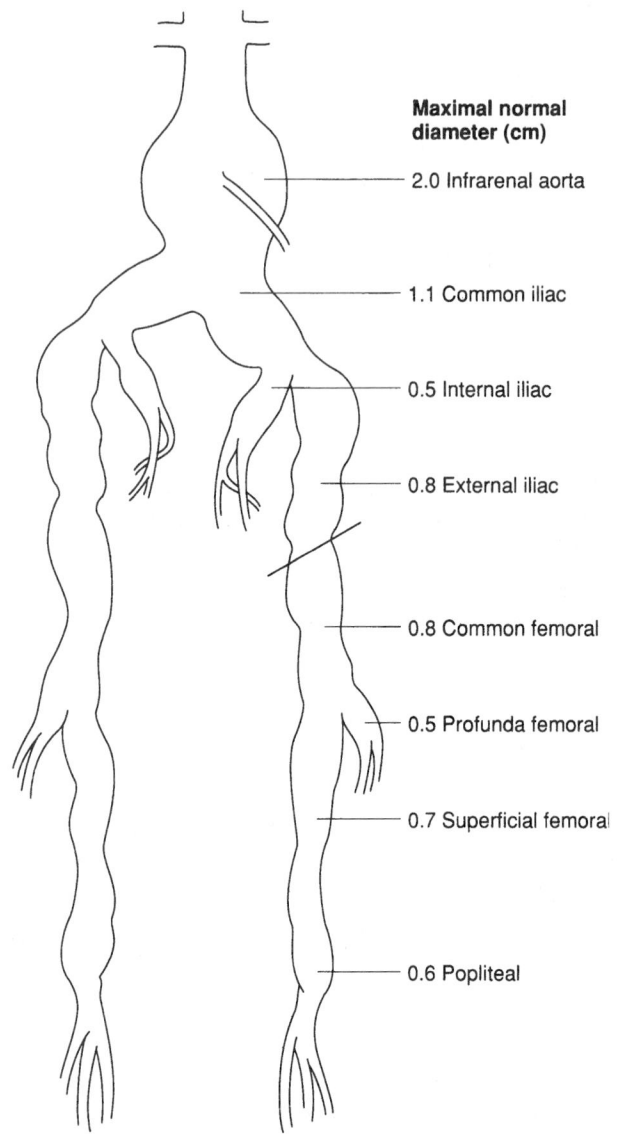

Maximal normal diameter (cm)

- 2.0 Infrarenal aorta
- 1.1 Common iliac
- 0.5 Internal iliac
- 0.8 External iliac
- 0.8 Common femoral
- 0.5 Profunda femoral
- 0.7 Superficial femoral
- 0.6 Popliteal

Figure 86-1. Normal arteriographic sizes of arteries. An aneurysm is defined as a 50% increase in the diameter of the vessel (After Hollier LH, Stanson AW, Gloviczki P, et al. Arteriomegaly: classification and morbid implications of diffuse aneurysmal disease. Surgery 1983;93:700)

BIOCHEMISTRY

Proteins

Elastin and collagen are deficient in AAA, leading to a breakdown of the extracellular matrix (ECM) of the wall of the aorta, which causes weakening and dilatation.

Elastin

Human tissues do not generate much new elastin after the first decade of life. If elastin is not synthesized properly early in development or if it is broken down, the body has limited capacity to synthesize new elastin to replace it.

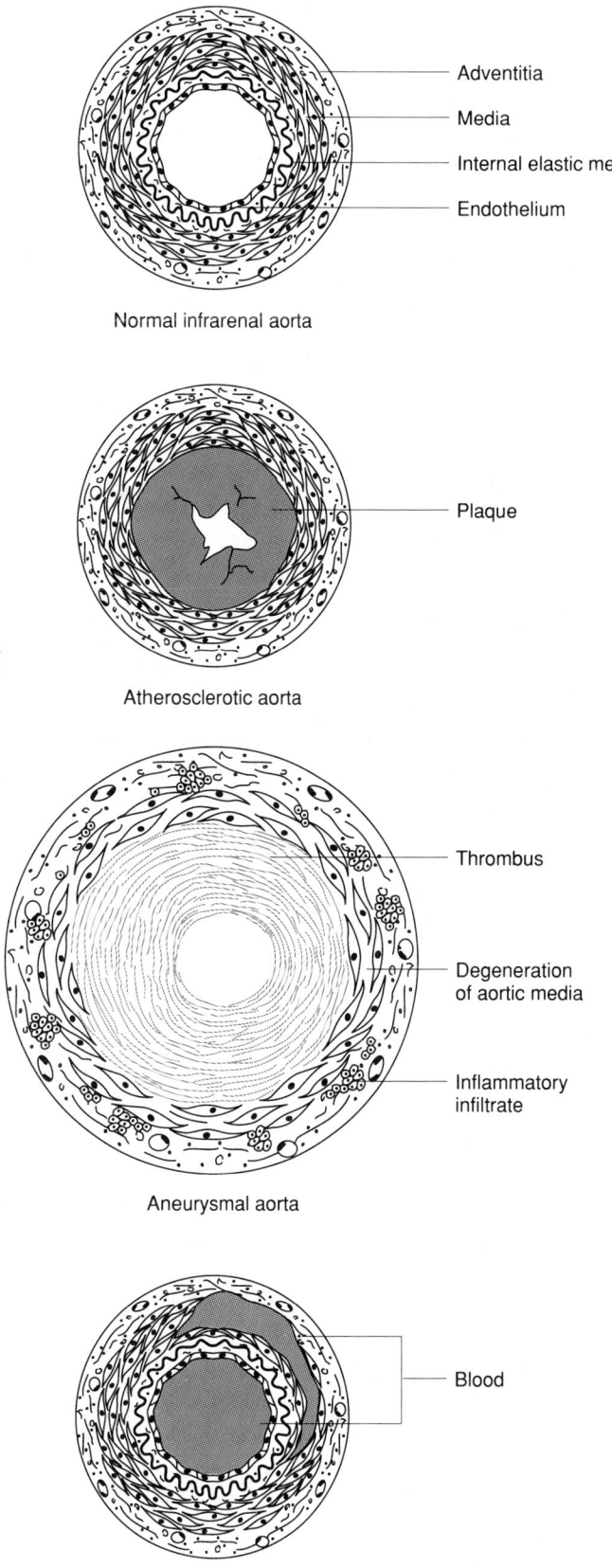

Adventitia

Media

Internal elastic membrane

Endothelium

Normal infrarenal aorta

Plaque

Atherosclerotic aorta

Thrombus

Degeneration
of aortic media

Inflammatory
infiltrate

Aneurysmal aorta

Blood

Aortic dissection

Figure 86-2. Schematic representation of the normal
aorta with three distinct layers—intima, media, and adventitia. Atherosclerosis results in intimal thickening secondary to the formation of plaque. An aneurysm is dilation of an artery with degeneration of the media. The inner
lining is a layer of thrombus. Aortic dissection results
from an intimal tear and a consequent plane of blood
cleaving the media.

Elastin can extend to two to three times its resting length and quickly return to its original length. AAA tissue has less ability to recoil than does normal tissue. Skin, ligaments, lung, and the walls of arteries are rich in elastin.

The elastin molecule is characterized by its lysine cross links. Glycine makes up about one third of the amino acids of elastin. Proline makes up about 11% of elastin, but elastin has little hydroxyproline and no hydroxylysine. Elastin is rich in nonpolar amino acids, such as alanine, valine, leucine, and isoleucine, which may contribute to its insolubility along with its extensive cross linking through lysine residues.

The half-life of elastin is 70 years. Elastin is synthesized by mesenchymal cells, such as smooth muscle cells, chondroblasts, mesothelial cells, fibroblasts, and myofibroblasts.

In the aortic media, elastin is arrayed in lamellae separated by smooth muscle cells. In most mammals the number of lamellae is directly proportional to the load the aorta bears. In humans, however, there are fewer lamellae than expected, which may explain why the abdominal aorta is the most frequent site of aneurysms in humans.

Collagen

The fibrillar collagens are a family of structural proteins of the ECM with repetitive sequences of amino acids in the format Gly-X-Y. The amino acid in the X position is frequently proline, and the amino acid in the Y position is frequently hydroxyproline. About 1000 amino acids long, the backbone forms a left-handed helix called an α chain. Three of these chains are coiled around each other after a right-handed twist to form a procollagen molecule.

The glycine at every third residue is important in the stability of collagen. Glycine, a small, flexible amino acid, is the only one that can fit in the turns of the coil. A mutation that changes this amino acid to another results in a conformational change that reduces the thermal stability of the molecule.

The tensile strength of collagen is four times that of elastin. Collagen contributes to the tensile strength of the aorta, and its failure probably is important in the development of AAA. Failure of collagen is a sentinel event in the chain of causal factors that result in aneurysmal dilatation. Elastin bears the load at small diameters, but as arterial diameter increases, it is collagen that prevents progression to aneurysmal proportions.

Fibrillin

Fibrillin makes up the microfibrillar structure of the ECM. The microfibrillar structure appears to act as the scaffolding for the deposition of elastin during elastogenesis. Fibrillin mutations cause Marfan syndrome. Considering the potential importance of a change in the scaffolding for elastin throughout the aorta and the occasional association of Marfan syndrome with AAA, fibrillin should be considered a candidate gene in AAA disease.

Other Extracellular Matrix Proteins

The ECM appears to be active in many functions, including response to injury, filtration of solutions, inflammatory states, the clotting cascade, and host defenses against spread of tumor and infection. Matrix components such as laminin, glycosaminoglycans, proteoglycans, and fibronectin may be important in the development of AAA.

Proteases

Elastase and collagenase activity are increased in AAA tissue. Patients with AAA who smoke have elevated blood elastolytic activity and decreased serum antiproteolytic activity. The elastolytic activity may be attributed to a serine protease from smooth muscle cells. Inhibition of the principal elastase with EDTA suggests metalloproteolytic activity. Collagenolytic activity seems to be elevated in ruptured AAA or explant cultures, but not in nonruptured AAA.

The matrix metalloproteinases (MMPs) are a family of extracellular proteinases that digest components of the matrix. They break down collagens, elastin, fibronectin, laminin, and proteoglycans. These proteinases are important in inflammatory states, organogenesis, and tumor invasion. They can be synthesized by macrophages, mesenchymal cells, and vascular smooth muscle cells. MMP3 (stomelysin) is present in AAA tissue and may participate in the pathogenesis of AAA.

Plasmin

Plasmin may be important in the pathogenesis of AAA. Macrophages can be induced to secrete plasminogen activator. Plasmin degrades the ECM and activates MMP9, MMP3, and MMP1. Tissue plasminogen activator is elevated in AAA and induces secretion of MMP9 by macrophages.

Protease Inhibitors

In the development of emphysema, smoking causes methylation and inactivation of the active site of α_1-antitrypsin, an important serum antiprotease. Smoking may participate in AAA in a similar way. It causes overactivity of proteases and weakens the ECM. An important risk factor for rupture of AAA appears to be the degree of concomitant chronic obstructive pulmonary disease (COPD).

Two inhibitors are specific for members of the MMP family: tissue inhibitor of metalloproteinase (TIMP) 1 and TIMP-2. Both are small glycosylated proteins produced by cells of the ECM, 30% of the molecular weight being attributed to carbohydrate. MMPs are secreted in complexes with TIMP in the ECM. Immunoreactive TIMP is reduced in AAA tissue, but its gene expression appears to be normal in dermal fibroblasts from patients with AAA.

INFLAMMATION

T lymphocytes, B lymphocytes, and macrophages are present in aneurysmal adventitia. Macrophages are present in aortas with aneurysms and atherosclerotic occlusive disease, but T lymphocytes are less frequent in normal or occluded vessels.

The lymphocytes in aneurysmal tissue secrete cytokines, including γ-interferon, tumor necrosis factor α (TNFα), and interleukins (ILs). These factors increase macrophage proteolytic activity and potentiate aneurysmal dilatation and rupture.

A COMPREHENSIVE THEORY
Human Genetics

A comprehensive theory of the pathogenesis of AAA must encompass genetic, mechanical, and environmental contributions. Many aortic aneurysms are familial, so genetic factors may be important in pathogenesis. The familial predisposition and preponderance of male over female patients suggest that AAA is an inherited disorder. The risk for AAA among first-degree relatives of aneurysm patients is six times that of the general population. Identifying a female family member with an aneurysm marks families at high risk for fatal ruptured aneurysm. The prevalence of clinically significant AAA (>4 cm diameter) is 2% to 3%. The prevalence of a previously undiagnosed AAA in first-degree relatives of AAA patients is much higher.

Pedigree analyses have not led to a unified interpretation of the mode of inheritance. If a single aneurysm gene exists, it is likely autosomal, but X-linked inheritance is possible if there is molecular heterogeneity. Statistical evaluation supports recessive inheritance.

Candidate Genes

Because of the extensive connective tissue matrix remodeling in AAA vessels, a search is being conducted for the genes involved in synthesis and degradation of connective tissue proteins. Genetic loci that code for haptoglobin, cholesterol-ester transfer protein, α_1-antitrypsin, type III collagen, TIMP, elastin, and fibrillin have been suggested. Fig. 86-3 shows some proved and possible interactions that

contribute to disruption of the ECM and eventual development of an aneurysm.

APPROACHES TO INTERVENTION

Early detection is the first step toward preventing AAA disease. If the AAA gene is identified, a screening test, such as a polymerase chain reaction on salivary DNA, may help identify patients with a genetic susceptibility before the disease is expressed. Once the population at risk is identified, patients can be followed with serial ultrasound examinations.

Detection of the presence of inflammatory cells, with induction of proteases and production of cytokines, may be another approach. Soluble cytokines down-regulate proteolytic inhibitory mechanisms and matrix synthesis. It may be possible that therapy as simple as the use of aspirin, or another antiinflammatory agent, may block some of the inflammatory responses that potentiate matrix destruction.

When the antigen responsible for the antibody response in the aneurysmal wall is identified, it may be possible to induce tolerance in patients. This approach is used for patients with rheumatoid arthritis.

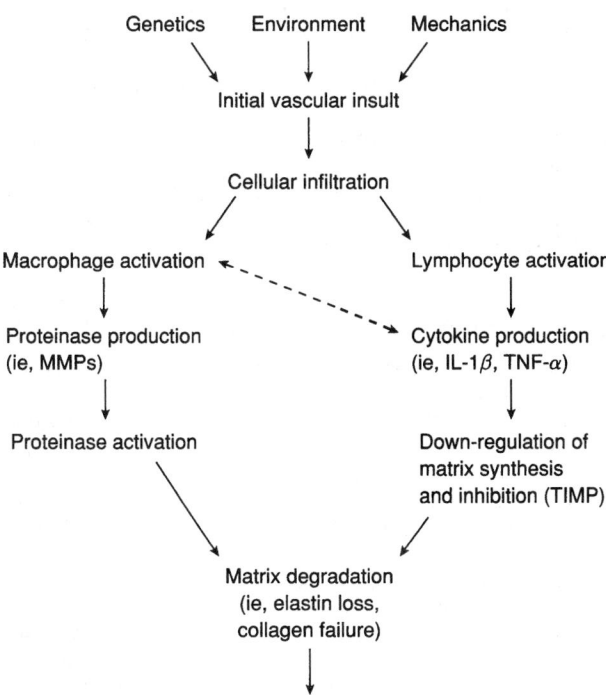

Figure 86-3. This schematic represents an overview of numerous influences on the expression of aneurysm disease. We believe that a genetic susceptibility will eventually be discovered to be the necessary cause of abdominal aortic aneurysms, with environmental factors such as smoking and mechanical factors such as hypertension being potential contributing causes. An initial injury occurs, triggering an inflammatory response that results in a chain of causative events, eventually resulting in matrix degradation and failure of the tensile properties of collagen that prevent aneurysms from occurring under normal conditions.

SUGGESTED READING

Baxter BT, Mcgee GS, Shively VP, et al. Elastin content, crosslinks, and mRNA in normal and aneurysmal human aorta. J Vasc Surg 1992;16:192.

Gadowsky GR, Pilcher DB, Ricci MA. Abdominal aortic aneurysm expansion rate: effect of size and beta-adrenergic blockade. J Vasc Surg 1994;19:727.

Gandhi R, Keller S, Cantor J, et al. Analysis of elastin crosslinks in the insoluble matrix of aneurysmal abdominal aorta. Surgery 1994;115:617.

Irizarry E, Newman KM, Gandhi RH, et al. Demonstration of interstitial collagenase in abdominal aortic aneurysm disease. J Surg Res 1993;54:437.

Pearce WH, Sweis I, Yao JST, McCarthy WJ, Koch AE. Interleukin-1β and tumor necrosis factor-α release in normal and diseased human infrarenal aortas. J Vasc Surg 1992;16:784.

Reilly JM, Brophy CM, Tilson MD. Characterization of an elastase from aneurysmal aorta which degrades intact aortic elastin. Ann Vasc Surg 1992;6:499.

St. Jean PL, Ferrell RE, Majmunder PP, Steed DL, Webster MW. Abdominal aortic aneurysm (AAA): association with α-antitrypsin, haptoglobin, and type III collagen. J Cardiovasc Surg 1991;32:38.

Tilson MD, Reilly JM, Brophy CM, Webster EL, Barnett TR. Expression and sequence of the gene for tissue inhibitor of metalloproteinases in patients with abdominal aortic aneurysms. J Vasc Surg 1993;18:266.

Webster MW, McAuley CE, Steed DL, Miller DD, Evans CH. Collagen stability and collagenolytic activity in the normal and aneurysmal human abdominal aorta. Am J Surg 1991; 161:635.

White JV, Haas K, Phillips S, Comerota AJ. Adventitial elastolysis is a primary event in aneurysm formation. J Vasc Surg 1993;17:371.

ESSENTIALS OF SURGERY: SCIENTIFIC PRINCIPLES AND PRACTICE,
edited by Lazar J. Greenfield, Michael W. Mulholland, Keith T. Oldham, Gerald B. Zelenock,
and Keith D. Lillemoe. Lippincott–Raven Publishers, Philadelphia, © 1997.

CHAPTER 87

EXTRACRANIAL CAROTID, INNOMINATE, SUBCLAVIAN, AND AXILLARY ANEURYSMS

PATRICK J. O'HARA

GENERAL CONSIDERATIONS

Aneurysmal degeneration of the innominate, extracranial carotid, subclavian, and axillary arteries is rare.

Anatomy

Fig. 87-1 shows the normal anatomy and development of the aortic arch and brachiocephalic arterial system. Variations in the origins of the arteries that originate from the aortic arch are not unusual. Causes of aneurysms in descending order of frequency are summarized in Table 87-1.

Pathophysiology

Rupture is rare. When it does occur it has catastrophic consequences. Depending on the location, size, and rate of expansion of an aneurysm, symptoms of nerve, tracheal, esophageal, or venous compression from a mass effect may occur. The most threatening aspect of these aneurysms is the propensity for embolism and thrombosis, which can lead to end-organ ischemia or infarction. *Extracranial carotid* aneurysms may produce focal cerebrovascular symptoms; *subclavian and axillary* aneurysms are associated with upper extremity ischemic symptoms; emboli from *innominate* aneurysms may cause right hemispheric or right upper extremity ischemic symptoms.

Therapeutic Objectives

Preservation of life and neurologic function
Preservation or restoration of end-organ function
Elimination or exclusion of the embolic source
Maintenance of perfusion by means of resection and arterial reconstruction or ligation and bypass

CAROTID ANEURYSMS

Although aneurysmal degeneration of the intracranial carotid arteries and their branches is frequent, *extracranial* carotid aneurysms are uncommon. Most involve the common and internal carotid arteries. The most common causes of extracranial carotid aneurysms are atherosclerosis and trauma. Other causes include infection, cystic medial necrosis, fibromuscular dysplasia, congenital anomalies, and pseudoaneurysms following trauma and surgery.

Clinical Manifestations

Symptomatic extracranial carotid aneurysms most commonly present with stroke, focal transient ischemic attacks (TIAs), amaurosis fugax, or evidence of retinal infarction.

These result from embolization from these lesions. Rupture is uncommon. Associated abdominal aortic and peripheral arterial aneurysms may be present. Other symptoms include focal neurologic symptoms, a pulsatile neck mass with or without discomfort, dysphagia, respiratory stridor, Horner syndrome, and symptoms of cranial nerve compression, probably from the mass effect of large aneurysms.

Diagnosis

The history is important but is seldom sufficient to confirm the diagnosis of extracranial carotid aneurysm. The presence of a *pulsatile mass* in the neck at physical examination suggests aneurysmal disease. The most frequent explanation for this finding is a prominent, tortuous carotid artery, common in elderly, hypertensive women. The differential diagnosis includes carotid body tumor, lymphadenopathy, cystic hygroma, salivary gland tumor, metastatic tumor, cervical lymphoma, lipoma, peritonsillar abscesses, and brachial cleft cysts. A careful examination often is sufficient to differentiate these entities from an aneurysm, and *duplex scanning* usually provides the definitive diagnosis.

If carotid duplex scanning confirms the presence of an aneurysm, or if the diagnosis is still in doubt, intraarterial *digital subtraction angiography* (DSA) of the arch and both carotid arteries with intracranial filming is required. Until the diagnosis of carotid aneurysm is ruled out, incision and drainage or biopsy of a neck mass is unwise because of risk for hemorrhage, which may be profuse and difficult to control.

Management

Atherosclerotic extracranial carotid artery aneurysms are associated with a high ipsilateral stroke rate if managed nonoperatively. Because of risk for neurologic morbidity, patients with extracranial carotid aneurysms are treated when the diagnosis is made.

Extracranial carotid aneurysms are managed by means of direct reconstruction. The methods vary according to local anatomy. Often, the internal carotid artery is sufficiently redundant to allow resection of the aneurysm and primary anastomosis (Fig. 87-2). Fusiform aneurysms that involve the carotid bifurcation can be managed with resection, end-to-end anastomosis of the internal and common carotid arteries, and reimplantation of the external carotid artery (Fig. 87-3). When insufficient redundant internal carotid artery remains to allow primary anastomosis, a saphenous vein interposition graft may be used in a variety of configurations (Fig. 87-4). Synthetic grafts can be used, but autogenous reconstruction is preferred. Intraluminal shunting may be required during carotid artery reconstruction. The graft can be threaded over the shunt, allowing better alignment, and avoiding the problem of kinking due to excessive graft length.

Aneurysmorrhaphy or resection with patch angioplasty may be an alternative, especially in the management of saccular aneurysms. If interposition grafting or patch angioplasty is required, autogenous saphenous vein is used, although redundant internal carotid artery may be used as autogenous patch material. In the absence of adequate autogenous graft material, synthetic prostheses may be used.

AXILLOSUBCLAVIAN ANEURYSMS

Aneurysms of the subclavian and axillary arteries are unusual. Axillosubclavian aneurysms are most commonly caused by trauma or atherosclerosis, although other less

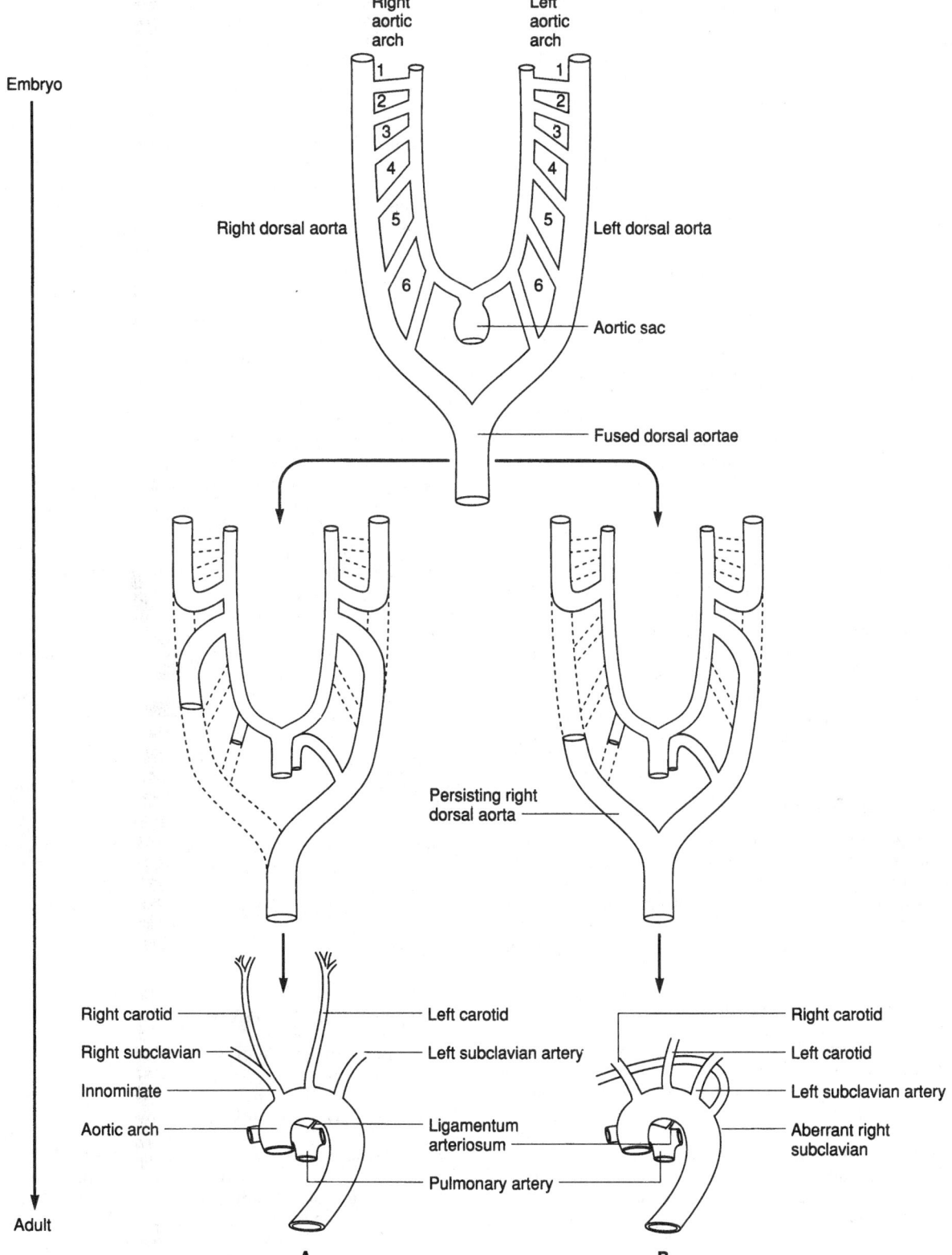

Figure 87-1. Diagrammatic representation of the embryologic development and anatomy of the aortic arch and brachiocephalic arterial systems. (*A*) Normal pattern. (*B*) Anomalous origin of the right subclavian artery. (After Langman J. Arterial system. In: Medical embryology. Baltimore, Williams & Wilkins, 1963:171)

Table 87-1. **CAUSES OF ANEURYSMS**

Artery	Cause
Brachiocephalic	Atherosclerosis
	Trauma
	Infection
Carotid	Atherosclerosis
	Trauma, penetrating or nonpenetrating
	Infection
	Dissection
	Connective tissue disease
	Fibromuscular disease
Axillosubclavian	Atherosclerosis
	Chronic trauma and extrinsic compression
	Chronic injury to arterial wall
	Cervical rib
	Fibrous band at thoracic outlet
	Improper crutch use
Subclavian	Aberrant right subclavian artery
	Medical degeneration
	Fibromuscular disease
	Arteritis
	Congenital anomalies
Mycotic	Infection of arterial puncture site associated with parenteral drug abuse

common causes, such as infection (especially syphilis in the past), arteritis, medial degeneration, fibromuscular disease, and congenital anomalies, account for some aneurysms. Most traumatic aneurysms are caused by chronic pressure that causes intimal damage and poststenotic dilatation. In the subclavian region, the usual cause is thoracic outlet obstruction related to cervical ribs or other causes of thoracic outlet syndrome. In the axillary region, improper long-term use of crutches can cause axillary artery aneurysms.

Clinical Manifestations

Although some axillosubclavian aneurysms are asymptomatic, most cause pain. A pulsatile mass usually is detected at physical examination. Symptoms of arterial occlusion, presumably due to thrombosis or embolism, occur in a large number of patients with true aneurysms. Acute expansion and rupture are ominous signs that may lead to death.

Diagnosis

A careful *history and physical examination* coupled with a high index of suspicion yields the diagnosis in most instances. Aneurysms in other locations must be sought. In the nonemergency setting, upper extremity *noninvasive arterial studies* may be used if there are symptoms of ischemia or embolism to document small-vessel involvement. *Radiographs* of the cervical spine are obtained to identify cervical ribs. *Ultrasound* examination may be helpful in evaluating the extrathoracic subclavian and axillary arteries with respect to dilatation and intimal injury. *Arteriography* is mandatory to confirm the diagnosis and define the extent of the arterial involvement and the state of the outflow bed. It includes arch and full runoff views, if the patient's condition allows.

Management

Because of the substantial risk to life and limb associated with axillosubclavian aneurysms, surgical repair is indicated if the patient's general medical condition allows. The surgical objectives are:

- Control or prevention of hemorrhage
- Removal of an embolic source
- Elimination of the underlying cause of the aneurysm
- Elimination of the aneurysmal mass effect
- Establishment of distal arterial perfusion

The surgical procedure depends on the cause, size, and location of the aneurysm. The aneurysm is resected and end-to-end anastomosis performed. Arterial interposition grafting or bypass is common (Fig. 87-5). Autogenous saphenous vein is used as graft material, but vein availability or size discrepancy may dictate use of a synthetic graft. A supraclavicular incision is usually required for proximal control, and the distal aspect may necessitate an infraclavicular incision. The clavicle may be divided if necessary but is repaired if possible, because symptoms of shoulder instability may occur.

Aneurysms confined to the proximal right subclavian artery are corrected through a median sternotomy; those involving the proximal left subclavian artery may be approached through a left thoracotomy. If thoracic outlet compromise is an etiologic factor, it is managed with concomitant decompression. Cervical and first rib resection may be performed through the supraclavicular incision.

Adjunctive peripheral embolectomy may be needed. If an associated vasospastic disorder is present or if symptomatic irretrievable small vessel emboli are present, sympathectomy may be performed. The role of perioperative thrombolytic therapy in this setting is undefined. This type of therapy carries a risk for hemorrhage, but it may be a consideration in the treatment of patients with small vessel embolism and limb-threatening ischemia unresponsive to conventional therapy.

Arterial ligation may be possible in the management of infected aneurysms or in other situations in which reconstruction is not feasible, but it is accompanied by a high incidence of effort-related upper extremity ischemic symptoms. Axilloaxillary bypass may be used in this unusual situation.

The rare aberrant right subclavian artery aneurysm is probably best managed by means of preliminary extra-anatomic bypass to the right subclavian artery followed by left thoracotomy for ligation of the aneurysm. It is difficult to control the origin of the aberrant right subclavian artery from a right thoracotomy or median sternotomy (Fig. 87-6).

INNOMINATE ANEURYSMS

Innominate artery aneurysms are unusual.

Clinical Manifestations

Patients with innominate artery aneurysms have chest discomfort, hoarseness caused by recurrent laryngeal nerve dysfunction, dysphagia, upper extremity or CMS embolic symptoms, or may have no symptoms. Many innominate artery aneurysms are detected during preoperative evaluation for repair of an abdominal aortic aneurysm or investigation of a mediastinal mass.

Diagnosis

The diagnosis is suggested when *chest radiography* reveals a mediastinal mass. Magnetic resonance imaging (MRI) or contrast-enhanced computed tomography (CT) of the chest helps differentiate aneurysm from tumor mass. *Arch aortography* confirms the pathologic arterial anatomy.

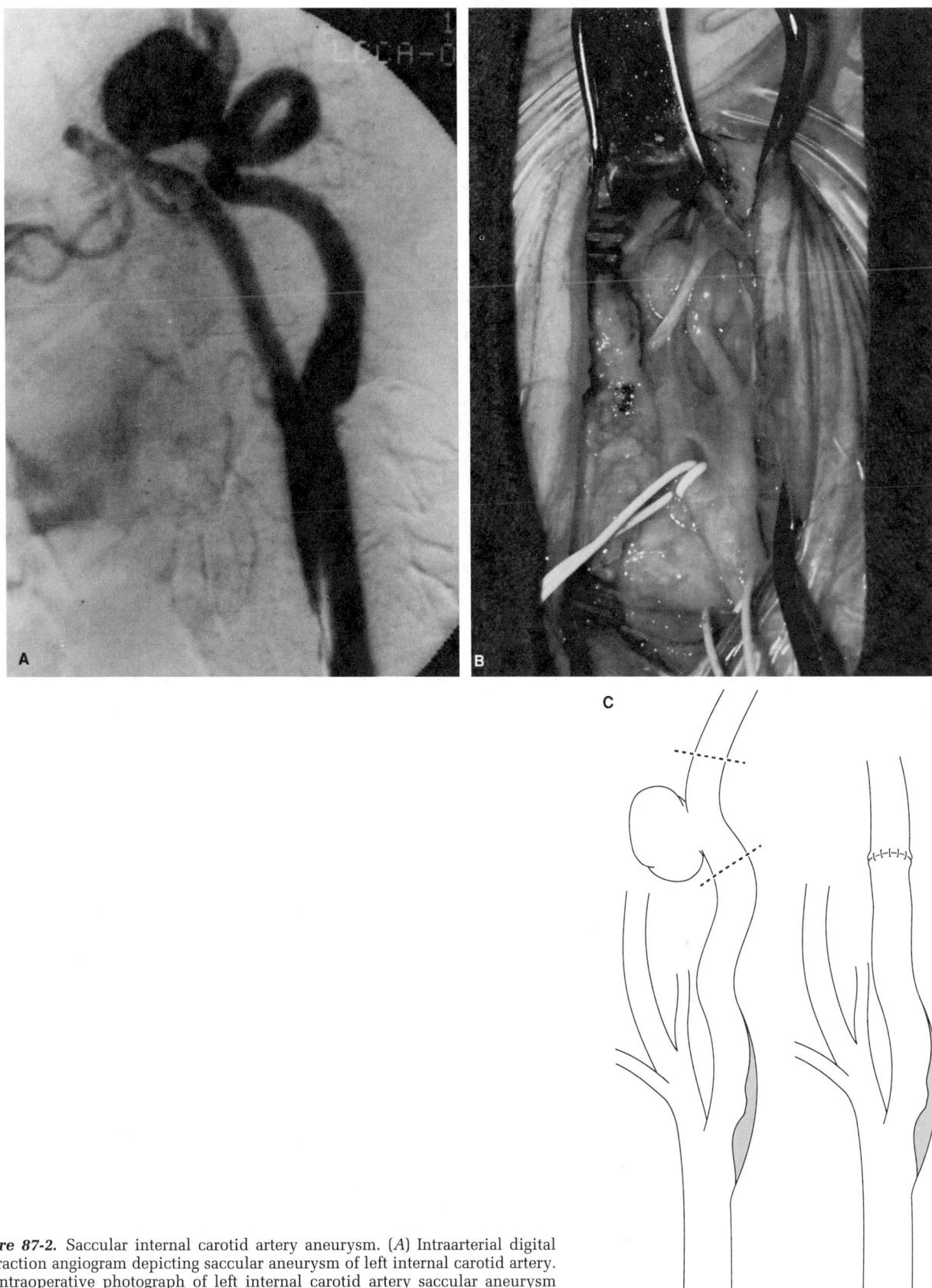

Figure 87-2. Saccular internal carotid artery aneurysm. (*A*) Intraarterial digital subtraction angiogram depicting saccular aneurysm of left internal carotid artery. (*B*) Intraoperative photograph of left internal carotid artery saccular aneurysm distal to hypoglossal nerve in the same patient. (*C*) Operative diagram depicting resection of left internal carotid saccular aneurysm with end-to-end arterial carotid anastomosis in the same patient.

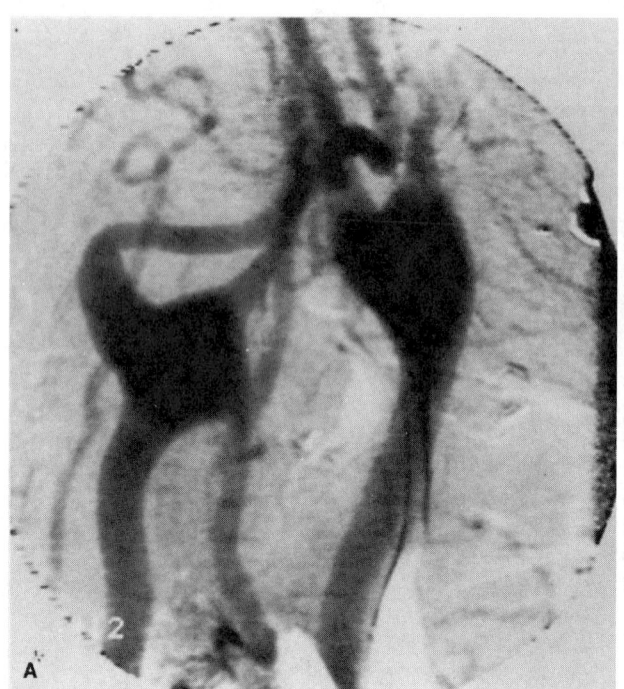

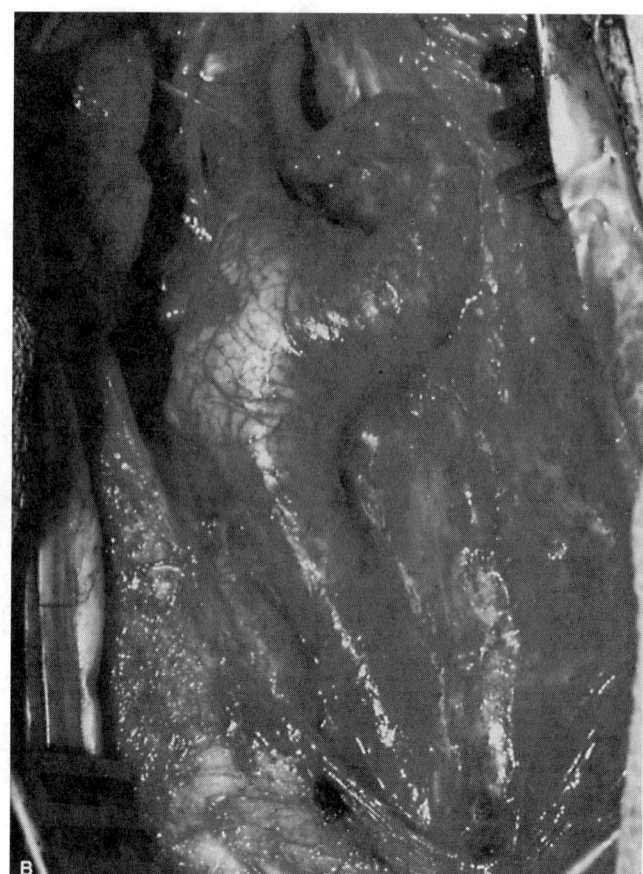

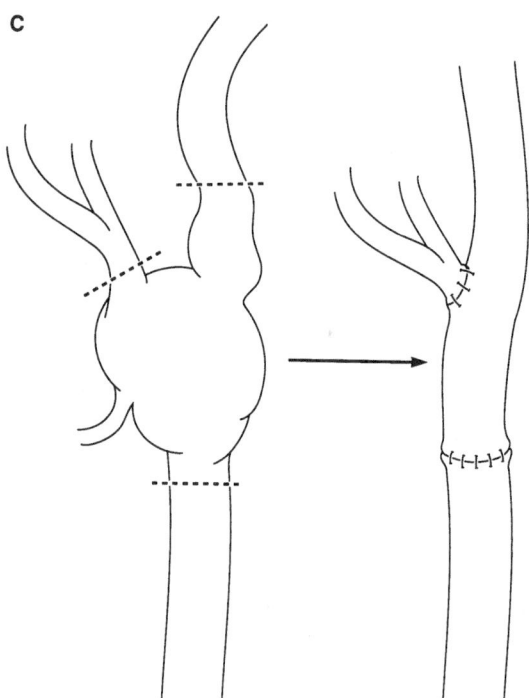

Figure 87-3. Fusiform internal carotid artery aneurysm. (*A*) Good-quality intravenous digital subtraction angiogram depicting bilateral fusiform carotid bifurcation aneurysms. (*B*) Intraoperative photograph of fusiform left carotid bifurcation aneurysm. (*C*) Operative diagram depicting resection of the fusiform left internal carotid aneurysm with end-to-end anastomosis of the internal and common carotid arteries and reimplantation of the external carotid artery.

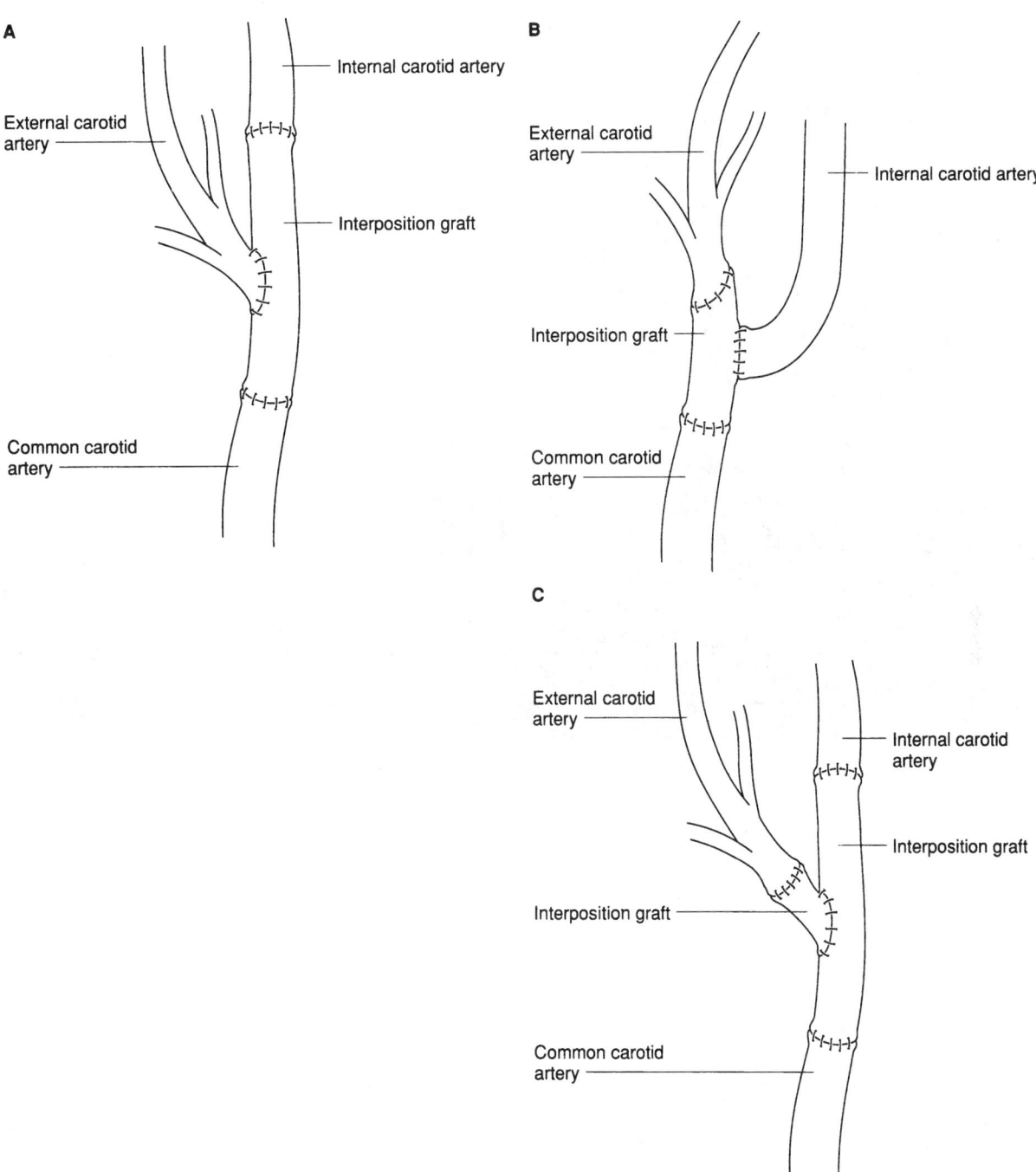

Figure 87-4. Diagrammatic representation of surgical management of extracranial carotid aneurysms with use of saphenous vein interposition grafting. (*A*) Internal carotid artery (ICA) replacement with external carotid artery (ECA) reimplantation. (*B*) ECA replacement with ICA reimplantation. (*C*) Both ICA and ECA replaced with interposition grafts. (After Painter TA, Hertzer NR, Beven EG, O'Hara PJ. Extracranial carotid aneurysms: report of six cases and review of the literature. J Vasc Surg 1985;2:312)

Management

Because of the risks of embolism and rupture, surgical repair is indicated, especially if the aneurysm is symptomatic and large or enlarging, and surgical risk is acceptable. Therapy involves excision of the aneurysm and restoration of both upper extremity and cerebral perfusion. Sometimes it may be acceptable to restore flow only to the right carotid artery.

The aneurysm can be approached through a median sternotomy, which can be extended along the anterior bor-der of the right sternocleidomastoid muscle for additional exposure. The aneurysmal innominate artery is replaced with a synthetic interposition graft or a bifurcated graft to the right common carotid and subclavian arteries. An alternative procedure is autogenous saphenous vein grafting from the aorta to the right subclavian artery and from the aorta to the right common carotid artery, if vein size is adequate.

Cardiopulmonary bypass is not required for elective innominate aneurysm repair but may be necessary in the

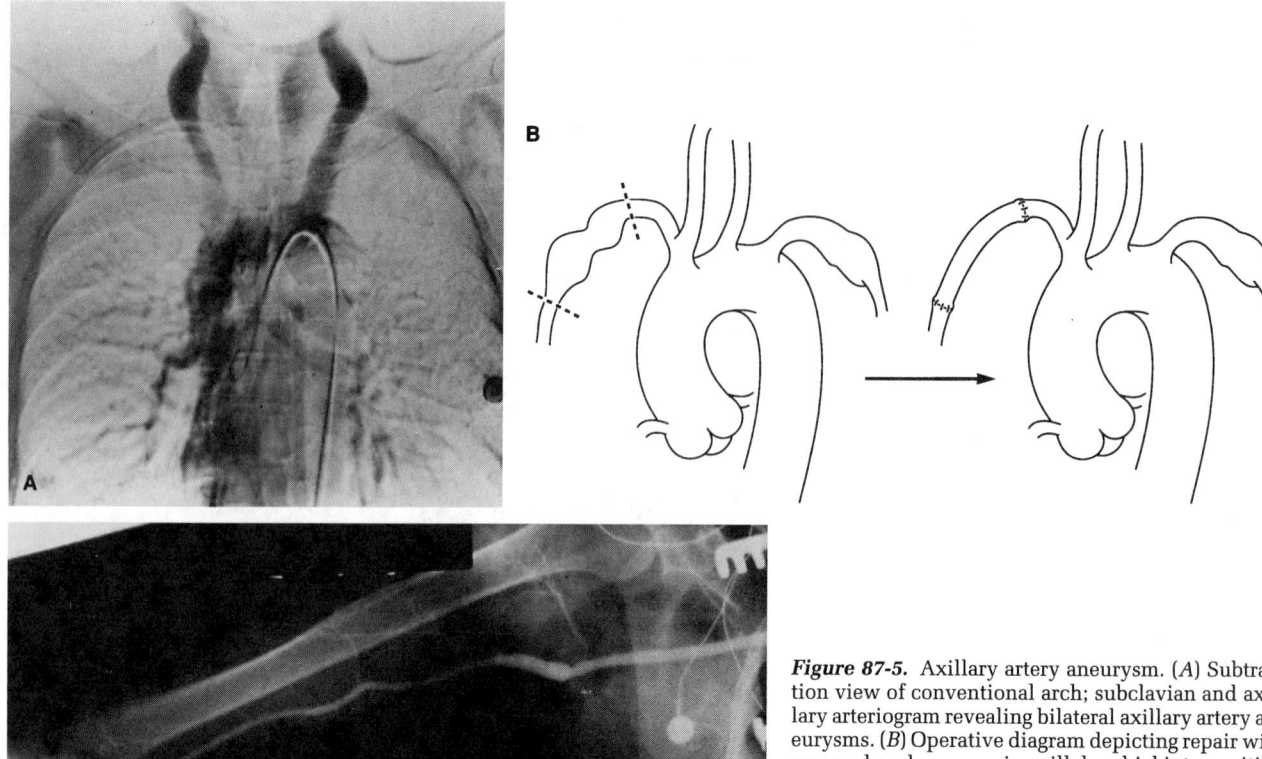

Figure 87-5. Axillary artery aneurysm. (A) Subtraction view of conventional arch; subclavian and axillary arteriogram revealing bilateral axillary artery aneurysms. (B) Operative diagram depicting repair with reversed saphenous vein axillobrachial interposition graft. (C) Intraoperative completion right axillobrachial arteriogram revealing functioning interposition graft.

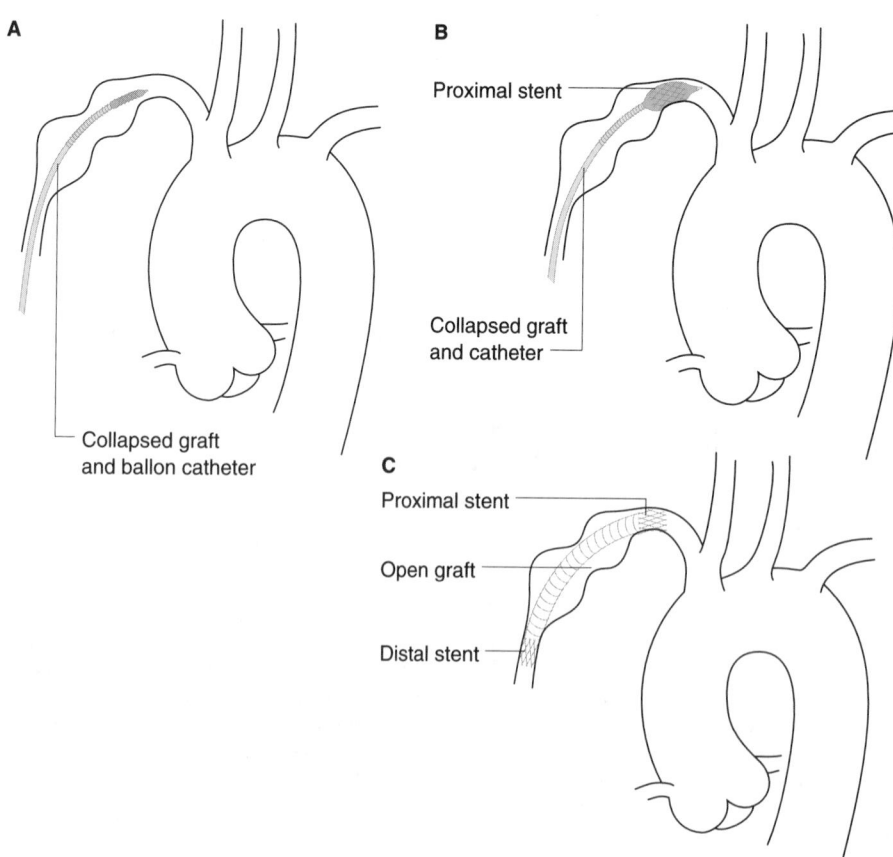

Figure 87-6. Intraluminal stent-graft placement for treatment of an axillosubclavian aneurysm. (A) Catheter delivery of the stent-graft. (B) Balloon deployment of the proximal stent to anchor the graft proximally. (C) Graft in place after deployment of the distal anchoring stent.

event of rupture. Ligation of the innominate artery is well-tolerated by the upper extremity, but cerebral injury may occur after occlusion of the common carotid artery. Ligation is rarely performed and is much less preferable than direct reconstruction.

SUGGESTED READING

Bower TC, Pairolero PC, Hallett JW, et al. Brachiocephalic aneurysm: the case for early recognition and repair. Ann Vasc Surg 1991;5:125.

Kieffer E, Bahnini A, Koskas F. Aberrant subclavian artery: surgical treatment in thirty-three adult patients. J Vasc Surg 1994;19:100.

Marin ML, Veith FJ, Panetta TF, et al. Transluminally placed endovascular stented graft repair for arterial trauma. J Vasc Surg 1994;20:446.

May J, White G, Waugh R, Yu W, Harris J. Transluminal placement of a prosthetic graft-stent device for treatment of subclavian artery aneurysm. J Vasc Surg 1993;18:1056.

Neumayer LA, Bull DA, Hunter GC, et al. Atherosclerotic aneurysms of the axillary artery. J Cardiovasc Surg 1992;33:172.

Parodi JC, Palmaz JC, Barone HD. Transfemoral intraluminal graft implantation for abdominal aortic aneurysms. Ann Vasc Surg 1991;5:491.

Sayers RD, Thompson MM, Bell PRF. Endovascular stenting of abdominal aortic aneurysms. Eur J Vasc Surg 1993;7:225.

Verkroost MW, Hamerlijnck RP, Vermeulen FE. Surgical management of aneurysms at the origin of an aberrant right subclavian artery. J Thorac Cardiovasc Surg 1994;107:1469.

ESSENTIALS OF SURGERY: SCIENTIFIC PRINCIPLES AND PRACTICE, edited by Lazar J. Greenfield, Michael W. Mulholland, Keith T. Oldham, Gerald B. Zelenock, and Keith D. Lillemoe. Lippincott–Raven Publishers, Philadelphia, © 1997.

CHAPTER 88

THORACIC, THORACOABDOMINAL, AND ABDOMINAL AORTIC ANEURYSMS

R. SCOTT MITCHELL, DANIEL J. REDDY, CALVIN B. ERNST, ALEXANDER D. SHEPARD, AND JERRY GOLDSTONE

True aneurysms of the aorta are expansions or dilatations of the aorta that involve all three layers of the wall (intima, media, and adventitia). They can be fusiform or saccular in configuration. False aneurysms can cause aortic enlargement and exhibit intimal and medial disruption; luminal blood is contained only by adventitial layers and surrounding reactive fibrosis.

Aortic ulcerations suggest penetration, excavation, or erosion of luminal blood into the aortic wall. Aortic dissection implies proximal or distal progression of the column of blood within the aortic wall. Ulcerations and dissection may or may not be associated with aortic enlargement. Clinical manifestation of aortic disease depends on the site of involved aorta and the underlying pathologic process.

Aortic aneurysms are caused by:

Atherosclerosis
Connective tissue degeneration (Marfan syndrome, Ehlers-Danlos syndrome)
Aortic dissection

THORACIC AORTIC ANEURYSMS

Arteriosclerotic Aneurysms

Aneurysmal disease of the thoracic aorta occurs mainly among elderly people. The aneurysms usually are asymptomatic and are discovered on routine chest radiographs or during evaluation for another medical problem. The descending aorta is involved more commonly than the ascending aorta. The family history often reveals a relative with a thoracic aortic aneurysm.

Diagnosis

Once aneurysmal dilatation of the aorta has begun, it progresses. Hypertension contributes to continued expansion. Symptomatic aneurysms >10 cm in diameter are likely to rupture.

A chest radiograph can alert the clinician to the presence of an aneurysm, but computed tomography (CT) and magnetic resonance imaging (MRI) allow accurate sizing of the aneurysm and can help differentiate chronic dissection and true arteriosclerotic or degenerative aneurysms. Once an aneurysm is suspected, imaging of the entire thoracic and abdominal aorta is performed because multiple aneurysms can exist.

Surgical Management

Indications for surgical treatment are:

Signs and symptoms of rapid expansion (chest pain, hemoptysis, hematemesis, hoarseness, stridor)
Aneurysm >7 cm in diameter
Aneurysm more than twice the diameter of normal adjacent aorta
Rapid increase in size of the aneurysm

Once the necessity for an operation is determined and a cardiac evaluation is completed, the aneurysm is replaced with an interposition graft (Fig. 88-1). Repair of an *ascending* aortic aneurysm is accomplished through a median sternotomy. Diseased aorta is replaced from the sinotubular ridge to the level of the innominate artery and, if necessary, the transverse aortic arch. Surgical repair of *descending* thoracic aortic aneurysms is performed through a left posterolateral thoracotomy. After distal and proximal cross-clamping, full-thickness cuffs of aorta are developed, and an interposition graft is sutured in place. Some surgeons repair descending aortic aneurysms while the patient is undergoing left heart bypass. Others use the "clamp and go" technique or temporary shunts or bypasses.

Degenerative Aneurysms

Diagnosis

Unlike arteriosclerotic aneurysms, aortic aneurysms of Marfan syndrome begin at the level of the aortic annulus, involve the coronary sinuses and the supracoronary aorta, and necessitate replacement of the entire aortic root. These changes may not be seen on chest radiographs (Fig. 88-2). Echocardiography, CT, or MRI is needed.

Surgical Management

Cardiac deaths account for almost all early deaths of persons with Marfan syndrome. Most of these deaths are due to aortic root dilatation or aortic dissection. Because of this danger, prophylactic aortic root replacement is performed for aneurysmal dilatation >6 cm.

Methods of surgical repair of a Marfan aorta involve: (1) sewing a valved conduit directly onto the aortic annulus, and (2) circumferential dissection of the coronary ostia

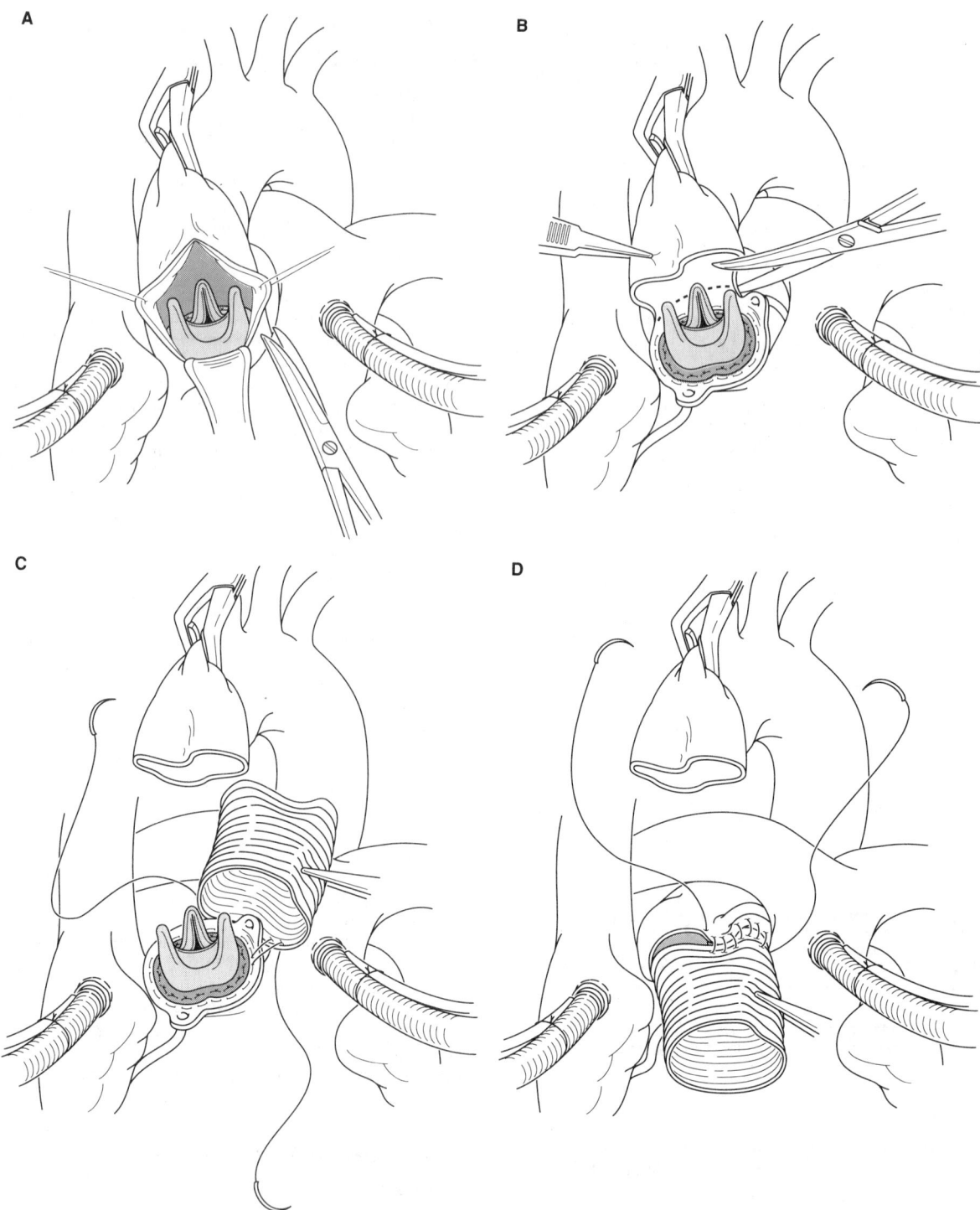

Figure 88-1. (*A*) Operative repair of ascending aortic aneurysm without degenerative aortic disease. Valve replacement, if indicated, is performed after cardiac arrest with cardioplegia and during continuous topical hypothermia. (*B*) A full-thickness cuff of proximal aorta is developed by meticulous dissection of the aorta off the pulmonary artery, and the aorta is transected just distal to the coronary ostia. (*C*) The posterior suture line begins to the left of the left main coronary ostium, and proceeds rightward, over the ostium. Meticulous hemostasis is mandatory, because repair sutures in this area can narrow the left main coronary artery. (*D*) Completion of the posterior suture line demonstrates the exposure attained by extensive mobilization of the aorta and pulmonary artery. (*E*) The anterior suture line may compromise the right coronary artery in the atrioventricular groove. (*F*) Careful measurement of graft length ensures a tension-free distal anastomosis. (After Frist WH, Miller DC. Repair of ascending aortic aneurysms and dissections. J Cardiac Surg 1986;1:33) (*continues*)

E   F

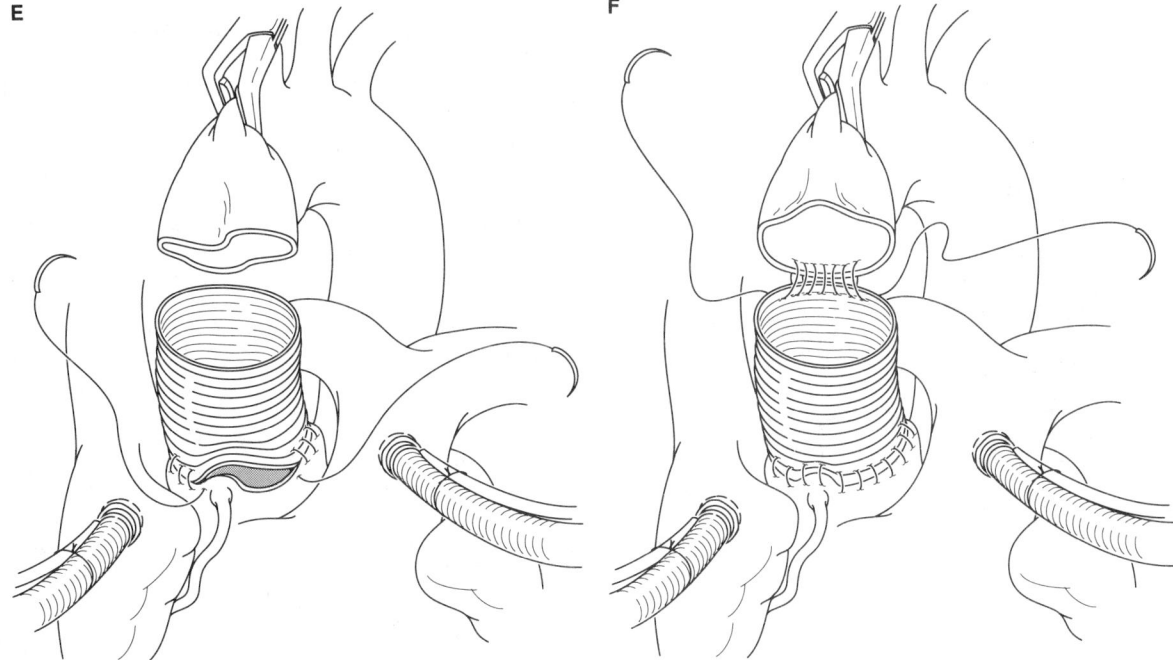

Figure 88-1. (*Continued*)

with buttons of aortic tissue. These buttons are anastomosed to the ascending graft in an end-to-side manner and often are buttressed with a circular pledget (Fig. 88-3). The distal anastomosis is to the completely transected aorta proximal to the innominate artery.

Aortic Dissention

The most important feature of acute aortic dissection is involvement or lack of involvement of the ascending aorta. Neither the exact location of the tear nor the distal extent of the dissection is as important to subsequent clinical behavior.

Diagnosis

The signs and symptoms of acute aortic dissection mimic those of more common illnesses. Most patients experience sudden, severe, sharp retrosternal or intrascapular pain, which may migrate. Others have entirely silent dissection, the diagnosis becoming apparent only after the onset of a secondary effect, such as congestive heart failure due to aortic regurgitation or limb ischemia due to arterial

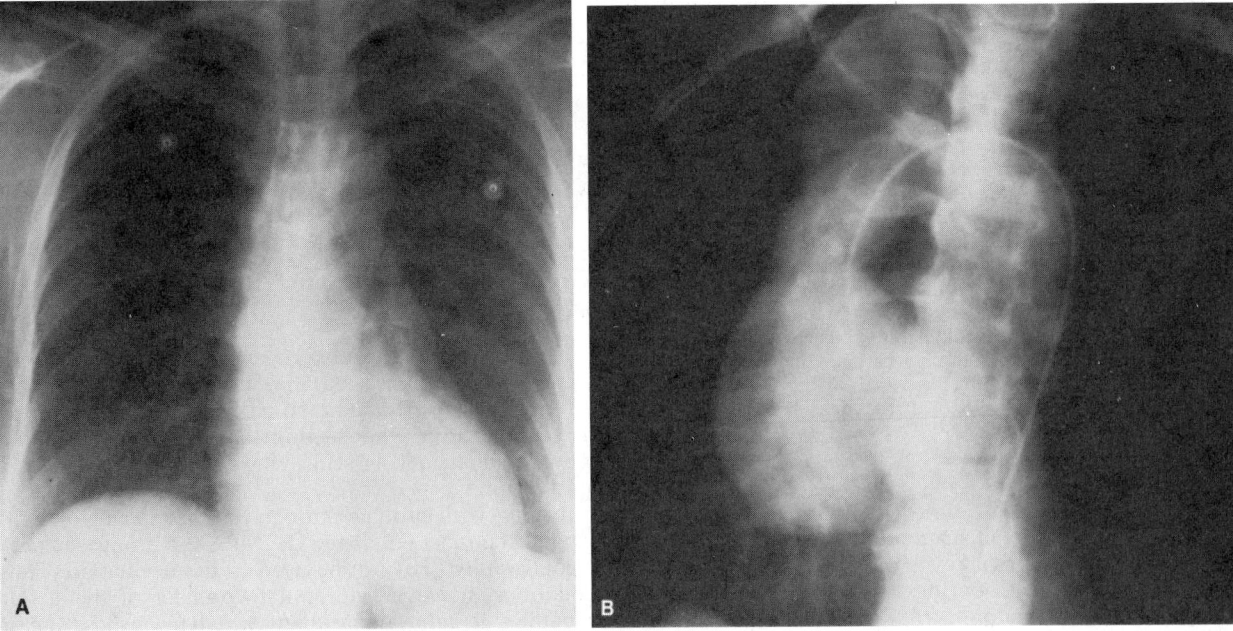

Figure 88-2. (*A*) Dilation of the proximal aorta may be hidden by mediastinal structures on routine posteroanterior chest radiograph. (*B*) Aortography reveals dilatation of the entire ascending aorta, including the coronary sinuses, and aortic regurgitation.

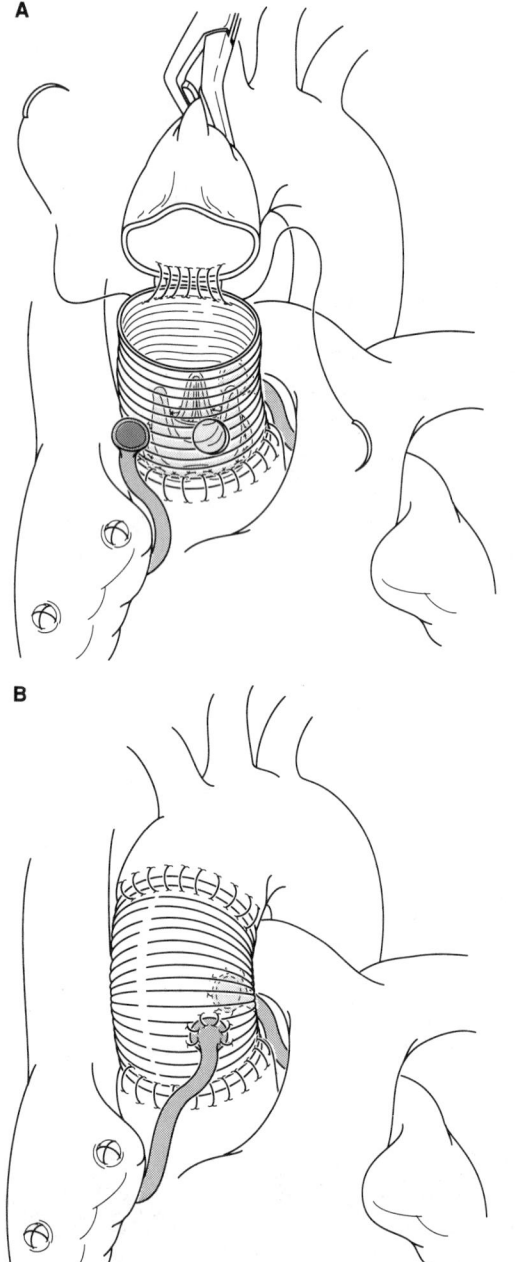

A

B

Figure 88-3. (*A*) Replacement of the aortic root is accomplished with a valved conduit anastomosed directly to the aortic annulus. The left coronary anastomosis is already complete, performed as an end-to-side anastomosis of a full-thickness aortic button before completion of the distal anastomosis. The full-thickness right coronary anastomosis is completed after the distal anastomosis to allow proper positioning without torsion or tension. (*B*) The completed repair, with reimplanted right and left coronary anastomoses. Circular Teflon felt bolsters may be necessary if the aortic tissues are unduly friable. (After Frist WH, Miller DC. Repair of ascending aortic aneurysms and dissections. J Cardiac Surg 1986;1:33)

occlusion. A high index of suspicion for seemingly unrelated signs and symptoms is key to timely diagnosis, which is critical to avoid death during the first 24 to 48 hours after acute aortic dissection.

A careful history and physical examination can produce subtle clues to the diagnosis; a new murmur of aortic regurgitation or an absent pulse can provoke further evaluation.

Contrast-enhanced dynamic CT, MRI, biplane aortography and cineangiography, and multiplanar transesophageal echocardiography all provide enough information to allow initial therapeutic decisions. At times, more than one diagnostic study may be needed for precise therapeutic planning.

Management

Hemodynamic stabilization, with particular attention to control of hypertension to levels just adequate for maintenance of cerebral, myocardial, and renal perfusion, is the immediate goal. After stabilization and diagnosis, treatment is directed at correction of the life-threatening aspects of the dissection. For dissection involving the *ascending aorta* (type A), this involves replacement of the supracoronary aorta to prevent rupture of the proximal root into the pericardium with subsequent tamponade. For patients with acute dissection of the *descending aorta* (type B), management is variable and the timing of intervention is somewhat controversial. Surgical treatment of young patients at good risk is aggressive to prevent proximal extension of the dissection, resect the intimal tear, and direct flow into the distal true lumen.

Surgical Procedure

The *ascending aorta* is approached through a median sternotomy. The distal aorta is manipulated to allow a full-thickness end-to-end anastomosis (Fig. 88-4). The distal graft is clamped just proximal to the anastomosis, and arterial perfusion is repositioned into the distal graft to allow antegrade perfusion. The proximal anastomosis and aortic valve repairs are made during this period of systemic rewarming.

Surgical repair of dissection of the *descending aorta* is accomplished through a left posterolateral thoracotomy. Only a short segment of aorta, the most severely affected, is resected, unless a known single intimal tear exists more distally. After intimal and adventitial continuity is reestablished with an interposed medial layer of prosthetic material, an interposition graft is sewn to full-thickness cuffs.

Trauma

Trauma is the most common cause of nondegenerative disease of the thoracic aorta. During sudden deceleration, the untethered aortic arch and descending aorta flex anteriorly, stretching the aorta against the ligamentum, with resultant partial or complete circumferential intimal disruption. For patients who survive this acute event, the rupture is partially contained by the aortic adventitia and pleura, but risk for hemorrhage stays high. Early diagnosis is essential.

Diagnosis

Aortic injury is suspected whenever there is a history of sudden deceleration, severe chest injury, multiple posterior rib fractures, thoracic spinal fracture, or fracture of the scapula. Aortic transection can exist in patients with known sudden deceleration who have no other signs of chest trauma.

Imaging with biplane aortography or cineangiography, dynamic contrast-enhanced CT, MRI, and intravascular ultrasonography (US) can be used in the evaluation. These modalities, however, necessitate transfer of the patient from the emergency department, which means loss of monitoring capabilities and risk for hemodynamic instability and catastrophic hemorrhage. Multiplane transesophageal echocardiography may be used as an alternative.

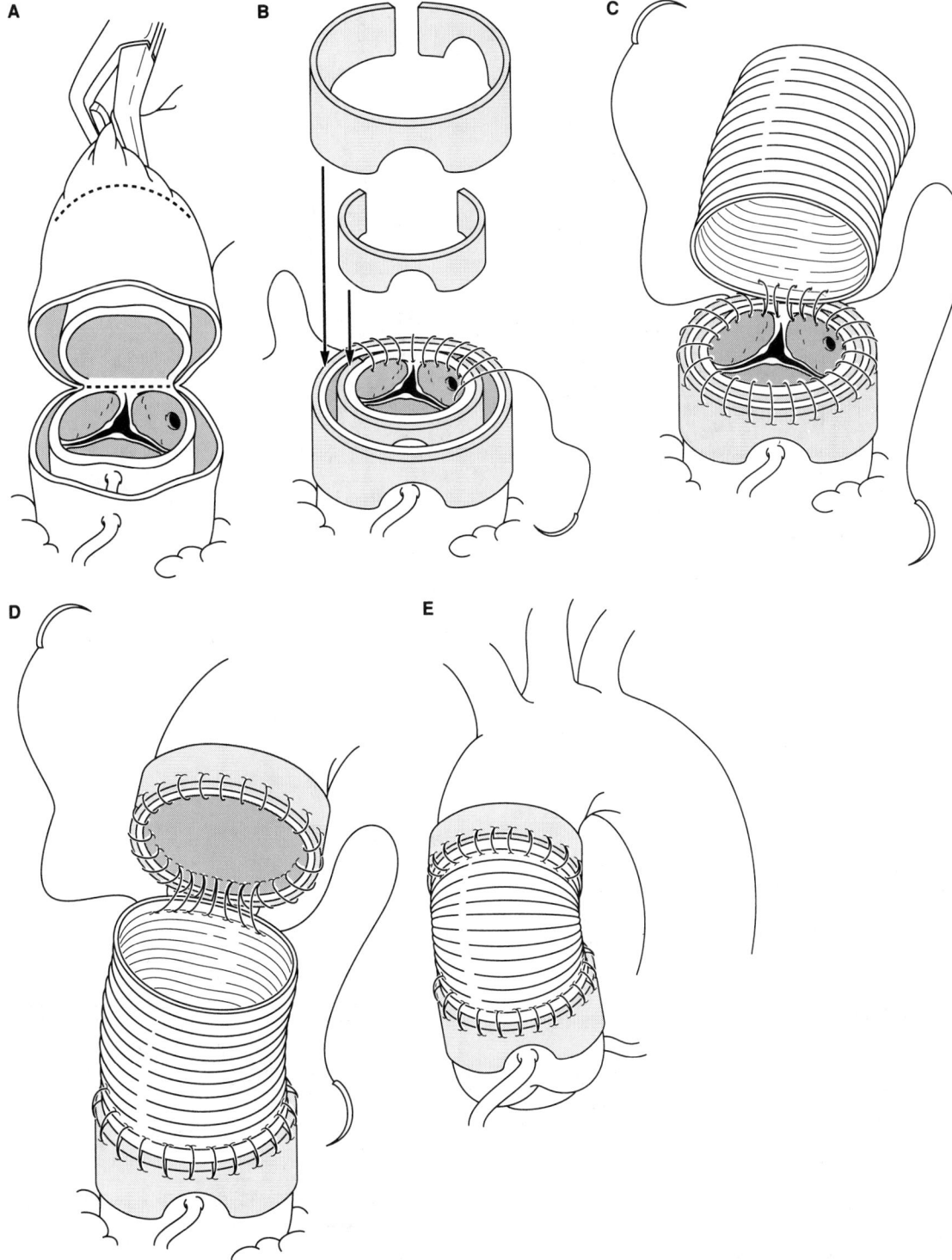

Figure 88-4. (*A*) Acute aortic dissection involving the ascending aorta. The false lumen, septum, and involvement of the right coronary are apparent. (*B*) A strip of Teflon felt is carefully tailored to obliterate the false lumen between the intima and adventitia, extending proximally to the aortic annulus. A second layer of felt can be used as an adventitial support if the vessel is particularly fragile. (*C*) Having preserved the native aortic valve, the proximal anastomosis is constructed end to end with full-thickness bites. (*D*) The distal false lumen is similarly obliterated, and a full-thickness anastomosis is constructed end to end. (*E*) Completed repair after ascending aortic dissection.

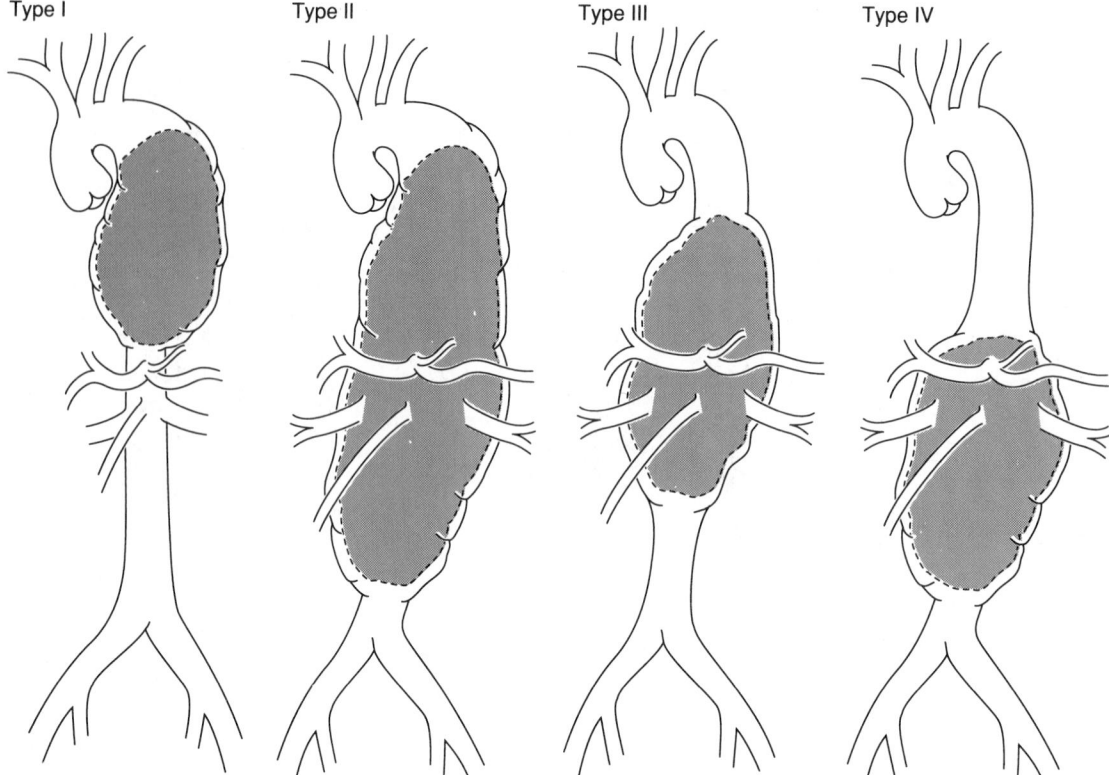

Figure 88-5. Four types of thoracoabdominal aortic aneurysms. (After Ernst CB, Reddy DJ. Thoracoabdominal aortic aneurysm. In: Haimovici H, Callow AD, DePalma RE, et al, eds. Vascular surgery: principles and practice, ed. 3. Norwalk, CT, Appleton & Lange, 1989:613)

Surgical Management

Surgical exposure is gained through a left posterolateral thoracotomy, and proximal and distal control of the aorta is obtained. Repair is then accomplished by means of direct-suture anastomosis or an interposition graft.

THORACOABDOMINAL AORTIC ANEURYSMS

Thoracoabdominal aortic aneurysms (TAAAs) are unusual. TAAAs may rupture, erode into adjacent structures, and initiate peripheral embolism. The aneurysm can be fusiform or saccular. A classification of TAAA is provided in Fig. 88-5 and Table 88-1.

Diagnosis

Symptoms

TAAA must be identified before complications develop. Although a large abdominal component of a TAAA may be palpable, the cephalad extent of the aneurysm may be indistinct. Some asymptomatic TAAAs are identified on chest radiographs, US scans, or CT scans of the chest or abdomen during evaluation of other problems. TAAAs <5 cm in diameter are usually asymptomatic. As they enlarge, most TAAAs become symptomatic before they rupture. Clinical manifestations include expansion, rupture, embo-

---

Table 88-1. CLASSIFICATION OF THORACOABDOMINAL AORTIC ANEURYSMS

Type	Extent of Involvement
I	Most of the descending thoracic aorta and upper abdominal aorta down to the celiac axis
II	Most extensive, most or all of the descending and abdominal aorta from the left subclavian artery to the abdominal aortic bifurcation
III	Distal half of the descending aorta and most of the abdominal aorta, including the celiac, superior mesenteric, and renal arteries
IV	Only the abdominal aorta, including the origins of all visceral vessels

---

Table 88-2. SYMPTOMS OF THORACOABDOMINAL AORTIC ANEURYSMS

Common Symptoms
Pain in the chest, back, abdomen, or flank

Additional Symptoms
Renal insufficiency or accelerated hypertension due to renal artery involvement
Paraparesis or paraplegia due to spinal cord ischemia
Acute leg ischemia due to distal embolism of aneurysmal contents

Uncommon Symptoms
Compression of the airway or esophagus
Hoarseness due to compression of the recurrent laryngeal nerve
Hematemesis or hemoptysis with profound hypovolemic shock due to erosion of a TAAA into the digestive or pulmonary tract
Diffuse intravascular coagulation
Consumptive coagulopathy

lism, and thrombosis. The symptoms of TAAA are listed in Table 88-2.

The differential diagnosis of TAAA includes perforated viscus, acute cholecystitis, colonic diverticulitis, angina pectoris, acute myocardial infarction, esophagitis with cardiospasm, esophageal perforation, vertebral osteoarthritis, pulmonary embolus, pneumonia, aortic dissection, and urinary tract disease.

Imaging

Both CT and aortography are needed for evaluation of most TAAAs. CT provides the best information about the size and extent of the aneurysm. Aortography with selective visceral arteriography outlines the visceral vascular and spinal cord circulation. MRI may be used for noninvasive diagnosis and classification of TAAAs. Transaxial images allow one to determine aneurysm diameter and length, extent of luminal thrombus, and amount of atherosclerotic occlusive disease. Parasagittal MRI can show the proximal and distal limits of the aneurysm.

Management

Whether repair of a TAAA is performed depends on extent of aneurysmal involvement and the patient's condition. Small aneurysms in patients at high risk can be cautiously followed. Large aneurysms in patients at low risk are repaired. The guideline is that repair is performed when the aneurysm diameter is at least twice the diameter of the uninvolved aorta.

The principles of surgical repair are removal of the aneurysm from the circulation and rapid reconstruction of the visceral vessels (the celiac, superior mesenteric, and renal arteries).

Surgical Technique

A posterolateral thoracoabdominal incision is used (Fig. 88-6). Some surgeons use no heparin, shunt, bypass, circulatory arrest, hypothermia, renal cooling, or vessel perfusion technique. Others use a variety of adjuncts to maximize visceral and spinal cord protection.

After the proximal aortic clamp is placed, the aorta is opened posterolaterally throughout the length of the aneurysm (Fig. 88-7). Laminated clot and intra-aneurysmal debris are removed. After the ostia of the visceral vessels are identified, balloon occlusion catheters are placed into these branches and gently inflated to control back-bleeding. Back-bleeding from the distal aorta is controlled with gentle external pressure, a clamp, or placement of intraluminal balloons in the distal aorta or iliac arteries.

An end-to-end anastomosis is made between the graft and the *proximal* end of the aorta. Identifiable intercostal vessels are reimplanted into elliptical holes in the graft. The graft is clamped distal to the reimplanted intercostal vessels and the aortic clamp is slowly removed. Additional elliptical holes are cut in the prosthesis to accommodate the visceral vessels. The celiac, superior mesenteric, and right renal arteries usually can be reimplanted as a single button containing all three ostia. Sometimes the left renal artery can be reimplanted with the other visceral vessels, but usually it is reimplanted separately.

After visceral vessel reconstruction, the proximal clamp is temporarily released to flush out debris. A second clamp is placed beneath the reconstructed visceral vessels, and the proximal occluding clamp is slowly released to test the integrity of the anastomoses. The occlusion balloon catheters are deflated and removed one by one, restoring

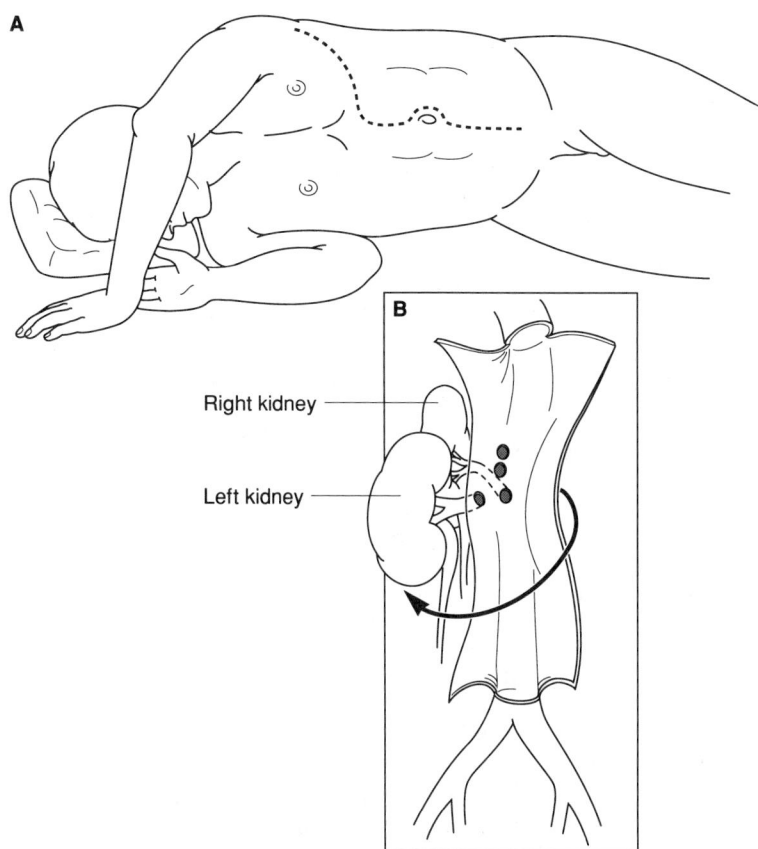

Figure 88-6. Incision and operative approach for a thoracoabdominal aortic aneurysm. (*A*) The patient lies in the right lateral semidecubitus position. The chest incision is made anywhere from the sixth the the ninth interspace, depending on the type of aneurysm. The retroperitoneal structures and left kidney are mobilized to the right. (*B*) Open aneurysm with ostia of the visceral vessels seen. (After Ernst CB, Reddy DJ. Thoracoabdominal aortic aneurysm. In: Haimovici H, Callow AD, DePalma RE, et al, eds. Vascular surgery: principles and practice, ed 3. Norwalk, CT, Appleton & Lange, 1989:618)

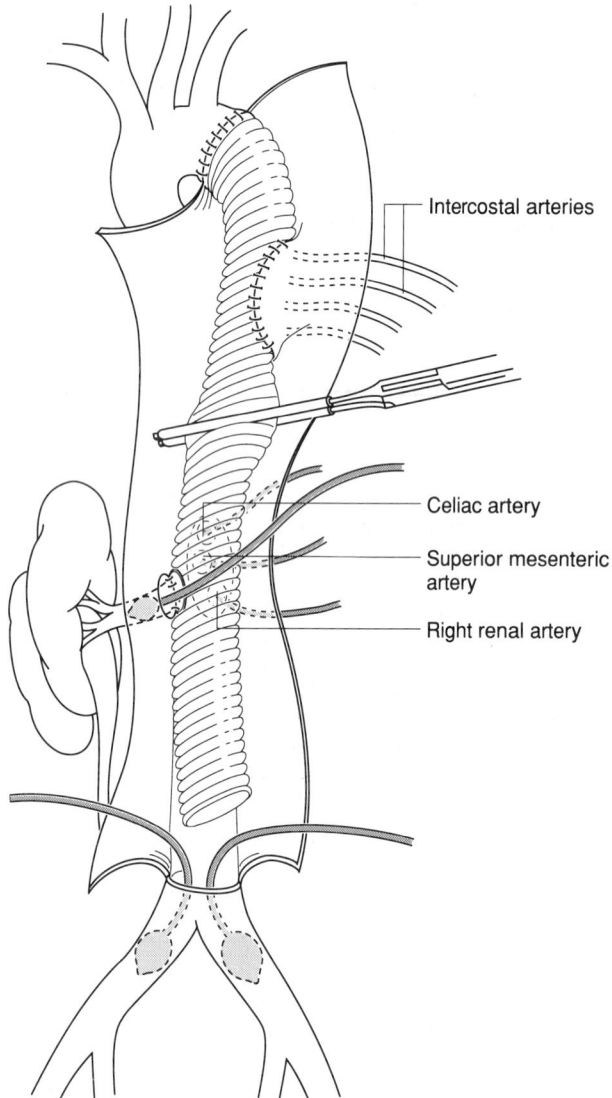

Figure 88-7. Various operative maneuvers used in the repair of thoracoabdominal aortic aneurysms. Intercostal arteries are implanted into the Dacron graft and reperfused before completion of the renal and gut anastomoses. The graft is clamped distal to the intercostal repairs, and the celiac, superior mesenteric, and right renal arteries are implanted as a single unit into the graft. The left renal artery reconstruction follows separately. The kidneys and intestine are reperfused before the distal aortic anastomosis is begun. Balloon occlusion catheters minimize back bleeding during the anastomosis. (After Ernst CB, Reddy DJ. Thoracoabdominal aortic aneurysm. In: Haimovici H, Callow AD, DePalma RE, et al, eds. Vascular surgery: principles and practice, ed 3. Norwalk, CT, Appleton & Lange, 1989:619)

blood flow to the visceral vessels. Flow to visceral vessels is confirmed.

Depending on the extent of aneurysmal involvement, the *distal* anastomosis is constructed end-to-end to the aorta immediately proximal to the bifurcation. If disease extends into the iliac vessels, a separate bifurcated graft is anastomosed to the aortic graft, and the distal anastomoses are made to the common iliac or to the common femoral arteries.

Complications

Complications after TAAA repair include postoperative bleeding, respiratory insufficiency, renal failure, and spinal cord ischemia with paraparesis or paraplegia.

ABDOMINAL AORTIC ANEURYSMS

Aneurysms of the abdominal aorta are the most common arterial aneurysms encountered in clinical practice. Most abdominal aortic aneurysms (AAAs) are discovered in patients without symptoms during evaluation of an unrelated problem. Although aneurysms can cause symptoms and serious consequences because of thrombosis or distal embolism, rupture is the most serious risk. The larger the aneurysm, the greater is the risk for rupture. It is impossible, however, to predict when even a small aneurysm will rupture. Other aneurysms can coexist, including common or internal iliac aneurysms and femoropopliteal aneurysms.

Classification

A classification of AAAs is provided in Fig. 88-8 and Table 88-3. The importance of classification lies in the implications for surgical management. Infrarenal aneurysms require only infrarenal aortic cross-clamping and infrarenal repair, whereas juxtarenal aneurysms require suprarenal clamping, but the proximal aortic anastomosis is at or just below the renal arteries. Pararenal aneurysms require suprarenal clamping and construction of the proximal aortic anastomosis necessitates attention to maintenance of the patency of the renal arteries.

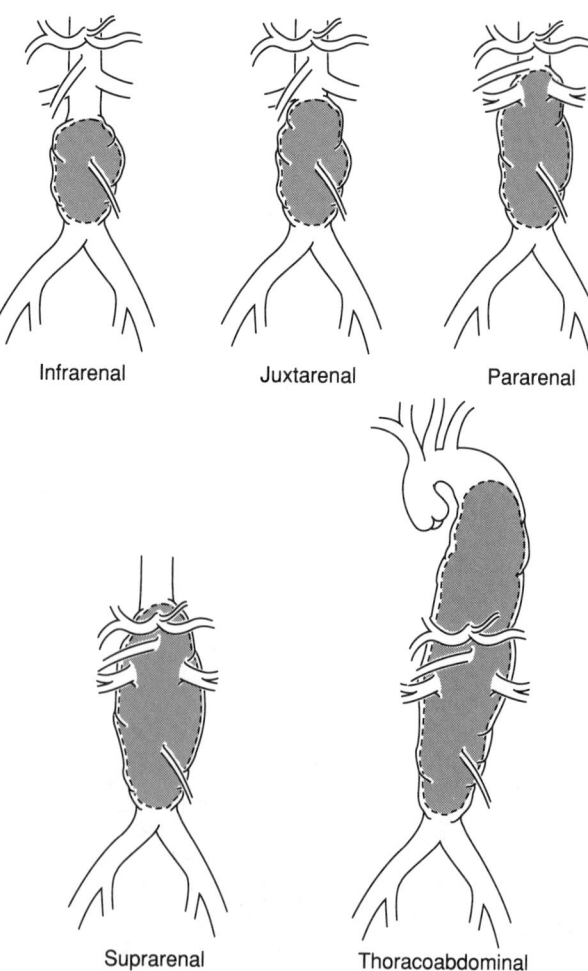

Figure 88-8. Classification of abdominal aortic aneurysms.

Table 88-3. CLASSIFICATION OF ABDOMINAL AORTIC ANEURYSMS

Type	Extent of Involvement
Infrarenal	Below origin of renal arteries, almost always fusiform
Juxtarenal	No normal segment of infrarenal aorta and renal arteries not involved
Pararenal	Cephalad extension to involve the renal artery origin but not the superior mesenteric artery, a type of suprarenal aortic aneurysm

Diagnosis

Symptoms

Most infrarenal AAAs are not symptomatic when diagnosed. They are discovered during a routine physical examination or during an imaging study performed for another reason (upper GI series, barium enema, IV pyelogram, lumbosacral spine radiographs, or abdominal CT or US examination). Some aneurysms are detected during an unrelated abdominal operation or by a patient who notices prominent abdominal pulsation.

When symptoms are associated with AAA, they may be due to rupture or expansion, pressure on adjacent structures, distal embolism, thrombosis, or dissection.

The clinical manifestations of ruptured aortic aneurysm are severe, mild, or diffuse abdominal pain, shock, and a pulsatile abdominal mass. The pain may be more prominent in the back or flank or may radiate to the groin or thigh. The severity of the shock varies from mild to profound, depending on the amount and rapidity of blood loss, and may last for a few minutes or >24 hours. The pain of an expanding, but intact, aneurysm may closely mimic that of a ruptured aneurysm. The pain is severe, constant, and unaffected by position. Hypotension and shock do not usually occur in the absence of rupture.

The diverse and nonspecific nature of the pain caused by expanding and leaking aneurysms often leads to errors and delays in diagnosis. Catastrophic rupture in the midst of a diagnostic procedure is a well-known occurrence. A patient with a contained rupture may arrive in the emergency department describing angina pectoris, a result of blood loss and reflex tachycardia, and be rapidly transferred to a coronary care unit without the abdominal examination that would identify the true cause of the chest pain. Most diagnostic errors are due to failure to palpate the expanding and pulsatile epigastric aneurysmal mass.

The abrupt onset of severe pain in the back, flank, or abdomen is characteristic of aneurysmal rupture or acute expansion. The nature and duration of symptoms varies with the type of rupture. Small tears of the aneurysm wall may result in a small leak that seals temporarily with minimal blood loss. This is usually followed within a few hours by frank rupture, which usually produces a medical emergency, although chronic, contained ruptures also can occur. Rupture most often occurs in the posterolateral aortic wall into the retroperitoneal space and, less commonly, into the free peritoneal cavity. Large aneurysms can erode the spine and cause severe back pain in the absence of rupture. Compression of adjacent intestine can cause early satiety and even nausea and vomiting.

Physical Examination

Physical examination alone establishes the correct diagnosis of AAA 5 cm in diameter in most instances, but determination of aneurysmal size by means of palpation is imprecise. Obesity, ascites, and lack of patient cooperation impair detection of an aneurysm at physical examination. Tumors or cystic lesions adjacent to the aorta, unusual aortic tortuosity, and excessive lumbar lordosis can lead to an erroneous diagnosis of an aneurysm. The expansile nature of a pulsatile mass is the key element in deciding whether a palpable abdominal mass is an aneurysm.

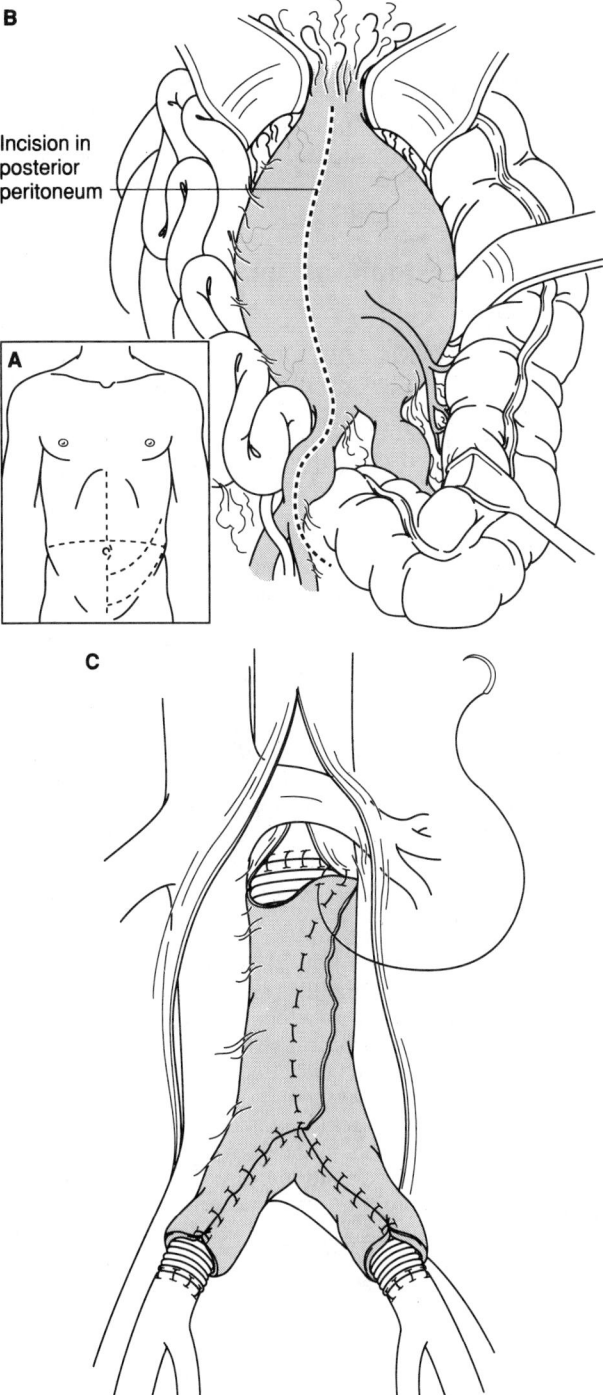

Figure 88-9. Operative repair of abdominal aortic aneurysm. (*A*) Suitable incisions. (*B*) Dissected aneurysm showing line of incision into aneurysm sac. (*C*) Closure of aneurysm wall over prosthetic graft.

Imaging

The oldest objective method of identifying an aneurysm is to obtain plain abdominal and lateral spinal radiographs. In many instances enough calcium is visible in the aortic wall to allow diagnosis of an aneurysm.

Aortic aneurysms also can be visualized with US, CT, and MRI. US is used to establish the diagnosis and to determine the size of abdominal and peripheral aneurysms. US is useful in differentiating a tortuous aorta from an aneurysm, but it is not reliable in defining the relation between AAA and the renal arteries. CT provides reliable information about the size of the entire aorta, including the thoracic aorta, so the size and extent of an aneurysm can be measured. MRI and MR angiography (MRA) are used to differentiate arteries and veins from viscera and other surrounding tissue.

Aortography is used to define the extent of aneurysm formation, especially suprarenal and iliac involvement, and to delineate associated aneurysmal and stenotic lesions involving renal and visceral arteries.

Repair of Abdominal Aortic Aneurysm

Indications

The primary objective of surgical treatment of AAA is to prevent the mortality and morbidity associated with rupture.

Emergency operation is performed on almost all patients with known or suspected rupture, regardless of the size of the aneurysm or the patient's age. An urgent or emergency operation also is indicated for most symptomatic aneurysms.

Elective aneurysm repair is used to treat patients without symptoms with aneurysms >5 cm in diameter who are at acceptable surgical risk and who have an estimated life expectancy >2 years. Elective operation may be prudent for aneurysms <5 cm diameter in patients at good risk. Aneurysms 4 to 5 cm in diameter that show enlargement on serial imaging studies also are repaired.

Patients at high risk (eg, the elderly and those with nonreconstructible coronary disease) with small aneurysms undergo observation until the aneurysm becomes symptomatic or large. Patients at high risk with large aneurysms undergo a thorough evaluation of the condition that puts them at high risk.

Surgical Technique

The choice of incision (Fig. 88-9) is based on extent of the aneurysm, status of the iliac arteries, degree of obesity and pulmonary disease, previous abdominal operations, need to inspect intraperitoneal structures, and speed with which the aorta must be controlled. The aorta is exposed in the retroperitoneum to the left of the midline.

Regardless of the infrarenal extent of an aortic aneurysm, graft replacement begins just below the renal arteries to prevent recurrent aortic abnormalities. If the aorta is especially weak or friable, the sutures can be supported with prosthetic felt pledgets. The degree of disease in the iliac arteries determines the distal extent of the graft. Most patients are treated with a straight tube (aortoaortic) graft.

If the iliac arteries are involved with extensive aneurysmal or occlusive disease, the distal anastomosis can be at the level of the distal common iliac or even the femoral arteries.

For *ruptured aneurysms*, the priority is to gain proximal control of the aorta. If the rupture is contained, proximal aortic control is achieved at the level of the supraceliac aorta through the lesser omentum. The hematoma can be entered and the clamp repositioned distally after the aortic neck is identified. Caution must be exercised to avoid injury to major veins.

With free intraperitoneal rupture, the aorta can be quickly compressed at the diaphragm without formal dissection of this area. An infrarenal aortic clamp or an intraluminal aortic balloon occluding catheter can be substituted as soon as possible. After bleeding is controlled, blood and volume are replenished before attempts are made to restore flow to the lower extremities. Heparin is avoided for ruptured aneurysms, since bleeding and coagulopathy often are associated with massive blood loss and replacement.

Complications of Aortic Aneurysm Repair

The most frequent cause of death is myocardial dysfunction, which is usually ischemic in origin. Nonfatal MI also is common. Other complications are hemorrhage, declamping hypotension, renal failure, injury to the intestine or ureters, GI complications of which ischemia of the left colon and rectum is the most severe, paraplegia, ischemia of the lower extremities, microembolism, and infection of the prosthetic graft.

SUGGESTED READING

Cambria RP, Brewster DC, Abbott WM, et al. Transperitoneal versus retroperitoneal approach for aortic reconstruction: a randomized, prospective study. J Vasc Surg 1990;11:314.

Cartier R, Orszulak TA, Pairolero PC, et al. Circulatory support during crossclamping of the descending thoracic aorta. J Thorac Cardiovasc Surg 1990;99:1038.

Chang BB, Shan DJ, Paty PS, et al. Can the retroperitoneal approach be used for ruptured abdominal aortic aneurysms? J Vasc Surg 1990;11:326.

Coselli JS, Crawford ES, Williams TW, et al. Treatment of postoperative infection of ascending aorta and transverse arch, including use of viable omentum and muscle flaps. Ann Thorac Surg 1990;50:868.

Crawford ES, Svensson LG, Hess KR, et al. A prospective randomized study of cerebrospinal fluid drainage to prevent paraplegia after high risk surgery on the thoracoabdominal aorta. J Vasc Surg 1991;13:36.

Cronenwett JL, Sargent SK, Wall, et al. Variables that effect the expansion rate and outcome of small abdominal aortic aneurysms. J Vasc Surg 1990;11:260.

Golden MA, Whittemore AD, Donaldson MC, et al. Selective evaluation and management of coronary artery disease in patients undergoing repair of abdominal aortic aneurysms: a sixteen-year experience. Ann Surg 1990;212:415.

Greenhalgh RM, Mannick JA, Powell JT, eds. The cause and management of aneurysms. Philadelphia, WB Saunders, 1990:351.

Safi HJ, Bartoli S, Hess KR, et al. Neurologic deficit in patients at high risk with thoracoabdominal aortic aneurysms: the role of cerebral spinal fluid drainage and distal aortic perfusion. J Vasc Surg 1994; 20:434.

ESSENTIALS OF SURGERY: SCIENTIFIC PRINCIPLES AND PRACTICE,
edited by Lazar J. Greenfield, Michael W. Mulholland, Keith T. Oldham, Gerald B. Zelenock,
and Keith D. Lillemoe. Lippincott–Raven Publishers, Philadelphia, © 1997.

CHAPTER 89

SPLANCHNIC ARTERY ANEURYSMS

JAMES C. STANLEY

Splanchnic artery aneurysms are uncommon, but the frequent use of arteriography, computed tomography (CT), and ultrasonography (US) has led to increasing recognition of these lesions. Most splanchnic aneurysms are incidental findings at arteriography, CT, US, or magnetic resonance imaging (MRI) for nonvascular disorders. A large number present surgical emergencies, often resulting in death. Arteriosclerosis appears to be a secondary event rather than an etiologic factor in most of these aneurysms. The location, frequency, likelihood of rupture, and treatment of splanchnic artery aneurysms are summarized in Table 89-1. The radiologic appearance is shown in Figures 89-1 through 89-5.

The following factors contribute to the development of *splenic artery aneurysms:*

- Medial fibrodysplasia
- Multiple pregnancies
- Portal hypertension and splenomegaly

Pregnancy is an important risk factor for rupture of a splenic artery aneurysm. Almost all aneurysms recognized during pregnancy rupture, usually leading to death. Pregnancy-related rupture occurs most often during the third trimester.

Causes of *hepatic artery aneurysms* include:

- Medial degeneration
- Trauma and infection
- Arterial injury during invasive percutaneous diagnostic and therapeutic procedures that involve penetration of the liver
- Systemic arteriopathy, such as periarteritis nodosa

Few hepatic artery aneurysms are symptomatic. When they become symptomatic, most present with right upper quadrant or epigastric pain. Rapid expansion of these aneurysms may cause severe discomfort similar to that of acute pancreatitis. Large aneurysms cause obstructive jaundice, although most hepatic artery aneurysms are too small to compress the major bile ducts. These lesions rarely present as pulsatile abdominal masses.

Infection from a cardiac source is the most common cause of *aneurysms of the proximal superior mesenteric artery* (SMA). Nonhemolytic streptococci and many common pathogens that accompany parenteral substance abuse cause bacterial endocarditis and are the underlying source of infection. Many of these aneurysms are associated with intramural dissection. SMA aneurysms also may be caused by medial degeneration, periarterial inflammation, and trauma. Although many SMA aneurysms are asymptomatic, a large number cause abdominal discomfort, often suggestive of intestinal angina.

Most *celiac artery aneurysms* are associated with medial degeneration. Most celiac artery aneurysms are asymptomatic or associated with vague abdominal discomfort.

Gastric and gastroepiploic artery aneurysms occur as a result of periarterial inflammation or medial degeneration. Often there is a history of peptic ulcer disease. Most of these aneurysms are symptomatic when recognized, frequently presenting emergencies.

Aneurysms of the jejunal, ileal, and colic arteries usually are caused by acquired medial defects. A large number of mycotic aneurysms affect these vessels, developing as the sequela of infected emboli that originate from subacute bacterial endocarditis. Periarteritis nodosa is a common underlying cause of multiple aneurysms that affect these intestinal branch arteries.

Pancreatic and pancreatoduodenal artery aneurysms are associated with pancreatitis-related vascular necrosis or vessel erosion by an adjacent pancreatic pseudocyst. Medial degeneration and trauma are less common causes. These peripancreatic aneurysms often are difficult to diagnose and manage. Most are associated with epigastric pain and discomfort, which may be due to underlying pancreatic inflammatory disease.

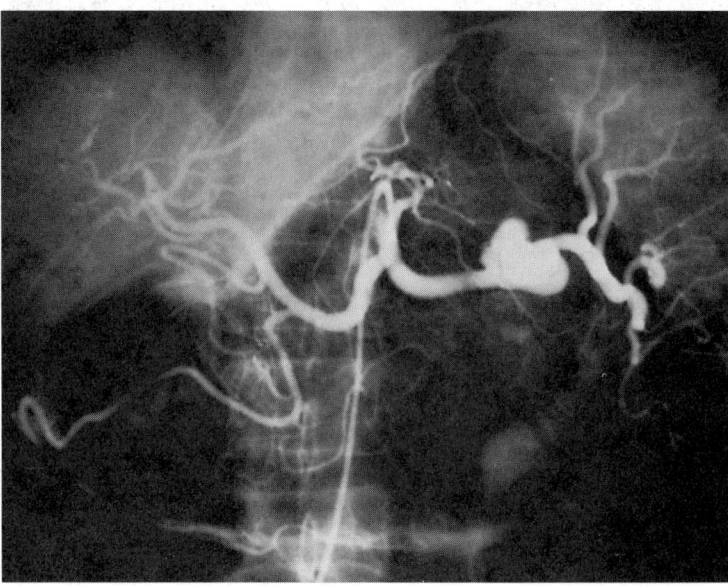

Figure 89-1. Splenic artery aneurysm. Arteriogram documents a pancreatitis-related aneurysm affecting the mid-splenic artery. (Stanley JC, Frey CF, Miller TA, et al. Major arterial hemorrhage: a complication of pancreatic pseudocysts and chronic pancreatitis. Arch Surg 1976;111:435)

Table 89-1. SPLANCHNIC ARTERY MACROANEURYSMS

Aneurysm Location	Frequency Within Splanchnic Circulation	Male/ Female Ratio	Frequency of Reported Rupture	Mortality Rate With Rupture	Treatment
Splenic artery	60%	1:4	2% (bland aneurysms)	25% (bland aneurysms); during pregnancy— 70% maternal and 75% fetal	Splenectomy; aneurysm exclusion or excision without splenectomy
Hepatic artery	20%	2:1	20%	35%	Aneurysmectomy with and without hepatic artery reconstruction; hepatic territory resection; transcatheter aneurysm obliteration
Superior mesenteric artery	5.5%	1:1	Uncommon (thrombosis more common)	50%	Aneurysmectomy with superior mesenteric artery reconstruction; ligation if collateral circulation is adequate
Celiac artery	4%	1:1	13%	50%	Aneurysmectomy with celiac artery reconstruction; ligation if circulation is adequate
Gastric and gastroepiploic arteries	4%	3:1	90%	70%	Aneurysm excision with involved gastric tissue; ligation if extramural
Pancreaticoduodenal, pancreatic, and gastroduodenal arteries	3.5%	4:1	75% Inflammatory 50% Noninflammatory	50%	Aneurysm excision with false aneurysms (pseudocyst-related); pancreatic resection; ligation if extrapancreatic
Jejunal, ileal, and colic arteries	3%	1:1	30%	20%	Aneurysm excision with involved intestine; ligation if extramural

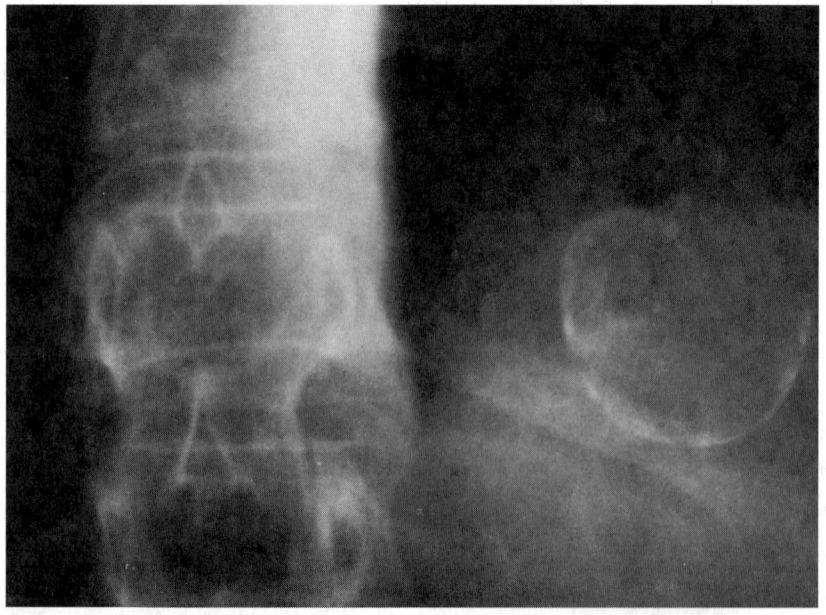

Figure 89-2. Splenic artery aneurysm. Curvilinear signet ring-like calcification in the left upper quandrant characteristic of a splenic artery aneurysms. (Stanley JC, Thompson NW, Fry WJ. Splanchnic artery aneurysms. Arch Surg 1970;101:689)

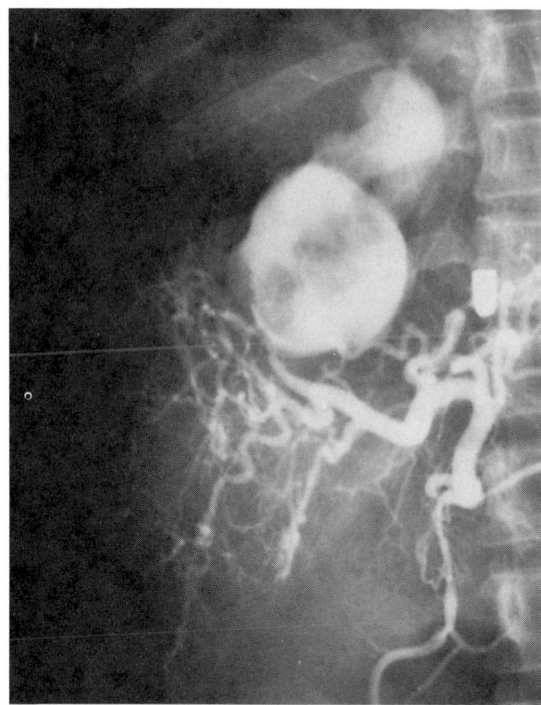

Figure 89-3. Traumatic hepatic artery aneurysm. Blunt abdominal injury and gunshot wounds cause most traumatic lesions. (Whitehouse WM Jr, Graham LM, Stanley JC. Aneurysms of the celiac, hepatic, and splenic arteries. In: Bergan JJ, Yao JST, eds. Aneurysms: diagnosis and treatment. New York, Grune & Stratton, 1981:405)

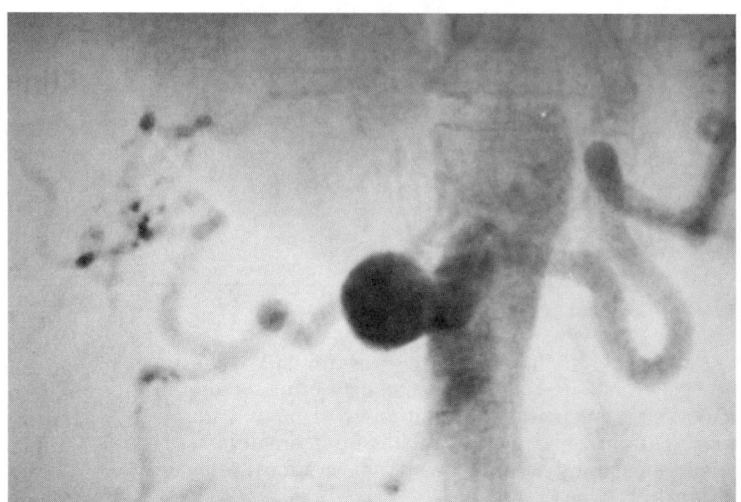

Figure 89-4. Celiac artery aneurysm. Aortogram reveals saccular aneurysm that exhibited medial degenerative changes and secondary arteriosclerosis. (Stanley JC, Whitehouse WM Jr. Aneurysms of the splanchnic and renal arteries. In: Bergan JJ, Yao JST, eds. Surgery of the aorta and its body branches. Orlando, Grune & Stratton, 1979:497)

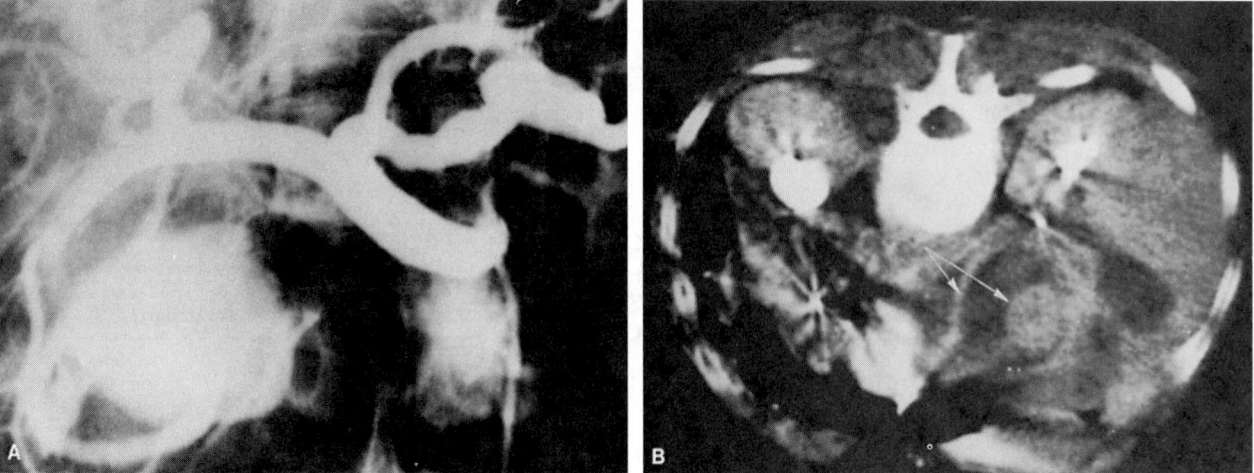

Figure 89-5. Gastroduodenal artery aneurysm. (*A*) Selective celiac arteriogram. (*B*) CT scan of a pancreatic pseudocyst (*short arrow*) containing the aneurysm (*long arrow*). (Eckhauser FE, Stanley JC, Zelenock GB, et al. Gastroduodenal and pancreaticoduodenal artery aneurysms: a complication of pancreatitis causing spontaneous gastrointestinal hemorrhage. Surgery 1980;88:335)

SUGGESTED READING

Chiou AC, Josephs LG, Menzoian JO. Inferior pancreaticoduodenal artery aneurysm: report of a case and review of the literature. J Vasc Surg 1993;17:784.

Hashizume M, Ohta M, Veno K, et al. Laparoscopic ligation of splenic artery aneurysm. Surgery 1993;113:352.

Iyomasa S, Matsuzaki Y, Hiei K, et al. Pancreaticoduodenal artery aneurysm: a case report and review of the literature. J Vasc Surg 1995;22:161.

Okazaki M, Higashihara H, Ono H, et al. Percutaneous embolization of ruptured splanchnic artery pseudoaneurysms. Acta Radiologica 1991;32:349.

Salam TA, Lumsden AB, Martin LG, et al. Nonoperative management of visceral aneurysms and pseudoaneurysms. Am J Surg 1992;164:215.

Stanley JC, Zelenock GB. Splanchnic artery aneurysms. In: Rutherford RB, ed. Vascular surgery, ed 3. Philadelphia, WB Saunders, 1995:1124.

Stauffer JT, Weinman MD, Bynum TE. Hemobilia in a patient with multiple hepatic artery aneurysms: a case report and review of the literature. Am J Gastroenterol 1989;84:59.

Wagner WH, Cossman DV, Treiman RL, et al. Hemosuccus pancreaticus from intraductal rupture of a primary splenic artery aneurysm. J Vasc Surg 1994;19:158.

ESSENTIALS OF SURGERY: SCIENTIFIC PRINCIPLES AND PRACTICE, edited by Lazar J. Greenfield, Michael W. Mulholland, Keith T. Oldham, Gerald B. Zelenock, and Keith D. Lillemoe. Lippincott–Raven Publishers, Philadelphia, © 1997.

CHAPTER 90

RENAL ARTERIAL ANEURYSMS

JAMES C. STANLEY

Aneurysms of the renal artery are unusual. The types are: true renal arterial aneurysms, dissecting renal arterial aneurysms, aneurysmal dilatation with medial fibrodysplastic disease, and arteritis-related microaneurysms. True aneurysms and dissecting aneurysms are most relevant to clinical practice (Table 90-1).

TRUE RENAL ARTERIAL ANEURYSMS

True renal arterial aneurysms are usually located at renal arterial bifurcations (Fig. 90-1). Most are saccular. The average diameter of true aneurysms is 1.3 cm. Almost all are extraparenchymal, a large portion of these occurring at first- or second-order branchings of the main renal artery.

There are two histologic categories of true renal arterial aneurysm. The first type appears to be associated with a congenital *elastic tissue defect* or medial degenerative process. The lesions are characterized by: internal elastic lamina fragmentation, excessive accumulation of collagen and other ground substances, a paucity of elastic tissue, and a loss of recognizable medial smooth muscle.

The second type exhibits *arteriosclerosis*. The lesions are characterized by: hemorrhage, calcium deposition, collections of cholesterol, necrotic debris, and a matrix of fibrous tissue.

The atheromatous changes often occur at irregular intervals in these aneurysms. The intervening areas are composed of thin, collagenous acellular fibrous tissue. Severe arteriosclerosis of the adjacent renal artery is uncommon.

Both congenital and acquired factors appear to contribute to the formation of true renal arterial aneurysms. The increase in frequency of aneurysms with age appears to be a sequela of loss of integrity of the elastic tissue at these weakened branchings.

Blood pressure elevations occur in most patients with renal arterial aneurysms and may have a role in aneurysm development. Increased mural tension, especially in the presence of preexisting internal elastic deficiencies at bifurcations, may further compromise the structural integrity of the renal artery.

Clinical Manifestations

The clinical manifestations of intact renal arterial aneurysms are poorly defined. Most aneurysms appear to be asymptomatic. Aneurysmal expansion, compression of nearby structures, and renal infarction from dislodged thrombus may cause flank or abdominal pain. Hematuria and abdominal bruits are attributed to some of these lesions, but in most instances, these findings result from nonaneurysmal disease. Although quite rare, covert rupture of renal arterial aneurysms into an adjacent vein may be associated with hematuria and hypertension.

Embolization of aneurysmal thrombus or thrombotic occlusion of an adjacent artery rarely may result in renal ischemia and renovascular hypertension. Atheromatous plaque ulceration within large aneurysmal sacs may predispose to embolic complications. If the renal segment affected by embolization is totally infarcted, the patient may not have hypertension. If the tissue simply becomes hypoperfused, however, it may be the source of considerable renin and the cause of severe secondary hypertension.

Renal arterial occlusive disease in the vicinity of aneurysms may account for some secondary hypertension. As-

Table 90-1. **TRUE AND DISSECTING RENAL ARTERY ANEURYSMS**

Lesion	Males/Females	Contributing Factors	Rate of Rupture	Mortality With Rupture	Treatment
True aneurysm	1/1.2	Congenital defects Arterial fibrodysplasia Hypertension	3%	10% (during pregnancy— 55% maternal, 85% fetal)	Aneurysmectomy with renal artery reconstruction Aneurysmorrhaphy Nephrectomy for ruptured aneurysms
Dissecting aneurysm	10/1	Blunt trauma Arterial catheterization Arterial fibrodysplasia Arteriosclerosis	Uncommon	Undefined	Renal artery reconstruction

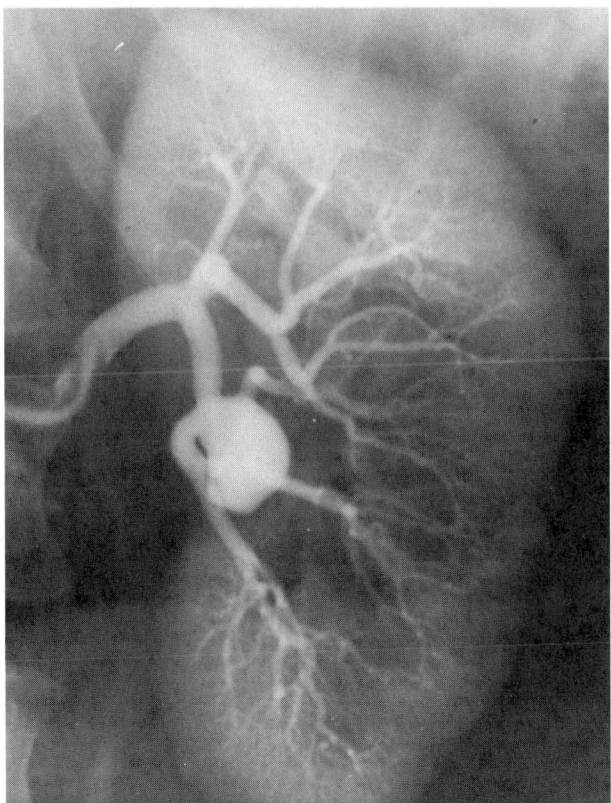

Figure 90-1. Renal artery aneurysm at a second-order branch. (Stanley JC, Whitehouse WM Jr. Renal artery macroaneurysms. In: Bergan JJ, Yao JST, eds. Aneurysms. New York, Grune & Stratton 1982:417)

sessment of renin activity, with determination of renal-systemic renin indices for patients with hypertension and isolated renal arterial aneurysms, may establish the presence of renovascular hypertension.

Rupture is the most serious complication of renal arterial aneurysms. Exsanguinating hemorrhage from a ruptured renal arterial aneurysm is rare. Loss of a kidney is a near universal outcome of rupture. Overt extraparenchymal rupture occurs in some patients with these lesions, and covert rupture causing renal arteriovenous fistulas occurs in others.

Rupture of renal arterial aneurysms during pregnancy is a serious problem. Rupture during pregnancy does not appear to be related to age, increased blood pressure, or number of pregnancies. Rupture of renal arterial aneurysm carries high fetal and maternal mortality rates.

High risk for rupture of a renal arterial aneurysm is attributed to large aneurysm size, absence of calcification, and high blood pressure. These factors are not always relevant, however. Overt rupture often can occur in patients with normal blood pressure, as can calcific atherosclerotic aneurysms. Size is of limited value as an indicator of rupture potential, but large size still is a logical reason to assign greater risk for rupture.

Management

The following are the indications for surgical treatment of true renal arterial aneurysms: symptomatic aneurysmal expansion, aneurysms with coexisting functionally important renal arterial stenosis causing secondary hypertension, aneurysms with thrombus, particularly if distal em-

bolization is evident, aneurysms in women who want to bear children, and aneurysms >1.5 cm in diameter if the patient is otherwise healthy.

The objective of surgical therapy is to eliminate the aneurysm without losing the kidney or compromising its function. Renal arterial reconstruction after aneurysmectomy is complex. Most aneurysms are best approached by way of transabdominal, extraperitoneal exposure of the renal vessels after medial displacement of the overlying colon and foregut viscera.

Large aneurysms of the main renal artery can be excised with simple primary closure of the artery, but excision of smaller aneurysms often necessitates arterial closure with a vein patch. Reconstruction is with autogenous saphenous vein or internal iliac artery as aortorenal grafts for aneurysms at the bifurcation, especially those associated with stenoses.

Aneurysmectomy with reimplantation of the involved vessel or vessels into normal adjacent or proximal renal artery is appropriate for many first- and second-order branch aneurysms (Fig. 90-2). Renal arterial aneurysms 2 to 3 mm in diameter may be plicated by means of closed aneurysmorrhaphy. These small aneurysms often are encountered as incidental lesions in the management of larger aneurysms.

Nephrectomy is the usual therapy for ruptured aneurysms. Arterial reconstruction is performed when the kidney is not irreparably injured from ischemia due to rupture. Partial nephrectomy may be performed when aneurysmal erosion has occurred into adjacent veins, causing a chronic arteriovenous fistula. Acute arteriovenous fistulas can be managed with local excision and arterial reconstruction. Interventional arteriography with transcatheter embolization may be an alternative to subtotal nephrectomy for aneurysms not amenable to conventional aneurysmectomy and vascular reconstruction.

Patients with renal arterial aneurysms not treated surgically undergo long-term follow-up care. Serial ultrasonography (US), computed tomography (CT), and magnetic resonance imaging (MRI) are useful in establishing the stability of an aneurysm. Arteriography can be performed on patients with symptoms of aneurysmal expansion, hematuria, or hypertension. Because of the relatively low incidence of complications attending most renal arterial aneurysms, noninvasive studies performed on a regular basis are favored over repeated arteriographic examinations.

DISSECTING RENAL ARTERIAL ANEURYSMS

Isolated renal arterial dissection causing aneurysms is rare. Dissecting aneurysms are classified into two categories: (1) those due to blunt abdominal trauma or intraluminal catheter-induced injury, and (2) those occurring spontaneously (Fig. 90-3).

Nearly one third of renal arterial dissections are bilateral. Blood viscosity, shear forces, and flow turbulence contribute to the propagation of all dissections, but inadequate structural integrity due to injury or disease initiates the dissection.

Blunt abdominal trauma contributes to renal arterial dissection by two specific mechanisms: (1) violent displacement of the kidney with deceleration causing marked stretching of the artery with fracture of the intima, which is the least elastic vessel wall component. This commonly results in subintimal dissection, and (2) compression of the renal arteries against the vertebrae.

Iatrogenic catheter-related renal arterial injury during arteriography is another cause of dissection. These dissec-

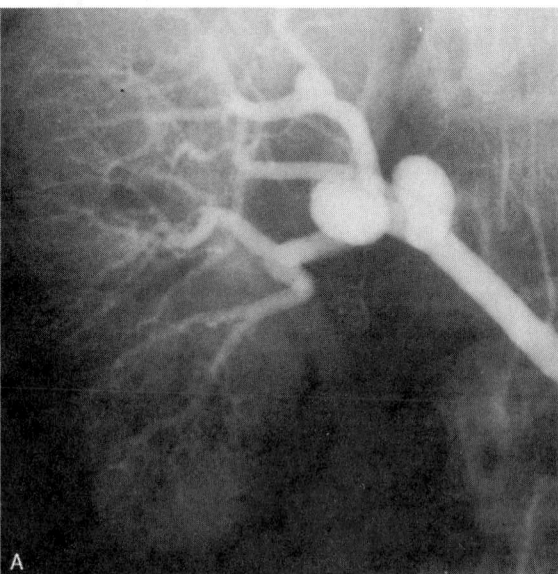 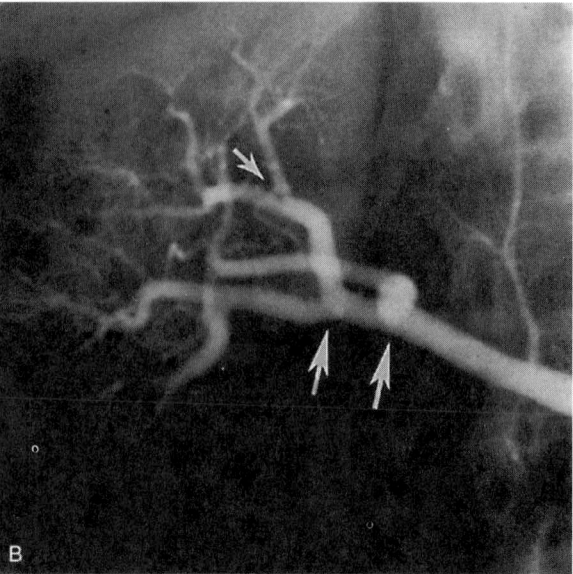

Figure 90-2. Renal artery aneurysms involving multiple segmental artery branchings (*A*). Surgical treatment included aneurysmectomy and end-to-side reimplantation (*large arrows*) of segmental vessels into the adjacent artery and closed aneurysmorrhaphy (*small arrow*) (*B*). (Stanley JC. Renal artery aneurysms and dissections. In: Veith FJ, ed. Current critical problems in vascular surgery, vol 3. St Louis, Quality Medical Publishing, 1991;311)

tions are more likely to affect arteriosclerotic arteries than dysplastic renal arteries and usually occur within the inner media or subintimal tissues. Dissections accompanying therapeutic catheterization during balloon angioplasty are common, although few cause critical narrowing or occlusion of the renal artery.

Primary or spontaneous dissections causing pseudoaneurysms affect the renal arteries more than any other pe-

ripheral artery. Most are related to coexistent arteriosclerotic or dysplastic renovascular disease. Spontaneous dissections usually occur within the outer media adjacent to the external elastic lamina (Fig. 90-4). They occur less commonly within the central media. Often, these dissections are attributed to rupture of abnormal vasa vasorum.

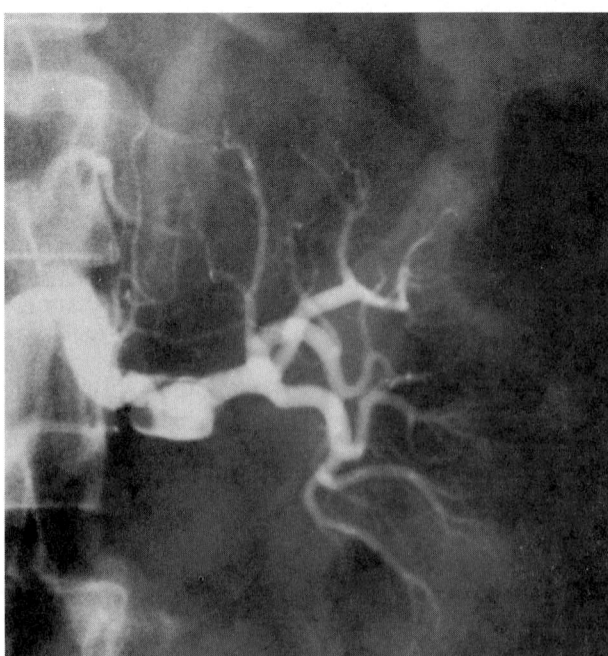

Figure 90-3. Saccular dissecting main renal artery aneurysm. (Gewertz BL, Stanley JC, Fry WJ. Renal artery dissections. Arch Surg 1977;112:409)

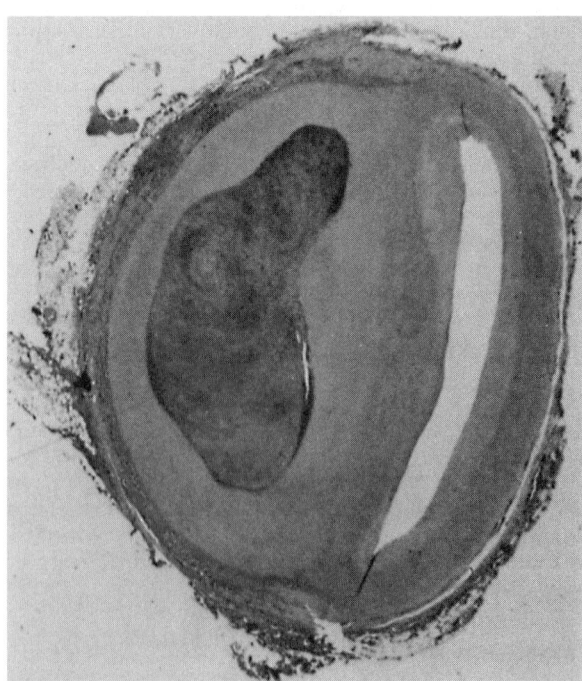

Figure 90-4. Dissection exhibiting deep mural hematoma and compression of adjacent lumen (hematoxylin-eosin, ×60). (Stanley JC. Pathologic basis of macrovascular renal artery disease. In: Stanley JC, Ernst CB, Fry WJ, eds. Renovascular hypertension. WB Saunders, Philadelphia, 1984:46)

It is possible that the dissecting intramural hematoma increases medial ischemia and contributes to further aneurysm formation. Spontaneous renal arterial dissections usually affect proximal vessels and terminate at branchings.

Clinical Manifestations

Clinical manifestations of renal arterial dissection are pain, hematuria, and elevated blood pressure. Chronic renal arterial dissection usually is associated with renovascular hypertension or impaired renal function. Some dissections may be self-limited, asymptomatic, and of no functional importance.

Incorrect initial clinical diagnosis is common. Intravenous pyelography is used to examine patients who may have serious renal hilar injuries, including dissecting aneurysms. Some patients with documented renal arterial injury have falsely normal excretory urograms. Minor perirenal hematomas and cortical contusions can impair excretion of contrast material. Intravenous urography is deferred in favor of early arteriography.

Arteriography is necessary to diagnose and define the extent of renal arterial dissection. Dissection is diagnosed when all of the following are recognized: luminal irregularities with aneurysmal dilatation or saccular dissection associated with segmental stenosis, extension of the dissection to the first renal arterial branching, cuffing at branchings, and variable degrees of reversibility on serial arteriograms.

Management

Trauma-related dissection warrants emergency primary arterial reconstruction, once hemodynamic narrowing or occlusion of the main renal artery or a major segmental branch is recognized. Delayed repair is necessary for less obvious trauma-related injuries if hypertension persists or renal function deteriorates. Spontaneous dissecting aneurysms, when acute, are easier to manage than traumatic lesions. Surgical therapy is begun soon after hemodynamically significant stenoses or occlusions are recognized. Surgical intervention also is used to manage chronic spontaneous dissection associated with severe renovascular hypertension or deteriorating renal function.

Kidney preservation is important for patients with renal arterial dissection. If the patient has sustained blunt abdominal trauma, the other renal artery also may be damaged. Nephrectomy must be avoided. Although many dissections are not amenable to surgical repair, arterial reconstruction in the form of aortorenal bypass with autogenous saphenous vein or hypogastric artery allows kidney salvage.

SUGGESTED READING

Dayton B, Helgerson RB, Sollinger HW, et al. Ruptured renal artery aneurysm in a pregnant uninephric patient: successful ex vivo repair and autotransplantation. Surgery 1990;107:708.

Dzsinich C, Gloviczki P, McKusick MA, et al. Surgical management of renal artery aneurysm. Cardiovasc Surg 1993;3:243.

Reilly LM, Cuningham CG, Maggisano R, et al. The role of arterial reconstruction in spontaneous renal artery dissection. J Vasc Surg 1991;14:468.

Rijbroek A, Dijk AV, Roex AJM. Rupture of renal artery aneurysm during pregnancy. Eur J Vasc Surg 1994;8:375.

Sarkar R, Coran A, Lindenauer SM, et al. Arterial aneurysms in children: a clinicopathologic classification. J Vasc Surg 1991;13:47.

Stanley JC, Messina LM, Wakefield TW, et al. Renal artery recon-

struction. In: Bergan JJ, Yao JST, eds. Techniques in arterial surgery. Philadelphia, WB Saunders, 1990:247.

Stanley JC, Zelenock GB, Messina LM, et al. Pediatric renovascular hypertension: a thirty-year experience of operative treatment. J Vasc Surg 1995;21:212.

ESSENTIALS OF SURGERY: SCIENTIFIC PRINCIPLES AND PRACTICE, edited by Lazar J. Greenfield, Michael W. Mulholland, Keith T. Oldham, Gerald B. Zelenock, and Keith D. Lillemoe. Lippincott–Raven Publishers, Philadelphia, © 1997.

CHAPTER 91

FEMORAL AND POPLITEAL ANEURYSMS

CHARLES L. MESH AND LINDA M. GRAHAM

PERIPHERAL ANEURYSMS

Incidence

Femoral and popliteal artery aneurysms are the most frequent peripheral aneurysms. A large percentage of patients with peripheral aneurysms have concomitant abdominal aortic aneurysms. Men have arteriosclerotic femoral and popliteal artery aneurysms far more frequently than women, in a ratio of about 20:1.

Pathogenesis

Most true femoral and popliteal aneurysms are of arteriosclerotic cause; false aneurysms are related to surgical intervention or trauma. The frequency of peripheral aneurysms is increasing as the average age of the population increases and as iatrogenic and violent arterial trauma become more common.

The cause of arteriosclerotic aneurysms of the femoral and popliteal vessels is not clear. One factor appears to be turbulent flow past a relative stenosis. At the femoral level, this causes poststenotic dilatation beyond the inguinal ligament. At the popliteal level, dilatation occurs distal to the tendinous hiatus of the adductor magnus muscle. Arterial wall fatigue due to vibration and turbulence proximal to a major branching, or to stress and kinking during hip and knee flexion, also can contribute to aneurysm formation. The predilection among men suggests aneurysm formation may be due, in part, to a sex-linked, genetic abnormality. Enhanced collagen synthesis, relative elastin dilution, and disturbed architecture in aneurysms explain the multiplicity of peripheral aneurysms as a reflection of a systemic abnormality in the arterial wall.

Clinical Manifestations

Femoral and popliteal aneurysms are frequently asymptomatic incidental findings during a routine physical examination. When symptomatic, the aneurysms cause lower extremity ischemia due to thrombosis or distal embolization. Local pain may be caused by enlargement. Leg pain and edema can result from compression of the adjacent nerve and vein.

FEMORAL ARTERY ANEURYSMS

Femoral artery aneurysms can jeopardize the viability of the leg if thrombosis, embolization, or rupture occurs. The aneurysms often are associated with limb-threatening popliteal aneurysms and life-threatening abdominal aortic aneurysms. Rare femoral aneurysms develop, secondary to connective tissue disorders.

Arteriosclerotic Aneurysms

A small percentage of patients with abdominal aortic aneurysms have femoral aneurysms, and a large percentage of patients with femoral artery aneurysms have abdominal aortic aneurysms. Multiple aneurysms are common among patients with femoral artery aneurysms.

Femoral aneurysms frequently involve the common femoral artery. They can be classified as follows:

Type I, limited to the common femoral artery
Type II, involving the orifice of the deep femoral (profunda femoris) artery

Isolated lesions of the deep femoral artery are rare, difficult to diagnose when asymptomatic, and, thus, are prone to rupture.

Clinical Manifestations

Most patients with arteriosclerotic femoral artery aneurysms are men in the seventh decade of life. Patients have the usual risk factors for atherosclerosis: cigarette smoking, hypertension, and diabetes mellitus. Cardiovascular disease is common with the clinical manifestations of coronary artery and cerebrovascular disease.

The clinical features of femoral artery aneurysms range from no symptoms to severe ischemia of the lower extremity. Although just under half of patients do not have symptoms at the time of diagnosis, most seek treatment because of local symptoms or symptoms of lower extremity ischemia. Local pain or a groin mass is the only symptom in some patients. Lower extremity venous disease is present in some patients, and in half of these, it is attributable to venous obstruction by the femoral artery aneurysm. A large number of patients have claudication, rest pain, or gangrene.

Femoral artery aneurysms can be complicated by embolism, thrombosis, or rupture. Peripheral microembolization can produce signs as mild as spotty discoloration of the toes, and as severe as peripheral gangrene, or it may be diagnosed unexpectedly at angiography. Although embolism occurs with some femoral aneurysms, the femoral artery may not be the source of the emboli because many patients have a concomitant popliteal aneurysm. Some patients with arteriosclerotic femoral artery aneurysms have acute, and some have chronic thrombosis. Some lesions rupture.

Diagnosis

The diagnosis of femoral aneurysm is suggested by the finding of a pulsatile groin mass at physical examination. Although a radiograph of the region sometimes depicts the calcified rim of an aneurysm, only ultrasonography (US), computed tomography (CT), and magnetic resonance imaging (MRI) are reliable in the diagnosis of femoral artery aneurysms. These modalities are used to define the size of the femoral artery and to exclude the presence of associated aneurysmal disease in the distal aorta and popliteal arteries. The diagnostic accuracy of arteriography is limited because it only outlines the residual lumen and may miss large aneurysms filled with mural thrombus. Arteriography is used to define the anatomy of the femoral region

and distal vasculature for planning surgical therapy (Fig. 91-1).

Treatment

All symptomatic femoral aneurysms are managed surgically. Asymptomatic aneurysms >2.5 cm in diameter are repaired unless the patient is at prohibitive risk for surgical intervention. If management is to be nonsurgical, the size of the aneurysm is documented, and the patient undergoes serial examinations and duplex scanning.

Femoral artery aneurysms usually are approached through a vertical groin incision. Unusually large aneurysms or ruptured aneurysms necessitate proximal control of the external iliac artery through a retroperitoneal approach. After proximal and distal arterial control is obtained, the aneurysmal sac is opened and the atheromatous debris removed. Small aneurysms can be excised, but routine excision of large aneurysms is not recommended. If the superficial femoral artery is chronically occluded and the patient has minimal symptoms, interposition grafting to the deep femoral artery is performed. If recent emboli or in situ thrombosis occlude the outflow tract, catheter thromboembolectomy, thrombolytic therapy, or both are useful.

Femoral artery aneurysms can be associated with concomitant occlusive disease or other aneurysms. Patients with multiple asymptomatic aneurysms undergo staged treatment. Life-threatening aortoiliac aneurysms are managed before limb-threatening femoral and popliteal aneurysms. A femoral aneurysm can be managed during aortofemoral bypass if the distal anastomosis is made beyond the aneurysm or into a femoral interposition graft. For patients with severe lower extremity ischemia, the femoral aneurysm is managed with an interposition graft.

Anastomotic Pseudoaneurysms

Anastomotic aneurysms result from a disrupted suture line between a graft and the host artery. They are a late (>6 years) complication of bypass procedures. Anasto-

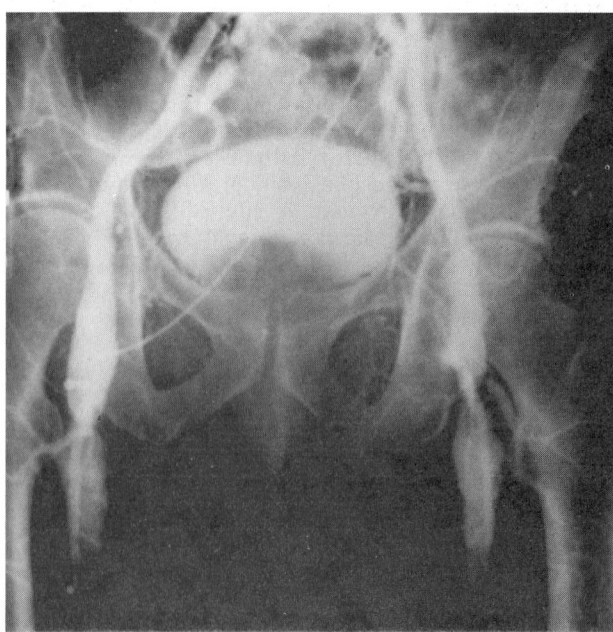

Figure 91-1. Arteriogram demonstrating bilateral femoral artery aneurysms that extend into the superficial femoral arteries. Unlike many patients with femoral artery aneurysms, this patient did not have associated aortic or popliteal aneurysms.

motic aneurysms at the femoral artery account for most of these lesions, and false aneurysms develop in a small number of femoral anastomoses. After aortofemoral bypass, some femoral anastomoses are complicated by pseudoaneurysm. After infrainguinal bypass, aneurysms develop more often in synthetic anastomoses than autogenous venous anastomoses.

Pathogenesis

Factors that contribute to anastomotic aneurysm formation include weakness of the arterial wall, type of graft material, type of suture, presence of infection, method of anastomotic construction, and stress on the suture line from hypertension, leg motion, or excess tension on the graft limb. Progressive atherosclerotic degeneration of the recipient artery also can cause anastomotic aneurysms. False aneurysms are more common with synthetic grafts than with saphenous vein grafts.

Although most anastomotic aneurysms are not accompanied by overt graft infection, occult infection with coagulase-negative *Staphylococcus* organisms may be important in the development of anastomotic aneurysms. Hypertension, joint motion, or excessive tension on the graft limb can stress the suture line and cause anastomotic disruption.

Clinical Manifestations

Femoral anastomotic aneurysms usually present as a pulsatile groin mass sometimes accompanied by pain, redness, or symptoms of venous obstruction. Acute complications of anastomotic aneurysms include hemorrhage, embolism, and occlusion. When false aneurysms accompany graft sepsis, the signs occur early in the postoperative period.

Diagnosis

The diagnosis of a false aneurysm is usually made at physical examination when a pulsatile groin mass is detected in a patient who has undergone a femoral arterial reconstructive procedure. The differential diagnosis includes other nonpulsatile groin masses (hernia, lymphocele, and abscess) through which pulsation from a normal femoral artery is felt. The presence of an anastomotic femoral aneurysm necessitates a search for other anastomotic aneurysms. Some patients have multiple lesions, and the presence of multiple lesions implies infection. Complete evaluation of an anastomotic aneurysm includes US, CT, or MRI of all anastomoses of the involved graft. Angiography is performed before repair of the anastomotic aneurysm to define the proximal and distal arterial anatomy (Fig. 91-2).

Treatment

Because of the progressive nature of anastomotic aneurysms, surgical treatment is undertaken for all lesions except small (<2 cm in diameter), asymptomatic aneurysms in patients at high risk. The principles of surgical treatment include proximal and distal control and replacement of the aneurysmal segment. Securing proximal control may require division of the inguinal ligament to isolate the graft limb. Distal control is obtained with intraluminal balloon occlusion catheters, or the superficial and deep femoral arteries can be controlled with dissection distal to the previous exposure. After débridement of the damaged artery, an interposition graft is placed between the limb of the prosthetic graft and the healthy artery. Cultures of the graft and vessel wall are performed to exclude infection as the cause of the aneurysmal degeneration. If there is obvious infection, graft sepsis is managed by means of removal of all infected prosthetic material.

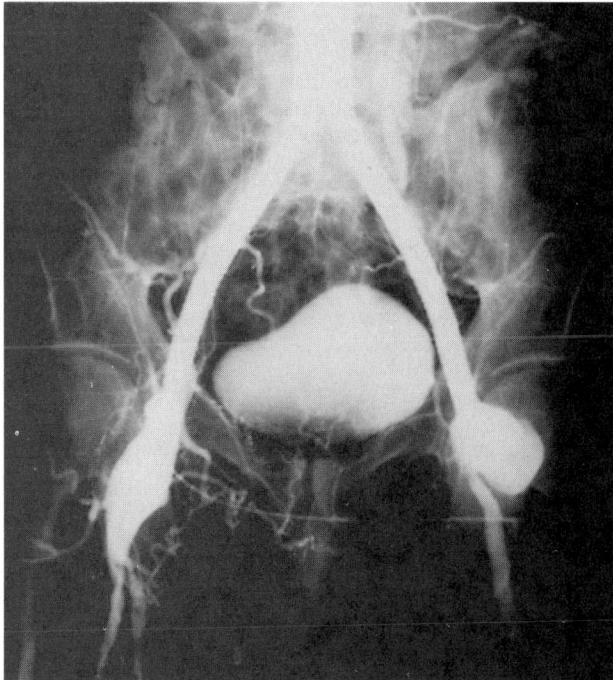

Figure 91-2. Arteriogram demonstrating bilateral femoral anastomotic aneurysms after an aortofemoral bypass and a left femoropopliteal bypass.

Catheter-Induced Pseudoaneurysms

The femoral artery is the preferred site of arterial access for diagnostic angiography and interventional endovascular therapy. Because these techniques require prolonged arterial cannulation, large-bore sheaths, and anticoagulation, arterial complications are expected.

Pathogenesis

Pseudoaneurysms are collections of blood in continuity with the arterial system not enclosed by all three layers of the arterial wall. Under normal circumstances, arterial wall defects produced by catheter insertion are sealed by hemostasis aided by direct application of pressure, and the arterial wall repairs itself. When hemostasis is unsuccessful, blood under arterial pressure leaks from the artery, dissects surrounding tissue planes, and forms a pseudoaneurysm. The lesion is perceived at physical examination as a pulsatile mass. The gross findings at operation are a blood-filled, fibrous capsule in continuity with the arterial lumen and a catheter-sized mural defect. Symptoms are caused by rupture of the lesion or compression of surrounding structures.

Diagnosis

The diagnosis of catheter-induced pseudoaneurysm is suggested when a pulsatile groin mass is found after femoral arterial catheterization. The differential diagnosis includes hematoma, lymphadenopathy, and abscess. CT, MRI, or conventional or color-flow duplex US is used to delineate the lesion.

Natural History

Thrombosis is unlikely in patients taking anticoagulants or those with pseudoaneurysms >1.8 cm in diameter. Thrombi develop spontaneously in groin pseudoaneurysms.

Treatment

Early surgical repair is mandatory for all catheter-induced pseudoaneurysms that are expanding, compressing adjacent nerves, or compromising the skin. For other lesions, if an ultrasonographer skilled in the technique is available, obliteration with US-guided compression can be attempted.

Mycotic Aneurysms

A mycotic aneurysm is any infected aneurysm. Mycotic femoral aneurysms usually are complications of trauma due to parenteral drug abuse or invasive medical procedures.

Pathogenesis

Mycotic aneurysms have one of four causes:

1. Septic emboli from bacterial endocarditis lodge in normal arteries and cause infection that weakens the arterial wall and aneurysm formation
2. During an episode of bacteremia, microorganisms lodge in a preexisting atherosclerotic plaque or aneurysm, multiply, and cause aneurysmal degeneration
3. Bacteria spread from a local abscess, and the inflammatory process destroys the arterial wall and produces a pseudoaneurysm
4. Trauma to the artery with concomitant contamination causes formation of an infected pseudoaneurysm

Staphylococcus, Salmonella, Escherichia coli, and *Proteus* organisms are the most frequent isolates. *Staphylococcus aureus* organisms are recovered from a large percentage of patients with mycotic femoral artery aneurysms due to trauma and drug abuse.

Clinical Manifestations

Patients with mycotic femoral aneurysms have chills, fever, and a tender, enlarging, pulsatile groin mass. Lower extremity edema may be caused by venous obstruction. Some patients have a history of intravenous drug use, recent penetrating trauma, or bacterial endocarditis. Local signs of infection, such as erythema, warmth, and tenderness, are found at physical examination. Evidence of septic embolization may include petechial skin lesions, splinter hemorrhages, cutaneous abscesses, or signs of septic arthritis. A small sentinel bleed may herald impending free rupture and uncontrollable, life-threatening hemorrhage.

Diagnosis

The diagnosis of mycotic femoral aneurysm is straightforward, but differentiation of an abscess adjacent to the femoral artery from a femoral mycotic aneurysm can be difficult. For patients with a pulsatile groin mass, laboratory findings, including leukocytosis, elevated erythrocyte sedimentation rate, and positive blood cultures suggest, but are not specific for, a mycotic aneurysm. US, CT (Fig. 91-3), and MRI are helpful but cannot be used to differentiate infected from uninfected aneurysms. Arteriography may help confirm the presence of an aneurysm, but it is more important in delineating the proximal and distal arterial anatomy for surgical intervention. The diagnosis of mycotic aneurysm can be confirmed only at operation with the demonstration of organisms on Gram stain, or with positive cultures of the wall of the aneurysm.

Treatment

All mycotic femoral aneurysms are treated surgically. They are life- and limb-threatening because they can expand and rupture. The goals of treatment are eradication of infection and restoration of distal circulation.

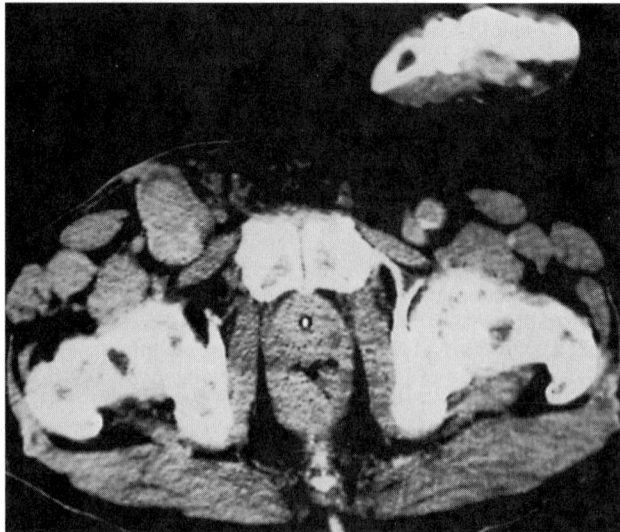

Figure 91-3. CT scan of an infected right femoral anastomotic aneurysm diagnosed 5 years after aortofemoral graft placement.

The complexity of the operation varies with the location and extent of the aneurysm. Retroperitoneal exposure of the distal external iliac artery is preferred for large or proximal femoral lesions. An infected femoral artery aneurysm confined to the common, superficial, or deep femoral artery can be excised with proximal and distal arterial ligation. Amputation is unusual when an isolated arterial segment is ligated without reconstruction.

Infection that involves the femoral artery bifurcation necessitating multiple arterial resections is associated with lower extremity ischemia, followed by gradual improvement as collateral circulation increases. About one third of patients need an amputation if the limb is not urgently revascularized. Patients whose sepsis can be controlled at the initial procedure by means of excision of the aneurysm and aggressive débridement of adjacent tissue, can undergo immediate revascularization with an autogenous saphenous vein graft. The bypass is covered with a sartorius muscle flap.

Patients whose sepsis cannot be locally controlled at the initial arterial resection cannot undergo in situ reconstruction. If limb-threatening ischemia persists for 24 hours after arterial ligation, revascularization through uninfected tissue planes via the lateral femoral or obturator route is undertaken to avoid amputation. Use of prosthetic material is avoided. Antibiotics are begun preoperatively, modified according to sensitivities from intraoperative cultures, and continued for at least 6 weeks.

POPLITEAL ARTERY ANEURYSMS

Popliteal artery aneurysms are the most common arteriosclerotic peripheral aneurysm. Multiple aneurysms often accompany popliteal aneurysms. Extrapopliteal degeneration occurs in more than half of patients, and abdominal aortic and femoral lesions occur in just less than half. A large number of patients have bilateral popliteal aneurysms, and abdominal aortic aneurysms occur in a large number of these patients. Popliteal artery aneurysms are prone to limb-threatening complications.

Clinical Manifestations

Almost all patients with popliteal aneurysmal degeneration are men; most are in the seventh decade of life. Because risk factors for atherosclerosis (smoking, hypertension, diabetes mellitus) are common among these patients, so are other cardiovascular and cerebrovascular diseases.

About half of patients have no symptoms at the time of diagnosis. Symptoms that do occur are those of limb ischemia, such as claudication, rest pain, or gangrene. Blue-toe syndrome is a reliable sign of microembolization. Nonischemic signs and symptoms are a popliteal mass and local pain, leg swelling, or phlebitis due to compression of adjacent nerves or veins.

Natural History

Popliteal artery aneurysms may be complicated by thrombosis, embolism, or rupture. Thrombosis and embolization cause obliteration of the distal tibial blood vessels. One fourth of patients with these complications need an early amputation. Rupture is rare. Hemorrhage usually is confined to the popliteal space and does not preclude arterial reconstruction.

Diagnosis

For most patients with popliteal aneurysms, palpation of the popliteal space with the knee flexed reveals a pulsatile mass. Small aneurysms may not be palpable. If thrombosis has occurred, only a nonpulsatile mass may be felt. Radiographs of the knee that demonstrate mural calcium suggest but do not confirm the diagnosis. Only US, CT, or MRI can be used to exclude the other lesions in the differential diagnosis of a mass in the popliteal fossa (tumor, Baker cyst) and to confirm the presence of a popliteal artery aneurysm.

Once the diagnosis of popliteal artery aneurysm is made, a search for associated, life-threatening aortic and limb-threatening peripheral aneurysms must be undertaken. Because abdominal aortic aneurysms can be missed during physical examination, CT and MRI are performed. Angiographic findings can be misleading because of the presence of intraluminal thrombus. Once repair is planned, however, angiography is essential to define the patency of the distal blood vessels (Fig. 91-4).

Treatment

Early surgical treatment is recommended because of the high incidence of complications. Operation is deferred only when a patient is at inordinately high surgical risk or has a limited life expectancy because of malignant disease.

The goals of surgical treatment are to eliminate the risk for complications and to restore adequate lower extremity blood flow. If there are multiple aneurysms, life-threatening aortic aneurysms are managed first and then limb-threatening popliteal aneurysms are repaired.

Most popliteal artery aneurysms are easily exposed through medial thigh and calf incisions. For lesions confined to the popliteal fossa, the posterior approach is effective. Most aneurysms are left in situ, bypassed, and then ligated. The conduit of choice is reversed saphenous vein harvested from the thigh. The proximal and distal anastomoses may be end to end or end to side. When end-to-side anastomosis is chosen, the aneurysm must be excluded from the circulation by means of proximal and distal ligation. When the distal popliteal and proximal tibial vessels are occluded with recent emboli, they may be cleared with a balloon catheter, intraoperative thrombolytic therapy, or both. Bypass grafts to the distal tibial vessels may be necessary.

If the aneurysm is large and causes local symptoms, the sac is opened, the thrombus evacuated, and the redundant portion of the wall removed. Obliterative endoaneurysmorrhaphy avoids trauma to the popliteal veins. For exten-

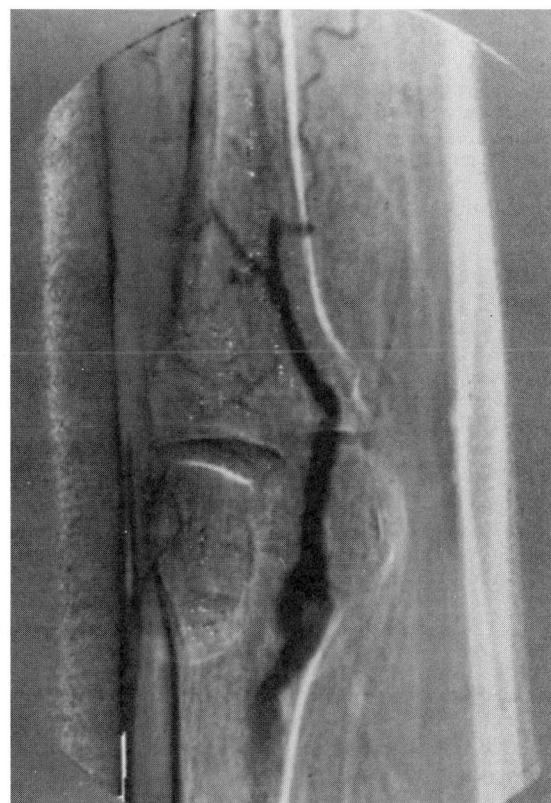

Figure 91-4. Arteriogram demonstrating a popliteal aneurysm associated with occlusion of the outflow tract, presumably from repeated episodes of embolism. A bypass to the distal posterior tibial artery was successful.

sive femoral and popliteal aneurysms, in situ saphenous vein bypass, combined with proximal and distal aneurysmal ligation preserves arterial continuity and avoids the risk for venous and neurologic injury associated with graft tunneling adjacent to large popliteal aneurysms.

Treatment of a patient with an acutely ischemic extremity and a thrombosed popliteal aneurysm is controversial. Recommendations range from thrombolysis in all ischemic extremities with a popliteal artery aneurysm, to thrombolysis only in extremities with thrombosed popliteal artery aneurysms and no runoff. Because thrombolysis may unmask a runoff vessel suitable for distal bypass, it is useful as a diagnostic adjuvant to angiography.

SUGGESTED READING

Baxter BT, Halloran BG. Matrix protein metabolism in abdominal aortic aneurysms. In: Yao JST, Pearce WH, eds. Aneurysms: new findings and treatments. Norwalk CT, Appleton & Lange, 1994:25.

Carpenter JP, Barker CF, Roberts B, Berkowitz HD, Lusk EJ, Perloff LJ. Popliteal artery aneurysms: current management and outcome. J Vasc Surg 1994;19:65.

Cox GS, Young JR, Gray BR, Grubb MW, Hertzer NR. Ultrasound-guided compression repair of postcatheterization pseudoaneurysms: results of treatment in one hundred cases . J Vasc Surg 1994;19:683.

Kent KC, McArdle CR, Kennedy B, Baim DS, Anninos E, Skillman JJ. A prospective study of the clinical outcome of femoral pseudoaneurysms and arteriovenous fistulas induced by arterial puncture. J Vasc Surg 1993;17:125.

Kresowik TF, Khoury MD, Miller BV, et al. A prospective study of the incidence and natural history of femoral vascular complications after percutaneous transluminal coronary angioplasty. J Vasc Surg 1991;13:328.

Lancashire MJR, Torrie EPH, Gallard RB. Popliteal aneurysms identified by intra-arterial streptokinase: a changing pattern of presentation. Br J Surg 1990;77:1388.

Messina LM, Brothers TE, Wakefield TW. Clinical characteristics and surgical management of vascular complications in patients undergoing cardiac catheterization: interventional versus diagnostic procedures. J Vasc Surg 1991;13:593.

Seabrook GR, Schmidtt DD, Bandyk DF, Edmiston CE, Krepel CJ, Towne JB. Anastomotic femoral pseudoaneurysm: an investigation of occult infection as an etiologic factor. J Vasc Surg 1990;11:629.

Shortell CK, DeWeese JA, Ouriel K, Green RM. Popliteal artery aneurysms: a 25-year surgical experience. J Vasc Surg 1991;14:771.

Varga ZA, Locke-Edmunds JC, Baird RN. A multicenter study of popliteal aneurysms. J Vasc Surg 1994;20:171.

ESSENTIALS OF SURGERY: SCIENTIFIC PRINCIPLES AND PRACTICE, edited by Lazar J. Greenfield, Michael W. Mulholland, Keith T. Oldham, Gerald B. Zelenock, and Keith D. Lillemoe. Lippincott–Raven Publishers, Philadelphia, © 1997.

CHAPTER 92

VASCULAR MALFORMATION AND ARTERIOVENOUS FISTULA

S. MARTIN LINDENAUER

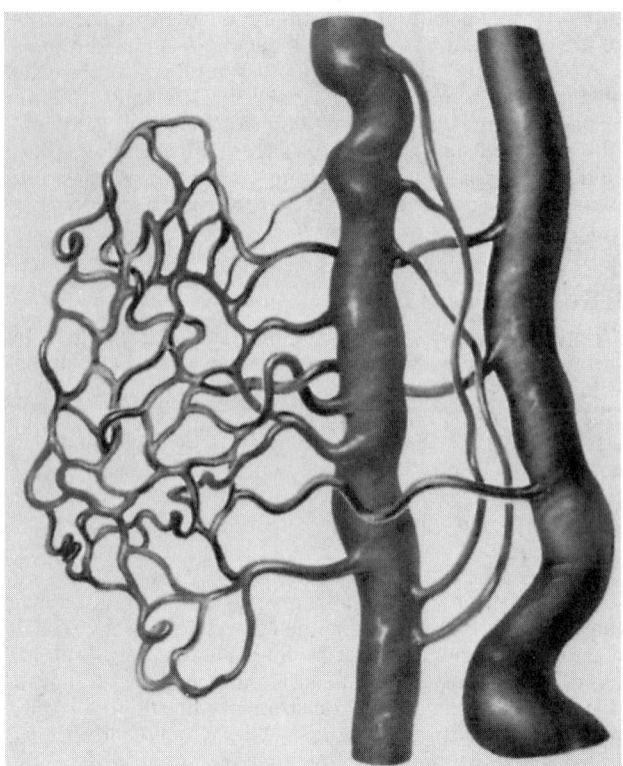

Figure 92-1. Artist's rendition of multiple connections between an artery and vein in a congenital arteriovenous fistula (Malan E, ed. Vascular malformations. Milan, Carlo Erba Foundation, 1974:34)

An *arteriovenous (AV) fistula* is an abnormal connection between an artery and vein that bypasses a capillary bed. *Aquired AV fistula* is almost always caused by penetrating trauma such as a stab or bullet wound or needle, or trocar injury during percutaneous diagnostic and therapeutic cardiac and radiographic procedures. Acquired AV fistula also may be nontraumatic, caused by erosion of an aneurysmal artery into an adjacent vein or by infection or a neoplasm. An acquired AV connection is usually single, but sometimes a second or third communication is present.

Acquired AV fistula usually causes early dilatation of the artery and vein leading to and from the fistula site. The extent of dilatation is related to the size of the fistula, location (central vs peripheral), and duration. A fistula of long duration is associated with degenerative changes in the proximal arterial wall and premature arteriosclerosis and calcification. Despite elimination of the fistula, aneurysmal dilatation and late rupture of the dilated artery proximal to the fistula occur.

A *congenital AV fistula* may not be apparent at birth. It is differentiated from acquired AV fistula by multiple connections that are sometimes too numerous to count (Fig. 92-1). Congenital abnormalities that do not have multiple connections are cardiac atrial and ventricular septal defects, patent ductus arteriosus, and rare peripheral AV malformations with a solitary connection.

AV fistulas sometimes are constructed for *therapeutic* purposes, such as vascular access for hemodialysis, chemotherapy, and long-term parenteral nutrition. AV fistulas also can be established to enhance the patency of a low-flow distal bypass and in venous reconstruction.

HEMODYNAMIC ALTERATIONS

The abnormal hemodynamics of AV fistula cause local, peripheral, and systemic effects, all of which are influenced by the size of the fistulous connection and its location and duration. Central AV fistulas produce heart failure; distal AV fistulas cause ischemia. Congenital AV fistulas produce less dramatic peripheral and systemic manifestations than acquired fistulas.

The predominant feature of AV fistula is a decrease in peripheral vascular resistance produced by bypass of the capillary bed distal to the fistulous connection. The length and diameter of the fistula influence the degree of reduction in peripheral resistance. Peripheral resistance is inversely proportional to the diameter of the connection in an AV fistula. The multiple small connections of a congenital AV fistula usually do not lower peripheral resistance.

Local Hemodynamic Effects

Changes in Volume and Flow

Overall flow through the proximal part of the artery increases, and the reversed flow of normal diastole is absent. Although systolic and diastolic flow increase, a greater increase in diastolic flow markedly reduces pulsatility. Flow in the proximal vein increases and becomes pulsatile, coinciding with arterial systole and diastole. This is usually most evident close to the fistulous connection and becomes less prominent away from the connection.

Flow in the *proximal artery* is toward the fistula; flow in the *proximal vein* is proximal. After several weeks, arterial and venous collateral circulation develops around the fistula. Flow in the *distal artery and vein* may be proximal or distal, depending on the anatomic arrangement, and it can change over time. The direction of venous flow distal to the fistula changes as the venous valves become incompetent.

With a small AV fistula with minimal arterial collateral circulation, flow in the distal artery continues antegrade. With a large chronic AV fistula, the well-developed arterial collaterals that bypass the fistula allow reversal of flow in the distal artery. Sometimes the flow in the artery distal to the AV fistula is stagnant, depending on the balance between peripheral resistance and the degree of arterial collateral development. Retrograde distal arterial flow contributes to the peripheral ischemia that occurs with AV fistula.

Pressure Changes

Arterial pressure may be normal in the proximal artery. When the fistulous connection is large and associated with increased volume flow and decreased peripheral resistance, arterial pressure may be lower than normal. As the proximal artery dilates, pressure increases and can become greater than in a normal artery at a comparable location.

The pressure in the distal artery of an AV fistula is reduced in association with retrograde arterial flow. The decreased distal pressure is offset by the collateral vessels that develop. Increased collateral flow decreases arterial outflow resistance and increases flow reversal in the distal artery (Fig. 92-2).

Because of the nature of venous capacitance, pressure in the vein proximal to an AV fistula rises minimally despite the large increase in volume flow. The pressure in the distal vein rises acutely when the venous valves are competent. Over time, distal venous resistance decreases because of dilatation and venous valve incompetence. The

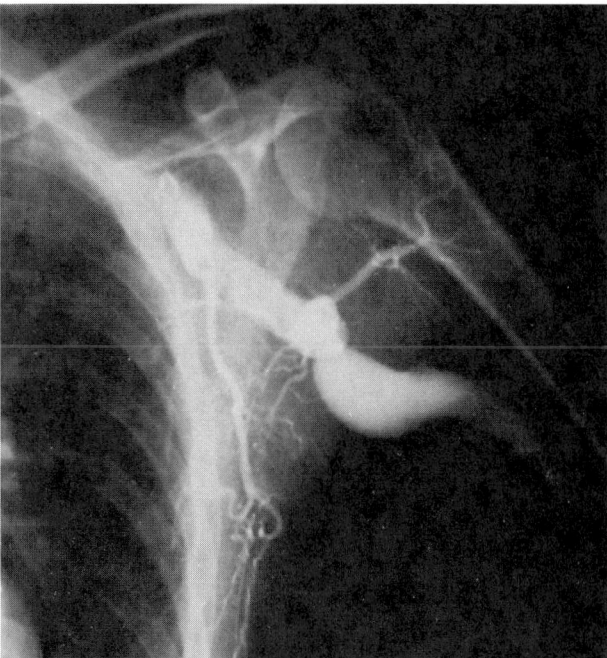

Figure 92-3. Radiograph of an axillary artery aneurysm proximal to a brachial arteriovenous fistula of 21 years' duration. (Lindenauer SM, Thompson NW, Kraft RO, Fry WJ. Late complications of traumatic arteriovenous fistulas. Surg Gynecol Obstet 1969;192:526)

varicosities that result may be the feature that brings the abnormality to clinical attention.

Turbulence

A unique characteristic of AV fistula is the thrill and bruit produced by the turbulent flow and resultant wall vibration in this unusual hemodynamic environment. It is similar but usually more marked than the turbulence in the area of bifurcations, aneurysms, and abrupt changes in lumen diameter.

Dilatation

In clinically apparent AV fistulas, the characteristic change in the proximal artery and draining vein is dilatation. Over time, this leads to structural changes in the arterial wall. Sometimes the structural damage can result in aneurysm formation, which occurs even after the fistula is disconnected (Fig. 92-3). Dilated proximal vein becomes elongated, tortuous, and thickened (Fig. 92-4). It is in this setting that venous aneurysm occurs (Fig. 92-5).

Infection

Venous wall exposed to the forceful jet of arterial blood at the fistula site is damaged and can be the locus of bacterial endarteritis.

Valvular Incompetence

Dilatation of the distal vein can be progressive, and the valves in the deep system and perforating and superficial venous valves become incompetent. A serious consequence is development of venous varicosities, chronic venous valvular insufficiency, and chronic venous ulceration. When distal arterial insufficiency is associated with an uncorrected AV fistula, the ulcer can have arterial and venous components. Correction of the fistula can eliminate the arterial component, but the chronic venous changes usually are not reversible.

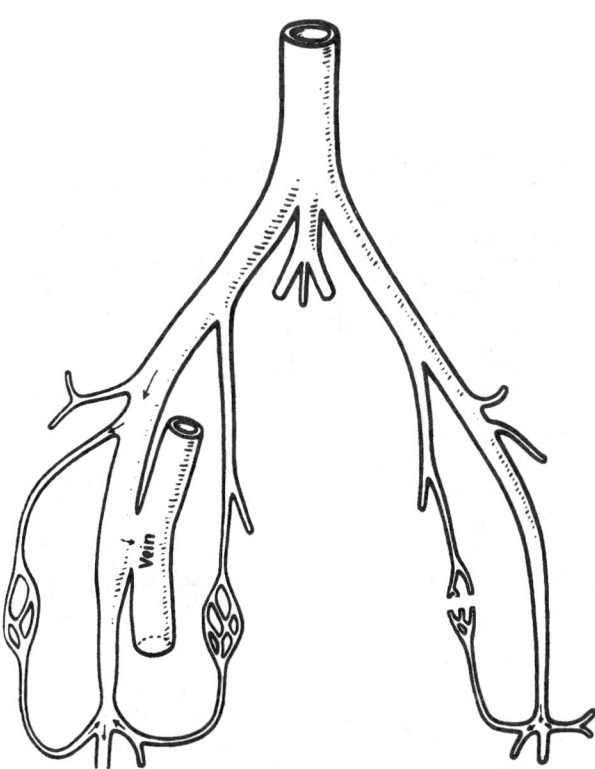

Figure 92-2. Illustration of collateral formation around a femoral arteriovenous fistula that is contributing to flow reversal in the arterial segment distal to the fistula. (Holman E. Abnormal arteriovenous connections. Springfield, IL, Charles C Thomas, 1968:62)

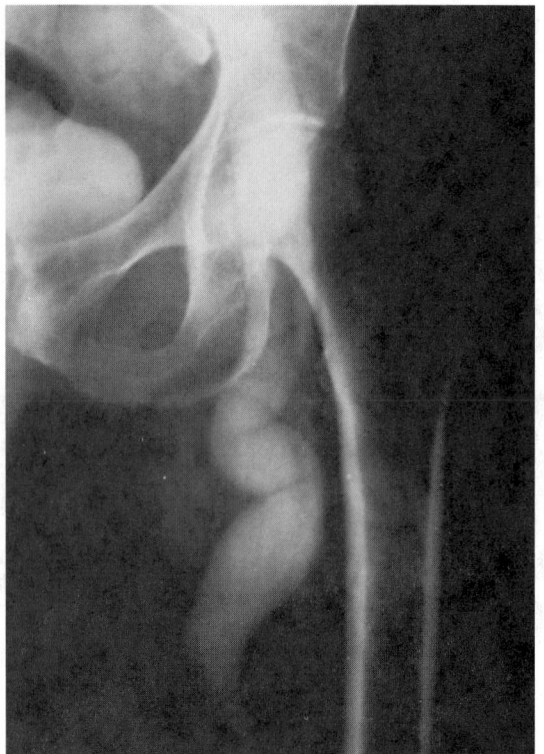

Figure 92-4. Radiograph of dilated and tortuous ileofemoral vein proximal to a chronic arteriovenous fistula.

Aneurysm

Depending on anatomic arrangement, an abnormal AV connection can enlarge and form a frank aneurysm (AV aneurysm), which may calcify.

Systemic Hemodynamic Effects

Changes in Cardiac Output and Stroke Volume

The most important systemic abnormality of AV fistula is a drop in total peripheral vascular resistance. The systemic response is an increase in cardiac output achieved with an increase in heart rate and stroke volume. The enhanced stroke volume is related to greater venous return and larger total blood volume.

The increase in cardiac output in the presence of an AV fistula occurs almost immediately and rapidly reaches maximal level. Abrupt compression or occlusion of an AV fistula rapidly decreases cardiac output. With a large fistula, the increase in cardiac output may not equal the increased flow through the fistula. In this situation systemic arterial flow decreases as a result of peripheral vasoconstriction. If this compensatory mechanism is insufficient, systemic arterial pressure can fall, and high-output cardiac failure occurs. This is typical with acute aortocaval fistula, as can occur with erosion of an aortic aneurysm into the inferior vena cava. Most AV fistulas are peripheral and small, so the changes are less severe.

The increase in cardiac output is due to an increase in stroke volume, and heart rate may be only minimally elevated. With peripheral AV fistula, the proximal artery or the fistula itself may be occluded by external pressure, resulting in a decrease in heart rate (Branham sign). Compression of the fistula causes a slight rise in systemic arterial pressure. The bradycardia can be abolished with atropine.

The increased stroke volume contributing to elevated cardiac output with an AV fistula is associated with increased venous return. It may also reflect enhanced cardiac contractility due to elevated catecholamine levels and adrenergic stimulation.

Cardiomegaly

Cardiomegaly is almost always present in patients with a hemodynamically significant AV fistula. The degree of cardiomegaly is related to the size of the fistula and its duration. Cardiomegaly is far more with acquired fistula than with congenital fistula. Cardiomegaly reverses when the fistula is eliminated. The increase in cardiac size represents dilatation and hypertrophy.

Change in Total Blood Volume

The increase in total blood volume with a large AV fistula correlates with the size of the fistula and the increase in cardiac output. The increase in total blood volume is due to a disproportionate increase in plasma volume. This occurs through the normal sodium- and water-retaining mechanisms activated in response to the fistula, in which systemic arterial pressure changes stimulate the renin-angiotensin-aldosterone system. Congestive heart failure (CHF) occurs with all large, chronic AV fistulas. Closure of the fistula is associated with urinary diuresis. High-output CHF seldom occurs in patients with congenital AV fistulas.

SIGNS AND SYMPTOMS

There is almost always a history of *penetrating injury.* There may be evidence of prior injury in the form of a cutaneous scar at the site of the fistula. A pulsating mass, *vibration,* or buzzing sound can be felt and sensed by the patient. The site of the fistula is warm, and the extremity distal to the fistula is cool.

Arterial circulation distal to an AV fistula is invariably

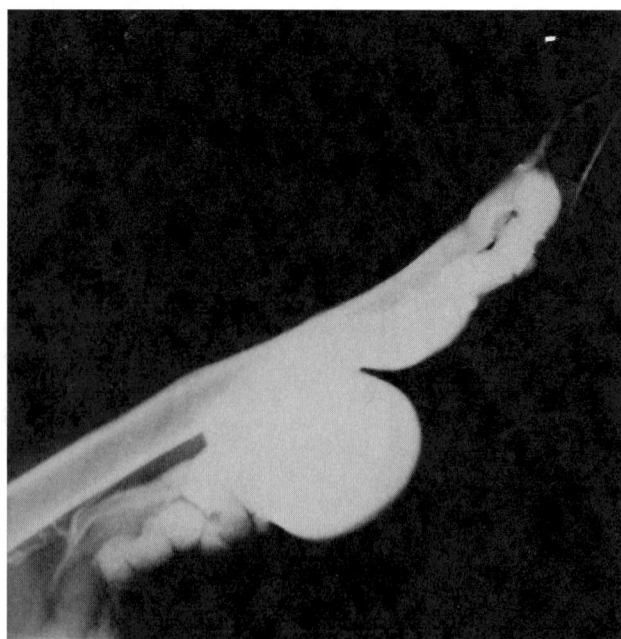

Figure 92-5. Radiograph of a brachial venous aneurysm proximal to a chronic antecubital arteriovenous fistula. (Thompson NW, Lindenauer SM. Central venous aneurysm and arteriovenous fistula. Ann Surg 1969;170:853)

diminished, and venous return is impaired. The signs are edema, diminished pulses, pallor, and varicosities. There may be pain, symptoms of intermittent claudication, paresthesia, cutaneous ulceration, or frank gangrene of the digits.

A loud *murmur* is usually heard directly over the fistula, and a thrill often is present. The loudness and duration of the murmur are equal during systole and diastole (machinery murmur). There may be systolic accentuation.

The veins distal to the fistula, particularly in the leg, are dilated and varicose and demonstrate incompetent valves. There may be an increase in limb girth. In young children, extremity AV fistula can cause limb length inequality. The veins in the region of the fistula may pulsate and exhibit a thrill and murmur.

Compression of the artery proximal to the fistula or compression of the fistulous connection produces a decrease in heart rate (Branham sign).

DIAGNOSIS

Vascular Laboratory

The decrease in arterial pressure distal to an AV fistula in an extremity can be measured with a *Doppler velocity meter*. Additional evidence of an AV fistula is an increase in distal arterial pressure with manual compression of the fistula and an immediate increase in pulse volume. If flow in the distal artery is reversed, compression just distal to the suspected AV fistula causes an increase in arterial pressure in the distal extremity. Distal arterial pressure also increases with compression at the proximal or distal vein.

Plethysmographic measurements of limb or digital volume distal to a suspected AV fistula usually are decreased. Doppler flow velocity is high in the artery proximal to an AV fistula, and the quality of the signal is different.

Direct measurement of *skin temperature* with a thermistor documents low temperature distal to the fistula and high temperature in the area of the fistula.

Oxygen saturation in the venous blood draining an AV fistula is usually elevated compared with the venous oxygen saturation of the other limb.

Increased cardiac output can be measured with *thermal dilution* techniques. Compression of the fistulous connection decreases cardiac output, and the amount of the difference is a good estimate of volume flow through the fistula.

Technetium-labeled albumin microspheres injected into the proximal artery pass through an AV fistula and are trapped in the lung, where they can be monitored with an external gamma detector. The fraction of microspheres detected over the lung provides qualitative assessment of volume flow through the fistula. This technique may be used to differentiate congenital AV fistulas from congenital anomalies in which an AV component is minimal or absent.

Imaging

The most important modality for diagnosis and management of AV fistula is *arteriography*. It provides information about the precise site, number, and size of fistulous connections and indicates functional status of the abnormality and extent of collateral circulation (Fig. 92-6).

Duplex scanning can help identify increased flow velocity and the enlarged artery and vein leading to a peripheral fistula.

Computed tomography (CT) with contrast enhancement is used to demonstrate the sometimes troublesome multiple connections present in muscle and bone in a congenital fistula. Congenital fistulas can be visualized with *magnetic resonance imaging* (MRI). MRI allows precise anatomic localization and provides details concerning the size and extent of a congenital AV fistula. The relation to specific muscle groups, bones, and vascular structures can be determined. The MRI appearance of a congenital AV fistula consists of dilated tortuous vessels infiltrating or replacing involved tissues. Although enlarged vessels are present, the exact arteries and veins supplying and draining the lesion often cannot be ascertained.

MANAGEMENT

Acquired AV Fistulas

The goal of management is preservation of arterial flow. Because of complications such as progressive cardiomegaly and high-output CHF, treatment is undertaken as soon as the diagnosis is made. This can be accomplished with percutaneous embolization, surgical excision, or a combination of both.

The arterial defect usually can be closed primarily. A vein patch is used if primary closure would compromise the arterial lumen. Adjacent soft tissue is interposed over the suture line to provide a buttress to avoid recurrence of the fistula. Doppler ultrasound (US) examination is performed during surgical excision to ascertain the presence of residual fistulous connections.

Fistulas that present difficulty in surgical closure can be eliminated by means of arterial embolization. Emboli are injected so that they lodge at the site of the fistulous connection. Embolization is used in wounds caused by shotgun blasts with multiple injuries to the femoral arterial system. Fistulas between the hypogastric artery and vein may be difficult to control and can be dealt with by means of embolization. Complications of embolization include distal ischemia, infarction, embolization to an undesired artery, and transvenous migration with pulmonary embolism.

Congenital AV Fistulas

Therapy for congenital AV fistulas is difficult because of the many connections and the propensity of some fistulas to infiltrate muscle and bone. Inactive microscopic connections that cannot be seen at gross inspection often are left behind and account for the invariable recurrence. Ligation of major feeding vessels may result in peripheral ischemia and limits the opportunity to embolize such fistulas percutaneously. Most congenital AV fistulas are managed conservatively unless they are small, well-localized, and accessible.

Percutaneous embolization or surgical management of congenital AV fistulas is reserved for pressing indications, such as ulceration, bleeding, cardiac failure, or excessive limb growth in a prepubertal child. Compulsive attempts to remove all of the fistula can result in an ischemic or nonfunctional extremity, excessive hemorrhage, or unnecessary amputation. Recurrence of a congenital fistula is not failure of therapy but is inevitable.

Aortocaval Fistula

Occlusion of the inferior vena cava is important to prevent thromboembolism or air embolus and to control vena caval bleeding. After vena caval control, the aneurysm is opened, and the fistula is identified by the venous blood coming from an orifice in the side of the cava. Once the vena cava is repaired, aneurysm resection is performed. After fistula repair, cardiac and other manifestations of the AV fistula clear rapidly.

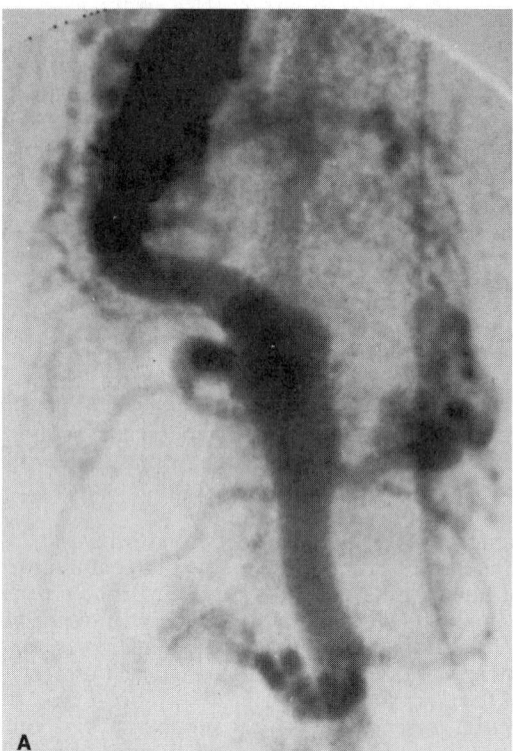 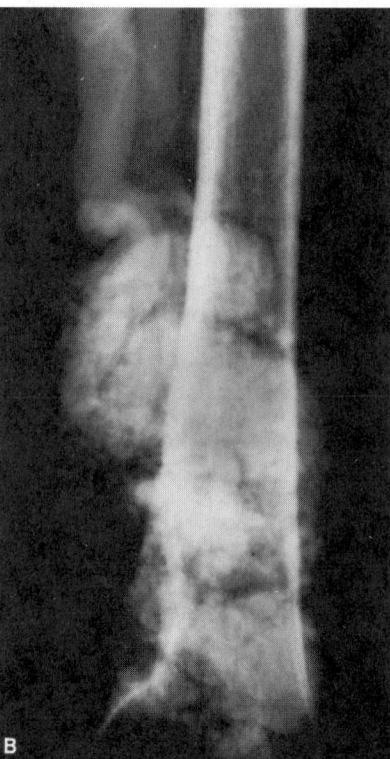

Figure 92-6. (*A*) Radiograph taken during the early phase of arteriography of congenital arteriovenous fistula of distal thigh, showing multiple abnormal dilated and tortuous arteries. (*B*) Radiograph from the later phase of arteriography in the same patient. There is a mass of abnormal vascular channels, and simultaneous visualization of the dilated proximal artery and vein is possible.

Fistulas Due to Femoral Artery Catheterization

B-mode gray-scale ultrasonography with color-flow Doppler imaging is used to diagnose AV fistula of the femoral vessels. The fistula can then be managed by means of manual external compression of the fistula track with the ultrasound transducer. Because many femoral AV fistulas due to catheterization close spontaneously, operation is reserved for lesions that enlarge or exhibit continued patency after 2 months. Femoral AV fistulas can be repaired by means of endovascular placement of an intraluminal graft-covered stent.

Complications of AV Fistulas for Hemodialysis

Depending on the size and the location of the fistula, troublesome distal ischemia or frank rest pain may be present. Treatment involves decreasing the amount of fistula flow by means of constriction of arterial inflow with a band of prosthetic material. An easy way to determine the degree of constriction necessary to relieve the ischemia is to monitor the distal artery while constricting the proximal artery until distal retrograde flow is eliminated.

Some patients with heart disease have CHF as a result of an AV fistula established for hemodialysis. Cardiac output may be decreased by means of reduction of fistula flow volume.

Some patients experience excessive swelling of the hand or fingers after establishment of a fistula at the wrist. The fistula may have been too large at the time it was made or may have enlarged. The increased venous pressure causing the swelling and discomfort often subsides. If it does not, the fistula is removed and normal arterial and venous continuity is restored.

Permanent Occlusive Devices

A variety of permanent occlusive devices may be introduced percutaneously to occlude traumatic or congenital AV fistulas. They are used as primary treatment and as an adjunct to surgical therapy. Materials include metal coils, detachable balloons, thrombin-soaked gelatin foam, autologous muscle, alcohol, and liquid acrylic adhesive.

VASCULAR MALFORMATIONS

Congenital vascular malformations (CVMs) are divided into those that are primarily venous and those in which an AV fistula is present. Both may include a lymphatic component. AV malformations are subdivided into those that contain overt large hyperdynamic AV connections and those that are small and functionally hypodynamic. Hyperdynamic AV malformations can be diffuse and appear to cross natural tissue boundaries and invade muscle and bone. Hypodynamic malformations are well-circumscribed.

Etiology

CVMs result from arrest of the normal embryologic development of the vascular system. The factors that cause abnormal development of peripheral arteries and veins are not known. Potential exogenous causes include viral infection and effects of medication. With few exceptions, the cause of the abnormal persistence of AV connections, capillary angiomas, or venous agenesis is unknown. The cause of associated phenomena such as increased bone length, and increased extremity girth with CVMs also is unknown.

CVMs are rare. CVMs that are primarily AV have different biologic and pathophysiologic features and prognosis and therapy from those of traumatic or acquired AV fistulas. Congenital AV malformations are present from birth and represent abnormal vascular development or an arrest in normal development. The AV connections are multiple, yet they seldom produce serious systemic effects. The malformations may be diffuse or circumscribed. At arteriography, the lesions demonstrate rapid blood flow and sometimes AV shunting. They look like a vascular neoplasm with a parenchymal appearance.

The bony and soft tissue hypertrophy that often occurs with congenital AV malformations may be caused by altered hemodynamics or may represent an additional primary component. These lesions are equally distributed between boys and girls. They are several times more common in the lower extremity than the upper. Congenital AV malformations are present at birth but are not always clinically evident. Unlike hemangioma of infancy, they seldom undergo spontaneous involution.

Signs and Symptoms

Cutaneous AV malformations can present with a mass, discoloration of the skin, enlarged veins, unequal limb length and girth, or hemorrhage or ulceration. It is unclear what stimuli may activate dormant lesions, but the hormonal changes of puberty or pregnancy coincide with clinical recognition and exacerbation of these lesions. Although these lesions look like they invade adjacent tissues, there is no histologic evidence of cellular proliferation or other evidence of neoplasia.

In addition to the lower extremities, congenital AV malformations occur in the pelvis and head. They also may affect the viscera but are usually clinically silent. The most common presenting features of visceral AV malformations are hemoptysis, hematuria, hematemesis, and melena.

Only rarely do large, hyperdynamic AV malformations cause changes in cardiac output or other local or systemic hemodynamic abnormalities. The lesion may be warm, and if there is an AV component, the mass does not decrease with elevation and is more firm than a venous anomaly. Sometimes there may be pulsating veins and a thrill and bruit. If there is hemodynamic alteration, the area distal to the lesion may be cool with diminished pulses. Arterial ischemia and ulceration, chronic venous stasis changes, and venous ulceration may occur.

Patients may be aware of heaviness, throbbing, pulsation, and vibration and may feel increased local warmth. The extremity may exhibit a striking increase in length and girth resulting from hypertrophy of bony and soft tissue. Cortical bone may thicken. Bony defects are present on plain radiographs when there is involvement and erosion of bony tissue.

The cutaneous manifestations are striking—a mass of dilated vessels and extremely large venous varicosities. Venous pulsations may be visible. A cutaneous hemangioma may be present and vary in extent and appearance. There may be gross distortion of the contour of the limb. Varicosities may not become apparent until a child begins to stand and walk. The varicosities are atypical in location and appearance. Limb hypertrophy, varicosities, and a hemangioma of the skin may be present with or without a demonstrable AV fistula. Absence of deep veins or AV communication corresponds to Klippel-Trenaunay syndrome.

The Branham sign (slowing of the pulse with compression of the AV communication of the major proximal artery) may be elicited. Because of multiple connections, it may be difficult to compress the appropriate vessels. When muscle and bone are involved, compression is not feasible.

Localized hypoactive microfistulous AV malformations present as an asymptomatic localized mass, and the vascular nature may not be apparent until they are excised.

The dilated veins sometimes present are cutaneous hemangiomas.

Only rarely do congenital AV malformations produce cardiac manifestations.

Diagnosis

The diagnosis of a congenital AV malformation can be made on the basis of signs and symptoms, but arteriography is essential to delineate the number, location, and extent of the abnormalities (Fig. 92-7). Arteriography always is performed if therapeutic intervention is considered. It shows one or more dilated proximal arteries and draining veins and the multiple fistulous connections. It may be difficult or impossible to differentiate arteries, veins, or connecting channels. In a hypodynamic fistula, the only abnormality may be early venous opacification. Other indirect arteriographic findings suggestive of hypodynamic microfistulous AV malformation are increased flow through afferent arterial trunks and accumulation of contrast medium in the area of the suspected fistula.

MRI can help determine the character of blood flow and define the anatomy of the lesion and involvement of muscle and bone. Slow-flow venous malformations can be differentiated from high-flow AV fistulas with MRI.

The abnormal vascular spaces of a venous malformation can be visualized with closed-system venography. Venous oxygen saturation draining an AV malformation is usually elevated in relation to the uninvolved extremity.

Treatment

Management of all CVMs is conservative. Asymptomatic lesions require no therapy and usually exhibit no progression. The main form of conservative therapy is elastic support hose, which can reduce flow through AV malformations. Indications for surgical therapy include hemorrhage,

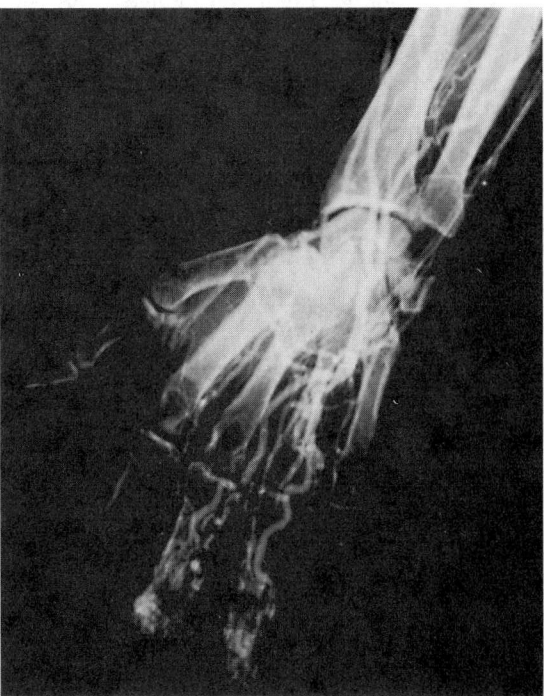

Figure 92-7. Radiograph of congenital arteriovenous fistulas confined to the distal portions of the third and fourth fingers of a young man.

ischemia, CHF, nonhealing ulcers, functional impairment, and limb-length inequality.

Bleeding in the gastrointestinal and urinary tracts may be the source of chronic anemia, which can be occult and necessitate a diligent search and extirpation. If the abnormal vessels can be localized at angiography, embolization can be performed. Initial embolization can make surgical excision easier, less extensive, or not necessary. Any intervention is temporary because AV malformations always recur.

Complex AV malformations in the pelvis are usually impossible to remove and are associated with blood loss and injury to vital structures, such as the ureter, bladder, rectum, and pelvic nerves. Although safer and easier, percutaneous embolization, if too extensive, can result in ischemic necrosis of vital organs. Permanent embolic materials, such as stainless steel coils, tissue adhesive, polyvinyl alcohol particles, and detachable balloons, can be used. Care must be taken that occlusion of large-caliber feeding vessels does not preclude embolization. Complications of embolization include passage through an AV communication resulting in pulmonary embolism, embolization of normal tissue, and ischemic neuritis.

Hypoactive AV malformations that are small, localized, and not hemodynamically significant can be difficult to diagnose before removal. They usually present as an asymptomatic subcutaneous mass, and excision is necessary for histologic examination and diagnosis. Once the nature of the mass is identified, further excision is not required because recurrence is common and the presence of the lesion is not associated with long-term undesirable effects.

Cutaneous hemangiomas present at birth as an isolated lesion often regress by the age of 5 or 6 years. They simply require observation. Some, however, exhibit rapid or atypical growth or are associated with thrombocytopenia. Therapy is surgical excision or embolization, if possible. Heparin, corticosteriods, or antifibrinolytic agents can be used.

The rare CVM that involves a joint can be troublesome for a young, active person with recurrent episodes of hemarthrosis. Excision may limit joint function, so therapy is limited to embolization and avoidance of contact sports.

CVMs cause limb lengthening. Small discrepancies can be managed with special footwear. Marked leg-length inequality can cause a pelvic tilt and low back pain. If it not be corrected with a shoe insert, the discrepancy may require epiphysiodesis of the affected leg to slow the rate of growth.

Klippel–Trenaunay Syndrome

Klippel–Trenaunay syndrome is a congenital venous anomaly. It is usually confined to one leg with varying degrees of venous varicosities. A cutaneous hemangioma or port wine stain is present. The hemangioma has a variegated irregular margin and often involves the buttock and lower back but seldom crosses the midline of the lower trunk. Increased length and girth of the affected extremity are common. The lesion is present at birth but may become manifest only when the child begins to stand or walk. The syndrome occurs equally among boys and girls as an isolated anomaly. It does not occur in siblings or other family members.

There may be a varying amount of lymphatic involvement. The deep venous system may be absent or abnormal. Arteriography does not show an AV fistula. The presence of a congenital AV fistula associated with Klippel–Trenaunay triad (varicosities, cutaneous hemangioma, and hypertrophy) is more properly designated Parkes–Weber syndrome.

Plain radiographs of the extremities usually demonstrate phleboliths (round calcified nodules within dilated veins). The lesion may be extensive on CT scans or MRI. The cavernous hemangioma or the varicosities of Klippel–Trenaunay syndrome also can be visualized by means of direct percutaneous puncture.

The lesions of Klippel–Trenaunay syndrome seldom cause symptoms. They are managed conservatively with elastic hose. If there is a large, troublesome lymphatic component, intermittent use of a pneumatic compression device may provide relief. In the absence of a deep venous system, removal of superficial veins can worsen symptoms and is avoided.

SUGGESTED READING

Allen BT, Munn JS, Stervern SL, et al. Selective non-operative management of pseudoaneurysms and arteriovenous fistulae complicating femoral artery catheterization. J Cardiovasc Surg 1992;33:440.
DeSouza NM, Reidy JF. Embolization with detachable balloons: applications outside the head. Clin Radiol 1992;46:170.
Fellmeth BD, Roberts AC, Bookstein JJ, et al. Postangiographic femoral artery injuries: nonsurgical repair with US-guided compression. Radiology 1991;178:671.
Kent KC, McArdel CR, Kennedy B, Baim DS, Anninos E, Skillman JJ. A prospective study of the clinical outcome of femoral pseudoaneurysms and arteriovenous fistulas induced by arterial puncture. J Vasc Surg 1993;17:125.
Kwan E, Hieshima GB, Higashida RT, Halbach VV, Wolpert SM. Interventional neuroradiology in neuro-ophthalmology. J Clin Neuroophthalmol 1989;9:83.
Lindenauer SM. Treatment of venous aneurysms. In: Ernst CB, Stanley JC, eds. Current therapy in vascular surgery, ed 2. Toronto, Decker, 1991:1019.
Marin ML, Veith FJ, Panetta TF, et al. Percutaneous transfemoral insertion of a stented graft to repair a traumatic femoral arteriovenous fistula. J Vasc Surg 1993;18:299.
Peeters FL, Kromhout JG, Reekers JA, Koster PA. Treatment of solitary arteriovenous fistulas. Surgery 1991;109:220.
Redmond PL, Kumpe DA. Embolization of an intrahepatic arterioportal fistula: case report and review of the literature. Cardiovasc Intervent Radiol 1988;11:274.
Silverman RA. Hemangiomas and vascular malformations. Pediatr Clin North Am 1991;38:811.

ESSENTIALS OF SURGERY: SCIENTIFIC PRINCIPLES AND PRACTICE,
edited by Lazar J. Greenfield, Michael W. Mulholland, Keith T. Oldham, Gerald B. Zelenock,
and Keith D. Lillemoe. Lippincott–Raven Publishers, Philadelphia, © 1997.

CHAPTER 93

VENOUS PHYSIOLOGY AND DISORDERS OF THE SUPERFICIAL AND DEEP VEINS

THOMAS W. WAKEFIELD AND LAZAR J. GREENFIELD

ANATOMY

Superficial Veins

The *greater saphenous vein* begins anterior to the medial malleolus where superficial veins draining the medial aspect of the dorsum of the foot join veins from the medial aspect of the sole. The greater saphenous vein travels just under the skin in a straight line on the anteromedial aspect of the lower leg 1 to 2 cm posterior to the tibia and passes along the medial aspect of the knee. It continues in a straight line to the thigh, where it joins the femoral vein 2 to 4 cm lateral to the pubic tubercle and inferior to the inguinal ligament at the fossa ovalis (Fig. 93-1).

The *superficial external pudendal vein* joins the saphenous vein medially, although the arrangement of this branch and other superficial saphenous tributaries is not constant. The saphenous vein receives a number of tributaries that drain the posteromedial and anterolateral aspects of the leg. The greater saphenous vein may exist as two separate trunks that join to form a single vein at the origin and termination.

The *lesser saphenous vein* originates behind the lateral malleolus from the confluence of veins draining the lateral aspect of the foot. It curves toward the midline of the posterior calf and ascends in a straight line to join the popliteal vein behind the knee near the head of the gastrocnemius muscle, although it can terminate above the level of the knee crease. The lesser saphenous vein lies just below the skin. It may continue upward in the posterior region of the thigh and connect with tributaries of the greater saphenous vein.

Veins of the Foot

The greater and lesser saphenous veins are joined in the foot by the *superficial dorsal venous arch*. The deep veins of the sole are the *lateral* and *medial plantar veins*. They are joined through communicating veins to a cutaneous arch and come together to form the *posterior tibial vein* (Fig. 93-2). Multiple communicating veins connect the superficial to the deep veins in the foot.

Deep Veins

The deep veins of the lower leg are *venae comitantes* that accompany the anterior tibial, posterior tibial, and peroneal arteries. Each deep vein consists of two or three venae comitantes adjacent to the artery with multiple connections that cross and surround the artery. The anterior tibial venous drainage originates on the dorsum of the foot and lies in the anterior compartment of the calf next to the interosseous membrane.

The *posterior tibial veins,* which drain the superficial and deep plantar veins, are inferior to the medial malleolus and follow the posterior tibial artery. The *peroneal veins* lie directly behind and medial to the fibula and ascend along the peroneal artery (Fig. 93-3). These deep veins of the calf have frequent interconnections. The soleus muscle sinusoids have no valves and are called *venous lakes.* The venous lakes in the calf are a common site of early thrombus formation. They coalesce to join the posterior tibial and peroneal veins. These sinusoids are less apparent in the gastrocnemius muscle, where the veins tend to be linear and have valves.

The paired venae comitantes merge to form single trunks that unite at the knee to form the *popliteal vein.* Sometimes the junction occurs above the knee, resulting in a dual popliteal venous system. The popliteal vein continues proximally as the *superficial femoral vein* close to the superficial femoral artery in the adductor canal. It is joined below the inguinal ligament by the deep femoral (profunda femoris) vein and continues as the common femoral vein.

The *deep femoral vein* frequently connects directly or through tributary veins to the popliteal vein. The anatomy of the popliteal and femoral veins is variable, and duplication is common. The *common femoral vein* runs medial to the common femoral artery under the inguinal ligament and continues as the external iliac vein. The greater saphenous vein usually joins the common femoral vein 2 to 4 cm proximal to the junction of the deep and superficial femoral veins at the fossa ovalis.

The *external iliac vein* is the continuation in the pelvis of the common femoral vein. It is joined at the level of the sacroiliac joint by the *internal iliac vein* (hypogastric), which drains the pelvis. The internal iliac veins form a large collateral network in the pelvis that includes connections with the gluteal, obturator, and internal pudendal veins, a large number of unnamed vessels, and multiple extrapelvic collateral pathways.

The *common iliac veins* originate from the joining of the external and internal iliac veins. They ascend medially and join to the right of the fifth lumbar vertebra and the aorta to form the inferior vena cava (IVC). The *right common iliac vein* ascends in an almost straight line to the IVC. The *left common iliac vein* is transversely oriented

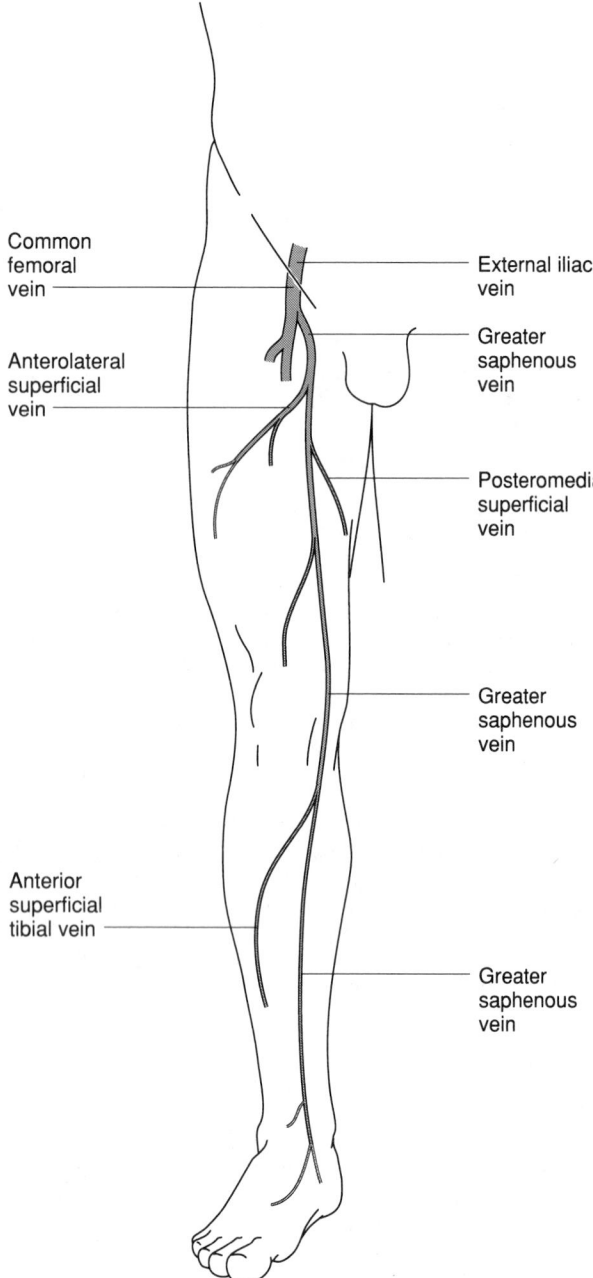

Figure 93-1. Greater saphenous vein and its branches.

and joins the right iliac vein at an angle of about 90°. The left common iliac vein may be compressed between the lumbosacral spine posteriorly and the anterior crossing of the right common iliac artery.

The *inferior vena cava* ascends from the level of the fifth lumbar vertebra and ends at the right atrium. It lies to the right of the midline and lateral to the aorta and receives a number of paired *lumbar veins* that connect with the vertebral and paravertebral venous plexus. At the level of the L-1 to L-2 interspace, the *renal veins* join the IVC. More proximally, the *hepatic veins* join the IVC. The IVC may be duplicated below the level of the renal veins, a left-sided cava draining into the left renal vein, which joins to form a single proximal IVC. The incidence of IVC and renal vein anomalies is high.

Collateral circulation around an obstructed IVC occurs through many pathways, including the vertebral plexus,

gonadal veins, ureteral veins, the azygos system, and the extensive superficial collaterals, which include the superficial epigastric, circumflex iliac veins, and the lateral thoracic and intercostal veins.

Important communicating veins exist at the termination of the greater and lesser saphenous veins where they join the deep venous system in the popliteal fossa and in the fossa ovalis. The *perforating veins* of the lower leg are important in venous disease and chronic venous insufficiency (CVI), especially the three or four perforating veins at the level of the medial and lateral malleolus. Other perforating veins are located in the upper medial calf and along the posterolateral aspect of the lower leg, connecting the lesser saphenous vein with the deep veins of the calf. A small number of communications exist in the mid-thigh between the greater saphenous vein and the superficial femoral vein. The locations of perforating veins can be determined only with venous duplex imaging or venography.

Venous Valves

Venous valves direct the flow of blood to the heart and prevent valvular reflux. These valves consist of two thin, delicate cusps composed of an intimal fold with a small amount of connective tissue between the leaves of the fold. Venous valves are numerous in the distal part of the leg, decrease in number in the proximal portion, and do not exist in the vena cava. Loss of valvular function in the leg leads to venous hypertension.

Valves in the deep veins of the thigh vary in number and position. There are a few constant valves, however (Table 93-1).

Valves are oriented so that they direct venous flow from the superficial to the deep system. In the deep system they direct flow from the foot to the heart. They prevent reflux of blood from the higher pressure deep venous circulation into the superficial saphenous system. The valves in these perforating veins lie both deep and superficial to the muscle fascia.

PHYSIOLOGY

Foot vein pressure is influenced by posture—supine or erect. Measured when a person is *supine,* venous pressure is the residual kinetic energy of the heart reduced by capillary and arteriolar resistance. This residual pressure is about 15 mmHg and causes a pressure gradient of 13 to 15 mmHg in the return of blood to the heart (right atrial pressure usually is 0 to 2 mmHg). When foot vein pressure is measured with the person *standing,* the hydrostatic pressure caused by the weight of the column of blood that extends from the heart to the foot must be included. Foot vein pressure for the upright posture is the sum of hydrostatic pressure and kinetic pressure (15 mmHg). For a person 6 feet (180 cm) tall, hydrostatic pressure is about 100 mmHg, so when the person is standing, the pressure measured in a foot vein is about 115 mmHg.

The vein wall is composed of collagen, elastic tissue, and smooth muscle fibers. The smooth muscle fibers are responsible for active venous tone. Venous capacity is influenced by variations in transmural pressure and, to a lesser extent, by the contractility of the smooth muscle in the venous wall. This is particularly true when the veins are collapsed and transmural pressure is low. When there is additional filling, the veins assume a circular configuration, and smooth muscle venous tone assumes greater importance in regulating venous volume.

The venous system can accommodate wide variations in volume with little change in pressure. This ability allows

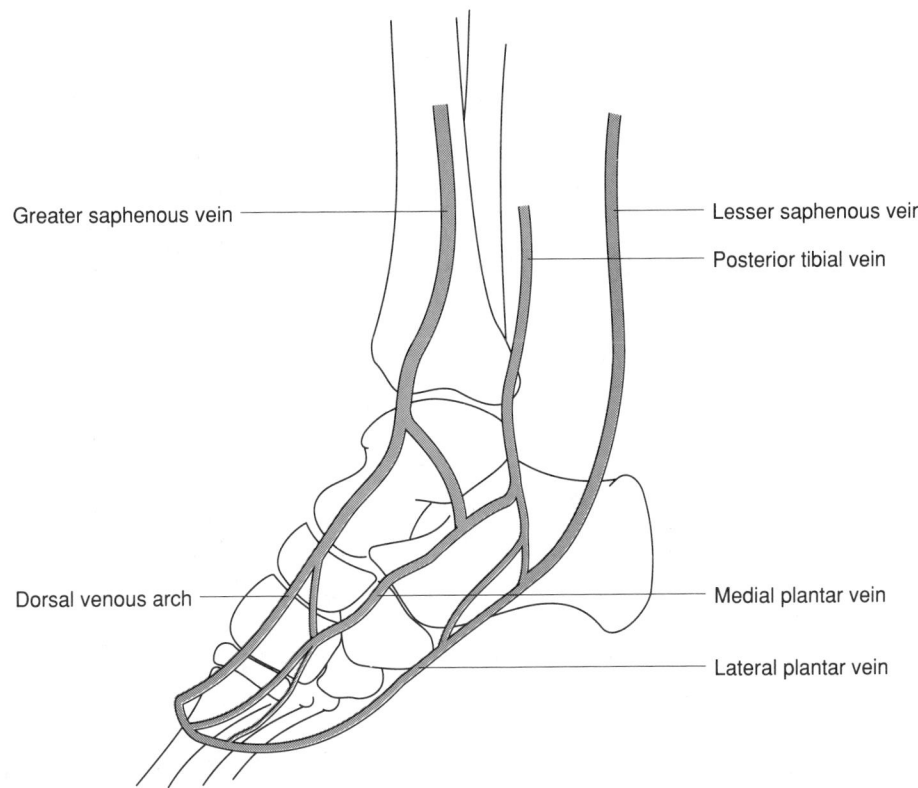

Figure 93-2. Veins of the foot.

alteration in blood volume with minimal change in central venous pressure. When venous capacitance is exceeded, central venous pressure rises substantially.

Empty veins are flat. As they fill, they change from elliptical to circular in cross section. Initially, there is little resistance to flow as veins distend and their shape changes. During early filling, as veins assume a circular configuration, more blood can be accommodated with little increase in venous pressure. Once veins assume a circular configuration, the pressure per unit volume increases rapidly and reaches a plateau. Transmural pressure, which causes distention, is the difference between the intraluminal pressure and the external tissue pressure. With outflow obstruction, a small volume increase causes a disproportionate increase in pressure in the veins. Venous flow is affected by respiration, body position, calf muscle pump function, and arterial circulation. For example, flow is at its minimum during peak inspiration. The bicuspid venous valves direct flow of venous blood toward the heart and prevent reflux (Fig. 93-4).

The valve cusps are easily engaged by retrograde blood flow, and because valve diameter is slightly greater than luminal diameter, a tight seal ensures prevention of valvular reflux. A crucial set of valves exist in the perforating veins.

Normal veins can accommodate large volume changes with only small pressure changes. With calf muscle pump dysfunction, venous pressures do not normalize but remain elevated. This chronic state of elevated venous pressure (venous hypertension) leads to CVI. Venous claudication occurs when the iliofemoral venous segment is obstructed by thrombosis that has not lysed and when collaterals develop inadequately around the obstruction. With exercise, the deep venous system fills but does not empty, and the thigh and leg become heavy and painful with a bursting sensation.

DISORDERS OF THE SUPERFICIAL VEINS

Varicose veins occur when venous valves become incompetent, producing distention and tortosity. *Primary* varicose veins occur spontaneously in the absence of deep venous involvement. *Secondary* varicose veins originate as the outward manifestation of CVI. More women than men have varicose veins. Among women varicose veins are associated with obesity, lack of physical activity, hypertension, and late menopause. Among men varicose veins are associated with smoking and lack of physical activity.

Nonsurgical Treatment

Therapy for varicose veins involves management of CVI—elastic stocking *support,* periodic leg *elevation,* and *exercise* while wearing the elastic stockings. The stockings prevent additional distention of superficial veins.

Injection sclerotherapy may be indicated for small varicosities but is more frequent for telangiectactic ("spider") veins. Indications for injection sclerotherapy include:

- Pain over a varicose or telangiectactic vein
- Symptoms of CVI (especially before or during menstruation)
- Previous thrombophlebitis in small varicose veins
- Bleeding from a varicose or spider vein
- Trophic changes related to a spider vein

Contraindications to injection sclerotherapy include:

- Active thrombophlebitis
- Pregnancy during the first and second trimester
- Lactation and 3 months thereafter
- Severe leg edema
- Inability to participate in physical activity after treatment

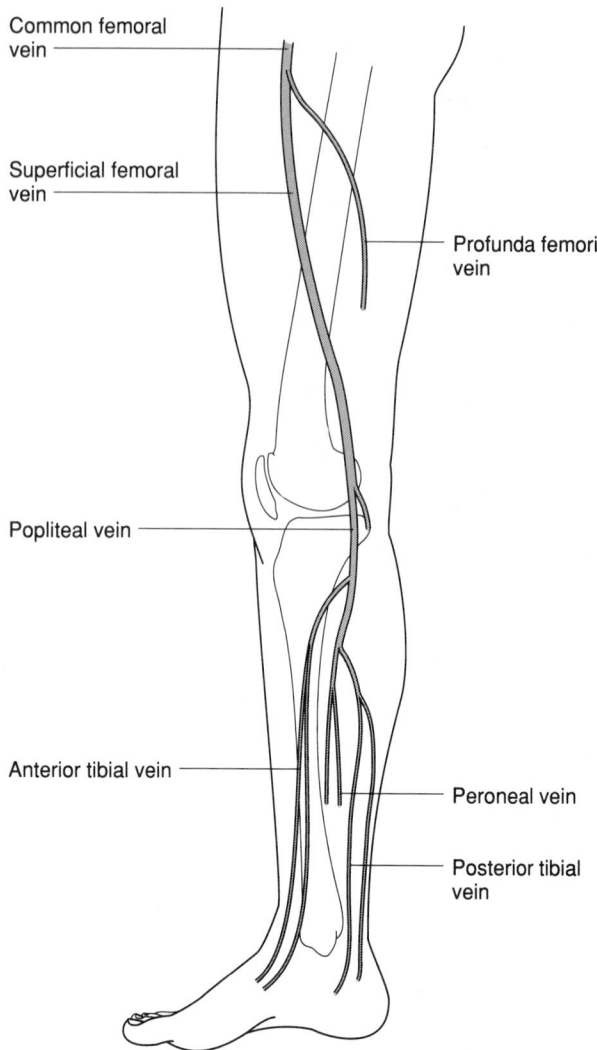

Figure 93-3. Deep veins of the lower leg.

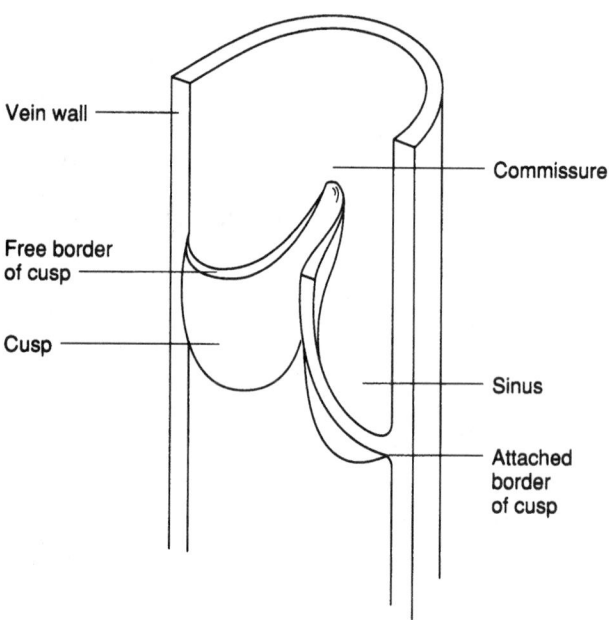

Figure 93-4. Structure of a venous valve.

- A condition that necessitates bedrest
- Severe arterial occlusive disease
- Inability to wear bandages after treatment
- Goal of cosmetic effect if there are no symptoms

Surgical Treatment

Preoperative Testing

An intact deep venous system is documented with venous ultrasound duplex imaging. Photoplethysmography (PPG), may be indicated to help predict the success of

Table 93-1. VALVES WITH A CONSTANT LOCATION

Vein	Location
Common femoral	Just distal to the junction with the deep femoral vein
Popliteal	Just distal to the adductor hiatus
Greater and lesser saphenous systems	Proximal end of the greater saphenous vein just at or slightly distal to its junction with the common femoral vein
Perforating veins	Between the superficial and deep veins

varicose vein removal and the need for postoperative elastic support. If CVI is present, the patient is instructed to use CVI management (support, elevation, exercise). Indications for surgical treatment are:

- Pain over the varicosities (as opposed to the discomfort of deep venous insufficiency)
- Superficial thrombophlebitis in the varicosities
- Erosion of the skin with bleeding
- Disabling edema with or without subcutaneous cellulitis
- Induration or lipodermatosclerosis
- Manifestations of CVI (especially ulceration)

Contraindications to surgical treatment are:

- Goal is cosmetic improvement only
- Varicose veins due to CVI from deep venous insufficiency in which the CVI is causing the symptoms
- Varicose veins associated with chronic diseases such as degenerative arthritis, arterial occlusive disease, neurogenic syndromes, lymphedema, congestive heart failure, or obesity
- Varicose veins associated with an arteriovenous (AV) fistula or congenital venous abnormality

Surgical Procedures

One of the following operations is used:

- Selective vein removal
- High ligation with perforator interruption
- Stab evulsion phlebectomy

In stab evulsion phlebectomy, after high ligation of the greater saphenous vein, small stab wounds are made along the varicosities. Hooks are used to remove the varicosities. For secondary varicosities, larger incisions and interruption and ligation of perforating veins are needed. For secondary varicosities in which varicose clusters are related to deep venous insufficiency and perforator incompetence, high ligation usually is not necessary. *Complications* include hematoma, infection, sural nerve irritation (from lesser saphenous stripping), and saphenous nerve irritation (minimized by removing the stripper from proximal to distal).

DISORDERS OF THE DEEP VEINS

CVI is a consequence of deep venous thrombosis (DVT) or congenital or hereditary venous valvular incompetence. Other causes include cavernous hemangioma, congenital AV fistula, and pelvic tumors.

With valvular incompetence, the standing column of blood produces elevated venous pressures. Patients with CVI have little if any reduction in venous pressure during exercise. With venous obstruction, venous pressure may actually rise with exercise. After exercise, venous pressure returns much faster than it should, so the lower leg and ankle (gaiter) region is exposed to chronically elevated venous pressures.

The changes of CVI (stasis pigmentation, stasis dermatitis, and ulceration) occur in the gaiter area for two reasons: (1) incompetent perforating veins produce extreme venous hypertension in the ankle region; (2) the ankle has little soft-tissue support. Elevated venous pressures cause edema from plasma fluid constituents in the interstitial space and build-up of plasma proteins and red blood cells. These constituents produce low-grade inflammation, the red cells break down to produce hemosiderin, a blue-brown pigment, and the subcutaneous tissues become scarred and fibrotic. Because of fibrosis in the subcutaneous tissue, skin perfusion decreases, causing skin ischemia, which facilitates ulceration.

Symptoms of CVI begin with edema, which usually occurs at and below the ankle without involving the forefoot or toes. It usually responds well to leg elevation. The edema is worse at night than in the morning, and eventually dermatitis, stasis pigmentation, induration, and ulceration occur. Other causes of ulceration must be differentiated from venous ulceration (Table 93-2). Along with aching, fatigue, itching, night cramps, and swelling, some patients describe venous claudication. This is caused by incomplete and poor recanalization of the venous system after extensive occlusive DVT.

Nonsurgical Treatment

Venous insufficiency is an incurable but manageable problem. Most changes of CVI in the leg are caused by chronic swelling. Elastic compression stockings improve but do not prevent swelling. *Elevating the legs* above the heart level, as patients with CVI are directed to do two to three times a day, is important to decrease venous hypertension.

The patient puts on *elastic support* hose before arising in the morning and removes them before going to sleep at night. The manner in which elastic compression improves the symptoms of CVI is not clear. External compression may restore competence of the dilated valve or may affect the venoarterial reflex. *Exercise* such as walking and bicycling *with elastic support* and swimming and water exercise are excellent for patients with CVI. If stasis ulceration develops, it usually improves with leg elevation and local wound care, especially with *occlusive dressings*.

Surgical Treatment

Most patients with CVI do not need *surgical treatment*. Some, however, do benefit from surgical therapy.

Preoperative Testing

The diagnosis of CVI must be confirmed. Noninvasive laboratory studies include complete venous Doppler exams, PPG, and air plethysmography (APG). PPG is qualita-

Table 93-2. DIFFERENTIATION OF ULCERS

Type of Ulcer	Characteristics
Venous	Large and irregular in outline
	Shallow, moist granulation base
	Occur in gaiter area
	Involved in areas of skin with stasis dermatitis and stasis pigmentation
Neurotrophic	Painless
	Bleed with manipulation
	Deep, indolent, surrounded by chronic inflammatory tissue reaction that appears as a callous
	Usually located over pressure points, commonly the plantar surface of the first and fifth metatarsal heads
	Common among patients with long-standing neuropathy
Ischemic	Extremely painful
	Associated with rest pain in the distal forefoot
	When chronic are circumscribed
	Ulcer base often has poorly developed, grayish granulation tissue
	Surrounding skin pale and mottled
	Débridement causes little bleeding

tive but not quantitative; APG is quantitative. *APG* is used to measure many physiologic processes in the lower leg at one time, including venous obstruction, venous reflux, and calf muscle pump function. *Duplex imaging* of the closing times of individual venous valves indicates venous reflux.

After the vascular laboratory tests, ascending *phlebography* is used to assess the patency of the tibial, popliteal, superficial femoral, common femoral, iliac, IVC, and perforating veins. Descending phlebography provides visual information about the function of the valves.

The following indications for surgical treatment:

Ligation of Perforating Veins
Indications
* *Recurrent* or recalcitrant venous ulcers when there are large incompetent perforating veins under the area of ulceration
* Persistent pain in the region of a previous venous ulcer with an underlying incompetent perforating vein and repeated failure of skin graft healing in an area of venous ulceration

Contraindications
* Absence of an appropriate perforator under the ulcer
* Stasis disease of the skin and subcutaneous tissue so severe that the incision for the procedure is not expected to heal

Vein or Valve Reconstruction
Indications
* Venous claudication associated with venous outflow obstruction
* Symptoms of venous reflux (severe aching, fatigue, and swelling)
* Recurrent venous ulceration from venous obstruction or reflux not responsive to conservative therapy or perforator ligation
* Combined superficial and deep venous insufficiency so severe that the symptoms cannot be relieved with a superficial venous operation alone
* Failure of conservative therapy to relieve severe symptoms of deep venous insufficiency

Contraindications
* Venous obstruction seen at phlebography but not symptomatic

- CVI not controlled with aggressive conservative management
- Symptoms associated with chronic disease such as degenerative arthritis or peripheral vascular occlusive disease of nonvenous origin
- Symptoms of CVI that cannot be documented with anatomic or physiologic tests

Surgical Procedures

Bypass of Venous Obstruction

There are two types: femorofemoral and saphenopopliteal. For both bypasses, concomitant procedures such as perforator ligation, saphenous vein stripping, and construction of distal AV fistulas can be performed (the last if prosthetic conduits are used). In both procedures, the saphenous vein used as a conduit tends to dilate over time.

Valve Restoration

Methods are:
- Valvuloplasty
- Venous segment transposition
- Venous valvular autotransplantation
- External banding
- Venous wall plication
- A substitute valve operation with use of a polymeric silicone tendon spacer behind the knee

SUGGESTED READING

Bergan JJ, Yao JST, eds. Venous disorders. Philadelphia, WB Saunders, 1991:137.

Chang BB, Paty PSK, Shah DM, et al. The lesser saphenous vein: an unappreciated source of autogenous vein. J Vasc Surg 1992;15:152.

Cordts PR, Hanrahan LM, Rodriguez AA, et al. A prospective, randomized trial of unna's boot versus duoderm CGF hydroactive dressing plus compression in management of venous leg ulcers. J Vasc Surg 1992;15:480.

Eriksson I. Reconstructive surgery for deep vein valve incompetence in the lower limb. Eur J Vasc Surg 1990;4:211.

Goren G, Yellin AE. Ambulatory stab evulsion phlebectomy for truncal varicose veins. Am J Surg 1991;162:166.

Hammarsten J, Pedersen P, Cederlund C-G, et al. Long saphenous vein saving surgery for varicose veins: a longterm follow-up. Eur J Vasc Surg 1990;4:361.

Markel A, Manzo RA, Bergelin RO, et al. Valvular reflux after deep venous thrombosis: incidence and time of occurrence. J Vasc Surg 1992;15:377.

Sarin S, Scurr JH, Coleridge Smith JD. Mechanism of action of external compression on venous function. Br J Surg 1992; 79:499.

Wilkinson LS, Bunker C, Edwards JCW, et al. Leukocytes: their role in the etiopathogenesis of skin damage in venous disease. J Vasc Surg 1993;17:669.

Zierler RE, Strandness DE Jr. Hemodynamics for the vascular surgeon. In: Moore WS, ed. Vascular surgery: a comprehensive review, ed 4. Philadelphia, WB Saunders, 1993:179.

ESSENTIALS OF SURGERY: SCIENTIFIC PRINCIPLES AND PRACTICE,
edited by Lazar J. Greenfield, Michael W. Mulholland, Keith T. Oldham, Gerald B. Zelenock,
and Keith D. Lillemoe. Lippincott–Raven Publishers, Philadelphia, © 1997.

CHAPTER 94

VENOUS THROMBOSIS AND PULMONARY THROMBOEMBOLISM

LAZAR J. GREENFIELD

Factors that lead to deep venous thrombosis (DVT) are changes in the vessel wall, stasis, and prothrombotic changes in the blood—the Virchow triad. Other risk factors are: age >40 years, male sex, obesity, malignant disease, history of DVT or pulmonary embolism, any operation >2 hours, pregnancy, oral contraceptive use, nephrotic syndrome, lupus anticoagulant, dysfibrinogenemia, inherited deficiency or disorder or protein (C deficiency or resistance), antithrombin III or plasminogen, and drug abuse.

The soleal venous valve sinuses are the typical site of formation of a nidus of thrombus. Thrombus begins with a small accumulation of platelets on the vessel wall. Some thrombi propagate without obstructing flow and develop a long floating tail that can break loose from its tenuous anchor within the valvular sinus. This sequence of events is the most dangerous aspect of DVT, because pulmonary embolism can and does occur without premonitory signs or symptoms at the point of origin. Some thrombi propagate and attach to the opposite wall, obstructing venous flow and producing retrograde thrombosis and signs of venous stasis in the extremity (Fig. 94-1). As distal venous pressure increases, edema develops subcutaneously and in the confines of the deep fascia, producing pain.

DIAGNOSIS

The *clinical features* of venous thrombosis of the larger deep veins of the lower extremity are insidious development of pain, extensive pitting edema, and blanching (phlegmasia alba dolens). DVT develops in pregnancy (milk leg) when the uterus as well as the right common iliac artery compresses the left common iliac vein against the pelvic brim.

Mechanical changes occur in conjunction with hormonal effects that enhance coagulation and relaxation of the venous wall. Arterial flow is normal, and the blanching results from subcutaneous edema. Other factors that affect the left iliac vein include an overdistended bladder, pelvic tumors, and congenital or acquired webs within the vein. These factors explain the preponderance of left over right iliac vein involvement.

If venous thrombosis obstructs most of the venous return of an extremity, venous hypertension impairs arterial flow and produces phlegmasia cerulea dolens; the color change is due to circulatory stagnation. Symptoms begin with development of paresthesia and progress to loss of sensory and motor function. At this stage, venous gangrene is likely unless blood flow is restored.

The *physical findings* in DVT are determined by the level of venous obstruction. Edema and discoloration occur below the level of occlusion. The clinical findings are nonspecific and are mimicked by cellulitis, trauma, and other inflammatory disorders.

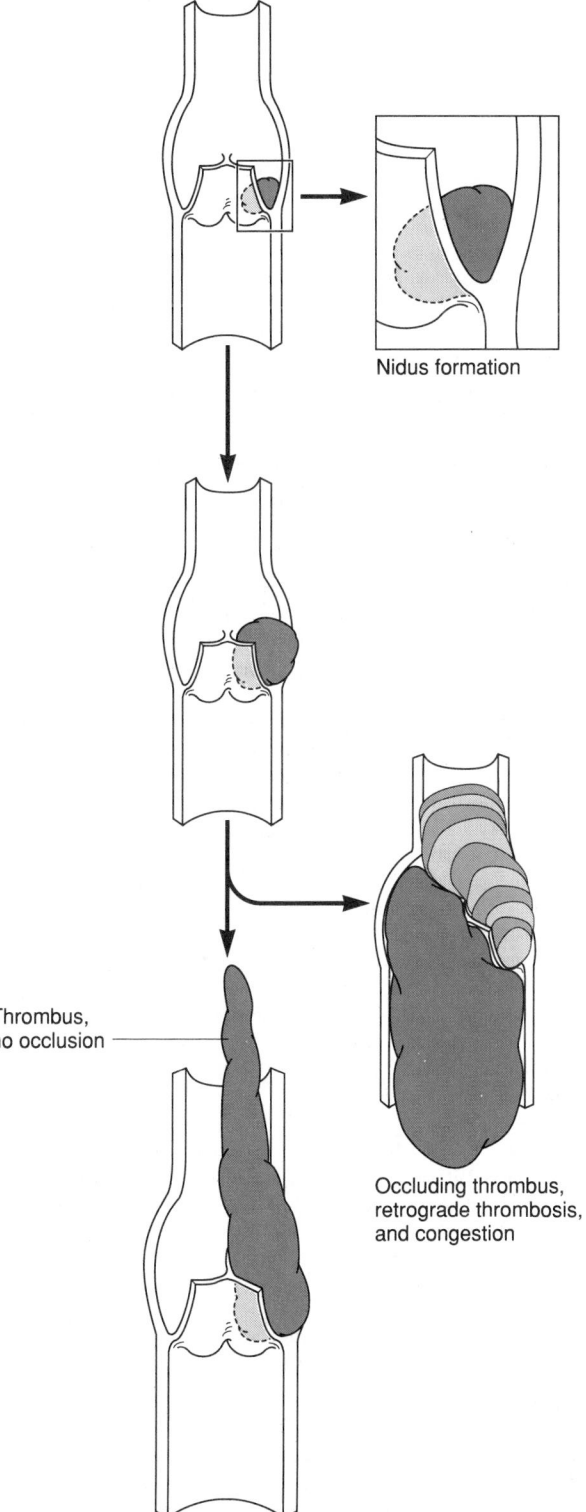

Figure 94-1. The nidus of thrombus that forms in a valvular sinus can lyse or continue to propagate. If it propagates without obstructing the lumen, it remains clinically silent and is susceptible to detachment, producing pulmonary thromboembolism. If it propagates to obstruct the lumen, it is likely to produce venous hypertension, retrograde thrombosis, and symptoms of deep venous thrombosis.

Venography

Venography was the standard for diagnosis of DVT. Contrast medium is injected into a vein in the foot. A tourniquet on the lower leg promotes filling of the deep venous system. An abnormal examination is lack of filling in the deep system with passage of contrast medium into the superficial system or demonstration of discrete filling defects (Fig. 94-2). Venography can be performed with isotope rather than contrast material and with use of a γ-scintillation counter to record flow pattern.

Ultrasound

Venous flow can be assessed with a combination of Doppler analysis and B-mode ultrasonography (US) (*duplex study*). Color-enhanced Doppler imaging adds to the speed and accuracy of the measurements. A duplex examination is the most appropriate initial screening test for suspected DVT; a normal examination safely excludes the diagnosis of DVT in the area studied.

A *Doppler probe alone* can be used to detect DVT. Lack of augmentation of flow with distal compression or release of compression proximal to the probe suggests venous thrombi. A normal Doppler study is reassuring, but abnormal or equivocal findings must be confirmed with B-mode US or contrast venography. A normal study is not reassuring when pulmonary thromboembolism is suspected—the thrombus may have left the extremity.

B-mode US allows direct visualization of venous valvular movement, accelerated blood flow in the presence of a thrombus, and imaging of the thrombus itself. Fresh thrombi are not echogenic but can be identified when pres-

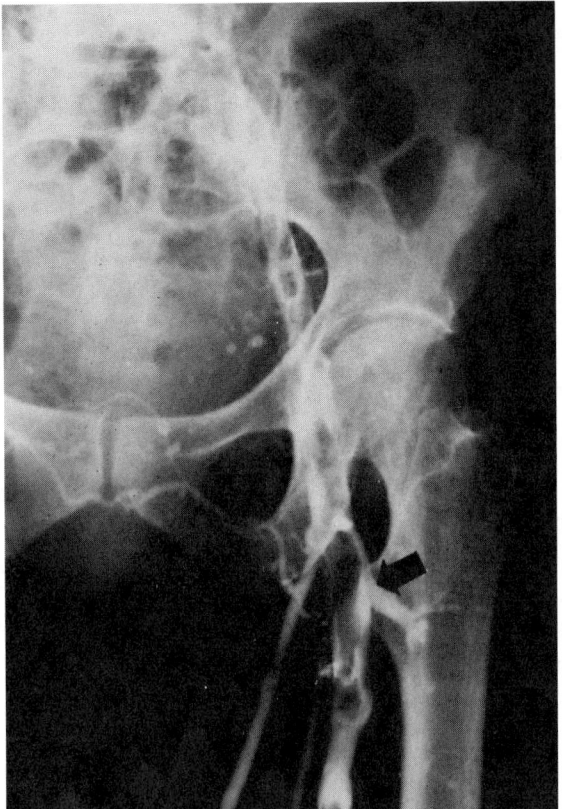

Figure 94-2. Contrast venogram showing a filling defect produced by thrombus within the femoral vein (*arrow*) and extension into the iliac veins.

sure of the probe does not compress the walls of the vein. The affected vein is larger than expected and can be compared with the vein in the opposite extremity. Chronic thrombi are echogenic and heterogeneous, and have an irregular surface (Fig. 94-3).

Impedance Plethysmography

Impedance plethysmography is used to measure the volume response of an extremity to temporary occlusion of the venous system. The diagnosis of venous thrombosis depends on changes in venous capacitance and on rate of emptying after release of the occlusion. Prolongation of the outflow wave suggests venous thrombosis. This technique does not show calf venous thrombosis or define a new abnormality in patients with old postthrombotic sequelae. Strain-gauge plethysmography is used to measure leg volume and can be used in place of the impedance technique. Accuracy depends on the absence of conditions such as cardiac failure, constrictive pericarditis, hypotension, arterial insufficiency, and external compression of veins.

Assay of Fibrin and Fibrinogen Products

Degradation of intravascular fibrin can be detected by means of measurement of the plasma products of lysis of fibrin or fibrinogen by means of radioimmunoassay. The findings are not specific for acute venous thrombosis.

PROPHYLAXIS

For surgical patients <40 years of age, risk for DVT is low. Prophylaxis is leg elevation and early walking with or without graduated compression stockings. For surgical patients older than 40 years risk is moderate, and prophy-

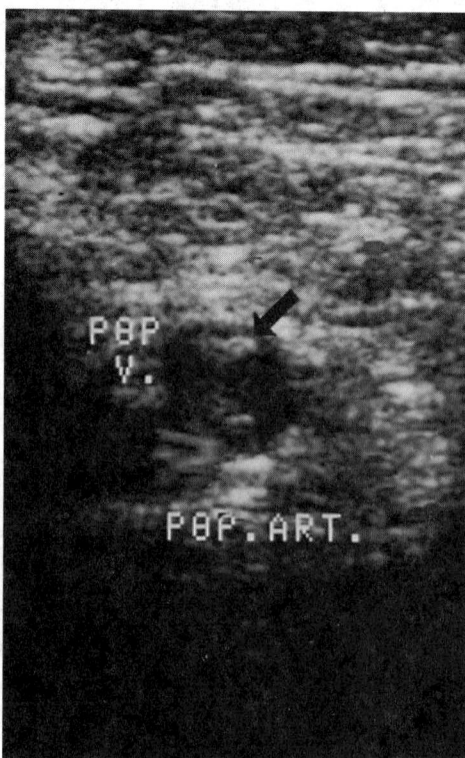

Figure 94-3. B-mode ultrasound image of the popliteal vein, showing an echogenic mature thrombus within the lumen (*arrow*).

laxis is intermittent pneumatic compression or low-dose heparin administered subcutaneously twice a day. Patients older than 40 and obese, with malignant disease, a history of DVT, or severe trauma need protection such as low-dose heparin, intermittent pneumatic compression, oral anticoagulants, or dextran.

MEDICAL TREATMENT

Treatment of a patient with DVT has three objectives: minimization of risk for pulmonary embolism, limiting further thrombosis, and facilitating resolution of existing thrombi to avoid the post-thrombotic syndrome.

The patient remains at bed rest with the foot of the bed elevated. Pain, swelling, and tenderness resolve over 4 to 5 days with anticoagulation, when walking with elastic stocking support is allowed. Standing still and sitting are prohibited to avoid venous pressure and stasis.

Anticoagulation

Systemic anticoagulation is provided first with heparin and then with warfarin for prolonged protection against recurrent thrombosis. Heparin neutralizes thrombin, inhibits thromboplastin, and reduces the platelet release reaction.

Problems associated with heparin include bleeding, thrombocytopenia, hypersensitivity, arterial thromboembolism, and osteoporosis. Arterial thromboembolism can complicate heparin administration and is common among the elderly. It occurs after 7 to 10 days of therapy and is associated with thrombocytopenia. *This complication can be fatal.* Heparin is discontinued immediately.

Oral administration of anticoagulants is begun soon after initiation of heparin therapy because it usually takes several days for prothrombin time (PT) to come within therapeutic range. A maintenance dose is preferable to a large loading dose. This avoids suppression of the natural anticoagulant, protein C. Coumarin derivatives block synthesis of several vitamin K-dependent clotting factors, and a PT longer than the suggested range is associated with bleeding complications. Administration of fresh frozen plasma rather than vitamin K usually restores PT.

After an episode of acute DVT, anticoagulation is maintained for a minimum of 3 months. Because drugs (eg, barbiturates) interact with coumarin derivatives, regular monitoring of PT is essential after the patient leaves the hospital. Oral anticoagulants are teratogenic and cannot be used during pregnancy or if pregnancy is being planned. Heparin is used during pregnancy.

Fibrinolysis

Fibrinolytic agents such as tissue plasminogen activator (tPA), streptokinase, and urokinase are used to activate the intrinsic plasmin system. They are, however, associated with hemorrhagic complications. Some patients treated with streptokinase have allergic reactions that vary from urticaria to anaphylaxis. Streptokinase offers no advantage over heparin in the treatment of recurrent venous thrombosis or thrombosis present >72 hours.

Lytic agents are contraindicated after an operation or trauma. Silent pulmonary embolism can occur in patients treated with tPA. Even when thrombolysis is complete, preservation of valvular function is not ensured. Catheter-directed thrombolysis with direct infusion of urokinase into the thrombus may provide lysis with minimal risk for complications.

SURGICAL APPROACHES

Surgical Thrombectomy

Thrombi are removed from the deep veins of the leg via the common femoral vein. Fogarty venous balloon catheters are used for extraction of the proximal thrombus, and an elastic wrap is used for milking the extremity to extrude the distal thrombus (Fig. 94-4). The procedure is used for limb salvage in the presence of phlegmasia cerulea dolens and impending venous gangrene.

Vena Caval Interruption

Indications
- Recurrent thromboembolism despite adequate anticoagulation
- DVT or documented thromboembolism if anticoagulation is contraindicated
- Complication of anticoagulation that forces discontinuation of therapy
- Recurrent pulmonary embolism with pulmonary hypertension and cor pulmonale
- Following pulmonary embolectomy for massive pulmonary embolism
- Device or ligation failure with recurrent embolism

Relative indications
- Occlusion of more than half of the pulmonary vascular bed and patient cannot tolerate additional embolism
- Propagating iliofemoral thrombus despite anticoagulation
- High risk and a large free-floating iliofemoral thrombus on venogram

Insertion

A Greenfield filter maintains patency after trapping emboli and allows continued flow to avoid stasis and facilitate lysis of the embolus. The filter is inserted percutaneously through the jugular or femoral vein. It is placed above the renal veins when necessary for embolism control (eg, when thrombus is within the renal veins or vena cava itself) or in the superior vena cava.

Complications

The complications of use of a filter range from minimal wound hematoma due to early resumption of anticoagulation, to lethal migration of some devices into the pulmonary artery. The most common complication is misplacement. When the filter is misplaced below the diaphragm, the patient has inadequate protection, but the location (renal or iliac vein) does not pose a circulatory problem because the filter is expected to remain patent.

Some patients have recurrent embolism after filter placement. The recurrence may be from a source of thrombus outside the filtered flow, such as the pelvic veins by way of the ovarian vein, the upper extremities, or the right atrium. Recurrent embolism is an indication for inferior venacavography to evaluate the filter for entrapped and propagating proximal thrombus. This problem is rare and can be managed with thrombolytic therapy if the amount of thrombus is small or with placement of a second filter in the suprarenal vena cava.

Capture of a large embolus within a filter can suddenly occlude the vena cava and cause a precipitous fall in blood pressure. In a patient with a known pulmonary embolism, this event can be mistaken for recurrent pulmonary embolism. *The results are disastrous if vasopressor therapy is initiated rather than fluid volume replacement.* Functional hypovolemia due to caval occlusion can be differentiated from right ventricular overload due to recurrent pulmonary embolism at the bedside by means of measurement of central venous pressure and arterial oxygen tension. A patient with vena caval occlusion responds dramatically to volume resuscitation.

PULMONARY THROMBOEMBOLISM

The most serious complication of DVT is pulmonary thromboembolism. The diagnosis can be confused with myocardial infarction (MI), pneumothorax, sepsis, or pneumonia. The disorder ranges from asymptomatic minor embolism to sudden death from massive embolism.

Pathophysiology

Although DVT precedes pulmonary embolism, a large number of patients do not have signs of venous thrombosis. Most pulmonary emboli originate from the veins of the lower extremity; the others originate in the right side of the heart or other veins. Emboli from a recent thrombus tend to be multiple, fragmenting in the right side of the heart or during impaction into the pulmonary vascular bed. Older thrombi contain laminated fibrin layers that make them solid and difficult to lyse.

Once an embolus lodges and interrupts pulmonary blood flow, the ratio of regional ventilation to perfusion increases. The lung responds with bronchoconstriction to reduce the mismatched ventilation. This response is mediated by a local reduction in carbon dioxide output. Serotonin from platelets that adhere to the embolus may contribute to the bronchoconstriction. Because heparin inhibits release of serotonin, it is administered early. Other vasoactive agents (bradykinin, histamine, prostaglandins) are also released from platelets, and the net effect is a reduction in size of peripheral airways, lung volume, and static pulmonary compliance.

The hypoxemia that characterizes embolism appears to be due to an increased alveolar–arterial oxygen gradient

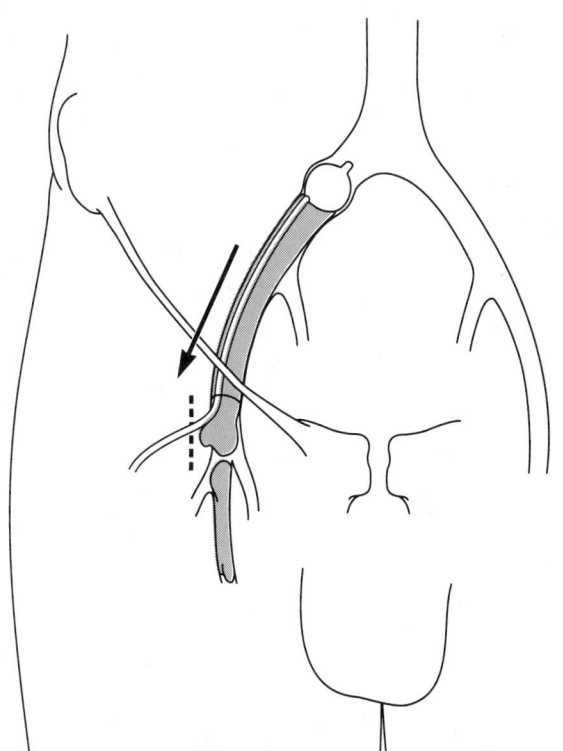

Figure 94-4. The Fogarty balloon catheter technique of venous thrombectomy allows evacuation of thrombus in the iliofemoral system proximal to the incision. Distal thrombus is evacuated by an elastic wrap that squeezes the thrombus proximally.

and reduced mixed venous P_{O_2}. Such shunting is possible if a patent foramen ovale opens in the presence of elevated right atrial pressures. Such an opening can allow passage of a venous embolus into the systemic circulation (paradoxic embolism). Although there may be some improvement in P_{aO_2} after supplemental oxygen is administered, the effects usually are minimal. The return of pulmonary blood flow effected by embolectomy restores respiratory gas exchange, but the ischemia can cause loss of capillary integrity and interstitial pulmonary edema or overt pulmonary hemorrhage.

Pulmonary infarction as a consequence of embolism is rare. It is associated with problems of poor systemic perfusion, such as shock and congestive heart failure. Symptoms include pleuritic chest pain, dyspnea, cough, and hemoptysis. Signs include fever, tachycardia, splinting, and sometimes a friction rub. There is usually prominent leukocytosis, an elevated lactic dehydrogenase level, and hyperbilirubinemia. A wedge-shaped area of density usually is present on chest radiographs.

The pulmonary vascular and cardiac effects of embolism are a direct consequence of the degree of filling of the pulmonary vascular bed. Occlusion of >30% of the vascular tree is required to elevate mean pulmonary artery pressure; >50% occlusion is required to reduce systemic arterial pressure. The degree of pulmonary hypertension is usually proportional to the extent of angiographic vascular occlusion.

Diagnosis

Clinical Presentation

The signs and symptoms (Table 94-1) of an embolic episode depend on the quantity of embolus and, to a lesser extent, on the cardiopulmonary status of the patient. The patient experiences sudden chest pain, cough, dyspnea, tachypnea, and marked anxiety. The patient has tachycardia, an increased pulmonary second sound, cyanosis, prominent jugular veins, and varying degrees of collapse. There can be wheezing, pleural friction rub, splinting of the chest wall, rales, low-grade fever, ventricular gallop, and wide splitting of the pulmonic second sound. When present, hemoptysis occurs late in the course of the disease and represents pulmonary infarction.

The differential diagnosis of pulmonary embolism includes esophageal perforation, pneumonia, septic shock, and MI, all of which are life-threatening. Laboratory studies are not specific in the differential diagnosis. A white blood cell count <15,000/μL (15' 10^9/L) can help rule out pneumonitis when a pulmonary infiltrate is present.

Electrocardiography

The most common ECG findings associated with pulmonary embolism are nonspecific ST-segment and T-wave changes. More specific signs of right ventricular overload such as the often quoted S_1-Q_3-T_3 pattern seldom occur. The primary value of the ECG is to exclude MI. The finding of MI, however, does not exclude the diagnosis of pulmonary embolism; a lung scan or pulmonary angiogram may be needed to clarify the problem.

Chest Radiography

Chest radiography helps exclude other possibilities, such as pneumonia, pneumothorax, esophageal perforation, or congestive heart failure. It is crucial in the interpretation of a lung scan because radiographic density or evidence of chronic lung or cardiac disease makes a perfusion defect less likely to represent pulmonary embolism.

Arterial Blood Gases

Frequent measurement of blood gases and pH can support the diagnosis of pulmonary embolism. Most patients have hypoxemia with P_{aO_2} <60 mmHg. The reduction in P_{aO_2} that follows severe embolism is the most discriminating finding. If concurrent hypoxemia and hypocarbia are not present, the diagnosis of embolism in a severely ill patient is unlikely.

Central Venous Pressure

For a patient with systemic hypotension, central venous pressure measurement can supply valuable information. The venous catheter also provides access for administration of drugs and fluids. A low central venous pressure virtually excludes pulmonary embolism as the cause of the hypotension. Elevated right ventricular filling pressures can be transient as hemodynamic accommodation occurs. In subacute or chronic embolism, central venous pressure can be normal.

Lung Scan

If blood pressure and a normal chest radiograph are normal, a lung scan can be performed. Validity increases as the size of the perfusion defect approaches lobar distribution. Smaller peripheral perfusion defects are difficult to interpret, because pneumonitis, atelectasis, or other ventilation abnormalities alter pulmonary perfusion. A normal lung scan usually excludes the diagnosis of pulmonary embolism.

Pulmonary Vascular Imaging

Selective pulmonary arteriography is the most accurate method of confirming the presence, size, and distribution of pulmonary emboli. A series of radiographs outline areas of decreased perfusion and usually show filling defects or the rounded trailing edge of impacted emboli (Fig. 94-5). Straight cutoffs of the smaller pulmonary arteries are difficult to interpret, particularly if there is associated chronic lung disease, which tends to obliterate pulmonary vessels. Pulmonary arterial pressures can be measured before injection of the contrast material. A normal pulmonary angiogram excludes the diagnosis of pulmonary embolism.

Dynamic contrast-enhanced *magnetic resonance angiography* allows multiplanar, rapid, dynamic visualization of the pulmonary arteries. It is an accurate method for detecting pulmonary embolism in the proximal portions of

---

Table 94-1. CLINICAL MANIFESTATIONS OF MAJOR PULMONARY EMBOLISM

Clinical Manifestations	Prevalence (%)
SYMPTOMS	
Dyspnea	80
Apprehension	60
Pleural pain	60
Cough	50
Hemoptysis	27
Syncope	22
SIGNS	
Tachypnea	88
Tachycardia	63
Accentuated P_2	60
Rales	51
S_3 or S_4	47
Pleural rub	17

(Data from Urokinase Pulmonary Embolism Trial. A national cooperative study. Circulation 1973;14[Suppl II]:86)

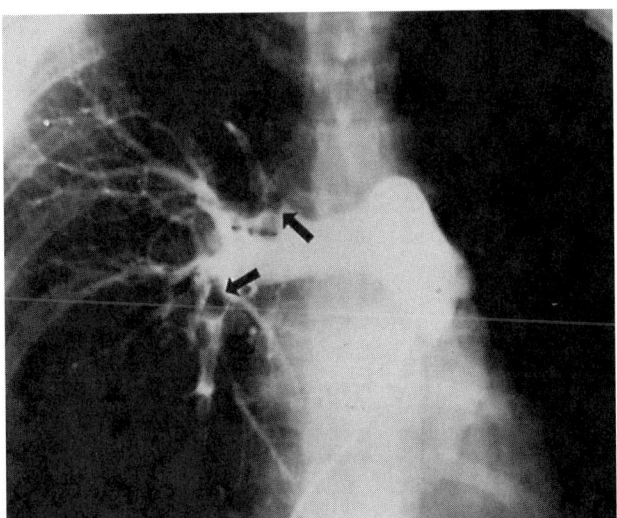

Figure 94-5. Pulmonary arteriogram demonstrating no flow to the left lung and filling defects in the right lower and upper lobar pulmonary arteries (*arrows*).

the pulmonary arteries. It does not help detect peripheral thromboembolism.

Transesophageal echocardiography can be performed at the bedside under emergency circumstances. It can be used to make or exclude the diagnosis of massive pulmonary embolism.

Management

Anticoagulation

Embolism can be classified into four grades of severity (Table 94-2). *Minor embolism* is managed with anticoagulants alone. Heparin is selected for initial treatment in a dose designed to lengthen partial thromboplastin time (PTT) to at least twice normal. Oral anticoagulation therapy usually is begun at the same time as heparin therapy to allow the drugs several days to overlap as PT enters the therapeutic range.

Thrombolytic Therapy

The advantage of thrombolytic therapy may be to improve the resolution of *major thromboembolism*. A patient who is not in shock and who has no contraindication to thrombolytic therapy would probably benefit from its use.

Plasminogen activators include streptokinase, urokinase, and tPA. The drugs are administered by means of IV infusion after a loading dose. The beneficial effects on

thromboembolism usually occur in 12 to 24 hours. Hemorrhagic side effects can occur with use of streptokinase and urokinase, and they may necessitate transfusion. Use of streptokinase is associated with allergic reactions, fever, and adult respiratory distress syndrome.

Management of Pulmonary Hypertension

Pulmonary emboli can accumulate gradually over a prolonged period if they do not undergo lysis and obliteration of the pulmonary vascular bed. Pulmonary hypertension results from the changes in the pulmonary vascular bed. The presentation can be subtle with only dyspnea or syncope on exertion, but a loud P_2 and right-sided strain are present on an ECG. The sequence can occur without respiratory symptoms. The patient may benefit from a vena caval filter to prevent further embolism. When acute cardiopulmonary decompensation occurs after embolism, embolectomy is not feasible. Some patients can undergo delayed thrombectomy or heart–lung transplantation.

Pulmonary Embolectomy

After a *massive embolism* causes systemic hypotension, survival may be only a matter of minutes. Initial management is full heparinization and administration of inotropic drugs to support the circulation while the diagnosis is confirmed with angiography. Dopamine or isoproterenol can be used for initial circulatory support.

If the patient responds to heparin sodium and does not require vasopressors to maintain systemic blood pressure or urine output, careful monitoring is essential to determine whether anticoagulation alone can control the disorder. A vena caval filter can be inserted.

Partial circulatory bypass under local anesthesia through the femoral artery and vein can provide initial support to allow general anesthesia (Fig. 94-6). Once the sternotomy is accomplished, the partial bypass can be converted to total bypass by means of a superior vena caval catheter. The pulmonary emboli can be removed through a pulmonary arteriotomy (Fig. 94-7).

Open pulmonary embolectomy is effective, but it has a high mortality rate. The most serious complication is uncontrollable pulmonary parenchymal hemorrhage, which can follow restoration of pulmonary perfusion. Open pulmonary embolectomy is used to treat patients who need closed cardiac massage to maintain blood pressure or when catheter embolectomy does not remove thrombi.

Transvenous Catheter Embolectomy

An alternative to open embolectomy during cardiopulmonary bypass is transvenous removal of pulmonary emboli under local anesthesia (Figs. 94-8, 94-9). Emboli cannot be removed if impacted >72 hours. A Greenfield vena

Table 94-2. STRATIFICATION OF PULMONARY THROMBOEMBOLISM

Category	Signs and Symptoms	Gases	PA Occlusion (%)	Hemodynamics
Minor	Anxiety Hyperventilation	$P_aO_2 < 80$ mmHg $P_aCO_2 < 35$ mmHg	20–30	Tachycardia
Major	Dyspnea Collapse	$P_aO_2 < 65$ mmHg $P_aCO_2 < 30$ mmHg	30–50	CVP elevated; PA pressure > 20 mmHg; responds to resuscitation
Massive	Dyspnea Shock	$P_aO_2 < 50$ mmHg $P_aCO_2 < 30$ mmHg	>50	CVP elevated; PA pressure > 25 mmHg; requires pressors, inotropes
Chronic	Dyspnea Syncope	$P_aO_2 < 70$ mmHg P_aCO_2 30–40 mmHg	>50	CVP elevated; PA pressure > 40 mmHg; fixed low cardiac output

CVP, central venous pressure; PA, pulmonary artery.

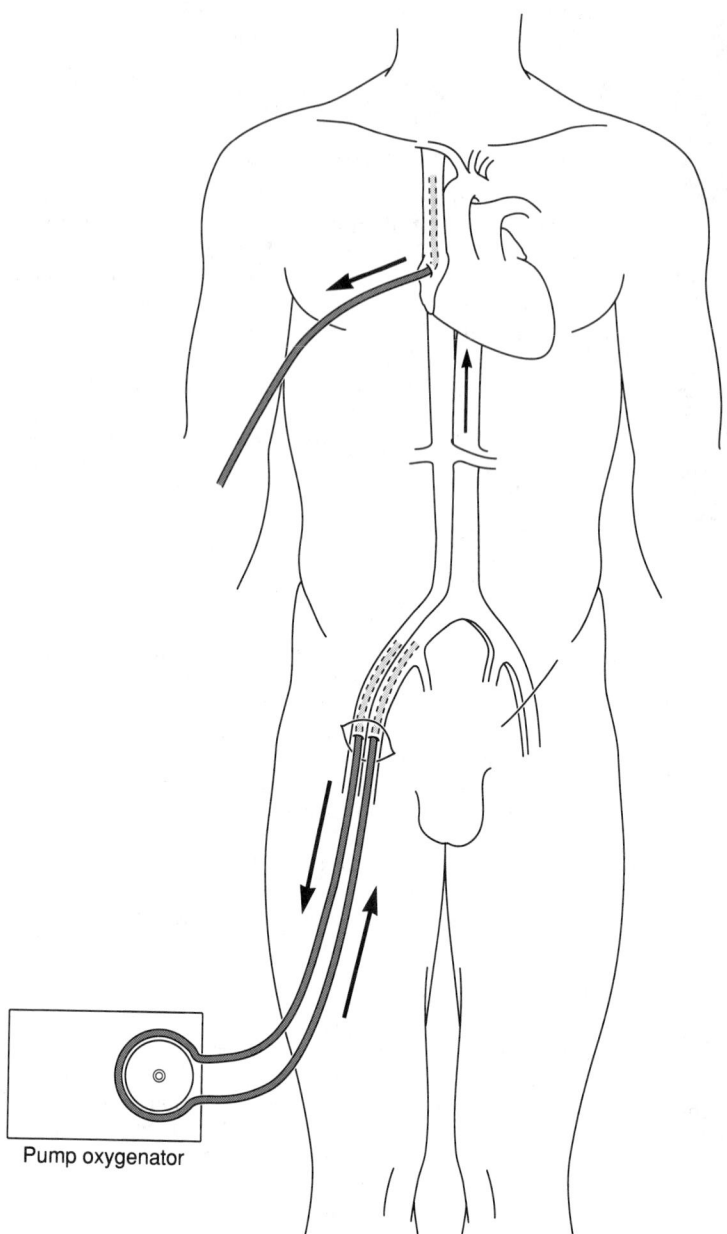

Figure 94-6. For a deteriorating patient with massive pulmonary embolism and systemic hypotension, circulatory support can be achieved by cannulation of the femoral artery and vein under local anesthesia for partial cardiopulmonary bypass. The patient can then tolerate general anesthesia and sternotomy, which allows insertion of a superior vena caval cannula for total bypass and pulmonary embolectomy (see Fig. 94-7).

Pump oxygenator

caval filter can be placed after removal of sufficient emboli to produce near-normal hemodynamics to protect patients from recurrent embolism.

Management of Chronic Pulmonary Embolism and Pulmonary Hypertension

Recurrent thromboembolism can lead to progressive obliteration of the pulmonary vascular bed if the thrombi do not undergo lysis. The resultant pulmonary hypertension produces exertional dyspnea and signs of right heart strain with cor pulmonale. With progression of right heart overload, tricuspid insufficiency can develop. This disorder can be difficult to differentiate from primary pulmonary hypertension.

Open thrombectomy for chronic pulmonary artery occlusion is a means of improving pulmonary blood flow. For the procedure to be feasible, the occlusion must involve the proximal portion of the pulmonary arterial tree, and the distal bed must be patent.

OTHER TYPES OF VENOUS THROMBOSIS

Thrombophlebitis

Thrombophlebitis is a disorder of the superficial veins characterized by aseptic local inflammation. In the upper extremity the usual cause is IV infusion of acidic fluid or prolonged cannulation. In the lower extremity the usual cause is varicose veins. Risk for venous thrombosis due to injection of contrast material can be minimized by means of washout of the contrast material with heparinized saline solution.

Thrombophlebitis Migrans

Thrombophlebitis migrans (recurrent superficial thrombophlebitis) is associated with malignant visceral tumors, systemic collagen vascular disease, and blood dyscrasias. The deep veins and visceral veins may be involved.

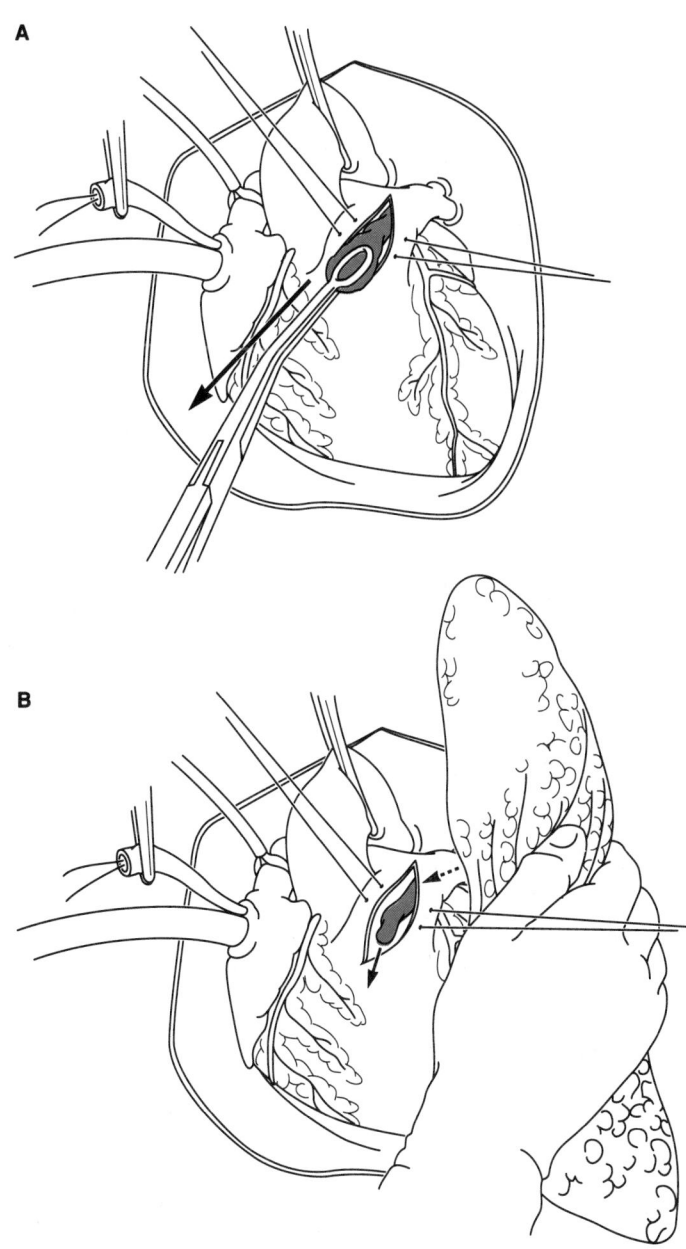

Figure 94-7. (*A*) A patient with massive pulmonary embolism on total cardiopulmonary bypass (see Fig. 94-8) can undergo pulmonary embolectomy through the opened main pulmonary artery. (*B*) More peripheral emboli can be retrieved by balloon embolectomy and compression of the lung.

Subclavian Venous Thrombosis

Subclavian venous thrombosis is often caused by an indwelling catheter. It can also occur as a primary event in a young, athletic person (effort thrombosis), presumably as a result of injury at the thoracic outlet. Late treatment is elevation and anticoagulation. Venous insufficiency and discomfort with exercise can persist. Pulmonary thromboembolism can result from these thrombi.

Use of the axillary and subclavian veins for diagnostic and therapeutic procedures can cause traumatic and foreign body thrombosis. Often these thrombi are asymptomatic because of gradual onset, short-segment involvement, or only partial occlusion. Thrombolytic therapy can be considered for any acute subclavian venous thrombosis within 3 to 4 days of onset. If the thrombus lyses, a contrast venogram is obtained to outline any anatomic site of compression that can be managed surgically.

Direct thrombectomy can be performed through a first rib or medial clavicular excision. This procedure is considered for young patients and people who perform manual labor. Thrombectomy is performed in conjunction with construction of an ipsilateral arteriovenous fistula for angioaccess if there is proximal venous thrombosis.

Abdominal Venous Thrombosis

Thrombosis of the inferior vena cava can result from tumor invasion or propagating thrombus from the iliac veins or ligation, plication, or insertion of occluding caval devices.

Thrombosis of the *renal vein* is associated with the nephrotic syndrome. It can be a source of thromboembolism and is managed by means of suprarenal placement of a Greenfield filter.

Portal venous thrombosis occurs in neonates because of propagating septic thrombophlebitis of the umbilical vein. Collateral development leads to esophageal varices. Thrombosis of the portal, hepatic, splenic, or superior mesenteric vein in an adult is associated with hepatic cirrhosis.

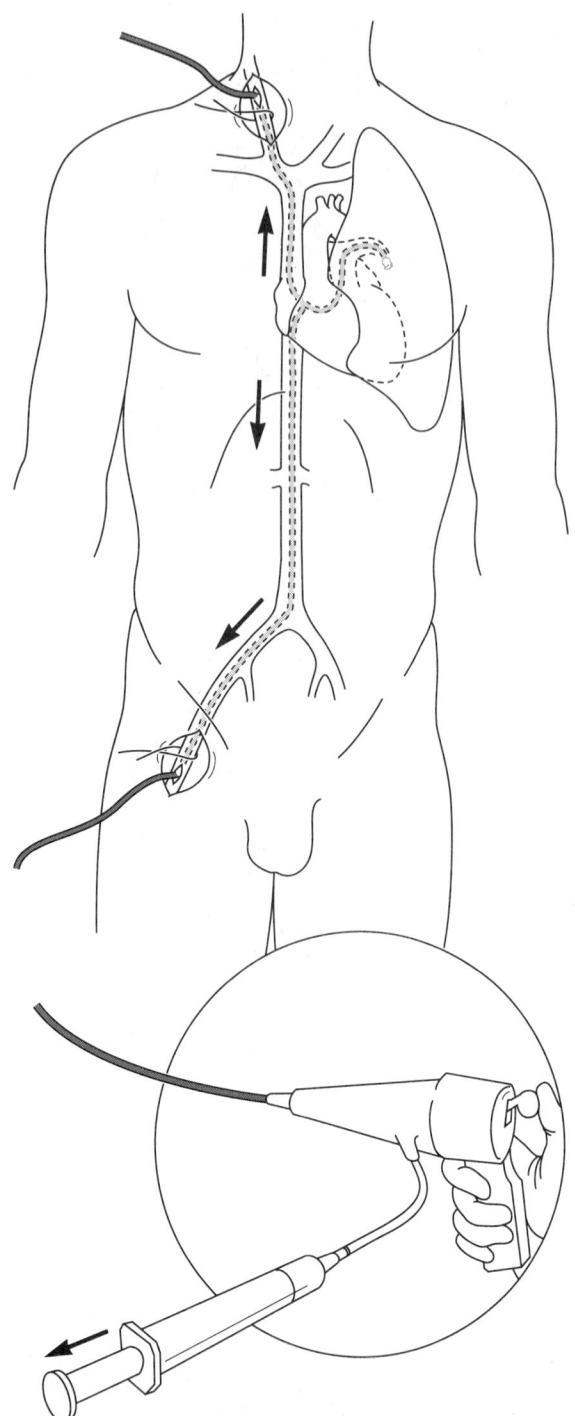

Figure 94-8. Access for catheter pulmonary embolectomy can be obtained under local anesthesia from either the right jugular vein or the femoral vein. The steerable cup-catheter is then positioned under fluoroscopy in proximity to the embolus. Syringe suction is applied to capture the embolus within the cup, which is then withdrawn.

Thrombosis of *mesenteric or omental veins* can simulate an acute abdomen but usually results in prolonged ileus rather than intestinal infarction.

Hepatic venous thrombosis (Budd–Chiari syndrome) produces massive hepatomegaly, ascites, and liver failure. Treatment is a side-to-side portacaval shunt for decompression of the liver or liver transplantation.

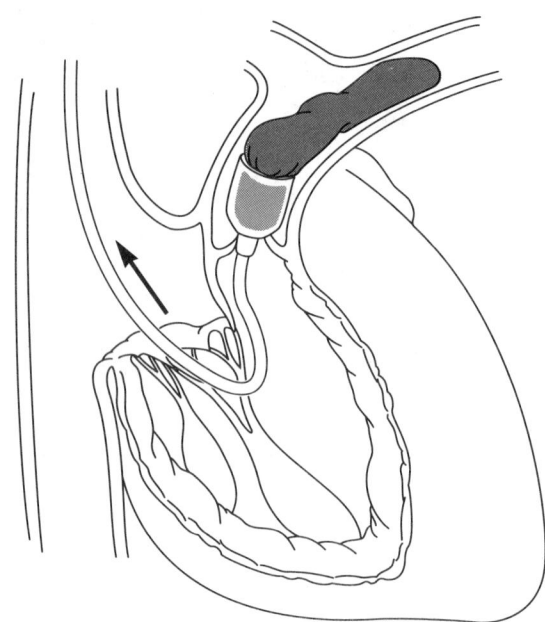

Figure 94-9. Once the embolus is captured within the embolectomy catheter cup (see Fig. 94-8), the catheter is withdrawn while syringe suction is maintained to hold on to the embolus.

The development of pelvic sepsis after abortion, tubal infection, or puerperal sepsis can lead to septic thrombophlebitis of the *pelvic veins* and septic thromboembolism. Management is drainage or excision of the abscess and antibiotic therapy. A Greenfield filter also can be used, if necessary.

SUGGESTED READING

Clagett GP. Prevention of postoperative venous thromboembolism: an update. Am J Surg 1994;168:515.

Greenfield LJ, Proctor MC, Williams DM, Wakefield TW. Long-term experience with transvenous catheter pulmonary embolectomy. J Vasc Surg 1993;18:450.

Imperiale TF, Speroff T. A meta-analysis of methods to prevent venous thromboembolism following total hip replacement. JAMA 1994;271:1780.

Moliterno DJ, Lange RA, Gerard RD, Willard JE, Lackner C, Hillis LD. Influence of intranasal cocaine on plasma constituents associated with endogenous thrombosis and thrombolysis. Am J Med 1994;96:492.

Moser KM, Fedullo PF, LittleJohn JK, Crawford R. Frequent asymptomatic pulmonary embolism in patients with deep venous thrombosis. JAMA 1994;271:223.

Quinn RJ, Nour R, Butler SP, et al. Pulmonary embolism in patients with intermediate probability lung scans: diagnosis with Doppler venous US and D-dimer measurement. Radiology 1994;190:509.

Semba CP, Dake MD. Iliofemoral deep venous thrombosis: aggressive therapy with catheter-directed thrombolysis. Radiology 1994;191:487.

Sreeram N, Cheriex EC, Smeets JLRM, Gorgels AP, Wellens HJJ. Value of the 12-lead electrocardiogram at hospital admission in the diagnosis of pulmonary embolism. Am J Cardiol 1994;73:298.

Sullivan TM, Martinez BD, Lemmon G, Clark PM, Schwartz RA, Bondy B. Clinical experience with the Greenfield filter in 193 patients and description of a new technique for operative insertion. J Am Coll Surg 1994;178:117.

Voorberg J, Roelse J, Koopman R, et al. Association of idiopathic venous thromboembolism with single point-mutation at Arg[506] of factor V. Lancet 1994;343:1535.

ESSENTIALS OF SURGERY: SCIENTIFIC PRINCIPLES AND PRACTICE,
edited by Lazar J. Greenfield, Michael W. Mulholland, Keith T. Oldham, Gerald B. Zelenock,
and Keith D. Lillemoe. Lippincott–Raven Publishers, Philadelphia, © 1997.

CHAPTER 95

CHRONIC VENOUS INSUFFICIENCY

LAZAR J. GREENFIELD

Chronic venous insufficiency is a disabling disorder that produces aching, edema, and ulceration in the lower extremities. About 5% of the population has stasis changes in the lower leg, and more than 500,000 people suffer chronic venous ulcers.

PATHOPHYSIOLOGY

When a person is standing, large hydrostatic pressure loads oppose the return of venous blood from the lower extremities. Venous valves support hydrostatic pressure, facilitating unidirectional venous return in response to pumping by the calf muscles. These bicuspid valves also direct flow from the superficial veins into the deep venous system by way of the perforating veins. Valvular incompetence in the superficial veins produces varicose veins, and venous malformations can cause skin changes and venous insufficiency.

In the absence of normal venous valvular function, chronic venous insufficiency is caused by reflux of blood into the superficial system through incompetent perforating veins. This reflux is compounded by muscle contraction, which pushes blood distally within the incompetent deep system. Walking then does not produce a normal decrease in venous pressure; instead it causes ambulatory venous hypertension.

Under normal circumstances it takes more than 20 to 30 seconds after cessation of exercise for venous pressure to return to resting levels by means of distal refill. In chronic venous insufficiency, proximal reflux causes a rapid increase in pressure after exercise stops. Lack of valvular function usually is caused by damage due to venous thrombosis with or without proximal venous obstruction; it also may be due to congenital absence of valves.

Chronic venous hypertension increases hydrostatic pressure at the capillary level, causing transudation of fluid and protein and diapedesis of erythrocytes. Hemosiderin from these erythrocytes causes typical brownish skin pigmentation. Excessive melanocyte activity due to chronic inflammation may contribute to the discoloration. Chronic dermatitis (*venous eczema*) develops and produces pruritus. The histologic features are increased capillary proliferation, fat necrosis, and fibrosis in skin and subcutaneous tissue (*lipodermatosclerosis*). The condition may even progress to calcification, which is seen on radiographs.

The capillaries show perivascular layering with fibrin and fibrinogen, a result of increased extravasation in the presence of venous hypertension. Fibrinolysis in the area is impaired because of decreased levels of fibrinolytic activator and the presence of a fibrinolytic inhibitor. The latter is a primary systemic defect that occurs in patients with a history of deep venous thrombosis (DVT). The pericapillary fibrin layer may act as a barrier to oxygen transport to the cells, resulting in slow tissue death and replacement by scar tissue. At the least, it impairs wound healing. A more recent concept is that leukocyte trapping with stasis,

obstruction to flow, extravasation of toxic products, and anoxia produce inflammation and tissue necrosis.

Although the lymphatic vessels in the area of lipodermatosclerosis may be abnormally permeable, total lymphatic return from an extremity with venous hypertension is two or three times normal. The lymphatic contribution to the disorder is caused by changes in skin and subcutaneous tissues. Venous ulcers usually occur on the medial aspect of the leg above the ankle, where venous pressure is highest close to a perforating vein. The skin around the ulcer is indurated, and there may be adjacent cellulitis.

If venous obstruction persists after an episode of DVT or for any other mechanical reason, persistent lower extremity edema may be complicated by disabling pain with exercise. This venous claudication is produced by elevated interstitial pressure in the muscle and fascial compartments of the extremity from the hyperemia of exercise. Extensive subcutaneous venous collaterals over the leg and trunk are demonstrated with venography. Segmental arterial pressure is measured to ensure there is no arterial insufficiency.

DIAGNOSIS

A patient with the possible diagnosis of chronic venous insufficiency is examined in both the upright and supine positions, and the location of edema is recorded. Venous stasis can be differentiated from lymphedema according to whether the foot and toes are involved; such involvement is a characteristic of lymphedema. Venous stasis edema begins at the ankle and extends to involve the lower leg and sometimes the thigh. Superficial varicosities may or may not be present depending on the competence of perforating veins. Venous ulcers usually occur on the posteromedial aspect of the lower leg but may occur on the lateral aspect or in multiple locations.

Noninvasive Studies

Often the diagnosis of chronic venous insufficiency is made on the basis of patient history and examination. The value of noninvasive venous studies is that they allow one to confirm the diagnosis, measure the extent of the disorder, establish a baseline from which to measure future changes, and determine which patients may be candidates for a corrective procedure.

Photoplethysmography

At photoplethysmography infrared light (805 nm) is used to measure the rate of venous capillary refill in the skin after emptying after exercise. The volume of cutaneous blood changes in proportion to ambulatory venous pressure, showing rapid refilling in the presence of reflux. Photoplethysmography cannot be used to measure blood flow.

A probe is fixed to the medial aspect of the calf 10 to 12.5 cm above the medial malleolus. A tourniquet can be used to differentiate superficial from deep venous insufficiency but not to isolate the level of deep venous valve dysfunction. The patient sits with his or her feet resting on the floor and performs heel raises without weight bearing. The refilling time is measured in seconds or to 50% maximum (Fig. 95-1).

Outflow Plethysmography

Venous volume of the lower extremity can be measured by means of impedance, strain-gauge, or air plethysmography (APG). Application of a proximal tourniquet with compression above resting venous pressure increases leg volume as the leg becomes congested. With release of

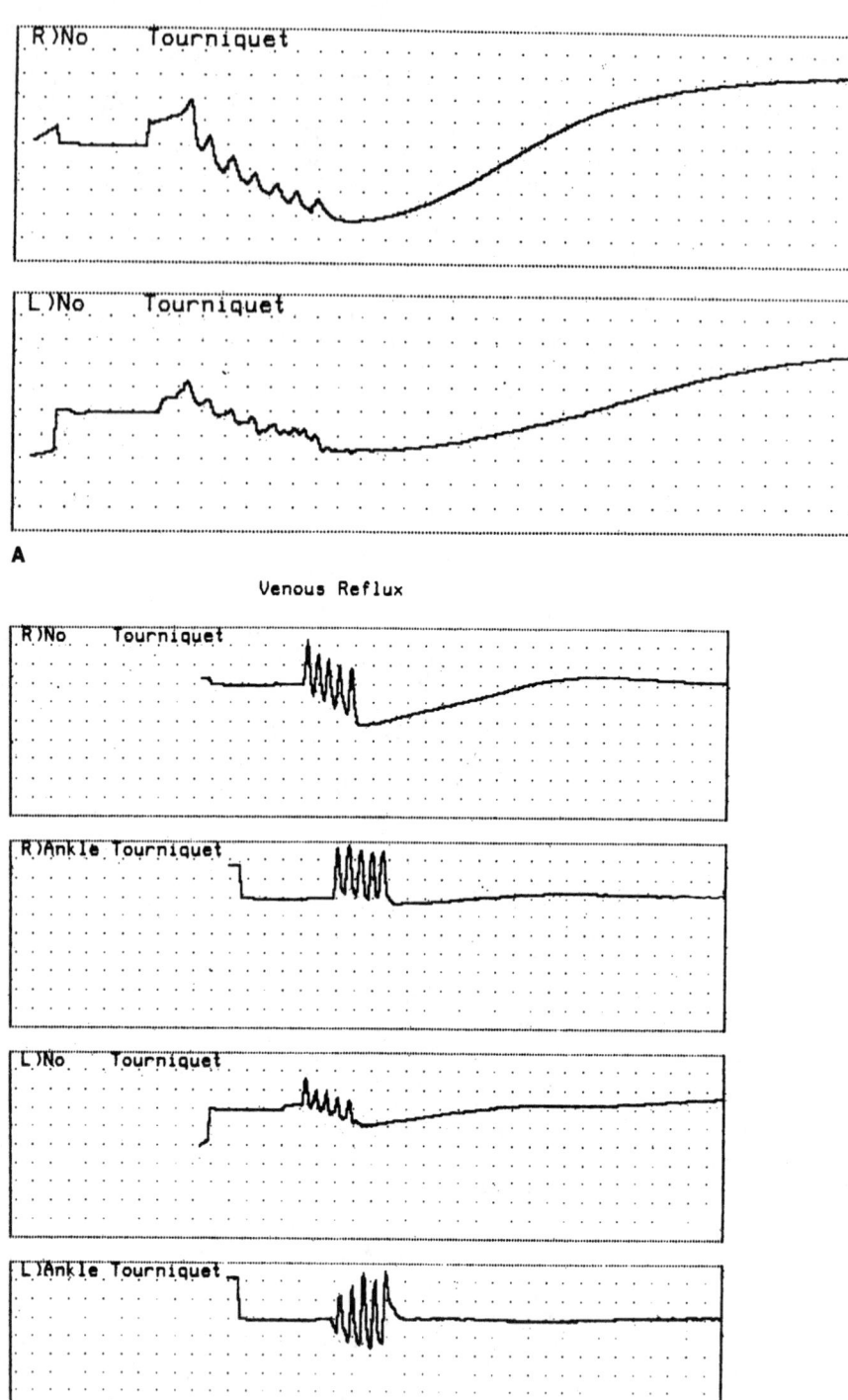

Figure 95-1. (A) Photoplethysmographic (PPG) tracing showing decreases in cutaneous blood volume with calf muscle exercise followed by gradual recovery over 18 seconds as a normal response in both lower extremities in the absence of a tourniquet. (B) PPG tracing showing deep venous insufficiency in both lower extremities as reflected by minimal decreases in cutaneous blood volume with exercise and rapid refilling time (10 seconds) unimproved by the addition of a tourniquet.

the tourniquet, there should be a rapid return to baseline with a 50% reduction within 2 seconds. Any obstruction to venous return, intraluminal or extraluminal, retards outflow and prolongs emptying time.

APG is the most valuable test of venous function because it is a measurement of calf venous volume changes in response to active and passive maneuvers in the supine and erect positions. The venous filling index is a measurement of the volume of blood that refluxes into the calf as the

best index of overall valvular incompetence. Calf ejection fraction and residual volume fraction are measurements of calf muscle pump effectiveness and residual volume in the calf after 10 heel raises.

Doppler Study

A bidirectional Doppler ultrasound examination is used to assess direction of flow in accessible veins, such as the saphenous, femoral, and popliteal. Accelerated flow pro-

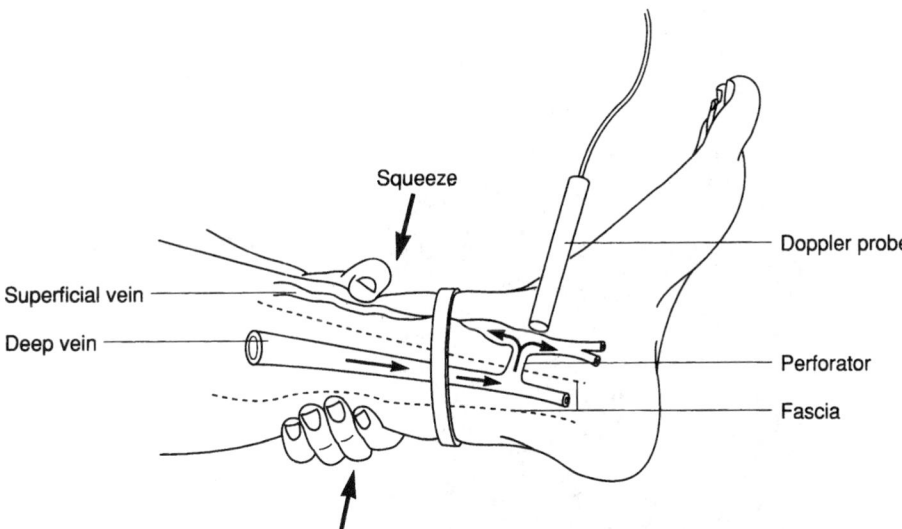

Figure 95-2. The bidirectional Doppler probe detects incompetent perforating veins when superficial venous flow is arrested by the tourniquet and deep venous pressure is increased by squeezing the leg above the tourniquet. Reflux also depends on incompetence of the deep vein valves.

duced with transient obstruction above the level insonated or with compression below confirms patency and the absence of an obstructing thrombus. Reversal of flow occurs when the valves are incompetent. False-positive results can occur when collateral veins are insonated. Incompetent perforator veins can be identified with use of a tourniquet and compression above the tourniquet to test the competency of the deep system (Fig. 95-2).

Duplex Colorflow Scan

Duplex scans combine B-mode ultrasound imaging and pulsed Doppler analysis of flow. It allows accurate assessment of both superficial and deep venous systems in chronic venous insufficiency. The addition of color flow study allows imaging of forward or reverse flow in real time. When rapid inflation and deflation cuffs are used in the standing position, the major veins can be interrogated and the extent of reflux documented according to duration, peak, and reverse blood flow velocities after cuff deflation. Knowledge of venous diameter allows quantitative estimation of reflux. It is used to measure the effectiveness of venous valvular reconstruction. Combining duplex evaluation with APG provides a physiologic approach to the definition and location of the venous disorder (Fig. 95-3).

Invasive Studies

Contrast Venography

Contrast venography is used to determine the presence or absence of normal or abnormal valves, the extent of abnormality of the veins, and the estimated amount of ve-

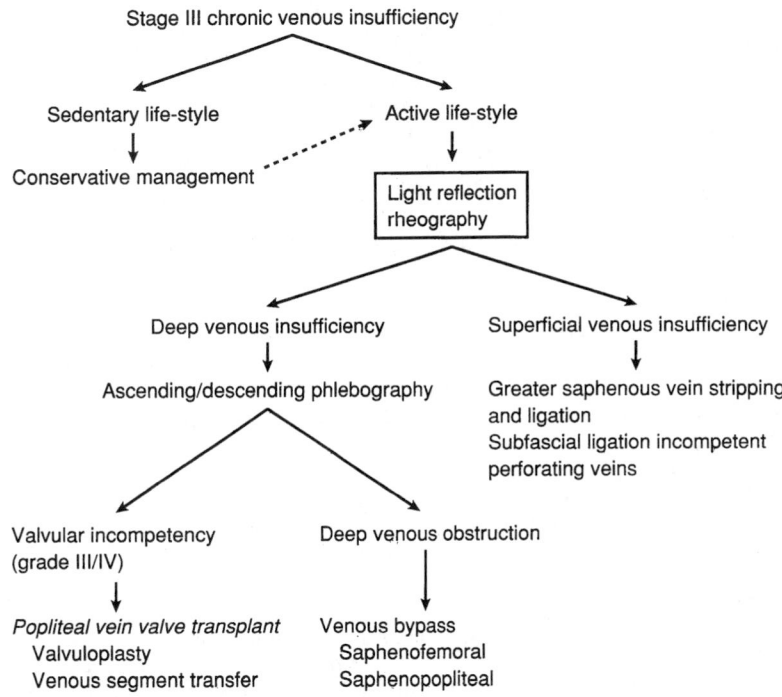

Figure 95-3. Algorithm for the management of chronic venous insufficiency using air plethysmography and duplex scanning. (After Ernst CB, Stanley JC. Current therapy in vascular surgery, ed 3. St Louis, CV Mosby, 1995:918)

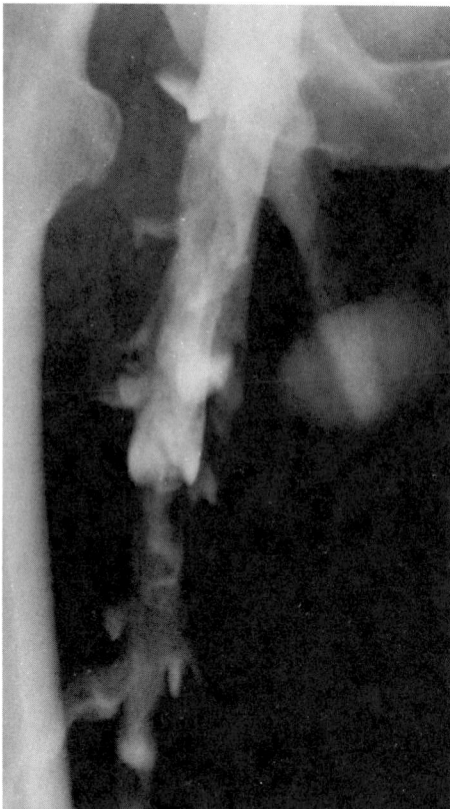

Figure 95-4. Contrast venography can be used to measure venous reflux by proximal injection while the patient is tilted upright or is increasing venous pressure by the Valsalva maneuver. Contrast medium was injected above the inguinal ligament in this case, which shows reflux into both superficial and profunda veins, indicating valvular incompetence. The most severe grade of reflux occurs when contrast is seen below the knee.

nous reflux. Reflux is induced by means of table tilting or injection of contrast medium into an iliac vein while the patient does a Valsalva maneuver. Reflux is graded according to how far distally the contrast material is seen; the most severe grade is contrast material below the level of the knee (Fig. 95-4). In addition to descending venography, ascending venography is performed by means of injection of contrast medium into the foot to demonstrate the status of veins below the knee for evidence of thrombus, recanalized veins, and incompetent perforating veins. Contrast medium can be thrombogenic unless it is washed out of the extremity with a flush of heparinized saline solution. Nonionic contrast materials of lower osmolality are less thrombogenic.

Ambulatory Venous Pressure

Ambulatory venous pressure is measured by means of venipuncture on the dorsum of the foot. Calf exercise by means of heel raises normally reduces venous pressure and is followed by gradual refilling. Without normal valves or an effective calf pump, the pressure drop is diminished and the rate of refilling is rapid, producing a short recovery time. Ambulatory venous pressure correlates with stasis ulceration when the pressure is >60 mmHg. The risk of ulceration is negligible if the pressure can be maintained <45 mmHg.

MANAGEMENT

The foundation of management of chronic venous insufficiency is patient education and graded support with elastic stockings. The patient needs to understand the hydro-

static effects of standing and the advantages of elevating the legs above heart level. The optimal elastic stocking is calf length with a compression pressure of 30 to 50 mmHg at the ankle. The stockings are fitted when the legs are not edematous. Patients are instructed to put on the stockings each day when they arise after the legs have been elevated overnight.

Primary Venous Incompetence

Congenital absence of venous valves is a rare abnormality that can occur in both upper and lower extremities. Valve ring dilatation with valvular incompetence is more

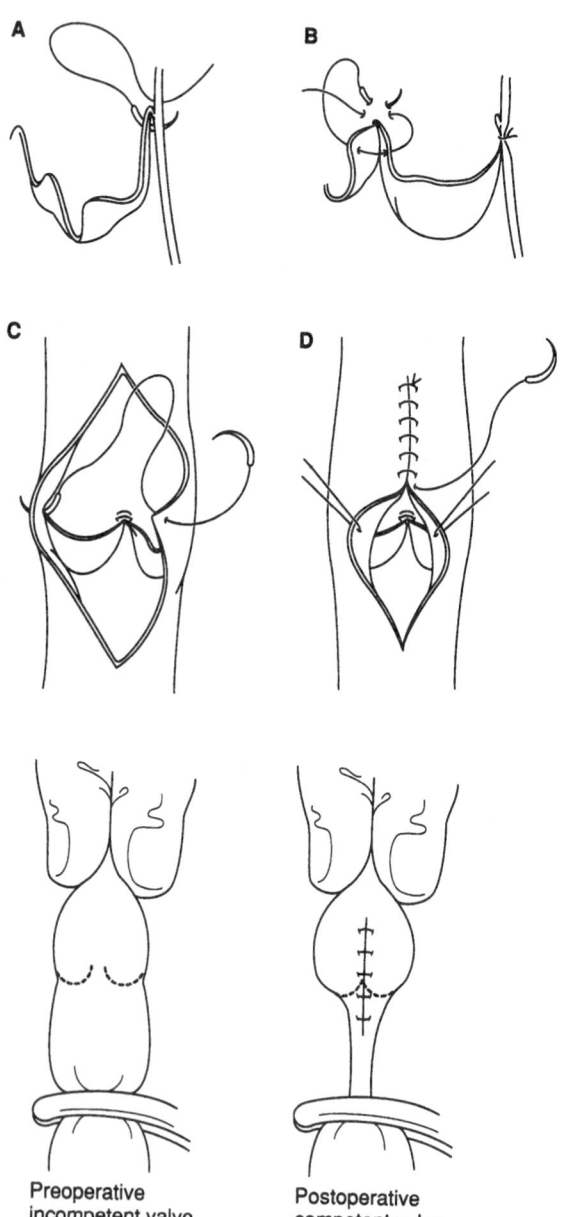

Preoperative incompetent valve   Postoperative competent valve

Figure 95-5. (*A* and *B*) Direct repair of an incompetent floppy valve can be accomplished by shortening the face edges of the valve cusp at the commissures. (*C*) To achieve this access, it is necessary to open the vein precisely at one commissure. (*D*) After closure, the competency of the valve can be tested by proximal compression of the distally occluded vein. (After Bergan J, Yao J, eds. Operative techniques in vascular surgery. Orlando, Grune & Stratton, 1980)

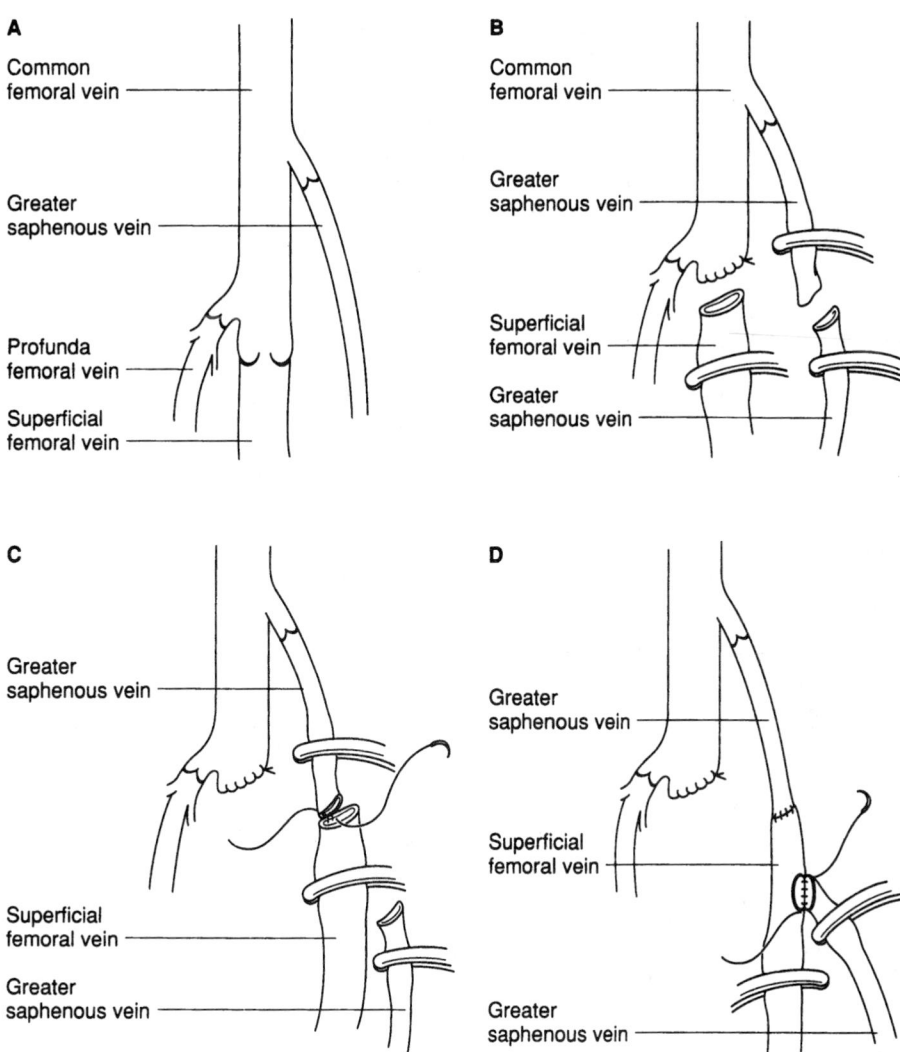

Figure 95-6. Functional venous competency can be restored by transposing an incompetent superficial femoral vein (SFV; *A*) to the divided greater saphenous vein (GSV; *B* and *C*), which has a competent proximal valve. The distal GSV is then reattached to the SFV (*D*). (After Bergan J, Yao J, eds. Operative techniques in vascular surgery. Orlando, FL, Grune & Stratton, 1980)

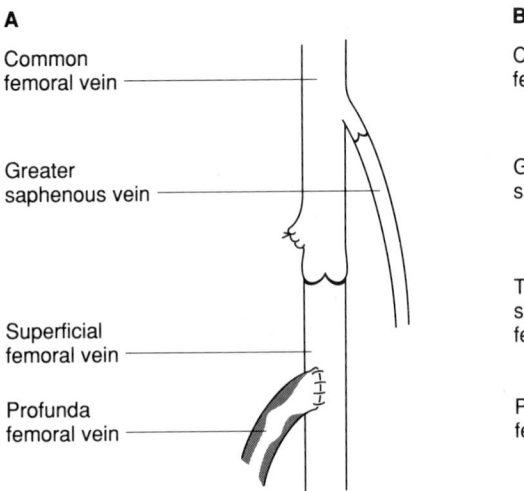
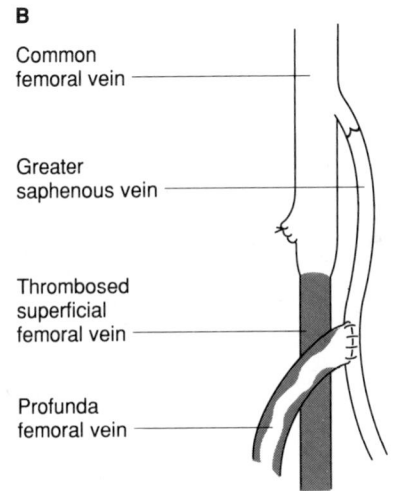

Figure 95-7. The transposition procedure can also be used with a stenotic and incompetent profunda femoral vein (*A*) attached to a competent superficial femoral vein (*B*) or, if that vein is thrombosed, to the competent greater saphenous vein (*B*).

common in superficial than deep veins. It can occur during overdistention of the vein (eg, distal to an arteriovenous fistula or during pregnancy). Changes in the valves that produce thickening or fixation usually are postthrombotic, but these changes occur without a history of venous thrombosis and may be due to other, unknown abnormal events.

Primary venous valve prolapse due to a floppy valve appears to result from a congenital abnormality that leads to lengthening of the free edge of the valve cusp. This allows the valve to evert, rendering it incompetent. In this situation, it may be possible to repair the valve with a plication technique that restores normal length and support for the valve leaflet (Fig. 95-5).

If there are no suitable valves, vein segment transfer or transposition with autologous venous valve transplantation can be attempted. In the transposition procedure, a vein segment in the extremity with normal valvular function is identified and becomes the recipient of flow from the incompetent vein when it is implanted distal to the competent valve. For example, an incompetent superficial femoral vein can be divided and reattached to a competent greater saphenous vein to take advantage of the valvular support in the saphenous system (Fig. 95-6). Combinations of vein transpositions can be used with or without associated valvular repairs (Fig. 95-7). Lack of an adjacent, available, competent vein is an indication for venous valve transplantation. This procedure is considered investigational.

Venous Ulceration

Chronic venous stasis ulcers tend to remain unhealed for many years. With standard therapy of paste bandages and elastic compression, most heal. The others are managed with split-thickness skin grafts with or without ligation of adjacent perforating veins. The ulcers have a high rate of recurrence, however, depending on how well the patient maintains elastic stocking support. The best results are obtained with a totally occlusive dressing combined with graded elastic support. Antibacterial agents, antiseptics, or enzymes are not needed in the management of stasis ulcers. When skin grafts are used, it is advisable to fenestrate the graft or to use mesh or pinch grafts to allow evacuation of serous wound drainage.

The patient remains at bed rest until the ulcer is completely healed. The most useful measures to prevent ulcer recurrence include saphenous vein ligation when this system is incompetent, ligation of perforating veins, permanent elastic stocking support, and use of stanozolol to enhance fibrinolytic activity.

Venous Obstruction

Most venous obstruction is postthrombotic, although the same clinical features can be produced by tumors in the pelvis and by structural changes such as iliac artery compression of the left common iliac vein. Because collateral circulation usually improves over time, few patients undergo bypass procedures. If needed, the most common procedure is saphenous vein crossover grafting (Fig. 95-8). The saphenous vein is mobilized from the normal contralateral extremity, divided distally, tunneled suprapubically, and anastomosed to the femoral vein. Because of the high failure rate with this procedure, some surgeons use prosthetic graft material for the bypass.

Because prosthetic grafts are thrombogenic in the venous system, a temporary arteriovenous fistula often is used to promote flow and patency until a compatible graft lining is developed. Venous bypass of the inferior vena cava with externally supported PTFE grafts is an example. External ring support of the graft is necessary to prevent compression by abdominal pressure. An arteriovenous fistula is needed for the graft to remain patent.

When venous bypass is being considered with a fistula, the ankle-arm pressure index should be >0.75 to avoid arterial insufficiency, and the fistula diameter should not be >4 mm to avoid distal venous hypertension, valvular damage, and overload of cardiac output. Arteriovenous fistulas also dilate collateral veins, which remain effective when the fistula is closed after 2 or 3 months. Closure of the fistula is facilitated by leaving a ligature around the fistula in the subcutaneous tissue, where it can be retrieved under local anesthesia, or percutaneous radiological procedures may be used for permanent occlusion, usually by an occlusive balloon.

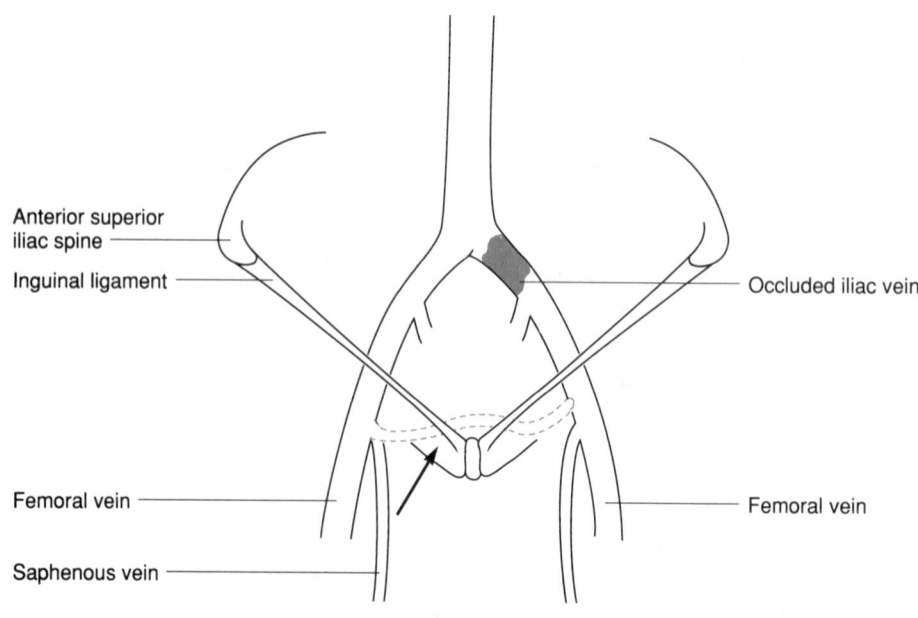

Anterior superior iliac spine

Inguinal ligament

Occluded iliac vein

Femoral vein

Femoral vein

Saphenous vein

Figure 95-8. Chronic iliofemoral venous obstruction can be relieved by using the saphenous vein from the contralateral normal leg as a bypass graft. The vein is mobilized and divided distally, then tunneled behind the pubis (*arrow*) for attachment to the obstructed femoral vein.

SUGGESTED READING

Browse NL, Burnand KG, Thomas ML, eds. Diseases of the veins: pathology, diagnosis and treatment. London, Edward Arnold, 1988.

Husni EA. Reconstruction of veins: the need for objectivity. J Cardiovasc Surg 1983;24:525.

ESSENTIALS OF SURGERY: SCIENTIFIC PRINCIPLES AND PRACTICE,
edited by Lazar J. Greenfield, Michael W. Mulholland, Keith T. Oldham, Gerald B. Zelenock, and Keith D. Lillemoe. Lippincott–Raven Publishers, Philadelphia, © 1997.

CHAPTER 96

LYMPHATIC SYSTEM DISORDERS

LAZAR J. GREENFIELD

ANATOMY AND FUNCTION

There are paired lymph sacs in the neck and lumbar region by the sixth week of gestation and a developing cisterna chyli by the eighth week. Communicating channels connect these systems to form the thoracic duct by means of merger of the right lymphatic duct with the left across the fourth to sixth thoracic vertebrae to connect with and drain into the left subclavian vein. Smaller lymphatic ducts drain into the right subclavian vein.

Developmental arrest or abnormalities result in primary *hypoplasia* or absence of ducts and lymph nodes. Abnormal growth of jugular lymph sacs produces unilocular or multilocular lymph cysts called *cystic hygromas*. These cysts occur most often in the neck but also occur in the axilla, mediastinum, retroperitoneum, and intestinal mesentery. *Hyperplastic* changes can occur and produce lymphangiomas with or without other vascular malformations.

Lymphatic capillaries collect fluid and protein from the extravascular spaces. This is a great responsibility because >50% of the circulating albumin is lost into the interstitial space every 24 hours. During this period, as much as 1.8 kg of lymph is returned to the venous system. In addition to the proteins that cannot be reabsorbed by the venules, red cells, bacteria, and other large particles are evacuated only through the lymphatics. This permeability is facilitated by the absence of a basement membrane beneath the lymphatic endothelial cells. Lymphatic capillaries are present beneath the epidermis in the superficial dermis. These vessels drain into valved channels in the deep dermis and subdermal tissues, forming larger channels that follow the vascular pathways superficial to the deep fascia. Lymphatics are present in the intermuscular fascia, but they are absent in muscle, tendon, cartilage, brain, and cornea.

Lymph is transported via afferent vessels to regional *lymph nodes,* the size of which varies according to function and activity (Fig. 96-1). Within the medullary sinuses of the node, circulating lymphocytes are replaced, and initial contact between foreign material and the immune system is made. *Efferent* lymph leaves the node via hilar channels. These channels are less numerous than the *afferent* channels, which enter the convex side of the node.

In addition to direct thoracic duct drainage into the subclavian vein, there are other lymphovenous communications within nodes and in peripheral vessels. Central lymphatic flow is promoted by the lymphatic valves and muscular contraction in the ducts. The rate and force of the contractions are determined by filling pressures (preload) and outflow resistance (afterload). Pressures >40 mmHg can be generated, and an obstructed lymphatic vessel can show pressures >60 mmHg because there is not a good collateral system for lymphatics.

PATHOPHYSIOLOGY

Lymphedema results from obstruction of lymph ducts as a result of developmental defects (primary) or acquired disorders (secondary). The effect of inadequate lymph drainage in the tissues is an increase in protein and fluid accumulation, additional fluid being retained by the osmotic effect of the protein. Protein content in edema fluid increases from a normal 0.1 to 0.5 g/dL to an abnormal 1 to 5 g/dL, which stimulates tissue fibrosis in the subcutaneous tissue, skin thickening, and hyperkeratosis.

The microlymphatics of human skin show network enlargement in primary lymphedema of late onset, whereas they are aplastic or ectatic in congenital lymphedema. Although the edema is initially soft and pitting, it becomes indurated and rubbery with time and progresses to involve the entire extremity. Lymphedema can be differentiated from venous stasis edema because there is usually no hyperpigmentation or ulceration in lymphedema, and the edema does not decrease appreciably with overnight elevation. It is more common for lymphedema to involve the dorsum of the foot and toes and to be associated with recurrent episodes of cellulitis and lymphangitis after trivial trauma. The latter complication presents with erythema, pain, and red streaks on the extremity. Lymphangitis may be accompanied by systemic signs of infection, typically by β-hemolytic streptococci.

The most common serious complication of lymphedema is *lymphangiosarcoma,* which usually affects the upper extremity of a patient with chronic lymphedema after mastectomy for carcinoma. Multiple, raised, bluish red or purple lesions occur in the skin or subcutaneous tissue and can progress to an ulcerating mass lesion if untreated. Lymphangiosarcoma has a poor prognosis; most patients die of the disease in less than 2 years. The tumor can occur on the lower extremity as a nonhealing ulcer with hemorrhagic nodules. A biopsy must be performed on any suspicious nonhealing lesion.

Because lymphedema occurs as a result of an abnormality of the lymphatic system, use of the term is restricted to situations in which other causes of edema are excluded or a specific lymphatic abnormality is demonstrated. The presence of bilateral, dependent, pitting edema usually indicates a renal or cardiac cause. Other generalized hypoproteinemias are idiopathic or occur with malnutrition, cirrhosis, and protein-losing enteropathy. Venous disease is the most likely cause of unilateral edema.

DIAGNOSIS

A patient with lymphedema has swelling and fatigue. Limb size increases during the day and decreases at night but is never normal. It is important to determine whether there is a family history of primary lymphedema and whether the patient has visited any countries where filariasis is endemic. Weight loss and diarrhea suggest small-intestinal lymphangiectasia.

Examination shows lymphedema to be firm and rubbery but nonpitting. Lymph vesicles that contain fluid with a high protein concentration may be present. Complications of lymphedema, such as infection, cellulitis, erythema, and hyperkeratosis, may be present. It is important to document limb size to identify isolated limb gigantism and

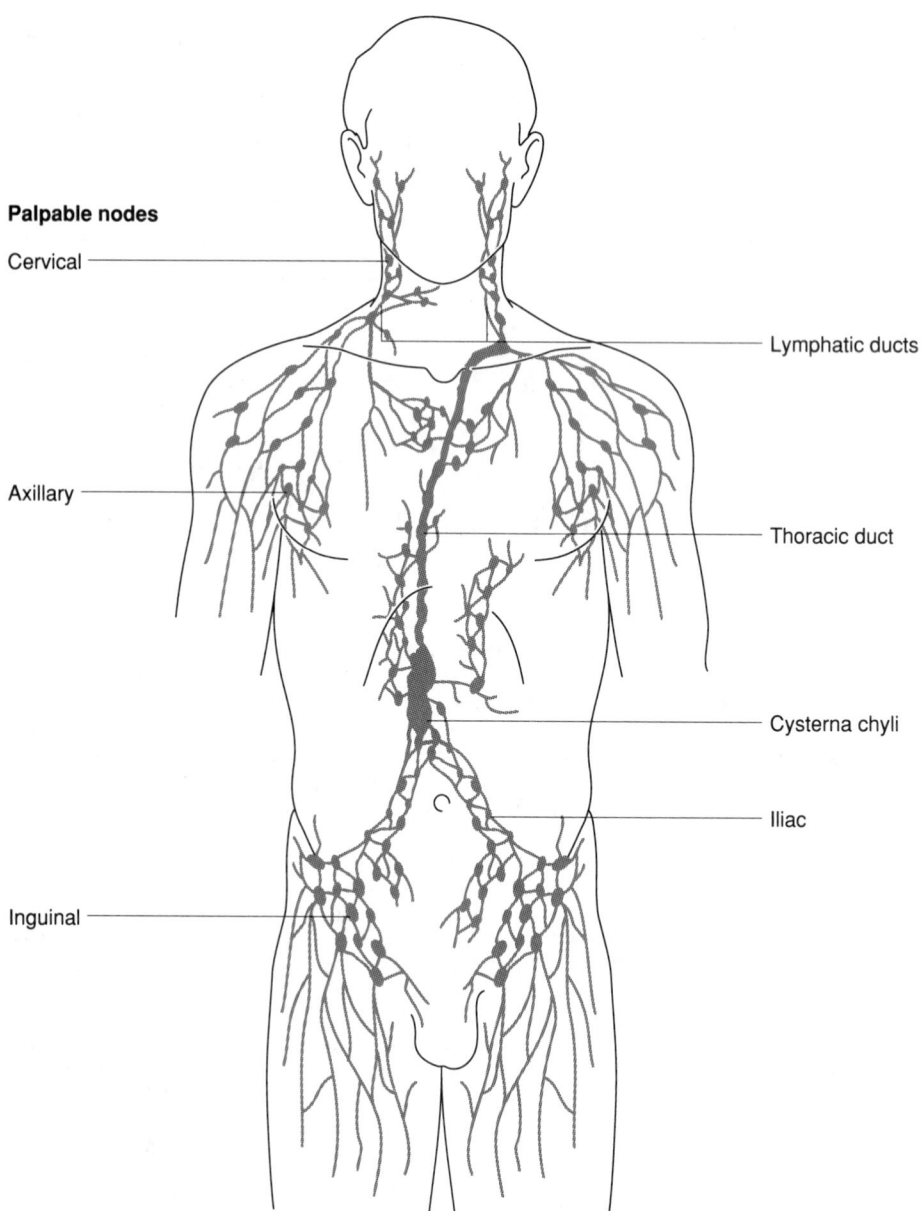

Palpable nodes

Cervical

Lymphatic ducts

Axillary

Thoracic duct

Cysterna chyli

Iliac

Inguinal

Figure 96-1. Major lymph node groups and collecting ducts. (After Basmajian JV. Primary anatomy, ed 7. Baltimore, Williams & Wilkins, 1976:293)

Klippel–Trenaunay–Weber syndrome, which may have hypoplastic lymphatics in addition to venous abnormality, capillary nevus, and limb elongation. The patient is examined for upper extremity and genital lymphedema, hydroceles, and amelogenesis imperfecta.

The *differential diagnosis* of lower extremity edema includes systemic disorders such as congestive heart failure and acute and chronic venous abnormality. In congestive heart failure, there is a generalized increase in venous pressure with distended neck veins and an enlarged liver. Whether a patient has venous disease is resolved by means of a noninvasive duplex examination with Doppler and B-mode ultrasound imaging. In the absence of these disorders, the patient usually is treated on the basis of the clinical diagnosis of lymphedema. Only rarely is it necessary to confirm the diagnosis with lymphatic visualization.

Lymphatic Visualization

Dye Injection

A highly diffusible dye, such as patent blue or sky blue, is injected 0.2 mL at a time subcutaneously into each interdigital web. Massaging the skin and moving the joints usu-

ally defines a network of fine intradermal lymphatics. If the collecting vessels are obstructed or inadequate, the dye diffuses through the dermal lymphatics to produce a marbled appearance called *dermal backflow*.

Radiographic Lymphography

It is possible to cannulate a lymphatic visualized by means of dye injection and to inject oily contrast medium (Lipiodol). This is a meticulous and tedious procedure and may require general anesthesia. If the lymphatics in the foot are not usable, it is possible to cannulate lymphatics adjacent to groin nodes or to inject the node directly. With adequate visualization the lymphatics in the extremity can be identified. They often appear as parallel tracks of uniform size that bifurcate as they proceed proximally, unlike the venous system (Fig. 96-2). Some dilatation at the level of the valves is normal.

Radionuclide Lymphatic Clearance

Radionuclide scanning with human serum albumin labeled with radioactive iodine or technetium-99m colloid can be used to monitor lymphatic clearance by means of

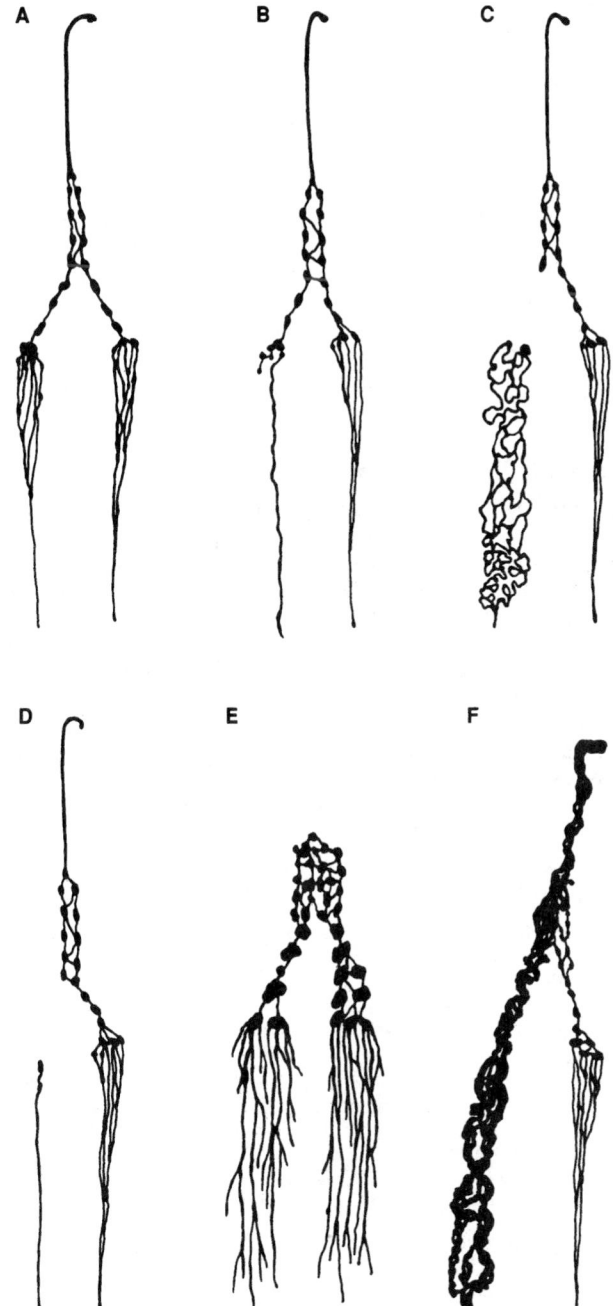

Figure 96-2. Diagrammatic representation of lymphographic patterns from feet to thoracic duct as seen in a normal person (*A*), in distal hypoplasia (*B*, right lower extremity), in proximal hypoplasia with distal distention (*C*, right limb), in combined proximal and distal hypoplasia (*D*), in bilateral hyperplasia (*E*), and in megalymphatics (*F*) often seen with a large, incompetent thoracic duct. (After Kinmonth JP. The lymphatics: surgery, lymphography and diseases of the chyle and lymph systems, ed 2. London, Edward Arnold, 1982:134)

serial scanning. The technique is simpler than conventional lymphography. The disadvantages are haziness of the scan, radiation dosage, and distribution of radionuclide into the extracellular fluid, making calculation of clearance dependent on leg volume.

Analysis of Tissue Fluid

Tissue fluid or lymph can be aspirated or collected from a tube in the subcutaneous tissues, but analysis contributes little to the diagnosis of lymphedema.

TRAUMA

The lymphatics are delicate vessels vulnerable to operative and penetrating trauma. Disruption of larger lymphatic ducts can cause pseudocysts, fistulas, or lymph collection in body cavities such as pleura, pericardium, or peritoneum.

Lymphocysts

Pseudocysts that form after an operation or trauma are called *lymphocysts*. They can enlarge progressively, producing pressure symptoms. Lymphocysts typically occur after radical node dissection and kidney transplantation. Some cysts involute or respond to aspiration, but most cysts must be explored and the draining ducts suture ligated. Identification of the ducts is facilitated by distal subcutaneous injection of blue dye. Wound drainage and a pressure dressing enhance healing of the area.

Thoracic Duct Trauma

Injury to the thoracic duct is usually the result of operative or penetrating trauma and produces chylothorax. Initial management is thoracostomy tube drainage. The volume of chylous drainage is reduced with an elemental diet and administration of medium-chain triglycerides. If the lung does not expand or if drainage persists for more than 1 week, thoracotomy is performed to ligate the thoracic duct. The thoracic duct is identified by means of preoperative administration of milk and cream or intraoperative injection of blue dye into the distal wall of the esophagus. Chylopericardium can be managed similarly, although it usually responds to external drainage and dietary control.

Chylous Ascites and Chyluria

Chylous ascites usually occurs as a result of congenital abnormalities or malignant tumors involving the retroperitoneum. It does not often result from trauma. Proximal obstruction of the thoracic duct may cause persistent leakage and make spontaneous closure unlikely. Lymphography may be necessary to clarify the situation if a congenital abnormality is suspected. Management is similar to that of chylothorax. *Chyluria* can result from filariasis or congenital abnormalities and is diagnosed with the finding of milky urine. Lymphangiography is used to define the anatomy for operative correction.

CLASSIFICATION OF LYMPHEDEMA

Primary lymphedema is classified structurally into *hyperplasia* and *hypoplasia* (see Fig. 96-2).

Primary lymphedema
Primary hypoplastic
    Distal hypoplasia or aplasia
    Proximal hypoplasia
    Proximal and distal hypoplasia
Primary hyperplastic
    Bilateral hyperplasia
    Megalymphatic
Secondary lymphedema
    Malignant neoplasia
    Radiation
    Trauma or surgical excision
    Inflammation or parasitic invasion
    Paralysis

Primary lymphedema usually is hypoplastic. Subgroups are defined according to lymphographic findings. Patients with *distal hypoplasia* have a mild, nonprogressive form of the disorder, if the proximal pathways are normal. Most patients are women. The onset usually is at puberty (lymphedema praecox); 10% of cases are present at birth (congenital lymphedema), and 10% occur after age 35 (lymphedema tarda). In *proximal hypoplasia,* lymphedema involves the entire extremity. It occurs with equal frequency among men and women. The combination of proximal and distal hypoplasia has features of both types and usually is progressive.

Primary *hyperplastic* lymphedemas are uncommon. Bilateral hyperplasia usually is recognized as diffuse capillary angiomata on the lateral aspects of the feet. Lymphography shows dilated lymphatics with normal valves. *Megalymphatics* have valves; in this condition chylous reflux can produce chylorrhea, skin vesicles, or chyluria.

The most common cause of *secondary lymphedema* in the United States is malignant disease metastatic to lymph nodes. Another common cause is surgical removal of nodes, especially when combined with radiation therapy, which produces lymphatic fibrosis. In tropical and subtropical countries, filariasis is the most common cause of secondary lymphedema, producing elephantiasis. Other infective or chemical agents (eg, silica) can enter the lymphatic system by means of barefoot walking and cause fibrosis of lymphatics and lymph nodes.

MANAGEMENT OF LYMPHEDEMA

Conservative Treatment

There are anatomic and physiologic limitations to the management of lymphedema. Physiologically, diuretic removal of fluid is not as effective in lymphedema as in edema due to other causes because of the residual protein in lymphedema. Anatomically, fibrosis produces irreversible changes in subcutaneous tissues. The management objectives are to control edema, avoid cellulitis and lymphangitis, and maintain healthy skin.

To *control edema,* the leg is elevated, and sequential pneumatic compression boots are used to massage the leg. Once the leg has reached optimal size, the patient is fitted with firm elastic stockings. For lymphedema, a full-length leotard is worn. The stockings are removed at night, and the foot of the bed is elevated 6 to 8 inches to maintain the pressure gradient from leg to right atrium. For more severe forms of the disorder, 2 to 3 days of hospitalization is recommended with use of a high-pressure pneumatic compression pump to reduce the size of the extremity.

Red streaking up the leg and the onset of pain and swelling usually indicate early *cellulitis* or *lymphangitis.* The causative organisms usually are staphylococci or β-hemolytic streptococci. Patients must be treated vigorously, usually with intravenous antibiotics. The extremity is immobilized, and warm, moist compresses are applied to provide symptomatic relief. Without treatment, the infection can obliterate more lymphatics and produce fever, malaise, nausea, and vomiting.

Skin problems include eczema and ulcers. Eczema usu-ally responds to hydrocortisone cream. Topical and systemic antifungal agents may be necessary for chronic infections, particularly between the toes. Ulceration is unusual, in contrast to the stasis edema of venous insufficiency, although fissures and lymph fistulas may develop and necessitate surgical excision.

Secondary lymphedemas may lend themselves to management of the underlying disorder. Diethylcarbamazine is used for filariasis, and appropriate antibiotics are used for tuberculosis or lymphogranuloma venereum. In rare cases of long-standing secondary lymphedema, lymphangiosarcoma can develop, appearing as a raised blue or reddish nodule. Satellite tumors and early metastases can develop if the lymphangiosarcoma is not recognized and widely excised. Treatment with benzopyrone is under investigation.

Surgical Treatment

Only 10% to 15% of patients with primary lymphedema are candidates for operative treatment, which usually is directed at reducing leg size. The indication for operation is functional rather than cosmetic improvement. The appearance of the extremity even after a successful debulking procedure is still abnormal. The best results are obtained when the bulk of the extremity has severely impaired movement or when there have been recurrent attacks of cellulitis. In the procedure used most often, skin flaps are raised to allow excision of the underlying subcutaneous tissues. Procedures involving lymphaticovenous anastomoses, microlymphatic bypass, or liposuction curettage are under investigation.

SUGGESTED READING

Casley-Smith JR, Morgan RG, Piller NB. Treatment of lymphedema of the arms and legs with 5,6-benzo-(alpha)-pyrone. N Engl J Med 1993;329:1158.

Gloviczki P, Fisher J, Hollier LH, et al. Microsurgical lymphovenous anastomosis for treatment of lymphedema: a critical review. J Vasc Surg 1988;7:647.

Huang G-K, Ru-Qi H, Zong-Zhao L, Yao-Liang S, Tie-De L, Gong-Ping P. Microlymphaticovenous anastomosis in the treatment of lower limb obstructive lymphedema: analysis of 91 cases. Plast Reconstr Surg 1985;76:671.

Ji YZ, Zheng JH, Chen JN, Wu ZD. Microsurgery in the treatment of chyluria and scrotal lymphangial fistula. Br J Urol 1993; 72:952.

Kinmonth JB. The lymphatics: surgery, lymphography and diseases of the chyle and lymph systems, ed 2. London, Edward Arnold, 1982.

Louton RB, Terranova WA. The use of suction curettage as adjunct to the management of lymphedema. Ann Plast Surg 1989; 22:354.

Pappas CJ, O'Donnell TF Jr. Long term results of compression treatment for lymphedema. J Vasc Surg 1992;16:555.

O'Brien BM, Mellow CG, Khazanchi RK, et al. Long term results after microlymphatico-venous anastomoses for treatment of obstructive lymphedema. Plast Reconstr Surg 1990;85:562.

Servelle M. Surgical treatment of lymphedema: a report on 652 cases. Surgery 1987;101:485.

PEDIATRICS

ESSENTIALS OF SURGERY: SCIENTIFIC PRINCIPLES AND PRACTICE,
edited by Lazar J. Greenfield, Michael W. Mulholland, Keith T. Oldham, Gerald B. Zelenock,
and Keith D. Lillemoe. Lippincott–Raven Publishers, Philadelphia, © 1997.

CHAPTER 97

NEONATAL AND PEDIATRIC PHYSIOLOGY

SAMUEL M. MAHAFFEY

The physiologic responses of children to injury or operation vary according to maturation (the functional state of development of various organ systems), anatomic abnormalities, and underlying metabolic disorders. The physiologic processes of neonates are closer to those of fetuses than those of adults.

GROWTH AND MATURATION

High-Risk Pregnancy, Premature Birth, and Intrauterine Growth

A newborn infant's condition is categorized by birthweight: Low birthweight, <2500 g; very low birthweight, <1500 g; small for gestational age, <10th percentile for the population; large for gestational age, >90th percentile for the population; appropriate for gestational age, 10th to 90th percentile; and intrauterine growth retardation (IUGR), restriction of fetal growth.

Prematurity is gestational age at birth <37 weeks. Complications of prematurity account for 85% of fetal deaths.

Postnatal Growth and Development

Deviation in somatic growth may be the first indication of functional abnormality. During the first year of life, healthy infants have a 200% increase in weight and a 50% increase in length. Genetic and environmental factors, such as parental size, nutritional status, overall health status, and socioeconomic factors, may determine the rate of postnatal growth.

Growth in stature is largely controlled by hormones and growth factors. Growth hormone, or somatotropin, is essential for the balanced growth of the body to normal adult size. Insulin also influences fetal and neonatal growth. Thyroid hormones have direct metabolic effects and effects due to induction of genes that affect cell growth and function.

Nutrient Requirements

An adequate supply of nutrients is essential to fulfill resting energy requirements, provide for growth, and provide necessary metabolic intermediates.

Water

Optimal water intake is a function of obligatory water loss and the amount retained for somatic growth. Fetal body water content is a function of fetal growth rate and the relative proportion of fat to fat-free body mass. The percentage of water content and the ratio of intracellular to extracellular water decrease during fetal development.

Postnatal water requirements include insensible water loss, urine loss, and accretion of lean body mass. Insensible water loss is caused by evaporation from the lung and skin and averages 1.5 to 3 g/kg/h. A premature infant's thin skin barrier and large body surface area-to-mass ratio enhance evaporative water loss.

Total daily water requirement, assuming an insensible loss of 50 mL/kg/d and a growth requirement of 15 mL/kg/d, is 100 mL per 100 kcal ingested.

Energy

Energy expenditure is expressed in kilocalories per kilogram of body weight. Expressed in this manner, the energy expenditure of neonates (50 kcal/kg/d) is about twice that of adults (25 kcal/kg/d).

Energy requirements are determined according to the relation

Energy balance = Energy intake − Energy expenditure

This seemingly simple equation has many components that make accurate measurement of energy balance extremely difficult. Determination of metabolizable energy depends on accurate measurement of energy intake and loss, including losses in urine and stool.

The main component of energy expenditure is *resting metabolic rate*, which is measured during the period of quiet inactivity in the postabsorptive state. It is a more practical measurement than basal metabolic rate, which is almost impossible to measure for neonates. Other determinants of energy expenditure include dietary intake, ambient temperature, activity, and the energy cost of growth. Because infants sleep 80% to 90% of the time, their energy requirements for physical activity are proportionally lower than those of adults. Activity is estimated to contribute about 10% to energy expenditure in the neonatal period.

The total energy cost of growth consists of a storage component (the energy value of the substrates retained) and an energy expenditure component (the energy required for absorption, metabolism, and assimilation). Neither the total energy cost of growth nor the energy expenditure component can be measured directly. The estimated energy cost of growth in neonates is 1.2 to 6 kcal/g.

For premature infants, recommended *energy intake* varies from 90 to 160 kcal/kg/d, so energy requirements also vary. Energy is provided as dietary carbohydrate and lipid. There are two methods for estimating *carbohydrate requirements*:

1. Examine the intake of healthy breastfed infants. Overall lactose intake is 7.5 to 10 g/kg/d, or about 40% of total energy intake in the first 4 months.

2. Measure fasting glucose release by a constant isotope tracer infusion method. Glucose production by term newborn is 4 to 6 mg/kg/min (5.8 to 8.6 g/kg/d) and is similar for a premature infant. This method yields a minimal glucose requirement and does not take into account requirements for growth.

Another consideration is the relative contribution of carbohydrate to overall energy intake. High carbohydrate to low fat ratios result in high rates of energy expenditure and decreased nitrogen retention; low carbohydrate to high fat ratios result in excessive fat deposition. A balanced ratio (about 40% carbohydrate) provides the highest rate of nitrogen retention.

Dietary *lipid* is a source of energy, a source of essential fatty acids, a component of structural membranes, and a carrier for fat-soluble vitamins. Lipids are carried in the bloodstream by lipoproteins and are cleared by lipoprotein lipase. Reduced activity of this enzyme may account for the inability of neonates (especially premature and small-for-gestational-age neonates) to clear large fat loads. Recommended daily *lipid requirement* is a total intake of 3.3 g of dietary lipid per 100 kcal, of which 1% is $\omega6$ fatty acids. Requirements for premature infants may be considerably higher.

Human milk, although variable in fat content and fatty acid profile because of maternal dietary intake, contains appropriate amounts of linoleic acid and long chain fatty acids, which are important for central nervous system (CNS) development. The fat content of formulas fed to premature infants, however, is based on vegetable oils. Although infants who are fed these preparations are at little risk for fatty acid deficiency, the metabolic pathway necessary for accretion of long-chain fatty acids into the CNS may be lacking.

Protein

Protein requirement is estimated as follows:

1. Base the requirement on growth. This gives a broad requirement for a specific population, or

2. Base the requirement on the quantity of protein needed for growth plus the quantity needed to replace inevitable losses. Inevitable losses in urine, feces, skin, and secretions are estimated at 0.4 to 0.9 g/kg/d. Based on this method, estimated protein requirements are: 2.5 g/kg/d for newborns 1.25 g/kg/d at 1 year, and 2.5 to 3.9 g/kg/d for premature infants weighing <2.5 kg.
3. Base the requirement on normalization of plasma amino acid profiles with the assumption that breast-fed infants exhibit ideal plasma amino acid concentrations (the standard for premature infants remains controversial). This method is used in the design of parenteral amino acid solutions.

Vitamins

Water-soluble vitamins function as enzyme cofactors, and requirements depend on energy intake and energy use. The fat-soluble vitamins A, D, E, and K participate primarily in cell differentiation and growth. Vitamin functions, deficiency states, and requirements are summarized in Table 97-1.

Trace Elements and Minerals

About 99% of all *calcium* is located in the skeleton, about one third of this in a readily exchangeable pool with the extracellular fluid. By term, a newborn accumulates 20 to 30 g of elemental calcium, 80% in the last trimester. Signs of pathologic hypocalcemia among newborns include irritability, jitteriness, tremors, seizures, and nonspecific symptoms that suggest sepsis. Preterm infants are deficient in calcium and phosphorus because they miss the peak period of skeletal mineralization, and this is often complicated by inadequate supply postnatally.

Important trace elements (<0.01% of body weight) include iron, iodine, fluoride, zinc, copper, manganese, chromium, molybdenum, selenium, and cobalt. These elements are cofactors for metal ion-activated enzymes, constituents of metalloenzymes, and constituents of other proteins.

Table 97-1. VITAMIN REQUIREMENTS AND FUNCTIONS

Vitamin	Recommended Intake*	Function	Deficiency State
Ascorbic acid	8 mg	Hydroxylation reactions, including carnitine and collagen	Scurvy
Thiamine	40 μg	Coenzyme in oxidative decarboxylation	Beriberi
Riboflavin	60 μg	Electron transport	Stomatitis, glossitis, cheilosis, seborrheic dermatitis
Vitamin B$_6$	35 μg	Interconversions of amino acids, synthesis of heme, metabolic reactions (brain)	Anemia, CNS abnormalities, vomiting, diarrhea
Niacin	0.8 mg NE	Metabolic intermediate (NAD, NADP)	Pellagra
Biotin	1.5 μg	Coenzyme	Dermatitis, conjunctivitis, seizures, ataxia, hearing loss, developmental delay
Pantothenic acid	0.3 mg	Integral part of coenzyme A	Cardiovascular instability, lethargy, depression
Vitamin B$_{12}$	0.5 μg†	Synthesis of nucleotides, methyl transfers	Megaloblastic anemia, neurologic changes
Folate	50 μg†	Acceptor and donor of one-carbon units in amino acid and nucleotide metabolism	Hypersegmentation of neutrophils, megaloblastic changes, poor growth
Vitamin D	400 IU†	Stimulates absorption of Ca and P	Rickets
Vitamin A	420 μg†	Growth and differentiation of epithelial tissues; vision	Night blindness, keratoconjunctivitis, dermatitis and growth failure
Vitamin E	0.5 mg α-TE	Antioxidant	

NE, niacin equivalent; α-TE, α-tocopherol equivalent.
* Minimum units per 100 kcal/d.
† Units/d.
(Committee on Nutrition, American Academy of Pediatrics. Nutritional needs of low-birth-weight infants. Pediatrics 1985;75:976)

Clinical Considerations

Enteral Feeding

The composition and use of human milk and infant formulas are summarized in Table 97-2. Consumed in adequate quantities, breast milk from a well-nourished mother is sufficient in all nutrients, with the possible exception of vitamins D and K, fluoride, and iron. Standard infant formulas are adequate for infants who are not breastfed. Specialized formulas are modified for use in specific clinical situations such as intolerance to standard formula; malabsorption of a component (such as fat malabsorption due to deficiency of pancreatic enzymes or bile salts); or inborn errors of metabolism (phenylketonuria, tyrosinemia, homocystinuria).

Healthy term newborns nipple feed on demand every 3 to 4 hours. Preterm infants suck a nipple but rarely have a coordinated suck and swallow until after 33 weeks' gestation. Gavage feedings are given to infants who have an immature suck and swallow or a medical condition that precludes nipple feeding. Intragastric feedings are given every 3 to 4 hours to term infants and more often to premature infants; they also may be given by continuous infusion.

Parenteral Nutrition

Parenteral nutrition is needed when the gastrointestinal (GI) tract cannot provide adequate digestion and absorption of nutrients. The objective of total parenteral nutrition (TPN) is a normal rate of growth and body composition with minimal morbidity. The solutions are administered into the central circulation through an indwelling central venous catheter. Peripheral parenteral nutrition is used to treat patients who can take some enteral nutrition or who have a short-term requirement for parenteral nutrition (<2 weeks).

Nutritional assessment before initiation of support involves physical examination and assessment of growth curves, anthropometrics, immune function, and visceral proteins such as albumin and transferrin. A number of technical and metabolic complications are associated with parenteral nutrition (Table 97-3), so monitoring continues during therapy (Table 97-4).

Nutrient requirements for TPN vary with patient age, baseline nutritional status, and energy expenditure. Lipid emulsions are used as an energy source and for prevention of essential fatty deficiency.

THERMOREGULATION

After birth, heat transfer from infant to environment occurs through the following mechanisms: Conduction, the direct transfer of heat between solid bodies; convection, the transfer of heat from the skin to the surrounding air; radiation heat loss, due to the emission of electromagnetic energy from the body, a function of temperature; and evaporation, similar to convection, except water rather than heated air is transported from the skin surface.

The components of the temperature regulation mechanism are intact in term neonates. Premature infants are at risk for temperature instability and cold stress. Tempera-

Table 97-2. COMPOSITION AND USE OF INFANT FORMULAS

Formula	Distribution of Calories	Carbohydrate Source	Protein Source	Fat Source	Osmolality	Use
HUMAN MILK AND STANDARD INFANT FORMULAS						
Human milk	Carbohydrate 38% Protein 7% Fat 55%	Lactose	Whey 80% Casein 20%	Human milk fat	300	Normal infants, premature infants
Enfamil, SMA	Carbohydrate 41%–43% Protein 9% Fat 48%–50%	Lactose	Nonfat cow's milk, whey Whey 60% Casein 40%	Coconut, soy, oleo, or safflower	278–305	Normal infants
Similac	Carbohydrate 43% Protein 9% Fat 48%	Lactose	Nonfat cow's milk Casein 82% Whey 18%	Coconut, soy	290	Normal infants
SOY-BASED INFANT FORMULAS						
Isomil Nursoy Prosobee	Carbohydrate 40% Protein 12%–13% Fat 47%–48%	Corn syrup solids, sucrose, or both	Soy isolate	Soy, coconut, corn, or safflower	150–296	Intolerance of lactose or cow's milk proteins
SPECIFIC-USE INFANT FORMULAS						
Nutramigen	Carbohydrate 54% Protein 11% Fat 35%	Corn syrup solids, corn starch	Casein hydrolysate	Corn oil	320	Lactose or cow's milk protein intolerance; malabsorption syndromes
Pregestimil	Carbohydrate 41% Protein 11% Fat 40%	Corn syrup solids, glucose, tapioca starch	Casein hydrolysate	MCT 60% Corn oil 20% Safflower 20%	300	Malabsorption syndromes; short gut
Portagen	Carbohydrate 46% Protein 14% Fat 40%	Corn syrup solids, sucrose	Sodium caseinate	MCT 88% Corn 12%	220	Malabsorption
Alimentum	Carbohydrate 41% Protein 11% Fat 48%	Surcrose, tapioca starch	Casein hydrolysate	MCT 50% Safflower, soy	370	

MCT, medium-chain triglycerides.

Table 97-3. COMPLICATIONS OF TOTAL PARENTERAL NUTRITION

PROBLEMS RELATED TO CENTRAL VENOUS CATHETER

Infection
Air embolism
Catheter malposition
  Pericardial effusion
  Pleural effusion

METABOLIC COMPLICATIONS

Fluid overload
Hyperglycemia
Hypoglycemia
Electrolyte imbalance
Nutritional deficiencies
Hyperlipidemia
Rickets
Cholestasis, which may lead to chronic liver dysfunction

COMPLICATIONS DUE TO USE OF LIPID EMULSION

Allergy to egg protein
Hyperphosphatemia
Thrombocytopenia
Deposition of fat emboli in the pulmonary capillaries
Kernicterus (fatty acids produced by hydrolysis may displace bilirubin
    from albumin-binding sites)

ture stabilization is provided with an incubator or a radiant warmer.

CARDIOVASCULAR PHYSIOLOGY

Fetal Circulation

In the fetal circulation, the placenta is the organ of gas exchange, the source of substrate, and the vehicle of removal of end products. Blood returning to the right ventricle is desaturated and low in substrate concentration. Right ventricular output is directed to the umbilical–placental circulation. Blood flowing to the left ventricle is saturated and high in substrate. Left ventricular output delivers oxygen to the fetal body through various streaming patterns (Fig. 97-1).

Desaturated blood returning to the heart from the brain

Table 97-4. MONITORING NUTRITIONAL SUPPORT

ASSESSMENT AT INITIATION OF NUTRITIONAL SUPPORT AND DAILY

Body weight
Intake and output
Chemstrips or urinalysis for glucose and ketones
Medication changes
Serum electrolytes (until stable)

ASSESSMENT AT INITIATION OF NUTRITIONAL SUPPORT AND WEEKLY*

Serum electrolytes, calcium, magnesium, and potassium
Serum albumin
Total or direct bilirubin
Alkaline phosphatase
Hepatic transaminases
Complete blood count

ASSESSMENT AS INDICATED

Trace elements (zinc, copper, iron)
Ammonia

* Every 2 to 4 weeks if long-term and stable.

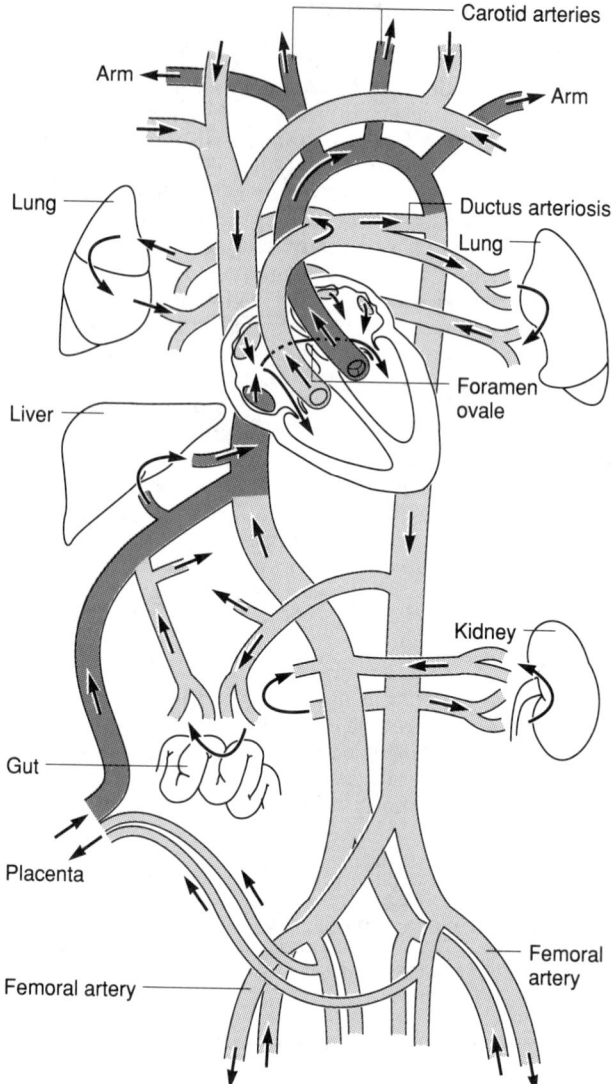

Figure 97-1. Persistent fetal circulation.

and upper body (through the superior vena cava) and the heart (through the coronary sinus) flows through the atrium and across the tricuspid valve into the right ventricle. Blood in the inferior vena cava is derived from two sources: (1) desaturated blood from the lower body and splanchnic circulation, which largely flows across the tricuspid valve into the right ventricle, and (2) oxygenated and substrate laden blood from the umbilical–placental circulation, which enters the inferior vena cava from the ductus venosus. This blood streams along the medial aspect of the inferior vena cava and is directed across the foramen ovale into the left atrium.

Because pulmonary vascular resistance (PVR) is high, only a fraction of right ventricular output flows to the lungs. The remaining right ventricular output flows across the ductus arteriosus to the descending aorta. About one third of this blood flows to the fetal body; the rest of the blood flows to the placenta for oxygenation and substrate uptake.

Transitional Circulation

The following changes in central blood flow begin at birth:

- the lungs expand, resulting in increased pulmonary blood flow and increased arterial oxygen tension

- PVR decreases, initially because of mechanical factors
- continued decreases are related to prostaglandin release or local changes in P_{O_2} or P_{CO_2}
- pulmonary venous return increases
- left atrial pressure exceeds right atrial pressure
- the foramen ovale closes
- the ductus arteriosus begins to close
- ventricular output increases, reflecting enhanced left ventricular filling from increased pulmonary venous return
- right ventricular work decreases
- left ventricular work increases, causing hypertrophy of the ventricle
- in both ventricles, ventricular filling shifts from late to early diastole.

Monitoring and Hemodynamic Assessment

Table 97-5 summarizes normal vital signs. The following procedures are routine critical care measures and are performed for any size infant: arterial catheterization, central venous catheterization, pulmonary artery catheterization, and venous oxygen saturation monitoring (venous oximetry).

In fetuses and neonates, maximum rate of rise of ventricular pressure (dP/dt_{max}) is positively affected by increase in heart rate, as in adults. Immature and adult myocardium respond to inotropic agents in a similar way, depending on changes in afterload, heart rate, and end-diastolic volume. Immature myocardium, however, shortens more slowly against the same load and by a smaller amount than adult myocardium.

Persistent Pulmonary Hypertension of the Newborn

A number of in utero and perinatal insults cause reestablishment of a fetal circulatory pattern in newborns. This results in shunting of unsaturated blood from the pulmonary circulation to the systemic circulation through a patent ductus arteriosus or foramen ovale. The pulmonary hypertension increases right ventricular strain and causes right ventricular failure. Buckling of the interventricular septum into the left ventricle impedes filling of the left ventricle, leading to biventricular failure. The combined effects of decreased cardiac output and arterial desaturation decrease oxygen delivery to the tissues and cause cellular oxidative metabolism to fail.

Pulmonary hypertension resulting in right-to-left shunting often causes a vicious circle of progressive hypoxia and worsening pulmonary hypertension, which can be fatal.

Management involves lowering PVR, including alkalosis and hyperventilation. The effect of alkalinization does not appear to be sustained, and the high ventilatory pressures required to achieve hyperventilation often cause barotrauma. An increase in both alveolar oxygen concentration ($P_{A_{O_2}}$) and arterial oxygen ($P_{a_{O_2}}$), by increasing inspired oxygen concentration, can reduce PVR.

RESPIRATORY PHYSIOLOGY

Lung growth is influenced by intrathoracic space, lung liquid volume and pressure, and amniotic fluid volume. *Structural maturation* of the lung involves multiplication and thinning of the alveolar walls. *Biochemical maturation* of the lung involves maturation of the surfactant system, which is mediated by adrenocorticotropin, cortisol, thyroid, and other hormones.

Respiratory Mechanics and Gas Exchange

In healthy children and adults, *functional residual capacity* (FRC) is well above *closing capacity.* In infants, closing capacity exceeds FRC, which explains in part the frequency with which respiratory disease of children progresses to acute respiratory failure. In diseases characterized by low FRC (pulmonary edema, respiratory distress syndrome, pneumonitis), respiratory therapy is designed to increase lung volume toward normal FRC (continuous positive airway pressure [CPAP] or positive end-expiratory pressure [PEEP]). Conditions resulting in increased closing capacity (bronchiolitis, asthma) are managed with bronchodilators and control of pulmonary secretions.

Decreased lung compliance is the most striking abnormality in respiratory distress syndrome. For gas flow to occur, a pressure gradient must be generated to overcome the nonelastic airway resistance of the lungs. Resistance is defined by the pressure gradient required to generate flow of gas.

In adults and older children, the peripheral airways have a large cross-sectional area, and only 20% of the total airway resistance is contributed by airways <2 mm. Small airway disease may produce little change in total airway resistance. In infants and young children, small airways account for about half of total airway resistance, and diseases that alter small airways (eg, bronchiolitis) can cause alterations in resistance and obstruction of gas flow.

Surfactant

The interface produced by the interaction of respiratory gases with the surface cells of the respiratory epithelium establishes a region of high surface tension. The surfactant

Table 97-5. NORMAL RANGE OF VITAL SIGNS

Age	Heart Rate (beats/min)	Systolic Blood Pressure (mmHg)	Diastolic Blood Pressure (mmHg)	Respiratory Rate (breaths/min)
Premature infant				
1 kg	120–140	36–58	18–38	40
3 kg	120–140	50–72	26–46	40
Term infant	120	65–80	30–50	40
0–12 mo*	100–120	105	65	40
1–6 yr*	100	105–110	70	30
6–12 yr*	80	110–125	70–80	20

* 90th percentile.
(Adapted from Horan MJ. Report of the Second Task Force on Blood Pressure Control in Children—1987. Pediatrics 1987;79:1)

complex lowers surface tension and stabilizes the alveolus to prevent atelectasis. Phospholipid synthesis and secretion and expression of surfactant proteins increase during gestation. The phosphatidylcholine content of amniotic fluid increases during the last trimester. The ratio of lecithin (phosphatidylcholine) to sphingomyelin (L/S ratio) is used to assess respiratory distress syndrome.

Surfactant deficiency is the main pathophysiologic factor in neonatal respiratory distress syndrome. Therapy is exogenous surfactant replacement. Several types of replacement surfactants are available, including surfactant obtained by lung lavage (which cannot be sterilized), surfactant from amniotic fluid (difficult to harvest enough for widespread use), and organic extracts of surfactant. Phospholipids, such as artificial lung-expanding compound, also can be used.

Evaluation of Respiratory Function

The clinical signs of impending respiratory failure are increased respiratory rate, altered respiratory pattern (including deep, shallow, or irregular breaths), use of accessory muscles, nasal flaring, and expiratory grunting. Auscultation of the chest may help define the nature and location of pulmonary disorders.

A *chest radiograph* is used to evaluate abnormal pulmonary function. *Pulse oximetry* is used to determine oxygen saturation. *Capnography* is the graphic display of airway CO_2 during the respiratory cycle. The maximum CO_2 during exhalation is the end-tidal CO_2. In healthy people, end-tidal CO_2 closely approximates P_aCO_2. Bedside *measurement of respiratory mechanics* allows continuous display of gas flow, airway pressures, delivered tidal volume, calculated compliance, airway resistance, and time constants of the lung. Adequacy of gas exchange is evaluated with *blood gases.*

Neonatal Ventilation

Neonatal ventilators are flow controlled, time triggered, time cycled, and pressure controlled. They provide continuous flow at preset values and a square wave flow pattern (Fig. 97-2). This pattern may increase risk for barotrauma in patients with immature lungs and abnormal lung parenchyma. The ventilators have an option for volume-controlled synchronized intermittent mandatory ventilation.

Pediatric Ventilation

Pediatric ventilators are similar to those for adults but are used at lower ranges of flow and volume.

Nonconventional Modes of Ventilation

High-Frequency Ventilation

Low tidal volumes and high ventilatory rates minimize the effects of high airway pressures.

High-Frequency Jet Ventilation. A high-pressure air and oxygen source generates gas flow. A solenoid valve interrupts gas flow, regulating the frequency of ventilation. A specially designed endotracheal tube is required. A second ventilator is required to provide PEEP and sigh breaths. The primary physiologic advantage is reduction in peak airway pressures compared with conventional positive-pressure ventilation.

High-Frequency Oscillatory Ventilation. A piston diaphragm oscillator alternates positive and negative pressures in the airway. High-frequency oscillatory ventilation is used to treat infants with respiratory distress syndrome.

RENAL PHYSIOLOGY

Renal Function

Total renal blood flow (% of cardiac output) throughout life is: fetus, 2% to 3%; first month of postnatal life, 6% to 18%; adults, 20% to 25%. Intrarenal blood flow also changes. Blood flow to the outer cortex increases with centrifugal development of the kidney (ie, from medulla to cortex). Glomerular filtration (GFR) is lower in fetuses and preterm infants than in term infants. GFR in very-low-birthweight infants is only about 40 mL/h, compared with 300 mL/h in term infants. An abrupt increase in GFR occurs with changes in renal blood flow at completion of nephrogenesis (34 to 36 weeks postconception). The increase occurs whether nephrogenesis is completed in utero or after birth.

Fractional excretion of sodium (FE_{Na}) is useful in assessment of renal function. There appears to be a steady decline in FE_{Na} during the transition from fetal to postnatal life: infants <34 weeks gestation, 3.3%; 34 to 37 weeks gestation, 1.2%; term, 0.4%.

Urinary sodium losses may be high in preterm infants, particularly those who are critically ill. Immaturity of tubular function may contribute to alterations in acid-base balance, particularly the development of a metabolic acidosis and difficulty handling acid load.

Neonates handle water load well, achieving maximal dilution of urine (30 to 50 mOsm/L). Ability to concentrate the urine, however, is limited to 400 to 600 mOsm/L.

In addition to immaturity of renal function, extrarenal factors are considered in correction of fluid and electrolyte abnormalities. For example, positive-pressure ventilation and CPAP impair renal perfusion and glomerular filtration.

Fluid Spaces

Total body water is distributed between the intracellular and extracellular spaces. The extracellular space has two compartments: plasma (intravascular) and interstitial (extravascular). The intracellular space includes red blood cell (RBC) volume and the water content of all the noncirculating cells. Plasma and RBC volumes constitute total blood volume.

In the early fetal period, water constitutes about 95% of the fetus, 80% at 7 months, and 75% at term. Water redistributes among the compartments as the percentage of the body that is extracellular fluid sharply declines, and there is a gradual rise in the percentage of intracellular fluid. This changing distribution continues throughout the neonatal period. Total body water content decreases until about 9 months of age, when it reaches 62%; intracellular water reaches its maximum at 43% of body weight, and extracellular fluid declines to 30% of body weight.

Blood volume is larger in fetuses than newborns; about one third of fetal blood volume is contained within the placenta and cord. Blood volume in term newborns is about 80 mL/kg.

Hydrops fetalis is accumulation of excess fluid in a fetus.

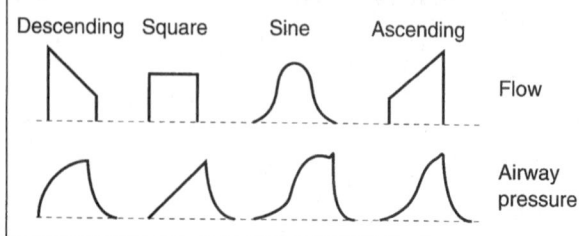

Figure 97-2. Waveform patterns in positive-pressure ventilation.

It produces generalized edema, ascites, and pleural and pericardial effusions. Hydrops fetalis is the end stage of severe alloimmune hemolytic anemia (erythroblastosis fetalis), usually due to maternofetal incompatibility for the D antigen in the Rh system. For some infants, intrauterine transfusion of packed RBCs into the umbilical vessels may reverse hydrops.

Fluid and Electrolyte Management

Assessment

Assessment is summarized in Table 97-6. The number of wet diapers in 24 hours is a guideline. Fluid and electrolyte therapy is divided into maintenance requirements, correction of existing deficits, and replacement of ongoing losses. The plan must be reevaluated often and modified when necessary. Evaluation includes a review of vital signs, urine output, input and output, weight, and laboratory findings.

Maintenance

Maintenance requirements are summarized in Table 97-7. For older infants and children, water requirements are calculated on the basis of body weight: 100 mL/kg/24 h (first 10 kg) + 50 mL/kg/24 h (second 10 kg) + 20 mL/kg/24 h (>20 kg).

Correction of Existing Deficits or Excesses

Correction of existing deficits or excesses requires assimilation of the history, physical findings, and laboratory studies to assess the magnitude of water and electrolyte loss or excess and to determine the composition of the replacement fluid.

Sodium. *Water intoxication* may be due to excessive *intake* of free water (eg, freshwater drowning) or inappropriate *retention* of free water (eg, secretion of antidiuretic hormone [ADH] after head injury). Therapy is water restriction.

A *large decrease in total body water* relative to Na$^+$ results in volume *contraction* and hypernatremia. Common

Table 97-7. MAINTANENCE WATER AND ELECTROLYTE REQUIREMENTS

	Holliday-Segar Method*	Body Surface Area Method
Water	<10 kg: 100 mL/kg 10–20 kg: 1000 mL + 50 mL/kg over 10 >20 kg: 1500 mL + 20 mL/kg over 20	1500–1800 mL/m^2/24 h
Sodium	3 mEq/100 mL H$_2$O/24 h	30–50 mEq/m^2/24 h
Potassium	2 mEq/100 mL H$_2$O/24 h	20–40 mEq/m^2/24 h

* Caloric expenditure estimates based on body weight alone; assumes 100 mL H$_2$O is required for each 100 kcal metabolized.

causes are inadequate free water intake or failure of tubular reabsorption of free water (usually due to inadequate ADH, or diabetes insipidus). Therapy depends on the cause; free water intake is increased or exogenous ADH is administered. *Increased total body Na$^+$* relative to total body water results in volume *expansion* and hypernatremia. The common cause is excessive Na$^+$ intake, often through unintentional administration (eg, some antibiotics contain large amounts of Na$^+$). Therapy is Na$^+$ restriction.

Sodium deficit relative to total body water results in *hyponatremia* and volume contraction. Causes include inadequate replacement of sodium losses and increased sodium excretion due to diuretic therapy.

Potassium. *Hypokalemia* results from increased renal potassium loss during diuretic therapy. Other causes are inadequate intake, unreplaced GI losses, and alkalosis. Hypokalemia can cause hypotonia, tetany, decreased concentrating ability. and ECG changes. Therapy is modification of diuretic therapy and oral or IV K$^+$ supplementation.

False hyperkalemia is common, the result of hemolysis of the sample when blood is withdrawn through small-gauge needles. *True hyperkalemia* is associated with renal insufficiency, excessive potassium intake, use of potassium-sparing diuretics, severe acidosis, and ECG changes. Hyperkalemia often occurs in critical illness and with massive cellular injury. Treatment includes cessation of potassium supplements, use of a cation exchange resin, administration of supplemental Ca^{2+}, administration of glucose and insulin, or alkalinization with sodium bicarbonate.

Acidosis. Acidosis due to inadequate oxygen delivery is corrected by improving oxygen delivery. Administration of sodium bicarbonate is reserved for refractory acidosis (pH <7.10) or correction of unreplaced loss of bicarbonate in the urine (renal tubular acidosis, carbonic anhydrase inhibition) or from the GI tract (diarrhea, excessive ostomy output, fistula).

Replacement of Ongoing Losses

Fluid is lost from nasogastric tubes, thoracostomy tubes, drains, diarrhea, ostomies, GI fistulas, biliary or pancreatic drainage, or leakage of peritoneal fluid (abdominal wall defects). The losses are replaced on a milliliter by milliliter basis with a fluid of comparable composition (Table 97-8). The fluid lost to the third space is essentially plasma, so the replacement solution must be comparable in composition: balanced salt or colloid solution.

HEPATIC PHYSIOLOGY

About 70% to 80% of the total hepatic blood flow in utero is contributed by the highly oxygenated blood of the umbilical vein. The rest is unsaturated blood from the

Table 97-6. ASSESSMENT OF VOLUME STATUS

HISTORY

Underlying illnesses
Nature, magnitude, and duration of fluid loss
Therapeutic interventions

PHYSICAL EXAMINATION

Mild to Moderate Volume Depletion (<10%)

Mild tachycardia
Dry mucous membranes and tears
Concentrated urine and oliguria
Decreased skin turgor
Sunken eyeballs and fontanelle

Severe Volume Depletion (>10%)

Increased severity of above signs
Hypotension
Absent or poor-quality peripheral pulse
Delayed capillary refill
Cool, clammy skin
Anuria
Depressed mentation

Table 97-8. **COMPOSITION OF BODY FLUIDS**

Source	Na⁺ (mEq/L)	K⁺ (mEq/L)	Cl⁻ (mEq/L)	HCO₃⁻ (mEq/L)	Protein (g/dL)	Suggested Replacement
Gastric	20–80	5–20	100–150	—	—	0.45% NaCl + 10 mEq/L Cl
Pancreatic	120–140	5–15	40–80	115	—	LR or 0.45% NaCl + 50 mEq/L NaHCO₃
Bile	120–140	5–15	80–120	100–115	—	LR or 0.45% NaCl + 50 mEq/L NaHCO₃
Ileostomy	45–135	3–15	20–115	30–50	—	LR or 0.45% NaCl + 25 mEq/L NaHCO₃
Diarrhea	10–90	10–80	10–110	30–50	—	LR or 0.45% NaCl + 25 mEq/L NaHCO₃
Pleural or peritoneal	140	5	100	25	6–8	LR + 5% albumin or plasmanate

LR, lactated Ringer solution.

portal vein and a negligible contribution from the hepatic artery.

After formation during the first trimester, the liver grows linearly throughout the rest of gestation. Bile secretory function is low during fetal life, and metabolic and secretory functions related to bile acid metabolism continue to be immature in neonates, predisposing infants to cholestasis. A number of hepatic enzyme systems are functionally immature in term infants and almost nonexistent in extremely premature infants.

Enzyme Function and Pharmacokinetics

A number of factors affect metabolism and elimination of drugs in newborns. The apparent volume of distribution of drugs is altered by differences in total body water and the low percentage of body fat. These differences influence the loading doses of drugs. Qualitative and quantitative differences in plasma proteins influence protein binding and the availability of free drug to an infant. Immature glomerular and tubular function influence renal elimination of drugs. Immature hepatic enzyme systems influence biotransformation reactions, which affect elimination of any drug that cannot be excreted in unchanged form.

Drugs that cannot undergo biotransformation must be excreted unchanged by the kidney. Renal elimination is influenced by the functional immaturity of the kidney, including decreased renal blood flow, decreased GFR, and immature tubular function. Aminoglycoside antibiotics are not metabolized and are excreted unchanged, primarily by glomerular filtration. This prolongs the serum half-life of these drugs, which is directly related to gestational age, postnatal age, and creatinine clearance.

Bilirubin Metabolism

Hyperbilirubinemia is common among newborns and is usually benign. High levels of unconjugated bilirubin, however, result in deposition of unbound bilirubin in the CNS and CNS toxicity (kernicterus). Therapy is required when the level of unconjugated bilirubin is rising rapidly or approaching toxic levels. Phototherapy is the initial treatment. Absorption of a photon of light results in photochemical conversion of the bilirubin molecule. If the level of unconjugated bilirubin continues to rise, exchange transfusion may be required.

Breast feeding is associated with neonatal hyperbilirubinemia. Decreased fluid intake, inhibition of hepatic bilirubin excretion that may be present in breast milk, and enhanced intestinal resorption of bilirubin are possible mechanisms.

DEVELOPMENTAL IMMUNOLOGY AND INFECTION

Development of the Immune System

Development of the immune system begins early in gestation and is not complete until after birth. The *structural* (organized tissues, including thymus, bone marrow, spleen, mucosa-associated immune tissue, and peripheral lymph nodes) and *circulating* (lymphocytes, macrophages, neutrophils, eosinophils, and mast cells) components of the mature immune system are present at birth, but a neonate's and an adult's immune systems have important functional differences.

In term newborns, differences are due to immunologic immaturity and lack of previous antigen exposure. Extremely premature infants are immunologically immature and immunologically incompetent because of inadequate development of the structural, cellular, and humoral components of the immune system. This translates to a 60-fold higher prevalence of sepsis among premature infants than among term infants.

Phagocytic activity and, thus, inflammatory responses are limited in term newborns. Although peripheral granulocyte counts in healthy newborns exceed those of normal adults, the storage pool is relatively small. Neonatal granulocytes also have defective chemotaxis in response to inflammatory mediators and microbicidal activity, particularly in stressed newborns.

Maternal Transfer of Humoral Immunity

Throughout gestation, humoral immunity is passively transferred to the fetus in the form of *IgG*. Late in gestation, IgG is actively transferred to achieve serum levels that exceed maternal levels. Small amounts of *IgM* are present in the fetus early in gestation, and small amounts are synthesized by a healthy fetus. In the absence of congenital infection, IgM levels remain low but increase rapidly after birth.

Neonates benefit immunologically from breastfeeding. Human colostrum and breast milk contain an array of cellular and humoral elements important in immune competence, including T and B lymphocytes, phagocytic cells, immunoglobulins, complement components, interferon, and other microbial inhibitors.

Neonatal Sepsis

Neonatal sepsis is a generalized bacterial infection accompanied by a positive blood culture during the first month of life. Maternal infection can be transmitted transplacentally (maternal bacteremia or viremia), by direct contamination of the amniotic fluid after prolonged rupture of membranes, or during passage through the birth canal.

The *signs and symptoms* of neonatal sepsis are subtle. Early signs include lethargy, irritability, temperature instability, change in respiratory pattern, or change in feeding pattern. Hematologic changes include thrombocytopenia, leukocytosis, and leukopenia. Hemodynamic changes are late manifestations. Fever and leukocytosis often do not occur among neonates.

Management involves obtaining cultures (including cerebrospinal fluid) and prompt initiation of antibiotic therapy based on the suspected organism, usually ampicillin or an antistaphylococcal agent with an aminoglycoside.

Most neonatal *viral infections* are acquired transplacentally. Congenital infections from the TORCH complex (toxoplasmosis, rubella, cytomegalovirus, and herpesvirus) often present with hepatosplenomegaly, a petechial rash, thrombocytopenia, and CNS manifestations such as calcifications and seizures. The human immunodeficiency virus (HIV) also is transmitted vertically.

SUGGESTED READING

Christensen RD, Brown MS. Effect on neutrophil kinetics and serum opsonic capacity of intravenous administration of immune globulin to neonates with clinical signs of early-onset sepsis. J Pediatr 1991;118:606.

DiFiore JW, Fauza DO, Wilson JM. Experimental fetal tracheal ligation reverses the structural and physiological effects of pulmonary hypoplasia in congenital diaphragmatic hernia. J Pediatr Surg 1994;29:248.

Fonkalsrud EW, Krummel TM, eds. Infections and immunologic disorders in pediatric surgery. Philadelphia, WB Saunders, 1993.

Gordon JB, Martinez FR, Keller PA, Tod ML, Madden JA. Differing effects of acute and prolonged alkalosis on hypoxic pulmonary vasoconstriction. Am Rev Respir Dis 1993;148:1651.

McIntyre NR, Li-Ing Ho. Effects of initial flow rate and breath termination criteria on pressure support ventilation. Chest 1991;99:134.

Polin RA, Fox WW, eds. Fetal and neonatal physiology. Philadelphia, WB Saunders, 1992.

Rau JL. Inspiratory flow patterns: the shape of ventilation. Respir Care 1993;38:132.

Roberts JD, Lang P, Bigatello LM, Vlahakes GJ, Zapol WM. Inhaled nitric oxide in congenital heart disease. Circulation 1993;87:447.

ESSENTIALS OF SURGERY: SCIENTIFIC PRINCIPLES AND PRACTICE, edited by Lazar J. Greenfield, Michael W. Mulholland, Keith T. Oldham, Gerald B. Zelenock, and Keith D. Lillemoe. Lippincott–Raven Publishers, Philadelphia, © 1997.

CHAPTER 98

PEDIATRIC HEAD AND NECK

JOHN R. WESLEY

AIRWAY OBSTRUCTION

Congenital Obstruction

The *signs* of respiratory distress in an infant are restlessness followed by tachypnea, chest wall retraction, and cardiorespiratory arrest. It is crucial to *establish an adequate airway* and to provide respiratory support while proceeding with the diagnostic evaluation. Establishment of an airway may include simple positioning of the infant, endotracheal intubation, or, in extreme situations, tracheostomy.

Diagnostic evaluation includes history, physical examination, chest radiography, arterial blood gases, and passage of a nasogastric tube with a radiopaque marker.

Clinical findings in upper airway obstruction are similar for diverse causes such as nasal encephalocele and choanal atresia. Tachypnea and suprasternal, intercostal, and costal margin retraction are prominent, but there is no apparent difficulty exhaling, and voice and cry are normal.

Emergency management consists of placement of an oropharyngeal airway. A tracheostomy may be necessary until nasal airway obstruction is corrected by means of division of the septum that occludes the posterior nares or by means of excision of a nasopharyngeal mass.

Airway obstruction at the level of the oral cavity may be caused by macroglossia due to muscular hypertrophy or to diffuse involvement by lymphangioma, neurofibromatosis, or hemangiopericytoma. Micrognathia may cause airway obstruction, particularly during feeding. Most infants respond to being placed in the prone position, which allows the posterior prolapsed tongue to fall forward. Cysts or tumors of the pharynx may produce a lesion large enough to obstruct the glottis.

The trachea and larynx may become obstructed by tumors or cysts that originate in the neck. Hemangiomas, lymphangiomas, cystic hygromas, and teratomas are the most common cervical tumors in infants and children. Emergency management of these lesions frequently requires placement of an endotracheal tube, which can be difficult if the larynx is displaced.

After the airway is stabilized, *additional diagnostic evaluation* includes neck and chest radiographs, computed tomography (CT), or magnetic resonance imaging (MRI), ultrasonography, and laryngobronchoscopy.

Tumors and cysts are *excised*. Hemangiomas may involute with time or be removed by means of endoscopic laser resection.

Acquired Obstruction

Foreign body aspiration (see Chap. 99) and *acute epiglottitis* are common causes of acquired airway obstruction in the pediatric age group. *Haemophilus influenzae* type B is nearly always the cause of acute epiglottitis. Most patients have an elevated temperature and an increased pulse and respiratory rate. Prolonged inspiratory stridor worsens with the supine position. The child usually sits erect, is anxious and drooling, and becomes increasingly exhausted because of air hunger.

No attempt is made to visualize the larynx outside the operating room because of risk for sudden airway occlusion with respiratory and cardiac arrest. If the child's condition allows, lateral neck *radiographs* with soft-tissue technique are obtained to confirm the presence of a swollen epiglottis. These radiographs are used to rule out other causes of acute airway obstruction, particularly foreign bodies in the hypopharynx, larynx, and trachea.

Conventional therapy is short-term endotracheal intubation performed in the operating room with general anesthesia and a tracheostomy tray at the ready. The inflammation resolves rapidly with intravenous antibiotics, and intubation is seldom required beyond 3 days.

BRANCHIAL CLEFT REMNANTS

Cysts, sinuses, and fistulas of the neck derived from branchial cleft remnants are common among children.

Anatomy and Embryology

The region of the neck in an embryo is a series of ridges (*branchial arches*) and furrows (*branchial clefts*) (Fig. 98-1). The arches coalesce during development, and part

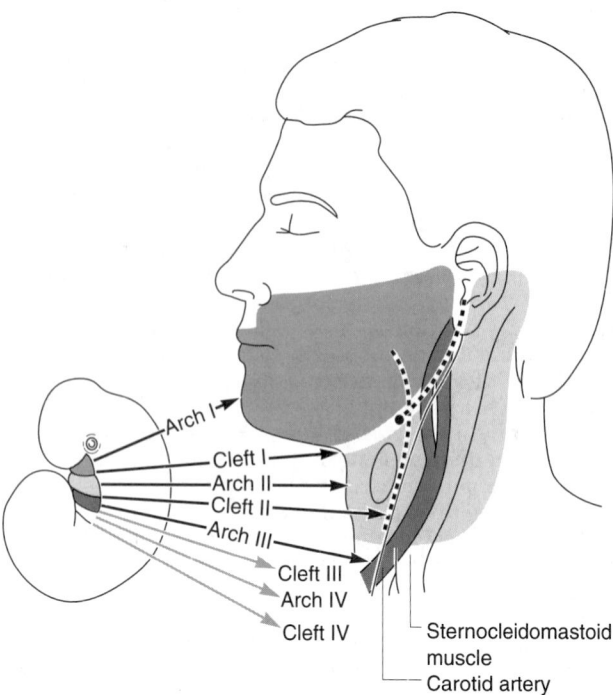

Figure 98-1. Derivation of various areas of the head and neck from the branchial arches and clefts of the embryo.

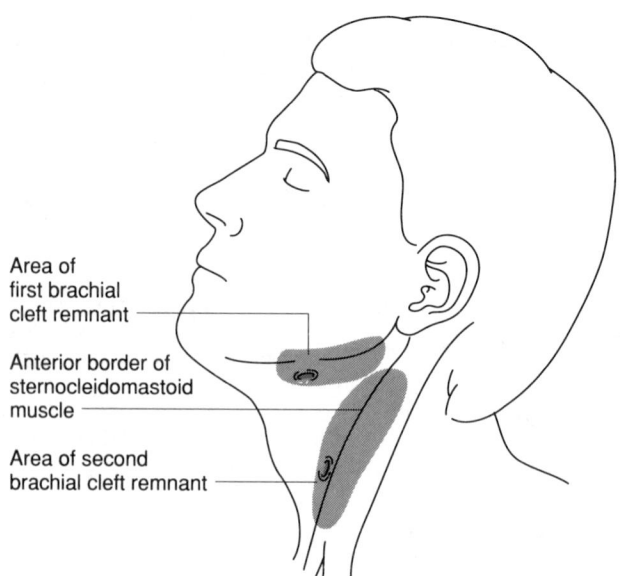

Figure 98-2. Areas of the neck in which cysts and sinuses from the first and second branchial clefts are usually found.

of the first branchial cleft remains open as the eustachian tube and auditory canal. The second branchial cleft closes completely; however, either branchial cleft may form a sinus track or cyst during coalescence (Fig. 98-2). Cysts or infections that originate from the third or fourth branchial arch and cleft are rare (Fig. 98-3).

Clinical Issues

First branchial cleft lesions appear as a sinus opening near the angle of the mandible. Second branchial cleft anomalies, which are more common, appear as a pinpoint opening on the anterior border of the sternocleidomastoid muscle, one fourth to one third of its length cephalad from the sternum. Attention is usually drawn to the defects because of the appearance of small drops of clear fluid at the opening of the track or infection in the track. The anomaly may be unilateral or bilateral. Less frequently, an oval mass overlies the surface of the parotid gland (first branchial cleft) or is situated anterior to the upper portion of the sternocleidomastoid muscle (second branchial cleft).

Cysts or sinuses that originate from the third or fourth branchial arch or cleft appear as air-containing inflamed lateral neck masses in neonates or as acute suppurative thyroiditis in infants or children. A barium examination may demonstrate the presence of a pyriform sinus fistula,

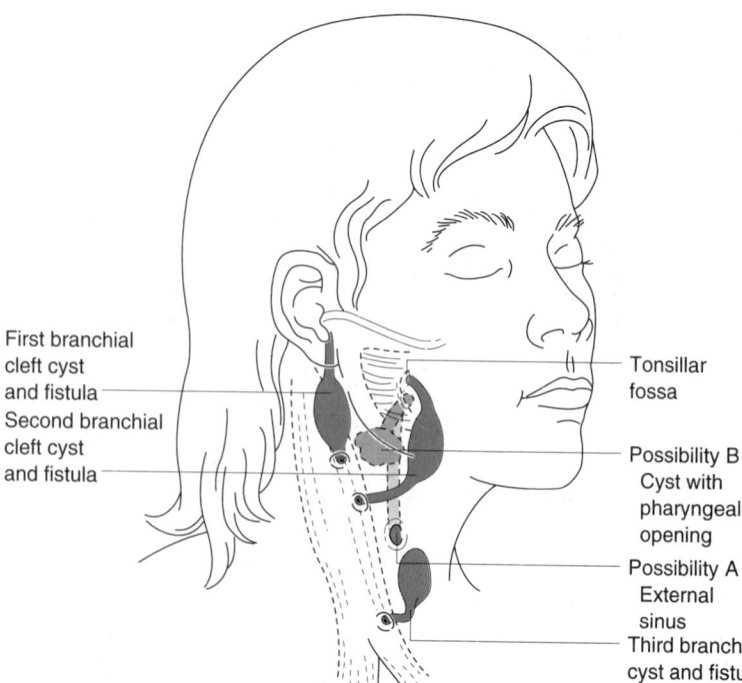

Figure 98-3. Types of first, second, and third branchial cleft remnants. Sinuses and fistulas are seen most often in infants and young children, whereas cysts usually appear at a later age.

particularly after a course of antibiotics and resolution of the surrounding inflammation. CT is useful in the diagnosis of lesions of third or fourth branchial cleft origin. If imaging is not successful, the next time inflammation occurs, compression of a pus-filled cyst during endoscopy may reveal the origin of the fistula as pus exudes from the pyriform sinus.

Operative Considerations

Treatment is surgical excision. The operation may be performed at any age. If active infection is present, a course of antibiotics is administered before excision.

The operation for *second branchial cleft* lesions begins with an elliptic transverse incision at the sinus opening and cephalad dissection of the track. Dissection is kept on the tract to avoid injury to structures such as the internal jugular vein, the internal or external carotid arteries, and the hypoglossal nerve. The tonsillar fossa is the endpoint of dissection. The sinus tract is suture ligated and divided (Fig. 98-4).

Cysts and sinuses of the *first branchial cleft* are less common than cysts of the second branchial cleft and are often misdiagnosed, incompletely removed, and subject to repeated infection. The sinus tract opening appears just beneath the center of the body of the mandible. The tract consists of stratified squamous epithelium, which may contain hair follicles, and extends upward behind the angle of the mandible to end at the cartilage of the external auditory canal (Fig. 98-5).

Repeated infection often leads to the diagnosis of a first branchial cleft cyst or sinus, but the cyst or sinus must be drained and infection managed with antibiotics before excision is attempted. An elliptic incision is made around the opening of the sinus, and dissection of the tract is carried upward to the lower portion of the auditory canal. Care is taken to avoid injury to the facial nerve, particularly the mandibular branch.

If the dissection is performed carefully and the lesion is not infected, it is not necessary to leave a drain after excision of a first or second branchial cleft anomaly. Failure to excise the cyst or sinus completely may lead to recurrence.

For all *third or fourth branchial lesions,* acute infection is managed first, and surgical extirpation follows. Exploration of the neck with excision of the entire tract to the level of the pyriform sinus is necessary to prevent recurrence. Endoscopy at the start of the operation may enable cannulation of the tract from above, which greatly facilitates localization of the tract during excision. Extreme caution is exercised to preserve the external branch of the superior laryngeal nerve. The tract usually passes inferior and external to the recurrent laryngeal nerve along the trachea to the superior pole of the thyroid. Thyroid lobectomy or resection of the superior pole is performed as indicated by the extent of the cyst (Fig. 98-6).

Other *minor branchial arch remnants* consist of a small cartilaginous mass that appears in the subcutaneous tissue along the lower anterior border of the sternocleidomastoid muscle. The lesion is usually visible and palpable, and bilateral occurrence is common. An accompanying sinus or cyst rarely occurs, and infection is uncommon. Excision may be performed for cosmetic reasons or may be delayed indefinitely.

Preauricular sinuses or pits are common. Asymptomatic lesions require no treatment. Draining sinuses and infected cysts require antibiotic treatment, incision and drainage for failure to resolve, and later excision to prevent recurrence.

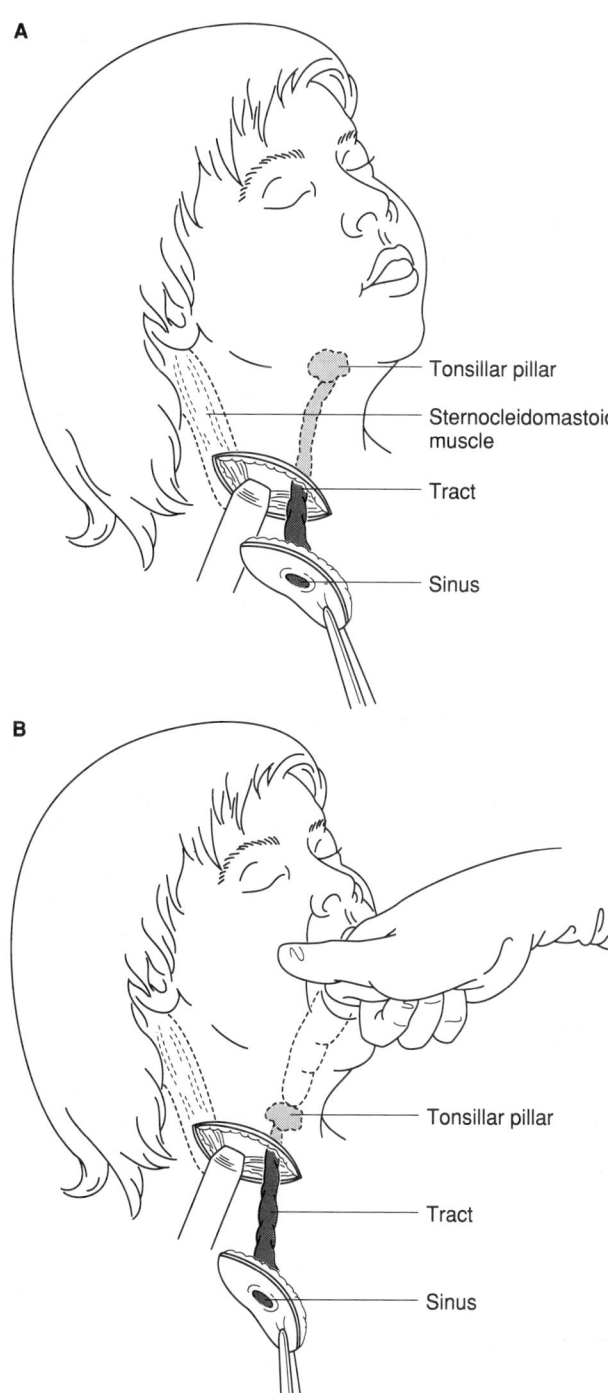

Figure 98-4. (*A*) Single incision in the lower part of the neck with the sinus tract developed to usual length. (*B*) The anesthesiologist's finger depresses the tonsillar fossa, facilitating complete dissection of the sinus tract through the single incision.

THYROGLOSSAL DUCT
Anatomy and Embryology

Thyroglossal duct cysts (or remnants) are lesions that originate from elements of the thyroglossal duct tract from the descent of the thyroid gland from the foramen cecum at the base of the tongue (Fig. 98-7). These lesions usually appear in late infancy or early childhood and are rarely apparent at birth. They are typically located in the hyoid

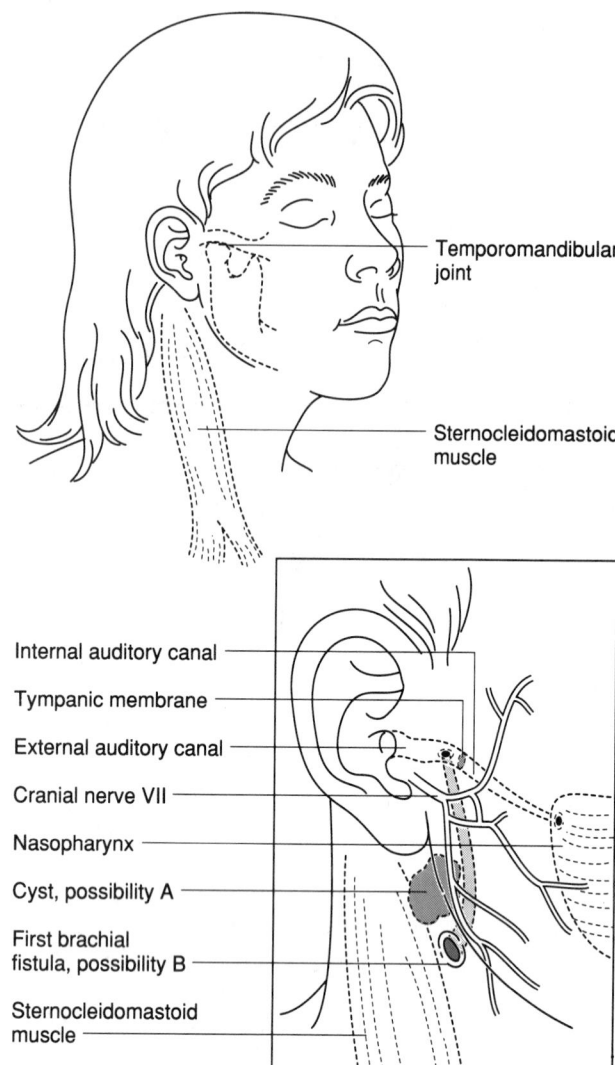

Figure 98-5. Relations of cyst or sinus of the first branchial cleft. Note especially the proximity to the facial nerve and external auditory canal.

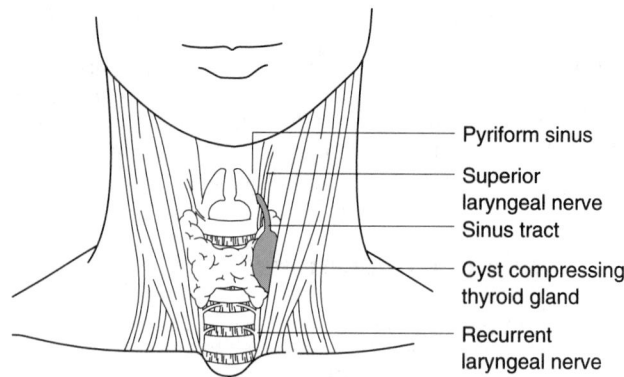

Figure 98-6. Relations of the third or fourth branchial cleft cyst or sinus to the thyroid gland and pyriform sinus.

the tip of the submandibular gland due to extension of the dissection too far lateral or failure to identify and resect the entire proximal midline tract at the base of the tongue. Subsequent infection is managed initially with antibiotics. Complete resolution often follows, obviating a second surgical procedure.

A low neck mass near the midline may be a cervical thymic cyst or bronchogenic cyst. Ultrasound or CT scans show whether the mass is cystic or solid and help determine whether the mass extends into the mediastinum. Complete surgical removal is indicated.

LYMPHANGIOMA AND CYSTIC HYGROMA

Anatomy and Embryology

About the sixth week of gestation, a system of clefts develops in the cervical mesenchyme and forms lymph channels. These channels give rise to lymph sacs that form cervical lymph nodes and lymphatics, ultimately draining into the internal jugular venous system. If portions of these lymphatic channels do not develop communications with the internal jugular system, masses of disorganized, dilated lymph channels form. These are *lymphangiomas*. They oc-

area of the neck in or just off the midline, although they may be present anywhere from the submental area to the upper trachea.

Clinical Issues

Thyroglossal duct cysts may be asymptomatic or appear as an acutely infected midline neck mass. When acute infection is the presentation, therapy with antibiotics that cover oral flora, such as amoxicillin, is instituted. Failure of resolution with 7 to 10 days of antibiotics necessitates incision and drainage of the infected cyst followed by excision when the infection resolves.

Operative Considerations

Successful surgical treatment involves removal of the cyst, its entire tract, and the central component of the hyoid bone. The proximal tract is suture ligated. Failure to remove the center of the hyoid bone and perform a complete excision results in a recurrence rate of about 50%. If a proper excision is done, recurrence indicates injury to

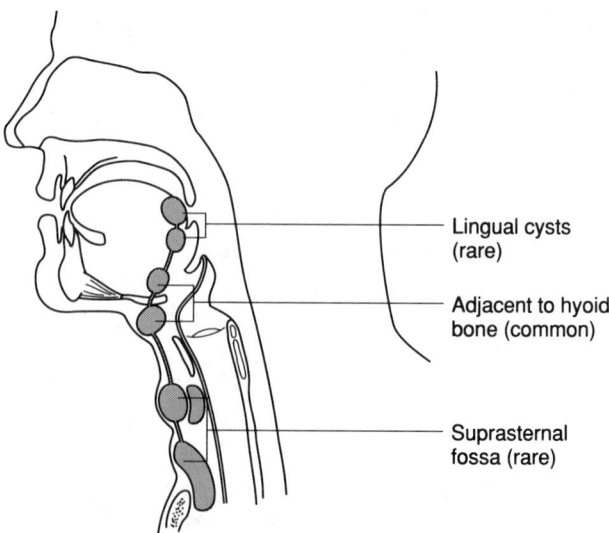

Figure 98-7. Locations of thyroglossal duct cysts.

cur in the lateral cervical and submandibular region along the jugular chain of lymphatics. They can be a few centimeters in diameter or massive tumor-like lesions that extend into the mediastinum. Large lesions with dilated cystic lymphatic channels are often called *cystic hygromas.*

Clinical Issues

Most cystic hygromas are present at birth. They may be diagnosed prenatally with ultrasonography. These lesions are generally soft, fluctuant, and multiloculated. In newborns cystic hygromas may compromise the airway and obstruct the esophagus and pharynx. If there is hypopharyngeal or supraglottic involvement, endotracheal intubation may be difficult. In extreme situations, early tracheostomy may be required.

Although small lesions may be missed at birth, most cystic hygromas are diagnosed by the age of 2 years. As lymph accumulates, the lesions may grow. Dramatic enlargement may occur hours or days after acute occlusion of draining lymphatics or acute hemorrhage into the lesion. Although a small lesion may be confused with hemangioma or a branchial cleft cyst, ultrasonography demonstrates the cystic multiloculated character of the lesion, and radionuclide scans or angiography can confirm its vascularity. Spontaneous regression of these lesions is unusual but may occur after acute inflammation.

Operative Considerations

Definitive surgical excision is indicated. Most lymphangiomas and cystic hygromas are readily excised. Large cystic hygromas may extend across tissue planes, infiltrate muscle, distort nerves and vessels, or otherwise involve vital structures that cannot be resected. When complete resection is not possible, the lesions are unroofed and drained with the expectation of recurrence and additional surgical excision.

LYMPHADENOPATHY

Palpable lymph nodes are common during childhood. The nodes most commonly enlarged are cervical, followed by occipital and submandibular nodes. The location of lymphadenopathy varies with age; the occipital nodes are most commonly affected in infants and the cervical nodes most commonly in older children.

Acute suppurative lymphadenitis related to bacterial pathogens is straightforward to diagnose. An infectious illness, such as an upper respiratory infection, pharyngitis, or facial rash, usually occurs. The nodes enlarge rapidly and are tender, and erythema of the overlying skin occurs. Fever and an elevated white blood cell count with a left shift occur. Fluctuant nodes can be aspirated with a large-bore needle to obtain material for culture. Removal of the necrotic infected material at aspiration often hastens resolution and may obviate incision and drainage.

Subacute inflammation of nodes is difficult to diagnose and manage. The nodes often are deep, may appear suddenly, or may enlarge slowly over days and weeks. If present, tenderness is minimal, and there may be no systemic signs. Lymph node hyperplasia can occur in response to any viral or bacterial infection and may not respond to antibiotics.

The most common causes of subacute inflammation of nodes in the United States are atypical *mycobacterial* infection and cat-scratch disease. Atypical mycobacterial enters through the oral pharynx and is not associated with pulmonary findings. A first-strength tuberculosis skin test (purified protein derivative) is often negative, but an intermediate-strength test may be positive.

It is common for pediatricians to encounter *asymptomatic lymph node enlargement* and not be able to determine the cause. A reasonable first response is to prescribe a 5 to 10 day course of an antibiotic to which *Streptococcus* and most *Staphylococcus* organisms are sensitive. If the adenopathy does not resolve in 2 to 3 weeks, the patient undergoes excisional biopsy. An enlarged nonsuppurative lymph node that does not resolve after a short course of antibiotics is considered lymphoma until proved otherwise with a biopsy.

Operative Considerations

Excisional lymph node biopsy is performed in the operating room with general anesthesia so that deep dissection can be performed to obtain the most involved lymph node. Samples of the node are subjected to bacterial, viral, fungal, and mycobacterial culture. Lymph nodes that may be infected with atypical mycobacterial organisms must be completely excised, or a draining fistula may result. A child with multiple enlarged nonsuppurative lymph nodes is examined by means of appropriate serum assays for infectious mononucleosis and other diseases associated with Epstein–Barr virus. If these tests are negative, Hodgkin disease or non-Hodgkin lymphoma is likely.

HEMANGIOMA

Hemangiomas occur anywhere on the head and neck and fall into one of three classifications:

1. Capillary, which have a substantial dermal component
2. Cavernous, which are primarily subcutaneous
3. Mixed

Any dermal capillary component helps one confirm by means of inspection that the underlying lesion is a hemangioma. A flow-directional ultrasound scan may show the vascular component of a complex mass when the tell-tale dermal component is missing.

Clinical Issues

Hemangiomas often grow rapidly during the first 6 to 12 months of life, after which they stabilize and begin to involute. The natural history generally is spontaneous resolution by means of thrombosis and epithelialization. The capillary component changes from bright red to gray as regression occurs. Most patients with hemangiomas of the head and neck can be treated with watchful waiting and reassurance that resolution is probable. Periodic clinic visits ensure detection of a hemangioma that begins to interfere with function by deforming an eyelid or obstructing an ear canal.

Treatment

Lesions that grow uncontrollably, present physiologic problems, or impair function are managed first with a course of steroids. If medical management is unsuccessful, careful surgical excision may be required. Some superficial lesions can be managed with laser therapy. Medical therapy with α-interferon and other anti-angiogneic factor is now becoming feasible.

SUGGESTED READING

Filston HC. Common lumps and bumps of the neck in infants and children. Pediatr Ann 1989;18:180.

Kinnefors A, Olofsson J. Acute epiglottitis in children: experiences with tracheostomy and intubation. Clin Otolaryngol 1983;8:25.

Miller D, Hill JL, Sun CC, O'Brien DS, Haller JA Jr. The diagnosis and management of pyriform sinus fistulae in infants and young children. J Pediatr Surg 1983;18:377.

Oon TT, Gilchrest BA. Laser therapy for selected cutaneous vascular lesions in the pediatric population: a review. Pediatrics 1988;82:652.

Orchard PJ, Smith CN, Woods WG, Day DL, Dehner LP, Shapiro R. Treatment of hemangioendotheliomas with alpha interferon. Lancet 1989;2:565.

Rosenfeld RM, Biller HF. Fourth branchial pouch sinus: diagnosis and treatment. Otolaryngol Head Neck Surg 1991;105:44.

ESSENTIALS OF SURGERY: SCIENTIFIC PRINCIPLES AND PRACTICE,
edited by Lazar J. Greenfield, Michael W. Mulholland, Keith T. Oldham, Gerald B. Zelenock, and Keith D. Lillemoe. Lippincott–Raven Publishers, Philadelphia, © 1997.

CHAPTER 99

PEDIATRIC THORAX

ARNOLD G. CORAN AND KEITH T. OLDHAM

CHEST WALL, LUNG, AND MEDIASTINUM

Chest Wall Deformities

Generally, congenital deformities of the chest wall cause cosmetic and psychologic problems rather than physiologic disability. Pulmonary and cardiac functional abnormalities rarely occur.

Pectus Excavatum and Pectus Carinatum

Pectus excavatum is the most frequent chest wall abnormality. It is characterized by a posterior curve in the body of the sternum, beginning at the manubrium and extending to the xiphoid (Fig. 99-1). Rapid growth of the costal carti-

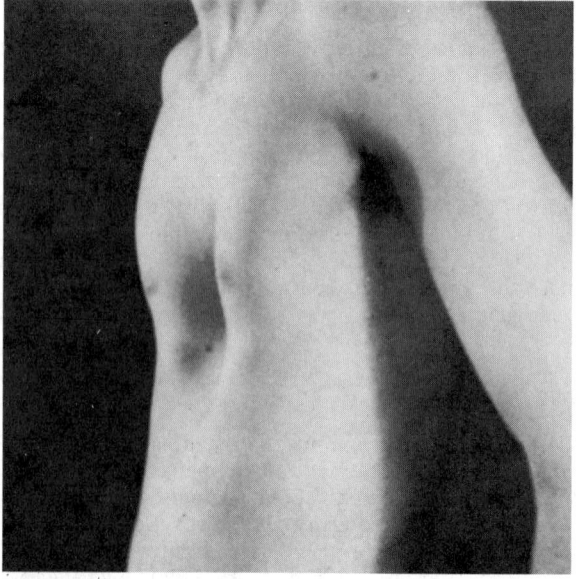

Figure 99-1. Typical pectus excavatum deformity.

lages during development causes the sternum to buckle. Pectus excavatum is present at birth and progresses during childhood. By adolescence, a stoop-shouldered posture is frequent. Concurrent scoliosis is corrected after pectus excavatum repair. Marfan syndrome is an associated disorder.

Repair is best undertaken in late childhood or adolescence. The procedure involves detachment of the muscles from the sternum; resection of the deformed costal cartilages, usually three through seven; fracture, elevation, and stabilization of the sternum; placement of a strut; and reattachment of the muscles.

Pectus carinatum (pigeon breast) occurs much less frequently than pectus excavatum. Excessively rapid growth of the costal cartilages causes elevation of the sternum. Surgical repair of pectus carinatum is similar to that of pectus excavatum, but the sternum is depressed to achieve the neutral position. There is no need for a sternal strut.

Sternal Clefts

Congenital sternal clefts are caused by failure of midline fusion of the paired sternal bands. The most common form of sternal cleft is a defect in the superior portion of the sternum, extending to but not including the xiphoid. These defects are extremely rare. Although the defects are asymptomatic, repair protects underlying mediastinal structures. Repair is undertaken immediately after birth. It consists of subcutaneous mobilization and midline approximation of the fibrocartilaginous sternal bars. If necessary, synthetic material or autogenous cartilage may be used to close the sternal defect.

Poland Syndrome

Features of Poland syndrome include absence of the sternal portions of the pectoralis major muscle, the pectoralis minor muscle, and portions of the serratus anterior and external oblique muscles; hand deformities, usually syndactyly and absence of the phalanges; hypoplasia of the nipple, breast, and subcutaneous tissue; absence or deformity of costal cartilages two through five; and hairlessness of the axilla on the affected side. The syndrome is asymptomatic.

The surgical approach to the chest deformity of Poland syndrome is similar to that for pectus excavatum and pectus carinatum. The tendency of the sternum to rotate in an axial plane toward the affected side, however, necessitates placement of a substernal strut. In girls, a mammary implant is required after puberty to compensate for asymmetry or absence of the breast.

CYSTS AND TUMORS

Congenital Cystic Disease of the Lung

Types of abnormality include: pulmonary sequestrations, cystic adenomatoid malformations, congenital lobar overinflation, and bronchogenic cysts.

Diagnosis

Children with congenital cystic disease of the lung have symptoms due to either recurrent infection in the cyst or adjacent lung, or compression and collapse of adjacent bronchi and lung tissue and respiratory distress. Extralobar sequestrations are often asymptomatic, as are most bronchogenic cysts. Congenital lobar overinflation may cause marked air-trapping and respiratory distress within the first 48 hours of life.

Plain radiography is the first imaging study when cystic lesions are suspected or respiratory symptoms occur. Computed tomography (CT) can help differentiate cystic from

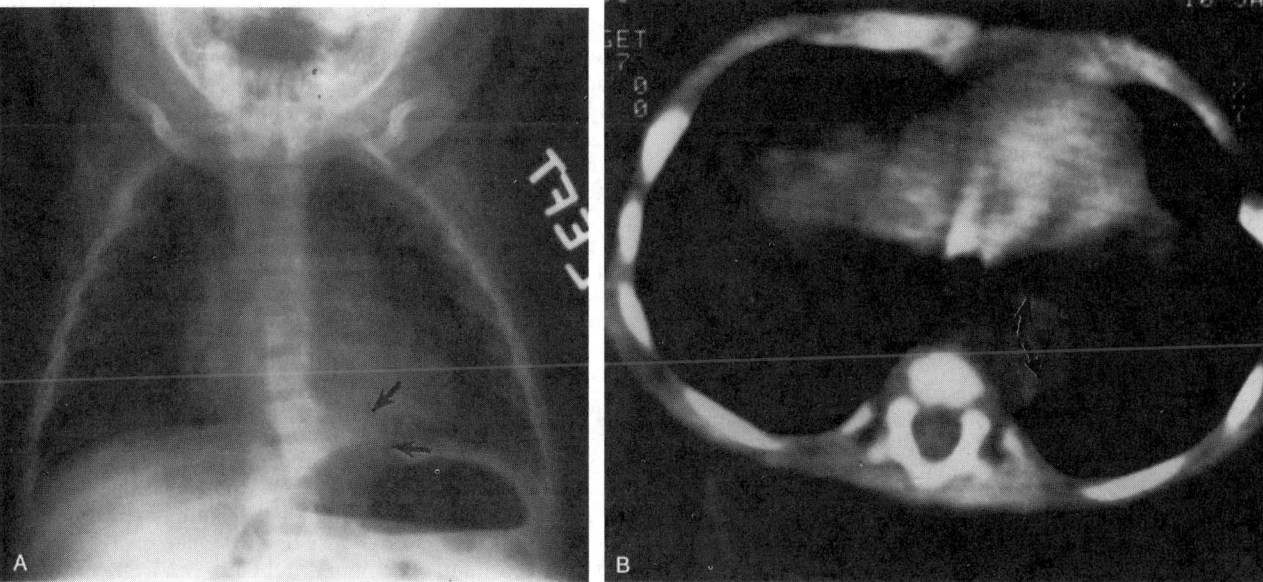

Figure 99-2. (*A*) Plain chest radiograph of a child with a mediastinal bronchogenic cyst (*arrows*). (*B*) CT appearance of the same lesion (*arrows*). (Courtesy of Don Frush, MD, Duke University Medical Center, Durham)

solid components in a radiopaque lung mass (Fig. 99-2). This is the single most useful diagnostic study. When a soft tissue or water-dense mass is adjacent to the chest wall, ultrasonography (US) can help identify the lesion (Fig. 99-3). CT and US overlap in diagnostic efficacy. Prenatal US diagnosis is routine.

Barium esophagography is performed on patients with dysphagia and may show abnormal communication with the gastrointestinal (GI) tract. Segmentation anomalies of the spine suggest a neurenteric cyst. Thoracic and upper abdominal aortography may be useful to demonstrate an anomalous systemic arterial vessel with a pulmonary sequestration; however, this is rarely necessary in contemporary practice. Digital subtraction angiography or Doppler-ultrasound may demonstrate the vascular anatomy.

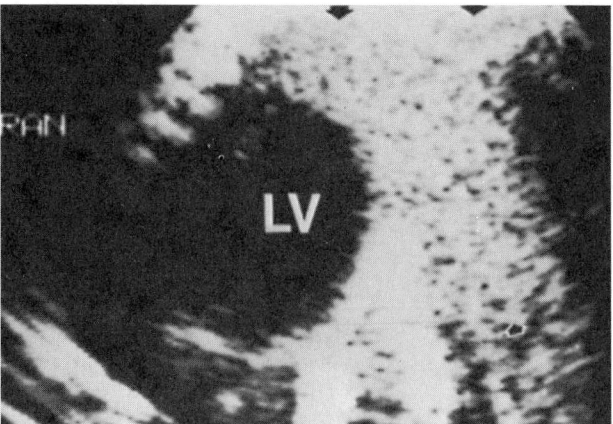

Figure 99-3. Transverse ultrasound scan through the left hemithorax of a patient with cystic adenomatoid malformation, showing a solid echogenic mass (*arrows*) adjacent to the heart. LV, left ventricle. (Wesley JR, Heidelberger KP, DiPietro MA, et al. Diagnosis and management of congenital cystic disease of the lung in children. J Pediatr Surg 1986;21:205)

Treatment

An infant with symptomatic congenital cystic disease of the lung undergoes immediate surgical treatment. Asymptomatic pulmonary cysts must be removed because they can become infected and because of a rare association with malignant neoplasms. Any cyst that is enlarging on serial chest radiographs is resected because of risk of compression of adjacent heart or lungs and cardiac or respiratory compromise. Congenital cysts infected at the time of diagnosis are removed when tissue levels of broad-spectrum antibiotics are established.

Surgical management includes complete lobectomy for patients with intralobar pulmonary sequestration and cystic adenomatoid malformation. Extralobar pulmonary sequestrations may be associated with a diaphragmatic hernia, and the surgeon keeps this in mind when operating for either condition. Children with congenital lobar overinflation undergo complete resection of the affected lobe. Emergency thoracotomy is occasionally necessary to relieve the compression of the adjacent lung tissue, heart, and great veins to prevent cardiopulmonary collapse.

Cysts of the Mediastinum

Although most cysts and tumors of the mediastinum are asymptomatic, resection usually is required. When present, symptoms include chest pain, cough, respiratory distress, hemoptysis, and dysphagia. Common cystic lesions are thymic cysts, enterogenous cysts, dermoid cysts, pericardial cysts, and cystic lymphangioma (cystic hygroma).

Lung Tumors

Primary Tumors

Bronchial adenomas are the most common primary lung tumors among children, but they are quite rare. They are low-grade adenocarcinomas that are classified as carcinoids, cylindromas, mucoepidermoid tumors, or bronchomucous gland adenomas. Carcinoid tumors are the most

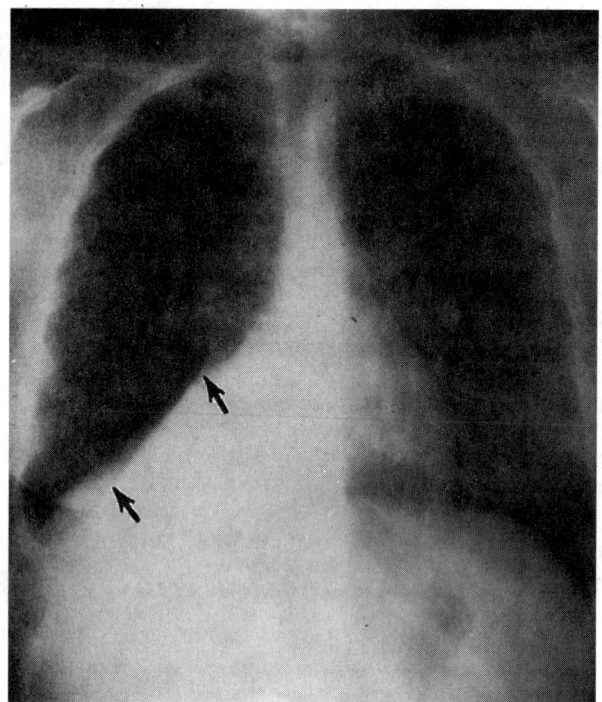

Figure 99-4. Chest radiograph of a 15-year-old girl with a 3-week history of refractory pneumonia. Right middle and lower lobe collapse is obvious (*arrows*). At bronchoscopy, this patient had a nearly completely obstructing carcinoid tumor of the bronchus intermedius.

choscopy, but most adenomas necessitate pulmonary resection, usually lobectomy, for complete removal. Some bronchial adenomas show evidence of malignancy through local invasion and metastases to regional nodes. Bronchial carcinoids may respond to radiation therapy.

Bronchogenic carcinoma of the lung is extremely rare among children. The diagnosis is rarely established until the disease is widespread. Cough and dyspnea associated with pleural effusion are the common presenting symptoms. With early discovery, tumor resection for cure is possible.

Pulmonary blastoma is a malignant lung tumor composed of cells that resemble fetal lung. The site is almost always in the periphery of the lung.

Other rare malignant tumors of the lung among children include neurofibrosarcoma, embryoma, mesothelioma, fibrosarcoma, rhabdomyosarcoma, and endothelial sarcoma. Lobectomy or pneumonectomy is performed if the disease is localized.

Benign tumors of the lung are rare among children. The most common are pulmonary hamartomas or chondromas. These occur in the periphery of the lung and are composed of fibrous tissue, adipose tissue, bronchial epithelium, and cartilage. They are usually asymptomatic but can cause bronchial obstruction. If symptomatic, they can be managed with limited wedge resection. The usual surgical indication is needed to establish a diagnosis. Other benign tumors of the lung among children include leiomyoma, leiomyoblastoma, and mucus gland adenoma. Surgical resection is required to relieve symptoms or establish the diagnosis.

Metastatic Tumors

Lung metastases are most common in children with Wilms tumor and osteogenic sarcoma. If metastases are present at the initial diagnosis of Wilms tumor, therapy is nephrectomy with chemotherapy and radiation therapy. Surgical removal of the metastatic lung tumor is undertaken if the pulmonary metastases remain or recur after initial treatment. Adjuvant chemotherapy for osteogenic sarcoma reduces the likelihood of pulmonary metastases. Therapy includes an aggressive surgical approach to pul-

common bronchial adenomas. Adenomas originate in a primary or secondary bronchus and produce persistent cough, hemoptysis, and bronchial obstruction with secondary pulmonary infection and atelectasis.

Chest radiographs may show pneumonia, atelectasis, or air-trapping (Fig. 99-4). The most important diagnostic test is bronchoscopy. Because these tumors are friable and prone to bleed, endobronchial biopsy must be done with great care. Some carcinoids have been removed at bron-

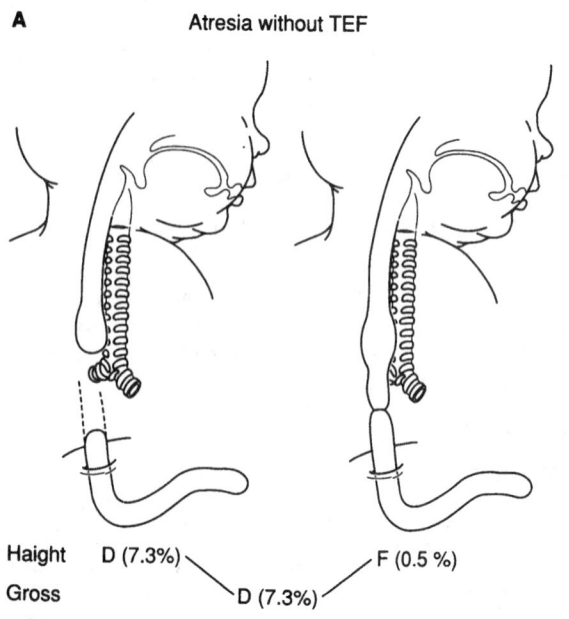

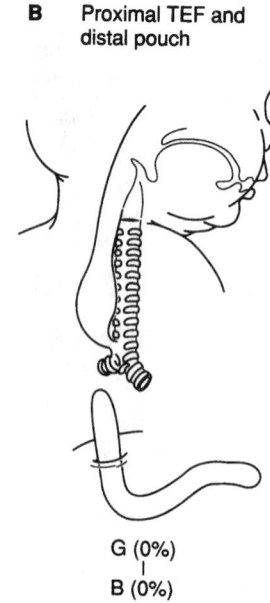

A Atresia without TEF

Haight   D (7.3%)   F (0.5 %)
Gross   D (7.3%)

B Proximal TEF and distal pouch

G (0%)
B (0%)

Figure 99-5. The anatomy of the possible variants of esophageal atresia (EA) and tracheoesophageal fistula (TEF). Both the Haight and the Gross classification systems are shown, with approximate incidence of occurrence. (After Manning PB, Morgan RA, Coran AG, et al. Fifty years' experience with esophageal atresia and tracheoesophageal fistula. Ann Surg 1986;204:446)

monary metastases after chemotherapy and resection of the primary tumor.

Mediastinal Tumors

Mediastinal tumors include lymphomas, neurogenic tumors (benign ganglioneuroma and neurofibroma, malignant neuroblastoma), teratomas, thymomas, and a variety of rare lesions. Some children with Hodgkin lymphoma have an anterior mediastinal mass. Cough, respiratory obstruction, or superior vena cava syndrome may be the presenting symptom. Cervical adenopathy also is present. Management is surgical extirpation except for the lymphomas in which biopsy and chemotherapy with or without chemotherapy is done .

CONGENITAL ABNORMALITIES OF THE TRACHEA AND ESOPHAGUS
Esophageal Atresia and Tracheoesophageal Fistula

The anatomic variations of esophageal atresia and tracheoesophageal fistula are shown in Fig. 99-5.

Pathophysiology

Respiratory symptoms develop soon after birth. Esophageal atresia prevents normal swallowing and results in accumulation of saliva in the proximal esophageal pouch, and aspiration occurs. Because esophageal atresia and tracheoesophageal fistula are asymptomatic at birth, the child is fed, but vomiting and aspiration occur.

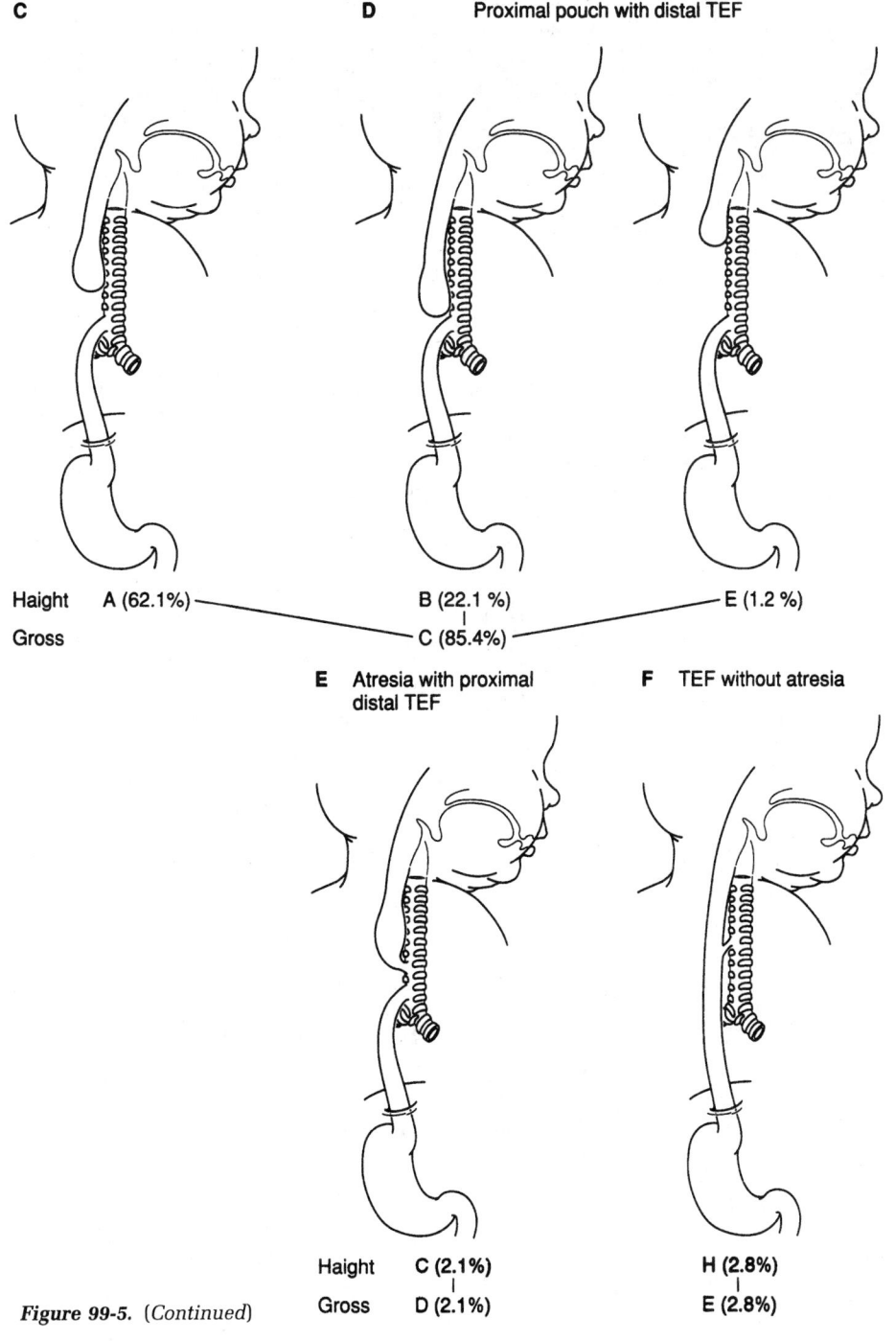

Figure 99-5. (*Continued*)

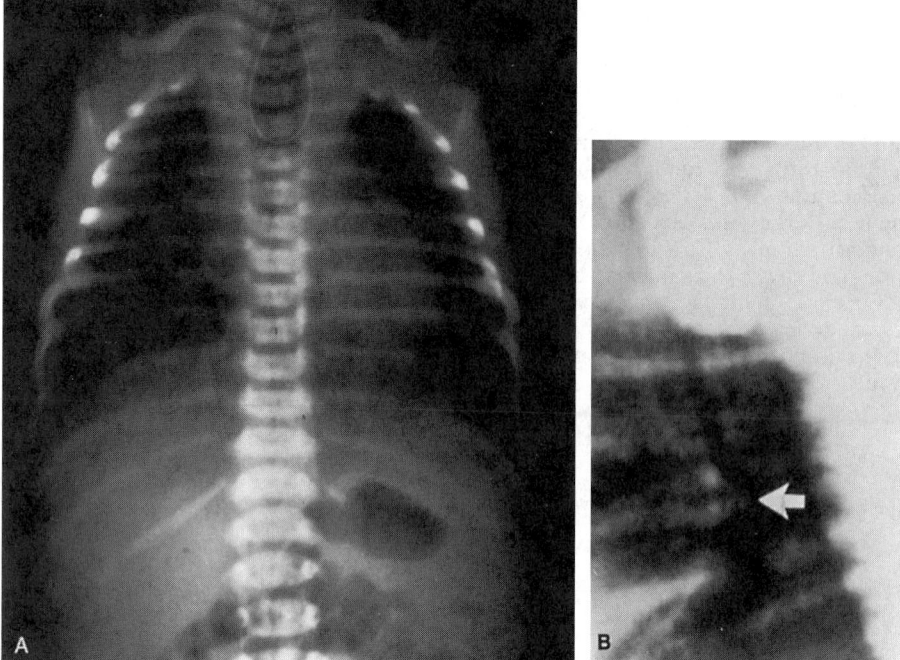

Figure 99-6. Chest radiographs of an infant with esophageal atresia and distal tracheoesophageal fistula. (*A*) The nasogastric tube can be seen coiled in the blind proximal esophageal pouch. (*B*) Air is visible within the fistula (*arrow*). (*B* from Coran AG. Congenital abnormalities of the esophagus. In: Zuidema GD, Orringer MD, eds. Shackelford's surgery of the alimentary tract, ed 2. Philadelphia, WB Saunders, 1990)

The distal tracheoesophageal fistula produces the most serious physiologic disturbances. Because most newborns have free gastroesophageal reflux, gastric secretions reflux unimpeded into the tracheobronchial tree and generate acid-induced pneumonitis. This is exacerbated by gastric distention caused by passage of air from the trachea into the fistula and into the stomach with each breath. This distention sometimes is so severe that it limits excursion of the diaphragm and impairs ventilation.

Associated anomalies vary from skeletal deformities to uncorrectable cardiac defects. The most common associated anomalies are cardiac abnormalities and imperforate anus. Every newborn with an imperforate anus is examined for the presence of esophageal atresia and vice versa.

Diagnosis

Maternal polyhydramnios is a feature of the history of patients with esophageal atresia. With prenatal US screening, this anomaly often is detected before delivery. After delivery, infants with esophageal atresia drool and accumulate excessive secretions in the posterior pharynx. Choking, coughing, and cyanosis occur, especially with feedings.

The simplest way to establish the diagnosis of esophageal atresia is to attempt to pass a catheter through the mouth or nose into the stomach. If the tube encounters obstruction, a plain radiograph in the frontal and lateral projections is used to document the atresia (Fig. 99-6). Contrast-enhanced radiographs are obtained to confirm the diagnosis. The abdomen is examined by means of plain radiography to determine whether intestinal gas is present. A gasless abdomen confirms the diagnosis of esophageal atresia without tracheoesophageal fistula.

Children with isolated tracheoesophageal fistula are usually several months of age at diagnosis. The history includes recurrent respiratory symptoms, such as pneumo-

nia and choking with feedings. Cine esophagography with barium shows communication between the trachea and esophagus. If a contrast study is normal but clinical suspicion is high, simultaneous bronchoscopy and esophagoscopy are performed.

Preoperative Treatment

Preoperative treatment involves prevention of aspiration and reflux and management of pneumonitis. A sump catheter is placed into the upper pouch, the infant is placed in an upright position, and if necessary, gastrostomy is performed under local anesthesia. The infant is given broad-spectrum antibiotics and kept in an upright position until the operation, which may not take place until several weeks after birth.

Surgical Treatment

The goal of surgical therapy is to correct the anomaly with one operation. This includes division of the tracheoesophageal fistula and primary esophagoesophagostomy. Infants at high risk who have esophageal atresia and tracheoesophageal fistula receive a gastrostomy for gastric decompression, proximal esophageal suction, and parenteral nutrition. Once the infant's condition is stable, extrapleural thoracotomy is used for division of the fistula and primary repair of the esophageal atresia. This is ordinarily done promptly after birth.

Complications

Three major complications are related to the esophageal anastomosis/leak, stricture, and recurrent fistula.

Two other postoperative conditions that are not technical complications are gastroesophageal reflux and tracheomalacia.

Laryngotracheoesophageal Cleft

Laryngotracheoesophageal cleft is a rare anomaly that probably is an extreme form of tracheoesophageal fistula. There are three forms of cleft: Type I, limited to the larynx; Type II, partial cleft of esophagus and trachea; and Type III, complete cleft extending from larynx to tracheal carina.

The most common symptom of laryngotracheoesophageal cleft is respiratory distress with feeding. Hoarseness, stridor, cyanosis, and aspiration pneumonia are important but nonspecific signs. The most effective way to define the anomaly is with rigid bronchoscopy. Management is surgical repair. Postoperative laryngeal instability may necessitate prolonged intubation.

Congenital Esophageal Stenosis

Congenital stenosis of the esophagus is rare. It is usually related to abnormal tissue in the esophageal wall that contains respiratory epithelium and cartilage. The abnormality may take the form of a congenital web or diaphragm in the middle to lower third of the esophagus. Stenosis occurs with esophageal atresia with or without tracheoesophageal fistula.

Children with congenital esophageal stenosis begin having symptoms when solid foods are introduced into the diet. The diagnosis can be made with a barium swallow radiographic examination and confirmed with esophagoscopy. Initial management is repeated dilation, especially for diaphragms or webs. Esophageal stenosis associated with abnormal remnants of respiratory tissue often necessitates segmental resection.

Esophageal Duplications

A variety of epithelium-lined cysts appear in the mediastinum. Enterogenous cysts (esophageal duplications) account for about one fourth of these cysts. They occur in the posterior mediastinum and are covered by intestinal muscular wall. They are lined with intestinal epithelium, often gastric epithelium, and sometimes ciliated respiratory epithelium. Some cysts may be attached to or communicate with the spinal canal (*neurenteric cysts*). They usually have no communication with the lumen of the esophagus and are filled with mucoid-type material. The presence of gastric epithelium can cause acid-peptic ulceration of the cysts with substernal pain, erosion into the bronchus or esophagus, and pulmonary hemorrhage. Most symptoms result from compression of adjacent viscera. The lesions are excised by means of dissection of the cyst from the adjacent esophagus.

Vascular Rings

Vascular rings, a rare cause of esophageal obstruction, result from faulty development of the aortic arch. Rings are complete or incomplete and obstruct the trachea, the esophagus, or both. Treatment is surgical division of the aortic arch and the fibrous tissue around the trachea and *esophagus.*

Congenital Tracheal Stenosis

Congenital stenosis of the distal trachea is fatal if not repaired. Failure of tracheal growth can range from mild, generalized hypoplasia to specific stenosis to pulmonary agenesis. Most forms are associated with complete tracheal rings at the level of the stenosis and disorganization of cartilage formation. The diagnosis is confirmed at bronchoscopy. Therapy depends on the anatomy of the lesion. Segmental stenoses are managed by means of resection and end-to-end anastomosis. Longer stenoses are managed with rib, pericardial, or synthetic grafts.

Foreign Bodies of the Tracheobronchial Tree

Clinical Features

Peanuts are the single most common foreign body aspirated into the tracheobronchial tree. They are particularly troublesome because they produce an inflammatory reaction and because they become soft, necessitating piecemeal removal. Other common foreign bodies include carrots, popcorn, toy parts, pins, wood, paper, and plastic.

The signs and symptoms of tracheobronchial foreign bodies are listed in Table 99-1. A history that suggests aspiration of a foreign body is adequate indication for bronchoscopy. Physical examination demonstrates wheezing or decreased breath sounds over one hemithorax. Inspiratory and expiratory chest radiographs demonstrate hyperinflation on the affected side.

Management

When the diagnosis is confirmed or the history is indicative, immediate rigid bronchoscopy is performed. Most bronchial foreign bodies can be extracted with an optical forceps. If this technique is unsuccessful, a flexible wire grasper or Fogarty catheter can be used, especially if the foreign body has migrated into a segmental bronchus. When the foreign body cannot be visualized, fluoroscopy is used to guide a flexible wire grasper to the foreign body.

CONGENITAL ABNORMALITIES OF THE DIAPHRAGM

Congenital diaphragmatic abnormalities may result from fusion defects or muscularization defects. Abnormalities of muscularization may be focal or involve an entire hemidiaphragm. The result is that a portion of the diaphragm does not have enough substance to prevent herniation of abdominal viscera into the thorax. Involvement of the entire hemidiaphragm produces diaphragmatic eventration. A focal muscularization defect may yield a posterolateral Bochdalek hernia, with a sac of pleura and peritoneum, or a parasternal Morgagni hernia (Fig. 99-7).

Table 99-1. CLINICAL FINDINGS OF TRACHEOBRONCHIAL FOREIGN BODIES

Signs and Symptoms	Incidence (%)
SYMPTOMS	
Cough	70
Wheezing	50
Dyspnea	30
Fever	20
Emesis	6
Pain	6
SIGNS	
Unilateral decreased breath sounds	50
Unilateral wheezing	45
Rhonchi	10
Cyanosis	10
Pneumonia	6

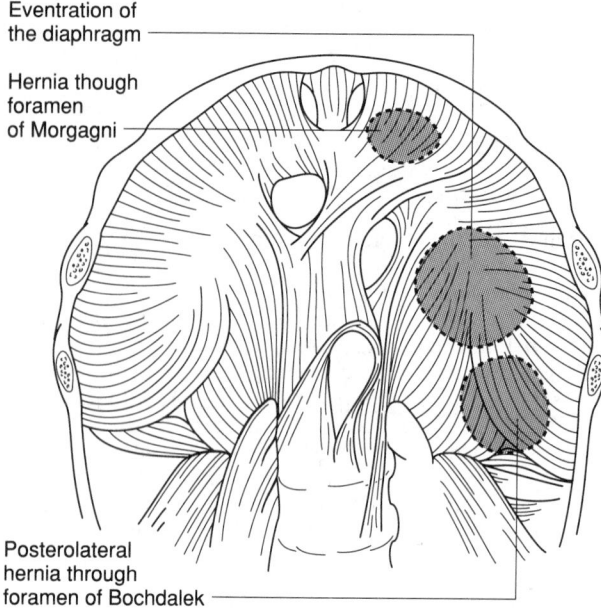

Eventration of
the diaphragm

Hernia though
foramen
of Morgagni

Posterolateral
hernia through
foramen of Bochdalek

Figure 99-7. Locations of congenital diaphragmatic defects.

Anatomy

A normal diaphragm (Fig. 99-8) is composed of striated muscle that originates in the chest and body walls at the thoracic outlet and inserts into the central tendon. Apertures allow passage of the inferior vena cava, aorta, and esophagus between the thorax and the abdomen. The arterial blood supply is through superior and inferior phrenic arteries, usually directly from the aorta, and the musculophrenic and pericardiophrenic arteries. Venous drainage follows the arterial supply, with drainage primarily into the inferior vena cava or azygous vein on the right and into the adrenal or renal and hemiazygous veins on the left.

Innervation is by the phrenic nerve and minor contributions from the lower thoracic nerves. Phrenic nerve injuries and neuromuscular disorders may produce diaphragmatic paralysis and necessitate surgical plication of the diaphragm.

Congenital Diaphragmatic (Bochdalek) Hernia

Anatomy and Physiology

Excluding esophageal hiatal hernia, a posterolateral defect at the foramen of Bochdalek is the most common congenital diaphragmatic hernia (CDH). The usual left-sided hernia contains small intestine, spleen, stomach, and colon; hernias on the right contain liver and possibly intestine (Fig. 99-9). The defect includes a ventral and medial leaf of diaphragm with a smaller, posterior muscular portion enveloped by pleura and peritoneum. A hernial sac may be present.

Defects range from a hernia 1 to 2 cm in diameter to complete agenesis of the hemidiaphragm. Prognosis is related not to the size of the defect but to the degree of pulmonary hypoplasia. Hernias associated with polyhydramnios, those occurring early in gestation, and those with more intrathoracic liver or intestine cause more severe pulmonary hypoplasia. After parturition, respiration is accompanied by air swallowing, which distends the intestine, exacerbating displacement of abdominal viscera into the thorax. Decompression of the GI tract is essential.

Diagnosis

Many diaphragmatic hernias are now discovered during prenatal US examinations. Options include termination of the pregnancy, delivery with ventilatory support and cardiopulmonary bypass available for the infant, and in utero repair of the defect.

After delivery, diaphragmatic hernias are detected because the infant experiences severe respiratory distress in the delivery suite or within the first few hours of life. If symptoms develop more than 24 hours after delivery or there are no symptoms when the hernia is discovered, repair is uneventful.

Many infants become unstable at or soon after birth. The infant's abdomen is scaphoid and the ipsilateral chest is prominent because of the intrathoracic, air-filled intestine. The cardiac impulse is displaced, usually to the right. Breath sounds are diminished or absent on the side of the hernia. The diagnosis is confirmed with a plain chest radiograph. Air-filled loops of intrathoracic intestine with a paucity of abdominal intestine, a nasogastric tube within an intrathoracic stomach, a small ipsilateral lung, no diaphragmatic silhouette, and a contralateral mediastinal shift are characteristic. It is occasionally difficult to differentiate these features from those of primary pulmonary disease. A barium upper GI tract series resolves the uncertainty in these instances.

Associated Anomalies

The most important abnormalities associated with diaphragmatic hernia are cardiovascular. Ventricular septal defects and aortic coarctation are common, but any cardiac or great vessel anomaly can occur. About 20% to 25% of children with diaphragmatic hernias have anomalies of the heart or great vessels. Cardiac US screening examinations are routine. Every infant with a diaphragmatic hernia has a patent ductus arteriosus because of pulmonary arterial hypertension. Central nervous system malformations, gastroesophageal reflux, pulmonary sequestration, chromosomal abnormalities (trisomy 13 and 18), and other rare anomalies also occur with diaphragmatic hernia.

Medical Management

All posterolateral diaphragmatic hernias in infants are repaired surgically, but surgical repair alone does not resolve the respiratory failure. Medical treatment emphasizes respiratory support and careful selection of the optimal time for surgical repair.

Preoperative management involves: nasogastric tube decompression of the intrathoracic intestine, prompt endotracheal intubation and ventilatory support by means of permissive hypercapnia, paralysis and fentanyl-induced anesthesia to ensure total control of ventilation and reduce pulmonary arterial pressure, administration of vasodilators and inotropic agents, and monitoring of arterial blood gases with a preductal sampling site and a postductal site for assessment of the degree of right-to-left shunting through the ductus arteriosus.

Infants with diaphragmatic hernias have considerable variation in degree of respiratory distress. Some appear simply to have inadequate alveolar surface area for gas exchange; these newborns die soon after birth regardless of treatment. Most have one or more periods of adequate gas exchange, which implies the presence of adequate alveolar surface area and suggests respiratory failure may be reversible. This in turn implicates pulmonary artery hypertension as a key pathophysiologic event.

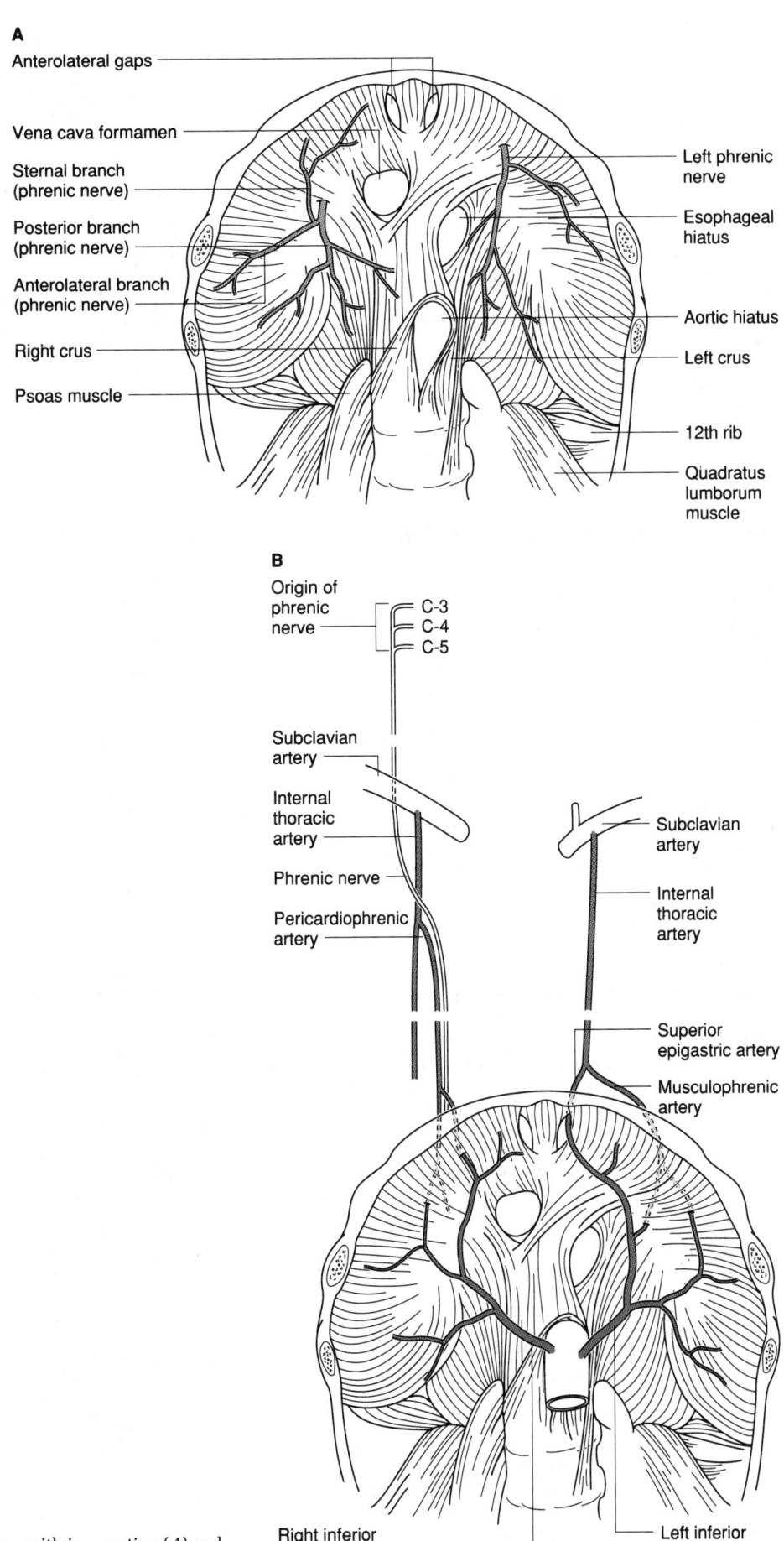

Figure 99-8. Intact normal diaphragm with innervation (*A*) and arterial blood supply (*B*).

Surgical Management

A transabdominal approach through a left subcostal incision is done. The herniated viscera are reduced with gentle traction, and suture repair of the defect is performed. Large diaphragmatic defects may require a transversus abdominis muscle flap, deformation of the chest wall, or insertion of prosthetic material for closure. A small peritoneal cavity resulting from in utero displacement of the abdominal viscera may present an abdominal wall closure problem similar to that of omphalocele or gastroschisis. Stretching the abdominal wall musculature is usually sufficient to effect closure; prosthetic material or a staged closure may be required. If chest tubes are used, water seal or minimal suction drainage must be provided to avoid acute mediastinal shifts.

Evolving strategies in the management of CDH include: extracorporeal membrane oxygenation, high-frequency ventilation, in utero repair of diaphragmatic hernia, pulmonary transplantation, and liquid ventilation.

Morgagni Diaphragmatic Hernias

Morgagni diaphragmatic hernia results from a defect in the anterior retrosternal muscle at one or sometimes both minor apertures where the superior epigastric arteries traverse the diaphragm. The location is parasternal rather than midline (Fig. 99-7). It is a rare, asymptomatic abnormality usually found at the time of diagnostic imaging for unrelated reasons. Air-filled viscera in the mediastinum are seen on plain chest radiographs. Because of the lack of symptoms, patients are older than those with Bochdalek hernias. The hernia most often contains liver, but transverse colon, stomach, and small intestine may be present. Incarceration of hollow viscera accounts for symptoms that do occur. Surgical repair involves a transabdominal approach, reduction of involved viscera, and simple suture closure of the diaphragm to the posterior sheath of the rectus abdominis muscle.

Eventration of the Diaphragm

Diaphragmatic eventration is defined as abnormal elevation of a portion of an intact diaphragm. It usually involves an entire hemidiaphragm but may be focal. *Congenital* eventration is associated with an embryonic defect in muscularization that yields an intact membranous diaphragm with an inadequate or abnormal muscular component. *Acquired* eventration is associated with neuromuscular dysfunction of the diaphragm due to injury to the phrenic nerve or trauma, inflammation, or local neoplastic invasion. Patients with acquired eventration have a normally formed but paralyzed hemidiaphragm, which undergoes muscular atrophy with time.

Many of these patients have asymptomatic eventration that is never discovered. The defect more commonly involves the left hemidiaphragm. Fluoroscopy or US is used to differentiate eventration from diaphragmatic hernia. A barium upper GI radiographic series may be needed. Symptoms among older children and adults are related to compression of the ipsilateral lung or displacement of the stomach into the chest with gastroesophageal reflux or gastric outlet obstruction. Infants may have respiratory failure due to impaired function of the diaphragm. Patients with symptoms benefit from surgical stabilization of the dia-

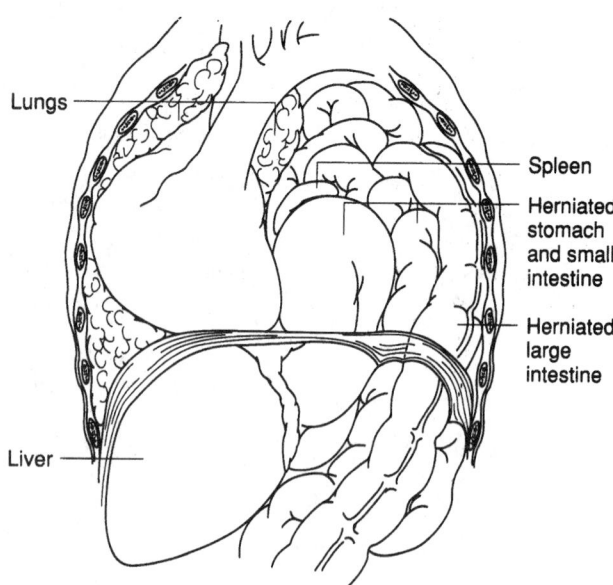

Figure 99-9. Left posterolateral diaphragmatic hernia. The anatomic relations are taken directly from a photograph of a postmortem examination. The stomach, spleen, small intestine, and colon occupy the left hemithorax. Particularly notable are the severe bilateral pulmonary hypoplasia and the mediastinal shift into the right hemithorax.

phragm; patients with asymptomatic eventration undergo observation.

The surgical approach may be through the abdomen or chest. For unilateral eventration, transthoracic exposure is preferred. Surgical management is suture plication of the diaphragm with fixation in an expiratory position.

SUGGESTED READING

Adolph V, Flageole H, Perreaultt T, et al. Repair of congenital diaphragmatic hernia after weaning from extracorporeal membrane oxygenation. J Pediatr Surg 1995;30:349.

Budorick NE, Pretorius DH, Leopold GR, et al. Spontaneous improvement of intrathoracic masses diagnosed in utero. J Ultrasound Med 1992;11:653.

Coughlin JP, Drucker DE, Cullen ML, et al. Delayed repair of congenital diaphragmatic hernia. Am Surg 1993;59:90.

Dolkart LA, Reimers FT, Helmuth WV, et al. Antenatal diagnosis of pulmonary sequestration: a review. Obstet Gynecol Surv 1992;47:515.

Harrison MR, Adzick NS, Estes JM, et al. A prospective study of the outcome for fetuses with diaphragmatic hernia. JAMA 1994;271:382.

Rodgers BM. Thoracoscopy. In: Holcomb GW III, ed. Pediatric endoscopic surgery. Norwalk, Appleton & Lange, 1994:103.

Stein SM, Cox JL, Hernanz-Schulman M, et al. Pediatric chest disease: evaluation by computerized tomography, magnetic resonance imaging, and ultrasonography. Southern Med J 1992;85:735.

Van Meurs KP, Rhine WD, Benitz WE, et al. Lobar lung transplantation as a treatment for congenital diaphragmatic hernia. J Pediatr Surg 1994;29:1557.

Wilson JM, Fauza DO, Lund DP, et al. Antenatal diagnosis of isolated congenital diaphragmatic hernia is not an indicator of outcome. J Pediatr Surg 1994;29:815.

Wung JT, Sahni R, Moffitt ST, et al. Congenital diaphragmatic hernia: survival treated with very delayed surgery, spontaneous respiration, and no chest tube. J Pediatr Surg 1995;30:406.

ESSENTIALS OF SURGERY: SCIENTIFIC PRINCIPLES AND PRACTICE,
edited by Lazar J. Greenfield, Michael W. Mulholland, Keith T. Oldham, Gerald B. Zelenock,
and Keith D. Lillemoe. Lippincott–Raven Publishers, Philadelphia, © 1997.

CHAPTER 100

PEDIATRIC ABDOMEN

JOHN R. WESLEY, KEITH T. OLDHAM,
AND ARNOLD G. CORAN

ABDOMINAL WALL DEFECTS

Gastroschisis and Omphalocele

Gastroschisis and omphalocele are congenital abdominal wall defects which are differentiated in Table 100-1. Immediately after birth the stomach is aspirated and a nasogastric (NG) tube is placed to reduce intestinal distention. The herniated viscera are wrapped with saline-soaked gauze and covered with a plastic drape to prevent heat loss. Surgical correction involves reduction of the herniated viscera and primary closure of the abdomen if possible. If not, staged reduction and secondary closure are done.

Umbilical Hernia

Most congenital umbilical hernias close spontaneously in the first 3 years of life.

Inguinal Hernia

Inguinal hernias are repaired as an elective outpatient procedure under general anesthesia. Because inguinal hernias in infants and children can often be bilateral, exploration of the contralateral groin is often done. Incarcerated hernias are reduced, and elective repair is performed promptly.

Hydrocele

Communicating hydroceles are similar to indirect inguinal hernias and are managed as such. Noncommunicating hydroceles typically resolve spontaneously by 1 year of age and are usually asymptomatic.

GASTROINTESTINAL DISORDERS IN CHILDREN

Neonatal Intestinal Obstruction

The main clinical manifestation of neonatal intestinal obstruction is bilious vomiting, often in conjunction with abdominal distention. Table 100-2 summarizes the diagnoses.

Intestinal Atresia or Stenosis

The forms of intestinal atresia are depicted in Fig. 100-1. Almost all infants with congenital jejunoileal obstructions have complete atresia. Colonic atresia is rare.

Diagnosis. Congenital intestinal obstruction is detectable with prenatal ultrasonography (US). Maternal polyhydramnios is an indication for prenatal US. The postnatal presentation of small-intestinal obstruction includes bilious vomiting, abdominal distention, and failure to pass meconium. At physical examination loops of proximal intestine are palpated through the abdominal wall. If there is complete congenital intestinal obstruction distal to the ampulla of Vater, the rectum contains white mucus rather than bile-stained meconium. After the history and physical examination, plain abdominal radiographs are obtained. A barium enema examination is used to confirm the diagnosis.

Management. Therapy for congenital intestinal obstruction is surgical. The strategy is to reestablish intestinal continuity and preserve as much length and normal anatomy as possible.

Congenital Duodenal Obstruction (Duodenal Atresia or Stenosis and Annular Pancreas)

A large percentage of infants with congenital duodenal obstruction also have trisomy 21. A karyotype is obtained for infants born with duodenal obstruction. A preoperative cardiac US examination also is performed to evaluate the possibility of congenital heart disease.

Diagnosis. Feeding intolerance and bilious vomiting in the first 24 to 48 hours of life are characteristic of congenital duodenal obstruction. Malformations proximal to the ampulla of Vater cause nonbilious vomiting. At physical examination, gastric peristaltic waves may be visible through the abdominal wall, and the stomach may be palpable. The small intestine is collapsed and gasless.

Maternal polyhydramnios is characteristic of congenital duodenal obstruction, and prenatal US diagnosis is reliable. The postpartum diagnostic evaluation for duodenal obstruction begins and may conclude with plain abdominal radiographs. Any uncertainty is resolved immediately with an upper GI series.

Table 100-1. **COMPARISON OF GASTROSCHISIS AND OMPHALOCELE**

Characteristic	Gastroschisis	Omphalocele
Defect size	2–3 cm	2–15 cm
Sac	Never	Always; may be torn, with remnants
Umbilical cord	Left of defect, on abdominal wall	Attached to sac
Herniated viscera	Small bowel; occasionally stomach, colon	Small bowel, colon, stomach, liver
Malrotation	Yes	Yes
Quality of bowel	Edematous, stiff, with inflammatory exudate	Normal
Alimentation	Delayed	Normal
Associated anomalies	Uncommon (10%)	Common (50%)

Table 100-2. **NEONATAL INTESTINAL OBSTRUCTION**

Diagnosis	History	Physical Examination	Relevant Studies
Intestinal atresia or stenosis	Bilious vomiting	Abdominal distention Acholic meconium	Plain radiograph Barium enema
Congenital duodenal obstruction	Bilious vomiting	Gastric distention Trisomy 21	Plain radiograph Upper GI study
Imperforate anus	Failure to pass meconium Bilious vomiting (late)	Abdominal distention Nonpatent anus	Evaluate for VATER syndrome and cardiac anomalies
Necrotizing enterocolitis	High-risk, premature infant Bilious vomiting	Abdominal distention Guaiac-positive stool	Plain radiograph Contrast studies contraindicated
Meconium ileus	Bilious vomiting Cystic fibrosis	Abdominal distention Acholic meconium	Plain radiograph Barium enema
Malrotation	Full-term, healthy infant Bilious vomiting	No abdominal distention	Plain radiograph Upper GI study Barium enema
Hirschsprung disease	Bilious vomiting Delayed passage of meconium Family history	Abdominal distention Trisomy 21	Barium enema Suction rectal biopsy
Uncommon causes of neonatal obstruction (intussusception, Meckel diverticulum duplications)	Variable	Incarcerated hernia Mass	Variable
Medical conditions associated with bilious vomiting and ileus	Variable	Variable	Sepsis Hypothyroidism Meconium plug syndrome Others

Management. After completion of the preoperative cardiac evaluation and management of any urgent medical problems, prompt surgical correction of congenital duodenal obstructions is undertaken. The goals are restoration of intestinal continuity as simply as possible without sacrificing intestinal length or absorptive area. The operation involves bypass of the obstructing lesion by means of duodenoduodenostomy.

Anorectal Malformations (Imperforate Anus)

The two common variants in boys are low imperforate anus with a perineal fistula and high anorectal agenesis with a rectoprostatic urethral fistula. In girls the rectal pouch is usually low and is most commonly associated with a fistula to the perineal body or the vaginal vestibule. The division between *high* and *low* is the pubococcygeal line. Abnormalities associated with anorectal malformations are the VATER associations, (Vertebral anomalies, Anorectal malformations, TracheoEsophageal fistula, Renal or lower genitourinary tract malformations), and cardiac anomalies, and limb and other skeletal anomalies.

Diagnosis. These malformations are apparent at birth when the infant undergoes a physical examination that includes inspection of the perineum and digital rectal examination. The signs and symptoms are those of intestinal obstruction. A bucket-handle skin bridge in the area of the anus suggests a low lesion. Signs of high malformation include the absence of normal anal skin features and the absence of external sphincter contraction with cutaneous stimulation. Abnormal gluteal contour produces a flat-bottom appearance. Among girls, almost all low malformations have a perineal or vaginal vestibular fistula.

The goal of diagnostic evaluation is to classify the abnormality as high or low. Diagnostic needle aspiration is performed on a possible fistula site or covered anus. Aspiration of meconium into the syringe localizes the rectum or fistula. Low lesions are estimated to be within 1 to 1.5 cm

of the perineum; other malformations are high. US is a very helpful tool to define the anatomic relations. Preoperative evaluation includes assessment of upper and lower urinary tracts with renal US and voiding cystourethrography in addition to imaging of the spine.

Management. Treatment of anorectal malformations is always surgical, but it is not a matter of life-threatening urgency. Low malformations are repaired in the newborn period and do not require a proximal diverting colostomy. High or indeterminate anorectal malformations necessitate diverting colostomy. The colostomy may be placed in the sigmoid or transverse colon as long as the site provides enough distal length for pull-through of the rectal pouch to the perineum. The functional outcome is usually excellent for low lesions. For high lesions, few patients are normal although most are socially functional. Formal reconstruction follows and a variety of techniques are employed.

Necrotizing Enterocolitis (NEC)

Neonatal NEC is an idiopathic condition characterized by mucosal intestinal injury that progresses to transmural intestinal necrosis. Conditions that occur with NEC include respiratory failure, sepsis, hypothermia, hypotension, acidosis, hypoxemia, and structural cardiac defects. Many clinical factors determine a premature infant's response to a variety of intestinal (mucosal) stresses (Fig. 100-2).

Diagnosis. The clinical signs of NEC include abdominal distention, bilious vomiting, and occult or gross blood in the stool. The infant is premature, has other medical problems, and has had feedings initiated recently. Table 100-3 shows the staging of NEC. The radiographic finding of pneumatosis intestinalis confirms the diagnosis.

Nonsurgical Management. Almost all infants with NEC can be treated nonsurgically. Initial management consists of NG decompression, broad-spectrum antibiotics,

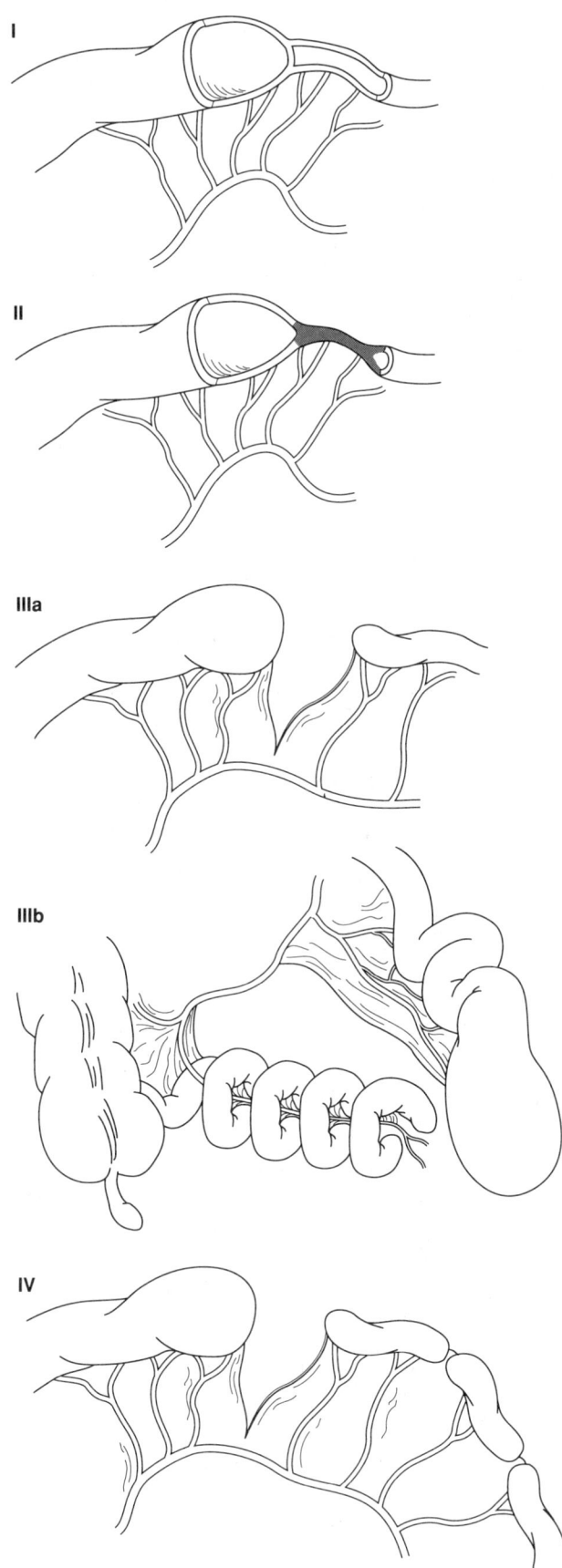

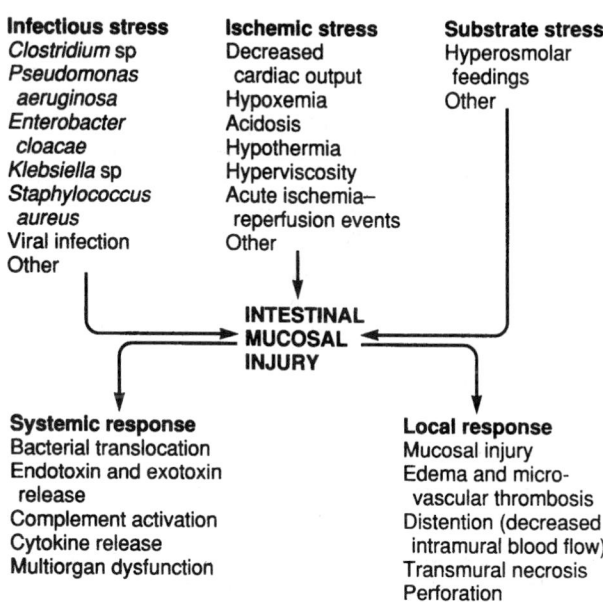

Figure 100-2. Schematic summary of the pathogenesis of necrotizing enterocolitis.

and correction of hypoxemia, hypotension, acidosis, fluid and electrolyte disorders, and any other reversible medical problems. Optimization of cardiac function may necessitate surgical closure of a patent ductus arteriosus. Monitoring for progression of the disease and perforation includes plain abdominal radiographs every 6 to 8 hours to screen

---

Table 100-3. NECROTIZING ENTEROCOLITIS

STAGE I (SUSPECTED)

Any one or more historical factors producing perinatal stress
Systemic manifestations
   Temperature instability
   Lethargy
   Apnea
   Bradycardia
Gastrointestinal manifestations
   Poor feeding
   Increasing pregavage residuals
   Emesis (may be bilious or test positive for occult blood)
   Mild abdominal distention
   Occult blood in stool (no fissure)
Abdominal radiographs showing distention with mild ileus

STAGE II (DEFINITE)

Any one or more historical factors
Above signs and symptoms, *plus*
   Persistent occult or gross gastrointestinal bleeding
   Marked abdominal distention
Abdominal radiographs showing significant intestinal distention
    with:
   Ileus
   Small bowel separation (edema in bowel wall or peritoneal fluid)
   Pneumatosis intestinalis
   Portal vein gas

STAGE III (ADVANCED)

Any one or more historical factors
Above signs and symptoms, *plus*
   Deterioration of vital signs
   Evidence of septic shock
   Marked gastrointestinal hemorrhage
Abdominal radiographs showing pneumoperitoneum in addition to
   findings listed for stage II

(Bell MJ, Kosloske A, Benton C, et al. Neonatal necrotizing enterocolitis in infancy: prevention of perforation. J Pediatr Surg 1973;8:6013)

Figure 100-1. Classification of intestinal atresias. Type I, muscular continuity with a complete web. Type II, mesentery intact, fibrous cord. Type IIIa, discontinuous muscle and mesentery. Type IIIb, apple-peel deformity. Type IV, multiple atresias.

for pneumoperitoneum, serial physical examinations, platelet counts, lactate levels, and arterial blood gases.

Indications to abandon medical therapy are intestinal perforation or refractory sepsis. Perforation is documented as pneumoperitoneum on plain radiographs. Evidence of persistent or progressive sepsis is thrombocytopenia, acidosis, hypoxemia, temperature instability, bradycardia, hypoglycemia, neutropenia, portal vein gas, and abdominal wall erythema or crepitus.

Surgical Management. The indication for surgical intervention is dead intestine, with or without perforation. Segmental resection of nonviable intestine can be performed with proximal and distal exteriorization. The ileocecal valve is preserved if possible, and every effort is made to conserve intestinal length.

Meconium Ileus

Meconium ileus results in obstruction of the small intestine in neonates with cystic fibrosis.

Diagnosis. Meconium ileus can be detected with prenatal US and fetal DNA screening in known kindreds. After birth, signs and symptoms are abdominal distention and bilious vomiting, usually beginning on the first day of life. Physical examination shows doughy loops of palpable distended intestine filled with meconium. Rectal examination shows white mucus or thick gray meconium without bile. Plain radiographs show multiple distended loops of intestine. Prenatal spillage of sterile meconium causes intraperitoneal calcifications. Imaging continues with a contrast enema, which shows a small, unused colon. Reflux of contrast material into the terminal ileum confirms the presence of intraluminal meconium concretions adjacent to the ileocecal valve. With a family history of cystic fibrosis and plain radiographs, contrast enema findings confirm the diagnosis of meconium ileus.

Nonsurgical Management. Nonsurgical relief of distal small-intestinal obstruction by means of enemas is possible in most instances. Long-term management includes pancreatic enzyme replacement, aggressive nutritional support, periodic enemas if obstructive symptoms develop, and avoidance of intravascular volume or sodium chloride depletion.

Surgical Management. Inability to relieve the ileal obstruction with enema irrigation and development of complications are indications for surgical management of meconium ileus. For persistent obstruction with simple ileus, the goal is to disimpact the terminal ileum and evacuate the meconium from the small intestine. This is done by means of enterotomy or enterostomy with direct irrigation as needed. Simple closure is performed. Segmental intestinal resection may be necessary if marginal or compromised intestine is found.

Complications of meconium ileus include segmental volvulus, atresia, stenosis, intestinal necrosis, perforation, and meconium cyst formation. In these circumstances, nonviable, stenotic, or perforated intestine is resected and intestinal continuity reestablished. If medical problems or established peritonitis preclude primary anastomosis, the proximal and distal intestine are exteriorized. The stomas are closed immediately after resolution of the underlying problem. Appendectomy is performed, and the entire small intestine is inspected for patency.

Meconium Plug Syndrome. Meconium plug syndrome is characterized by plugs of *normal* meconium that obstruct the colon or rectum, typically in a preterm infant. The colon is of normal caliber. Rectal examination may deliver the plug. The diagnosis is confirmed with contrast enema, which may also be therapeutic by irrigating the colon and rectum. Meconium plug syndrome can be associated with meconium ileus and Hirschsprung disease, so cystic fibrosis screening and suction rectal biopsy are performed.

Malrotation

The discovery of malrotation usually results from clinical evidence of duodenal obstruction or midgut volvulus. The signs and symptoms include gastric and proximal duodenal distention with bilious vomiting. Most malrotations are discovered in the first month of life, and almost all occur among children younger than 1 year. Patients usually do not have other medical problems.

Diagnosis. Radiographic findings of malrotation include a distended stomach and proximal duodenal bulb with little or no small-intestinal air. An upper GI series is the second and conclusive imaging study and almost always helps differentiate malrotation from duodenal atresia and stenosis. Malposition of the duodenojejunal junction to the right of the midline is diagnostic.

Management. Malrotation in neonates is managed surgically. Assessment, resuscitation, and preoperative preparation are concurrent, and the diagnosis of malrotation is followed immediately by laparotomy. The goals of surgical repair are to relieve the midgut volvulus and divide the Ladd bands to relieve extrinsic compression and obstruction of the distal duodenum. Appendectomy is performed, and mesocolic hernias are corrected.

Congenital Aganglionosis (Hirschsprung Disease)

Hirschsprung disease is characterized by migratory arrest of neuroblasts within the intestine, resulting in ineffective peristalsis. The common clinical outcomes are incomplete distal intestinal obstruction or enterocolitis in neonates (manifested by abdominal distention and bilious vomiting) and chronic constipation in an older child.

Diagnosis. Every effort is made to establish the diagnosis of Hirschsprung disease in the newborn period by means of plain abdominal radiographs, barium enema, anorectal manometry, and rectal biopsy.

Management. Surgical decompression is initiated as soon as Hirschsprung disease is detected. Proximal diversion is obtained with a colostomy (or enterostomy if necessary) in normal, ganglionated intestine. The colostomy is usually a loop to preserve marginal collateral vessels for pull-through. The strategy is to provide diversion until about 9 to 12 months of age or in older children until the colon is decompressed to normal caliber. After this, a definitive pull-through procedure is performed. Recent evidence suggests equivalent outcomes using primary neonatal pull-through without colostomy.

Enterocolitis. Some children with Hirschsprung disease have enterocolitis, and this may be the initial clinical presentation. The early clinical presentation of Hirschsprung enterocolitis includes fever, abdominal distention, and diarrhea, which may be explosive, distinctively malodorous, and bloody. Systemic sepsis, transmural intestinal necrosis, and perforation are later findings. The clinical progression can be rapidly fatal. Treatment of Hirschsprung enterocolitis consists of intravenous (IV) fluid resuscitation, broad-spectrum antibiotics, possibly colonic irrigation, and intestinal decompression.

OTHER CHILDHOOD GASTROINTESTINAL DISORDERS

Hypertrophic Pyloric Stenosis

The pathogenesis of infantile hypertrophic pyloric stenosis is unknown. Focal nitric oxide synthetase deficiency in the pylorus probably is responsible. There is a familial predisposition.

Diagnosis

The history is nonbilious, projectile vomiting in an infant 4 to 6 weeks of age. The vomiting occurs within minutes of feeding and is progressive. Cessation of feedings eliminates the vomiting. The infant appears well and feeds eagerly until late in the course. The pathognomonic physical finding is a palpable, firm, mobile, pyloric "olive" in the right upper quadrant or epigastrium. Late clinical features include intravascular volume depletion and hypokalemic, hypochloremic metabolic alkalosis.

The history and physical examination provide enough evidence to proceed with surgical exploration. If imaging is needed, a barium upper GI series and US examination are performed.

Management

Treatment of pyloric muscular hypertrophy is pyloromyotomy, a single longitudinal incision in the hypertrophied pyloric muscle.

Intussusception

Intussusception is invagination of a proximal segment of intestine into an adjacent distal segment (Fig. 100-3). Intussusception usually originates in the small intestine at or near the ileocecal valve, causing passage of the terminal ileum through the valve into the colon (ileocolic intussusception). Usually no intrinsic anatomic abnormality is found, although many associations occur (Table 100-4).

A consequence of intussusception is progressive edema and inflammation leading to intestinal obstruction. Incarceration, strangulation, and perforation of the intussusceptum are serious problems. The intussuscipiens is rarely compromised.

Diagnosis

The diagnosis of intussusception can be established with the history: an otherwise healthy infant 3 months to 3 years of age experiences sudden and severe colicky abdominal pain. Between bouts of colic, the infant is often lethargic or sleepy. Intractable vomiting and abdominal distention develop after 24 hours. Volume depletion may become profound. Guaiac-positive stool is present in almost all infants with intussusception. Hematochezia is less common, but blood mixed with mucus (currant-jelly stool) may be passed. Physical findings include a palpable, sausage-shaped mass in the right upper quadrant. The intussusceptum may be palpable at rectal examination and may prolapse through the anus. US examination demonstrates a mass with two lumens that resembles a bull's eye. Air and contrast enemas are diagnostic of ileocolic intussusception.

Nonsurgical Management

Hydrostatic or pneumaticreduction is accomplished with enema instillation of barium or air as long as progressive reduction is achieved. Reduction is confirmed with demonstration of free flow of contrast material into the terminal small intestine. Lack of flow suggests incomplete reduction and mandates surgical exploration.

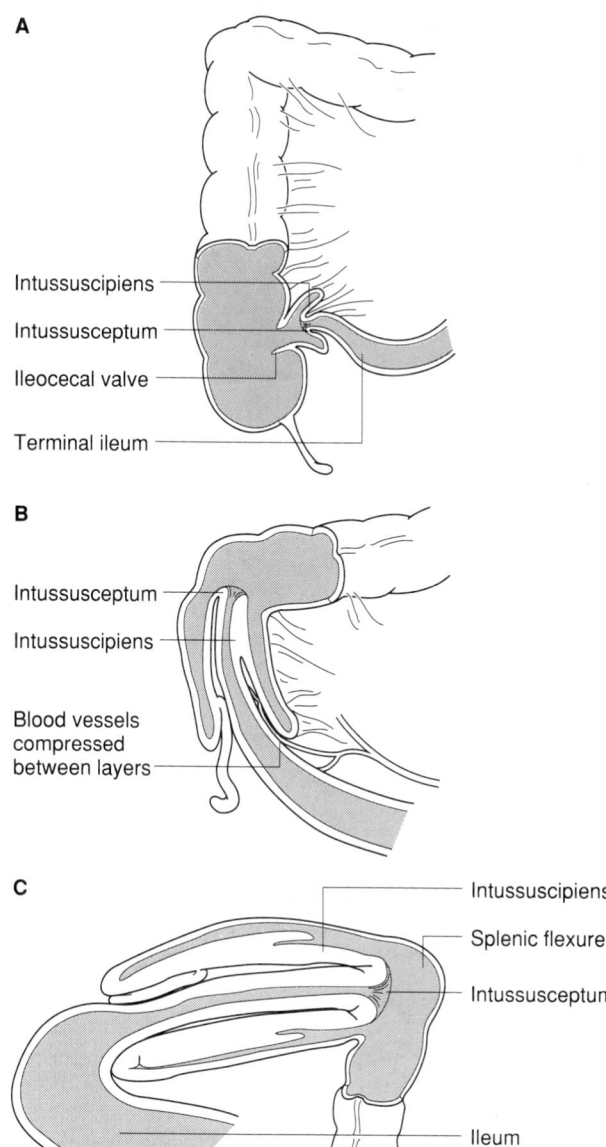

Figure 100-3. Ileocolic intussusception.

Surgical Management

Immediate laparotomy is needed for failed or uncertain enema reduction of intussusception. Spontaneous reduction occurs in some children during surgical preparation. Exploration to confirm the reduction is sufficient. If intussusception persists and the intestine is viable, manual reduction is undertaken. If this cannot be done, or if the intestine is clearly necrotic, segmental resection and primary anastomosis are performed. Appendectomy is performed.

Meckel Diverticulum

The most frequent congenital anomaly of the GI tract is Meckel diverticulum, which results from persistence of the embryonic yolk stalk. Most Meckel diverticula are asymptomatic throughout life. Most that do become symptomatic do so before the age of 2 years. Hemorrhage, acute diverticulitis, perforation, and small-intestinal obstruction or intussusception are the presenting signs.

Table 100-4. PREDISPOSING FACTORS TO THE DEVELOPMENT OF INTUSSUSCEPTION

ANATOMIC LEAD POINTS

Meckel's diverticulum
Polyp
Hypertrophied Peyer patch
Appendix
Duplication or enteric cyst
Lymphoma
Other neoplasm
Ectopic pancreas

ASSOCIATED INFECTIONS

Adenovirus
Rotovirus
Others

BLEEDING DISORDERS*

Henoch-Schönlein purpura
Hemophilia
Leukemia

TRAUMA*

Blunt abdominal trauma
Major retroperitoneal operative procedures

OTHER

Cystic fibrosis

* These factors are more likely to be associated with small bowel-to-small bowel intussusception than with ileocolic intussusception.

Management

The development of clinical symptoms of Meckel diverticulum is an absolute indication for surgical management. Treatment is simple excision.

Foreign Bodies

Foreign bodies entrapped in the esophagus are removed endoscopically. Objects that pass the gastroesophageal junction usually are eliminated in the stool.

Guidelines for endoscopic removal of GI foreign bodies are:

1. Symptoms suggesting perforation, obstruction, or intestinal injury (pain, vomiting, fever, peritonitis)
2. Failure of an object to pass from the stomach into the small intestine within 3 to 4 weeks
3. Ingestion of exceptionally long or sharp objects or an object judged unlikely to transverse the pylorus
4. Failure of a foreign body to continue to progress distally. One week or more in a fixed position suggests erosion and perforation.
5. Ingestion of batteries, particularly alkaline disc batteries

Gastrointestinal Hemorrhage

Tables 100-5 and 100-6 summarize sites and sources of GI hemorrhage. Source and site of GI hemorrhage are identified with pediatric fiberoptic endoscopy, arteriography, and radionuclide imaging. Newborns, infants, and children with minimal lower GI hemorrhage undergo simple digital rectal examination and anoscopy. Management depends on the cause of hemorrhage.

Cystic Duplications

Cystic duplications may exist anywhere in the GI tract, but the most common location is the ileum, particularly near the ileocecal valve. Cystic duplications are usually asymptomatic masses found incidentally during abdominal US and CT and GI contrast studies. Treatment is simple excision of mediastinal or rectal cysts without resection of adjacent intestine. In the small intestine short segmental resections with primary anastomoses are needed.

Tubular Duplications

Tubular duplications may occur anywhere in the GI tract but are most likely to occur in the terminal ileum and colon. Anatomic features include a shared blood supply and a common wall with the functional intestine. Communication between lumens is common. The lesion may involve long segments of ileum or colon. Malformations involving the entire colon and rectum are associated with genitourinary anomalies, particularly doubling of the external genitalia or bladder. These abnormalities probably

Table 100-5. CAUSES OF UPPER GASTROINTESTINAL HEMORRHAGE*

Patient Age Group	Common Causes	Less Common Causes
Neonate (0–30 d)	1. Gastritis 2. Esophagitis 3. Ingested maternal blood 4. Peptic ulcer	1. Iatrogenic trauma 2. Primary coagulopathy 3. Vascular malformations (hemangioma, telangiectasia, arteriovenous malformations) 4. Nasal or pharyngeal bleeding 5. Miscellaneous structural abnormalities (leiomyoma, gastric polyp, duplications)
Infant (30 d to 1 yr)	1. Gastritis 2. Esophagitis 3. Peptic ulcer	Same as for neonate, with addition of: 1. Drugs (salicylates, steroids) 2. Foreign body or caustic ingestion 3. Esophageal varices
Child (1–12 yr)	1. Esophageal varices 2. Esophagitis 3. Peptic ulcer	Same as for infant, with addition of: 1. Acquired thrombocytopenia (chemotherapy)
Older child and adolescent (12 yr to adulthood)	1. Esophageal varices 2. Esophagitis 3. Peptic ulcer	Same as for child

* Order of appearance approximates clinical frequency
(Modified from Oldham KT, Lobe TE. Gastrointestinal hemorrhage in children. Pediatr Clin North Am 1985;32:1247)

Table 100-6. CAUSE OF LOWER GASTROINTESTINAL HEMORRHAGE*

Patient Age Group	Common Causes	Less Common Causes
Neonate (0–30 d)	1. Benign anorectal lesions (anal fissure) 2. Upper GI hemorrhage 3. Milk allergy 4. Necrotizing enterocolitis 5. Midgut volvulus 6. Incarcerated hernia	1. Iatrogenic trauma 2. Primary coagulopathy 3. Vascular malformations 4. Enterocolitis (Hirschsprung disease, others) 5. Miscellaneous structural abnormalities (lymphoma, duplication, lymphangiectasia)
Infant (30 d to 1 yr)	1. Benign anorectal lesions 2. Idiopathic intussusception 3. Meckel diverticulum 4. Infectious diarrhea 5. Upper GI hemorrhage 6. Milk allergy	Same as for neonate, with addition of: 1. Acquired thrombocytopenia (drug-induced, aplastic anemia, disseminated intravascular coagulation, sepsis) 2. Ingestion of red foodstuffs (guaiac test mandatory)
Child (1–12 yr)	1. Benign anorectal lesions 2. Juvenile polyps 3. Intussusception 4. Meckel diverticulum 5. Infectious diarrhea 6. Upper GI hemorrhage	Same as for infant, with addition of: 1. Juvenile polyposis coli 2. Familial polyposis coli 3. Hemolytic–uremic syndrome 4. Henoch-Schönlein purpura 5. Systemic vasculitis (dermatomyositis, lupus) 6. Acquired thrombocytopenia (as above plus idiopathic thrombocytopenic purpura)
Older child and adolescent (12 yr to adulthood)	1. Juvenile polyps 2. Benign anorectal lesions 3. Inflammatory bowel disease 4. Upper GI hemorrhage	Same as for child, but: 1. Henoch-Schönlein purpura and hemolytic–uremic syndrome less likely 2. Meckel diverticulum

* Order of appearance approximates clinical frequency
(Modified from Oldham KT, Lobe TE. Gastrointestinal hemorrhage in children. Pediatr Clin North Am 1985;32:1247)

represent aborted embryologic twinning. Clinical presentations include peptic ulceration and obstruction. Treatment may require marsupialization with submucosal stripping of the epithelium or if obstruction is present distal enteroenterostomy.

Mesenteric and Omental Cysts

Mesenteric and omental cysts are rare cystic malformations caused by sequestration of embryonic lymphatic tissue within the mesentery or omentum. A history of abdominal pain and a soft, mobile abdominal mass at physical examination are the most important findings. Mesenteric and omental cysts may remain asymptomatic and be discovered incidentally during a routine physical examination or diagnostic imaging for unrelated reasons. Hemorrhage, obstruction, volvulus, cyst rupture, and infection are other presentations. US and CT depict all these lesions. Peripheral calcifications and recent hemorrhage may be diagnostic during imaging. Treatment consists of simple cyst excision if possible, and if necessary for mesenteric cysts, resection of adjacent intestine.

Primary Peritonitis

Peritonitis develops rapidly. Signs and symptoms are fever, vomiting, diffuse tenderness, involuntary guarding, and rigidity. Leukocytosis is characteristic, and ileus is apparent on plain radiographs.

Children with indwelling peritoneal catheters or shunts can be treated with broad-spectrum antibiotics, although removal of the device may be necessary. For those with ascites or nephrosis, diagnostic paracentesis is essential. The fluid is evaluated immediately by Gram stain and culture. Gram-positive peritonitis may be managed with antimicrobial agents. Gram-negative or mixed flora raises the question of GI tract perforation, particularly appendicitis, and cannot be resolved safely without surgical exploration. If the appendix is normal, the surgical objectives are to obtain appropriate cultures and Gram stain of the peritoneal fluid and establish whether intestinal perforation is responsible for the peritonitis. This necessitates complete exploration of the peritoneal cavity. The appendix is removed. Surgical lesions to be excluded at exploration are perforated appendix or Meckel diverticulum, perforated duodenal ulcer, and acute pancreatitis.

Ascites

Ascites is characterized by abdominal distention with bulging flanks. The diagnosis is confirmed with US or CT. Prenatal diagnosis is possible. The causes of neonatal and childhood ascites are listed in Tables 103-7 and 103-8.

Diagnosis begins with paracentesis and examination of the ascitic fluid. The characteristics of the ascitic fluid determine evaluation and treatment. Without a diagnosis from the initial fluid examination, imaging includes echo-

Table 100-7. COMMON CAUSES OF NEONATAL ASCITES

Maternal–fetal Rh incompatibility (now rare)
Structural malformations
  Urinary obstructions
  Congenital heart disease
  Malrotation, duplications, cysts (associated with intestinal volvulus)
  Biliary perforation
  Ovarian ascites
  Pulmonary abnormalities
Chylous ascites
Hematologic disorders
  α-Thalassemia
Infection
  Toxoplasmosis
  Cytomegalovirus
  Others
α_1-Antitrypsin deficiency
Idiopathic

Table 100-8. CHARACTERISTICS AND CAUSES OF CHILDHOOD ASCITES

SEROUS ASCITES
Cirrhosis
Budd-Chiari syndrome
Nephrosis
Right-sided heart failure
Postoperative ascites (after renal transplantation, peritoneal dialysis, ventriculoperitoneal shunts)
α_1-Antitrypsin deficiency
Other rare metabolic diseases

CHYLOUS ASCITES
Malrotation with volvulus
Small bowel obstruction
Incarcerated hernia
Lymphangioma
Trauma (including surgical trauma)

BILIARY ASCITES
Neonatal bile duct perforation
Cystic fibrosis
Biliary atresia
Hepatitis
Cytomegalovirus infection

URINARY ASCITES (7:1 MALE PREDOMINANCE)
Urinary obstruction
Posterior urethral valves
Bladder perforation
Ureterocele
Neurogenic bladder

PANCREATIC ASCITES
Acute pancreatitis (drugs, trauma, gallstones, infection)
Pancreatic pseudocysts

OVARIAN ASCITES
Cysts (torsion, rupture)
Tumors

MALIGNANT ASCITES
Any intraperitoneal neoplasm

IDIOPATHIC

---

cardiography, abdominal CT or US, and a voiding cystourethrogram.

The diagnosis dictates treatment. For example, neonatal biliary ascites may be caused by spontaneous bile duct perforation. The infant may have cystic fibrosis with transient bile plugging. The perforation is found at the junction of the cystic duct and common bile duct. External drainage is performed. Intractable ascites is managed with peritoneovenous shunting.

Rectal Prolapse

Spontaneous prolapse of the rectum may occur at or near the time of toilet training. Associations include straining at stool for any reason, cystic fibrosis, colorectal polyps, Hirschsprung disease, sacral neuropathy, and congenital anorectal malformations. Most children with rectal prolapse, however, have no associated abnormalities.

The diagnosis of rectal prolapse often depends entirely on the history given by the parents. They describe protrusion of mucosa or full-thickness rectum through the anus occurs. The only other lesion with a similar appearance is intussusception with passage of the intussusceptum through the anus. Children with rectal prolapse rarely have other symptoms. The rectal examination is diagnostic. If the prolapsed intestine is an intussusceptum, a finger can

be placed adjacent to it within the rectum. This is not possible with rectal prolapse.

Nonsurgical management is manual reduction, stool softeners, parental instruction, and taping of the buttocks. The prolapse usually resolves spontaneously resolution over a period of weeks, and surgical treatment is not indicated generally.

PEDIATRIC LIVER

Tumors of the Liver

Primary liver tumors are uncommon in children. The types and incidence of liver tumors are listed in Table 100-9. The most common presenting feature of pediatric liver neoplasms is an asymptomatic abdominal mass. Other symptoms, such as pain, hemorrhage, precocious puberty, and hypertension, are rare. Evaluation of a liver mass includes a plain radiograph of the abdomen to determine whether calcification is present. This finding suggests echinococcal disease. CT and MRI of the abdomen are the definitive diagnostic tests. Laparotomy or laparoscopy is necessary to establish the diagnosis and allow resection or other therapy.

PEDIATRIC BILIARY TRACT

Biliary tract disease among infants and children includes congenital, neoplastic, inflammatory, infectious, and gallstone-related disorders. Two problems unique to children are biliary atresia and congenital cystic disease of the biliary tract (choledochal cysts).

Biliary Atresia

The pathogenesis of biliary atresia is unknown. Patients are anicteric term infants without maternal or perinatal difficulties. The cardinal manifestation of the disease is progressive neonatal jaundice with onset in the first weeks of life. Infants with biliary atresia usually have a normal physical examination except for the icterus and perhaps mild hepatosplenomegaly. Feeding intolerance, growth

Table 100-9. INCIDENCE OF LIVER TUMORS IN CHILDHOOD

Tumor Type	Incidence (%)
BENIGN	
Vascular tumors	13
Hemangioma	9
Hemangioendothelioma	4
Mesenchymal hamartoma	6
Focal nodular hyperplasia	2
Adenoma	2
Teratoma	2
Other	3
MALIGNANT	
Hepatoblastoma	43
Hepatocellular carcinoma	23
Malignant mesenchymal tumor	4
Sarcoma	2
Embryonal rhabdomyosarcoma	1
Angiosarcoma	1

(Adapted from Dehner LP. Hepatic tumors in the pediatric age group: a distinctive clinicopathologic spectrum. In: Rosenberg HS, Bolande RP. Perspectives in pediatric pathology. Chicago, Year Book, 1978)

failure, and portal hypertension or fat-soluble vitamin deficiency are late findings of biliary atresia.

The jaundice of biliary atresia is not to be confused with the self-limited neonatal physiologic jaundice that affects many newborns. If there is doubt, prompt laparotomy, liver biopsy, and operative cholangiography are performed. The following modalities also may be used: radioisotope scanning, US, liver biopsy, and screening for α_1-antitrypsin deficiency.

Biliary atresia is managed by means of portoenterostomy or hepatic transplantation. Medical therapy is used *only* for postoperative management of chronic liver disease.

Congenital Cystic Disorders of the Biliary Tract

The consequences of choledochal cysts are obstruction to bile flow or compression of adjacent viscera. Obstructive jaundice is the presenting finding. Liver injury is usually reversible. Other findings may be gallstone formation, acute bacterial cholangitis, acute pancreatitis, portal hypertension, and adenocarcinoma of the biliary tract.

Diagnosis

Diagnosis is possible with perinatal US screening or after the development of obstructive jaundice. Physical examination may demonstrate hepatomegaly or evidence of portal hypertension. Imaging includes technetium scans, US, upper GI series, CT, or MRI. Percutaneous transhepatic cholangiography is used to define intrahepatic biliary tract anatomy.

Management

Cystic disease of the biliary tree always is managed with surgical intervention. The operation depends on the anatomic abnormality. Surgical procedures begin with cholangiography. Cholecystectomy is followed by cyst excision or sphincteroplasty. Reconstuction generally entails Roux en Y jejunal drainage.

PEDIATRIC PANCREAS
Acute Pancreatitis

Acute pancreatitis is the most common disorder of the pancreas among infants and children. Most childhood acute pancreatitis is idiopathic, posttraumatic, or due to use of immunosuppressive agents, especially high-dose corticosteroids.

Diagnosis

The diagnosis of acute pancreatitis is based on the presence of epigastric abdominal pain, fever, leukocytosis, and elevated plasma levels of amylase and lipase. Amylase-to-creatinine clearance ratio may improve diagnostic accuracy. US, CT, and MRI show evidence of edema and enlargement of the pancreas. US may show ductal dilatation.

Management

Management includes pain relief, parenteral fluids, parenteral nutrition, and pancreatic rest with NG decompression. If hypocalcemia occurs, calcium supplementation is provided. Almost all children with pancreatitis have simple edematous pancreatitis. Parenteral nutrition and ventilatory support are provided as necessary. Surgical therapy is reserved for complications.

Pancreas Divisum

Pancreas divisum is an anatomic variation that occurs when the dorsal and ventral pancreatic ducts do not fuse normally. ERCP is necessary to establish the diagnosis.

A diagnosis of pancreas divisum can be made with this demonstration of two separate, parallel ductal systems. Surgical treatment is sphincteroplasty of the accessory duct and cholecystectomy.

Pancreatic Cysts

Pseudocysts of the pancreas usually occur after trauma in children. Symptoms include epigastric pain associated with nausea, vomiting, and weight loss. The cyst is often palpable at abdominal examination. The diagnosis is made with US, CT, or MRI. Therapy in most instances is external drainage.

Except for posttraumatic pseudocysts, pancreatic cysts are rare among children. These cysts can be congenital, retention, neoplastic, or parasitic. Management is drainage or excision, depending on the type of cyst.

Pancreatic Neoplasms

Malignant pancreatic neoplasms are rare among children. Islet cell carcinoma is most common, followed by adenocarcinoma. These tumors almost always present as an asymptomatic abdominal mass, although obstructive jaundice may occur if the tumor is in the head of the pancreas. Therapy for local disease is resection with partial pancreatectomy or total pancreatectomy. Pancreatoduodenectomy can be performed if it allows complete resection of the tumor.

Endocrine Lesions of the Pancreas
Zollinger–Ellison Syndrome

Zollinger–Ellison syndrome is extremely rare among children. The symptoms are severe ulcer diathesis due to marked gastric hypersecretion. The diagnosis is confirmed by demonstration of elevated levels of gastrin in the serum. Treatment is resection of the gastrinoma and administration of histamine (H2) antagonists such as cimetidine and ranitidine. Omeprazole also can be used. If the gastrinoma of the pancreas cannot be resected, total gastrectomy is performed.

Gastrinomas and Zollinger–Ellison syndrome may be part of the multiple endocrine neoplasia syndrome. Almost all these patients have hyperparathyroidism. Other associated lesions are gastrinoma of the pancreas, pituitary adenoma, adrenocortical hyperplasia, and rarely, insulinoma.

Hypoglycemia

Most infants with refractory hypoglycemia have hyperinsulinemia. Most cases of hyperinsulinemia in the first 2 years of life are due to nesidioblastosis. Hyperinsulinemia due to islet cell adenoma, carcinoma, or hyperplasia is more common among older children. Infants with nesidioblastosis usually have symptomatic hypoglycemia. Frank seizures or other neurologic symptoms also can occur. These children have fasting blood glucose levels <40 mg/dL (2.2 mmol/L). Nesidioblastosis is associated with multiple endocrine neoplasia syndrome, and this possibility must be investigated.

Organic hyperinsulinemia is likely if the Whipple triad is demonstrated: (1) mental status changes or dizziness precipitated by fasting or exercise; (2) fasting blood glucose concentrations <40 mg/dL (2.2 mmol/L); and (3) symptoms relieved by oral or IV administration of glucose. The diagnosis is confirmed with simultaneous measurement of plasma insulin and glucose levels with the finding of an insulin level inappropriately high for the level of blood glucose.

Infants with nesidioblastosis initially are treated with maintenance of blood glucose levels >40 mg/dL (2.2 mmol/L) by means of infusion of hypertonic glucose solution through a permanent central venous catheter. Definitive management of nesidioblastosis may necessitate pancreatic resection. If islet cell adenoma is found, it is removed without further resection of the pancreas. Intraoperative US examination of the pancreas is performed. If no adenoma is found, the patient is assumed to have nesidioblastosis or islet cell hyperplasia. The next step is 95% pancreatectomy with preservation of the spleen. If a child is hypoglycemic after a 95% pancreatectomy, a 99% or near-total pancreatectomy with preservation of the duodenum is required.

SUGGESTED READING

A-Kader HH, Nowicki MJ, Kuramoto KI, Baroudy B, Zeldis JB, Balistreri WF. Evaluation of the role of hepatitis C virus in biliary atresia. Pediatr Infect Dis J 1994;13:657.

Cilley RE, Statter MB, Hirschl RB, Coran AG. Definitive treatment of Hirschprung's disease in the newborn with a one-stage procedure. Surgery 1994;115:551.

Georgeson KE, Fuenfer MM, Hardin WD. Primary laparoscopic pull-through for Hirschprung's disease in infants and children. J Pediatr Surg 1995;30:1017.

Grosfeld JL, Rescorla FJ, Skinner MA, West KW, Scherer LR. The spectrum of biliary tract disorders in infants and children: experience with 300 cases. Arch Surg 1994;129:513.

Lipsett PA, Pitt HA, Colombani PM, Boitnott JK, Cameron JL. Choledochal cyst disease: a changing pattern of presentation. Ann Surg 1994;220:644.

Morgan LJ, Shocat SJ, Hartman GE. Peritoneal drainage as primary management of perforated NEC in the very low birth weight infant. J Pediatr Surg 1994;29:30.

Otte JB, de Ville de Goyet J, Reding R, et al. Sequential treatment of biliary atresia with Kasai portoenterostomy and liver transplantation: a review. Hepatology 1994;20:41S.

Ryckman F, Fischer R, Pedersen S, et al. Improved survival in biliary atresia patients in the present era of liver transplantation. J Pediatr Surg 1993;28:382.

Tan CE, Davenport M, Driver M, Howard ER. Does the morphology of the extrahepatic biliary remnants in biliary atresia influence survival? A review of 205 cases. J Pediatr Surg 1994;29:1459.

Tomita R, Munakata K, Kurosu Y, Tanjoh K. A role of nitric oxide in Hirschprung's disease. J Pediatr Surg 1995;30:437.

ESSENTIALS OF SURGERY: SCIENTIFIC PRINCIPLES AND PRACTICE,
edited by Lazar J. Greenfield, Michael W. Mulholland, Keith T. Oldham, Gerald B. Zelenock, and Keith D. Lillemoe. Lippincott–Raven Publishers, Philadelphia, © 1997.

CHAPTER 101

PEDIATRIC GENITOURINARY SYSTEM

DAVID A. BLOOM, MICHAEL L. RITCHEY, AND ARNOLD G. CORAN

KIDNEY

Renal Agenesis

Unilateral renal agenesis (solitary kidney) is detected in the first few years of life during evaluation for multiple-system abnormalities. Renal function is minimally affected. Infants with *bilateral* renal agenesis, facial dysmorphia, pulmonary hypoplasia, and orthopedic abnormalities (Potter syndrome) are stillborn or soon die of respiratory or renal failure.

Renal Ectopy

Ectopic kidneys lie outside the renal fossa but inside the retroperitoneal space. The most common location of an ectopic kidney is the pelvis opposite the sacrum or below the aortic bifurcation. Intrathoracic kidney occurs when some or all of a kidney extends above the diaphragm.

Diagnosis

Ectopic kidneys can be difficult to visualize and are easily overlooked during excretory urography because they often overlie bony structures. Oblique plain radiographs may help establish this diagnosis. An ectopic kidney can be readily identified with ultrasonography (US) or computed tomography (CT). Most patients have no symptoms.

Management

The most common problem with renal ectopy is congenital ureteropelvic junction (UPJ) obstruction. Most of these patients need dismembered pyeloplasty. Because renal stones may develop in ectopic kidneys, screening studies are routine. Stones are removed by means of extracorporeal shock-wave lithotripsy or endourologic technique. Because the contralateral kidney may be abnormal, every effort is made to preserve an ectopic kidney.

Horseshoe Kidney

Unusual radiographic images result from fusion of two or more renal masses. Horseshoe kidney is the most common renal fusion abnormality. The two renal masses join at the midline, usually at the lower poles. The isthmus that connects the two kidneys consists of renal parenchyma or fibrous tissue, and the horseshoe kidney usually is low in the abdomen with an isthmus below the junction of the inferior mesenteric artery and aorta. Horseshoe kidney does not adversely affect survival. Clinical problems are caused by hydronephrosis, urinary tract infection (UTI), or urolithiasis. Adenocarcinoma and Wilms tumor can be associated with horseshoe kidney.

Diagnosis

Horseshoe kidney is diagnosed with excretory urography. The function of the isthmus parenchyma can be assessed with radionuclide imaging.

Management

Surgical correction of the UPJ obstruction is required, usually in the form of a dismembered pyeloplasty or an endocrinological approach.

Cystic Disease

Renal cystic disease is congenital or acquired. *Multicystic dysplastic kidney* is the most common form in infants and usually is unilateral. Cysts vary in size and do not communicate. The differential diagnosis is obstructive hydronephrosis.

Diagnosis

US evaluation is diagnostic. Isotopic renal scans show lack of function in a multicystic dysplastic kidney. Imaging of the rest of the urinary tract may exclude contralateral renal abnormalities and vesicoureteral reflux (VUR).

Management

US surveillance and nephrectomy is recommended for disease that does not regress or for symptomatic lesions, which are rare. *Autosomal recessive polycystic kidney disease* is a congenital disorder that affects both kidneys. It becomes evident at birth or later in childhood. All patients have liver disease, ranging from biliary ectasia to congenital hepatic fibrosis.

Diagnosis

The usual neonatal presentation is bilateral, massive flank masses that do not transilluminate. Renal US shows uniform echogenicity. Intravenous urography demonstrates a classic sun-ray pattern caused by streaking of contrast filled collecting tubules.

Autosomal dominant polycystic kidney disease, a relatively common genetic disease, is diagnosed in adulthood. It may present in childhood, although the initial course may be deceptively benign. The presence of even one renal cyst in a child whose family carries autosomal dominant polycystic kidney disease suggests the disease.

Ureteropelvic Junction Obstruction

UPJ obstruction is the most common cause of neonatal hydronephrosis. Causes include failure of recanalization of the fetal ureter; lack of peristaltic wave propagation due to microscopic derangement of the muscle bundles and increased intramural collagen deposition; or extrinsic obstruction by aberrant vessels, kinks in the proximal ureter, or adherent bands.

Diagnosis

Antenatal US evidence of hydronephrosis suggests asymptomatic UPJ obstruction. Signs and symptoms of UPJ obstruction later in life include abdominal mass, pain, hematuria, infection, or renal stones. Evaluation begins with abdominal US. Excretory urography sometimes is necessary to define the renal anatomy. Diuretic renography or antegrade perfusion measurement (Whitaker test) allows assessment of obstruction.

Management

Dependent drainage of the renal pelvis by dismembered pyeloplasty with resection of the obstructing segment is standard, although endoscopic techniques to achieve drainage have been developed recently.

URETER

Megaureter

Megaureter is a large, dilated ureter. An *obstructed megaureter,* congenital or acquired, is blocked at a narrow segment *proximal* to the ureterovesical junction. Increased collagen deposition, muscular deficiency, and a thickened circular band of muscle at the narrowed segment impair propagation of peristalsis and distend the proximal ureter.

A *nonrefluxing, nonobstructed megaureter* has a narrowed *distal* ureteral segment. There is variable dilatation of the proximal ureter. This condition may be caused by obstruction or reflux that resolves spontaneously.

Diagnosis

Symptoms are UTI, hematuria, and abdominal pain. Antenatal US provides the first clue. Diuretic renography helps differentiate nonobstructed from obstructed megaureter.

Management

Patients with asymptomatic megaureter may not need aggressive treatment. Intervention, however, can prevent further functional deterioration. Surgical management consists of reimplantation of the ureter into the bladder after excision of the obstructing segment. Tailoring the ureter by means of partial excision or imbrication may be combined with reimplantation to diminish reflux.

Ureteral Duplication

Duplication of the ureter is the most common urinary tract abnormality (Fig. 101-1). In complete duplication, two ipsilateral ureteral orifices enter the bladder. In bifid systems, duplication is incomplete, and two proximal ureters unite so that only one distal ureter enters the bladder. The most common associated disorder is VUR.

Diagnosis

UTI is the most common presentation. Girls may have urinary incontinence. The ureteral orifice may be in the uterus, cervix, or vagina, so vaginal discharge is another presenting symptom. Symptoms may not occur until adult life.

Management

Surgical management of ureteral duplication is similar to that of VUR and megaureter.

Ureterocele

Ureterocele is congenital cystic dilatation of the distal ureter. It may occur with ureteral duplication or alone (*simple ureterocele*) and may be an asymptomatic incidental finding in an adult. Simple ureterocele can present with obstruction, calculi, infection, reflux, or lack of renal function. Ectopic ureterocele can occur with ureteral duplica-

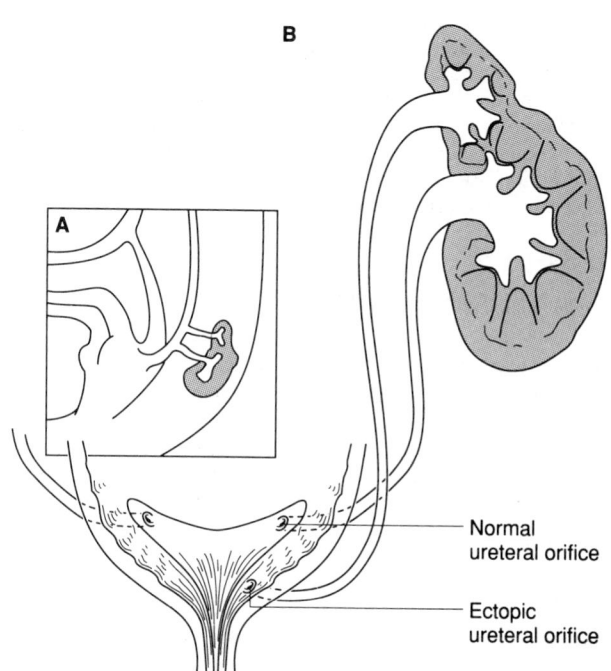

Figure 101-1. Ureteral duplication. The proposed embryology of two ureteral buds (*A*) and complete duplication with abnormal upper pole and ectopic ureteral orifice (*B*) are shown.

tion. It is characterized by entry of the ureterocele into the bladder neck or urethra.

The most common presentation of ureterocele is UTI. The renal segment involved is likely to have decreased or absent function because of dysplasia, obstruction, and infection. Obstruction of the lower renal segment can occur from compression by the dilated upper-pole ureter or the ureterocele. Reflux is likely in the lower ureter. The bladder outlet may also be obstructed by a ureterocele, which can prolapse into the urethra.

Management

Decompression of the ureterocele from above (pyelopyelostomy or upper-pole nephrectomy) or from below (by means of transurethral incision) is the initial therapeutic step. One third of patients may need correction of reflux or excision of an upper-pole ureteral stump.

Vesicoureteral Reflux

Primary VUR is a congenital abnormality of the ureterovesical junction. Renal scarring in children with VUR can occur from recurrent UTI. Reflux of infected urine causes renal cortical damage. Reflux of sterile urine is probably not harmful in the presence of normal bladder pressure. Reflux nephropathy is the result of renal scarring that occurs with reflux. Patients with reflux nephropathy are at risk for hypertension.

Diagnosis

Children with UTI undergo voiding cystography.

Management

Most children with VUR are treated without surgical intervention. Reflux resolves with time, particularly in children with low-grade VUR. The goal of nonsurgical management is prevention of UTI during the months or years it may take to outgrow the reflux.

When medical therapy fails or if the child does not outgrow reflux, a variety of surgical techniques are done to make a long subepithelial tunnel in the bladder wall with good muscular backing (Fig. 101-2). The ureter can be approached intravesically or extravesically. If a ureter is dilated, its diameter must be reduced to achieve an acceptable ureteral width-to-length ratio of 1 to 4. This can be done by means of excision of the redundant portion or by a variety of imbrication techniques.

Endoscopic correction of reflux consists of subureteral injection of collagen or another material to buttress the ureterovesical junction. Subtrigonal injection therapy for reflux is not as successful as surgical reconstruction, but it is less invasive.

BLADDER

Urachal Abnormalities

The urachus extends from the umbilicus to the anterior bladder wall. It becomes a solid cord during gestation, but a potential space may remain and become occluded by desquamated epithelium. *Failure of closure* produces a patent urachus with a communication between the bladder and umbilicus. This occurs in patients with bladder outlet obstruction and produces a wet umbilicus.

Diagnosis

The diagnosis is confirmed with radiography (cystogram).

Management

Spontaneous closure is possible, but excision of the tract and surgical closure of the bladder usually are necessary.

Cysts along the course of the urachus are caused by epithelial degeneration and desquamation.

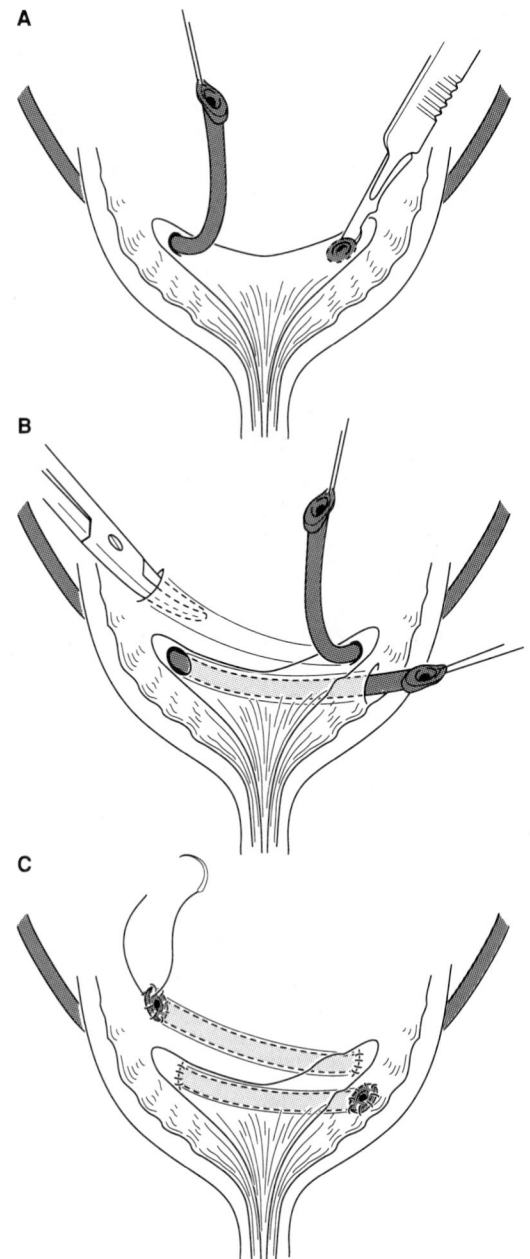

Figure 101-2. Ureteroneocystostomy (cross-trigonal reimplant).

Diagnosis

Symptoms, which may not develop until late childhood or adulthood, are suprapubic pain, tenderness, and a palpable mass. US is used to image the lesions.

Management

Treatment is incision and drainage followed by excision after any infection has resolved.

A *urachal sinus* occurs when a urachal cyst dissects into the umbilicus causing periumbilical inflammation and drainage.

Management

Therapy is surgical resection of the cyst and sinus with surgical closure of the bladder.

Neurogenic Bladder

Spinal dysraphism, the most common cause of neurogenic bladder in children, encompasses abnormalities ranging from occult dermal sinus and cord lipoma to visible myelomeningocele (MMC). Complications of neurogenic vesical dysfunction (infection, hydronephrosis, renal failure) are preventable. Leak-point pressure is a reliable predictor of risk for renal deterioration. The primary goal for children with MMC is to maintain safe intravesical pressures. Spontaneous voiding in these patients is unusual, and they are often incontinent. Bladder storage and outlet resistance are inadequate.

Diagnosis

A newborn is examined to identify risk for renal damage. Children with leakage at low intravesical pressures need treatment before the urinary tract is damaged.

Management

Initial treatment is intermittent catheterization and pharmacologic therapy. If bladder storage capability cannot be improved with anticholinergic therapy, an operation is necessary to achieve safe urine storage and continence. Intestinal and gastric segments, dilated ureters, and detrusor excision can augment bladder capacity. Sequelae of enterocystoplasty include electrolyte abnormalities, mucus production, stone formation, spontaneous perforation, and tumor formation. Bladder outlet resistance can be improved with bladder neck reconstruction, an artificial urinary sphincter, pubovesical sling, urethral suspension, and injection of collagen.

PENIS AND URETHRA

The external genitalia are morphologically identical in both sexes until the 50-mm crown-to-rump stage (about the ninth fetal week). After this the penis becomes morphologically distinct from the clitoris.

Prepuce

The foreskin of most infants cannot be fully retracted. During the first 5 years of life, intermittent erection and progressive accumulation of desquamated residue gradually separate the inner epithelial surface of prepuce from glans. *Keratin pearls* that accumulate between the glans and inner prepuce are normal in infancy and early childhood. Keratin pearls are sterile and best left alone or gently wiped away when they come to the surface. Forcible retraction of the foreskin is inadvisable.

Circumcision usually is a matter of family choice. *Circumcision is encouraged* for infants with a history of urinary infection or VUR to decrease risk for ascending infection. *Circumcision is discouraged* for infants with hypospadias, chordee, penoscrotal webbing to preserve the foreskin for use in reconstruction.

Phimosis is fibrotic contraction of the preputial aperture that makes retraction impossible. It is different from normal inability to retract the fused prepuce of an infant. Iatrogenic injury when someone forcibly retracts an infant's prepuce is a common cause of phimosis. Preputial injury leads to cicatrix formation, which narrows the preputial aperture. Normal erections or manual retraction of the foreskin may crack or tear the narrow aperture, leading to further scarring or infection. Severe phimosis can impede urinary flow. Circumcision or dorsal slit is an effective solution to phimosis.

Paraphimosis is entrapment of a phimotic prepuce proximal to the coronal margin. It causes lymphatic congestion, but venous congestion and arterial compromise may follow. Careful and persistent manual decompression usually solves the problem, but in unusual instances, emergency circumcision is necessary.

Hypospadias

Hypospadias is a developmental abnormality in which the urethra opens onto the ventral aspect of the penis. It is classified according to the position of the urethral meatus/glanular, coronal, midshaft, penoscrotal, scrotal, or perineal. Mild degree of chordee may be present. Some boys with hypospadias have cryptorchidism. A child with severe hypospadias and an undescended testicle may have an intersex disorder.

Management

Repair is performed after 6 months of age. A vascularized pedicled flap is used if skin flaps are necessary for urethral reconstruction. Severe hypospadias, especially with penoscrotal transposition, may be managed with staged reconstruction. If there is not enough penile skin, free grafts (skin, oral mucosa or bladder epithelium) can be used. Complications after reconstruction include urethrocutaneous fistula and stenosis or stricture of the neourethra.

Epispadias

Epispadias is an abnormality in which the urethra opens onto the dorsal aspect of the penis proximal to the tip of the glans. Dorsal chordee occurs. Bladder neck insufficiency and urinary incontinence can occur.

Management

Epispadias, dorsal chordee, and bladder neck incompetence are corrected surgically.

Posterior Urethral Valves

Posterior urethral valves cause neonatal urinary obstruction. The condition occurs only in boys. The obstructing lesion is a membrane or valvular leaflet in the distal prostatic urethra. Neonatal presentation includes a flank mass, urinary retention, urinary ascites, sepsis, azotemia, and a dysmorphic urinary tract. Older children have hematuria, obstructive voiding symptoms, enuresis, or infection.

Diagnosis

Blood chemistries, US, and voiding cystourethrography are done.

Management

Electrolyte imbalances and acidosis are corrected. Initial decompression of the urinary tract is accomplished with catheter drainage, possibly in the prenatal period. This is followed by endoscopic valve ablation. Cutaneous vesicostomy may allow an antegrade approach to later valve ablation. High urinary diversion and renal biopsy are necessary for persistent renal insufficiency.

TESTIS
Undescended Testis

If testicular descent has not occurred by 1 year of age, it is unlikely. Testes that remain undescended have a reduced number of germ cells and are at risk for malignant change. This risk probably is not altered by surgical relocation in the scrotum (orchiopexy), but a scrotal position enables self-examination.

Most undescended testes are ectopic. They have descended through the internal ring, inguinal canal, and external ring but have become trapped in a pocket (superficial pouch of Denis Brown) between the Scarpa fascia and external oblique fascia. Some undescended testes are in the inguinal canal.

Diagnosis

Undescended testes must be differentiated from retractile testes. At examination a retractile testis seem to be situated above the scrotum, but gentle and persistent manipulation brings the testis into the scrotum, where it stays if the patient is relaxed. Some ectopic undescended testes can be maneuvered into the scrotum, but once released, they ascend.

If the testis cannot be palpated, the inguinal canal is explored. If the testis still is not found or absence is proved with identification of blind-ending spermatic vessels, the search is expanded to the peritoneal cavity. Laparoscopy can be useful in this regard.

Management

Orchiopexy is performed after 1 year of age. Orchiectomy is recommended if this is uncorrected beyond puberty. Epididymal configuration can be abnormal in boys with undescended testes (Fig. 101-3). Abnormal or unattached genital ducts make fertility in that testis unlikely. These features are mentioned to the family and described in the operative note.

Torsion

Torsion is the most common pediatric scrotal emergency. In newborns, spermatic cord torsion occurs high on the cord. The loose connection of tunica vaginalis to the scrotum allows the entire scrotal content to twist (*extravaginal torsion*). This may occur before birth or in the immediately perinatal period.

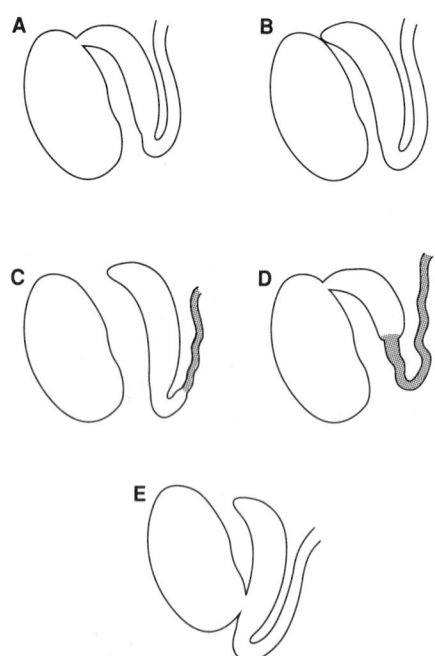

Figure 101-3. Epididymal anomalies in undescended testes. (*A*) Tenuous attachment of head of epididymis to the testis. (*B*) Complete separation of the epididymis from the testis. (*C*) Detached epididymis and atretic vas deferens. (*D*) Tenuous attachment of head. Atretic body and vasal atresia. (*E*) Section of head but partial attachment of body of epididymis tail.

Management

As the involved testis is virtually never salvageable in this situation, the main advantage to prompt exploration is the opportunity to anchor the contralateral testis and decrease the likelihood of contralateral torsion later.

Intravaginal torsion is twisting of the spermatic cord distal to the insertion of the tunica vaginalis. This is the usual form of cord torsion in older children, adolescents, and young adults. Torsion is extremely painful. It causes loss of the testis unless relieved immediately. A delay of >6 hours before surgical intervention makes salvage unlikely.

Management

Manual detorsion after parenteral administration of narcotics is a temporizing technique. Definitive therapy is surgical detorsion with contralateral fixation. A frankly necrotic testis is removed; an ischemic testis is untwisted and assessed for viability. It is best to try to preserve a twisted testis if there is evidence of viability.

Some boys have *transient or intermittent torsion.* They have acute scrotal pain, perhaps with swelling and erythema, that resolves within minutes or hours. Some young men with definitive torsion and a completely ischemic testis have a history of previous intermittent scrotal pain. This pattern of torsion and detorsion is an indication for elective bilateral orchiopexy.

Torsion of a gonadal appendage may cause as much pain as primary testicular torsion. Affected structures are the testicular appendix (a müllerian duct remnant) and epididymal appendages.

Diagnosis

Examination may show tender focal subcutaneous induration or a visible blue dot near the upper pole of the testis.

Management

If torsion of an appendix testis is recognized at examination, surgical treatment is not necessary. If a confident diagnosis cannot be made, exploration is necessary to exclude torsion of the spermatic cord.

US is performed after *trauma* to assess the integrity of the tunica albuginea or identify a testicular mass. Nuclear scans sometimes are useful. If scrotal pain and swelling occur in boys, torsion must be excluded. History and physical examination usually determine the need for surgical exploration. A diagnosis other than torsion must be made with absolute confidence.

Prepubertal Testis Tumors

Prepubertal testis tumors make up only a small portion of testis tumors. The usual lesion is a yolk sac tumor, which is a variant of embryonal-cell carcinoma. The tumors present with painless enlargement of a testis. The typical age of discovery is 2 years.

Management

Orchiectomy with removal of the spermatic cord is recommended with subsequent monitoring of serum α-fetoprotein level for relapse.

INTERSEX ABNORMALITIES

Gender assignment in the presence of ambiguous genitalia must be resolved in the newborn period. Reconstruction is performed if necessary. Deviation from this approach can cause severe emotional disability for child and family.

Normal sexual development during gestation requires

Table 101-1. DIFFERENTIATION OF FOUR MAJOR INTERSEX ABNORMALITIES

	Female Pseudohermaphroditism	True Hermaphroditism	Male Pseudohermaphroditism	Mixed Gonadal Dysgenesis
Buccal smear (Barr bodies)	Positive	Positive	Negative	Negative
Karyotype	XX	XX	XY	XO/XY
Urinary steroids	Positive	Negative	Negative	Negative
Gonads	Normal ovaries	Testis, ovary, ovatestis	Testes	Dysgenetic and streak ovaries

correct chromosome complement and composition, proper migration of germ cells from the yolk sac to the urogenital ridge for initial induction of the gonad, appropriate hormonal production by the gonad, and proper response by the target organs to the secreted hormones. A defect in any one of these steps can cause ambiguous genitalia. The abnormalities have four categories/female pseudohermaphroditism, male pseudohermaphroditism, true hermaphroditism, and mixed gonadal dysgenesis.

Diagnosis

Symmetry of the gonads and the presence or absence of Barr bodies on a buccal smear allow the differentiation among the four entities with a high degree of accuracy (Table 101-1).

Evaluation for ambiguous genitalia includes:

- Physical examination that includes a rectal examination to check for a uterus, vaginal examination, and consideration of phallus size and shape
- Family history to determine if other family members have a similar disorder. Congenital adrenal hyperplasia (CAH) is suggested if female relatives died in infancy
- Evaluation of drug ingestion during pregnancy (especially androgenic agents such as progesterone)
- Karyotype
- Urinary steroid measurements
- Serum electrolytes
- Retrograde genitogram to demonstrate the location of the vaginal entrance into the urogenital sinus
- Sometimes laparotomy or laparoscopy is required for definitive sex identification, especially with true hermaphroditism.

Surgical Considerations

Most infants with ambiguous genitalia are assigned female sex because regardless of genotype, an inadequate phallus cannot be corrected surgically. The exception is a genetic male with severe penoscrotal hypospadias and bilateral undescended testes but a functional phallus, who is reared as a boy. The timing of surgical reconstruction is a balance between the psychologic advantages of surgical intervention early in life and the technical limitations imposed by the small size of the structures. The current trend is toward early reconstruction.

VAGINAL ABNORMALITIES

Vaginal Atresia

- Complete—fallopian tubes are normal; uterus is bicornuate and rudimentary

- Distal—cervix, uterus, fallopian tubes are normal (Fig. 101-4)
- Proximal—fallopian tubes and uterus are normal, but cervix is abnormal (Fig. 101-5)

Diagnosis

Hydrocolpos or hydrometrocolpos may occur in infancy if the vagina or vagina and uterus fill with mucus. At menarche, hematocolpos or hematometrocolpos occur when the vagina fills with menstrual blood. The patient may have a large abdominal mass. In distal vaginal atresia, episodic abdominal pain occurs at menarche. Amenorrhea is expected.

Management

Hydrocolpos, hydrometrocolpos, hematocolpos, and hematometrocolpos associated with *distal* vaginal atresia can be managed with a perineal procedure in which the

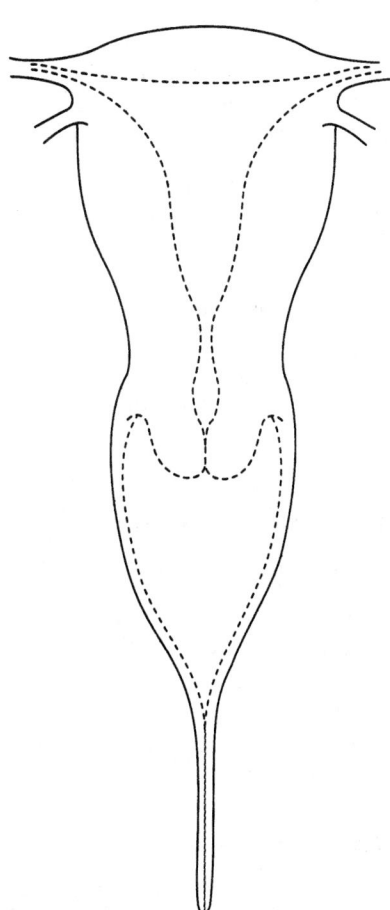

Figure 101-4. Distal vaginal atresia.

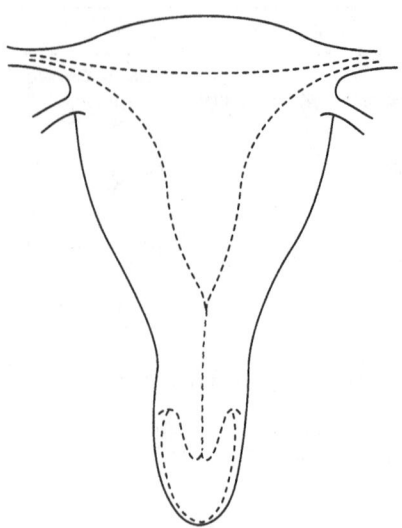

Figure 101-5. Proximal vaginal atresia with associated cervical atresia.

distal vaginal atresia or imperforate hymen is opened and drained. If these entities are associated with a *proximal* vaginal atresia, laparotomy is needed to drain the uterus and vagina and to approximate the distal vagina to the perineum. Vaginal replacement is with skin grafts or vascularized intestine.

Urogenital Sinus Defects

Urogenital sinus abnormalities occur when the urethra and vagina do not separate normally. The rectum is normal, and the uterus is bicornuate.

Management

Most commonly, repair with perineal cut-back vaginoplasty is feasible. When the vaginal entity is high in the sinus, vaginal pull-through is needed.

Cloacal Abnormalities

A cloacal abnormality is the lack of a separate opening for vagina and rectum. The labia are flat, and the phallus is small. The genotype may be male or female. Most patients are reared as girls.

Management

Surgical management depends on whether there is vaginal agenesis or proximal or distal vaginal atresia. The rectal and vaginal abnormalities are repaired.

UTERINE ABNORMALITIES

Uterine abnormalities rarely cause symptoms during childhood, and few patients have symptoms during adolescence. Most problems are related to infertility or complications of pregnancy and labor.

Atresia of the Cervix

The cervix forms as a solid cord of tissue between the uterine corpus above and the vagina below. When menstruation begins, hematometra forms above it.

Management

Dilation and incision when necessary are performed to drain the hematometra.

True Hypoplasia

In this condition, the cervix does not attain normal size, and its length and development are not proportional to those of the short and relatively small corpus. Severe hypoplasia causes failure of uterine growth beyond an early fetal stage. When present, the uterus is a small cord of tissue, usually without a cavity. Patients have amenorrhea with normally functioning ovaries, normal sexual characteristics, and cyclic breast changes.

Management

Hormonal therapy is not effective in promoting uterine growth in true hypoplasia. If the uterus is hypoplastic because of a lack of ovarian stimulation, hormonal replacement therapy in this situation (often given because of amenorrhea) enlarges these organs.

Aplasia

True uterine aplasia is rare. Although the uterus appears absent, inspection reveals thin cords extending from the ends of the uterine tubes medially along the superior surface of the broad ligaments. The ovaries are normal but may be displaced laterally toward the pelvic brim. Uterine tubes are poorly developed or aplastic. Vaginal agenesis is always present if there is a true agenesis of the uterus. There often are abnormalities of the lower urogenital tract as well.

Duplication

The genital folds do not unite normally, in this circumstance, resulting in a complete bicornuate uterus (two cervices) or simple duplication of the uterine body (Fig. 101-6).

ABNORMALITIES OF THE FALLOPIAN TUBES

Abnormalities of the fallopian tubes can cause sterility and problems of pregnancy. Small supernumerary or accessory tubes attached to the fimbriated ends or communicating with the isthmic or ampullar portions of the tubes are common and may be found when a child is operated on for another pelvic condition. Accessory tubes cause no problems and need not be disturbed.

Introital Problems

Labial Fusion

Midline adherence of the labia minora is relatively common. Usually is asymptomatic, incomplete, and flimsy. Time or mild lateral tension normalizes the opening. If the fusion interferes with micturition and precludes easy separation, an incision is made and the skin edges are sutured. A short course of topical estrogens prevents readhesion.

Urethral Prolapse

A distended, inflamed urethral meatus appears for no obvious reason. The condition usually causes minimal symptoms, and voiding is not compromised. The lesions regress with time and use of topical agents, but excision

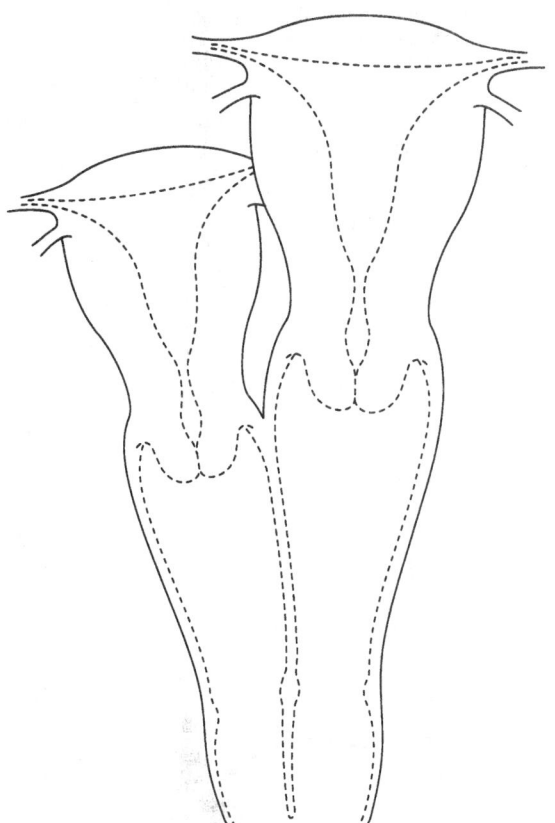

Figure 101-6. Duplication of the vagina and uterus.

sometimes is necessary. Differential diagnosis includes trauma, sexual abuse, urethral caruncle, and prolapsed ureterocele.

Sexual Abuse

This may lead to consequences in terms of genitourinary function and structure. A perineal and introital examination may reveal a widened introitus or asymmetry of the hymenal margin.

SUGGESTED READING

Bloom, DA, McGuire EJ, Lapides J. A brief history of urethral catheterization. J Urol 1994;151:317.

Bloom DA, Ritchey ML, Manzoni G. Laparoscopy for the nonpalpable testis. In: Holcomb GW III, ed. Pediatric endoscopic surgery. Norwalk, CT, Appleton & Lange, 1994:41.

Bloom DA, Sanvordenker JK. Genitourinary manifestations of sexual abuse in children. Adv Urol 1993;6:1.

Coran AG, Polley TZ Jr. Surgical management of ambiguous genitalia in the infant and child. J Pediatr Surg 1991;26:812.

Donahue PK, Gustafson ML. Early one-stage surgical reconstruction of high vaginal atresia. J Pediatr Surg 1994;29:352.

Donahue PK, Powell DM, Lee MM. Clinical management of intersex abnormalities. Curr Probl Surg 1991;27:15.

Kennelly MJ, Bloom DA, Ritchey ML, et al: Outcome analysis of bilateral Cohen cross-trigonal ureteroneocystostomy. Urology 1995;46:393.

Leonard MP, Canning DA, Epstein JI, et al. Local tissue reaction to the subureteral injection of glutaraldehyde cross-linked bovine collagen in humans. J Urol 1990;143:1209.

Wesley JR, Coran AG. Intestinal vaginoplasty for congenital absence of the vagina. J Pediatr Surg 1992;27:985.

ESSENTIALS OF SURGERY: SCIENTIFIC PRINCIPLES AND PRACTICE, edited by Lazar J. Greenfield, Michael W. Mulholland, Keith T. Oldham, Gerald B. Zelenock, and Keith D. Lillemoe. Lippincott–Raven Publishers, Philadelphia, © 1997.

CHAPTER 102

CHILDHOOD TUMORS

MICHAEL P. LAQUAGLIA

The incidence of pediatric solid tumors is shown in Fig. 102-1.

NEUROBLASTOMA

Neuroblastoma is the most common extracranial solid tumor and the most common abdominal malignant tumor of childhood. Girls and boys are affected almost equally. The median age at diagnosis is 2 years; most children are younger than 4 years. Neuroblastoma metastasizes to regional lymph nodes and distant sites, especially bone marrow and cortical bone. The liver and rarely the lungs also can be sites of metastasis.

Presentation

The clinical presentation of neuroblastoma depends on site of origin, age at diagnosis, and biologic aggressiveness of the tumor. More children younger than 1 year have cervical or pelvic tumors than do older children.

The most common presentation of neuroblastoma is an abdominal tumor that is hard and fixed. The tumor originates from the sympathetic nerves or, most commonly, the adrenal gland. Regional nodes often are involved along the aorta. The involved nodes can be bulky and may extend distally to the aortic bifurcation and proximally into the mediastinum, overshadowing the primary tumor. Patients with metastatic or large bulky tumors, especially if older than 1 year, may appear ill or be anemic.

The following syndromes are associated with neuroblastoma: periorbital ecchymoses (raccoon eyes), opsoclonus-myoclonus syndrome, and secretory diarrhea syndrome.

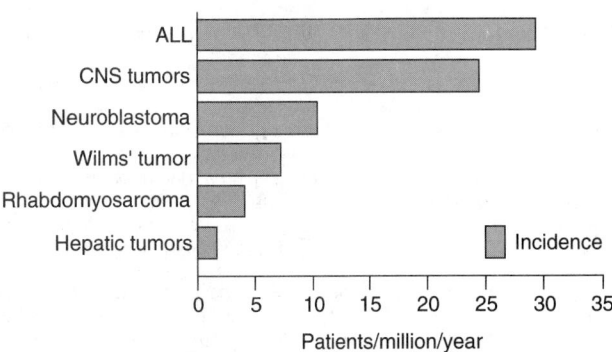

Figure 102-1. The incidence of childhood malignancies. Brain (CNS) tumors are the most common solid tumor in children. Neuroblastoma is the most common solid tumor treated by general pediatric surgeons. ALL, acute lymphocytic leukemia.

Table 102-1. **INTERNATIONAL STAGING CRITERIA FOR NEUROBLASTOMA**

Stage	Criteria	3-Year Survival Rate (%)	
		Overall	Relapse free
1	Localized tumor confined to site of origin; complete gross resection with or without microscopic margin; all identifiable regional nodes negative, including contralateral	97	88
2A	Unilateral tumor with incomplete gross excision; nodes negative	87	72
2B	Unilateral tumor with incomplete or complete gross excision with positive ipsilateral but negative contralateral nodes	86	63
3	Infiltration across the midline with or without regional nodal involvement; unilateral tumor with positive contralateral nodes; midline tumor with bilateral nodal involvement	62	58
4	Distant metastases to lymph nodes (4N), bone, bone marrow, liver, or other organs	<40	<40
4S	Localized primary tumor as described for stage 1 or 2 with distant metastases limited to liver, skin, and bone marrow (<10% involvement)	~75	~75

Table 102-2. **RISK STATUS DETERMINANTS IN NEUROBLASTOMA**

Parameter	Low Risk	High Risk
Age	<1 yr (especially <6 mo)	>1 yr at diagnosis
Stage	1, 2A, 2B, 4S	3, 4
Shimada classification	Favorable	Unfavorable
N-myc amplification	<3 copies	>3 Copies
Expression of TRK gene	trk Expressed	No trk expression
Flow cytometry	Hyperdiploid, triploid	Diploid
Cytogenetics	No 1p abnormality	1p Deletion
Ferritin at diagnosis	<142 ng/mL	≥142 ng/mL
Lactic dehydrogenase	≤1500 U/mL	>1500 U/mL
Neuron-specific enolase	≤100 ng/mL	>100 ng/mL

Table 102-3. **WILMS TUMOR–ASSOCIATED SYNDROMES AND CONDITIONS**

Syndrome	Syndrome Components	Wilms Tumor Risk
Beckwith-Wiedemann	Macroglossia, somatic gigantism, visceromegaly, hypoglycemia, abdominal wall defects	About 5% (500-fold increase)
WAGR	Wilms tumor, aniridia, ambiguous genitalia, mental retardation, WT1 deletion	40%–50% (40,000-fold to 50,000-fold increase)
Neurofibromatosis	Cafe-au-lait spots, plexiform neurofibromas, predisposition to multiple tumors	About 0.26% (26-fold increase)
Denys-Drash	Pseudohermaphroditism, glomerulopathy, gonadal tumors or dysgenesis	About 60%–70% (60,000-fold to 70,000-fold increase)
Perlman familial nephroblastomatosis	Bilateral renal hamartomas, macrosomia, islet cell hypertrophy, unusual facies, mental retardation	About 60%
Genital anomalies	Cryptorchidism, hypospadias, gonadal dysgenesis, pseudohermaphroditism	Increased

There is an increased risk of nephroblastoma in patients with the Denys-Drash and Perlman syndromes, but these are very rare, with less than 10 cases of Perlman syndrome reported. The incidence of Wilms tumor in the general population is 1 in 10000; therefore, the incidence of Wilms tumor in Beckwith-Wiedemann syndrome is 5/100 ÷ 1/10000, which is a 500-fold increase.

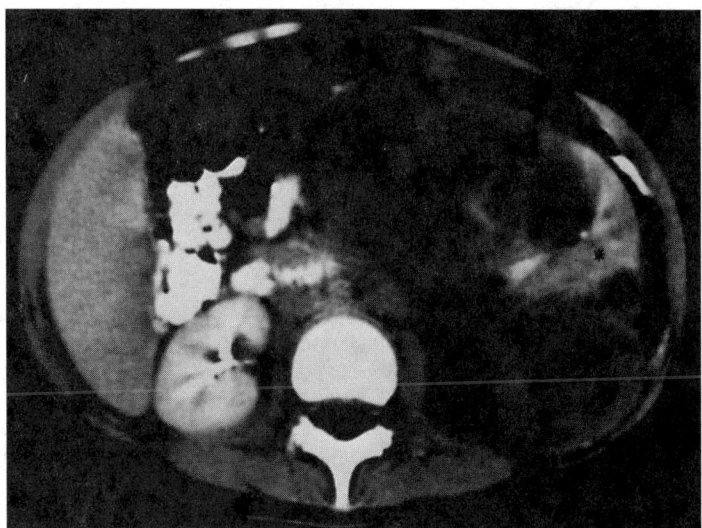

Figure 102-2. Initial CT scan of a child with a left-sided Wilms tumor. The distortion of the calyceal system is characteristic of intrinsic renal tumor. A kidney (*asterisk*) is identifiable.

Diagnosis

Evaluation is directed at delineation of tumor extent in the primary site and identification of metastatic deposits. The primary site is usually evaluated with *computed tomography* (CT) or *magnetic resonance imaging* (MRI). CT is performed with gastrointestinal (GI) and IV contrast material. This is true even for cervical and thoracic primaries so that the position and course of the pharynx and esophagus can be determined. The volume scanned includes the primary tumor and the regional lymphatics. The lower chest is included in scans of cervical primaries, the upper abdomen and lower neck in thoracic tumors, and the entire abdomen, pelvis, and lower chest for abdominal primaries.

Bone scans or *skeletal surgery* are routine to detect bone or bone marrow involvement. Plain *chest radiographs* are used to identify pulmonary metastases. If pulmonary metastases are present, a Doppler *ultrasound* (US) examination is used to identify intracaval tumor extension.

Radionuclide scans are performed to assess metastatic sites and as a baseline for evaluation of therapeutic response in the primary site.

A *24-hour urine* collection for measurement of epinephrine and norepinephrine degradation products (metanephrine, dopamine, and vanillymandelic acid) is used for diagnosis, These tumor markers are also used to assess therapeutic response.

Diagnosis of neuroblastoma entails histologic confirmation by means of direct tumor *biopsy* or demonstration of malignant cells in bone marrow samples. Bone marrow is assessed with *bone marrow aspiration* at four iliac crest sites and *bone biopsy* at two.

Staging

The staging of neuroblastoma is shown in Table 102-1. Table 102-2 lists criteria to estimate high and low risk. Risk assignment is important because it determines therapy.

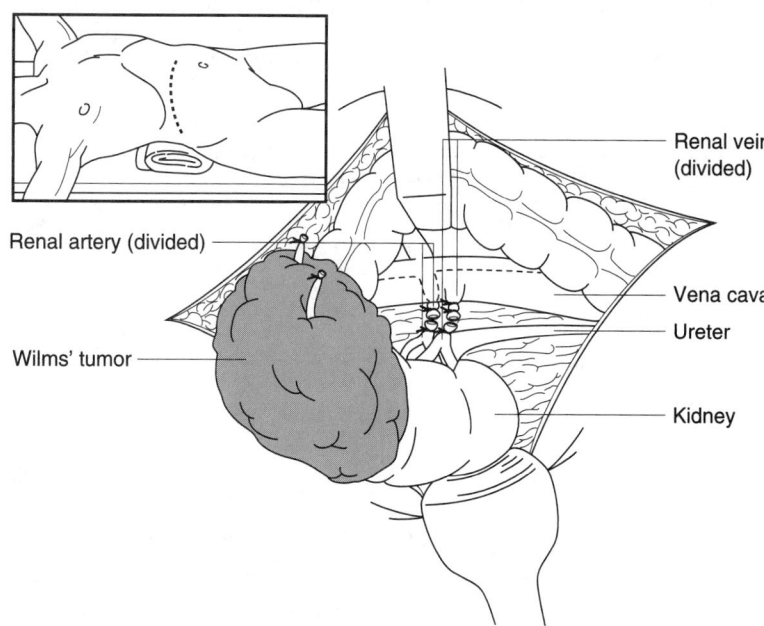

Figure 102-3. Operative approach to resection of a right renal Wilms tumor.

Table 102-4. STAGING CRITERIA FOR WILMS TUMOR

Wilms Tumor Staging System*		4-Year Survival Rate (%)
Stage 1	Tumor limited to kidney and completely excised; surface intact with no evidence of rupture	97
Stage 2	Tumor extends beyond kidney but completely excised; infiltration through the renal capsule, or extension into vessels outside the kidney substance, or local open biopsy or spillage confined to the flank; no residual tumor	95
Stage 3	Residual nonhematogenous tumor	91
Stage 4	Hematogenous metastases to lung, liver, bone, brain, etc.	78
Stage 5	Bilateral renal involvement at diagnosis	Same as for highest stage unilateral

* Survival based on outcome for favorable histology patients in the National Wilms' Tumor Study-3.

Management

Management of neuroblastoma depends on degree of risk. Patients with low-risk tumors do not need chemo- or radiation therapy. Resection of the primary lesion to confirm the diagnosis and obtain biologic markers is followed by observation. Serial imaging studies of the primary and possible metastatic sites are performed. Urinary catecholamines should fall to normal levels and stay there.

The initial operation for high-risk lesions is confined to acquisition of tissue, staging, and placement of a vascular access device. After four or five cycles of chemotherapy, a second-look operation is performed. Complete gross resection is the goal of second-look procedures. The approach is dictated by the properties of the primary tumor. For upper abdominal lesions, especially those involving midline branches of the abdominal aorta or the vena cava, thoracoabdominal exposure is helpful and well-tolerated. The goal of resection is complete vascular dissection. This encompasses the primary lesion and all involved regional nodes.

Chemotherapy for neuroblastoma entails high-dose in-

tensities of multiple agents. *Dose intensity* is defined as the drug dose normalized to surface area divided by the time interval over which it is administered. There is no universally accepted chemotherapy regimen.

WILMS TUMOR

Wilms tumor occurs almost equally among boys and girls. The peak incidence is 2 to 3 years of age. Table 102-3 lists conditions associated with Wilms tumor. The presence of any of these conditions prompts evaluation to rule out Wilms tumor.

Diagnosis

Most Wilms tumors are first diagnosed after detection of an asymptomatic abdominal mass, which can attain great size. This usually occurs during a routine pediatric examination or while the children are being attended by a relative. Some patients have rapid abdominal enlargement associated with pain, fever, and gross hematuria. These symptoms are attributed to intratumoral hemorrhage and may accompany spontaneous rupture.

The following evaluation is used for nephroblastoma:

1. An *excretory urogram* to identify the tumor site, demonstrate pelvicalyceal distortion, thereby localizing the process to the kidney, and assess the function of the contralateral kidney. CT of the abdomen with IV and oral contrast enhancement can be substituted for excretory urography (Fig. 102-2).
2. Abdominal, real-time *Doppler US* examination to identify intracaval tumor extension, liver metastases, or enlarged retroperitoneal lymph nodes.
3. Posteroanterior and oblique plain radiographs of the chest to identify pulmonary metastases.

Management

Therapy for Wilms tumor is surgical resection (Fig. 102-3). Exceptions include extensive intracaval tumors that require cardiopulmonary bypass for extraction, clearly unresectable tumors with documented invasion of contiguous structures, and possibly bilateral tumors, especially if it is unclear which side is most heavily involved. For most patients, exploration and resection are performed through a wide transverse incision that allows inspection and palpation of the contralateral kidney.

The surgeon must pay strict attention to local tumor

Table 102-5. NON-WILMS RENAL TUMORS

Tumor	Characteristics	Management
Clear cell sarcoma	Metastasis to bone and brain Relapse and death common Often confused with Wilms tumor	Aggressive systemic chemotherapy in all stages Radical resection of primary tumor followed by postoperative chemotherapy Postoperative irradiation of tumor bed Follow-up care: serial chest radiographs and brain MRI and bone scans every 6 mo for at least 3 yr after treatment
Rhabdoid tumor	Rare maligant tumor of kidney, also occurs in mediastium or brain	Surgical,resection Local radition therapy Systemic chemotherapy
Congenital mesoblastic nephroma	Usually occurs in infants Usually follows a benign course Invasion into the renal parenchyma or perinephric soft tissue	Radical nephrectomy Systemic chemotherapy for densely cellular lesions of tumors with high mitotic indices in older patients
Renal cell carcinoma	Adenocarcinoma similar to that in older patients Sites of metastases include lung, liver, bone, pleura, and brain	Radical nephrectomy

Table 102-6. CONDITIONS ASSOCIATED WITH RHABDOMYOSARCOMA

Neurofibromatosis
Beckwith–Wiedemann syndrome
Li–Fraumeni syndrome
Congenital anomalies (genitourinary, central nervous system, and cardiovascular malformations)
Basal cell carcinoma

extent or tumor rupture and status of the regional periaortic, interaortocaval, paracaval, and perirenal lymph nodes. Complete sampling of the nodes is performed, as is careful assessment of the tumor margins and possible areas of metastases. Direct visualization and bimanual palpation of the contralateral kidney are performed, even when CT scans do not suggest involvement. The liver is carefully palpated and the peritoneal and diaphragmatic surfaces inspected for metastases. Currently, all patients who undergo resection of Wilms tumor also undergo postoperative chemotherapy.

Staging

Once imaging, surgical, and pathologic data are acquired, a tumor stage is assigned (Table 102-4).

NON-WILMS RENAL TUMORS OF CHILDHOOD AND ADOLESCENCE

The characteristics and management of non-Wilms renal tumors are summarized in Table 102-5.

RHABDOMYOSARCOMA

Rhabdomyosarcoma affects boys and girls about equally. Conditions associated with this tumor are listed in Table 102-6. Li-Fraumeni cancer family syndrome involves sarcoma, especially rhabdomyosarcoma, in association with breast, bone, or brain cancer; lung and laryngeal cancer; and adrenocortical neoplasia. In this syndrome, children with rhabdomyosarcoma have first-degree relatives with the other malignant tumors.

Table 102-7. PRESENTATION OF RHABDOMYOSARCOMA

Site	Symptom
Head and neck	Facial or cervical swelling
	Pain
	Skin discoloration
	Sinusitis or middle ear infection
	Epistaxis
	Proptosis
	Cranial nerve palsy
Urinary tract	Gross or microscopic hematuria
	Suprapubic mass
	Urinary tract infection or obstruction
Vaginal or uterine cervix	Friable polypoid mass that prolapses through the vaginal orifice and may hemorrhage
Paratesticular region	Hard mass found during adolescence
Extremities	Painless or painful expanding mass
	Limp
	Skin change
	Pathologic fractures

Sites of rhabdomyosarcoma include head and neck (orbit, infratemporal fossa), genitourinary tract, including perineum and perianal area, extremities, trunk (chest wall, paraspinal area), retroperitoneum, and biliary tract. Rhabdomyosarcoma has four main types: embryonal, alveolar, botryoid, and pleomorphic. Embryonal is the most common among children.

Diagnosis

The presentation of rhabdomyosarcoma depends on site (Table 102-7). The steps in diagnosis are presented in Table 102-8. Imaging includes CT (Fig. 102-4) and positron emission tomography (PET).

Staging

The TNM system is used to stage rhabdomyosarcoma (Table 102-9).

Management

Management of rhabdomyosarcoma includes multiagent chemotherapy, judicious resection, and radiation therapy. The intensity of therapy is tailored to risk for subsequent

Table 102-8. DIAGNOSTIC EVALUATION FOR SUSPECTED RHABDOMYOSARCOMA*

Examination or Test	Rationale
History and physical examination	Search for lymph nodes, size of primary mass, general condition, underlying conditions
Complete blood count	Bone marrow replacement associated with anemia or thrombocytopenia; bone marrow toxicity is the major side effect of chemotherapy
Electrolytes, renal and hepatic function tests, creatinine clearance	Renal toxicity associated with cisplatin and other alkylators; genitourinary tumors may obstruct ureters; hepatic toxicity with dactinomycin
Four-site bone marrow aspirations, two-site bone biopsies	Bone marrow metastases reported in up to 6% of patients at diagnosis (29% of stage 4 patients have marrow involvement); bone marrow assessment before chemotherapy
Bone scan	Possibility of bone and bone marrow metastases
CT of the primary site	Evaluation of tumor size, invasiveness, enlargement of regional nodes, and complicating ureteral, biliary, bowel, or airway patency
CT of possible metastatic sites	CT scanning of the lungs and liver should be done to rule out parenchymal metastases. CT scanning is superior to MR imaging in assessing the degree of bone destruction in paraspinal, extremity, and head and neck (base of skull) lesions.
MR imaging	MR imaging is done for the same rationale as CT scanning. It may give more detailed information regarding the extent of viable tumor (T2-weighted imaging) and the presence of hepatic metastases. It is also the most useful tool for evaluation of the epidural space in paraspinal or base of skull primaries.
Gallium scanning	Both the primary tumor and metastatic deposits may be identified by gallium scanning

* The same work-up is applicable to other high-grade sarcomas.

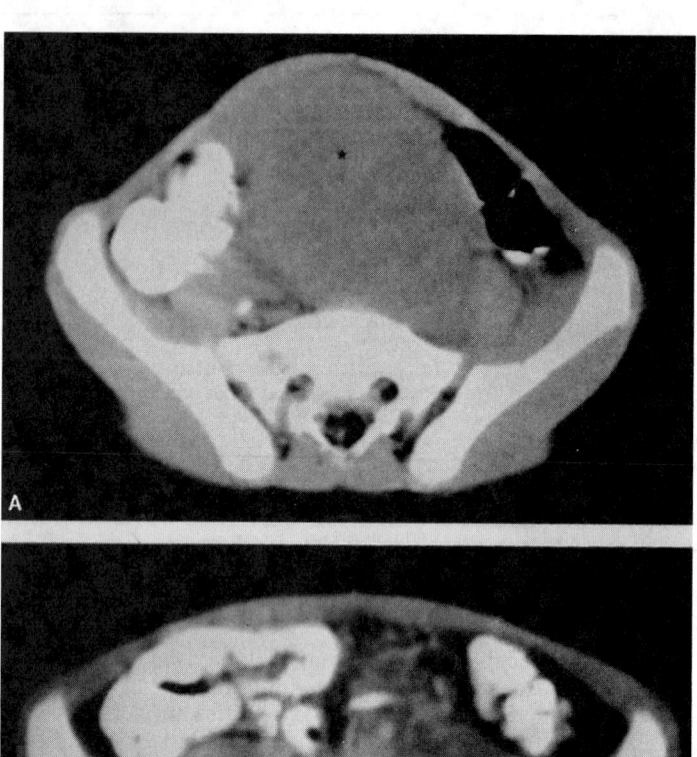

Figure 102-4. (*A*) Initial CT scan of a child with a large pelvic rhabdomyosarcoma. (*B*) CT scan of the same child after biopsy and cytoreductive chemotherapy. No tumor was demonstrable by diagnostic imaging.

relapse, which is a function of TNM stage. Agents are combined to limit drug resistance while attaining a synergistic antitumor effect.

Complete resection of primary tumors is undertaken before chemotherapy for small noninvasive lesions or after documented response with more formidable primary tumors. An example of the operative approach to lower extremity rhabdomyosarcoma involving anterior thigh muscles is depicted in Fig. 102-5. When chemotherapy results in complete or good tumor regression, external-beam irradiation may be used as a primary means of local control. Even in these circumstances, it is important to obtain biopsy specimens to document complete tumor eradication.

A debilitating or disfiguring operation is performed only if residual tumor is present after chemotherapy and radia-

tion therapy. Amputation of extremity rhabdomyosarcomas is performed only when lesions are bulky, invade bone or neurovascular structures, or are recurrent. Radical cystectomy is reserved for situations in which complete tumor eradication is not accomplished with chemotherapy and external-beam irradiation. External-beam radiation therapy of the primary site or involved regional nodes contributes to locoregional control.

NONRHABDOMYOMATOUS SOFT-TISSUE SARCOMAS

The characteristics and management of nonrhabdomyomatous soft tissue sarcomas are summarized in Table 102-10.

Table 102-9. TNM STAGING SYSTEM FOR RHABDOMYOSARCOMA

Clinical Stage	Invasiveness	Size	Status of Nodes	Distant Metastases
I	T1	a or b	N0	M0
II	T2	a or b	N0	M0
III	T1 or T2	a or b	N1	M0
IV	T1 or T2	a or b	N0 or N1	M1

T1, noninvasive; T2, invasive; Ta, ≤5 cm; Tb, >5 cm; N0, regional nodes negative; N1, nodes positive; M0, no distant metastases at diagnosis; M1, metastases present.

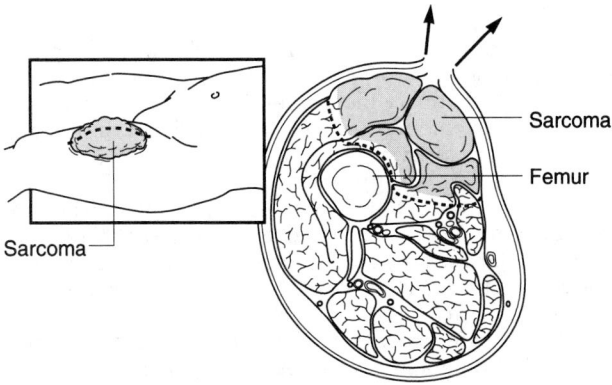

Figure 102-5. Technique for resection of a proximal lower-extremity rhabdomyosarcoma. Longitudinal incisions are always used. It is important to excise the tumor completely, with a surrounding 1- to 2-cm margin if feasible.

HEPATIC TUMORS

Presentation

Hepatocellular carcinoma is rare among children <4 years of age. The tumor lacks a distinct capsule and spreads diffusely through the liver in most patients, often with satellite nodules well-separated from the main tumor mass. Bilobar involvement occurs in most instances, and the umbilical fissure does not constitute a barrier to spread. Hepatocellular carcinoma is usually unresectable. Because of the association of hepatocellular carcinoma with hepatitis B infection, cirrhosis may be present in the surrounding nonneoplastic liver. This may preclude complete tumor resection if the volume of liver to be removed is likely to leave inadequate parenchyma for acceptable liver function.

Hepatoblastoma usually presents in the first 3 years of life. However, congenital presentation can occur, and the diagnosis has been made antenatally. Hepatoblastoma usually presents as a single, pseudoencapsulated lesion, often reaching large proportions before becoming clinically apparent. The tumor grows in an expansive way. If the umbilical fissure is not breached, successful extended resection

Table 102-10. NONRHABDOMYOMATOUS SOFT TISSUE SARCOMAS

Tumor	Characteristics	Management
Fibrosarcoma	Usually occur on extremities Hard, often infiltrating mass, maybe skin or deep fixation May invade bony or neural structures and metastasize to lung or liver	Initial trial of systemic chemotherapy Surgical resection with negative microscopic margins if possible without debility or deformity
Tendosynovial sarcoma	Lower extremity most common site of origin Metastasis to lung and pleura Present with enlarging extremity mass, pain	Surgical resection with clear microscopic margins, even if it involves amputation
Peripheral primitive neuroectodermal tumor (PNET)	Similar to Ewing sarcoma Most tumors localized at diagnosis Common sites of involvement include chest wall, pelvis, paraspinal areas, retroperitoneum, limbs, and abdomen Urinary catecholamines not elevated	Intensive multiagent chemotherapy followed by definitive resection
Desmoplastic small round cell tumor	Symptoms include abdominal or back pain, abdominal distention or mass, acute abdomen, intestinal, biliary, or ureteral obstruction, small nodules found in hernial sacs during repair	Systemic chemotherapy followed by exploratory laparotomy with resection of all gross disease and consolidation chemotherapy and external-beam radiation therapy to the primary site If diffuse peritoneal seeding is identified at diagnostic or second-look laparotomy or laparoscopy, total abdominal irradiation
Neurofibrosarcoma (neurogenic sarcoma, malignant schwannoma, malignant nerve sheath tumor, malignant neurilemoma)	Associated with von Recklinghausen disease (neurofibromatosis type I) Can be secondary tumors after external-beam radiation therapy Most common sites are extremity, retroperitoneum, and trunk Symptoms depend on location: pain, spontaneous hemothorax, perineal or perianal mass	Wide local excision followed by chemotherapy and irradiation
Leiomyosarcoma	Sites of involvement: GI and genitourinary tracts, retroperitoneum, lungs, pulmonary artery, vascular wall, popliteal artery, sinonasal area, peripheral soft tissues Lungs most common site of metastases Associated with von Recklinghausen disease and neurofibrosarcoma Presents with pain or GI bleeding	Complete surgical resection even if it involves amputation; chemo- and radiation therapy are ineffective
Liposarcoma	Extremely rare in childhood Most common sites are lower extremity, upper extremity, retroperitoneum Presents as a painless mass Metastasis uncommon	Complete surgical excision
Alveolar soft parts sarcoma	Rare Affects skeletal muscle and fascial planes Common sites are thigh and buttocks followed by abdominal and chest walls Metastatic to lung, bone, brain Relapses in distant sites; patients die of progressive disease	Surgical excision

Table 102-11. LABORATORY FINDINGS IN HEPATOBLASTOMA AND HEPTOCELLULAR CARCINOMA

Test	Finding
Liver function tests	Nonspecifically deranged in both tumors
Serum cholesterol level	Elevated in both
Serum α-fetoprotein (AFP)	Greatly elevated in hepatoblastoma
	Elevated among few patients with hepatocellular carcinoma and elevation not great

may be possible initially. Multicentricity or massive diffuse disease within the liver occurs in some patients. Cirrhosis of the surrounding liver is unusual.

Diagnosis

Symptoms

Children with *hepatoblastoma* have an abdominal mass or diffuse abdominal swelling. Often the child is in good health, and the lesion may be discovered by a parent or at a routine office visit. Symptoms such as pain, irritability, minor GI disturbances, fever, and pallor occur in a small number of patients. Hepatoblastoma can cause sexual precocity due to androgen synthesis, although this is rare.

Children and adolescents with *hepatocellular carcinoma* typically have a palpable abdominal mass, but it is rarely an incidental finding in a normal child. Pain is a frequent accompaniment. Constitutional disturbances, such as anorexia, malaise, nausea and vomiting, and weight loss are frequent.

With either hepatoblastoma or hepatocellular carcinoma jaundice is rare. A small number of patients have acute tumor rupture.

Laboratory Studies

The laboratory findings for hepatoblastoma and hepatocellular carcinoma are summarized in Table 102-11. Mild anemia is common in both tumors. Thrombocytosis often occurs with hepatoblastoma and sometimes occurs with hepatocellular carcinoma.

Imaging

Abdominal CT is performed for diagnostic discrimination and assessment of operability. The chest is included to identify pulmonary metastases. The typical appearance of *hepatoblastoma* is a solitary mass with lower attenuation than normal liver (Fig. 102-6). *Hepatocellular carcinoma* has a similar appearance but is more likely to be multifocal, invade the portal vein, and metastasize to draining lymph nodes. The two tumors cannot be differentiated on the basis of CT findings because the pattern of disease of either may be atypical. The diagnostic utility of MRI is similar to that of CT.

Plain radiographs and liver–spleen scans show abnormalities but do not assist in diagnosis or planning of therapy. Angiography is performed if embolization or infusion chemotherapy is being considered. Similar information is obtained with CT and MRI.

Abdominal US is probably the most useful screening tool for children with large livers. It allows one to differentiate between space-occupying lesions and diffuse hepatomegaly. Anatomic detail of the tumor margin is not delineated well enough for assessment of resectability. Doppler US is useful for evaluation of patency of the inferior vena cava and hepatic veins, but extreme compression of these vessels may prevent useful interpretation.

Staging

The staging and risk status for hepatoblastoma is shown in Table 102-12.

Management

Hepatoblastoma

Complete surgical resection is the objective of therapy for hepatoblastoma. Most patients have resectable tumors, although this often requires cytoreduction chemotherapy initially. Extensive anatomic resection usually is required, depending on tumor location and extent. As much as 85% of the hepatic substance may be removed with full and rapid regeneration despite postoperative chemotherapy.

Some patients with hepatoblastoma have inoperable tumors. Bilaterality, diffuse multicentricity and metastatic lesions may preclude resection. Various techniques are

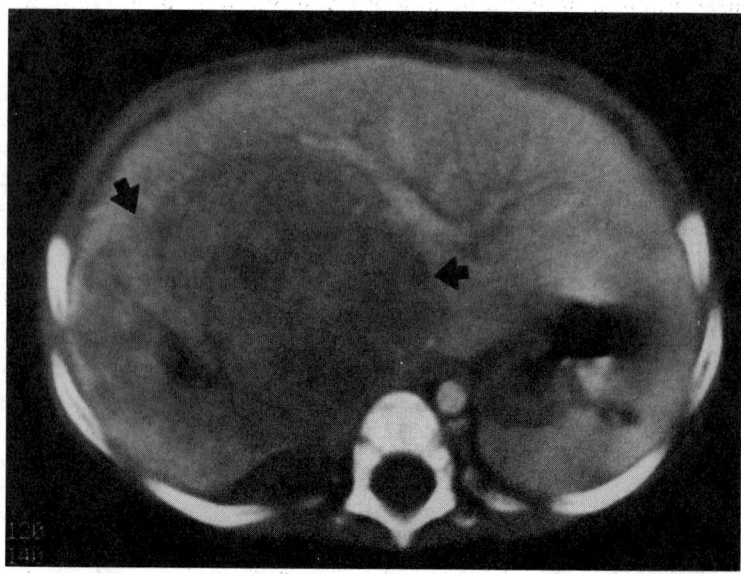

Figure 102-6. CT scan of a 2-year-old child with a large right lobar hepatoblastoma (*arrows*). Despite the large size, these lesions can often be completely resected before chemotherapy. Hepatocellular carcinoma, in contrast, often involves multiple hepatic segments, and there is a significant incidence of extrahepatic extension.

Table 102-12. RELATION OF STAGING TO PROGNOSIS FOR HEPATOBLASTOMA

Clinical Group	Criteria	Relative Risk for Death of Disease
I	Complete resection of tumor as initial treatment, irrespective of resectional technique	0.16
IIA	Complete resection after irradiation or chemotherapy	0.57*
IIB	Residual disease confined to one lobe	—
III	Disease involving both hepatic lobes	2.87
IIIB	Regional nodal involvement	—
IV	Distant metastases, irrespective of the extent of the hepatic tumor	3.51

* Relative risk was assessed for stage II and III patients collectively. The relative risk is compared with other stages.

used to increase resectability rate. These include preoperative chemotherapy, profound hypothermia with circulatory arrest, and total hepatic vascular occlusion. These maneuvers are useful in selected instances. For truly unresectable disease, aside from transplantation, management is chemotherapy. The role of radiation therapy is not clearly defined.

Hepatocellular Carcinoma

Complete surgical resection is a prerequisite for cure of hepatocellular carcinoma in children. Patients with incompletely resected tumors do not survive. Although patients undergoing resection survive longer than those who do not, the gain is small because of high local and systemic relapse rates. The overall prognosis is poor.

SUGGESTED READING

Crist W, Gehan EA, Ragab AH, et al. The Third Intergroup Rhabdomyosarcoma Study. J Clin Oncol 1995;13:610.

Green DM, Breslow M, Beckwith JB, et al. Treatment outcomes in patients less than two years of age with small stage I favorable histology Wilms' tumor: a National Wilms' Tumor study. J Clin Oncol 1993;11:91.

Hupperets PS, Havenith MG, Blijham GH. Recurrent adult nephroblastoma: long-term remission after surgery plus adjuvant high-dose chemotherapy, radiation therapy, and allogeneic bone marrow transplantation. Cancer 1992;69:2990.

Kushner BH, La Quaglia MP, Bonilla MA, et al. Highly effective induction therapy for stage 4 neuroblastoma in children over 1 year of age. J Clin Oncol 1994;12:2607.

La Quaglia MP, Heller G, Ghavimi F, Casper ES, Vlamis V, Hajdu S, Brennan MF. The effect of age at diagnosis on outcome in rhabdomyosarcoma. Cancer 1994;73:109.

Nakagawara A, Arima-Nakagawara M, Scavarda NJ, et al. Association between high levels of expression of the TRK gene and favorable outcome in human neuroblastoma. N Engl J Med 1993;328:847.

Ng EH, Pollock RE, Munsell MF, Atkinson EN, Rosenthal MM. Prognostic factors influencing survival in gastrointestinal leiomyosarcomas: implications for surgical management and staging. Ann Surg 1992;215:68.

Ni Y, Chang M, Hsu H, et al. Hepatocellular carcinoma in childhood: clinical manifestations and prognosis. Cancer 1991;68:1737.

Pizzo PA, Poplack DG, eds. Principles and practice of pediatric oncology. Philadelphia, JB Lippincott, 1993.

Ritchey ML, Kelalis PP, Breslow NB, et al. Surgical complications after nephrectomy for Wilms' tumor: a report from the National Wilms' Tumor Study-3. Surg Gynecol Obstet 1992;175:507.

ESSENTIALS OF SURGERY: SCIENTIFIC PRINCIPLES AND PRACTICE,
edited by Lazar J. Greenfield, Michael W. Mulholland, Keith T. Oldham, Gerald B. Zelenock,
and Keith D. Lillemoe. Lippincott–Raven Publishers, Philadelphia, © 1997.

CHAPTER 103

ORTHOPEDIC SURGERY

LARRY S. MATTHEWS, STEVEN A. GOLDSTEIN, BRIAN J.
SENNETT, AND FELIX H. SAVOIE

FRACTURES

The objectives of fracture management are anatomic reduction and fixation stability. Simple fractures in adults, particularly fractures of the upper extremities, are treated with cast immobilizationn. Most fractures in children are treated with cast immobilization, avoiding the hazards of surgical intervention. Fracture repair and extensive remodeling occur rapidly in children because of the systemic effects of biochemical factors related to the accelerated bone formation associated with growth. When open reduction and internal fixation treatment are needed, the following principles are followed: maximal maintenance of periosteal and vascular tissue without compromise of stability, anatomic reduction and fixation stability, use of strong biocompatible implants, fixation constructs that minimize load shielding of the underlying bone, and maintenance of maximal soft tissue coverage and interposition between the device and skin surface.

Factors that affect progression of healing after a fracture include age, nutritional status, presence of soft tissue trauma, and mechanical stability. Long-term clinical success depends on the location of the fracture (diaphyseal, metaphyseasl, or intraarticular), degree of comminution, and potential for healing and remodeling.

With a simple fracture and loss of structureal stability, bleeding into the area is followed by an early inflammatory response and a proliferation of cells. Mesenchymal cells dominate the region, and necrotic tissue undergoes phagocytosis. This early phase is followed by invasion of new arterioles and capillaries, followed by cellular differentiation into fibrocartilage and other collagen-producing fibroblasts. Repair continues by means of a combination of mechanisms: endochondral ossification, which involves a cartilage intermediate stage, direct bone apposition, and primary healing involving acceleration of remodeling across a stable, securely reduced fracture line.

The occurrence and distribution of the mechanisms depends on the stability of the fracture during treatment and on fracture location. The more unstable the fracture, the more involved is the endochondral mechanism in repair and the greater is the cross-sectional area of callus. The biologic process seems to be driven by the need to establish mechanical integrity as quickly as possible.

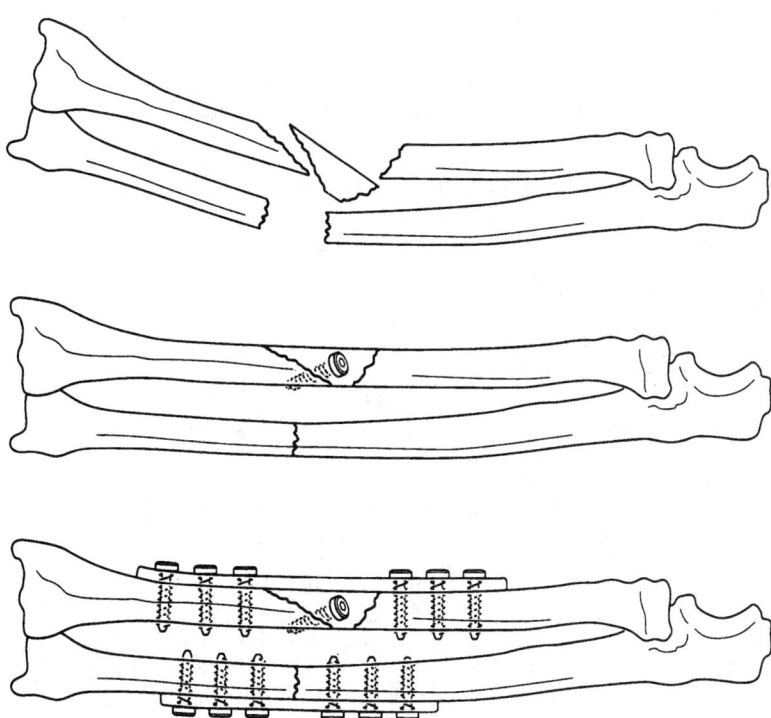

Figure 103-1. Internal fixation for a comminuted fracture of both bones of the forearm. The fractures were reduced with a combination of interfragmentary screws and compression plates and screws.

751

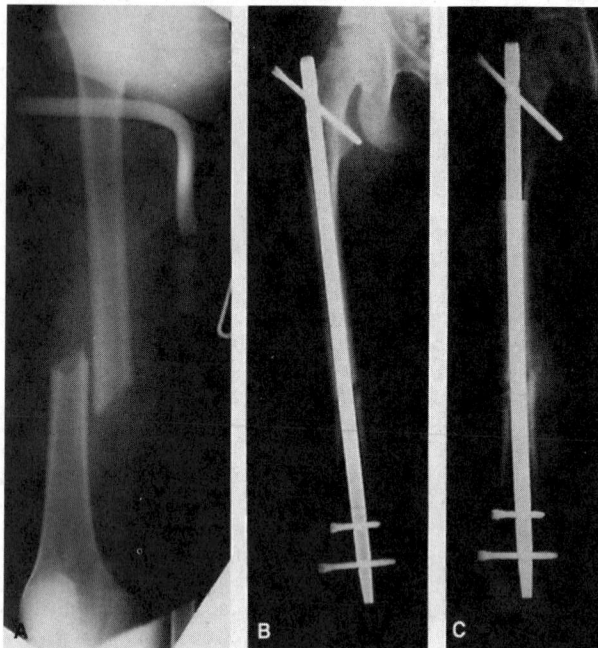

Figure 103-2. (*A*) Radiograph of a femoral shaft fracture with significant comminution. (*B*) The fracture was reduced with traction during surgery and was stabilized with an interlocking intermedullary nail. (*C*) The fracture healed rapidly, and both length and anatomic position were preserved.

The management of fractures involves wound care, geometric reassembly of the parts, and stable maintenance of the geometry during healing. Soft tissue transfer, local transposition of muscle tissue, and free tissue transfer allow fracture-site coverage with viable tissue. Management after multiple trauma is stable fixation, early bone grafting, and skin coverage in association with systemic support and antibiotic prophylaxis.

Fixation

A large array of plates, screws, and related devices are used to reconstruct unstable fractures. Motion at a fracture site may lead to malunion or nonunion (Fig. 103-1).

Open reduction, internal fixation, and implantation of *plates* are used to manage *metaphyseal fractures,* especially of the forearm and hand. Bone and implant are considered a single composite structure. Because a fracture fixation plate is rigid stainless steel, the combined structure is resistant to deformation. The implant shields the bone from the load normally transmitted through it.

Intramedullary *rods* are used to manage *diaphyseal fractures,* especially of the tibia, femur, and humerus. Intramedullary fixation allows early weight bearing and requires minimal immobilization of the joints above and below the fracture. Little long-term remodeling (loss of bone) occurs. Rehabilitation is rapid, and blood loss is minimal. Fractures close to the metaphyseal and diaphyseal junctions can be managed with intramedullary rods without compromise of rotational stability. When intramedullary fixation is used to manage segmented or comminuted fractures or other unstable fractures with proximal and distal bone loss, interlocking allows surgical reestablishment of the bone compartment and limb length (Fig. 103-2). The device can maintain length until the fracture heals.

Fractures Involving Joint Surfaces

Fractures that extend into joints are managed by means of open anatomic reduction and internal fixation. Most such fractures involve the tibial plateau (Fig. 103-3) or the radius in the wrist.

Restoration of normal acetabular geometry allows opposing articular cartilages to bear loads and slide past each other normally. Restoration of the fracture fragments frequently leads to normal ligamentous geometry and to normal joint kinematics. The healed, reduced, and nearly anatomic bony pelvis around the hip socket provides a base for total hip replacement.

LIMB-LENGTH DISCREPANCY

Limb-length discrepancy can be caused by polio, childhood trauma, genetic defect, or other causes. Management involves fixation of the proximal and distal portions of the involved bone, usually the femur or tibia, by means of an encircling metal hoop and multiple small-diameter pins

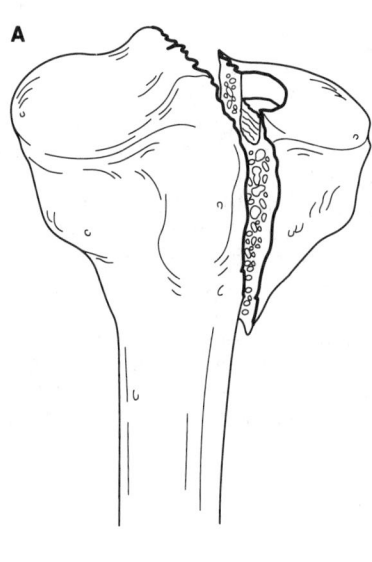

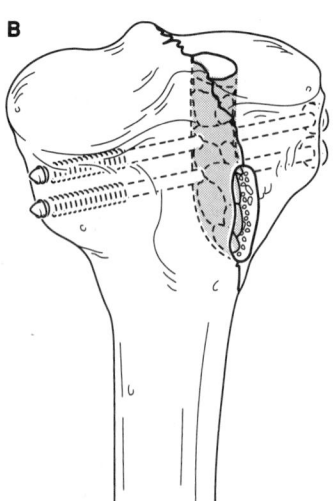

Figure 103-3. (*A*) Fracture of the lateral tibial plateau with significant inferior and lateral displacement and a punched-down region. (*B*) Accurate reduction, elevation of the punched-down region, support of the bone graft through a cortical window, and secure fixation should improve the chances for long-term joint function.

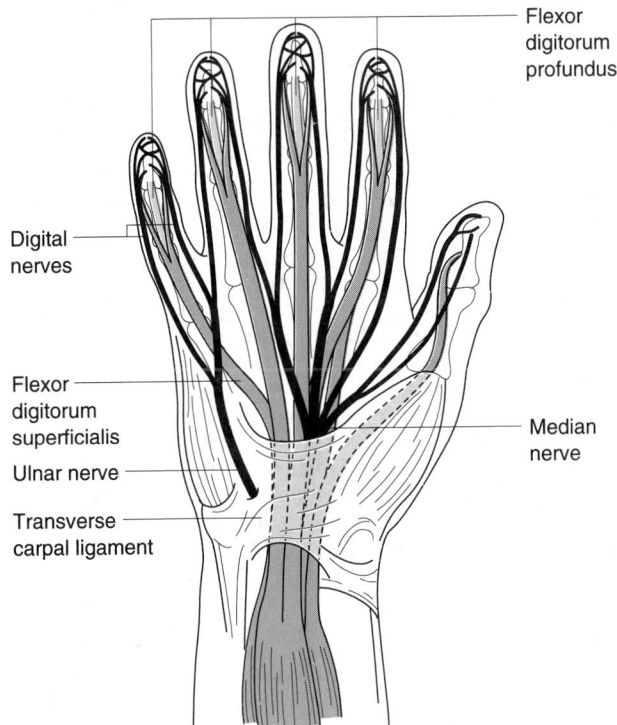

Figure 103-4. Volar anatomy of the hand and wrist.

Labels (clockwise from top): Flexor digitorum profundus; Digital nerves; Flexor digitorum superficialis; Ulnar nerve; Transverse carpal ligament; Median nerve

under strong tension. Two or more pins may be placed through the bone at almost any location. Pin placement is performed closed under image-intensifier control.

Metaphyseal corticotomy is performed through one or more small incisions with minimal damage to the periosteum and metaphyseal trabecular bone. After selective cortical weakening, the bone is broken so that the planes of the fracture are minimally separated. A threaded extension mechanism is used to distract the segments of the bone proximal and distal to the corticotomy. The usual rate of distraction is four evenly spaced 0.25-mm adjustments per day. As the fracture separates with time, a striated density of immature bone is evident on radiographs. The rate of distraction is adjusted to maintain lengthening during production of new bone between the bone segments. Continued weight bearing leads to a maturation of new bone. When sufficient strength of the new bone is achieved, the frame is removed.

MECHANICALLY DAMAGED JOINTS

Total Joint Replacement Arthroplasty

Many diseases, posttraumatic states, and conditions damage the joints and cause pain and disability (osteoarthritis or degenerative joint disease, rheumatoid arthritis, osteonecrosis, posttraumatic arthritis). These can be managed with total joint replacement arthroplasty. Hip and knee replacement are the most common procedures. The principles of joint implantation involve:

- Use of high fatigue-strength biocompatible metallic alloys

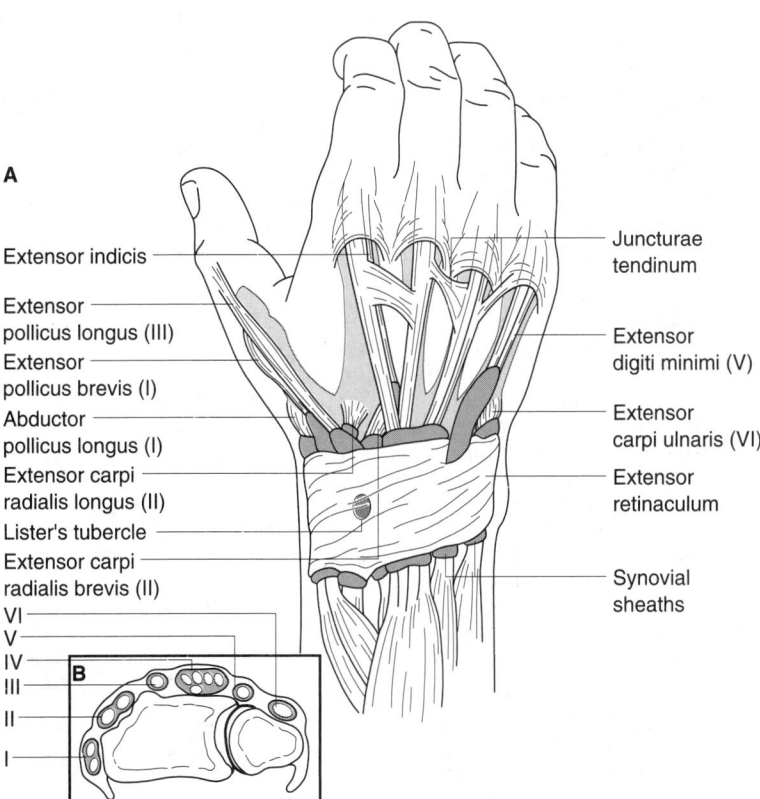

Figure 103-5. Dorsal anatomy of the wrist. (*A*) The extensor tendons are divided into six compartments by the extensor retinaculum as they course across the dorsum of the wrist. (*B*) Cross-sectional view illustrates the compartmentalization and the relation to the radius and ulna.

Labels (left side): Extensor indicis; Extensor pollicus longus (III); Extensor pollicus brevis (I); Abductor pollicus longus (I); Extensor carpi radialis longus (II); Lister's tubercle; Extensor carpi radialis brevis (II); VI; V; IV; III; II; I

Labels (right side): Juncturae tendinum; Extensor digiti minimi (V); Extensor carpi ulnaris (VI); Extensor retinaculum; Synovial sheaths

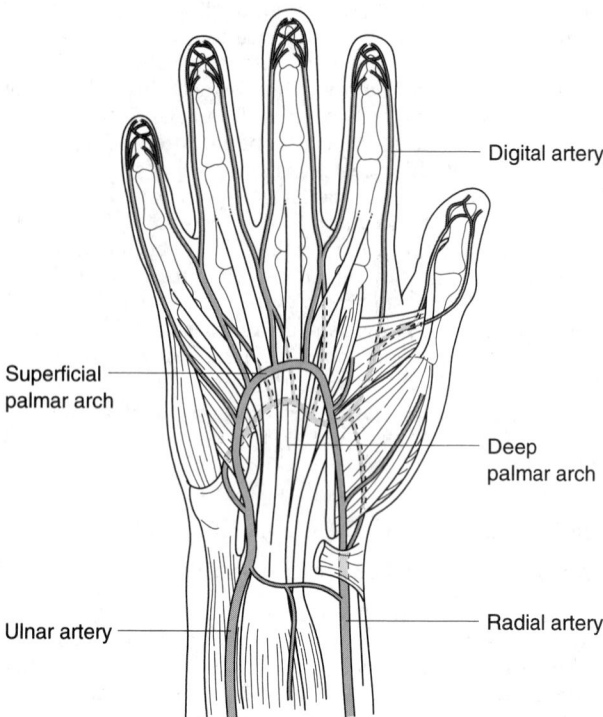

Figure 103-6. Blood supply to the hand. The vascular supply to the hand is through the radial and ulnar arteries. The deep palmar arch arises predominantly from the radial artery, and the superficial arch arises mainly from the ulnar artery. Digital arteries arise from the palmar arches.

- Low-friction articulating surfaces made from polished metal alloys opposed to a polyethylene-matched surface
- Articular surface designs that provide nearly normal ranges of motion while minimizing constraints that might subject the interface surfaces to high mechanical stresses
- Use of smooth geometric shapes that match the anatomic regions in which they are implanted
- Use of surgical instrumentation to provide consistent alignment and fit of the components in the recipient bones, and optimal bone surface preparation (removal of debris, reduction in bleeding) to improve penetration and interdigitation of the cement for more durable fixation

Total knee and hip prostheses have a fixation life expectancy of about 15 years for most patients. Because revision procedures are much less successful than the initial operation, total joint replacement is most appropriate for patients 60 years and older.

The most important failure of total joint arthroplasty is aseptic mechanical loosening at the interface between the bone, cement, and implant. Factors that contribute to loosening include excess weight, high activity level, component misalignment, and breakdown of the cement interface.

ARTHROSCOPY AND SPORTS MEDICINE

Arthroscopy is the most effective method for diagnosing and managing injuries to the ligaments of the knee. The technique is being investigated for use on the shoulder and wrist.

Complete tears of the anterior cruciate ligament cause anteroposterior instability that stress other knee structures, particularly under fully loaded, flexed, and rotational motion. Often there is a secondary tear of the medial or lateral meniscus, increased instability, and early development of posttraumatic degenerative arthritis. Arthroscopy allows immediate and certain diagnosis of anterior cruciate ligament tears and is valuable in surgical reconstruction of function. During an arthroscopic procedure bone-ligament-bone grafts can be placed in an anatomic location. These ligament grafts may be obtained from the patellar tendon or from autologous sources. The increased stability often is considerable, allowing patients to return to high-level sports activities.

The small size of the arthroscopic incision, clear visualization of the interior of the joint, and ability to perform definitive surgical correction with minimal damage to other structures allow almost immediate rehabilitation. Muscular atrophy due to extensive immobilization and lack of weight bearing is prevented. The neuromuscular coordination and skills important to athletes and workers are not lost.

EVALUATION OF HAND INJURIES

The muscles, nerves, and blood vessels of the hand are depicted in Figs. 103-4, 103-5, and 103-6.

A thorough history is obtained that includes the presenting symptoms, evolution of the problem, and aggravating and relieving factors. Age, sex, hand dominance, occupation, medical history, and preexisting conditions are recorded.

Physical examination includes evaluation of the neck, shoulder, elbow, forearm, wrist, and hand. Range of motion, strength, overall body habitus, muscle wasting, hypertrophy, deformities, skin changes, and areas of tenderness are evaluated. Capillary refill in the presence or absence of normal sweating patterns is evaluated, as is the sensibility of the digits.

Radiographic examination is essential and is performed on all injured extremities, regardless of the presenting symptom. Advanced testing such as electromyography, nerve conduction studies, technetium bone scanning, computed tomography, or magnetic resonance imaging can be used in the evaluation of a painful wrist and hand. Selective injections may help determine the cause of pain.

SUGGESTED READING

Green DP, ed. Operative hand surgery. New York, Churchill Livingstone, 1993.

Hungerford DS, Krackow KA, Kenna RV. Cementless total knee replacement in patients 50 years old and under. Orthop Clin North Am 1989;20:131.

Joyce ME, Terek RM, Jingushi S, Bolander ME. Role of transforming growth factor β in fracture repair. Ann NY Acad Sci 1990;593:107.

Martin RB, Burr DB. Structure, function and adaptation of compact bone. New York, Raven Press, 1989.

Mow VC, Ratcliffe A, Wood SLY, eds. Biomechanics of diarthrodial joints. New York, Springer-Verlag, 1990.

Poehling GG. Arthroscopy of the wrist and elbow. New York, Raven Press, 1994.

Rockwood CH, Green DP, eds. Fractures in adults, ed 3. Philadelphia, JB Lippincott, 1991.

Scuderi GR, Insall JN, Windsor RE, Moran MC. Survivorship of cemented knee replacements. J Bone Joint Surg [Br] 1989; 71:798.

Whipple TL. Arthroscopic surgery: the wrist. Philadelphia, JB Lippincott, 1992.

ESSENTIALS OF SURGERY: SCIENTIFIC PRINCIPLES AND PRACTICE,
edited by Lazar J. Greenfield, Michael W. Mulholland, Keith T. Oldham, Gerald B. Zelenock,
and Keith D. Lillemoe. Lippincott–Raven Publishers, Philadelphia, © 1997.

CHAPTER 104

CENTRAL NERVOUS SYSTEM

JULIAN T. HOFF AND MICHAEL F. BOLAND

The history and physical examination are the foundation of neurosurgical diagnosis. Headache, altered consciousness, memory impairment, speech difficulty, visual disturbance, weakness, paresthesia, and incoordination are symptoms of central nervous system (CNS) disease. The examination includes:

Assessment of mental status
Thorough cranial nerve testing
Optic funduscopy
Motor, sensory, and reflex testing

Details in the history suggest a cause (trauma, neoplasm, vascular disease, infection, degenerative disease, metabolic disorder), and neurologic examination localizes the lesion.

DIAGNOSTIC STUDIES

Studies helpful in neurosurgical diagnosis include plain-film radiography and tomography, myelography, arteriography, computed tomography (CT), magnetic resonance imaging (MRI), ultrasonography (US), electromyography (EMG) and nerve conduction velocity testing, evoked potentials (visual, auditory, and somatosensory), positron emission tomography (PET), and electroencephalography (EEG).

TRAUMA

Most accidents involving motor vehicles and falls include injury to the brain and spinal cord and the surrounding structures.

Scalp Injury

Scalp injury can cause serious hemorrhage and shock if not treated promptly. Bleeding usually can be controlled with a simple pressure dressing, firm finger pressure, or hemostats applied to the galea (aponeurosis of the scalp). Scalp wounds are closed as soon as possible. Simple scalp lacerations are débrided, copiously irrigated, and closed primarily. Lacerations that overlie a depressed fracture or a penetrating wound of the skull require débridement in the operating room.

Skull Fracture

Skull fractures are classified according to:

1. Whether the skin overlying the fracture is intact (closed) or disrupted (open or compound)
2. Whether there is a single fracture line (linear), several fractures radiating from a central point (stellate), or fragmentation of bone (comminuted)
3. Whether the edges of the fracture line are driven below the level of the surrounding bone (depressed) or not (nondepressed)

Simple skull fractures (linear, stellate, or comminuted) require no treatment. Depressed skull fractures often necessitate surgical elevation of the bone fragments. Open skull fractures also necessitate surgical intervention.

Any leakage of cerebrospinal fluid (CSF) is managed expectantly. Traumatic CSF leakage usually stops in 7 to 10 days. If leaking persists, lumbar CSF drainage can be performed to seal the leak, lowering CSF volume and intracranial pressure (ICP).

Brain Injury

Injury to the brain is caused by the rapid deceleration, acceleration, and rotation from a blow to the head. The initial impact can produce neuronal and axonal disruption, which constitutes the primary injury. Intracranial hematoma, cerebral edema, hypoxia, hypotension, hydrocephalus, or endocrine disturbance are secondary injuries.

Elevated ICP contributes to secondary brain injury by reducing cerebral perfusion pressure, which is the difference between mean arterial blood pressure and cerebral venous pressure. For clinically relevant purposes, cerebral venous pressure is identical to ICP. When ICP increases and mean arterial blood pressure remains stable, cerebral perfusion pressure decreases. When cerebral perfusion pressure falls to <70 mmHg, cerebral blood flow is compromised.

Rapid clinical assessment is essential. The Glasgow Coma Scale (Table 104-1) is used to determine neurologic status. The initial neurologic examination determines whether diagnostic testing is indicated. Patients without headache, lethargy, or a focal neurologic deficit are not likely to have a secondary injury, and imaging studies are not indicated. Patients with symptoms with or without a focal deficit undergo CT of the head. If CT does not show a lesion despite high clinical suspicion, carotid and cerebral angiography can help delineate a vascular abnormality.

After emergency surgical removal of any traumatic cerebral mass lesion, the goals of medical management are normalization of cerebral perfusion pressure and prevention of secondary injury to the already damaged brain. ICP monitoring may be indicated, especially for patients with marked depression or deterioration in neurologic function. Comatose patients who require emergency surgical treatment (abdominal, thoracic, orthopedic) also are monitored. Medical management consists of:

Table 104-1. GLASGOW COMA SCALE*

Parameter	Score
EYE OPENING	
Spontaneously	4
To voice stimulus	3
To pain	2
No eye opening	1
MOTOR RESPONSE	
Follows commands	6
Localizes a pain stimulus	5
Withdraws from pain	4
Flexor posturing to pain	3
Extensor posturing to pain	2
No response to pain	1
VERBAL RESPONSE	
Oriented	5
Confused	4
Inappropriate words	3
Incomprehensible sounds	2
No sounds	1

* The Glasgow Coma Scale assigns a numeric value to the responses in each of three categories with the score equal to the sum of the three responses.

- Head elevation
- Sedation
- Moderate hyperventilation
- Prophylactic use of anticonvulsants
- Mild dehydration with judicious sodium replacement
- Prompt management of SIADH (syndrome of inappropriate antidiuretic hormone secretion)
- Management of hyperthermia

If ICP remains elevated despite these measures, mannitol and furosemide are used to reduce cerebral edema. Deep sedation with narcotics and use of paralyzing agents such as pancuronium or atracurium can be helpful.

Epidural Hematoma

Any patient with a history of a blow to the head followed by unconsciousness undergoes CT. If an epidural hematoma (Fig. 104-1) is found, emergency craniotomy is indicated. If the CT scan is normal, the patient can be discharged. A reliable person is instructed to awaken the patient frequently during the next 24 hours to be certain the patient remains arousable.

Subdural Hematoma

Acute subdural hematomas are associated with severe head injury and originate from a combination of torn bridging veins, disruption of cortical arteries, and laceration of the cortex. The hematoma is imaged with CT (Fig. 104-2). *Subacute* subdural hematomas become apparent several days after injury and are associated with progressive lethargy, confusion, hemiparesis, or other hemispheric deficits. Removal of the hematoma usually produces striking improvement. *Chronic* subdural hematomas originate from tears in bridging veins, often after a minor head injury. These lesions are more common among infants and the elderly. Symptoms include progressive mental status changes with or without hemiparesis or aphasia. Treatment consists of burr hole drainage. Craniotomy may be necessary if the fluid reaccumulates.

Spinal Cord Injury

Traumatic injury to the spinal cord can result from vertebral fracture, fracture or subluxation, hyperextension of the cervical spine in the presence of a narrow spinal canal,

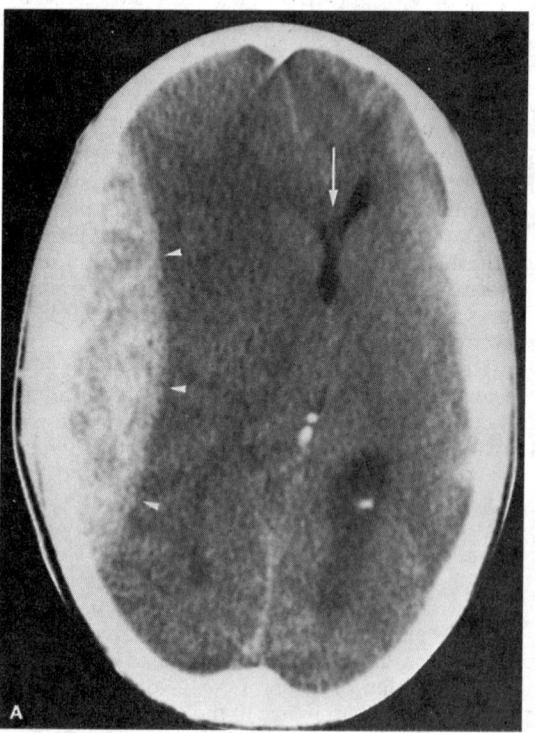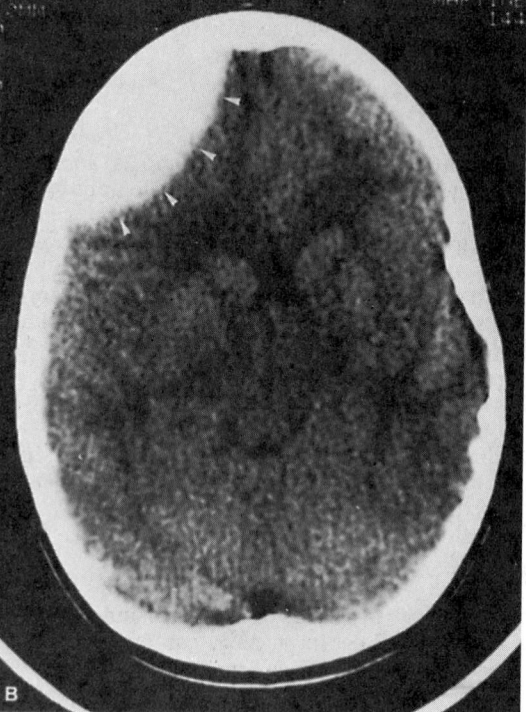

Figure 104-1. Two examples of acute epidural hematoma imaged by noncontrast CT. The increased attenuation of the lenticular-shaped mass (*arrowheads*) indicates that it is an acute lesion within the epidural space. There is a marked midline shift in *A* (*arrow*) compared with *B*. The patient in *A* was comatose and had little brain-stem function on examination. The patient in *B* was awake and conversant.

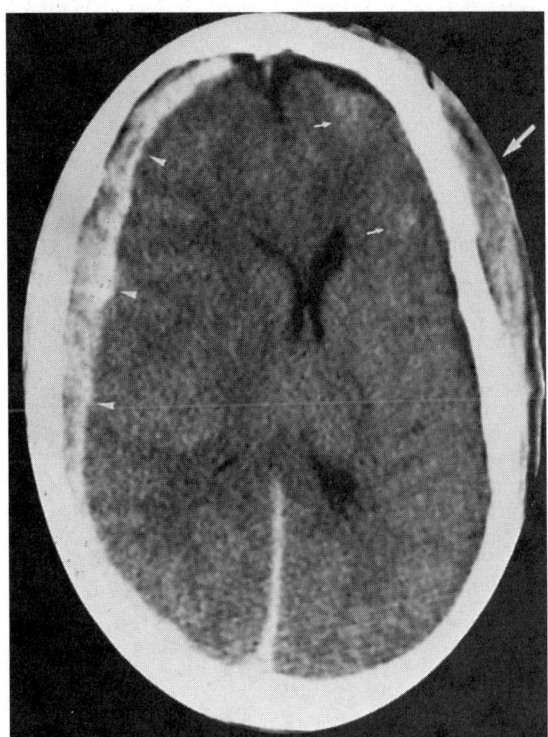

Figure 104-2. Acute subdural hematoma imaged by noncontrast CT. The high-attenuation, crescent-shaped lesion (*arrowheads*) indicates acute hemorrhage within the subdural space. Scalp swelling is visible on the contralateral side (*large arrow*), suggesting that the hematoma is due to a contrecoup injury. There are small hemorrhagic contusions in the contralateral frontal lobe as well (*small arrows*). These often accompany subdural hematomas in head trauma and signify severe injury. Midline shift is apparent.

herniation of intervertebral disc material into the canal, and penetrating injuries such as gunshots or stabbings. Neurologic involvement ranges from mild and transient to severe and permanent. Clinical findings include spinal tenderness, extremity weakness, numbness or paresthesia, respiratory embarrassment, and hypotension.

Complete lesions (total loss of function below the level of injury) are transections of the cord. Acute transections are characterized by arreflexia, flaccidity, anesthesia, and autonomic paralysis below the level of the lesion. Incomplete lesions are summarized in Fig. 104-3.

In addition to neurologic deficit, acute spinal cord injury is accompanied by many systemic responses:

- Cessation of respiratory efforts (damage above C-3)
- Insufficient tidal volumes (injury involving C-4 to C-6) that cause progressive hypoxia and carbon dioxide retention, which lead to airway obstruction, atelectasis, and pneumonia
- Ileus with gastric distention
- Bladder distention
- Hypotension (cord injury above T-5)
- Tachycardia in response to hypotension
- Bradycardia when the cervical cord is damaged and sympathetic input to the heart is lost

Once the patient's condition is hemodynamically stable, spinal radiographs are essential, but only while the patient remains immobilized on a backboard with a hard cervical collar firmly secured. If no abnormality is found despite a neurologic deficit that localizes the spinal cord level, MRI or myelography followed by CT is performed to look for

traumatic intervertebral disc rupture or spinal epidural hematoma.

The goals of treatment are to:

- Correct spinal alignment
- Protect undamaged neural tissue
- Restore function to reversibly damaged neural tissue
- Achieve permanent spinal stability

Reduction and immobilization of any fracture or dislocation must receive top priority to meet these objectives. Routine administration of systemic corticosteroids (dexamethasone) is helpful in spinal cord injury.

Indications for early *operation* for spinal cord injury are:

- Inability to reduce the fracture or dislocation with closed methods
- Neurologic deterioration in a patient with an initially incomplete cord lesion
- Severe compression of the spinal cord by an intraspinal mass visualized at myelography or MRI
- Penetrating injury with or without CSF leak

Open wounds, such as stab and gunshot wounds, are débrided and closed whether the cord injury is complete or incomplete. Early operation to stabilize the spine is warranted.

Peripheral Nerve Injury

Neuropraxia is temporary loss of function without axonal injury; structural damage does not occur (eg, a foot goes to sleep after crossing the legs). *Axonotmesis* is disruption of the axon with preservation of the axon sheath. Regeneration of the proximal axon occurs, but functional recovery depends on the amount of healthy proximal axon remaining after injury. *Neurotmesis* is disruption of both the axon and axon sheath with corresponding loss of function and is caused by transection of a nerve. Regeneration occurs, but function rarely returns to normal.

Sensory and motor changes correspond to the peripheral nerve involved. History and neurologic examination localize the site of injury. Radiographs of the injury site help find fractures or foreign bodies. Treatment of a lacerated nerve consists of primary repair when the wound is clean and uncomplicated, as in stab wounds, lacerations from glass, and surgical incisions. Secondary or delayed repair is indicated when the wound is dirty or complicated.

NEOPLASMS

Intracranial Tumors

Intracranial tumors exert both local and generalized effects by their presence within a closed bony structure. They originate from within or on the surface of a noncompliant brain. The local influence of a tumor consists of irritative or destructive effects. *Focal seizures* occur because of irritation of adjacent cortex. A *focal neurologic deficit* develops because of compressive forces on nearby functional brain. More generalized effects are raised ICP due to the presence of the abnormal mass. This may be obstructive hydrocephalus, tumor hemorrhage, or cerebral edema, or it may simply be the result of the added volume imparted by the tumor in the closed bony compartment of the skull. The effects can be manifested as headache, occasional nausea and vomiting, decreased level of consciousness, and slowed cognitive function. Table 104-2 shows the classification of intracranial tumors.

About one fourth of intracranial tumors are metastases. Malignant cells invade the CNS hematogenously and tend to lodge at the junction between the gray and white matter.

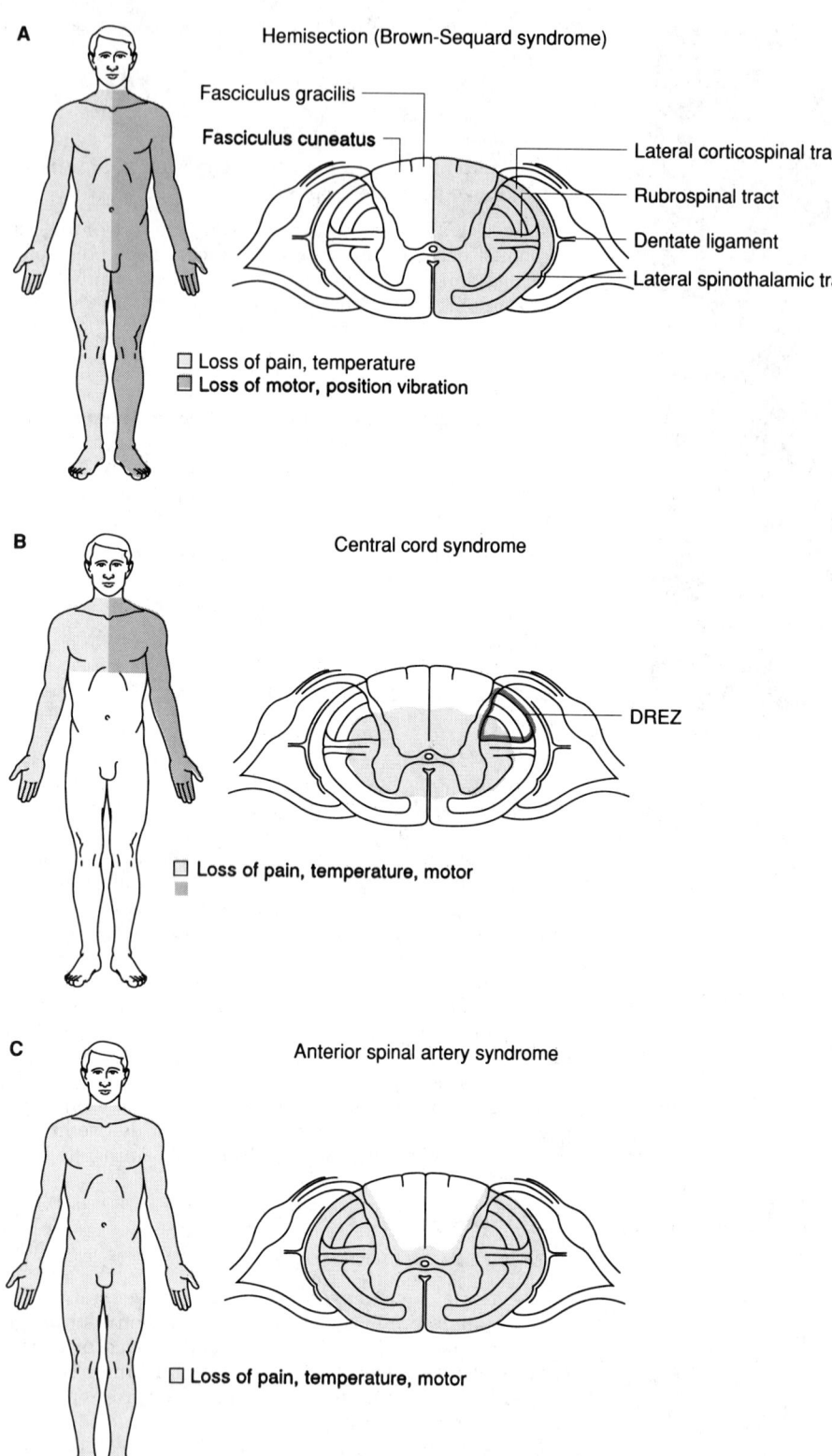

A Hemisection (Brown-Sequard syndrome)

Fasciculus gracilis

Fasciculus cuneatus

Lateral corticospinal tract

Rubrospinal tract

Dentate ligament

Lateral spinothalamic tract

☐ Loss of pain, temperature
▨ Loss of motor, position vibration

B Central cord syndrome

DREZ

☐ Loss of pain, temperature, motor
▨

C Anterior spinal artery syndrome

☐ Loss of pain, temperature, motor

Figure 104-3. Schematic cross sections of the spinal cord, showing hemisection (*A*), central cord syndrome lesion (*B*), and anterior spinal artery syndrome lesion (*C*). The figure diagrams demonstrate the neurologic deficits. DREZ, dorsal route entry zone.

Metastatic tumors occur singly or multiply and can involve almost any portion of the brain or, less commonly, the spinal cord. Although any neoplasm can metastasize, the most common primary sites are the lung, breast, kidney, testis, colon, and skin. Symptoms are related to site of metastasis. The symptoms include headache, mental status changes, seizures, and hemiparesis.

Metastatic lesions are imaged with CT but can mimic other lesions such as meningioma, abscesses, primary brain tumors, and aneurysms. MRI helps narrow the differential diagnosis. If metastasis is suspected, an extensive evaluation is conducted to find the primary source. If the primary site is not identified, an excisional biopsy is indicated.

Table 104-2. WORLD HEALTH ORGANIZATION BRAIN TUMOR CLASSIFICATION (ABRIDGED)

TUMORS OF NEUROEPITHELIAL TISSUE

Astrocytic tumor
  Astrocytoma
  Pilocytic astrocytoma
  Subependymal giant cell astrocytoma
  Astroblastoma
Oligodendroglial tumor
  Oligodendroglioma
  Mixed oligoastrocytoma
Ependymal and choroid plexus tumor
  Ependymoma
    Myxopapillary ependymoma
    Subependymoma
  Choroid plexus papilloma
Pineal cell tumor
  Pineocytoma
  Pineoblastoma
Neuronal tumor
  Gangliocytoma
  Ganglioglioma
  Ganglioneuroblastoma
  Neuroblastoma
Poorly differentiated and embryonic tumor
  Glioblastoma
  Medulloblastoma
  Gliomatosis cerebri

NERVE SHEATH TUMORS

Neurilemmoma
Neurofibroma

TUMORS OF MENINGEAL AND RELATED TISSUES

Meningioma
Meningeal sarcoma
Xanthomatous tumor

PRIMARY LYMPHOMA AND BLOOD VESSEL TUMORS

Hemangioblastoma

GERM CELL TUMORS

Germinoma
Embryonal cell carcinoma
Teratoma

OTHER TUMORS AND TUMOR-LIKE LESIONS

Craniopharyngioma
Rathke cleft cyst
Epidermoid
Dermoid
Colloid cyst
Lipoma
Choristoma
Vascular malformations
  Capillary telangiectasia
  Cavernous hemangioma
  Arteriovenous malformation
  Venous malformation

TUMORS OF THE ANTERIOR PITUITARY

Pituitary adenoma
Pituitary adenocarcinoma

LOCAL EXTENSION FROM REGIONAL TUMORS

Glomus jugulare tumor
Chordoma
Chondroma
Chondrosarcoma
Adenoid cystic carcinoma

METASTATIC TUMORS

UNCLASSIFIED TUMORS

A symptomatic, solitary lesion that is surgically accessible is removed. Surgical therapy is not undertaken for multiple lesions or patients who have severe primary disease. Treatment also includes preoperative dexamethasone, as for any brain or spinal cord tumor, to reduce adjacent brain edema. Whole-brain irradiation is almost always indicated. Stereotactic radiosurgery may be helpful.

Tumor metastasis to the leptomeninges (meningeal carcinomatosis) is common, particularly in childhood leukemias and in adults with lymphoma, breast and lung cancer, and melanoma. Analysis of the CSF is usually critical, often revealing an increased opening pressure, elevated white cell count and protein levels, and decreased glucose. There may or may not be identifiable malignant cells, but cytologic examination is always performed. Treatment of meningeal carcinomatosis is radiation therapy and intraventricular chemotherapy.

Spinal Tumors

Spinal tumors are classified as intradural or extradural. Intradural tumors are almost always primary CNS tumors. Most extradural tumors are metastatic or primary bone tumors of the spine. Most intradural spinal neoplasms are benign and can often be totally excised.

The definitive study for spinal tumors is MRI, although abnormal plain radiographs and myelograms can be diagnostic. Plain radiographs may show widening of the interpeduncular distance, bony erosion, enlargement of the neural foramina, or a paraspinous mass. Myelography helps determine the relation between the tumor and the spinal cord and dura. Postmyelogram CT can further define that relation.

The following are the most common spinal cord tumors:

Neurilemmoma and neurofibroma
Meningioma
Ependymoma
Astrocytoma
Hemangioblastoma
Lipoma
Dermoids
Metastatic Tumor

About one fourth of spinal neoplasms are metastatic in origin, and most appear in an extradural location. Common primary sites include breast, lung, prostate, and kidney. Treatment is surgical decompression with biopsy if the primary site is not known or if the neurologic decline is rapid. Otherwise, local radiation therapy is given. Other extradural malignant tumors include lymphoma, myeloma, plasmacytoma, chordoma, and osteogenic sarcoma. When bone destruction or surgical decompression renders the spine unstable, surgical stabilization is necessary.

Peripheral Nerve Tumors

The peripheral nervous system includes the peripheral and cranial nerves, spinal roots, and autonomic nervous system. Tumors can originate from any of these elements. Common tumors are schwannoma, neurofibroma, and malignant nerve sheath tumor. Unusual tumors include gan-

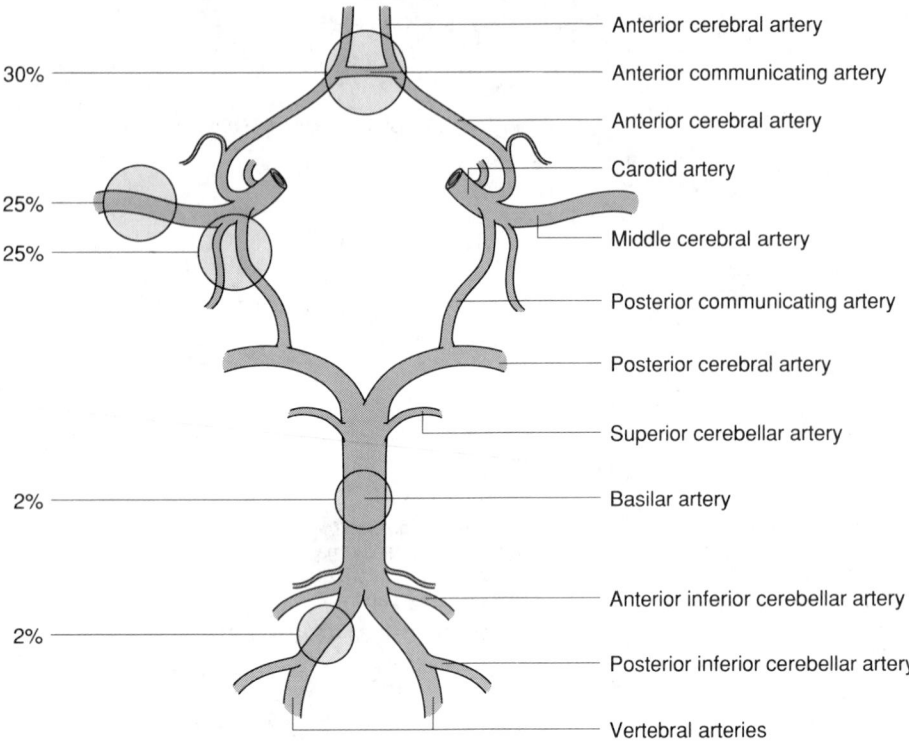

30%

25%
25%

2%

2%

Anterior cerebral artery
Anterior communicating artery
Anterior cerebral artery
Carotid artery
Middle cerebral artery
Posterior communicating artery
Posterior cerebral artery
Superior cerebellar artery
Basilar artery
Anterior inferior cerebellar artery
Posterior inferior cerebellar artery
Vertebral arteries

Figure 104-4. Locations of aneurysms of the circle of Willis and their relative occurrence.

gliogliomas, neuroblastomas, paragangliomas, chemodectomas, and pheochromocytomas.

CEREBROVASCULAR DISEASE
Ischemic Vascular Disease (Stroke)

Ischemia can be the result of (1) diminished flow due to stenosis or occlusion of major arteries, or (2) transient or permanent occlusion of small arterioles by intravascular emboli. The most common cause of stenosis or occlusion of large vessels is atherosclerosis. Arterial emboli usually originate from atherosclerotic ulceration in the region of the carotid bifurcation or from sources within the heart.

There is no effective medical or surgical therapy for a completed stroke. The goal of surgical intervention is to identify stroke-prone patients and reduce their risk for cerebral ischemia. These patients often have a history of transient ischemic attacks (TIAs).

Carotid endarterectomy is indicated when ipsilateral symptoms of cerebral ischemia or amaurosis fugax exist and angiography shows severe stenosis (>75%) or ulceration in the accessible portions of the common and proximal internal carotid arteries. The procedure consists of opening the affected portion of the carotid artery under systemic heparinization and removing the atherosclerotic plaque.

Intracranial Aneurysms

Intracranial aneurysms are diseased dilatations of the cerebral arteries. Their walls consist of ballooned-out intima, media, and adventitia with a variable degree of intraluminal or mural thrombus. Most are congenital and evolve and develop throughout life. They can become atherosclerotic. Aneurysms are found at the bifurcations of the main vessels of the circle of Willis (Fig. 104-4). Many patients with aneurysms have multiple aneurysms, and a few have an arteriovenous malformation (AVM).

Patients with intracranial aneurysms most commonly present with signs and symptoms of subarachnoid hemorrhage (SAH). The grading of severity of SAH is shown in Table 104-3. The diagnosis of SAH is made clinically and confirmed when CT scans show blood in the subarachnoid spaces or lumbar puncture reveals bloody CSF with xanthochromia.

Therapy for aneurysms is microsurgical dissection and obliteration, usually by placement of a metallic clip on the neck of the aneurysm by means of craniotomy.

The most serious and least understood complication of aneurysmal rupture is cerebral vasospasm. This occurs within 4 to 7 days of hemorrhage and results in narrowing of adjacent cerebral arteries. Because there is no effective way to reverse vasospasm, and calcium-channel blockers may not prevent its development, treatment is to increase

Table 104-3. GRADING OF SEVERITY OF SUBARACHNOID HEMORRHAGE

Grade	Severity
I	No symptoms or minimal headache
	Slight nuchal rigidity
II	Moderate to severe headache
	Nuchal rigidity
	No neurologic deficit other than a cranial nerve palsy
III	Lethargy
	Confusion
	Mild focal neurologic deficit
IV	Stupor
	Moderate to severe hemiparesis
	Possible early decerebrate posturing
	Vegetative disturbances
V	Deep coma
	Decerebrate posturing
	Moribund appearance

cerebral blood flow to overcome the spasm. This is accomplished by increasing systemic blood pressure, often by means of inotropic support and intravascular volume expansion, usually with colloid and red cell transfusion.

Arteriovenous Malformations

Arteriovenous malformations occur in the CNS as congenital abnormalities in which blood is directly shunted from arteries to veins. AVMs can be detected with contrast-enhanced CT. Configuration and extent are delineated with MRI. Lumbar puncture may be necessary if SAH is suspected clinically but not verified with CT. For all AVMs, complete cerebral angiography must be undertaken to define the extent of the malformation.

Management of AVM depends on the size and location of the lesion, the presenting symptom, and the age and condition of the patient. An AVM that has bled is surgically excised if possible. If the patient has seizures, the treatment decision is more difficult. If the patient is young and the malformation is readily accessible, surgical resection is performed, especially when the seizures are refractory to medical treatment. The operation involves microsurgical dissection and resection of the entire malformation, not simple ligation of feeding arteries.

Brain Hemorrhage

Spontaneous hemorrhage is associated with systemic hypertension. Although brain hemorrhage is often devastating, it can be surprisingly well-tolerated. CT delineates the hemorrhage, allows assessment of ventricular size and presence of edema, and often suggests the cause of the hemorrhage (eg, AVM, tumor, aneurysm).

Management of brain hemorrhage can be medical or surgical depending on the size of the lesion, its location, and the condition of the patient. Surgical resection is performed if a hematoma is >3 cm in diameter or if the patient's condition is deteriorating neurologically, no matter what the size of the hematoma. Cerebellar hematomas are removed. Medical management is directed at keeping ICP under control.

DEGENERATIVE DISEASE OF THE SPINE

If the nucleus of an intervertebral disc extrudes (herniates) through the annulus, adjacent neural structures may be compressed. In the cervical and thoracic spine, compression of the spinal cord can result in paraparesis or quadriparesis. At all levels, compression of a spinal root can cause weakness and sensory loss in structures innervated by the root. The severity of the clinical syndrome depends on the site and severity of compression by the displaced disc fragment. Sometimes the annulus and adjacent ligament hold, preventing complete extrusion of the fragmented disc. The annulus stretches only enough to allow the disc to bulge into the spinal canal or foramina.

Often the nucleus does not extrude but simply fragments in response to the forces exerted on the spinal column. This is intensified by concomitant dehydration of the disc with loss of elasticity as it ages. The disc space gradually narrows, the joint becomes loose, and the cartilaginous end plates of the adjacent vertebral bodies abut and wear more quickly. Bony spurs (osteophytes) develop at the joint in reaction to the increased mobility and decreased elasticity.

Formation of osteophytes around the joints of vertebrae is *spondylosis,* a common disorder that may be a normal process of aging. If an osteophyte forms in a neural foramen, the nerve root passing through can be chronically irritated and compressed. If the osteophyte develops within the cervical or lumbar canal, the cord or cauda equina can be compromised. Thoracic spine osteophytes causing neurologic dysfunction are rare.

Management of degenerative disease of the spine is summarized in Table 104-4.

INFECTION

The CNS can be infected by viruses, bacteria, and fungi and infested by parasites. Types of infection and infestation treatment are summarized in Table 104-5.

CONGENITAL AND DEVELOPMENTAL ABNORMALITIES

The common neurologic congenital malformations are:

- Arnold–Chiari malformation
- Dandy–Walker malformation
- Spinal dysraphism (spina bifida)
  Meningocele
  Myelomeningocele
  Lipomyelomeningocele
  Diastematomyelia
  Dermal sinus
  Myeloschisis

Dysraphism

Therapy for *spinal dysraphism* is surgical. Meningoceles are excised, and the skin is closed primarily after watertight closure of the posterior meningeal defect. Myelomeningoceles and myeloschises are closed as soon as possible to reduce risk for superficial infection and meningitis. Surgical repair is undertaken within 36 hours. The goal is to preserve as much neural tissue as possible, untether the spinal cord from surrounding soft tissue, and close the dura to prevent CSF leakage. Surgical repair of *cranial dysraphism* involves early resection of malformed and devitalized brain with dural closure.

Hydrocephalus

Hydrocephalus is an increase in the amount of CSF within the ventricular system. It is almost always due to a decrease in the absorption of fluid. In *communicating* hydrocephalus, the ventricular system continues to com-

Table 104-4. MANAGEMENT OF DEGENERATIVE DISEASE OF THE SPINE

Location	Medical Therapy	Surgical Therapy
Cervical	Immobilization of the neck with soft or hard cervical collar	Anterior: discectomy with or without bone graft fusion
	Analgesics	Posterior: laminectomy or foraminotomy, or both
	Muscle relaxants	
	Local heat	
	Physical therapy	
Thoracic Lumbar	None	Removal of disc fragment
	Bed rest	Partial laminectomy and removal of disc fragment
	Local heat	
	Analgesics	Foraminectomy if there is osteophyte formation
	Skeletal muscle relaxants	
	Physical therapy	

Table 104-5. **TYPES OF CNS INFECTION AND TREATMENT**

Type of Infection	Treatment
Bacterial Infections	
Subgaleal abscess	Open drainage
	Débridement
	Systemic antibiotics
Osteomyelitis	Drainage
	Débridement of infected bone
	Antibiotics for a prolonged period (6 wk)
Epidural abscess	Broad antibiotic coverage until the offending agent is identified
	Specific antibiotic therapy for a prolonged period (up to 6 wk)
	Surgical drainage when neurologic deficits progress despite aggressive medical therapy
Intracranial subdural empyema	Craniotomy with débridement, drainage, and IV antibiotics
Spinal subdural empyema	Emergency surgical drainage and prolonged antibiotic administration
Meningitis	Broad-spectrum IV antibiotics immediately
	Single-agent antibiotic therapy once culture results are known
Brain abscess	Drainage of the purulent material with simultaneous IV administration of antibiotics
	Craniotomy with evacuation and removal of abscess wall if necessary
Postoperative infection	Antibiotics, removal of artificial material
Fungal Infections	Long-term, systemic antifungal chemotherapy
	Surgical intervention for drainage of abscesses and resection of symptomatic mass lesions
	Ventricular shunt for hydrocephalus
Parasitic Infections	Prevention
Cysticercosis (*Taenia solium*, pork tapeworm)	
Echinococcosis (hydatid disease, *Echinococcus granulosus*, dog tapeworm)	

municate with the subarachnoid spaces outside the brain through the fourth ventricular foramina of Luschka and Magendie. In *noncommunicating* (obstructive) hydrocephalus it does not. The causes of hydrocephalus are listed in Table 104-6. Regardless of cause, the treatment of hydrocephalus is the same—removal of the cause (eg, tumor) or a shunting procedure to divert accumulated CSF.

Craniosynostosis

Craniosynostosis is premature closure of one or more cranial sutures; it becomes apparent in the first 6 months of life. When one suture fuses prematurely, the brain is not compressed to a deleterious degree, but the skull develops in an abnormal shape. If more sutures are fused, the brain can be damaged because of restricted growth. Therapy for craniosynostosis is surgical opening of the entire length of the affected suture. This is done as soon as possible after diagnosis. For multiple suture involvement,

Table 104-6. **CAUSES OF HYDROCEPHALUS**

Congenital
  Arnold–Chiari malformation
  Dandy–Walker malformation
  Aqueductal atresia or stenosis
  Developmental cyst
  Encephalocele
  Neoplasm
Acquired
  Infectious meningitis
  Infectious ventriculitis
  Late-onset aqueductal stenosis
  Intraventricular hemorrhage
  Subarachnoid hemorrhage
  Neoplasm

prompt treatment allows early skull expansion to accommodate brain growth.

NEUROSURGICAL MANAGEMENT OF PAIN

Most neurosurgical patients have pain as their primary symptom or as a secondary manifestation of disease. Pain can be categorized as an *acute* process, such as arm pain from a herniated cervical disc, or a *chronic* process, such as extremity pain from an invasive neoplasm. For most acute pain states, the cause can be identified and treated, but for chronic pain there is often no ready solution.

Cerebrum

Few painful states warrant procedures involving the cerebral hemispheres or deep brain nuclei.

Cranial Nerves

Trigeminal neuralgia (tic douloureux) is a common neuropathic painful condition. It presents as intermittent, shocklike pain in one or more divisions of one trigeminal nerve. It involves the second (maxillary) or third (mandibular) divisions of the nerve, or both, and rarely is bilateral. The pain usually lasts for seconds, is severe, and can be incapacitating. It is often triggered by touching the face, talking, or chewing. The pain can be present for weeks or months and then spontaneously disappear, only to return with increased severity. Most patients can be treated with phenytoin or carbamazepine, but eventually many need surgical treatment. Some patients have a posterior fossa tumor as the cause of the pain, so evaluation includes CT or MRI.

Surgical therapy is retrogasserian rhizotomy by an open surgical approach subtemporally or through the posterior

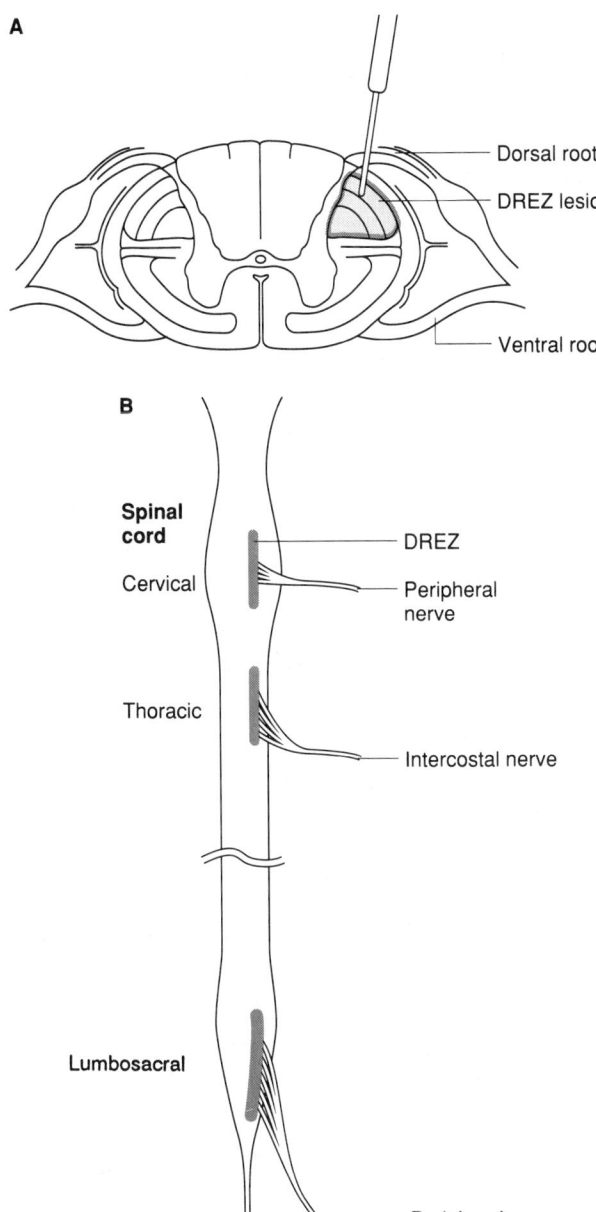

A

Dorsal root

DREZ lesion

Ventral root

B

Spinal cord

Cervical

DREZ

Peripheral nerve

Thoracic

Intercostal nerve

Lumbosacral

Peripheral nerve

Figure 104-5. Location of dorsal root entry zone for placement of dorsal root entry zone (DREZ) lesion.

fossa or a percutaneous approach by means of a radiofrequency electrode through the foramen ovale.

Brain Stem

Trigeminal tractotomy is used to manage unrelenting head and neck pain due to invasive malignant tumors.

Spinal Cord

Operations for chronic pain that involve the spinal cord are:

- Cordotomy-obliterates the spinothalamic tract
- Ablative lesions at the dorsal root entry zones (DREZ) of the spinal cord (Fig. 104-5)
- Dorsal rhizotomy-open through a laminectomy or percutaneous by means of radiofrequency thermocoagulation
- Dorsal root ganglionectomy
- Intrathecal administration of morphine
- Nonablative neuromodulation-transcutaneous stimulation that blocks nerve conduction of pain impulses

Peripheral Nerve

Pain from partial or complete nerve injury usually involves the sensory distribution of the nerve but can include an entire extremity. With partial or complete peripheral nerve transection, a painful *neuroma* can form. Treatment is excision of the neuroma, with prevention of recurrent formation by burying the nerve end in bone or muscle or by wrapping it in prosthetic material. Neuromodulation techniques also can be used.

A patient who has undergone an amputation may have chronic pain in the remaining portion of the limb at the site of the amputation (*stump pain*) or in the nonexistent amputated portion (*phantom pain*). Therapy for stump pain involves resection of neuromas, regional sympathectomy, cordotomy, and neuromodulation. Management of phantom pain includes the treatments for stump pain. DREZ lesions also may bring relief.

Major causalgia is related to partial injury of the sciatic or median nerves. Symptoms begin in the distribution of the affected nerve but can progress to involve the entire extremity. The extremity becomes swollen, warm, erythematous, and sensitive to touch. With time, it becomes cool and pale. Constant, burning pain develops and persists; the limb can become useless. Treatment is disruption of the sympathetic nerve supply to the extremity. This can be accomplished temporarily by means of chemical sympathectomy with local anesthetic or permanently by means of surgical sympathectomy.

Less severe and more easily managed pain originates from chronic compression of selected peripheral nerves. The most common conditions are carpal tunnel syndrome and compression of the ulnar nerve at the elbow. Treatment is surgical decompression of the involved nerve.

SUGGESTED READING

Apuzzo MLJ. Brain injury: complications, avoidance and management. New York, Churchill Livingstone, 1993.

Crockard A, Hayward R, Hoff JT, eds. Neurosurgery: the scientific basis of clinical practice, ed 2. Boston, Blackwell Scientific, 1992.

Errico TJ, Bauer RD, Waugh T, eds. Spinal trauma. Philadelphia, JB Lippincott, 1991.

McLaurin RL, Venes JL, Schut L, Epstein F, eds. Pediatric neurosurgery: surgery of the developing nervous system, ed 2. Philadelphia, WB Saunders, 1989.

Ojemann RG, Heros RC, Crowell RM, eds. Surgical management of cerebrovascular disease, ed 2. Baltimore, Williams & Wilkins, 1988.

Russell DS, Rubinstein LJ. Pathology of tumors of the nervous system, ed 5. Baltimore, Williams & Wilkins, 1989.

Youmans JR, ed. Neurological surgery: a comprehensive reference guide to the diagnosis and management of neurosurgical problems, ed 3. Philadelphia, WB Saunders, 1990.

ESSENTIALS OF SURGERY: SCIENTIFIC PRINCIPLES AND PRACTICE,
edited by Lazar J. Greenfield, Michael W. Mulholland, Keith T. Oldham, Gerald B. Zelenock,
and Keith D. Lillemoe. Lippincott–Raven Publishers, Philadelphia, © 1997.

CHAPTER 105

MALE ANATOMY AND PHYSIOLOGY

H. BARTON GROSSMAN, WILLIAM D. BELVILLE,
GARY J. FAERBER, JOHN W. KONNAK, AND DANA A. OHL

BLADDER AND URETHRA

The bladder is a composite of complex muscular fascicles that relax to accommodate urine and contract to expel it. At the base of the bladder is the trigone, composed of specialized smooth muscle, where the ureters terminate. Most of the urinary tract lining is transitional epithelium.

The two basic functions of the bladder are to store and empty urine, normally at low pressure. If the bladder loses its low-pressure storage ability, the ureters may be adversely affected in the delivery of their peristaltic load. If high pressure is sustained, ureteral dysfunction develops.

Bladder and sphincter control is the result of complex interaction between the central and peripheral nervous systems. During normal filling, the bladder relaxes and the smooth muscle sphincters contract. During normal bladder contraction during voiding, both striated and smooth muscle sphincter activity cease. The initial event that triggers a normal voiding cycle is relaxation of the striated (voluntary) sphincter.

Obstructive Uropathy

Anatomic

When the bladder outlet is obstructed, usually by benign prostatic hyertrophy (BPH), bladder pressure increases and flow rate decreases. Over time, obstruction adversely affects bladder storage function and ability to empty completely. Progressively high bladder pressure may be asymptomatic (silent prostatism). If sustained, high pressure may induce failure of ureteral emptying and transmit high pressure to the kidney. The result is compromised renal function, which may occur without noticeable reduction in urine output. Management is simple prostatectomy or intermittent catheterization. Laser, microwave, cryotherapy and radiowave treatments are under investigation.

Neurogenic

Neurogenic obstructive uropathy begins as failure to empty because the bladder is areflexic or is contracting against a (dyssynergic) contracting sphincter. In neurologic injury, the balance between pelvic peripheral nerves and the central nervous system is lost. If the patient is not treated, this functional obstruction leads to progressive loss of bladder compliance and problems include reflux, stasis, stones, infection, and renal failure. If the patient is treated with intermittent catheterization, sphincterotomy, vesicostomy, or suprapubic or Foley catheterization, these sequelae can be prevented in the short term. Long-term tube management, however, is associated with severe complications.

Urinary Incontinence

Urinary incontinence, excluding rare congenital anomalies and fistulas, is due to bladder or urethral dysfunction, alone or in combination. The bladder may be the primary source of incontinence because of hyperreflexia or inadequate storage ability that is volitional or idiopathic. Detrusor instability (hyperreflexia) may occur early in prostatic obstruction or result from an underlying, often subclinical neurologic cause. A regimen of anticholinergic medication (imipramine or oxybutynin) and a regular voiding schedule often achieves continence.

IMPOTENCE

Pathogenesis

Impotence is caused by interference with the normal vascular, neurologic, psychologic, endothelial, and hormonal mechanisms of erection. Causes of impotence include:

Diabetic neuropathy and vascular disease
Renal failure
Cirrhosis of the liver
Drugs (alcohol, cimetidine, atenolol, clonidine, diazepam)
Arteriosclerotic disease
Failure of the venous occlusive mechanism
Trauma
Neurologic disease (multiple sclerosis)
Spinal cord injury
Radical pelvic operations (radical prostatectomy)

Diagnosis

History

A sexual history is important. Impotence that is intermittent or of sudden onset may be psychogenic. This is especially true if the patient has normal morning erections or adequate erections with masturbation. Organic impotence is usually gradual in onset and progression; the patient is often unable to achieve a normal erection under any circumstance. A history of diabetes, hypertension, arteriosclerotic disease, or neurologic problems may suggest the cause. A list of medications is obtained, and drug and alcohol use determined.

Physical Examination

Physical examination for impotence includes evaluation of body habitus and detailed examination of the genitalia. A neurologic examination is performed, and peripheral pulses are evaluated.

Laboratory Tests

Initial laboratory studies include serum levels of testosterone, prolactin, and serum lipids and a screening test for diabetes. Depending on the results of the initial evaluation, the following studies may be indicated.

Nocturnal Penile Tumescence Testing

Men with psychogenic impotence often have a normal pattern of nocturnal erections during the rapid eye movement stage of sleep. Those with organic impotence have an abnormal or absent response. A simple screening test uses a snap gauge consisting of a cuff connected to bands that break if the penis expands. This can indicate whether nocturnal erections occur but does not give the pattern or duration of erection. Formal tumescence testing may be performed in a sleep laboratory or with a portable testing device. Devices produce a graph of frequency, duration, and quality of erection.

Vascular Testing

Penile blood flow can be estimated with Doppler determination of penile systolic blood pressure by use of a penile cuff or plethysmography. A normal study does not rule out vasculogenic impotence, but consistently low values can suggest this as a cause. The penis is flaccid during vascular testing, so the results do not reflect the increase in blood flow needed to cause an erection. Direct corporal injection with papaverine, a smooth muscle relaxant, or PGE_1 bypasses psychogenic and neurologic factors and produces an erection if the blood flow to the penis is normal. A poor or absent response can indicate vasculogenic impotence due to arterial insufficiency or venous leak.

A quantitative increase in the diameter of the central arteries can be documented with duplex ultrasonography (US). If arterial disease is suspected, superselective pelvic arteriography with injection of vasoactive agents is necessary to document the extent and nature of the disease. Venous leak may manifest increased diastolic flow at duplex US. If a venous leak is suspected, cavernosometry and cavernosography are performed.

Hormonal Studies

Low serum testosterone may indicate hypogonadism. Elevated prolactin can indicate a pituitary neoplasm, and appropriate cerebral studies are conducted.

Management

Nonsurgical Therapy

Most psychogenic and mild organic impotence responds to nonspecific measures, such as use of yohimbine, reassurance, and sexual counseling.

Intracorporal papaverine or PGE_1 injection can be used as primary therapy or to reassure the patient that the erectile mechanism is normal. Patients with neurogenic impotence often have dramatic results with papaverine injection. Patients with mild vasculogenic impotence, diabetes, or nonspecific impotence also can undergo injection therapy. Side effects of papaverine injection include priapism, fibrous plaques at the injection site, and liver toxicity.

About half of all patients with decreased serum testosterone levels respond to intramuscular or transdermal testosterone. Oral testosterone is not used because of liver toxicity and unpredictable serum levels.

Vacuum devices consist of a cylinder that fits around the penis and seals at the pubic skin. A pump is used to make a vacuum in the cylinder, which sucks blood into the penis, producing an erection. An elastic band is placed tightly around the base of the penis to maintain the erection. The vacuum is released and the cylinder removed. Complications include penile numbness and pain, failure of ejaculation, and petechiae.

Surgical Therapy

Penile implants can be used to treat any type of intractable impotence, but they are usually reserved for patients with diabetes or vascular or neurologic dysfunction who do not respond to conservative measures. Young patients with arteriogenic vascular impotence who have localized vascular lesions may undergo penile revascularization.

MALE-FACTOR INFERTILITY

Infertility is the inability of a couple to conceive within 1 year of unprotected intercourse.

Diagnosis

History

A complete medical history is taken. Special attention is directed at a history of fertility or infertility, current sexual practices, and understanding of the menstrual cycle and ovulation. Sometimes a cursory review of physiology and adjustment of intercourse timing are all that is needed to solve an infertility problem.

The patient is asked about congenital anomalies, systemic illness, operations (especially herniorrhaphy and bladder or scrotal procedures), and infections of or trauma to the genital and urinary tracts. Exposure to spermatogenic toxins is discerned. Common toxins are marijuana, anabolic steroids, chemotherapeutic agents, pesticides, and cleaning solvents.

The urologist treating the man interviews the woman to assess her fertility history and menstrual cycle and screen for ovulatory problems.

Physical Examination

A physical examination is performed with attention to the genital organs. Body habitus and secondary sex characteristics should be typical male type. The testes should be at least 4 cm long and moderately firm in consistency. Presence or absence of vas deferens can be determined with physical examination alone. The epididymis should be present and not indurated.

The patient is examined standing and during a Valsalva maneuver to find a varicocele. Varicoceles usually are present on the left but may be bilateral and should disappear

Table 105-1. NORMAL SEMEN PARAMETERS

Volume	2–5 mL
Sperm concentration	$>20 \times 10^6$/mL
Total sperm	$>60 \times 10^6$
Motility	>60%
Forward progression	>75%
Normal morphology	>60%
Fructose	Present
Agglutination	Absent
White blood cells	<5 WBCs/HPF

Table 105-2. CAUSES OF MALE-FACTOR INFERTILITY AND THEIR MANAGEMENT

Cause	Management
Complete testicular failure	None
Oligospermia	Clomiphene, intrauterine insemination, in vitro fertilization (IVF)
Oligoasthenospermia	
Varicocele	Occlusion of internal spermatic system with surgical or angiographic technique (laparoscopic ligation, microsurgical approaches)
Excurrent ductal obstruction	Microsurgical aspiration of epididymal sperm with IVF of partner oocytes
Acquired ductal obstruction	Microsurgical vasovasostomy and vasoepididymostomy to bypass vas deferens and epididymal obstructions
	Transurethral resection of ejaculatory duct orifice
Endocrine disorders	Administration of exogenous gonadotropins or pulsatile gonadotropin-releasing hormone infusion pump
Low testosterone levels	Exogenous testosterone by injection or testosterone patch
Antisperm antibodies	Corticosteroids
	Methods to decrease the numbers of sperm necessary to achieve pregnancy (insemination, in vitro fertilization)
Ejaculatory dysfunction	Reassurance, yohimbine, sexual counseling, papaverine injection
Psychogenic premature ejaculation, idiopathic primary anejaculation	
Retrograde ejaculation	Retrieval of sperm from the urine, sperm washing, artificial insemination
Complete neurogenic anejaculation	Rectal probe electrical stimulation of ejaculatory organs, artificial insemination
Cryptorchidism	Orchiopexy early in life
Chromosomal abnormalities	None

when the patient lies supine. Rectal examination is performed to assess the prostate and seminal vesicles.

Semen Analysis

A semen specimen is collected at least 2 days but no more than 5 days after the last ejaculation. Standards are based on minimal values consistent with fertility (Table 105-1). It is important to evaluate at least three semen specimens before instituting therapy. *Azoospermia* is the absence of sperm in the ejaculate. *Oligospermia* is a low sperm count. *Asthenospermia* is low motility in the sperm sample. *Teratospermia* is a high percentage of morphologically abnormal sperm.

Laboratory Tests. Other tests include:
Serum levels of FSH, LH, and testosterone
Biopsy and vasography
Direct immunobead test to detect antisperm antibodies
Sperm penetration assay
Postcoital test

Specific Disorders and Management

The causes of male-factor infertility and their management are summarized in Table 105-2.

URINARY LITHIASIS
Calculus Formation

The composition of kidney stones is summarized in Table 105-3. Several theories of stone formation exist:

Table 105-3. TYPES OF KIDNEY STONES

Stone Composition	Frequency (%)	Radiographic Appearance
Calcium oxalate ± calcium phosphate	75	Opaque
Pure calcium phosphate	7	Opaque
Magnesium ammonium phosphate (struvite)	12	Opaque
Uric acid	7	Lucent
Cystine	2	Opaque to radiolucent

Nucleation theory—stone formation is initiated by the presence of a crystal or foreign body, which in supersaturated urine promotes the growth of crystal lattice
Matrix theory—an organic matrix of urinary proteins acts as a nidus for crystal deposition
Inhibitor theory—substances in the urine prevent crystal formation, aggregation, or both. Inhibitors include pyrophosphate, citrate, magnesium, glycosaminoglycans, acidic glycopeptides, and small RNA fragments.

Diagnosis

Renal stones may or may not be painful. If present, pain is dull and localizes to the flank. Sometimes renal stones are associated with a urinary tract infection. *Ureteral* stones present precipitously with ureteral colic (severe flank pain radiating to the groin, nausea, vomiting). Ureteral stones in the intravesical ureter cause urgency and frequency.

Urinalysis shows gross or microscopic hematuria and sometimes pyuria, but some patients may have completely acellular urinalysis. Patients with abdominal pain undergo both abdominal *radiography* and urinalysis. Almost all urinary stones are radiopaque and identifiable with plain abdominal radiographs unless they are very small or over bony structures.

Management

Most stones *pass spontaneously* with the aid of increased hydration and analgesics. Calculi <4 mm wide are likely to pass spontaneously, stones >6 mm are not. Three areas in the urinary tract impede stone passage—the ureteropelvic junction, the site where the ureter crosses the iliac vessels, and the ureterovesical junction.

Conditions that lead to stone formation are listed in Table 105-4. In an evaluation for nephrolithiasis, it is important to ask about the presence of any of these conditions. All stones passed are retrieved for analysis. Patients passing their first stone have serum calcium and creatinine measured and urinalysis performed in addition to stone analysis.

If the stone is calcium oxalate and serum calcium level

Table 105-4. CONDITIONS LEADING TO URINARY LITHIASIS

INCREASED URINARY CALCIUM

Excess dietary calcium
Vitamin D toxicity
Resorptive hypercalciuria
    Prolonged immobilization
    Hyperparathyroidism
Absorptive hypercalciuria
Renal leak
Idiopathy

INCREASED SERUM CALCIUM

Hyperparathyroidism
Sarcoidosis
Vitamin D toxicity
Cushing syndrome
Milk-alkali syndrome
Thyrotoxicosis
Addison disease

INCREASED URINARY OXALATE

Excess dietary oxalate
Excess vitamin C
Gastrointestinal disorders
    Short-gut syndrome
    Gastric plication for obesity
    Small bowel resection
    Ulcerative colitis
    Regional enteritis

INCREASED URINARY URIC ACID

Excess dietary purine
Drug-induced
    Probenicid
    Sulfinpyrazone
    Salicylates
Myeloproliferative disorders
Type I glycogen storage disease
Chronic dehydration states

INCREASED URINARY CYSTINE

Autosomal recessive cystinuria

is normal, no further treatment is necessary other than encouraging the patient to increase fluid intake. Any patient with stones of uric acid, calcium phosphate, cystine, or struvite is at high risk for continued stone formation and undergoes metabolic evaluation. Patients with recurrent or enlarging stones, including calcium oxalate stones, undergoes metabolic evaluation.

Extracorporeal shockwave lithotripsy (ESWL) involves generation of a shock wave, focusing of a sound wave, and imaging of the stone. Patients are submersed in a water bath or coupled to the machine via a water cushion. When the shock waves strike the stone, they undergo reflection and refraction, resulting in compressive and tensile forces that fragment the stone. Localization is achieved with fluoroscopy or US.

Complications of ESWL are rare. The most common is ureteral obstruction by stone fragments, which necessitates additional ESWL, ureteroscopic stone retrieval, or stent placement. Contraindications to ESWL are uncorrected coagulopathy, distal anatomic obstruction that precludes passage of stone fragments, uncontrolled urinary tract infection, pregnancy, and technical problems related to patient size and body habitus.

Stones can be removed by means of percutaneous *endoscopic* renal and ureteroscopic techniques. Ultrasonic, electrohydraulic, and laser probes fragment stones under visual guidance through rigid or flexible instruments. Per-

cutaneous lithotripsy, alone or in combination with ESWL, is almost always successful.

BLADDER CANCER

Bladder cancer has a strong male prevalence.

Diagnosis and Staging

The hallmark of bladder cancer is gross painless hematuria. However, microscopic hematuria also may be the first indicator of this disease. Some patients have irritative symptoms, such as frequency and dysuria. These can be caused by advanced local disease or carcinoma in situ. Urine cytology is effective for screening patients with irritative symptoms. The staging of bladder cancer is illustrated in Fig. 105-1.

Excretory *urography* is performed because the renal pelves and ureters are at risk for urothelial neoplasia. *Cystoscopy* often is diagnostic and therapeutic because superficial tumors are easily excised or fulgurated through endoscopic instruments. Patients with locally advanced tumors undergo evaluation for metastases that consists of *chest radiography* and computed tomography (CT) of the abdomen and pelvis.

Management

Most patients with bladder cancer present with local disease. Some superficial tumors progress to invasive disease. Multifocal and recurrent tumors are managed with intravesical chemotherapy and transurethral resection. Agents include thiotepa, doxorubicin, mitomycin C, and bacillus Calmette-Guerin (BCG).

Locally advanced tumors are managed with radical cystectomy (cystoprostatectomy in men) and urinary diversion. Radiation therapy is associated with a high rate of local recurrence. Patients for whom radiation therapy does not work, often can be treated with cystectomy. Chemotherapy involves cisplatin-based multidrug therapy before (neoadjuvant) cystectomy, after (adjuvant) cystectomy, and with radiation therapy.

Ileal conduit diversion is still common, but alternative methods more closely approximate the reservoir function of the bladder. The operation includes use of intestine (large, small, or both) to make a pouch, a method to decrease the pressure in the pouch to avoid the use of intact segments of intestine, a mechanism to avoid reflux of urine into the ureters, and a mechanism to achieve continence. When the urinary pouch drains to the abdominal wall (eg, Kock pouch), intermittent catheterization is substituted for voiding. When the urinary pouch is anastomosed to the urethra, voiding is accomplished with abdominal straining.

Metastatic bladder cancer is treated with systemic chemotherapy with cisplatin-based regimens.

CARCINOMA OF THE URETER AND RENAL PELVIS

The diagnosis of tumors in the ureter and renal pelvis is made with excretory urography and urine cytology. Urine cytology is helpful when the tumors are high grade. Some transitional cell carcinomas of the ureter or renal pelvis can be managed with endoscopy. Other low-grade, noninvasive upper tract tumors are managed with local resection or nephroureterectomy. High-grade or invasive tumors are managed with nephroureterectomy. It is important to remove the entire ureter, including the ureteral orifice, be-

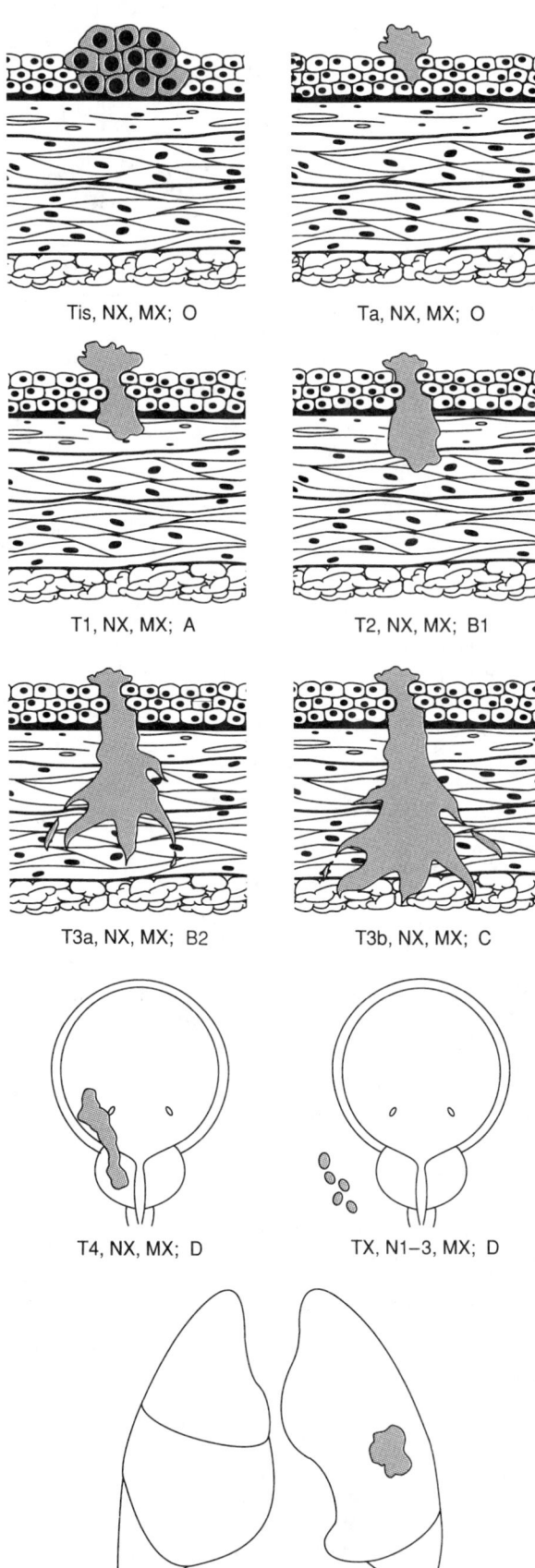

Figure 105-1. Staging of bladder cancer. Both the TNM (American Joint Commission on Cancer, ed 3) and the Jewett systems are shown.

cause of risk for recurrent cancer in the ureteral stump. Follow-up care includes excretory urography, cystoscopy, and urine cytology.

RENAL NEOPLASMS
Renal Cell Carcinoma

The most common malignant neoplasm of the renal parenchyma is renal cell carcinoma (hypernephroma). No definite cause is identified, but a genetic abnormality may be responsible. Multifocal bilateral tumors are associated with von Hippel-Lindau disease. Other possible causes are exposure to cadmium and lead, tobacco use, and renal failure.

Renal cell carcinoma is often clinically silent until late in its course. The growth rate of the tumors varies, and they may be large before symptoms or metastases occur. The triad of flank pain, palpable mass, and hematuria is associated with advanced disease. Renal carcinoma can produce a variety of hormone or hormone-like substances (eg, erythropoietin, renin, and parathormone) and may present with a variety of symptoms including anemia, hypertension, fever, erythrocytosis, abnormalities in liver function tests, and symptoms associated with metastatic disease. Many tumors are discovered incidentally when diagnostic studies such as intravenous urography, CT, or US are performed for other reasons.

Diagnosis and Staging

The staging of renal cell carcinoma is based on extent of disease (Fig. 105-2). The tumors have a predilection for growth into the renal veins and extension into the vena cava. Tumor thrombi may extend into the right atrium. Perihilar and periaortic nodal involvement occurs. Tumor cells have ready access to the venous circulation, so hematogenous metastases occur. The common sites are lung, bone, liver, brain, adrenal gland, and other kidney.

Excretory urography provides a good renal image with superior detail of the collecting system. Renal masses such as benign cysts or renal cell carcinomas appear to distort the renal outline or collecting system. The main differential diagnosis of a renal mass at excretory urography is renal cyst and solid tumor such as renal cell carcinoma. *CT* is used for differentiation. *Renal US* may be used to confirm the cystic nature of the mass. If the mass appears to be solid, *CT* or *angiography* may be used to characterize it. CT can demonstrate a solid mass, which becomes more dense or enhances with administration of contrast material. Hilar or periaortic lymphadenopathy or liver metastasis may be demonstrated, and the renal vein and vena cava can often be evaluated for tumor extension.

Selective renal angiography shows tumor vessels, arteriovenous fistulas, venous lakes, and tumor staining. *Vena cavography* is used to evaluate vena caval and renal vein involvement. *MRI* is a noninvasive method of defining the extent of venous involvement.

To stage the tumor, a *chest radiograph* or *chest CT* is used to evaluate pulmonary metastases. A *bone scan* may be performed to rule out osseous metastases.

Management

Surgical excision is the primary mode of therapy for renal cell carcinoma. *Radical nephrectomy* is the standard against which less radical procedures are judged. If vena caval extension of tumor reaches beyond the hepatic veins or into the right atrium, cardiopulmonary bypass with hypothermia and total circulatory arrest is used to aid tumor

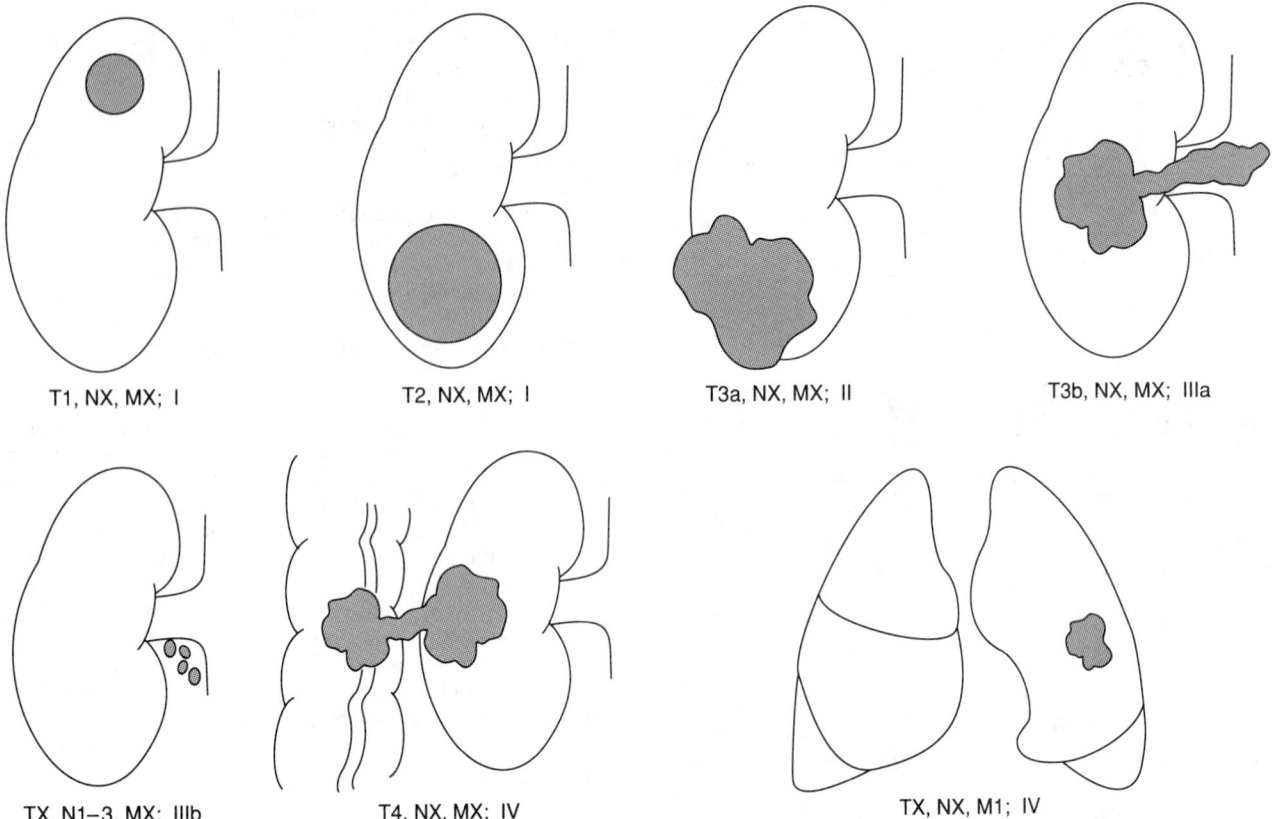

Figure 105-2. Staging of renal cancer. Both the TNM (American Joint Commission on Cancer, ed 3) and the Robson systems are shown.

excision in a bloodless field. Preoperative angioinfarction may aid nephrectomy when the tumors are large or extend into the vena cava. Resection of solitary metastases in lung, liver, bone, and other organs is considered.

Partial nephrectomy can be used for small bilateral tumors or to treat patients with a solitary kidney or poor renal function. Therapy for metastasis, including radiation and chemotherapy, is ineffective. Immunotherapy with interferon, interleukin-2, and lymphokine-activated killer cells can be tried.

Other Renal Neoplasms

Benign tumors include angiomyolipoma and oncocytoma. Renal sarcomas include leiomyosarcoma, liposarcoma, and hemangiopericytoma. Although angiomyolipoma does not metastasize, it can occur in multiple sites, grow to a large size, and bleed. Small tumors may be found if they have classic imaging characteristics. Oncocytomas are considered benign, but are difficult to differentiate from renal cell carcinoma. If the diagnosis is suspected and the lesion is small, partial nephrectomy or enucleation is considered. Renal sarcomas are malignant tumors with similar findings to renal cell carcinoma and are treated by means of radical nephrectomy.

PROSTATE CANCER

Adenocarcinoma of the prostate is the most common noncutaneous malignant tumor among men. Prostate cancer is a disease of older men. Other than age, there are few apparent etiologic factors. Testosterone supports growth

of the tumor, but there is no evidence that testosterone causes prostate cancer.

Prostate cancer grows slowly and has a long latent period. The disease originates in the periphery of the gland and progresses within the gland, through the capsule, and into the seminal vesicles. The main metastatic sites are the regional lymph nodes and the osseous skeleton. Staging is summarized in Fig. 105-3.

Detection

Early prostate cancer has few symptoms. Obstructive symptoms may occur, but they are similar to those of BPH: decreasing urinary stream, frequency, and nocturia. Bone pain, weight loss, and fatigue, are signs of advanced disease.

Three modalities are used in early detection of prostate cancer: digital rectal examination, serum prostate-specific antigen (PSA), and transrectal US of the prostate.

Tumors usually arise in the posterior lobe of the prostate in the sonographic peripheral zone. This area is readily palpable on *digital rectal examination*. Early prostate cancer presents as a small firm nodule in or at the periphery of the gland. The differential diagnosis includes prostatic calculi, granulomas, and BPH. Prostate biopsy is required to confirm the diagnosis.

At *transrectal US* prostate cancer appears as a hypoechoic lesion in the peripheral zone. Suspicious areas at US must be confirmed with biopsy.

Serum PSA is elevated in most men with cancer, but some men with BPH also have an elevated PSA. The use of PSA alone as a screening test for prostate cancer is con-

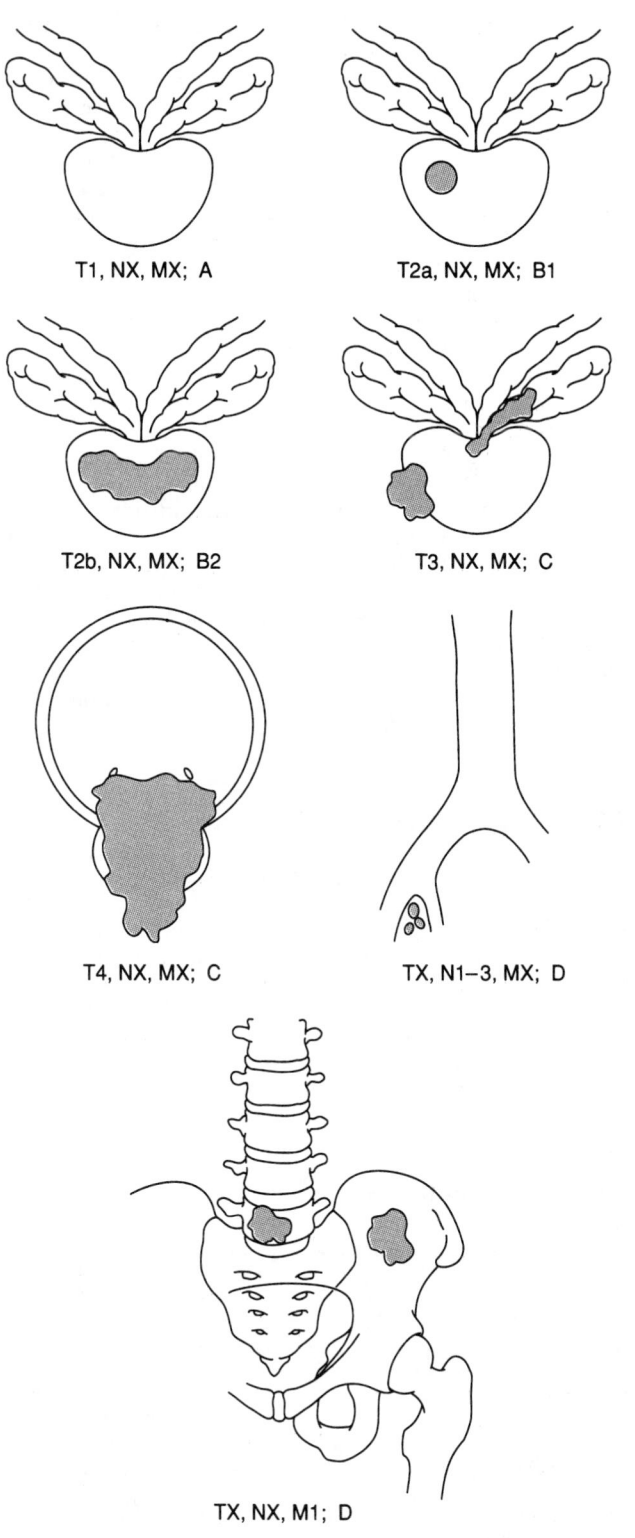

Figure 105-3. Staging of prostate cancer. Both the TNM (American Joint Commission on Cancer, ed 3) and the Jewett systems are shown.

troversial. PSA testing with digital rectal examination is reliable.

Management

Management of prostate cancer depends on whether the disease is localized or advanced beyond the prostate. Because prostate cancer advances slowly, the morbidity of

therapy may exceed the therapeutic benefit for elderly and debilitated patients.

If the tumor is confined in the prostatic capsule (stage A or B), treatment options include *radical prostatectomy,* external beam radiation therapy, and radioactive implants. Node dissection can be performed for staging. In patients likely to have positive nodes, laparoscopic pelvic node

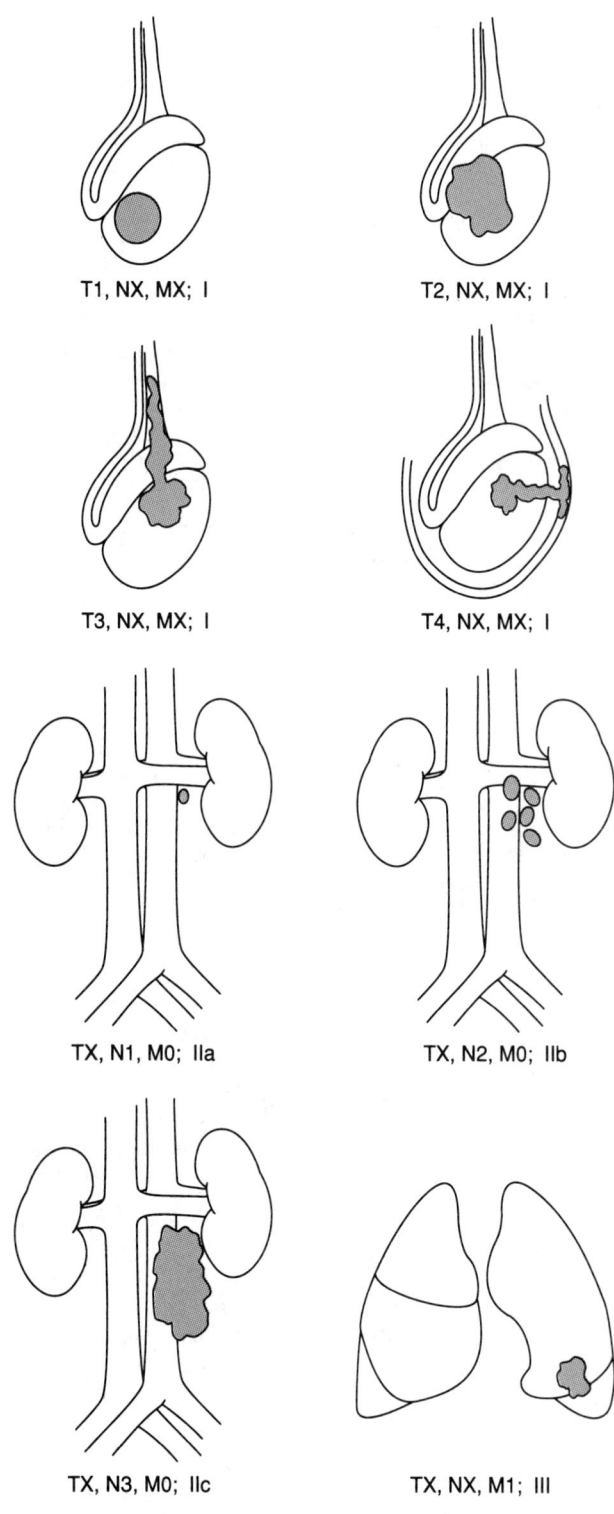

Figure 105-4. Staging of testis cancer. Both the TNM (American Joint Commission on Cancer, ed 3) and a commonly used descriptive system are listed.

dissection or dissection through an abbreviated incision can be performed. The complications of radical prostatectomy are impotence and incontinence.

Interstitial radiation implantation is associated with fewer complications than conventional radiation therapy but has a high local failure rate.

Hormonal ablation can be attempted in the management of advanced prostate cancer. Androgen ablation brings about improvement in almost all patients and regression in some.

Follow-Up Care

Prostatic carcinoma has a slow rate of progression, and recurrences may not be manifest for years after treatment. After treatment, patients are examined every 6 months with digital rectal examination and a PSA test. After radical prostatectomy, PSA levels should be zero. If the level is not zero, bone scanning and other imaging studies are performed. A rise in PSA usually indicates local recurrence or metastatic disease. If local recurrence is suspected, biopsy can be performed and hormonal ablation or salvage prostatectomy considered depending on the pathologic and clinical findings. If PSA stabilizes at a low level, biopsy is not performed for 1 year. A positive biopsy after 2 years suggests persistent or recurrent disease.

Follow-up care of patients with advanced disease includes examinations every 6 months. The patient is asked about bone pain, weight loss, and fatigue. PSA and renal function tests are performed. Relapse is reflected in a rise in PSA followed by symptoms of metastatic disease. Bone pain is palliated with local radiation therapy or treatment with strontium 89.

TESTIS CANCER

The most common malignant neoplasms of the testis originate from the germ cells. Histologic manifestations include choriocarcinoma, embryonal cell carcinoma, endodermal sinus tumor, seminoma, and teratoma. For therapeutic purposes the tumors are divided into seminomas and nonseminomas.

Diagnosis

The usual presenting *symptom* is testicular enlargement that may be associated with mild discomfort. Scrotal *US* may be helpful, particularly when physical examination is difficult, for example, in the presence of a large hydrocele. The diagnostic and therapeutic procedure for any suspected testis carcinoma is *inguinal exploration with orchiectomy* if the surgical findings confirm the presence of a testicular mass.

The *tumor markers* α-fetoprotein (AFP) and the β-subunit of human chorionic gonadotropin (β-hCG) contribute both to the diagnosis and follow-up care for testis cancer. Radiologic evaluation of metastases is accomplished with CT of the chest, abdomen, and pelvis. Lymphangiography also can be performed. Tumor markers and radiologic evaluation are used in tumor staging (Fig. 105-4).

Management

Seminomas are highly responsive to radiation. When bulky retroperitoneal or distant metastases are present, cisplatin-based combination chemotherapy is administered.

The management of *nonseminomatous tumors* is controversial. *Stage 1* tumors are treated with retroperitoneal lymphadenectomy. A nerve-sparing operation can be attempted to preserve antegrade ejaculation. An alternative strategy is observation without therapeutic intervention. The rationale depends on accurate staging of tumors and administration of effective therapy at the first sign of recurrence. Patients who elect observation undergo monthly tumor-marker measurements and chest radiographs for 2 years. Abdominal CT is repeated at least every 3 months during this period.

Stage 2 nonseminomatous tumors <5 cm in diameter are managed by means of retroperitoneal lymphadenectomy. Adjuvant therapy (cisplatin-based chemotherapy) is effective but may not be required. *Bulky stage 2 and stage 3* nonseminomatous tumors are initially treated with cisplatin-based chemotherapy. Three or four cycles of chemotherapy are administered, and restaging is performed. Evidence of residual disease with normalization of tumor markers is an indication for surgical excision. The finding of residual cancer indicates the need for additional chemotherapy. A frequent pathologic finding in this circumstance is benign teratoma, which may result from eradication of the malignant elements of the tumor by means of chemotherapy. When benign teratoma or necrotic tumor is found, the patient need only be examined with periodic tumor markers and chest radiography.

RETROPERITONEAL TUMORS

Although primary retroperitoneal tumors are uncommon, most are malignant. These tumors occur most commonly in the fifth and sixth decades of life, and typically are lymphoma or sarcoma. Most benign lesions are congenital cystic lesions and lipomas. The types of tumors are:

Extragonadal germ cell tumors
Metastatic retroperitoneal tumors
Benign retroperitoneal conditions

SUGGESTED READING

Benson M, Whang I, Olsson C, McMahon D, Cooner W. The use of prostate specific antigen density to enhance the predictive value of intermediate levels of serum prostate specific antigen. J Urol 1992;147:817.

Coe FL, Parks JH, Asplin JR. The pathogenesis and treatment of kidney stones. N Engl J Med 1992;327:1142.

Dalbagni G, Presti J, Reuter V, Fair WR, Cordon-Cardo C. Genetic alterations in bladder cancer. Lancet 1993;342:469.

Gnarra JR, Tory K, Weng Y, et al. Mutations of the VHL tumor suppressor gene in renal carcinoma. Nature Genet 1994;7:85.

Grossman HB, Schwartz SL, Konnak JW. Ureteroscopic treatment of urothelial carcinoma of the ureter and renal pelvis. J Urol 1992;148:275.

Johansson J, Adami H, Anderson S, Bergstrom R, Holmberg L, Krusemo U. High 10-year survival rate in patients with early, untreated prostate cancer. JAMA 1992;267:2191.

Miyao N, Tsai YC, Lerner SP, et al. Role of chromosome 9 in human bladder cancer. Cancer Res 1993;53:4066.

Oesterling JE, Jacobsen S, Chute C, et al. Serum prostate-specific antigen in a community-based population on healthy men: establishment of age-specific reference ranges. JAMA 1993;270:860.

Thrasher J, Paulson D. Prognostic factors in renal cell carcinoma. Urol Clin North Am 1993;20:247.

Wirth M. Immunotherapy for metastatic renal cell carcinoma. Urol Clin North Am 1993;20:283.

ESSENTIALS OF SURGERY: SCIENTIFIC PRINCIPLES AND PRACTICE,
edited by Lazar J. Greenfield, Michael W. Mulholland, Keith T. Oldham, Gerald B. Zelenock,
and Keith D. Lillemoe. Lippincott–Raven Publishers, Philadelphia, © 1997.

CHAPTER 106

FEMALE GENITAL SYSTEM

W. GLENN HURT AND DAVID E. SOPER

VULVA

Vulvar Intraepithelial Neoplasia

Vulvar intraepithelial neoplasia (VIN) is usually asymptomatic, but it can cause pruritus. It often is associated with human papillomavirus (HPV) infection. VIN appears as white, red, or deeply pigmented lesions that can have a papular or macular configuration and can be unifocally or multifocally distributed.

Diagnosis

Application of 5% acetic acid and colposcopic examination of the vulva help detect the lesions. The locations of all lesions are documented, and biopsy specimens are obtained. VIN is graded according to its squamous cell atypia: VIN-1, mild dysplasia; VIN-2, moderate dysplasia; and VIN-3, severe dysplasia or carcinoma in situ.

Management

Therapy for VIN is local excision, CO_2 laser vaporization, or for extensive involvement, skinning vulvectomy.

Vulvar Carcinoma

Almost all vulvar cancers are squamous cell carcinoma, the rest are melanoma, sarcoma, Bartholin gland adenocarcinoma or carcinoma, Paget disease of the vulva, or basal cell carcinoma. Except for sarcomas, these cancers usually occur among women 55 years of age. Patients with HPV infection and granulomatous disease are at risk for vulvar carcinoma. Vulvar carcinoma often is surrounded by an area of VIN.

Diagnosis

Biopsy is required for definitive diagnosis. The International Federation of Gynecology and Obstetrics (FIGO) recommends surgical staging of vulvar cancer (Table 106-1).

Management

- *Unilateral microinvasive carcinoma* (<2 cm in diameter, <1 mm invasion, without vascular or lymphatic space involvement)—wide local excision without node dissection
- *Unilateral invasive carcinoma*—depending on location, radical vulvectomy with unilateral inguinal-femoral lymphadenectomy
- *Others*—radical vulvectomy with bilateral inguinal-femoral lymphadenectomy
- *Melanoma, sarcoma, Bartholin gland carcinoma*—radical vulvectomy and bilateral inguinofemoral lymphadenectomy, possibly abdominoperineal resection of Bartholin gland carcinomas because of pararectal and sacral lymphatic drainage
- *Paget disease*—without underlying adenocarcinoma, wide local excision; with underlying adenocarcinoma, radical vulvectomy and bilateral inguinofemoral lymphadenectomy

- *Basal cell carcinoma*—wide local excision
- *Bartholin Gland Abscess*

Bartholin gland adenitis or abscess is caused by an infection that contains bacteria similar to vaginal flora. *Neisseria gonorrhoeae* and *Chlamydia trachomatis* also can cause Bartholin gland infection.

Management

Therapy for acute adenitis is broad-spectrum antibiotics and sitz baths. Therapy for abscesses is incision and drainage near the site of the occluded duct and antibiotics. When the Bartholin duct is obstructed, mucoid secretion collects and causes cystic dilatation. Therapy is placement of a drainage catheter or marsupialization of the gland. Recurrent Bartholin cysts and abscesses may necessitate excision of the gland. If any Bartholin gland is nodular or has findings that suggest carcinoma, an incisional or excisional biopsy is performed.

Necrotizing Fasciitis

Necrotizing fasciitis is a life-threatening infection of the superficial fascia and fat. It is usually limited to the lower extremities, abdominal wall, and vulva. The condition most often affects women with diabetes or atherosclerosis, those undergoing long-term therapy with steroids or nonsteroidal antiinflammatory drugs (NSAIDs), and those with autoimmune diseases.

Necrotizing fasciitis is caused by *Streptococcus pyogenes* with or without *Staphylococcus aureus* or by anaerobic and facultative aerobic bacteria. The infection usually starts as a small skin lesion. It can remain quiescent for weeks, or it can be fulminant with rapid extension along tissue planes.

Diagnosis

Criteria for diagnosis include: extensive necrosis of superficial fascia with widespread involvement of the surrounding tissues; moderate to severe systemic toxic reaction, including altered mental status; absence of major vascular occlusion; and pathologic examination of débrided tissue showing intense leukocytic infiltration, focal necrosis of fascia and surrounding tissues, and microvascular thrombosis.

An incisional biopsy with removal of at least 1 cc of subcutaneous tissue and frozen section evaluation helps differentiate necrotizing fasciitis from nonspecific ulcers, abscesses, or ischemic necrosis.

Management

> Correction of anemia
> Restoration of fluid and electrolyte balance
> Institution of broad-spectrum antibiotic therapy
> Extensive surgical débridement

Frozen section biopsies may be helpful in determining tissue involvement and in establishing surgical margins. Gram stains and cultures (aerobic and anaerobic) are performed on the resected tissue. After débridement, the wound is packed with povidone-iodine-impregnated gauze and the patient is transferred to an intensive care unit.

VAGINA

Vaginal Intraepithelial Neoplasia

Vaginal intraepithelial neoplasia (VAIN) is usually asymptomatic. It is detected with an abnormal Papanicolaou (Pap) smear. The lesion is usually located in the upper

Table 106-1. STAGING OF GYNECOLOGIC CANCER AS RECOMMENDED BY THE INTERNATIONAL FEDERATION OF GYNECOLOGY AND OBSTETRICS

Stage	Description	Stage	Description
VULVAR CANCER		IIIA	No extension to pelvic wall
0		IIIB	Extension to pelvic wall or hydronephrosis of nonfunctioning kidney
Tis	Carcinoma in situ; intraepithelial carcinoma	IV	Carcinoma beyond true pelvis or involving mucosa of bladder or rectum
I		IVA	Spread to adjacent organs
T1, N0, M0	Tumor confined to vulva or perineum, 2 cm or less in greatest dimension. No nodal metastasis	IVB	Spread to distant organs
II		**UTERINE CORPUS CANCER**	
T2, N0, M0	Tumor confined to vulva or perineum, more than 2 cm in greatest dimension. No nodal metastasis	IA G123	Tumor limited to endometrium
		IB G123	Invasion to less than half the myometrium
III		IC G123	Invasion to more than half the myometrium
T3, N0, M0	Tumor of any size with:	IIA G123	Endocervical glandular involvement only
T3, N1, M0	(1) Adjacent spread to lower urethra, vagina, anus, *or*	IIB G123	Cervical stromal invasion
T1, N1, M0	(2) Unilateral regional lymph node metastasis	IIIA G123	Tumor invades serosa or adnexa, or presence of positive peritoneal cytology
T2, N1, M0		IIIB G123	Vaginal metastases
IVA		IIIC G123	Metastases to pelvic or paraaortic lymph nodes
T1, N2, M0	Tumor invades any of the following:	IVA G123	Tumor invasion of bladder or bowel mucosa
T2, N2, M0	Upper urethra, bladder mucosa, rectal mucosa, pelvic bone, or	IVB	Distant metastases including intraabdominal or inguinal lymph nodes
T3, N2, M0	bilateral regional node metastasis		
T4, any N, M0		**Note**	
IVB		G1	5% or less of a nonsquamous or nonmorular solid growth pattern
Any T, any N, M1	Any distant metastasis including pelvic lymph nodes	G2	6%–50% of a nonsquamous or nonmorular solid growth pattern
Note		G3	More than 50% of a nonsquamous or nonmorular solid growth pattern
N (regional lymph nodes)			
N0	No lymph node metastasis	**OVARIAN CANCER**	
N1	Unilateral regional lymph node metastasis		Growth limited to ovaries
N2	Bilateral regional lymph node metastasis	I	One ovary; no tumor on external surfaces; capsule intact; no ascites present containing malignant cells
		IA	
M (distant metastasis)		IB	Both ovaries; no tumor on external surfaces; capsules intact; no ascites present containing malignant cells
M0	No clinical metastasis	IC	IA or IB but with tumor on surface of one or both ovaries; or with capsule ruptured; or with ascites containing malignant cells or with positive peritoneal washings
M1	Distant metastasis (including pelvic lymph node metastasis)		Growth involving one or both ovaries with pelvic extension
VAGINAL CANCER		II	Extension or metastases to uterus or fallopian tubes
0	Carcinoma in situ; intraepithelial carcinoma	IIA	Extension to other pelvic tissues
I	Carcinoma limited to vaginal mucosa	IIB	IIA or IIB but with tumor on surface of one or both ovaries; or with capsules ruptured; or with ascites containing malignant cells or with positive peritoneal washings
II	Carcinoma involving subvaginal tissue but not onto pelvic wall	IIC	
III	Carcinoma onto pelvic wall or pubic symphysis	III	Tumor involving one or both ovaries with peritoneal implants outside pelvis or positive retroperitoneal or inguinal nodes; superficial liver metastases; tumor limited to pelvis but with histologically verified malignant extension to small bowel or omentum
IV	Carcinoma beyond true pelvis; involvement of bladder or rectal mucosa		
CERVICAL CANCER		IIIA	Tumor limited to true pelvis with negative nodes but with histologically confirmed seeding of peritoneal surfaces
0	Carcinoma in situ; intraepithelial carcinoma	IIIB	Tumor limited to one or both ovaries with histologically confirmed implants of peritoneal surfaces, none greater than 2 cm in diameter; nodes negative
I	Carcinoma confined to cervix	IIIC	Abdominal implants greater than 2 cm in diameter or positive retroperitoneal or inguinal nodes
IA	Preclinical carcinoma; diagnosed microscopically	IV	Growth involving one or both ovaries with distant metastasis; pleural effusion with positive cytology; parenchymal liver metastasis
IA1	Minimal microscopic evidence of stromal invasion		
IA2	Microscopic invasion from base of epithelium of 5 mm or less and lateral spread of 7 mm or less	**INVASIVE GESTATIONAL TROPHOBLASTIC NEOPLASIA**	
IB	Lesions of greater dimensions than stage IA2		Tumor confined to uterine corpus
II	Carcinoma beyond cervix but not to pelvic wall. Cancer involves vagina but not lower third	I	Tumor to adnexa but limited to genital structures
IIA	Obvious parametrial involvement	II	Tumor to lungs with or without genital involvement
IIB	Obvious parametrial involvement	III	Metastasis to other sites
III	Carcinoma to pelvic wall. No cancer-free space between tumor and pelvic wall. Tumro involves lower third of vagina. Hydronephrosis or nonfunctioning kidney not due to another cause	IV	

third of the vagina. VAIN tends to be multifocal and is often associated with HPV infection and neoplasia of the cervix or vulva.

Diagnosis

Colposcopy helps identify abnormal vaginal epithelium. Biopsy is performed on epithelial abnormalities.

Management

Therapy is CO_2 laser vaporization, excision of isolated lesions, or application of 5% 5-fluorouracil cream. Long-term follow-up care is necessary because VAIN recurs and is associated with malignant tumors of the lower genital tract.

Vaginal Carcinoma

Primary vaginal cancer is rare. Most vaginal cancers are extension or metastases from cancers of the uterus or vulva. Mean age at diagnosis is 65 years. Most vaginal cancer is squamous cell carcinoma. Adenocarcinoma, sarcoma, endodermal sinus tumors, or melanoma can exist anywhere along the vaginal canal.

Diagnosis

Cytologic smears and biopsies of tissue that looks or feels abnormal are used to detect asymptomatic lesions. Abnormal vaginal discharge and painless bleeding are the most common presenting signs. Vaginal cancer spreads primarily by direct extension and lymphatic dissemination. The location of the lesion determines paravaginal and lymph node involvement. FIGO recommends clinical staging of vaginal cancer (Table 106-1).

Management

Surgical therapy has limited use in the management of vaginal cancer. Radiation therapy is recommended for most invasive squamous cell carcinomas and adenocarcinomas of the vagina. Therapy for primary vaginal sarcomas, endodermal sinus tumors, and melanomas is surgical. Postoperative radiation therapy or chemotherapy may be needed.

Pelvic Organ Prolapse

Pelvic organ prolapse occurs as a result of weaknesses within the pelvic organ support system and the vagina. Contributing factors include pregnancy and childbirth; increased intraabdominal pressure associated with chronic respiratory diseases, abdominal masses, ascites, or obesity; postmenopausal atrophy; congenital tissue weakness; and iatrogenic factors, such as inadequate surgical intervention for correction of pelvic support defects.

Symptoms include pelvic pressure, bearing-down sensation, sacral backache, coital difficulty, protrusion from the vagina, spotting and ulceration of the prolapsed tissues, urinary urgency and frequency, urinary incontinence, voiding difficulties or retention, and difficult defecation.

Diagnosis

The diagnosis of prolapse is suggested by history and confirmed at pelvic examination. A catheter is inserted to determine urinary residual as an indicator of bladder emptying efficiency and to obtain a urine specimen for urinalysis and culture. During the pelvic examination cytologic smears are obtained, and estrogen status is ascertained by means of inspection of the vaginal epithelium for rugae. Repeated replacement of prolapsed organs and observation of their descent during Valsalva maneuvers help determine areas of weakness within the pelvic support system and the extent to which each of the pelvic organs is involved. The maximum degree of descent of the anterior, apical, and posterior vaginal walls is documented.

Management

Therapy for prolapse is surgical. However, a pessary can be used to reduce and support the pelvic organs of patients who are at poor operative risk or who refuse surgical therapy. The operation is aimed at correction of the specific weakness within the pelvic support system or vagina. Procedures include vaginal hysterectomy with or without salpingo-oophorectomy, posterior culdoplasty, anterior colporrhaphy, posterior colporrhaphy, enterocele repair, perineoplasty, retropubic urethropexy-colposuspension, or sacrospinous ligament fixation of the vaginal vault.

UTERUS

Abnormal Cervical Cytology

A squamous intraepithelial lesion (SIL) can be classified as low grade (SIL-LG) or high grade (SIL-HG). The diagnosis of atypical squamous cells of undetermined significance (ASCUS) reflects uncertainty about whether the patient has SIL. Cytologic findings resulting in the diagnosis of ASCUS can be due to reactive or reparative changes, infection, or early neoplasia.

SILs (neoplasia or dysplasia) are asymptomatic conditions caused by abnormal maturation of the squamous epithelium of the squamocolumnar junction of the cervix. Risk factors include adolescent coitus, multiple sexual partners, and giving birth before 20 years of age. Cervical infection with HPV appears to be an etiologic factor.

Diagnosis

SILs are detected with a Pap smear and are diagnosed by means of colposcopy, ectocervical biopsy, and endocervical curettage. Cervical conization is recommended if any of the following exists: disagreement about the grade of the lesion at cytologic screening and colposcopic biopsy, endocervical curettage showing SIL, cytologic abnormality without colposcopically visible lesion, microinvasive carcinoma on directed biopsy, and the need to remove a neoplasm to preserve childbearing potential.

Management

Therapy is based on cytologic, colposcopic, and histologic agreement about the grade of SIL and the location and limits of all lesions. An algorithm for the management of abnormal cervical cytology is shown in Fig. 106-1. The rate of progression of SIL-LG is considered minimal. A finding of SIL-HG places the patient at risk for invasive cancer if not adequately controlled. SIL-HG must be eradicated by means of cryotherapy or CO_2 laser vaporization. Hysterectomy is reserved for patients with SIL-HG who have completed childbearing or have other gynecologic reasons for hysterectomy. Follow-up care is provided to detect persistence or recurrence to prevent the development of invasive carcinoma of the cervix.

Cervical Carcinoma

The mean age at diagnosis of cervical carcinoma is 52 years. Almost all invasive cervical carcinoma is squamous cell; the rest is adenocarcinoma. Common signs include bloody vaginal discharge, postcoital spotting, and metrorrhagia. Advanced disease can cause pelvic and leg pain, dysuria, hematuria, obstipation, and rectal bleeding. Cervical lesions can be exophytic, ulcerative, or endophytic.

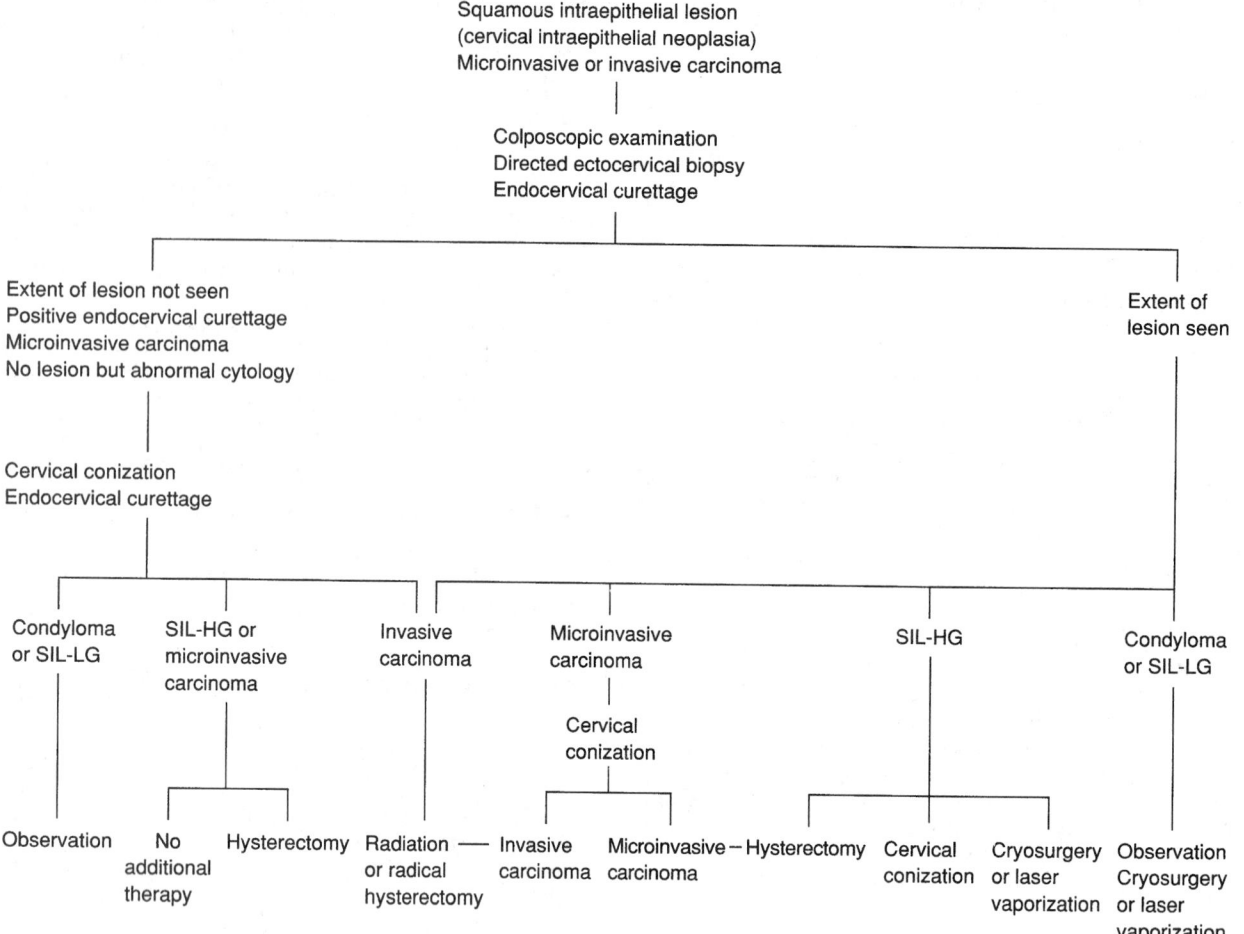

Figure 106-1. Management of abnormal cervical cytology. When the Bethesda system is used to report cervical cytology, low-grade squamous intraepithelial lesion (SIL-LG) should be considered the same as cervical intraepithelial neoplasia 1, and high grade squamous intraepithelial lesion (SIL-HG) the same as cervical epithelial neoplasia 2 and 3. Conization can be performed by cold knife (scapel), loop electrosurgical excision procedure, or laser. Frequent follow-up examinations are indicated after therapy for cervical neoplasia.

Cervical cancer spreads by direct extension to the parametrial tissues, vagina, rectum, bladder, and regional pelvic lymph node chains. FIGO recommends clinical staging of cervical cancer (Table 106-1).

Management

Microinvasive carcinoma of the cervix, which has a depth of invasion of ≤3 mm, no confluent tongues of invasive disease, and no lymphatic or vascular invasion, has an incidence of pelvic lymph node metastasis <1%. Therapy is conization or simple extrafascial hysterectomy.

Therapy for *invasive* cervical carcinoma is determined by the patient's age, health status, and stage of disease: *Stage I and IIA*—radical hysterectomy and pelvic lymphadenectomy (obturator, internal iliac, and iliac nodes) or a combination of intracavitary and external radiation therapy allows preservation of the ovaries and is likely to leave a coitally functional vagina.

Stage IIB, III, and IV—radiation therapy.

Endometrial Hyperplasia

Chronic, unopposed estrogen stimulation of the endometrium due to anovulation, estrogen-producing tumors, or estrogen administration causes endometrial hyperpla-

sia. Tamoxifen, used as therapy for breast cancer, contributes to development of endometrial polyps, hyperplasia, and carcinoma. Atypical adenomatous hyperplasia (complex atypical hyperplasia) is considered to be a premalignant condition when it occurs in perimenopausal women.

Management

Adenomatous endometrial hyperplasia without atypia in a premenopausal woman is treated with cyclic progestin for 6 months. Endometrial sampling is performed 3 months into therapy to prove resolution of hyperplasia. Periodic sampling is performed after therapy to detect recurrence. Perimenopausal and postmenopausal women who have adenomatous endometrial hyperplasia with atypia are advised to undergo hysterectomy because of risk for endometrial cancer. Postmenopausal patients at poor surgical risk can undergo progestin therapy.

Endometrial Carcinoma

Endometrial carcinoma is the most common malignant tumor of the female genital tract. It is most often an adenocarcinoma. Median age at diagnosis is 60 years. Risk factors include nulliparity, obesity, delayed menopause, chronic anovulation, and unopposed postmenopausal estrogen therapy. The most common sign is menometrorrhagia or postmenopausal bleeding.

Diagnosis

Diagnosis is made by means of outpatient endometrial sampling or uterine curettage. The prognosis of endometrial carcinoma is determined by histologic type, degree of cellular differentiation, extent of myometrial invasion, and presence or absence of node metastases. FIGO recommends surgical and pathologic staging of uterine corpus cancer (Table 106-1).

Management

- *Stage I*—Surgical intervention. At operation, a peritoneal cytologic sample is obtained, and extrafascial abdominal hysterectomy and bilateral salpingo-oophorectomy are performed. Patients with poorly differentiated endometrial carcinoma, more than superficial myometrial invasion, or extension into the cervix undergo selective pelvic and periaortic lymphadenectomy to determine prognosis and to aid in treatment planning (adjuvant radiation therapy). These patients may also benefit from postoperative radiation therapy.
- *Stage II*—Radical hysterectomy, bilateral salpingo-oophorectomy, and pelvic and periaortic lymphadenectomy, *or*
- External radiation therapy and abdominal extrafascial hysterectomy with bilateral salpingo-oophorectomy
- *Stage III or IV*—Radiation or surgical therapy, or both, and progestin or chemotherapy, or both

Uterine Sarcoma

Uterine sarcomas are derived from the endometrium, myometrium, or, rarely, the vascular and connective tissues. They are usually detected in women 55 to 60 years of age. Sarcomas cause uterine enlargement, abnormal uterine bleeding, and pelvic pain. Therapy for uterine sarcoma is abdominal hysterectomy with bilateral salpingo-oophorectomy.

Abnormal Uterine Bleeding

The endometrium is exquisitely sensitive to circulating levels of estrogen and progesterone. The physician must determine if abnormal bleeding is the result of endocrine or anatomic factors.

Diagnosis

Most abnormal uterine bleeding among women <40 years old who have normal pelvic examinations is due to anovulation. Administration of medroxyprogesterone usually corrects abnormal bleeding. If it does not, hysteroscopy and endometrial sampling are performed.

Hysteroscopy is performed in the early proliferative phase. Visualization of the uterine cavity allows differentiation between field abnormality and focal lesion, such as a submucous leiomyoma, endometrial polyp, or carcinoma. Endometrial sampling allows determination of the presence or absence of endometrial hyperplasia or carcinoma within the uterus. Endometrial sampling during the luteal phase allows documentation of ovulation.

Management

Laser vaporization and electrical cauterization of the endometrium are used to obliterate the endometrial cavity in menorrhagia when the patient does not respond to hormonal therapy and does not want a hysterectomy, provided the possibility of cancer or other anatomic abnormal-

ity is eliminated. Patients who have small submucous leiomyomas or polyps and whose overall uterine size does not warrant hysterectomy may undergo hysteroscopic resection of the lesion.

Patients who want to maintain childbearing potential and whose abnormal bleeding is due to leiomyomas can be treated with gonadotropin-releasing hormone (GnRH) analog therapy to shrink the leiomyoma before hysteroscopic or laparoscopic resection or laparotomy with myectomy. Patients who have completed childbearing and whose anatomic lesions are causing bleeding that does not respond to conservative therapy may undergo hysterectomy. When uterine, tubal, or ovarian cancer or cancer metastatic to these organs is the cause of abnormal uterine bleeding, hysterectomy is recommended.

Leiomyoma

Twenty-five percent of women in the reproductive years have uterine leiomyomas. Most tumors are asymptomatic, but some cause abnormal bleeding, pelvic pressure, and pain. Large leiomyomas can interfere with bladder and bowel function. Rare leiomyomas may contribute to abortion or premature labor.

Management

Risk for malignant degeneration is extremely low and is not an indication for surgical therapy. Myomectomy is indicated when the patient wants to maintain childbearing potential and a leiomyoma appears to be the cause of bleeding, pain, or loss of pregnancy. Preoperative administration of GnRH analog over a period of 2 to 3 months reduces overall uterine size and may facilitate endoscopic resection of leiomyomas or myomectomy at laparotomy. Hysterectomy may be indicated for asymptomatic leiomyomas when the uterus is larger than it would be at 12 to 14 weeks' gestation or when there is rapid growth of the leiomyoma, which suggests malignant disease. Hysterectomy may be indicated if the leiomyoma causes bleeding or pain despite conservative therapy.

Tubal Carcinoma

Tubal carcinoma accounts for a minute portion of malignant tumors of the female genital tract. Mean age at diagnosis is 55 years. Symptoms are watery vaginal discharge, uterine bleeding, and pelvic pain. There may be an adnexal mass.

Diagnosis

The diagnosis is rarely made preoperatively. The tumor is staged as if it were ovarian cancer (Table 106-1).

Management

Treatment is surgical. A peritoneal cytologic sample is obtained, and abdominal hysterectomy, bilateral salpingo-oophorectomy, selective periaortic lymphadenectomy, and partial omentectomy are performed. Postoperative radiation therapy or chemotherapy may be indicated.

Ascending Genital Infections

Mucopurulent Endocervicitis

Mucopurulent endocervicitis is caused by *C trachomatis, N gonorrhoeae,* or both. Diagnosis is based on the finding of yellow or green endocervical exudate on a white swab in association with cervical erythema, edema, and friability of the zone of ectopy. In pregnancy, mucopurulent cervicitis can contribute to premature delivery, post-partum endometritis, and infection in the neonate.

Pelvic Inflammatory Disease

Pelvic inflammatory disease (PID) involves the spread of microorganisms in the endocervix through the endometrial cavity to the fallopian tubes and into the peritoneal cavity. Ascent of bacteria may be caused by canalicular spread, spermatozoal transport of organisms, retrograde menstruation, douching, or iatrogenic manipulation during endometrial biopsy, hysterosalpingography, dilation and curettage, or insertion of an intrauterine device. The presence of bacterial vaginosis, a disorder of vaginal flora characterized by an overgrowth of anaerobic bacteria, may facilitate ascent of sexually transmitted and other aerobic pathogens. The microorganisms most often associated with PID are *N gonorrhoeae*, *C trachomatis*, and *Haemophilus influenzae*. The long-term consequences of PID include tubal factor infertility, ectopic pregnancy, and chronic pelvic pain.

Diagnosis. Criteria for the clinical diagnosis of PID are: lower abdominal pain, bilateral adnexal tenderness at bimanual pelvic examination, and vaginal leukorrhea (microscopy of a wet mount of vaginal contents revealing a large number of inflammatory cells).

Microscopic examination is used to exclude PID in a woman with abdominal pain. Adjunctive diagnostic criteria include leukocytosis, elevated C-reactive protein or erythrocyte sedimentation rate, temperature >38°C, or palpable adnexal complex. Endometrial biopsy revealing plasma cell endometritis is helpful in confirming the presence of upper genital tract inflammation. Laparoscopic findings include tubal hyperemia, edema, and a sticky exudate.

Management. Laparoscopy is recommended for patients with a questionable diagnosis or if antibiotic treatment fails. At laparoscopy, there appears to be therapeutic benefit to removal of free pus from the peritoneal cavity, drainage of pyosalpinx, and lysis of adhesions. Guidelines for the treatment of PID are given in Table 106-2.

Tuboovarian Abscess

Tuboovarian abscesses are the most severe form of PID. These lesions involve loculations of pus in and about the tubes, ovaries, and intestine.

Management. Most abscesses can be treated with antibiotics alone. If a patient in her reproductive years has a tuboovarian abscess at laparotomy, therapy is irrigation and drainage without extirpation of the adnexa in conjunction with broad-spectrum antibiotic therapy. Patients who do not respond to antibiotic therapy need laparotomy and drainage of the abscess or unilateral adnexectomy.

Toxic Shock Syndrome

Staphylococcal Toxic Shock Syndrome

The toxic shock syndrome (TSS) associated with *Staph aureus* infection is fever, diffuse or palmar erythroderma progressing to peripheral desquamation, mucous membrane hyperemia, vomiting, and diarrhea. Multiple organ system dysfunction with rapid progression to hypotension and shock occurs in severe instances. Menstrual TSS occurs in young (16 to 30 years) women who use highly absorbent tampons. Nonmenstrual causes are surgical wound infection, postpartum infection, and nonsurgical infection such as mastitis.

Table 106-2. *1993 CDC GUIDELINES FOR TREATMENT OF PID*

OUTPATIENT TREATMENT

Regimen A

Cefoxitin, 2 g IM, plus probenecid, 1 g PO concurrently, or ceftriaxone, 250 mg IM, or equivalent cephalosporin

plus

Doxycycline, 100 mg PO bid for 14 d

Regimen B

Ofloxacin, 400 mg PO bid for 14 d

plus

Either clindamycin, 450 mg PO qid, or metronidazole, 500 mg PO bid for 14 d

INPATIENT TREATMENT

Regimen A

Cefoxitin, 2 g IV q6h, or cefotetan,* 2 g IV q12h

plus

Doxycycline, 100 mg q12h PO or IV

Regimen B

Clindamycin, 900 mg IV q8h

plus

Gentamicin, 2 mg/kg loading dose IV or IM, followed by a 1.5-mg/kg maintenance dose q8h

NOTE

One of the above regimens is given for at least 48 hr after the patient clinically improves.

After discharge from the hospital, continue doxycycline, 100 mg PO bid for a total of 14 d, or clindamycin, 450 mg PO qid for a total of 14 d.

---

* Other cephalosporins that provide adequate gonococcal, other facultative gram-negative aerobic, and anaerobic coverage—such as ceftizoxime, cefotaxime, and ceftriaxone—may be used in appropriate doses.

Reproduced from Centers for Disease Control. 1993 sexually transmitted diseases treatment guidelines. MMWR 1993;42:75.

Streptococcal TSS

The organism involved with streptococcal TSS is *S pyogenes*. Mucous membranes serve as the source of the microorganism without manifesting signs of a symptomatic infection. Tissue invasion occurs, and shock, multiorgan failure, and tissue destruction can ensue. Streptococcal TSS occurs in septic abortion, postpartum endomyometritis, necrotizing fasciitis, and postoperative infection. A rash is not a prominent presenting sign.

Clostridial TSS

TSS associated with *Clostridium sordellii* infection is characterized by sudden onset of weakness, nausea, and vomiting followed by progressive refractory hypotension with local and spreading edema. It is differentiated from staphylococcal TSS by the absence of *Staph aureus*, fever, and rash. Clostridial TSS occurs most commonly in patients with episiotomy infection, and is associated with postpartum infection, wound infection, vaginal foreign body, and degenerating cervical myoma. The pathogenesis involves production of edema-producing *Clostridium difficile*-like toxins by *C. sordellii*.

Diagnosis

Considerations during the physical examination of a patient who may have TSS include removal of tampons, sponges, or other foreign bodies from the vagina. Culture is performed on the mucous membranes (oropharynx, vagina), blood, focal lesions or sources (endometrium), and urine.

Management

All patients with TSS have an evolving clinical course that results in shock. Management involves physiologic support, broad-spectrum antimicrobial therapy, and sometimes surgical intervention. Once the diagnosis is clarified, specific antimicrobial treatment is initiated. Fluid replacement to correct hypotension and physiologic monitoring in an intensive care unit are required. Immunoglobulin therapy may be possible.

OVARY

Characteristics of benign versus malignant ovarian neoplasms are listed in Table 106-3. Ultrasonography (US), computed tomography (CT), or magnetic resonance imaging (MRI) can be used to determine the characteristics of ovarian neoplasms. For women in the reproductive years, asymptomatic unilateral, unilocular ovarian cysts <10 cm in diameter are observed for 6 to 8 weeks for resolution. In postmenopausal women, asymptomatic unilateral, unilocular ovarian cysts <5 cm in diameter are rarely malignant. Complex (septa, internal papillations, or solid components) or solid ovarian enlargements at any age are likely to be malignant and necessitate prompt investigation. An algorithm for the management of adnexal masses is shown in Fig. 106-2.

Benign Neoplasms of the Ovary

Physiologic Cysts

Follicular and corpus luteum cysts are common among women of reproductive age. Because oral contraceptives suppress ovulation, these cysts should not develop in pa-

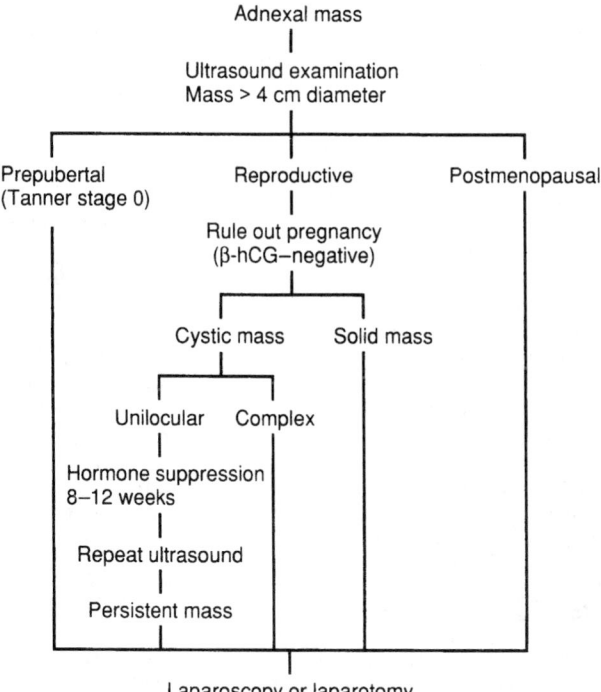

Figure 106-2. Management of adnexal mass.

tients taking oral contraceptives. If unilateral, unilocular cysts develop in women of reproductive age not taking oral contraceptives, contraceptives can be prescribed for two or three cycles to allow resolution of the cysts and prevent new cysts. Unilateral, unilocular cysts >10 cm in diameter are not likely to disappear and warrant a shorter period of observation.

Theca-Lutein Cysts

Theca-lutein cysts can develop during ovarian stimulation, gestational trophoblastic disease, or pregnancy. They are bilateral and complex and sometimes associated with ascites. They resolve with cessation of ovarian stimulation or termination of pregnancy.

Benign Cystic Teratomas

Benign cystic teratomas (dermoids) are common in the reproductive years. They can contain calcifications and are often bilateral. Pelvic radiographs, US, and CT are helpful in establishing a preoperative diagnosis. Ovarian cystectomy is performed to preserve ovarian function. If the teratoma is unilateral, the opposite ovary is inspected. If the second ovary is abnormal, a biopsy specimen is obtained. *Biopsy is not performed on a normal contralateral ovary.* Perimenopausal and postmenopausal women with cystic teratomas undergo bilateral oophorectomy.

Cystadenomas

Serous or mucinous cystadenomas are common, benign epithelial ovarian tumors. Therapy is cystectomy or oophorectomy. Intraoperative frozen section evaluation is important to determine whether the cysts contain malignant tissue. Postmenopausal women undergo hysterectomy and bilateral salpingo-oophorectomy.

Fibromas, Thecomas, Brenner Tumors

Fibromas, thecomas, and Brenner tumors of the ovary are indistinguishable at operation. They are differentiated on the basis of histologic findings. Most are benign. Ther-

Table 106-3. CHARACTERISTICS OF BENIGN VERSUS MALIGNANT OVARIAN TUMORS

Characteristic	Benign	Malignant
CLINICAL FINDINGS		
Unilateral	+++	+
Bilateral	+	+++
Cystic	+++	+
Solid	+	+++
Mobile	+++	+
Fixed	+	+++
Irregular	+	+++
Smooth	+++	+
Excrescences	−	+++
Ascites	+	+++
Cul-de-sac nodules	+	+++
Rapid growth rate	+	+++
SONOGRAPHIC FINDINGS		
Thick septa	+	+++
Internal solid parts	+	+++
Indefinite margins	+	+++
Ascites	+	+++
Matted loops of bowel	+	+++
CT FINDINGS		
Enlarged retroperitoneal nodes	−	+++
SERUM ASSAY FINDINGS		
Elevated CA-125	+	+++

(Shingleton HM, Hurt WG. Postreproductive gynecology. New York, Churchill Livingstone, 1990; modified from DiSaia PJ, Creasman WT. Clinical gynecologic oncology, ed 3. St Louis, CV Mosby, 1989)

apy is oophorectomy during the reproductive years or hysterectomy and bilateral salpingo-oophorectomy during the perimenopausal and postmenopausal years.

Endometriomas

Endometriosis most commonly involves the ovaries (half are bilateral); it can also involve the uterosacral ligaments, rectovaginal septum, sigmoid colon, lower genital tract, pelvic peritoneum, small intestine, bladder, and ureters. Endometriomas also may implant in laparotomy or episiotomy scars or more distant sites, such as umbilicus, pleura, or extremities.

During operations for endometriosis, every attempt is made to remove all evidence of disease. If ovarian tissue is preserved, postoperative progesterone, danazol, or GnRH analog therapy can be prescribed to suppress growth of residual implants. For extensive endometriosis, when childbearing is complete, and for perimenopausal and postmenopausal women, therapy for endometriosis is hysterectomy with bilateral salpingo-oophorectomy and hormone replacement therapy.

Ovarian Carcinoma

One in 70 women has ovarian cancer. Risk factors include: advanced age, decreased fertility, first-degree relative with ovarian, colon, breast, or endometrial cancer, Peutz-Jeghers syndrome, and Turner syndrome with XO/XY mosaicism.

Although ovarian cancer can occur at any age, germ cell tumors are more common among adolescents, and epithelial tumors are more common among postmenopausal women. The older the patient, the more likely she is to have advanced disease.

Diagnosis

Ovarian cancer presents with abdominal swelling, pain, gastrointestinal symptoms, and an adnexal mass. Evaluation consists of a hemogram, serum chemistries, and assessment of tumor antigens, including CA-125, α-fetoprotein, and the β-subunit of hCG. CA-125 is more likely to be elevated with epithelial ovarian tumors; β-hCG with malignant teratomas, choriocarcinomas, and embryonal carcinomas; and α-fetoprotein with endodermal sinus tumors and embryonal carcinomas. These tumor markers are more helpful in detecting persistent or recurrent disease than in establishing a preoperative diagnosis. Abdominal CT, intravenous urography, radiographic evaluation of the upper and lower gastrointestinal tracts, and proctosigmoidoscopy may be performed. The diagnosis of type of malignant tumors of the ovary depends on histologic evaluation.

Management

Surgical therapy for malignant tumors of the ovary includes abdominal hysterectomy, bilateral salpingo-oophorectomy, partial omentectomy, selective periaortic and pelvic lymphadenectomy, and tumor cytoreduction. FIGO recommends surgical staging of ovarian cancer (Table 106-1). Staging of epithelial cancers is mandatory. For adolescents and women of reproductive age, it may be possible to preserve childbearing potential if the malignant disease is limited to one ovary. Patients treated in this manner are observed closely and can benefit from abdominal hysterectomy with removal of the remaining ovary after childbearing is complete.

The need for intraoperative instillation of radioactive substances, postoperative chemotherapy, or radiation therapy is individualized according to histologic diagnosis and grade of tumor, stage of disease, and overall condition and prognosis.

Therapy for advanced-stage malignant tumors of the ovary is removal of the uterus, tubes, ovaries, and omentum and cytoreduction (tumor debulking) of as much of the disease as is reasonable. Cytoreductive surgical therapy improves response to chemo- and radiation therapy.

PREGNANCY-RELATED CONDITIONS

Abortion

Fifteen percent of pregnancies end in spontaneous abortion. Abortion can be caused by maternal or fetal factors, but most are due to chromosomal abnormalities in the fetus.

Diagnosis

Vaginal bleeding and lower abdominal cramping are the most common symptoms of abortion.

Management

Therapy for uterine bleeding without cervical dilatation (threatened abortion) is expectant. Quantitative β-hCG determinations and US examinations are used to determine the course of the pregnancy. If the cervix is dilated or the patient gives a history of passage of tissue, incomplete abortion probably has occurred, and uterine suction curettage is needed to prevent further bleeding and infection. US can help confirm the absence of a viable pregnancy in these patients.

Ectopic Pregnancy

Factors contributing to ectopic pregnancy include PID, infertility treatments (tubal operation, ovulation induction), and use of intrauterine contraceptive devices.

Diagnosis

All women with lower abdominal pain and irregular or absent menstrual periods are examined for possible ectopic pregnancy. Ectopic pregnancy is associated with abnormally rising serum β-hCG levels and inability to detect an intrauterine gestational sac or fetus with US.

Management

An algorithm for the management of ectopic pregnancies is presented in Fig. 106-3. Some small, uncomplicated, unruptured ectopic pregnancies can be managed with medical therapy (methotrexate). Most tubal ectopic pregnancies are diagnosed and managed with salpingostomy or salpingectomy by means of laparoscopy or minilaparotomy. Laparotomy is reserved for patients whose condition is hemodynamically unstable or who have advanced pregnancies. Patients who want to maintain childbearing potential undergo the most conservative procedure that allows removal of the ectopic pregnancy and preserves the integrity of the fallopian tubes.

Gestational Trophoblastic Neoplasia

Gestational trophoblastic neoplasia is a spectrum of pregnancy-related tumors that includes hydatidiform mole, invasive mole, and choriocarcinoma. These tumors appear to be the result of abnormal fertilization. They are derived exclusively from fetal tissue, cytotrophoblast, and syncytiotrophoblast but can invade maternal tissues and secrete hCG.

Invasive disease (invasive mole or choriocarcinoma) can follow any gestational event/hydatidiform mole, delivery

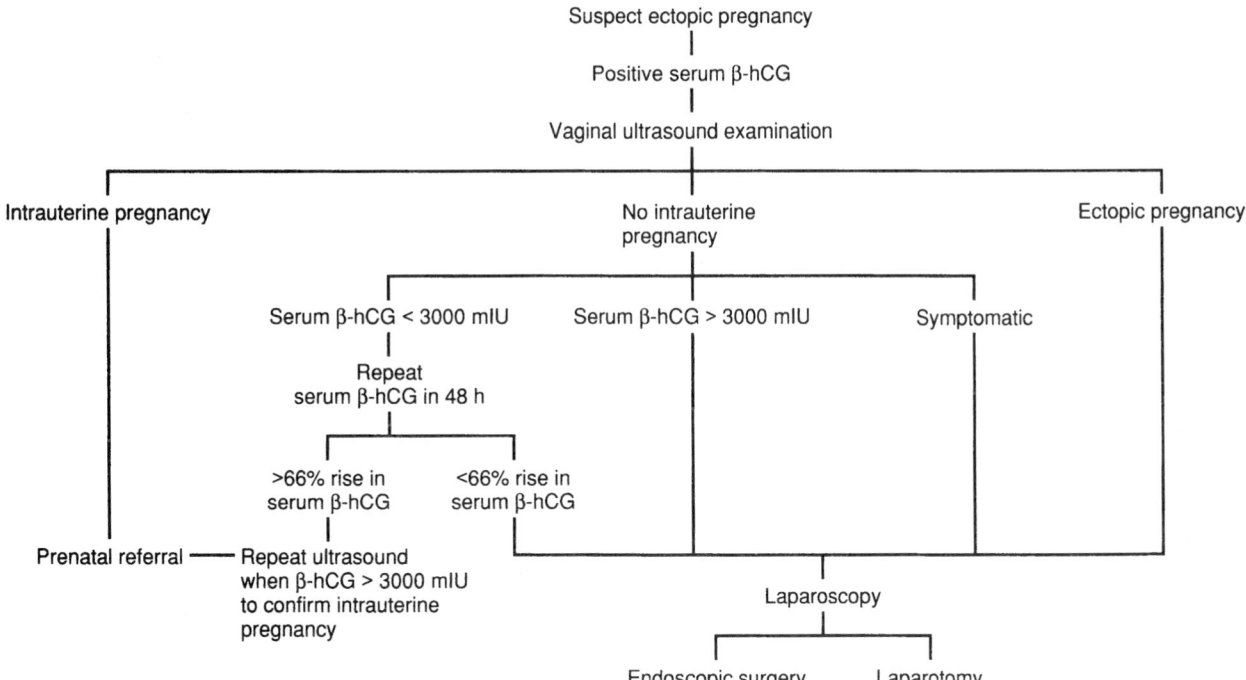

Figure 106-3. Management of suspected ectopic pregnancy. The level of serum β-hCG at which intrauterine pregnancy is detected by vaginal ultrasound examination can vary according to institution.

of intrauterine pregnancy, abortion, or ectopic pregnancy. It can be localized to the uterus or metastasize throughout the body. FIGO recommends clinical staging of invasive gestational trophoblastic neoplasia (Table 106-1).

Diagnosis

Clinical findings are irregular uterine bleeding and a uterus that is larger than expected for gestational age but contains no fetus. Pretreatment evaluation includes hemogram, serum chemistries, quantitative serum β-hCG measurement, chest radiograph, pelvic US, and CT of head, abdomen, and pelvis to document metastases. Histologic diagnosis is not required when the patient has an elevated β-hCG and no evidence of gestation.

Management

Therapy for *noninvasive disease* (hydatidiform mole) is suction curettage. Abdominal hysterectomy is an option only if childbearing is complete. Follow-up care includes weekly serum β-hCG determinations until the level stays within normal levels then monthly measurements for 6 months. During this follow-up period, strict contraception (use of oral contraceptives) is advised. Therapy for persistent or recurrent noninvasive disease is single-agent chemotherapy (methotrexate or actinomycin D).

Therapy for *Stage I* disease is single-agent chemotherapy (methotrexate or actinomycin D) or combination chemotherapy for resistant disease (etoposide, methotrexate, actinomycin D, cyclophosphamide, vincristine). Therapy for

Stage II, III, and IV disease is combination chemotherapy and whole-brain radiation therapy for metastasis to the brain. Systematic follow-up care includes weekly quantitative serum β-hCG determinations until normal for 3 consecutive weeks, then monthly determinations for 12 to 24 months. During this follow-up period, strict contraception is advised. Resistant disease may necessitate combination chemotherapy and, rarely, surgical resection of localized disease (uterine, pulmonary, hepatic, brain).

SUGGESTED READING

Centers for Disease Control. 1993 sexually transmitted diseases treatment guidelines. MMWR 1993;42:75.

DiSaia PJ, Creasman WT. Clinical gynecologic oncology, ed 4. St Louis, CV Mosby, 1993.

Holmes KK, Mardh PA, Sparling PF, et al. Sexually transmitted diseases, ed 2. New York, McGraw-Hill, 1990.

Olt G, Berchuck A, Bast RC Jr. The role of tumor markers in gynecologic oncology. Obstet Gynecol Surv 1990;45:570.

Pastorek JG. Obstetric and gynecologic infectious disease. New York, Raven, 1994.

Shingleton HM, Hurt WG. Postreproductive gynecology. New York, Churchill Livingstone, 1990.

Soper DE, Brockwell NJ, Dalton HP, Johnson D. Observations concerning the microbial etiology of acute salpingitis. Am J Obstet Gynecol 1994;170:1008.

Speroff L, Glass RH, Kase NG. Clinical gynecologic endocrinology and infertility, ed 5. Baltimore, Williams & Wilkins, 1994.

Sweet RL, Gibbs RS. Infectious diseases of the female genital tract, ed 2. Baltimore, Williams & Wilkins, 1990.

ESSENTIALS OF SURGERY: SCIENTIFIC PRINCIPLES AND PRACTICE,
edited by Lazar J. Greenfield, Michael W. Mulholland, Keith T. Oldham, Gerald B. Zelenock,
and Keith D. Lillemoe. Lippincott–Raven Publishers, Philadelphia, © 1997.

CHAPTER 107

CUTANEOUS NEOPLASMS

ALFRED E. CHANG, TIMOTHY M. JOHNSON,
AND RILEY S. REES

MELANOMA

Epidemiology and Etiology

Most patients with melanoma have a fair complexion and a tendency to sunburn rather than tan. Melanoma is rare among African Americans and Asian Americans, suggesting that skin pigment plays a protective role. The incidence of melanoma is subject to geographic and ethnic variation. Populations close to the equator have a high prevalence of melanoma. Increases in frequency of melanoma at different body sites are consistent with changes in clothing habits. The rising incidence of melanoma may be related to exposure to ultraviolet radiation (UVR) from sunlight.

A group at risk for melanoma are people with *dysplastic nevi*. Dysplastic nevi are acquired lesions of the skin that are usually larger than common nevi. Dysplastic nevi can appear anywhere on the body but are most common on the torso. Concentration on covered areas, such as buttocks, breasts, and scalp, is a distribution different from acquired nevi. Melanoma can originate within a preexisting dysplastic nevus or de novo. Dysplastic nevi occur in the general population (sporadic form) and in melanoma-prone families (familial form).

Congenital nevi also are associated with development of melanoma. These lesions are categorized as small (<1.5 cm diameter), medium (1.5 to 20 cm diameter), or large (>20 cm diameter). Almost all are small. Large congenital nevi are associated with a 5% to 20% lifetime risk for melanoma. It is unclear to what extent melanoma develops in small and medium congenital nevi.

Large congenital nevi vary greatly in size and occupy a large part of the body surface. Clinical features include a grossly irregular surface, increased pigmentation with shades of brown, and hypertrichosis. Management of large congenital nevi is individualized on the basis of technical difficulty, cosmetic factors, and risk for melanoma.

Genetics

Some cutaneous melanomas occur with a familial predisposition. An autosomal-dominant model of transmission with variable penetrance apparently is responsible for hereditary melanoma. Melanoma genesis may involve two or more genes as well as environmental factors. The chro-mosomes most commonly mutated in melanoma are 1, 6, 7, 9, and 10.

Clinical Diagnosis and Classification

Early detection by means of visual inspection leads to diagnosis and cure if attention is paid to the following clinical features:

1. Color. Brown or black lesions may contain shades of white, red, or blue. Shades of blue are the most ominous.
2. Angular notching at the perimeter of the lesion
3. Irregular elevations on the surface

Another indication of malignancy is enlargement, darkening, bleeding, or ulceration of a pigmented lesion. None of these clinical signs is pathognomonic. Any lesion with these characteristics is excised for biopsy.

Melanomas are classified into four categories on the basis of growth patterns and clinical characteristics: lentigo maligna melanomas, superficial spreading melanomas, nodular melanomas, and acral lentiginous melanomas.

Lentigo maligna melanomas are the least aggressive of the four types. They occur on the sun-exposed areas of the head and neck and the dorsum of the hands. The median age at diagnosis is 70 years, and most patients are women. The lesions are large (>3 cm diameter), flat, and tan with areas of dark brown or black pigmentation in some parts and areas of regression in others. There is radial growth of abnormal melanocytes in the epidermis with minimal invasion into the papillary dermis. This radial growth precedes vertical growth and invasion into the papillary dermis by many years. If only radial growth occurs, the lesion is lentigo maligna (Hutchinson freckle), not malignant melanoma. Vertical growth is associated with a focal area of elevation that may be darker or lighter than the surrounding lentigo maligna.

Superficial spreading melanomas account for most cutaneous melanomas and are of intermediate malignancy compared with other types. The lesions originate in a preexisting nevus. The peak incidence is the fifth decade of life, with equal distribution between the sexes. There are radial and vertical growth phases. The radial growth phase is characterized by the presence of melanoma tumor cells in the epidermis and papillary dermis and development of a raised, irregular surface on the skin. Vertical growth into the deeper layers of skin is associated with increasing nodularity of the lesion and greater potential for metastasis. Superficial spreading melanomas are characterized by variation in color, irregular borders, and irregular surface.

Nodular melanomas are the most aggressive of the four types of melanoma. Median age at diagnosis is 50 years, and the lesions occur twice as often among men as women. The lesions originate from uninvolved skin rather than a preexisting nevus. Nodular melanomas are bluish black, are more consistent in color than the other types, and have smooth borders. They are almost exclusively characterized by a vertical growth phase invading the deeper layers of

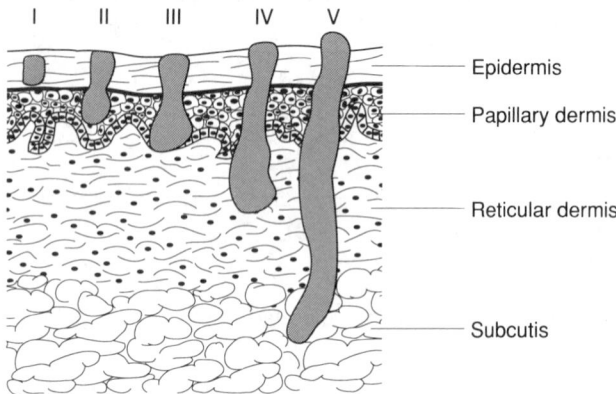

Figure 107-1. The Clark levels of invasion.

skin and often the subcutis. Lack of a radial growth phase can make early diagnosis difficult.

Acral lentiginous melanoma is a variant of melanoma that occurs on the palms and soles and in subungual locations. Acral lentiginous melanoma affects a small percentage of Caucasians with melanoma and a large percentage of dark-pigmented peoples (African Americasns, Hispanics, Asian Americans) with melanoma. Diagnosis usually is made in the sixth decade of life. These lesions are characterized by a radial growth phase, usually of long duration, followed by a nodular, vertical growth phase associated with metastatic potential. In the radial growth the lesion is flat with color variation. In subungual locations, lesions in this phase are irregular, tan-brown streaks in the nail that originate from the base of the nail bed. Most subungual melanomas involve the great toe or thumb, and they can be confused with subungual hematomas.

Staging and Prognostic Factors

Microstaging

Clark Level (Fig. 107-1).

- Level I—All tumor cells are confined to the epidermis with no invasion through the basement membrane (melanoma in situ)
- Level II—Tumor cells penetrate through the basement membrane into the papillary dermis but do not extend to the reticular dermis
- Level III—Tumor cells fill the papillary dermis and abut the reticular dermis but do not invade it
- Level IV—Tumor cells extend into the reticular dermis
- Level V—Tumor cells invade the subcutaneous tissues

Breslow Depth of Invasion. The primary tumor is classified according to thickness, measured with an ocular micrometer, from the top of the granular layer to the base of the tumor. There is an inverse correlation between tumor thickness and survival. Tumor thickness conveys more prognostic information than Clark level of invasion.

Regional Lymph Node Involvement

The presence of regional lymph node metastases is associated with poor prognosis. The more lymph nodes involved, the less likely is long-term survival.

Clinical and Pathologic Staging

The American Joint Committee on Cancer (AJCC) system classifies clinically localized melanomas according to thickness of the lesion (Table 107-1):

- Stage IA—<0.75 mm thick
- Stage IB—0.76 to 1.5 mm thick
- Stage IIA—1.51 to 4 mm thick
- Stage IIB—>4 mm thick
- Stage III—regional nodal involvement
- Stage IV—evidence of disseminated metastases

Clinically localized, thin lesions are AJCC stages IA and IB, intermediate-thickness lesions are AJCC stage IIA, and thick melanomas are AJCC stage IIB.

Prognostic Factors

Factors that allow prediction of survival in the AJCC system are tumor microstaging, nodal status, and presence of distant metastases. The anatomic location of melanomas also is a prognostic indicator (Table 107-2).

Women with melanomas have a better survival rate than men. The sex distribution of melanoma is summarized in Table 107-3. The presence of ulceration within a melanoma appears to be associated with poor prognosis. Men have a higher proportion of ulcerated lesions than women. Although ulceration appears to correlate with thickness of the melanoma, the presence of ulceration is an independent prognostic factor.

Histologic characteristics of localized melanomas can help establish prognosis. Melanomas are described according to growth phase. Lesions in the radial growth phase are nontumorigenic and associated with an excellent

Table 107-1. AMERICAN JOINT COMMISSION ON CANCER MELANOMA STAGING SYSTEM, 1985

TNM DEFINITIONS

Primary Tumor

TX	Unknown, cannot be assessed
T0	Atypical melanocytic hyperplasia in situ, Clark I
T1	Clark II, 0.75 mm or smaller
T2	Clark III, 0.76–1.5 mm
T3	Clark IV, 1.51–4 mm
T4	Clark V, larger than 4 mm or satellites within 2 cm of primary tumor

Regional Lymph Node Involvement

NX	Unknown, cannot be assessed
N0	Negative
N1	One regional node station, nodes mobile, 5 cm in diameter or smaller, or negative nodes and fewer than five in-transit metastases
N2	More than one node station positive, nodes larger than 5 cm or fixed, more than five in-transit metastases, or any metastases with positive nodes

Distant Metastasis

MX	Unknown, cannot be assessed
M0	None
M1	Skin or subcutaneous tissue beyond the primary nodal area
M2	Visceral

STAGE GROUPING

Stage IA	T1, N0, M0
Stage IB	T2, N0, M0
Stage IIA	T3, N0, M0
Stage IIB	T4, N0, M0
Stage III	Any T, N1, M0
Stage IV	Any T, N2, M0, or any T, any N, M1–2

Table 107-2. SURVIVAL OF AJC CLINICAL STAGE I AND II MELANOMA PATIENTS IN RELATION TO TUMOR LOCATION

Thickness (mm)	Survival Rate (%)*				
	Extremities	Hands or Feet	Head and Neck	Trunk†	BANS
<0.85	100	100	100	100	98
0.85–1.69	100	100	100	97	78
1.7–3.64	86	60	64	77	58
≥3.65	83	0	65	12	33

BANS, upper back, posterolateral arm, posterior and lateral neck, and posterior scalp.
* 7.5-year acturial survival rates of 598 AJC clinical stage I and II patients. (Day CL, Mihm MC, Lew RA, et al. Cutaneous malignant melanoma: prognostic guidelines for physicians and patients. CA Cancer J Clin 1982;32:113.)
† Non-BANS truncal melanomas.

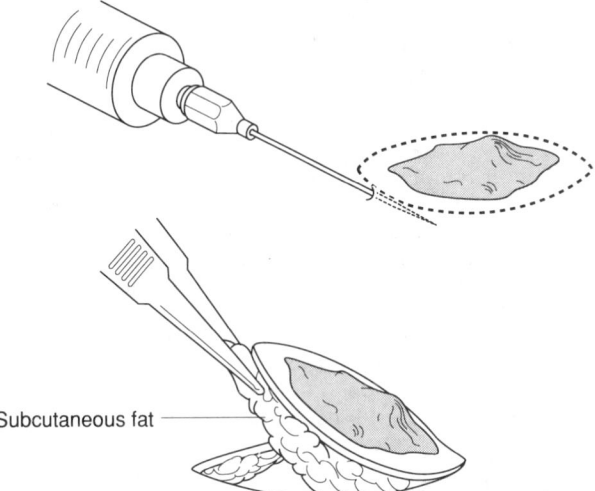

Figure 107-2. Techniques for biopsy of melanoma. (After Urist MM, Balch CM, Milton GW. Surgical management of primary melanoma. In: Balch CM, Milton GW, eds. Cutaneous melanoma. Philadelphia, JB Lippincott, 1985:74)

prognosis. Lesions with evidence of a vertical growth phase are likely to be tumorigenic. The vertical growth phase is the presence of larger aggregates of tumor cells within the papillary dermis, often markedly different in pigment from cells in the radial growth phase and associated with increased mitotic cells.

Therapy for Primary Melanoma

Biopsy

For melanoma, tumor thickness most accurately determines therapy and prognosis. A full-thickness biopsy to the adipose tissue is required for any lesion that may be melanoma. If a melanoma is transected with a partial-thickness shave biopsy, the ability to obtain an accurate measurement of tumor thickness is lost. *A superficial shave biopsy is never performed for a suspicious pigmented lesion.* Before biopsy, a morphologic description of the lesion is recorded, and a photograph is taken for complete documentation. A Wood lamp can be used to delineate subclinical pigment extension.

Excisional biopsy (Fig. 107-2) with 1 to 2 mm margins is performed to provide a total specimen for histologic interpretation and microstaging. Permanent sections are used for diagnosis; frozen sections are not used in the microstaging of primary melanoma. If the lesion is a melanoma, excisional biopsy is the first stage of a two-stage procedure. The second stage is reexcision to the underlying muscle fascia with 0.5 to 3 cm margins, depending on tumor thickness.

For lesions too large for complete excision and those situated where the amount of skin is critical for functional or cosmetic results, an *incisional biopsy* may be performed with a scalpel or punch tool 4 to 6 mm in diameter. Incisional biopsies for melanoma do not increase risk for metastasis or affect patient survival. They are performed on the most raised or most pigmented area of the lesion. Several punch biopsy specimens can be obtained from different areas of lesions with multiple morphologic features.

Excisional or incisional saucerization biopsy can be used for melanoma. One disadvantage of saucerization biopsy is risk for bacterial colonization in the wound during healing.

Surgical Excision of Primary Melanoma

For melanoma in situ, excision of normal skin 0.5 cm around the lesion or biopsy site is acceptable for local control. For invasive cutaneous melanoma, wide excision of the primary tumor or biopsy site is advocated for optimal local control.

Risk for local recurrence correlates more with thickness of melanoma than with margin of excision. Local recurrence after excision of melanomas <1 mm thick is rare regardless of the margin. Excision margins of 1 cm provide excellent local control for lesions <1 mm thick; 2-cm margins are sufficient for intermediate-thickness lesions. For lesions >4 mm thick, excision margins of at least 3 cm are needed (Table 107-4).

Site of the melanoma can affect extent of excision. Facial lesions cannot be excised if the margin is >1 cm. Therapy for subungual melanomas always is amputation, usually at the metatarsophalangeal or metacarpophalangeal joint.

Table 107-3. DISTRIBUTION OF MELANOMAS WITH RESPECT TO GENDER

Location	Occurrence (%)	
	Men	Women
Scalp	7	3
Face	12	9
Neck	5	3
Arm	13	19
Front of body	16	8
Back of body	36	23
Leg	9	31
Sole of foot	2	4

Table 107-4. SURGICAL MARGINS FOR MELANOMA EXCISIONS

Melanoma Thickness (mm)	Margin (cm)
In situ	0.5
<1	1
1–4	2
>4	3

Management of Regional Metastatic Melanoma

Lymphadenectomy

Surgical excision of metastases to regional lymph nodes is the only potentially curative therapy. For patients not cured with lymphadenectomy, resection can avoid pain associated with tumor enlargement, skin breakdown, and tumor necrosis. Most patients who seek treatment because of melanoma have localized disease; only a small percentage have clinical evidence of nodal metastases; and an even smaller percentage have distant metastases. Rarely is a diagnosis of melanoma made in the absence of a definable primary lesion. Surgical excision of clinically positive lymph nodes is *therapeutic lymph node dissection.* This elective lymph node dissection (ELND) is one of the most controversial procedures in surgical oncology.

Site-Specific Considerations

The nodal drainage areas accessible for surgical excision include ilioinguinal, axillary, cervical, and parotid regions. With truncal melanomas, or if the tumor is located in the midline, the primary nodal drainage may not be obvious. Lymphatic vessels from the upper half of the body drain to the axilla, and those from the lower half of the torso drain into the inguinal region. Some melanomas of the upper torso drain to the supraclavicular region.

Two contiguous, node-bearing regions exist in the ilioinguinal area. The first is composed of the superficial femoral nodes within the femoral triangle; the second contains the deep nodes above the inguinal ligament along the iliac and obturator vessels. Removal of the femoral nodes is superficial groin dissection, and removal of the iliac and obturator nodes is deep groin dissection (Fig. 107-3). The iliac and obturator nodes can be removed during superficial groin dissection.

Axillary dissection includes removal of lymph nodes lateral, beneath, and medial to the pectoralis minor muscle. The axillary lymph node region is contiguous with the supraclavicular node region. Evidence of supraclavicular nodal involvement is not uncommon if bulky axillary disease is present. There is no satisfactory procedure to remove contiguous involved axillary and supraclavicular lymph nodes. In these situations, axillary dissection is considered only for palliation.

Melanomas originating on the scalp or face anterior to the pinna of the ear and superior to the commissure of the lip metastasize to the parotid region. Lesions inferior to the commissure of the lip spread to the cervical region. Melanomas on the posterior scalp behind the pinna usually spread to occipital and posterior cervical lymph nodes. Radical neck dissection to remove the cervical nodes is performed in combination with a superficial parotid node dissection for anterior facial melanomas.

Adjuvant Therapy

Patients who undergo lymphadenectomy for AJCC stage III disease are at high risk for recurrent disease. No effective adjuvant therapy exists to treat these patients or those who undergo surgical excision for localized deep melanomas. Interferon-α and tumor vaccines are being investigated.

Management of Disseminated Melanoma

Follow-up care for patients with AJCC stage I, II, or III melanoma rendered tumor-free with surgical treatment includes regular interviews and physical examinations. Yearly chest radiographs and liver function studies may

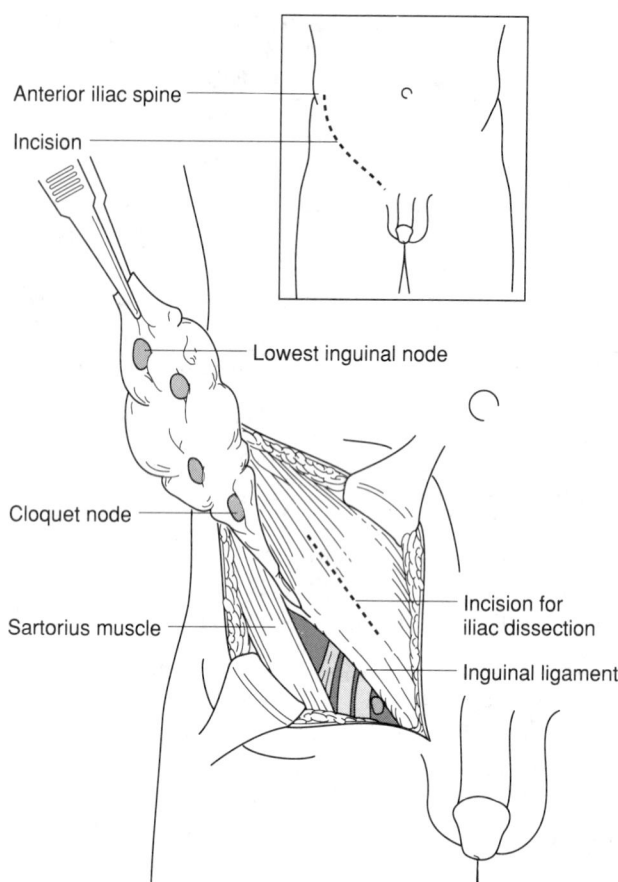

Figure 107-3. Technique of groin dissection.

be used to evaluate visceral disease. Lactic dehydrogenase levels are checked. Attention is directed at any gastrointestinal (GI) or central nervous system symptoms.

Melanoma can disseminate to any organ. The most common sites of recurrence are skin, subcutaneous tissues, distant lymph nodes, and visceral sites. Common visceral sites of metastasis are lung, liver, brain, bone, and GI tract. Most patients who die with disseminated disease have multiple organ involvement. The cause of death is respiratory failure or brain complications.

Surgical excision of recurrent melanoma can be used as palliation for patients with isolated recurrences in the skin, central nervous system, lung, or GI tract. Surgical excision of solitary brain metastases provides palliation and better quality of life than brain irradiation. Resection of isolated pulmonary metastases or subcutaneous recurrences is not considered curative but can lengthen disease-free survival. GI lesions causing obstruction or bleeding are managed with resection or bypass to relieve these symptoms.

Melanoma may respond to *radiation therapy.* Radiation therapy also is used for palliation of bone pain due to metastatic disease or brain metastasis.

Melanoma is responsive to few *chemotherapeutic drugs.* The agents tried are DTIC and the nitrosoureas.

Melanoma may be responsive to *immunotherapy* with interleukin-2 (IL-2), tumor vaccine, or monoclonal antibodies. *Gene therapy* is under investigation.

NONMELANOMA SKIN TUMORS

Nonmelanoma basal (BCC) and squamous cell (SCC) carcinomas are the most common types of malignant tumors. The tumors are mainly of epithelial origin. Etiologic factors for BCC and SCC are: chronic exposure to UVR, light complexion, exposure to chemical carcinogens, human papillomavirus (HPV) infection, chronic radiodermatitis, trauma, and chronic scarring disorders, such as lupus erythematosus.

Basal Cell Carcinoma

BCC is the most common form of skin cancer. These epithelial-derived tumors are classified according to clinical appearance, histologic pattern, and biologic behavior. Although BCCs rarely metastasize, they are characterized by slow but relentless and destructive local invasion that results in high morbidity without treatment. Subclinical local invasion may be deep, extensive, and asymmetric with finger-like extensions several centimeters beyond the clinical borders.

The most common type of BCC is the *ulcerative,* well-circumscribed nodular variety. These tumors often present as pearly papules or nodules with telangiectasia. They may be pruritic and sometimes bleed. With time, the center ulcerates to produce peripheral rolled borders (rodent ulcers). Some lesions are deeply pigmented and nodular and can be confused with melanoma. The histologic features of these BCCs are isolated areas of basaloid tumor islands originating from the epidermis with peripheral palisading of nuclei and stromal retraction. Sometimes BCC has histologic features of squamous metaplasia with keratinization. These tumors have basosquamous differentiation and can become aggressive and develop regional lymphatic spread.

Most difficult to treat with surgical excision is BCC with an *aggressive growth pattern* (morpheaform, sclerosing, or fibrosing BCC). These tumors are flat and scarlike. They are likely to recur because isolated, finger-like fronds of basal cell tumor cells may deeply invade surrounding structures well beyond the margins of the lesion.

Superficial BCCs are scaly, pink to red lesions. They often are confused with psoriasis or other eczematous, scaly conditions.

Squamous Cell Carcinoma

SCC is the second most common form of skin cancer. It is derived from epithelial keratinocytes. The tumors can deeply invade surrounding structures or metastasize to regional lymph nodes, so they must be recognized and treated aggressively. Precursor lesions to invasive SCC include actinic keratoses and Bowen disease. SCC begins as an erythematous papulonodule with overlying keratotic crust or ulceration. The lesions can progress to ulceration with surrounding erythema with or without a keratotic center. SCC shows malignant degeneration of epithelial cells with differentiation toward keratin formation.

Ulcerative SCC is an aggressive malignant skin tumor that has central ulceration and raised borders. These tumors can originate in actinic damaged skin, solar keratoses, cutaneous horns, burn scars, or chronic wounds. The lesions infiltrate widely and can spread to regional lymphatic vessels. On the head and neck, they metastasize to the periparotid, jugular digastric, or midjugular lymph nodes. If these tumors spread to the regional lymph nodes, the prognosis is poor. Tumors that originate in chronic wounds or burn scars exhibit particularly aggressive behavior.

Factors that determine high risk for local recurrence, extensive subclinical invasion, and metastasis include: diameter >2 cm, invasion to or below the reticular dermis, poorly differentiated histologic pattern, rapid growth, origin (scar, radiation, chronic ulcer, sinus tract), anatomic site (central face, ear, lip, embryonic fusion planes), host immunosuppression, neurotropism, and recurrence after previous treatment.

Other Tumors

Hundreds of cutaneous tumors exist. Three tumors in the differential diagnosis of BCC are Merkel cell carcinoma, microcystic adnexal carcinoma, and sebaceous gland carcinoma.

Merkel cell carcinoma is a malignant neuroendocrine tumor with features of epithelial differentiation. Merkel cell carcinoma is biologically aggressive and carries high risk for local recurrence and regional and systemic metastasis. Merkel cell carcinoma is a red to purple papulonodule or indurated plaque. Tumors originate on the head and neck, extremities, and torso. Merkel cell carcinoma is a small cell tumor with characteristic positive immunocytochemical staining for neuron-specific enolase, cytokeratin, and neurofilament protein. A chest radiograph is indicated to rule out metastatic oat cell carcinoma, which may be similar in clinical and histologic appearance. Treatment is wide local excision with adjuvant radiation to the primary site and the draining nodal groups. Frequent follow-up examinations for local, regional, or distant recurrence are warranted.

Microcystic adnexal carcinoma is a rare cutaneous neoplasm with follicular and eccrine differentiation characterized by invasive, relentless, and destructive local growth. Risk for neurotropism and local recurrence is high. Microcystic adnexal carcinoma occurs primarily on the head and neck as a slowly enlarging, white to pink papuloplaque. Local invasion through the underlying muscle is common. The use of Mohs excision combined with permanent horizontal sectioning from the final normal Mohs specimens offers the greatest likelihood of cure.

Sebaceous gland carcinoma is a rare malignant tumor derived from adnexal epitheliumof sebaceous glands. The tumor can originate on ocular or extraocular sites. It usually presents as a yellowish to pink, slowly growing papulonodule on the eyelid. Local recurrence after surgical excision is frequent. Adjuvant radiation therapy is beneficial.

Surgical Treatment of Nonmelanoma Skin Cancers

A skin biopsy must be performed before any treatment of skin cancer. Most nonmelanoma skin cancers respond to curettage and electrodesiccation, cryosurgery, radiation therapy, or surgical resection. Many skin cancers can be removed with elliptical excisions that follow skin tension lines. Curettage before excision is often helpful to delineate subclinical tumor extension for BCC and SCC. Margins for low-risk SCC are 0.5 to 1 cm. Margins for low-risk BCC are 0.3 to 0.5 cm.

Mohs excision may be used to manage BCCs and SCCs

Table 107-5. RECONSTRUCTION AFTER SURGICAL EXCISION OF SKIN CANCER

Location	Type of Reconstruction
Face	Full-thickness skin grafts, local skin flaps
Nose, eyelid	Full-thickness skin grafts from preauricular area, retroauricular area, or neck
Torso, limbs	Skin grafts, skin flaps
Hand	Cross-finger flaps, groin flaps, reverse radial forearm flaps, or free tissue transfer

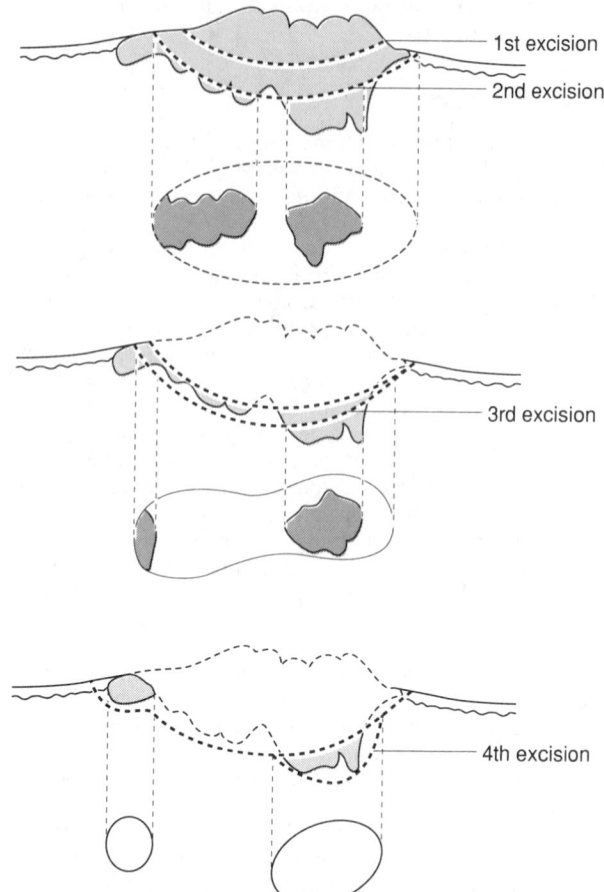

Figure 107-4. Mohs micrographic surgical technique.

Mohs Micrographic Excision

Mohs micrographic excision is used for management of high-risk nonmelanoma skin cancers. It is performed under local anesthesia as an outpatient procedure. After removal of all gross tumor, a thin layer of tissue is excised. The tissue is mapped, color-coded for orientation, and subjected to frozen-section processing. The specimen is flexible and flattened, with the beveled peripheral skin edge placed in the same horizontal plane with the deep margin. In this plane, the deep and peripheral margins are examined in one horizontal cut by means of frozen-section analysis with total margin control. After histologic interpretation of the frozen-section specimens, the precise anatomic location of any residual tumor can be identified. The process is repeated until all margins are tumor-free (Fig. 107-4). Soft tissue reconstruction is performed the same day.

Mohs excision is performed for nonmelanomas with a high risk for recurrence after conventional therapy and tumors for which conservation of normal tissue is important. Risk factors for recurrence after conventional therapy are: recurrent tumor, diameter >2 cm, location on the central face, eyelid, or ear, aggressive histologic growth pattern of BCC, poorly differentiated SCC, microcystic adnexal carcinoma, dermatofibroma sarcoma protuberans, tumor with poorly defined clinical margins, neurotropism, immunosuppressed patient with SCC, tumor in site of radiation, and incompletely excised tumor.

Tumors for which maximal conservation of tissue may be important include tumors on the eyelid, nose, ear, lip, digit, or genitalia and tumors of young patients.

Adjuvant Radiation Therapy

Radiation therapy may be used for primary management of small, low-risk nonmelanoma skin cancers. For cutaneous SCC with many risk factors and for those with extensive neurotropism, adjuvant prophylactic radiation therapy to the primary site and the primary draining lymph nodes may decrease risk for local recurrence and regional nodal metastasis. Prophylactic adjuvant radiation therapy is considered for highly aggressive, deeply invasive BCC that exhibits extensive neurotropism.

that exhibit high risk. If Mohs excision is not available, excision is performed with careful frozen-section control with permanent-section confirmation.

Regional lymphadenectomy is performed if clinically positive nodes are evident.

Reconstructive therapy for skin cancer is complex because of the sites involved (Table 107-5). Split-thickness grafts are used only for massive defects when prognosis or functional class is poor. For very high-risk nonmelanoma skin cancers, split-thickness skin grafting may be necessary to monitor tumor recurrence. Definitive reconstruction can be performed later.

SUGGESTED READING

Balch CM, Urist MM, Karakousis CP, et al. Efficacy of 2 cm surgical margins for intermediate thickness melanomas (1 to 4 mm): results of a multi-institutional randomized surgical trial. Ann Surg 1993;218:262.

Cox AL, Skipper J, Chen Y, et al. Identification of a peptide recognized by five melanoma-specific human cytotoxic T cell lines. Science 1994;264:716.

Hieken TJ, Rauth S, Ronan SG, et al. Hereditary melanoma. Surg Oncol Clin North Am 1994;3:563.

Johnson TM, Rowe DE, Nelson BR, et al. Squamous cell carcinoma of the skin (excluding lip and oral mucosa). J Am Acad Dermatol 1992;26:467.

Johnson TM, Tromovich TA, Swanson NA. Combined curettage and excision: a treatment for primary basal cell carcinoma. J Am Acad Dermatol 1991;24:613.

Lienard D, Ewalenko P, Delmotte J-J, et al. High-dose recombinant tumor necrosis factor alpha in combination with interferon gamma and melphalan in isolation perfusion of the limbs for melanoma and sarcoma. J Clin Oncol 1992;10:52.

Miller AR, McBride WH, Hunt K, et al. Cytokine-mediated gene therapy for cancer. Ann Surg Oncol 1994;1:436.

Rosenberg SA, Yannelli JR, Yang JC, et al. Treatment of patients with metastatic melanoma with autologous tumor-infiltrating lymphocytes and interleukin 2. J Natl Cancer Inst 1994;86:1159.

Smith SP, Foley EH, Grande PJ. Use of Mohs surgery to establish quantitative proof of heightened tumor spread in basal cell carcinoma recurrent following radiotherapy. J Dermatol Surg Oncol 1990;16:1012.

Trent JM, Meyskens FL, Salmon SE, et al. Relation of cytogenetic abnormalities and clinical outcome in metastatic melanoma. N Engl J Med 1990;322:1508.

ESSENTIALS OF SURGERY: SCIENTIFIC PRINCIPLES AND PRACTICE,
edited by Lazar J. Greenfield, Michael W. Mulholland, Keith T. Oldham, Gerald B. Zelenock,
and Keith D. Lillemoe. Lippincott–Raven Publishers, Philadelphia, © 1997.

CHAPTER 108

SARCOMAS OF BONE AND SOFT TISSUE

VERNON K. SONDAK

Sarcomas originate from mesoderm-derived elements— bone, cartilage, connective tissue, fat, and muscle. Sarcomas behave in a similar way wherever they originate. However, the site of origin of sarcoma does affect treatment and outcome.

EPIDEMIOLOGY

Sarcomas occur among all age groups. Most patients with sarcoma have no identifiable predisposing factor, genetic or environmental. Traumatic injury does not seem to predispose to sarcoma. All patients with soft tissue or bony tumors are asked about trauma because malignant disease must be differentiated from benign posttraumatic lesions.

Sarcoma is connected with the following conditions:

- Radiation exposure—therapeutic (Fig. 108-1) or occupational
- Exposure to chemicals, such as arsenic and vinyl chloride
- Exposure to herbicides containing dioxin
- Human immunodeficiency virus (HIV-1) infection (Kaposi sarcoma)
- Long-standing lymphedema of an extremity
- Neurofibromatosis type 1 (von Recklinghausen disease)
- Retinoblastoma
- Li-Fraumeni syndrome

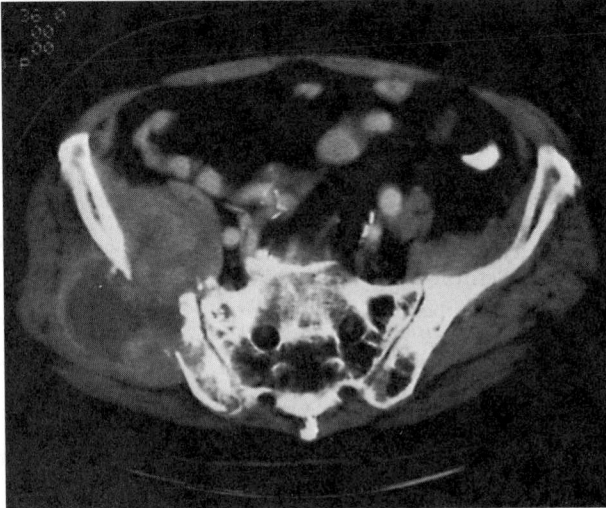

Figure 108-1. Osteosarcoma of the iliac bone that occurred 7 years after radiation therapy for cancer of the prostate and 30 years after radiation therapy for testicular cancer. The lesion was unresectable and associated with severe pain and lower extremity edema. The patient received significant palliation from two courses of intraarterial doxorubicin, after which the blood supply to the tumor was occluded by transcatheter embolization.

PATHOLOGIC CLASSIFICATION

Sarcomas are classified according to type of tissue formed by the tumor (histogenic classification) rather than type of tissue in which the tumor originates. A malignant tumor originating within skeletal muscle but composed of malignant smooth muscle cells is a *leiomyosarcoma*, not a rhabdomyosarcoma. Bone tumors are not called osteosarcomas unless the malignant cells clearly produce osteoid. Some bone tumors produce cartilage (*chondrosarcoma*); a few are *fibrosarcoma* or another histologic type. Some soft tissue neoplasms produce bone or cartilage (*extraosseous osteosarcoma* or *chondrosarcoma*). Table 108-1 lists the types of benign and malignant soft tissue tumors. Table 108-2 lists the relative frequency of the sarcomas.

Histologic type is not as important in prognosis and therapy as histologic grade. Histologic grade is based on degree of cellular atypia, frequency of mitotic figures, and presence or absence of spontaneous tumor necrosis:

- *Low-grade*—little cellular atypia, few mitoses, no tumor necrosis
- *Intermediate-grade*—atypia, numerous mitoses, little or no tumor necrosis
- *High-grade*—necrosis in addition to atypia and frequent mitotic figures

Cytogenetic aberrations occur in a number of soft tissue sarcomas, and some of these may be specific for certain histologic types. For example, the *MDR1* (multidrug-resistance) gene is present in more untreated sarcomas than other tumor types. Presence of this gene correlates with resistance to a number of cytotoxic drugs, many of which are routinely used in sarcoma chemotherapy.

DIAGNOSIS AND STAGING OF SOFT TISSUE SARCOMAS

Delays before definitive diagnosis are common among patients with sarcoma. Many patients undergo prolonged treatment for chronic hematomas or pulled muscles. If a soft tissue mass appears with no history of trauma or persists beyond 6 weeks after local trauma, biopsy is performed.

Soft tissue sarcoma of the extremity, trunk, head, and neck presents as a painless mass. Retroperitoneal sarcomas present as a palpable mass in association with abdominal fullness, early satiety, or vague abdominal pain. Biopsy is performed for all soft tissue masses >5 cm and for any new, enlarging, or symptomatic lesions. Small, subcutaneous lesions that have not changed for many years may be safely observed.

Biopsy

Excisional biopsy is performed on small soft tissue masses (<3 to 5 cm in greatest diameter). With these lesions risk for malignancy is low, and complete excision does not jeopardize treatment in the event a sarcoma is found. For all other soft tissue masses, incisional biopsy is performed (Fig. 108-2).

Fine-needle aspiration cytologic examination is used in the diagnosis of some soft tissue lesions. Computed tomography (CT)-guided fine-needle aspiration is helpful in the diagnosis of intra-abdominal and retroperitoneal tumors, but is rarely needed for extremity sarcomas. Fine-needle aspiration minimizes risk for tumor spillage in the peritoneal cavity that can accompany open surgical biopsy of a retroperitoneal sarcoma.

Table 108-1. HISTOGENIC CLASSIFICATION SCHEME FOR BENIGN AND MALIGNANT SOFT TISSUE TUMORS

Tissue Formed (Histogenesis)	Benign Soft Tissue Tumor	Malignant Soft Tissue Tumor
Fat	Lipoma	Liposarcoma
Fibrous tissue	Fibroma	Fibrosarcoma
Skeletal muscle	Rhabdomyoma	Rhabdomyosarcoma
Smooth muscle	Leiomyoma	Leiomyosarcoma
Bone	Osteoma	Osteosarcoma
Cartilage	Chondroma	Chondrosarcoma
Synovium	Synovioma	Synovial sarcoma
Blood vessel	Hemangioma	Angiosarcoma; malignant hemangiopericytoma
Lymphatics	Lymphangioma	Lymphangiosarcoma
Nerve	Neurofibroma	Neurifibrosarcoma
Mesothelium	Benign mesothelioma	Malignant mesothelioma
Tissue histiocyte	Benign fibrous histiocytoma	Malignant fibrous histiocytoma
Pluripotent	None recognized	Malignant mesenchymoma
Uncertain	None recognized	Ewing sarcoma; alveolar soft parts sarcoma; epithelioid sarcoma

Staging and Metastatic Evaluation

Once the diagnosis of sarcoma is made, the extent of the primary tumor is assessed and the presence or absence of metastatic disease determined. Staging is based on clinical and histologic information (Table 108-3). After tumor grade, tumor size is next in prognostic importance. The larger the primary sarcoma, the greater is the risk for metastasis and death. Superficial tumors (entirely above the muscular fascia) have a more favorable prognosis than deep tumors. Diameter 5 cm, location deep to the fascia, and high histologic grade are unfavorable factors. Stage is based on number of unfavorable factors.

The initial evaluation must provide information about the extent of the primary tumor. CT or magnetic resonance imaging (MRI) is used. These studies allow definition of the primary tumor in relation to bone, muscle, neurovascular structures, and adjacent organs. This is critical information in treatment planning.

Plain radiographs and radionuclide bone scans provide information about invasion of bone by tumor (Fig. 108-3), but these studies are not important in the evaluation of a primary soft tissue sarcoma. Sarcomas have a characteristic arteriographic appearance, with prominent neovascularity and displacement of normal vessels. Angiography is rarely necessary for extremity lesions, but it may be helpful for retroperitoneal tumors. Magnetic resonance angiography also is helpful (Fig. 108-4).

Regional lymph node involvement is uncommon in soft tissue sarcomas. When node involvement occurs, it conveys essentially the same prognosis as distant metastatic disease and is classified as stage IV. Nearly all patients with nodal involvement have high-grade primary sarcomas (Fig. 108-5). The most common site of metastases is the lungs. All patients with newly diagnosed soft tissue sarcoma undergo chest radiography and CT to search for pulmonary metastases. For intra-abdominal or retroperitoneal tumors, CT includes the liver.

MANAGEMENT OF EXTREMITY SOFT TISSUE SARCOMAS

The most common site of origin of sarcomas is the leg (Table 108-4), usually the muscles of the thigh. The proximal upper extremity also is a common location.

Surgical Therapy

Extremity sarcomas are managed with limb-sparing surgical approaches. Radical amputation (amputation at least one joint above the most proximal extent of tumor) is reserved for patients who cannot undergo limb-sparing approaches, usually because of bony invasion or large tumor size, or for those who have a recurrence after a previous limb-sparing operation. Compartment excision is performed when the tumor is large but only when it is confined to one compartment (Fig. 108-6).

Most limb-sparing protocols include wide local excision as the definitive surgical procedure. Wide local excision involves gross total removal of the tumor with a wide margin of normal tissue, but no attempt is made to resect an entire muscle compartment (Fig. 108-7). A margin of 3 to 5 cm of normal tissue is obtained proximally and distally. On the lateral and deep margins, at least one grossly uninvolved fascial plane is resected en bloc with the tumor whenever possible. For large or deep-seated tumors, periosteum or adventitia may be the deep margin. Vascular structures can be resected and reconstructed with grafts. Nerves, such as the sciatic nerve, sometimes are sacrificed. When low-grade lesions are resected, major vessels or nerves are not removed with the tumor.

Table 108-2. RELATIVE FREQUENCY OF HISTOLOGIC TYPES OF SOFT TISSUE SARCOMAS IN ADULTS (ALL SITES)

Histologic Type	Percentage
Malignant fibrous histiocytoma	25.9
Liposarcoma	17.7
Leiomyosarcoma	14.8
Fibrosarcoma	6.6
Neurofibrosarcoma	4.0
Synovial sarcoma	3.6
Rhabdomyosarcoma	3.6
Angiosarcoma	2.9
Extraskeletal chondrosarcoma	1.2
Malignant mesenchymoma	1.0
Extraskeletal osteosarcoma	0.6
Unclassified	5.4
Other	12.7

(Modified from Lawrence W Jr., Donegan WL, Natarajan A, et al. Adult soft tissue sarcomas: a pattern of care survey of the American College of Surgeons. Ann Surg 1987;205:349)

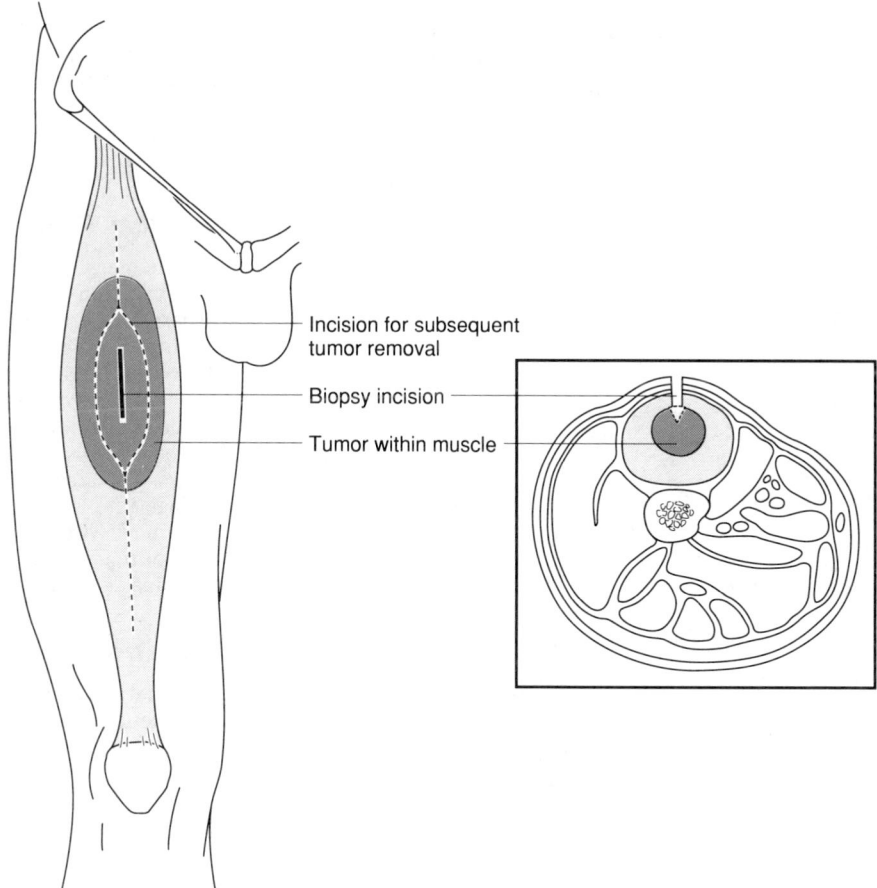

Figure 108-2. Technique for biopsy of an extremity soft tissue mass suspected of being a sarcoma. The incision should be oriented along the long axis of the extremity, at the point where the lesion is closest to the surface, and situated so that it can be readily excised along with the tumor if a diagnosis of sarcoma is made. There should be no raising of flaps or disturbance of tissue planes superficial to the tumor. The mass should not be enucleated within the pseudocapsule; rather, incisional biopsy leaving the bulk of the lesion undisturbed should be carried out. Before wound closure, hemostasis should be achieved to avoid a hematoma, which could disseminate tumor cells through normal tissue planes. Drains are not used routinely.

Radiation Therapy

For patients with small, low-grade tumors, wide local excision alone is associated with a low rate of local recurrence. Other patients who undergo surgical excision also undergo radiation therapy to improve chances for local control. Radiation can be effective primary therapy for extremity sarcoma if a patient refuses or cannot tolerate surgical therapy.

Limb-Sparing Therapy

There is no standard limb-sparing protocol. The following principles form the basis for therapy.

Wide resection is performed. The tumor and its pseudocapsule are not entered during the definitive excision. Patients treated after excisional biopsy undergo wide reexcision, even if they have no clinical or radiographic evidence of residual tumor. Ideal margins are 3 to 5 cm in all directions, but at least one uninvolved fascial plane must be taken. Major nerves or vascular structures can be taken to achieve wide excision of high-grade lesions. Low-grade sarcomas close to major nerves and vessels can be dissected safely off these structures.

Therapy for resected *low-grade* sarcoma of the extremity is postoperative radiation if the margins of resection are narrow or are compromised to preserve neurovascular structures. If a wide margin is obtained around a small, low-grade sarcoma, observation without radiation may be appropriate. Therapy for *intermediate-* and *high-grade* extremity sarcomas almost always is multimodality therapy. Wide excision plus postoperative radiation is appropriate for tumors <10 cm in diameter if preoperative evaluation reveals that a satisfactory surgical margin can be obtained. For tumors >10 cm, or for fixed sarcomas on an extremity, limb-sparing treatment entails preoperative treatment of the tumor. Radiation alone or with chemotherapy can be used to treat these patients. Amputation is reserved for tumors that extensively surround or involve bone or that recur after limb-sparing therapy and cannot be re-resected locally.

Chemotherapy

Chemotherapy before surgical resection is called *neoadjuvant chemotherapy*. Intra-arterial and intravenous infusions of doxorubicin are used preoperatively to manage extremity sarcomas. Combination chemotherapy with doxorubicin-containing regimens also is administered preoperatively. An alternative is isolated limb perfusion, particularly for large or recurrent sarcomas. Neoadjuvant systemic chemotherapy is part of the management of osteosarcomas but not soft tissue tumors.

The main cause of death among patients with soft tissue sarcoma is distant metastatic disease, particularly among patients with high-grade tumors or extremity lesions. As local control rates improve, emphasis is placed on eradicating metastatic disease with postoperative *adjuvant systemic chemotherapy*. Doxorubicin is used as single-agent adjuvant chemotherapy for high-grade extremity sarcomas.

MANAGEMENT OF RETROPERITONEAL SARCOMA

Most patients with retroperitoneal sarcomas, even low-grade tumors, die of the disease, often with locally recurrent tumor. The poor outcome is related to inability to

Table 108-3. AMERICAN JOINT COMMISSION ON CANCER GTNM CLASSIFICATION AND STAGE GROUPING OF SOFT TISSUE SARCOMAS

Stage	Description
TUMOR GRADE	
G1	Well differentiated
G2	Moderately well differentiated
G3	Poorly differentiated
G4	Undifferentiated
PRIMARY TUMOR	
T1	Tumor ≤ 5 cm in greatest diameter
T2	Tumor > 5 cm in greatest diameter
REGIONAL LYMPH NODE INVOLVEMENT	
N0	No known metastases to lymph nodes
N1	Verified metastases to lymph nodes
DISTANT METASTASIS	
M0	No known distant metastasis
M1	Known distant metastasis
STAGE GROUPING	
Stage IA	G1, T1, N0, M0
Stage IB	G1, T2, N0, M0
Stage IIA	G2, T1, N0, M0
Stage IIB	G2, T2, N0, M0
Stage IIIA	G3–4, T1, N0, M0
Stage IIIB	G3–4, T2, N0, M0
Stage IVA	Any G, any T, N1, M0
Stage IVB	Any G, any T, any N, M1

(Modified from Beahrs OH, Henson DE, Hutter RVP, Kennedy BJ. Manual for staging of cancer, ed 4. Philadelphia, JB Lippincott, 1992:132)

diagnose these tumors at an early stage. Retroperitoneal tumors rarely cause symptoms until they become large, and even then symptoms are vague and nonspecific. Abdominal pain, weight loss, early satiety, and nausea and vomiting are the common symptoms. An abdominal mass usually can be felt. Some patients with retroperitoneal sarcoma have hypoglycemia simulating insulinoma.

Surgical Therapy

Wide margins of resection are difficult to achieve. Complete excision of all gross tumor is essential for long-term disease-free survival, but this is achievable only about half the time. To remove all gross tumor, concomitant resection of adjacent organs is required (Table 108-5).

When a retroperitoneal sarcoma is encountered unexpectedly at laparotomy, careful incisional biopsy is performed with minimal disruption of surrounding tissue planes. The area of the biopsy is isolated to prevent tumor spillage into the peritoneal cavity. When the diagnosis is confirmed, wide excision can be performed. A transperitoneal approach allows more complete resection than a flank approach.

Radiation Therapy

Irradiation of macroscopic residual tumor in the retroperitoneum usually is unsuccessful, emphasizing the importance of complete surgical resection. Radiation can be used as postoperative adjuvant therapy. Tissue tolerance of radiation is much lower in the abdomen and retroperitoneum than the extremities. Intraoperative radiation therapy can be attempted to limit normal tissue toxicity. This approach allows one to move the intestine and other sensitive structures out of the field while a single high dose of radiation is administered directly to the tumor bed.

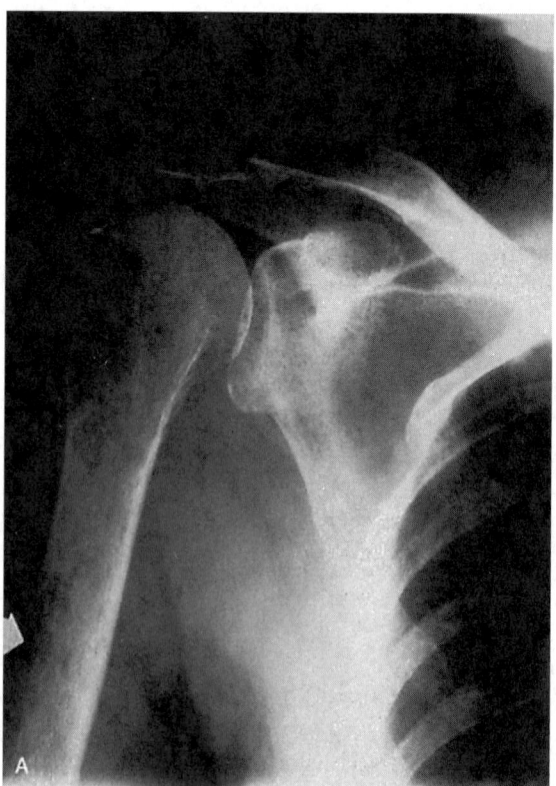

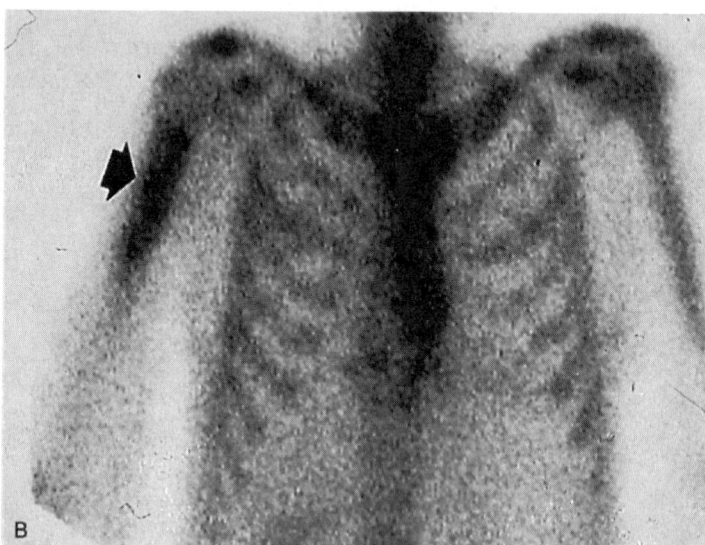

Figure 108-3. (A) Plain radiograph of the proximal humerus and shoulder joint, showing bony destruction (*arrow*) secondary to a large, high-grade soft tissue sarcoma adjacent to the humerus. (B) Radionuclide bone scan in the same patient reveals a much greater degree of involvement (*arrow*).

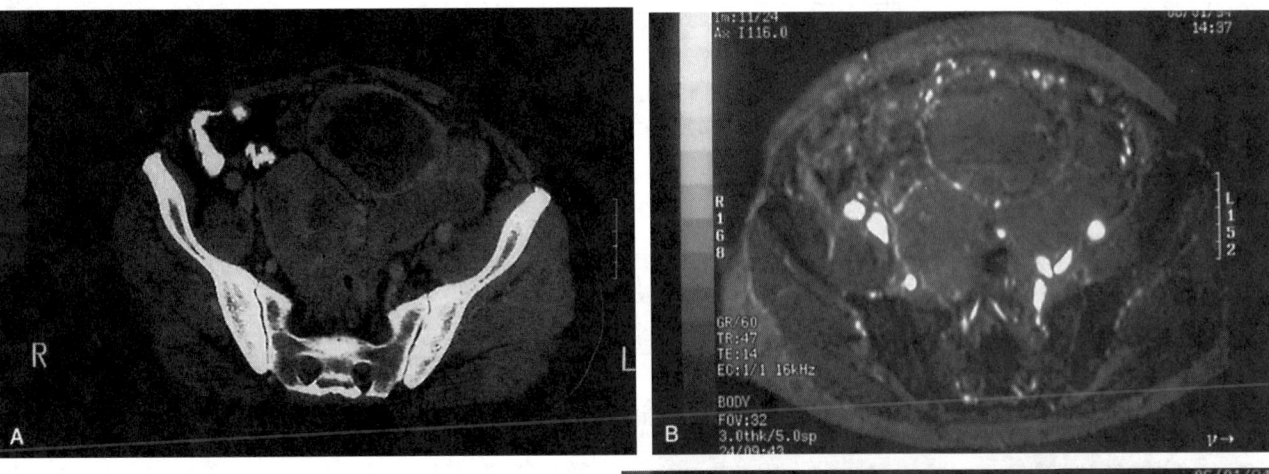

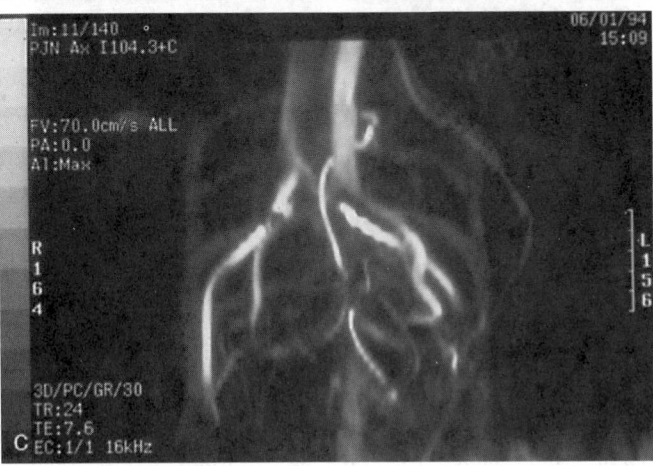

Figure 108-4. (*A*) CT scan of a large, high-grade pelvic sarcoma. There are multiple lobulations of tumor, with areas of spontaneous necrosis and a fluid-fluid level. The iliac vessels cannot be clearly distinguished as separate from the tumor mass. (*B*) MR angiogram of the same region revealing the iliac arteries and veins as prominent white spots against the dark background of tumor. (*C*) Planar reconstruction demonstrating the distal aorta and vena cava and the iliac arteries and veins. The MR angiogram suggested the vessels were free of involvement, as indeed was the case at the time of resection.

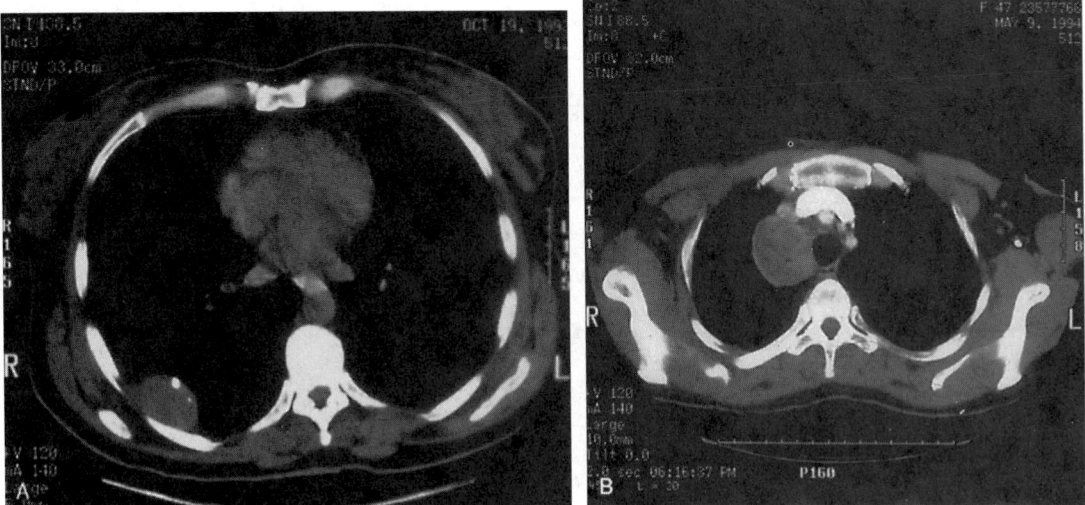

Figure 108-5. (*A*) High-grade malignant fibrous histiocytoma of the pleura. This tumor was treated with chest wall resection and postoperative radiation. (*B*) A follow-up CT scan 7 months later revealed mediastinal adenopathy, which was subsequently confirmed to represent nodal metastasis from sarcoma.

Table 108-4. SITE OF ORIGIN OF SOFT TISSUE SARCOMAS IN ADULTS

Anatomic Site	Percentage
Lower extremity	46.4
Trunk	17.9
Upper extremity	13.1
Retroperitoneum	12.5
Head and neck	8.9
Mediastinum	1.3

(Lawrence W Jr., Donegan WL, Natarajan A, et al. Adult soft tissue sarcomas: a pattern of care survey of the American College of Surgeons. Ann Surg 1987;205:349)

Chemotherapy

Aggressive systemic chemotherapy is poorly tolerated by patients who have just undergone resection of multiple organs. Preoperative intraarterial chemotherapy is limited because most retroperitoneal tumors do not have a single feeder vessel.

DIAGNOSIS AND MANAGEMENT OF DESMOID TUMORS

Desmoid tumors are unusual soft tissue lesions similar to low-grade soft tissue sarcomas. Desmoids almost never metastasize even after multiple local recurrences. A desmoid tumor presents as an enlarging, often painless, soft tissue mass. Clinically and radiographically there is no way to differentiate desmoid tumor from soft tissue sarcoma. Wide excision is the mainstay of treatment, but local recurrence after surgical treatment is common. Death due to desmoid tumor is rare. The tumors do not metastasize, but they do undergo local recurrence in critical areas such as the neck. Little is known about the cause of desmoid tumors. They occur mainly in two settings/pregnancy and familial adenomatous polyposis.

Nonsurgical therapy for desmoid tumors is hormonal therapy with tamoxifen; nonsteroidal antiinflammatory drugs (NSAIDs), especially sulindac; radiation therapy as primary treatment and postoperative adjuvant therapy; or cytotoxic chemotherapy.

The *surgical approach* to sporadic desmoid tumors is resection with a histologically negative margin if possible but without sacrifice of major neurovascular structures or adjacent organs unless absolutely necessary. If pathologic analysis of the resected specimen reveals tumor close to the surgical margin, reexcision is performed or postoperative radiation is administered. Unresectable or recurrent desmoids and those associated with familial polyposis are treated first with a combination of tamoxifen and sulindac. Resection or radiation therapy is used if this therapy fails or to eliminate residual disease after partial responses. Chemotherapy is a last resort.

DIAGNOSIS AND MANAGEMENT OF PRIMARY BONE SARCOMAS

Primary sarcomas of bone pose some unique challenges, but in many ways their behavior is similar to that of soft tissue sarcomas. Most malignant tumors of bone are metastatic from another site or are of hematologic origin (lymphoma or myeloma). Primary bone sarcomas include the following:

- *Spindle-cell bone sarcomas*—osteosarcomas, chondrosarcomas, fibrosarcomas, and malignant fibrous histiocytomas

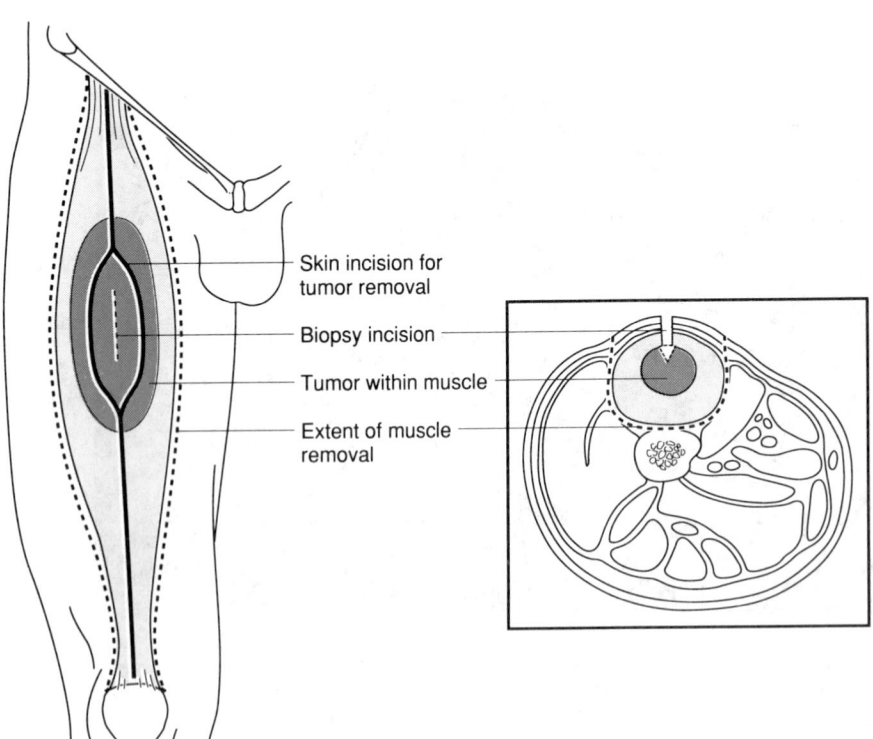

Skin incision for tumor removal

Biopsy incision

Tumor within muscle

Extent of muscle removal

Figure 108-6. Compartment excision involves removal of the entire muscle group in which the tumor arises from origin to insertion. The skin incision frequently crosses one or even two joint spaces. Many large soft tissue sarcomas are not confined to a single muscular compartment.

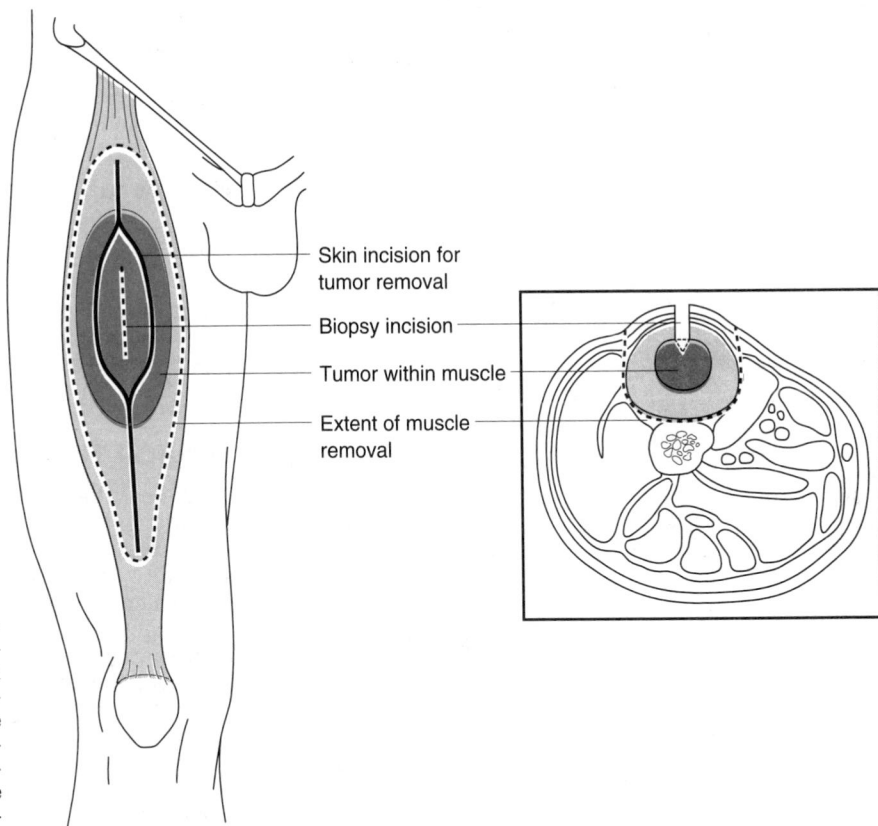

Skin incision for
tumor removal

Biopsy incision

Tumor within muscle

Extent of muscle
removal

Figure 108-7. Wide local excision involves removal of the tumor with a margin of normal tissue: 3 to 5 cm is obtained proximally and distally, and on the lateral and deep margins, at least one grossly uninvolved fascial plane is resected en bloc with the tumor. No attempt is made to resect an entire muscle compartment. If necessary, major vascular structures or nerves may be resected.

- *Small round-cell sarcomas*—osseous Ewing sarcoma, primitive neuroectodermal tumor of bone

Osteosarcomas are the most common primary bone sarcomas. They occur most commonly around the knee, in the distal femur or proximal tibia, but they can occur in any bone (Table 108-6). Osteosarcomas originate in the metaphyseal ends of the bone. Most osteosarcomas occur in childhood and adolescence, but a second peak occurs after 60 years of age. The second peak corresponds to osteosarcomas originating in bones affected by Paget disease, a common predisposing condition for osteosarcoma.

The staging of osteosarcomas is shown in Table 108-7. Most osteosarcomas are stage IIB (high-grade, tumor invasion beyond cortex, no nodal or distant metastases). Involvement of regional lymph nodes is rare at presentation. Pulmonary metastases are the most common site of distant spread and may be discovered in as many as one fourth of patients at presentation. Bone metastases are not

uncommon in osteosarcoma, but they are less frequent than lung metastases.

Clinical Evaluation

A painful mass is the most common presenting symptom of extremity osteosarcoma. The tumor also may present as a painless mass, particularly when it originates in the axial skeleton. Motion is limited when the tumor originates near or involves a joint. A history of trauma is not uncommon, but traumatic injury is not linked to sarcoma development. Some patients have a pathologic fracture of the involved bone.

Plain radiographs of the affected bone are the first step in evaluation of osteosarcoma. High-grade osteosarcomas cause rapid destruction of bone with new bone formation and periosteal reaction. These changes appear on radiographs as an extensive, poorly defined bony lesion often with an extraosseous component (Fig. 108-8). Codman triangles, indicative of periosteal reaction, are characteristic but not pathognomonic of osteosarcoma.

Table 108-5. **ORGANS RESECTED IN CONTINUITY WITH A PRIMARY RETROPERITONEAL SARCOMA**

Organ Resected	Percentages of Operations
Kidney	46
Colon	24
Pancreas	15
Spleen	10
Major vessels (vena cava, iliac artery, or vein)	10

(Jacques DP, Coit DG, Hajdu SI, Brennan MF. Management of primary and recurrent soft-tissue sarcoma of the retroperitoneum. Ann Surg 1990;212:51)

Table 108-6. **SITE OF ORIGIN OF OSTEOSARCOMAS**

Anatomic Site	Percentage
Lower extremity	77.6
Upper extremity	12.9
Pelvis	6.0
Shoulder	2.6
Vertebrae	0.8

(Modified from Eilber F, et al. Management of stage IIB osteogenic sarcoma: experience at the University of California, Los Angeles. Cancer Treat Symp 1985;3:118)

Table 108-7. AMERICAN JOINT COMMISSION ON CANCER GTNM CLASSIFICATION AND STAGE GROUPING OF OSTEOSARCOMAS

Stage	Description
TUMOR GRADE	
GX	Grade cannot be assessed
G1	Well differentiated
G2	Moderately well differentiated
G3	Poorly differentiated
G4	Undifferentiated
PRIMARY TUMOR	
TX	Primary tumor cannot be assessed
T0	No evidence of primary tumor
T1	Tumor confined within the cortex
T2	Tumor invades beyond the cortex
LYMPH NODE INVOLVEMENT	
NX	Regional lymph nodes cannot be assessed
N0	No regional lymph node metastasis
N1	Regional lymph node metastasis
DISTANT METASTASIS	
MX	Presence of distant metastasis cannot be assessed
M0	No distant metastasis
M1	Distant metastasis
STAGE GROUPING	
Stage IA	G1, T1, N0, M0
	G2, T1, N0, M0
Stage IB	G1, T2, N0, M0
	G2, T2, N0, M0
Stage IIA	G3, T1, N0, M0
	G4, T1, N0, M0
Stage IIB	G3, T2, N0, M0
	G4, T2, N0, M0
Stage III	Not defined
Stage IVA	Any G, any T, N1, M0
Stage IVB	Any G, any T, any N, M1

(Modified from Beahrs OH, Henson DE, Hutter RVP, et al. Manual for Staging of Cancer, ed 4. Philadelphia, JB Lippincott, 1992)

If a radiograph suggests osteosarcoma, additional radiologic evaluation is conducted before biopsy. CT is the most important modality in the evaluation of bone sarcoma. It allows assessment of degree of bony destruction, extent of soft tissue involvement, and relation of the tumor to adjacent neurovascular structures. The entire affected bone, including the joints above and below the tumor, is visualized. Chest CT shows evidence of pulmonary metastases too small to be seen on chest radiographs.

MRI is an adjunct to CT for some patients, particularly those considering limb-sparing surgical therapy. The definition of marrow involvement by tumor allows accurate planning of the proximal extent of tumor resection.

Angiography, which defines the relation of tumor to vessels, is not needed unless intraarterial chemotherapy is administered.

Radionuclide bone scans with technetium-99m pyrophosphate can help identify distant metastases to other bones and define skip areas of involvement within the bone of origin. Gallium-67 and thallium-201 scans may be useful for assessing the response of a primary osteosarcoma to preoperative chemotherapy. PET and MRI spectroscopy also can be performed.

Biopsy

After the radiologic evaluation to establish the extent of the bony lesion, incisional biopsy is performed. The biopsy incision is planned to not jeopardize limb sparing. A verti-

cal incision, oriented along the long axis of the extremity, is always used for arm or leg tumors. For tumors close to the knee, the incision is placed medially or laterally. When the primary tumor is in the pelvis or shoulder girdle, the biopsy site is included in the definitive surgical incision.

Preoperative Chemotherapy

Preoperative (neoadjuvant) chemotherapy is standard for osteosarcoma. Preoperative chemotherapy makes limb-sparing surgical therapy more successful by decreasing the extent of soft tissue involvement and allowing time for manufacture of a bone replacement. Tumor response to preoperative chemotherapy may identify patients who need intensive postoperative chemotherapy.

Surgical Therapy

Surgical therapy for extremity osteosarcoma is radical amputation or by en bloc resection with limb sparing. Limb-sparing approaches are considered for patients with extremity sarcomas and no evidence of neurovascular involvement. Patients with pathologic fractures are at high risk for local recurrence and cannot undergo limb-sparing treatment. All limb-sparing protocols for osteosarcoma entail preoperative chemotherapy.

Essential to limb-sparing operations is complete removal of the affected bone and soft tissues. The biopsy site is taken in continuity with the tumor, and the adjacent joint is resected. A proximal bone margin of 6 to 7 cm is taken beyond the highest area of abnormality on preoperative scans. Even if pretreatment induces tumor shrinkage, the operation removes all areas of disease. The marrow at the level of bony transection is removed by curettage, and frozen-section analysis is performed to verify the proximal

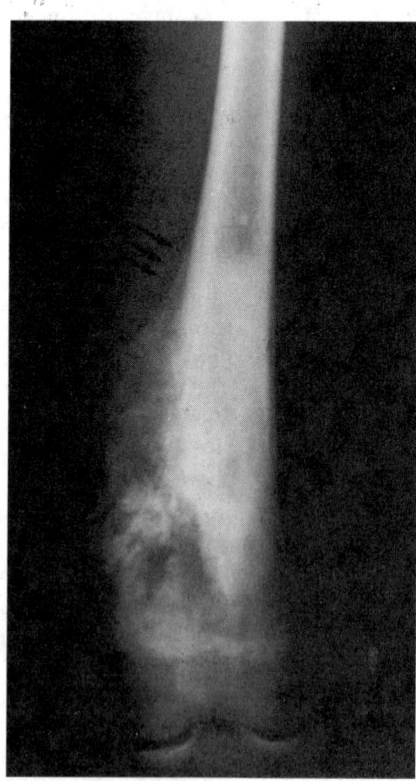

Figure 108-8. Plain radiograph of the femur showing a high-grade osteosarcoma. The tumor is an ill-defined destructive lesion with an extensive soft tissue component. Codman triangles are present (*arrows*).

bone margin. For extensive lesions of the femur, the entire femur is resected in a limb-sparing procedure. Reconstruction after resection of extremity osteosarcoma includes autografts, cadaveric allografts, or simple arthrodeses.

Some pelvic osteosarcomas can be resected with limb sparing. Small or low-grade tumors of the pelvis can be removed by means of internal hemipelvectomy. Almost the entire hemipelvis and hip joint can be resected, leaving the neurovascular supply to the leg intact. Although the leg is shortened, weight bearing is possible because of fibrous adhesion of the femur to the resection site. Allograft reconstruction of the hemipelvis can be done to shorten the time until full weight bearing is possible.

Postoperative Chemotherapy

Preoperative chemotherapy does not replace postoperative therapy but may influence the duration and type of postoperative chemotherapy.

MANAGEMENT OF CHILDHOOD SOFT TISSUE SARCOMAS

Treatment of children with osteosarcoma is similar to that of adults. Soft tissue sarcomas, however, may necessitate different treatment of children. This is largely the result of the differing tumor types in children. Spindle-cell sarcomas, such as fibrosarcoma, malignant fibrous histiocytoma, and liposarcoma, are relatively rare among children. When they do occur, they behave identically to those in adults and are managed similarly. Small-cell sarcomas, which are poorly differentiated, high-grade, aggressive tumors, account for most childhood soft tissue sarcomas. Rhabdomyosarcoma is the prototypical small-cell sarcoma. Extraosseous Ewing sarcoma and primitive neuroectodermal tumor account for most of the other tumors. Small-cell sarcomas are more sensitive to chemotherapy than most spindle-cell sarcomas.

Rhabdomyosarcoma tends to occur in three anatomic sites:

- Head and neck, including orbit and paranasal sinuses (most common)
- Genitourinary tract
- Extremities

Most patients are <5 years of age, although a second peak occurs in adolescence involving mainly boys with pelvic and paratesticular primary tumors. There are three subtypes of rhabdomyosarcoma:

- Embryonal (most common)
- Alveolar
- Botryoid

Besides chemosensitivity, childhood rhabdomyosarcomas differ from adult sarcomas in the following ways:

- Lymph node metastases are more common than in adult sarcomas
- Primary tumors are often locally extensive and invasive and often lack the pseudocapsule of spindle-cell sarcomas
- Head and neck primaries can invade into the base of the skull or even into the brain

Surgical therapy has a limited role in rhabdomyosarcoma. The initial surgical procedure is incisional biopsy with the incision placed in a way that does not complicate excision. Chemotherapy and local irradiation are the main therapy, especially for rhabdomyosarcomas of the head and neck or pelvis.

MANAGEMENT OF RECURRENT AND METASTATIC SARCOMAS

Many adults and children with locally recurrent or even metastatic sarcomas can be cured with aggressive surgical therapy often combined with radiation and chemotherapy. All patients with sarcoma undergo observation for recurrence. For high-grade lesions, follow-up care is directed at detection of local recurrence and metastases. It includes periodic physical examinations and chest radiographs plus CT of the primary site and lungs at least once a year for 5 years. Low-grade lesions rarely metastasize in the absence of local recurrence, and follow-up evaluation is focused on the original tumor site. Low-grade sarcoma can recur 20 years after the original resection, so follow-up care must be long-term.

Local Recurrence

If a patient initially treated with surgical therapy alone experiences local recurrence, multimodality treatment is provided with repeat resection, radiation, and sometimes chemotherapy. Patients with recurrences after surgical therapy and radiation are likely to need radical amputation to control recurrence in an extremity but still can undergo salvage operations. Local recurrence of retroperitoneal sarcoma, particularly low-grade tumors, sometimes can be resected, but cure is not likely.

Distant Metastases

The lungs are the most frequent site of distant spread of sarcomas and are often the only site of metastasis. Patients with three or fewer metastases, long doubling time of the metastatic tumors, and unilateral disease have the best prognosis after surgical resection. Patients lacking one or all of these factors can undergo curative resection. Preoperative or postoperative adjuvant chemotherapy can improve outcomes for patients undergoing complete resection of pulmonary metastases, especially from osteosarcomas.

Patients with unresectable pulmonary metastases or with extrapulmonary metastases are treated with cytotoxic chemotherapy. Radiation therapy may be useful as palliation for some patients with bony or cerebral metastases.

SUGGESTED READING

Arca MJ, Sondak VK, Chang AE. Diagnostic procedures and pretreatment evaluation of soft tissue sarcomas. Semin Surg Oncol 1994;10:323.

Eilber FR, Eckardt JJ, Rosen G, et al. Neoadjuvant chemotherapy and radiotherapy in the multidisciplinary management of soft tissue sarcomas of the extremity. Surg Oncol Clin North Am 1993;2:611.

Greenblatt MS, Bennett WP, Hollstein M, et al. Mutations in the p53 tumor suppressor gene: clues to cancer etiology and molecular pathogenesis. Cancer Res 1994;54:4855.

McGuire SM, McGuire AL, McGuire MH. The genetic risk factors for bone and soft tissue tumors. Surg Oncol Clin North Am 1994;3:599.

Meyers PA, Heller G, Healey J, et al. Chemotherapy for nonmetastatic osteogenic sarcoma: the Memorial Sloan-Kettering experience. J Clin Oncol 1992;10:5.

Putnam JB, Roth JA. Resection of sarcomatous pulmonary metastases. Surg Oncol Clin North Am 1993;2:673.

Sindelar WF, Kinsella TJ, Chen PW, et al. Intraoperative radiotherapy in retroperitoneal sarcomas: final results of a prospective, randomized clinical trial. Arch Surg 1993;128:402.

Skinner KA, Eilber FR, Holmes EC, et al. Surgical treatment and chemotherapy for pulmonary metastases from osteosarcoma. Arch Surg 1992;127:1065.

Sondak VK, Leonard JA Jr, Robertson JM, et al. Limb-sparing surgery for extremity soft tissue sarcomas: functional and reha-

bilitation considerations. Surg Oncol Clin North Am 1993;
2:657.

Zalupski MM, Ryan JR, Hussein ME, et al. Systemic adjuvant
chemotherapy for soft tissue sarcomas of the extremities. Surg
Oncol Clin North Am 1993;2:621.

ESSENTIALS OF SURGERY: SCIENTIFIC PRINCIPLES AND PRACTICE,
edited by Lazar J. Greenfield, Michael W. Mulholland, Keith T. Oldham, Gerald B. Zelenock,
and Keith D. Lillemoe. Lippincott–Raven Publishers, Philadelphia, © 1997.

CHAPTER 109

RECONSTRUCTIVE PLASTIC SURGERY

L. SCOTT LEVIN

Foremost among the principles of plastic surgery is the concept of replacing like with like. New tissues of adequate vascularity and dimension are transferred to areas of deficiency. A flap of local or regional tissue is capped on a vascular pedicle that supplies the different components of the flap. If rearrangement of local tissue or regional tissue is not possible, free tissue transfer is used. With this approach, autologous tissue, including muscle, skin, bone, and fascia is transplanted to substitute for tissue that is removed.

Plastic surgery is divided into aesthetic surgery and reconstructive surgery, which often overlap. Aesthetic surgery takes what is normal and improves it in appearance. Reconstructive surgery restores what is normal after injury, congenital abnormality, or ablation.

WOUND PRINCIPLES

Delicate tissue handling leads to improved wound healing, diminished scar formation, and less distortion. Understanding of the blood supply to all tissues is paramount. Tissue ischemia causes cell death, and necrosis causes fibrosis and possibly infection of the wound and compromised healing. Pathologic conditions of wound healing such as hypertrophic scars or keloids can result if tissue-handling principles are violated.

Wounds closed under excess tension can widen and

A

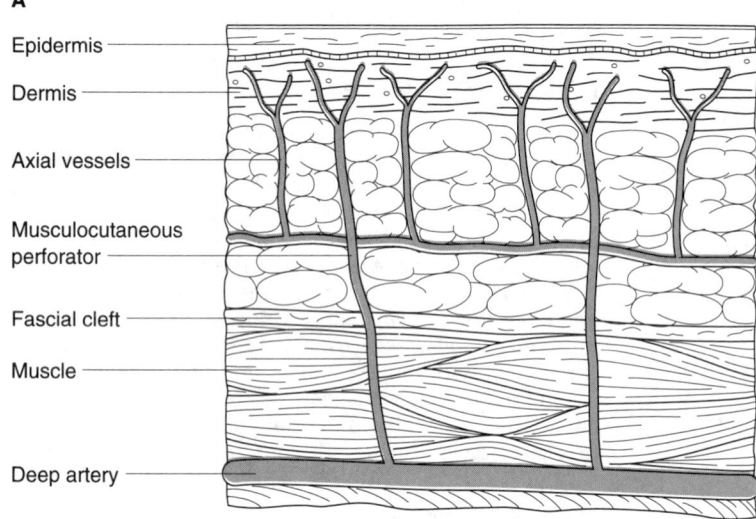

Epidermis
Dermis
Axial vessels
Musculocutaneous perforator
Fascial cleft
Muscle
Deep artery

B

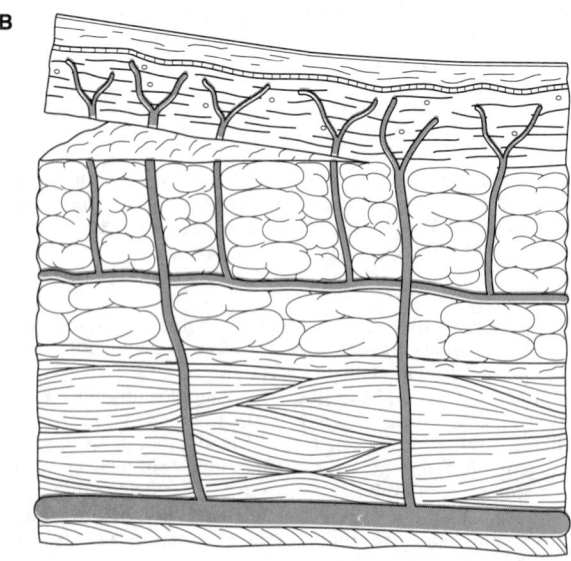

C

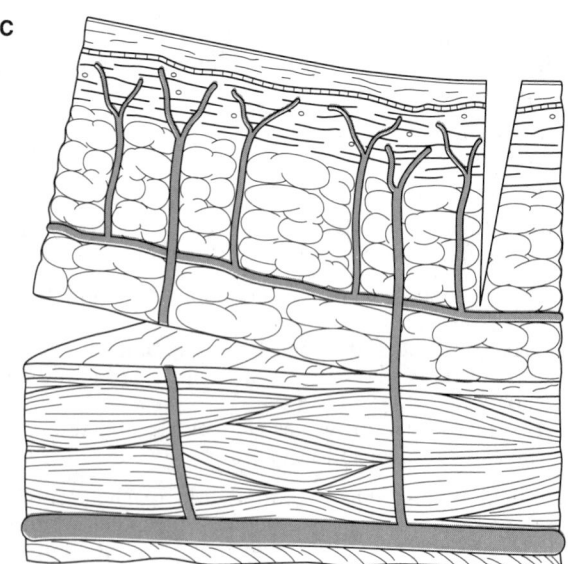

Figure 109-1. Flaps are classified by their vascular supply. (*A*) Normal blood supply to the skin. (*B*) Rotation or transposition flap. (*C*) Island flap with its blood supply.

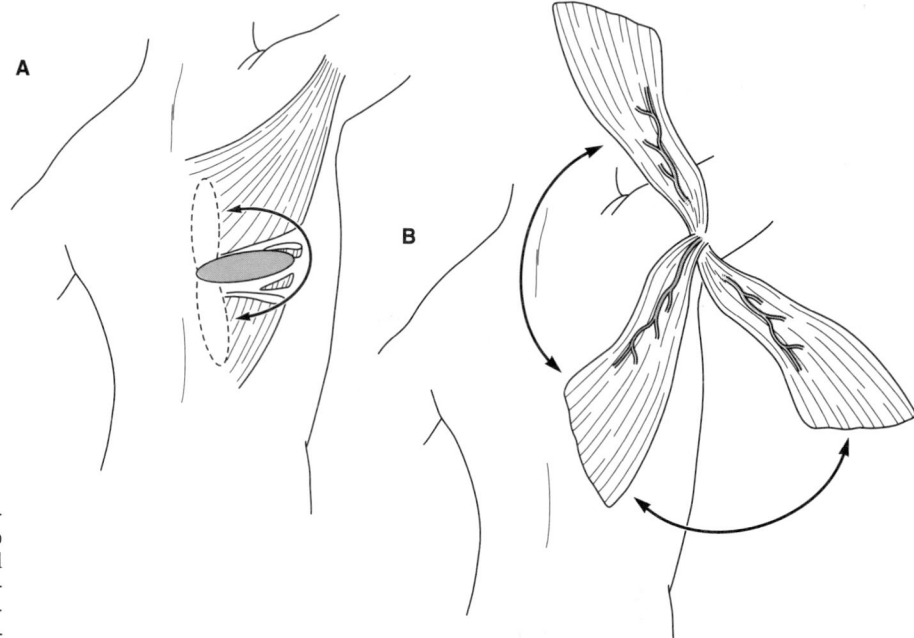

Figure 109-2. Two variations of a latissimus dorsi rotation flap. (*A*) Flap rotation arc for a skin paddle based on the posterior intercostal perforators. (*B*) Arc of rotation for a musculocutaneous flap based on the thoracodorsal artery.

thicken. *Hypertrophic scars* are thickened that do not extend beyond the borders of the original scar. *Keloids* are proliferative thickening; they extend beyond the boundary of the scar. Management of hypertrophic scarring is excision of the scar and closure of the wound under less tension with finer sutures. Because keloids can recur, resection and repair is accompanied by an adjunct such as radiation therapy or local steroid injection.

Conditions that contribute to poor wound healing include steroid dependency, previous irradiation, diabetes, peripheral vascular disease, ulcerative colitis, Crohn's disease, intrinsic lung disease, and rheumatoid arthritis. Oncology, transplant, and other immunosuppressed patients often have wound-healing problems. They also often have nutritional deficiencies. Vitamin A counteracts the catabolic effects of steroids to improve wound healing. It is given routinely as a supplement in the perioperative period to patients taking steroids.

The effects of irradiation linger for many years, and must be considered in planning incisions and flaps. This problem is notable among patients with malignant tumors of the head and neck. These patients benefit from early collaborative surgical planning because additional soft tissue may have to be placed after tumor resection. Reconstruction after extremity soft tissue sarcoma resection or head and neck tumor therapy can be difficult without prospective planning. Irradiated tissues have diminished blood flow and impaired venolymphatic drainage and are subject to infection and wound breakdown.

In the care of patients with diabetes or arterial insufficiency who undergo vascular bypass procedures, angioplasty, or endarterectomy, wound problems may occur at the site of vascular repair or saphenous vein harvest. These patients have impaired tissue blood flow and may have concomitant risk factors such as tobacco use. If the wounds do not respond to conservative care, excision and skin

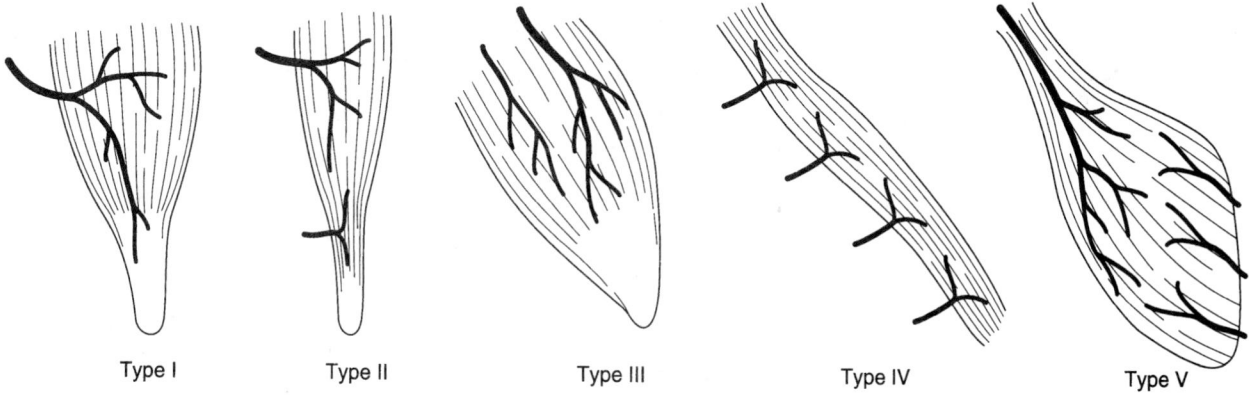

Type I   Type II   Type III   Type IV   Type V

Figure 109-3. Muscle vascular anatomy (flap types I to V). (After Mathes SA, Nahai F. Clinical application for muscle and musculo-cutaneous flaps. St Louis, CV Mosby, 1992:3)

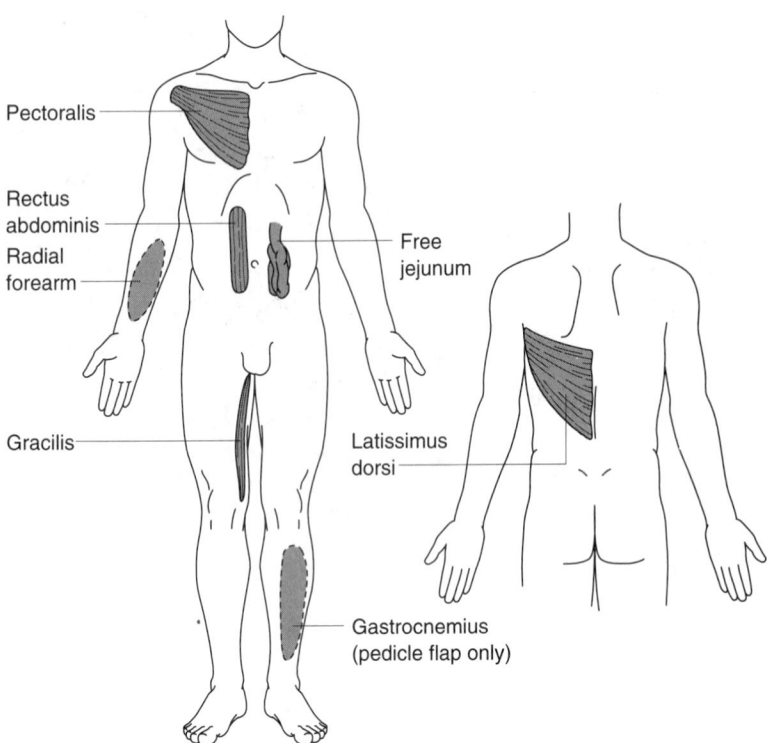

Figure 109-4. Locations of commonly used flaps.

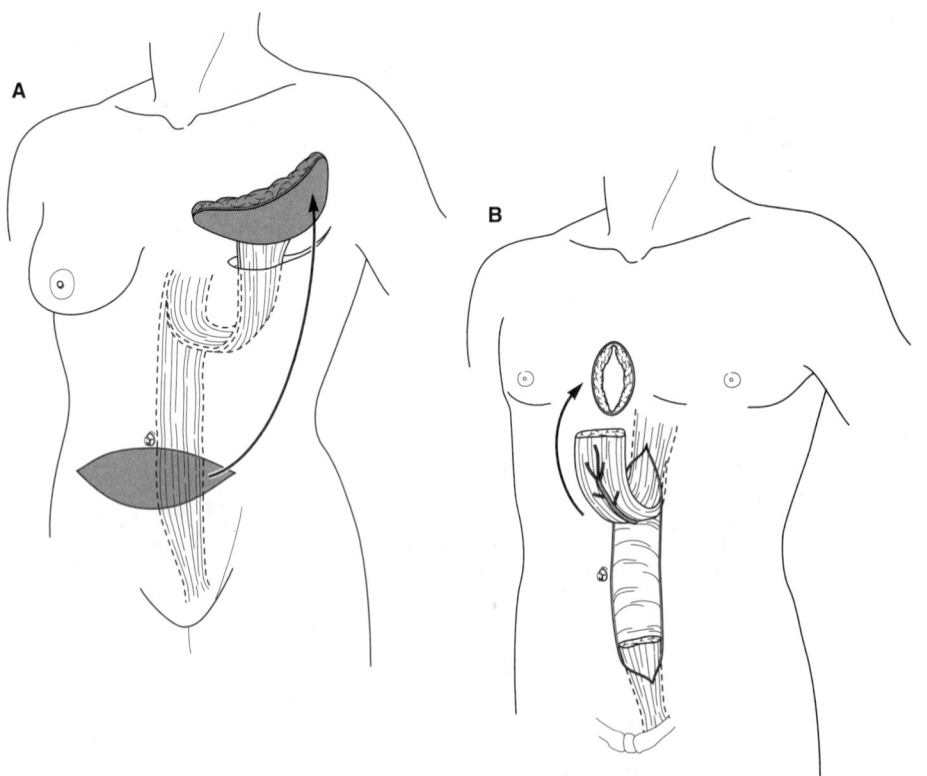

Figure 109-5. Examples of tissue transposition. (*A*) Rectus abdominis muscle flap with skin island. (*B*) Rectus abdominis muscle transposition used to close a local deficiency.

grafting are considered, provided that the wound bed has clean granulation tissue capable of accepting a graft.

PRINCIPLES OF THE FLAP

Flaps are classified based on vascular supply and excursion.

Blood Supply

Skin territories are fed by direct cutaneous arteries, septal perforators, or arterioles from subjacent muscles (Fig. 109-1).

An example of *direct cutaneous* blood supply is the deltopectoral flap, fed by the second, third, or fourth intercostal perforators from the internal mammary artery. A *musculocutaneous* flap has skin perforators from the underlying muscle, which is supplied by a vascular pedicle. An example is a latissimus dorsi flap (Fig. 109-2), in which the skin is supplied by perforating vessels from the latissimus dorsi muscle, and the muscle is supplied by the thoracodorsal artery and venae comitantes.

Muscle flaps (Fig. 109-3) are categorized in the following manner:

- Type I flaps have a single major vascular pedicle
- Type II flaps have one major vascular pedicle and one minor pedicle
- Type III flaps have a dominant vascular pedicle and smaller segmental pedicle
- Type IV flaps have multiple pedicles
- Type V flaps have one major and several small minor pedicles

A *fasciocutaneous* flap has skin supplied by perforators. The perforators pass to the surface along fascial septa and between adjacent muscle bellies and arborize at the deep fascia to form a plexus. Branches from the plexus supply subcutaneous tissue and dermis. An example is the radial forearm flap used in reconstruction of the hand.

Among the most commonly used *tissue transfers* (Fig. 109-4) are:

- Groin and scapular skin flaps
- Latissimus dorsi, trapezius, pectoralis, rectus abdominis, gracilis, hamstring, gastrocnemius and soleus muscle flaps
- Radial forearm and lateral arm fasciocutaneous flaps

Excursion

A *transposition flap* is composed of tissue moved to an adjacent area of deficiency. The defect is covered by means of a skin graft or local rearrangement of adjacent tissues (Fig. 109-5).

An *advancement flap* is lifted on its blood supply and advanced into an adjacent defect. An example is the V-Y flap used for ischial pressure sores.

Island pedicle flaps are made when a block of tissue is raised on an artery and venae comitantes and transposed over longer distances. The radial forearm flap for hand or upper extremity coverage is an example.

A *free flap,* or free tissue transplantation, is a flap isolated on the artery and venae comitantes to a block of tissue, removed from the blood supply, and transplanted to another site with microsurgical technique. These flaps often contain muscle, skin, bones, or a combination of these elements (*composite flaps*).

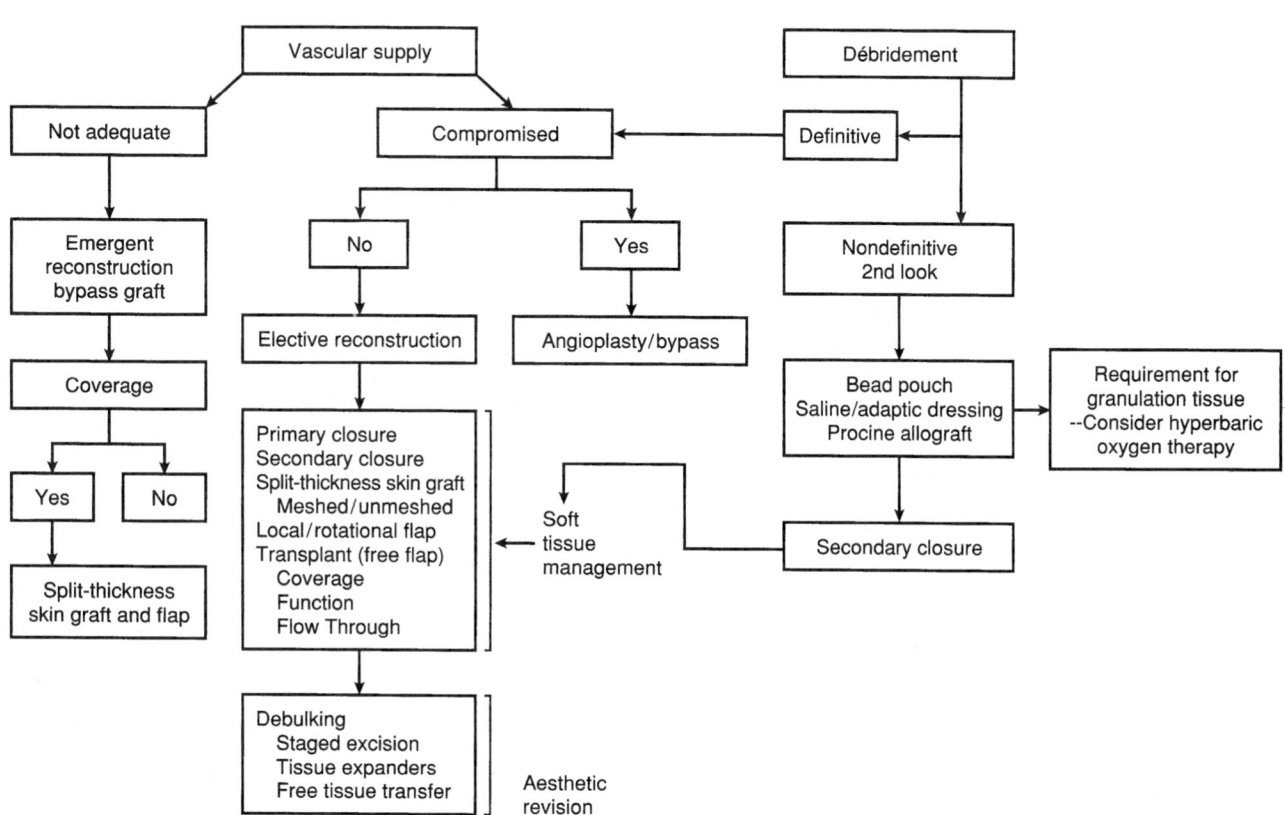

Figure 109-6. Reconstructive ladder for soft tissue defects. (After Levin LS. The reconstructive ladder: soft tissue principles for orthopaedic surgeons. Tech Orthop 1995;10:88)

RECONSTRUCTIVE LADDER

Most wounds are closed by *primary closure.* In the presence of infection or contamination, *delayed primary closure* is used. This involves primary wound approximation 1 to 5 days after wounding. Healing by *secondary intention* allows small open areas or small wounds to heal spontaneously. This approach avoids trapping of bacteria as wound contraction and epithelialization occur. For larger defects, *skin grafting* can be performed, provided the bed is appropriate to receive a graft. Grafting is performed on clean granulation tissue with adequate vascular inflow for anastomosis.

When skin grafting is not satisfactory or when a cavity must be filled, a *local rotation* procedure with a muscle or fasciocutaneous flap is used. *Tissue expansion* also is an option in this situation. At the highest rung on the reconstructive ladder (Fig. 109-6) is *free tissue transfer.* Almost any tissue can be transplanted, including intestine, muscle, skin, bone, and fascia. Composite flaps provide and restore form and function.

SUGGESTED READING

Barwick WJ, Goldberg JA, Scully SP, Harrelson JM. Vascularized tissue transfer for closure of irradiated wounds after soft tissue sarcoma resection. Ann Surg 1992;216:591.

Cohen M, ed. Mastery of plastic and reconstructive surgery. Boston, Little, Brown, 1994.

Georgiade GS, Georgiade NG, Barwick WJ, et al, eds. Textbook of plastic, maxillofacial and reconstructive surgery, ed 2. Baltimore, Williams & Wilkins, 1992.

Jones TR, Lee G, Emami B, Strasberg S. Free colon transfer for resurfacing large oral cavity defects. Plast Reconstr Surg 1995;96:1092.

Mathes SH, Nahai F. Clinical application for muscle and musculocutaneous flaps. St. Louis, Mosby, 1992.

O'Brien BM. Long term results after microlymphaticovenous anastomoses for the treatment of obstructive lymphedema. Plast Reconstr Surg 1990;85:562.

Shestak KC, Myers EN, Ramasastry SS, Jones NF, Johnson JT. Vascularized free tissue transfer in head and neck surgery. Am J Otolaryngol 1993;14:148.

Rockwell WB, Cohen IK, Ehrlick HP. Keloids and hypertrophic scars: a comprehensive review. Plast Reconstr Surg 1989;84:827.

SUBJECT INDEX

Page numbers followed by *f* indicate illustrations; *t* following a page number indicates tabular material.

A

Abdomen, acute, 398–401
  in children, 401*t*
  nonsurgical causes of, 401*t*
Abdominal aorta, anatomy of, 615*f*
Abdominal aortic aneurysm
  classification of, 658*f*
  intraluminal prosthesis for treatment of, 586*f*
  operating repair of, 660*f*
  real-time B-mode scan of, 549*f*
  in 74-year-old man, 563*f*
Abdominal esophagus, 155
Abdominal hemorrhage
  initial management of, 88*f*
Abdominal injury
  injury scale scoring system for, 85*t*
  diagnostic algorithm for, 87*f*
Abdominal pain, Crohn's disease and, 225
Abdominal pain map, 399*f*
Abdominal scintigraphy, 365
Abdominal wall
  hernia of, 383, 385–388
  musculature of, 385*f*
  posterolateral muscles of, 386*t*
Abdominoperineal resection, 354
  extent of surgery in, 351*f*
Above-knee amputation, 639*f*
  preoperative level selection for, 637*t*
Abscess(es). *See also specific type of abscess*
  management of, Crohn's disease and, 226–227
Absent pulse, 528
Absorption
  by gallbladder, 305
  in small intestine, 214-216
Absorptive cell, 210
Abuse, 97*t*. *See also* Child abuse
Acalculous cholecystitis, 308–309
Accidental injury. *See also* Trauma
  elective surgery and, 16*t*
Acetylcholine, 493
Acetylcholine receptor, 8*f*
Acetylsalicyclic acid (ASA), 192
Achalasia, 161–162

  manometry and, 164*f*
  radiographic appearance of, 162
  symptoms and signs of, 162
Acid–base balance, 76–82
  disturbances in, 80–82
Acid ingestion, 170
Acinar cell, 238
Acinic cell carcinoma, 151
Acquired AV fistula, 672
Acquired eventration, 724
Acquired hepatic cyst, 293
Acquired immunodeficiency syndrome (AIDS), 60
  rectal disease and, 380–381
  infections and, 60*t*
  hepatic infection and, 282
Acquired tracheoesophageal fistula, 173
Acral lentiginous melanoma, 784
Acromegaly, treatment of, 436*f*
Actinomycin D, 122*t*
Activated clotting time (ACT), 34, 36
Activated partial thromboplastin time (APTT), 36
Active transport, 305
Acute abdomen
  differential diagnosis of, 401*t*
  nonsurgical causes of, 401*t*
Acute abdominal pain in immunocompromised patient, 402*t*
Acute anal fissure, 377
Acute aortic dissection of ascending aorta, 656*f*
Acute arterial embolism, 529*t*
Acute arterial thrombosis, 529*t*
Acute cholecystitis, 307
Acute deep venous thrombosis, 568*f*
Acute edematous pancreatitis, 245*t*
Acute epidural hematoma, 756*f*
Acute epiglottitis, 711
Acute gastrointestinal hemorrhage, 359–366
Acute hemorrhage from esophageal varices, 364*f*
Acute hepatic failure, 281–282
Acute lower gastrointestinal hemorrhage
  differential diagnosis of, 360*t*

  evaluation of, 361*f*
Acute metabolic acidosis, 81
Acute mitral regurgitation, 499
Acute myocardial infarction, 35
  pattern of evolution of ECG in, 496*f*
Acute pancreatitis, 242, 323
  clinical associations with, 243, 244*t*
  complications of, 243
  diagnosis of, 244-245
  incidence of, 243
  infectious causes linked to development of, 244*t*
  pathology of, 242
  pathophysiology of, 242–243
  presentation of, 243–244
  pancreatic abscess and, 246
  pancreatic pseudocysts and, 246
  treatment of, 245–246
Acute-phase proteins, regulation of, by cytokines, 39*t*
Acute-phase response, inflammation and, 45
Acute postoperative pain management, 107–108
Acute pulmonary embolism, 567
  renal transplantation and, 569*f*
Acute rejection of hepatic transplant, 140
Acute renal failure (ARF)
  management of, 73–75
Acute respiratory distress syndrome (ARDS), 37
Acute subdural hematoma, 757*f*
  in child, 756
Acute suppurative lymphadenitis, 715
Acute upper gastrointestinal hemorrhage
  differential diagnosis of, 360*t*
  evaluation of, 361*f*
Adaptor protein, 14*f*
Addison disease, 66
Adenine, 8
Adeno-associated virus (AAV), 132
Adenocarcinoma, 151. *See also specific sites and types*
  ductal, 254